Commissioning Editor: Miranda Bromage
Development Editor: Rachel Robson
Project Supervisor: Mark Sanderson

Fetal Medicine: Basic Science and Clinical Practice

edited by

Charles H. Rodeck DSc FRCOG FRCPath FMedSci
Professor and Head, Department of Obstetrics and Gynaecology,
University College London, London, UK

and

Martin J. Whittle MD FRCOG FRCP(Glas)
Professor and Head, Division of Reproductive and Child Health,
Birmingham Women's Hospital, Edgbaston, Birmingham, UK

CHURCHILL LIVINGSTONE
LONDON • EDINBURGH • NEW YORK • PHILADELPHIA • SYDNEY • TORONTO

CHURCHILL LIVINGSTONE
An imprint of Harcourt Brace and Company Limited

First published 1999

ISBN 0–4430–5357X

British Library Cataloguing in Publication Data
A catalogue record for this book is available from the British Library

Library of Congress Cataloging in Publication Data
A catalog record for this book is available from the Library of Congress

Note
Medical knowledge is constantly changing. As new information becomes available, changes in treatment, procedures, equipment and the use of drugs become necessary. The editors/authors/contributors and the publishers have, as far as it is possible, taken care to ensure that the information given in this text is accurate and up-to-date. However, readers are strongly advised to confirm that the information, especially with regard to drug usage, complies with the latest legislation and standards of practice.

Typeset by Phoenix Photosetting, Chatham, Kent, UK
Printed in China

The
Publisher's
policy is to use
paper manufactured
from sustainable forests
II

Foreword

Twenty years ago texts dealing with embryology and fetal development were based on information provided by pathological examination. Today, through ultrasound and, occasionally, endoscopic visualization, fetal treatment and behaviour can be monitored dynamically. Twenty years ago it was a feat to culture fetal cells from amniotic fluid to enable the diagnosis of major chromosomal abnormalities. Today, through technology that has had an exponential course, the genetic makeup of a fetus can be microanalysed to the point where few inherited diseases elude diagnosis.

Until recently, one could do little to salvage fetuses whose mothers had severe medical complications of pregnancy or when there was intrinsic fetal disease. Diabetes, Rh disease, alloimmune thrombocytopenia, hypertension and some infections are no longer having the same devastating effect on perinatal mortality and morbidity. Clearly, better methods of fetal surveillance bolstered appreciably by the advent of Doppler investigation of the fetal arterial and venous circulations are responsible for improved fetal salvage. The very newest technology involving three-dimensional ultrasound is even rendering the minute placental circulation accessible to *in vivo* investigation. The diagnostic and therapeutic techniques themselves, while decreasing perinatal mortality, actually are dwarfed simply by the extensive knowledge that has been gained over the last two decades about the nature of the conditions threatening today's fetuses – knowledge that translates into improvements on the quality of life throughout an individual's life span.

The editors, pioneers in their own right, have assembled an impressive group of authors who have comprehensively explored the smallest details of fetal disease. From the individual amino acid sequences in heritable disease to the techniques to free fetal limbs from an amniotic band, the book provides an up-to-date compendium of knowledge regarding current fetal medicine.

John Hobbins

Preface

The demise of the large textbook has been repeatedly announced, yet it has failed to happen – why? Perhaps because they provide a summation of knowledge and define a discipline. We believe that this book, the first devoted to Fetal Medicine, fulfils these functions. We thought it essential to include the relevant basic science because the rate of increase in information is outstripping the ability of clinicians to keep up. New scientific terminolgy and language pose barriers to understanding which we hope that this book will help to overcome.

In such a multidisciplinary field it has been impossible to be all-inclusive: we have preferred to be selective, including only core subjects. In embryology, topics were chosen to illustrate scientific principles, and in neonatology, for their immediate relevance to the fetus. After some initial reluctance, maternal medicine was excluded. Although currently most feto-maternal subspecialists work in both fields, it is likely that a separation will occur in the near future and there are numerous excellent texts dealing with maternal medicine.

We make no apology for some overlap and repetition in a number of the chapters. This has given authors the freedom to express differing views and to develop their own themes, thus maintaining the internal consistency of their chapters. Neither do we apologise for not imposing either cis- or trans-atlantic spelling. That would seem parochial in comparison to the theme of the book and its global authorship and readership.

The development of this book has taken over 10 years, partly due to a series of upheavals in the publishing world. Much credit for its conception must go to the persuasive and persistent charm of Sylvia Hull. Others who have helped to nurture it include Lucy Gardner, Antonia Seymour, Prudence Daniels, Deborah Russell, and most recently Miranda Bromage and Rachel Robson, and they deserve our gratitude. Most of all, we thank our contributors. Their time (much of it doubtless after midnight), expertise and perseverence have provided us with superb chapters.

CHARLES H. RODECK MARTIN J. WHITTLE

Contents

Contributors

Lenore Abramsky
Genetic Associate, Department of Medical and Community Genetics, Imperial College School of Medicine, London, UK

Matteo Adinolfi MD PhD FRCP
Professor of Developmental Immunology, Department of Obstetrics and Gynaecology, University College London, London, UK

Zarko Alfirevic MD MRCOG
Senior Lecturer, Department of Obstetrics and Gynaecology, University of Liverpool, UK

Douglas G. Altman PhD
Head, ICRF Medical Statistics Group, Centre for Statistics in Medicine, Institute of Health Sciences, Headington, Oxford, UK

S. Arulkumaran FRCS FRCOG PhD
Professor of Obstetrics and Gynaecology, School of Human Development, University of Nottingham, Derby City General Hospital, Derby, UK

M.C. Aubry MD
Maternité, Hôpital Necker Enfants Malade, Paris, France

Albert Aynsley-Green MA DPhil MBBS FRCP(Lond) FRCP(Edin) FRCPCH
Nuffield Professor of Child Health, Institute of Child Health, University of London, London, UK

David Barton PhD DipRCPath
Chief Scientist and Lecturer in Molecular Genetics, National Centre for Medical Genetics, Our Lady's Hospital for Sick Children, Crumlin, Dublin, Ireland

Beryl R. Benacerraf MD
Clinical Professor of Obstetrics and Gynecology; Clinical Professor of Radiology; Director of Obstetrical Ultrasound, Massachusetts General Hospital, Harvard Medical School, Boston; Diagnostic Ultrasound Associates, PC, Boston, USA

Susan Bewley MA MRCOG
Director of Obstetrics, Department of Obstetrics and Gynaecology, Guy's and St Thomas's Hospitals, London, UK

Johanne Bitzer MD
Associate Professor and Chief, Division for Gynecologic Social Medicine and Psychosomatics, University Women's Hospital, Basel, Switzerland

Harm-Gerd Blaas MD PhD
Department of Obstetrics and Gynecology, Trondheim University Hospital, National Centre of Fetal Medicine, Trondheim, Norway

Catherine Bobrow MBChB
Research Fellow, Fetal Medicine Research Unit, Bristol University, St Michael's Hospital, Bristol, UK

Robert A. Brace PhD
Professor of Reproductive Medicine, Division of Perinatal Medicine, Department of Reproductive Medicine, University of California, San Diego, California, USA

David J. H. Brock BA PhD FRCPath FRCPE FRSE
Emeritus Professor of Human Genetics, Human Genetics Unit, Molecular Medicine Centre, Western General Hospital, Edinburgh, UK

Geoffrey Brown BSc PhD
Reader in Cellular Immunology and Co-Director, LRF Differentiation Programme, Division of Immunity and Infection, The Medical School, University of Birmingham, Edgbaston, Birmingham, UK

Thue Bryndorf MD
Section of Clinical Genetics, Department of Obstetrics and Gynecology, Juliane Marie Center, Rigshospitalet, Copenhagen, Denmark

Carlos Carreño MD
Florida Institute for Fetal Diagnosis and Therapy, Tampa, USA

Jean Chapple MBChB MCommHFFPHM FRCP MFFP DRCOG DCH
Consultant in Perinatal Epidemiology, Kensington, Chelsea and Westminster Health Authority and Honorary Senior Lecturer, Department of Epidemiology and Public Health, Imperial College School of Medicine, London, UK

Malcolm L. Chiswick MD FRCP(Lond) FRCPCH DCH
Professor of Child Health and Paediatrics, University of Manchester; Consultant Paediatrician, St Mary's Hospital for Women and Children, Manchester, UK

Lyn S. Chitty PhD MRCOG
Fetal Medicine Unit, Obstetric Hospital, University College Hospital, London, UK

S. Chua MMed MRCOG
Department of Obstetrics and Gynaecology, National University Hospital, Singapore

Phillipa M. Clark BM RCPCH DCH FRACP MD
Research Fellow and Developmental Paediatrician, Department of Paediatrics, University of Auckland, Auckland, New Zealand

Patricia Collins BSc PhD
Lecturer, Department of Human Morphology, Biomedical Sciences Building, University of Southampton, Southampton, UK

Joshua A. Copel MD
Professor and Section Head, Department of Obstetrics and Gynecology, Yale University School of Medicine, New Haven, USA

F. Daïkha-Dahmane MD PhD
Praticien Hospitalier, Laboratoire de Biologie du Dévelopement, Hôpital Robert Debré, Paris, France

Anne Deans MBBS MRCGP MRCOG
Consultant Obstetrician and Gynaecologist, Frimley Park Hospital and University College Hospital, London, UK

Joy Delhanty PhD FRCPath
Professor of Human Genetics, Department of Obstetrics and Gynaecology, Royal Free and University College London, London, UK

Mark Denbow MBBS
Division of Paediatrics, Obstetrics and Gynaecology, Institute of Obstetrics and Gynaecology, Imperial College of Medicine, Queen Charlotte's and Chelsea Hospital, London, UK

Sanjeev Deshpande MD FRCPCH
Consultant Neonatologist, Royal Shrewsbury Hospital, Shrewsbury, UK

Miodrag Dodic MD PhD
Research Officer, Howard Florey Institute, University of Melbourne, Parkville, Victoria, Australia

Marc Dommergues MD
Praticien Hospitalier, Maternité, Hôpital Antoine Béclère, Clamart, France

Mark T. Drayson BSc MBChB PhD MRCPath
Senior Lecturer, Division of Immunology and Infection, The Medical School, University of Birmingham, Edgbaston, Birmingham, UK

Yves Dumez MD
Professor, Maternité Hôpital Necker Enfants-Malades, Paris, France

Robin A. J. Eady DSc(Med) FRCP
Professor of Experimental Dermatopathology and Head, Department of Cell and Molecular Pathology, St John's Institute of Dermatology, King's, Guy's and St Thomas' School of Medicine, St Thomas' Hospital, London, UK

Sturla H. Eik-Nes MD PhD
Department of Obstetrics and Gynecology, Trondheim University Hospital, National Centre for Fetal Medicine, Trondheim, Norway

Sherman Elias MD
Professor and Head, Department of Obstetrics and Gynecology, University of Chicago, Chicago, Illinois, USA

Hazem El-Refaey MD MRCOG
Senior Lecturer and Honorary Consultant, Imperial College School of Medicine, Chelsea and Westminster Hospital, London, UK

Mark I. Evans MD
Charlotte B. Failing Professor, Acting Chairman and Specialist-in-Chief of Obstetrics and Gynecology; Professor of Molecular Medicine and Genetics; Professor of Pathology; Director, Division of Reproductive Genetics; Director, Center for Fetal Diagnosis and Therapy; Director, Human Genetics Program, Department of Obs/Gyn, Hutzel Hospital, Detroit, Michigan, USA

Nick Evans DM
Department of Neonatal Medicine, Royal Prince Alfred Hospital, Sydney, Australia

Sharon F. Evans MSc PhD AStat
Senior Biostatistician, Head, Biostatistics and Study Design, Women's and Infants' Research Foundation, King Edward Memorial Hospital, Perth, Australia

Leslie J. Fairbairn BSc PhD
Paterson Institute for Cancer Research, Christie Hospital, Withington, Manchester, UK

Anne C. Ferguson-Smith PhD
Department of Anatomy, University of Cambridge, Cambridge, UK

Nicholas Fisk FRACOG DDU FRCOG
Department of Obstetrics and Gynaecology, Division of Paediatrics, Obstetrics and Gynaecology, Institute of Obstetrics and Gynaecology, Imperial College of Medicine, Queen Charlotte's and Chelsea Hospital, London, UK

Alan W. Flake MD
Professor of Pediatric Surgery and Director, Department of Surgery, Children's Hospital of Philadelphia, Philadelphia, USA

Alan H. Friedman MD
Assistant Professor, Pediatrics, Department of Pediatrics, Yale University School of Medicine, New Haven, USA

Jocelyn D. Glazier PhD
Department of Child Health, University of Manchester, St Mary's Hospital, Manchester, UK

Peter D. Gluckman CNZM MBChB MMedSc DSc FRACP FRSNZ
Professor of Paediatric and Perinatal Biology, Research Centre for Developmental Medicine and Biology, and Dean, Faculty of Medicine, University of Auckland, Auckland, New Zealand

Stephen J. Gould MBBS BSc FRCPath
Consultant Paediatric Pathologist, Women's Centre, John Radcliffe Hospital, Headington, Oxford, UK

Keith Greene MD FRCOG
Director of Plymouth Perinatal Research Group, University of Plymouth; Consultant Obstetrician and Gynaecologist, Derriford Hospital, Plymouth, UK

Alistair J. Gunn MBChB PhD FRACP
Department of Paediatrics, Faculty of Medicine and Health Sciences, University of Auckland, Auckland, New Zealand

James E. Haddow MD
Vice President/Medical Director, Foundation for Blood Research, Scarborough, Maine, USA

Victor K. M. Han MD FRCPC FRCP
MRC Group in Fetal and Neonatal Health and Development, The Child Health Research Institute and The Lawson Research Institute, University of Western Ontario London, Ontario, Canada

Jane E. Harding MBChB DPhil FRACP
Professor of Neonatology, Department of Paediatrics, Auckland, New Zealand

Richard Harding PhD DSc
Department of Physiology, Monash University, Clayton, Victoria, Australia

Joyce Harper PhD
Senior Lecturer in Preimplantation Genetics, Department of Obstetrics and Gynaecology, University College London, London, UK

Brendan Harrington MA MBChB MD MRCP MRCPCH
Consultant Paediatrician, Department of Paediatrics, Wrexham Maelor Hospital, Wrexham, UK

Jane M. Hawdon PhD FRCP FRCPCH
Consultant Neonatologist, Neonatal Unit, Obstetric Hospital, University College London Hospitals, London, UK

David Henderson-Smart MD FRACP
Department of Neonatal Medicine, King George V Hospital for Mothers and Babies, Camperdown, New South Wales, Australia

Lyndon M. Hill MD
Professor of Obstetrics and Gynecology, Department of Obstetrics, Gynecology and Reproductive Sciences; Medical Director, Ultrasound Department, Magee-Womens Hospital, Pittsburgh, USA

Eric P. Hoffmann PhD
Director, Center for Genetic Medicine, Children's National Medical Center, Washington DC, USA

G. Justus Hofmeyr MD MRCOG
Department of Obstetrics and Gynaecology, Coronation Hospital and University of the Witwatersrand, Johannesburg, South Africa

Wolfgang Holzgreve MD
Professor and Chairman, Department of Obstetrics and Gynaecology, University of Basel, Basel, Switzerland

Stuart B. Hooper PhD
Department of Physiology, Monash University, Clayton, Victoria, Australia

James C. Huhta MD
Medical Director, Noninvasive Laboratories, Pediatric Cardiology, Tampa Children's Hospital; Clinical Professor of Pediatrics, University of South Florida, School of Medicine, Florida, USA

Eric Jauniaux MD PhD
Reader in Obstetrics and Gynaecology, Department of Obstetrics and Gynaecology, University College London, London, UK

Phillippe Jeanty MD PhD
Director, Ultrasound Department, Women's Health Alliance, Nashville, USA

Pam Johnson MD MRCGP MRCOG
Senior Lecturer/Honorary Consultant Obstetrician, Institute of Obstetrics and Gynecology, Queen Charlotte's and Chelsea Hospital, London, UK

Hayley Johnston BSc
Howard Florey Institute, University of Melbourne, Parkville, Victoria, Australia

P. Kaminopetros MRCOG
Clinical Research Fellow, Department of Obstetrics and Gynaecology, University College London, London, UK

Humphrey H. H. Kanhai MD PhD
Professor of Maternal/Fetal Medicine, Head, Department of Obstetrics, Leiden University Medical Centre, Leiden, The Netherlands

Peter Kaufmann MD
Professor of Anatomy, Chairman and Head, Department of Anatomy II, University of Technology, Medical Faculty, Aachen, Germany

Ashley King MA MD MRCP MRCPath
Associate Lecturer, Research Group in Reproductive Immunobiology, Department of Pathology, University of Cambridge, Cambridge, UK

Mary King RDMS
Department of Pediatric, General and Thoracic Surgery, The Children's Hospital of Philadelphia, Philadelphia, USA

John Kingdom MD FRCS MRCOG
Associate Professor, Maternal-Fetal Division, Department of Obstetrics and Gynecology, Mount Sinai Hospital, University of Toronto, Toronto, Canada

Wim J. Kleijer PhD
Department of Clinical Genetics, Erasmus Medical Centre, Rotterdam, The Netherlands

Charles S. Kleinman MD
Professor, Pediatrics, Diagnostic Imaging and Obstetrics and Gynecology; Section Head, Pediatric Cardiology, Department of Pediatrics, Yale University School of Medicine, New Haven, USA

Eric L. Krivchenia MS CGC
Genetic Counselling Coordinator, Division of Reproductive Genetics, Department of Ob/Gyn, Hutzel Hospital, Detroit, Michigan, USA

Michel R. A. Lalloz BSc PhD
Clinical Scientist/Honorary Senior Lecturer, Department of Haematological Medicine, King's College Hospital, London, UK

Anthony D. Lander PhD FRCS DCH
Senior Lecturer, Paediatric Surgery, Institute of Child Health, University of Birmingham and Birmingham Children's Hospital, Birmingham, UK

Linda S. Lashford
Young Oncology Unit, Christie Hospital, Withington, Manchester, UK

D. Mark Layton MBBS FRCP FRCPCH
South Thames Regional Centre for Prenatal Diagnosis of Blood Disorders, Department of Haematological Medicine, King's College Hospital, London, UK

Pamela Lewis MD
Department of Obstetrics and Gynecology, Wayne State University, Hutzel Hospital, Detroit, Michigan, USA

Y. W. Loke MA MD
Reader in Reproductive Immunopathology, Research Group in Reproductive Immunobiology, Department of Pathology, University of Cambridge, Cambridge, UK

Josefine Lorenzen PhD
Clinic for Psychotherapy and Psychosomatics, Essen, Germany

Stephen Lortat-Jacob MD
Praticien Hospitalier, Service de Chirurgie Infantile, Hôpital Necker Enfants-Malades, Paris, France

Stephen J. Lye PhD
Samuel Lunenfeld Research Institute, Mount Sinai Hospital, Toronto, Canada

John A. McGrath MD MRCP
Senior Lecturer in Dermatological Molecular Genetics, Department of Cell and Molecular Pathology, St John's Institute of Dermatology, King's, Guy's and St Thomas' School of Medicine, St Thomas' Hospital, London, UK

D. Mahieu-Caputo MD
Maternité, Antoine Béclère, Clamart, France

Maurice J. Mahoney MD JD
Professor of Genetics, Pediatrics, and Obstetrics and Gynecology, Yale University School of Medicine, New Haven, USA

Neil Marlow MBBS DM FRCP FRCPCH
Professor of Neonatal Medicine, Department of Child Health, University Hospital, Queen's Medical Centre, Nottingham, UK

Peter Miny MD
Professor and Vice Chair, Department of Medical Genetics, University of Basel, Basel, Switzerland

Bernadette Modell PhD FRCP FRCOG
Professor of Community Genetics, Department of Primary Care and Population Sciences, Royal Free and University College Medical School, London, UK

Michael Modell MBBS FRCP FRCGP
Professor of Primary Care, Department of Primary Care and Population Sciences, Royal Free and University College Medical School, London, UK

Karen Moritz BSc MSc
Howard Florey Institute, University of Melbourne, Parkville, Victoria, Australia

Susan M. B. Morton BSc MBChB
Commonwealth Scholar, Epidemiology Unit, London School of Hygiene and Tropical Medicine, London, UK

Françoise Muller MD PhD
Maître de Conférence des Universités, Hôpital Ambroise Paré, Boulogne, France

James P. Neilson BSc MD FRCOG
Professor of Obstetrics and Gynaecology, Department of Obstetrics and Gynaecology, University of Liverpool, Liverpool, UK

John P. Newnham MBBS MD FRCOG FRANZCOG DDU CMFM
Professor, Maternal Fetal Medicine, University of Western Australia; Director, Women's and Infants' Research Foundation, King Edward Memorial Hospital, Perth, Australia

Kypros H. Nicolaides MBBS MRCOG
Harris Birthright Research Centre for Fetal Medicine, King's College Hospital Medical School, London, UK

Umberto Nicolini MD
Associate Professor of Obstetrics and Gynaecology, Head of Obstetrics and Gynaecology, University of Rome, 'Tor Vergata', Milan, Italy

C. Nihoul-Fékété MD
Professor, Service de Chirurgie Infantile, Hôpital Necker Enfants-Malades, Paris, France

Jan G. Nijhuis MD PhD
Department of Obstetrics and Gynaecology, Maastricht, Academic Hospital Maastricht, The Netherlands

Joan M. Noble RGN Dip PHN
Divisional Administrator, Wolfson Institute of Preventive Medicine, St Bartholomew's and the Royal London School of Medicine and Dentistry, Queen Mary and Westfield College, London, UK

Penelope L. Noble MBBS BSc MRCOG
Harris Birthright Research Centre for Fetal Medicine, King's College Hospital Medical School, London, UK

Patrick O'Brien MRCOG
Consultant Obstetrician and Gynaecologist, Obstetric Hospital, University College London Hospitals, London, UK

John M. Old PhD FRCPath
Head of Laboratory, National Haemoglobinopathy Reference Service, Institute of Molecular Medicine, John Radcliffe Hospital, Headington, Oxford, UK

Glenn E. Palomaki BS
Director, Biometry, Foundation for Blood Research, Scarborough, Maine, USA

Donald M. Peebles MA MD MRCOG
Senior Lecturer, Department of Obstetrics and Gynecology, University College London, London, UK

Arianne Peers BSc
Howard Florey Institute, University of Melbourne, Parkville, Victoria, Australia

John Philip MD
Professor, Section of Clinical Genetics, Department of Obstetrics and Gynaecology, Juliane Marie Center, Rigshospitalet, Copenhagen, Denmark

Gianluigi Pilu MD
Consultant in Obstetrics and Gynaecology, Department of Obstetrics and Gynaecology, University of Bologna, Bologna, Italy

Leendert Porcelijn MD
CLB, Sanquin Blood Supply Foundation, Amsterdam, The Netherlands

Rubén A. Quintero MD
Florida Institute for Fetal Diagnosis and Therapy, Tampa, Florida, USA

Bryan Richardson MD FRCS(C)
Professor, Department of Obstetrics and Gynecology and Physiology, University of Western Ontario, Faculty of Medicine; Director, MRC Group in Fetal and Neonatal Health and Development, London, Ontario, Canada

Charles H. Rodeck MBBS BSc DSc(Med) FRCOG FRCPath FMedSci
Professor and Head, Department of Obstetrics and Gynaecology, University College London, London, UK

Juan G. Rodriguez MD
Research Fellow, Fetal Medicine Research Unit, Bristol University, St Michael's Hospital, Bristol, UK

Roberto Romero MD
Chief, Perinatology Research Branch, NICHD/NIH; Professor of Obstetrics and Gynecology, Wayne State University School of Medicine, Hutzel Hospital, Detroit, USA

Nick Rutter MD FRCP
Professor of Paediatric Medicine, Department of Child Health, Queens Medical Centre, Nottingham City Hospital, Nottingham, UK

Paul T. Sharpe BA PhD
Professor, Department of Craniofacial Development, Guy's Hospital, London, UK

Colin P. Sibley PhD
Professor, Department of Child Health, University of Manchester, St Mary's Hospital, Manchester, UK

Joe Leigh Simpson MD
Chairman and Professor, Department of Obstetrics and Gynecology; Professor, Department of Molecular and Human Genetics, Baylor College of Medicine, Houston, Texas, USA

Peter W. Soothill MBBS MD MRCOG
Professor of Maternal and Fetal Medicine, Fetal Medicine Research Unit, Bristol University, St Michael's Hospital, Bristol, UK

Athina P. Souka MD
Harris Birthright Research Centre for Fetal Medicine, King's College Hospital Medical School, London, UK

Daniel V. Surbek MD
Attending Physician, Department of Obstetrics and Gynecology, University of Basel, Basel, Switzerland

Sevgi Tercanli MD
Attending Physician, Ultrasound Division, Department of Obstetrics and Gynecology, University of Basel, Basel, Switzerland

Kent L. Thornburg PhD
Professor, Department of Physiology and Pharmacology; Director, Congenital Heart Research Center, Oregon Health Sciences University, Portland, USA

J. Guy Thorpe-Beeston MA MD MRCOG
Consultant in Obstetrics and Fetal Medicine, Chelsea and Westminster Hospital, London, UK

Brian Trudinger MD FRACOG FRANZCOG
Department of Obstetrics and Gynecology, University of Sydney at Westmead Hospital, Westmead, Australia

Mark Turner BSc MBChB MRCP MRCPCH DRCOG
Department of Child Health, University of Manchester, St Mary's Hospital, Manchester, UK

Nicholas J. Wald MBBS FRCP FRCOG DSc(Med) FFPHM
Professor, Department of Environmental and Preventive Medicine, Wolfson Institute of Preventive Medicine, St Bartholomew's and the Royal London School of Medicine and Dentistry, Queen Mary and Westfield College, London, UK

Martin P. Ward Platt MBChB MD FRCP FRCPH
Consultant Paediatrician and Senior Lecturer in Child Health, Royal Victoria Infirmary, Newcastle-upon-Tyne, UK

Carl P. Weiner MD
Professor and Chair, Department of Obstetrics and Gynecology, University of Maryland Medical System, Baltimore, USA

Martin J. Whittle MD FRCOG FRCP(Glas)
Professor and Head, Division of Reproductive and Child Health, Birmingham Women's Hospital, Edgbaston, Birmingham, UK

E. Marelyn Wintour PhD DSc
Senior Principal Research Fellow, Howard Florey Institute, University of Melbourne, Parkville, Victoria, Australia

Dennis C. Wood RDMS RCPT
Coordinator, Fetal Cardiology, Maternal-Fetal Medicine, Department of Obstetrics and Gynecology; Instructor, Jefferson Ultrasound Research and Education Institute, Thomas Jefferson University, Philadelphia, USA

Nicholas Wood MBChB MRCP MRCPCH
Clinical Research Fellow, Department of Child Health, University Hospital, Queen's Medical Centre, Nottingham, UK

Michael Wyldes MBChB MRCOG MA
Consultant Obstetrician and Gynaecologist, Princess of Wales Maternity Unit, Birmingham Heartlands Hospital, Birmingham, UK

Jerome Yankowitz MD
Director, Division of Maternal–Fetal Medicine and Fetal Diagnosis and Treatment Unit, Department of Obstetrics and Gynecology, University of Iowa Hospitals and Clinics, Iowa City, USA

Yuval Yaron MD
Division of Reproductive Genetics, Department of Obstetrics and Gynecology, Hutzel Hospital, Detroit, Michigan, USA

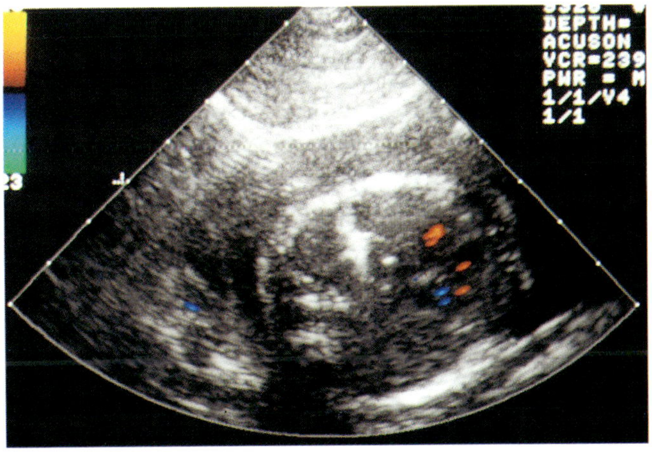

Plate 36.1 Technique of ultrasound-guided fetal liver biopsy in the second trimester of pregnancy. Sonogram obtained during fetal liver biopsy. Note tip of the special needle in the fetal liver.

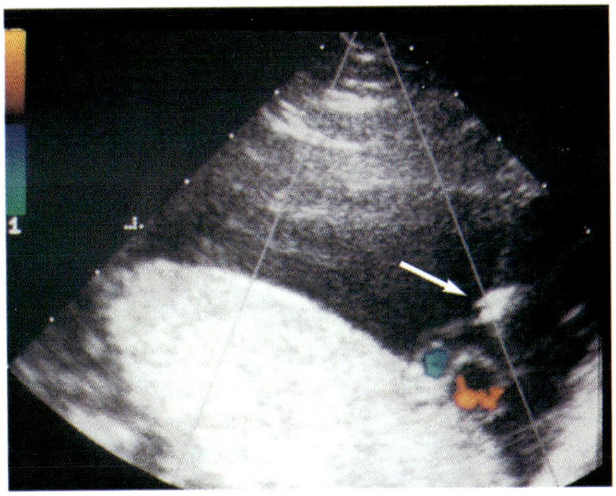

(a)

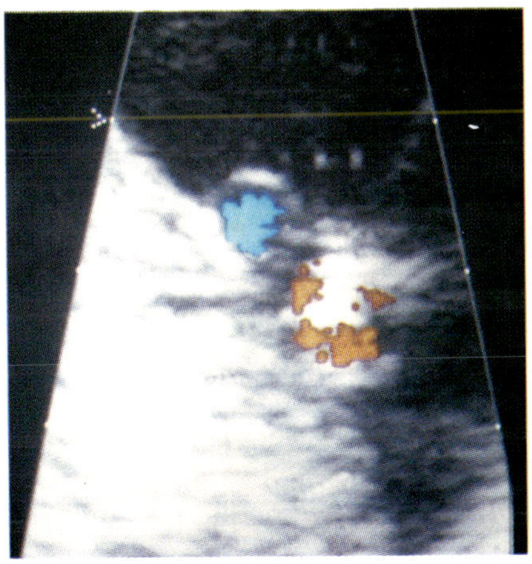

(b)

Plate 36.2 Cordocentesis technique. (a) Sonogram showing needle approaching the umbilical cord. (b) Sonogram showing tip of the needle in the umbilical vein.

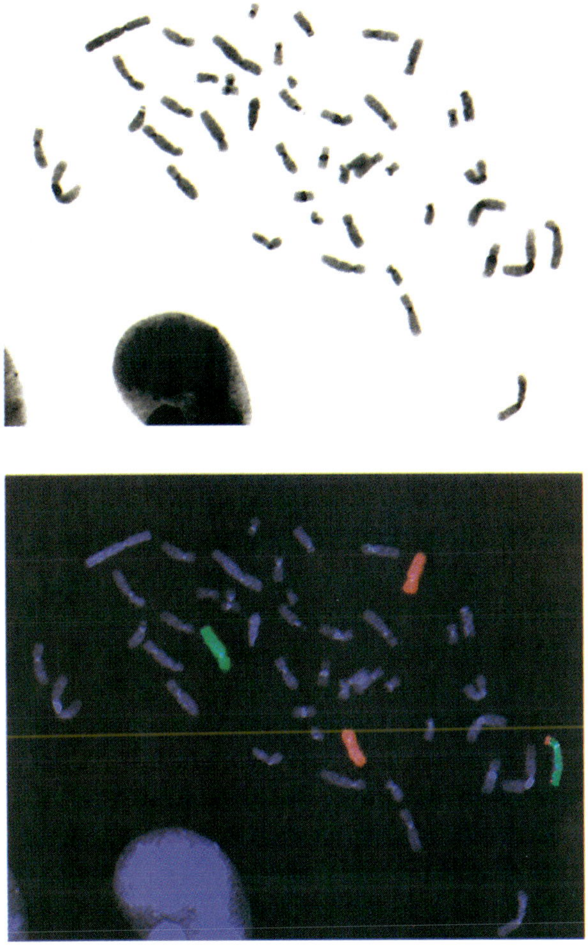

Plate 37.1 This metaphase from a prenatal amnionsample is stained with whole chromosome painting probes (Oncor coatasome). Chromosome 4 is green, chromosome 8 is red. One green chromosome (4) is carrying an extra red (8) piece of DNA, while the red chromosomes (8) have no extra green, i.e. an unbalanced translocation. This was suspected when the Giemsa banded chromosomes were analysed. The balanced translocation (illustrated in Plate 37.2) was known to be present in the father. Break points derived from Giemsa banded karyotype (not shown). The karyotype is 46, XX, ish der (4) t (4;8) (q15.3;p22) pat (wcp4+, wcp8+).

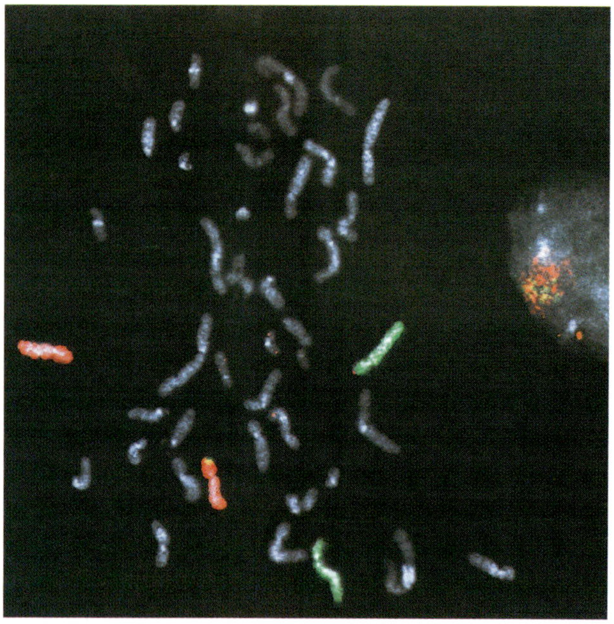

Plate 37.2 This is a metaphase from a blood sample from the father of the fetus whose karyotype is seen in Plate 37.1. One of the red chromosomes (8) is carrying a green piece of DNA (4). One of the green chromosomes (4) is carrying a red piece (8). This may also be seen on the Giemsa banded karyotype, from which break points are derived (not shown). The karyotype is 46, XY. ish t (4;8) (p15.3;p11) (wcp4+, wcp8+; wcp4+, wcp8+).

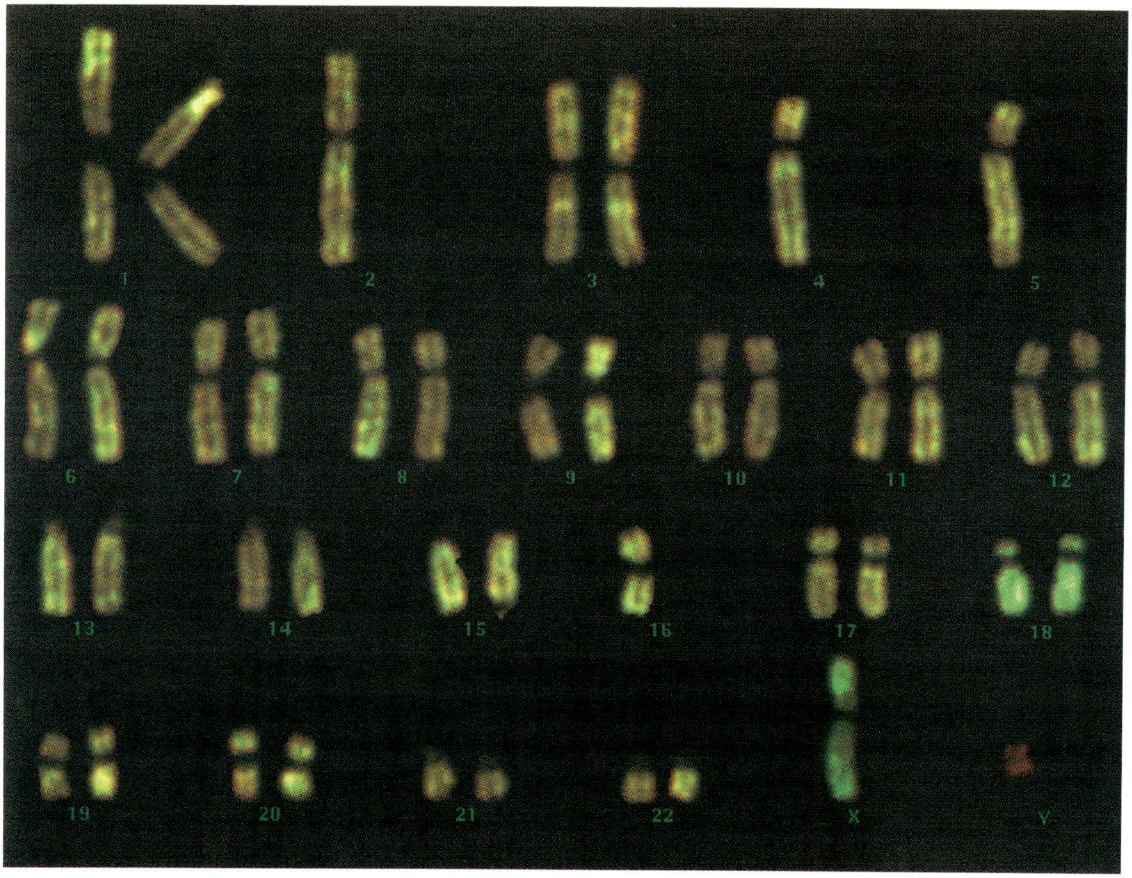

Plate 37.3 Comparative genomic hybridization. Normal metaphase chromosomes were hybridized with DNA from a chorionic villus sample labelled with green fluorochrome and DNA from a healthy individual labelled with red fluorochrome. All autosomes (1–22) except chromosomes 18 show equal intensities of the two fluorochromes. The green colour of the two chromosomes 18 indicate that chromosome 18 is overrepresented in the chorionic villus sample relative to the normal sample. The X chromosome is green and the Y chromosome is red because the chorionic villus sample is from a female and the normal DNA is from a male.

Plate 37.4 Fluorescence in situ hybridization on interphase blood cells from a newborn child with trisomy 18. The hybridization was performed with a locus specific probe for chromosome 18.

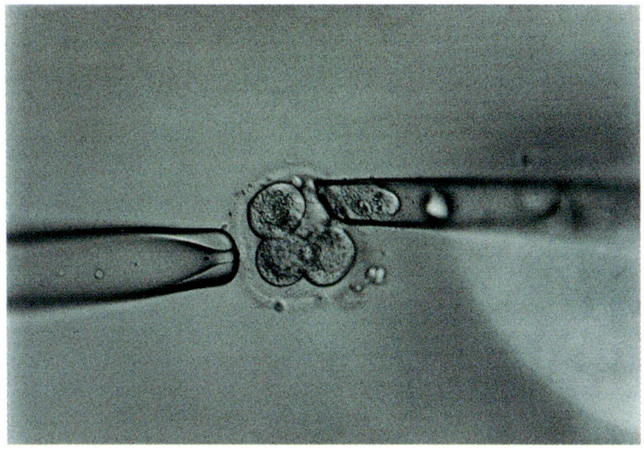

(a)

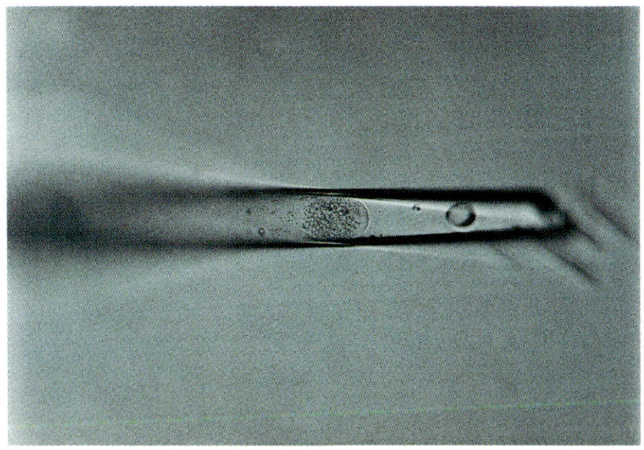

(b)

Plate 39.1 (a) Cleavage stage embryo biopsy. (b) Blastomere aspiration. The blastomere can be seen in the capillary tube.

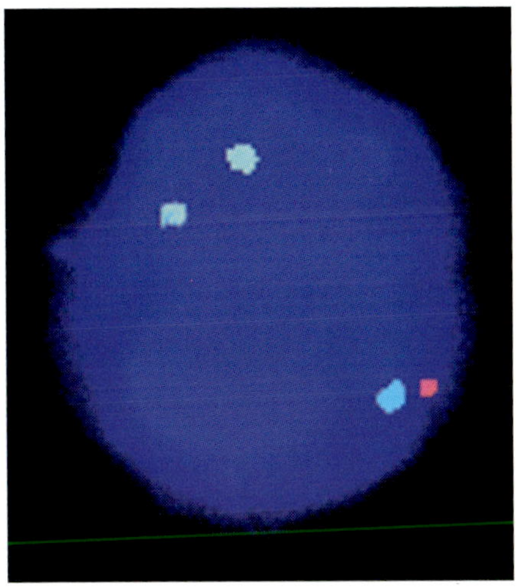

Plate 39.2 Fluorescent in situ hybridization on a blastomere from a patient carrying a 18:21 translocation. Probes were used for the centromeric region of chromosome 18 (aqua), 18q telomeric probe (red) and 21q22.2 (green). The blastomere is monosomy 18 as there is only one aqua and one red signal.

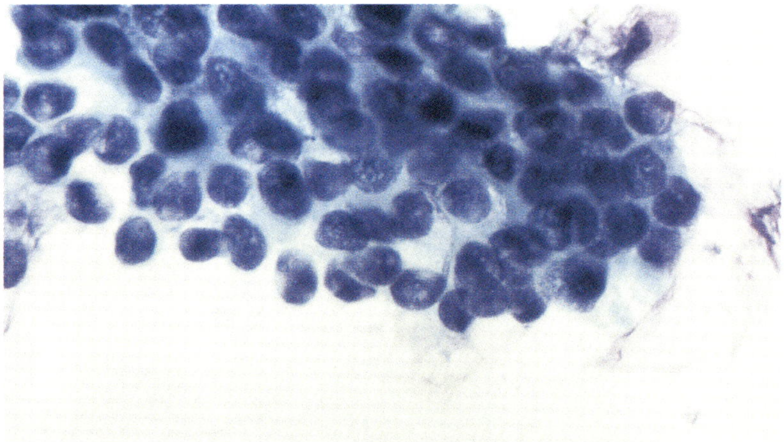

(a)

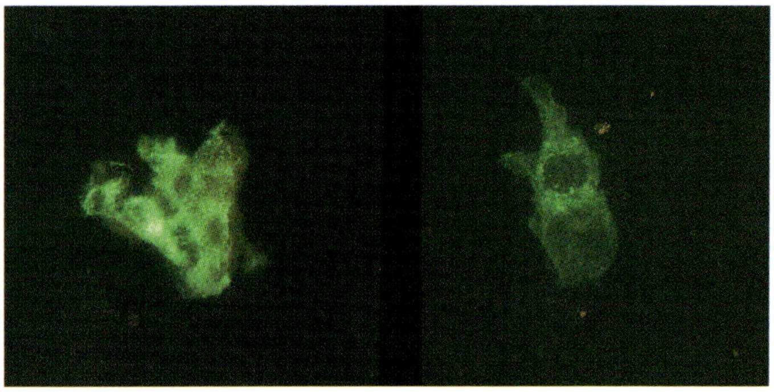

(b)

Plate 40.1 (a) Trophoblastic clump found in cervical mucus. (b) Trophoblastic cells stained with fluorescent-labelled monoclonal antibody against placental antigens (F1.41).

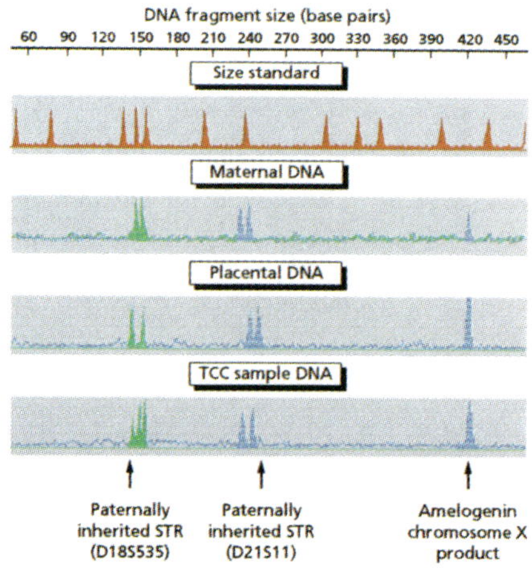

Plate 40.2 Peaks of fluorescent intensity indicate products of PCR, separated by capillary electrophoresis. DNA from the transcervical cell sample clearly displays the paternally inherited STR from both the D21S11 and the D18S535 markers. The chromosome Y amelogenin PCR product (252 base pairs) is absent from both placental and TCC DNA, indicating the fetus to be female.

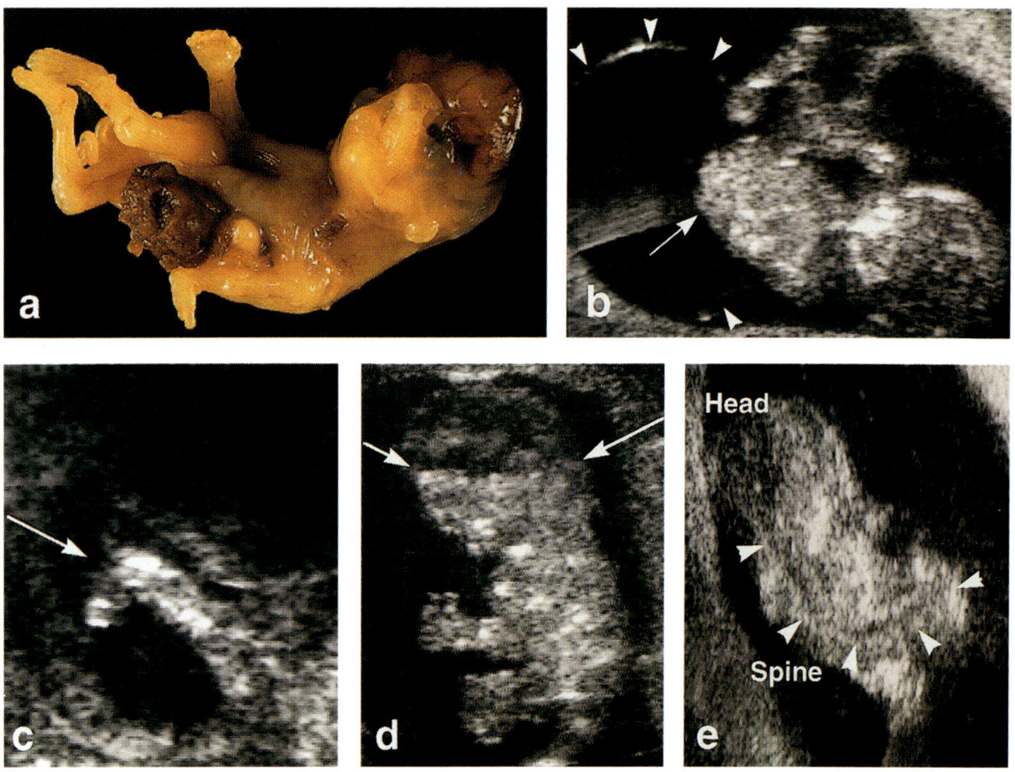

Plate 49.1 Ultrasound images of a maldeveloped embryo at 9 weeks (CRL 27 mm), which was aborted spontaneously at 10 weeks. (a) Postabortem photograph: A large thoracoabdominal defect is visible. The body is distorted. One arm is malformed. The amniotic adhesions have lead to facial defects, the cranial vault consists of only a membrane. This is an acrania. (b) The abdominal content (arrow) lies in a cystic cavity (arrow heads). (c) The arrow points at the disrupted arm (compare with (a)). (d) Ultrasound picture of the head: The arrows point at the demarcation between the cranial basis and the abnormal vault. The brain cavities are not visible. (e) The arrow heads point at the distorted spine.

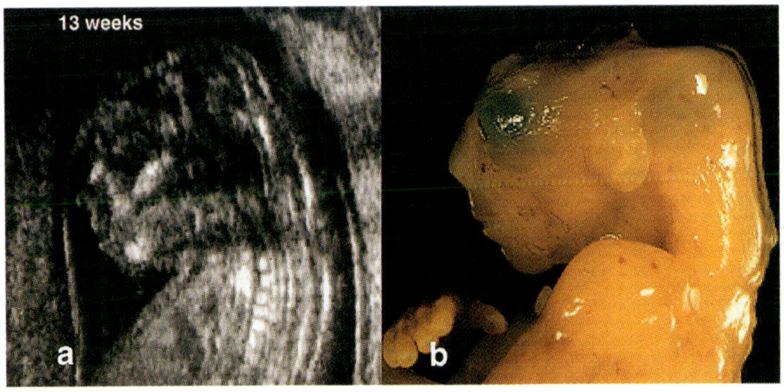

Plate 49.2 Sagittal section through the head of a 13-week-old anencephalic fetus. (a) Ultrasound image. (b) Postabortem photograph.

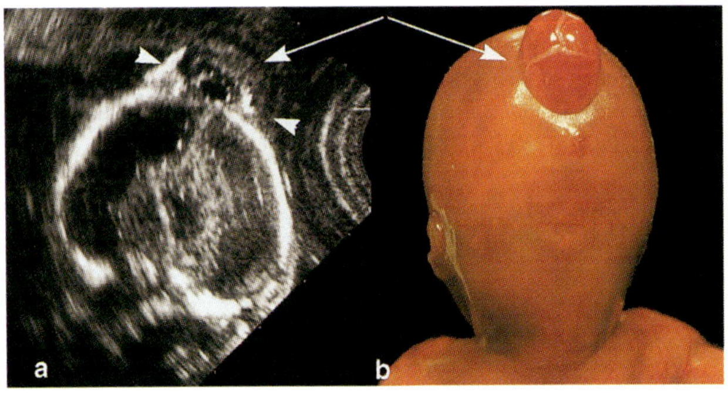

Plate 49.3 (a) Ultrasound picture and (b) postabortem photograph of the fetus with COMS at 17 weeks (Fig. 49.11). The encephalocele (arrows) originates from the mesencephalon.

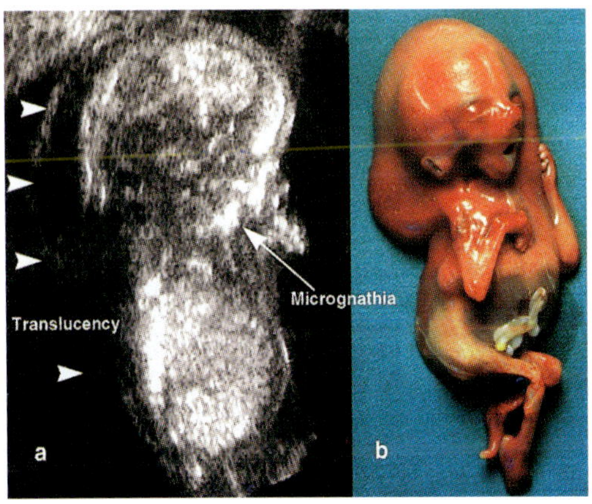

Plate 49.4 (a) 12-week-old fetus with lethal multiple pterygium syndrome. The fetus had micrognathia (long arrow) and nuchal translucency (arrow heads). The extremities had contractures. (b) Postabortem photograph of a 17-week-old fetus with the same diagnosis. Note the contractures and the pterygia.

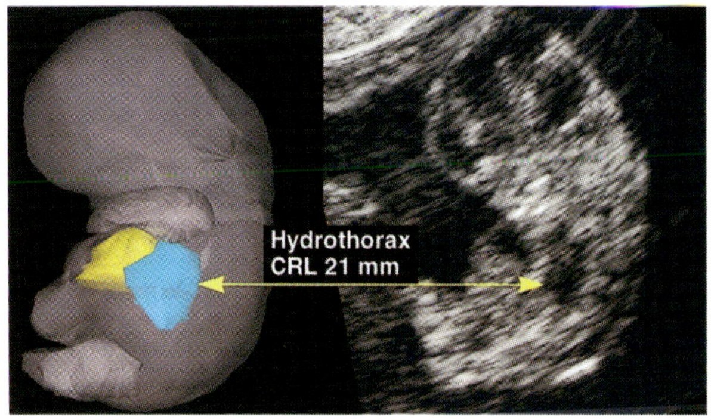

Plate 49.5 Three-dimensional reconstruction of a hydropic embryo, CRL 21 mm, with general edema and hydrothorax. The embryo died a few days after the examination. The 3D image shows the swollen appearance of this embryo, the fluid in the pleural cavity (blue) and the heart (yellow). The volumes were: embryo 1278 mm^3, pleural cavities 151 mm^3, and heart 22 mm^3.

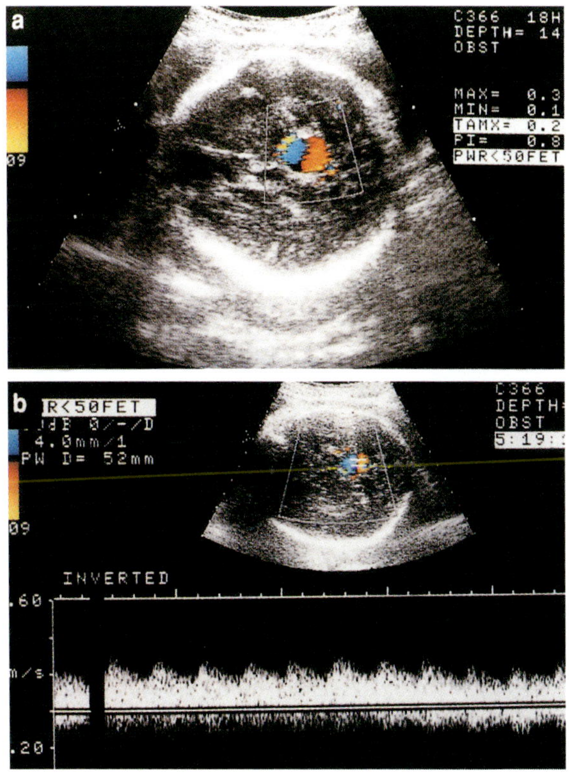

Plate 50.1 Colour Doppler ultrasonography of arteriovenous malformation involving the vein of Galen at 35 weeks' gestation. (a) Colour flow imaging clearly demonstrates the vascular nature of the lesion. (b) Pulsed Doppler demonstrates turbulent flow within the vessel. (From Sepulveda, W. et al. (1995) *Ultrasound Obstet. Gynecol.* **6**, 282–286. Used by permission.)

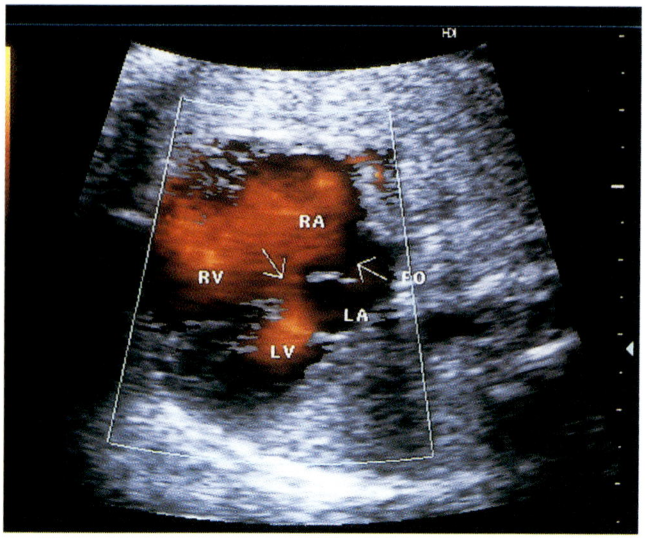

Plate 51.1 Color power angiography image of same fetus as Fig. 51.3 showing flow across the primum atrial septal defect in addition to flow across the foramen ovale. There was a minimal ventricular septal defect, so flow is not seen below the level of the atrioventricular valves. (FO = foramen ovale.)

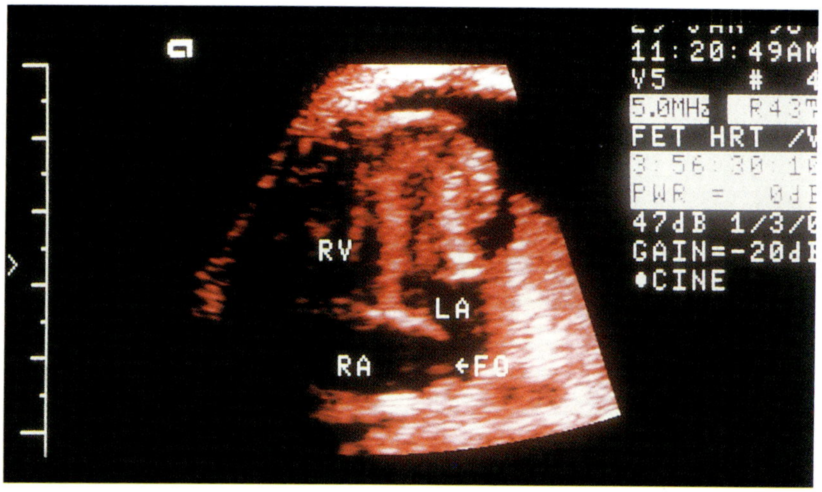

Plate 51.2 Apical four chamber view of fetus with hypoplastic left ventricle. Note discrepancy in atrial and ventricular sizes and displacement of the interatrial septum towards the left. (FO = foramen ovale.)

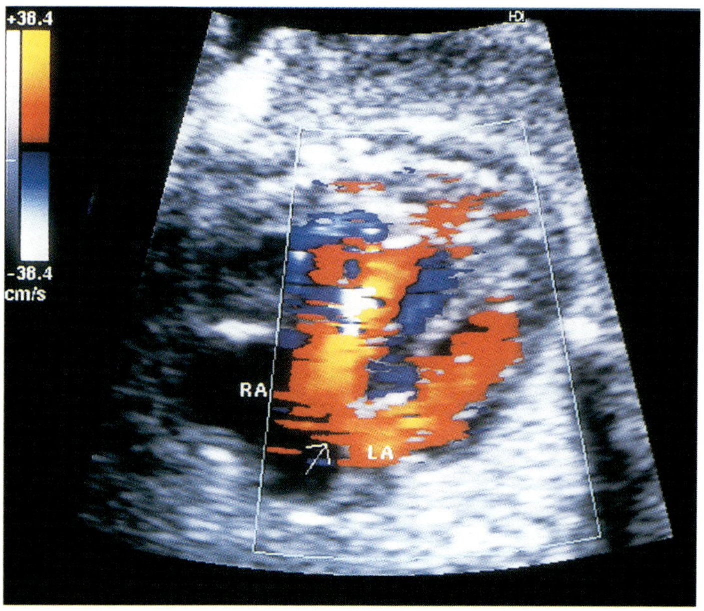

Plate 51.3 Colour Doppler flow mapping (CDFM) of same fetus as Plate 51.2 demonstrating reversal of normal flow across the foramen ovale (arrow), from left atrium (LA) to right (RA).

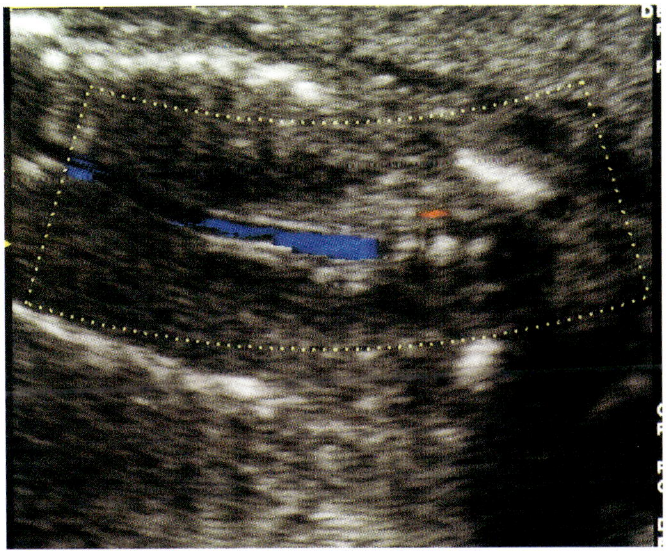

Plate 53.1 Bilateral renal agenesis at 22 weeks. The aorta is imaged by coloured flow mapping, but not the renal artery.

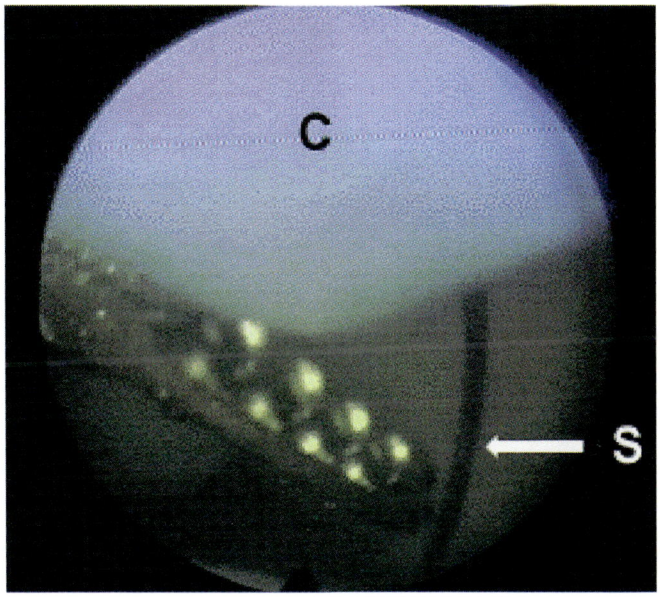

Plate 57.2 Technique to perform the umbilical cord ligation. The suture material is placed underneath the umbilical cord. The end of the suture is retrieved on the other side of the cord. A loop around the cord has been performed with a single instrument. These steps are performed best under endoscopic guidance, but may be accomplished under sonographic guidance alone in selected cases. (C = umbilical cord; S = suture.)

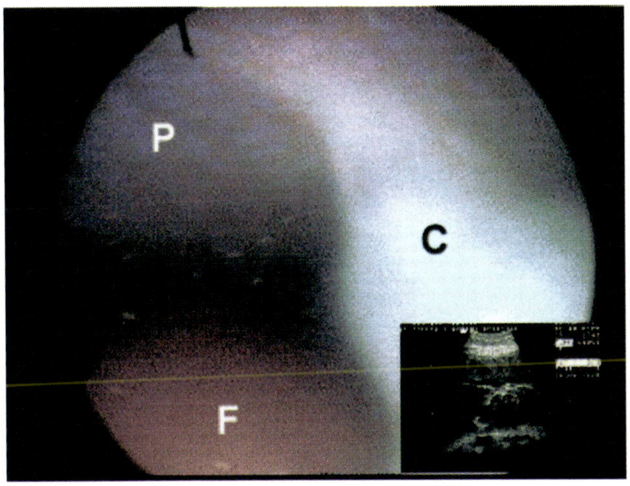

Plate 57.1 Simultaneous display of sonographic and endoscopic images in a single monitor using a videomixer. Coordination of the operating instruments is greatly facilitated. (C = Umbilical cord; P = placenta; F = fetus.)

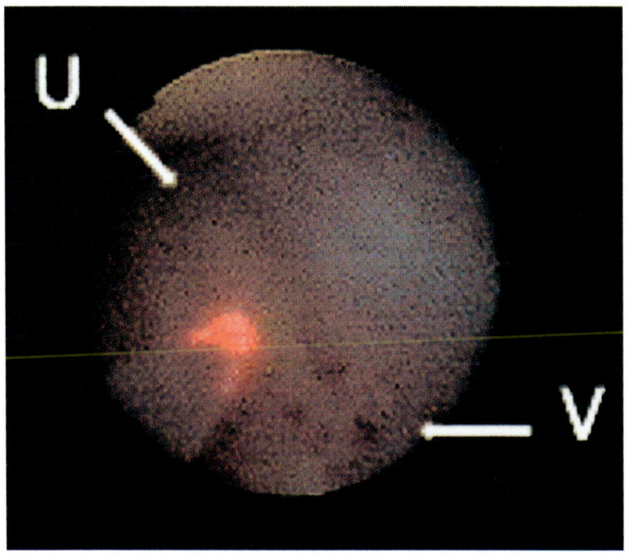

Plate 57.3 In utero endoscopic ablation of posterior urethral valves. The YAG-laser fibre is being fired against the valve. Completion of the ablation of the valves is accomplished with gentle rotation of the endoscope. Urethral permeability is confirmed with vesicoinfusion. (U = urethra; V = verumontanum.)

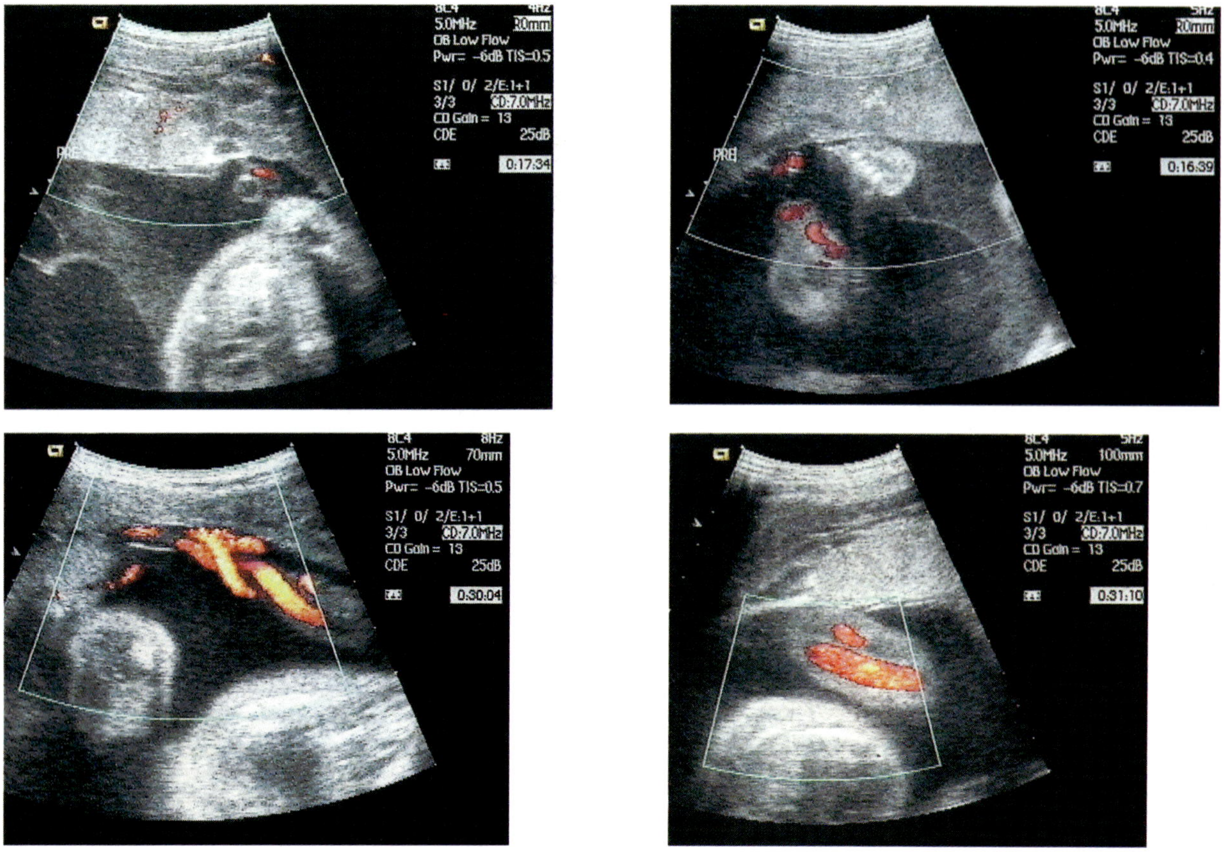

Plate 65.1 Demonstration of intertwin transfusion in a monochorionic twin pair. Microbubble contrast is seen following injection into the intrahepatic vein of the first twin, with enhancement seen within the cardiac chambers of the cotwin shortly afterwards. (Reproduced with permission from Denbow M, Blomly M, Cosgrove D & Fisk N. (1997) Ultrasound microbubble contrast angiography in monochorionic twin fetuses. *Lancet* **349**, 773.)

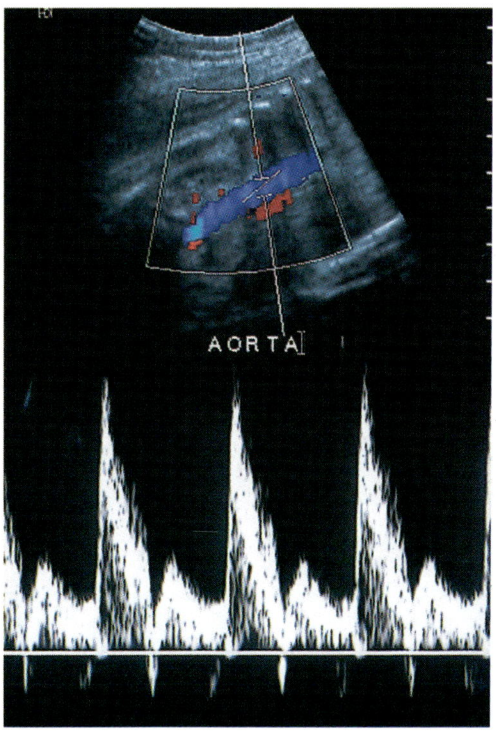

Plate 72.1 The aortic FVW recorded from the descending thoracic aorta.

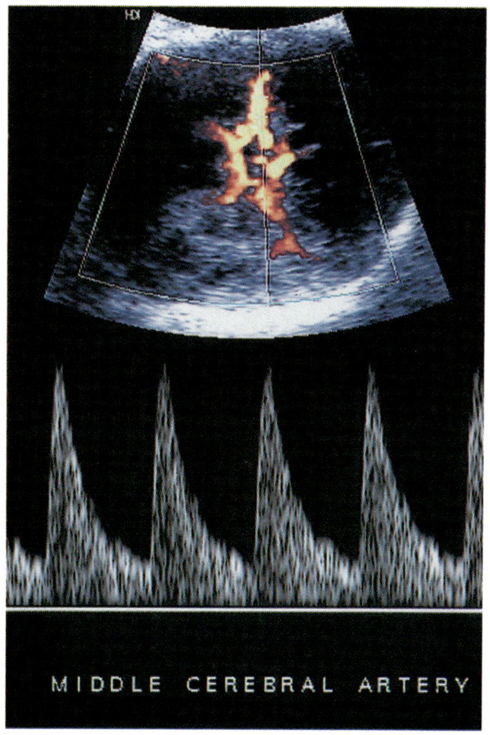

Plate 72.2 The circle of Willis is readily seen using colour power angiography in a transverse view of the fetal head. The FVW is readily recorded from the middle cerebral artery.

SECTION 1

Cell, molecular and reproductive biology

Early concepts and terminology

1

P. Collins

Traditional accounts of embryology rely on familiarity with the germ layer concept developed in the latter years of the 19th century. All students are acquainted with ectoderm, endoderm and mesoderm layers and accept the grouping of mature tissues and systems with these layers. However, as we, at the end of the 20th century, approach the 21st it seems an apposite time to review the usage of our old terminology and the assumptions which have developed as a consequence, and move forward stating our present knowledge base using the most appropriate language with which to express our existing concepts and hypotheses.

The transitory nature of our conceptual frameworks is acknowledged. We know that the 'snapshots' of knowledge in textbooks may be outdated by the time of publication and are now more likely to turn to the Internet to find the latest publications on a topic. However, the language we use to describe even the most recent findings is still rooted in the past and in many ways hinders our ability to explain developmental processes.

The rapid advances in developmental biology which have increased our understanding of embryological processes have elucidated many cell lines each of which give rise to parts of the embryo, each cell type being important in different stages of development. The relatively new methods of cell study, e.g. inter alia, cloning cells taken from early and later stages of development, and production of chimeric embryos where cells from, for example, quail embryos are substituted for cells in chick embryos, have compounded the problem of how to describe cell populations in early embryos so as to marry the older embryological terminology everyone is familiar with to the newer, more specialised, vocabulary of developmental biology.

It has been suggested that to cope with the complex and often conflicting terminologies in embryology, nomenclature relating to the histological appearance of cells is more helpful than the older traditional concepts[1–3]. Indeed the advances in embryology now make it increasingly difficult to relate older and newer language. This first chapter will give a brief account of the way the older terminology developed and move on to explain the usage of the more recent terminologies.

The origin of the traditional language of embryology

The traditional language of embryology comes from work and concepts generated between 1830 and 1900, when, in the mid-1800s, the theory of evolution was being formulated. Ernst Haeckel[4] (1874), particularly, promoted a concept which stated that embryos would pass through all the previous evolutionary stages, resembling a series of extant or extinct adult animals as they recapitulated evolution during development. Thus Haeckel designated a *blastula* stage of development, where a sphere or bilaminar layer of embryonic cells were present, and a later *gastrula* stage achieved after the blastula cells had invaginated to produce more than one or two layers. It is from Haeckel we have the term *gastrulation* to describe the process where cells initially on the embryonic surface move inside the embryo to produce intraembryonic cell populations.

At this time the instruments for examining embryos were rudimentary and the cell theory was still relatively young. Scientists of the day saw layers of tissue rather than the individual cells composing the layers. Even in those studies where it is clear from the publications that cells could be seen, distinctions between early embryonic cell types probably could not be made with the instruments available. The concepts thus generated by these early embryologists were products of their time, dependent on the methods of experiment and observation customary when they were formulated.

During the process of gastrulation cells from the outside of the embryo move to the interior and become organised in specific sites. The concept of three main or *germ layers* was formulated by von Baer[5] (1828) and promoted by the Hertwig brothers[6] (1879–83) who supported the doctrine that three germ layers were found in all animal embryos. The layers of adult two layered creatures had been named *ectoderm* and *endoderm* by Allman[7] (1855), and later the term *mesoderm* was introduced to describe both the structure that intervened between the ectoderm (exoderm) and endoderm (entoderm) of triploblastic animals, and the corresponding embryonic middle layer[4] (Haeckel 1871, 1874). At the same time the more specific embryological terms *epiblast*, *mesoblast* and *hypoblast* were used by Balfour[8] (1873) in his studies on chick embryos. Thus for most of the 20th century, textbooks have supported a notion that the tissues of the developed body are derived from one of the three germ layers. Whilst this is not untrue in simplistic terms, the accent on three layers has obfuscated the dynamic differentiation processes occurring in embryos and hindered much description of what can be seen histologically.

A similar process occurred with the description of external embryonic form. Von Baer noted that all vertebrate embryos pass through externally similar stages and Haeckel published a series of drawings demonstrating remarkable similarity between embryos which go on to become very dissimilar adults. This latter concept has remained unchallenged for over a century. Recent examination of Haeckel's pictures, together with a clear analysis of the developmental stages of various organs in each embryo has revealed a story much closer to the Emperor's new clothes. Richardson[9] notes that drawings by contemporaries of Haeckel show much more accurate interpretations of mammalian embryos of the same developmental stage with clear differences between them. He notes that Haeckel's drawings have given a misleading view of embryonic development. Thus the idea of one stage of development where all vertebrate are the same, promoted extensively at the turn of the century and repeated unchallenged nearly to this day, has again obfuscated what really occurs in a number of vertebrate embryos and has hindered our search for what is actually present in embryos by limiting our language and expectations.

A description of the developmentally based terminology which recent textbooks of embryology embrace follows, outlining the initial derivation and fate of the early cell lines. As can be seen, the complexities of development now require a redefining of the older terminologies and the introduction of new ones to describe the changes taking place and the cell types involved.

Recent nomenclature of early development and specification of cell origin

The initial zygote cleaves into a number of cells which, because of their position and experiences, have different fates. The earliest positions of cells in the morula will influence the first decision between trophoblastic cells, which will give rise to the placenta and membranes, or embryonic cells. The initial embryonic cells, which are arranged as a disc, are collectively termed *epiblast*. These cells will produce all of the embryonic cell lines and some extraembryonic cell lines. The epiblast cells are supported by an underlying *hypoblast* layer of extraembryonic cells which will later become sequestered into the yolk sac wall. An interaction between epiblast and hypoblast gives rise to the *primitive streak*, a region of cell proliferation and movement, that defines the cranio-caudal axis of the embryo. Passage through the primitive streak will confer a fate onto cells specified by the position of invagination or the time of invagination (Lawson *et al.*[10]). Predictive fate maps of the epiblast have been constructed from data on the differentiative fate of cells taken from different regions of the embryonic disc and cloned (Fig. 1.1).

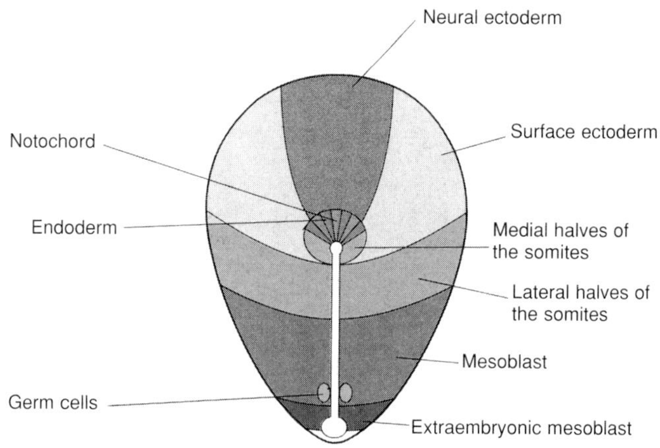

Fig. 1.1 Predictive fates of the epiblast cell population at the time the primitive streak is present. (From Gray's Anatomy, 38th edition, Edinburgh: Churchill Livingstone, 1995, p. 143.)

The primitive streak extends from near the centre of the embryonic disc, where it forms the *primitive node*, a curved ridge of cells, to the edge of the disc close to the stalk connecting the embryo to the developing placenta. Passage through the primitive node gives rise to the axial cell populations, the *notochord* and the *medial halves of the somites*, and also to the *endoderm* which spreads out beneath the epiblast displacing the hypoblast laterally into the yolk sac wall. Passage through the rostral portion of the primitive streak, however, produces the *lateral halves of the somites* and the middle portion of the streak produces the *lateral plate cells* (Selleck & Stern[11,12]). The next caudal portion of the primitive streak gives rise to the *primordial germ cells*. These are sequestered in the extraembryonic tissues very early on in development and do not return to the embryo until the early gonads have formed. The most caudal portion of the streak contributes cells to the *extraembryonic tissue*.

Once these cells have passed through the primitive streak the remaining epiblast contains cells populations which will become the surface epithelium of the embryo (this still retains the term 'ectoderm') and the neuroepithelium of the embryo which will form the central, peripheral and autonomic nervous systems. This population is termed 'neurectoderm' prior to neurulation; it is found in front of the primitive node.

The cells within the epiblast are epithelial, when they pass through the primitive streak they undergo a change in morphology allowing them to migrate. This new migratory population is initially termed *mesoblast* (Collins & Billet[3]; Nakatsuji[13]). All of the early migratory cells derived from ingression through the primitive streak revert to epithelia when they arrive at their final destinations and subsequently form proliferative centres. Cells produced from these early germinal epithelia form populations described as *mesenchyme* further subdivided according to their position in the embryo. Special populations of mesenchyme also develop from the neural epithelium. At the margins of the neural plate are clusters of neuroepithelial cells termed *neural crest cells*. These cells will form the peripheral nervous system in the trunk and head and an extensive mesenchymal population in the head, often termed 'ectomesenchyme'. The neural crest is found only in vertebrates; it is considered to be an evolutionary advance allowing the development of special sense organs within complex facial structures.

The production of migrating cells from the primitive streak and the development of the neurectoderm which undergoes neurulation (see p. 70) forming the central nervous system, dramatically changes the shape of the embryonic disc causing reflection of the edge of the disc which is displaced to a ventral position with the newly formed neural tube being dorsal. This early head and tail flexion with corresponding lateral flexion produces the body plan or *Bauplan* and thus a recognisable embryo. Of the developmental studies which have been undertaken over the years in a range of vertebrate species very few correlate the developmental state of internal organs with external characteristics. Richardson[9], in a study of heterochrony, a change in developmental timing during evolution, has correlated the time of appearance of a number of features to somite number, which is seen as an arbitrary way of expressing developmental age of embryos. This method of investigation allows comparison of the order of development of internal features between a number of embryos and greatly aids our thinking of evolution and development.

Animal models of development

Embryological studies have concentrated on a relatively few species which are easily accessible. Thus chick and quail development has been extensively researched as has *Xenopus* and other amphibians. Mammalian embryos are difficult to access and difficult to culture for long periods of time; however, the development of the mouse and rat has been closely studied. Although some human material has been used for study of very early embryonic development, work is not permitted after 14 days when the primitive streak is formed. Within the last ten years, identification of common DNA sequences in vertebrates and invertebrates has meant that embryological processes are now being followed in many species and the findings are equally relevant to human embryos (see p. 49).

The use of diverse species for research means that knowledge about the differences in early development between these species is important. All avian embryos develop from a blastoderm or flattened layer of epiblast above a vast yolk. Mice and rats have folded embryonic regions with the epiblast on the inner surface and the hypoblast on the outer convex surface. During head and tail folding in the mouse, morphological movements alter the embryonic body from a position where the head and tail are in close proximity with the dorsal region fully extended to one where the dorsal region is fully flexed. In human embryos, the embryonic area is disc shaped similar to avia and although a degree of extension occurs as neurulation proceeds the extreme extension, as in the mouse, does not occur.

Much confusion in the literature arises because of the difference in nomenclature of axes in animal and human studies. In animals the axes are described as dorsal/ventral (back to front), lateral/lateral (side to side) and anterior/posterior (nose to tail), and these descriptions are used for embryos. In adult humans, however, the convention for these same axes is posterior/anterior, lateral/lateral and cranial/caudal and this terminology is used variably for human embryos. Much disorientation results from moving from descriptions of human embryos to animal embryos without bearing these terminological differences in mind. The latter descriptors, for the human, are used in this section (for a discussion of left-right development see p. 59).

REFERENCES

1. Løvtrup S. Epigenetic mechanisms in the early amphibian embryo: cell differentiation and morphogenetic elements. *Biol Rev* **38**:91–130, 1983.
2. Løvtrup S. An introduction to the new evolutionary paradigm. In *Beyond Neo-Darwinism* Ma-Wan Ho & PT Saunders. (eds) London: Academic Press, 1984.
3. Collins P, Billett ES. The terminology of early development: history, concepts and current usage. *Clin Anat* **8**:418–425, 1995.
4. Haeckel E. The gastrea theory, phylogenetic classification of the animal kingdom and the homology of the germ lamellae (trans. E.O. Wright). *Quart J Micr Sci* **14**:142–165, 223–247, 1874.
5. Von Baer KE. *Entwicklingsgeschichte der Tiere: Beobachtung und Reflexion.* Konigsberg: Bontrager, 1828.
6. Hertwig WAO, Hertwig R. Studies on the germ layers. In *Naturwissenschaften*, pp. 13–16, Jena: Zeit. 1879–83.
7. Allman GJ. On the structure and development of *Myriothela*. *Phil Trans Roy Soc London* **165**(2):549–575, 1855.
8. Balfour FM. The development and growth of the layers of the blastoderm. *Quart J Micr Sci* **13**:266–276, 1873.
9. Richardson MK. Heterochrony and the phylotypic period. *Develop Biol* **172**:412–421, 1995.
10. Lawson KA, Meneses JJ, Pederson RA. Clonal analysis of epiblast fate

during germ layer formation in the mouse embryo. *Development* **113**:891–911, 1991.
11. Selleck MA, Stern CD. Fate mapping and cell lineage analysis of Hensen's node in the chick embryo. *Development* **112**:615–626, 1991.
12. Selleck MA, Stern CD. Commitment of mesoderm cells in Hensen's node of the chick embryo to notochord and somite. *Development* **114**:403–415, 1992.
13. Nakatsuji N. Development of postimplantation mouse embryos: unexplored field rich in unanswered questions. *Devel Growth Differ* **35**:489–499, 1992.

Genomic imprinting

2

A.C. Ferguson-Smith

Introduction

A fertilized egg inherits a haploid set of chromosomes from both the egg and the sperm. However, in mammals these maternal and paternal gametes do not contribute equal genetic functions to the developing diploid embryo. This functional difference between the two sets of parental chromosomes is due to a process called 'genomic imprinting'. Genomic imprinting is a mechanism that differentially 'marks' the maternally and paternally inherited chromosome homologues and results in particular genes being expressed or repressed in response to this parent-specific modification. Because the imprint affects gene activity, some imprinted genes are expressed only from the maternally inherited chromosome and others are expressed only from the paternally inherited chromosome as is illustrated schematically in Fig. 2.1. It is not known why such a process evolved and the precise mechanisms involved in the regulation of imprinted genes is not yet fully understood. However, it follows that the dosage of an imprinted gene can be doubled or lost completely if there is a unipaternal duplication or deficiency involving the gene or chromosomal region in which it resides (Fig. 2.1). This can have profound effects on embryonic development.

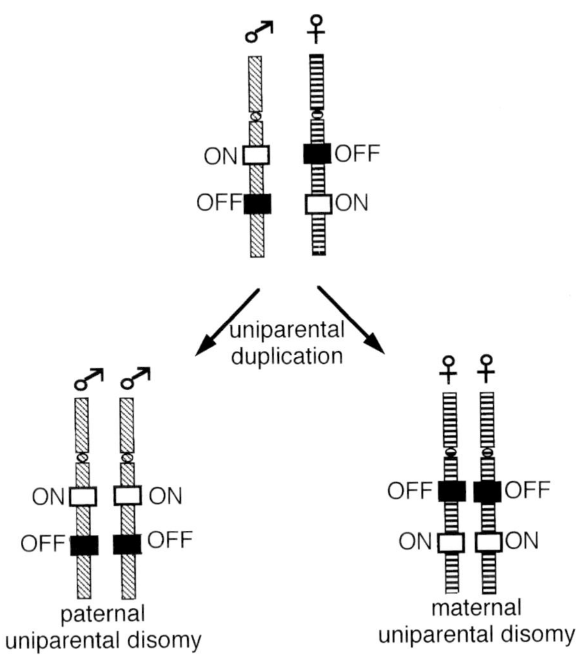

Fig. 2.1

Developmental consequences of imprinting

Genomic imprinting ensures the requirement for both a mother and a father to produce normal mammalian offspring as shown by the failure of bimaternal and bipaternal conceptuses to complete embryogenesis[1,2]. Parthenogenesis, the development of an egg without fertilization by a sperm, is successful in some lower organisms. However, it is clear that parthenogenetic eutherian mammals cannot survive to term. In the mouse, parthenogenesis, to create a diploid maternal egg, can be induced experimentally. Parthenogenetic embryos will survive to midgestation and appear morphologically relatively normal although growth retarded. The extraembryonic tissues, however, are extremely underdeveloped and do not proliferate properly. Gynogenetic embryos, also containing a diploid maternal contribution though from two different mothers, exhibit the same properties as parthenogenones. Diploid paternal androgenetic conceptuses are made by replacing the female pronucleus in a newly fertilized egg with a second male pronucleus from another egg. These embryos fare worse than parthenogenones, with very poor development of the embryo which rarely develops beyond the four-somite stage. In contrast to the parthenogenones, the extraembryonic tissues are well developed though not completely normal.[1,2] In this respect, the androgenone is reminiscent of the complete hydatidiform mole in humans. These conceptuses contain a genome derived solely from paternal chromosomes. The mole resembles a mass of cytotrophoblast without any embryonic components[3]. Thus it appears that the parental genomes have reciprocal functions in early embryogenesis, with the presence of a paternal genome generally being important for the development of the extraembryonic lineages and the maternal genome being required for the development of the embryonal components at these early stages. This reflects the properties of imprinted genes whose activities are either doubled or lost in the uniparental conceptuses.

The androgenetic and parthenogenetic cells appear to have reciprocal properties later in development too, as is evident from the analysis of chimaeric mice, which contain normal cells as well as some androgenetic or parthenogenetic cells. The presence of normal cells 'rescues' the early lethality seen in complete parthenogenetic and androgenetic embryos. Indeed, parthenogenetic/normal chimaeras survive to term and are viable and fertile. They exhibit growth retardation but otherwise appear normal. Within the chimera, however the parthenogenetic cells prefer to populate cells of ectodermal origin such as neural tissue and are rarer in mesodermal lineages such as skeletal muscle[4,5]. Androgenetic cells are also rescued by the presence of normal cells in androgenetic/normal chimeras. However, they will only survive to term if the contribution of androgenetic cells is low. Unlike the parthenogenetic cells in chimeras, the androgenetic cells have a preference for mesodermal lineages and are rarely found in neural tissue. A high percentage of androgenetic cells in the mesodermal lineages giving rise to the axial skeleton, results in rib deformity characterised by apparent overproliferation of costal cartilages in addition to abnormalities of the vertebral column[6,7]. These chimeric studies illustrate that imprinted genes have a role to play in the regulation of embryonic growth and in the normal development of particular lineages. These findings are reminiscent of some of the clinical phenotypes observed in imprinted disorders in man (see later) and indicate that the mouse continues to be a good model system to investigate the molecular and developmental functions of imprinting in development and disease.

Genetic studies of genomic imprinting in the mouse

It has been shown through extensive genetic studies by Cattanach and his colleagues, that the requirement for both parental genomes is limited to a subset of chromosomes[8,9]. This has become evident from mouse-breeding experiments which result in embryos carrying uniparental duplications and corresponding deficiencies of whole chromosomes (uniparental disomy – UPD) or particular chromosomal regions. These duplications represent a subset of the whole genome duplications seen in the parthenogenetic and androgenetic embryos. UPD (Fig. 2.1) found in all cells, is usually due to meiotic non-disjunction events giving rise to unbalanced gametes in both parents. This can be generated experimentally by interbreeding mouse lines harbouring chromosome translocations, but in man is extremely rare. In man, somatic mosaicism with UPD is more common, and often arises through mitotic events causing reduction to disomy of a trisomic conception. Nonetheless, if imprinted genes reside on the affected chromosome then phenotypic effects caused by the altered dosage of imprinted genes may occur (Fig. 2.1). By systematically generating conceptuses harbouring uniparental duplications spanning different chromosomal regions, Cattanach *et al.* have shown that mouse chromosomes 2, 6, 7, 11, 12, 17 and 18 are imprinted (mice have 19 pairs of autosomes and 1 pair of sex chromosomes) and hence the biparental requirement applies to a subset of the genome[8]. On perturbation of the parental origin of these chromosomes, quite severe phenotypes are observed, including lethality, growth effects and behavioural anomalies[9]. This indicates that imprinted genes reside within these regions; however, it does not rule out the presence of imprinted genes elsewhere, which cause more subtle effects when their dosage is perturbed by uniparental duplication. Around 90% of the imprinted genes identified to date map to the regions identified in these genetic studies.

Evidence of genomic imprinting in man

It became evident that imprinting had clinical implications through the study of patients with disorders that exhibit parental-origin effects in their patterns of inheritance. There are now several syndromes which are recognised as imprinting disorders and imprinting mutations have been implicated in the genesis of some tumours, notably Wilms' tumour and familial glomus tumours. Many of these disorders, which proved puzzling at first, show a normal autosomal dominant pattern of inheritance from a parent of one sex. However, offspring of an affected individual of the opposite sex are completely unaffected (see Fig. 2.2). The disorder re-manifests itself in a subsequent generation after inheritance through a phenotypically normal carrier individual of the appropriate sex. Males and females are equally affected which clearly distinguishes an imprinting pedigree from that of a sex-linked disorder. A pedigree showing parental-origin specific inheritance is shown in Fig. 2.2. For example, benign familial glomus tumours show autosomal dominant inheritance but are only manifest in individuals inheriting the mutant gene from their fathers. This is an example of an imprinted tumour syndrome showing familial inheritance of the type shown in Fig. 2.2[10]. Other imprinted disorders have been associated with a significant level of UPD. To date, all human chromosomes involved in these syndromes show evolutionary conservation

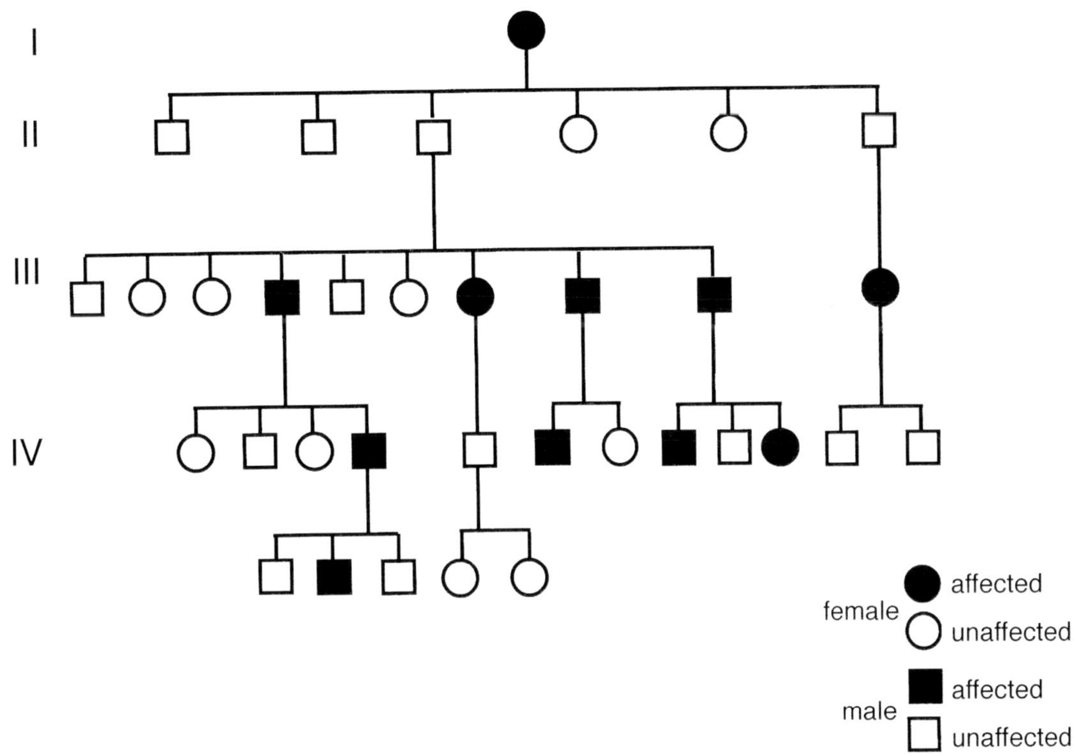

Fig. 2.2

with those in the mouse identified as imprinted chromosomes (see above). Examples of these relationships are given in Table 2.1 which lists human disorders for which there exists good evidence for imprinting through pedigree analysis and/or the significant presence of UPD.

Two regions associated with imprinted diseases have been the subject of intense scrutiny. Beckwith–Wiedemann syndrome (BWS) is a fetal overgrowth disorder associated with multi-organ hyperplasia and an increased incidence of childhood tumours[11,12]. Genetic linkage studies have mapped BWS to human chromosome 11p15.5. Familial BWS (15%) is inherited as an autosomal dominant trait exhibiting parental origin effects. A small number of these patients (2–3%) have cytogenetic abnormalities of 11p15. These abnormalities are predominantly maternally inherited inversions and balanced translocations or paternally derived duplications involving 11p. The majority of cases are sporadic with about 20% of these having paternal isodisomy of chromosome 11. Detailed analysis of these patients has demonstrated that UPD in BWS arises as a mitotic event in the zygote and thus patients are

TABLE 2.1
Human genetic disorders with imprinting effects

Disease	Chromosomal localisation	Parental-origin effect	Reference
Transient neonatal diabetes	6	Paternal duplication/UPD	37
Growth retardation	7	Maternal UPD	38
Beckwith–Wiedemann syndrome and Wilms' tumour	11p	Maternal mutation inheritance paternal duplication/UPD	11, 12, 14, 16
Hereditary glomus tumours	11q	Paternal inheritance of mutation	10, 39
Prader–Willi syndrome	15q11–13	Paternal inheritance of mutation maternal UPD	19, 20, 21, 24
Angelman syndrome	15q11–13	Maternal inheritance of mutation paternal UPD	18, 20–24
mUPD14 syndrome	14	Maternal UPD	40, 41

mosaic for UPD and normal lineages. In the mouse, the conserved chromosomal region is on chromosome 7 and is known to contain a least six imprinted genes, five of which have been shown to be imprinted on human chromosome 11p. One good candidate gene which may be involved in BWS is the insulin-like growth factor II gene (*IGF2*) which is expressed from the paternally inherited chromosome and repressed when maternally inherited[13]. Individuals with paternal disomy involving 11p, express a double dose of this growth factor[14]. A second imprinted gene, *p57KIP2*, which is believed to function as a negative regulator of cell growth, is located nearby and reciprocally imprinted to *IGF2* with the maternal allele being active and the paternal allele repressed[15]. Absence of activity of this gene may also be involved in BWS[16]. As in humans, chimaeric mice with some normal cells and cells containing the paternal uniparental duplication of this region of chromosome 7 show fetal overgrowth reminiscent of BWS[17]. Thus the aetiology of the disease might be explained by an excess of an imprinted growth promoting factor expressed from the paternally inherited allele (such as *IGF2*) or a deficiency of a growth repressor expressed from the maternal allele (such as *p57KIP2*). Currently, one cannot rule out a role for both of these genes and perhaps others in BWS.

The second well-studied imprinted disease region is on human chromosome 15q11–13 which is involved in two distinct imprinted neurological disorders, the Prader–Willi syndrome (PWS) and Angelman syndrome (AS)[18–20]. PWS is characterised by mild-to-moderate mental retardation, hypotonia and neonatal failure to thrive followed by hyperphagia and obesity after the neonatal period. Other clinical features include short stature, small hands and feet and behavioral

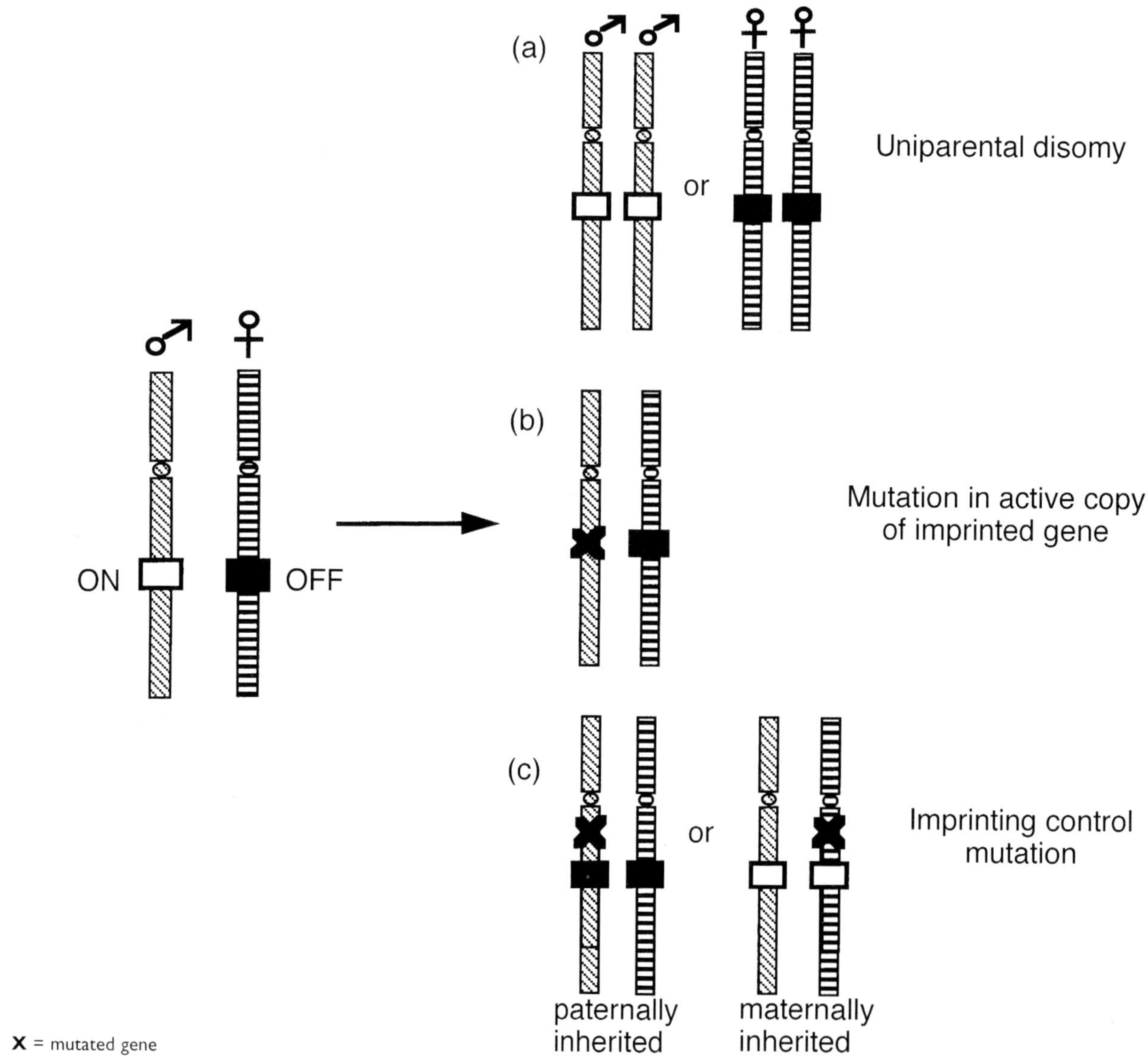

Fig. 2.3

disorders. Seventy per cent of patients with PWS have a deletion in 15q which is exclusively paternal in origin. Twenty-nine per cent have maternal UPD for chromosome 15. Intriguingly, 1% carry a defect that affects the ability of the region to appropriately imprint and thus the transcriptional machinery of the cell is fooled into believing that the paternally inherited chromosome is maternal (see later). The syndrome has therefore been attributed to loss of product of a paternally expressed gene or genes. Angelman syndrome is a distinct disorder mapping to the same region. Its clinical features include severe mental retardation, absence of speech, ataxia and a happy disposition associated with inappropriate bouts of laughter. AS patients are hyperactive and are prone to seizures. In contrast to PWS, 75% of cases are due to deletions that are exclusively maternal in origin; 1% are associated with paternal UPD for chromosome 15 and 4% are caused by a defect in the imprinting mechanism acting over a large region, as in PWS[21]. The remaining 20% of AS cases cannot be explained by UPD, deletion or imprinting mutation and are attributed to mutation in a single maternally expressed/paternally repressed gene[22,23]. To date only one such gene has been identified – UBE3A, a ubiquitin protein ligase[24]. Extensive molecular analysis, predominantly of the regions deleted in PWS/AS patients, has led to the identification of a cluster of at least five transcripts that are expressed solely from the paternally inherited chromosome but as yet a role for these transcripts in the disorders has not been determined[24]. The characterisation of the mutations that affect the mechanism of imprinting has led to the proposal that an imprinting centre (IC) exists in the region that plays a key role in marking the two parental chromosomes. Understanding how the IC regulates imprinting is an exciting challenge[25,26]

Hence in man, at least three types of mutations in an imprinted region can cause a disorder showing parental origin effects (Fig. 2.3). First, uniparental disomy (or mosaicism for UPD) or uniparental duplication including trisomy, which alters the dosage of an imprinted gene or genes (as imprinted genes appear to be clustered) can have clinical consequences, as seen for example in BWS (Fig. 2.3a). Second, as is the case for hereditary glomus tumours, a mutation in the imprinted gene itself can cause a non-functional gene product, or a complete absence of gene product because the other allele is already inactivated by imprinting (Fig. 2.3b). Third, a mutation can occur that affects the ability of the gene or region to appropriately imprint. This type of mutation which affects the imprinting mechanism, may not necessarily be in the gene itself but may be close by or quite far away, and have effects on several imprinted genes over a distance (Fig. 2.3c). This is the case for the IC mutations identified in the PWS/AS region.

Mechanisms of imprinting

The mechanism causing parental-origin dependent gene expression must allow the transcriptional machinery of the cell to distinguish between two chromosomal homologues and differentially act on one or the other. The imprint is believed to be initiated during gametogenesis and then acted upon in the zygote and developing conceptus to affect developmental gene activity. It is therefore likely that the imprint is a modification to the DNA and/or chromatin which must have the following properties:

- It must be able to affect the transcription of the gene.
- It must be heritable in somatic cells over many cell divisions and not lost during chromosome replication. This renders the imprint stable and allows it to have parental-origin specific memory. This step is known as 'maintenance'.
- Most importantly, the imprints must be erased in the male and female germ lines during gametogenesis to allow new imprints to be set down which are specific to the parental origin of the newly formed gametes. The process is outlined schematically in Fig. 2.4.

There are only a few recognised mammalian gene modifications that might fulfil the above criteria. By far the best studied is DNA methylation. DNA methylation of CpG-dinucleotides (5-methyl cytosine) is known to affect gene activity[27]. Indeed, methylation of CpG-rich regulatory portions of genes, for example on the inactive X-chromosomes

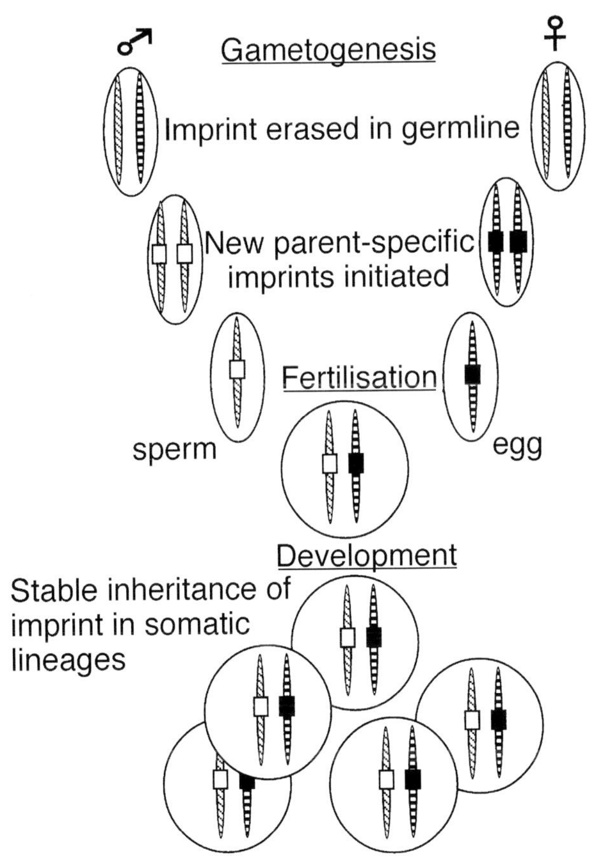

Fig. 2.4

in females, have long been associated with gene inactivity[28]. More recently, it has been shown that imprinted genes contain regions that are differentially methylated on the two parental chromosomes. However, sometimes the methylation is associated with the inactive allele[29,30] and sometimes with the active allele[31,32]. In the absence of the DNA methyltransferase gene, which encodes the methylating enzyme, the imprint is lost from somatic cells and imprinted gene activity is perturbed[33]. Thus, methylation is involved, at least, in the maintenance of imprinting. Whether methylation is the germline imprinting initiator remains to be proven. However, several differences in methylation have been found in the DNA of eggs and sperm in imprinted regions, which suggest that CpG-methylation may have a role to play in the earliest imprinting events.

The role of other modifications in the imprinting process currently remains unclear, mainly because few others involved in transcriptional control have been identified. It is apparent that many imprinted genes show differences in their chromatin structure between the active and inactive alleles[29,34]. However, in the case of imprinting, the relationship, if any, between a region's chromatin conformation and its methylation status is not understood. It is now well documented that modifications to chromatin-associated proteins, notably acetylation of core histones, have key roles to play in the regulation of gene expression and it is possible that these may be involved in the imprinting mechanism[35]. It is likely, however, that there are several steps involved in building an imprint which may include more that just short-range modifications of gene promoters. It seems that the imprints are acting over larger domains, perhaps to provide a particular chromatin context within which individual gene can be further modified. We can be sure that these contexts must differ between the two parental homologues.

As more imprinted genes are being discovered and parental origin-specific modifications associated with them are being characterised, we can start to understand both the developmental role and the mechanisms of genomic imprinting. However, the story may be quite a complex one. Some genes are showing imprinting in only a subset of tissues[36]. In addition, genes imprinted in the mouse may not necessarily be imprinted in man. The importance of imprinted genes in mammalian development is evident from the identification and study of mutations exhibiting parental origin effects in their patterns of inheritance. However, we are a long way from understanding the molecular basis and evolutionary reason for this intriguing phenomenon.

REFERENCES

1. Barton SC, Surani MA, Norris ML. Role of maternal and paternal genomes in mouse development. *Nature* **311**:374–376, 1984.
2. McGrath J, Solter D. Completion of mouse embryogenesis requires both maternal and paternal genomes. *Cell* **37**:170–183, 1984.
3. Bagshawe KD, Lawler SD. Unmasking moles. *Brit J of Obs & Gynae* **89**:255–259, 1982.
4. Fundele R, Norris ML, Barton SC, et al. Systematic elimination of parthenogenetic cells in mouse chimaeras. *Development* **106**:20–35, 1989.
5. Fundele R, Norris M, Barton S, et al. Temporal and spatial selection against parthenogenetic cells during development of fetal chimaeras. *Development* **108**:203–211, 1990.
6. Barton S, Ferguson-Smith A, Fundele R, Surani MA. Influence of paternally imprinted genes on development. *Development* **113**:679–688, 1991.
7. Mann J, Gadi I, Harbison M, Abbondanzo S, Stewart C. Androgenetic mouse embryonic stem cells are pluripotent and cause skeletal defects in chimaeras. *Cell* **62**:251–260, 1991.
8. Cattanach BM, Beechey CV. Genetic imprinting map. *Mouse Genome* **94**:96–99, 1996.
9. Cattanach B, Jones J. Genetic imprinting in the mouse: Implications for gene regulation. *J Inher Metab Dis* **17**:403–420, 1994.
10. Van der Mey AGL, Maaswinkel-Mooy PD, et al. Genomic imprinting in hereditary glomus tumours: evidence for a new genetic theory. *Lancet*, Dec 2, 1291–1294, 1989.
11. Wiedemann H. Tumours and hemihypertrophy associated with Wiedemann–Beckwith syndrome. *Eur J Pediatr* **141**:129, 1983.
12. Elliot M, Maher ER. Beckwith–Wiedemann Syndrome. *J Med Genet* **7**:560–564, 1994.
13. DeChiara TM, Robertson EJ, Efstratiadis A. Parental imprinting of the mouse insulin-like growth factor II gene. *Cell* **64**:849–859, 1991.
14. Weksberg R, Shen DR, Fei Y-L, Song QL, Squire J. Disruption of insulin-like growth factor 2 imprinting in Beckwith–Wiedemann syndrome. *Nature Genetics* **5**:143–150, 1993.
15. Matsuoka S, Thompson J, Edwards M, et al. Imprinting of the gene encoding the human cyclin-dependent kinase inhibitor, p57KIP2, on human chromosome 11p15. *Proc Natl Acad Sci (USA)* **93**:3026–3030, 1996.
16. Hatada I, Ohashi H, Fukushima Y, et al. An imprinted gene p57KIP2 is mutated in Beckwith–Wiedemann syndrome. *Nature Genet* **14**:171–173, 1996.
17. Ferguson-Smith AC, Cattanach BM, Barton SC, Beechey CV, Surani MA. Embryological and molecular investigation of parental imprinting on mouse chromosome 7. *Nature* **351**:667–670, 1991.
18. Angelman H. 'Puppet children' A report of three cases. *Develop Med Child Neurol* **7**:681–688, 1965.
19. Ledbetter D, Riccardi V, Airhart S, et al. Deletions of chromosome 15 as a cause of the Prader–Willi Syndrome. *New Engl J Med* **304**:325–329, 1981.
20. Knoll J, Nicolls R, Magenis RE. Angelman and Prader–Willi Syndrome share a common chromosome 15 deletion but differ in parental origin of the deletion. *Am J Med Genet* **32**:285–290, 1989.
21. Buiting K, Saitoh S, Gross S. Inherited microdeletions in the Angelman and Prader–Willi syndromes define an imprinting center on human chromosome 15. *Nature Genet* **9**:395–400, 1995.
22. Magenis RE, Brown M, Lacy D, Budden S, LaFranchi, S. Is Angelman syndrome an alternate result of del(15)(q11q13)? *Am J Med Genet* **28**:829–838, 1981.
23. Malcolm S, Clayton-Smith J, Nichols M, et al. Uniparental paternal disomy in Angelman's syndrome. *Lancet* **337**:694–697, 1991.
24. Jiang YH, Tsai TF, Bressler J, Beaudet AL. Imprinting in Angelman and Prader–Willi syndromes. *Curr Opin Genet Dev* **8**(3):334–342, 1998.
25. Dittrich B, Buiting K, Korn B, et al. Imprint switching on human chromosome 15 may involve alternative transcripts of the SNRPN gene. *Nature Genet* **14**:163–170, 1996.
26. Ferguson-Smith AC. Imprinting moves to the centre. *Nature Genet* **14**:119–121, 1996.
27. Bird A. CpG-rich islands and the function of DNA methylation. *Nature* **321**:209–213, 1986.
28. Riggs A, Pfeiffer G. X-chromosome inactivation and cell memory. *Trends Genet* **14**:9–25, 1992.
29. Ferguson-Smith AC, Sasaki H, Cattanach BM, Surani MA. Parental-

origin specific epigenetic modification of the mouse *H19* gene. *Nature* **362**:751–755, 1993.
30. Bartolomei M, Webber A, Brunkow M, Tilghman S. Epigenetic mechanisms underlying the imprinting of the mouse *H19* gene. *Genes Devel* **7**:1663–1673, 1993.
31. Sasaki H, Jones P, Chaillet JR, et al. Parental imprinting: potentially active chromatin of the repressed maternal allele of the mouse Igf2 gene. *Genes Devel* **6**:1843–1856, 1992.
32. Stoger R, Kubicka P, Liu C-G, et al. Maternal-specific methylation of the imprinted mouse *Igf2r* locus identifies the expressed locus as carrying the imprinting signal. *Cell* **73**:61–71, 1993.
33. Li E, Beard C, Jaenisch R. Role for DNA methylation in genomic imprinting. *Nature* **366**:362–365, 1993.
34. Feil R, Handel M, Allen N, Reik W. Chromatin structure and imprinting. *Dev Genet* **17**:240–252, 1995.
35. O'Neill L, Turner B. Histone acetylation in chromatin and chromosomes. *Seminars in Cell Biology* **6**:229–236, 1995.
36. Giddings SJ, King CD, Harman KW, Flood JF, Carnaghi LR. Allele specific inactivation of insulin 1 and 2, in the mouse yolk sac, indicates imprinting. *Nature Genetics* **6**:310–313, 1994.
37. Temple IK, James R, Crolla J, et al. An imprinted gene(s) for diabetes. *Nature Genetics* **9**:110–112, 1995.
38. Ledbetter D, Engel E. Uniparental disomy in humans: development of an imprinting map and its implications for prenatal diagnosis. *Human Mol Genet* **4**:1757–1764, 1995.
39. McCaffrey T, Meyer F, Michels V, Piepgras D, Marion M. Familial paragangliomas of the head and neck. *Arch Otolaryngol Head Neck Surg* **120**:1211–1216, 1994.
40. Temple IK, Cockwell T, Hassold T, Pettay D, Jacobs P. Maternal uniparental disomy for chromosome 14. *J Med Genet* **28**:511–514, 1991.
41. Healey S, Powell F, Battersby M, Tench G, McGill J. Distinct phenotype in maternal uniparental disomy of chromosome 14. *Am J Hum Genet* **51**:147–149, 1994.

Staging embryos in development

3

P. Collins

Introduction

Estimations concerning the length of time an embryo or fetus has been *in utero* are based initially on information from the mother on the date of her last menstrual period and subsequently on observation of the embryo or fetus *in utero* by means of ultrasonography. Knowledge about what external and internal structures would normally be developing at a particular time during early gestation has been generated over the years from study of miscarried or aborted embryos, studies of animal embryos of known gestational age, and now more recently from ultrasonographic data. Decisions about the health or ill health of the embryo or fetus may be based on comparison of its developmental status with examples found in embryonic staging series.

A variety of staging systems for human embryos were devised in the early years of this century. To enhance this information, studies on other animals were also performed and externally similar stages compared. However, devising a staging system is very different from describing a day-by-day account of development. It will be clearer to explain how developmental stages for animal embryos have been constructed and then compare this to the ways staging schemes for human embryos were derived.

Chick stage series

Chick development was described by Hamburger and Hamilton[1]; republished by Sanes[2] and Hamilton[3]) as a series of 46 stages. In this series fertilized eggs were maintained at 39.4°C and embryos were examined over the 20-day incubation. Because development is continuous, dividing it up into stages is a very arbitrary process. It is like seeing the action in a movie only by viewing a succession of freeze-frame images; to show others the story a representative number of images must be selected, but which ones? For the chick series the major factors were that stages could be identified unequivocally by one or more external morphological features and that successive stages were spaced as closely as possible. Dozens of embryos of the same chronological age were examined to look for the slightest differences in a range of external features. The features under consideration changed as development proceeded and the speed of change varied during the incubation. In the first weeks, the changes in the embryos were so rapid that the stages are only hours apart, whereas in the second half of the incubation the stages are a day apart. Thus stages one to seven occur during the first 24 hours of incubation; the somites appear and are used as external features between 23 hours (stage 7) and 53 hours (stage 14). After this time limb buds and pharyngeal arches are used especially.

The internal characteristics of the chick embryos were not described so development of particular organs was not initially related to the external features. However, the Hamburger & Hamilton series of stages is supported by extensive photographs of each stage so that correlation of external features with internal structures identified in subsequent studies is possible.

Hamburger produced similar staging series for *Ambystoma*, *Triturus taeniatus* and *T. cristatus*, species of salamander. Since that time, series have been produced for many reptiles and amphibians. These studies are arduous and time consuming but provide the most valuable hard data on the timing of embryonic development. All of the early series were on amphibian, avian or reptile embryos which are easily accessible throughout incubation. However, the incubation temperature will effect the speed of gestation and in the case of reptile embryos will have an effect on the sex of the offspring. In turtles, male embryos result from cool incubations, whereas females arise from warmer temperatures; the opposite occurs in the gecko. In most reptiles intermediate temperature incubations result in development of both males and females.

Mammalian embryos have proved much more inaccessible for study. In laboratory species, gestation in days is universally used as a guide to developmental status, thus the staging is based on chronology rather than external features although descriptive terms are often also used to indicate the stage.

Human stage series

Human embryonic stages are, like the chick stages, universally based on the apparent morphological state of development of the embryo, not on either chronological age or on size. The supposed age of a human embryo is only dubiously estimated from the menstrual history. There is considerable variability in both premenstrual and postmenstrual phases of the menstrual cycle, on top of which there are great possibilities for error in correctly identifying menstruation or erroneously interpreting its absence. The concept of 'postovulatory age' has been used[4] referring to the length of time since the last ovulation before pregnancy began. This is predicated on the very close interval between the time of ovulation and the time of fertilization.

The first comparative description of human embryos is attributed to Wilhelm His (Snr), who with the use of fixation, sectioning and reconstruction of sections provided the first insights into internal morphology at different ages. Human embryos were first placed in a staged series by Mall[5], founder of the Department of Embryology of the Carnegie Institution of Washington. Mall arranged 266 human embryos into a series of 14 stages on the basis of their external form. The embryos ranged from 2 to 25 mm in length. His work was continued by George Streeter[6,7,8,9] who concentrated on embryos initially up to 32 mm greatest length.

Embryos in the Carnegie Collection were received already in fixative. The greatest length of the embryos, measured with callipers without any attempt to straighten the natural curvature, was recorded usually after two weeks in 10% formalin; this was to standardise any shrinkage caused by fixation. Tables of embryonic length correlated to stage and predicted age were produced. These were based on fixed embryos graded as excellent. In each stage the greatest length may vary by 4 mm within the embryonic period.

All of the embryos were photographed, wax embedded and serially sectioned, the sections were examined and drawings and reconstructions made. Observations were made about the degree of development of a range of internal organs and these were correlated with the external characteristics. No one criterion could place a particular embryo within one stage or another. The stage was estimated from examination of a number of key structures throughout the body. Where human embryos of particular stages were not available, comparison to the development of macaque embryos was made. Now it is known that such comparisons are not warranted. Embryos were assigned to 'horizons' based on these examinations and their ages were thus estimated. Streeter believed such estimations could be ± 1 day for any given stage. So whereas in the chick stage series, the investigators knew the time of incubation and made decisions about whether an embryo demonstrated sufficient external characteristics to warrant inclusion in a particular stage, human embryos were grouped according to similar characteristics and the series was used to infer age. This becomes increasingly difficult as development proceeds and variation in the rate of development or in the size of different embryos becomes more marked.

The strength of Streeter's studies is that portions of embryonic material can often be staged by reference to his work, e.g. he correlated the development of the semi-circular canals to the length of the Mullerian or paramesonephric ducts, such that when the Mullerian duct is up to one-third of the way to the cloaca one semi-circular canal is present, when the duct is two-thirds of the way to the cloaca two ducts are present, and when the duct reaches the cloaca all the semi-circular ducts are present. Thus a particular stage is not an alternative way of indicating the developmental age of an embryo; a stage conveys the developmental status of many of the systems in concert.

Streeter originally designated the time periods 'horizons'; however, this has now been superseded by 'stage' which is common for other developmental description. His system of stages (now the basis for the Carnegie staging system) range from 1 to 23 over a developmental period from fertilization to 8 postovulatory weeks. Streeter ended the series at stage 23 using the onset of marrow formation in the humerus as the marker for the end of the embryonic and the beginning of the fetal period of development. Embryos at stage 23 are approximately 30 mm long (range 27–31 mm) and 56 postovulatory days. This correlation of size and age at the end of the embryonic period has been confirmed ultrasonically[10].

Streeter's work has been continued by Ronan O'Rahilly who has published extensively on human development. A most inestimable monograph with Fabiola Muller[4] revises Streeter's stages, incorporates O'Rahilly's continuation of his work, and includes a detailed catalogue of the Carnegie Collection. Each stage is clearly illustrated with external photographs, drawings, reconstructions and histology of internal details.

WHAT IS CONSIDERED 'NORMAL' IN HUMAN EMBRYOS?

A note of caution about existing human stage series must be made. Six hundred embryos were sectioned and examined to arrive at the Carnegie staging system yet the majority of those were listed as normal. Collections of miscarriages usually contain a large incidence of chromosomally abnormal embryos. The very young embryos in the Carnegie Collection were obtained from hysterectomies and later ones were often received with a scanty background history. Variations and anomalies in individual organs were noted in some embryos. However, the techniques were not available at the time this series was developed, the early 1900s, to check for chromosomal or gene abnormalities. It is suggested that at least 15% of all recognized pregnancies will abort before 12 weeks gestation (see below for explanation of the timescale referred to) and of these 40% will be due to chromosome abnormalities. Thus collections of miscarried pregnancies can be inferred to contain many abnormal embryos.

Similar problems of examining early embryos and predicting what their status would have been at term occur in embryo studies when investigating teratogenic insult. Low level teratogens may affect some developing systems and not others in individual embryos. When examining a mammalian embryo removed during development the final outcome of the teratogen on that embryo cannot be predicted with certainty. On the one hand the embryo might have developed to term with sufficient catch up growth to reduce the apparent severity of the condition; on the other hand, the embryo might not have sufficient cell populations to recover from the insult and might have died the following week had the experiment continued. The younger the embryos in such studies, the harder it is to make these predictions.

MOLECULAR MARKERS AND STAGING SYSTEMS

The importance of correlating internal features with external characteristics in embryo series cannot be underestimated, and we should be grateful to the early human embryologists for providing such detailed data. It is now realised that similar external embryonic features of different vertebrate species do not indicate similar internal stages of development[11]. Correlating chick embryos of stage 21 with rat embryos of day 12 and human embryos of stage 14 because the external characteristics look similar does not mean that, for example, the lungs are at the same stage of development in these embryos. This latter consideration has become increasingly important with the advent of molecular biology. Stages of development can now be reinterpreted as the time at which specific gene expression is seen in certain tissues. Because many genes are conserved between vertebrates and because deletion of some genes can cause morphological or developmental anomalies, the effects of gene deletion in mouse embryos is now being studied and correlated with known human conditions displaying the similar gene defects and resulting signs and symptoms. Indeed, many genes are being experimentally removed from the mouse genome in the hope of mimicking a human anomalous condition. However, this approach assumes that the development of any one system either operates in isolation from other systems such that inducers of one population do not have any effect on a distant one, or that all systems in mouse and human are developing along the same timescale.

To correlate gene expression with morphology seems to be the next step forward and accurate staging systems are fundamental to this approach. The leap from species to species is more problematical. The observation that internal and external development is not in any synchronisation between vertebrate groups has lead to the investigation of heterochrony, a change in developmental timing during evolution[11]. If the time at which a range of developmental events occur in *Homo sapiens* during the somite period is plotted against these same events in other species, it can be seen that although, for

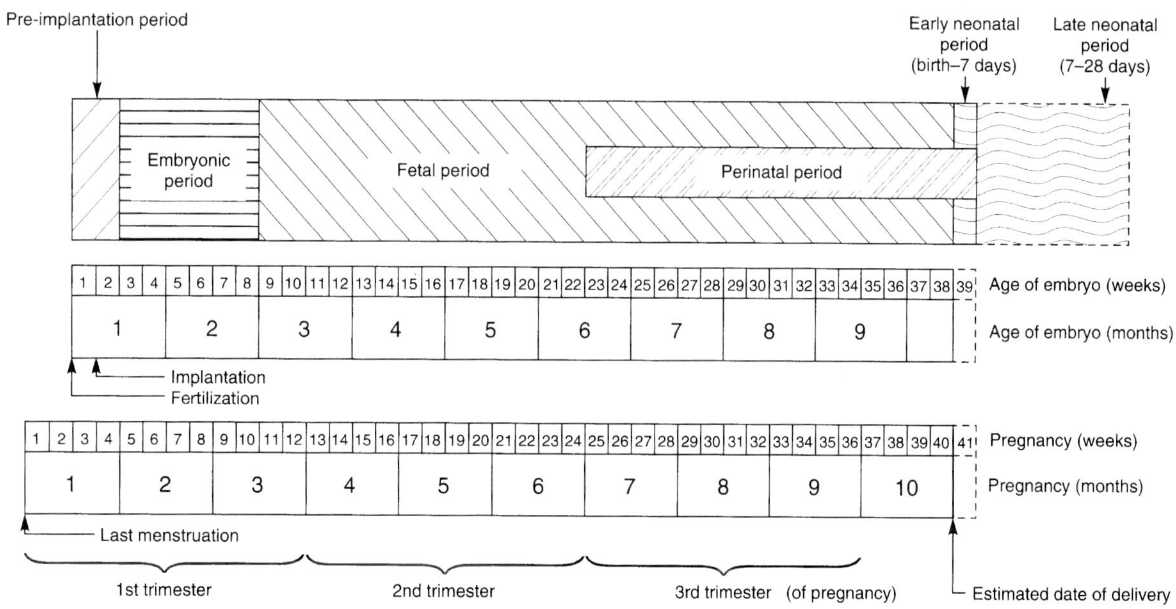

Fig. 3.1 The two times scales used to depict human development. Embryonic development, in the upper scale, is counted from fertilization (or from ovulation, i.e. in postovulatory days)[3]. The clinical estimation of pregnancy is counted from the last menstrual period and is shown on the lower scale. Note that there is a two-week discrepancy between these scales. The perinatal period is very long as it includes all of the preterm deliveries. (From Gray's Anatomy, 38th edition, Edinburgh: Churchill Livingstone, 1995, p. 344.)

example, the heart primordia in many species arise early, the appearance of the nasal placodes may be earlier or later than in *Homo sapiens*. It is not yet clear whether the development of any one system also requires background feedback about the stage of development of other systems for its successful completion.

OBSTETRIC STAGING SCHEMES

Use of the Carnegie staging scheme with reference to individual stages presupposes the adoption of that timescale of development. So, suggesting an embryo is at stage 17, implies that it is six weeks postovulation. In this scale development averages 266 days, or 9.5 months.

The obstetric timescale is involved in estimating a day of delivery and then assessing the fetus to see if it seems appropriately aged to deliver at that time. The commencement of gestation is determined *clinically* by counting from the date of the last menstrual period. Estimated in this manner a pregnancy averages 280 days, or 10 lunar months (40 weeks). Examination of Fig. 3.1 where both scales are depicted shows the two-week discrepancy between these scales. Generally, books written for obstetricians or fetal physicians will use the lower, obstetric scale, whereas embryology books will use the upper, embryological scale.

There is little information about the growth of the fetus from weeks 9 to 20 (embryonic timescale), and the interaction between developing systems at this time. Yet today it is not uncommon for fetuses to be born at ages equivalent to 19 or 20 embryonic weeks and survive. At these stages, estimations of fetal age become less important than estimations of fetal maturity. There are a number of tables showing the

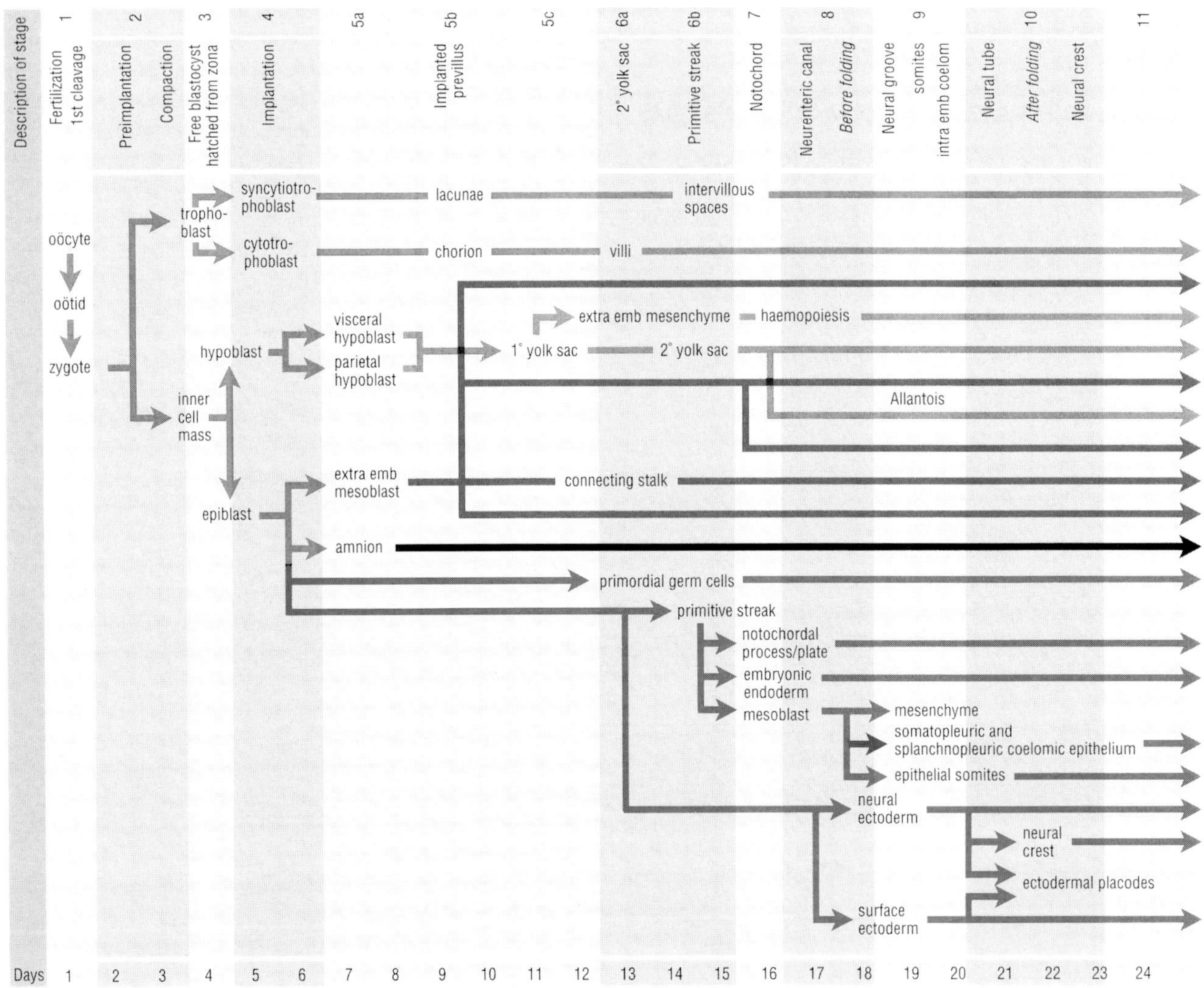

Fig. 3.2 Chart to show the development processes occurring during the first 10 stages of development. In the early stages a series of binary choices determine the cell lineages. Generally the earliest stages are concerned with formation of the extraembryonic tissues, whereas the later stages see the formation of embryonic tissues. (From Gray's Anatomy, 38th edition, Edinburgh: Churchill Livingstone, 1995, p. 140.)

expected range of length and weight correlated to obstetric gestation weeks.

MAIN STAGES IN THE EMBRYONIC PERIOD

Embryonic development is not apparent before stage 6. Stages 1–5 are concerned with setting up the cell populations for implantation; most of the cell lines generated are extraembryonic and involved in establishing the placenta and fetal membranes. In stage 6a the primordial germ cells are sequestered into the extraembryonic mesoblast and in stage 6b the primitive streak appears. From this time, intraembryonic cell populations are generated and it is the morphological movements of these populations which produces a recognisable embryo. Figure 3.2 shows stages 1–11 matched to estimated age. The proliferation of cells at the primitive streak occurs through stages 7 and 8, when the notochord is first evident, and provides cell populations which pass within the embryo. By stage 9 the neural populations are becoming defined and result in neurulation and the beginning of somite formation, more clearly seen in stage 10 which typically has 7–12 pairs of somites. The formation of the neural plate and the beginnings of its rostral fusion contribute to the morphological movements of head folding, where the cardiac area, which was rostral to the neural epithelium, becomes ventral and forms a boundary of the cranial intestinal portal. Stages 6b to 10 are concerned with embryogenesis when morphogenetic movements affecting the whole embryo move widely dispersed cell populations closer and into their relevant positions for local interactive processes to commence. The stage 11 embryo is at the gateway of organogenesis and all body systems can be seen to originate from this point.

THE STAGE 11 EMBRYO, BODY PLAN STAGE

The criterion for stage 11 is the presence of 13–20 pairs of somites (Fig. 3.3); during this stage the rostral neuropore will close. Fusion occurs from the rhombencephalon rostrally towards the mesencephalon and from the region of the future optic chiasma towards the mesencephalic roof. The optic primordia have begun evagination towards the surface ectoderm. The otic vesicle which will invaginate and give rise to the inner ear (cochlea and semicircular ducts) has not yet formed but the surface epithelium has thickened and begun

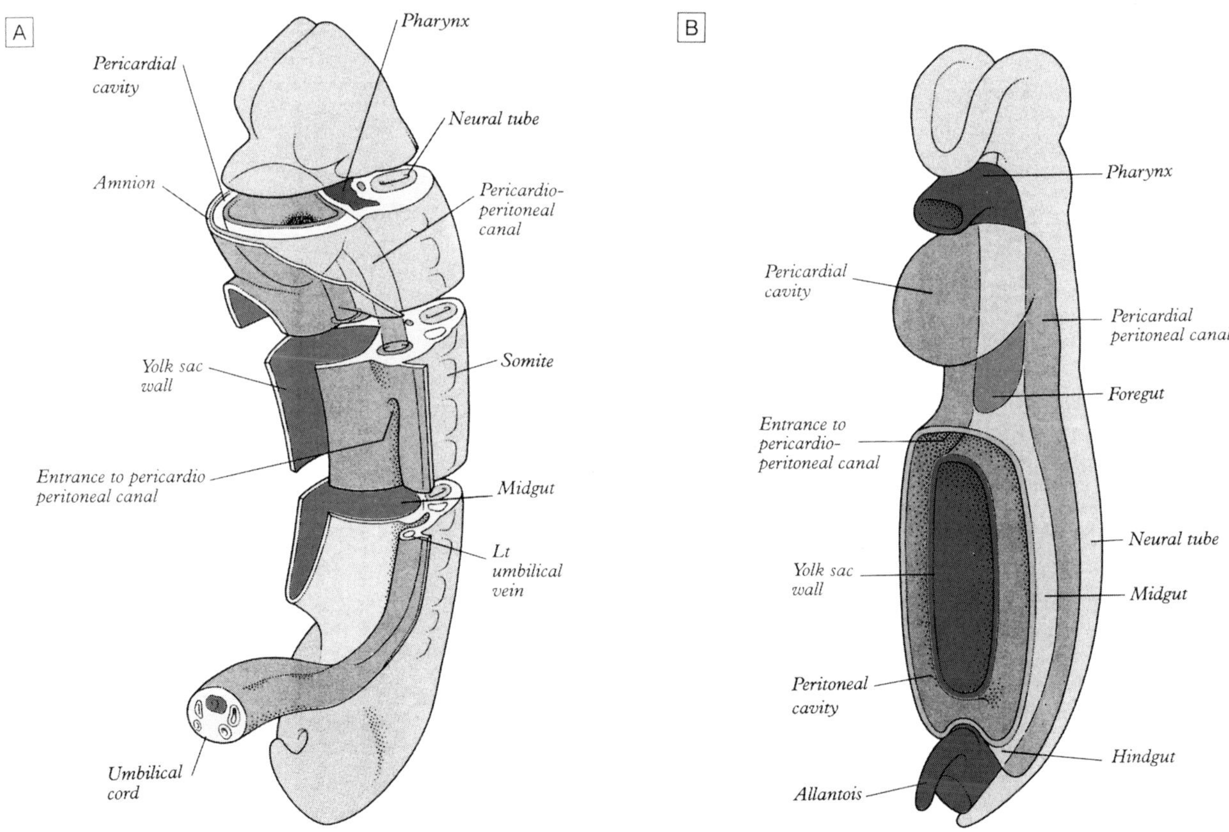

Fig. 3.3 (A) Diagram of a stage-11 embryo with the position of the intra-embryonic coelom indicated (after Streeter). (B) Diagram of three major epithelial populations within a stage-11 embryo, viewed from a ventrolateral position. The neural tube lies dorsal to the gut; ventrally the intraembryonic coelom crosses the midline at the level of the foregut and hindgut, but is lateral to the midgut and a portion of the foregut. (From Gray's Anatomy, 38th edition, Edinburgh: Churchill Livingstone, 1995, p. 151.)

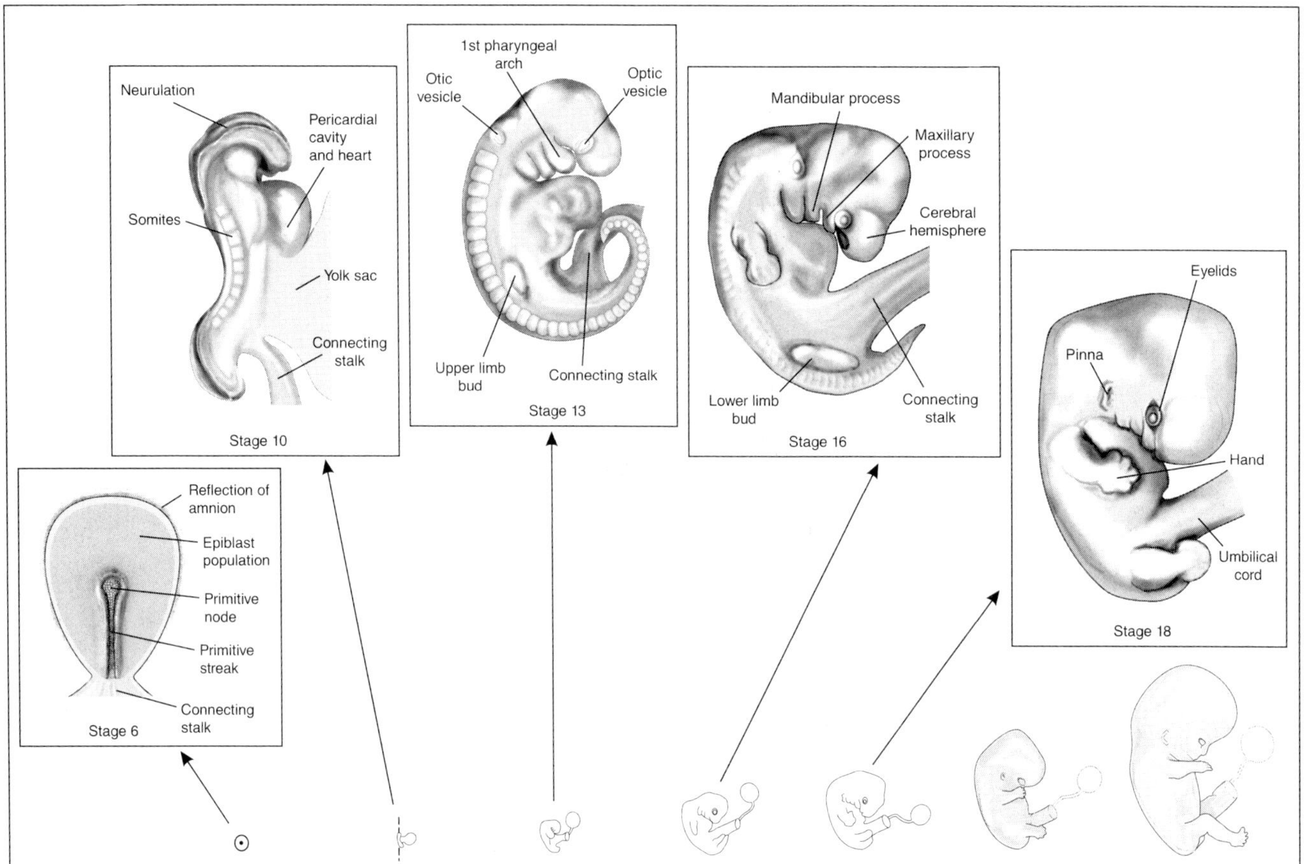

Stage	6	10	13	16	18	20	23
Size (mm)	0.4	1.5–3	4–6	8–11	13–17	21–23	28–30
Age (Days)	14 First missed period	22	28	37 Second missed period	44	50–51	56.5

Fig. 3.4 Diagram showing the external appearance and size of embryos between stages 6 and 23. Early in development external features are used to describe the stage, e.g. somites, pharyngeal arches or limb buds.

to invaginate. Around the developing pharynx the mandibular processes are present but the maxillary processes have yet to arise. The second pharyngeal arch, the hyoid, is present but not the third. Ventral to the foregut is the heart, this develops very precociously and is seen in stage 9 embryos as tube-like with a united ventricular portion but still separate atrial components. The specialised cells of the coelom, which will give rise to the myocardium, can be identified as can the matrix produced locally between the endocardium and the myocardium. Cardiac contractions commence at the beginning of stage 10 when the heart has a recognisable ventricle, bulbus cordis and arterial trunk, and a cardiac loop can be distinguished; the organ is already asymmetrical. By stage 11, the sinus venosus, atria, left and right ventricles, truncus arteriosus and substantial dorsal aortae can be identified. The heart is connected to a range of endothelial vessels and plexuses which are most mature cranially and still forming caudally. The fluid in the vascular system contains relatively few cells. It ebbs and flows because of the pulsations of the myocardium which also cause movement of fluid in the intraembryonic coelom. These combined circulations are sufficient to provide nutrient supply to the embryonic tissues.

The intraembryonic coelom is especially important at this stage of development. The coelom arises from confluent spaces which appear in the embryo from stage 9. As head folding occurs these spaces coalesce to form a horseshoe-shaped cavity within the embryonic body, which passes between the endoderm of the gut and the ectoderm of the body wall on each side of the developing fore- and midgut, and meets in the midline beneath the rostral neuropore as the future pericardial cavity. The ends of the horseshoe are in wide communication with the extraembryonic coelom

Week	1	2	3	4	5	6	7	8	9	10	11	12
Crown-Rump Length: mm.			2	4	10	13	18	30				55
External appearance			Head & tail folding	pharyngeal arches		upper lip palate		digits on hand external ear	eyelids fuse			
Nervous system			neurulation first neural crest cells	otic vesicle optic cup		anterior lobe pituitary	posterior lobe pituitary membranous labyrinth					
Respiratory				trachea lung buds	primary bronchi			futher division of bronchi				
Gut			fore-mid hind-gut	thyroid liver urorectal septum	pharyngeal pouches dorsal & ventral pancreas	rotation of stomach		midgut loop rotating				midgut loop returns to abdomen
Kidney				mesonephroe mesonephric duct ureteric bud		major calyces	metanephric nephrons	minor calyces	kidneys ascend			
Genital			germ cells in allantoic wall	indifferent gonad		Mullerian ducts testis differentiating external genitalia indifferent			uterus & uterine tubes vagina		testis at inguinal canal prostate external genitalia differeniating	
Cardiovascular			primitive vascular system heart tube	septum primum heart beats	septation of ventricles spleen			septum secundum				
Musculoskeletal			somite period 20 days......	forelimb bud	......30 days forelimb digit rays hind limb bud		cartilaginous part of skull		membranous part of skull			

Fig. 3.5 Timetable of development. The development of individual systems can be seen progressing from left to right. The relative status of different systems can be seen by looking from top to bottom at a particular time. (From Gray's Anatomy, 38th edition, Edinburgh: Churchill Livingstone, 1995, p. 334.)

around the embryo and within the chorion. The walls of the coelom are composed of germinal epithelia which provide mesenchymal cell populations for the connective tissues and smooth muscle of the respiratory and gastrointestinal tracts, the body wall and especially the heart. The myocardium arises directly from the dorsal pericardial wall in the folded embryo. The ventral pericardial wall will give rise to the serous, parietal pericardial layer.

The foregut develops as the head fold elevates and the pericardial cavity swings ventrally. It is flattened dorsoventrally, extending laterally to form the pharyngeal pouches. The buccopharyngeal membrane is present at this stage and may begin to rupture. There is only small indication of the future respiratory primordium. The liver is represented by the septum transversum mesenchyme and underlying endoderm but the latter is still widely connected to the yolk sac. The nephric system consists of a solid nephrogenic cord lateral to somites 8–13. The cloacal membrane is situated ventrally after tail folding just caudal to the connecting stalk which passes to the developing placenta. The primordial germ cells can be identified in the embryo at stage 11. They are initially in the mesenchyme around the yolk sac and allantoic walls. With tail folding they are brought into the body cavity with the hindgut epithelium and surrounding mesenchyme and then by amoeboid movement and by growth displacement they migrate dorsocranially. They do not reach the gonads until stage 15, some nine days later, when the local cell population are developed sufficiently to receive them.

During stage 11, the most important epithelial layers attain their position, i.e. surface epithelium, notochord, neural epithelium, somites, gut epithelium and the lining of the coelomic cavity (Fig. 3.3). The germinal epithelia of the somites and the coelomic cavity then generate extensive mesenchymal populations at the same time that the neural crest mesenchyme cells are migrating within the head and neck. Finally, each epithelium is surrounded and supported by different mesenchymal populations, i.e. the neural tube and notochord are surrounded by neural crest mesenchyme in the head and somatopleuric mesenchyme in the trunk. The gut epithelium is surrounded by splanchnopleuric mesenchyme which becomes specialised particularly around the respiratory diverticulum. The surface ectoderm is supported by somatopleuric mesenchyme in the trunk and by neural crest mesenchyme in the head. The coelomic epithelia themselves produce specialised epithelial populations which give rise to the gonads, adrenal medulla and the lining of the uterine tubes; these epithelia are all supported by local mesenchyme. Angiogenic mesenchyme is found throughout the embryo from stage 9. It is capable of extensive migration and differentiates into endothelium or blood cells throughout the

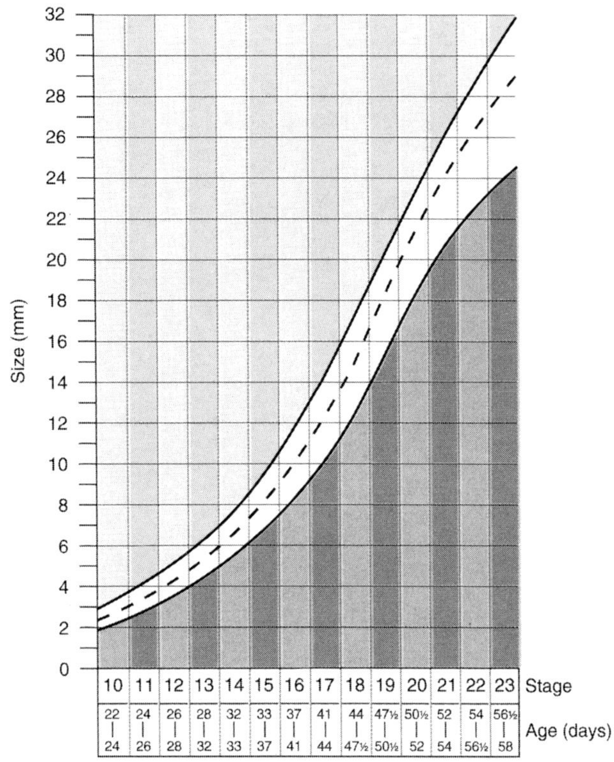

Fig. 3.6 Chart of development stages 10–23 illustrating the range of size embryos attain within the two-day period of a 'stage'[3,7]. (From Gray's Anatomy, 38th edition, p. 135.)

embryo. Angiogenic mesenchyme is found within the endodermal and splanchnopleuric layers but never within ectoderm derived tissues.

Stage 11 may be considered to be the body plan stage. To achieve it genes functioning across the whole embryo are in operation. As stage 11 fades into stage 12, organogenesis is underway and the epithelial/mesenchymal interactions which result in all development are now operating along local lines. Diversity of differentiative outcomes is now possible by upregulation of specific genes in specific regions of the embryo.

Between stage 11 and stage 23, a period of about 32 days, the embryo grows in length from 3 mm to 30 mm. It passes from a general vertebrate embryo to a fully formed but immature human. Figure 3.4 illustrates the dramatic increase in size and developmental status during this time. Figure 3.5 shows the progress in individual systems across the timescale. Although Streeter closed the embryonic period at 56.5 days the time cut off is arbitrary, the processes established at that time continue into fetal life and where further growth and maturation proceeds to term and beyond into childhood. Figure 3.6 correlates the stage and age of embryos to length throughout the embryonic period.

REFERENCES

1. Hamburger V, Hamilton HL. A series of normal stages in the development of the chick embryo. *J Morphol* **88**:49–92, 1951, and *Develop Dynamics* **195**:231–272, 1992.
2. Sanes JR. On the republication of the Hamburger–Hamilton stage series. *Develop Dynamics* **195**:229–230, 1992.
3. Hamilton V. Afterword: The stage series in the chick embryo. *Develop Dynamics* **195**:273–275, 1992.
4. O'Rahilly R, Muller F. *Development stages in human embryos*. Publication 637. Carnegie Institution of Washington, 1987.
5. Mall FP. On stages in the development of human embryos from 2 to 25 mm long. *Anat Anz* **46**:78–84, 1914.
6. Streeter GL. Developmental horizons in human embryos. Description of age group XIII, embryos about 4 or 5 millimeters long, and age group XIV, period of indentation of the lens vesicle. Carnegie Institution of Washington Publication 557. *Contrib Embryol* **31**:27–63, 1945.
7. Streeter GL. Developmental horizons in human embryos. Description of age groups XV, XVI, XVII, and XVIII, being the third issue of a survey of the Carnegie Collection. Carnegie Institution of Washington Publication 575. *Contrib Embryol* **32**:133–203, 1948.
8. Streeter GL. Developmental horizons in human embryos. Description of age groups XIX, XX, XXI, XXII, and XXIII, being the fifth issue of a survey of the Carnegie Collection (prepared for publication by CH. Heuser & GW Corner). Carnegie Institution of Washington Publication 592. *Contrib Embryol* **34**:165–196, 1951.
9. Streeter GL. Developmental horizons in human embryos. Description of age group XI, 13 to 20 somites, and age group XII, 21 to 29 somites. Carnegie Institution of Washington. Publication 541. *Contrib Embryol* **30**:211–245, 1942.
10. Drumm JE, O'Rahilly R. The assessment of prenatal age from the crown–rump length determined ultrasonically. *Am J Anat* **148**:555–560, 1977.
11. Richardson MK. Heterochrony and the phylotypic period. *Develop Biol* **172**:412–421, 1995.

Embryonic tissues

4

P. Collins

Introduction

Two early tissues can be seen in embryos. Cells are arranged either as epithelia or as mesenchyme. Both cell types have the usual plasma membrane and internal organelles seen in all cells.

PLASMA MEMBRANE

The plasma membrane of the cells contains vast numbers of proteins which may reside within the bilipid layer or protrude intracellularly and/or extracellularly. Those proteins which project exteriorly are covered with carbohydrates as glycoproteins or proteoglycans and contribute to the *glycocalyx* of the cell (Fig. 4.1). The glycocalyx also contains glycoproteins

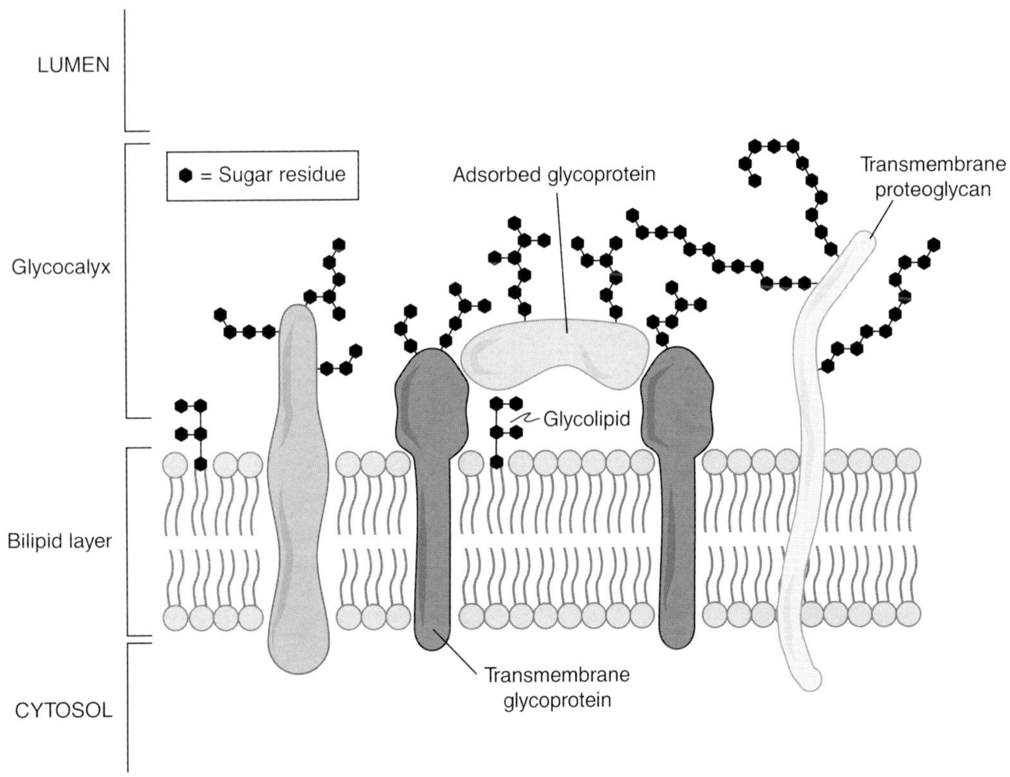

Fig. 4.1 The glycocalyx is synthesized by epithelial cells. It is a feltwork of glycoproteins on the luminal aspect of an epithelium. It is the interface for communication between the lumen of a tube or body cavity and the cells.

and proteoglycans which have been secreted into the extracellular space around the cells and then absorbed onto the cell surface. Thus it is difficult to specify exactly where a cell plasma membrane ends and the surrounding extracellular matrix begins. The glycocalyx is fundamental in cell–cell and cell–matrix communication. Cells place specific protein and carbohydrate groups into the glycocalyx when touching and adhering to other cells, when displaying cell markers to other cells, in blood clotting cascades and in inflammatory responses.

The membrane systems within the embryonic cells, i.e. nucleus, mitochondria, endoplasmic reticulum, Golgi apparatus, lysosomes and secretory vesicles, are supported within the cytoplasm by a range of cytoskeletal elements which also allow cells to maintain surface specialisations (microvilli), to change shape (as in the movements of endocytosis and exocytosis), to move in specific directions and (with the glycocalyx molecules) to adhere strongly to a substrate when movement ceases.

THE CYTOSKELETON

The cytoskeleton is a highly dynamic network of protein filaments that extends throughout the cell. As it also allows the cell to move or move portions of its plasma membrane, the cytoskeleton is less like a bony framework and more like a moveable muscular system. Three types of protein filaments produce the diverse range of cytoskeletal elements, *actin filaments*, *microtubules* and *intermediate filaments* (Fig. 4.2); these are synthesized from actin, tubulin and a range of fibrous proteins, e.g. vimentin, laminin, respectively.

ACTIN FILAMENTS

Actin filaments are polar structures composed of globular molecules of actin arranged as a helix. They work in networks and bundles, often found just beneath the plasma membrane where they crosslink to form the cell cortex. Actin filaments are used to change the shape of the plasma membrane, moving it outwards in projections or inwards in invaginations. Discrete bundles of actin, anchored into the cortex, can produce thin spiky protrusions of the plasma membrane, microvilli, whereas sheet-like extensions of the membrane (lamellipodia) are supported by continuous flattened bundles of actin similarly anchored. Conversely, actin filaments can pull portions of the membrane inwards in the formation of endocytotic vesicles or in cell division. Here, contractile bundles of actin associated with the motor protein myosin form. Although myosin is most familiar in muscle fibres, non-muscle cells contain various myosin proteins. Contractile bundles of actin filaments and myosin filaments are synthesized for specific functions and then disassembled, e.g. during cell division after chromosomal separation the plasma membrane constricts to the middle of the cell allowing two daughter cells to separate. Such assemblies of actin and myosin are also found in development, near the apical surface of epithelial cells where they play a role in folding of epithelial sheets, and in mesenchyme where they can form stress fibres which allow the cells to exert tension on the extracellular matrix.

MICROTUBULES

Microtubules are long, hollow cylinders composed of the globular protein tubulin. They are much more rigid than actin

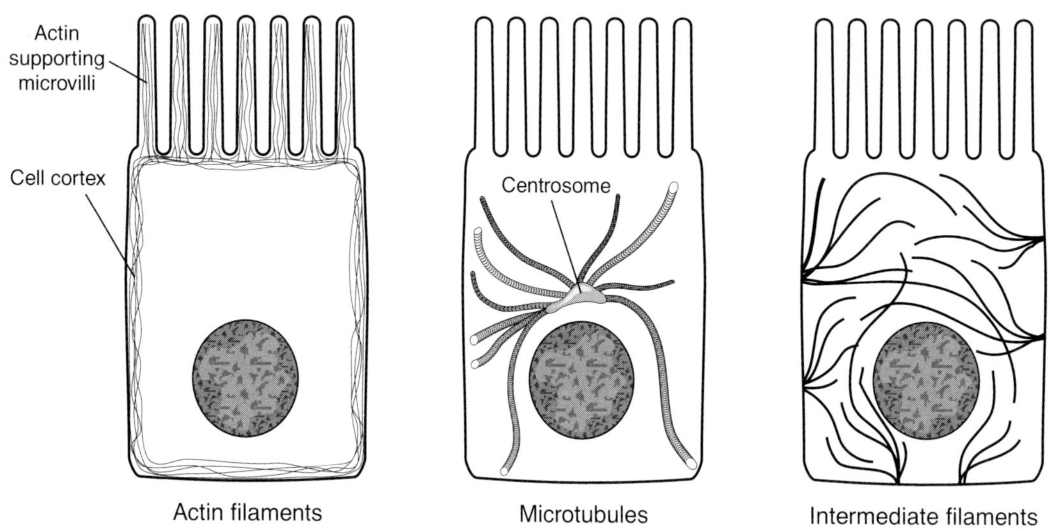

Fig. 4.2 Three types of cytoskeletal elements within a cell allow the cell to maintain a shape or move it.

filaments. Microtubules emanate from the centre of the cell in a region termed the centrosome. They lengthen by adding tubulin to the proximal end of each microtubule while subunits are lost from the distal end. The centrosome offers a focus and region of stabilization for the proximal ends of the hundreds of microtubules in a cell; it also contains the two centrioles which are used by the cell when dividing. Vast numbers of microtubules extend in all directions to the plasma membrane and seem to ensure that the centrosome is at the centre of the cell. From this position the microtubule array sites the other cellular organelles and holds them in place using a range of contact proteins. Should the cell touch another cell, there may be internal movements of the organelles driven by the microtubules resulting in repositioning of the centrosome. Microtubules display a dynamic instability, with new subgroups being added or subtracted very rapidly. The turnover of distal units can be slowed by contact with proteins close to the plasma membrane; this allows cells to maintain a particular shape and polarity. Microtubules are also used in cell-surface specialisations where they form the basis of cilia in the familiar 9+2 arrangement of nine microtubule doublets around a pair of single microtubules.

INTERMEDIATE FILAMENTS

Intermediate filaments are made of a variety of proteins all formed from highly elongated fibrous molecules. They are arranged as rope-like fibres which span each cell often from one cell junction to another. They are termed intermediate filaments because their apparent diameter on electron microscopy is between that of actin filaments and thick myosin filaments. Specific varieties of intermediate filaments are present in epithelial and mesenchymal cells. Epithelial cells contain keratin filaments whereas mesenchymal cells have vimentin and vimentin-related filaments and in those cells which will develop a myogenic lineage, desmin filaments are seen. Neuroepithelial cells develop neurofilaments and glial fibrillary acidic protein filaments are seen in astrocytes.

Epithelia

Cells composing epithelia are polarised with apical and basal surfaces. The apical surface commonly displays specialised features such as microvilli whereas the basal surface is the site of extracellular protein deposition in the form of a basal lamina. Laterally, the cells contact their neighbours via varieties of juxtaluminal junctional complexes which bridge the narrow intercellular clefts.

BASAL LAMINA

Basal laminae are thin flexible sheets of extracellular matrix which are made by and underlie epithelial cells (Fig. 4.3). Basal laminae are also found surrounding individual muscle cells, fat cells and Schwann cells. The presence or absence of a basal lamina beneath an epithelium during development is of consequence. Basal laminae organise the proteins in adjacent cell membranes, they induce cell differentiation and cell metabolism, they serve as routes for cell migration and can influence cell polarity in those cells that touch them; they can change with time during development and thus can maintain a developmental impetus.

The basal lamina is described in electron microscopic studies as having an electron lucent layer, the *lamina lucida* or *rara*, closest to the basal surface of the cell and an electron-dense layer, the *lamina densa* below. If the epithelial layer rests on underlying mesenchyme, a layer of collagen fibrils connects the basal lamina to the underlying tissue, sometimes with specialised anchoring collagen fibrils. The strength of this connection is important for development and growth. Many textbooks do not distinguish between the basal lamina as described above and the *basement membrane*, a thicker layer which includes the basal lamina and extracellular components of the underlying connective-tissue matrix.

Embryonic basal laminae are composed chiefly of *laminin*. Later, other extracellular molecules such as *type IV collagen*, *perlecan* and *entactin* (see below) contribute to the feltwork of the layer (Fig. 4.3). In some regions of the body, basal laminae form specialised structures or units which have a specific function during development or in adult life. An example of this arrangement is seen in tooth development, where initially ameloblasts and odontoblasts are separated by a basal lamina. The ameloblasts deposit enamel directly onto one side of this basal lamina and the odontoblasts deposit dentine onto the other (see p. 33); in this way the tooth is formed. In both the kidney and the lung the basal lamina from the specialised cells of the organ abuts directly onto the endothelial basal lamina producing a selectively permeable barrier. In the kidney, this is the glomerular basement membrane.

In development the basal lamina acts as a selective barrier to the movement of cells and migrating cells will move along basal laminae but not through them. Cells beneath an epithelial layer see only the basal lamina which the overlying cells produce. Changes in the local basal laminal composition is one way by which the epithelial cells can communicate with the cells migrating beneath them. In adult tissues the basal lamina permits the movement of macrophages, lymphocytes and nerve processes and plays an important part in tissue regeneration after injury.

CELL–CELL JUNCTIONS

Juxtaposed cells usually do not touch. For contact to be established, the cells produce specific molecules which promote the development of a *cell–cell junction* between them (Fig. 4.4). Junctional complexes allow sheets of epithelial cells to act in concert in maintaining a barrier, or in producing alterations in the overall epithelial morphology; they also permit cell–cell communication and are in this respect

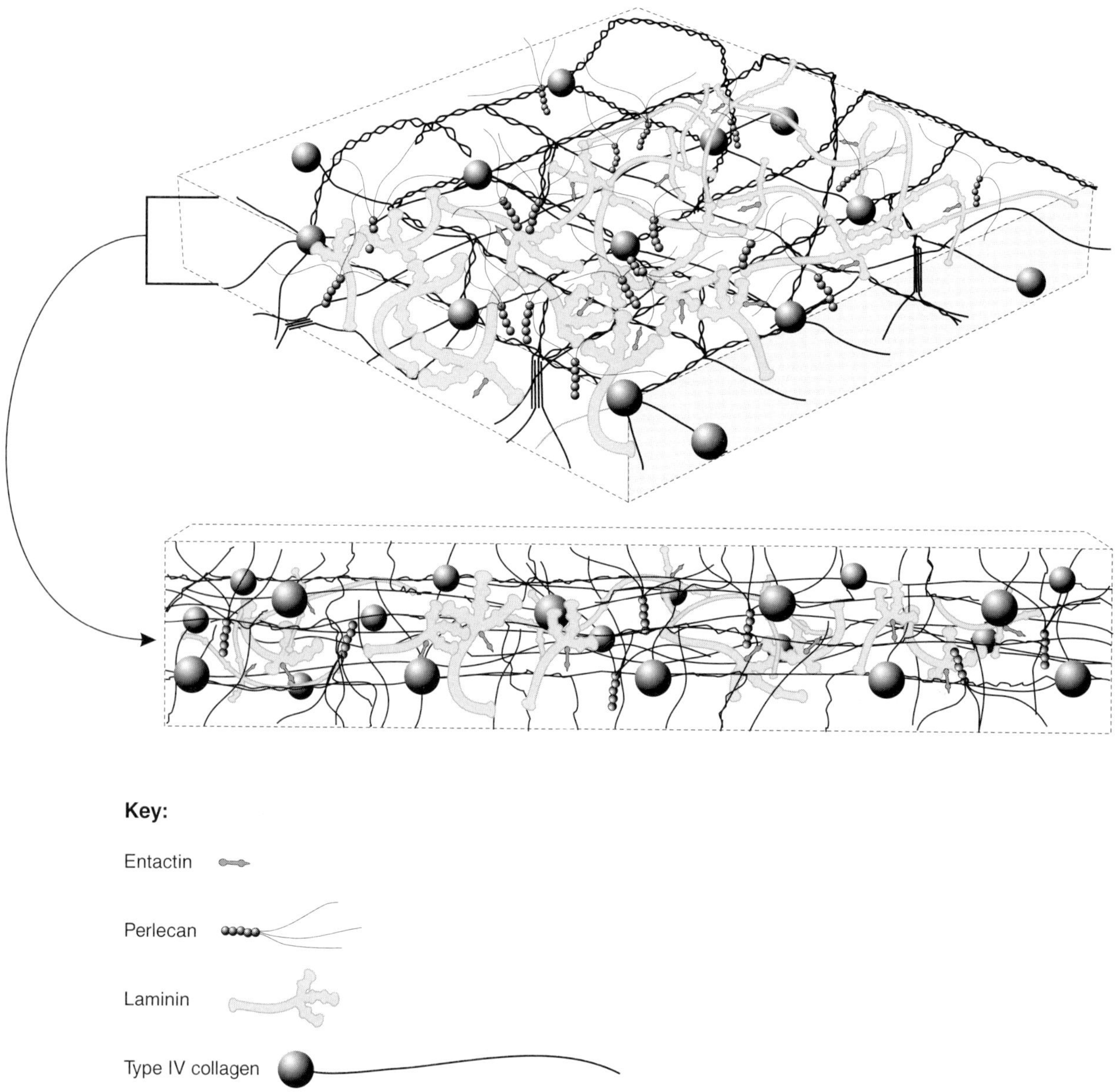

Fig. 4.3 A basal lamina is synthesized by epithelial cells. It is a feltwork of proteins which attach to the epithelial cells and provide an attachment for underlying cells. It is the interface for communication between the extracellular space and the cells.

especially important in development. Cell junctions are classified into three main groups: (i) *tight junctions*, which prevent leakage of molecules between cells from one side of a sheet of cells to the other; (ii) *anchoring junctions*, where the neighbouring cell membranes attach and are supported by cytoskeletal elements within the cells, either actin or intermediate filaments – this type of junction also anchors epithelial cells to the extracellular matrix; (iii) *communicating junctions* mediate the passage of electrical or chemical signals from one cell to another.

The formation of these junctional complexes is dependent on a range of cell adhesion molecules (see Fig. 4.4). In cell–cell anchoring junctions (adhesion belts and desmosomes) the cell adhesion molecules (CAMs) involved are termed *cadherins*; they are attached intracellularly to intermediate or actin filaments in the cell cortex. The latter run parallel to the plasma membrane; thus the actin bundles of adjacent cells are linked. Concomitant contraction of the actin bundles will result in narrowing of the apices of the epithelial cells and rolling of the epithelial layer into a deep groove or a tube.

Epithelial cells contact the underlying basal lamina by different types of anchoring junctions (hemidesomosomes and focal contacts). In these cases, the transmembrane linker pro-

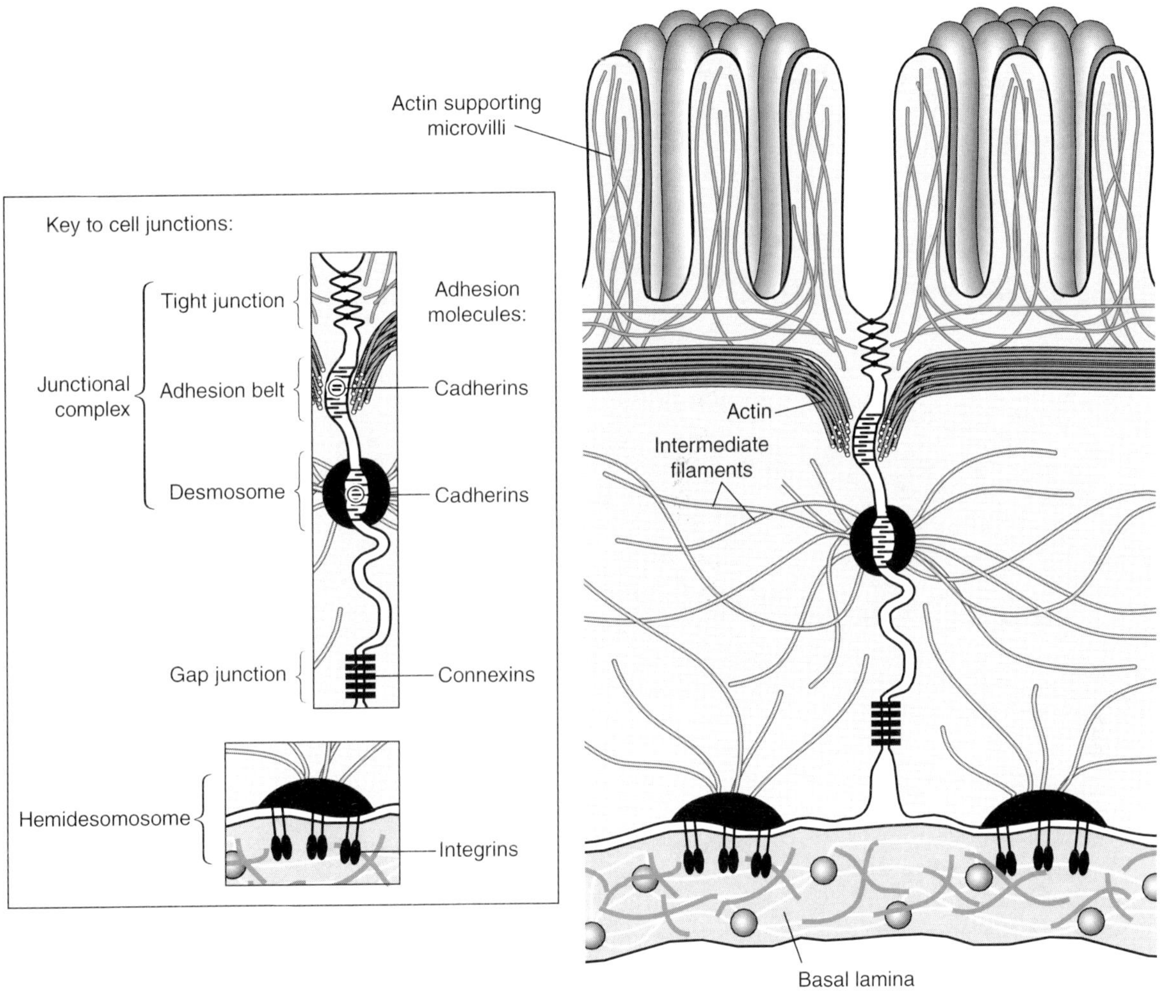

Fig. 4.4 Junctions complexes form between epithelial cells preventing passage between cells, permitting communication between cells, and joining cells to each other and to the basal lamina. Junctions are supported by adhesion molecules and the cytoskeletal elements within the cells.

teins belong to the *integrin* family of extracellular matrix receptors. Cytoskeletal filaments support the connection of the integrin within the cell membrane to the matrix.

Communication between adjacent epithelial cells is mediated by *gap junctions*. In forming a gap junction, each cell contributes six identical protein subunits (called connexins) which form a structure, similar to an old-fashioned cotton reel, termed a *connexon*. This is situated across the bilaminar membrane with the thicker rims extending into the extracellular and intracellular spaces. Each connexon is capable of opening and closing, thus controlling the gap. When two connexons from adjacent cells are aligned, a tubular connection is made between the cells. Each gap junction is really a cluster of apposed connexons which each permit molecules smaller than 1000 daltons to pass through them. In early embryos, most cells are electrically coupled to one another by gap junctions. Later in development, epithelial cells synthesize gap junctions at particular stages when it is inferred that information is passing from cell to cell. When gap junctions are removed, there is often a difference in differentiation in the cellular progeny. Gap junctions are seen in adult tissues, e.g. connecting cardiac myocytes to permit transmission of the electrical signals of the cardiac cycle.

Mesenchymal cells

Mesenchymal cells, in contrast to epithelial cells, have no polarity, thus no directional surface specialisations. They have junctional complexes which are not juxtaluminal and they produce extensive extracellular matrix molecules and fibres from the whole cell surface (Fig. 4.5). As development proceeds, proliferating mesenchymal populations begin to differentiate. This is often first seen by the upregulation of specific mRNA in the cell or in the production of different extracellular matrix molecules by selected progeny.

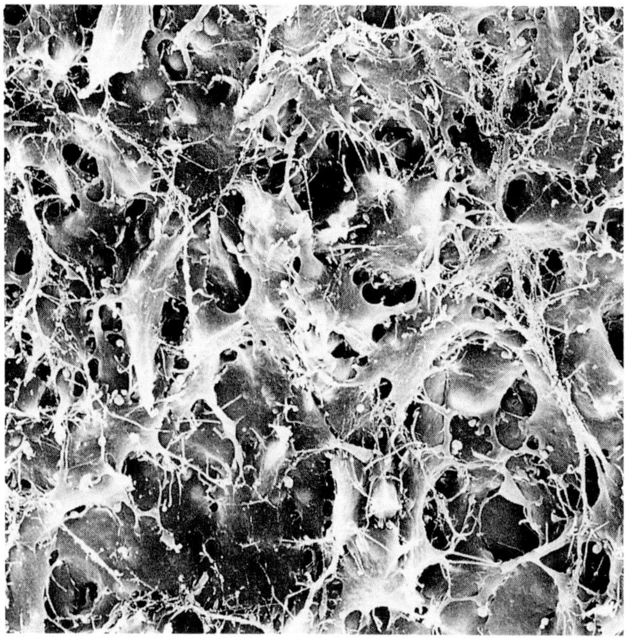

Fig. 4.5 SEM of mesenchyme cells. Mesenchyme cells have no polarity. They control the space around them by their synthesis of extracellular matrix. (Photograph by Dr P. Collins.)

EXTRACELLULAR MATRIX

A substantial part of the developing embryo is made up of extracellular matrix. This name is given to the vast array of complex molecules which are secreted locally by mesenchymal cells and assembled into networks which structure the spaces between the embryonic cells. In early development, mesenchymal populations are composed of migrating epithelial cells and mesenchymal cells generated from germinal epithelia. It is the latter group which will give rise to the range of connective tissues seen in the adult. Connective tissues form the architectural framework of the body and it is the matrices which determine the tissue's physical properties, i.e. in bone, cartilage or fascia. It is variation in the constituents and amount of the matrix molecules which gives the diversity of connective tissues (Fig. 4.6).

There are two main classes of extracellular matrix molecules, *glycosaminoglycans* (GAGs) which may be linked covalently to proteins as *proteoglycans*, and *fibrous proteins*, e.g. *collagen*, *elastin*, *laminin* and *fibronectin*. The glycosaminoglycan and proteoglycan molecules form a highly hydrated gel-like ground substance into which the fibrous proteins are embedded.

Four main groups of GAGs have been described: (i) hyaluronic acid; (ii) chondroitin sulphate and dermatan sulphate; (iii) heparan sulphate and heparin; (iv) keratan sulphate. Hyaluronic acid is the most simple GAG. It is especially abundant in embryos where it fills the spaces between cells and because of its level of hydration becomes turgid and generally resists compression. By synthesizing hyaluronic acid cells can open up migration pathways or support epithelia which is undergoing morphological change. The other GAGs, which are more complex that hyaluronic acid, have much shorter disaccharide chains, contain sulphated sugars and are usually bound to a protein core forming proteoglycans. Aggregates of hyaluronate and proteoglycans can make huge molecules which occupy a volume equivalent to a bacterium.

Within tissues, GAGs can form gels of varying pore size and thus act as filters regulating the movement of molecules according to their size or charge. The heparan sulphate proteoglycan *perlecan* is found in the basal lamina of the kidney glomerulus and functions as a filter in the glomerular basement membrane. Proteoglycans which bind various growth factors act as reservoirs for messages which can be positioned in the matrix by cells at one stage to be read by cells developing later. GAGs and proteoglycans associate with the fibrous proteins in the matrix and provide support between the fibres.

Collagens form the major fibrous proteins in the matrix, So far, about 15 types of collagen have been described, each made from a range of basic α-chains and each encoded by a separate gene. Each collagen molecule is made from three α-chains wound around one another like a rope. The main types of collagen found in connective tissue are types, I, II, III, V and XI. These types aggregate into the huge hawser-like bundles which can be seen on electron microscopy. Collagen types IX and XII are smaller and link the larger fibres to one another and to other matrix molecules. Types IV and VII are found in the basal laminae where type IV forms the feltwork of the mature basal lamina and VII forms the anchoring structures which attach the basal lamina to the underlying matrix. Collagen is used to provide the initial matrices for cartilage and bone and is particularly seen in tendons and ligaments. In these cases, the amount of GAGs is reduced and the collagen fibres are aligned by the fibroblasts in response to the direction of the stresses acting on the collagen. In this way, the connective tissues of the body are responsive to the physical demands placed upon them. Anomalies of collagen synthesis can give rise to diseases in life, for example the condition osteogenesis imperfecta is caused by mutations in type I collagen production, leading to bones which are brittle and fracture with little stress; mutations in type II collagen lead to disorders of cartilage.

Elastin is composed of short elastin proteins which are crosslinked so that when relaxed, the fibres are randomly coiled but when stretched each elastin molecule can expand so contributing to the overall effect. Elastic fibres are at least five times more extensible than a rubber band of the same cross-sectional area. Usually collagen fibres are interwoven with elastic fibres to prevent overstretching and damage.

Laminin is one of the first extracellular proteins synthesized in the embryo, forming most of the early basal laminae. Each molecule is shaped like an asymmetric cross. Molecules join together to form a feltwork often supported by smaller entactin molecules.

Fibronectin is an adhesive protein which helps cells attach to

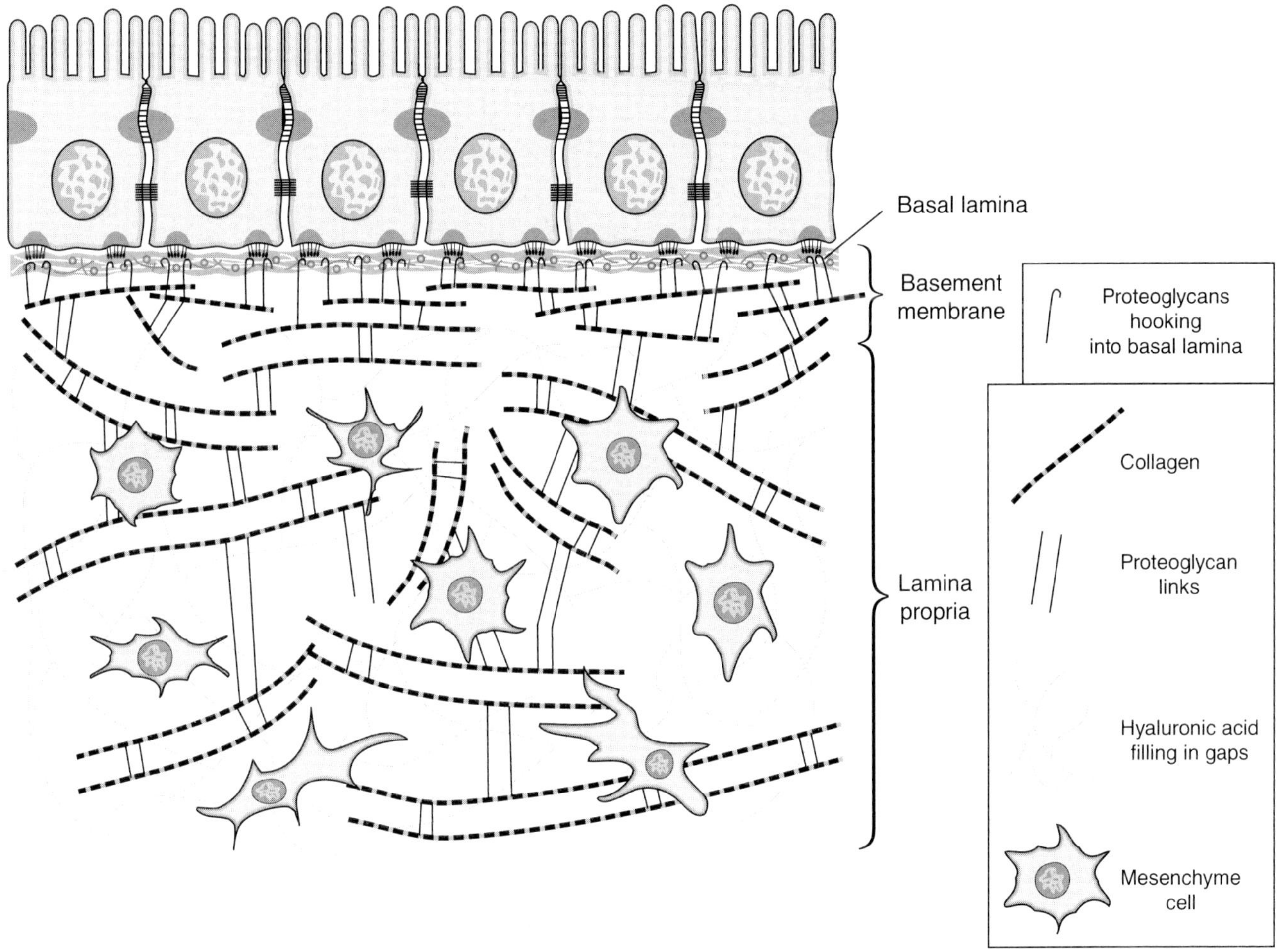

Fig. 4.6 Mesenchyme cells and extracellular matrix forming a lamina propria beneath an epithelium. The mesenchyme cells synthesize collagens, proteoglycans and glycosaminoglycans as a framework and add other proteins, e.g. fibronectin, as necessary. Extracellular matrix is attached to a basal lamina forming a basement membrane.

the matrix. Generally contact with fibronectin causes cells to move. It has been shown in culture that neural crest cells will preferentially migrate along fibronectin-rich substrates, and within three-dimensional cultures migrating cells can achieve their greatest speeds migrating along fibronectin pathways. It is interesting to note that bonding with fibronectin does not necessarily fix a cell to one position within the matrix so contacts with this protein are made and then released with ease.

CELL–MATRIX JUNCTIONS

Cells interact with the extracellular matrix molecules via protein receptors or co-receptors in the plasma membrane. *Syndecans* are proteoglycan co-receptors which span the plasma membrane. The extracellular part carries chondroitin sulphate and heparan sulphate chains while the intracellular domain interacts with the cell cortex actin filaments. *Integrins* are receptor proteins which bind to and respond to the extracellular matrix information. Again an extracellular receptor site binds with matrix molecules, especially fibronectin and laminin; intracellularly the integrin binds to the actin or intermediate filaments. When the integrins in the cell membrane contact a matrix molecule, e.g. fibronectin, the orientation of the fibronectin will cause alignment of the actin cytoskeleton and a reorientation of the cell itself. Later, when the cells are depositing extracellular matrix molecules, the actin cytoskeleton will exert forces to orient the matrix molecules in a similar configuration. Thus the interaction between matrix molecules and cells and then cells and matrix can drive development and propagate order from cell to cell.

The cell–matrix junctions permit communications within the embryo just as gap junctions permit communications between cells. However, the cell–matrix mechanisms allow messages to be left in the matrix which may indicate migration routes or halt migrating cells and suggest a differentiation pathway. The matrix information system can thus control the temporal pattern of development.

Transformation from epithelium to mesenchyme

The two embryonic states of epithelial tissue and mesenchyme are not necessarily immutable and transition from epithelia to mesenchyme and vice versa occurs during development. However, such a change requires a temporal or external inductive agent and causes dramatic upregulation and synthesis of a whole variety of special intra- and extracellular molecules as described above. Generally, in the embryo epithelial cells seem to derive from existing epithelial populations whereas mesenchymal cells are produced initially from proliferative (germinal) epithelia and then later by amplifying mitoses within the mesenchymal population (see p. 21). Changes from one cell state to another are considered important in development.

The early migrating cells derived from the primitive streak have a mesenchymal morphology yet will become epithelial when they reach their destinations forming the somites, the somatopleuric and splanchnopleuric epithelial lining the intraembryonic coelom, including the lining of the pericardial cavity. All of these epithelia become germinal centres which produce further mesenchymal populations. However, an additional group of invaginating mesenchymal cells derived from the neural crest never revert to epithelia. Angiogenic mesenchyme, which is believed to arise from extraembryonic sources initially, is especially proliferative and capable of great migration within the embryo; it differentiates into endothelium throughout early development. A small subset of endothelial cells in the heart are induced to transform back to mesenchyme at the atrioventricular canal and the proximal outflow tract. This may be the only example of a mesenchymal population derived from an endothelial lineage[1]; the cells retain expression of an endothelial marker.

Tissue interactions

In order for the information carried in the genome of an embryo to be expressed, the cells produced by mitotic division must be able to contact and respond to each other; this process occurs locally by the construction of gap junctions (see above). However, as an embryo grows, it is composed of more and more cell populations which become differentiated into *tissues* and separated by the matrix molecules they produce. In these more complex situations, the tissues have a repertoire of communication methods which require both epithelial and mesenchymal arrangements and their matrices working in concert. From a starting point of an early embryo at the body plan stage, all of the basic organs arise through interactions between close epithelial populations (plus their basal laminae), epithelia and mesenchyme (with the extracellular matrix), and between differentiating mesechymal populations. The basic interactions are the same. Such sequential spatial and temporal reciprocal interactions have been termed *epigenetic cascades*[2].

PERMISSIVE INTERACTIONS

It has been shown by experimental study that neither epithelia nor mesenchyme will grow alone – each needs the other for DNA synthesis and mitosis to occur. However, in many cases it is not the cell bodies that are required. Epithelial cells will grow in culture as long as there is some sort of mesenchymal extract in the medium, and mesenchymal cells will grow in culture as long as they can contact a basal lamina. Thus in both cases, factors in the matrix which have arisen from the cell population are enough to support growth. These basic requirements of development are termed *permissive interactions*. The supporting tissue may not be that usually present in development and indeed much research time has been spent in investigating which mesenchymal tissues would support growth of specific epithelia and vice versa. However, in many cases, although growth was maintained in these experiments development would not proceed at all or in the normal manner. For such development more information is needed from the reciprocating tissues, and such information could enable both tissues to change in a manner that neither of them could do without the information. This is the basis of *instructive interactions*.

INSTRUCTIVE INTERACTIONS

Wessells[3] proposed four general principles which can be seen in most instructive interactions:

- In the presence of tissue A, responding tissue B develops in a certain way.
- In the absence of tissue A, responding tissue B does not develop in that way.
- In the absence of tissue A, but in the presence of tissue C, tissue B does not develop in that way.
- In the presence of tissue A, a tissue D, which would normally develop differently, is changed to develop like B.

Thus in an instructive interaction one tissue induces another to respond in a specific way. If the target tissue can respond to the inductive signal it is called *competent*. If the target tissue does not respond it is described as *non-competent*. Non-competence may be because the tissue has previously responded to a earlier inductive signal which has restricted its repertoire of possible responses. As development proceeds, more and more cell populations will become non-competent as they differentiate.

Inductive interactions may be more or less complicated: only the induced tissue may change or both tissues may change and participate, as in morphogenesis, or, more commonly, several reciprocal inductive interactions may be required over a prolonged period of developmental time before a specific organ or tissue will form.

Epithelial–mesenchymal interactions

The instructive interactions between epithelia and mesenchyme produce the general morphological changes which are seen in every system throughout embryogenesis. They are a subset of embryonic tissue interactions occurring between epithelial tissue and specific subdivisions of mesenchymal tissue which arise during differentiation. These interactions provide a mechanism for coordinating and fine tuning the mitotic rates and differentiative abilities of the two tissues. A range of interactions occurring in different systems of the embryo are described.

BRANCHING MORPHOGENESIS

Most organs, from lungs to kidneys, initially develop a main duct from which branches arise often dichotomously; later these mature into typical patterns seen in the fully formed organ. The mechanism of branching morphogenesis is therefore similar in a variety of systems. Although the early descriptions of this process described only the morphogenesis, now the specific matrix molecules involved during the interaction have been identified (Fig. 4.7).

At the tip of a proliferating duct, the epithelium and its basal lamina is in contact with the underlying mesenchymal cells and their extracellular matrix molecules. Local production of hyaluronidase by the mesenchyme breaks down the basal lamina and promotes proliferation of the epithelium. Cleft production is initiated by the mesenchyme which produces type III collagen fibrils within putative clefts. The collagen acts to protect the basal lamina from the effects of the hyaluronidase and the overlying epithelia have a locally reduced mitotic rate. The region of rapid mitoses at the tip of the acinus is thus split into two and two branches develop from this point. If the type III collagen is removed from the cleft, branching does not occur; if excess collagen is not removed, supernumerary clefts appear. Note that this interaction may occur with any epithelial type and any subpopulation of mesenchyme.

NEURAL ECTODERM AND SURFACE ECTODERM INTERACTIONS

The above interactions are clearly seen in formation of the lens of the eye. The optic cup is an outgrowth of the diencephalon of the brain. As the cup approaches the overlying surface ectoderm, it induces a local change. The ectoderm cells become narrower at the apical region causing the sheet of cells to curve and move towards the optic cup. Ultimately, a small lens vesicle invaginates and the unaffected surface ectoderm becomes confluent over the structure. If the optic cup is removed no lens vesicle develops. If the optic cup is removed and placed beneath a different portion of surface ectoderm a similar lens vesicle is induced (Fig. 4.8).

NEURAL ECTODERM AND NEURAL CREST MESENCHYME INTERACTIONS: THE 'FLY-PAPER MODEL' OF SKULL DEVELOPMENT

The subtle interplay between the mesenchyme and the epithelial basal lamina is demonstrated in the fly-paper model of skull development[4]. Here, an interaction occurs between the neuroectoderm of the neural tube and the surrounding neural crest mesenchyme. The neuroepithelium will display fibronectin amongst other fibrous proteins in the basal lamina. This will ensure the migration of the neural crest over the

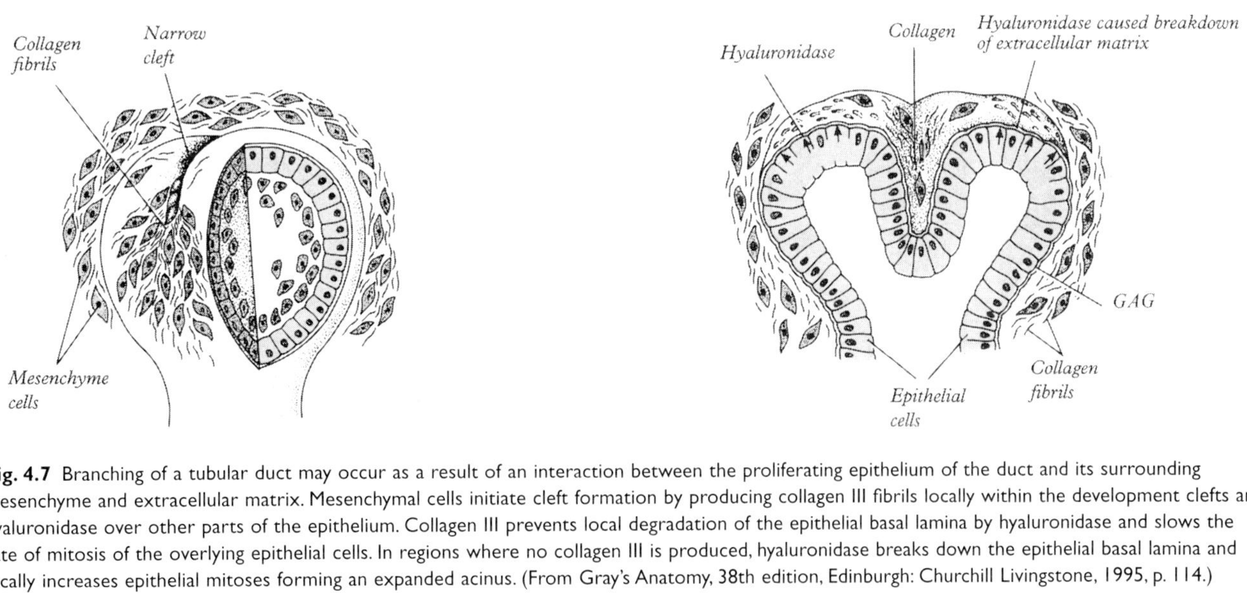

Fig. 4.7 Branching of a tubular duct may occur as a result of an interaction between the proliferating epithelium of the duct and its surrounding mesenchyme and extracellular matrix. Mesenchymal cells initiate cleft formation by producing collagen III fibrils locally within the development clefts and hyaluronidase over other parts of the epithelium. Collagen III prevents local degradation of the epithelial basal lamina by hyaluronidase and slows the rate of mitosis of the overlying epithelial cells. In regions where no collagen III is produced, hyaluronidase breaks down the epithelial basal lamina and locally increases epithelial mitoses forming an expanded acinus. (From Gray's Anatomy, 38th edition, Edinburgh: Churchill Livingstone, 1995, p. 114.)

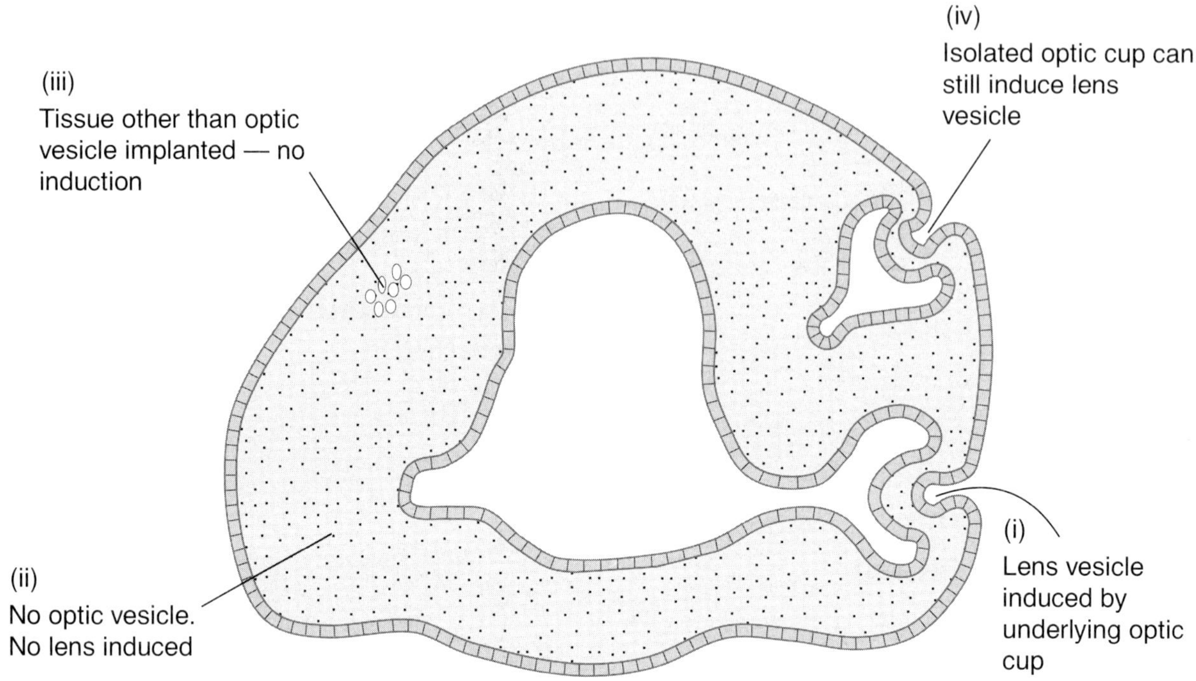

Fig. 4.8 Induction of the lens vesicle by the optic cup. This illustrates clearly the four general principles of an instructive interaction. (After Wessells[3].)

neural tube and into the developing face. As development proceeds, the neuroepithelium transiently expresses type II collagen in the basal lamina on the basal aspect of the neural tube, around the olfactory regions, around the optic cups prior to and during lens invagination, around the otic vesicles which will form the inner ear, and on the basal and lateral surfaces of the diencephalon, mesencephalon and rhombencephalon. The notochord also expresses type II collagen in its basal lamina. Some time after the type II collagen has been removed from the basal laminae, neural crest mesenchyme

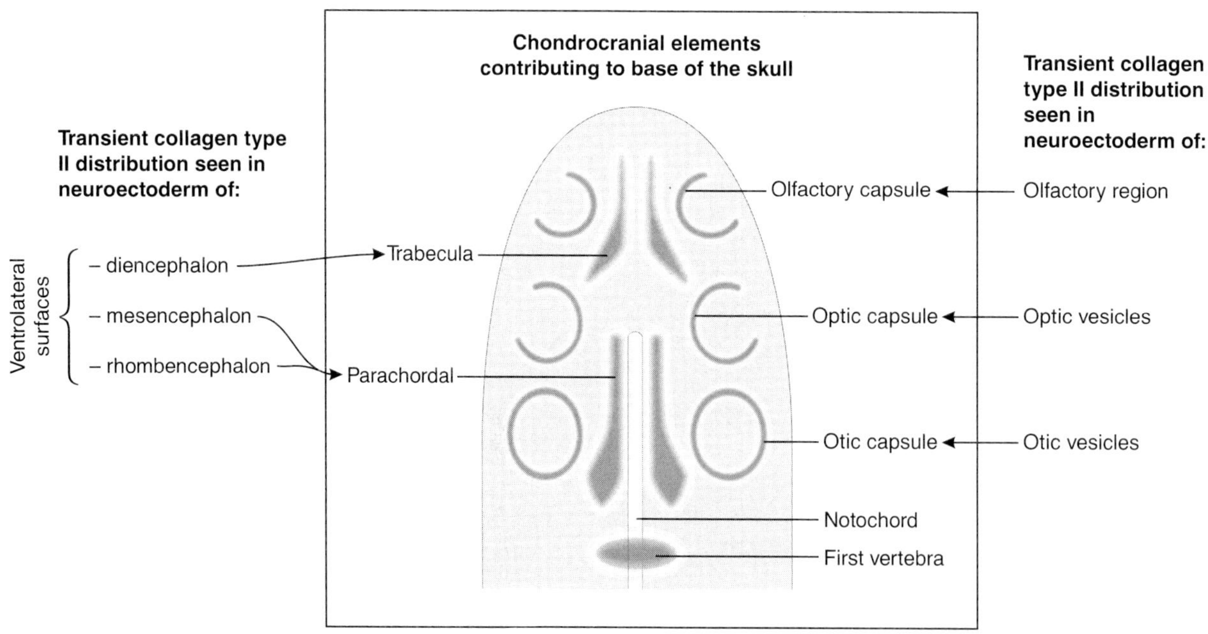

Fig. 4.9 Transient expression of type II collagen in the basal lamina of the neuroepithelium causes mesenchyme cells which touch it to upregulate their own synthesis of type II collagen and differentiate along a chondrogenic pathway. The pattern of expression in the neuroectoderm determines the form of the chondrocranium. (From Thorogood[4] with permission.)

adjacent to the regions listed commence synthesis of type II collagen and ultimately differentiate along a chondrogenic pathway. It seems as if the type II collagen in the basal lamina affects those cells which contact it and cause their upregulation of type II collagen. The pattern of the expression of type II collagen in the basal laminae determines the form of the chondrocranium (Fig. 4.9). Slight alterations in the pattern of expression could have profound effects on the shape and form of the chondrocranium perhaps producing the diversity of skull shapes seen in vertebrates.

SURFACE ECTODERM AND NEURAL CREST INTERACTIONS

A further example of a reciprocal tissue interactions can be seen in mammalian tooth development summarised in Fig. 4.10 (from Lumsden[5]). Tooth development begins along the *dental lamina* of the premaxilla, maxillae and mandible. The epithelium proliferates to form an *enamel organ* under the influence of the neural crest mesenchyme which forms a *dental papilla*; together this unit is a tooth bud or germ. The enamel organ induces the dental papilla mesenchyme to become *odontoblasts*; these cells then induce the epithelial cells to differentiate into *ameloblasts*. The tooth is formed by matrix deposition each side of the epithelial basal lamina, enamel one side and dentine the other.

The neural crest mesenchyme is responsible for patterning development of the pharyngeal arches including tooth formation. Dental papilla mesenchyme is able to induce the formation of teeth in nonoral epithelium, and can specify the type of tooth produced, i.e. incisor or molar. If cranial neural crest is cultured alone it will differentiate into cartilage. When it is recombined with limb epithelium then cartilage and bone will form. However, if cranial neural crest is recombined with mandibular epithelium, salivary islands, hair and teeth form as well as cartilage and bone, indicating that the mandibular epithelium is essential and specific for the development of teeth.

Early recombination (9–11.5 days of development) of mouse mandibular epithelium (first arch) and hyoid mesenchyme (second arch) results in teeth in 90% of cases, this shows that the dental lamina epithelium can induce tooth development in the head neural crest mesenchyme. The reverse recombination, early second arch epithelium and mandibular arch mesenchyme does not produce teeth, indicating that it is only the first arch epithelium which has this property. However, later recombination experiments (11.5–12 days of development), with second arch epithelium

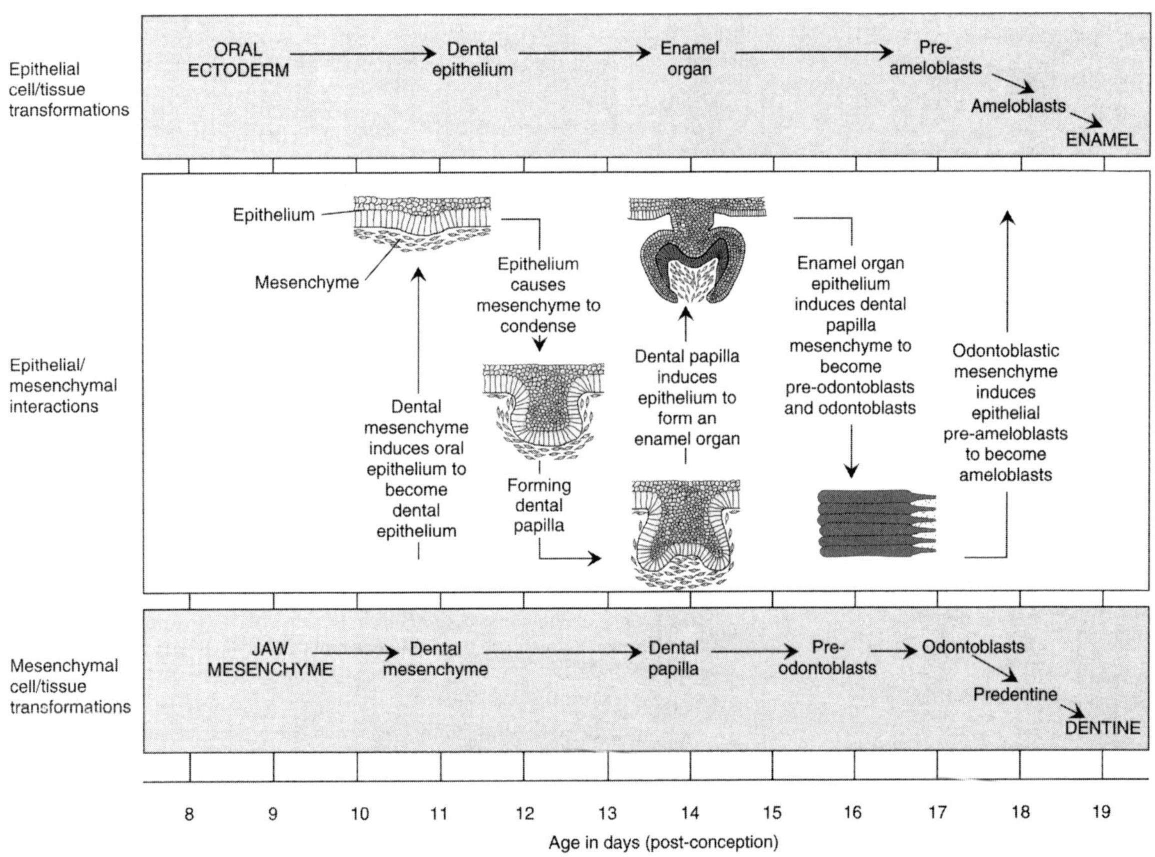

Fig. 4.10 An example of reciprocal tissue interaction in mammalian tooth development. The sequence of epithelial–mesenchymal interactions involved in the development of teeth in the embryonic mouse. E8–19 represent age in days after conception. (From Gray's Anatomy, 38th edition, Edinburgh: Churchill Livingstone, 1995, p. 111. After Lumsden[5].)

and first arch mesenchyme, will produce teeth. In this case the neural crest mesenchyme has already been induced along a dental lineage[6].

The local specification of particular teeth can be changed experimentally. If presumptive incisor region of the mandibular epithelium is recombined with predetermined molar papillae from post-day 12 tooth germs, the shape of the teeth can be redefined by the epithelium and incisiform teeth develop.

The interaction between oral epithelium and neural crest mesenchyme will operate across species, thus recombination of dental mesenchyme from 16–18-day mouse with oral epithelium from the mandibular epithelium of the chick resulted in tooth formation[7]. This is the more surprising as chicks do not normally develop teeth.

SURFACE ECTODERM AND SOMATOPLEURIC MESENCHYMAL INTERACTIONS IN THE LIMB

The tissues involved in limb development arise from a ridge along the flank of the embryo. Interaction of specialized regions of the *somatopleuric mesenchyme* with the overlying ectoderm gives rise to local, thickened regions of surface ectoderm and proliferation of the underlying mesenchyme. At these sites the ectoderm forms a longitudinal ridge of high columnar cells, the *apical ectodermal ridge (AER)* and the specialized somatopleuric mesenchyme maintains its growth. The AER and underlying mesenchyme together are termed the *progress zone* and the limb grows meristematically from this point, i.e. proliferation produces the next distal portion of limb. These two populations require each other. Only the apical ectodermal ridge can promote limb outgrowth and only limb mesenchyme will result in limb development. Positional values are assigned to the proliferating epithelial and mesenchymal populations by the progress zone thus first the humerus is developed, then the radius and ulna, then the carpals and so on (Fig. 4.11).

Within the portion of the limb which has received its positional value the mesenchyme instructs the overlying ectoderm about the appropriate epidermal structure to develop. Parts of a chick hind limb develop different characteristics with feathers on the thigh and scales on the leg. If mesenchyme from the thigh is transplanted beneath the leg, feathers will develop instead of the normal scales. This type of experiment has been repeated recombining neck ectoderm which will not normally develop feathers with thigh mesenchyme, in this case the epidermis will develop feathers.

If thigh mesenchyme is inserted beneath the apical ectodermal ridge of a developing wing which is at the stage to assign radius and ulna, two things occur. Firstly, information from the apical ectodermal ridge about the age of the limb will override the 'thighness' of the mesenchyme and it will express leg characteristics appropriate to the developmental time of the wing. Thus the proximal limb characteristics are replaced by distal ones. Secondly, the wing epithelium is reassigned to develop leg characteristics by the mesenchyme. Thus the limb develops a fibula and tibia and the epidermis displays scales. This latter experiment show the reciprocal nature of inductive interactions with both tissues giving and responding to information.

Positional information which cause the development of the axes of the limb are controlled by both mesenchyme and epithelium. A subset of mesenchyme situated at the postaxial border of the limb bud termed the *zone of polarising activity (ZPA)*. controls the cranio-caudal axis of the limb, i.e. where the thumb develops. Active substances released at this region will cause a number five digit to form, the little finger (Fig. 4.11). The reducing influence of this substance allows development of digits four, three, two and then the thumb to develop. However, even if this system is disrupted by mixing the mesenchyme up within the limb producing five equally structured digits, the limb still displays dorsal and ventral surfaces. The inductive influence for dorsal/ventral patterning is specified by the ectodermal epithelium.

ENDODERM AND SPLANCHNOPLEURIC MESENCHYME INTERACTIONS IN THE LUNG

The respiratory tree derives from interactions between endodermal epithelium and surrounding splanchnopleuric mesenchyme. The trachea arises from the pharynx as a midline, ventral diverticulum which grows causally then bifurcates into the primary bronchi which expand dorsally on each side of the oesophagus. Originally splanchnopleuric mesenchyme surrounding the pharynx envelopes both the oesophagus and the trachea; however, the proximity of the lung buds to the pericardio-peritoneal canals which will later give rise to the pleural cavities provides a different mesenchymal population. Proliferation of the adjacent *splanchnopleuric coelomic epithelium* (of the primary pleural cavities) provides *investing mesenchyme* around the developing trachea and lung buds from stage 13 of development. The proliferative activity decreases in stage 14 and the mesenchyme becomes arranged in zones around the developing endoderm. This investing mesenchyme contains a mixed population of cells, that which will pattern the endodermal epithelium, a subpopulation of angiogenic mesenchyme which may migrate in to form the endothelial networks surrounding the air sacs, and splanchnopleuric mesenchyme which will give rise to the smooth muscle cells which surround both the respiratory tubes and the blood vessels. The splachnopleuric coelomic epithelium will after its proliferative phase give rise to the visceral pleura.

The control of the branching pattern of the respiratory tree resides with the *splanchnopleuric mesenchyme*. Recombination of tracheal mesenchyme with bronchial respiratory endoderm causes an inhibition of bronchial branching, whereas recombination of bronchial mesenchyme with tracheal epithelium will induce bronchial outgrowths from the trachea[3,8]. Initially the tracheal mesenchyme is continuous

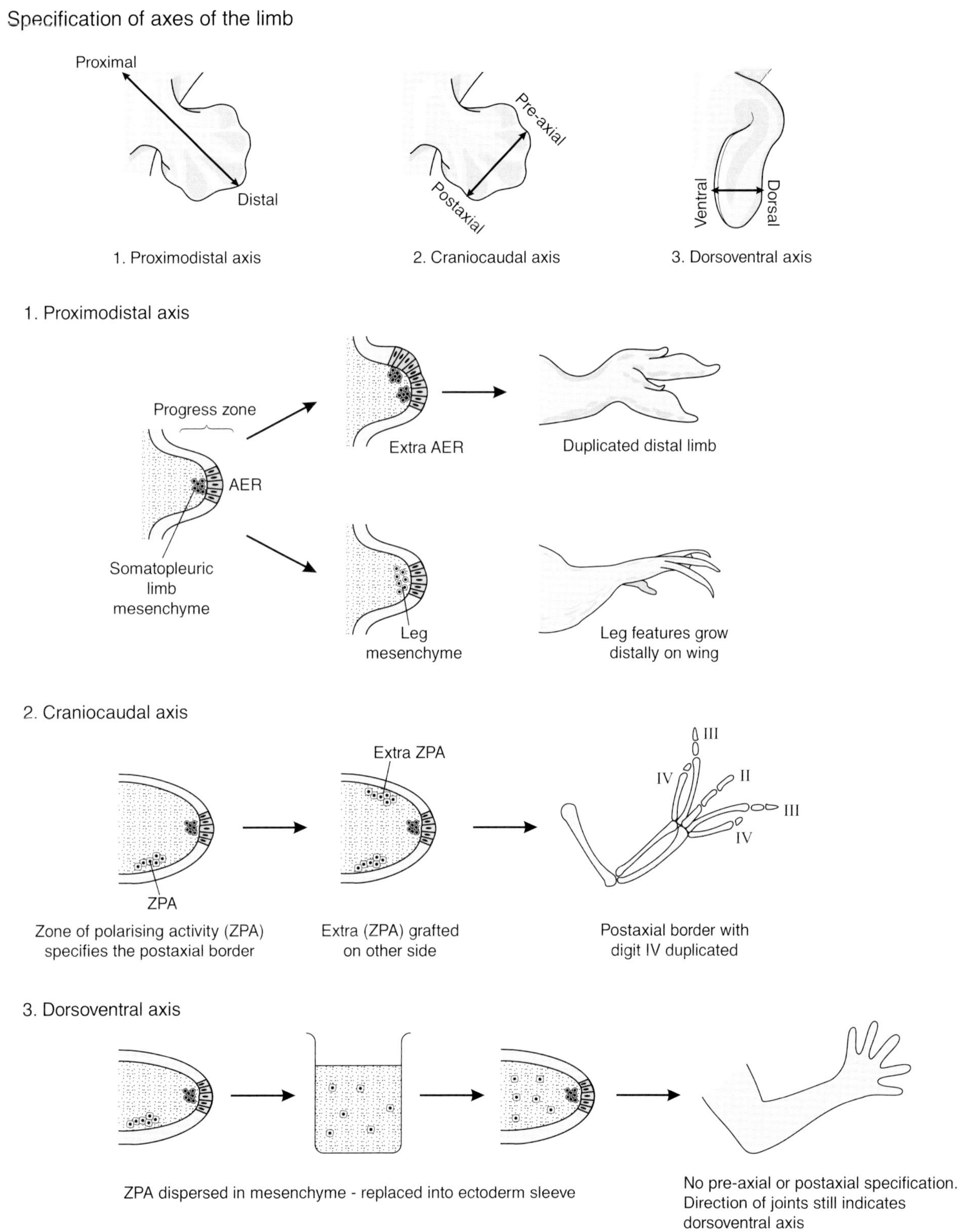

Fig. 4.11 The three axes of the limb are specified by different interactions. The proximodistal axis is specified by the progress zone, the craniocaudal axis by the zone of polarising activity, and the dorsoventral axis by the ectoderm of the limb. The pattern of development within the limb and the ectodermal specialisations are controlled by the limb mesenchyme.

with that surrounding the ventral wall of the oesophagus, but with lengthening and division of the tracheal bud and deviation of the lung buds dorsally, each bud becomes surrounded by its own specific mesenchyme thus permitting regional differences between the lungs, i.e. the number of lobes, or the degree of growth and maturity of a particular lung. Each lung develops by a process of dichotomous branching as described in branching morphogenesis. *Tenascin*, an extracellular matrix molecule (also known as hexabrachion or cytotactin), is present in the budding and distal tip regions, but absent in the clefts. Conversely, fibronectin is found in the clefts and along the sides of the developing bronchi, but not on the budding and distal tips[9].

ENDODERM AND SPLANCHNOPLEURIC MESENCHYME INTERACTIONS IN THE GASTROINTESTINAL TRACT

LIVER

The liver is a very precocious embryonic organ, functioning as the main centre for haemopoiesis in the fetus. It develops from an endodermal evagination of the foregut and from the septum transversum mesenchyme, a region of unsplit lateral plate mesenchyme at the very rostral edge of the disc prior to head folding. The development of the liver is intimately related to the development of the heart as the vitelline, followed by the umbilical veins, are disrupted by the septum transversum to form a hepatic plexus the forerunner of the hepatic sinusoids.

Endodermal epithelial cells from the foregut proliferate and extend as lines of epithelial cells into the septum transversum mesenchyme. Contact of endodermal epithelium with the mesenchymal cells induces them to form blood islands and endothelium. The advance of the endodermal epithelial cells promotes the conversion of more and more septum transversum mesenchyme into endothelium and blood cells with only a little remaining to form the scanty (human) liver capsule and interlobular connective tissue.

The morphogenesis of the liver lobes are patterned by the septum transversum mesenchyme and both endoderm and septum transversum mesenchyme are required for normal liver development. If a mechanical barrier is inserted across the mesenchymal hepatic area just caudal to the endodermal outgrowth, liver tissue will develop normally cranial to the barrier where it is in contact with the endoderm. However, caudal to the barrier, the mesenchyme will form endothelial cells and hepatic lobes, but there will be no hepatocytes present.

Experiments in which either the epithelium or the mesenchyme is changed will not result in liver development, e.g. cephalic and somitic mesenchyme do not promote the differentiation of hepatic endoderm, and intestinal endoderm cells combined with hepatic mesenchyme will not differentiate into hepatocytes. However, all derivatives of the lateral plate mesenchyme, both somatopleuric and splanchnopleuric mesenchyme can promote the differentiation of hepatic endoderm, although not so strongly as hepatic mesenchyme, and lateral plate mesenchyme will form blood sinusoids under these conditions. It is inferred that matrix or cell surface properties are common throughout the lateral plate mesenchyme but are different from axial mesenchymal cells[10].

GASTRIC MUCOSA

Within the gastrointestinal tract, the local organisation of the mucosa and smooth muscle layers is under the control of the local splanchnopleuric mesenchyme. Recombination experiments of chick gut epithelium and mouse mesenchyme and vice versa show that the patterning of the intestinal villi will be determined by the underlying mesenchyme. However, the epithelial cells will produce enzymes associated with the relevant species, i.e. mouse epithelium will produce lactase and chick epithelium sucrase, regardless of the origin of the underlying mesenchyme[11].

INTRAEMBRYONIC MESODERM AND INTERMEDIATE MESENCHYME INTERACTIONS

The metanephric kidney develops from three sources, an evagination of the mesonephric duct, the *ureteric bud*, a local condensation of mesenchyme termed the *metanephric blastema*, and *angiogenic mesenchyme* which migrates into the metanephric blastema slightly later to produce the glomeruli and vasa recta[12–14]. It may also be the case that innervation is necessary for metanephric kidney induction.

During embryonic development, functional mesonephric kidneys develop but are remodelled in male embryos as parts of the reproductive tracts. The mesonephric kidneys develop on the posterior abdominal wall and extend ultimately from the pleural region to the lumbar, with both development and regression proceeding in a craniocaudal progression. However, in the metanephric kidney, a proportion of the mesenchyme remains as stem cells which continue to divide and enter the nephrogenic pathway later as individual collecting ducts lengthen. Thus the temporal development of the metanephric kidney is patterned radially with the outer cortex being the last part to be formed.

In each kidney a ureteric bud arises as a diverticulum from the mesonephric duct and grows dorsally to enter the metanephric mesenchymal population. The bud bifurcates when it comes into contact with the metanephric blastema as a result of local extracellular matrix molecule synthesis by the mesenchyme. Both chondroitin sulphate proteoglycan synthesis and chondroitin sulphate glycosaminoglycan processing are necessary for this and consequent branching of the ureteric bud[15]. Subsequent divisions of the ureteric bud and the mesenchyme form the gross structure of the kidney with *major* and *minor calyces*; the distal branches of the ureteric ducts will form the *collecting ducts* of the kidney. As the collecting ducts elongate, the metanephric mesenchyme condenses around them. The ureteric bud undergoes a further series of bifurcations within the surrounding metanephric mesenchyme, forming smaller *ureteric ducts*. The metanephric mesenchyme condenses around the dividing ducts into smaller condensations which then undergo a mesenchyme to epithelium transformation forming vesicles. To initiate this transformation, the cells cease production of mesenchymal matrix molecules and commence production of epithelial ones. This has been demonstrated in tissue culture.

Initially, syndecan can be detected between the mesenchymal cells in the condensate. The cells cease expression of the cadherin N-CAM, fibronectin and collagen I and commence production of the cadherin L-CAM (also called uvomorulin) and the basal laminal constituents laminin and collagen IV. The mesenchymal clusters thus convert to small groups of epithelial cells which undergo complex morphogenetic changes (Fig. 4.12). Each epithelial group elongates, forms a comma-shaped, then an S-shaped body, which elongates further. It then fuses to a branch of the ureteric duct at its distal end while expanding as a dilated sac at the proximal end. The sac involutes with local cellular differentiation such that the outer cells become the *parietal glomerular cells*, while the inner ones become *visceral epithelial podocytes*. The podocytes develop in close proximity to invading capillaries which derive from local angiogenic mesenchyme[16]; this third source of mesenchyme produces the endothelial and mesangial cells within the glomerulus. Both the metanephric-derived podocytes and the angiogenic mesenchyme produce fibronectin and other components of the glomerular basal lamina. The isoforms of type IV collagen within this layer follow a specific programme of maturation which occurs as the filtration of macromolecules from the plasma becomes restricted[17].

Interestingly, although the interactions in kidney development were usually focused on the induction of metanephric mesenchyme by the ureteric bud epithelium, it had been noted that when cultured across a filter the inductive stimulus was quite weak. In contrast, fragments of spinal cord were found to be very potent inducers of metanephric mesenchyme, initiating epithelialisation. This suggested that perhaps nerves arriving at the interaction site during development were of some importance. Indeed, it has been shown that blocking nerve growth factor receptor mRNA in the developing kidney, not only prevents receptor synthesis, but that nephrogenesis is also completely halted[18].

OTHER CELLS TYPES AFFECTING OR AFFECTED BY LOCAL INTERACTIONS

It seems that the basic epithelial–mesenchymal interaction may not be so basic or simple after all. Whereas initial observations were made on cultured embryos later studies were made on cultured embryonic explants which could be perturbed in some manner. The range of inductive tissues was ascertained, using other mesenchymes or epithelia from the same embryo, from different embryos of the same species and even from different species. Now it seems that the homogeneity of the mesenchymes under examination may have been assumed. The presence of angiogenic mesenchyme may be fundamental for some interactions. This mesenchyme is seen close to endodermal epithelia but not ectodermal. It is not clear whether angiogenic mesenchyme arises from endodermal populations inside the embryo. However, it is clear that it does arise extraembryonically from the parietal hypoblast. Embryonic angioblasts are highly invasive, moving in every direction throughout embryonic mesenchymal tissue. It may be that these cells make a contribution to the interactive processes, especially in those organs where close proximity of endothelia to specialised cells is a feature.

Similarly, the innervation of blood vessels, glandular cells and myoepthelial cells may need to be achieved early in development, at the time of the early interactions. Indeed, the condition Hirschsprung's disease which results in a failure of neural crest cells to colonise the gut appropriately and form local constituents of the enteric nervous system, is thought to occur because of disordered basal laminal molecules. The enteric nervous system arises from neural crest cells at somite levels 1–7 and from 28 onwards. Normally the crest cells invade the splanchnopleuric mesenchyme around the endoderm and site themselves in the putative submucosal and myogenic layers. The splanchnopleuric mesenchyme will develop into both the lamina propria connective tissue lineages and the smooth muscle cells of the muscularis mucosa and the muscularis propria. Hirschsprung's disease is characterised by a dilated segment of colon proximally and lack of peristalsis in the segment distal to the dilation. Infants with this condition show delay in the passage of meconium, constipation; vomiting and abdominal distension. A mouse model has been investigated which demonstrates the same pathology and symptoms[19]. In the normal mouse laminin and type IV collagen are found beneath the mucosal and serosal epithelia and around the blood vessels. In the mutant mouse there is a broad zone of these basal laminal proteins around the entire outer gut mesenchyme with increase in the amount of laminin, type IV collagen and heparan sulphate, specifically in the aganglionic portion of bowel. It is suggested that the overabundance of basal laminal components prevents the neural crest cells from penetrating the gut wall; their new position outside the gut does not confer on them the environmental stimuli for enteric nerve differentiation. Consequently, these crest cells differentiate into autonomic ganglia and nerves similar to the parasympathetic nerves which normally modulate enteric nervous system activity. This system demonstrates the importance of local mesenchymal and extracellular matrix activity for the normal induction of neurons as well as epithelial cells.

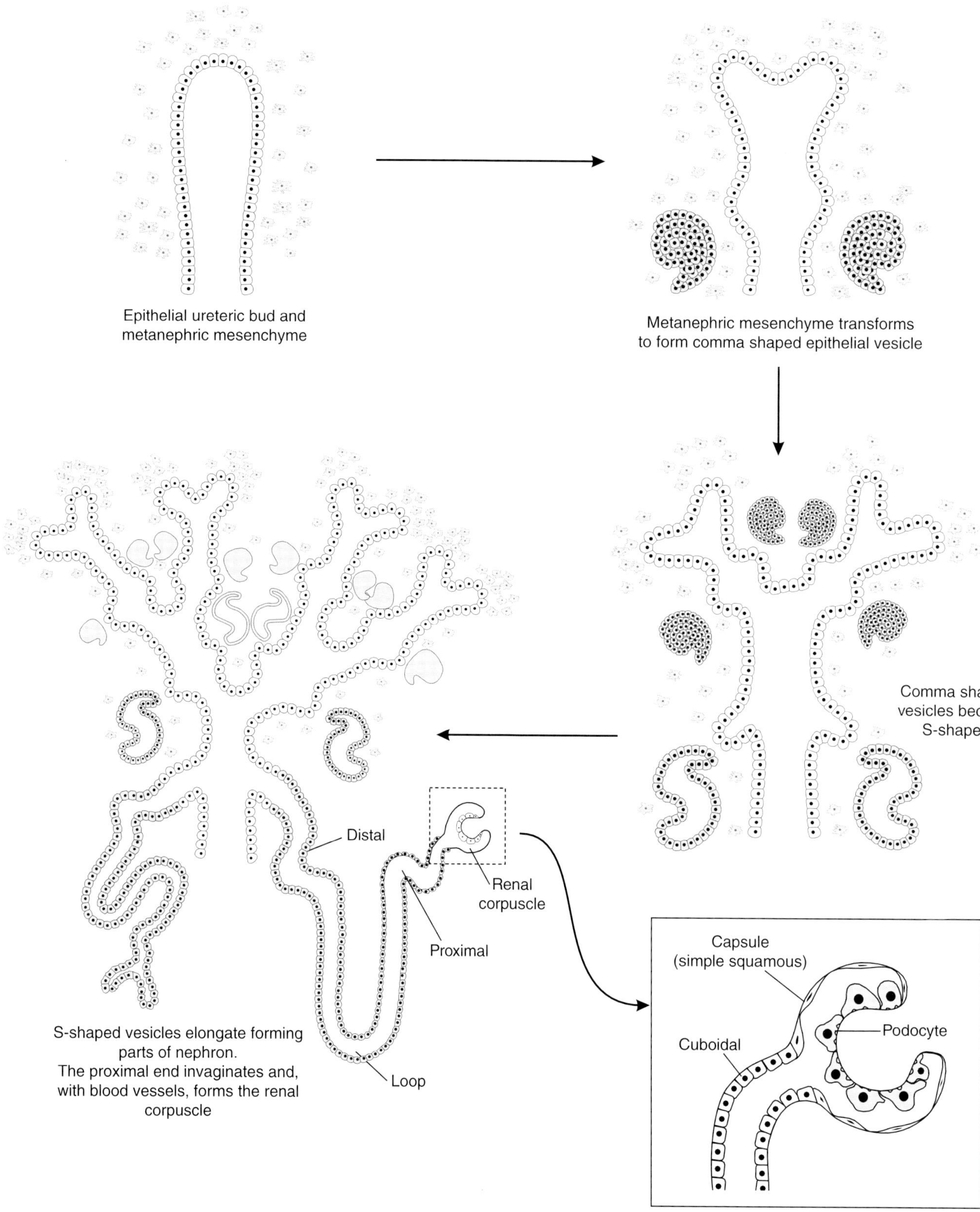

Fig. 4.12 In the developing kidney there is a mesenchyme-to-epithelial transformation. The epithelial ureteric bud forms the collecting ducts in the kidney. It induces the metanephric mesenchyme to transform into local epithelial vesicles which develop into the nephrons.

REFERENCES

1. Markwald RR, Mjaatvedt CH, Krug EL, Sinning AR Interactions in heart development. Role of cardiac edherons in cushion tissue formation. *Ann NY Acad Sci* **588**:13–25, 1990.
2. Hall BK. *Evolutionary Developmental Biology*. London: Chapman and Hall, 1992.
3. Wessells NK. *Tissue Interactions and Development*. Menlo Park, CA: Benjamin/Cummings, 1977.
4. Thorogood P. The developmental specification of the vertebrate skull. *Development* **103** (Suppl.) 141–153, 1988.
5. Lumsden AGS. Neural crest contribution to tooth development in the mammalian embryo. In *Developmental and Evolutionary Aspects of the Neural Crest* (ed. P.F.A. Maderson) pp. 261–300, New York: Wiley, 1987.
6. Kollar EJ, Mina M. Role of the early epithelium in the patterning of the teeth and Meckel's cartilage. *J Craniofac Genet Dev Biol* **11**:223–228, 1991.
7. Kollar EJ, Fisher C. Tooth induction in chick epithelium: expression of quiescent genes for enamel synthesis. *Science* **207**:993–995, 1980.
8. Hilfer SR, Rayner RM, Brown JW. Mesenchymal control of branching pattern in the fetal mouse lung. *Tissue Cell* **127**:523–538, 1985.
9. Abbott LA, Lester SM, Erickson CA. Changes in mesenchymal cell-shape, matrix collagen and tenascin accompany bud formation in the early chick embryo. *Anat Embryol* **183**:299–311, 1992.
10. Le Douarin N. An experimental analysis of liver development. *Med Biol* **53**:427–455, 1975.
11. Haffen K, Kedinger M, Simon-Assmann P. Cell contact dependent regulation of enterocyte differentiation. In *Human Gastrointestinal Development* (ed. E. Lebenthal). New York: Raven Press, 1989.
12. Grobstein C. Inductive interaction in the development of the mouse metanephros. *J Exp Zool* **130**:319–340, 1955.
13. Saxen L, Koskimies O, Lahti A, Miettinen H, Rapola J, Wartiovarra J. Differentiation of kidney mesenchyme in an experimental model system. *J Adv Morphogen* **7**:251–293, 1968.
14. Saxen L. Failure to demonstrate tubule induction in a heterologous mesenchyme. *Dev Biol* **23**:511–523, 1970.
15. Fouser L, Avner ED. Normal and abnormal nephrogenesis. *Am J Kidney Dis* **21**:64–70, 1993.
16. Ekblom P, Sariola H, Karkinen-Jaaskelainen M, Saxen L. The origin of the glomerular endothelium. *Cell Differentiation* **11**:35–39, 1982.
17. Bard JBL, Woolf AS. Nephrogenesis and the development of renal disease. *Neurol Dial Transplant* **7**:563–572, 1992.
18. Sariola H, Saarma M, Sainio K., *et al.* Dependence of kidney morphogenesis on the expression of nerve growth factor receptor. *Science* **254**:571–573, 1991.
19. Gershon MD. Phenotypic expression by neural crest-derived precursors of enteric neurons and glia. In *Developmental and Evolutionary Aspects of the Neural Crest* (ed. P.F.A Maderson) New York: John Wiley, 1987.

Cellular mechanisms in development

5

P. Collins

Introduction

The earliest cells of the embryo are described as 'totipotent' indicating that they have the capacity to differentiate into any cell type in the body. The pathways cells take to differentiation depend on the regulation of the genes within the cell and the interaction of the cell with its environment and neighbours. Information from these other sources will cause shifts in the differentiative fate of the cell's progeny.

All embryonic cell populations are initially receptive to inductive signals. They respond by becoming '*committed*' to a particular pathway of development which thus restricts their ability to respond to further inductive influences, i.e. they become '*restricted*'. After a series of restrictions cells are said to become '*determined*'. Determined cells are programmed to complete a process of development which will lead to differentiation. The determined state is a heritable characteristic of cells and can be passed on to progeny, it is stable and not dependent on environmental factors; the differentiated state is usually not heritable, it is often dependent on environmental conditions and it may prevent further cell division.

The state of determination or differentiation may be assessed by studying cells in culture. For example, melanocytes display the black pigment melanin. If melanocytes are cultured without the tyrosine needed to synthesize melanin, the cells will become pale and no longer appear differentiated. When the tyrosine is replaced into the culture medium, the cells will once more synthesize melanin and return to their differentiated state, illustrating that they maintained their determination despite not being able to display their differentiation. Similar cultures of cells taken from embryos at different stages of development will reveal which types of protein the cells are capable of synthesizing and thus their level of determination or differentiation. Cell proteins have been classified as 'basic', or 'housekeeping proteins', if they are considered essential for cellular metabolism, and are termed 'primary', as are the genes which regulate them. As cells become determined, they synthesize proteins appropriate to their cell group, e.g. liver and kidney cells, but not myocytes, produce arginase; this class of protein is termed 'secondary'. Finally, at the most differentiated state cells produce 'tertiary' proteins (also called 'luxury proteins') specific to their needs, e.g. haemoglobin in erythrocytes. This range of proteins, primary, secondary and tertiary are an expression of stages of determination and differentiation and are coded by a range of genes.

PROLIFERATIVE AND QUANTAL MITOSES

Within a mesenchymal population, cell divisions will both increase the total numbers of cells but also provide the foci for changes in determination. In normal cell division, sometimes described as proliferative, transient amplifying, or multiplicative mitoses, progeny similar to the parents are produced. In some situations, e.g. as a response to a local inductive influence, the cells will enter a *quantal cell cycle* where the outcome is a *quantal mitosis* which increases the restriction of their progeny. The progeny then continue in amplifying mitoses at the progressive level of determination. It is at these quantal mitoses that binary choices are made in the embryo.

STEM CELLS AND PROGENITOR CELLS

Within a proliferating cell population, instead of a division producing two progeny with increased determination, the mitosis may produce one determined progeny and another cell with the same state of determination as the parent. This latter cell can reproduce again passing on an increased state of determination to only one offspring. This type of division has been termed 'asymmetric' in contrast to the 'symmetrical' proliferating mitoses. Stem cells are seen in development and in adult life, for example in the bone marrow or in the gut epithelium.

Progenitor cells are those which are already determined to some extent. They may individually follow their differentiation pathway or may proliferate producing more similarly determined progenitor cells. In this case, no stem cell can be identified; all cells seem capable of either differentiation of continued mitosis. An example would be populations of migrating myoblasts in the embryonic limb bud.

TERMINAL DIFFERENTIATION

The differentiative fates of cells within embryos may be to become long-living lymphoblasts or neuroblasts, but may just as well be to undergo programmed cell death, also called 'apoptosis'. Apoptosis is a mechanism whereby cells bequeath their organelles to neighbouring cells without releasing any cellular fragments which might stimulate an inflammatory response. Apoptosis occurs in the adult state as well as in embryos. In organogenesis, apoptosis allows for some slack in the system. More cells than may be needed are produced by amplifying mitosis, later the cells are supported by the local extracellular matrix or by innervation or blood supply. Those cells which are in excess and cannot be supported by these means will undergo apoptosis. This proposition has been supported by study of the nematode *Caenorhabditis elegans* which suggests that a cell death programme is normally 'on' in all cells, and that cell death is prevented by an overriding 'survival' programme (reviewed by Raff[1]). As different tissues might be expected to produce different sets of survival factors, a cell in an abnormal location deprived of its specific signals required for survival would die.

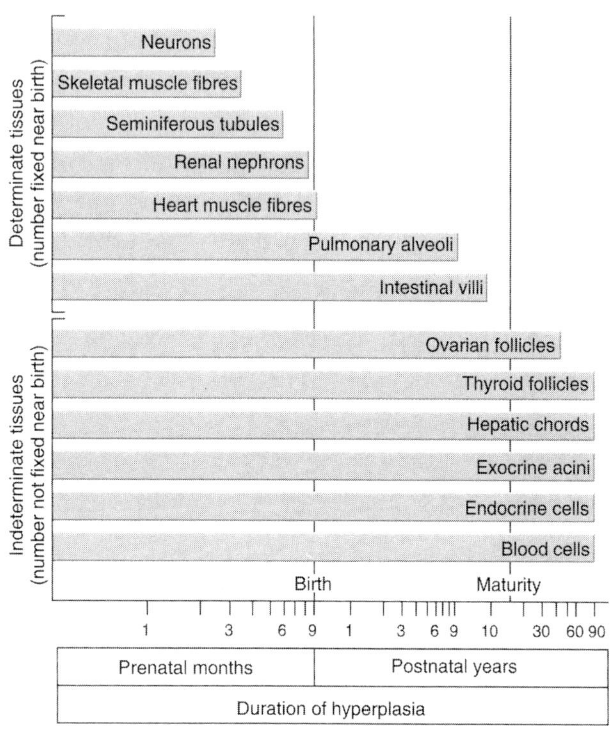

Fig. 5.1 The duration of multiplicative growth for various human tissues (After Gilbert SF. *Developmental Biology*, Sinauer Associates, MA, 1992).

The times at which cells cease proliferative mitoses and become differentiated is different for different tissues (Fig. 5.1). Although some tissues will all enter determined pathways and differentiation before birth, other cells retain the ability to divide, e.g. as stem cells, or if environmental conditions changes, as in a wound, are able to revert temporarily to the determined state, affect a repair and then differentiate once again.

Regulation of growth in development

The effects of regulation are well established but the mechanisms underlying such regulation are not yet understood. There is a strong underlying presumption that the embryo, by some mechanism, has an indication of its own size and how big it should be for a particular developmental stage. Homeostatic mechanisms are deployed in order to seek and maintain this 'target size' in embryos where naturally occurring or experimental perturbations cause it to depart from the normal growth curve.

It is observed that embryos are usually of a similar size and that division of a single embryo into two, as in twinning, or fusion of two or more embryos into a giant embryo will both result in normal development. Thus the embryo as a whole is able to regulate its size and its overall cell number and this regulation extends into fetal life and infancy.

The processes involved here have not yet been elucidated, however, in development two ends of a spectrum of control seem to be in operation. In twins, embryos are formed which are approximately half the normal size. The proportions within each are normal and by the second trimester of pregnancy each is comparable to a singleton fetus[2]. Thus each embryo and fetus undergoes a higher than normal growth rate to attain this size. In the fusion experiments, aggregates of 16 eight-cell stage mouse embryos will result in normal-sized chimeric fetuses which will develop to term. Here, downward regulation in size occurs shortly after implantation, between the appearance of the amniotic cavity and the primitive streak. It seems to involve a lengthening of the cell cycle during the period[2] and thus is a slower than normal growth rate. In both examples, twinning and embryo fusion, the regulation of size occurs before the onset of organogenesis and it may be that at this stage evaluation of the status of the embryo is made before organogenesis proceeds.

Local perturbations of embryonic tissue, where a region or regions are removed will result in compensatory catch-up growth without disturbing the pattern or the proportions of the fully formed embryo. However, later disruptions of portions of embryo may deplete specific cell populations and result in abnormalities either at the site of deletion, or more often at locations different from the site of the primary insult[2,3]. This implies that the depleted cell population would migrate but be unable to undergo sufficient multiplicative growth to form structures in its final location.

Embryonic regulation seems not to be the same as regeneration in adult or fetal tissues[4]. Regeneration involves the reestablishment of regional differences in the newly formed replacement parts, while regulation involves the reestablishment of a fate map on a partial domain of uncommitted tissue[4]. Regeneration occurs in many lower organisms, e.g. the replacement of a whole severed limb or tail, or appropriate part in adult amphibia, and in regeneration of liver after resection in humans. In general, regeneration follows one of two main types, '*morphallaxis*', in which the whole reforms by rearrangement and differentiation of the existing tissues without further growth, and '*epimorphosis*' in which there is new growth of blastemal tissue, which subsequently matures into the full regenerate. Regeneration involves similar positional signalling cues to normal development, and may share some similar morphogens, e.g. retinoic acid and its receptors. An interesting form of embryonic response, which is midway between embryonic regulation and regeneration is the phenomenon of scar-free dermal embryonic wound healing[5,6].

GENOMIC REGULATION OF SIZE

Growth beyond that instructed by the genome is only possible if the genome itself has been altered. In a series of experiments to illustrated the specific effects of growth hormone, the gene for rat growth hormone was isolated and combined with a mouse gene which regulates serum zinc levels as a promoter. The combined gene was introduced into mouse pronuclei shortly before fertilization. This resulted in transgenic mice with both genes within their chromosomes. Postnatally some of the transgenic mice were fed a diet which included zinc supplement. This switched on the rat growth hormone gene inducing synthesis of rat growth hormone from the liver. The transgenic mice became up to 80% larger than their litter mates, with all of their organs in proportion[7].

MATERNAL REGULATION OF SIZE

The above experiments show that the species-specific genome is regulating the size of the embryo and fetus and that different species, and therefore genes, will set growth to different levels. A further complexity on growth *in utero*, however, is that fetal growth and ultimate birth weight is affected by the maternal environment. The rate of growth of fetuses slows from about 36 to 40 weeks due to the limiting influence of the maternal uterus. This effect was demonstrated many years ago by the crossing of large Shire horses with Shetland ponies. A Shire mare crossed with a Shetland delivered a foal of similar size to a pure-bred Shire foal, and a Shetland mare crossed with a Shire delivered a foal only a third as large, similar in size to a Shetland foal[8]. Both cross breed of foal attained sizes much larger than pure Shetlands but smaller than pure-bred Shires.

Growth is therefore regulated by many factors at different stages of development: intrinsic regulatory genes in early development, maternal influences nearer term and the species specificity of growth hormones in infancy.

The cell cycle

Determination, differentiation and development, in general, all result from a series of interactions in which information from one cell is presented to another and as a consequence the behaviour of one or both cells is changed. Earlier embryonic studies described the changes in shape which were seen in development and then how these might be modified by experimentation. In these cases, cell populations and morphogenetic movements were observed. Recently, the cues which cause such changes and movements have been investigated as molecular biology has allowed identification of proteins within the cell, the mRNA which indicates the synthesis of such proteins, and latterly isolation and synthesis of individual genes. Through such studies, some of the drivers and checks of development can be studied.

An increase in cell restriction begins with a quantal cell division, thus the mechanisms of mitosis need to be examined. Cells which are undergoing amplifying mitoses pass through a cell cycle which lasts for 12 hours or more. The cell cycle is traditionally divided into four phases, of which the most dramatic is mitosis and cell division (Fig. 5.2). The phases of the cell cycle are noted by the letters M for mitosis and G_1, S and G_2 for the interphase. During mitosis, the cell packs up most of its organelles, the centrioles duplicate and move to each end of the cell and begin synthesis of microtubules which are arranged as the mitotic spindle, and the chromatin in the nucleus condenses into the chromosomes.

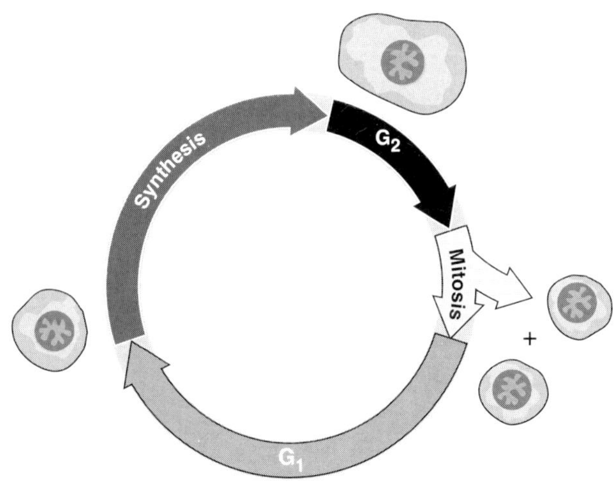

Fig. 5.2 The four stages of the cell cycle. After cell division (mitosis) the cell grows continuously until the next mitosis. The phases G_1, G_2 and S are parts of interphase. (If the cell is not dividing it enters G_0.)

As the cell has already replicated its DNA, the chromosomes which become visible at metaphase are duplicated but held together at the centromere. The nuclear membrane breaks down, the chromosomes gather at the equator of the cell and are drawn apart towards the poles of the spindle, where they decondense and re-form intact nuclei. The cell cytoplasm divides by cytokinesis, an event which is viewed as the end of the M phase.

G_1 is the time period during which the cell grows until it is large enough to begin DNA synthesis. It may move along to S phase (synthesis) once it has reached an appropriate size and if the environmental conditions are favourable. If the cell is not yet committed to DNA replication, or is going to follow a differentiation pathway, the cell can step out of the cycle into G_0 for days, weeks or longer before resuming proliferation. The majority of cells in the adult are in G_0. The S phase marks replication of the nuclear DNA and is followed by G_2 which is the time taken for further growth. At the end of G_2 the cell must be of sufficient size, have replicated all its DNA, and be in a suitable environment before it can continue into mitosis. Signals from the cells or from the environment can prevent the cell moving from one phase to another.

The cycle itself is driven by complexes of cyclins, so called because they undergo synthesis and degradation in each division cycle of the cell. The cyclins bind to cyclin-dependent protein kinases (Cdk) to trigger mitosis and to trigger DNA replication. They thus provide a checkpoint for exit from G_1 and entry into S phase and exit from G_2 and entry into M phase.

In early embryonic cell divisions the zygote and blastomeres are very large. Growth is not required at this time and the cleavage divisions operate to restore the nuclear to cytoplasm ratio producing cells of typical size. Under these conditions, cells pass through M phase and S phase in quick succession. After each division, the cell progeny are half the size of the parent. Later, the cycle lengthens and various control systems come into operation. It is important that the rate of passage through the S phase allows completion of DNA replication. Should a cell enter M phase before replication is complete, it will die. The cell cycle control system receives a feedback signal from incompletely replicated DNA which will prevent movement to the G_2 phase. Similar protective mechanisms ensure that DNA is only replicated once during S phase.

Cytokines and growth factors

As a result of experiments to find the most appropriate media for maintaining the proliferation of cells in culture, two families of 'factors' were identified, arising initially from lymphocytes and from platelets. Culture of lymphocytes and macrophages revealed a family of factors within the supernatant which was able to facilitate cell–cell communication and proliferation. These soluble factors were isolated and collectively termed *cytokines*. The cytokines include: 10 subtypes of *interleukin (IL)* which cause in the main T and B cell proliferation; three types of *interferon (IFN)* which are mainly anti viral in nature; *tumour necrosis factor (TNF)* α and β which are cytotoxic; *transforming growth factor β (TGFβ)* which inhibits T- and B-cell proliferation; and *granulocyte-macrophage colony-stimulating factor (GM-CSF)* with factors for granulocytes and macrophages individually, which promote growth. The proliferative actions of cytokines are mediated by specific cell receptors on the surface of target cells.

Culture of mammalian cells was found to be more successful with blood serum added to the medium rather than plasma. Serum is the fluid which remains after blood has clotted whereas plasma is obtained by removing the cells without permitting clotting to occur. The difference between these two fluids was the presence of factors released from platelets as the blood clotted. Experiment showed that an extract of platelets alone added to the medium would support cell-culture proliferation, and the extract was termed a *growth factor*. The particular growth factor from the platelets was shown to be a protein and named *platelet-derived growth factor* or *PDGF*. For PDGF to have an effect on a target cell, the cell must display an appropriate receptor protein on its surface as in the action of cytokines. Receptor proteins for cytokines and growth factors are part of the cell glycocalyx along with *inter alia* cell adhesion molecules and integrins (see pp. 23 and 27).

Large families of growth factors have now been identified, not all of them proteins; steroid hormones which act on intracellular receptor protein are an example. Growth factors have been divided into broad- and narrow-specificity classes or families. PDGF is a broad-specificity factor as is *epidermal growth factor (EGF)*. PDGF acts on fibroblasts, smooth-muscle cells and neuroglial cells, while EGF acts on epidermal cells and on many embryonic epithelia. Other broad-specificity growth factors are: the *insulin-like growth factors (IGFI, IGFII)* (previously termed 'somatomedins'), stimulating cell metabolism and with other growth factors stimulating cell proliferation; *fibroblast growth factor (FGF)* with subgroups, again being inductive in embryos; and *transforming growth factor β (TGFβ)* having been identified in lymphocytes and also grouped as a cytokine, yet being produced widely by many cell types. The TGFβ family also includes activins and bone morphogenetic proteins (BMPs), which similar to TGFβ, may suppress growth as well as stimulate it.

Of the narrow-specificity factors, *nerve growth factor (NGF)* and related *brain-derived neurotrophic factor (BDNF)*, and neurotrophins 3 and 4 promote survival of neurons; *erythropoietin* promotes proliferation and differentiation of erythrocytes; and *interleukin-3 (IL-3)* and related *haemopoietic colony-stimulating factors (CSFs)*, which are also classed as cytokines, stimulate proliferation of blood cell precursors.

Cytokines and growth factors can signal a wide variety of cellular effects as indicated above, including stimulation or inhibition of growth, differentiation, migration etc.[9] Because each family is so large, and because there are a similarly extensive number of receptors, the possible signalling combinations are considerable. Often, a single growth factor can bind with varying affinities to individual receptor family members. Some of these receptors are monogamous, recognising only one isoform of the growth factor, whereas others are polygamous, recognising all isoforms. The effects of any individual growth factor may therefore depend on which receptor isoform, or ratio of isoform receptors, are displayed on the cell surface. It is now clear that developmental information resides, not in any single molecule, but rather in the combination of molecules, to which a cell is exposed. Thus, varying combinations of growth factors, in varying concentrations can elicit quite different effects on similar cells[10].

Growth factors and cytokines can be delivered to and act upon cells in a variety of fashions: by contact between epithelial and mesenchyme cells either directly or via matrix molecules, and within mesenchymal populations by endocrine, autocrine, paracrine, intracrine, juxtacrine and matricrine methods (Figs 5.3 and 5.4). When released many growth factors are in a latent form, e.g. associated with a propeptide (latency-associated peptide) in the case of TGFβ[11,12] or attached to a binding protein, in the case of insulin-like growth factors. Activity of the growth factor is dependent on dissociation from the binding protein or the latency-associated protein. Such activation mechanisms may involve specific proteases and/or conformational changes in the latency-associated complex, by binding, for example, to a different receptor (in the case of TGFβ, binding of mannose-6-phosphate residues on the latency-associated peptide, to the mannose-6-phosphate/IGFII receptor).[12]

The specific activity of various growth factors may also equally depend on stabilisation of the growth factor at the receptor by an accessory molecule. A good example of this is the delivery and stabilisation of the activity of FGF2 by heparin sulphate proteoglycan[13]. Such complexity in the signalling system means that for most developing organs, there is at present only a rudimentary knowledge of the specifics of which combinations of signals give rise to which kinds of differentiation.

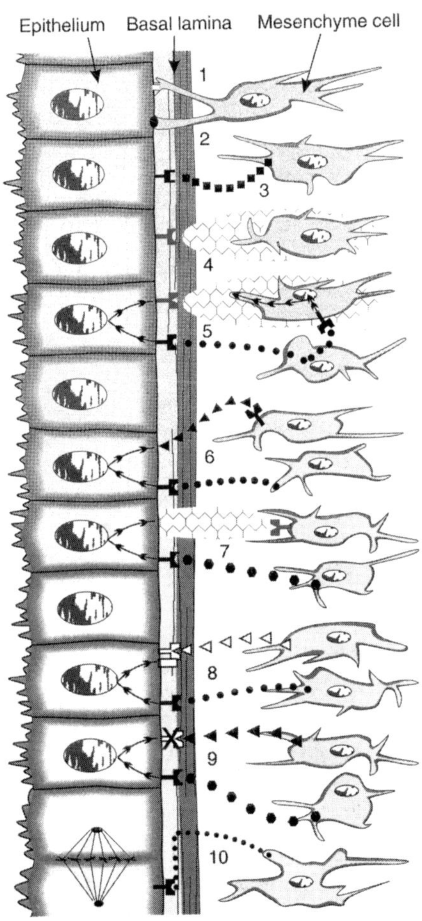

1 Direct cell-cell contact by gap junctions.

2 Cell-cell contact by cell adhesion molecules.

3 A soluble factor (growth factor) reacting with a receptor for that factor on the epithelial cells.

4 Extracellular matrix molecule secreted by the mesenchyme cells interacting with a receptor on the epithelial cell.

5 A soluble factor (growth factor) secreted by a mesenchymal cell having a biphasic action interacting (i) with a receptor on an epithelial cell, causing it to express a specific extracellular matrix molecule receptor; (ii) with a receptor on a mesenchyme cell, causing it to secrete a specific extracellular matrix molecule which then interacts with the induced epithelial receptor.

6 A soluble factor (growth factor) secreted by a mesenchyme cell interacting with a receptor on an epithelial cell causing it to express a receptor, or secrete a factor, which interacts with another factor synthesized, or receptor expressed, by another mesenchyme cell.

7 A soluble factor secreted by a mesenchyme cell interacting with a receptor on an epithelial cell causing it to synthesize an extracellular matrix molecule (or a receptor for such a molecule) which then interacts with a specific receptor for that molecule on another mesenchyme cell.

8 A soluble factor secreted from a mesenchyme cell interacting with a receptor on an epithelial cell causing it to synthesize a molecule which stabilises or enhances the interaction between a mesenchymal derived factor and its epithelial receptor.

9 A soluble factor secreted by a mesenchyme cell interacting with a receptor on an epithelial cell causing the inhibition of synthesis/assembly of a factor or receptor.

10 A soluble factor secreted by a mesenchyme cell binding to the extracellular matrix of the basal lamina where it remains active and subsequently interacts with a receptor on an epithelial cell which appears at a later developmental time.

Fig. 5.3 The many ways by which mesenchyme cells can signal to epithelial cells. Precisely the same mechanisms can operate in reverse, i.e. epithelium to mesenchyme. (From Gray's Anatomy, 38th edition, Edinburgh: Churchill Livingstone, 1995, p. 112.)

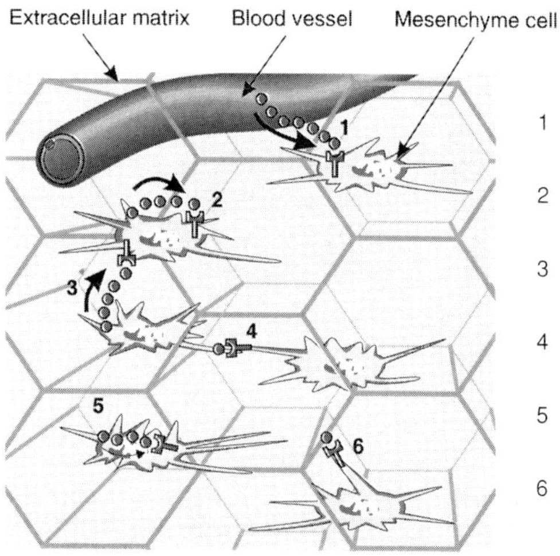

1 **Endocrine** Delivery of growth factor by the bloodstream from a distant biosynthetic site to the target mesenchyme cell.

2 **Autocrine** Synthesis of growth factor by the cell, its secretion, binding and activation of a surface receptor elsewhere on its own surface.

3 **Paracrine** Synthesis of growth factor by the cell, its secretion and diffusion to an adjacent cell (or group of cells) where it binds to and activates a cell surface receptor.

4 **Juxtacrine** Synthesis of growth factor by the cell. The growth factor remains on the cell surface and binds to and activates a receptor on an immediately adjacent cell.

5 **Intracrine** Synthesis of growth factor within the cytoplasm of the cell. The growth factor moves to the nucleus and binds and activates its own nuclear receptors.

6 **Matricrine** Synthesis and export of growth factor from the cell. The growth factor binds to the extracellular matrix where it remains active and subsequently binds to and activates a receptor for that growth factor on the same or a different cell.

Fig. 5.4 Cells can also communicate by the reception, production and growth factors. A typical embryonic mesenchyme cell could produce growth factors in this way. (From Gray's Anatomy, 38th edition, Edinburgh: Churchill Livingstone, 1995, p. 113.)

Most growth factors and cytokines exert their action by binding to cell-surface receptors: However, it is now known that some signalling molecules can pass through the target-cell plasma membrane and once inside the cell, directly regulate the activity of intracellular proteins. A particularly local phenomenon is seen with the gas nitric oxide (NO). NO is made by the enzyme nitric oxide synthase within a cell and diffuses out of the cell where it is produced and passes directly into neighbouring cells. The local action of NO is ensured by its short half-life of about 5–10 seconds. The effect of NO is seen in relaxation of the tunica media of blood vessels. Signals from sympathetic nerves cause acetylcholine release; this in turn induces the endothelial cells to synthesize NO which then signals the smooth-muscle cells to relax.

GROWTH FACTORS AND CYTOKINES IN ACTION

Whereas in previous years, experiments focused on recombinant studies and interactions, interest is now directed at finding expression of various genes, transcription factors, cytokines and growth factors within the embryo at different stages. Responses to deletion of specific gene action, or application of cytokines and growth factors at inappropriate times and places in the embryo are also being studied. Because interactions now seem to be driven by complex cascades of many growth factors, each study can only add a small piece to the jigsaw. As yet, there are too few pieces in place to see what the picture is going to look like.

The factors which are driving development, i.e. genes and their proteins, have been identified in a wide range of developing organisms. Mammalian growth factors or related molecules have now been demonstrated in birds, fish, amphibians and the fruit fly *Drosophila*, indicating conservation of developmental genes and processes throughout evolution. For example, transforming growth factor β is one of the largest families with at least 24 members. TGFβ-related genes have been identified in *Drosophila*, and bone morphogenetic protein-4 has been found in *Xenopus* and mouse. Much research is now directed at elucidating the effects of gene knockout, or application of growth factors in a range of embryos to see if the coping mechanisms are similar in these species. Should this be the case, it may suggest great conservation of developmental processes during evolution.

A range of such interactions from a number of developing systems will be presented to give the flavour of the research now underway to elucidate the mechanisms of development.

Members of the FGF family and TGFβ family (principally activins) are involved in signalling mesoblast induction[10], e.g. isolated amphibian blastocoel roofs (animals caps) treated with activin form dorsomedial mesoderm structures whereas treatment with FGF results in ventral components; activin alone (in the absence of hypoblast) will induce primitive streak formation in the chick epiblast. Palatal differentiation into nasal pseudostratified ciliated columnar cells, oral stratified squamous cells, or medial edge epithelial cell adhesion and migration by the underlying mesenchyme appears to be signalled by a variety of growth factors, e.g. transforming growth factor-α[14–17].

The diverse range of growth factors and their receptors, and their importance in developmental processes has been discussed by Ferguson[18]. He argues that the numerous growth factors and their receptors interact to give a smooth temporal integration of developmental events. Thus one growth factor may alter the synthesis of another growth factor, or its receptor[17]. If the signalling systems are both hierarchical and functionally redundant, with each developmental event having a window of operational viability that may be achieved by a principal mechanism with a number of parallel backup mechanisms, then, if there were a disturbance in any one system, its effects would be minimised by a parallel backup system. Thus whilst one main mechanism for developmental processes might be sought, this may not necessarily be the way that evolution has optimised embryonic development. Survival of the embryo may be considered the driving force behind evolution, with generation of phenotypic variation also an important phylogenetic force. Ferguson[18] suggests that both of these may be achieved by utilising developmental mechanisms which are quite slack, with appropriate backups, or self-balancing programmes, which ensure smooth development of the embryo, its survival and the generation of variation.

GROWTH FACTORS IN THE CARDIOVASCULAR SYSTEM

In the early embryo, the embryonic aortic arches III, IV and VI are formed from angiogenic mesenchyme. These vessels display smooth muscle in the tunica media fairly early on, which may be derived from local splanchnopleuric mesenchyme. Later, these arches become surrounded by early and late populations of neural crest mesenchyme which invade the tunica media. The later population differentiates into an elastogenic phenotype in a downstream progression around the vessels, from the truncus arteriosus to the aortic arch arteries until all of them are elastogenic. At the same time the original smooth-muscle cells disappear along the great vessels to their first branch point[19]. The mediae of those vessels which do not receive a contribution from the neural crest, e.g. the intrapulmonary arteries or the subclavian arteries, continue to accumulate layers of smooth muscle derived from the original surrounding mesenchyme. Ablation of the cardiac neural crest leads to changes in the embryonic aortic arch vessels, they may be absent, too large, too small, or aberrant in their connections and there is loss of bilateral symmetry. There is a significant decrease in the quantity of mesenchyme around these vessels resulting in direct apposition of endothelium and pharyngeal endodermal epithelium[20]. Those vessels not receiving neural crest cells, i.e. the ductus arteriosus (VIth aortic arch artery) and the pulmonary arteries have a muscular tunica media and not an elastic media as the other arch arteries.

It has been recently suggested that retinoic acid (RA) may play a role in inducing and maintaining smooth-muscle differentiation in the developing ductus arteriosus. Transgenic mice which will express β-galactoside (β-Gal) in response to endogenous RA signals during development were studied. β-Gal was observed in the ductus arteriosus throughout fetal development, persisting in the neonate until the ductus is closed. Although this expression was very intense in the ductus arteriosus, it was absent or minimal in the pulmonary trunk and aortic arch. By 17.5 days of development, β-Gal was expressed in the tunia media. Immunostaining of adult smooth-muscle myosin showed that, while SM1 is expressed in all embryonic vessels, SM2 is precociously expressed in the ductus as early as 15.5 days and its expression continues into the neonatal period colocalized with β-Gal[21].

REFERENCES

1. Raff RA. Evolution of development decisions and morphogenesis: the view from two camps. *Development* (Supplement), 15–22, 1992.
2. Snow MML. Environmental influences on fetal growth: effects and consequences. In *Fetal Growth* (eds F. Sharp, R.B. Fraser & R.D.G. Milner), pp. 115–125. London: Royal College of Obstetricians & Gynaecologists Press, 1989.
3. McKee GJ, Ferguson MWJ. The effects of mesencephalic neural crest cell extirpation on the development of chick embryos. *J Anat* **139**:491–512, 1984.
4. Slack JMW. *From Egg to Embryo*, 2nd edn. Cambridge: Cambridge University Press, 1991.
5. Whitby DJ, Ferguson MWJ. The extracellular matrix of lip wounds in fetal, neonatal and adult mice. *Development* **112**:651–668, 1991.
6. Whitby DJ, Ferguson MWJ. Immunohistochemical localisation of growth factors in fetal wound healing. *Develop Biol* **147**:207–215, 1991.
7. Palmiter RD, Brinster RL, Hann RE, Trumbauer ME, Rosenfeld MG, Brinberg NC, Evan RM. Dramatic growth of mice that develop from eggs microinjected with metallothionein growth hormone fusion genes. *Nature* **300**:611–615, 1982.
8. Walton A, Hammond J. The maternal effects of growth and information in Shire horse–Shetland pony crosses. *Proc R Soc London Ser B Biol Sci* **125**:311–335, 1938.
9. Sporn MB, Roberts AS. *Peptide Growth Factors and their Receptors*, Vols 1 and 2. Berlin: Springer-Verlag, 1990.
10. Jessell TM, Melton DA. Diffusable factors in vertebrate embryonic induction. *Cell* **68**:257–270, 1992.
11. Miyazono K, Ichijo M, Heldin CH. Transforming growth factor β latent forms, binding proteins and receptors. *Growth Factors* **8**:11–22, 1993.
12. Taipale J, Miyazono K, Heldin CN, Keski-Oja J. Latent transforming growth factor β_1 associates to fibrillant extracellular matrix and TGFβ binding proteins. *J Cell Biol* **124**:171–181, 1994.
13. Walker A, Turnbull JE, Gallagher JT. Specific heparan sulphate saccharides mediate the activity of basic fibroblast growth factor. *J Biol Chem* **269**:931–935, 1994.
14. Dixon MJ, Garner J, Ferguson MWJ. Immunolocalisation of EGF, EGF receptor and TGFα during murine palatogenesis *in vivo* and *in vitro*. *Anat Embryol* **184**:83–91, 1991.
15. Brunet CL, Sharpe PM, Ferguson MWJ. Inhibition of $TGF\beta_3$ (but not $TGF\beta_1$, or $TGF\beta_2$) activity prevents normal mouse embryonic palate fusion. *Int J Devel Biol* **39**:345–355, 1995.
16. Ferguson MWJ, Sharpe PM, Thomas BL, Beck F. Differential expression of insulin like growth factors I and II mRNA, peptide and binding protein, during mouse palate development comparison with TGFβ peptide distribution. *J Anat* **181**:219–238, 1992.
17. Sharpe PM, Foreman DM, Brunet CL, Ferguson MWJ. Localisation of acidic and basic fibroblast growth factor during mouse palate development and their effects on mouse palate mesenchyme cells *in vitro*. *Roux's Arch Devel Biol* **202**:132–143, 1993.
18. Ferguson MWJ. Craniofacial malformations: towards a molecular understanding. *Nature Genetics* **6**:329–330, 1994.
19. Rosenquist TH, Beall AC. Elastogenic cells in the developing cardiovascular system: smooth muscle, nonmuscle and cardiac neural crest. *Ann NY Acad Sci* **588**:106–119, 1990.
20. Bockman DE, Redmond ME, Kirby ML. Altered development of pharyngeal arch vessels after neural crest ablation. *Ann NY Acad Sci* **588**:296–304, 1990.
21. Colbert MC, Kirby ML, Robbins J. Endogenous retinoic acid signaling colocalizes with advance expression of the adult smooth muscle myosin heavy chain isoform during development of the ductus arteriosus. *Circ Res* **78**:790–798, 1996.

Homeobox genes and the determination of the embryonic body plan

6

P.T. Sharpe

Introduction

One of the great remaining mysteries in biology is how 'form' (morphology) is generated during embryogenesis, faithfully reproducing the body plan each successive generation. The fact that morphology is inherited means that the overall control must reside at the level of the gene, and since the advent of gene cloning in the 1970s, the search has been on to identify genes involved in regulating the development of the embryonic body plan. Not surprisingly, it appears that even the simplest and most basic aspects of embryonic morphology involve complex interactions requiring many different genes.

From studies carried out during the last ten years, two central themes have emerged: (i) that the molecular control of embryonic morphology has been highly conserved in evolution, even between invertebrates and vertebrates, and (ii) that this control involves families of genes coding for proteins that act as regulators of gene transcription. The vast majority of our current understanding of the genes involved in mammalian embryogenesis come from genetic studies in flies.

The homeobox

The fruit fly *Drosophila melanogaster* has for several decades been one of the biologist's organisms of choice for studying development. *Drosophila* has a rapid breeding cycle, a simple anatomy and mutations can be generated easily. Thus, rapid progress in understanding fly development was made well in advance of vertebrate development.

The *Drosophila* embryo, larva and adult fly, have a distinct head and a distinct tail region with repeating segmental units in between. Three segments form the thorax, with a further eight segments forming the abdomen. After the segments have been established in development, the characteristic structure of each segment is specified by a homeotic gene. The different developmental fates of successive segments along the embryo are thus specified by cranio-caudal expression of successive homeotic genes.

In *Drosophila*, most of the homeotic genes are clustered in two complexes on chromosome 3. The Antennapedia complex (Antp) contains five homeotic genes, and the Bithorax complex (BX-C) contains three homeotic genes. These clusters are together termed the homeotic complex (HOMC). Interestingly, the relative order of the genes along the chromosome is reflected in their functional domains in development. Thus 'head' genes are located at one end of the Antennapedia complex and, moving along the chromosome to the Bithorax complex, genes are involved in thorax and finally abdominal development are found; this feature is known as colinearity (Fig. 6.1).

Homeotic mutations in *Drosophila* are characterised by conversion of one body part into another. The Antennapedia (Antp) mutation, for example, has a phenotype where legs replace antennae on the fly's head. The genes mutated in homeotic mutants were cloned from the early 1980s. It was found that homeotic genes, although different from each other, all have a consistent stretch of DNA, 180 basepairs long, which codes for 60 amino acids[1]. This region of homology was termed the homeobox ('homeo' = homeotic, 'box' = conserved motif) and analysis of the amino acid sequence recognised that this region was likely to form a helix–turn–helix configuration in the protein. Helix–turn–helix motifs had been known for some time to have DNA binding properties in prokaryotic proteins and the assumption, later confirmed, was that homeotic proteins bind to DNA and act as regulators of gene transcription[2,3].

However, the homeotic genes are only one small, specialised group of genes in flies that have a homeobox. By using the homeobox sequence (i.e. the specific 180 basepair sequence) as a hybridisation probe, many other genes

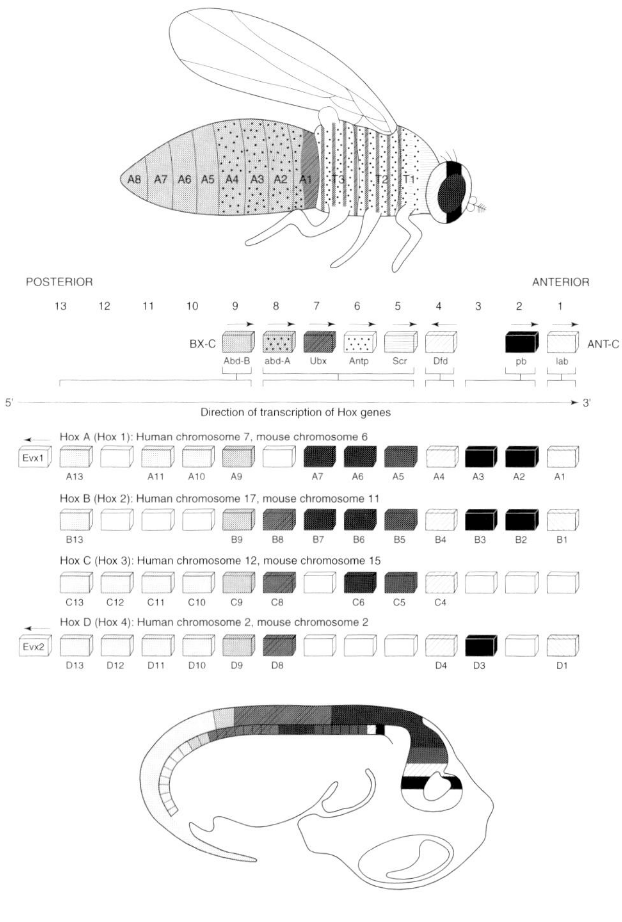

Fig. 6.1 Diagrammatic representation of the genetic relationships between an adult *Drosophila* (top) and a mammalian embryo (bottom). Each shaded box in the top row indicates a homeotic gene in *Drosophila*; the distribution of the genes is shown in the same shades on the adult fly. The shaded boxes in the lower four rows indicate the Hox genes identified in the mammalian embryo. The open boxes correspond to expected positions of genes, based on the genes discovered in other clusters, but no genes have been found to exist in these positions. The expression of these genes is shown on the mammalian embryo. The colinearity between gene position and embryonic expression can be seen. Since production of this figure a 39th Hox gene, *Hoxb-13* was identified. (Adapted from Zeltser, L., Despan, C. and Heintz N. *Hoxb-13*: a new Hox gene in a distant region of the HOXB cluster maintains colinearity. *Development* (1996) **122**: 2475–2484.)

containing the homeobox have been identified, all of which to date have been found to be expressed during embryogenesis (see below). The homeobox is thus a much used DNA-binding motif and homeobox genes constitute a large multigene family. There are other types of DNA binding motif found in transcriptional regulatory proteins. These large multigene families include *inter alia* those named zinc finger, HMG-box, helix–loop–helix, winged helix and MADs-box. It seems that once an efficient DNA binding sequence appeared in evolution, it was repeatedly duplicated many times resulting in many genes with a relatively small number of different motif types.

Vertebrate hox genes

Around 1984, biologists started to search for the existence of genes containing the *Drosophila* homeobox in vertebrates. It was reasoned that since the homeobox was highly conserved between homeotic genes it might also have been conserved during evolution in genes that play key control roles in vertebrate development. The first such gene identified was in *Xenopus* and was rapidly followed by cloning of several genes in mice[4]. The murine genes were found to have homeobox sequences that were very similar to those in *Drosophila* homeotic genes. Such genes were termed Hox genes (note the use of lower case here). When their genomic organisation was studied, it was discovered that the murine Hox genes were clustered together on four chromosomal locations. Similar arrangements have been identified in humans where the genes are termed HOX (note upper case to distinguish human genes).

The nomenclature of Hox genes has undergone two major revisions since 1984 as more genes were cloned and the relationships between Hox genes and homeotic genes were established. The term 'Hox' is now reserved exclusively for genes that are most related by homeobox sequence to the homeotic genes and are part of the four clusters in vertebrates. In mice and humans, the clusters are named A, B, C, D. The four chromosomal locations are denoted by letter, thus: cluster A is on mouse chromosome 6, human chromosome 7; cluster B is on mouse chromosome 11, human chromosome 17; cluster C is on mouse chromosome 15, human chromosome 12; and cluster D on mouse chromosome 2, human chromosome 2. Individual genes are named according to chromosome and relative position in the cluster with respect to their cognates in other clusters, i.e. Hoxa-1, Hoxa-2, Hoxb-1, Hoxb-2 etc[5,6]. This nomenclature thus reflects the evolutionary origins of the clusters which had a single common ancestor with homeotic genes in invertebrates and which have undergone serial duplication to produce four clusters in mammals (Fig. 6.1).

The standardisation of Hox gene nomenclature was initiated by *Drosophila* developmental biologists when it became apparent that groups of Hox genes were related to individual homeotic genes by homeobox sequence, cluster position and expression. Thus the embryonic expression of Hox genes in mammals also displays colinearity with position in the clusters. Genes expressed rostrally are located at the 3′ ends of clusters, whereas genes expressed in more caudal domains are located at the 5′ ends of clusters[7–9] (Fig. 6.2). Thus the homeotic gene *labial*, a gene required for head development is most closely related to the Hox A genes. These genes, e.g. *labial, Hoxa-1, -b-1, -d-1* constitute a cognate group, with the Hox genes referred to as paralogues.

(a) 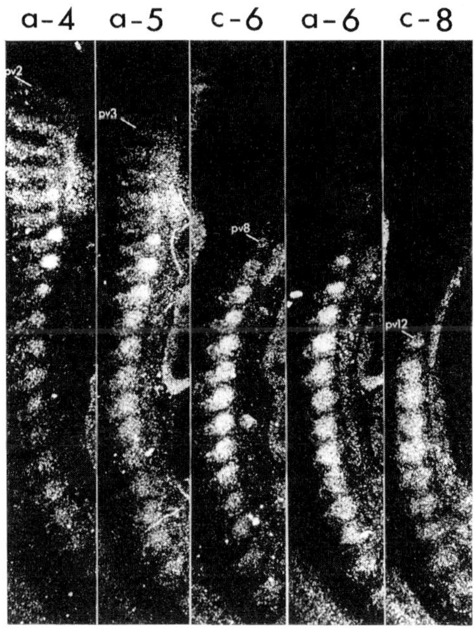

(b) 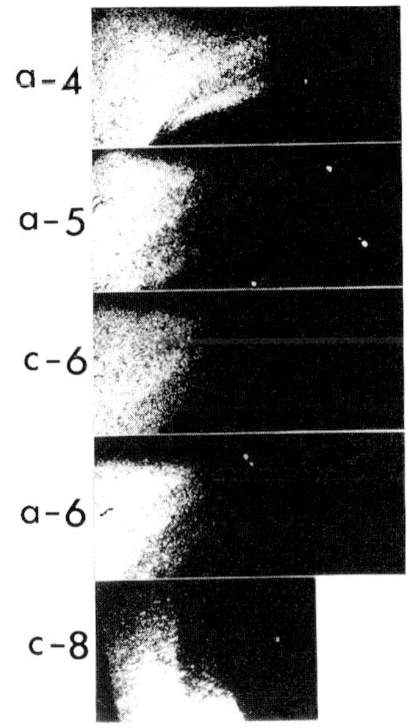

Fig. 6.2 (a) Serial parasagittal sections through a mouse embryo with *in situ* hybridisation of five types of Hox gene showing which ones are expressed in the prevertebrae of the embryo. (b) Adjacent section through the same animal at higher magnification showing the expression of the Hox genes in the nervous system. Expression of *Hoxc-6* marks the junction between the neural tube (spinal cord) and the hindbrain (rhombencephalon).

COLINEARITY

The remarkable evolutionary conservation of colinearity is so far unique in biology and, given that mice and *Drosophila* represent two extremes of the animal kingdom, suggests that a common set of genes grouped together into a cluster underlies the development of all multicellular animals. It is assumed that such conservation must imply that colinearity is essential for correct functioning of the genes, although there is little hard evidence to support this. The position of a Hox gene in its cluster is, however, important for correct regulation since placing a gene in a different position alters its expression[10]. This and other data has led to the suggestion that colinearity, i.e. sequential expression in embryos and general position, is some form of cellular memory involving proteins that make stretches of chromosome accessible or inaccessible for transcription[11]. Thus, for example, the mouse gene *Bmi-1* is a member of a group of proteins related to the *Drosophila* gene *Polycomb* which is known to have a role in controlling the expression of homeotic genes[12]. When *Bmi-1* is overexpressed in transgenic mouse embryos, expression of several Hox genes is shifted in a caudal direction in the somites and is accompanied by rostral transformations in the identities of subsequent vertebral bodies[13] (Fig. 6.3). Similarly, mice lacking *Bmi-1*, by gene knock out, show caudal transformations of vertebrae which are accompanied by rostral shifts in Hox gene expression[14]. All Hox genes are expressed in the developing nervous system and somites; colinearity is most obvious in the rostral boundaries of expression in these tissues. Rostral expression boundaries in the nervous system and in the somites are offset due to the rapid growth of the head shortly after gastrulation, so that nervous system boundaries are more rostrally placed than somite boundaries (Fig. 6.3). Colinearity is also observed in other non-axial tissues where Hox genes are expressed such as the developing limbs and the genitourinary organs. Development of these organs mainly involves expression of the more 5′ Hox genes particularly those of the Hoxd complex.

In developing limbs, there are striking overlapping colinear domains of the 5′ Hoxd genes *Hoxd-9, -d-10, -d-11, -d-12* and *-d-13* that change as the limb bud develops[15,16]. These genes appear to play a role in controlling rates of growth of specific areas of developing cartilage and bone in the digits (see below). Hoxd genes are also expressed in a colinear fashion in the developing genitourinary tract and at the caudal somatic (rather than autonomic) end of the digestive tract. Gene knock-out analysis has confirmed a role for these genes in development of these organs.

Because of the overlapping domains of Hox gene expression, it has been proposed that they function in specifying axial positions in the embryo in a combinatorial fashion. An alternate view is that the co-expression of Hox genes may represent functional redundancy between genes and that the different Hox gene paralogues can determine the same axial phenotypes.

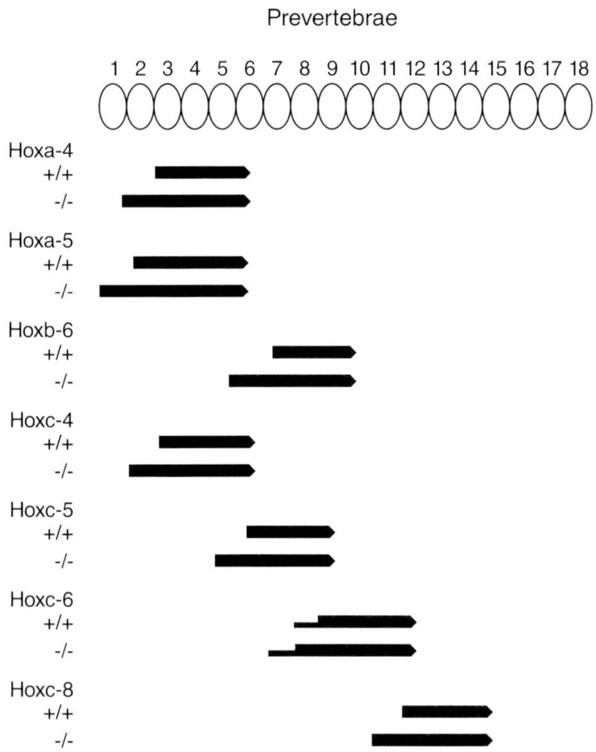

Fig. 6.3 Schematic representation of the rostral boundaries of Hox genes in *Bmi-1* –/– and *Bmi-1* +/+ embryos. The ellipses at the top of the diagram indicate prevertebrae numbered from C1, the future atlas. The black arrows show the Hox expression domains with the left-hand end located at the rostral expression boundary. The caudal boundaries of Hox gene expression are less well defined and their positions, marked by the arrowheads, are arbitrarily chosen. The partially truncated black arrows showing *Hoxc-6* expression indicate that in these experiments no sharp rostral boundary could be distinguished. Adapted from van der Lugt *et al*[12].

Function of Hox genes

The function of Hox genes in terms of morphology (rather than biochemistry) has been studied most extensively by targeted gene disruption in transgenic mice (gene knock-out). Almost all Hox genes have now been knocked out and in some cases two or even three genes have been knocked out in the same animal. Four generalisations can be made from the results of these knock-outs.

1. There is limited redundancy of function between the different Hox genes. Thus every knock-out of an individual Hox gene has some detectable phenotype.
2. A common feature of all the phenotypes of the Hox gene knock-outs are abnormalities of the development of the axial skeleton.
3. Abnormalities in embryonic development observed in Hox gene knock-outs relate to the rostral position of the domain of expression of each individual gene.
4. Although many Hox genes are expressed in the developing nervous system, few abnormalities in nervous system development have been detected in the knock-outs.

Knock-outs of all individual Hox genes have produced obvious phenotypes, demonstrating each gene has some non-redundant function. The common feature of these phenotypes is abnormalities in development of prevertebrae (i.e. structures derived from the rearrangement of the somites, combining the caudal half of one somite and the cranial half of the somite below). These abnormalities take various forms including transformation, additions or deletions, but the common feature is that the actual level of the defect exhibits colinearity. Thus 3′ genes produce defects in more cranial prevertebrae than 5′ genes[17]. Other phenotypes are observed in knock-outs, particularly of the more caudal genes which affect limb development and development of the genitourinary tract and the cloacal region. Colinearity is preserved in all these abnormalities in different tissues. Thus, regardless of the embryonic tissue, the relationships between gene order and function are always maintained.

LIMB BONE DEVELOPMENT

The overlapping expression domains of the more 5′ Hoxa and Hoxd genes suggested a role in pattern formation of the bones of the limbs. Targeted mutations in several of the genes has confirmed a requirement for these for normal limb development but has also shown their role to be complex.

Mutations in *Hoxd-11* and *Hoxd-13* result in regional malformation in the bones of the limbs and although the last bones to form are the most severely affected the malformations are not polarised but rather suggestive of defects in localised cell proliferation[18–21]. Similarly, mutations in *Hoxa-11* show bone malformation characteristic of proliferation defects rather than patterning[18]. The extent to which these mutation affect limb bones is different; thus *Hoxd-11* has affects from the distal tips of the radius and ulna to the digits, *Hoxd-13* affects the carpals, metacarpals and digits and *Hoxa-11* affects the radius, ulna and carpals of the forelimb only. Mutations in *Hoxa-13* do, however, show obvious patterning defects where the pre-axial digits of both limbs fail to develop and there is altered morphogenesis of some carpal and tarsal bones.

In order to understand better the complex requirements for these genes, double and triple mutations have been generated. Mice lacking function of *Hoxa-11* and *Hoxd-11* have only a vestige of the ulna and radius and the extent of the defects is related to the number of functional alleles of each gene[22]. Significantly in the double homozygous mutants the forelimbs are more affected than the hindlimbs suggesting that there may be compensation by other Hox genes such as *Hoxc-11* which is strongly expressed in the hindlimbs.

A simple model for these observations is that different paralogous groups of 5′ Hox genes are responsible for development of different limb bones. Thus Hox-10 genes would be responsible for outgrowth and formation of the humerus and femur, the Hox-11 genes for outgrowth and formation of the radius, ulna, tibia and fibula[17]. The mechanism of action might involve regulation of cell proliferation as well as specifying cell identities.

AXIAL SKELETON DEVELOPMENT

Every Hox gene probably contributes to the formation of the axial skeleton and the considerable overlap in expression of the genes in the developing prevertebrae means there is great potential for overlap of function such that loss of function of one Hox gene can be masked by presence of another.

The results of mutations in all Hox genes are consistent with a role in modifying a common vertebral unit (module) and thus specifying the identity of each vertebra. The type of vertebral anomaly produced by Hox gene mutation is variable; both cranial and caudal transformations of vertebral morphology are observed as well as abnormalities that cannot be interpreted as either cranial or caudal transformations. In mice with mutation in *Hoxd-3* or *Hoxb-4* the IInd cervical vertebra (C2) is transformed into a Ist cervical vertebra (C1) whereas when *Hoxa-5* is mutated the VIIth cervical vertebra is transformed into one resembling a thoracic vertebra, complete with ribs[23–25].

Combining Hox gene mutations results in defects which are more severe than the total of the individual abnormalities. Mutations in *Hoxa-4*, *Hoxb-4* and *Hoxd-4* (triple knock-out) result in multiple cervical vertebrae developing with characteristics of C1, suggesting that C1 represents a 'ground state' for all cervical vertebrae and that the role of Hox-4 genes is to specify the phenotype of individual cervical vertebrae[26]. However, mutation of *Hoxa-3* and *Hoxd-3* (double mutations) result in C1 being deleted altogether[27]. An interpretation of these data is that Hox genes control local cell proliferation of precursor cells and when multiple genes are deleted, the proliferation rates are so drastically affected that the structure fails to develop. If proliferation is only slowed down as in the case of single-gene mutations, then the proliferating cells may find themselves in new positions as surrounding cells divide at higher rate and they then develop according to their new positions.

CLOACAL REGION

Hoxd-13 and *Hoxd-12* are both expressed in the terminal part of the developing hindgut in murine embryos in presumptive smooth muscle which will give rise to the circular and longitudinal muscles. Mutation in either of these Hox genes results in abnormal morphology of the internal sphincter with the longitudinal muscle layer being severely reduced or absent[28].

Hox genes and pharyngeal arch development

Hox gene expression is intimately related to the development of the rhombomeres in the developing hindbrain (see Chapter 8). Rhombomeres act as lineage restrictions (segments) during neural development and the expression of Hox genes at these boundaries has implied that the genes may have a role in specifying different neuronal populations in the developing brain[29]. Significantly, the expression of Hox genes in the cranial neural crest cells which arise in segmental patterns from the hindbrain rhombomeres has been observed[30,31]. Thus Hox gene expression domains in rhombomeres are preserved in cranial neural crest cells. Since cranial neural crest cells contribute mesenchymal populations to the developing pharyngeal arches it is possible that Hox expression has a role in patterning the arch structures and derivatives.

Functional evidence for a role in pharyngeal arch development from gene knock-out studies is rather weak in that mutations in Hox genes expressed in cranial neural crest do not always appear to result in major abnormalities in structures derived from these cells. However, mutations in *Hoxa-2*, which is expressed up to the rhombomere 1/2 boundary, display a complete lack of second pharyngeal arch structures and formation in their place of first arch structures[32]. Mice with mutations in *Hoxa-3* have deficiencies in several organs derived from pharyngeal arches and/or pouches such as the thymus, parathyroids and carotid arteries, whereas *Hoxa-3/d-3* double mutants have laryngeal cartilage defects[27,33].

Retinoic acid and Hox gene expression

The teratogenic effects of retinoic acid (RA), a derivative of vitamin A, have been extensively studied for over 25 years. Mammalian embryos exposed to excess retinoic acid show abnormalities of many different organs, the most striking being craniofacial and limb defects (reviewed by Morriss-Kay[34]). An intriguing feature of craniofacial RA teratogenesis is that the abnormalities produced appear to originate from abnormal development of the hindbrain. Hox gene expression in cultures of embryonic carcinoma cells (EC cells) is sensitive to exogenous RA concentrations, where the sensitivity reflects colinearity, i.e. cranial genes are activated by lower concentrations of RA than more caudal genes. These observations have led to the conclusion that RA exerts its teratogenic effects on craniofacial development by altering Hox gene expression[35]. By looking at the expression of Hox genes in the developing hindbrain of embryos exposed to excess RA it is clear that RA alters Hox gene expression in a way that correlates with the defects observed. Thus RA induces a transformation of rhombomeres 2/3 into a 4/5 identity, with a corresponding transformation of the trigeminal motor nerve into one with a facial identity[36]. Neural crest cells derived from rhombomeres 2/3 also appear to be caudally transformed, since they express Hox genes corresponding to rhombomeres 4/5.

Similar effects of excess RA on vertebral and limb development have also been shown to be consistent with RA affecting Hox gene expression. In the normal limb Hox gene expression consists of overlapping domains of the caudal Hoxd genes (*Hoxd-9–Hoxd-13*) and results in the normal digit pattern. Implantation of RA-soaked beads into the preaxial border of the developing limb results in a mirror-image duplication of the digit pattern. This is explained by the RA diffusing through the limb to produce a morphometric gradient of opposite orientation to the endogenous gradient produced by the zone of polarising activity (ZPA) at the postaxial border (see p. 34). Expression of Hoxd genes in these RA implanted limbs is also duplicated in a mirror-image fashion consistent with a role in determining the digit pattern[15]. Caudal transformations of vertebrae along the complete body axis observed with RA administration are also postulated to result from alteration of Hox gene expression[37].

Human HOX gene mutations

It was not until 1996 that the first mutation in a HOX gene was reported to be the cause of a human malformation. Mutations in the HOXD-13 were found in patients with the limb deformity, synpolydactyly. Synpolydactyly is an autosomal dominant disorder characterised by webbing between the fingers and toes and digit duplications (Fig. 6.4).

The first indication that HOXD genes might be linked to synpolydactyly came from mapping studies localising the disorder to 2q31[38]. This was followed by two independent reports showing duplication of polyalanine stretches in the putative HOXD-13 protein in synpolydactyly patients[39–41].

Because the synpolydactyly phenotype differs from that in the *Hoxd-13* knock-out mice it has been argued that the extension of alanines in the HOXD-13 protein probably creates a gain of functional mutation. However, it has subsequently been shown that when *Hoxd-13*, *Hoxd-12* and *Hoxd-11* are mutated together in mice the phenotype produced is very reminiscent of human synpolydactyly[42]. This suggests that the polyalanine extension in HOXD-13 is producing a protein that in some way results in inactivation of the HOXD-12 and HOXD-11 proteins.

Non-Hox homeobox genes

Hox genes represent only one particular group of genes having homeoboxes and there are many more homeobox genes that are not clustered and which are only related to Hox genes by virtue of having a homeobox. These homeobox genes are called by a variety of names (e.g. *Msx*, *Mox*, *Dlx*,

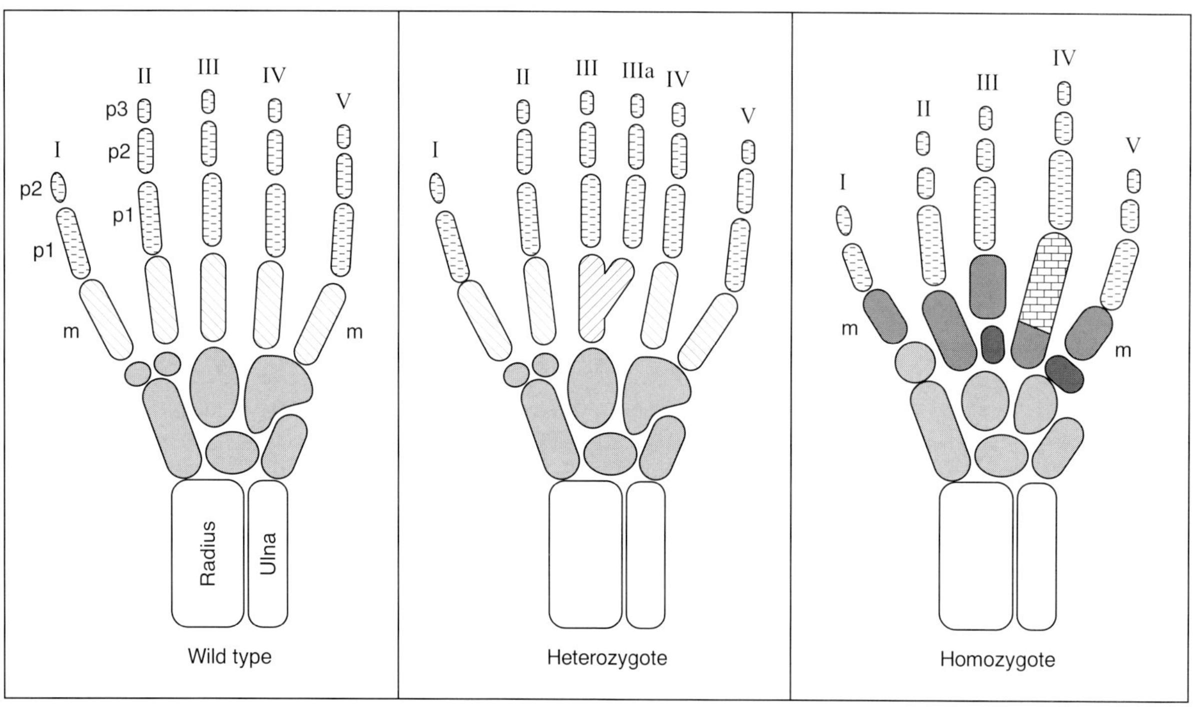

Fig. 6.4 Examples of the hand skeletons from individuals heterozygous or homozygous for the HOXD-13 mutation responsible for synpolydactyly. The hand on the left shows the normal arrangement. The heterozygote shows branching of metacarpal III which consequently produces an extra digit; the digit structure is unaltered. The homozygote causes anomalies of the carpal bones, conversion of metacarpals to carpal-like bones and extra carpal bones; the digit number and structure is not affected. Reproduced with permission from Sharpe[41].

Otx, *Emx*, *Goosecoid* etc.) and have widely varied expression patterns in embryos, too numerous to be covered here. A common feature of many of these genes is that on the whole their expression is unrelated to the craniocaudal expression of the Hox genes and they are often highly restricted to particular cells in developing organs. Many of these genes are related to individual *Drosophila* homeobox genes but in vertebrates they are duplicated to varying extents. Thus *Drosophila* has a single *msh* gene whereas mammals have three msh-related genes, *Msx-1*, *Msx-2* and *Msx-3*[43–48]. Similarly in *Drosophila*, *Distal-less* (*D1*) gene has a least seven related genes (*Dlx-1* to -7) in mammals[49–53] It is probable that duplication of these genes occurred progressively during evolution of more complex body plans, again demonstrating a link between morphology and homeobox genes.

Several of these homeobox genes have been shown to be mutated in human disorders. The murine *Msx-1* gene which was originally shown to be required to correct tooth development in knock-out mice has subsequently been linked to tooth agenesis in humans with identification of a missense mutation in the homeodomain of *MSX1*[54,55]. Mutations in the *EMX2* homeobox gene, which in murine embryos is expressed in a discrete domain in the developing forebrain, have been reported in patients with severe schizencephaly, a rare congenital disorder characterised by clefts in the cerebral hemispheres[56].

Pax genes

A group of genes related to homeobox genes are the PAX genes, so called because they contain a DNA-binding domain similar to that found in the *Drosophila* segmentation *paired* gene (reviewed by Hastie[57] and Gruss & Walther[58]) A total of nine PAX genes have been identified and four of these, *Pax-3*, *Pax-4*, *Pax-6* and *Pax-7* as well as containing a 'paired-box' also contain a homeobox[59,60]. PAX genes have proved to be particularly interesting largely because two of them, *PAX-3* and *PAX-6*, have been shown to be the genes that are mutated in two human genetic diseases, Waardenburg's syndrome (*PAX-3*)[61,62] and Aniridia (*PAX-6*)[63–65]. Waardenburg's syndrome is responsible for 2–3% of total congenital deafness and accompanying features include dystrophic canthorum, and pigmentary disturbances such as frontal white blaze of hair. These abnormalities are in tissues derived from neural crest-derived cells which express *PAX-3*. The Aniridia phenotype is a failure of iris and retinal development which correlates with the sites of *PAX-6* expression. Both these conditions are autosomal dominant and thus loss of function of only one copy of the gene via mutation produces the phenotype. This suggests that the concentration of PAX proteins during development is important. Both Waardenburg's and Aniridia have equivalent mutations in mice, namely *Splotch* (Waardenburg) and *Small eye* (aniridia) caused by mutation in the *Pax-3*[66] and *Pax-6*[67] genes, respectively. In common with the transgenic mutations in Hox genes, the Pax mutations only produce abnormalities in a subset of tissues where they are expressed. Thus although both genes are expressed in the developing CNS, no major abnormalities are seen here in the mutants.

Links between the other members of the PAX gene family and mouse/human mutations are being investigated and one gene, *Pax-1*, is the cause of the mouse *undulated* mutation which is a defect in vertebra formation. No human equivalent of undulated has been identified[68].

'Deep' homology

During the last ten years, developmental biologists have become familiar with the conservation of developmentally regulated genes between invertebrates and mammals. Indeed it is this conservation that is a major driving force behind much of today's research into the development of both invertebrates and vertebrates. Conservation of gene (protein) sequences over many millions of years of evolution has been an accepted phenomenon for many years, e.g. genes involved in processes common to all species such as energy metabolism and ribosome structure. When vertebrate homeobox genes were first identified, there was much scepticism amongst developmental biologists that these genes would play a similar role in vertebrate embryogenesis to homeotic genes in flies. At that time, the accepted dogma was that since invertebrate and vertebrate embryology was so different, there would be little if any similarities in molecular mechanisms. The years since then have seen a remarkable change in thinking and our understanding of the evolution of developmental mechanisms and embryogenesis has changed dramatically.

The first suggestions that molecular mechanisms controlling important developmental processes might be conserved came from the conservation of Hox and homeotic gene colinearity. The extent of the similarities between Hox and homeotic gene sequences, organisation, expression and function provided a strong argument that Hox and HOM proteins had similar regulatory roles in fly and mammalian development. A further level of conservation was realised when it was demonstrated that the regulation of Hox and HOM genes was also conserved. Regulatory regions of the *Drosophila Deformed* homeotic gene were shown to be able to reproduce expression of the cognate murine genes in transgenic mouse embryos[69].

Confirmation of functional equivalence of Hox and HOM genes has been provided by experiments showing that the *Drosophila labial* homeotic mutation could be rescued in transgenic flies by expressing the vertebrate *labial* orthologue, *Hoxb-1*[70]. Although the way invertebrate and vertebrate embryos develop can be very different, for example contrast fly development which involves metamorphosis with human development, there is at least some level of basic functional conservation of Hox and HOM genes in determination of the craniocaudal body axis.

The development and structure of invertebrate and vertebrate organs bear little if any resemblance to each other. There are many examples of organs which, although serving similar functions, are very different structures. For example, the compound eye of flies and the human eye are both photoreceptors and any similarities end there. Morphologically they are completely different and it has always been naturally assumed that there is no evolutionary relationship between the two. This view has now been severely questioned and, unlikely as it may seem, it is probable that evolution of the compound eye and the human eye are linked. The clues to this remarkable suggestion have come from studies of the molecular control of development of eyes in flies and humans. The requirement for the *PAX-6* gene for normal human eye development has already been described. A mutation identified in *Drosophila* called *eyeless* has the obvious phenotype of no eyes. When the gene for *eyeless* was cloned and sequenced, it was found to relate highly to the human *PAX-6* gene. Moreover, if the *eyeless* gene is ectopically expressed in transgenic flies, ectopic eyes are induced indicating that eyeless is a master control gene for eye development[71]. Other examples of this phenomenon of 'deep' homology are also now being observed. Development of the fly heart and the mammalian heart both require the expression of the same gene called *tinman* in flies and *Nkx2.5* in mammals. Development of the appendages in flies (wings, legs, etc.) requires many of the same genes identified as having key roles in development of vertebrate limbs[72–74].

The identification of development control genes in vertebrates and invertebrates is not only starting to provide a detailed understanding of how embryogenesis is controlled but also unmasks hitherto unprecedented links between molecules and morphological change in evolution. The discovery of the homeobox has thus proved to be a landmark in developmental biology as important as the discovery of the structure of DNA was to molecular biology. The ever increasing number of genes that are being identified for human malformation syndromes which were originally cloned by homology with *Drosophila* genes emphasizes the importance of studying development in both invertebrates and vertebrates.

Acknowledgements

I am grateful to Anthony Graham for critically reading this chapter. Work in the author's laboratory is supported by the MRC and the Human Frontier Science Programme.

REFERENCES

1. Gehring WJ. Homeoboxes and the study of development. *Science* **236**:1245–1252, 1987.
2. Sherperd JCW, McGinnis E, Carrasco AE, DeRobertis EM, Gehring WJ. Fly and frog homeo domains show homology with yeast mating type regulatory proteins. *Nature* **310**:70–71, 1984.
3. Levine M, Hoey T. Homeobox proteins as sequence-specific transcription factors. *Cell* **55**:537–540, 1988.
4. Carrasco AE, McGinnis W, Gehring WJ, De Robertis EM. Cloning of a *Xenopus laevis* gene expressed during early embryogenesis that codes for a peptide region homologous to *Drosophila* homeotic genes. *Cell* **37**:409–414, 1984.
5. Scott MP. Vertebrate homeobox gene nomenclature. *Cell* **71**:551–553, 1992.
6. Duboule D. *Guidebook to the homeobox genes*. Oxford: Sambrook and Tooze Publications, 1994.
7. Graham A, Papalopulu N, Krumlauf R. The murine and *Drosophila* homeobox clusters have common features of organisation and expression. *Cell* **57**:367–378, 1989.
8. Gaunt SJ, Sharpe PT, Duboule D. Spatially restricted domains of homeo-gene transcripts in mouse embryos: relation to a segmented body plan. *Development* (Supplement) **104**:169–179, 1988.
9. Duboule D, Dollé P. The structural and functional organization of the murine HOX gene family resembles that of *Drosophila* homeotic genes. *EMBO J* **8**:1497–1505, 1989.
10. van der Hoeven F, Zákány J, Duboule D. Gene transpositions in the *HoxD* complex reveal a hierarchy of regulatory controls. *Cell* **85**:1025–1035, 1996.
11. Gaunt SJ, Singh PB. Homeogene expression patterns and chromosomal imprinting. *TIG* **6**(7):208–212, 1990.
12. van der Lugt NMT, Alkema M, Berns A, Deschamps J. The *Polycomb*-group homolog Bmi-1 is a regulator of murine *Hox* gene expression. *Mech Dev* **58**:153–164, 1996.
13. Alkema MJ, van der Lugt NMT, Bobeldijk RC, Berns A, van Lohuizen M. Transformation of axial skeleton due to overexpression of *bmi-1* in transgenic mice. *Nature* **374**:724–727, 1995.
14. van der Lugt NMT, Domen I, Linders K. *et al.* Posterior transformation, neurological abnormalities, and severe hematopoietic defects in mice with a targeted deletion of the *bmi-1* proto-oncogene. *Genes Dev* **8**:757–769, 1994.
15. Izpisua-Belmonte J-C, Tickle C, Dollé P, Wolpert L, Duboule D. Expression of homeobox Hox-4 genes and the specification of position in chick wing development. *Nature* **350**:585–589, 1991.
16. Nelson CE, Morgan BA, Burke AC. *et al.* Analysis of *Hox* gene expression in the chick limb bud. *Development* **122**:1449–1466, 1996.
17. Capecchi MR. Function of homeobox genes in skeletal development. *Ann NY Acad Sci* **785**:34–37, 1996.
18. Small KM, Potter SS. Homeotic transformations and limb defects in *Hoxa-11* mutant mice. *Genes Dev* **7**:2318–2328, 1993.
19. Dollé P, Dierich M, Le Meur T, Schimmang B, Schuhbaur B, Chambon P, Duboule D. Disruption of the *Hoxd-13* gene induces localised heterochrony leading to mice with neotenic limbs. *Cell* **75**:431–441, 1993.
20. Davis AP, Capecchi MR. Axial homeosis and appendicular skeleton defects in mice with a targeted disruption of *hoxd-11*. *Development* **120**:2187–2198, 1994.
21. Fromental-Ramain C, Warot X, Messadecq N, LeMeur M, Dollé P, Chambon P. *Hoxa-13* and *Hoxd-13* play a crucial role in the patterning of the limb autopod. *Development* **122**:2997–3011, 1996.
22. Davis AP, Witte DP, Hsieh-Li HM, Potter SS, Capecchi MR. Absence of radius and ulna in mice lacking *hoxa-11* and *Hoxd-11*. *Nature* **375**:791–795, 1995.
23. Condie BG, Capecchi MR. Mice homozygous for a targeted disruption of *Hoxd-3 (Hox-4.1)* exhibits anterior transformations of the first and second cervical vertebrae, the atlas and the axis. *Development* **119**:579–595, 1993.
24. Ramirez-Solis R, Zheng H, Whiting J, Krumlauf R, Bradley A. *Hoxb-4* (*Hox 2.6*) mutant mice show homeotic transformation of a cervical vertebra and defects in the closure of the sternal rudiments. *Cell* **73**:279–294, 1993.
25. Jeannotte L, Lemieux M, Charron J, Poirier F, Robertson EJ. Specification of axial identity in the mouse: role of the *Hoxa-5* (*Hox1.3*) gene. *Gene Dev* **7**:2085–2096, 1993.

26. Horan GS, Ramirez-Solis R, Featherstone MS, Wolgemuth DJ, Bradley A, Behringer RR. Compound mutants for the paralogous hoxa-4, hoxb-4, and hoxd-4 genes show more complete homeotic transformations and a dose-dependent increase in the number of vertebrae transformed. *Genes Dev* **9**:1667–1677, 1995.
27. Condie BG, Capecchi MR. Mice with targeted disruptions in the paralogous genes hoxa-3 and hoxd-3 reveal synergistic interactions [published erratum appears in *Nature* (1994), **371**(6497), 537]. *Nature* **370**:(6487), 304–307, 1994.
28. Kondon T, Dollé P, Zákány J, Duboule D. Function of posterior *HoxD* genes in the morphogenesis of the anal sphincter. *Development* **122**:2651–2659, 1996.
29. Lumsden A, Keynes R. Segmental patterns of neuronal development in the chick hindbrain. *Nature* **337**:424–428, 1989.
30. Lumsden A, Sprawson N, Graham A. Segmental origin and migration of neural crest cells in the hindbrain region of the chick embryo. *Development* **113**:1281–1291, 1991.
31. Prince V, Lumsden A. Hoxa-2 expression in normal and transposed rhombomeres: independent regulation in the neural tube and neural crest. *Development* **120**:911–923, 1994.
32. Rijli F, Mark M, Lakkaraju S, Dierich A, Dollé P, Chambon P. A homeotic transformation is generated in the rostral branchial region of the head by disruption of Hoxa-2 which acts as a selector gene. *Cell* **75**:1333–1349, 1993.
33. Chisaka O, Capecchi MR. Regionally restricted developmental defects resulting from targeted disruption of the mouse homeobox gene *hox-1.5*. *Nature* **350**:473–479, 1991.
34. Morriss-Kay G. Retinoic acid and craniofacial development: molecules and morphogenesis. *Bioessays* **15**:9–15, 1993.
35. Simeone A, Acampora D, Arcioni L, Andrews PW, Boncinelli E, Mavilio F. Sequential activation of HOX2 homeobox genes by retinoic acid in human embryonic carcinoma cells. *Nature* **346**:763–766, 1990.
36. Marshall H, Nonchev S, Sham MH, Muchamore I, Lumsden A, Krumlauf R. Retinoic acid alters hindbrain Hox code and induces transformation of rhombomeres 2/3 into a 4/5 identity. *Nature* **360**:737–741, 1992.
37. Kessell M, Gruss P. Homeotic transformations of murine prevertebrae and concomitant alteration of Hox codes induced by retinoic acid. *Cell* **67**:89–104, 1991.
38. Sarfarazi M, Akarsu AN, Sayli BS. Localization of the syndactyly type II (synpolydactyly) locus to 2q31 region and identification of tight linkage to HOXD8 intragenic marker. *Hum Mol Gen* **4**(8):1453–1458, 1995.
39. Akarsu AN, Stoilov I, Yilmaz E, Sayli BS, Sarfarazi M. Genomic structure of *HOXD13* gene: a nine polyalanine duplication causes synpolydactyly in two unrelated families. *Hum Mol Gen* **5**(7):945–952, 1996.
40. Muragaki Y, Mundlos S, Upton J, Olsen BR. Altered growth and branching patterns in synopolydactyly caused by mutations in HOXD13. *Science* **272**:548–551, 1996.
41. Sharpe PT. Hox gene mutations – the wait is over. *Nature Medicine* **2**:748–749, 1996.
42. Zákány J, Duboule D. Synpolydactyly in mice with a targeted deficiency in the *HoxD* complex. *Nature* **384**:69–71, 1996.
43. Holland PWH. Cloning and evolutionary analysis of msh-like homeobox genes from mouse, zebrafish and ascidian. *Gene* **98**:253–257, 1991.
44. Hill RE, Jones FI, Rees AR *et al.* A new family of mouse homeobox containing genes: molecular structure, chromosomal location and developmental expression. *Genes Dev* **3**:26–37, 1989.
45. Robert B, Sassoon D, Jaqu B, Gehring W, Buckingham M. Hox-7, a mouse homeobox gene with a novel pattern of expression during embryogenesis. *EMBO J* **8**:91–100, 1989.
46. MacKenzie A, Ferguson MWJ, Sharpe PT. Hox-7 expression during murine craniofacial development. *Development* **113**:601–611, 1991.
47. MacKenzie A, Ferguson MWJ, Sharpe PT. Expression patterns of the homeobox gene, Hox-8 in the mouse embryo suggest a role in specifying tooth initiation and shape. *Development* **115**:403–420, 1992.
48. Shimeld SM, McKay IJ, Sharpe PT. The murine homeobox gene Msx-3 shows highly restricted expression in the developing neural tube. *Mechs Dev* **55**:201–210, 1996.
49. Cohen SM, Bronner G, Kuttner F, Jurgens G, Jackle H. Distal-less encodes a homeodomain protein required for limb development in *Drosophila*. *Nature* **338**:432–434, 1989.
50. Price M, Lemaistre M, Pischetola M, Di Lauro R, Duboule D. A mouse gene related to Distal-less shows expression in the developing forebrain. *Nature* **351**:748–750, 1991.
51. Porteus MH, Bulfone A, Ciaranello RD, Rubenstein JLR. Isolation and characterisation of a novel cDNA clone encoding a homeodomain that is developmentally expressed in the ventral forebrain. *Neuron* **7**:221–229, 1991.
52. Robinson GW, Wray S, Mahon KA. Spatially restricted expression of a member of a new family of murine Distal-less homeobox genes in the developing forebrain. *New Biologist* **3**:1183–1194, 1991.
53. Stock DW, Ellies DL, Zhao Z, Ekker M, Ruddles FH, Weiss KM. The evolution of the vertebrate Dlx gene family. *Proc Natl Acad Sci USA* **93**:10858–10863, 1996.
54. Satokata I, Maas R. Msx1 deficient mice exhibit cleft palate and abnormalities of craniofacial and tooth development. *Nature Genetics* **6**:348–356, 1994.
55. Vastardis H, Karimbux N, Guthua SW, Seidman JG, Seidman CE. A human MSX1 homeodomain missense mutation causes selective tooth agenesis. *Nature Genetics* **13**:417–421, 1996.
56. Brunelli S, Faiella A, Capra V, Nigro V, Simeone A, Cama A, Boncinelli E. Germline mutations in the homeobox gene *EMX2* in patients with severe schizencephaly. *Nature Genetics* **12**:94–96, 1996.
57. Hastie N. Pax in our time. *Curr Biol* **1**:342–344, 1991.
58. Gruss P, Walther C. Pax in development. *Cell* **69**:719–722, 1992.
59. Walther C, Guenet J-L, Simon D. *et al.* Pax: A murine multigene family of paired box containing genes. *Genomics* **11**:424–434, 1991.
60. Stapleton P, Weith A, Urbanek P, Kozmik Z, Busslinger M. Chromosomal localisation of seven PAX genes and cloning of a novel family member, PAX-9. *Nature Genetics* **3**:292–298, 1993.
61. Baldwin CT, Hoth HF, Amos JA, da-Silva EO, Milunsky A. An exonic mutation in the HuP2 paired domain gene causes Waardenburg's syndrome. *Nature* **355**:637–638, 1992.
62. Tassabehji M, Read AP, Newton VE, Harris R, Balling R, Gruss P, Strachan T. Waardenburg's syndrome patients have mutations in the human homologue of the Pax-3 paired box gene. *Nature* **355**:635–636, 1992.
63. Ton CCT, Hirvonen H, Miwa H, *et al.* Positional cloning and characterisation of a paired box and homeobox-containing gene from the Aniridia region. *Cell* **67**:1059–1074, 1991.
64. Jordan T, Hanson I, Zaletayev D, Hodgson S, Prosser J, Seawright A, Hastie N, van Heyningen V. The human PAX6 gene is mutated in two patients with aniridia. *Nature Genetics* **1**:328–332, 1992.
65. Strachan T, Read AP. PAX genes. *Curr Opin Genet Dev* **4**:427–438, 1994.
66. Epstein D, Vekemans M, Gros P. Splotch (Sp2H), a mutation affecting development of the mouse neural tube, shows a deletion within the paired homeodomain of Pax-3. *Cell* **67**:767–774, 1991.
67. Hill RE, Favor J, Hogan BLM. *et al.* Mouse *Small eye* results from mutations in a paired-like homeobox-containing gene. *Nature* **354**:522–525, 1991.
68. Balling R, Deutsch U, Gruss P. Undulated, a mutation affecting the development of the mouse skeleton has a mutation in the paired box of Pax-1. *Cell* **55**:531–535, 1988.
69. Awgulewitsch A, Jacobs D. *Deformed* autoregulartory element from *Drosophila* functions in a conserved manner in transgenic mice. *Nature* **358**:341–344, 1992.
70. Lutz B, Lu H-C, Eichele G, Miller D, Kaufman TC. Rescue of *Drosophila labial* null mutant by the chicken ortholog *Hoxb-1* demonstrates that the function of *Hox* genes is phylogenetically conserved. *Genes Dev* **10**:176–184, 1996.
71. Halder G, Callaerts P, Gehring WJ. Induction of ectopic eyes by targeted expression of the *eyeless* gene in *Drosophila*. *Science* **267**:1788–1792, 1995.
72. Kim Y, Nirenberg M. *Drosophila* NK-homeobox genes. *Proc Nat Acad Sci USA* **86**:7716–7720, 1989.
73. Bodmer R. The gene *tinman* is required for specification of the heart and visceral muscles in *Drosophila*. *Development* **118**:719–729, 1993.
74. Harvey RP. *NK-2* homeobox genes and heart development. *Dev Biol* **178**:203–216, 1996.

The embryology of left-right: defects of situs in the embryo

7

A.D. Lander

Handed left–right asymmetries and defects of situs

The body appears to be symmetrical from the outside but the viscera exhibit the following handed lateral asymmetries: the cardiac apex, aortic arch, stomach and spleen lie to the left; the liver, gall bladder, vena cava, and greater lung lobation are found on the right. In addition, in humans the small bowel mesentery runs from a stable left-sided cephalad attachment to a stable caudal position on the right. An unpaired asymmetric organ may have one of three arrangements; solitus (the usual arrangement); inversus (mirror-image arrangement); or ambiguous (indeterminate). With paired organs that differ from their contralateral partner, such as atria, bronchi and lung lobes, the arrangement may similarly be either usual or mirror-image, but in addition, two situations of symmetry can occur. For example, there may be the same number of lung lobes on each side, or both atria may have the same sidedness, as assessed best by the atrial appendages, either both left- or both right-sided in appearance. Such arrangements are called isomerisms.

Many of the terms used to describe patterns of defects of situs including cardiac segmental situs are poorly defined and unhelpful. One set of consistent terms is as follows: 'situs solitus' describes the usual arrangement; 'situs inversus' refers to a perfect mirror-image arrangement and 'heterotaxy' refers to any other arrangement including discordant inversions and isomerisms. Often not all the asymmetries have been assessed and so 'global solitus' and 'global inversus' may be appropriate terms. Between 1 in 7000 and 1 in 12 000 people have global situs inversus, the sex ratio is equal[1] and about 25% of these have primary ciliary dyskinesia (PCD).

Care should be used with the following terms: 'dextrocardia' means that the majority of the heart is in the right chest, 'mesocardia' that it is centrally placed and 'laevocardia' that it lies mostly in the left chest. 'Dextrocardia' is therefore not necessarily a perfect mirror-image heart; indeed there are often abnormal atrioventricular and ventriculoarterial connections. Two other terms are used: 'dextroversion' to imply a right pointing apex in an otherwise normally connected heart[2] and 'dextroposition' to refer to an otherwise normal heart with a malposition due to pathology such as a diaphragmatic hernia.

Defects of situs attributable to defective left–right development include congenital heart defects (CHD) exhibiting one or more of the following; atrial inversion or isomerism, atrioventricular (AV) discordance, ventriculoarterial (VA) discordance or a sinistral ventricular loop. These defects of segmental cardiac situs co-associate and are associated with non-cardiac defects of situs. For example, a sinistral loop with AV and VA discordance (congenitally corrected transposition of the great arteries in global solitus) is seen with asplenia[3,4]. Ventriculoarterial discordance with a dextral loop (transposition of the great arteries – TGA) has been widely associated with other defects of situs[3,5–7] and is seen in PCD[8,9] and amongst the anomalies of diabetic embryopathy (see below). Bartelings and Gittenberger-de-Groot[10] believe there to be a mirror-image formation of the columns of the aortopulmonary septum in TGA.

Non-cardiac defects of situs include: polysplenia, asplenia, preduodenal portal vein (PDPV), annular pancreas, some unusual arrangements of bronchial branching and lung lobation and anomalies of the major vessels and gastrointestinal mesenteric attachments. These rare anomalies also co-associate strengthening a belief in a common aetiology. However, malrotation of the duodenojejunal (DJ) flexure, which is frequently responsible for neonatal intestinal obstruction and volvulus, is also often seen without other defects of situs. In these instances, the anomaly appears to arise from inadequate lateralization of the DJ flexure rather than from a primary defect of distinguishing left from right.

Heterotaxias include so many permutations of sidedness of the asymmetric organs that stochastic developmental mechanisms seem likely. For example, discordance between bronchial and atrial situs occurs[11], asplenia is reported with inverted atria and bronchi[12], and right bronchial isomerism is reported with polysplenia[13]. However, there is not complete independence of sidedness and some patterns of defects of situs are more common than others, for example, the atrial isomerisms.

Atrial isomerism

Left atrial isomerism is associated with left bronchial isomerism, bilateral anterior caval veins, azygos continuation of the posterior caval vein, an ambiguous atrioventricular connection, but a relatively normal ventriculoarterial junction. The majority have multiple spleens and abnormal lateralisation of the abdominal viscera including a short pancreas and a third have a confluent suprahepatic venous channel connecting the hepatic veins to the atrium. The pulmonary venous connections are normal often with two pulmonary veins on each side.

Right atrial isomerism is associated with right isomerism of the lungs and bronchi, bilateral anterior caval drainage. Total anomalous pulmonary venous drainage including anomalous drainage via a narrow sinus in the roof of the atrium is seen. There is always absence of the coronary sinus, and often a common atrioventricular valve, double inlet or ambiguous atrioventricular connection and abnormal ventriculoarterial connection and pulmonary obstruction. The majority have asplenia.

It should be remembered that the atrial isomerisms are associated with midgut malrotation and should receive a contrast study shortly after birth[14–16].

Unlike the atria, the left and right ventricular primordia are not paired since the left ventricle arises from the caudal heart tube and the right from the rostral heart tube. It is looping that places the ventricles laterally. Being non-paired midline structures, ventricular isomerism cannot exist.

Twins and congenital heart defects

In conjoined twins there is a widely held belief that defects of situs are common in the right-sided twin, but the picture is complex. Defects of cardiac situs occur in about half of right-sided twins in both dicephalus[17–21] and thoracopagus[22–24]. An excess of right isomerisms in the right twin may suggest that a property of right-sidedness is fixed in the right twin[25]. However, defects include both left and right isomerisms and discordant inversions. In addition the left twin is not immune to defects of situs. There is a paucity of CHD in craniopagus twins[26–31] suggesting that defects of situs in conjoining may be limited to interactions between neighbouring organisers/antero-posterior axes, perhaps related to the morphogens recently found to be asymmetric in the region of the node or organiser[32]. The incidence of defects of situs with pre-primitive streak stage separation in monozygotic twins is not clear[33].

Anomalies in non-lateralised organs associated with defects of situs

One in ten cases of extrahepatic biliary atresia (EHBA) have polysplenia[34–37] when the following anomalies are also frequently seen: azygos continuation of the posterior vena cava, midgut malrotation, PDPV and hepatic arterial anomalies. These have consequences for portoenterostmy and orthotopic liver transplantation[36,38]. Patients are more likely to be female and have fewer cardiac defects than if they had polysplenia alone[34,39]. EHBA has also been seen with asplenia[40,41] and in PCD[42–44]. The implication is that these cases of EHBA have an early aetiology. In PCD dysmotile cilia account for the pathology in the lungs, ears and sinuses, but the association with random global situs is difficult to explain. Other associations include renal-hepatic-pancreatic-dysplasia[45–49], agnathia and hydrocephalus.

Aetiology of defects of situs

Genetic and environmental factors play a role. Autosomal recessive[50], X-linked[51,52] and possible autosomal dominant[53,54] pedigrees have been described. In animals teratogens can cause situs inversus, sometimes alone[55] but mostly with other anomalies[56,57]. In humans[42,58–61] and some strains of mice[62], defects of situs are seen in diabetic embryopathy. A mitochondrial production of superoxide anion fuelled by pyruvate and amino acids affects situs in rodent embryos cultured from primitive streak stages[63]. This may model the defects of situs seen with maternal diabetes since the level of pyruvate[64] and some amino acids[65], are often raised even with good glycaemic control. The implications are that diabetic embryopathy has an early onset and that vigorous total metabolic control might be beneficial. A mechanical or pharmacological hepatoportal delivery of insulin should correct the biochemistry and may reduce these anomalies.

PCD is a heterogeneous collection of autosomal recessive ciliary dyskinesias in which most commonly there is a defect in the ciliary protein, dynein. Afzelius[66] suggested that orientated cilia might establish visceral handedness, and cells with single cilia have been noted in the ventral murine node and early notochord[67]. However, these cilia are immotile[68] and motile cilia do not appear until after the lateral asymmetries are established. Since dynein is also an intracellular motor protein it may be involved in the establishment of situs. Alternatively since the orientation of cilia in PCD shows greater variance than normal[69] it may be that a common mechanism is responsible for both the orientation of laterally asymmetric information and also for ciliary orientation.

Animal models provide clues to left–right development

Many of the handed lateral asymmetries are invariant morphological features of vertebrates, and since vertebrates share similar mechanisms for AP development they are also more likely to share mechanisms in left–right development than for these to have converged during evolution. One consequence of this homology is that it restricts developmental hypotheses to those that are compatible with the known development of the other vertebrates. Furthermore, it gives us greater faith in the findings from more accessible systems such as *Xenopus* and chick. Von Baer[70] (1828) observed that intervertebrate morphological structural similarity was greatest during early organogenesis. This homology is present even earlier, during gastrulation, but the variability in morphology before this time, for example during cleavage, may preclude these stages from a role in left–right specification. That amphibia and many fish develop away from their mothers suggests that the maternal environment does not provide the handed information, a hypothesis supported by murine experiments[25].

The murine autosomal recessive allele inversus viscerum (iv)[71], causes random global situs with a few discordant inversions and atrial isomerisms[72]. The anomalies include annular pancreas, PDPV, cardiac defects and abnormal spleens. The *iv* mutation lies on mouse chromosome 12 (syntenic to human chromosome 14q3)[73,74], and the gene codes for a component of a dynein molecule named left–right dynein (lrd)[75]. Interestingly, lrd mRNA is found in the ventral cells of the murine node before any asymmetric gene expression is evident.

A recessive mutation *inv* on chromosome 4 in a transgenic mouse OVE210, exhibits nearly 100% global inversus[76]. The defect is fatal and homozygotes die before 7 days of age with renal tubular cystic dysplasia and jaundice with near normal liver histology. The condition does not model the rare human renal–hepatic–pancreatic dysplasia frequently seen with global inversus. Interestingly, these embryos behave like +/+ siblings in optimised whole-embryo culture from primitive streak stages (personal observation).

Asymmetries in gene expression

An early morphological asymmetry is a dextral bulging of the heart tube (see Fig. 7.1), but asymmetries in gene expression precede this and are found during gastrulation. The gastrulating embryo consists of a bilaminar germ disc, a caudal primitive streak and a node at the cranial end of the streak. Handed asymmetries in gene expression are reported in the early somite period in the chick[32,77] and in *Xenopus*[78]. Recent findings in the chick suggest that a right-sided activin βB source induces expression of the activin type IIa receptor cActRIIa which suppresses a gene called Sonic hedgehog (*Shh*), initially found throughout the node so restricting it to its left half.

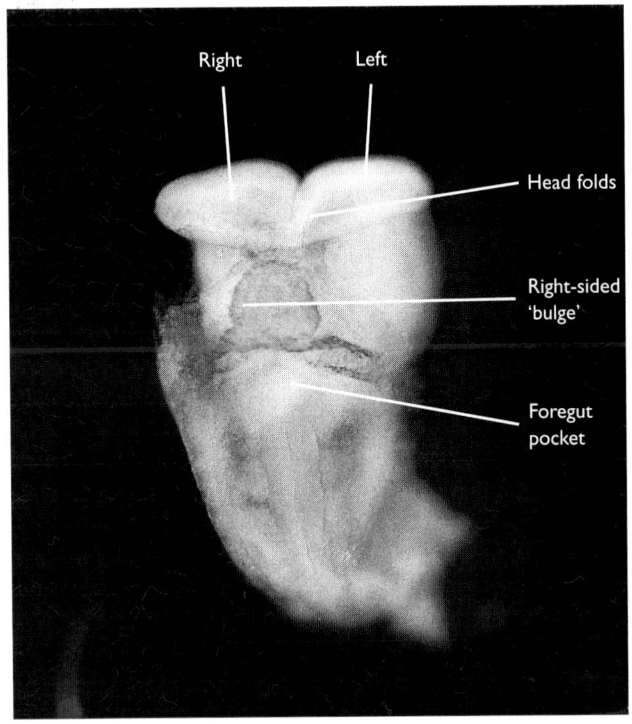

Fig. 7.1 Rat heart at six-somite stage stained with antimyosin antibody illustrating the early morphological asymmetry of a bulging of the heart tube to the right which precedes looping.

Whilst the first somites form *cNR-1* (a chick transforming growth factor-β (TGFβ) family member related to mouse *nodal*), which had been symmetrically expressed in the primitive streak appears just anterior and lateral to the node in left-sided lateral mesoderm. This asymmetric *cNR-1* expression is induced by *Shh*. *HNF3β* also becomes upregulated in the left side of the streak just posterior to the node but its role is unclear. In the right lateral plate mesoderm in the chick another gene *cSR-1* is expressed whose disruption with antisense oligonucleotides leads to random global situs[79].

Some similar genes are found in other vertebrates. In mouse, *nodal* and in *Xenopus*, *xNR-1* are expressed in left-sided lateral plate mesoderm. Interestingly in the mouse, another gene coding for a TGFβ protein has similar expression to *nodal* but is also found in the left half of the ventral neural tube up to the mid-brain level. This is surprising since no asymmetry in these structures is evident.

Lefty and *nodal* asymmetries are in register with global situs being inverted in *inv/inv* mice and randomised in *iv/iv* mice[78]. These genes are thus 'downstream' of the defects in these mutants. Furthermore, these mutants exhibit a caudalised anterior boundary of *nodal* and *lefty* expression[80] perhaps accounting for the CHD seen in these mice. The two genes are expressed adjacent to the cardiac inflow primordia and might act through some signalling mechanism to influence subsequent heart looping.

The roles of the activin receptor and *Shh* steps in the mouse and *Xenopus* are not as clear (see King and Brown[81]) but in *Xenopus* maternal *Vg1* gene expression may be right-sided and induce the activin-like activity[82].

The important unanswered developmental question is, what induces these asymmetries in gene expression? Since lrd dynein has been found in the node and is abnormal in *iv/iv* mice could this play a role? Dyneins are motor proteins which carry other molecules towards the minus ends of microtubules. The dynein's role may be to move molecular signals that activate other genes on the node's left-hand side, or to carry signals that repress them to the right-hand side. If this were so it still remains to ask, how do the microtubules get oriented?

Theoretical models

Positional information may be universal and it may be that it is the rules of interpretation that vary between species[83]. The evidence supports this view for the AP axis and for some the presence of a Hox code is the quintessential feature of an 'animal'[84]. For example, from the third thoracic segment, which expresses the *Ultrabithorax (Ubx)* gene, the butterfly develops wings[85,86] whereas *Drosophila* develops halteres[87,88].

Left–right positional information might also be universal. Isolated discordant inversions, such as the left-sided azygos vein in rodents and the inverted gonadal asymmetries seen between mammals and birds, may be due to variations in the interpretation of positional information rather than due to alterations of the positional information itself.

The cerebral asymmetries of function are also handed with only about 7–10% of people, irrespective of global situs, being left-handed (see Lander and Brown[89]. Cerebral asymmetry may underlie the neurobiology of language and may develop by mechanisms homologous to those that establish visceral situs[90]. A recent meta-analysis of sibships supports a locus in the X–Y homologous region of the sex chromosomes being involved in cerebral asymmetry[91].

Chirality in embryos

The gradual allocation of groups of cells to more narrowly defined fates, begs two questions: 'What is the nature of the information by which cells are chosen by position?' and 'What are the molecular and cellular events that constitute the specification or change in cell fate?' The events that constitute changes in cell fate during left–right development will be similar to those involved in other changes of cell fate, but the informative mechanism by which position is chosen that leads to left being distinguished from right will be unique amongst mechanisms that provide positional information. The generation of bilateral symmetry or of random asymmetries does not require left to be distinguished from right. A left/right agnostic cobbler could make a pair of shoes but could not satisfy a request to provide only left shoes. This is the enigma of knowing left from right.

Handed left–right asymmetries thus require a chiral referent to prescribe a direction to a laterally asymmetric specification of cell fate during development. The nature of this referent is of particular interest because it acts upon a unique symmetry breaking event that is necessarily fundamentally different from those events that act to polarise the anteroposterior and the dorsoventral axes. The available chiral referents include all handed macromolecules whose chirality ultimately derives from the L-amino acids and D-sugars. This makes inverted laterally asymmetric specification by mirror-image molecular chirality most unlikely. The referent and its informative pathway are thus thought to interact with the laterally asymmetric information to prescribe to it a direction. They are otherwise thought to be independent phenomena. The laterally asymmetric information leads to laterally asymmetric specification and situs. These three – information, specification and subsequently situs – are usually conceived to be in register with one another, and to be inverted in inversus. But, as will be shown, this need not be the case.

Left–right agnosia

Faith in left–right agnosia in the aetiology of inversion is strong[25,66,92–98], but the body plan inversion should then be a perfect situs inversus or solitus at random, and this is not seen. For example, though both PCD and *iv/iv* exhibit random global situs both frequently exhibit minor defects of situs that may not be equally distributed to global solitus and inversus. To account for this, the following model is suggested. A chiral referent establishes chiral information as a gradient in [X] across the embryo. This gradient acts at the bifurcation point of a second asymmetry in [Y] via a mechanism which when defective in PCD and *iv/iv* mice leads to randomisation of [Y] and random global situs. In both PCD and *iv/iv* mice the asymmetry in [X] is still present and is developmentally active. It is in register with global situs in solitus and against it in inversus leading to the biology of the two conditions being at variance under mirror-image reflection.

The two-morphogen model

The following model accommodates a spectrum of defects of situs. Bilateral symmetry is broken by the chiral referent and a stable asymmetry is established in register with it. It is suggested that these processes are insensitive to known teratogenic or genetic insults. Two morphogen gradients are then set up with this primary asymmetry. The ratio of the concentrations of these two morphogens is informative leading to left- or right-sided cell fate specification. Lateral asymmetry is

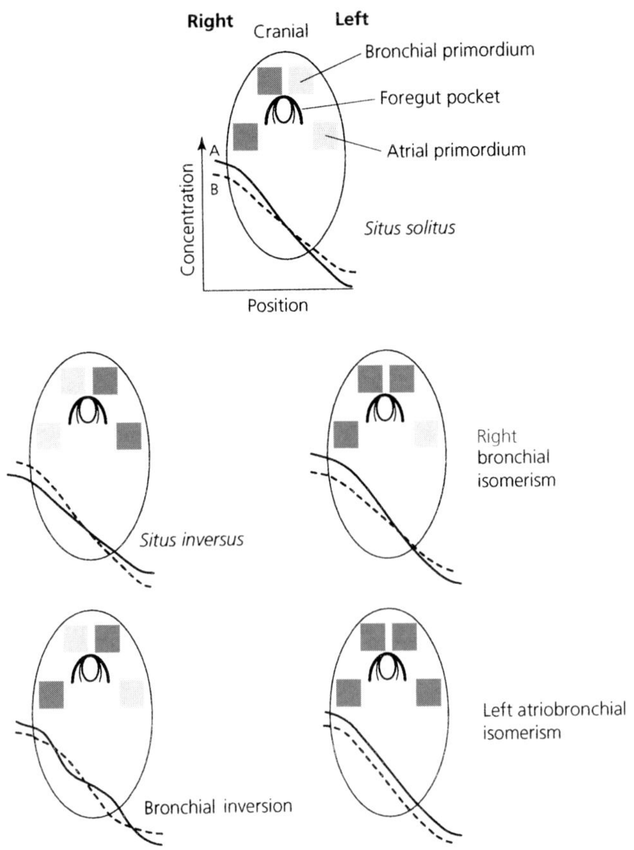

Fig. 7.2 The two-gradient model. Two morphogen gradients, A and B, are set up by a primary asymmetry. The sidedness of a primordium is right-sided if in that region the concentration of A is > B and left-sided if A is < B. Though the primary asymmetry in the gradients of A and B remains unaltered *situs inversus* and other anomalies of situs can be specified. Some anomalies with their gradients are illustrated above.

prescribed by different ratios either side of the midline (see Fig. 7.2).

This model does not require a loss or inversion of the chiral information to explain inversions, so allowing 100% inversions as in *inv/inv* mice. Furthermore, relatively minor alterations in initial conditions, perhaps even due to biological noise, can account for a collection of defects of situs including the lateral isomerisms. Also, one parameter can be varied to account for left or right isomerisms without requiring other defects of situs to be generated, as may be seen in some families. Importantly, the laterally asymmetric information underlying situs solitus is not the mirror-image of the laterally asymmetric information underlying situs inversus. 'Randomisation' is modelled with nearly indistinguishable gradients so allowing a role for stochastic factors. Thus in half the progeny the gradient prescribes solitus and in half inversus. The proximity of the gradients allows biological noise to result in occasional defects of situs. The phenotype of the double homozygote (*iv/iv, inv/inv*) is accounted for by *iv/iv* always approximating the gradients. About 7% of people are left-handed even if they have global situs inversus. It is possible that the primary handed asymmetry that underlies situs in this model may also underlie the handed cerebral asymmetries that play a role in the neurobiology of language.

Chaotic development

Schrödinger speculated that the ability of living organisms to generate order and avoid complete chaos was linked to the aperiodicity of crystal DNA. This is true, though the chaos avoided is not that of chaotic dynamics, which are deterministic[99], but that of complete randomness. In contrast, Turing[100] persuasively tells us that it is the complete randomness of fluctuations that rescues blastocysts from persistent spherical symmetry into the generation of pattern. However, these fluctuations cannot rescue us from chiral agnosia.

Turing's[100] reaction–diffusion model predicts random laterally asymmetric information but he suggested that a chiral referent at the moment of instability is all that is needed to account for the absence of bilateral symmetry. The chiral boundary conditions for this model were formally applied by Almirantis and Nicolis[94], confirming that, at the point where the system bifurcates, a shallow chiral gradient can be amplified many times. Furthermore, these dynamics raise the possibility that the direction in which the symmetry breaks could be reversed without reversing the chiral referent or its downstream action at the bifurcation point simply by altering the kinetics of the reactions.

It appears to be an assumption of much of 'molecular biology' that an understanding of large-scale biological phenomena would automatically follow from an understanding of the structure and reactions of the molecular components, even to the point where development might be computable from a knowledge of the genome and a knowledge of cell biology. In neither physical chemistry nor engineering has this reductionist philosophy been completely successful, where for example intermediate phenomenological concepts such as surface tension, viscosity, vapour pressure, enthalpy, entropy, temperature etc. are needed to describe and predict large-scale phenomena. There may be statistical analogies for these concepts based upon molecular models, but in general large-scale phenomena are not deducible from the molecular rules. Therefore, the inability to predict large-scale phenomena might not disappear with a greater understanding of the molecular nuts and bolts. One might argue that these intermediate concepts do exist, for example growth, cleavage, cell movement including invagination, differentiation, cell death, fate maps, induction, positional information and lateral inhibition. If they do exist, symmetry might be considered among their number. Each time an embryonic axis appears the system has progressed to a lower order of symmetry. At one time there is symmetry and then there is asymmetry. These are discrete events. It happens at least once for each axis. There is loss of spherical symmetry with the establishment of a dorso-ventral axis in the blastocyst, loss of radial symmetry with the establishment of the primitive streak in the gastrulating epiblast, and loss of bilateral symmetry evident when the heart loop bulges to one side.

Non-codeable molecular events

Unlike those animals which have maternally prescribed asymmetry from their earliest formation, such as *Drosophila*, the spherically symmetrical blastula must require fluctuation to break symmetry and these are small-scale phenomena that cannot be genetically coded. As Turing[100] observed, the spherical blastula has deviations from perfect symmetry that might not be regarded as important since the deviations vary greatly from blastula to blastula and the developed organisms are barely distinguishable. Yet if perfect spherical symmetry is assumed, whatever reactions and diffusions occur it will remain spherically symmetrical for ever, and quite unable to make a vertebrate. The breaking of bilateral symmetry is special, however, because it is handed and requires a chiral referent.

It is proposed that a system might exist that is sensitive enough to initial conditions to allow a control that permits the sort of amplification of orientated molecular chirality to organ handedness that is sought. Such a system under other initial conditions may also be unstable and unpredictable resulting in chaotic phenotypes or defects of situs. Further, the lateral isomerisms might be modelled as either the retention of symmetry or perhaps in a novel way as the re-acquisition of symmetry through symmetry-increasing phenomena.

Usually stresses that force systems away from equilibrium lower spatial symmetry whilst increasing the complexity of the dynamics. Less widely recognised are symmetry-increasing bifurcations in which further stresses on asymmetric chaotic states lead to higher order symmetry. So perhaps a case can be made for the isomerisms being a re-acquisition of symmetry, when stresses increase further. Such a model would allow a specific stress to induce inversions with one level of stress and isomerisms with a greater stress, so allowing one genetic defect to be associated with a number of phenotypes. Such dynamics might also explain the absence of a system with perfect random lateral asymmetries. The nuts and bolts of these dynamics are open to speculation but Turing-like bifurcations have been described in microtubular formation[101] giving precedent to the concept.

References

1. Baker-Cohen KF. Visceral and vascular transposition in fishes, and a comparison with similar anomalies in man. *Am J Anat* **109**:37–55, 1961.
2. Silverman NH. Echocardiographic anatomy. In Silverman, NH. (ed) *Pediatric Echocardiography*, pp. 1–34. Baltimore, MA: Williams & Wilkins 1993.
3. Rose V, Izukawa T, Moes CAF. Syndromes of asplenia and polysplenia. A review of cardiac and non-cardiac malformations in 60 cases with special reference to diagnosis and prognosis. *Br Heart J* **37**:840–851, 1975.
4. Solomon MH, Winn KJ, White RD, Bulkley BH, Kelly DT, Gott VL, Hutchins GM. Kartagener's syndrome with corrected transposition. Conducting system studies and coronary arterial occlusion complicating valvular replacement. *Chest* **69**:677–680, 1976.
5. Ivemark BI. Implications of agenesis of the spleen on the pathogenesis of cono-truncus anomalies in childhood. An analysis of the heart malformations in the splenic agenesis syndrome with fourteen new cases. *Acta Pediatrica* **44**:1–110, 1955.
6. Simpson J, Zellweger H. Familial occurrence of Ivemark syndrome with splenic hypoplasia and asplenia in sibs. *J Med Genet* **10**:303–304, 1973.
7. Zlotogora J, Elian E. Asplenia and polysplenia syndromes with abnormalities of lateralisation in a sibship. *J Med Genet* **18**:301–302, 1981.
8. Holmes LB, Blennerhassett JB, Austen KF. A reappraisal of Kartagener's syndrome. *Am J Med Sci* **255**:13–28, 1968.
9. Dickey LB. Kartagener's syndrome in children. *Dis Chest* **23**:657–666, 1953.
10. Bartelings MM, Gittenburger-de Groot AC. Morphogenetic considerations on congenital malformation of the outflow tract. II. Complete transposition of the great arteries and double outlet right ventricle. *Int J Cardiol* **33**:5–26, 1991.
11. Burn J, Coffey R, Allan LD, Robinson P, Pembrey ME, Macartney FJ. Isomerism: a genetic analysis. In *Pediatric Cardiology* (eds E.F. Doyle, M.A. Engle, W.M. Gersony, W.J. Rashkind & N.S. Talner) pp. 1126–1128. New York: Springer-Verlag, 1986.
12. Tunaoglu FS, Olgunturk R, Gucuyener K, Demirsoy S, Uzami:s C. Unusual variation of asplenia syndrome. *Jap Heart J* **32**:859–865, 1991.
13. Moerman P, Verbeken E, Fryns JP, Goddeeris P, Lauweryns JM. Associations of Meckel syndrome with M-anisosplenia in one patient. *Clin Genet* **22**:143–147, 1982.
14. Sharland MR, Chowcat NL, Qureshi SA, Drake DP. Intestinal obstruction caused by malrotation of the gut in atrial isomerism. *Arch Dis Child* **64**:1623–1624, 1989.
15. Chang J, Brueckner M, Touloukian RJ. Intestinal rotation and fixation abnormalities in heterotaxia: early detection and management. *J Pediatr Surg* **28**:1281–1284, 1993.
16. Moller JH, Amplatz K, Wolfson J. Malrotation of the bowel in patients with congenital heart disease associated with splenic anomalies. *Radiology* **99**:393–398, 1971.
17. Siebert JR, Machin GA, Sperber GH. Anatomic findings in dicephalic conjoined twins: implications for morphogenesis. *Teratology* **40**:305–310, 1989.
18. Cunniff C, Jones KL, Jones MC, Saunders B, Shepard T, Benirschke K. Laterality defects in conjoined twins: implications for normal asymmetry in human embryogenesis [see comments]. *Am J Med Genet* **31**:669–677, 1988.
19. Denny F, France N, Lloyd G, Sinclair L. A dicephalic monster (dicephalus isodiplopterata). *Clin Pediatr* **8**:27–31, 1969.
20. Gerlis LM, Seo JW, Ho SY, Chi JG. Morphology of the cardiovascular system in conjoined twins: spatial and sequential segmental arrangements in 36 cases. [Review]. *Teratology* **47**:91–108, 1993.
21. Seo JW, Lee YS, Chi JG. Cross-sectional illustration on major types of conjoined twins. *J Korean Med Sci* **3**:19–25, 1988.
22. Seo JW, Shin SS, Chi JG. Cardiovascular system in conjoined twins: an analysis of 14 Korean cases. *Teratology* **32**:151–161, 1985.
23. Barth RA, Filly RA, Goldberg JD, Moore P, Silverman NH. Conjoined twins: prenatal diagnosis and assessment of associated malformations [published erratum appears in *Radiology* **178**(1), 287, 1991]. *Radiology* **177**:201–207, 1990.
24. Ho SY, Frescura C, Thiene G. Isomerism of the left atrial appendage and left lung in conjoined twins. *Int J Cardiol* **27**:277–279, 1990.

25. Brown NA, Wolpert L. The development of handedness in left/right asymmetry. *Development* **109**:1–9, 1990.
26. Winston KR, Rockoff MA, Mulliken JB, Strand RD, Murray JE. Surgical division of craniopagi. [Review.] *Neurosurgery* **21**:782–791, 1987.
27. Winston KR. Craniopagi: anatomical characteristics and classification. [Review.] *Neurosurgery* **21**:769–781, 1987.
28. Gaist G, Piazza G, Galassi E, Cavina C, Salvioli GP. Craniopagus twins. An unsuccessful separation and a clinical review of the entity. *Childs Nervous System* **3**:327–333, 1987.
29. Bucholz RD, Yoon KW, Shively RE. Temporoparietal craniopagus. Case report and review of the literature. *J Neurosurg* **66**:72–79, 1987.
30. Cameron DE, Reitz BA, Carson BS. *et al.* Separation of craniopagus Siamese twins using cardiopulmonary bypass and hypothermic circulatory arrest. *J Thorac Cardiovasc Surg* **98**(Pt 2):961–967, 1989.
31. Pertuiset B, Lafourcade J, Viars P, Nicoletis C, Metzger J, Ancri D, Kasuo U, Lasselin M. [Successful separation in 1974 of craniopagus twins united at the vertex. Indications, technics, follow-up after 14 years]. [French]. *Neuro-Chirurgie* **35**:177–185, 1989.
32. Levin M, Johnson RL, Stern CD, Kuehn M, Tabin C. A molecular pathway determining left–right asymmetry in chick embryogenesis. *Cell* **82**:803–814, 1995.
33. Burn J. Disturbance of morphological laterality in humans. *Ciba Foundation Symp* **162**:282–296, 1991.
34. Dimmick JE, Bove KE, McAdams AJ. Extrahepatic biliary atresia and the polysplenia syndrome. *J Pediatr* **86**:644–645, 1975.
35. Chandra RS. Biliary atresia and other structural anomalies in the congenital polysplenia syndrome. *J Pediatr* **85**:649–655, 1974.
36. Abramson SJ, Berdon WE, Altman RP, Amodio JB, Levy J. Biliary atresia and noncardiac polysplenic syndrome: US and surgical considerations. *Radiology* **163**:377–379, 1987.
37. Carmi R, Magee CA, Neill CA, Karrer FM. Extrahepatic biliary atresia and associated anomalies: etiologic heterogeneity suggested by distinctive patterns of associations. *Am J Med Genet* **45**:683–693, 1993.
38. Brun P, Bauthier F, Boucher D, Brunelle F. Ultrasound findings in biliary atresia in children. *Ann Radiol* **28**:259–263, 1985.
39. Falchetti D, de Carvalho FB, Clapuyt P, de Ville de Goyet J, de Hemptinne B, Claus D, Otte JB. Liver transplantation in children with biliary atresia and polysplenia syndrome. *J Pediatr Surg* **26**:528–531, 1991.
40. Silveira TR, Salzano FM, Howard ER, Mowat AP. Extrahepatic biliary atresia and twinning. [Review.] *Brazilian J Med Biol Res* **24**:67–71, 1991.
41. Miyamoto M, Kajimoto T. Associated anomalies in biliary atresia patients. In *Biliary Atresia and its Related Disorders – Proceedings of an International Symposium*, (ed. M. Kasai) pp. 13–18. Amsterdam: Excerpta Medica, 1983.
42. Davenport M, Savage M, Mowat AP, Howard ER. Biliary atresia splenic malformation syndrome: an etiologic and prognostic subgroup. *Surgery* **113**:662–668, 1993.
43. Teichberg S, Markowitz J, Silverberg M, Aiges H, Schneider K, Khan E, Daum F. Abnormal cilia in a child with the polysplenia syndrome and extrahepatic biliary atresia. *J Pediatr* **100**:399–401, 1982.
44. Gershoni-Baruch R, Gottfried E, Pery M, Sahin A, Etzioni A. Immotile cilia syndrome including polysplenia, situs inversus, and extrahepatic biliary atresia. *Am J Med Genet* **33**:390–393, 1989.
45. Franco V, Aragona F. Association of specific syndromes with renal cystic disease. *Hum Pathol* **20**:496, 1989.
46. Crawfurd MA. Renal dysplasia and asplenia in two sibs. *Clin Genet* **14**:338–344, 1978.
47. Lurie IW, Kirillova IA, Novikova IV, Burakovski IV. Renal–hepatic–pancreatic dysplasia and its variants. *Genet Couns* **2**:17–20, 1991.
48. Yoshikawa Y, Watanabe T, Kato N. Bilateral renal dysplasia accompanied by pancreatic fibrosis, meconium ileus, and situs inversus totalis. *Acta Pathol Japonica* **31**:845–852, 1981.
49. Hiraoka K, Haratake J, Horie A, Miyagawa T. Bilateral renal dysplasia, pancreatic fibrosis, intrahepatic biliary dysgenesis, and situs inversus totalis in a boy. *Hum Pathol* **19**:871–873, 1988.
50. Arnold GL, Bixler D, Girod D. Probable autosomal recessive inheritance of polysplenia, situs inversus and cardiac defects in an Amish family. *Am J Med Genet* **16**:35–42, 1983.
51. Mathias RS, Lacro RV, Jones K. X-linked laterality sequence: situs inversus, complex cardiac defects, splenic defects. *Am J Med Genet* **28**:111–116, 1987.
52. Casey B, Devoto M, Jones KL, Ballabio A. Mapping a gene for familial situs abnormalities to human chromosome Xq24–q27. 1. *Nature Genet* **5**:403–407, 1993.
53. Niikawa N, Kohsaka S, Mizumoto M, Hamada I, Kajii T. Familial clustering of situs inversus totalis, and asplenia and polysplenia syndromes. *Am J Med Genet* **16**:43–47, 1983.
54. Warkany J. *Congenital Malformations: Notes and Comments*. Chicago: Year Book Medical Publishers Inc, 1971.
55. Fujinaga M, Maze M, Hoffman BB, Baden JM. Activation of α_1-adrenergic receptors modulates the control of left/right sidedness in rat embryos. *Dev Biol* **150**:419–421, 1992.
56. Wilson JG, Jordon HC, Brent RL. Effects of irradiation on embryonic development. II. X-rays on the ninth day of gestation in the rat. *Am J Anat* **92**:153–188, 1953.
57. Fujinaga M, Baden JM, Yhap EO, Mazze RI. Reproductive and teratogenic effects of nitrous oxide, isoflurance and their combination in Sprague–Dawley rats. *Anesthesiology* **67**:960–964, 1987.
58. Kucera J. Rate and type of congenital anomalies among offspring of diabetic mothers. *J Reprod Med* **7**:61–70, 1971.
59. Magee CA, Lurie I, Kuehl K, Ferencz C, Loffredo C. Looping anomalies of the heart and great vessels; associated risk factors. *Teratology (Ter Soc Abs)* **49**:(Abs 35), 372, 1994.
60. Rowland TW, Hubbell JP, Nadas AS. Congenital heart disease in infants of diabetic mothers. *J Pediatr.* **83**:815–820, 1973.
61. Dunn V, Nixon GW, Jaffe RB, Condon VR. Infants of diabetic mothers: radiographic manifestations. *Am J Roentgenol* **137**:123–128, 1981.
62. Morishima M, Ando M, Takao A. Visceroatrial heterotaxy syndrome in the *NOD* mouse with special reference to atrial situs. *Teratology* **44**:91–100, 1991.
63. Lander A, Brown NA. Culture-induced inversion of heart looping in pre-somite rat embryos is reduced by either superoxide dismutase or α-cyano-4-hydroxycinnamic acid. *Teratology (Ter Soc Abs)* **49**:(P10), 387, 1994.
64. Shishko PI, Kovalev PA, Goncharov VG, Zajarny IU. Comparison of peripheral and portal (via the umbilical vein) routes of insulin infusion in IDDM patients. *Diabetes* **41**:1042–1049, 1992.
65. Carlsten A, Hallgren B, Jagenburg R, Svanborg A, Werkö L. Amino acids and free fatty acids in plasma in diabetes. I. The effect of insulin on the arterial levels. *Acta Med Scand* **179**:361–370, 1966.
66. Afzelius BA. A human syndrome caused by immotile cilia. *Science* **193**:317–319, 1976.
67. Fujimoto H, Yanagisawa KO. Defects in the archenteron of mouse embryos homozygous for the T-mutation. *Differentiation* **25**:44–47, 1983.
68. Bellomo D, Lander A, Harragan I, Brown NA. Cell proliferation in mammalian gastrulation: the ventral node and notochord are relatively quiescent. *Dev Dyn* **205**:471–485, 1996.
69. Rautiainen M, Collan Y, Nuutinen J, Afzelius BA. Ciliary orientation in the 'immotile cilia' syndrome. *Eur Arch Otorhinolaryngol.* **247**:100–103, 1990.
70. von Baer KE. *Entwicklungsgeschichte der Tiere: Beobachtung und Reflexion.* Königsberg: Bornträger, 1828.
71. Hummel KP, Chapman DB. Visceral inversion and associated anomalies in the mouse. *J Hered* **50**:9–13, 1959.
72. Seo JW, Brown NA, Ho SY, Anderson RH. Abnormal laterality and congenital cardiac anomalies: relations of visceral and cardiac morphologies in the *iv/iv* mouse. *Circulation* **86**:642–650, 1992.
73. Brueckner M, D'Eustachio P, Horwich AL. Linkage mapping of a mouse gene, *iv*, that controls left–right asymmetry of the heart and viscera. *Proc Natl Acad Sci USA* **86**:5035–5038, 1989.
74. de Meeus A, Alonso S, Demaille J, Bouvagnet P. A detailed linkage map of subtelomeric murine chromosome 12 region including the situs inversus mutation locus IV. *Mamm Genome* **3**:637–643, 1992.
75. Supp DM, Witte DP, Potter SS, Brueckner M. Mutation of an axonemal dynein affects left–right asymmetry in inversus viscerum mice. *Nature* **389**:963–966, 1997.
76. Yokoyama T, Copeland NG, Jenkins NA, Montgomery CA, Elder FFB, Overbeek PA. Reversal of left–right asymmetry: a situs inversus mutation. *Science* **260**:679–682, 1993.

77. Levin M, Pagan S, Roberts DJ, Cooke J, Kuehn MR, Tabin CJ. Left/right patterning signals and the independent regulation of different aspects of situs in the chick embryo. *Dev Biol* **189**:57–67, 1997.
78. Lowe LA, Supp DM, Sampath K, Yokoyama T, Wright CV, Potter SS, Overbeek P, Kuehn MR. Conserved left–right asymmetry of nodal expression and alterations in murine situs inversus. *Nature* **381**:158–161, 1996.
79. Isaac A, Sargent M, Cooke J. Control of vertebrate left–right asymmetry by a snail related zinc finger gene. *Science* **275**:1301–1304, 1997.
80. Collignon J, Varlet I, Robertson EJ. Relationship between asymmetric nodal expression and the direction of embryonic turning. *Nature* **381**:155–158, 1996.
81. King T, Brown NA. Embryonic asymmetry: Left TGF β at the right time? *Curr Biol* **7**:212–215, 1997.
82. Hyatt BA, Lohr JL, Yost HJ. Initiation of vertebrate left–right axis formation by maternal Vg1. *Nature* **384**:62–65, 1996.
83. Wolpert L. Positional information and pattern formation. *Curr Top Dev Biol* **6**:183–224, 1971.
84. Slack JMW, Holland PWH, Graham CF. The zootype and the phylotypic stage. *Nature* **361**:490–492, 1993.
85. Warren RW, Nagy L, Selegue J, Gates J, Carroll S. Evolution of homeotic gene regulation and function in flies and butterflies [see comments] [published erratum appears in *Nature* (1995) **373**(6513), 451]. *Nature* **372**:458–461, 1994.
86. Warren RW, Nagy L, Selegue J, Gates J, Carroll S. Evolution of homeotic gene regulation and function in flies and butterflies. *Nature* **373**:451, 1995.
87. Lawrence PA, Sampedro J. *Drosophila* segmentation: after the first three hours. *Development* **119**:971–976, 1993.
88. Lawrence PA. *The Making of a Fly: The Genetics of Animal Design*. Oxford: Blackwell Scientific Publications, 1992.
89. Lander A, Brown NA. Abnormalities of lateralization. In *Gray's Anatomy*, 38th edn., pp. 119–121, 1995.
90. McManus IC. The inheritance of left-handedness. *Ciba Foundation Symposium* **162**:251–267, 1991.
91. Corballis MC, Lee K, McManus IC, Crow TJ. Location of the handedness gene on the X and Y chromosomes. *Am J Med Genetics* **67**:50–52, 1996.
92. Layton WM. Random determination of a developmental process: reversal of normal visceral asymmetry in the mouse. *J Hered* **67**:336–338, 1976.
93. Moreno A, Murphy EA. Inheritance of Kartagener syndrome. *Am J Med Genet* **8**:305–313, 1981.
94. Almirantis Y, Nicolis G. Morphogenesis in an asymmetric medium. *Bull Math Biol* **49**:519–538, 1987.
95. Almirantis Y. Left–right asymmetry in vertebrates. *Bioessays* **17**:79–83, 1995.
96. Wilhelmi H. Experimentelle untersuchungen über situs inversus viscerum. *Arch f Entwcklngsmech d Organ* **48**:517–532, 1921.
97. Oppenheimer JM. Asymmetry revisited. *Am Zool* **14**:867–879, 1974.
98. Wehrmaker A. Right–left asymmetry and situs inversus in *Triturus alpestris*. *Wilhelm Roux Arch Entwmech Org* **163**:1–32, 1969.
99. May RM. Simple mathematical models with very complicated dynamics [erratum: Figures 2 and 3 should be transposed but the captions were correct]. *Nature* **261**:459–467, 1976.
100. Turing AM. The chemical basis of morphogenesis. *Phil Trans R Soc B* **237**:37–72, 1952.
101. Tabony J. Morphological bifurcations involving reaction–diffusion processes during microtubule formation. *Science* **264**:245–248, 1994.

Development of the head

8

P. Collins

Introduction

The human head contains the neural tissue necessary for our cognition, coupled with a complex grouping of special sense organs for our perception. There is a vast array of touch and temperature receptors which allow the examination of the local environment with great discrimination and a range of small muscles in the face and the tongue which can be used with exquisite control. Movements of the facial and oral musculature form part of our rich non-verbal communication repertoire, and integration of the skeletal and visceral functions in this region permits the range of reflexes which keep us alive and able to interact in our prescribed social contexts. Complex control of this region occurs in the newborn. Indeed, the sucking and swallowing reflexes seen in the neonate and preterm infant require the coordination of most of the twelve cranial nerves. Within the first couple of feeds, the full-term neonate can suck at a rate of once per second, swallow after five or six sucks, and breathe during every second or third suck. Milk crosses the pharynx en route to the oesophagus, and air passes in and out of the nasopharynx and lungs without apparent interruption of breathing and swallowing. Throughout this operation there is little significant misdirection of fluids into the trachea or air into the stomach[1].

The ease with which suckling is established in the neonate is a reflection of the match between the skull shape and palatal development at birth, and the mammary apparatus of the mother. Generally, vertebrate neonates have rounded skulls which assist passage along the birth canal, and relatively short faces which facilitate ease of suckling. It is only after weaning that the range of vertebrate skulls are expressed as in the elongated snouts of the ant eater and the tapir. The ability of the vertebrate skull to produce such a range of variation from what appears to be a basic plan is due to the recruitment of a novel mesenchymal population in the vertebrates alone, the neural crest.

The successful development of the head with all its component parts is due to the accurate expression of genes throughout all of the tissues of the head, from the neuro-epithelia, surface ectoderm and endodermal epithelia, to the neural crest, somitic and angiogenic mesenchymal populations.

Development of the head is often dealt with by linear descriptions of individual systems, e.g. nervous system, gastrointestial system, etc. While this approach is helpful for understanding the cranial portions of these systems, it does not convey the interaction and complexity which is seen in head development. This chapter is an attempt to bring together all these aspects so that the integration of the systems in this region can be appreciated. The range of interrelated structures developing in concert in the head can be seen in Fig. 8.1. The developmental processes occurring within the head will be presented with some of the more recent findings from experimental investigations.

Formation of the neural population

Specification of the neural population begins at gastrulation when the primitive streak forms[1a]. Cells which proliferate and invaginate at the most rostral end of the streak, the *primitive node* (Hensen's node) form the *notochordal process*, also termed the 'head process' (rather misleadingly), chordamesoderm, or chorda. From this same position a surface population of neural ectodermal cells proliferate in concert with the notochordal cells. Both populations are suggested to arise from a common progenitor cell[2]. Forward migration of both the notochordal cells and the overlying midline neural ectodermal cells is matched and continues rostrally until the cells contact the prechordal plate, a localised thickening of the first endodermal population to ingress at the primitive node. The prechordal

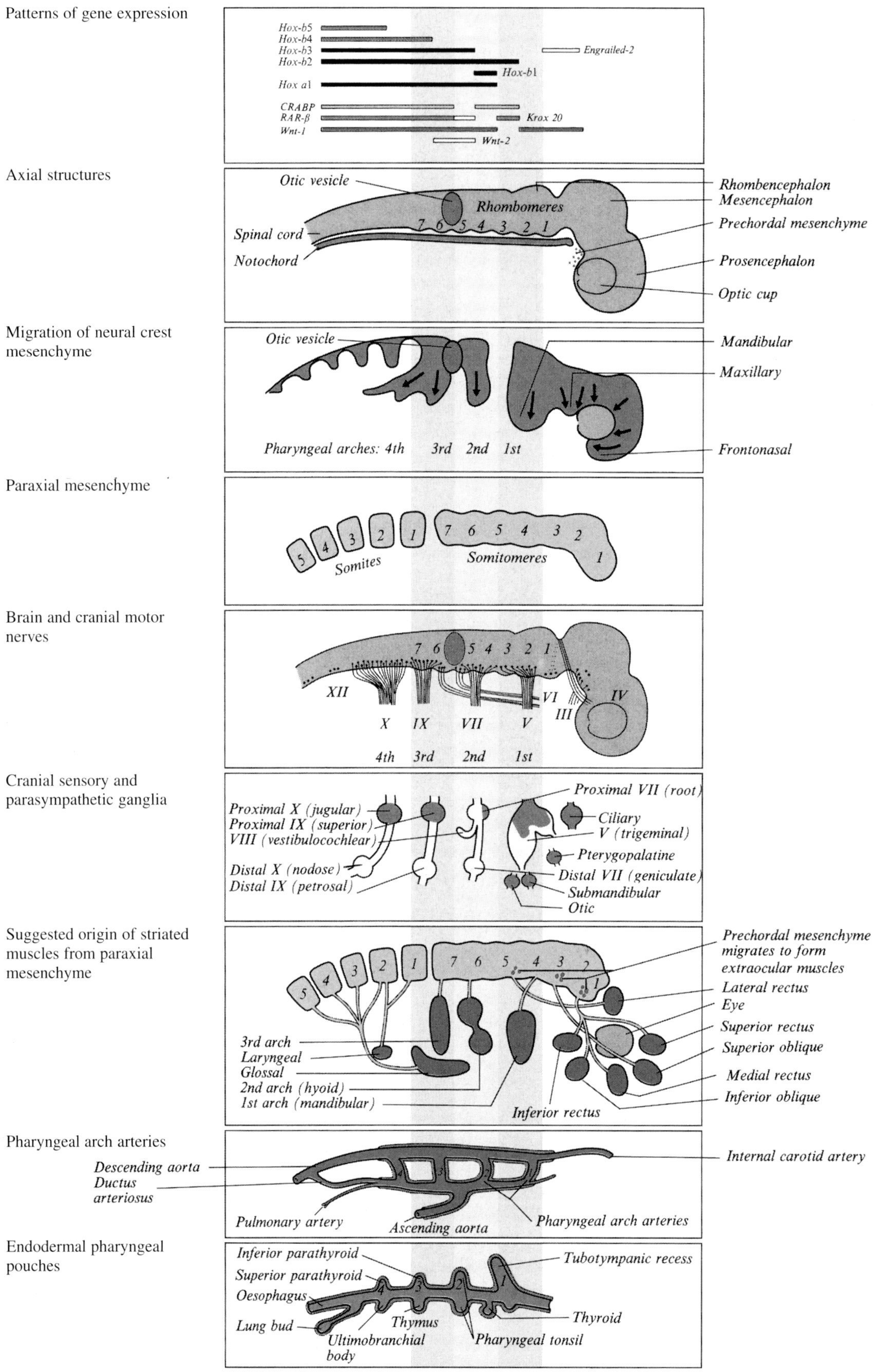
Patterns of gene expression
Hox-b5
Hox-b4
Hox-b3
Hox-b2
Engrailed-2
Hox-b1
Hox a1
CRABP
RAR-β
Krox 20
Wnt-1
Wnt-2
Axial structures
Otic vesicle
Rhombomeres
7 6 5 4 3 2 1
Spinal cord
Notochord
Rhombencephalon
Mesencephalon
Prechordal mesenchyme
Prosencephalon
Optic cup
Migration of neural crest mesenchyme
Otic vesicle
Mandibular
Maxillary
Pharyngeal arches: 4th 3rd 2nd 1st
Frontonasal
Paraxial mesenchyme
5 4 3 2 1
Somites
7 6 5 4 3 2 1
Somitomeres
Brain and cranial motor nerves
7 6 5 4 3 2 1
XII
VI
IV
III
X IX VII V
4th 3rd 2nd 1st
Cranial sensory and parasympathetic ganglia
Proximal X (jugular)
Proximal IX (superior)
VIII (vestibulocochlear)
Distal X (nodose)
Distal IX (petrosal)
Proximal VII (root)
Ciliary
V (trigeminal)
Pterygopalatine
Distal VII (geniculate)
Submandibular
Otic
Suggested origin of striated muscles from paraxial mesenchyme
5 4 3 2 1
7 6 5 4 3 2 1
3rd arch
Laryngeal
Glossal
2nd arch (hyoid)
1st arch (mandibular)
Inferior rectus
Prechordal mesenchyme migrates to form extraocular muscles
Lateral rectus
Eye
Superior rectus
Superior oblique
Medial rectus
Inferior oblique
Pharyngeal arch arteries
Descending aorta
Ductus arteriosus
Pulmonary artery
Ascending aorta
Pharyngeal arch arteries
Internal carotid artery
Endodermal pharyngeal pouches
Inferior parathyroid
Superior parathyroid
Oesophagus
Lung bud
Thymus
Ultimobranchial body
Tubotympanic recess
Thyroid
Pharyngeal tonsil

plate can be thought of as the site of the future buccopharyngeal membrane, but has other characteristics (see below).

At the onset of primitive streak formation, the putative neural population occupies a zone at the rostral end of the embryonic disc (see Fig. 1.1). After streak formation and the invagination of the notochordal process and the prechordal plate, the neural ectoderm forms a neural plate which is widest at its rostral end, tapering caudally to a narrower zone. The neural plate does not extend to the edges of the embryonic disc, it is surrounded by surface ectoderm. The midline cells of the neural plate match the length of, and are in contact with, the notochordal process. The edges of the plate are raised as folds and distinct from the surface ectoderm. Prior to neurulation, only the brain and cervical regions of the nervous system are represented within the neural plate. As the embryo grows, cells are added to the caudal end of the neural plate matching the increase in notochordal length. The most caudal region of the neural tube develops by a different mechanism (see below).

Three distinct neural populations arise from this early arrangement of neural ectoderm:

- The precursors of the central nervous system.
- The precursors of the peripheral nervous system.
- The ectodermal placodes.

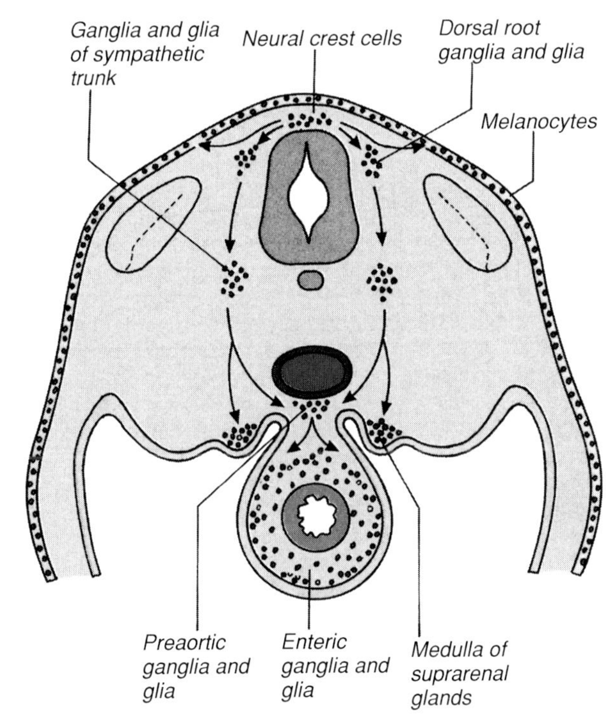

Fig. 8.2 Diagram showing the migration routes taken by neural crest cells in the trunk. (From Gray's Anatomy, 38th edition, Edinburgh: Churchill Livingstone, 1995, p. 234.)

The precursors of the central nervous system arise from the neural plate excluding the edges. The cells produce populations of neurons and glia. The peripheral nervous system arises from populations of cells in the neural folds at the edges of the neural plate, the so-called neural crest. Neural crest cells give rise to all the peripheral ganglia, somatic sensory and autonomic, and their supporting glia, including the neurons and glia of the enteric nervous system (Fig. 8.2). They further produce the cells of the adrenal medulla and melanocytes which later invade the developing epidermis. The ectodermal placodes are neural cells which remain within the surface ectoderm of the head after neurulation to invaginate later. They contribute to the sensory ganglia of the cranial nerves and the epithelium of the inner ear (Fig. 8.3). Some placodal cells, e.g. those forming the olfactory mucosa, are found in the neural folds in local regions where typical crest cells are absent.

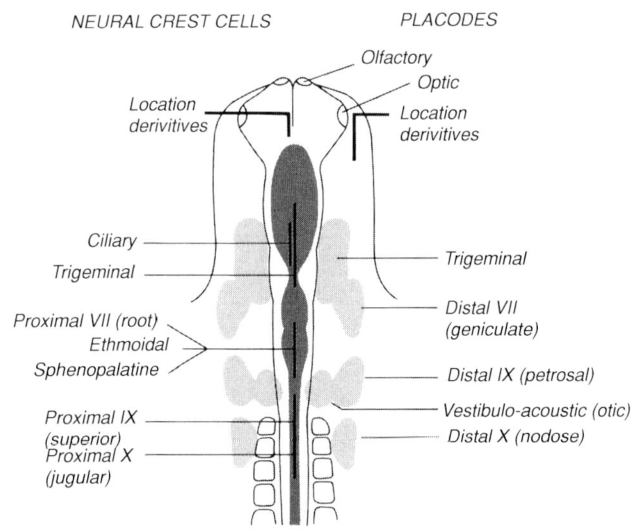

Fig. 8.3 Diagram indicating the contribution of neural crest cells and placodal cells to the ganglia in the head. (From Gray's Anatomy, 38th edition, Edinburgh: Churchill Livingstone, 1995, p. 225.)

Contribution of the early neural crest to the head

At the time of neurulation, the neural crest cells occupy a zone at the outermost edges of the neural plate, adjacent to the surface ectoderm. When neural epithelial fusion occurs, the crest cells invaginate deep to the surface ectoderm and begin their migration around the forming neural tube. Non-neuronal migratory neural crest cells are produced along the neural axis rostrally as far as the diencephalon, a position corresponding

Fig. 8.1 Schema illustrating the organization of the head and pharynx in an embryo at about stage 14. The individual tissue components have been separated but are aligned in register through the numbered zones (after Noden[11]). (From Gray's Anatomy, 38th edition, Edinburgh: Churchill Livingstone, 1995, p. 286.)

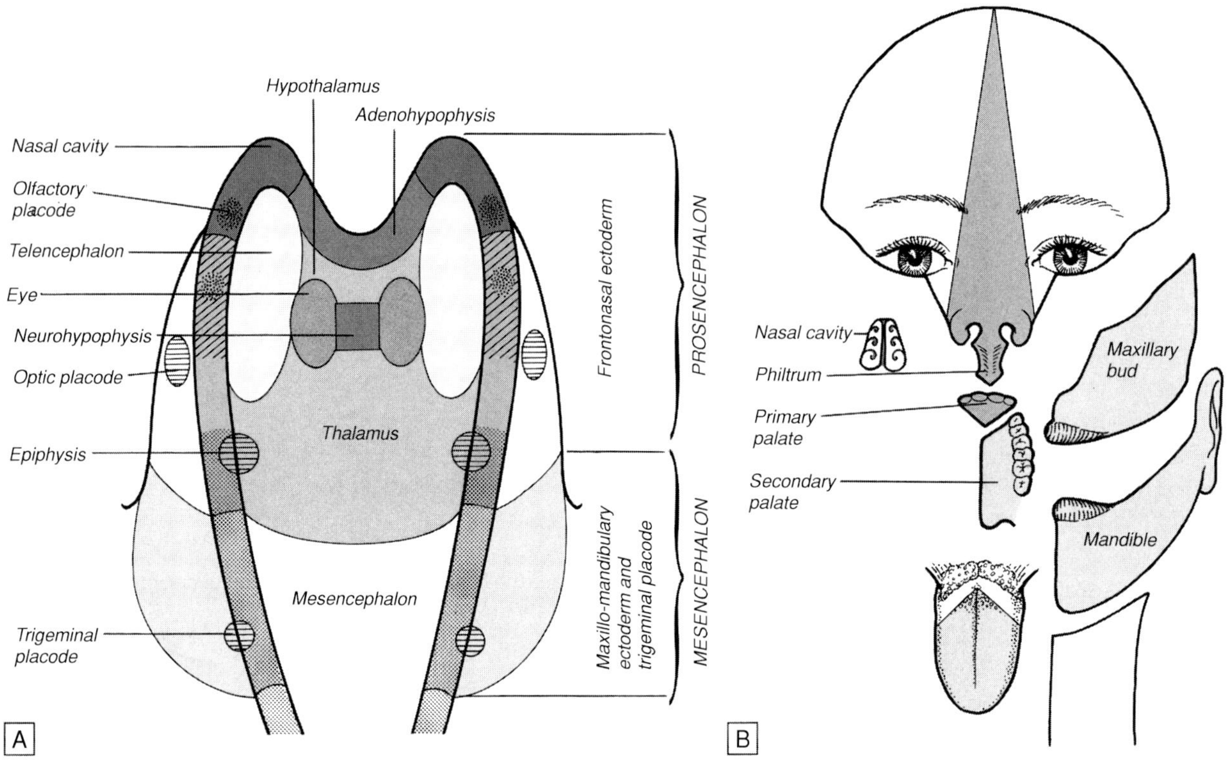

Fig. 8.4 Fate map of the rostral region of the neural primordium as established by the quail–chick chimera system. (A) The various territories yielding rostral head are indicated on the neural plate and neural fold of a 1–3 somite embryo. (B) The results obtained in the avian embryo have been extrapolated to the human head. Thus, the rostral neural fold area yields the epithelium of the rostral roof of the mouth, the nasal cavities and part of the frontal area. (From Gray's Anatomy, 38th edition, Edinburgh: Churchill Livingstone, 1995, p. 222.)

to the extent of the neural floor plate and notochord. Cells arising from the neural fold rostral to this level give rise to the hypophyseal placode, i.e. the future Rathke's pouch, the olfactory placodes and associated nasal epithelium, including the roof of the nasopharynx and the skin of the frontonasal area (Fig. 8.4). The non-neuronal neural crest provides a significant mesenchymal population in the head and neck.

Paraxial mesenchyme and the neural tube

The neural plate is supported by underlying mesoblast populations which are invaginating through the primitive streak. When neurulation begins, the underlying paraxial mesenchymal population undergoes segmentation to form somites (see below). The process of somitogenesis occurs in concert with neural tube closure. Failure of neurulation will result in incomplete development of the somites and anomalous development of the vertebrae at that level, e.g. spina bifida.

Neurulation

The neural plate extends much further laterally in the head region than in the trunk. The rapid growth of the plate and underlying mesoblast promotes the ventral movement of the edges of the embryonic disc and neurulation. Neurulation begins at about 19 post-ovulatory (p.o.) days (stage 9 see p. 5) when the neural epithelial cells become elongated and then wedge shaped as a result of changes in the conformation of their cytoskeletal elements. The underlying mesoblast and extracellular matrix provide support for the elevating folds and surface ectoderm and assist the alignment of the neural layers as they approach and fuse. Neural tube fusion begins in the hindbrain or upper cervical region at about 22–23 p.o. days (stage 10). This is primary neurulation. It extends both rostrally and caudally until only small neuropores remain open at each end. The rostral neuropore closes in the middle of the fourth week and the caudal neuropore closes slightly later. Secondary neurulation occurs in the lumbosacral region of the spinal cord, involving cavitation of a single mass of cells.

Formation of the notochord

The first cell lines which invaginate through the rostral end of the primitive streak form a *notochordal process*. This is a flat plate of epithelial cells which form the roof of the secondary yolk sac, the notochordal cells being in contact with laterally placed endodermal cells which are invaginating contemporaneously. The notochord separates from the endoderm by a mechanism similar to neurulation, i.e. the cells become wedge shaped and the population forms a groove followed by a tube with the edges opposing and fusing.

The notochord separates from the alimentary tract early in development. However, the last region to contain a notochordal process is the pharynx. Here the notochordal process remains within the endodermal layer until stage 11. It may be that this arrangement facilitates interactions in this region as, whereas in the cervical and more caudal regions the notochord is involved in sclerotome formation, rostrally the unsegmented paraxial mesenchyme overlying the pharyngeal region may receive different inductive information to initiate its differentiation into skull components; perhaps the later retention of the notochordal process in the pharynx promotes this.

Earlier works identified a mesenchymal population referred to as *prechordal mesenchyme* which was suggested to be part of the prechordal plate (see below). However, more recent experimental studies have shown that immediately after its formation the notochordal process is composed of determined myogenic cells[3]; later, myogenic cells are not present. As development proceeds the posterior portion of the notochordal process becomes transformed into the notochord proper, whereas the prechordal cells retain a mesenchymal morphology and myogenic fate. Orthotopic grafting has demonstrated that these cells later join the more laterally

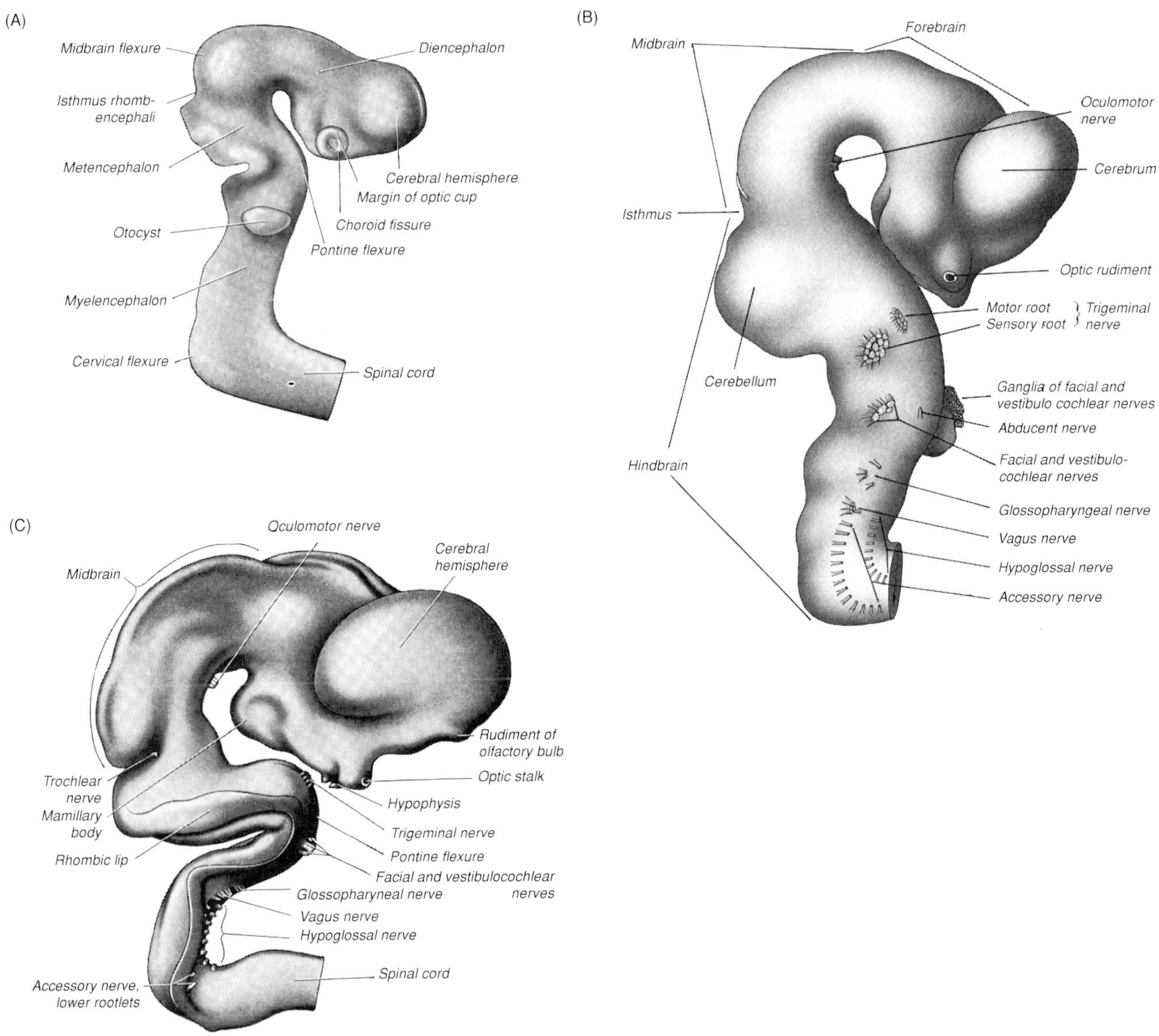

Fig. 8.5 (A) The right side of the brain of a human embryo, 9 mm long. (Drawn from a model by His.) (B) The brain of a human embryo about 10.2 mm long: right lateral surface. (From a model by His.) (C) The right side of the brain of a human embryo, 13.6 mm long. The roof of the hindbrain has been removed. (From a model by His.) (From Gray's Anatomy, 38th edition, Edinburgh: Churchill Livingstone, 1995, p. 220.)

placed paraxial mesenchyme and finally migrate to become the oculomotor musculature of the eyes (see below).

Early development of the brain

Even prior to closure of the neural tube, the neural plate is much more extensive at its rostral end. Here, elevation of the neural folds produces three deep, slit-like putative brain vesicles. The *prosencephalon*, or forebrain, the *mesencephalon* or midbrain and the *rhombencephalon* or hindbrain, continuous caudally with the spinal cord. Later the roof of the rhombencephalon thins and becomes covered with non-neural tissue. As a result of relatively unequal growth occurring in each of these brain regions three flexures appear in the brain; two flexures are concave ventrally with corresponding flexures of the head, e.g. the mesencephalic flexure at the rostral end of the notochord and the cephalic flexure at the junction of the hindbrain and spinal cord. The third flexure has its convexity directed ventrally at the level of the future pons.

With the development of the flexures the original three brain vesicles enlarge allowing some further subdivision. The rhombencephalon is subdivided by the pontine flexure into the metencephalon rostrally which will give rise to the pons and cerebellum, and the myelencephalon caudally which will give rise to the medulla oblongata. The mesencephalon remains undivided; however, the prosencephalon is divided into two parts, the telencephalon, from which paired, lateral evagination will develop into the cerebral hemispheres, and the diencephalon which will form the lateral walls of the IIIrd ventricle (Fig. 8.5).

Rhombomeres

Prior to the development of the brain vesicles a series of eight bulges can be seen in the walls of the rhombencephalon, these are termed *rhombomeres*. They constitute the primary patterning units in this region. Single-cell labelling experiments have shown that cells within rhombomeres form segregated non-mixing populations. Rhombomeres can be seen for only a short period of time in early development. However, it is thought that during this period, morphogenetic specification of the neural crest arising from the rhombencephalon occurs (Fig. 8.6). Neural crest cells from rhombomeres 1 and 2 contribute to the trigeminal ganglion, crest cells from rhombomere 4 contribute to the facial and vestibuloacoustic ganglion, while crest cells from rhombomere 6 contribute to the superior petrosal ganglion. There are no contributions to the ganglia from rhombomeres 3 and 5. As well as contributing to the somatic sensory ganglia, the neural crest cells also give rise to the parasympathetic ganglia in the head, the ciliary and pterygopalatine ganglia in the frontonasal region, and the otic and submandibular ganglia within the first arch (Fig. 8.1). Within the neck, neural crest cells give rise to the cervical ganglia of the sympathetic trunk.

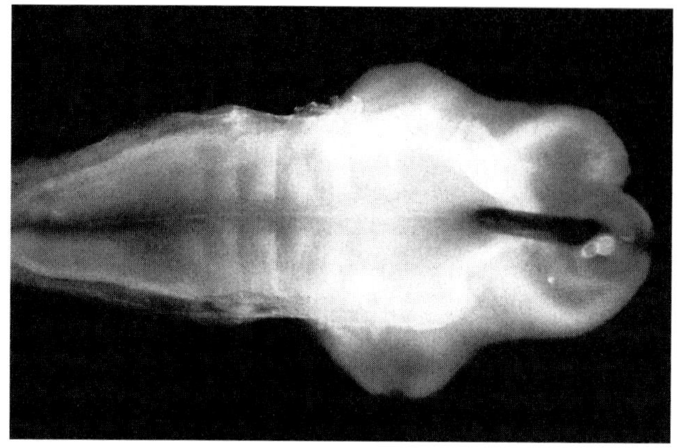

Fig. 8.6 Photograph showing rhombomeric segmentation (Photograph supplied by Prof. A. Lumsden. From Gray's Anatomy, 38th edition, Edinburgh: Churchill Livingstone, 1995, p. 225.)

Expression of genes in the Hox a, b, c and d clusters have been studied in a number of vertebrates. Hox genes are expressed in the rhombomeres and also in neural crest arising at the same level. When neural crest migration is complete the same set of Hox genes is activated in the surface ectoderm[4] (see p. 79 and Fig. 8.7).

Patterning in the early neural tube

The close relationship between the notochord and neural floor plate is maintained during neurulation and is necessary for the correct specification of the motor and sensory neurons in the spinal cord. Motor neurons differentiate ventrally very close to the floor plate whereas sensory neurons differentiate close to the roof plate. Experiments in the chick have shown that if the notochord is removed the neural floor plate is eliminated and normally dorsally placed, sensory neurones are produced, whereas if a notochord or a floor plate is grafted to the dorsal midline of the neural tube ectopic motor neurones are induced (Fig. 8.8).

Within the mesencephalon and rhombencephalon, the same organisation of cranial nerves is generally seen, the motor nerves being placed ventrally and the sensory inputs dorsally. With the widening of the rhombencephalic vesicle, the future IVth ventricle, this arrangement is more linear with the motor nerves arising medially and the sensory ones laterally. Thus the motor cranial nerves III, IV, VI and XII broadly parallel the organisation of the somatic motor neurons in the spinal cord. However, the mixed cranial nerves V, VII, IX and X which supply the pharyngeal arches exit more dorsally than the somatic motor nerves. This is suggested to be because of the effect of the locally migrating neural crest cells.

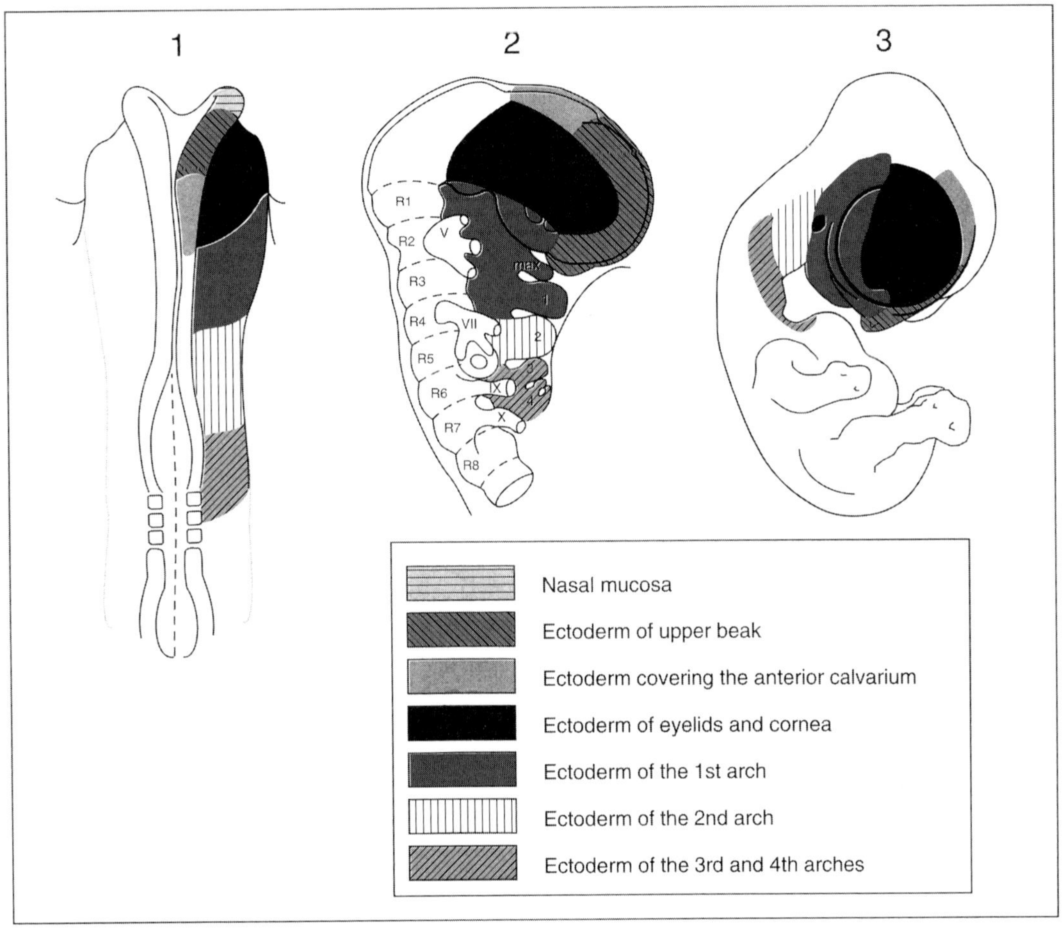

Fig. 8.7 Growth of the ectodermal territories in the chick from the 3-somite stage (1) to the 8-day embryo (3). In (2) the rhombomeres are indicated and the cranial nerves supplying the pharyngeal arches; there is no neural crest outflow from rhombomeres 3 and 5. V = trigeminal nerve; VII = facial nerve; IX = glossopharyngeal nerve; X = vagus nerve; Max = maxillary prominence; the pharyngeal arches are indicated 1–4. (Adapted from Couly, Le Pouarin 1990.)

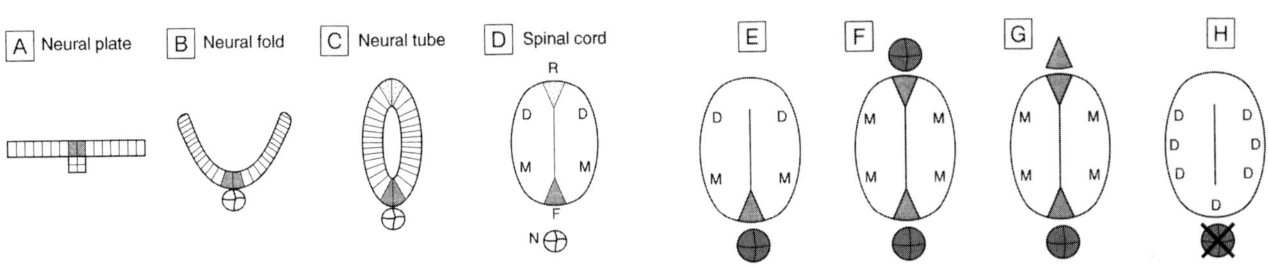

Fig. 8.8 (A–D) Diagrams to show successive stages in the development of the neural tube and spinal cord. (A) The neural plate consists of epithelial cells. Cells at the midline of the neural plate are contacted directly by the notochord. More lateral regions of the neural plate overlie the paraxial mesenchyme (not shown). (B) During neurulation, the neural plate bends at its midline elevating the lateral edges of the plate as the neural folds. Contact between the midline of the neural plate and the notochord is maintained at this stage. (C) The neural tube is formed when the dorsal tips of the neural folds fuse. Cells in the region of fusion form a specialized group of dorsal midline cells, the *roof plate*. (D) Cells at the ventral midline of the neural tube retain proximity to the notochord and differentiate into the *floor plate*. After neural tube closure neuroepithelial cells continue to proliferate and eventually differentiate into defined classes of neurons at different dorsoventral positions within the spinal cord. For example, sensory relay, commissural and other classes of dorsal neurons (D) differentiate near to the roof plate (R), and motor (M) neurons differentiate ventrally near to the floor plate (F), which by this time is no longer in contact with the notochord (N). (E–H) These figures summarize the results obtained from experiments in chick embryos in which a notochord or floor plate is grafted to the dorsal midline of the neural tube and in which the notochord is removed before neural tube closure. (E) The normal condition, showing the ventral location of motor neurons (M) and the dorsal location of sensory relay neurons (D). (F) Dorsal grafts of a notochord result in the induction of a floor plate at the dorsal midline and in the induction of ectopic dorsal motor neurons. (G) Dorsal grafts of a floor plate also result in the induction of a new floor plate at the dorsal midline and in the induction of ectopic dorsal motor neurons. (H) Removal of the notochord results in the elimination of the floor plate and the motor neurons and the expression of dorsal cells types (D) in the ventral region of the spinal cord. (After Jessell & Dodd 1992 with permission of W.B. Saunders.)

Predictive fate maps of the neural plate and neural crest

The close proximity of the neural plate and neural crest populations in the rostral end of the neural plate contribute, in many cases jointly, to structures of the special senses and face. Mapping the fate of cells in this region using chick–quail chimera experimentation has revealed what each part of the floor and adjacent neural folds become (see Fig. 8.4). From these studies, the elegant complexity of development can be appreciated. For example, the parts of the hypophysis develop adjacent to each other in the early neural epithelium. The part destined to be the neurohypophysis is found in the floor of the neural plate separated from the adenohypophysis by the hypothalamus. The adenohypophysis, in the rostral neural fold, will remain as an ectodermal placode after neurulation invaginating later as Rathke's pouch to join the neurohypophysis as it evaginates from the diencephalon. The nasal epithelium also arises from the rostral neural folds along with the special epithelium which will give rise to the olfactory placodes. These will form the sensory neurones of the Ist cranial nerve. Much of the frontonasal portion of the face also arises from the neural folds, which contribute both ectodermal and mesenchymal cells to this area.

Development of the skull

The skull has two distinct portions, the *neurocranium* which surrounds the brain and special sense organs, and the *viscerocranium* which includes the lower face and jaws, the palate, hyoid, epiglottis and larynx. The neurocranium is formed from paraxial mesenchyme from the first five somites, the unsegmented paraxial mesenchyme rostral to the first somite, and from neural crest. The viscerocranium is derived exclusively from neural crest mesenchyme.

Formation of somites from paraxial mesenchyme

Paraxial mesenchyme is derived from the early invagination of cells through the primitive node and streak. Cells ingressing through the primitive node form the medial portion of the paraxial mesenchyme, while cells ingressing through the rostral part of the streak form the lateral portion[5]. The paraxial mesenchyme extends rostrally to lie lateral to the notochord. From the lateral sides of the rhombencephalon, caudal to the otic vesicle, the paraxial mesenchyme undergoes segmentation to form the somites. Each somite is formed by the compaction of a cluster of paraxial mesenchymal cells and their transformation into an epithelial cuboid. The cells become polarised with respect to a central lumen, developing cilia on their apical surface. The cells are joined by tight junctions and produce a basal lamina. Processes from the somite cells pass through the basal lamina to contact the basal laminae of the neural tube and notochord.

Each somite can be described as having six facets like a cube and each facet has a slightly different fate. The fate of somites also varies depending on the position it occupies along the length of the embryo (Fig. 8.9). The ventromedial cells of the somite transform to mesenchyme and are termed the *sclerotome*. These cells migrate toward and with the sclerotome of the other side, surround the notochord; they will give rise to the bones, joints and ligaments of the vertebral column. There is a resegmentation of the sclerotomic mesenchyme with the caudal half of one pair of sclerotomes fusing with the cranial half of the pair of sclerotomes below to make a vertebral body initially then the components of the neural arch and spine later. The spinal nerves preferentially grow through the cranial half of the sclerotomes and the position of the spinal nerves specifies the location of the intervertebral discs.

The remaining cells of the somite are now termed the *epithelial plate of the somite*. They form a germinal epithelium which produces a number of discrete myogenic lineages. Myotomal cells form initially at the dorsomedial lip of the epithelial somite extending from the cranial to the caudal border. These dorsolateral cells will become the epaxial muscle mass which forms the muscles dorsal to the vertebrae, mainly the erector spinae group. They remain attached to each end of their somite so are finally attached to adjacent vertebrae. Myoblast populations also arise from the ventrolateral edge of specific somites; the occiptial somites produce cells which migrate to the tongue and somites opposite the limb buds give rise to the limb myoblasts. Both of these origins produce premitotic populations which proliferate as they migrate. The remaining epithelial plates of all the somites grow into the flank of the body where they fuse to form a premuscular mass which gives rise to the ventrolateral muscles of the body wall, the hypaxial muscles.

Neural crest around the developing brain

With closure of the neural tube populations of mesenchymal neural crest cells migrate around the brain to stream into the pharyngeal arches. Some cells remain covering the neural epithelium and give rise to the meninges and dermal bones of the cranial vault.

MENINGES

The meninges are usually divided in development into the pachymeninx (dura mater) and the leptomeninges (arachnoid layer, subarachnoid space with arachnoid cells and fibres, and pia mater). Pia mater is seen first as a network containing blood vessels on the surface of the neural tube extending to the mesencephalon by about day 27. Mesenchyme at the rostral end of the notochord extends into the mesencephalic

(A)

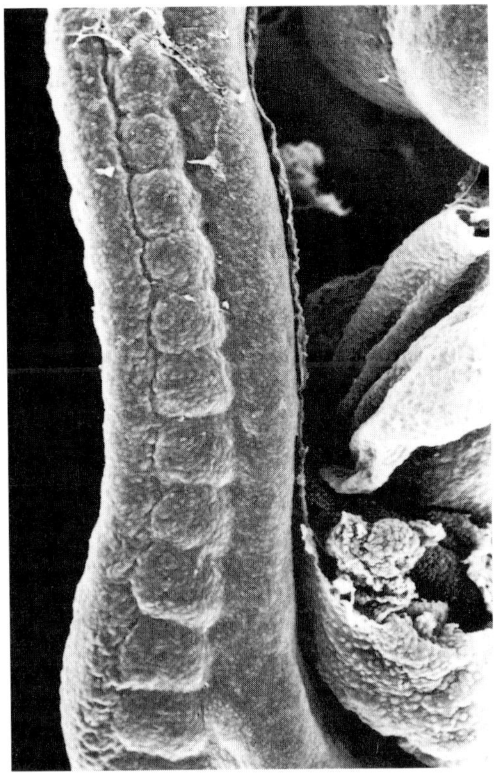

Fig. 8.9 (A) Scanning electron micrograph of a lateral view of an embryo showing the somites. The cranial somites are at the lower border and the more caudal somites are at the upper border. A change in size of the cranially more advanced somites is apparent. (Photograph by P. Collins)
(B) The stages of somitogenesis. Development proceeds in a craniocaudal progression. The more cranially placed somites (at the lower right of the figure) are further developed than those caudally placed (at the upper left of the figure). The stages in somitogenesis are given on the left of the figure; more detailed information is given on the right.

(B) *Somitogenesis*

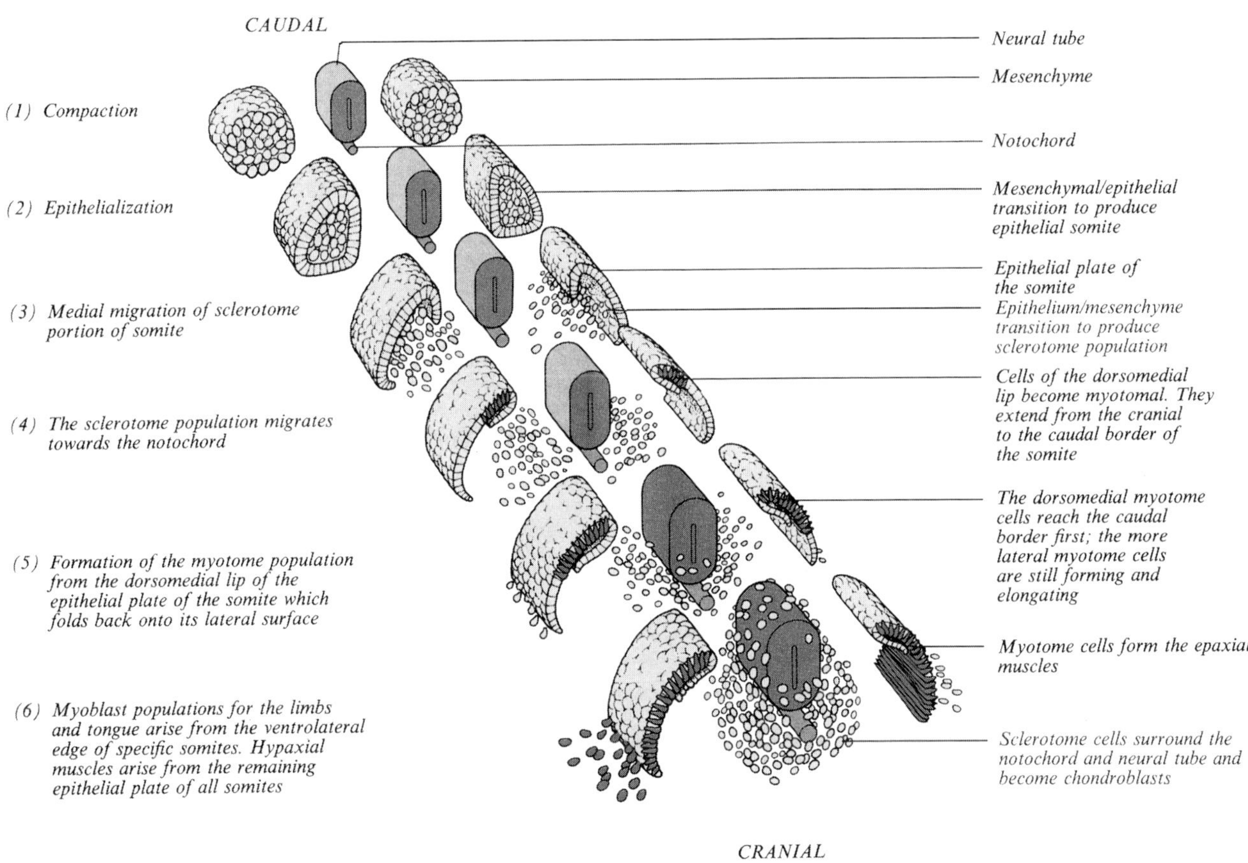

flexure and forms the anlage of the tentorium cerebelli. By 41 days, the dura mater can be seen around the basal regions of the brain and by 48 days the venous sinuses are developing within the dural layer. The dura is almost complete over the rhombencephalon and mesencephalon by 57 days but present only laterally around the prosencephalon. From this time, the subarachnoid spaces and cisterns are present and the arachnoid mater becomes separated from the dura mater by accumulation of CSF.

There is a relationship between the development of the cranial dura and the overlying skull which continues into postnatal life while the bones of the calvaria are still growing. The skull is formed from desmocranial mesenchyme (of neural crest origin) which supports ossification centres. Waves of osteodifferentiation move radially outward from these centres stopping when adjcent bones meet; regions where sutures will form. Once sutures have formed a second phase of development begins in which growth of the cranial bones continues at the sutural margins[6]. The presence of dura is not required for this initial suture morphogenesis; this appears to be controlled by mesenchymal cell proliferation and the extracellular matrix synthesis induced by the overlapping of advancing osteo-inductive fronts of calvarial bones. However, later, it has been shown experimentally that if the calvaria is removed the skull regenerates with sutures and bones developing in anatomically correct positions, suggesting that calvarial patterning is controlled by the dura. Transplantation of sutures in which the fetal dura is left intact results in a continuous fibrous suture between developing vault bones, whereas in transplants where the dura is removed bony fusion occurs. This suggests that once a suture has formed it serves as a primary site for cranial bone growth but requires constant interaction with the dura to avoid osseous obliteration[6].

SKULL

UPPER REGIONS OF THE SKULL

Neural crest arising caudal to the mid-diencephalon gives rise to the frontal, parietal bones, and the squamous parts of the temporal and occipital bones. All of these latter bones develop from membranous ossification via interactions with the meninges as described above.

BASE OF THE SKULL

The basal regions of the skull are preformed in cartilage derived, in some cases, from the unsegmented paraxial mesenchyme rostral to the otic vesicle. Meier[7] noted presegmental structures termed somitomeres each side of the rostral notochord, beneath the overlying neural plate and identified seven somitomeres using scanning electron microscopy. Using chick–quail chimeras is has been possible to follow the fate of this somitomeric mesenchyme demonstrating the mixed origin of the skull base from the evolutionarily more recent neural crest and the older unsegmented paraxial mesenchyme (see p. 82). In the midline most rostrally, the medial mesenchyme gives rise to the trabeculae cranii and the ethmoid complex; these are derived from neural crest. Next the hypophyseal cartilage arises from unsegmented paraxial mesenchyme which ossifies to form the postsphenoid part of the sphenoid bone (this also has a neural crest contribution in the chick[8]). Caudally, the parachordal cartilages arise from the unsegmented paraxial mesenchyme which condenses each side of the notochord. The latter fuse with the second to fourth occipital sclerotomes to form the clivus. The region of fusion of these elements corresponds to the spheno-occipital synchondrosis, which is the site of growth for up to 20 years of age. Extensions from the occipital sclerotomes on each side grow laterally and dorsally to encircle the brain stem and form the foramen magnum. Laterally, the otic capsules are formed from the first somite, medial paraxial mesenchyme and also from neural crest[8] (see also Fig. 4.9).

Development of the pharynx

So far, the development of the brain and notochord has been considered. Ventral to these structures are the foregut and the heart. In the unfolded embryo, the putative foregut region underlies the widest part of the neural plate, the region of the buccopharyngeal membrane, and the surface ectoderm to the rostral edge of the disc. In early studies, the term prechordal (prochordal) plate was used to describe a localized thickening of the endoderm rostral to the notochordal process, making this region analogous to the buccopharyngeal membrane. Because it is now known that the primitive streak gives rise to the entire endodermal population, it is reasonable to surmise that the earliest invaginating endodermal population provides cells for the head region and later invaginations provide cells for more caudal portions of the gastrointestinal tract. Thus, the earliest invaginating cells of the prechordal plate could give rise to all of the endodermal foregut.

Although head folding is usually described as a movement of the edge of the embryonic disc to a ventral position, the significant local proliferation of the epithelial populations, especially the neural tissue, means that a forward growth of the embryo occurs as a result of the expansion of the medial (now dorsal) portion of the embryonic disc. During this time, the endoderm forms an elongating tube with the proliferating prechordal region at the base.

After head folding, the early foregut is a cul-de-sac with one end open to the midgut and the cranial intestinal portal, and the other closed at the buccopharyngeal membrane. The roof or dorsal wall of the foregut contains the notochordal plate (the notochord proper forms after stage 11), and the floor or ventral wall of the foregut is in close contact with the developing heart, i.e. the angiogenic mesenchyme and coelomic epithelium which will form the endocardium, myocardium and pericardial cavity. The caudal portion of the foregut will give rise to the respiratory primordia and the oesophagus, while the rostral portion will provide the lining and special glands of the pharynx.

There is much we do not yet know about the cranial interface between the voluntary pharyngeal muscles and the involuntary muscles of the gastrointestinal tract. A new mesenchymal population between the endoderm and the paraxial mesenchyme of the somitomeres and occipital somites, has been identified[9]. It develops as a sparse layer in a rostrocaudal and lateromedial sequence, forming initially a fenestrated monolayer between developing blood vessels and the endoderm and later as a definitive layer between the notochord and the roof of the foregut. It is suggested that it is involved in the formation of the pharyngeal and oesophageal smooth muscle and connective tissue.

The buccopharyngeal membrane marks the division between the endoderm internally and ectoderm externally. As facial development proceeds the ectodermal surface of the buccopharyngeal membrane is found at the base of a hollow, the stomodeum. The structures of the face derive from the stomodeal walls and so are covered with epithelia entirely of ectodermal origin. The buccopharyngeal membrane breaks down during stage 12 and subsequent development blurs its original position which is best thought of as a zone passing from behind the eyes (the adenohypophysis invaginates just in front of the buccopharyngeal membrane) to the posterior part of the anterior two-thirds of the tongue.

With development of the pharyngeal arches (see below) the primitive rostral foregut becomes widened at the putative mouth, narrowing caudally. The foregut is compressed dorsoventrally and there is virtually no lateral wall. Between the arches the endoderm transiently contacts the overlying ectoderm forming inner and outer depressions where contact is established. Externally these depressions are termed pharyngeal clefts, internally pharyngeal pouches. The connection remains between the first cleft and pouch, as the tympanic membrane, but more caudal connections are lost. In some cases, the lower pouches develop dorsal and ventral portions with different fates. Thus the second pouch forms the palatine tonsil, the third pouch forms the thymus ventrally and the parathyroid III dorsally. The fourth pouch forms the parathyroid IV and an ultimobranchial body.

The pharyngeal endoderm is in contact with mesenchyme and epithelia from many sources and may itself be reciprocating in their development. It is intimately involved with neural crest mesenchyme, paraxial mesenchyme – both unsegmented and somitic – lateral plate mesenchyme (of the septum transversum just caudal to the heart), and angiogenic mesenchyme which forms the endocardium and endothelium; it is also associated with notochordal epithelium and cleft ectoderm. The development of the pharyngeal arches is thus likely to involve interactions with all of these sources.

THE PHARYNGEAL ARCHES

The face, pharynx and larynx arise from mesenchymal and epithelial populations arising from the rostral neural folds but especially from modification of a number of pharyngeal arches which encircle the early foregut. These structures were termed branchial or visceral arches but are now, in mammalian embryos, most often called pharyngeal arches (Fig. 8.10).

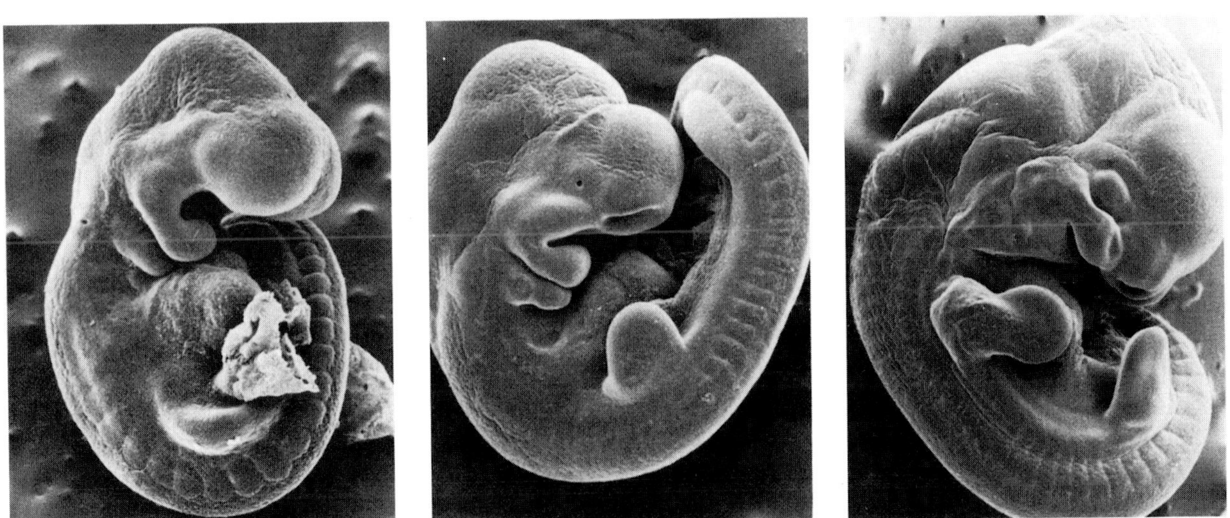

(A) (B) (C)

Fig. 8.10 Series of scanning electron micrographs of rat embryos at days 11, 12 and 13: lateral view. (A) Day 11, the pharyngula stage; the otic vesicle is still open but the lens vesicle has yet to invaginate; the first, second and third pharyngeal arches are present; an upper limb bud is present dorsal to the heart. (B) Day 12, the lens vesicle has invaginated but is still open; the maxillary prominence has developed and is beneath the eye; the upper limb is becoming paddle-shaped and the lower limb is present. (C) Day 13, the eyelids are beginning to develop; the maxillary prominence is merging with the lateral nasal prominence; both limb buds are well developed. The relative size and number of somites can be seen at each age. (Photographs by P. Collins) (From Gray's Anatomy, 38th edition, Edinburgh: Churchill Livingstone, 1995, p. 275.)

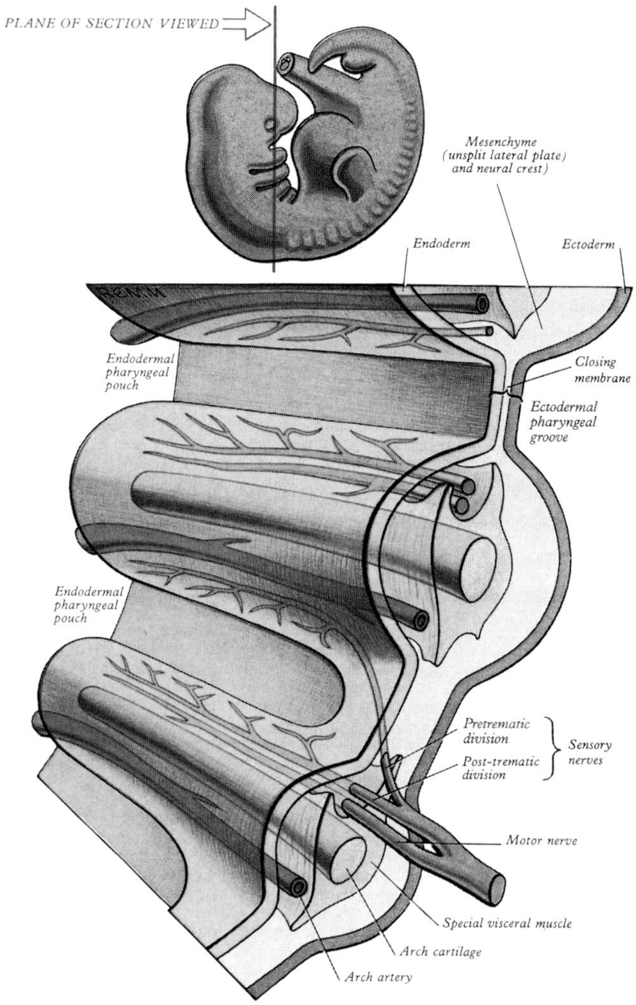

Fig. 8.11 Schema of developing pharyngeal region showing details of generalized pharyngeal constituents, including arches, endodermal pouches and ectodermal grooves. (From Gray's Anatomy, 38th edition, Edinburgh: Churchill Livingstone, 1995, p. 276.)

Five pharyngeal arches are seen in mammalian embryos classically numbered I, II, III, IV and VI; there is extensive evidence for not including arch V in the series. Each pharyngeal arch consists of an epithelial covering exteriorly and a mesenchymal core (Fig. 8.11). The epithelium is ectoderm externally and endoderm internally for arches II–VI, and ectoderm entirely for the first arch which is considered atypical. The mesenchyme within each arch arises from specific neural crest and paraxial populations. Angiogenic mesenchyme is found throughout the arches especially associated with the endoderm. Motor and sensory cranial nerves are associated with the epithelia and mesenchyme.

Each arch contains:

- specific epithelial structures from ectoderm or endoderm
- skeletal and connective tissue elements from neural crest mesenchyme
- striated muscle from paraxial mesenchyme
- an arch artery from angiogenic mesenchyme
- motor and sensory nerves innervating the arch

The final topographical arrangement of the tissues within each arch is patterned by Hox gene expression passed from the rhombomeres to the neural crest mesenchyme which migrates to the arches and to the ectoderm.

Origin of the skin covering the head and neck

The ectoderm covering the external aspects of the arches arises from regional territories which have been termed *ectomeres*. The most rostral neural fold gives rise to the epithelium of the nasal cavity while the prosencephalic neural fold produces the frontonasal epithelium and that of the forehead. The epithelium of the upper eyelid and cornea arises from the ectoderm covering the prosencephalon. The epithelia covering the first, second, third and fourth arches arise from the ectoderm on the lateral side of the head overlying the mesencephalon and rhomebcephalon (see Fig. 8.7). It is the epithelia covering the second arch which grow over the caudal arches giving the smooth surface of the neck. Platysma is pulled down with this portion of the arch and thus has superficial fascia both superficial and deep to the muscle.

Neural crest in the arches

The developmental pattern of each arch depends on the origin of the neural crest it contains. Neural crest cells migrate from the neural folds of the diencephalon caudally. They do not arise from the prosencephalic folds. The most rostral fold produces epithelium of the nasal cavities, the diencephalic folds give rise to frontonasal mesenchymal populations, while that from the mesencephalic folds, along with the upper rhombomeres, produce mesenchyme for the first arch. Crest cells from rhombomeres 1 and 2 contribute to the first arch mesenchyme, crest cells from rhombomere 4 produce second arch mesenchyme, while crest cells from rhombomere 6 produce third arch mesenchyme. All rhombomeres apart from 3 and 5 contribute migratory neural crest; it is suggested 3 and 5 do not because of a dominant negative effect exerted by the even-numbered rhombomeres.[10]

NEURAL CREST MESENCHYME PATTERNING IN THE ARCHES

The specification of the neural crest, concerning its function within the arches, occurs before it migrates from the neural folds. In grafting experiments, if first arch crest is grafted into the second arch, mandibular structures form suggesting that the differentiation pattern of the second arch surface ectoderm and paraxial mesenchyme is redefined by the new crest mesenchyme[11]. Similar findings are seen in the development of teeth which arise as an interaction between surface ectoderm and crest mesenchyme (see p. 33).

The axial homeobox genes Hox-a and Hox-b are initially expressed in the rhombomeres then subsequently in the neural crest from the point of origin, during migration and after migration has ceased. Each pharyngeal arch expresses a different combination of hox genes in the segment restricted manner[12]. Disruption of hox genes causes failure of normal crest cell proliferation and migration, producing anomalies similar to those seen in human neonates, e.g. DiGeorge's syndrome.

SKELETAL ELEMENTS

The earliest skeletal elements in each arch are cartilage precursors which in some cases are replaced by membranous bone. Thus Meckel's cartilage in the first arch becomes mainly ligamentous or absorbed into the mandible, and the second arch cartilage, Reichert's, similarly is reduced for much of its length to a ligament (stylohyoid). The auditory ossicles are initially formed in cartilage but later become ossified. The cartilaginous elements in arches four and six remain as cartilage. That in arch three combines with the second arch and ossifies as the hyoid bone.

It is interesting that, although the development of the cartilage elements of each arch had been described in the same way for many years, little is said about the origin of the epiglottic cartilage, despite its obvious importance in the functioning of the larynx. The epiglottis arises in the midline ventral to the larynx, in a region termed the hypobranchial eminence. Lateral to the laryngeal inlet are the ventral ends of the sixth arches in which arytenoid swellings appear; these later differentiate into the arytenoid and corniculate cartilages. Together the arytenoid swellings and the epiglottis reduce the opening into the larynx from a vertical slit to a T-shaped cleft. Later, the cuneiform cartilages differentiate from the epiglottic mesenchyme. It is likely that the epiglottis arises from neural crest mesenchyme, perhaps from fused ventral portions of the sixth arches which later separate from it. However, it has not been established that this is the case.

FACE

The face is formed from the first arch and the frontonasal process which does not contain any cartilage elements. The lower portion of the 'C'-shaped first arch containing Meckel's cartilage is termed a mandibular process. Each mandibular process grows first caudally then ventrally to meet and fuse with the process from the other side. (The term 'prominence' is also used to describe these mesenchymal and epithelial structures.) The mandible arises from these merged mesenchymal populations by intramembranous ossification. Rostrally mesenchyme from the diencephalic neural folds migrates around the olfactory placodes producing surface elevations on each side of the head termed the medial and lateral nasal swellings. The olfactory placodes are originally widely separated and coplanar with the surface ectoderm but, as the nasal swellings develop, they become depressed at the base of olfactory pits. The medial nasal swellings approach each other and extend caudally beyond the lateral nasal swellings. Extensions from the medial swellings into the roof of the stomodeum proliferate to form the premaxillary fields. The upper portion of the first arch, which contains the quadrate cartilage, is termed the maxillary process. Each maxillary process extends beneath the eye in a ventral direction and fuses with the lateral nasal swelling, the two being at first separated by a nasomaxillary groove (naso-optic furrow). The ectoderm between them gives rise to a solid cellular rod, which sinks into the mesenchyme. Its caudal end proliferates to contact the caudal part of the nasal wall, while its cranial end connects with the developing conjunctival sac. The epithelial rod becomes canalized to form the nasolacrimal duct.

PALATE

The maxillary processes extend medially during stage 17 (41 days) to produce palatine processes or shelves, which grow towards the midline and downwards, being separated by the developing tongue in the floor of the mouth. At this stage, the tip of the developing tongue is in contact with the cranial surface of the primitive palate, i.e. the stomodeal roof. During stage 23 (56–57 days), the palatine processes rapidly elevate, assuming a horizontal position which allows them to grow towards each other and fuse. The change in position occurs very rapidly caused by matrix changes. Hyaluronic acid is synthesized and accumulates causing swelling and expansion of the mesenchyme, and collagen fibrils are aligned with the mesenchymal cells. The epithelial populations each side of the palatal shelves restrain the swelling. In response to locally released acetylcholine and serotonin, the collagen fibrils and mesenchyme contract causing elevation of the shelves. Other factors also promote palatal elevation. At this time, there is extensive growth in head height rather than head width, there is growth of Meckel's cartilage which allows the tongue to lower into the developing mandible, and also mouth opening, tongue protrusion and hiccup movements have been noted.

The palatal shelves fuse with the premaxilla and with each other from front to back, and at the same time fuse with the free border of the nasal septum. The mesenchyme within the maxilla, premaxilla, and palatal shelves forms bone by intramembranous ossification. Interestingly, the patterning of the neural crest in the palate supports respiratory epithelium (pseudostratified, ciliated columnar epithelium) on the upper, nasal surface, and stratified squamous non-keratinising epithelium on the lower, oral surface.

Generally male palatal shelf elevation occurs 7 days before females, making congenital cleft palate more likely in female embryos. Such defects may be manifest as cleft lip when a maxillary process and lateral nasal process fail to fuse, or cleft palate if the maxillary processes do not fuse together. More severe conditions result from complete failure of fusion, with facial clefts resulting where the nasolacrimal duct persists as an open furrow. On the other hand, the philtrum (formed from the frontonasal process) may be a separate entity, continuous dorsally with the nasal septum but unattached to the palatine processes; in such cases the floor of the nasal cavity is deficient throughout its extent.

CONNECTIVE TISSUE ELEMENTS

Neural crest patterns and supports the development of all of the epithelia in the head and neck giving rise to the ectodermal and endodermal glands. The ectoderm gives rise to the teeth (see p. 33) and salivary glands whereas the endoderm with neural crest patterning produces the palatine and pharyngeal tonsils, the thyroid gland, the parathyroid glands, and the thymus. In all of the latter cases the pharyngeal endoderm provides the epithelial cell line which will produce appropriate cytodifferentiation. However, in the absence of neural crest, the endoderm epithelium is not supported or patterned correctly and only limited cytological differentiation of the epithelium occurs. Congenital lack of neural crest as in DiGeorge's syndrome is characterised by the absence (or near absence) of the thymus, parathyroids and thyroid glands.

In addition to patterning the development of the glands, interactions between the mesenchyme and surface epithelia persist which continue the maintenance of the differentiated epidermis. Thus the mucous membrane of the oral cavity differentiates and is maintained as stratified squamous non-keratinising epithelium, whereas the outer aspect of the face has stratified squamous keratising epithelium; the special epithelia of the lips delineates the junction between the two.

Paraxial mesenchyme in the arches – muscles in the head and neck

The fate of the unsegmented paraxial mesenchyme in the head (somitomeres) mirrors that of the somites. The medial mesenchyme forms bony and connective tissue and contributes to elements of the base of the skull, whereas the lateral mesenchyme gives rise to muscle producing the myoblastic lineages which migrate into the pharyngeal arches (Fig. 8.1). Figure 8.1 is based on studies by Noden and attributes somitomeres 4, 6, and 7 to supply the first second and third arches respectively. However, more recent studies by Trainor in the mouse[13] indicate a different destination for these premyoblastic populations. Thus Trainor suggests that somitomeres 2 and 3 give rise to the first arch muscle mass which forms the tensor tympani, tensor veli palatini, the masticatory muscles, including mylohyoid and the anterior belly of digastric. Somitomeres 4 and 5 give rise to the second arch muscle mass. The muscles derived from the second arch migrate extensively; stylohyoid, stapedius and the posterior belly of digastric remain attached to the hyoid skeleton, whereas the muscles of facial expression, platysma, the auricular muscles and epicranius all lose connection with it. The paraxial mesenchyme of somitomeres 6 and 7 migrate to the third arch forming stylopharyngeus, and somitomere 7 alone migrates to the fourth arch[13] forming cricothyroid. Somitomeric muscles have not been identified in the sixth arch in the mouse. It will be interesting to follow the update on the origin of these muscles.

The origin of the general musculature of the pharynx, soft palate and larynx has not yet been identified by immunological or chimeric studies. It is thought that myogenic mesenchyme from the third arch migrates into the palate, around the caudal margin of the auditory tube and into the palatopharyngeal arches. However, it is the case that animal studies of the development of this region may not give appropriate information as in the human the pharyngeal and laryngeal muscles are developed extensively for vocalisation.

The discovery that paraxial mesenchyme produces the musculature of the pharyngeal arches updates the older view that arch musculature was of a special lineage, arising *in situ*, termed branchial and innervated by special branchial efferent neurons. It will be many years before the identification of the origin of these muscles will be reflected in embryological texts, and more until a new nomenclature is in general use. As these muscles are the only group (so far identified) to derive from the unsegmented paraxial mesenchyme and be patterned by the neural crest mesenchyme, perhaps a continuance of their 'special' status can be tolerated. However, adherence to the old terminology in this region will hinder the understanding of this important area of development.

THE ORIGIN OF THE EXTRAOCULAR MUSCLES

The oculomotor muscles of the eye are typically described as being derived from 'pre-otic somites', and they are usually indicated close to the developing eye. The pre-otic somites are cavities seen in the developing head which were compared to the somites at their epithelial stage, just after compaction. Although a very early study described the development of oculomotor muscles arising from the prechordal mesenchyme, i.e. that migrating through the primitive streak just ahead of the notochord[14], it was not until chimeric experiments could be performed that this view was confirmed. It has now been demonstrated that the prechordal mesenchyme is displaced laterally at the time of head flexion and that the cells become associated with the more laterally place paraxial mesenchymal cells[3,15]. Some time later, this mesenchyme migrates to occupy the walls of the local head cysts where it differentiates into the premyoblastic populations for all the extrinsic ocular muscles. In Fig. 8.1 the prechordal mesenchyme is indicated with the axial structures and also with the somitomeric mesenchyme which will give rise to the pharyngeal arch musculature. The precursor myoblasts have been grouped with different somitomeres to correspond to the level from which their innervation arises.

Innervation of the head and arches

Chick–quail chimeras experimentation by Le Douarin and others has produced data on the contribution of the neural crest to the somatic and autonomic nervous systems. Neural crest cells migrate from the mesencephalon and rhombencephalon when 4–10 somites are present, i.e. corresponding to early neurulation[16,17]. These cells provide neural and glial cells for the cranial sensory nerves and for the autonomic ganglia.

Throughout the body, four major groups of crest cells have been identified as providing populations for the autonomic system. They are the cranial, vagal, trunk and lumbosacral crest. Within the head region cranial crest gives rise to the cranial parasympathetic ganglia, whereas vagal crest gives rise to the thoracic parasympathetic ganglia. The vagal crest region also provides neurons and glia for the enteric nervous system.

The ciliary ganglion is formed by crest cells from the caudal third of the mesencephalon and the rostral metencephalon which migrate close to the ophthalmic branch of the trigeminal nerve. The pterygopalatine ganglion arises from preotic myelencephalic crest and may receive contributions from the ganglia of the trigeminal and facial nerves. The submandibular ganglia and otic ganglia also derive from myelencephalic crest and may have contributions from the facial and glossopharyngeal cranial nerves respectively.

Vagal neural crest from the level of somites 1–7 migrate to the proximal and middle portions of the gut, with sacral neural crest cells supplying the distal gut. It is worth noting that the number of enteric neurons is believed to be of the same magnitude as the number of neurons in the spinal cord[18]. Much fewer preganglionic fibres modulate this system which can mediate its own reflex activity independent of control by the brain and spinal cord. The crest cells destined to become enteric neurons attain their axial value as they leave the neuraxis. If quail crest cells from the trunk are transplanted to the vagal regions of chick hosts they will produce embryos with entirely quail enteric nerves showing that the premigratory neural crest cells are not pre-patterned for specific axial levels. Once these cells reach their destination, they are thought to be regionally patterned by the local splanchnopleuric mesenchyme.

Some neural crest cells arising from a region between the midotic placode and the caudal limit of somite 3 have been termed cardiac neural crest cells. These cells migrate to pharyngeal arches III, IV and VI where they provide support for the embryonic arch arteries (see below), cells of the aorticopulmonary septum and truncus, and cells which give rise to the parasympathetic ganglia of the heart. Sensory innervation of the heart is from the inferior vagal ganglion, derived from the nodose placode.

The pharyngeal arches received motor and sensory axons from the cranial nerves. Nerves I, II, VII and VIII are associated with special senses, and there are special sense contributions from IX and X. Nerves III, IV and VI are motor and associated with the eye musculature. The arches are innervated by nerves V, VII, IX and X which supply arches I, II, III and IV respectively; branches of X supply arch VI. In each case the motor nerves are derived from the basal plate of the central nervous system and the sensory nerves from the neural crest cells located in the various somatic ganglia.

Angiogenic mesenchyme in the arches

The embryonic aortic arch arteries arise as paired bilateral vessels from a dilated aortic sac (the fused ventral aortae of lower animals), pass laterally around the pharynx within an arch, and join the right or left dorsal aorta as appropriate. As the embryo enlarges, the pharyngeal arches develop in sequence and blood passes into the arch artery. Thus during this stage of development, blood follows a succession of different pathways, to the first arch, then first and second arches, second and third arches, third and fourth arches and finally third, fourth and sixth aortic arches. Each sixth embryonic arch vessel is, from its inception, associated with a developing lung bud. When the aortico-pulmonary septum divides the truncus arteriosus into pulmonary trunk and ascending aorta, the sixth arch artery retains continuity with the former.

In the early embryo, the tunica media of the third, fourth, sixth arches and the dorsal aorta contains smooth muscle cells that are not elastogenic and not of neural crest origin. Some vessels, i.e. the intrapulmonary arteries and the subclavian arteries, continue to accumulate layers of smooth muscle derived from the surrounding mesenchyme. However, the remaining arch arteries become surrounded by neural crest very early in development. This initial crest population does not express smooth muscle or elastogenic antigens. Later, a larger population of crest cells migrates around the arch arteries and proceed to differentiate along an elastogenic pathway, proceeding from the truncus arteriosus downstream. At the same time, the original smooth muscle disappears along the developing great vessels to their first branch point[19]. In conditions where neural crest is absent or ablated, the embryonic aortic arch vessels may be absent, too large, too small or aberrant in their connections with loss of bilateral symmetry. There is a significant decrease in the quantity of mesenchyme around the vessels resulting in direct apposition of endothelium and pharyngeal endodermal epithelium[20].

The sixth arch artery, which becomes the ductus arteriosus on the left retains a muscular media and is not elastic as the other arch arteries[21]. Fetal and neonatal ductal tissue produce prostaglandin E_2 (PGE_2), prostaglandin I_2 (PGI_2) and prostaglandin $F_{2\alpha}$ ($PGF_{2\alpha}$) which inhibit the ability of the ductus to contract in response to oxygen. The increased oxygen tension after birth is thus one of the factors involved in ductal closure. Coarctation of the aorta is a condition in which the aorta is constricted just above (preductal) or below (postductal) the entrance of the ductus arteriosus. An abnormal disposition of a smooth muscle media around the aorta at this point could result from an imperfect migration of the cardiac neural crest to establish the usual elastogenic media. The result would be an abnormal constriction of the aorta after birth.

External features of head development

Structures composing the head can be first discerned in embryos of 22 p.o. days[22] (stage 10). Although little is obvious externally all the development described in this chapter is progressing. Neurulation begins at this stage and 4–12 pairs of somites are present. Facial development begins with the mandibular and hyoid arches becoming visible. However, the proximity of the rostral neural fold, the buccopharyngeal membrane and the heart primordium makes identification of these structures difficult. By 24 p.o. days (stage 11[22]) the neural tube has formed and brain vesicles are present. During this stage, the rostral neuropore will close. The mandibular and hyoid arches are enlarging as neural crest cells stream into them. This increase in mesenchymal population facilitates the invagination of the otic placode which commences.

By 26 p.o. days, three pharyngeal arches can be seen with deepening clefts between them where the surface ectoderm and pharyngeal endoderm are in contact. Dorsal and ventral portions of the arches can be discerned. The otic vesicle has invaginated and only a small opening is now present. The optic vesicle is evaginated from the diencephalon and approaching the surface ectoderm.

During stage 14 (32 p.o. days) the maxillary process can be seen, the lens has invaginated from the surface ectoderm and a small hole may remain on the surface. Stage 15 sees the cerebral evaginations. During stage 16 (37 p.o. days) the mandibular processes fuse across the midline and the maxillary processes meet with the lateral nasal swellings. In stage 17 (41 p.o. days) the medial nasal swellings move closer and extend caudal to the lateral nasal swellings, thus producing the premaxilla. They meet the medially moving maxillary processes during this period. Auricular hillocks can be identified at this stage and their development continues in stage 18 (44 p.o. days) forming the auricular pinna. The eyes are pigmented at this time and the edges of the eyelids can be identified at the edges of the globe. By stage 19 (47–48 p.o. days), the lower border of arch two has fused with the ectoderm on the cranial aspect of the pericardial region and the neck appears smooth. During stage 20 (50–51 p.o. days) the pinna is recognisable, the nostrils face anteriorly and the eyelids are covering the edges of the eyes. There is still a significant neck flexion and the mouth is in contact with the pericardial bulge. From this time to stage 23 (56–57 p.o. days) the embryo shows less cervical flexion and the lower border of the mandible gains contact with the pericardial bulge. By this stage, the eyelids have still not yet met and fused.

Evolution of the head

It is suggested that the evolution of the head has occurred because of the recruitment, by vertebrates, of a novel mesenchymal population in the head, the neural crest. Creatures such as the cephalocaudate *Amphioxus*, which do not have neural crest, develop via similar mechanisms throughout the cephalic end of their body and along the trunk. The developmental mechanisms which are seen in the vertebrate head are different from those in the trunk. This observation can be used to deduce that the vertebrate head evolved by a different route from the other axial structures, using different cell populations which do not respond to the usual inducers produced in the trunk.

A hypothesis of head evolution has been put forward by Gans and Northcutt[23] and Northcutt and Gans[24]. They propose that the rostral portion of the head, including the sense organs, prosencephalon, mesencephalon and surrounding skull is derived from the neuroectoderm. Certainly the neuroectoderm gives rise to the sense organs via a series of ectodermal placodes, often situated initially in the edges of the neural plate. This same region also give rise to a unique migratory mesenchyme population, the neural crest, which forms the 'prechordal' skull, i.e. that part rostral to the notochord[25].

The neural crest in the head fulfils a role similar to that of the somatic and splanchnopleuric mesenchymes within the trunk, i.e. it patterns the adjacent epithelia and intrinsic mesenchymal tissue. It is able to differentiate along a chondrogenic lineage in the head, a fate which cannot occur in the trunk, and can thus contribute to the base plan of the skull, which provides a template for the wide range of vertebrate head shapes, and to the modification of the pharyngeal arches into oral structures.

The vertebrate head also subsumes a number of somites into its caudal region. The *Agnathia* have no vertebral contribution to the skull, whereas amphibians and selachians incorporate three occipital somites, and in mammals all five occipital somites are included. This caudal enlargement contributes to the general increase in the volume of the skull around the expanding rhombencephalon at the same time as the neural crest is surrounding the prosencephalon rostrally.

Hox genes are expressed along the embryonic axis in invertebrate and vertebrate embryos. An *Amphioxus* gene has recently been shown to be homologous to a mouse hox gene. The rostral expression of this gene in amphioxus is at the level of the 4/5 somite boundary at the neurula stage. In the vertebrate embryo homologous gene expression corresponds to the rhombomere 4/5 boundary[26]. Holland *et al.*[26] propose that the structures expressing these genes in the two body plans are homologous, suggesting that the vertebrate head evolved by elaboration and expansion of a pre-existing cranial region rather than by production of a new rostral portion. In this hypothesis, the neural crest could have been utilised because it was a source of mesenchyme which could be modified and adapted without simultaneous reorganisation of the trunk.

Ultimately, the ability to compare the genetic drivers of development will assist in our future understanding of the evolutionary processes which produced the head, and detailed study of the embryonic tissue populations in the head will increase our understanding of the nature of craniofacial anomalies. We may predict that we will be looking for genetic correction of some of these defects in the future.

REFERENCES

1. Herbst JJ. Development of suck and swallow. In *Human Gastrointestinal Development* (ed. E. Lebethal), pp. 229–239. New York: Raven Press, 1989.

1a. Selleck MAJ, Stern CD. Commitment of mesoderm cells in Hensen's node of the chick embryo to notochord and somite. *Development* **114**:403–415, 1992.

2. Jessel TM, Bovolenta P, Placzek M, Tessier-Lavigne M, Dodd J. Polarity and patterning the neural tube: the origin and function of the floor plate. In *Cellular Basis of Morphogenesis CIBA Foundation Symposium 144* (ed. L. Wolpert), pp. 255–280. Chichester: John Wiley, 1989.

3. Wachtler F, Jacob M. Origin and development of the cranial skeletal muscles. *Bibl Anat* **29**:24–46, 1986.

4. Couly GF, Le Douarin NM. Head morphogenesis in embryonic avian chimeras: evidence for a segmental pattern in the ectoderm corresponding to the neuromeres. *Development* **108**:543–558, 1990.

5. Selleck MAJ, Stern CD. Fate mapping and cell lineage analysis of Hensen's node in the chick embryo. *Development* **112**:615–626, 1991.

6. Opperman LA, Sweeney TM, Redmon J, Persing JA, Ogle RC. Tissue interactions with underlying dura mater inhibit osseous obliteration of developing cranial sutures. *Dev. Dynamics* **198**:312–322, 1993.

7. Meier S. Development of the chick mesoblast. Formation of the embryonic axis and the establishment of the metameric pattern. *Dev Biol* **38**:73–90, 1979.

8. Couly GF, Coltey PM, Le Douarin NM. The triple origin of skull in higher vertebrates: a study in quail–chick chimeras. *Development* **117**:409–429, 1993.

9. Noden DM. Development of craniofacial blood vessels. *Issues Biomed* **14**:1–24, 1991.

10. Graham A, Heyman I, Lumsden A. Even-numbered rhombomeres control the apoptotic elimination of neural crest from odd-numbered rhombomeres in the chick hindbrain. *Development* **119**:233–245, 1993.

11. Noden DM. Interactions and fates of avian craniofacial mesenchyme. *Development* **103**(suppl):121–140, 1988.

12. Hunt P, Gulisano M, Cook M, Sham M, Faiella A, Wilkinson D, Boncinelli E, Krumlauf R. A distinct Hox code for the branchial region of the head. *Nature* **353**:861–864, 1991.

13. Trainor PA, Tan S, Tam PPL. Cranial paraxial mesoderm: regionalisation of cell fate and impact on craniofacial development in mouse embryos. *Development* **120**:2397–2408, 1994.

14. Adelmann HB. The development of the eye muscles in the chick. *J Morphol* **44**:29–87, 1927.

15. Christ B, Jacob M, Jacob HJ, Brand B, Wachtler F. Myogenesis: a problem of cell distribution and cell interactions. In *Somites in Developing Embryos. NATO ASI Series. Series A: Life Sciences* (eds R. Bellairs, D.A. Ede & J.W. Lash) pp. 261–275, 1986. New York: Plenum Press, 1986.

16. Nichols DH. Ultrastructure of neural crest formation in the midbrain/rostral hindbrain and preotic hindbrain regions of the mouse embryo. *Am J Anat* **179**:148–154, 1987.

17. Chan WY, Tam PPL. A morphological and experimental study of the mesencephalic neural crest cells in the mouse embryo using wheat germ agglutinin–gold conjugate as the cell marker. *Development* **102**:427–442, 1988.

18. Furness JB, Costa M. Types of nerves in the enteric nervous system. *Neuroscience* **5**:1–20, 1980.

19. Rosenquist TH, Beall AC. Elastogenic cells in the developing cardiovascular system: smooth muscle, nonmuscle and cardiac neural crest. *Ann NY Acad Sci* **588**:106–119, 1990.

20. Bockmann DE, Redmond ME, Kirby ML. Altered development of pharyngeal arch vessels after neural crest ablation. *Ann NY Acad Sci* **588**:296–304, 1990.

21. Ruiter DJ, Schlingermann RO, Reitveld FJR, de Wall MW. Monoclonal antibody-defined human endothelial antigens as vascular markers. *J Invest Dermatol* **93**:25S–32S, 1989.

22. O'Rahilly R, Muller F. *Developmental Stages in Human Embryos*. Washington: Carnegie Institution, 1987.

23. Gans C, Northcutt RG. Neural crest and the origin of vertebrates: a new head. *Science* **220**:268–274, 1983.

24. Northcutt RG, Gans C. The genesis of neural crest and epidermal placodes: a reinterpretation of vertebrate origins. *Q Rev Biol* **58**:1–28, 1983.

25. Couly GF, Coltey PM, Le Douarin NM. The developmental fate of the cephalic mesoderm in quail–chick chimeras. *Development* **114**:1–15, 1992.

26. Holland PWH, Holland LZ, Williams NA, Holland ND. An *Amphioxus* homeobox gene: sequence conservation, spatial expression during development and insights into vertebrate evolution. *Development* **116**:653–661, 1992.

SECTION

2

Fetal and placental physiology

Implantation

9

Y.W. Loke and A. King

Nidation

The initial event in implantation is achieved by contact and adhesion between the embryonic trophectoderm of the blastocyst and the uterine surface epithelium.[1] Because material from this early phase of the process is not readily available for study in humans, the mechanisms involved are not clearly understood. The apical surface of the uterine epithelium is generally considered to be repellant to cellular attachment most of the time and only becomes receptive at a specific period under the appropriate hormonal stimulus. This period of receptivity or 'implantation window' is estimated to be approximately seven days in humans. The stage of embryonic development must also coincide with this 'window' for implantation to occur. The small number of successful pregnancies achieved by *in vitro* fertilisation (IVF) relative to the high rate of successful fertilisation could be due to failure to synchronise the state of development of the blastocyst with this 'implantation window'.

There have been many attempts to identify the structural or phenotypic features of the surface uterine epithelium which may characterise the period of the 'window'. Ultrastructural changes, such as loss of microvilli, alteration of tight junctions and modification of the glycocalyx have been reported. Recently, characteristic structures known as 'pinopods' which are visualised by scanning electron microscopy of the uterine epithelium have been described to correlate with the time of implantation. Production of the mucin-type secretory glycoprotein, MUC-1, is observed to increase markedly in the secretory phase of the cycle. Since similar glycosaminoglycans can facilitate attachment and spreading of mouse blastocysts *in vitro*, this glycoprotein could play an important role in implantation. Variations in the expression of integrin subunits by the uterine surface epithelium are also thought to be associated with endometrial receptivity with these receptors binding to appropriate ligands synchronously expressed by the blastocyst.

Trophoblast populations

At the time when the blastocyst adheres to the epithelial lining of the uterine mucosa, it is surrounded by a layer of cells derived from the trophectoderm. As the blastocyst penetrates into the uterine mucosa, this layer differentiates into an outer multinucleated syncytiotrophoblast (primitive syncytium) and an inner layer of primitive mononuclear cytotrophoblast. Lacunae soon appear in the syncytium and these rapidly enlarge by fusing with each other. The uteroplacental circulation becomes established when this lacuna system erodes the uterine capillaries. The intervillous space of the definitive placenta is a derivation of these lacunae.

The subsequent differentiation of trophoblast occurs along two main pathways – villous and extravillous[2] (Fig. 9.1). The interaction of villous trophoblast is with maternal blood and its main function is transport of nutrients and oxygen to the fetus. Extravillous trophoblast is involved in the establishment of the placental blood supply and these are the trophoblast cells which contact maternal uterine tissues. At the tips of some chorionic villi, cytotrophoblast cells proliferate into solid masses of tissue known as cytotrophoblast columns which anchor these villi to the underlying decidua. From these columns individual trophoblast cells break off to invade the decidua. These interstitial trophoblast appear to move towards the decidual spiral arteries, encircling these vessels which then show endothelial swelling and a characteristic 'fibrinoid' destruction of the smooth muscle of the media. How trophoblast cells induce these changes in the vessel wall is presently unknown. When the trophoblast cells reach the decidual–myometrial junction, many of them become multinucleated and are now known as placental bed giant cells.

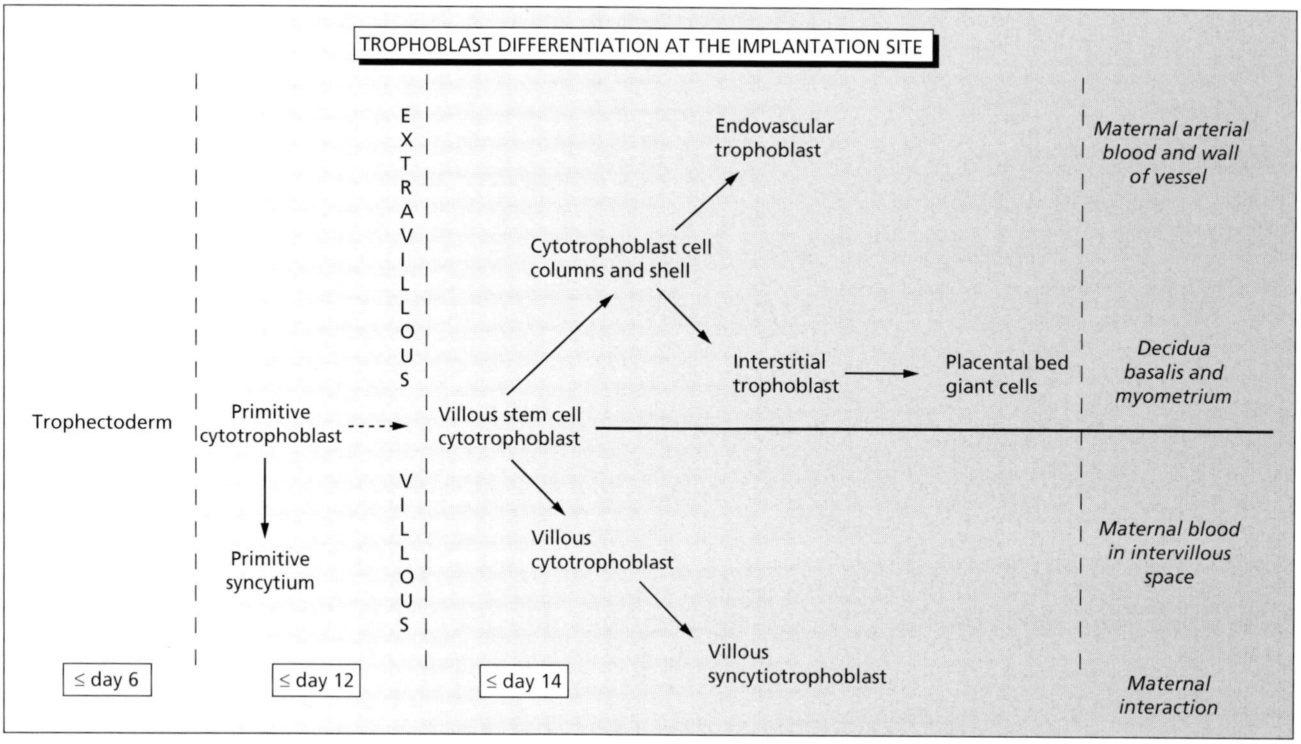

Fig. 9.1 Villous and extravillous pathways of trophoblast differentiation. (From Loke and King, *Human Implantation: Cell Biology and Immunology*, Cambridge University Press.)

These can be regarded as the end-point of the extravillous pathway of trophoblast differentiation.

Cytotrophoblast cells from the cell columns which lie over the openings of the decidual spiral arteries form a plug of cells which early in gestation appear to occlude the lumen of the vessels. Because of their situation, these trophoblast cells are known as endovascular trophoblast. From these plugs, trophoblast cells extend in a retrogade manner along the inner wall of the blood vessel rather like wax dripping down a candle, replacing the endothelial lining. Eventually, trophoblast cells become incorporated into the fibrinoid material of the vessel wall, but it is still uncertain whether these are derived mainly from endovascular trophoblast invading outwards through the wall or from interstitial trophoblast coming in from the decidua outside. Whatever the mechanism, this transformation of the spiral arteries by trophoblast is crucial to successful implantation because these changes convert the arteries from muscular vessels into flaccid sacs capable of transmitting the increased blood flow required for the developing feto-placental unit. Failure of this arterial transformation will result in reduced conductance and poor perfusion of the placenta which will affect the growth and development of the villous tree[3]. This in turn will lead to clinical conditions such as miscarriage, stillbirth, unexplained intrauterine growth retardation (IUGR) and pre-eclampsia.

Decidualisation

The uterine endometrial mucosa is transformed into decidua during pregnancy. Morphologically, the most obvious changes are seen in the stromal cells which become rounded and glycogen-rich. There is also infiltration by large numbers of bone-marrow-derived cells. These changes begin during the luteal phase of the menstrual cycle (pre-decidual change) but, if pregnancy occurs, decidualisation becomes more pronounced. Three layers can be discerned – an upper layer of decidua compacta subjacent to the surface epithelium, a middle layer of decidua spongiosa containing dilated glands and a basal layer from which regeneration of a new mucosa arises after menstruation or parturition. After implantation, decidua is found in three anatomical regions of the uterus. The decidua basalis lies beneath the developing placenta and it is this layer which is infiltrated by invading interstitial trophoblast. Overlying the embryo is the decidua capsularis which eventually fuses with the decidua parietalis which lines the uterus on the side away from the implantation site. This fusion, which occurs around the fourth month of gestation, completely obliterates the original uterine cavity, bringing the amniochorion overlying the capsular pole of the implanted embryo into direct contact with decidua parietalis. Thus, there are two points of contact between fetal and maternal tissues: one is between the amniochorion and decidua parietalis, and the other is between invading interstitial trophoblast and decidua basalis.

Unlike other species, such as rats, mice, guinea pigs and rabbits where decidualisation only begins at implantation, in humans this change has already begun at the late secretory phase of the normal menstrual cycle even in the absence of pregnancy, indicating that decidualisation is influenced by hormonal changes with oestrogen and progesterone being the major players. This conclusion is supported by the sequential expression of oestrogen receptors and progesterone receptors by cells of the human endometrium during the cycle. Both glandular and stromal cells of the endometrium increasingly express oestrogen receptors and progesterone receptors until the time of ovulation and expression then declines in the glands. Meanwhile, in the stroma, expression of progesterone receptors continues throughout the secretory phase and in early decidua.

Regarding the function of decidua, popular opinion favours the view that it facilitates implantation by providing an appropriate substrate for trophoblast migration and a fertile soil for nourishment of the developing fetus throughout gestation. However, it is also possible that decidua provides a restraining influence against overinvasion by trophoblast. This view is in accord with observations that in situations where decidualisation is inadequate, such as in ectopic pregnancies or implantation over a previous Caesarian section scar tissue, trophoblast invasion is unrestrained. It is likely that decidua provides a balance allowing migration of trophoblast but only to a certain depth. Thus, mammalian reproduction may be considered as a parental tug-of-war between the requirements of the fetus to derive as much nourishment as possible from the mother, and the defence of the mother to reduce this nutritional burden for the sake of her own health and for future pregnancies.

Trophoblast interaction with extracellular matrix

Cell migration is dependent on the expression of adhesion molecules which bind to matrix proteins in the extracellular environment. For example, the physiological migration of epithelial cells in wound healing and the pathological invasion of cancer cells require cell–matrix interaction. Trophoblast migration into decidua appears to utilise a similar mechanism. There are four families of adhesion molecules, of which the most important for adhesion to the extracellular matrix (ECM) is the family of integrins. These are transmembrane glycoproteins consisting of non-covalently associated α and β subunits. Different α and β subunits exist and the way they combine determines the ligand specificity of the integrin. For example, the heterodimers $\alpha1\beta1$ and $\alpha6\beta4$ are receptors for the ECM protein, laminin, while $\alpha5\beta1$, $\alpha4\beta1$ and $\alpha4\beta7$ bind fibronectin.

Using monoclonal antibodies specific for various subunits, the pattern of expression of integrins by different trophoblast populations at the implantation site is now well documented[4]. The $\alpha6\beta4$ integrin is seen on the layer of villous cytotrophoblast cells and is continued to be expressed by those cytotrophoblast cells of the cell columns nearest the villous core. This integrin disappears further out in the cell columns to be replaced by the heterodimer $\alpha5\beta1$ which is continued to be expressed by the interstitial trophoblast invading into decidua. Thus, there appears to be a downregulation of the $\alpha6\beta4$ laminin receptor with a concomitant upregulation of the $\alpha5\beta1$ fibronectin receptor as trophoblast invades the decidua. This observation is very similar to that seen during the healing of a skin wound where the sessile keratinocytes that form the normal epidermis express $\alpha6\beta4$ while those keratinocytes which migrate over to close the wound express $\alpha5\beta1$. In pre-eclampsia, trophoblast fails to downregulate $\beta4$ and to upregulate $\alpha1$ subunits as seen in normal pregnancy, indicating that disregulation of these integrins could be responsible for the inadequate trophoblast invasion of decidua associated with this pathological condition. What factors determine this switch from one integrin to another, however, are not known. Differential expression of other integrin subunits has also been demonstrated on trophoblast. For example, the $\alpha2$ subunit localises to cytotrophoblast cells at the base of the cell columns where many mitotic figures are seen. This is in accord with studies on other cellular systems where the $\alpha2\beta1$ integrin is frequently expressed strongly by rapidly proliferating cells.

Changes in the pattern of integrin expression as trophoblast migrates into decidua are accompanied by a parallel alteration in the production of ECM proteins. Fibronectin is not detected in the proximal part of the cytotrophoblast cell columns, but appears in the distal portion of the columns. This matrix protein is probably produced by trophoblast. However, the decidual stroma is also rich in fibronectin and it is thought that progesterone might be the stimulant for synthesis by decidual stromal cells as fibronectin is not a feature of non-pregnant endometrial stroma. There are several isoforms of fibronectin which are produced by alternative splicing of the precursor mRNA. The fibronectin synthesised by trophoblast appears to be the embryonic isoform similar to that used in cell migration during embryogenesis. Laminin, produced by stromal cells, is also found in great abundance in decidua. Both laminin and fibronectin show the unusual feature of being located as a distinct pericellular layer surrounding individual decidual stromal cells. Similar to fibronectin, the amount of laminin present varies throughout the menstrual cycle, with very little found during the proliferative phase followed by a gradual increase by the secretory phase and conspicuous quantities are laid down in decidua. The laminin molecule is made up of three genetically distinct chains α, β and γ linked together in a cross-shaped structure. A number of α, β and γ chains have been identified which can combine to give rise to seven different heterotrimers

TABLE 9.1
Laminin isoforms

Name	Chain composition
Laminin-1	$\alpha1\beta1\gamma1$
Laminin-2	$\alpha2\beta1\gamma1$
Laminin-3	$\alpha1\beta2\gamma1$
Laminin-4	$\alpha2\beta2\gamma1$
Laminin-5	$\alpha3\beta3\gamma2$
Laminin-6	$\alpha3\beta1\gamma1$
Laminin-7	$\alpha3\beta2\gamma1$

designated as LM1–7 (Table 9.1). Current opinion is that the laminin produced by decidual stromal cells is mainly LM-2 and LM-4. In contrast to the findings with laminin, collagen type VI is present as a dense microfibrillar network in the stroma of preimplantation endometrium, but is no longer detectable in decidua. This has led to the suggestion that the loss of collagen VI could result in the formation of a more flexible decidual matrix which would facilitate trophoblast invasion.

Binding to ECM proteins by integrins will transduce signals into the trophoblast cell via signalling pathways which include activation of protein tyrosine kinases, such as the focal adhesion kinase (FAK), pp. 125^{FAK}. In this way, interaction of trophoblast integrins with matrix proteins such as laminin and fibronectin could play an important role in influencing trophoblast behaviour during implantation.

Matrix degradation by trophoblast

Besides adhesion to ECM proteins via integrins, cellular migration also requires degradation of the matrix. This process involves the production of proteolytic enzymes by the migrating cell. The two main groups of enzymes are members of the plasminogen activator (PA) system of serine proteases and the family of matrix metalloproteinases (MMP). The MMP family is divided into three main classes based on their substrate specificities (Table 9.2): the collagenases, the gelatinases and the stromelysins. There is an intricate interaction between the PA and MMP systems, and together they can break down the major components of ECM. The activity of these proteases is subjected to close control by specific inhibitors. There are two inhibitors for PA (PAI) designated as PAI-1 and PAI-2, and two tissue inhibitors for MMP (TIMP) designated as TIMP-1 and TIMP-2.

Trophoblast cells possess proteolytic activity which can be demonstrated *in vitro* by their digestion of the surrounding matrix on which the cells are seeded[5]. Zymogram studies have shown that trophoblast cells produce a wide array of proteases, this production being greater in first-trimester trophoblast compared to trophoblast later in gestation which, therefore, mirrors the invasive capacity of early trophoblast.

TABLE 9.2
Members of the matrix metalloproteinase (MMP) family

Name	Extracellular matrix substrate
Collagenases	
MMP-1	Collagens I, II, III, VII, X
MMP-5	Collagens I, II, III
Gelatinases	
MMP-2	Gelatins, collagens IV, V, elastin
MMP-9	Gelatins, collagens IV, V, elastin
Stromelysins	
MMP-3	Proteoglycans, FN, LM, gelatin, collagens III, IV, V, X
MMP-10	Proteoglycans, FN, LM, gelatin, collagens III, IV, V, X
MMP-7	Proteoglycans, collagen IV, FN, gelatin, elastin

FN = fibronectin; LM = laminin.

These observations have led to the conclusion that PA, MMP, PAI and TIMP together provide an intricate network that controls matrix degradation during trophoblast invasion.

Endovascular trophoblast migration

This process appears to utilise a mechanism different from the one described for interstitial trophoblast invading decidua[4]. Here, members of the selectin family of adhesion molecules are involved. Three members of this family, L-, E- and P-selectins, have been identified. Unlike other adhesion molecules, selectins bind to carbohydrate ligands such as the blood group-related antigen Lewis X (Le^X) or its sialylated derivative sialyl-Le^X. Endovascular trophoblast expresses sialyl-Le^X and E- and P-selectins have been localised to vascular endothelial cells in decidua basalis but not decidua parietalis. Thus, the appropriate molecules are present for endovascular trophoblast to adhere to vascular endothelial cells. The fact that these selectins are observed only on endothelial cells of the decidua basalis suggests a local source of inductive signal for their expression. It is interesting to note that similar mechanisms are utilised by neutrophils migrating out from the circulation into an acute inflammatory site.

Trophoblast expression of major histocompatibility complex (MHC) antigens

MHC class I and class II antigens serve as important recognition molecules concerned with vertebrate immune responses. In humans, these antigens are also known as human leukocyte antigens (HLA). Class I antigens are expressed on nearly all nucleated cells and class II antigens on specialised cells involved in antigen presentation such as dendritic cells, macrophages and B cells. Both HLA class I and class II antigens are highly polymorphic and incompatibility for these

TABLE 9.3
Characteristics of HLA-C and HLA-G compared with HLA-A and HLA-B

HLA-C and HLA-G	HLA-A and HLA-B
Low surface expression	High surface expression
Few alleles	Many alleles
Polymorphism not concentrated at antigen-binding site	Polymorphism concentrated at antigen-binding site
Reactive T cells occasionally demonstrable to HLA-C but not to HLA-G	Reactive T cells readily demonstrable

antigens between donor and recipient is the basis of graft rejection.

No trophoblast cell populations express HLA class II antigens and villous trophoblast is also negative for HLA class I. However, extravillous trophoblast cells that invade decidua and interact with uterine tissues do express HLA class I antigens. Presently, there are six HLA class I loci which code for an expressed protein: three classical loci (HLA-A, -B and -C) and three non-classical loci (HLA-E, -F and -G). The antigens expressed by extravillous trophoblast are HLA-C and HLA-G. Thus, trophoblast is unusual compared to other cell types which express HLA-A, -B and -C. The expression of HLA-G appears to be restricted to extravillous trophoblast which suggests that it might have an important role to play in implantation.

The functions of HLA-C and HLA-G, however, have not yet been clearly defined. Both these antigens exhibit characteristics which are somewhat different from those of HLA-A and HLA-B (Table 9.3). From this it can be seen that HLA-C and -G are probably not important ligands for T cells and, therefore, are unlikely to stimulate a classical graft rejection response by the mother.[2]

Leukocyte populations in decidua

Analysis of the leukocyte populations in decidua has shown that the predominant cell type is natural killer (NK) cells rather than T or B cells. Many of these cells have prominent granules in their cytoplasm and are hence also referred to as large granular lymphocytes (LGL). They have the unusual phenotype of $CD56^{bright}$ $CD16^{-}$ which differentiates them from the classical NK cells in peripheral blood which are $CD56^{dim}$ $CD16^{+}$. The number of these NK cells in the uterine mucosa varies throughout the menstrual cycle. They are sparse during the proliferative phase, increase significantly by the secretory phase and remain in high numbers in decidua during the early part of gestation. This suggests that their recruitment is hormonally controlled. The numbers then decline as pregnancy progresses and only very few cells remain by term. During the first trimester, these NK cells are particularly abundant in the decidua basalis in close contact with invading trophoblast cells. This temporal and spatial association with the implanting placenta has led to the proposal that these decidual NK cells might play an important role in the control of trophoblast migration and differentiation[2].

Trophoblast–decidual NK cell interaction

There is recent and convincing evidence that NK cells in peripheral blood express receptors capable of recognising HLA class I molecules[6]. One family of receptors belongs to the immunoglobulin superfamily and are known as killer inhibitory receptors (KIR) because, in contrast to T cells, interaction of these NK cell receptors with HLA class I molecules leads to the transmission of negative signals that inhibit cytolysis of target cells. However, it has subsequently been shown that some members of this family can transmit positive signals leading to cytolysis or cytokine production. These receptors are, therefore, known as killer activatory receptors (KAR). Both KIR and KAR are transmembrane glycoproteins and it is their transmembrane and cytoplasmic domains which determine their activatory or inhibitory signalling roles. Another NK cell receptor family for HLA class I molecules has also been described, CD94. Unlike KIR/KAR, the CD94 family are type II membrane glycoproteins with an external lectin-like domain which forms heterodimers with another NK lectin, NKG2. Recent studies have confirmed that decidual NK cells also express both KIR/KAR and CD94 so that they are likely to utilise similar mechanisms of target cell recognition as peripheral blood NK cells.

Interestingly, the class I antigen which may be most influential to NK cell function is HLA-C and there is recent evidence that HLA-G might also be important. These are the two HLA class I molecules expressed by extravillous trophoblast (see above). Thus, the possibility

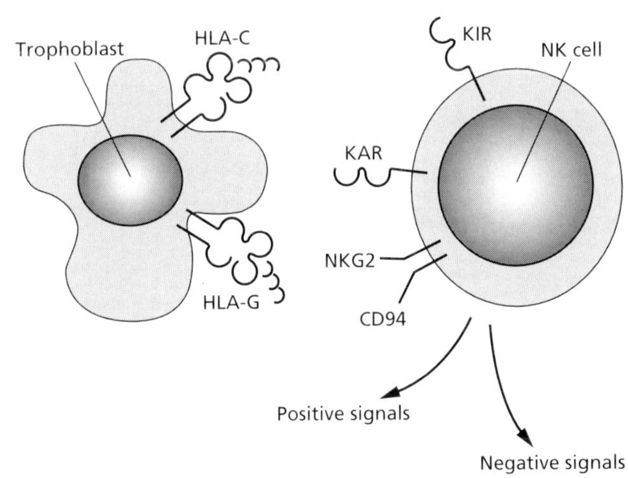

Fig. 9.2 HLA molecules expressed by extravillous trophoblast and their potential receptors on decidual NK cells. (From Loke and King, *Molecular Medicine Today*.)

arises that decidual NK cells could recognise HLA-C or HLA-G expressed by invading trophoblast resulting in the generation of an appropriate combination of positive or negative signals that would influence trophoblast behaviour during the process of implantation (Fig. 9.2). Certain combinations of this interaction might be less optimal than others leading to poor control of trophoblast invasion which is the cause of clinical conditions such as miscarriage, IUGR and pre-eclampsia. This would represent a form of allogeneic recognition that is fundamentally different to that seen in organ transplantation.

Conclusion

Elucidation of the molecular and cellular interactions occurring during placental implantation is essential for a clear understanding of what happens in the early stages of gestation. Correct implantation is required for proper placental and fetal growth. In addition, epidemiological data have shown that growth retardation *in utero* is associated with an increase in incidence of diseases in adult life. Thus, any dysregulation of this process will have far-reaching consequences.

REFERENCES

1. Aplin JD. The cell biology of human implantation. *Placenta* **17**:269–275, 1996.
2. Loke YW, King A. *Human Implantation: Cell Biology and Immunology*. Cambridge: Cambridge University Press, 1995.
3. Pijnenborg R. Trophoblast invasion. *Reprod Med Rev* **3**:53–73, 1994.
4. Burrows TD, King A, Loke YW. Trophoblast migration during human placental implantation. *Hum Reprod Update* **2**:307–321, 1996.
5. Cross JC, Werb Z, Fisher SJ. Implantation and the placenta: key pieces of the development puzzle. *Science* **266**:1508–1518, 1994.
6. Lanier LL, Philips JH. Inhibitory MHC class I receptors on NK cells and T cells. *Immunol Today* **17**:86–91, 1996.

Development of the placenta and its circulation

10

P. Kaufmann and J. Kingdom

Introduction

We have tried to entice the reader into areas in which placental biology and pathology directly impinge on their practice. In this way, we hope the content will prove useful for many of the ensuing chapters. More detailed anatomical and physiological information can be found in Benirschke and Kaufmann (1995)[1] and Knobil and Neill (1994)[2].

Macroscopy of the delivered placenta

The full-term human placenta is a disc-like, usually circular, organ normally inspected in its 'inverted' state from the fetal, or chorionic plate, surface. Macroscopic abnormalities, such as succenturiate lobes, velamentous cord insertion, or circumvallate margin, are identified from this aspect and occur in approximately 10% of cases at full-term[3]; in general, these abnormalities occur more frequently in pregnancies complicated by poor fetal growth and/or vaginal bleeding but they are of passing interest to the clinician since other factors dominate management. Nevertheless, experience in second trimester ultrasonographic examination of the placenta is increasing, with rare but clinically relevant problems, such as vasa praevia, being identified[4].

The appearances and weight of the delivered placenta, a highly vascularized organ, are strongly dependent upon the following: mode of delivery; timing of cord clamping; and degree of maternal blood loss from the intervillous space[1,5]. These considerations are important when considering epidemiological data relating placental weight to adult disease states, or when considering interpretation of morphological data describing structural differences between placentas from pathological situations (typically delivered by caesarean section) and controls (often delivered vaginally)[6]. Unbiased interpretation of microscopic placental appearances depends upon appropriate sampling (including all representative areas), tissue fixation and embedding. These considerations will be illustrated in due course.

The human placenta provides direct contact between maternal blood and the chorionic (fetal) villi – the haemochorial placenta (Fig. 10.1). It is radically different in structure, but not necessarily in function, from that of commonly employed animal models in perinatal physiology such as the sheep, which has an epithelio-chorial arrangement in which two additional anatomical layers separate maternal and fetal blood. It is the uniquely invasive properties of the extravillous trophoblast which result in the haemo-monochorial arrangement. This process of invasion is precisely controlled and it is the disordered extravillous trophoblast proliferation/migration which relates to major clinical conditions such as pre-eclampsia (inadequate invasion) or placenta accreta (excessive invasion).

The gross structure of the full-term placenta is illustrated in Fig. 10.1. The chorionic plate is a fibrous disc into which the umbilical arteries ramify as chorionic plate vessels in a dichotomous fashion, each penetrating the plate to enter the stem (truncus) of a villous tree, and accompanied by a vein draining oxygenated blood back towards the umbilical vein. The chorionic plate vessels are covered by the amniotic membrane which is normally glossy and can easily be peeled off. At the placental margin, the chorionic plate thickens to form a ring connecting the placenta with the chorion laeve; when this ring is undergrown by villous trees and the intervillous space, the membranes insert medial to the edge of the chorionic plate, in what is termed a circumvallate placenta.

Macroscopic evidence of intra-amniotic infection, such as cloudy yellow malodorous discoloration, or localized collections of discoloured amniotic fluid, should be sought when clinically relevant. Successful diagnosis of underlying cause is dependent upon collection of fluid/pus (for gas chromatography), a membrane roll (from rupture point to edge of placenta) and samples of placenta and cord into sterile

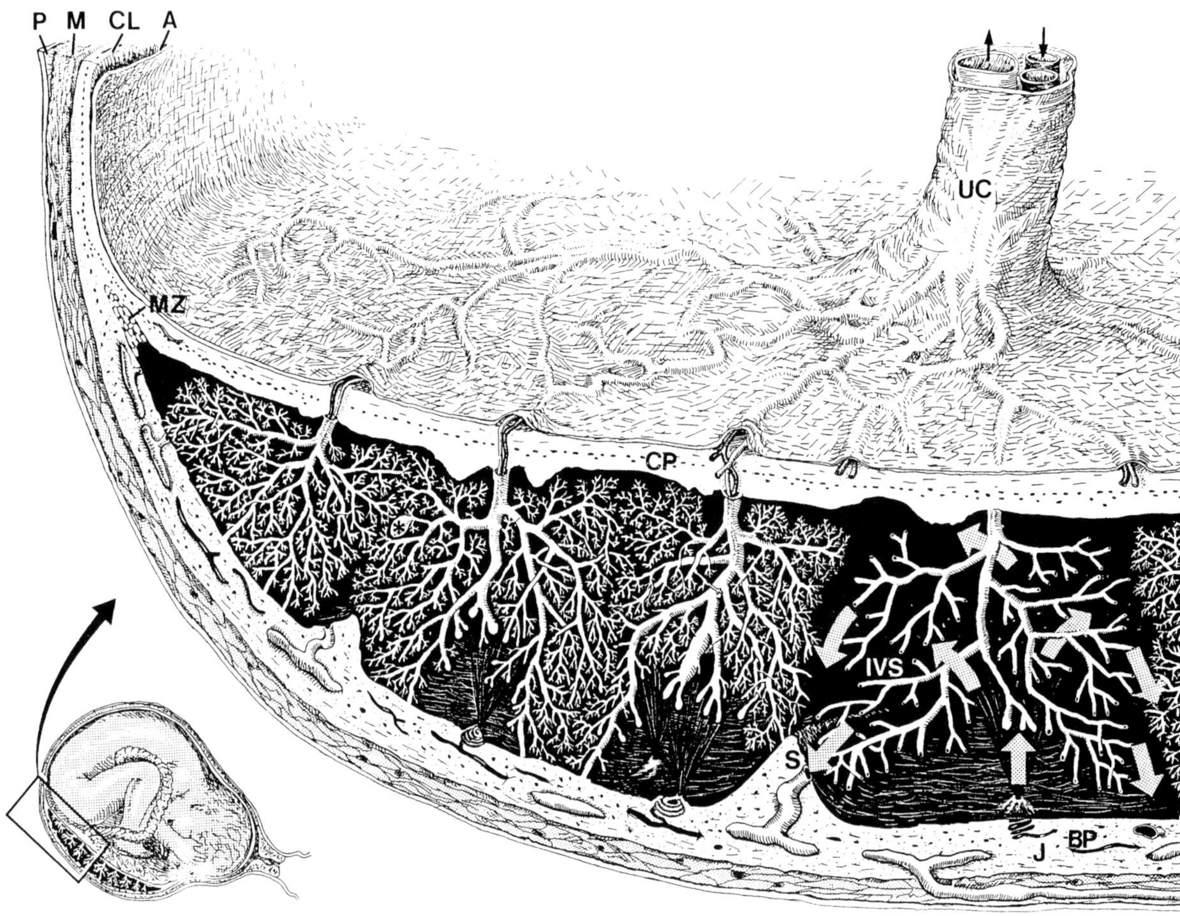

Fig. 10.1 Nearly mature human placenta *in situ*. CP = chorionic plate; IVS = intervillous space; P = serosa; M = myometrium; CL = chorion laeve; A = amnion; MZ = marginal zone between placenta and fetal membranes, with obliterated intervillous space and ghost villi; * = cell island; S = septum; J = junctional zone; BP = basal plate; UC = umbilical cord. From Kaufmann and Scheffen[120] with permission.

containers, prior to transport to the pathology department. Cloudy nodular discolorations of the amnion, amnion nodosum, are indicative of prolonged rupture of the membranes and oligohydramnios[1].

The maternal surface of the placenta (referred to as the basal plate) is an artificial surface in that delivery of the 'placenta' requires the organ to be cleaved through the basal plate (Fig. 10.1). In this sense, part of the trophoblast remains undelivered in the placental bed, normally regressing over the ensuing weeks. The basal plate is a heterogeneous mixture of trophoblastic and decidual cells, embedded in large amounts of extracellular debris, fibrinoid and blood clot. The basal surface is divided by a system of grooves into 10–40 elevated areas referred to as the maternal lobes of the placenta. These correspond approximately to the underlying arrangement of villous trees with three or four trees per lobe in the centre; small lobes at the periphery of the placenta are generally occupied only by a single villous tree. Only the latter correspond to what Schuhmann[7] described as a placentone: a villous tree together with its surrounding part of the intervillous space and its corresponding uteroplacental vessels (Fig. 10.2).

Terms such as 'fetal placenta' for the chorionic plate (including villous trees) and 'maternal placental' for the basal plate (including uteroplacental vessels invaded by trophoblast) are tempting from a clinical perspective, as will be discussed in relation to Doppler studies[8] However, since it is impossible to physically separate the fetal and maternal cellular constituents, this concept must be viewed with extreme caution.

The complex physiological arrangements, and disordered anatomy present under pathological circumstances, underscore the value of *in situ* studies as opposed to data acquired from dispersed (e.g. cell culture) or homogenized tissues (e.g. biochemistry). Furthermore, since many pathological states result in preterm delivery, it becomes essential to appreciate the developmental biology of this complex organ as outlined in the next section.

Placental development

The key stages of placental development, beginning with blastocyst attachment, are shown in Fig. 10.3. The initial stages

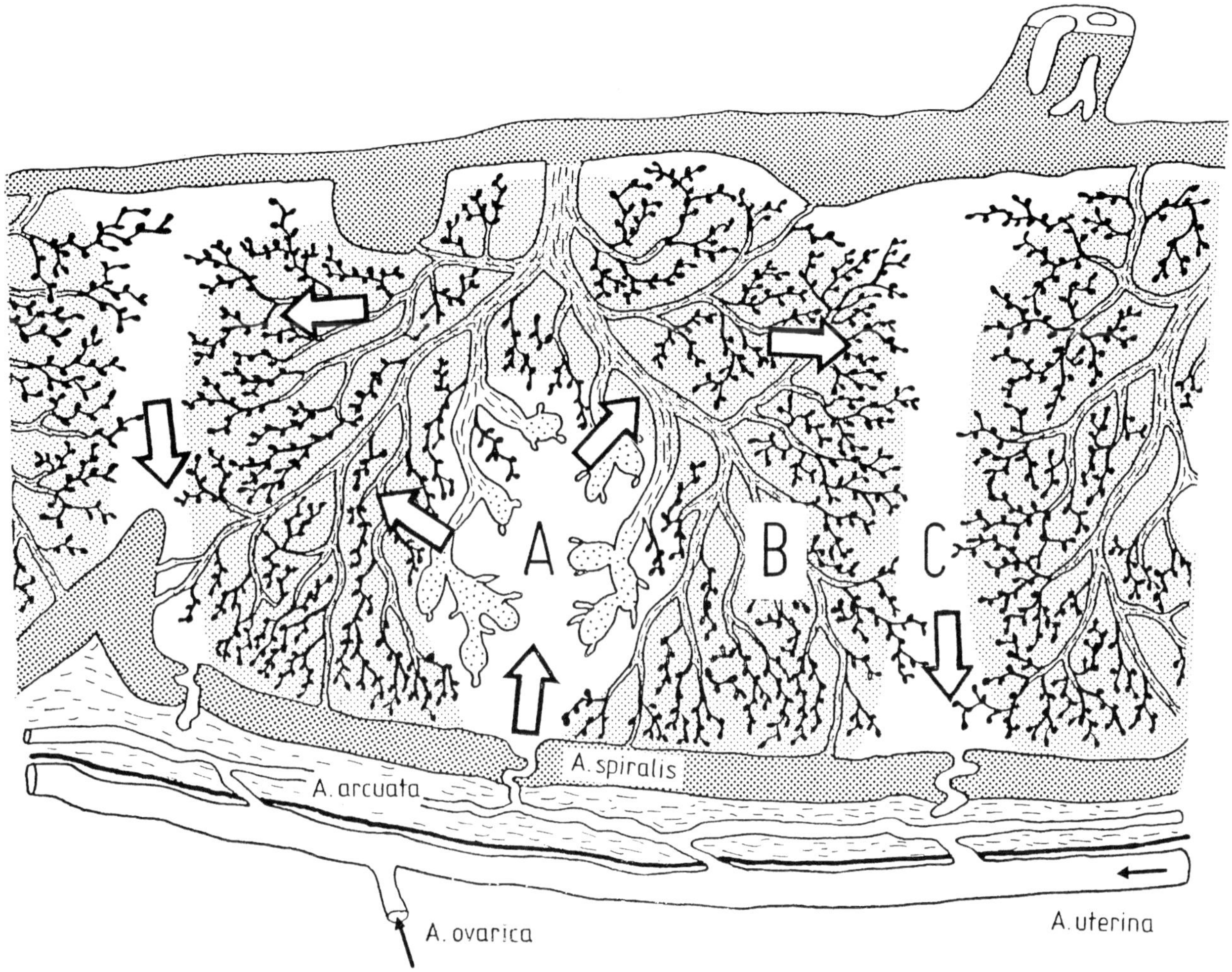

Fig. 10.2 Spatial relations between villous trees, single villous types, and the maternal bloodstream. A placentone is one villous tree together with the related part of the intervillous space. Maternal blood (arrows) enters the intervillous space in the centres of the villous trees (central cavity) (A) and leaves the intervillous space via wide clefts (C) between neighbouring villous trees. Modified from Kaufmann and Scheffen[120] with permission.

are concerned with embedding of the blastocyst, a collection of cells destined to form the embryo surrounded by a monolayer of cytotrophoblast, beneath the uterine epithelium (Fig. 10.3a,b). The cytotrophoblast in contact with the epithelium proliferates and fuses to form a syncytial layer which expands into the uterine stroma bringing the entire conceptus inside the uterine wall (Fig. 10.3c). Rapid expansion of the syncytiotrophoblast, due to multiplication of cytotrophoblast, takes place and lacunar spaces form within the syncytium which coalesces to form a loose network – the forerunner of the intervillous space. The remaining pillars of syncytiotrophoblast are known as trabeculae (Fig. 10.3c,d). Finger-like protrusions of the trophoblast into the lacunae, formed by underlying growth of cytotrophoblast, are the beginning of villous development – the primary villi. These are invaded by stroma, derived from the extra-embryonic mesenchyme, the future connective tissue of the placenta derived from the allantois, to begin the process of fetal vascularization (Fig. 10.3e). By day 20 post-fertilization, cells within this mesenchymal stroma organize to form primitive capillaries (Fig. 10.3f), while others form haemangioblastic stem cells[9]. The capillary system of the primitive villi connects proximally with those of the fetus (derived from the allantois) and a complete fetoplacental circulation is established by day 35 post-fertilization. Haematopoiesis is observed within newly-formed villous capillaries during the first trimester, following which this process becomes dominant in the fetal liver.

Development of the maternal, or intervillous, placental circulation proceeds in a different manner. As the trophoblastic shell invades the uterine stroma, it comes into contact with maternal capillaries (Fig. 10.3d). The leading edge is comprised of cytotrophoblast which has extended the full length of trabeculae destined to form anchoring villi (Fig. 10.3f). This arrangement allows cytotrophoblast to enter maternal capillaries, thereby preventing maternal haemorrhage into the stroma. The lacunar spaces of the syncytiotrophoblast initially contain maternal plasma, since maternal erythrocytes are not consistently identified within the intervillous space prior to 11 post-menstrual weeks of gestation[10]. This apparent lack of intervillous blood perfusion is supported by both

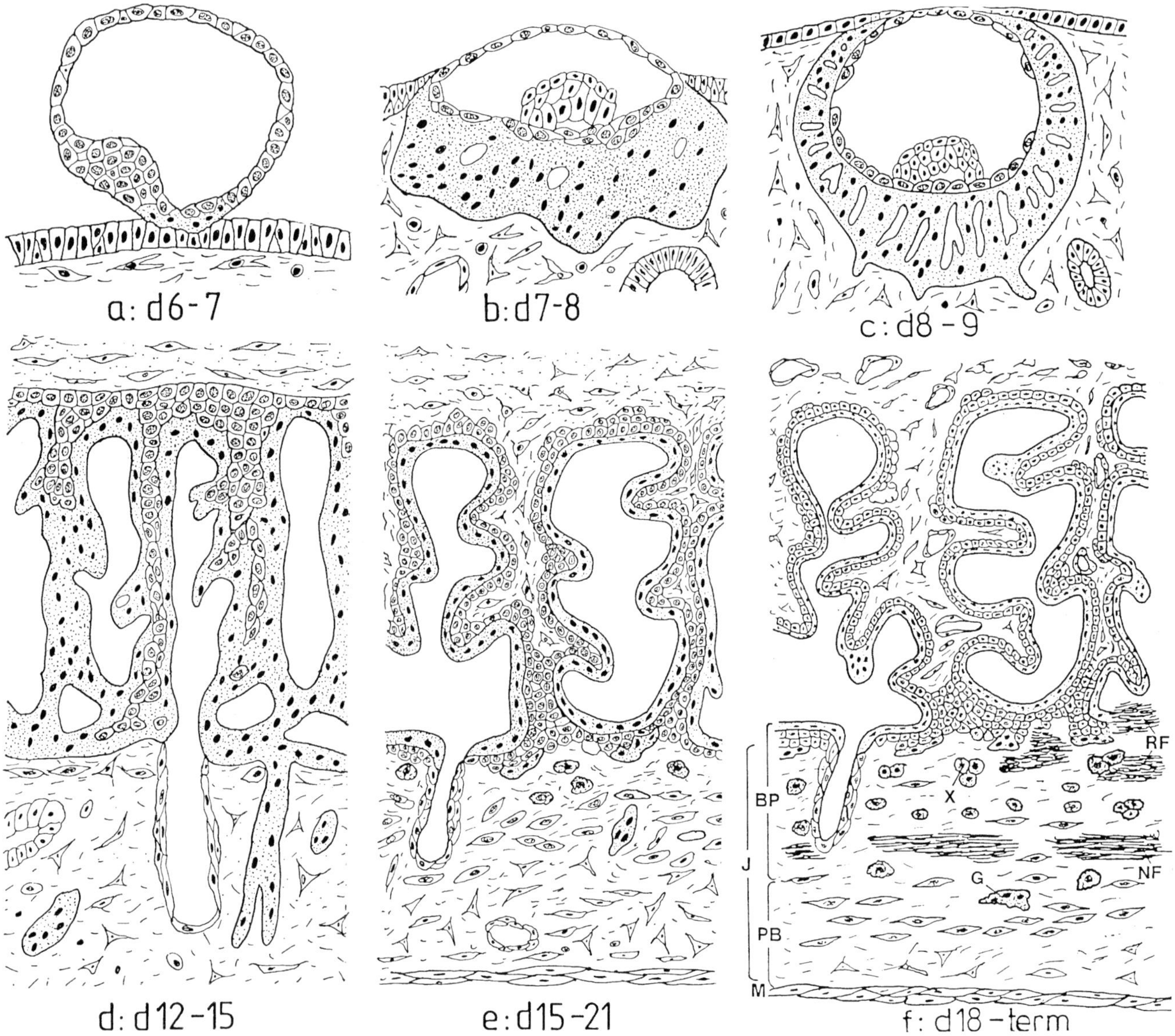

Fig. 10.3 Simplified drawings of the typical stages of early placental development. (a) Early invasion; (b) prelacunar stage; (c) lacunar stage; (d) transition from lacunar to primary villous stage; (e) secondary villous stage; (f) tertiary villous stage. E = endometrial epithelium; EB = embryoblast; CT = cytotrophoblast; ST = syncytiotrophoblast; EM = extra-embryonic mesoderm; CP = chorionic plate; T = trabeculae and primary villi; L = maternal blood lacunae; TS = trophoblastic shell; EV = endometrial vessel; D = decidua; RF = Rohr's fibrinoid; NF = Nitabuch's fibrinoid; G = trophoblastic giant cell; X = extravillous cytotrophoblast; BP = basal plate; PB = placental bed; J = junctional zone. Modified from Kaufmann and Scheffen[120] with permission.

angiographic studies, by transcervical endoscopic observations of the intervillous space[11], and by elegant studies which demonstrate an oxygen gradient between maternal stroma and villous placenta in the first trimester[12]. This arrangement appears to allow embryogenesis to take place in an environment which is hypoxic relative to maternal tissues, while at the same time protecting the developing conceptus from the risk of displacement by haemorrhage, i.e. spontaneous abortion, during early invasion of the stroma.

Towards the end of the first trimester, the existence of both a fetal and a maternal circulation results in a haemochorial arrangement whereby the two circulations are separated by the 'placental barrier', which is made up of the following layers (Fig. 10.4): (1) a continuous layer of syncytiotrophoblast, covering the villi and thus lining the intervillous space; (2) an initially (first trimester) complete, but later on (second and third trimester) discontinuous layer of cytotrophoblast; (3) a trophoblastic basal lamina; (4) connective tissue derived from the extra-embryonic mesoderm; and (5) fetal endothelium, which is surrounded by an endothelial basal lamina only in the last trimester. Throughout the following months of pregnancy, this barrier undergoes quantitative rather than qualitative changes; the syncytiotrophoblast is reduced in thickness from more than 20 μm to a mean of

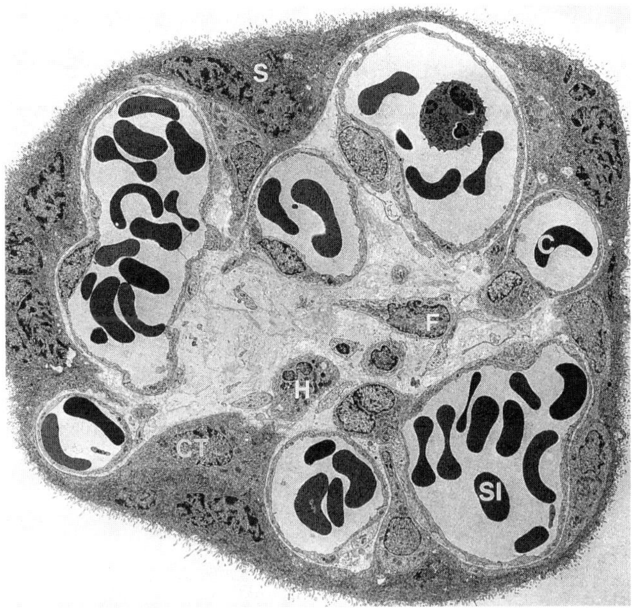

Fig. 10.4 Electron micrograph of a terminal villus from a fully mature placenta showing capillaries (C) and sinusoids (SI). The sparse connective tissue is composed of macrophages (H) and fibroblasts (F). S = syncytiotrophoblast; CT = cytotrophoblastic cell. × 1400. From ref. 122, with permission.

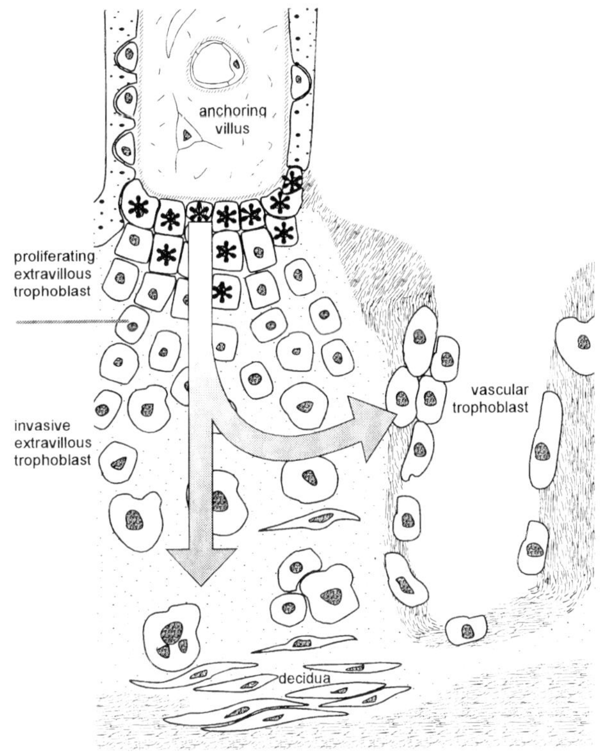

Fig. 10.5 Schematic drawing of a trophoblastic cell column connecting a villous stem (above) to the basal plate (below). Proliferating stem cells (*) of the extravillous trophoblast. The arrow symbolizes the invasive pathway. Fibrin-type fibrinoid (line shading). Extracellular matrix (light point shading).

3.5 μm[1]. The cytotrophoblast is rarified and, at full-term, can be found in only 20% of the villous surface. The mean villous diameter decreases, since the newly formed generations of villi are generally smaller than the previous generation and it follows that the fetal capillaries become located to the villous surface. These factors result in a reduction of the mean materno-fetal diffusion distance from between 50 and 100 μm in the first trimester, down to between 4 and 5 μm at full-term[1] – just one of the many aspects of placental differentiation designed to cope with the increasing metabolic demands of the rapidly growing fetus.

Trophoblast invasion and utero-placental vessels

Trophoblast invasion into the maternal tissues is not restricted to the process of implantation and early placentation; it is a continuous process serving a number of purposes. The so-called 'cell columns', at the base of the anchoring villi, connecting the villous trees to the basal plate, provide the cellular sources for this invasive process (Fig. 10.5). These cell columns do not contain stroma since they were not excavated by mesenchyme during formation of the villous trees. The cytotrophoblast cells composing these cell columns, together with similar structures in the chorionic plate and membranes, are collectively described as the extravillous trophoblast (EVT) (for review see Kaufmann and Castellucci[13]).

As can be seen in Fig. 10.5, the column of EVT cells resting on the basal plate should be viewed as a rapidly proliferating zone from which EVT migrates continuously into maternal tissues. However as soon as EVT cells leave this proliferative zone, they leave the cell division cycle and change to an invasive phenotype. Their pattern of integrin expression, secretion of proteolytic enzymes and production of extracellular matrix proteins is strikingly similar to that of malignant tumour cells[13]. Fortunately they differ in one fundamental aspect – they have lost their ability to proliferate. Because of this, the depth of invasion into maternal tissues is limited to their individual life span: where deportation into the maternal venous, or lymphatic, circulation occurs, metastatic growth is impossible since these cells have lost their ability to proliferate.

Invasion by EVT serves two very different purposes, namely adhesion of the placenta to the uterine wall and adaptation of uteroplacental arteries to the fetal requirements.

ADHESION OF THE PLACENTA

The invasive trophoblast cells secrete huge amounts of extracellular matrix (composed of laminins, collagen IV, fibronectins, vitronectin and heparan sulfate) known as matrix-type fibrinoid[14] into which they are embedded. The EVT cells adhere to the extracellular matrix via the surface expression of molecules known as integrins. Likewise, the endometrial stromal cells adhere via similar mechanisms; root-like projections of extravillous trophoblast, together with its associated matrix, penetrate deep into the myometrium, thereby ensuring perfect anchoring of the placenta. Adhesion of the placenta by the glue-like extracellular matrix[15] depends on the viability of the EVT expressing integrins; in this sense it is reversible at delivery. This anchoring process is essential, otherwise entry of maternal blood into the intervillous space at high velocity would shear off the chorionic plate.

The invasive nature of haemochorial placentation is precisely regulated under normal circumstances; when it occurs to excess, the EVT may invade deeply into (accreta) or through (percreta) the uterine wall, such that physiological separation of the placenta cannot occur. Conversely, a failure of this anchoring process predisposes to abruption, either during the antepartum period or during labour. However the mechanisms by which invasive behaviour of the EVT, or adhesive properties of the matrix, are disturbed in these conditions is not yet understood.

PHYSIOLOGICAL CHANGES OF UTEROPLACENTAL ARTERIES

The number of uteroplacental spiral arteries supplying the intervillous space becomes reduced as pregnancy advances, due to vascular obliteration such that, by term, the intervillous space is perfused by approximately one hundred spiral arteries[16]. However, intervillous blood flow increases considerably, largely due to a series of changes which occur throughout pregnancy, designed to meet the nutritional and metabolic demands of the growing fetus. These comprise terminal dilatation of the arteries as well as loss of elasticity and contractility of the arterial walls, well known physiological changes of the uteroplacental arteries in which there is replacement of the muscular media, its autonomic innervation and surrounding connective tissue cells by extravillous trophoblast[17]. Arterial dilatation is an important component of falling uteroplacental vascular impedance and these changes release the uteroplacental arteries from autonomic and local vasomotor influences upon vascular impedance, such that intervillous perfusion is limited by systemic arterial pressure. Differential regulation of uteroplacental blood flow by the mother is not possible. As an example, the insertion of an epidural anaesthetic during labour will result in a fall in uteroplacental perfusion, with predictable changes in fetal heart rate, unless both blood pressure and systemic vascular impedance are maintained by volume expansion and intravenous ephedrine.

The commonly prevailing view of uteroplacental arterial dilatation is one of vessel wall destruction[16–20]. This view has been challenged by several groups[21–23] who, based on studies in the human and guinea pig, concluded that dilatation precedes trophoblast-mediated destruction of the vessel wall. Recently, Nanaev *et al.* (1995)[24] have elucidated one mechanism by which extravillous trophoblast cells, approaching uteroplacental arteries in the guinea pig, induce vasodilatation – namely an intense co-expression of endothelial (eNOS) and macrophage nitric oxide synthase (mNOS) implying local generation of nitric oxide (NO). Once maximally dilated by the low levels of NO generated by eNOS, the media of the uteroplacental arteries may subsequently be destroyed by the cytotoxic properties of high levels generated by the macrophage isoform[24].

In humans, the process of uteroplacental dilatation and invasion begins in the central part of the placenta and spreads towards the periphery[25]. When the placenta is predominantly located on one side of the uterus, Doppler examination of the ipsilateral uteroplacental artery during the second trimester indicates lower impedance than the opposite side. The observation of high-impedance waveforms from the uteroplacental arteries, together with preservation of the early diastolic notch on the placental side of the uterus, is associated with complications of pregnancy such as pre-eclampsia, intrauterine growth restriction and abruption[8]. The non-invasive Doppler studies are supported by earlier histological studies demonstrating incomplete trophoblast invasion of spiral arteries in these conditions[25–29]. Recently animal data have become available exploring the relation between NOS activity and reproductive performance. Chwalisz, Garfield and coworkers[30–32] have shown that pre-eclampsia-like features, such as hypertension, proteinuria and intrauterine growth restriction can be induced in rats and guinea pigs by competitive inhibition of nitric oxide synthase (NOS) with L-nitroarginine methyl ester. Further studies, in particular of extravillous trophoblast using immunohistochemistry and *in situ* hybridization, are needed both in order to confirm the role of reduced extravillous nitric oxide secretion in the pathogenesis of pre-eclampsia and to elucidate the local and/or endocrine factors responsible for the control of NO secretion[33].

The uteroplacental veins, approximately 50–200 in number, drain the intervillous space from the margins of the fetal cotyledons, thus surrounding the basal parts of the villous trees (for review see Benirschke and Kaufmann[1]). In contrast to the arteries, the veins are only poorly invaded by extravillous trophoblast and obviously are not involved in the regulation of the intervillous blood flow.

Intervillous space and architecture of the villous trees

The human placenta is of the hemochorial, villous type, such that maternal blood does not circulate through clearly defined blood vessels. Rather than leaving the spiral arteries, maternal blood circulates through the diffuse intervillous space and flows directly between the villi (Figs 10.1 and 10.2). Most anatomical investigations of the intervillous space have been made on delivered placentas which in the absence of a perfusion pressure appears as a system of extremely narrow clefts. Using postpartum data for intervillous blood volume (23–38%) and villous surface area at term (11–13 m^2), the mean width of the intervillous space has been calculated as ranging from 16 to 32 µm[1].

The classic injection studies of spiral arteries by Wigglesworth[34] indicated that a majority of the 60–70 villous trees, branching from the chorionic plate, are maternally perfused from their centres thus creating hollow-centered structures (Fig. 10.2). This concept was substantiated by Schuhmann's description of the 50–100 maternal arterial inlets as being located near the centres of the villous trees[7,35]. The 50–200 maternal venous outlets per placenta are thought to be arranged around the periphery of the villous trees such that each villous tree is perfused in a centrifugal manner. This unit was called a 'placentone' by Schuhmann and Wehler[35].

The mature placenta should be viewed, in functional terms, as a loose aggregation of 40–60 placentones which, under *in vivo* conditions, are in contact and overlap with each other[1]. This concept is valid for the thicker, more central, regions of the placenta since structural borderlines like placental septa are generally absent[36]. As a result, the villous trees are more homogeneous in comparison with the peripheral placentones, which are more distinctly separated from each other and as a consequence exhibit typical structural differences between their central and their peripheral zones (Fig. 10.2).

According to Schuhmann and Wehler[35], the centres of typical placentones exhibit loosely arranged villi, mostly of the immature intermediate type (see below), providing a large intervillous space for the maternal arterial inlet (Fig. 10.2). Schuhmann[7] suggested that these central cavities are 'inflated' under *in vivo* conditions, and thus collapse rapidly after delivery. The radio-angiographic studies conducted on the rhesus monkey[37] and in the human[38] support the placentone concept; colour flow Doppler imaging can now be used to study intraplacental blood flow relationships.

The arterial jet flows rapidly upwards through the central cavity, dispersing in a centrifugal manner to perfuse the surrounding well developed and more densely packed villi of mature intermediate and terminal type (see below) as indicated in Fig. 10.1 and 10.2[39]. Neighbouring villous trees are separated by perilobular zones comprising a loose arrangement of mature intermediate and terminal villi (Fig. 10.2). These zones are the venous outflow area and are connected to the subchorial lake.

The concept of individually functioning placentones has important implications for blood-flow regulation. If the maternal spiral artery is ligated, degeneration of the villous tree will result[40]; this makes sense since it would be pointless for the fetus to perfuse villous trees which have no maternal supply. *In vitro* dual-circuit perfusion studies of intact human placental cotyledons clearly demonstrate that maternal hypoxia induces reversible vasoconstriction of the stem villous arterioles. We believe this phenomenon is physiological rather than pathological, ensuring optimal maternal–fetal perfusion overlap throughout the network of placentones.

Reduced intervillous perfusion will result in villous placental hypoxia since fetal perfusion continues to remove oxygen bound to fetal haemoglobin; in response to falling oxygen tension, the stem villous arterioles will constrict to reduce the rate of removal of oxygen until intervillous oxygen tension equilibrates again. Spiral artery thrombosis and obliteration is commonly found in later gestation, associated with villous degeneration and placental infarction since presumably the lack of intervillous perfusion leads to stem villous arterial thrombosis[41]. Nevertheless, the huge functional reserve of the term placenta ensures this degenerative process poses no threat to fetal oxygenation.

Basic villous structure

Placental villi are composed of a superficial layer of trophoblast which surrounds the villous stroma (Figs 10.4 and 10.6). The main component is an outer, complete layer of syncytiotrophoblast, generally uninterrupted, and thus completely lining the intervillous space where it is in direct contact with maternal blood. As a true syncytium, the syncytiotrophoblast has lost all generative potency. Its regeneration and growth depends on the existence of mononuclear cellular trophoblast referred to as villous cytotrophoblast or Langhans cells. The latter form a second layer between syncytiotrophoblast and villous stroma; a continuous monolayer in early pregnancy, becomes discontinuous with villous growth[42]. Direct analysis of karyotype by chorionic villous sampling depends upon rapid division of cytotrophoblast. Determination of fetal karyotype by culture of villous explants depends upon the slower multiplication of villous stromal cells; since these are derived from embryonic (allantoic) tissues, they more accurately reflect the karyotype in fetal tissues, hence the general preference for culture-based results[43].

From a functional perspective, fusion of newly formed cytotrophoblast into the outer syncytium results in the transfer of fresh organelles, enzyme systems and messenger RNA transcripts into the syncytium. Aged syncytial nuclei cluster together, known as 'syncytial knots', and protrude into the intervillous space, prior to release into the maternal circulation. Continued rejuvenation of the syncytial layer is essential in order to sustain the intense metabolic activity required for maternofetal transfer processes, secretory and endocrine functions. As gestation advances, this process of rejuvenation appears to slow down, since the ratio of cytotrophoblast to syncytial nuclei within individual terminal villi decreases as syncytial knots become more common. Reduced villous cytotrophoblast number and/or replication, leading to syncytial apoptosis and knot formation, is typical

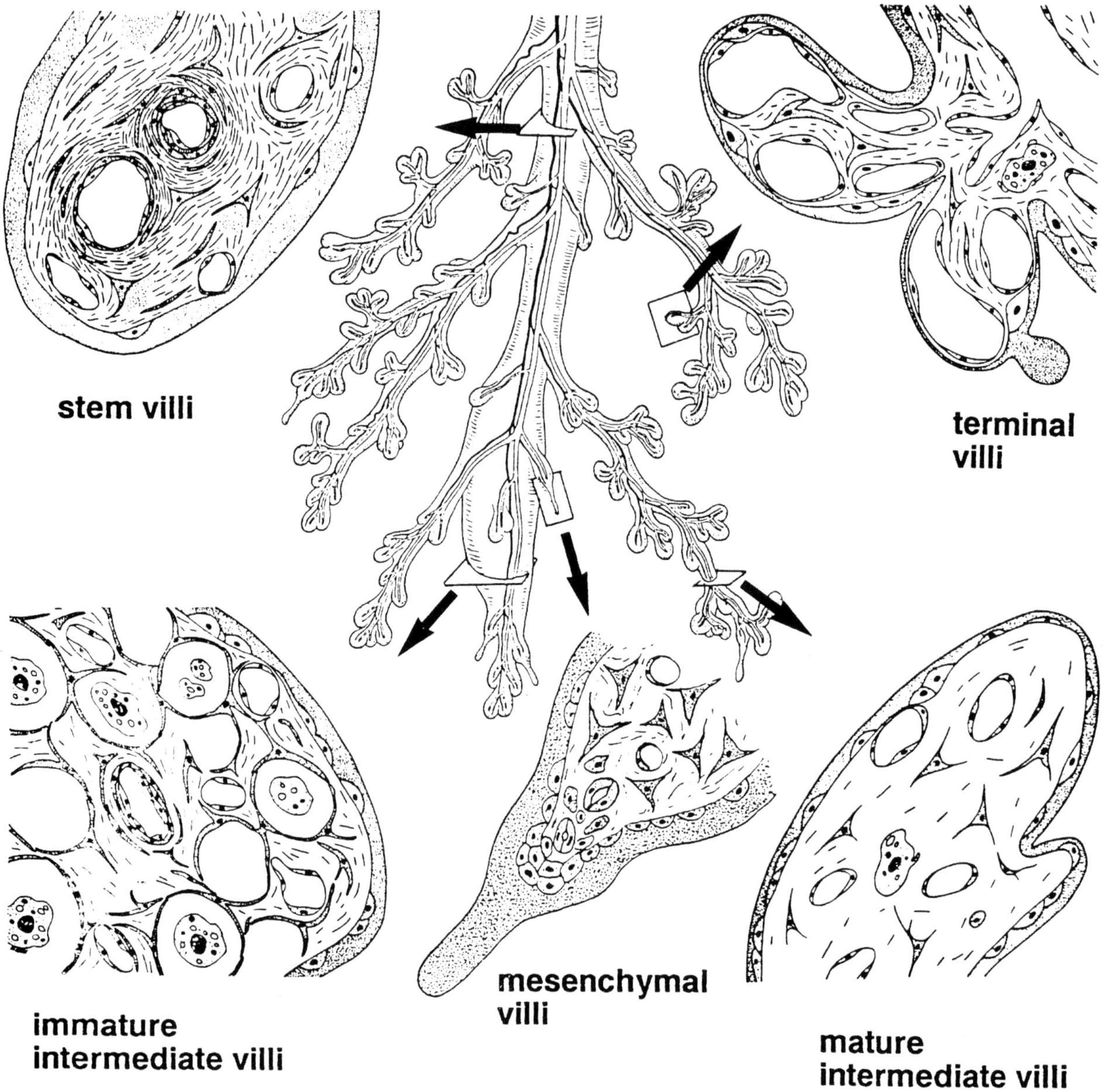

Fig. 10.6 Simplified representation of a peripheral part of a mature placental villous tree, together with typical cross-sections of the various villous types. For details cf. text. From Kaufmann[121], with permission.

in preterm placentas complicated by severe intrauterine growth restriction with abnormal umbilical artery Doppler flow studies, suggesting syncytiotrophoblastic insufficiency[44].

The fetal vessels within the villi comprise muscularized arteries and veins, not always easily distinguished[45], and appearing as capillaries in the peripheral mature intermediate and terminal villi, the latter providing a surface for gas exchange thought to exceed 10 m^2 (for review see Benirschke and Kaufmann[1]). The endothelium of the fetal capillaries acts as a passive filter, limiting macromolecular transfer across the vessel wall to molecules below 20 000 Da[46,47], though somewhat influenced by molecular charge[48,49]. The contractile cells that surround the walls of the larger vessels, i.e. arterioles and arteries, are of great interest clinically since reduced fetoplacental perfusion, detected by Doppler ultrasound examination of the umbilical arteries *in vivo*, is associated with poor fetal growth, fetal death and perinatal loss[50]. Since autonomic innervation has never been detected in the placenta[51] vasomotor regulation in the stem vessels must be controlled by paracrine events, local shear stress and from endocrine signals[52]. This will be addressed in detail below.

Connective tissue cells within the stroma are heterogeneous in nature, producing various connective-tissue fibres which increase the mechanical stability of the villous core. In addition, macrophages (Hofbauer cells) can be observed in varying numbers. The functions of these cells is uncertain. They are capable of producing a variety of growth factors known to be responsible for the regulation of growth and differentiation of all villous components[53]. Moreover, they express the CD4 antigen[54] which functions as the membrane receptor for infection by human immunodeficiency virus. Virus accumulation within the Hofbauer cells has been described[55], but it is still unknown how the virus passes the syncytiotrophoblast.

Integrity of the maternofetal barrier

Alpha-fetoprotein (AFP) is produced by the fetal liver. Its concentration in the fetal blood is 50 000 times higher than in the maternal blood due to the fact that the trophoblastic barrier is generally not permeable to proteins[56]. The introduction of mid-trimester maternal serum AFP screening programmes for the detection of fetal spina bifida led to the observation that elevated levels of AFP (generally greater than two multiples of the median (MOM) value for gestation) and no associated fetal malformation had an increased risk of adverse outcomes such as pre-eclampsia, intrauterine growth restriction and antepartum fetal death[57]. The implication is that increased placental permeability may lead to impaired pregnancy outcome. Abnormal Doppler studies of the uteroplacental vessels together with elevated AFP indicate pregnancies at highest risk[58]. Pregnancies complicated by pre-eclampsia have increased amounts of villous trophoblast fragments in uterine venous blood[59]. Villous repair following loss of trophoblast involves deposition of fibrin, and *in vitro* studies using horseradish peroxidase confirm these as sites of increased permeability, and so be responsible for the increased release of AFP into the maternal circulation[60]. In the normal term placenta, approximately 7% of the villous surface is covered by fibrin deposits which may be responsible for the passage of macromolecules.

Another paratrophoblastic transfer route for smaller molecules is provided by the transtrophoblastic channels, approximately 20 nm in diameter and seen only by electron microscopy[56,61–63]. These exist to allow transfer of water-soluble, lipophobic molecules with an effective molecular diameter <1.5 nm[62,63] and may be important for the regulation of fluid balance[56,64]. Under certain circumstances such as fetal hydrops, increased fetal venous pressure, or reduced fetal oncotic pressure, these channels dilate such that not only water, but also fetal proteins, may pass into the maternal circulation[56,61].

Villous development and villous types

The importance of appreciating villous development helps to determine the significance of the current literature concerning the pathophysiology of intrauterine growth restriction (see below). Each villous tree arises from the chorionic plate by a thick trunk (truncus chorii) which branches repeatedly; some subdivisions extend as far as the basal plate forming the anchoring villi, while the vast majority end freely in the intervillous space (Figs 10.1, 10.2 and 10.6). Five types of villi have been distinguished on the basis of their calibre, stromal characteristics and vessel structure[16,65–67] (Fig. 10.6).

1. Stem villi[16,65] (Fig. 10.6) represent the first 5–30 generations of unequal dichotomous branchings, and serve to give mechanical support to the villous trees. They range from about 100 μm to several millimetres in diameter and are characterized by a compact fibrous stroma containing centrally located arteries or larger arterioles, and veins or venules.
2. Long slender mature intermediate villi[65] (Fig. 10.6), ranging from 80 to 120 μm in diameter, arise from the ends of the end generation of stem villi. These are often gently curving, and terminal villi arise at intervals from the convex aspects of their surface. Internally, they consist of a loose stromal core, and embedded within this are narrow capillaries and occasional arterioles, characterized by a monolayer of contractile cells.
3. Terminal villi[16,65] (Figs 10.3, 10.6 and 10.7) are the final branches of the villous tree and, from a physiological viewpoint, are the most important component. They are short stubby protuberances, up to 200 μm in length with a diameter of 50–100 μm, arising from the surface of mature intermediate villi. Their characterizing feature is the high degree of capillarization – more than 50% of terminal villous volume is represented by capillaries. The thickness of the syncytiotrophoblast is not uniform over

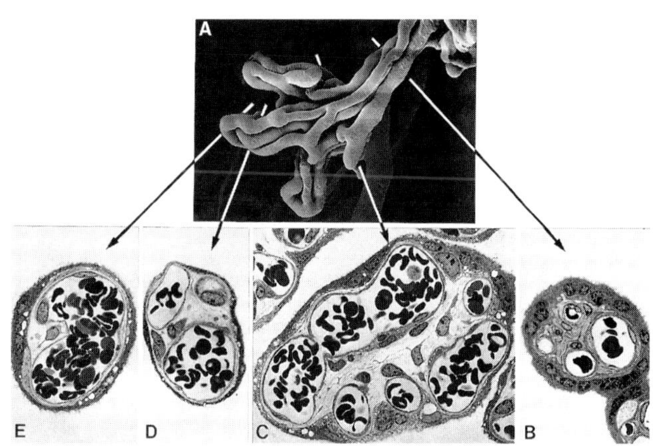

Fig. 10.7 Fetal vascularization of terminal villi. (A) Cast of vessels from a group of terminal villi. Corresponding semi-thin sections of the transition to a mature intermediate villus (B), the basis of the branching terminal villi (C), a single terminal villus near its tip (D), and a flat section of the terminal villous tip (E). These pictures demonstrate the structural variability of terminal villi; they all have in common that fetal capillaries and the highly dilated sinusoids amount to more than 50% of the stromal volume as long as postpartal collapse can be avoided by early fixation. × 300. From Kaufmann *et al.*[75], with permission.

the terminal villous surface – rather, there are areas where the trophoblast is extremely attenuated, devoid of syncytial nuclei, known as the 'vasculosyncytial membrane' (VSM). Underlying such areas are dilated segments of fetal capillaries referred to as 'sinusoids', where the diffusional distance between maternal and fetal plasma is reduced to as little as 0.5–2.0 μm (Fig. 10.4). The proportion of villous surface area occupied by VSM increases as gestational age advances towards term[66]. At other points on the villous surface, the syncytiotrophoblast is relatively thick containing clusters of syncytial nuclei. These are the most important sites of metabolic and endocrine activity.
Groups of degenerating nuclei protrude into the intervillous space as syncytial knots and sprouts and may break away (Fig. 10.8); the resulting syncytial globules are deported in the maternal blood, most becoming lodged in the pulmonary capillary bed. It has been estimated that up to 150 000 such globules enter the maternal circulation each day[69], a mechanism by which aged syncytial nuclei can be shed. This phenomenon may play a role in modifying the maternal immune system, although how this is achieved by tissue devoid of major histocompatibility complex (MHC) antigens remains uncertain.

4. Immature intermediate villi[65] (Fig. 10.6) represent peripheral continuations of stem villi that are in the process of development. Thus, whilst common in immature placentas, their distribution in the mature organ is generally limited to the central regions of the lobules, surrounding the central cavities, characteristically lacking in terminal villi (Fig. 10.2). These villi are recognized by the characteristically loose reticular meshwork in the stroma, in which numerous macrophages (Hofbauer cells) are found. Embedded amongst the stromal cells are arterioles and venules, confirming that these villi are the forerunners of stem villi. It is important that their presence in normal term pregnancy is recongnized, and that they are not incorrectly interpreted as oedematous villi.
5. Mesenchymal villi[70] (Fig. 10.6). These are again a transient population, seen predominantly in the earliest stages of pregnancy where they are the precursors of immature intermediate villi. In the more mature placenta they are inconspicuous, usually situated at the surfaces of immature intermediate villi where they represent the points of villous sprouting.

The development of the villous tree starts by the formation of syncytial or trophoblastic sprouts; in early gestation these are seen arising in an apparently random pattern from the surfaces of mesenchymal and immature intermediate villi[70,71] (Fig. 10.9). These primary villous sprouts are invaded centrally by cytotrophoblast, followed by a second central invasion by mesenchyme, to form secondary villi; the latter differentiates into stroma and capillaries resulting in tertiary (mesenchymal)

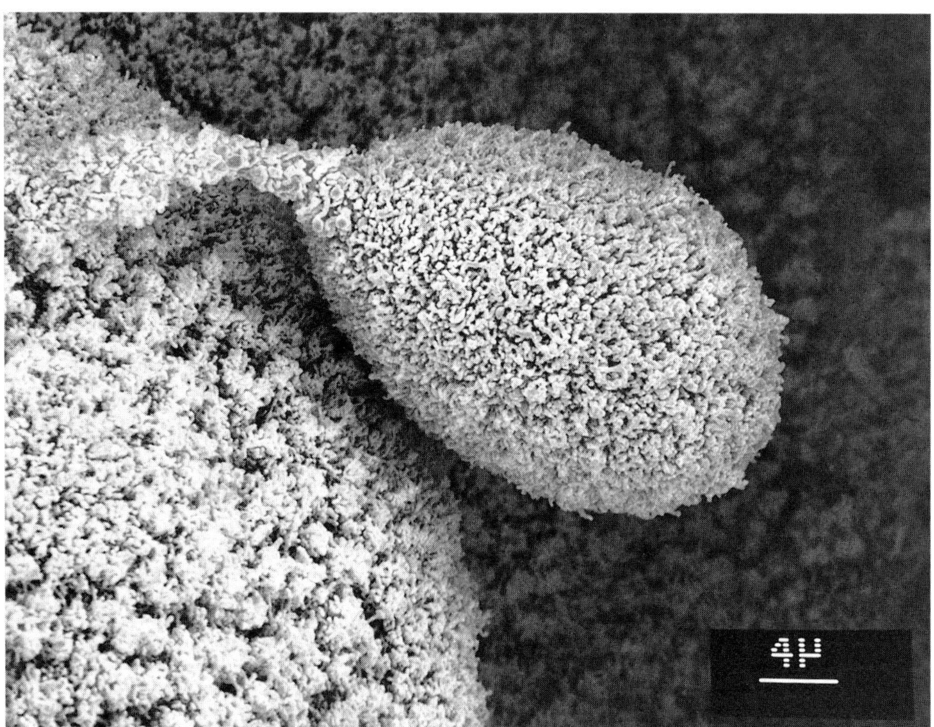

Fig. 10.8 Term placenta. A syncytial sprout (centre) is connected to a terminal villus (left) by a thin stalk and protrudes into the intervillous space (right). This type of sprout may detach and enter the maternal circulation. Scanning electron micrograph, × 2500.

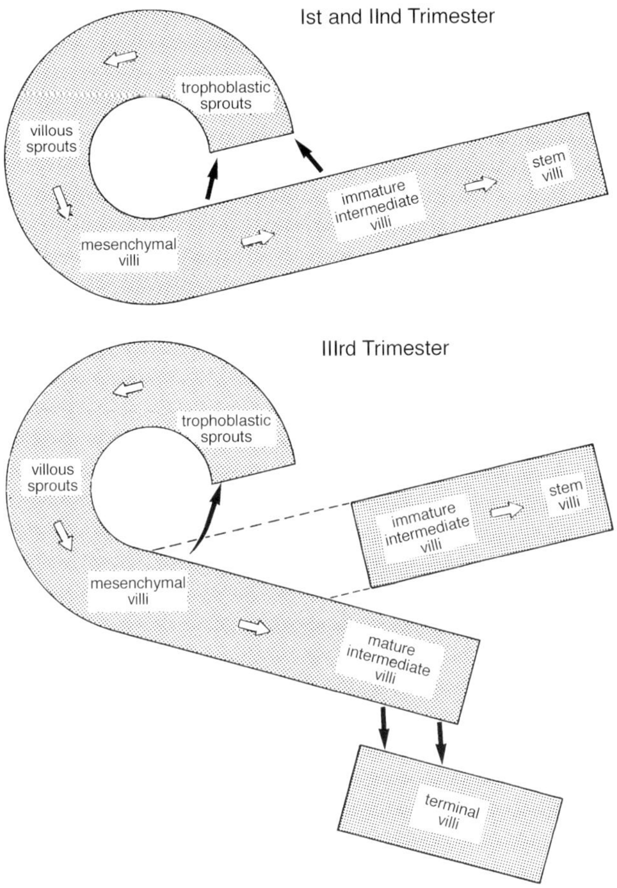

Fig. 10.9 Routes of villous development during early and late pregnancy. White arrows = transformation of one villous type into another. Black arrows = new production of villi or sprouts along the surface of other villi. Slightly modified from ref. 70, with permission.

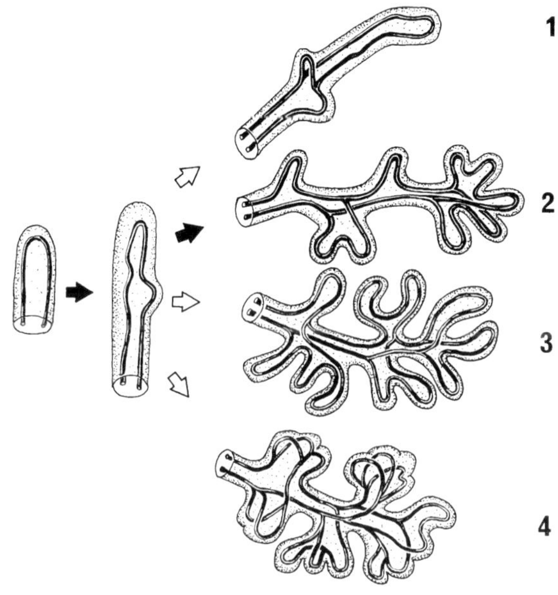

Fig. 10.10 Simplified diagram of the terminal villous development in relation to capillary growth. Varying degrees of imbalance between villous and capillary growth result in different types of terminal villous development, such as terminal villi deficiency (1), normal mature placenta (2), hypermaturity (3), and hypoxic hypervascularization, e.g. pre-eclampsia or maternal anemia (4), the conditions 1 and 3 are found e.g. in IUGR combined with AEDFV. From Kaufmann *et al.*[75], with permission.

villi, which in turn differentiate into immature intermediate villi[70]. New syncytial sprouts continue to form until the immature intermediate villi are themselves transformed into stem villi. This concept is important to appreciate because the clinical literature[72–74] erroneously refers to primary, secondary and tertiary stem villi; in truth, the number of generations of stem villi is variable, ranging from 5 to 30 generations, due to unequal dischotomous branchings and depending on the local activity of the immature intermediate villi.

Expansion of the villous trees is rapid during the first trimester so long as mesenchymal and immature intermediate villi, the actively growing villi, produce only new villi of their own type (Fig. 10.9). The situation changes gradually during the second trimester, when fetal growth accelerates and placental growth is slower.

By the onset of the third trimester, the immature villous types (mesenchymal and immature intermediate villi) are transformed into their mature counterparts (Fig. 10.9). In this way, growth of the villous trees slows down, but is directed towards production of terminal villi, the more functional component of the placenta.

Formation of terminal villi is thought to be the result of stimulated capillary growth[75,76]. Within mature intermediate villi, arterioles give way to long slender capillaries. Under normal conditions, elongation of these capillaries is increased during the third trimester and exceeds that of the containing villi (Fig. 10.10). As a result, capillary coils are formed, which protrude from the surface, raising an attenuated blister of trophoblast before them. In this way, terminal villi are formed, and the same capillary may run through several terminal villi in series before communicating with a venule. There are indications that the degree of capillarization and formation of terminal villi is regulated by oxygen partial pressure[77–79]. Different degrees of oxygen supply result in different types of terminal villous maldevelopment (Fig. 10.10)[75].

The switch in differentiation pathways (Fig. 10.9) at the start of the third trimester is of key importance in placental development[67,70]. If this takes place too early, then the organ stops growing too soon, differentiating prematurely such that the terminal villi are very densely packed due to a deficit of later generations of stem villi. The resulting placenta is highly mature, perfectly capillarized, but too small; a useful corollary is the reduction in adult height caused by premature maturation of the epiphyses. Alternatively, if the switch in placental development is delayed, then the placenta continues growing and is characterized by excessive size yet lacking mature terminal structures. This phenomenon may influence other factors besides fetal growth; villous structure in post-term placentas is characterized by villous immaturity, as if mature peripheral structures may somehow participate in the initiation of parturition[1].

Diagnostic problems with placental sampling

The average dimensions of a placentone is 2–4 cm, i.e. too large to be represented in individual sections for paraffin histology. As will be discussed in detail below, villous structure within a single placentone will vary from an immature central or growth zone, to the mature peripheral villi responsible for gas exchange (Figs 10.2 and 10.6). It becomes necessary to examine several sections to gain an accurate impression of villous development. Great emphasis has been placed on random systematic sampling of the placenta in relation to the chorionic surface[80]. However, since villous structure varies enormously within individual placentones, it is essential to ensure sections representative of the entire depth of placenta are examined, from chorionic to basal plates. Such technical considerations are of increasing importance, since there is a recent trend towards publication of morphological data in the clinical literature from a variety of disease states[44,45,81]. This problem is greater still when using small tissue samples, for example, by *in situ* biopsy at Caesarean section[82], or by chorionic villous sampling and in particular when using the electron microscopy techniques discussed below[44].

Physiology of fetoplacental blood flow

Fetal size, and thus oxygen and nutritional demands, rapidly outstrip growth of the placenta such that by term, 1 g of placenta supports 6 g of fetus. In order to meet these demands, the peripheral villous placenta differentiates such that by term the proportion of descending aortic blood flow entering the umbilical arteries is increased to 40%[83] and the diffusive capacity is increased 10-fold[68]. These alterations are almost wholly dependent upon the exponential elaboration of terminal villi in the second half of pregnancy[1]. As in the uteroplacental circulation, which becomes 'denervated' by trophoblast, so the villous tree remains free of fetal autonomic influences since it is devoid of nerves[51]. The fetoplacental circulation competes with the lower fetal body for aortic blood, receiving a large proportion through the development of low impedance.

Doppler studies of the umbilical arteries indicate a progressive fall in fetoplacental vascular impedance, reflected by increasing end-diastolic flow velocity[84]. During the first trimester, end-diastolic velocities are absent[85], becoming consistently present by 14 weeks of gestation. Thereafter the steady rise in end-diastolic velocity parallels differentiation of the villous tree into its mature form[85]. The relative importance of these fundamental anatomical changes is of great interest, implying that impedance is controlled by capillary angiogenesis (cf. the dramatic changes in capillarization throughout pregnancy, Fig. 10.10), as opposed to the theory that impedance is limited by changes in either density or vasomotor tone of stem villous arterioles[52].

VASOMOTOR INFLUENCES

The various endocrine and paracrine influences upon vascular tone of the fetoplacental vessels have been addressed in detail elsewhere[52,86]. However, while the umbilical arteries are easy to isolate and mount as ring preparations, their vasomotor responses are only directly relevant to obliteration of the fetoplacental circulation at birth[87]. Cell-culture studies, involving umbilical vein endothelial cells, are subject to the same criticisms. Dual-circuit placental perfusion, at least, is representative of villous vascular impedance; however, it is limited by gassing with 95% oxygen, resulting in tensions exceeding 300 mmHg, and by inferring that responses of healthy tissue to hypoxia are relevant to pathological circumstances. Myography of small, typically 150–200 μm, stem vessels, provides interesting physiological data[88,89] and although the technique is limited by selection bias, it is uniquely valuable since it provides data from pathological placentas, which are notoriously difficult to perfuse[90].

That any of these specific vasomotor mechanisms is responsible for the physiological fall in vascular impedance requires the demonstration that their activity changes appropriately during gestation. Functional atrial natriuretic peptide (ANP) receptors, mediating vasodilatation via guanylate cyclase, are increased in density at 28–40 weeks[91]. Total villous placental NOS activity was found to reduce as pregnancy advanced[92]. Obviously dual-circuit perfusion studies of placentas from spontaneous preterm births prior to 32 weeks' gestation would clarify, for example, the role of NO generation, or other vasodilators, in mediating the reduction in vascular impedance. Immunohistochemical studies, supported by appropriate Western blotting data, would similarly be very valuable in this context.

ANATOMICAL INFLUENCES

If the stem villous arterioles are normally maximally dilated, and we have no evidence to refute this possibility, total vascular impedance would be influenced by the sectional area and arrangement of the more distal capillaries. By contrast with systemic vascular beds, which have a relatively short distance between arterioles and venules, bridged by many parallel capillaries, so that impedance/flow is regulated by autonomically-innervated precapillary sphincters, the capillary bed of the peripheral villi is much longer (2000–4000 μm), less richly branched and is focally dilated into sinusoids within terminal villi (Figs 10.7 and 10.10). Since we do not know the *in vivo* contractile state of the stem villous arterioles, we cannot exclude the fact that falling fetoplacental vascular impedance is primarily due to anatomical changes within the peripheral capillaries.

Pathophysiology of intrauterine growth restriction

A proportion of small-for-gestational age fetuses, especially those recognized before 32 weeks of gestation, demonstrate features of intrauterine growth restriction (IUGR): increased head/abdomen circumference ratio, reduced amniotic fluid volume, vasodilatation of the middle cerebral artery and increased impedance to blood flow in the umbilical arteries[45]. In the more severe cases, end-diastolic velocities in the umbilical arteries are absent or even become reversed, which is associated with a perinatal loss rate of 40–70%[93]. Meta-analysis of randomized control trials in high-risk pregnancies suggests a modest benefit from the availability of umbilical artery Doppler[50], though this may be confined to those circumstances where absent end-diastolic flow velocity waveforms (AEDFV) are detected[94].

Animal studies, and predictions from computer models, suggest that the development of AEDFV in the umbilical arteries requires at least a fourfold increase in vascular impedance[95,96]. This needs to be borne in mind when interpreting the significance of differences in placental structure or in function between pathological cases and controls, the latter not always being matched for gestational age.

From a functional perspective, endothelial-dependent relaxation can be demonstrated in small stem villous vessels from IUGR placentas delivered following complications of AEDFV[90]. Circulating ANP and its functional vascular receptors are both increased under these circumstances[91], as is the umbilical artery plasma concentration of nitrites, an index of villous placental NOS activity[97]. However, homogenized villous tissues from IUGR placentas demonstrated reduced activity of eNOS[98]. The likely explanation is a combination of reduced trophoblast eNOS expression, due to increased apoptosis, and increased fetoplacental endothelial expression of eNOS[99]. The significance of these observations, and more importantly the clarification of the role of eNOS in generating AEDFV, will only become apparent once appropriate *in situ* studies, preferably including electron immunohistochemistry, are conducted in homogeneous study groups of sufficient sample size to permit useful conclusions.

Pathological studies of placentas from AEDFV pregnancies are more numerous than functional studies, largely due to the ease of tissue collection and routine embedding in paraffin. Interest in the pathological basis of AEDFV was generated by the important observations from Australia in 1985[72] indicating a reduction in the density of small stem arterioles in the 20–90 μm range. Others confirmed these findings[73,74] and embolization studies conducted in the sheep[95,100] led to the advancement of the 'obliteration theory', whereby the reduced density of stem arteries was assumed to be due to vessel loss by thrombosis involving fetal platelets[101]. The technical limitations of these paraffin studies were succinctly summarized by Burton and Jauniaux[102], but the developmental biology of peripheral villi[1] and of the need for correct sampling methods[80] are relatively new concepts. Immunohistochemical localization of actin within stem villi of AEDFV and control placentas failed to indicate any selective loss of even the smallest (10–25 μm) diameter vessels[45]. Bearing in mind the fourfold increase in impedance needed to generate AEDFV in the umbilical arteries, it seems unlikely, in the absence of intense vasoconstriction, that the principal pathology of AEDFV resides in stem arteries – however, this debate continues.

That the defect in AEDFV might reside beyond the stem villi has been suggested from morphometric data[81,103] and from the straightforward deduction that fetal hypoxia in IUGR[104] implies a defect in oxygen diffusion across the placenta – a function not assigned to stem villi. Detailed transmission electron microscopic (TEM) studies of terminal villi from AEDFV pregnancies, together with parallel immunohistochemical studies of stromal matrix proteins, indicated an abnormally mature trophoblast combined with stromal fibrosis, features suggestive of an elevation in local intervillous oxygen tension prior to delivery[44]. At first somewhat surprising, these data can be explained by a basic failure in transfer of oxygen from the intervillous space to the fetus[105]. Parallel scanning electron microscopic studies from placentas of pregnancies complicated by AEDFV, involving both terminal villi and their capillary casts, indicated reduced numbers of elongated and poorly branched villi[106]. These findings, which have important implications for maternal oxygen therapy in IUGR[107], support the notion that AEDFV can be primarily conferred at the level of the terminal villi. Finally, this disorder of villous maturation may account for the association between elevated levels of human chorionic gonadotrophin and adverse perinatal outcome[108], as is the case already mention for AFP.

IUGR in the presence of end-diastolic velocities in the umbilical arteries, or pre-eclampsia in the presence of normal umbilical artery Doppler waveforms, appears to be associated with increased villous branching capillarization (cf. Fig. 10.10) i.e. the opposite of what was found with AEDFV[1,109]. Under these circumstances, the defect in uteroplacental blood flow, represented by notched high-impedance Doppler waveforms, may be greater than the defect in fetoplacental blood flow, such that the intervillous space and peripheral villi become hypoxic relative to physiological conditions – a situation which would favour increased peripheral capillary growth.

The fetal membranes

Discussions on placental development have tended to focus on the invasive process of haemochorial placentation at the expense of the uterine capacity and membranes. As will be outlined, these latter structures are of increasing importance, both to understand the basis of premature rupture of the membranes[110–112] and to realize the potential of non-invasive prenatal diagnosis[113].

As can be seen in Fig. 10.1 and 10.3(c), the margins of the placenta are defined by regression of the early intervillous space; rather than proceeding through all stages of villous development, the constituent parts of the chorion (chorionic plate, early intervillous space and basal plate) fuse to form the chorion laeve. In this way, the mature discoid placenta arises from differentiation and growth of just 30% of the early blastocystic trophoblast.

The endocrine signals, both from the trophoblast and corpus luteum, transform the uterine endometrium into the decidua; increasing the diameter of the chorionic sac, containing the developing embryo, results in progressive bulging of overlying decidua (decidua capsularis) towards the opposing uterine wall (decidua parietalis) and thus gradual obliteration of the uterine cavity (Fig. 10.11).

Expansion of the chorionic sac occurs primarily as a result of fluid accumulation termed the 'coelomic fluid'. The amniotic vesicle forms within this sac, enlarging progressively to surround the developing embryo with which it fuses along the umbilical cord. The amniotic sac enlarges into the chorionic sac, progressively obliterating the coelomic cavity. By 12 weeks of gestation, the decidua capsularis starts fusing with the decidua parietalis. In week 17 this process is largely finished, thereby obliterating both the uterine and the coelomic cavities (Fig. 10.11).

The histological structure of mature fetal membranes following delivery, approximately 200–500 μm in diameter, are shown in Fig. 10.12. The amniotic epithelium should be viewed as an active structure. It participates in the regulation of amniotic fluid volume, in fetal acid–base balance through the abundant expression of carbonic anhydrase[114] and in uterine contractility, since it synthesizes contractile prostaglandins and endothelin[115]. Beneath it is a thin layer of amniotic mesoderm, resting on connective tissue below which is the cytotrophoblast of the chorion laeve (Fig. 10.12). Attached to the outer surface of the latter is part of the decidual layers (capsular and parietal) indicating that membrane separation takes place at this level, i.e. deeper than the original materno-fetal interface.

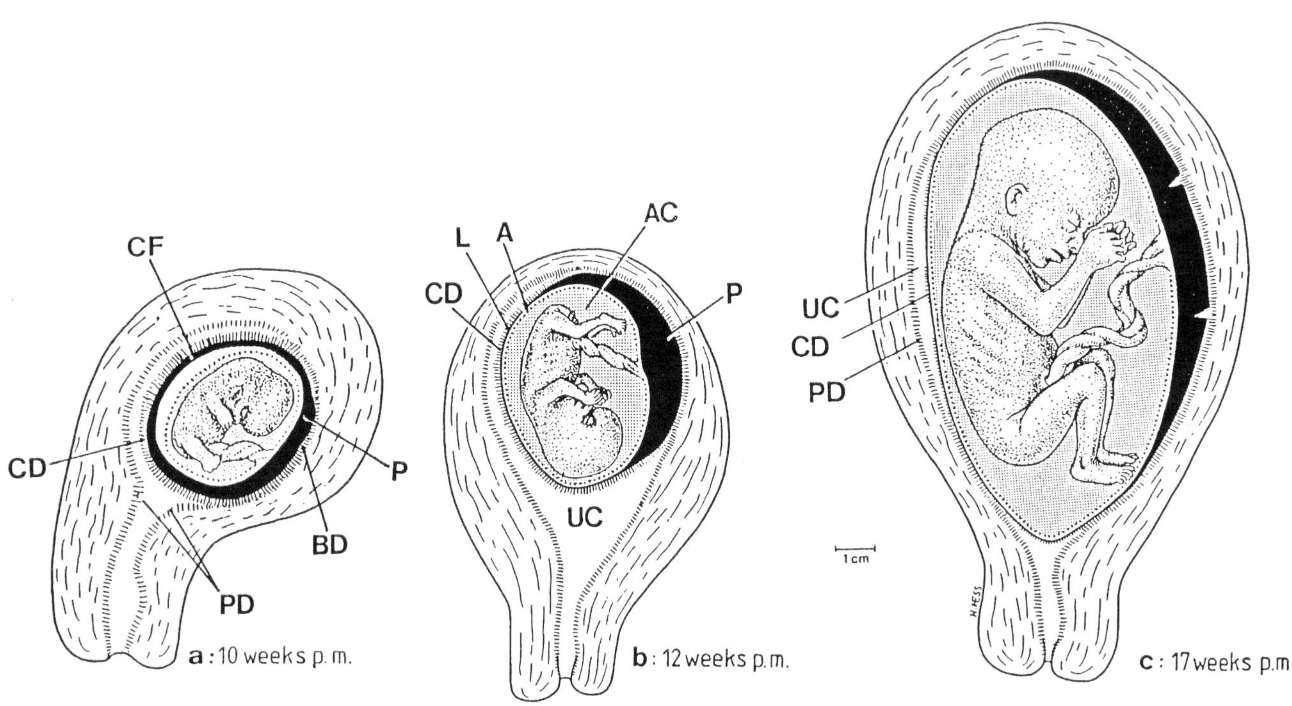

Fig. 10.11 Late stages of the development of the fetal membranes. (a) Up to 10 weeks p.m., the embryo is surrounded by the chorion frondosum (CF); its later specialization into chorion laeve and the placenta is indicated by a slight increase in thickness (P) only. The chorion frondosum is covered by the capsular decidua (CD), which is continuous with the basal decidua (BD) at the placental site, and with the parietal decidua (PD), which lines the uterine cavity. Amnion (dotted line) surrounds the embryo and is not fused in most places with the chorion frondosum. (b) Two weeks later (12th week p.m.), the original chorion frondosum has differentiated into the thick placenta (P) and the thinner fetal membranes that surround the inner amnionic cavity (AC). At this stage, the membranes are composed of inner amnion (A), intermediate chorion laeve (L), and outer capsular decidua (CD). Because of the embryo's small size, the uterine cavity (UC) is still largely open. (c) From 17 weeks on, the membranes come into close contact with the uterine wall. The remainder of the capsular decidua (CD) fuses with the parietal decidua (PD) and largely close the uterine cavity (UC). From then on, the chorion laeve contacts the parietal decidua. Modified from Becker *et al.*[122].

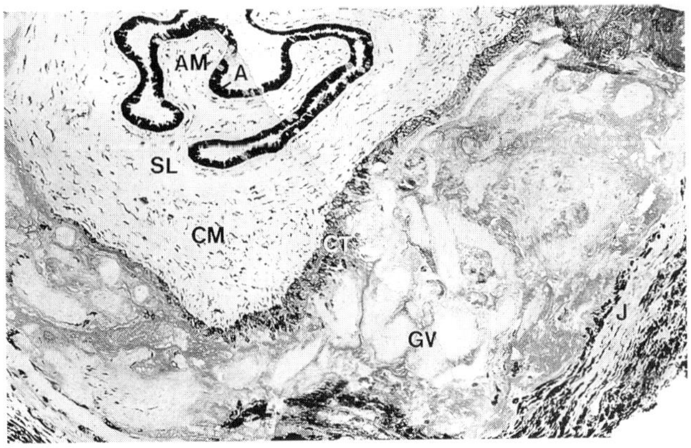

Fig. 10.12 Membranes near their lateral placental attachment, showing lactate dehdyrogenase activity as marker for vital cells. A = amnion; AM = amnion mesoderm; SL = spongy layer separating amnion and chorion laeve; CM = chorionic mesenchyme of the chorion laeve; CT = cytotrophoblast layer of the chorion laeve; GV = ghost villi as remnant from the former chorion frondosum; J = junctional zone, consisting of invasive trophoblast and decidua. Cryostat section, × 70. From Benirschke and Kaufmann[1], with permission.

PREMATURE RUPTURE OF THE MEMBRANES

The perinatal consequences of pre-eclampsia and IUGR are kept in perspective when one remembers that premature rupture of the membranes (PROM) and preterm labour (PTL) are jointly responsible for the majority of perinatal death and handicap. Malak and Bell demonstrated that fibrillin-containing microfibrils, rather than elastin fibres, are responsible for the elastic properties of the membranes at term[111]. Disruption of the connective tissue elements takes place at the site of spontaneous rupture[110], following which the rupture site extends by presumably mechanical means. Since uterine contractions and cervical effacement normally precede spontaneous rupture of the membranes, the process of parturition must somehow coordinate these events. PROM in the absence of uterine contractions suggests that pathological processes, such as the release of degrading enzymes by bacteria[116–118] are involved. *Mycoplasma* and *Ureaplasma* species are commonly isolated from the membranes or endocervix of patients with preterm PROM[119], but their presence does not guarantee membrane rupture. Further *in vitro* studies are needed in order to address this problem more effectively.

Concluding remarks

We hope the reader has appreciated the clinical relevance of human placental anatomy – from prenatal diagnosis within the first trimester uterine cavity to abnormal development of peripheral villi in pregnancies complicated by intrauterine growth restriction. We trust such information will stimulate continuing research into the structural biology of the placenta in the critical disease states which occupy much time amongst maternal–fetal medicine specialists.

REFERENCES

1. Benirschke K, Kaufmann P. *Pathology of the Human Placenta*. New York: Springer, 1995.
2. Knobil E, Neill JD. *The Physiology of Reproduction*. New York: Raven Press, 1994.
3. Torpin R. *The Human Placenta*. Springfield, IL: Charles C. Thomas, 1969.
4. Jauniaux E, Ramsay B, Campbell S. Ultrasonographic investigation of placental morphologic characteristics and size during the second trimester of pregnancy. *Am J Obstet Gynecol* **170**:130–137, 1994.
5. Bouw GM. Quantitative morphology of the placenta. I. Standarization of sampling. *Eur J Obstet Gynecol Reprod Biol* **6**:325–331, 1976.
6. Voigt S, Kaufmann P, Schweikhart G. Zur Abgrenzung normaler, artefizieller und pathologischer Strukturen in reifen menschlichen Plazentazotten. II. Morphometrische Untersuchungen zum Einfluss des Fixationsmodus. *Arch Gynecol* **226**:347–362, 1978.
7. Schuhmann RA. Plazenton: Begriff, Entstehung, funktionelle Anatomie. In *Die Plazenta des Menschen* (eds V. Becker, T.H. Schiebler & F. Kubli) pp. 199–207, Stuttgart: Thieme Verlag, 1981.
8. Bewley S, Cooper D, Campbell S. Doppler investigation of uteroplacental blood flow resistance in the second trimester: a screening study for pre-eclampsia and intrauterine growth retardation. *Br J Obstet Gynaecol* **98**:871–879, 1991.
9. Demir R, Kaufmann P, Castellucci M, Erbengi T, Kotowski A. Fetal vasculogenesis and angiogenesis in human placental villi. *Acta Anat Basel* **136**:190–203, 1989.
10. Hustin J, Schaaps JP, Lambotte R. Anatomical studies of the utero-placental vascularization in the first trimester of pregnancy. *Trophoblast Res* **3**:49–60, 1988.
11. Schaaps JP, Hustin J. *In vivo* aspect of the maternal–trophoblastic border during the first trimester of gestation. *Trophoblast Res* **3**:39–48, 1988.
12. Rodesch F, Simon P, Donner C, Jauniaux E. Oxygen measurements in endometrial and trophoblastic tissues during early pregnancy. *Obstet Gynecol* **80**:283–285, 1992.
13. Kaufmann P, Castellucci M. Extravillous trophoblast in the human placenta. *Trophoblast Res* **10**:21–65, 1997.
14. Frank HG, Malekzadeh F, Kertschanska S *et al.* Immunohistochemistry of two different types of placental fibrinoid. *Acta Anat Basel* **150**:55–68, 1994.
15. Feinberg RF, Kliman HJ, Lockwood CJ. Is oncofetal fibronectin a trophoblast glue for human implantation? *Am J Pathol* **138**:537–543, 1991.
16. Boyd JD, Hamilton WJ. *The Human Placenta*. Cambridge: Heffer, 1970.
17. Brosens IA, Robertson WB, Dixon HG. The physiological response of the vessels of the placental bed to normal pregnancy. *J Pathol Bacteriol* **93**:569–579, 1967.
18. Pijnenborg R, Dixon G, Robertson WB, Brosens IA. Trophoblastic invasion of human decidua from 8 to 18 weeks of pregnancy. *Placenta* **1**:3–19, 1980.
19. Pijnenborg R, Robertson WB, Brosens IA. The arterial migration of trophoblast in the uterus of the golden hamster, *Mesocricetus auratus*. *J Reprod Fertil* **40**:269–280, 1974.
20. Burrows TD, King A, Loke YW. Expression of adhesion molecules by endovascular trophoblast and decidual endothelial cells: implications for vascular invasion during implantation. *Placenta* **15**:21–33, 1994.
21. Pijnenborg R, Bland JM, Robertson WB, Brosens IA. Uteroplacental arterial changes related to interstitial trophoblast migration in early human pregnancy. *Placenta* **4**:397–413, 1983.
22. Moll W, Nienartowicz A, Hees H, Wrobel K-H, Lenz A. Blood flow regulation in the uteroplacental arteries. *Trophoblast Res* **3**:83–96, 1988.

23. Hees H, Moll W, Wrobel K-H, Hees I. Pregnancy-induced structural changes and trophoblastic invasion in the segmental mesometrial arteries of the guinea pig (*Cavia porcellus* L.). *Placenta* **8**:609–626, 1987.
24. Nanaev AK, Chwalisz K, Frank HG, Kohnen G, Hegele-Hartung C, Kaufmann P. Physiological dilation of uteroplacental arteries in the guinea pig depends on nitric oxide synthase activity extravillous trophoblast. *Cell Tissue Res* **282**:407–421, 1995.
25. Brosens IA. The uteroplacental vessels at term – the distribution and extent of physiological changes. *Trophoblast Res* **3**:61–67, 1988.
26. Brosens IA, Dixon HG, Robertson WB. Fetal growth retardation and the arteries of the placental bed. *Br J Obstet Gynaecol* **84**:656–663, 1977.
27. Brosens IA, Robertson WB, Dixon HG. The role of the spiral arteries in the pathogenesis of pre-eclampsia. *J Pathol* **101**:177–191, 1970.
28. Sheppard BL, Bonnar J. The maternal blood supply to the placenta in pregnancy complicated by intrauterine fetal growth retardation. *Trophoblast Res* **3**:69–82, 1988.
29. Khong TY, De Wolf F, Robertson WB, Brosens IA. Inadequate maternal vascular response to placentation in pregnancies complicated by pre-eclampsia and by small-for-gestational age infants. *Br J Obstet Gynaecol* **93**:1049–1059, 1986.
30. Garfield RE, Yallampalli C, Buhimschi I, Chwalisz K. Reversal of pre-eclampsia symptoms induced in rats by nitric oxide inhibition with L-arginine, steroid hormones and an endothelin antagonist. *Soc Gynecol Invest Chicago (III)*:Abstract No. 384, 1994.
31. Chwalisz K, Ciesla I, Garfield RE. Inhibition of nitric oxide (NO) synthesis induces preterm parturition and preeclampsia-like conditions in guinea pigs. *Soc Gynecol Invest* (Abstract), 1994.
32. Yallampalli C, Garfield RE. Inhibition of nitric oxide synthesis in rats during pregnancy produces signs similar to those of preeclampsia. *Am J Obstet Gynecol* **169**:1316–1320, 1993.
33. Yallampalli C, Byam Smith M, Nelson SO, Garfield RE. Steroid hormones modulate the production of nitric oxide and cGMP in the rat uterus. *Endocrinology* **134**:1971–1993, 1994.
34. Wigglesworth JS. Vascular organization of the human placenta. *Nature* **216**:1120–1121, 1967.
35. Schuhmann RA, Wehler V. [Histological differences of placental villi within materno-fetal circulation units. Contribution to the functional morphology of the placenta.] Histologische Unterschiede an Plazentazotten innerhalb der materno-fetalen Strömungseinheit: ein Beitrag zur funktionellen Morphologie der Plazenta. *Arch Gynecol* **210**:425–439, 1971.
36. Becker V, Jipp P. Über die Trophoblastschale der menschlichen Plazenta. *Geburtshilfe Frauenheilkd* **23**:466–474, 1963.
37. Ramsey EM, Corner, GWJ, Donner MW. Serial and cineradioangiographic visualization of maternal circulation in the primate (hemochorial) placenta. *Am J Obstet Gynecol* **86**:213–225, 1963.
38. Borell U, Fernström I, Westman A. Eine arteriographische Studie des Plazentarkreislaufs. *Geburtshilfe Frauenheilkd* **18**:1–9, 1958.
39. Moll W. Physiologie der maternen plazentaren Durchblutung. In *Die Plazenta des Menschen* (eds V. Becker, T.H. Schiebler & F. Kubli), pp. 172–194. Stuttgart: Thieme, 1981.
40. Wallenburg HCS, Hutchinson DL, Schuler HM, Stolte LAM, Janssens J. The pathogenesis of placental infarction. II. An experimental study in the rhesus monkey placenta. *Am J Obstet Gynecol* **116**:841–846, 1973.
41. McDermott M, Gillan JE. Chronic reduction in fetal blood flow is associated with placental infarction. *Placenta* **16**:165–170, 1995.
42. Simpson RA, Mayhew TM, Barnes PR. From 13 weeks to term, the trophoblast of human placenta grows by the continuous recruitment of new proliferative units: a study of nuclear number using the disector. *Placenta* **13**:501–512, 1992.
43. Wilkinshaug L, Roberts DJ, Morton CC. Confined placental mosaicism and intrauterine growth retardation: A case-control analysis of placentas at delivery. *Am J Obstet Gynecol* **172**:44–50, 1995.
44. Macara LM, Kingdom JCP, Kaufmann P *et al.* Structural analysis of placental terminal villi from pregnancies complicated by intrauterine growth restriction: failure of oxygen transport from the intervillous space to the fetus. *Placenta* **17**:37–41, 1996.
45. Macara L, Kingdom JCP, Kohnen G, Bowman AW, Greer IA, Kaufmann P. Elaboration of stem villous vessels in growth restricted pregnancies with abnormal umbilical artery Doppler waveforms. *Br J Obstet Gynaecol* **102**:807–812, 1995.
46. Sibley CP, Bauman KF, Firth JA. Permeability of the foetal capillary endothelium of the guinea-pig placenta to haem proteins of various molecular sizes. *Cell Tissue Res* **223**:165–178, 1982.
47. Sibley CP, Bauman KF, Firth JA. Ultrastructural tracer studies on the protein permeability of the guinea-pig placenta. *J Anat* **137**:787–826, 1983.
48. Firth JA, Bauman KF, Sibley CP. Permeability pathways in fetal placental capillaries. *Trophoblast Res* **3**:163–177, 1988.
49. Sibley CP, Bauman KF. Firth JA. Molecular charge as a determinant of macromolecule permeability across the fetal capillary endothelium of the guinea-pig placenta. *Cell Tissue Res* **229**:365–377, 1983.
50. Alfirevic Z, Neilson JP. Doppler ultrasonography in high-risk pregnancies: systematic review with meta-analysis. *Am J Obstet Gynecol* **172**:1379–1387, 1995.
51. Reilly FD, Russell PT. Neurohistochemical evidence supporting an absence of adrenergic and cholinergic innervation in the human placenta and umbilical cord. *Anat Rec* **188**:277–286, 1977.
52. Kingdom JCP, Burrell SJ, Kaufmann P. Pathology and clinical implications of abnormal umbilical artery Doppler waveforms. *Ultrasound Obstet Gynecol* **9**:271–286, 1997.
53. Castellucci M, Mühlhauser J, Zaccheo D. The Hofbauer cell: the macrophage of the human placenta. In *Immunobiology of Normal and Diabetic Pregnancy* (eds D. Andreani, G.D. Bompiani, U. Di Mario, W.P. Faulk & A. Galluzzo) pp. 135–144. New York: John Wiley, 1990.
54. Goldstein J, Braverman MB, Salafia CM, Buckley P. The phenotype of human placental macrophages and its variation with gestational age. *Am J Pathol* **135**:648–659, 1988.
55. Backe E, Jimenez E, Unger M, Schafer A, Jauniaux E, Vogel M. Demonstration of HIV-1 infected cells in human placenta by *in situ* hybridisation and immunostaining. *J Clin Pathol* **45**:871–874, 1992.
56. Kaufmann P, Schröder HJ, Leichtweiss HP. Fluid shift across the placenta. II. Fetomaternal transfer of horseradish peroxidase in the guinea pig. *Placenta* **3**:339–348, 1982.
57. Hamilton HP, Abdalla HI, Whitfield CR. Significance of raised maternal serum alpha-fetoprotein in singleton pregnancies with normally formed fetuses. *Obstet Gynecol* **65**:465–470, 1985.
58. Konchak PS, Bernstein IM, Capeless EL. Uterine artery Doppler velocimetry in the detection of adverse obstetric outcomes in women with unexplained elevated maternal serum alpha-fetoprotein levels. *Am J Obstet Gynecol* **173**:1115–1119, 1995.
59. Redman CWG. Current topic: pre-eclampsia and the placenta. *Placenta* **12**:301–308, 1991.
60. Brownbill P, Edwards D, Jones C, Mahendran D, Owen D, Sibley CP, Johnson R. Mechanisms of alphafetoprotein transfer in the perfused human placental cotyledon from uncomplicated pregnancy. *J Clin Invest* **96**:2220–2226, 1995.
61. Kertschanska S, Kosanke G, Kaufmann P. Is there morphological evidence for the existence of transtrophoblastic channels in human placental villi? *Trophoblast Res* **8**:581–596, 1994.
62. Stulc J, Friedrich R, Jiricka Z. Estimation of the equivalent pore dimensions in the rabbit placenta. *Life Sci* **18**:167–180, 1969.
63. Thornburg KL, Faber JJ. Transfer of hydrophilic molecules by placenta and yolk sac of the guinea pig. *Am J Physiol* **233**:C111–C124, 1977.
64. Schröder HJ, Nelson P, Power GG. Fluid shift across the placenta: I. The effect of dextran T40 in the isolated guinea-pig placenta. *Placenta* **3**:327–338, 1982.
65. Kaufmann P Sen DK, Schweikhart G. Classification of human placental villi. I. Histology. *Cell Tissue Res* **200**:409–423, 1979.
66. Sen DK, Kaufmann P, Schweikhart G. Classification of human placental villi. II. Morphometry. *Cell Tissue Res* **200**:425–434, 1979.
67. Kaufmann P. Development and differentiation of the human placental villous tree. *Bibl Anat* **22**:29–39, 1982.
68. Jackson MR, Mayhew TM, Boyd PA. Quantitative description of the elaboration and maturation of villi from 10 weeks of gestation to term. *Placenta* **13**:357–370, 1992.
69. Ikle A. Trophoblastzellen im strömenden Blut. *Schweiz Med Wochenschr* **91**:943–945, 1961.
70. Castellucci M, Scheper M, Scheffen I, Celona A, Kaufmann P. The development of the human placental villous tree. *Anat Embryol (Berlin)* **181**:117–128, 1990.
71. Burton GJ. The fine structure of the human placental villus as revealed by scanning electron microscopy. *Scan Microsc* **1**:1811–1828, 1987.

72. Giles WB, Trudinger BJ, Baird PJ. Fetal umbilical artery flow velocity waveforms and placental resistance: pathological correlation. *Br J Obstet Gynaecol* **92**:31–38, 1985.
73. McCowan LM, Mullen BM, Ritchie K. Umbilical artery flow velocity waveforms and the placental vascular bed. *Am J Obstet Gynecol* **157**:900–902, 1987.
74. Bracero LA, Beneck D, Kirshenbaum N, Peiffer M, Stalter P, Schulman H. Doppler velocimetry and placental disease. *Am J Obstet Gynecol* **161**:388–393, 1989.
75. Kaufmann P, Luckhardt M, Leiser R. Three-dimensional representation of the fetal vessel system in the human placenta. *Trophoblast Res* **3**:113–137, 1988.
76. Kaufmann P, Bruns U, Leiser R, Luckhardt M, Winterhager E. The fetal vascularisation of term human placental villi. II. Intermediate and terminal villi. *Anat Embryol (Berlin)* **173**:203–214, 1985.
77. Jackson MR, Mayhew TM, Haas JD. Morphometric studies on villi in human term placentae and the effects of altitude, ethnic grouping and sex of newborn. *Placenta* **8**:487–495, 1987.
78. Scheffen I, Kaufmann P, Philippens L, Leiser R, Geisen C, Mottaghy K. Alterations of the fetal capillary bed in the guinea pig placenta following long-term hypoxia. In *Oxygen Transfer to Tissue* (eds J. Piiper & T.K. Goldstick), pp. 779–790. New York: Plenum Press, 1990.
79. Bacon BJ, Gilbert RD, Kaufmann P, Smith AD, Trevino FT, Longo LD. Placental anatomy and diffusing capacity in guinea pigs following long-term maternal hypoxia. *Placenta* **5**:475–488, 1984.
80. Mayhew TM, Burton GJ. Methodological problems in placental morphometry: apologia for the use of stereology based on sound sampling practice. *Placenta* **9**:565–581, 1988.
81. Jackson MR, Walsh AJ, Morrow RJ, Mullen JBM, Lye SJ, Ritchie JW. Reduced placental villous tree elaboration in small-for-gestational-age pregnancies: Relationship with umbilical artery Doppler waveforms. *Am J Obstet Gynecol* **172**:518–525, 1995.
82. Schweikhart G, Kaufmann P. Zur Abgrenzung normaler, artefizieller und pathologischer Strukturen in reifen menschlichen Plazentazotten. I. Ultrastruktur des Syncytiotrophoblasten. *Arch Gynecol* **222**:213–230, 1977.
83. Eik Nes SH, Brubakk AO, Ulstein M. Measurement of human fetal blood flow. *Br Med J* **i**:283–284, 1980.
84. Hendricks S, Sarensen TK, Wong KY *et al.* Doppler umbilical artery waveform indices – normal values from fourteen to forty-two weeks. *Am J Obstet Gynecol* **161**:761–765, 1989.
85. Jauniaux E, Burton GJ, Moscoso G, Hustin J. Development of the early human placenta: a morphometric study. *Placenta* **12**:269–276, 1991.
86. Myatt L. Control of vascular resistance in the human placenta. *Placenta* **13**:329–341, 1992.
87. Templeton AGB, Whittle MJ, McGrath JC. The role of endogenous thromboxane in contractions to U46619, oxygen, 5-HT and 5-CT in the human isolated umbilical artery. *Br J Pharmacol* **103**:1079–1084, 1991.
88. McCarthy AL, Woolfson RG, Evans BJ, Davies DR, Raju SK, Poston L. Functional characteristics of small placental arteries. *Am J Obstet Gynecol* **170**:945–951, 1994.
89. Sabry S, Mondon F, Ferre F, Dinhxuan AT. *In vitro* contractile and relaxant responses of human resistance placental stem villi arteries of healthy parturients: Role of endothelium. *Fundam Clin Pharmacol* **9**:46–51, 1995.
90. McCarthy A, Patterson Brown S, Raju K, Poston L. Functional properties of small human placental arteries in relation to abnormal umbilical Doppler waveform analysis. *Placenta* **14**: A50 (Abstract), 1993.
91. Kingdom JCP, McQueen J, Ryan G, Connell JMC, Whittle MJ. Fetal vascular atrial natriuretic peptide receptors in human placenta – alteration in intrauterine growth retardation and preeclampsia. *Am J Obstet Gynecol* **170**:142–147, 1994.
92. Rutherford RAD, McCarthy A, Sullivan MHF, Elder MG, Polak JM, Wharton J. Nitric oxide synthase in human placenta and umbilical cord from normal intrauterine growth-retarded and pre-eclamptic pregnancies. *Br J Pharmacol* **116**:3099–3109, 1995.
93. Karsdorp VHM, Vanvugt JMG, Vangeijn HP *et al.* Clinical significance of absent or reversed end diastolic velocity waveforms in umbilical artery. *Lancet* **344**:1664–1668, 1994.
94. Pattinson RC, Norman K, Odendaal HJ. the role of Doppler velocimetry in the management of high risk pregnancies. *Br J Obstet Gynaecol* **101**:114–120, 1994.
95. Morrow RJ, Adamson SL, Bull SB, Ritchie JW. Effect of placental embolization on the umbilical arterial velocity waveform in fetal sheep. *Am J Obstet Gynecol* **161**:1055–1060, 1989.
96. Todros T, Guiot C, Pianta PG. Modelling the feto-placental circulation: 2. A continuous approach to explain normal and abnormal flow velocity waveforms in the umbilical arteries. *Ultrasound Med Biol* **18**:545–551, 1992.
97. Lyall F, Greer IA, Young A, Myatt L. Nitric oxide concentrations are increased in the feto-placental circulation in intrauterine growth restriction. *Placenta* **17**:165–168.
98. Morris NH, Sooranna SR, Learmont JG *et al.* Nitric oxide synthase activities in placental tissue from normotensive pre-eclamptic and growth retarded pregnancies. *Br J Obstet Gynaecol* **102**:711–714, 1995.
99. Myatt L, Eis ALW, Brockman DE, Greer IA, Lyall F. Endothelial nitric oxide synthase in placental villous tissue from normal, pre-eclamptic and intrauterine growth restricted pregnancies. *Hum Reprod* **12**:167–172, 1997.
100. Trudinger BJ, Stevens D, Conelly A *et al.* Flow velocity waveforms and the placental resistance: the effects of embolization of the umbilical circulation. *Am J Obstet Gynecol* **157**:1443–1449, 1987.
101. Wilcox GR, Trudinger BJ. Fetal platelet consumption: a feature of placental insufficiency. *Obstet Gynecol* **77**:616–621, 1991.
102. Burton GJ, Jauniaux E. Sonographic, sterological and Doppler flow velocimetric assessment of placental maturity. *Br J Obstet Gynaecol* **102**:818–825, 1995.
103. Hitschold T, Weiss E, Beck T, Hunterfering H, Berle P. Low target birth weight or growth retardation? Umbilical Doppler flow velocity waveforms and histometric analysis of fetoplacental vascular tree. *Am J Obstet Gynecol* **168**:1260–1264, 1993.
104. Nicolaides KH, Bilardo CM, Soothill PW, Campbell S. Absence of end-diastolic frequencies in the umbilical artery: a sign of fetal hypoxia and acidosis. *Br Med J* **297**:1026–1027, 1988.
105. Kingdom JCP, Kaufmann P. Oxygen and placental villous development: origins of fetal hypoxia. *Placenta* **18**:613–621, 1997.
106. Krebs C, Macara LM, Leiser R, Bowman AW, Greer IA, Kingdom JCP. Intrauterine growth restriction with absent end-diastolic flow velocity in the umbilical artery is associated with maldevelopment of the placental terminal villous tree. *Am J Obstet Gynecol* **175**:1534–1542, 1996.
107. Johanson R, Lindow SW, Vanderelst C, Jaquire Z, Vanderwesthuizen S, Tucker A. A prospective randomised comparison of the effect of continuous O_2 therapy and bedrest on fetuses with absent end-diastolic flow on umbilical artery Doppler waveform analysis. *Br J Obstet Gynaecol* **102**:662–665, 1995.
108. Wenstrom KD, Owen J, Boots LR, Dubard MB. Elevated second-trimester human chorionic gonadotropin levels in association with poor pregnancy outcome. *Am J Obstet Gynecol* **171**:1038–1041, 1994.
109. Todros T, Sciaronne A, Piccoli E, Guiot C, Kaufmann P, Kingdom J. Umbilical doppler waveforms and placental villous angiogenesis in pregnancies complicated by fetal growth restriction. *Obstet Gynecol* 1999 (in press).
110. Malak TM, Bell SC. Structural characteristics of term human fetal membranes: a novel zone of extreme morphological alteration within the rupture site. *Br J Obstet Gynaecol* **101**:375–386, 1994.
111. Malak TM, Bell SC. Distribution of fibrillin-containing microfibrils and elastin in human fetal membranes: a novel molecular basis for membrane elasticity. *Am J Obstet Gynecol* **171**:195–205, 1994.
112. Ockleford CD, Malak TM, Hubbard A, Bracken K, Burton SA, Bright NA. Confocal and conventional immunofluorescence and ultrastructural localisation of intracellular strength-giving components of human amniochorion. *J Anat* **183**:483–505, 1993.
113. Rodeck CH, Tutschek B, Sherlock J, Kingdom J. Methods for the transcervical collection of fetal cells during the first trimester of pregnancy. *Prenat Diagn* **15**:933–942, 1995.
114. Mühlhauser J, Crescimanno C, Rajaniemi H, Parkkila S, Castellucci M, Milovanow AS, Kaufmann P. Immunohistochemistry of carbonic anhydrase in human placenta and fetal membranes. *Histochemistry* **101**:91–98, 1994.
115. Sagawa N, Hasegawa M, Itoh H *et al.* Current topic: The role of amniotic endothelin in human pregnancy. *Placenta* **15**:565–575, 1994.

116. Draper D, McGregor J, Hall J, Jones W, Beutz M, Heine RP, Porreco R. Elevated protease activities in human amnion and chorion correlate with preterm premature rupture of membranes. *Am J Obstet Gynecol* **173**:1506–1512, 1995.
117. Mercer BM, Arheart KL. Antimicrobial therapy in expectant management of preterm premature rupture of the membranes. *Lancet* **346**:1271–1279, 1995.
118. Jackson RJ, Gates KL, Sheridan RJ, Lim DV. Degradation of amniotic collagen fibrils by group-B streptococci. *Curr Microbiol* **26**:141–145, 1993.
119. Hillier SL, Martius J, Krohn M, Kiviat N, Holmes KK, Eschenbach DA. A case-control study of chorioamnionic infection and histologic chorioamnionitis in prematurity. *N Engl J Med* **319**:972–978, 1988.
120. Kaufmann P, Scheffen I. Placental development. In *Neonatal and Fetal Medicine – Physiology and Pathophysiology* (eds R. Pollin & W. Fox) Orlando, FL: W.B. Saunders, 1992.
121. Kaufmann P. Basic morphology of the fetal and maternal circuits in the human placenta. *Contrib Gynecol Obstet* **13**:5–17, 1985.
122. Becker V, Schiebler TH, Kubli F. *Die Plazenta des Menschen*. Stuttgart: Georg Thieme, 1981.

Placental function in maternofetal exchange

11

J.D. Glazier, B. Harrington, C.P. Sibley and M. Turner

Introduction

In this chapter we have attempted to summarise current understanding of the mechanisms of transport by the placenta. A full description of placental transport would combine details of the physiological processes involved with information about the identities, properties and genetic control of the relevant molecular species. However, there is still much to be learnt before such a treatise will be possible. Transport by the human placenta may lead to solutes crossing to the fetal circulation. In this case, solutes must traverse the syncytiotrophoblast cell layer (microvillous/brush border plasma membrane, cytoplasm and basal plasma membrane) as well as connective tissue and fetal capillary endothelium (Fig. 11.1)[1]. Each of these elements may contribute independently to the transport properties of the placenta. While the syncytiotrophoblast is assumed to be the rate-limiting barrier and to have the major role in exchange of molecules up to the size of peptides and small proteins, and has been most extensively studied, the other components of the barrier are also certainly important, particularly as regards exchange of proteins and other macromolecules.[2]

It must be borne in mind that transport by components of the placenta does not always lead to transfer across the placenta, since some of the transport will satisfy the metabolic needs of the placenta itself (so-called 'housekeeping transport'). This can make it difficult to draw firm conclusions about the nature of transport pathways involved in maternofetal exchange. However, it is important to distinguish between the types of transport and note exactly which part of the placenta was used to derive experimental results because overall flux (rate of transfer) could have several components. Any attempt to manipulate transport in the clinical setting would require knowledge of the target transporter and any others that could compensate for the effects of the manipulation.

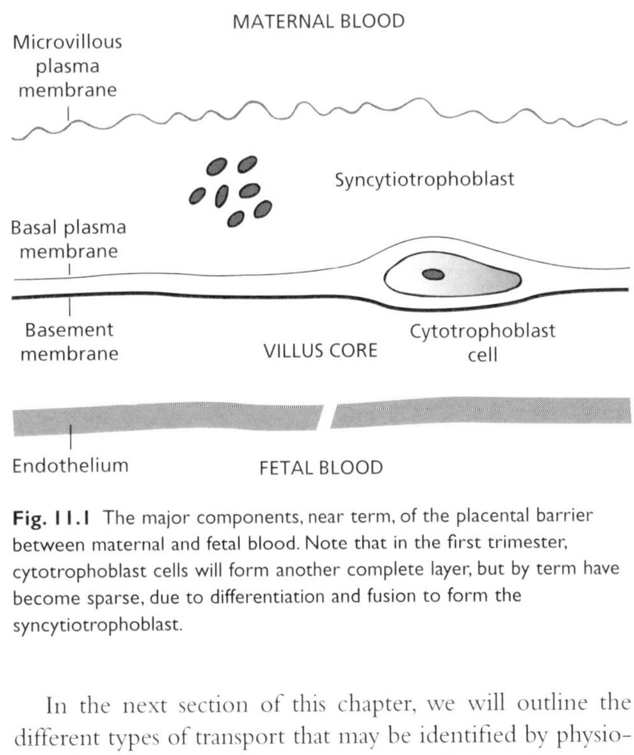

Fig. 11.1 The major components, near term, of the placental barrier between maternal and fetal blood. Note that in the first trimester, cytotrophoblast cells will form another complete layer, but by term have become sparse, due to differentiation and fusion to form the syncytiotrophoblast.

In the next section of this chapter, we will outline the different types of transport that may be identified by physiological means and outline some of the factors that could alter the magnitude of transport. In the subsequent sections we will focus on what is known about the transport of particular solutes or groups of solutes. The experimental techniques that have been used to study transfer across the human placenta are summarised in Tables 11.1 and 11.2. Complete characterisation of a transport mechanism should broadly include four sets of information: (i) the amount of substance transferred per unit time and per unit surface area, the flux, in both maternofetal and fetomaternal directions, the difference between the two giving the magnitude and direction of the net flux; (ii) the magnitude and factors controlling the driving force for the transfer of a substance, e.g.

TABLE 11.1
Preparations used for the study of human placental transfer mechanisms

Preparation*	Strengths	Weaknesses
Intact pregnancy		
Sampling at cordocentesis[160]	1. Direct data about transport	1. Only one time point 2. May be affected by the indication for cordocentesis
Maternal injection[33]	1. Indicates magnitude of fluxes 2. Inter-species comparisons	1. Ethical problems with some markers 2. Limited to just before planned delivery 3. Use of blockers not possible, thus details of transport cannot be elucidated
Perfused placenta (*in vitro*)[12,13]	1. Aims to mimic physiological situation 2. Dynamic control of all perfusates 3. Allows use of blockers to test transport hypotheses 4. Allows comparisons between molecules (e.g. of different size)	1. Artifactual leaks may make interpretation difficult. 2. Tissue quality may be degraded by prolonged perfusion
Membrane vesicles		
Microvillous[137]	1. Standardised preparation of isolated membrane 2. Control of both sides of the membrane possible 3. Allows use of blockers to test transport hypotheses	1. Irregularities in vesicle size and orientation 2. May indicate presence of a transport mechanism but not its importance
Basal[139]	As for microvillous membrane vesicles but not so widely used	1. Difficult to prepare
Placental fragments[167,168]	1. Physiological relationships preserved 2. Control of solutions	1. Non-syncytial elements may alter apparent rates of transport
Isolated villus[28]	1. Intact membranes with correct relationships	1. Other elements present
Cell culture (of cytotrophoblast)[66]	1. Standardised preparations 2. Full control of experimental conditions	1. Cells may not be the same as *in vivo* (e.g. degree of differentiation or polarisation)

*Example references only are given.

plasma concentrations along the length of the exchange surface and blood flow; (iii) the route of transfer, e.g. whether across the plasma membranes and through the cytosol (transcellular route) or via extracellular water-filled channels (paracellular route); (iv) the role and contribution of the placenta's own metabolic processes. Historically, measurement of flux was the focus of attention but more recently the focus has shifted to the cellular and molecular aspects of transport (see Tables 11.1 and 11.2). However, there is an ongoing requirement for the physiological relevance of individual mechanisms to be reconciled with overall flux and accretion.

A variety of species have been used to study placental transport but considerable care must be taken in extrapolating from these to the human because of the great diversity of placental morphology and function[3]. Nevertheless such animal studies can provide a useful base from which studies of the human placenta can be launched[4].

A more complete coverage of all the many facets of placental transfer and additional information may be obtained from other reviews[3,5].

Types of transport

The placental exchange barrier limits solute transfer to varying degrees. Lipophilic substances (e.g. oxygen) that dissolve readily in the plasma membrane will rapidly diffuse across the barrier[6]. On the other hand, for hydrophilic substances (e.g. sodium ions, amino acids), the placenta is a significant barrier to transfer. However, this barrier is not absolute because there are multiple pathways available for hydrophilic solutes to pass across the placental membranes. These pathways may be described as pores, channels, carriers (including co-transporters and exchangers), pumps and vesicular. These may be matched to mechanisms such as filtration (pores), diffusion

TABLE 11.2
Measurement methods used in transfer studies on the human placenta

Measurement*	Strengths	Weaknesses
Biochemical[71,160]	1. Objective 2. Well characterised	1. Measurement errors (e.g. elevated K^+ levels due to hypoxia/haemolysis 2. Sampling biases
Anthropometry (weight, etc.)	1. Objective 2. Some population standards available	1. Sample heterogeneity 2. Only one measurement, at end-point.
Markers		
(a) Radioisotopes as tracers in intact[33] and perfused[118] systems	1. Allows computation of magnitude of fluxes 2. Allows inter-species comparisons	1. Ethically unacceptable in human 2. Possibility of isotope effects
(b) Molecular species not present in large amounts *in vivo*, e.g. inulin or mannitol[8]	1. Not harmful	1. Substance may be metabolized in unpredictable manner
(c) Stable isotopes[203]	1. Not harmful	1. Possibility of isotope effects 2. Technologically demanding
Imaging, e.g. electron microscopy[15,16] ± markers	1. Allows localisation of transport processes	1. Only one static measurement per specimen 2. Imaging process may perturb transport process
Electrophysiology (i) microelectrode[28] (ii) patch clamp[64]	1. Allows characterisation of ion channels and comparison to other tissues	1. Technically demanding 2. Results may be ambiguous and require confirming by other methods
Solute-specific fluorescent dyes[88]	1. Specific 2. Non-radioactive 3. Should not interfere with physiological processes	1. Calibration 2. Membrane binding
Molecular[67,204]	1. Rapid screen for presence of transport proteins 2. Detailed structure of transporter protein provided 3. Understanding control of expression of transporter proteins	1. Gives no clue to function of transport proteins 2. Quantitation difficult

*Example references only are given.

(pores and channels), facilitated diffusion and secondary active transport (carriers), primary active transport (pumps) and endocytosis/exocytosis (vesicular).

Pores allow for the movement of solute and solvent through a paracellular pathway, such that the transported substances do not have to cross any plasma membranes in order to traverse a layer of tissue. Pores may allow transfer by diffusion of solute alone, or, by bulk flow, of solute and solvent together. The extent of diffusion through pores can be altered by changes in electrochemical gradients and, in the case of bulk flow, by changes in plasma hydrostatic and osmotic pressures[7]. Technical difficulties have prevented the assessment of all the relevant variables in the human placenta. However, there is clear physiological evidence, both *in vivo* and *in vitro*, that transfer through pores does occur in the human placenta[8,9–13] as well as in the placentas of several other species[14]. The morphological correlates of the pores across the syncytiotrophoblast are unclear, as superficial examination would suggest that there are no gaps to allow this paracellular transfer. However, recently, morphological evidence of pores has become available[15–17]. It is becoming increasingly clear that this paracellular route of transfer is quantitatively of major importance for the transfer of small hydrophilic solutes such as calcium ions and chloride ions[18,19]. Of course, the transcellular route through the syncytiotrophoblast, utilising channels and carriers, may well be qualitatively of greater importance, allowing fine tuning of net flux.

Channels are integral membrane proteins through which ions may diffuse down electrochemical gradients either into or out of cells. Although passive, the diffusion of solute through channels is selective, gated, saturable and may be functionally asymmetric[20]. These properties allow cells to modify the extent of inward and outward solute movements due to diffusion in response to homeostatic signals mediated by intracellular, autocrine, paracrine and endocrine agents and by effects at the genome. This probably allows a range of normal processes and a broad repertoire of reactions to abnormal processes.

Carriers are integral membrane proteins that selectively combine with a solute and can carry it from one side of the membrane to the other[21]. The combining site is only exposed to one side of the membrane at a time. Channels and carriers show different behaviours. In general terms, if a solute is added to the far side (the trans side) of the membrane then the combining site will be able to return to the near side (the cis side) more quickly than it would otherwise. The combining site will be on the near side more often and will remove solute more frequently. A carrier will thus carry more solute if it is 'trans stimulated' while a channel will not respond in this way[22]. Some carriers can transport more than one solute at a time. A cotransporter carries two solutes in the same direction, an exchanger swaps solutes. This allows cells to coordinate the movement of disparate solutes.

Pumps carry solutes against concentration gradients. This is called 'active transport' because energy (as ATP) is used up in the process[22]. A good example is the active extrusion of sodium by cells in exchange for potassium on the Na^+,K^+-ATPase (sodium pump). This is primary active transport. Carriers can harness the gradients generated by pumps by linking solute movements to sodium movements. This is secondary active transport which allows cells to move solutes against concentration gradients and thus to control their surroundings more subtly than if diffusion gradients were the only forces present.

Vesicles are formed on one side of an epithelium such as the syncytiotrophoblast by invagination of the plasma membrane and, on the opposite side of the cell, will fuse with the plasma membrane and open onto the extracellular space. Solute and water may be taken up into the forming vesicle by simple entrapment ('fluid phase' endocytosis) or solute may be taken up specifically by binding to receptors on the surface of the area of membrane about to vesiculate. Vesicles may move around the cytoplasm randomly by Brownian motion or may be directed by the cytoskeleton.

Factors affecting transport

Most placental transport is driven by diffusion, or modifications of this process. Factors affecting diffusion will thus affect the magnitude of transport. The rate of diffusion is determined by the concentration gradient across the barrier and the permeability of the barrier and its components. Different substances have different concentration gradients[3]. Permeability varies between solutes, according to their size, shape and lipophilicity. The permeability properties of the exchange barrier itself have been found to change over the course of gestation, at least in animals; in rats, guinea pigs and rabbits the permeability of the placenta to hydrophilic solutes increases towards term.[23–25] There may also be a switch over the course of gestation in the relative importance of diffusion and filtration as driving forces[26].

A potential difference (p.d.) across the exchange barrier will affect the transport of charged solutes. Potential differences between mother and fetus have been measured in some species[27] but it is unclear whether these are generated by the placenta. In humans, a p.d. has been measured both across the microvillous membrane and across the entire exchange barrier of isolated mature intermediate villi derived from term placentas, magnitude around 4 mV, fetal side negative[28]. *In vivo*, a small maternofetal p.d. was measured in women in the third trimester[29] of similar magnitude to that found *in vitro*[28]. However, at term there is reported to be no significant maternofetal p.d.[30].

The pattern and magnitude of blood flow affects transport[31]. If a substance, e.g. oxygen, crosses the membrane so quickly that it is gone as soon as it arrives, then the rate-limiting steps of transfer will be the rate at which it arrives and the rate at which it is taken away. Thus, if placental blood flow is deranged, oxygen delivery will be impaired. Furthermore, the pattern of blood flow will affect the efficiency of exchange. If the blood flows are in opposite directions (countercurrent flows) the exchange will be more efficient than if they are in the same direction (concurrent flows). The human placenta is thought to have an intermediate arrangement[31].

The placenta is a metabolically active organ and this will significantly affect the traffic of solutes such as oxygen, amino acids and carbohydrates[32]. Control of placental metabolism, as well as of transport, by hormonal, genetic or intrinsic means, by mother or fetus, is likely to be of considerable importance.

Finally, it should be noted that while the placenta shares many characteristics with other tissues, e.g. sodium pumps and intracellular signalling apparatus, we can identify features which are less prominent in other organs and these need to be mentioned as a background to any discussion of function or pathology. Firstly, the supply of some substances is vastly in excess of fetal accretion[33], while other fluxes are more obviously related to fetal requirements. Secondly, transport represents diverse phenomena; some substances, for example glucose, are transported by one or two mechanisms only and alterations in these mechanisms will be relatively easy to detect. Other substances, for example sodium, are transported by many specific mechanisms, none of which is dominant, and alterations in these systems will be more difficult to detect. Water flux, which is greater than for any other molecule[34], appears to be particularly complex. Stulc and Stulcova[35,36] have recently provided evidence that, in the rat, net water flux may be the balance of osmotic flow in the maternofetal direction following active transport of ions and bulk flow in the fetomaternal direction down a hydrostatic pressure gradient. Alteration in water transfer may thus reflect a wide range of changes and is therefore not simple to understand and will not be easy to manipulate.

Specific examples of transferred substances

RESPIRATORY GAS EXCHANGE

Gas exchange at the placenta is determined by the following factors:

(i) the concentration gradient of the gas across the placenta;
(ii) the gas-carrying capacities of fetal and maternal blood;
(iii) the rates of fetal and maternal placental blood flow;
(iv) the relative spatial orientation of the two blood flows; and
(v) the permeability properties and surface area of the membranes involved.

The contributions of these factors to oxygen transfer are reviewed comprehensively by Carter[37]. Membrane permeability and total surface area change over gestation but cannot respond to short-term perturbations and the relative orientation of blood flows is also fixed. Blood flow in the intervillous space is thought not to occur before 10–12 weeks[38] though this is still contentious[39]. Once intervillous blood flow is established, transfer processes seem to fit a cross-current model best. Blood flows and concentration gradients can change, in the short term, in normal physiological states and, in the long term, in abnormal states such as gestational diabetes, pre-eclampsia and intrauterine growth retardation.

OXYGEN SUPPLY

Throughout pregnancy fetal blood has a higher haemoglobin (Hb) concentration than maternal blood and a higher affinity for oxygen (O_2), due to a lower affinity for 2,3-diphosphoglycerate[40]. Fetal blood at term has an O_2-carrying capacity of 25 ml/dl whereas maternal blood can carry only 15 ml/dl. There are many ways of expressing O_2 exchange, but the crucial physiological variable is fetal O_2 uptake since this will determine the capacity for oxidative metabolism. In the sheep, for example, homeostatic mechanisms keep this variable remarkably constant in the face of wide variations in other variables (see above). It is not until fetal O_2 uptake drops below a critical level (0.6 mmol O_2/min/kg) that metabolic acidosis ensues. A small drop in umbilical artery O_2 content results in a large increase in the amount of O_2 transferred from mother to fetus. This is due to the relative characteristics of HbA and HbF O_2 dissociation curves for mother and fetus, respectively. The result of this relationship is that the single most important determinant of O_2 transfer from maternal to fetal blood is the O_2 content of blood perfusing the placenta from the umbilical arteries. This mechanism keeps fetal O_2 uptake relatively constant during short-term changes in umbilical and uterine blood flow via compensatory changes in fractional O_2 extraction[41,42]. Whilst responses to short-term hypoxia are seen in clinical situations such as cord compression, maternal exercise, fetal activity or uterine contractions, no effect on long-term outcome has been demonstrated. However, long-term hypoxia is important to fetal wellbeing; in fetal sheep, it leads to changes in metabolism and reduced growth[43,44]. The placenta consumes a significant proportion of the O_2 extracted from maternal blood (40% in the sheep)[43]. In short-term hypoxia, this proportion increases, maintaining placental O_2 consumption at the expense of fetal O_2 delivery[45]. However, in long-term hypoxia in fetal sheep, placental O_2 consumption falls to a greater extent than fetal O_2 consumption[46], indicating downregulation of oxidative metabolism in the placenta in response to chronically reduced O_2 supply.

CARBON DIOXIDE REMOVAL

Most carbon dioxide (CO_2) in the blood is hydrated to hydrogen ions (H^+) and bicarbonate (HCO_3^-)ions; this conversion is catalysed by carbonic anhydrase (CA) inside red blood cells. Some CO_2 is associated with deoxygenated Hb, as carbamino-Hb, and only a small amount is in solution. In the guinea pig, transfer of HCO_3^- relies on the presence of CA on both maternal and fetal facing trophoblast membranes[47], suggesting HCO_3^- must be converted back to CO_2 before transfer across the placenta. Carbon dioxide is lipid soluble and readily transferred across the placenta by simple diffusion. In the same study, a small amount of transfer of the HCO_3^- ion, in exchange for lactate or chloride ions, was seen when CA activity was inhibited with acetazolamide. Fetal plasma (umbilical vein) P_{CO_2} at term is between 38 and 45 mmHg[48] whereas maternal arterial P_{CO_2} is between 26 and 34 mmHg[49] (lower than pre-pregnancy values due to hyperventilation). This concentration gradient will therefore drive CO_2 transfer. However, as diffusion of the small, lipophilic CO_2 molecule is a rapid process, relative fetal and maternal placental blood flows are the critical determinants of its rate of transfer.

ACID–BASE BALANCE

The role of the placenta in fetal acid–base balance is poorly understood. Mechanisms for regulating acid–base status are a dynamic element of fetal metabolism. For example, as normal gestation proceeds the pH of blood in the umbilical vessels falls[50]. These changes do not occur in isolation. P_{O_2} also declines during normal gestation and fetal Hb rises[50].

Lactate is traditionally viewed as a by-product of anaerobic respiration. However, in the fetus, lactate may be an important source of energy for the fetus and the placenta even when oxygen and glucose supplies are adequate[51]. Umbilical venous lactate concentrations are higher than the umbilical arterial levels and both are higher than the levels in the maternal circulation[51]. This would suggest that lactate is secreted into both circulations by the placenta[52]. Small-for-gestational age (SGA) fetuses have lower umbilical arterial and venous P_{O_2} and pH values with higher P_{CO_2} and lactate values than in the normally grown fetus[50,52]. This elevated lactate concentration might suggest a reduced oxidative capacity in the SGA fetus; the lower P_{O_2} and raised P_{CO_2} are likely to be indicative of reduced placental blood flow.

UNIVALENT IONS

SODIUM

In the rat, there is good evidence that sodium is actively transported to the fetus[53]. Analysis of the classical data of Flexner and colleagues, obtained by *in vivo* measurements of ^{24}Na transfer[33], suggests that, whilst the bulk of sodium transfer to the fetus might be by passive means, the human placenta also does not act solely as a simple filter of sodium[4]. Several routes for transport of sodium have been demonstrated in human placental preparations, as listed below, and any passive movement will be modified by these. However, it is not yet understood which of these routes contribute to placental homeostasis and which to fetal growth. There is molecular and physiological evidence for the systems outlined below.

Sodium channels

There is functional evidence for sodium channels in the microvillous membrane of the human syncytiotrophoblast[54] and some molecular evidence for the presence of the 'epithelial sodium channel' (ENaC) in human placenta[55].

Na^+–H^+ exchange

Na^+/H^+ exchange across the placental microvillous membrane was first demonstrated by Balkovetz and colleagues[56] and confirmed by others[57,58]. Pharmacological data suggest that the microvillous membrane contains the NHE-1 isoform of the protein, which is thought to be involved in cellular housekeeping and that the basal membrane contains the NHE-2 isoform which is usually found on epithelia involved in secretion or absorption[59].

Na^+–amino acid co-transport

There is good evidence for these systems in the human placenta and this is covered in detail below.

Na^+,K^+-ATPase

The presence of a Na^+,K^+-ATPase (sodium pump) in human placental tissue has been confirmed by enzyme[60] and molecular[61,62] techniques. Comparison of isolated microvillous and basal membranes (Table 11.1) suggests that the bulk of the pump activity is on the basal membrane in the human syncytiotrophoblast. Such a location would allow for active transport of sodium to the fetus, whilst maintaining the electrochemical gradient for the transport of solutes into the syncytiotrophoblast utilising the sodium linked co-transporters.

CHLORIDE

A recent study using the *in situ* perfused human placental cotyledon suggests that the bulk of maternofetal chloride transfer is by passive diffusion but that transcellular routes do contribute a quantitatively small fraction[19]. Several such routes have been identified. The presence of chloride channels is suggested by measurement of electrodiffusion in microvillous membrane vesicles[54], by the inhibitory effect of chloride channel blockers on chloride uptake by vesicles[63] and by patch clamp studies[64–66]. These patch clamp studies have so far identified four chloride-selective conductances (channels) in the microvillous membrane of intact placental villi and/or cultured cytotrophoblast cells: a maxi-chloride channel (i.e. a channel with a large conductance)[64], a calcium-activated chloride conductance[66], a chloride conductance activated by hypotonic shock[66] and a small conductance channel which appears to be stimulated by ATP and cyclic AMP-dependent protein kinase[65]. The latter channel is likely to be the placental manifestation of the cystic fibrosis transmembrane conductance regulator, especially as its gene has been shown to be expressed in the placenta[67]. Besides these channels, there is also good evidence that there is a chloride–bicarbonate exchanger in the microvillous plasma membrane of the human placenta akin to that in the red cell[68,69].

POTASSIUM

The rat placenta actively transports potassium to the fetus[70] but it is not known whether this occurs in the human. Plasma potassium concentrations are usually found to be higher in fetus than in mother, but there is great risk of artefact in such measurements[71]. As already noted, Na^+,K^+-ATPase is present in the placenta and there appear to be potassium channels in the microvillous membrane[54,72–74]. However, Dancis and colleagues[75], using ^{86}Rb as a marker for potassium, found that although uptake of the radioisotope by placental fragments was inhibited by ouabain, the transfer across perfused placentas was unaffected. They took this to show that whilst the Na^+,K^+-ATPase is present and active on the cell membranes, it contributes only a small amount to transplacental flux. Thus it may be that, as with sodium and chloride, the bulk of maternofetal potassium transfer in the human is by paracellular diffusion.

DIVALENT IONS

Placental transport of calcium, magnesium and phosphorus involves common features. Firstly, transport from mother to fetus is against a concentration gradient, the concentration of each of these solutes being higher in fetal plasma compared with maternal[76,77]; this suggests that active transport mechanisms underlie the placental transfer of all three ions. Secondly, the net placental transport of each of the divalent ions increases over the last third of gestation, co-incident with the mineralisation of the fetal skeleton[76,78]. This coordinated gestational increase in placental transport, despite different transport mechanisms being involved for the individual ions, is remarkable. Unfortunately the means by which this coordination is brought about is not yet known.

CALCIUM

Fetal plasma concentrations of total and ionised calcium are higher than maternal and evidence to support active, transcellular placental calcium transport has come mainly from placental perfusion studies in a variety of species. These have demonstrated that (i) calcium accumulation occurs on the fetal side against an adverse maternal to fetal perfusate calcium concentration gradient[79–81], (ii) calcium transfer is reduced by the addition of metabolic inhibitors such as dinitrophenol and cyanide or by lowering the perfusate temperature[18,82–84] and (iii) calcium transfer, normalised for molecular size, is significantly higher than that of paracellular diffusional markers[82,83,85].

Transcellular transfer of calcium across the human placenta most likely involves three steps (Fig. 11.1), the first step being transport from the maternal blood to the trophoblastic cytosol across the microvillous plasma membrane of the syncytiotrophoblast. The electrochemical gradient for calcium movement across this plasma membrane is favourable. The median potential difference across the microvillous membrane, when measured *in vitro* was –22 mV (trophoblast negative[28]) and the intracellular 'free' (ionised) calcium concentration is likely to be of the order of 10^{-7} M[86–88], four orders of magnitude lower than the extracellular 'free' calcium concentration of 10^{-3} M in plasma. Studies using isolated microvillous plasma membrane vesicles from human term placenta have demonstrated that calcium uptake across this membrane is unaffected by the potential-dependent channel blockers verapamil and nifedipine, suggesting a lack of involvement of voltage-dependent calcium channels; calcium uptake was saturable and involved both high-affinity and low-affinity systems, respectively (K_m = 0.17 mM and 2.98 mM, according to Brunette and Leclerc[89], 18 μM and 1.5 mM according to Kamath and colleagues[90]), suggestive of facilitated diffusion mechanisms. At physiological concentrations, 'free' calcium entry will be predominantly by the lower affinity system, with some capacity to respond to changes in maternal calcaemia.

The second step in the transcellular transfer of calcium across the placenta involves translocation across the trophoblast cytosol, without generating marked fluctuations in intracellular calcium concentration. This is likely to be achieved in part by some compartmentalisation and buffering of intracellular calcium by organelles such as the endoplasmic reticulum, mitochondria, lysosomes and the nucleus[91,92]. The presence of various calcium-binding proteins will also have an impact. In particular the role of a 9 kDa calcium binding protein (calbindin-D_{9k}) has been the focus of many recent studies. This protein may serve not only as an intracellular calcium buffer[93], but also as a facilitator of calcium diffusion through the cytosol[94], at least as extrapolated from studies on the intestine.[95–97]. In rodent placenta, the expression of calbindin-D_{9k}[98–101] and mRNA for this protein[102–104] increases markedly over the last third of gestation. The temporal association between this gestational induction in calbindin-D_{9k} mRNA expression and the gestational increase in the unidirectional maternofetal clearance of calcium across this tissue[103] suggests that the protein is stoichiometrically involved in transplacental calcium transport and, at least in this species, is probably rate limiting. However, puzzlingly, in the human placenta, evidence is conflicting as to whether mRNA for calbindin-D_{9k} or the protein itself is or is not expressed[105–108].

The third step in the transcellular transfer of calcium across the placenta involves efflux of calcium from the trophoblast cytosol across the basal plasma membrane and hence across the fetal capillary endothelium into fetal plasma. As this step involves transport against a chemical gradient, an active mechanism is implicated. Indeed, the transfer of calcium across this membrane *in vitro* requires ATP[109,110] although ATP-independent, saturable mechanisms also exist involving facilitated diffusion and Na^+–Ca^{2+} exchange[110–112]. Messenger RNA for the calcium pump has been demonstrated in human and rat placenta[103,113] and a high-affinity calcium pump has been localised immunohistochemically to the fetal-facing plasma membrane in the placentas of these species[114]. The calcium pump is therefore positioned to mediate calcium efflux across these membranes into the fetal capillary. In rat placenta, the co-expression of calbindin-D_{9k} and the calcium pump may well be of functional significance as calbindin-D_{9k} can bind to the same domain of the calcium pump as calmodulin[115], the binding of which stimulates calcium pump activity.

MAGNESIUM

Both total and ultrafiltrable concentrations of magnesium in fetal plasma are higher than maternal[3]. Placental perfusion studies in the rat have provided clear evidence to support active, transcellular placental magnesium transport. These studies, in which the placenta is perfused *in situ* through the fetal circulation, have demonstrated that unidirectional maternofetal transfer of magnesium is significantly higher than that of paracellular diffusional markers[82,116,117] and is reduced by the addition of the metabolic inhibitor cyanide or by lowering the perfusate temperature[82]. These studies also indicate that the carrier mediating magnesium transfer is sodium-dependent as addition of amiloride and ouabain, or the removal of sodium from the perfusate, results in reduced transfer[117]. Concordant with this observation, others report reduced ^{28}Mg uptake from maternal plasma into rat fetuses following maternal injection of amiloride[118]. The molecular identity of the transporter involved in the placental transport of magnesium awaits elucidation, but the studies described are compatible with the presence of a Na^+–Mg^{2+} exchanger. It is not yet known whether a similar system operates in the human placenta.

PHOSPHORUS

Although fetal plasma concentrations of inorganic phosphate are higher than maternal, it is not known whether phosphorus is transported across the placenta in this form or as organic phosphate. Evidence for active, transcellular transport of inorganic phosphate has again mainly come from placental perfusion studies, this time in the guinea pig. Both the uptake and the unidirectional maternofetal transfer of inorganic phosphate across the perfused guinea pig placenta is sodium-dependent, and is reduced by anoxia and by the addition of the metabolic inhibitor cyanide[119,120]. Phosphate uptake into microvillous membrane vesicles from human placenta is stimulated by sodium[121], and is electrogenic, carrying two sodium ions for each phosphate[122], providing support for the involvement of a sodium–phosphate co-transporter and therefore of a transcellular route in this species.

CONTROL OF PLACENTAL TRANSPORT OF CALCIUM AND MAGNESIUM AND EFFECT OF DIABETES MELLITUS

Although, as mentioned above, the net transplacental flux of calcium, magnesium and phosphate must increase over gestation to account for mineralisation of the fetal skeleton, the regulatory factors involved in this are not known. Potential determinants of maternofetal flux include electrochemical gradients and hormonal control. The impact of an altered maternal concentration of these solutes on placental transport depends to some extent on the kinetics of the system involved. For instance, the K_m of transcellular maternofetal calcium transport across the human and rat placenta is 2.06 mM and 0.45 mM respectively[18,85]. From these kinetic parameters, calcium transport across the human placenta is unlikely to be saturated under physiological conditions, in contrast to the rat. It is therefore not surprising that dietary-induced maternal hypocalcaemia in humans leads to rickets in the infant[123] whereas in the rat chronic maternal hypocalcaemia does not have any effect on maternofetal calcium flux, or on fetal calcium accretion[124,125]. Similarly, maternal hypermagnesaemia leads to fetal hypermagnesaemia in the human[126], but has relatively little effect in the rat[127].

Abnormalities of placental calcium and magnesium transport in diabetes mellitus may provide clues to the normal hormonal control of these processes. This disease is associated with a reduced fetal/neonatal bone mineralisation in both human and rat pregnancy[128–130] indicative of a parallel reduction in the net placental flux of calcium, magnesium and phosphate. Supportive of this is the evidence that the unidirectional maternofetal flux of both calcium and magnesium is reduced in rat diabetic pregnancy and both these variables are normalised to control levels by insulin treatment[130]. Furthermore, the reduction in maternofetal calcium flux and the corrective effect of insulin mirrors the changes found in the expression of placental calbindin-D_{9k} mRNA[130]. Placental calcium pump mRNA levels, however, remain unaltered by diabetes or insulin treatment[131]. Although there is also a lowered maternal plasma concentration of 1,25-dihydroxyvitamin D_3, the active metabolite of vitamin D, associated with diabetic rat pregnancy[132], this alone cannot account for the depressed placental calbindin-D_{9k} mRNA expression or placental calcium flux as neither are dependent on maternal vitamin D[133,134]. The molecular mechanisms involved in the putative depression of mineral transport by the human diabetic placenta remain to be elucidated.

GLUCOSE

The concept of carrier-mediated sugar transport across the placenta was first proposed by Widdas[135], who demonstrated that passive diffusion alone could not account for the rate of glucose transport across the sheep placenta. Since then, several studies have confirmed the existence of a facilitated transplacental transport system for glucose, demonstrating this to be stereospecific, saturable and energy-independent in a variety of species[136]. In human placenta, uptake of radiolabelled D-glucose or methyl D-glucose, a non-metabolisable analogue, across the microvillous and basal plasma membranes of the syncytiotrophoblast was found to be rapid, stereospecific, Na^+-independent and inhibitable by cytochalasin B, phloretin and phlorizin[137–139]. Photoaffinity labelling with cytochalasin B demonstrated the glucose carrier in the microvillous membrane had a molecular weight of about 51 000–52 000 kDa[140,141], similar to the molecular weight of the GLUT family of Na^+-independent sugar transporters[142].

Antibodies against GLUT1, the isoform found in the erythrocyte, bind to a protein of 50 000–55 000 kDa in human placental homogonates[143–145] and immunolocalisation studies have demonstrated that GLUT1 is concentrated in the microvillous and basal plasma membranes of human syncytiotrophoblast[143,145]. Both first trimester and term human placenta showed greater GLUT1 immunoreactivity on the microvillous plasma membrane compared with the basal plasma membrane[144], and this difference in the relative abundance of GLUT1 between the two plasma membranes has been confirmed quantitatively by Western blotting[145,146]. This asymmetry in GLUT1 distribution together with the much greater surface area of the microvillous membrane may well result in syncytial glucose concentrations approaching maternal, providing a maximal gradient for transfer to the fetus. Another isoform, GLUT3, is also expressed by human placenta at mRNA level[147], but evidence for it at the protein level remains equivocal, with indications for its presence[148,149] and its absence[145,146]. Nevertheless, GLUT3 protein is expressed in significant amounts by the choriocarcinoma derived cell line,

JAr, perhaps suggesting an association in the placenta with rapidly dividing cells[150]. In support of this, a preliminary study has immunocytochemically localised GLUT3 on cytotrophoblast cells of first trimester placenta[151].

Both GLUT1 and GLUT3 are abundant in rat and mouse placenta at the mRNA and protein level, with co-expression of both isoforms by the labyrinthine zone, the area involved in maternofetal exchange[152–154]. Interestingly, the GLUT3 isoform, but not the GLUT1, is sensitive to prevailing maternal glucose concentrations, with upregulation of placental GLUT3 mRNA expression in the face of marked maternal hyperglycaemia in these species, but only in rat placenta is there an associated increase at the protein level of this isoform[153,154]. Conversely, GLUT1 expression is downregulated by glucose in isolated cytotrophoblast cells from human placenta[155].

The driving force for facilitated transport across the placenta is the maternofetal concentration gradient with fetal whole blood or plasma concentrations being lower than maternal in a variety of species[5,153–157]. From the K_m values for the glucose transporters in the microvillous and basal plasma membranes of the human syncytiotrophoblast, 31 mM[137] and 23 mM[139] respectively, it can be concluded that not only is transport likely to be linearly related to maternal concentration in the physiological range, but also that transplacental glucose transport will not be saturated under physiological conditions. In support of this, placental perfusion studies have demonstrated that saturation of glucose transport is only achieved at supraphysiological concentrations of glucose[158].

There is no good evidence for control of glucose transport across the placenta; what data there is has been reviewed by Sibley and Boyd[136] and Ingermann[158].

AMINO ACID TRANSPORT

The concentration of almost all amino acids is higher in umbilical venous blood than in maternal uterine arterial blood from mid-trimester onwards, implying active transport from mother to fetus across the syncytiotrophoblast[159,160]. In support of this, a wide range of amino acid transporters have now been characterised in the microvillous and basal plasma membranes of the syncytiotrophoblast (Table 11.3). Concentrations within placental tissue itself are higher than in either maternal or fetal serum[161,162] so the interesting question is how net flux from mother to the fetus occurs. To accumulate amino acids against the prevailing concentration gradient, within syncytiotrophoblast, many carriers rely on co-transport with sodium ions which have been pumped out of the syncytium in an energy-dependent process to create an electrochemical gradient. Asymmetric distribution of a carrier between the two membranes may be an important mechanism for promoting net flux towards the fetus. Thus the sodium ion gradient generated by Na^+, K^+-ATPase in relation to both maternal and fetal plasma promotes influx of those amino acids co-transported with this ion (sodium-dependent in Table 11.3). This concentration gradient created by specific carriers will be dissipated by the tendency for an amino acid to 'leak' back down its concentration gradient, via either simple or facilitated diffusion, into the maternal and fetal circulations. It has been demonstrated in the guinea pig that this backflow is markedly greater at the basal than microvillous membrane[163]. Additionally, there is evidence that a carrier may not behave in the same way in the microvillous membrane as it does when positioned in the basal membrane[164–166]. Whether this is due to a structural difference in the protein or modulation of its action is not known. How the accumulation of amino acids which are not co-transported with sodium is energised is not known.

REGULATORY MECHANISMS

Amino acid availability may be important since the synthesis of some carriers increases in the presence of low levels of substrate, e.g. System A[167]. High intracellular concentrations of

TABLE 11.3
Amino acid transport systems in the human placenta

System name	Membrane location	Amino acids (aa)	Reference
A	MVM + BM	neutral aa, MeAIB	205, 206
ASC	BM	Ala, Ser, Cys, anionic aa	206, 207
N	MVM	His, Gln	208
β	MVM	Tau	204, 209
X^-_{AG}	MVM + BM	Asp, Glu	207, 210
l	MVM + BM	Leu, BCH	205, 206
y^+	MVM + BM	Lys, Arg	165, 166, 206, 211
$b^{0,+}$	BM	Lys, Arg	165, 212
B^0	Unknown	Broad-specification	165, 212
y^+L	MVM	Lys, Arg	211

A carrier is designated with a capital letter if transport is Na^+-dependent. MeAIB and BCH are substrate analogues with greater specificities than naturally occurring amino acids for the given carrier, which have been developed to facilitate study of individual transporters. Abbreviations (other than standard three-letter amino acid codes): MeAIB, methylaminoisobutyric acid; BCH, 2-aminobicyclo [2,2,1]-heptane-2-carboxylic acid; MVM, microvillous membrane; BM, basal membrane.

amino acids have been shown to modulate carrier activity. For example, System A is inhibited but System 1 is stimulated[168]. The role of some extrinsic factors on amino acid transport have also been studied; in cultured human trophoblast cells uptake of aminoisobutyric acid (AIB, a non-metabolisable alanine analogue) is stimulated by insulin[169], insulin-like growth factor-I[170] and epidermal growth factor[171] and diminished, in the rat, by tumour necrosis factor-α[172]. Taurine transport is regulated by protein kinase C[173] and inhibited by calcium[174].

PATHOPHYSIOLOGICAL STATES

Cordocentesis has shown that fetal amino acid concentrations are lower in small-for-gestational age (SGA) fetuses than in appropriately grown (AGA) controls at mid-trimester and term[160]. Vesicle studies have shown that System A activity is lower in the microvillous membrane of term SGA babies compared to term AGA babies[175]. Whether these two facts represent cause and effect in growth retardation is unknown. Uterine artery ligation in the rat leads to growth-retarded fetuses and reduced amino acid transfer but no change in placental System A activity[176]. As, in this situation, the placenta is normal, these data imply that the reduced System A activity in human growth retardation might be the result of placental pathology, in agreement with morphological studies[177]. However, induction of growth retardation in rat fetuses by protein restricting the maternal diet is associated with a reduction in System A activity at both the microvillous and basal plasma membranes, whilst transport by System ASC is unaffected[178]. In the same study, System y^+ at both membranes and mRNA for System y^+ transporter protein were reduced. Maternal smoking, alcohol abuse and recreational drug use are recognised as causes of fetal growth retardation and there is evidence that these affect placental System A activity. Amino acid uptake in human and primate placentas seems relatively unaffected by acute ethanol exposure[179] but is depressed in primates by chronic exposure[180]. Experiments with placental villous fragments showed reduced uptake of amino acids in the presence of nicotine, other components of tobacco smoke and cocaine[181]. Human vesicle studies have failed to reproduce the effect of either ethanol or nicotine but do show a direct effect of cocaine[182], implying an intact cell structure is required for some effects but not others.

This picture of an association between reduced placental System A activity and poor fetal growth is, however, complicated by the finding that System A activity is also reduced in microvillous membrane vesicles prepared from the placentas of macrosomic babies born to diabetic women but not in placentas from AGA babies of diabetic women, compared to those from placentas from normal-sized babies born to normal women[183]. This indicates the complexity of the link between fetal size and amino acid transfer, at least for System A.

IMMUNOGLOBULIN G

In women, some passive immunity is conferred on the fetus by the selective transfer of immunoglobulin G (IgG) by the placenta. In species which carry a functioning yolk sac placenta to term, it is this epithelium which is predominantly involved in IgG transfer rather than the chorioallantoic placenta[184]. Studies on the mechanism of selective IgG transfer by the syncytiotrophoblast of the human chorioallantoic placenta have therefore been based on models derived from experiments on the yolk sac placenta[185]. The essentials of this model are that: (i) IgG destined for transfer to the fetus is taken up from maternal plasma by receptor-mediated endocytosis via specific Fc receptors in coated pits (specialised areas of plasma membrane which have a fuzzy electron-dense outline, under the electron microscope, due to a protein called clathrin) on the microvillous plasma membrane of the syncytiotrophoblast; (ii) Fc receptor bound IgG within coated vesicles, formed by invagination of the coated pits, is protected from digestion by lysosomes within the syncytiotrophoblast; (iii) vesicles containing undigested IgG fuse with the basal plasma membrane of the syncytiotrophoblast, exocytose and release the IgG into the interstitial space.

Studies in which IgG in the syncytiotrophoblast has been localised under the electron microscope, as well as biochemical experiments, mainly support the first part of the model described above[186–190], though not every study has found IgG in coated pits/vesicles[191]. Experimental evidence for the accuracy of parts (ii) and (iii) of the model is more equivocal; various intracellular compartments seem to contain IgG and direct evidence for exocytosis is weak[188–191].

Once IgG reaches the interstitial space on the fetal side of the syncytiotrophoblast, it still has to traverse the basement membrane and fetal capillary endothelium (Fig. 11.1). Although the former does not appear to present a significant barrier[188,191] the latter does; the available data suggest that transcytosis in vesicles is a more likely route of transfer across the endothelium than is diffusion through the lateral intercellular spaces between endothelial cells[188–190].

Therefore, much work remains to be done in order to fully characterise the mechanism of selective IgG transfer across the placenta.

DRUGS

Recent epidemiological studies have shown that many classes of drugs are taken during pregnancy, the most common being analgesics, anti-emetics, antibiotics, tranquillisers, antihistamines and diuretics[192]. Most drugs are considered to be transferred across the placenta by diffusion[193] and their rate of transplacental transfer will depend on their physico-chemical characteristics (lipophilicity, hydophilicity, molecular size, ionisation state), the degree to which they are bound by plasma proteins[193] and whether they have undergone biotransformation either in the maternal compartment or during transplacental transfer[194]. The potentially extremely serious consequences to the fetus of high maternal plasma concentrations of toxic lipophilic substances has recently been clearly demonstrated; Jacobson and Jacobson[195] found that *in utero* exposure to polychlorinated biphenyls has a long-term impact on intellectual function.

The most common approach to studying human placental transfer of drugs is to sample maternal and umbilical cord blood following a maternal bolus of drug administration. This technique, however suffers from some disadvantages, namely the measurements may not be made during a time frame where flux is unidirectional or maximal, often no reference tracer is included for comparison, it is difficult to evaluate the influence of maternal or placental metabolism, or the degree of drug binding to plasma proteins/placental tissue. Furthermore, placental drug transfer is only one of the factors involved in the consideration of pharmacokinetic data relating to drug concentration–time profiles in the fetus[196,197].

Other approaches such as the *in vitro* perfused human placental cotyledon technique have been useful in dissecting out the relative rates of transfer for drugs belonging to the same class. For instance, the more lipid soluble propanolol showed a threefold higher steady-state diffusion rate compared to the more hydrophilic atenolol, despite these being of a similar molecular weight[198]. The use of isolated microvillous membrane vesicles from human placenta has also provided mechanistic insights, with evidence of facilitated diffusion mechanisms for cephalosporin antibiotics[199], the antiviral drug gancyclovir[200] and corticosterone[201,202]. This latter technique has also been particularly useful in determining the direct effect of various drugs including those of abuse, such as cocaine, nicotine and ethanol, on the activity of several transporters in trophoblast plasma membranes (Table 11.4).

Acknowledgements

We are very grateful to Mrs Jean French for secretarial assistance.

TABLE 11.4
Effect of various drugs on some transporters in the microvillous (MVM) and basal (BM) plasma membranes of human syncytiotrophoblast

Membrane	Drug	Transporter	Effect	Reference
BM	Cimetidine, clonidine, amiloride	Na^+–H^+ exchanger	↓	59
	Cocaine	Alanine	↓	228
MVM	Salicylate	Sulphate	↓	213, 214
	Furosemide, bumetanide	Chloride	→	63, 215
	Furosemide, salicylate, bumetanide	Chloride	↓	68, 216
	Cimetidine, clonidine, loperamide, amiloride	Na^+/H^+ exchanger	↓	58, 215, 217, 220, 225
	Cocaine	Alanine	↓	182
	Cocaine, nicotine, cimetidine, salicylate, furosemide, indomethacin	Alanine	→ ↓	218
	Ethanol	Alanine	→	218, 219
	Nicotine/ethanol	AIB	→	221
	Imipramine, verapamil, propranolol, quinine, flurazepam, amiloride ritodrine, atropine, ranitidine, cimetidine, procainamide	Choline	↓	218, 222
	Clonidine, imipramine, amiloride	organic cation/H^+ exchanger	↓	223
	Probenecid, furosemide, indomethacin salicylate	p-aminohippurate	↓ →	224
	Fluoxetine, paroxetine	Serotonin	↓	226, 227

REFERENCES

1. Kaufmann P, Burton GJ. Anatomy and genesis of the placenta. In *The Physiology of Reproduction* 2nd edn. (eds E. Knobil & J.D. Neill). New York: Raven Press, 1994.
2. Firth JA, Leach L. Not trophoblast alone: a review of the contribution of the fetal microvasculature to transplacental exchange. *Placenta* **17**:89–96, 1996.
3. Morriss FH, Boyd RDH, Mahendran D. Placental transport. In *The Physiology of Reproduction* 2nd edn. (eds E. Knobil & J.D. Neill), p. 813. New York: Raven Press, 1994.
4. Sibley CP. Review article. Mechanisms of ion transfer by the rat placenta: a model for the human placenta? *Placenta* **15**:675–691, 1994.
5. Faber JJ, Thornburg KL. *Placental Physiology: Structure and Function of Fetomaternal Exchange*. New York: Raven Press, 1983.
6. Faber JJ, Hart FM. The rabbit placenta as an organ of diffusional exchange. *Circn Res* **19**:816–833, 1966.
7. Faber JJ, Anderson DF. Model study of placental water transfer and causes of fetal water diseases in sheep. *Am J Physiol* **258**:R1257–R1270, 1990.
8. Bain MD, Copas DK, Landon MJ, Stacey TE. *In vivo* permeability of the human placenta to inulin and mannitol. *J Physiol* **399**:313–319, 1988.
9. Bain MD, Copas DK, Taylor A, Landon MJ, Stacey TE. Permeability of the human placenta *in vivo* to four non-metabolized hydrophilic molecules. *J Physiol* **431**:505–513, 1990.
10. Willis DM, O'Grady JP, Faber JJ, Thornburg KL. Diffusion permeability of cyanocobalamin in human placenta. *Am J Physiol* **250**:R459–R464, 1986.

11. Thornburg KL, Burry KJ, King Adams A, Kirk EP, Faber JJ. Permeability of placenta to inulin. *Am J Obstet Gynecol* **158**:1165–1169, 1988.
12. Schneider H, Sodha RJ, Progler M, Young MPA. Permeability of the human placenta for hydrophilic substances studied in the isolated dually *in vitro* perfused lobe. *Contrib Gynecol Obstet* **13**:98–103, 1985.
13. Illsley NP, Hall S, Penfold P, Stacey TE. Diffusional permeability of the human placenta. *Contrib Gynecol Obstet* **13**:92–97, 1985.
14. Stulc J. Extracellular transport pathways in the haemochorial placenta. *Placenta* **10**:113–119, 1989.
15. Edwards D, Jones CJP, Sibley CP, Nelson DM. Paracellular permeability pathways in the human placenta. A qualitative and morphological study of maternal-fetal transfer of horseradish peroxidase. *Placenta* **14**:63–73, 1993.
16. Brownbill PD, Edwards D, Jones C *et al.* Mechanisms of alphafetoprotein transfer in the perfused human placental cotyledon from uncomplicated pregnancy. *J Clin Invest* **96**:2220–2226, 1995.
17. Kertschanska S, Kosanke G, Kaufmann P. Is there morphological evidence for the existence of transtrophoblastic channels in human placental villi? *Trophoblast Res.* **8**:581–596, 1994.
18. Stulc J, Stulcova B, Smid M, Sach I. Parallel mechanisms of Ca^{++} transfer across the perfused human placental cotyledon. *Am J Obstet Gynecol* **170**:162–167, 1994.
19. Doughty IM, Glazier JD, Greenwood SL, Boyd RDH, Sibley CP. Mechanisms of maternofetal chloride transfer across the *in vitro* perfused human placental cotyledon. *Am J Physiol* **40**:1107–1114, 1996.
20. Pappone PA, Cahalan MD. Ion permeation in cell membranes. In *Physiology of Membrane Disorders* (eds T.E. Andreoli *et al.*) New York: Plenum, 1985.
21. Macey RI. Mathematical models of membrane transport processes. In *Physiology of Membrane Disorders* (eds T.E. Andreoli *et al.*), p. 111. New York: Plenum, 1985.
22. Stein WD. *Channels, Carriers and Pumps: An Introduction to Membrane Transport*. San Diego CA: Academic Press, 1992.
23. Atkinson DE, Robinson NR, Sibley CP. Development of the passive permeability characteristics of the rat placenta during the last 3rd of gestation. *Am J Physiol* **261**:R1462–R1464, 1991.
24. King-Adams A, Read DL, Thornburg KL *et al. In vivo* placental permeability to hydrophilic solutes as a function of fetal weight in the guinea-pig. *Placenta* **9**:409–416, 1988.
25. Faber JJ. Transplacental clearances of inert hydrophilic tracers in rabbits of 18 days gestation. *Placenta* **16**:403–412, 1995.
26. Faber JJ. Diffusion permeability of the immature placenta of the rabbit embryo to inert hydrophilic molecules. *Am J Physiol* **265**:H1804–H1808, 1993.
27. MacNaughton TG, Power GG. Current topic: the maternal–fetal electrical potential differences; new findings and a perspective. *Placenta* **12**:185–197, 1991.
28. Greenwood SL, Boyd RDH, Sibley CP. Transtrophoblast and microvillous membrane potential difference in mature intermediate human placental villi. *Am J Physiol* **265**:C460–C466, 1993.
29. Stulc J, Svihovec J, Drabkova J *et al.* Electrical potential difference across the mid-term human placenta. *Acta Obstet Gynecol Scand* **57**:125–126, 1978.
30. Mellor DJ, Cockburn F, Lees MM, Blagden A. Distribution of ions and electrical potential differences between mother and fetus in the human at term. *J Obstet Gynaecol Br Commonw* **76**:993–998, 1969.
31. Schroeder HJ. Comparative aspects of placental exchange functions. *Eur J Obstet Gynaecol* **63**:81–90, 1995.
32. Battaglia FC, Meschia G. *An Introduction to Fetal Physiology*. Orlando, FL: Academic Press, 1986.
33. Flexner LB, Cowie DB, Hellman LM, Wilde WS, Vosburgh GJ. The permeability of the human placenta to sodium in normal and abnormal pregnancies and the supply of of sodium to the human fetus as determined with radioactive sodium. *Am J Obstet Gynecol* **55**:469–480, 1948.
34. Barcroft J. *Researches on Pre-natal Life*. Oxford: Blackwell Scientific Publications, 1946.
35. Stulc J, Stulcova B. Asymmetrical transfer of inert hydrophilic solutes across rat placenta. *Am J Physiol* **265**:R670–R675, 1993.
36. Stulc J, Stulcova J. Effect of NaCl load administered to the fetus on the bidirectional movement of ^{51}Cr-EDTA across rat placenta. *Am J Physiol* **220**:R984–R989, 1996.
37. Carter AM. Factors affecting gas transfer across the placenta and the oxygen supply to the fetus. *J Dev Physiol* **12**:305–322, 1989.
38. Jauniaux E, Jurkovic D, Campbell S. Current topic: *in vivo* investigation of the placental circulations by Doppler echography. *Placenta* **16**:323–331, 1995.
39. Moll W. Invited commentary: absence of intervillous blood flow in the first trimester of human pregnancy. *Placenta* **16**:333–334, 1995.
40. Banner CH, Ludwig I, Ludwig M. Different effects of 2,3-diphosphoglycerate and adenosine triphosphate on the oxygen affinity of adult and foetal human haemoglobin. *Life Sci* **7**:1339–1343, 1968.
41. Edelstone DI, Peticca BB, Goldblum LJ. Effects of maternal oxygen administration on fetal oxygenation during reductions in umbilical blood flow in fetal lambs. *Am J Obstet Gynecol* **152**:351–358, 1989.
42. Wilkening RB, Meschia G. Fetal oxygen uptake, oxygenation and acid–base balance as a function of uterine blood flow. *Am J Physiol* **244**:H749–H755, 1983.
43. Anderson DF, Parks CM, Faber JJ. Fetal O_2 consumption in sheep during controlled long-term reductions in umbilical blood flow. *Am J Physiol* **250**:H1037–H1042, 1986.
44. Jacobs R, Robinson JS, Owens JA, Falconer J, Webster MED. The effect of prolonged hypobaric hypoxia on growth of fetal sheep. *J Dev Physiol* **10**:97–112, 1988.
45. Gu W, Jones CT, Parer JT. Metabolic and cardiovascular effects on fetal sheep of sustained reduction of uterine blood flow. *J Physiol* **368**:109–129, 1985.
46. Owens JA, Falconer J, Robinson JS. Effect of restriction of placental growth on oxygen delivery to and consumption by the pregnant uterus and fetus. *J Dev Physiol* **9**:137–150, 1987.
47. Hatano H, Leichtweiss HP, Schroder H. Uptake of bicarbonate/CO_2 in the isolated guinea pig placenta. *Placenta* **10**:213–221, 1989.
48. Economides DL. Acid–base balance in the fetus. In *Scientific Essentials of Reproductive Medicine* (eds S.G., Hiller, H.C. Kitchener & J.P. Neilson), p. 376. London: WB Saunders, 1996.
49. Robson SC. Maternal respiratory and cardiovascular changes during pregnancy. In *Scientific Essentials of Reproductive Medicine* (eds S.G. Hiller, H.C. Kitchener & J.P. Neilson), p. 433. London: WB Saunders, 1996.
50. Soothill PW, Nicolaides KH, Rodeck CH, Campbell S. Effect of gestational age on fetal and intervillous blood gas and acid–base values in human pregnancy. *Fetal Ther* **1**:168–175, 1986.
51. Burd LI, Jones MD, Simmons MA, Makowski EL, Meschia G, Battaglia FC. Placental production and foetal utilization of lactate and pyruvate. *Nature* **254**:210–211, 1975.
52. Nicolaides KH, Economides DL, Soothill PW. Blood gases, pH and lactate in appropriate- and small-for-gestational-age fetuses. *Am J Obstet Gynecol* **161**:966–1001, 1989.
53. Stulc J, Stulcova B, Sibley CP. Evidence for active maternal–fetal transport of Na^+ across the placenta of the anaesthetized rat. *J Physiol* **470**:637–649, 1993.
54. Illsley NP, Sellers MC. Ionic conductances in the microvillous and basal membrane vesicles isolated from human placental syncytiotrophoblast. *Placenta* **1**:25–34, 1992.
55. McDonald FJ, Price MP, Snyder PM, Welsh MJ. Cloning and expression of the β and δ-subunits of the human epithelial sodium channel. *Am J Physiol* **268**:C1157–C1163, 1995.
56. Balkovetz DF, Leibach FH, Mahesh VB *et al.* Na^+/H^+ exchanger of human placental brush-border membrane: identification and characterization. *Am J Physiol* **251**:C852–C860, 1986.
57. Chipperfield AR, Langridge-Smith JE, Steele LW. Sodium entry into human placental microvillous (maternal) plasma membrane vesicles. *Q J Exp Physiol* **73**:399–411, 1988.
58. Glazier JD, Jones CJP, Sibley CP. Purification and Na^+ uptake by human placental microvillous membrane vesicles prepared by three different methods. *Biochim Biophys Acta* **945**:127–134, 1988.
59. Kulanthaivel P, Furesz TC, Moe AJ *et al.* Human placental syncytiotrophoblast expresses two pharmacologically distinguishable types of Na^+/H^+ exchangers, NHE-1 in the maternal facing (brush-border) membrane and NHE-2 in the fetal-facing (basal) membrane. *Biochem J* **284**:33–38, 1992.
60. Miller RK, Berndt WO. Evidence for $Mg2^+$-dependent Na^+ and K^+-activated ATPase and $Ca2^+$ ATPase in the human term placenta. *Proc Soc Exp Biol Med* **143**:118–122, 1973.

61. Chehab FF, Kan YW, Law M *et al.* Human placental Na^+, K^+-ATPase α subunit: cDNA cloning, tissue expression, DNA polymorphism and chromosomal localization. *Proc Nat Acad Sci* **84**:7901–7905, 1987.
62. Clarson LH, Glazier JS, Greenwood SL, Sibley CP. Activity and expression of Na^+/K^+-ATPase in human placental trophoblast cells in culture. *J Physiol* **497**:735–744, 1996.
63. Byrne S, Glazier JD, Greenwood SL *et al.* Chloride transport by human placental microvillous membrane vesicles. *Biochim Biophys Acta* **1153**:122–126, 1993.
64. Brown PD, Greenwood SL, Robinson J, Boyd RDH. Chloride channels of high conductance in the microvillous membrane of term human placenta. *Placenta* **14**:103–115, 1993.
65. Byrne S, Greenwood SL, Sibley CP. A chloride channel of small conductance in cytotrophoblast cells isolated from human term placenta. *Placenta* **16**:A10, 1995.
66. Kibble JD, Greenwood SL, Clarson LH, Sibley CP. A Ca^{2+}-activated whole-cell chloride conductance in human placental cytotrophoblast cells activated by a G-protein. *J Membrane Biol* **151**:131–138, 1996.
67. Mylona P, Glazier JD, Sides MK, Sibley CP. Expression of the cystic fibrosis (CF) and multidrug resistance (*MDR1*) genes during development and differentiation in the human placenta. *Hum Molec Reprod* **2**:101–106, 1996.
68. Shennan DB, Davis B, Boyd CAR. Chloride transport in human placental microvillous membrane vesicles. I. Evidence for anion exchange. *Pflugers Arch* **406**:60–64, 1986.
69. Grassl SM. Cl^-/HCO_3^- exchange in human placental brush border membrane vesicles. *J Biol Chem* **264**:11103–11106, 1989.
70. Mohammed T, Stulc J, Glazier JD, Boyd RDH, Sibley CP. Mechanisms of potassium transfer across the dually perfused rat placenta. *Am J Physiol* **265**:R341–R347, 1993.
71. Mohammed T, Maresh M, Sibley CP, Boyd RDH. Absent maternofetal potassium gradient at term. *Arch Dis Child* **65**:384–386, 1990.
72. Yamamoto T, Bkaily G, Belisle S. Inwardly rectifying currents in human term placental cells. *Pflugers Arch* **419**:421–423, 1991.
73. Greenwood SL, Brown PD, Edwards S, Sibley CP. Patch clamp studies of human placental cytotrophoblasts in culture. *Trophoblast Res* **7**:53–68, 1993.
74. Clarson LH, Greenwood SL, Sides MK, Sibley CP. Expression of an inwardly rectifying K^+ current in differentiated human cytotrophoblast cells. *J Physiol* **494**:32P, 1996.
75. Dancis J, Kammerman S, Jansen V, Levitz M. The effect of ouabain on placental transport of ^{86}Rb. *Placenta* **4**:351–360, 1983.
76. Husain SM, Mughal MZ. Mineral transport across the placenta. *Arch Dis Child* **67**:874–878, 1992.
77. Mughal MZ, Tsang RC. Calcium, phosphorus, and magnesium transport across the placenta. In *Fetal and Neonatal Physiology Volume II* (eds R.A. Polin & W.W. Fox), pp. 1735–1744. Philadelphia: W.B. Saunders, 1992.
78. Widdowson EM. Growth and composition of the fetus and newborn. In *Biology of Gestation Volume II. The Fetus and Neonate* (ed. N.S. Assali), pp. 1–49. New York: Academic Press, 1968.
79. Abramovich DR, Dacke CG, Elcock C, Page KR. Calcium transport across the isolated dually perfused human placental lobule. *J Physiol* **382**:397–410, 1987.
80. Twardock AR, Austin MK. Calcium transfer in perfused guinea pig placenta. *Am J Physiol* **219**:540–545, 1970.
81. Weatherley AJ, Ross R, Pickard DW, Care AD. The transfer of calcium during perfusion of the placenta in intact and thyroparathyroidectomized sheep. *Placenta* **4**:271–278, 1983.
82. Shaw AJ, Mughal MZ, Mohammed T, Maresh MJA, Sibley CP. Evidence for active maternofetal transfer of magnesium across the *in situ* perfused rat placenta. *Pediatr Res* **27**:622–625, 1990.
83. Štulc J, Štulcová B. Transport of calcium by the placenta of the rat. *J Physiol* **371**:1–16, 1986.
84. Williams JMA, Abramovich DR, Dacke CG, Mayhew TM, Page KR. Inhibitor action on placental calcium transport. *Calcif Tissue Int* **48**:7–12, 1991.
85. Štulc J, Štulcová B, Švihovec J. Transport of calcium across the dually perfused placenta of the rat. *J Physiol* **420**:295–311, 1990.
86. Juhlin C, Lundgren S, Johansson H *et al.* 500-Kilodalton calcium sensor regulating cytoplasmic Ca^{2+} in cytotrophoblast cells of human placenta. *J Biol Chem* **265**:8275–8279, 1990.
87. Bax C, Bax B, Bain M, Zaidi M. Ca^{2+} channels in human term trophoblast cells *in vitro*. A study using the Ca^{2+}-sensitive dye Fura 2. *Trophoblast Res* **8**:573–580, 1994.
88. Hellman P, Ridefelt P, Juhlin C, Åkerström G, Rastad J, Gylfe E. Parathyroid-like regulation of parathyroid hormone-related protein release and cytoplasmic calcium in cytotrophoblast cells of human placenta. *Arch Biochem Biophys* **293**:174–180, 1992.
89. Brunette MG, Leclerc M. Ca^{2+} transport through the brush border membrane of human placenta syncytiotrophoblasts. *Can J Physiol Pharmacol* **70**:835–842, 1992.
90. Kamath SG, Kelley LK, Friedman AF, Smith CH. Transport and binding in calcium uptake by microvillous membrane of human placenta. *Am J Physiol* **262**:C789–C794, 1992.
91. Croley TE. The intracellular localization of calcium within the mature human placental barrier. *Am J Obstet Gynecol* **117**:926–932, 1973.
92. van Kreel BK, van Dijk JP. Mechanisms involved in the transfer of calcium across the isolated guinea pigs placenta. *J Dev Physiol* **5**:155–165, 1983.
93. Christakos S, Gabrielides C, Rhoten WB. Vitamin D-dependent calcium binding proteins: Chemistry, distribution, functional considerations, and molecular biology. *Endocr Rev* **10**:3–26, 1989.
94. Feher JJ, Fullmer CS, Fritzsch GK. Comparison of the enhanced steady-state diffusion of calcium by calbindin-D_{9K} and calmodulin: possible importance in intestinal calcium absorption. *Cell Calcium* **10**:189–203, 1989.
95. Bronner F. Vitamin D-dependent active calcium transport: The role of CaBP. *Calcif Tissue Int* **43**:133–137, 1988.
96. Bronner F, Pansu D, Stein WD. An analysis of intestinal calcium transport across the rat intestine. *Am J Physiol* **250**:G561–G569, 1986.
97. Feher JJ, Fullmer CS, Wasserman RH. Role of facilitated diffusion of calcium by calbindin in intestinal calcium absorption. *Am J Physiol* **262**:C517–C526, 1992.
98. Bruns MEH, Fausto A, Avioli LV. Placental calcium binding protein in rats. Apparent identity with vitamin D-dependent calcium binding protein from rat intestine. *J Biol Chem* **253**:3186–3190, 1978.
99. Bruns MEH, Vollmer S, Wallshein V, Bruns DE. Vitamin D-dependent calcium-binding protein. Immunochemical studies and synthesis by placental tissue *in vitro J Biol Chem* **256**:4649–4653, 1981.
100. Delorme AC, Marche P, Garel JM. Vitamin D-dependent calcium-binding protein. Changes during gestation, prenatal and postnatal development in rats. *J Dev Physiol* **1**:181–194, 1979.
101. Mathieu CL, Burnett SH, Mills SE, Overpeck JG, Bruns DE, Bruns ME. Gestational changes in calbindin-D_{9K} in rat uterus, yolk sac, and placenta: Implications for maternal–fetal calcium transport and uterine muscle function. *Proc Natl Acad Sci USA* **86**:3433–3437, 1989.
102. de Maintenant F, Perret C, Brun P, Thomasset M. Expression of cholecalin (9000 MW cholecalciferol-induced CaBP) gene in rat duodenum and placenta during gestation. In *Vitamin D. A Chemical, Biochemical and Clinical Update* (ed. A.W. Norman), pp. 355–356. Berlin: Walter de Gruyter, 1985.
103. Glazier JD, Atkinson DE, Thornburg KL *et al.* Gestational changes in Ca^{2+} transport across rat placenta and mRNA for calbindin$_{9K}$ and Ca^{2+}-ATPase. *Am J Physiol* **263**:R930–R935, 1992.
104. Krisinger J, Dann JL, Jeung EB, Leung PCK. Calbindin-D_{9K} gene expression during pregnancy and lactation in the rat. *Mol Cell Endocrinol* **88**:119–128, 1992.
105. Brun P, Dupret JM, Perret C, Thomasset M, Mathieu H. Vitamin D-dependent calcium-binding proteins (CaBPs) in human fetuses: Comparative distribution of 9K CaBP mRNA and 28K CaBP during development. *Pediatr Res* **21**:362–367, 1987.
106. Howard A, Legon S, Spurr NK, Walters JRF. Molecular cloning and chromosomal assignment of human calbindin-D9K. *Biochem Biophys Res Commun* **185**:663–669, 1992.
107. Jeung EB, Krisinger J, Dann JL, Leung PCK. Molecular cloning of the full-length cDNA encoding the human calbindin-D_{9K}. *FEBS Lett* **307**:224–228, 1992.
108. Jeung EB, Leung PCK, Krisinger J. The human calbindin-D_{9K} gene. Complete structure and implications on steroid hormone regulation. *J Mol Biol* **235**:1231–1238, 1994.
109. Fisher GJ, Kelley LK, Smith CH. ATP-dependent calcium transport across basal plasma membranes of human placental trophoblast. *Am J Physiol* **252**:C38–C46, 1987.

110. Lafond J, Leclerc M, Brunette MG. Characterization of calcium transport by basal plasma membranes from human placental syncytiotrophoblast. *J Cellular Physiol* **148**:17–23, 1991.
111. Kamath SG, Smith CH. Na^+/Ca^{2+} exchange, Ca^{2+} binding, and electrogenic Ca^{2+} transport in plasma membranes of human placental syncytiotrophoblast. *Pediatr Res* **36**:461–467, 1994.
112. Kamath SG, Haider N, Smith CH. ATP independent calcium transport and binding by basal plasma membrane of human placenta. *Placenta* **15**:147–155, 1994.
113. Howard A, Legon S, Walters JRF. Plasma membrane calcium pump expression in human placenta and small intestine. *Biochem Biophys Res Commun* **183**:499–505, 1992.
114. Borke JL, Caride A, Verma AK *et al.* Calcium pump epitopes in placental trophoblast basal plasma membranes. *Am J Physiol* **257**:C341–C346, 1989.
115. James P, Vorherr T, Thulin E, Forsen S, Carafoli E. Identification and primary structure of a calbindin 9K binding domain in the plasma membrane Ca^{2+} pump. *FEBS Lett* **278**:155–159, 1991.
116. Shaw AJ, Mughal MZ, Maresh MJA, Sibley CP. Effects of two synthetic parathyroid hormone-related protein fragments on maternofetal transfer of calcium and magnesium and release of cyclic AMP by the *in-situ* perfused rat placenta. *J Endocrinol* **129**:399–404, 1991.
117. Shaw AJ, Mughal MZ, Maresh MJA, Sibley CP. Sodium-dependent magnesium transport across *in situ* perfused rat placenta. *Am J Physiol* **261**:R369–R372, 1991.
118. Günther T, Vormann J, Höllriegl V. Effects of amiloride and furosemide on ^{28}Mg transport into fetuses and maternal tissues of rats. *Mag Bull* **10**:34–37, 1988.
119. Štulc J, Štulcová B, Švihovec J. Uptake of inorganic phosphate by the maternal border of the guinea pig placenta. *Pflügers Arch* **395**:326–330, 1982.
120. Štulc J, Štulcová B. Transport of inorganic phosphate by the fetal border of the guinea-pig placenta perfused *in situ*. *Placenta* **5**:9–20, 1984.
121. Brunette MG, Allard S. Phosphate uptake by syncytial brush border membranes of the human placenta. *Pediatr Res* **19**:1179–1182, 1985.
122. Lajeunesse D, Brunette MG. Sodium gradient-dependent phosphate transport in placental brush border membrane vesicles. *Placenta* **9**:117–128, 1988.
123. Maxwell JP. Further studies of adult rickets (osteomalacia) and fetal rickets. *Proc Roy Soc Med* **28**:265, 1934.
124. Rasmussen P. Effect of calcium deprivation on rat dams on fetuses and newborn offspring. *Calcif Tissue Int* **38**:289–292, 1986.
125. Mughal MZ, Robinson NR, Sibley CP. The role of vitamin D status in maternofetal calcium exchange across the rat placenta. *J Physiol* **386**:22P, 1987.
126. Cruikshank DP, Pitkin RM, Reynolds WA, Williams GA, Hargis GK. Effects of magnesium sulfate treatment on perinatal calcium metabolism. I. Maternal and fetal responses. *Am J Obstet Gynecol* **134**:243–249, 1979.
127. Garel JM. Parathyroid hormone, calcitonin and mineral metabolism in the mammalian fetus and neonate. In *Perinatal Calcium and Phosphorus Metabolism* (eds M.F. Holick, T.K. Gray & C.S. Anast), p. 71. Amsterdam: Elsevier Science, 1983.
128. Mimouni F, Steichen JJ, Tsang RC, Hertzberg V, Miodovnik M. Decreased bone mineral content in infants of diabetic mothers. *Am J Perinatol* **5**:339–343, 1988.
129. Verhaeghe J, Bouillon, Nyomba BL, Lissens W, Van Assche FA. Vitamin D and bone mineral homeostasis during pregnancy in the diabetic BB rat. *Endocrinology* **118**:1019–1025, 1986.
130. Husain SM, Birdsey TJ, Glazier JD, Mughal MZ, Garland HO, Sibley CP. Effect of diabetes mellitus on maternofetal flux of calcium and magnesium and $calbindin_{9K}$ mRNA expression in rat placenta. *Pediatr Res* **35**:376–381, 1994.
131. Birdsey TJ, Clarson LH, Husain SM, Glazier JD, Garland HO, Sibley CP. CaATPase and $calbindin_{9K}$ mRNA expression in placenta of diabetic rats. *Proc Soc Gynecol Invest* **41**:P188, 1994.
132. Verhaeghe J, Thomasset M, Bréhier A, Van Assche FA, Bouillon R. $1,25(OH)_2D_3$ and Ca-binding protein in fetal rats: Relationship to the maternal vitamin D status. *Am J Physiol* **254**:E505–E512, 1988.
133. Brommage R, DeLuca HF. Placental transport of calcium and phosphorus is not regulated by vitamin D. *Am J Physiol* **246**:F526–F529, 1984.
134. Glazier JD, Mawer EB, Sibley CP. Calbindin-D_{9K} gene expression in rat chorioallantoic placenta is not regulated by 1,25-dihydroxyvitamin D_3. *Pediatr Res* **37**:720–725, 1995.
135. Widdas WF. Inability of diffusion to account for placental glucose transfer in the sheep and consideration of the kinetics of a possible carrier transfer. *J Physiol* **118**:23–39, 1952.
136. Sibley CP, Boyd RDH. Control of transfer across the mature placenta. In *Oxford Reviews of Reproductive Biology* Volume 10 (ed. J.R. Clarke), pp. 382–423. Oxford: OUP, 1988.
137. Johnson LW, Smith CH. Monosaccharide transport across microvillous membrane of human placenta. *Am J Physiol* **238**:C160–C168, 1980.
138. Bissonnette JM, Black JA, Wickham WK, Acott KM. Glucose uptake into plasma membrane vesicles from the maternal surface of human placenta. *J Membr Biol* **58**:75–80, 1981.
139. Johnson LW, Smith CH. Glucose transport across the basal plasma membrane of human placental syncytiotrophoblast. *Biochim Biophys Acta* **815**:44–50, 1985.
140. Johnson LW, Smith CH. Identification of the glucose transport protein of the microvillous membrane of human placenta by photoaffinity labelling. *Biochem Biophys Res Comm* **109**:408–413, 1982.
141. Bissonnette JM, Ingermann RL, Thornburg KL. Placental sugar transport. In *Carrier Mediated Transport of Solutes from Blood to Tissue* (eds D.L. Yudilevich & D.L. Mann) pp. 65–75. London: Longman, 1985.
142. Baldwin SA, Mammalian passive glucose transporters: members of a ubiquitous family of active and passive transport proteins. *Biochim Biophys Acta* **1154**:17–49, 1993.
143. Takata K, Kasahara T, Kasahara M, Ezaki O, Hirano H. Localization of the erythrocyte/HepG2-type glucose transporter (GLUT1) in human placental villi. *Cell Tissue Res* **267**:407–412, 1992.
144. Hahn T, Hartmann M, Blaschitz A, *et al.* Localisation of the high affinity facilitative glucose transporter protein GLUT1 in the placenta of human, marmoset monkey (*Callithrix jacchus*) and rat at different developmental stages. *Cell Tissue Res* **280**:49–57, 1995.
145. Barros LE, Yudilevich DL, Jarvis SM, Beaumont N, Baldwin S. Quantitation and immunolocalization of glucose transporters in the human placenta. *Placenta* **16**:623–633, 1995.
146. Jansson T, Wennergren M, Illsley NP. Glucose transporter protein expression in human placenta throughout gestation and in intrauterine growth retardation. *J Clin Endocrinol Metab* **77**:1554–1562, 1993.
147. Kayano T, Fukumoto H, Eddy RL *et al.* Evidence for a family of human glucose transporter-like proteins. Sequence and gene localization of a protein exprssed in fetal skeletal muscle and other tissues. *J Biol Chem* **263**:15245–15248, 1988.
148. Haber RS, Weinstein SP, O'Boyle E, Morgello S. Tissue distribution of the human GLUT3 glucose transporter. *Endocrinology* **132**:2538–2543, 1993.
149. Shepherd PR, Gould GW, Colville CA, McCoid SC, Gibbs EM, Kahn BB. Distribution of GLUT3 glucose transporter protein in human tissues. *Biochem Biophys Res Commun* **188**:149–154, 1992.
150. Clarson LH, Glazier JD, Sides MK, Sibley CP. Expression of the facilitated glucose transporters (GLUT 1 and GLUT 3) in human placental trophoblast derived cells. *Placenta* **18**:333–340, 1997.
151. Tadokoro C, Yoshimoto Y, Yamasaki M, Sakata M, Kurachi H. Localisation of human placental glucose transporter 1 (GLUT1) and glucose transporter 3 (GLUT3) during early pregnancy. *Placenta* **16**:A.16, 1996.
152. Zhou J, Bondy CA. Placental glucose transporter gene expression and metabolism in the rat. *J Clin Invest* **91**:845–852, 1993.
153. Devaskar SU, Devaskar UP, Schroeder RE, deMello D, Fiedorek FT, Mueckler M. Expression of genes involved in placental glucose uptake and transport in the nonobese diabetic mouse pregnancy. *Am J Obstet Gynecol* **171**:1316–1323, 1994.
154. Boileau P, Mrejen C, Girard, Hauguel-de Mouzon S. Overexpression of GLUT3 placental glucose transporter in diabetic rats. *J Clin Invest* **96**:309–317, 1995.
155. Hauguel-de Mouzon S, Leturque A, Alsat E, Loizeau M. Evain-Brion D, Girard J. Developmental expression of *Glut1* glucose transporter and *c-fos* genes in human placental cells. *Placenta* **15**:35–46, 1994.
156. Armentrout T, Katz S, Thornburg KL, Faber JJ. Osmotic flow through the placental barrier of chronically prepared sheep. *Am J Physiol* **233**:H466–H474, 1977.

157. Ashmead GG, Kalhan SC, Lazebnik N, Nuamah IF. Maternal – fetal substrate relationships in the third trimester in human pregnancy. *Gynecol Obstet Invest* **35**:18–22, 1993.
158. Ingermann RL. Control of placental glucose transfer. *Placenta* **8**:557–571, 1987.
159. Young M, Prenton MA. Maternal and fetal plasma amino acid concentrations during gestation and in retarded fetal growth. *Br J Obstet Gynaecol* **76**:333–334, 1969.
160. Cetin I, Marconi AM, Corbetta C, Lanfranchi A, Baggiani AM, Battaglia FC, Pardi G. Fetal amino acids in normal pregnancies and in pregnancies complicated by intrauterine growth retardation. *Early Hum Dev* **29**:183–186, 1992.
161. Pearse W, Sornson H. Free amino acids of normal and abnormal human placenta. *Am J Obstet Gynecol* **105**:696–701, 1969.
162. Sooranna S, Burston D, Ramsey B, Steer P. Free amino acid concentrations in human first and third trimester placental villi. *Placenta* **15**:747–751, 1994.
163. Eaton BM, Yudilevich DL. Uptake and asymmetric efflux of amino acids at maternal and fetal sides of placenta. *Am J Physiol* **241**:C106–C112, 1981.
164. Carstenson M, Leichtweiss H-P. L-alanine carriers at maternal and fetal surfaces of the guinea pig placenta trophoblast. *Gynecol Obstet Invest* **22**:172–185, 1986.
165. Furesz TC, Moe AJ, Smith CH. Two cationic amino acid transport systems in human placental basal plasma membranes. *Am J Physiol* **261** (*Cell Physiol* **30**):C246–C252, 1991.
166. Furesz TC, Moe AJ, Smith CH. Lysine uptake by human placental microvillous membrane: comparison of system y⁺ with basal membrane. *Am J Physiol* **268** (*Cell Physiol* **37**):C755–C761, 1995.
167. Smith CH, Depper R. Placental amino acid uptake. II. Tissue preincubation, fluid distribution and mechanisms of regulation. *Pediatr Res* **8**:697–703, 1974.
168. Steel RB, Smith CH, Kelley LK. Placental amino acid uptake. VI. Regulation by intracellular substrate. *Am J Physiol* **243** (*Cell Physiol* **12**):C46–C51, 1982.
169. Karl PI, Alpy KL, Fisher SE. Amino acid transport by the cultured human placental trophoblast: effect of insulin on AIB transport. *Am J Physiol* **262** (*Cell Physiol* **31**):C834–C839, 1992.
170. Karl P. Insulin-like growth factor 1 stimulates amino acid uptake by the cultured human placental trophoblast. *J Cell Physiol* **165**:83–88, 1995.
171. Bloxam DL, Bax BE, Bax CMR. Epidermal growth factor and insulin-like growth factor 1 differently influence the directional accumulation and transfer of 2-aminoisobutyric acid (AIB) by human placental trophoblast in two-sided culture. *Biochem Biophys Res Commun* **199**:922–929, 1994.
172. Carbo N, Lopez-Soriano F, Argiles J. Administration of tumour necrosis factor-α results in a decreased placental transfer of amino acids in the rat. *Endocrinology* **136**:3579–3584, 1995.
173. Kulanthaivel P, Cool DR, Ramamoorthy S, Mahesh VB, Leibach RH, Ganapathy V. Transport of taurine and its regulation by protein kinase C in JAr human placental choriocarcinoma cell line. *Biochem J* **277**:53–58, 1991.
174. Kulanthaivel P, Myamoto Y, Mahesh VB, Leibach RH, Ganapathy V. Inactivation of taurine transporter by calcium in purified human placental brush border membrane vesicles. *Placenta* **12**:327–340, 1991.
175. Mahendran D, Donnai P, Glazier JD, D'Souza SWD, Boyd RDH, Sibley C. Amino acid (System A) transporter activity in microvillous membrane vesicles from the placentas of appropriately grown and small for gestational age babies. *Pediatr Res* **34**:661–665, 1993.
176. Glazier JD, Sibley CP, Carter AM. Effect of fetal growth restriction on System A amino acid transporter activity in the maternal facing plasma membrane of rat syncytiotrophoblast. *Pediatr Res* **40**:325–329, 1996.
177. Macara L, Kingdom JCP, Kaufmann P *et al.* Structural analysis of placental terminal villi from growth restricted pregnancies with abnormal umbilical artery Doppler waveforms. *Placenta* **17**:37–48, 1996.
178. Malandro MS, Beveridge MJ, Kilberg MS, Novak DA. Effect of low-protein diet-induced intrauterine growth retardation on rat placental amino acid transport. *Am J Physiol* **271** (*Cell Physiol* **40**):C295–C303, 1996.
179. Fisher SE, Atkinson M, Holtzman I, David R, Van Thiel DH. Effect of ethanol upon placental uptake of amino acids. *Prog Biochem Pharmacol* **18**:216–223, 1981.
180. Fisher SE, Atkinson M, Jacobson S *et al.* Selective fetal malnutrition: the effect of *in vivo* ethanol exposure upon *in vitro* placental uptake of amino acids in the non-human primate. *Pediatr Res* **17**:704–707, 1983.
181. Barnwell SL, Sastry BVR. Depression of amino acid uptake in human placental villus by cocaine, morpine and nicotine. *Trophoblast Res* **1**:101–120, 1983.
182. Dicke JM, Verges DK, Polakoski KL. Cocaine inhibits alanine uptake by human microvillous membrane vesicles. *Am J Obstet Gynecol* **169**:515–521, 1993.
183. Kuruvilla AG, D'Souza SWD, Glazier JD, Mahendran D, Maresh MJ, Sibley CP. Altered activity of the System A amino acid transporter in microvillous membrane vesicles from placentas of macrosomic babies born to diabetic women. *J Clin Invest* **94**:689–695, 1994.
184. Thornburg KL, Faber JJ. Transfer of hydrophilic molecules by placenta and yolk sac of the guinea pig. *Am J Physiol* **233**:C111–C124, 1977.
185. Wilde AE. Endocytic mechanisms in protein transfer across the placenta. *Placenta* Supplement 1, 165–186, 1981.
186. Pearse BM. Coated vesicles from human placenta carry ferritin, transferrin and immunoglobulin G. *Proc Nat Acad Sci USA* **79**:451–455, 1982.
187. Ockleford CD, Clint JM. The uptake of IgG by human placental chorionic villi: a correlated autoradiographic and wide aperture counting study. *Placenta* **1**:91–111, 1980.
188. King BF. Absorption of peroxidase-conjugated immunoglobulin G by human placenta: an *in vitro* study. *Placenta* **3**:395–406, 1982.
189. Leach L, Eaton BM, Firth JA, Contractor SF. Immunogold localisation of endogenous immunoglobulin-G in ultrathin frozen sections of the human placenta. *Cell Tissue Res* **257**:603–607, 1989.
190. Leach L, Eaton BM, Firth JA, Contractor SF. Immunocytochemical and labelled tracer approaches to uptake and intracellular routing of immunoglobulin G (IgG) in the human placenta. *Histochem J* **23**:444–449, 1991.
191. Lin CT. Immunoelectron microscopic localization of immunoglobulin G in human placenta. *J Histochem Cytochem* **28**:339–346, 1980.
192. Bonati M, Bortolus R, Marchetti F, Romero M, Tognoni G. Drug use in pregnancy: an overview of epidemiological (drug utilization) studies. *Eur J Clin Pharmacol* **38**:325–328, 1990.
193. Crawford JS. The placenta, drugs and the fetus. In *Principles and Practice of Obstetric Anaethesia* 5th edn. (ed. J.S. Crawford), p. 132. Oxford: Blackwell, 1984.
194. Chao ST, Juchau MR. Placental drug metabolism. In *Teratogenesis and Reproductive Toxicology* (eds E.M. Johnson & D.M. Kochhar), pp. 31–48. Berlin: Springer-Verlag, 1983.
195. Jacobson JL, Jacobson SW. Intellectual impairment in children exposed to polychlorinated biphenyls *in utero*. *N Eng J Med* **335**:783–789, 1996.
196. Waddell WJ, Marlowe C. Transfer of drugs across the placenta. *Pharmac Ther* **14**:375–390, 1981.
197. Levy, G. Pharmokinetics of fetal and neonatal exposure to drugs. *Obstet Gynecol* **58**:9S–16S, 1981.
198. Schneider H, Proegler M. Placental transfer of β-adrenergic antagonists studied in an *in vitro* perfusion system of human placental tissue. *Am J Obstet Gynecol* **159**:42–47, 1988.
199. Kudo Y, Urabe T, Fujiwara A, Yamada K, Kawasaki T. Carrier-mediated transport system for cephalexin in human placental brush-border membrane vesicles. *Biochim Biophys Acta* **978**:313–318, 1989.
200. Henderson GI, Hu ZQ, Yang Y, *et al.* Ganciclovir transfer by human placenta and its effects on rat fetal cells. *Am J Med Sci* **306**:151–156, 1993.
201. Fant ME, Harbison RD, Harrison RW. Glucocorticoid uptake into human placental membrane vesicles. *J Biol Chem* **254**:6218–6221, 1979.
202. Fant ME, Yeakley J, Harrison RW. Evidence for carrier-mediated transport of glucocorticoids by human placental membrane vesicles. *Biochim Biophys Acta* **731**:415–420, 1983.
203. Chien PFW, Smith K, Watt PW, Scrimgeour CM, Taylor DJ, Rennie MJ. Protein turnover in the human fetus studied at term using stable isotope tracer amino acids. *Am J Physiol* **265**:E31–E35, 1993.
204. Ramammorthy S, Leibach FH, Mahesh VB, *et al.* Functional characterization and chromosomal localization of a cloned taurine transporter from human placenta. *Biochem J* **300**:893–900, 1994.

205. Johnson LE, Smith CH. Neutral amino acid transport systems of microvillous membrane of human placenta. *Am J Physiol* **254**:C773–C780, 1988.
206. Hoeltzli SD, Smith CH. Alanine transport systems in isolated basal plasma membrane of human placenta. *Am J Physiol* **256**:C630–C637, 1989.
207. Hoeltzli SD, Kelly LK, Moe AJ, Smith CH. Anionic amino acid transport systems in isolated basal plasma membrane of human placenta. *Am J Physiol* **259** (*Cell Physiol* **28**):C47–C55, 1990.
208. Karl PI, Tkaczevski H, Fisher SE. Characteristics of histidine uptake by human placental microvillous membrane vesicles. *Pediatr Res* **25**:19–26, 1989.
209. Karl PI, Fisher SE. Taurine transport by microvillous membrane vesicles, cultured trophoblasts and isolated perfused human placenta. *Am J Physiol* **258** (*Cell Physiol* **27**):C302–C308, 1990.
210. Moe AJ, Smith CH. Anionic amino acid uptake by microvillous membrane vesicles from human placenta. *Am J Physiol* **257** (*Cell Physiol* **26**):C1005–C1011, 1989.
211. Eleno N, Deves R, Boyd CAR. Kinetics and membrane potential dependence of cationic amino acid transport systems y^+ and y^+ L in human brush border membrane vesicles. *J Physiol* **479**:291–300, 1994.
212. Kekuda R, Prasad PD, Fei YJ *et al.* Cloning of the sodium-dependent, broad-scope, neutral amino acid transporter B^0 from a human placental choriocarcinoma cell line. *J Biol Chem* **271**:18657–18661, 1996.
213. Shennan DB, Boyd CAR. Human placental sulphate transport is strongly inhibited by salicylate. *Br J Obstet Gynecol* **93**:522–523, 1986.
214. Shennan DB, Russell TVN. Salicylate inhibits human placental sulphate transport *in vitro*. *Biochem Pharmacol* **41**:723–728, 1991.
215. Illsley NP, Jacobs MM. Control of the sodium–proton antiporter in human placental microvillous membranes by transport substrates. *Biochim Biophys Acta* **1029**:227–234, 1990.
216. Faller D, Ryan MP. Factors affecting chloride conductance in apical membrane vesicles of human placenta. *J Membr Biol* **130**:227–239, 1992.
217. Ganapathy V, Balkovetz DF, Miyamoto Y *et al.* Inhibition of human placental Na^+–H^+ exchanger by cimetidine. *J Pharmacol Exp Ther* **239**:192–197, 1986.
218. van der Aa EM, Peereboom-Stegeman JHJC, Russel FGM. Isolation of syncytial microvillous membrane vesicles from human term placenta and their application in drug–nutrient interaction studies. *J Pharmacol Toxicol Methods* **34**:47–56, 1995.
219. Asai M, Narita O, Kashiwamata S. Effects of acetaldehyde and/or ethanol on neutral amino acid transport systems in microvillous brush border membrane vesicles prepared from human placenta. *Experientia* **41**:1566–1568, 1985.
220. Balkovetz DE, Miyamoto Y, Tiruppathi C, Mahesh VB, Leibach FH, Ganapathy V. Inhibition of brush-border membrane Na^+–H^+ exchanger by loperamide. *J Pharmacol Exp Ther* **243**:150–154, 1987.
221. Schenker S, Johnson RF, Hays SE, Ganeshappa R, Henderson GI. Effects of nicotine and nicotine/ethanol on human placental amino acid transfer. *Alcohol* **6**:289–296, 1989.
222. Grassl SM. Choline transport in human placental brush-border membrane vesicles. *Biochim Biophys Acta* **1194**:203–213, 1994.
223. Ganapathy V, Ganapathy ME, Nair CN, Mahesh VB, Leibach FH. Evidence for an organic cation–proton antiport system in brush-border membranes isolated from the human term placenta. *J Biol Chem* **263**:4561–4568, 1988.
224. van der Aa EM, Meuwsen IJB, Boersen ACM, Wouterse AC, Peereboom-Stegeman JHJC, Russel FGM. *p*-Aminohippurate uptake by syncytial microvillous membrane vesicles of human term placenta. *Placenta* **15**:279–289, 1994.
225. Ganapathy ME, Leibach FH, Mahesh VB, Devoe LD, Ganapathy V. Interaction of clonidine with human placental Na^+–H^+ exchanger. *Biochem Pharmacol* **35**:3989–3994, 1986.
226. Cool DR, Leibach FH, Ganapathy V. High-affinity paroxetine binding to the human placental serotonin transporter. *Am J Physiol* **259**.C196–C204, 1990.
227. Cool DR, Leibach FH, Ganapathy V. Interaction of fluoxetine with the human placental serotonin transporter. *Biochem Pharmacol* **40**:2161–2167, 1990.
228. Dicke JM, Verges DK, Polakoski KL. The effects of cocaine on neutral amino acid uptake by human placental basal membrane vesicles. *Am J Obstet Gynecol* **171**:485–491, 1994.

Fetal growth and its regulation

12

V.K.M. Han

Introduction

Intrauterine growth restriction or retardation (IUGR) and prematurity are the two predominant causes of fetal and neonatal mortality and morbidity in perinatal–neonatal medicine today. The use of antenatal steroids, high-resolution ultrasound, and modern perinatal care, together with neonatal surfactant replacement therapy, alternative modes of ventilation in addition to conventional ventilation, and advanced neonatal nursing and supportive care, have made significant improvements in neonatal mortality and morbidity in premature newborns in the past two decades. With modern perinatal–neonatal care, some of the acute neonatal morbidities associated with IUGR pregnancies[1], such as birth asphyxia and biochemical disturbances, can be recognized, and to an extent prevented. The perinatal and neonatal outcomes have improved to a degree in term pregnancies that some have questioned the validity of the diagnosis of 'term IUGR'[2]. However, in spite of rapid development in technologies in the assessment and monitoring fetal health and growth, IUGR is still associated with a significantly higher perinatal mortality, particularly in preterm infants. The majority of the mortality occurs *in utero*, highlighting our deficiencies in the diagnosis of fetal health in IUGR fetuses, and in the knowledge of fetal growth and its adaptation to adverse maternal uteroplacental environment. In addition, recent epidemiologic data suggest that low-birthweight infants are more likely to develop diseases such as hypertension, coronary heart disease, stroke and diabetes in adulthood, indicating that the impact IUGR on the fetus may be long lasting[3,4]. This chapter will describe the basic cellular processes that are involved in the normal embryonic and fetal growth, and the biochemical and molecular mechanisms that regulate them.

Normal embryonic and fetal growth

Fetal growth is not a uniform progression of cell replication, but a series of fundamentally different anabolic processes, which are precisely integrated. Development prior to placental implantation involves rapid cell hyperplasia, cavitation, differentiation and pattern formation, which becomes apparent when primitive germ layers separate. Metabolism at this time is anaerobic, and cells communicate by cell–cell contacts and by the release of autocrine and paracrine factors, including growth factors. Implantation of the placenta allows aerobic respiration and the development of energy-expensive enzyme systems necessary for differentiative cell function. The appearance of a fetoplacental circulation improves the delivery of nutrients to the tissues, and consequently the rate of cell multiplication rises. In addition, the placenta acts as an endocrine organ influencing both fetal and maternal physiology, and also as an immunological barrier between the fetus and the mother to allow the 'foreign' fetus to develop within the maternal immunologic environment. During early embryonic development, the pattern of growth is largely dictated by the fetal genome, but as the body size increases, the fetus becomes constrained by maternal and environmental influences such as uterine blood flow, maternal size and maternal disease.

PREIMPLANTATION DEVELOPMENT

As the fertilized embryo (zygote) traverses the maternal tubal and uterine cavity, from the point of fertilization to its implantation site, the initial stages of embryonic development are being completed. These involve cellular multiplication to become a multicellular embryo and then cavitation to become a blastocoele. As the blastocoele is formed, the embryonic cells differentiate into an inner cell mass (future embryo) and the trophectoderm (future placenta). This first cellular differentiation process is extremely important in preparing the embryo for successful implantation. The zygote inherits transcripts from the oocyte cytoplasm (oogenic mRNA) and cytoplasmic DNA (mitochondrial), and the role of these maternal transcripts differs between species. In many, they are thought to be important in maintaining the continuity of basic cellular metabolic processes and cellular mitoses that occur in the initial development. As embryonic development proceeds, there is a switch from control by the maternal genome to the zygotic genome. In some organisms, this change is abrupt, whereas in others, it is gradual. In the mammalian embryo, such as the mouse, the amount of oogenic mRNA decreases dramatically during the two-cell stage, and is replaced by mRNAs of zygotic origin. In humans, the transition occurs later at the four-cell stage. Mitochondrial DNA is greatly amplified during oogenesis in preparation for the early stages of zygotic development as well. In the *Xenopus* oocyte, the nuclear to mitochondrial DNA ratio which is normally about 1 : 100 is reversed to 1 : 1 to 1 : 100 during oogenesis.

The molecular mechanisms that regulate these processes as well as those in the latter part of the preimplantation development include the activation of genes encoding cytoskeletal proteins, certain enzymes (e.g. arylsulfatase) and several transcriptional factors, which in turn regulate the expression of downstream genes including growth factors, intercellular recognition molecules, extracellular matrices, ion channels, etc. A coordinated expression of these genes at appropriate cellular sites is crucial for the successful implantation. In many species, proper development of the preimplantation embryo is influenced by the maternal tubal and uterine environment contributed by the molecules and peptides produced by the tubal and uterine endometrial glands.

Using reverse transcription polymerase chain reaction (RT-PCR), the presence of transcripts encoding growth factors, growth factor receptors, intercellular recognition molecules and extracellular matrix molecules has been demonstrated[5,6] indicating the role of these factors in the cellular processes occurring during preimplantation development as well as in preparing the embryo for the implantation process. Evidence from *in vitro* fertilization in humans suggests that the fertilized embryo prior to implantation requires specific nutrient and culture conditions in order to achieve successful implantation. How these manipulations can lead to short- and long-term behaviour of the zygotic genome is still unknown.

POSTIMPLANTATION DEVELOPMENT

Following implantation, the placenta and the embryo undergo concomitant development that occur somewhat independently of each other, but also closely related. Normally developed and functioning placenta is not only important for successful implantation but also to ensure that the pregnancy is continued to term and that the fetus achieves its growth potential. In addition, poorly implanted placenta owing to abnormal trophoblast function is now believed to be the underlying mechanism for diseases of pregnancy such as pre-eclampsia.

DEVELOPMENT OF THE PLACENTA

The development of the haemochorial placenta in the human is a complex process involving several embryonic cell types interacting with the maternal cells[7]. Following implantation, the trophoblast layer of the developing blastocyst penetrates the epithelium of the maternal endometrium, and makes contact with the underlying stroma and induces it to decidualize. The early trophoblast layer, the trophectoderm, is largely multinuclear. These cells are highly invasive, colonizing glands, degrading local extracellular matrix and endocytosing glandular secretory elements. As the maternal capillary spaces are invaded, membrane bound intracellular spaces (lacunae) appear within the trophectodermal cytoplasm, which is the earliest haemochorial contact. Beneath the trophectoderm is an inner stem cell layer of primitive mononuclear cytotrophoblasts which undergoes active proliferation and fusion with the overlying syncytium. During the third week after ovulation, villous core mesenchyme develops beneath the cytotrophoblasts and within it develop fetal blood vessels. At this stage, the essential components of the hemochorial interface are in place. The major route of nutrient supply to the growing embryo becomes the villous interface, with the solute transfer taking place across the syncytium from the mother to the embryo.

During the third post-ovulatory week, proliferating cytotrophoblasts at the tip of the villi penetrate the syncytium to make contact with the underlying maternal tissue. The extravillous trophoblast now ceases proliferation, but the invasion of the maternal stroma continues. Extravillous trophoblast migrates along the inner walls of the maternal spiral arteries that feed the intervillous space. The purpose of this invasion is to remodel the arterial walls with the loss of smooth muscle and associated elastic and collagenous extracellular matrix, so that the resistance to the flow of arterial blood into the intervillous spaces is reduced. The arteries are then allowed to expand, and the supply of nutrients to the growing fetus is both enhanced and made independent of the influence of maternal vasoconstrictors; thus the placental circulation becomes a privileged site. Placental perfusion is then independent of maternal autonomic control. This development is critical to ensure that the blood supply to the placenta is only under the influence of maternal perfusion pressure in the uterine artery. The outer layer of the non-villous areas of the placenta is also composed of non-invasive cytotrophoblasts abutting the maternal stroma, with some proliferation continuing up to term.

The development of a haemochorial placenta thus involves the formation (proliferation and differentiation) of motile and non-motile mononuclear trophoblast, alternating between faster and slower rates of proliferation, and further differentiation into various trophoblast populations. The signals responsible for the complex sequence of developmental events are not known. It is likely that all intercellular communicating molecules involved in embryogenesis, namely the growth factors, the cell adhesion molecules, the integrins and the extracellular matrix molecules have specific roles in the development of the placenta[8]. Recently, gene targeting has been utilized to delineate the role of growth factors, growth factor receptors, extracellular matrix proteins and integrins in placental development (see below).

DEVELOPMENT OF THE EMBRYO

Embryogenesis involves three major processes: morphogenesis (the mechanics of generating shape), pattern formation (how the fate of each cell is specified into different tissues and organs of the body) and differentiation (the specialization of cells into different phenotypes). Although most mammals have a similar number of cell types, the process that differentiates between species in terms of their functional characteristics is the pattern formation that spatially organizes the cells. Therefore the genetic make-up of the cell (lineage) together with the epigenetic mechanisms involving cell–cell, cell–matrix and cell–soluble factor interactions are important in the ultimate development of the tissues and organs.

Morphogenesis and pattern formation

Morphogenesis and pattern formation are regulated by bone morphogenetic proteins (BMPs)[9] and homeobox genes[10]. BMPs are members of the transforming growth factor-β (TGF-β) superfamily and were named as such because of their ability to induce formation of bone. In addition to their role in a wide variety of biological processes, BMPs have been shown to be important in several aspects of development, the most crucial of which is the role of active BMP signals to form the ventral side of the body in early pattern formation. The BMP signal (BMP-4 in particular) establishes ventral fates in both the ectoderm and mesoderm. In addition, the dorsal-inducing properties of the Spemann organizer is in part mediated by inhibiting the BMP signalling. Thus dorsal–ventral pattern formation has been suggested to be simply due to the presence or absence of BMP signalling, i.e. the presence of active BMP signal induces ventral fates and the absence generates dorsal fate.

Homeobox genes contain a common sequence element of 180 bp, the homeobox, which was first discovered in *Drosophila*. The homeobox encodes a 60-amino acid homeodomain that is responsible for sequence specific DNA binding of much larger homeodomain proteins. These proteins act as transcriptional factors which activate or repress target genes. In vertebrates, over 170 different homeobox genes have been cloned, which can be divided into (a) the clustered homeobox genes called *Hox* genes or class I homeobox genes, and (b) the non-clustered or divergent homeobox genes, e.g. *Pax, Msx, Emx, Reig* named after their homologues in the fly. There are at least 39 mammalian *Hox* genes that are organized in four clusters called *HoxA, HoxB, HoxC* and *HoxD*, each localized to a different chromosome (7, 17, 12 and 2, respectively) and comprising 9–11 genes. The individual *Hox* genes within the different cluster can be aligned with each other and with genes of the *Drosophila*. These genes are expressed as early as in the gastrula, and are localized to all three germ layers with the overlapping domains that extend from the caudal end of the embryo to a sharp anterior limit which is specific for each *Hox* gene. Based on transgenic and gene targeting studies in mice involving the *Hox* genes, the function of these genes have been identified. As a result of these gain- and loss-of-function mutations, it is now clear that, as in *Drosophila*, the mammalian *Hox* genes of the posterior are more dominant with respect to function over the more anterior acting ones. In general, *Hox* genes are important in the patterning of the axial skeleton, the appendicular skeleton, the reproductive and digestive tracts, the hindbrain, and a component of the development of the craniofacial region. More recent studies suggest that the vertebral or axial specification is more likely achieved by the functional co-operation of a 'combination' of *Hox* genes expressed at a given axial level than by the function of a single gene. The second type of homeobox genes, the non-cluster type, is involved in the craniofacial and forebrain development (*Otx, Pax* and *Emx*), hindbrain development (*En-1* and *En-2*), eye development (*Pax6*), and the development of many other organs such as kidney, heart, etc. Mutation of human homologues of both clustered (*Hox*) and non-clustered homeobox genes has been associated with different congenital syndromes, such as synpolydactly and hand–foot–genital syndrome (*HOXD13* and *HOXA13*), schizencephaly (*EMX2*), Reiger syndrome (*REIG*), and Boston-type craniosynostosis (*MSX2*), and may predispose the individual to cancer, such as acute myeloid leukaemia (*HOXA9*), pre-B-cell leukaemia (*PBX1*), T-cell leukaemia (*HOX11*) and rhabdomyosarcoma (*PAX3* and *PAX7*).

Cellular growth and differentiation

Once the general body plan has been specified, the development of embryonic tissues and organs is regulated by local interactions between the cells and their extracellular matrix, which determine further morphogenesis and differentiation. Cellular proliferation and differentiation are just two aspects of a complex process by which the conceptus (organs and tissues inclusive) increases in size and function (Fig. 12.1). In addition, considerable cell migration occurs in early embryogenesis to bring different cell types into intimate contact, which may at a certain phase of development lead to tissue induction (e.g. induction of mesoderm from ectoderm by endoderm). Following blastulation, epithelial–mesenchymal interactions become particularly important in shaping tissue morphology. With further proliferation, differentiation,

Development of the cardiovascular system

13

K.L. Thornburg

Cardiac development

Immediately following gastrulation, two specific areas of splanchnic mesoderm in the mammalian embryo become cardiac precursor cells[1]. As development proceeds, these areas fold beneath the embryo within the 'wings' of lateral tissue that enclose the space that will become primitive foregut (Fig. 13.1). During the folding process, these areas form bilateral heart tubes. Each has the potential to become a complete heart but instead, the two heart tubes come together on the ventral side of the embryo and fuse to make a complete single tube, marking the *fusion stage* (Fig. 13.1). This takes place on about day 21–22 postovulation in the human and represents the stage when cardiomyocytes become capable of beating.

As the tube matures, it becomes composed of three layers (inside to outside): endocardium, cardiac jelly and myocardium. The inner lumen containing blood is lined by endocardium which is surrounded by gelatinous cardiac jelly. The physiological role of cardiac jelly is unknown. The outside layer is muscle composed of primitive but already specialized working myocardium. At this stage, the tube already contains specific regions destined to become structures of the mature heart (Fig. 13.1D). These regions include, from top to bottom, truncus arteriosus, bulbus cordis, ventricle, atrium and sinus venosus. As soon as the vascular tree has formed a complete circuit, the heart begins to perform as a beating pump. Thus the heart, though primitive, is the first functioning organ of the body. The sequential segmental contraction of the heart tube at discrete points along the tube allows the wall thickenings to function as valves so that the heart operates as an efficient forward motion pump. The heart tube then grows in a fashion that causes the bulboventricular region to bulge rightward to form a right-handed loop as the heart forms an S-shaped structure (Fig. 13.1). The *looping stage* and is found in the 25–27-day embryo. At present, the physical and biological mechanisms that underlie the looping process are unknown.

The most complex part of heart formation is the *septation stage* in which all heart chambers and outflow tracts are formed. It is likely that many structural heart defects arise at this stage. The interatrial septum is formed by two migrating membranous tissue walls that form in succession between the right and left atria (Fig. 13.2). The first (septum primum) grows from the 'roof' of the atrium down to the 'floor' making a complete wall. This would prevent the necessary flow of blood from the right atrium to the left atrium, if it were not that a hole forms in the wall as it grows. A second wall (septum secundum) then grows from the roof along side the first septum but it does not grow completely to the floor. The combination of these two membranes form the foramen ovale and provide its flap valve properties.

The interventricular septum is formed internally from a trabecular ridge that originates at the point where the primitive ventricle and bulbis cordis join. Septal tissue forms from a compaction of trabecular tissue. The latter arises from endocardium that invades the cardiac jelly and grows toward the outer myocardial layer in the looping stage. As the jelly disappears, a complex network of spongy pockets (lacunae) and trabeculae is formed. The coalescence of the inner spongy layer gives rise to the interventricular ridge that eventually forms the muscular septum and the papillary muscles. During the septation stage, the interventricular septum slowly migrates in an upward direction toward the atria, leaving an open channel between the ventricles. As the heart matures and twists in shape, this interventricular channel is closed by a downward-growing membranous septum that arises from bulbar ridges and cushion tissue. A persistent 'hole' between the ventricles is the most common type of congenital heart defect when the membranous portion fails to grow.

The truncus arteriosus is the outflow vessel of the embryonic heart tube. It divides longitudinally to become the aorta that serves the body and the pulmonary artery that serves the lungs. The septation of the truncus into its component arteries is complicated because the two great vessels must twist

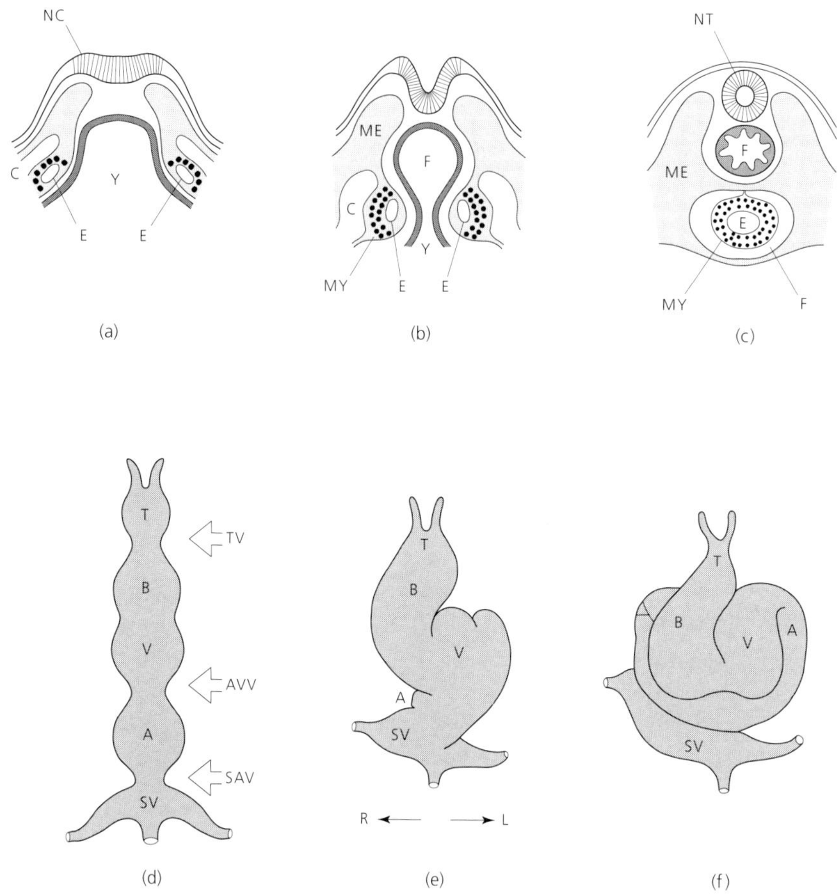

Fig. 13.1 Diagrams of transverse sections of embryos showing the development of the heart (a). Fusion of the paired endocardial and myoepicardial tubes (b) results in a single straight cardiac tube (c). C, Coelomic cavity; E, endocardial tubes; F, foregut; ME, mesoderm; MY, myocardium; P, pericardial cavity; NC, neural crest; NT neural tube; Y, yolk sac. Development of the heart. (d) Simple tubular heart. (e) Early looping – to the left side. (f) Established looping with definition of unseptated cardiac chambers. The *open arrows* indicate the valve sites. A, Atrium; AVV, atrioventricular valve; B, bulbus cordis; SAV, sinoatrial valve; SV, sinus venosus; T, truncus arteriosus; TV, truncal valve. After Reller *et al.*[1].

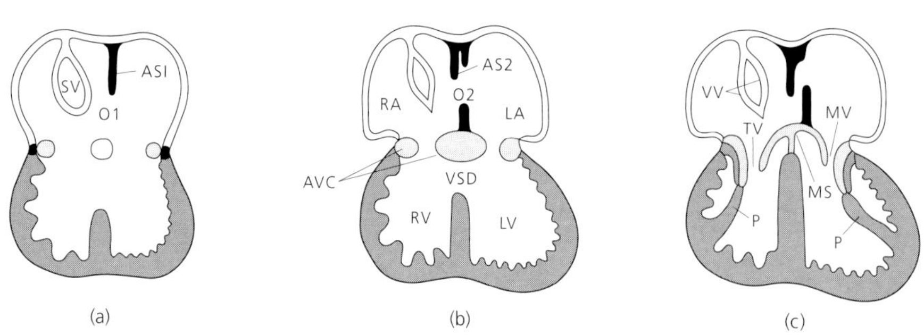

Fig. 13.2 Stages in cardiac chamber septation; the diagrams represent coronal sections of the heart. (a) Early stage – commencing atrial and ventricular septation. (b) Atrial ostium primum closed and ostium secundum forming; ventricular septation incomplete. (c) Septation complete and membranous septum formed. The atrioventricular valves have been formed by cushion tissue and delamination of myocardium. ASI, Atrial septum primum; AS2, atrial septum secundum; AVC, atrioventricular cushion; LA, left atrium; LV, left ventricle; MS, membranous septum; MV, mitral valve; O1, atrial ostium primum; O2, atrial ostium secundum; P, papillary muscles; RA, right atrium; RV, right ventricle; SV, sinus venosus; TV, tricuspid valve; VSD, ventricular septal defect; VV, venous valves. After Reller *et al.*[1].

upon themselves to match their proper circuits. A spiral septum is derived from two longitudinal ridges that spiral down the inside of the truncus and fuse within the bulbotruncal region of the heart (Fig. 13.3). The ridges gradually fuse along the entire outflow tract and form the two intertwining vessels. Truncal septation cannot occur unless the spiral septum is 'seeded' by neural crest cells that migrate from the neural tube, travel along the branchial clefts down to the truncus arteriosus and invade the regions of the spiral septum and the heart proper. When migration is impeded, a non-septated truncus arteriosus results (called 'persistent truncus arteriosus'), a defect often seen as part of the spectrum of cardiovascular congenital anomalies.

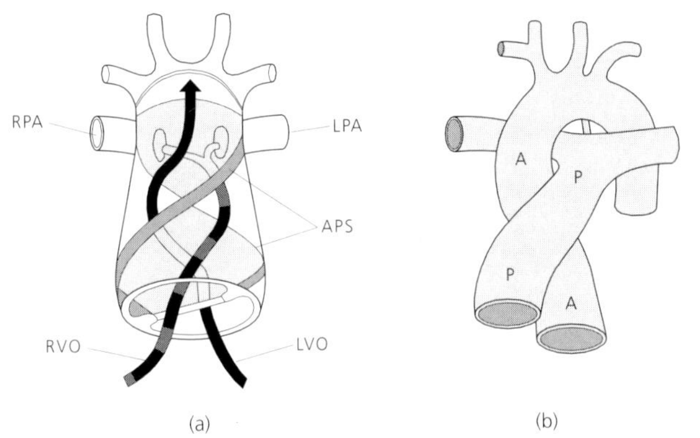

Fig. 13.3 Septation of the truncus arteriosus. (a) Diagram showing the spiral aorticopulmonary septum, which separates the systemic arterial flow (*solid dark line*) from the pulmonary arterial flow (*broken line*). (b), The mature pulmonary artery and aorta, after septation and separation, showing the persisting spiral relationship. A, Aorta; APS, aorticopulmonary septum; LPA, left pulmonary artery; LVO, left ventricular outflow pathway; P, pulmonary trunk; RPA, right pulmonary artery; RVO, right ventricular outflow pathway. After Reller *et al.*[1].

MATURE MYOCYTE

The histological arrangement within the mature cardiac myocyte is common to all mammals. Although some species have heart cells with unique features, even experts have difficulty in distinguishing the working myocyte of one species from the myocyte of another. The cell membrane of the cardiomyocyte, known as the sarcolemma, contains the proteins that propagate the action potential and other crucial homeostatic transport proteins[2]. As the myocyte matures, the sarcolemma invaginates at regular intervals and forms tubules that reach the interior of the cell. These are known as transverse tubules or T-tubules that carry the action potential to the cell interior. The most striking feature of the mature cell is its striated muscle pattern derived from the registry of contractile proteins that compose the muscle strands known as myofibrils. Myofibrils are composed of a series of sarcomeres, the individual contractile units of striated muscle (Fig. 13.4). The most easily visible protein strand is myosin, that composes the heavy strands (thick filaments) that run from the darkly stained Z-line toward the center of the sarcomere. Thin actin filaments are found in the center of the sarcomere reaching between the thick filaments, with which they overlap.

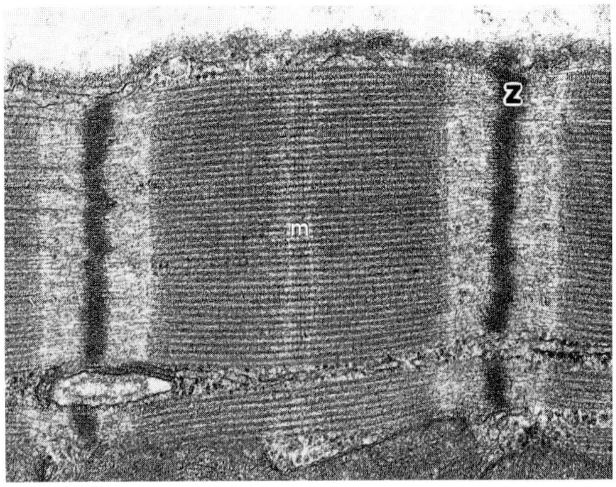

Fig. 13.4 Showing electron micrograph of a single sarcomere of a near term sheep heart. Note the Z-line (Z) and M-line (m). The heavy electron-dense line between Z-lines is the contractile protein, myosin. Courtesy K.L. Thornburg.

The mature cell is characterized by alternating layers of myofibrils and mitochondria. There hardly seems to be room for necessary organelles. Every mature cell has one or more nuclei and contains a complex inner network of membrane known as the sarcoplasmic reticulum (SR). SR forms special couplings near the sarcolemma (SL). It is generally accepted that small fluxes of Ca^{2+} traverse the SL in response to an action potential via voltage gated Ca^{2+} channels (dihydropyridine receptor). In response to the stimulation of the Ca^{2+} stores are released from the SR into the cytosol via ryanodine-sensitive release channels. Contraction proceeds as myosin and actin interact in the presence of activator Ca^{2+}.

Embryonic hearts have many attributes similar to mature hearts. They are capable of circulating blood even before the working cells have a distinct myocyte appearance. Embryonic hearts carry out the basic pump functions as expected from a mature heart in that they generate pressures (very low) with normal pressure waves (Fig. 13.5), they respond to preload and afterload and they control output via changes in venous flow, stroke volume and heart rate[3,4]. However, after looking at the ultrastructural features of the early cardiomyocyte, one is surprised at its functional capability. The immature contractile units (sarcomeres) are scarce, disorganized and are sometimes seen at odd angles with respect to the SL (Fig. 13.6). The amazing feature of all developing vertebrate hearts is the gradual increasing complexity of the heart cell, the cardiomyocyte, while it continues to carry out its work in providing kinetic energy to circulating blood.

Each species has its own rate of development and most fall into one of two categories: altricial or precocial. Altricial

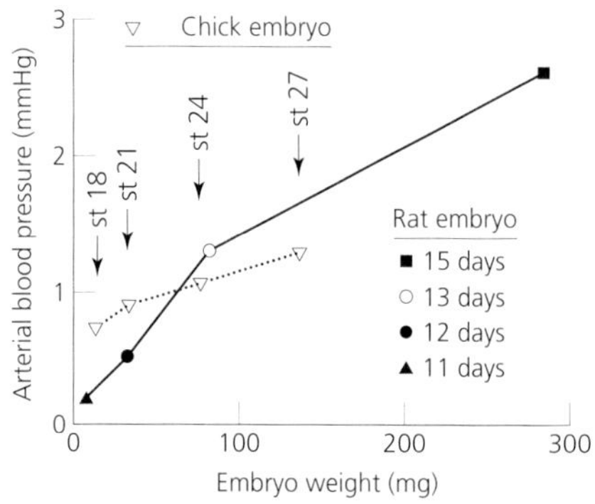

Fig. 13.5 Changes in blood pressure in chick and rat embryos with respect to wet weight of embryo. Stage (st) 18 is equivalent to 3 days; stage 21, 3.5 days; stage 24, 4.5 days; and stage 27, 5.5 days. After Nakazawa *et al.*[45].

animals are born in a very immature, dependent state at which time they often have their eyes closed and may have little fur. Rats and rabbits are examples. In contrast, precocial animals are born in a mature state. They are often on their feet within minutes of birth and some are even able to eat solid food within hours. Guinea pigs and most large mammals are examples. In general, altricial mammals are born with hearts that are histologically and functionally immature and most precocial animals have hearts that are rather mature by comparison. The immature fetal cell of either type of animal is characterized by its small size and histological arrangement where myofibrils are located only at the periphery of the cell; the central portion of the myocyte contains large fluid filled 'spaces' that contain mitochondria, Golgi apparatus, glycogen and polyribosomes. Figure 13.7 compares the ultrastructure of the immature cat heart with the adult cat heart.

MYOCYTE SIZE

Embryonic hearts grow by myocyte hyperplasia (cell division) in all species. In altricial species, this growth pattern continues over the life of the fetus. In rats, myocytes do not increase much in size after the early embryonic period throughout gestation. After birth rat myocytes undergo a terminal maturation process by which they become binucleate and cease to divide. Clubb and Bishop[5] have shown that the binucleation stage takes place during postnatal life so that about 50% of the

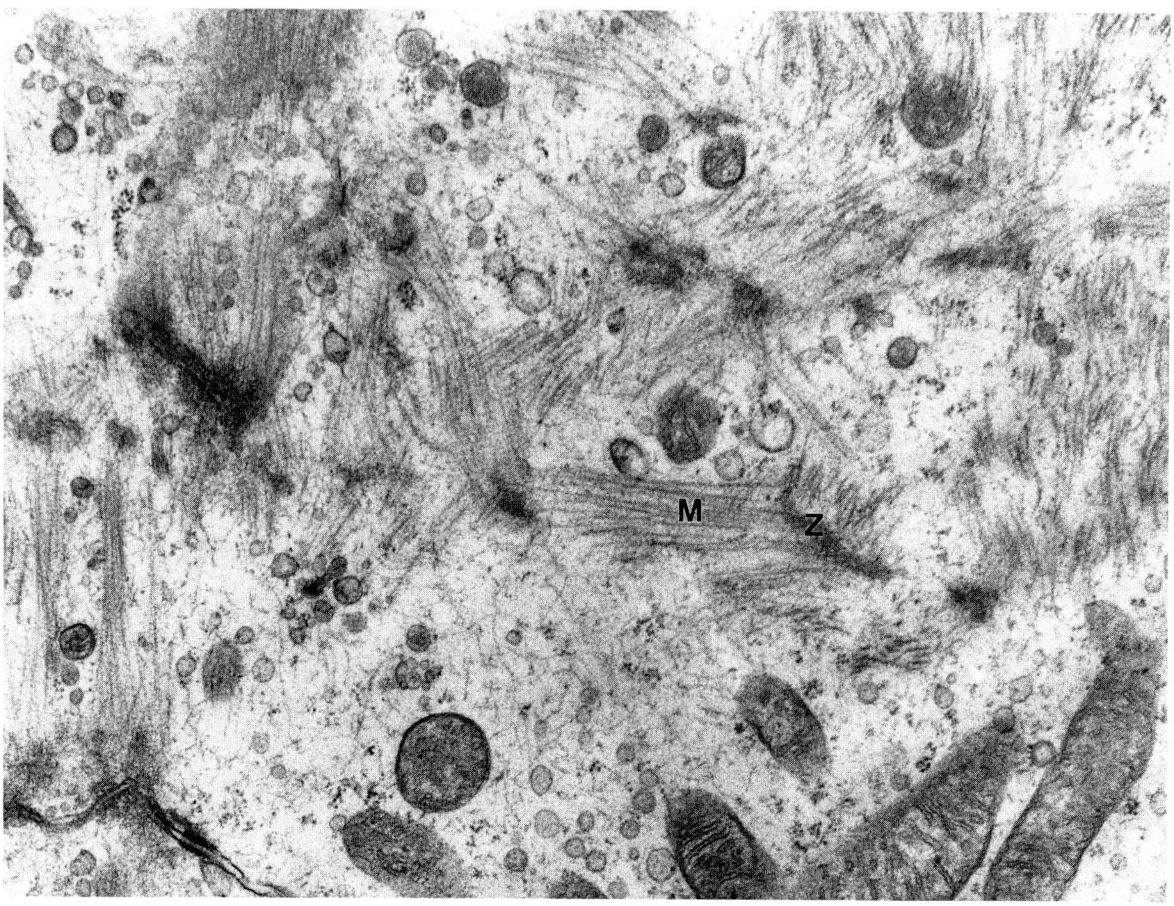

Fig. 13.6 Showing electron micrograph of an embryonic chick heart cell from postfusion stage. This cell is in early stages of sarcomerogenesis but is capable of contraction. Z, Z-line; M, contractile protein forming a myofibril. Courtesy K.L. Thornburg.

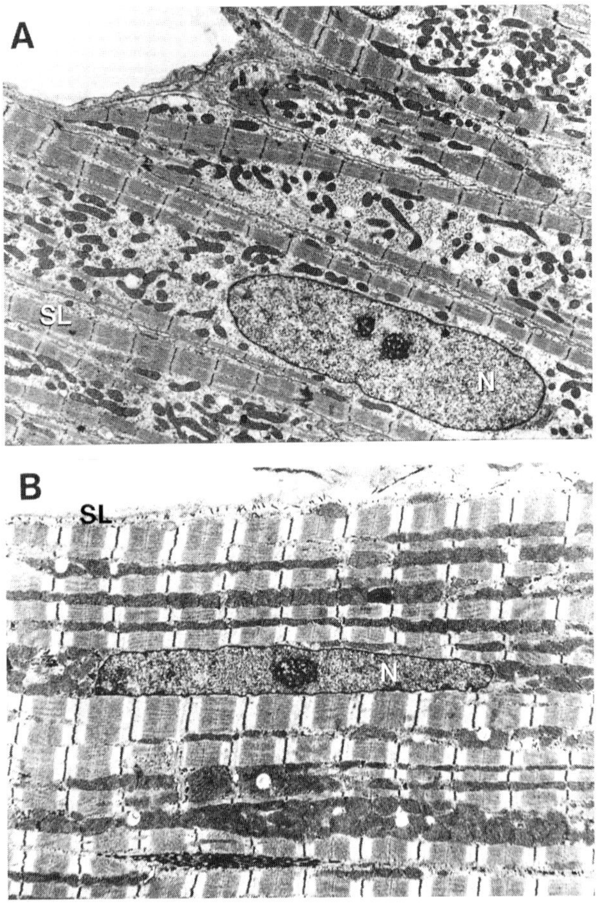

Fig. 13.7 Electron micrographs of heart muscle from immature cat. (A) In the neonatal cat five cells are seen separated by sarcolemma (SL). (B) In the adult heart, one cell is seen. Contractile material is found at the periphery in neonate cells but throughout the cytoplasm in the adult cell. The nucleus (N) in the neonate is centered within the cell and mitochondria are scattered throughout the central cytoplasm. In the adult, mitochondria are sandwiched between the layers of myofibrilla material. After Maylie[46].

cells are binucleate at 9 postnatal days. A similar process is found in all mammalian hearts[6]. The number of cells present in the heart at the stage of terminal maturation is the number that will be present in the heart for the life of the individual. The entire heart organ must grow considerably to keep up with the growth of the animal. For this growth, the chambers enlarge by increasing the dimensions and volume of the individual myocytes and by architectural rearrangement of the matrix scaffold.

FUNCTIONAL MATURATION OF THE MYOCYTE

As mentioned above, cardiomyocytes are able to contract as soon as functioning myofibrils are present while their morphology and biochemical development is primitive. One of the most important physiological features is the maturation of the Ca^{2+} transport and sequestration systems. The primitive myocyte has virtually no SR. The rate at which functional SR will be integrated into the cell is species dependent – the sheep has abundant SR at birth, the cat has almost none. Because SR is the storage site for most intracellular Ca^{2+}, the immature myocyte must acquire and extrude Ca^{2+} across the SL during systole and diastole, respectively, each and every beat. In the immature myocyte, it appears that Ca^{2+} enters the myocyte through voltage gated Ca^{2+} channels, in response to an action potential, in sufficient quantity to provide *activator* Ca^{2+} for each beat. The lack of internal Ca^{2+} storage places limitations on myocyte growth because the myocyte must not get so large that diffusion distances are rate limiting at fetal heart rates. Fetal cardiac myocytes are designed with small diameters in early fetal life and they grow only as SR is developed. The myocytes have important adaptations. Myofibrillar material is found only at the periphery of the cell in immature cells with direct access to Ca^{2+} fluxes crossing the SL each beat. As these cells mature, and SR and T tubules are manufactured by the cell, the myofibrillar material is placed more deeply within the cell. Table 13.1 shows the relative importance of SR and SL contributions to the rate of tension generation in developing myocardium of rabbits[7].

TABLE 13.1
Cardiac contraction in the rabbit*

Gestation (days)	Maximal developed tension (g/g cardiac muscle)	Percentage of cardiac muscle that is myofibril	Maximal developed tension (g/g cardiac muscle)
18	18	13%	1.4
21	22	15.3%	1.4
28	40	24.3%	1.6
New-born	68	39%	1.7
Adult	78	50%	1.6

*Adapted from Nakanishi *et al.*[7]

Adult circulation

Most physiology textbooks contain information only on adult organ function. However, the fetal cardiovascular system functions so differently from the adult that one cannot extrapolate directly from these textbooks. The differences are explained by differing anatomical, cytomorphological and biochemical characteristics. In the adult heart, the right and left ventricles beat in series with almost exactly the same stroke volume per beat, with small short-term differences being compensated by the Frank–Starling mechanism (discussed below). The adult right ventricle is designed to be a low pressure–volume pump that ejects blood through the inflated lungs with their vascular resistance some tenfold lower than that of the systemic circulation. The left ventricle, on the other hand, is designed to be a high-pressure pump for perfusing the systemic circulation. Further, because the adult circulation is in series, virtually all blood that returns to the heart is passed through the lung before returning to the systemic circuit.

The fetal circulation

Figure 13.8 shows the fetal circulatory arrangement that is quite different from that of the adult arrangement[8]. The fetal circulation is characterized by four shunts: (1) the umbilical circulation, (2) the ductus venosus, (3) the foramen ovale and (4) the ductus arteriosus. The *umbilical circulation* is a special vascular configuration that carries 40% of the fetal cardiac output to the placenta for gas exchange. The umbilical arteries arise at the caudal end of the dorsal aorta. Just beyond the branching of the external iliac arteries, the dorsal aorta becomes the common umbilical artery that serves mostly the umbilical arteries except for small branches to legs. In normal fetuses, the umbilical circulation is a low-resistance circuit. However, several pathological conditions are characterized by an increase in placental vascular resistance and the fetal heart must increase its workload substantially just to perfuse the placenta. The haemoglobin in blood returning to the fetus from the placental circulation is some 80% saturated with oxygen. Placental blood flows through the umbilical vein to the liver where a small portion oxygenates the liver but most flows through the second shunt, the *ductus venosus*, and joins desaturated blood from the lower body inferior vena cava (IVC). The ductus venosus is not found in the guinea pig[9]. The IVC courses through the diaphragm and bifurcates in the chest near the heart. Some 30–90% of the IVC flow (depending on species) is directed across the *foramen ovale* into the left atrium[9,10]. The foramen ovale is usually described in textbooks as a one-way flap valve between the atria that allows only right to left flow. In sheep, the foramen is a rather long windsock shaped membrane containing muscle fibres that originates as a branch of the IVC at the bifurcation, the crista terminalis. There is evidence that oxygenated blood from the placenta is preferentially directed to the left atrium via the foramen ovale[11] and that the flow through the foramen is highly dependent on the kinetic energy of the blood in the IVC[12]. The oxygenated blood entering the left heart via the foramen ovale is primarily delivered to heart and brain. Blood returning from the head and the lower body, flows through the right atrium and ventricle and is ejected into the main pulmonary artery. Most of the pulmonary arterial flow is directed across the *ductus arteriosus*, a shunt that connects the pulmonary artery with the descending aorta. Because the lungs are not inflated *in utero*, their vascular resistance is high and their oxygen flow needs low. In the fetus, desaturated blood flowing through the pulmonary artery joins blood from the aortic isthmus and travels down the descending aorta to the placenta for reoxygenation. The fetal shunts are crucial for survival of the fetus but after the placental circulation is abruptly disrupted at birth, they are no longer needed. All disappear shortly after birth. It is not uncommon in humans for the ductus arteriosus to remain open longer than desired and it is sometimes closed via a catheter-placed obstruction device or by surgical ligation.

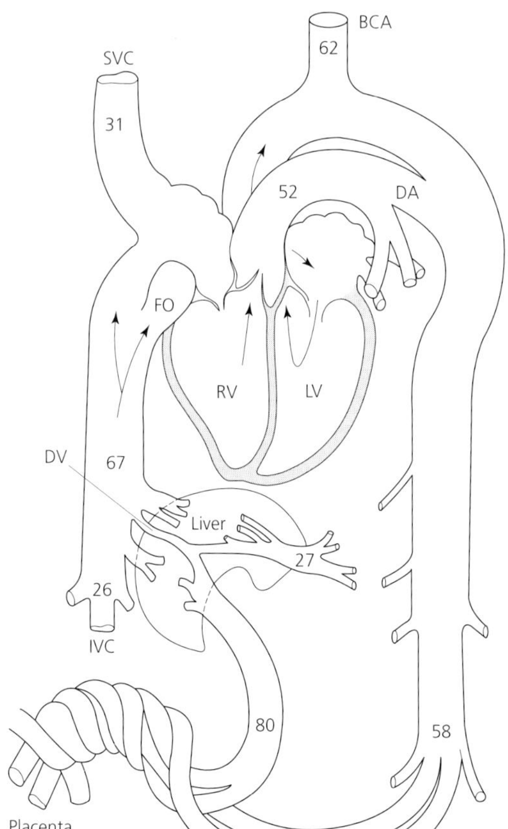

Fig. 13.8 Circulation of the mature fetal lamb. Numbers indicate mean oxygen saturation (%). RV, right ventricle; LV, left ventricle; SVC, superior vena cava; BCA, brachiocephalic artery; FO, foramen ovale; DA, ductus arteriosus; DV, ductus venosus, IVC, inferior vena cava. After Dawes[8].

Fetal haemodynamics

Flow through blood vessels is often described by the haemodynamic equivalent of Ohm's law,

$$\dot{Q} = \Delta P/R \qquad (13.1)$$

where $\dot{Q}$ is blood flow, ΔP the driving pressure ($P_{art} - P_{ven}$) and R the resistance to flow. This simple concept is mostly adequate for understanding the physics of the circulation in the fetus. However, it does not take into account the complex resistive forces that occur as a result of pulsatile flow and reflections of pulse waves from distant bifurcations. To take these factors into account, one can estimate the total impedance of the vascular tree using high fidelity measurements of pressure and flow at the pulmonary and aortic roots. The impedance is the total hindrance to the ejection of blood by the ventricle due to both vascular resistance and pulsatile flow[13]. There are recent studies examining impedance within the fetal circulation[14].

The regulation of blood flow in the fetus has been studied extensively. The advent of several techniques was prerequisite to the feasibility of performing these studies. Foremost was the chronic catheterization of sheep fetus[15]. Most of what we know about fetal cardiovascular physiology has been learned from this model. The microsphere technique has also been a very valuable tool because it allows the measurement of organ flows. In this technique, millions of plastic radiolabelled microspheres (~ 15 μm) are injected into the left ventricle where they mix and circulate according to blood flow distribution. The number of spheres that get trapped in an organ is proportional to the flow to that organ as determined by the numbers of spheres in a reference sample drawn at a known flow (e.g. Table 13.2). Electromagnetic flow sensors and later transonic and Doppler sensors have greatly expanded our capability to measure flows and flow velocities continuously within specific beds. Ultrasonic sonomicrometer piezoelectric crystals have been used extensively to obtain instantaneous dimensions of the heart[16,17], ductus arteriosus and other structures. Using sonomicrometry, pressure–dimension relation of the fetal heart can be determined under a variety of physiological conditions.

TABLE 13.2
Fetal organ blood flows in near term animals (ml/min/100 g)

Organ	Llama***	Guinea Pig*	Sheep**	(Percentage Biventricular output)
Brain	85		150	4%
Heart	165	165	265	3%
Lung			160	6%
Adrenals	330	385	395	0.1%
Kidney	95	110	245	3%
Placenta		125	140	40%
Carcass	8	20	15	35%

Modified from *Carter (1984)[9], **Teitel (1988)[43] and ***Llanos (1995)[44].

The haemodynamic features of the fetal circulation are also very different from those of the adult. The mean arterial pressure increases gradually over gestation and reaches ~50 mmHg in the mature fetus. Because of the unique fetal shunt system, the fetal ventricles eject against similar mean arterial pressures and are filled by similar filling pressures (3–5 mmHg) throughout fetal life. The arrangement of the arterial tree in the fetus may affect heart function. The right ventricle ejects into the pulmonary artery that feeds the low-resistance placental circulation. One might guess, therefore, that the impedance to ejection is less for the right ventricle than for the left ventricle which ejects into the circuit that perfuses the head and the smaller aortic isthmus (the segment between the brachiocephalic artery and ductus arteriosus).

FETAL CARDIAC OUTPUT

Because the two fetal ventricles pump in parallel rather than in series, the output of the heart is best expressed as the combined ventricular output. The biventricular output of the 'resting' sheep fetus is about 500 ml/min/kg and represents a flow that cares for the total oxygen needs of the fetal body. In contrast, an adult sheep has a cardiac output of about 150 ml/min/kg[18]. A near-term sheep fetus of 4 kg pumps about 2 l/min. The output of the human fetus at 38 weeks is also about 2 l/min as estimated from Doppler flow velocities and estimates of tricuspid and mitral valve cross-sectional areas[19]. In the sheep fetus, the right ventricle contributes about 60–70% of the cardiac output[10,20]. In the human fetus, the estimated contribution of the total cardiac output from the right ventricle is 55–60% near term[19].

It seems obvious that the heart cannot pump more than is returned to it through the veins. Indeed, the fetal heart and circulation are precisely coupled through mean atrial pressure so that venous return and cardiac output are equal. This coupling is complex because it involves regulating the fetal blood volume. The equilibrated pressure in the fetal circulation when the heart is at rest (mean systemic pressure) has been estimated[21] and is thought to be two times higher (~14 mmHg) than for adults. This may indicate that the fetal circulation is relatively 'over-filled' compared to the adult circulation. The difference between the mean systemic pressure and mean right atrial pressure is thought to estimate a driving pressure for venous flow back to the heart[22]. Therefore, the downstream pressure of venous return is also the filling pressure of the heart that operates on the Frank–Starling principle (below).

DISTRIBUTION OF CARDIAC OUTPUT

Blood flow is distributed to the organs of the fetal body according to the inherent vascular resistance of the organ in question and autoregulatory needs of the organ. It is not known how organs set their flow needs or how an organ acquires its unique autoregulatory capability. Table 13.2 shows weight specific flows for different organs under normoxemic conditions.

It is generally accepted that there is autoregulatory capability at the organ level in the fetus and that autoregulation is an important component of the blood-pressure regulation system[10]. Autoregulation, the tendency of an organ to keep its blood flow constant over a range of driving pressures, is thought to be the result of local metabolic control of vascular resistance at the arteriolar level to maintain oxygen delivery at an appropriate level. Nevertheless, there is considerable variation among organs in the direction and magnitude of blood-flow change with fluctuations in arterial oxygen content. The lungs vasodilate in the presence of increased oxygen content[23]. Other organs vasoconstrict. There are powerful organ-specific blood flow reallocations within the fetus during episodes of hypoxaemia. Blood flow to the heart, brain and adrenal glands are increased dramatically as flow to the fetal carcass is diminished (Fig. 13.9).

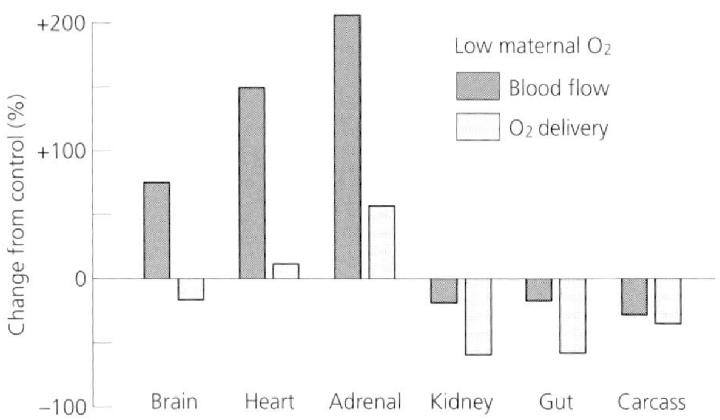

Fig. 13.9 Changes in blood flow and estimated oxygen deliveries to selected sheep fetal organs during an acute fetal hypoxaemic episode induced by allowing the ewe to breathe air containing a reduced fraction of oxygen (Cohn et al[47]). Oxygen deliveries were estimated from published relationships between organ flows and blood oxygen contents for various organs and the estimated contents from similar experiments in other laboratories (Longo et al[48,49] Peeters et al[50]; oxygen deliveries are only rough approximations. After Thornburg[51].

DETERMINANTS OF CARDIAC OUTPUT

Heart rate

Cardiac output is defined as the product of heart rate and stroke volume and each is regulated. The fetal heart normally beats at a rate set by the pacemaker in the sinoatrial node. The inherent beating rate of the heart increases during early embryonic life and then decreases over the life of the fetus being about 200/min by mid-gestation in sheep and 150/min at birth. Interestingly, fetuses of mammals of all sizes have about the same inherent heart rate. The decrease in rate with fetal age is largely due to increasing cholinergic parasympathetic tone as vagal innervation becomes established at the sinus node. Antagonism of the cholinergic muscarinic receptors by atropine returns the fetal heart to its inherent (~200/min) rate. Rapid pacing of the fetal heart decreases stroke volume as filling time decreases, but with output being different depending on which ventricle is being paced. There has been debate about whether heart rate or stroke volume holds the prominent place in the regulation of cardiac output *in vivo*. The issue is moot since both affect output and both depend on cooperation with the circulation via venous return.

Stroke volume

In the non-growing mammalian heart, there are three primary determinants of stroke volume: preload, afterload and contractility. In the immature heart, one must also consider chamber growth because over gestation it affects stroke volume more than is possible by the other three. Our knowledge about how each primary determinant affects the volume of blood ejected from the ventricle is derived from nearly a century of research on striated muscle and its application to the odd-shaped ventricles of the heart. Two primary properties of striated muscle apply to the function of the whole heart. The first is the length–active tension relationship (Fig. 13.10) and the second is the force–velocity relationship (Fig. 13.11).

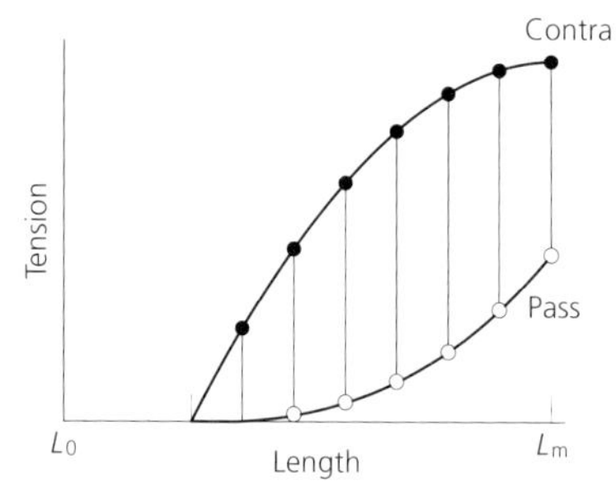

Fig. 13.10 The relationship of length to tension for passive (open circles) and contracting (closed circles) cardiac muscle strips is shown schematically. The vertical lines connect the diastolic length–tension point to the systolic length–tension point for an isometric contraction. L_0 is the unstressed muscle length and L_{max} is the muscle length that produces the maximum tension during isometric contraction. The rapid increase in active tension at muscle lengths above L_0 is the basis for the Frank–Starling mechanism. After Thornburg and Morton[52].

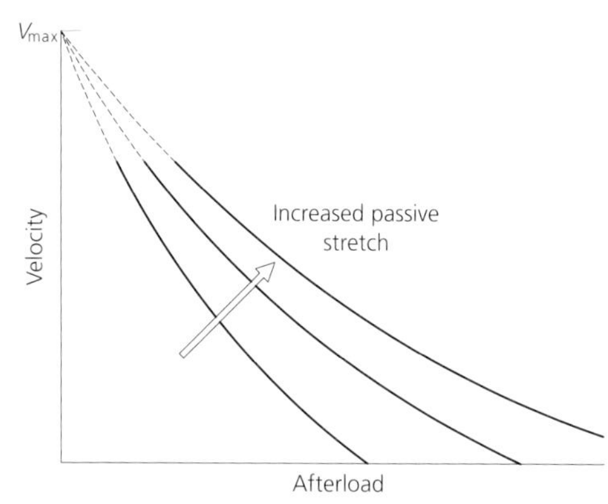

Fig. 13.11 The relationship of velocity of contraction to systolic tension or afterload is shown schematically for isotonically contracting cardiac muscle strips. Velocity and extent of contraction are inversely related to afterload. Increased preload or passive stretch and increased contractility increase velocity of shortening at any given afterload. V_{max} is the extrapolated intercept velocity at zero afterload and is relatively constant at different preloads allowing it to be used as an index of contractility. The reciprocal relationship between extent of shortening and afterload is the basis for the reciprocal relationship between arterial pressure and stroke volume. After Thornburg and Morton[52].

These properties have been nicely described by Braunwald *et al.*[24]. In all striated muscle, the active tension generated by contraction is increased as the muscle is stretched from its resting length (Fig. 13.10). This 'ascending' relationship holds until further increases in length no longer result in increased tension – a length referred to as L_{max}. Tension decreases with length thereafter forming a descending limb. The second property is the force–velocity relation (afterload–velocity relation). If the initial length of a muscle is kept constant, but the muscle is required to contract against increasing load, the velocity at which the muscle contracts will decrease as load increases until the muscle cannot contract at all (isometric tension) (Fig. 13.11). These two muscle properties have been studied in great detail, and while there are specific differences between cardiac and skeletal striated muscle, the general principles of striated muscle apply fully to cardiac muscle.

Preload

In the heart, the force per unit cross-sectional area present within the ventricular wall just before it contracts (end diastole) is called preload. End-diastolic pressure (EDP) or end-diastolic volume (EDV) are often used as surrogates for preload when force per unit cross-sectional area is unknown. From Fig. 13.10, one could predict that as preload increases and muscle fibres are lengthened, they would generate more tension. Thus, it follows that the fraction of the end-diastolic volume that is actually ejected each beat (ejection fraction) is a function of the transmural pressure across the ventricular wall that determines wall tension preceding that beat (preload). As end-diastolic volume increases, stroke volume increases. This has long been known as the Frank–Starling relation or as Starling's law of the heart which was originally stated as, 'The mechanical energy set free on passage from the resting to the contracted state is a function of the length of the muscle fibre, i.e. of the area of chemically active surfaces'[25].

Afterload

The second determinant of stroke volume is afterload, the force per cross-sectional area within the myocardium (wall stress) during contraction. Ventricular wall stress can be estimated using a simplified form of Laplace's law which states

$$S_w = \tfrac{1}{2}P_t\,(r/h) \qquad (13.2)$$

where S_w is wall stress (force per unit cross sectional area), P_t is transmural pressure, r is radius of curvature, h is wall thickness. From this relationship, one can see that the wall stress will increase in direct proportion to the radius of curvature (r) if wall thickness (h) is constant. From this equation, one can appreciate the physiological benefit of increasing wall thickness in response to pressure load (compensatory hypertrophy) because S_w decreases as wall thickness increases, making ejection easier.

Decreases in stroke volume with increased wall stress are explained by the force–velocity relationship discussed above (Fig. 13.11). One can see that as arterial blood pressure goes up, the heart has an increasing load against which it must eject its stroke volume. Pressure is the largest component of afterload. However, a more accurate estimate of afterload can be obtained from the total impedance of the vascular tree. As mentioned above, the vascular impedance is the additive resistive forces of mean and pulsatile flow components.

Contractility

When preload and afterload are kept constant, a ventricle can increase or decrease its ejection fraction through changes in contractility. Contractility (intropy) is the relative contractile state (strength) of the myocardium. Increases in contractility are usually the result of greater cytosolic Ca^{2+} concentrations during systole. However, the sensitivity of the contractile elements to Ca^{2+} ion and the ATPase activity of the myosin isoforms are also factors that affect contractility. Drugs that increase contractility are known as inotropic agents. Digitalis is an example. Increases in heart rate affect myocyte intracellular Ca^{2+} concentration and therefore alter contractility.

There are important differences between immature myocardium and adult myocardium with regard to contractile capability. Friedman[26] showed that fetal myocardium generates less tension per gram than does adult myocardium. Similarly, Nakanishi *et al.*[7] reported that the 18-day rabbit heart could generate about 18 g of tension for each gram of cardiac muscle, whereas the adult could generate nearly 78 g (Table 13.1). Such changes have been assumed to be largely due to the reduced proportion of the myocyte volume containing contractile material[26]. Contraction velocities of unloaded muscle from fetal and adult myocardium are about equal, suggesting that mature and immature sarcomeres behave similarly. However, this is now known to be more complex than originally thought and there may be genuine contractility increases with maturity.

There are differences in contraction velocity of cardiac muscle depending on which of several types of myosin is present. For example, alpha-myosin (V_1) has high ATPase activity whereas beta-myosin (V_3) has low ATPase activity. The ventricular myocardium of the rat switches from V_3 to V_1 in the postnatal period and again to V_3 in old age. V_3 is the prominent isoform in adult humans over the life of the individual. Therefore, it has not been possible to interpret changes in the contractile state with isoenzyme activity in humans.

Maylie *et al.*[27] have shown that anatomical maturity and functional maturity are correlates in the developing cat heart. However, Anderson and colleagues[17] used post-extrasystolic potentiation as an index of *in vitro* or *in vivo* contractility in sheep myocardium and argued that relative force or pressure generation rates (dF/dT or dP/dT) are suitable indices of contractility and are independent of contractile protein content. They demonstrated increases in potentiated pressure generation rates during the perinatal period in the sheep model and argued that the degree of potentiation represents an increase in contractility for the heart. It is difficult to know how their findings (that nicely characterize the development of the myocardium) fit with the finding that fractional shortening of the sheep heart is constant during the perinatal period except for a transient increase at birth. Therefore, it is not clear how their 'contractile reserve' translates into actual contractility under normal conditions. This interesting finding requires further study.

To what extent do preload, afterload and contractility determine stroke volume in the intact fetus? This question is often raised among physiologists and answers have come in various forms. The cardiac function curve is often used to investigate preload. The function curve is a plot of cardiac output, stroke volume or stroke work (stroke volume × driving pressure) against an index of ventricular filling (mean atrial pressure, end-diastolic pressure or end-diastolic volume)[28]. Function curves have been constructed for the whole heart of the fetus[21]. Figure 13.12 shows that as mean atrial pressure (above amniotic pressure) increases from a low level, cardiac output increases proportionately up the ascending limb until the plateau limb is reached, above which no further increases can be generated. The conclusion is that the fetus operates near the top of the curve and that there is very little 'preload reserve' on the plateau. When the fetal ventricles were studied independently, the same conclusion was reached for each ventricle[29,30]. Interestingly, the function curve of the right ventricle is situated well above the curve of the left ventricle. This indicates that for the same filling pressure, the stroke volume is greater for the right ventricle than for the left.

The shape of the function curve is interesting. When mean atrial pressure is referenced to amniotic fluid pressure, the true filling pressure is not being measured because such a pressure is not the ventricular transmural pressure, the pressure difference across the ventricular wall. A better estimate of transmural pressure should be obtained by placing a soft catheter or small balloon in the pericardial space, especially since the physical behavior of the catheter in that space is known[31]. The placement of a pericardial catheter does not much alter the shape of the function curve. However, because it is known that augmentation of end-diastolic volume inevitably leads to increased stroke volume, the plateau of the function curve evidently does not represent true increases in end-diastolic volume, even though the transmural pressure appears to increase. This points to the difficulty of measuring local transmural pressures at the freewall of the ventricle. The shape of the function curve, nevertheless, has physiological meaning. The fetus operates near the breakpoint of the function curve where the two limbs intersect. When such measurements are made in real time, the fetal heart is found to be 'crawling' up and down the function curve near the breakpoint every few minutes. This should not be surprising since these haemodynamic cues are undoubtedly important as heart growth signals. There is a need for new techniques to measure ventricular transmural pressure in the fetus under physiological conditions *in utero*.

It has long been known in adults that increased afterload decreases ventricular shortening velocity and ejection fraction. When afterload was increased in the fetus, it was found that the two ventricles responded very differently. Figure 13.13 shows the relationship between stroke volume and arterial pressure for each ventricle[32] as arterial pressure is increased by inflating an occluder around the descending aorta just beyond the ductus arteriosus. Note that the right ventricular stroke volume decreases rapidly with increasing pressure but that the left ventricular stroke volume decreases hardly at all. This indicates that the right ventricle is inherently unable to maintain its stroke volume in the face of

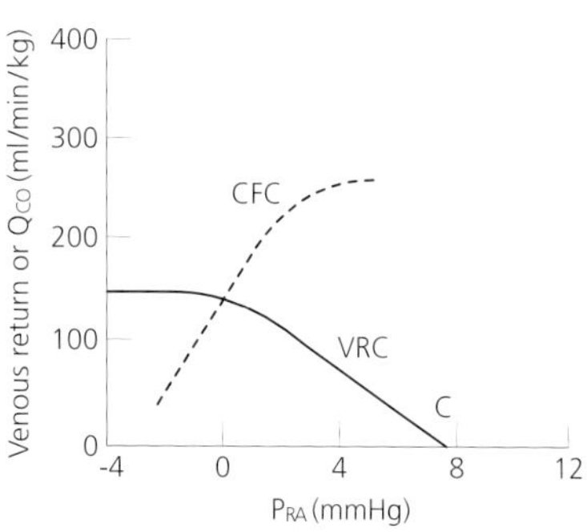

Fig. 13.12 Theoretical venous return curve (*VRC*) and cardiac function curve (*CFC*) for normal adults. Modified from Gilbert[21].

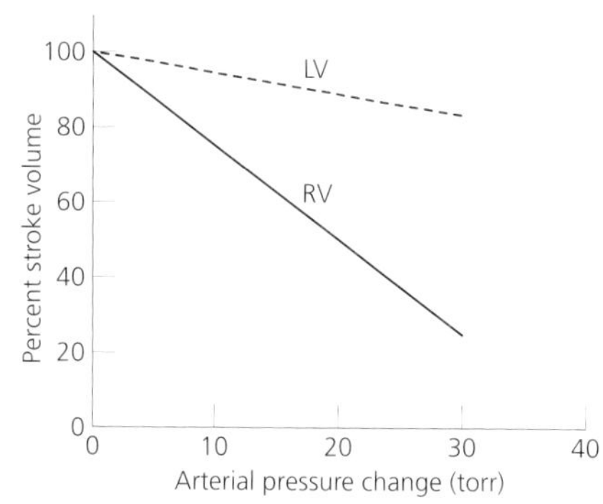

Fig. 13.13 The simultaneous average responses of the right and left ventricles to increased arterial pressure are shown for nine fetuses. Stroke volume is expressed as a percent of control value and arterial pressure as the increment above control. The linear regression coefficient for each ventricle was calculated, the average slope forced through 100% on the Y-axis and the lines extended through the pressure range studied. The right ventricular pressure sensitivity (−2.5 ± 1.4% stroke volume/torr) was more than fivefold the left ventricular pressure sensitivity (−0.5 ± 0.7% stroke volume/torr) ($p<0.001$). After Reller *et al.*[32].

increased arterial pressure. This 'afterload sensitivity' of the right ventricle is physiologically important because increases in arterial pressure from hypoxaemia or placenta growth abnormalities will preferentially affect the right ventricle and will change haemodynamic patterns in the fetus.

There is no convincing evidence that contractility of the fetal heart is normally regulated on a beat to beat basis, though in hypoxaemic fetuses, catecholamine concentrations may be high and direct inotropic stimulation of the myocardium is likely.

VENTRICULAR GEOMETRY

The fetal ventricles were long thought to be nearly identical in shape and function[33–35]. This impression likely came from the stark contrast between adult and fetal hearts. In adult hearts, the thin-walled right ventricle appears to be a crescent shaped add-on to the thick walled cylindrical left ventricle. In contrast, the fetal ventricles have nearly identical wall thicknesses and their cross-sectional views look similar in certain sections and echocardiographic images. Unfortunately, this impression is misleading. The fetal ventricles are sufficiently different in shape and architecture that their physiological function is importantly affected. This interventricular difference in form and function is further exaggerated with time during postnatal life (Fig. 13.14). The internal dimensions of the near term fetal ventricles have been determined for sheep[36] from hearts fixed at physiological filling pressures (Fig. 13.15) as have the component weights (Table 13.3). Several key physical features are important in understanding the physiological capabilities of the working heart *in utero*:

- The right ventricular chamber is some 30% larger than the left ventricular chamber. If we assume that filling pressures are about equal, as most studies have shown, and that ejection fractions are equal, this

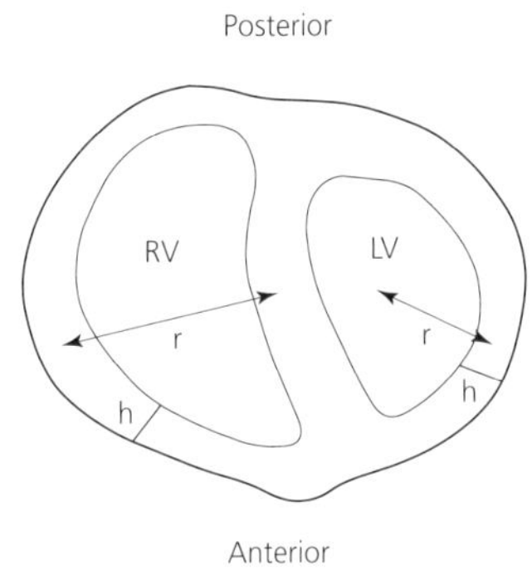

Fig. 13.15 Cross-sectional slice from a near-term fetal heart cut halfway between the apex and annulus. Note that the two ventricles are clearly distinguishable in shape at this stage of gestation. Even by inspection, one could estimate that the right ventricle has a larger radius of curvature than the left ventricle. (See Equation 13.2.) After Thornburg *et al.*[54].

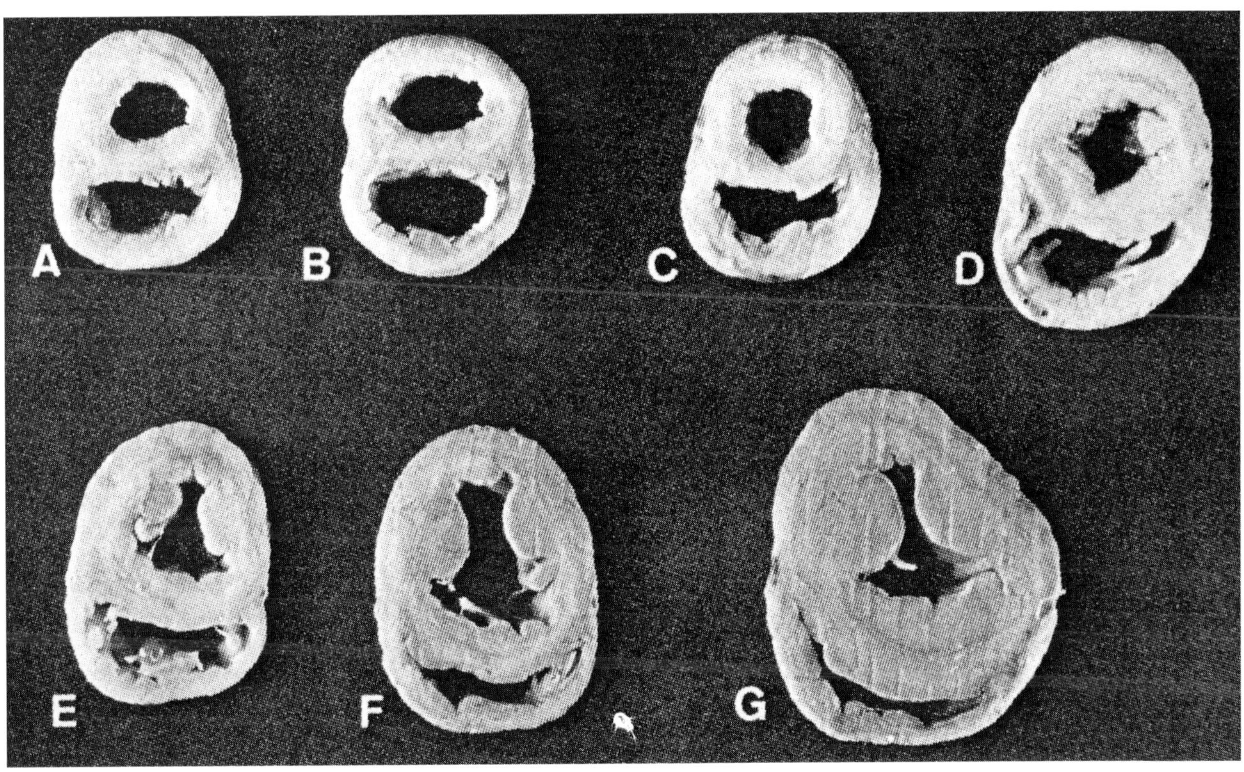

Fig. 13.14 Horizontal sections across the ventricles of pig hearts from 1 day to 9 weeks old with the left ventricle on the top of each slice. A = 1 day; B = 2 days; C = 3 days; D = 9 days; E = 18 days; F = 37 days; G = 9 weeks. After Versprille *et al.*[53].

TABLE 13.3
Heart mass for the 129-day sheep fetus (*n* = 44)

	Weight (g)	S.D.
Total atrial	3.1	0.9*
Total ventricular	16.0	4.8
Left ventricle	6.2	1.8
Right ventricle	5.8	1.9
Septum	4.0	1.2
Fetal mass	2.9 (kg)	0.8
Ventricular/fetal mass	5.5 (g/kg)	0.9
Dry/wet heart mass	0.17	0.02**

*n = 34; **n = 21.

finding explains the dominant right-ventricular stroke volume in the fetus.

- The meridional radius to wall thickness ratio is larger for the right ventricle than for the left[36]. For the middle section of the fetal heart (about one-half the distance between the apex and the annulus) the average radius of curvature for the right ventricle is 12.8 mm and 10.9 mm for the left ventricle. The wall thicknesses are about 3.0 mm and 4.2 mm respectively. The r/h of the right ventricle (4.5) compared to the smaller r/h (2.6) indicates that the right ventricle has a higher resting wall stress and is at a mechanical disadvantage compared to the left ventricle. This provides a physical explanation for ventricular differences in sensitivity to arterial pressure as predicted by Laplace's law (see Equation 13.2).

There are several pathological conditions where the right ventricle must carry the workload of the systemic circulation. This can be done more easily if the ventricle is conditioned by episodes of moderate pressure loading before being harnessed to the high resistance of the systemic circulation. The fetal sheep right ventricle has been studied to determine whether it is able compensate for increased pressure load over time by inflation of an occluder around the main pulmonary artery.[37] The mean pressure in the pulmonary artery was increased by about 10 mmHg above the usual 45–50 mmHg for a 10-day period. Function curves were generated to see if stroke volume was affected at any given filling pressure and the ventricle was tested to determine whether its ability to generate pressure was impaired. The outcome was interesting. Right ventricular wall thickness and weight were both increased. The pressure–volume curves of both ventricles were left shifted which means that the chamber volume was smaller for any given filling pressure (Fig. 13.16). If ejection fractions were unchanged, this would translate into a reduced stroke volume and depressed function curves. These data indicate that the fetal right ventricle adapts to a pressure load by increasing free wall thickness (a lesson already learned from mature hearts) but at the expense of the chamber volume. It would be interesting to know to what extent wall thickening would continue with continued load.

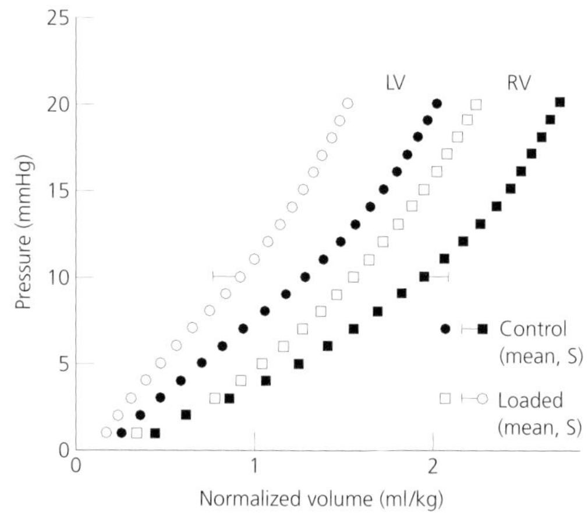

Fig. 13.16 Pressure–volume relations of K^+-arrested fetal hearts *in vitro*. Curves were made by rapidly infusing isotonic saline into left ventricular (LV) and right ventricular (RV) chambers through a plug in the valve annulus while simultaneous pressure measurements were made. Measurements are shown with the contralateral ventricle at 10 mmHg transmural pressure and the pericardium in place. After Pinson *et al.*[37].

Figure 13.17 shows the change in sensitivity to increasing arterial pressure following pressure loading. Note that the right ventricular stroke volume curve has dramatically decreased its slope so that the ventricle is able, after conditioning, to eject much more volume at any given pulmonary arterial pressure. Also note that r/h (see Equation 13.2) approaches that of the left ventricle and that the function of the two ventricles is now similar. Studies on the isolated heart following pulmonary arterial banding show that the left ventricle is also affected. The mechanisms that underlie contralateral ventricular effect are not known but changes in preload and ventricular interaction are likely.

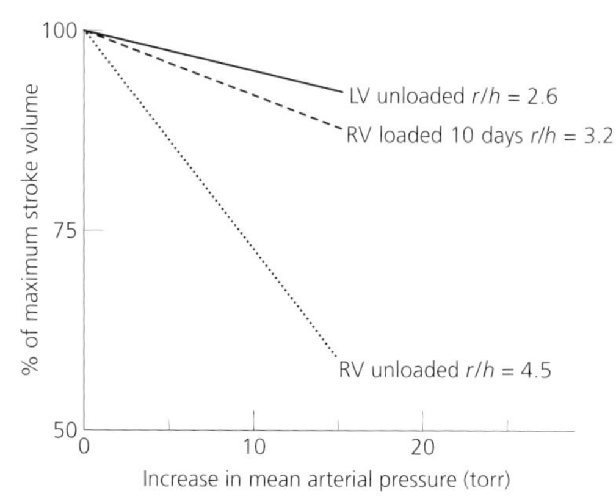

Fig. 13.17 Percentage change in right ventricular stroke volume of fetuses plotted as a function of increase in pulmonary artery pressure. The normal relationships between stroke volume and mean arterial pressure for the unloaded right ventricle (RV unloaded) and the unloaded left ventricle (LV unloaded) are taken from Fig. 13.13. The relationship between stroke volume and pulmonary arterial pressure after 10 days of mild pressure loading is shown as 'RV loaded 10 days'. Each curve is shown with its respective radius to wall thickness ratios which affect wall tension as shown in Equation 13.2. After Thornburg *et al.*[55].

REGULATION OF CORONARY FLOW

The flow of blood through the coronary circulation has been studied extensively in the adult but only little in immature hearts[38–40]. From studies of the mature heart, the concept of flow reserve has been helpful. When the heart is fully dilated by a pharmacological agent, coronary flow increases linearly with the driving pressure ($P_{art} - P_{cs}$), where P_{art} is the inflow pressure in the coronary artery and P_{cs} is the outflow pressure in the coronary sinus (the source of the outflow pressure is not known for sure) (Fig. 13.18). However, coronary flow at rest is only a fraction of its potential at any given pressure. In fact, if pressure is increased, the heart regulates oxygen delivery so precisely that flow increases very little over its autoregulatory range (the plateau in Fig. 13.18). The difference between the autoregulated flow and the flow at full dilation is the 'flow reserve', a value that depends on the pressure from which the curve is generated.

Coronary flow correlates best with oxygen consumption which in turn is affected by pressure and heart rate. In the sheep fetus, coronary flow can be measured using microspheres[38] and a cuff-type Doppler device that indicates flow–velocity[41]. The oxygen consumption of the heart is similar on a gram basis to the adult heart[38]. However, the oxygen content of the fetal arterial blood is half that of the adult. One, then, could expect that fetal coronary flow must be about twice that of the adult. In fetal sheep, the resting coronary flow is about 200 ml/min/100 g and coronary flow in adult animals ranges between 80 and 110 ml/min/100 g, as expected[18,41].

When the fetal sheep coronary circulation is dilated maximally with increasing doses of adenosine, the maximal right ventricular flow is about 600 ml/min 100 g at resting pressure[41]. The right ventricle was studied during gradual increases in pressure load as an occluder around the pulmonary artery was inflated in a near-term sheep[42]. Fetal coronary flow increased with increases in pressure load until mean pulmonary arterial pressure reached 80 mmHg, the point where the ventricle failed. At this pressure, right ventricular flow was ~400 ml/min/100 g, a value that was two-thirds less than flow during dilation with adenosine. This indicates that right ventricular work is not able to elicit a flow response to take full advantage of potential flow reserve even

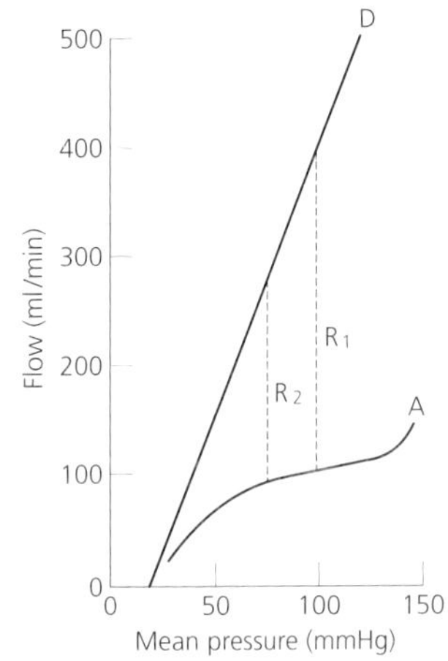

Fig. 13.18 Diagram of pressure–flow relationships in normal left ventricle during autoregulation (A) and maximal vasodilatation (D). R_1 and R_2 are the coronary flow reserves at mean coronary perfusing pressures of 75 and 100 mmHg when aortic pressure and heart rate are constant. After Hoffman[20a].

when the ventricle is failing. The fetal myocardium, like the adult myocardium, is not able to recruit all of its reserve under physiological conditions. However, the fetal heart appears to be especially equipped to handle hypoxaemic episodes *in utero*. When the fetus is made acutely hypoxaemic by the administration of low oxygen gas mixtures to the ewe, coronary flow increases with decreasing arterial oxygen content. At very low oxygen concentrations (<1 mM) flows in the myocardium are dramatic and may reach 1.6 l/min/100 g. Stroke volume is maintained at this level of oxygenation for short periods (~15 min).

Acknowledgements

I would like to thank my colleagues who have been co-investigators, technicians, and supporters. J. Job Faber, Debra Anderson, Mark J. Morton, Mark D. Reller, George D. Giraud, Antonio Barbera, John Bissonnette, James Metcalfe, C.Wright Pinson, Deborah Reid, David Wu, Mike Burson, Tom Green, Bob Webber, Pat Renwick, Linda Wolf, Lisa Rhuman, Zara Wanlass, Emily Gilster. From these, I have received more than I have given.

REFERENCES

1. Reller MD, McDonald RW, Gerlis LM, Thornburg KL. Cardiac embryology: basic review and clinical correlations [review]. *J Am Soc Echocardiogr* 4(5):519–532, 1991.
2. Katz AM. *Physiology of the Heart*, 2nd edn. New York: Raven Press, 1992.
3. Faber JJ, Green TJ, Thornburg KL. Embryonic stroke volume and cardiac output in the chick. *Dev Biol* **41**(1):14–21, 1974.
4. Keller BB. Overview: functional maturation and coupling of the embryonic cardiovascular system. In *Developmental Mechanisms of Heart Disease* (eds E.B. Clark, R.R. Markwald & A Takao), pp. 367–385. Armonk NY: Futura, 1995.
5. Clubb FJ, Bishop SP. Formation of binucleated myocardial cells in the neonatal rat: an index for growth hypertrophy. *Lab Invest* **50**:571–577, 1984.
6. Rakusan K. Cardiac growth, maturation, and aging. In *Growth of the Heart in Health and Disease* (ed. R. Zak), pp. 131–164. New York: Raven Press, 1984.
7. Nakanishi T, Seguchi M, Takao A. Development of the myocardial contractile system [review]. *Experientia* **44**(11–12):936–944, 1988.
8. Dawes GS. *Foetal and Neonatal Physiology*. Chicago: Year Book Medical Publishers. 1968.
9. Carter AM. The blood supply to the abdominal organs of the fetal guinea-pig. *J Dev Physiol* **6**:407–416, 1984.

10. Anderson DF, Bissonnette JM, Faber JJ, Thornburg KL. Central shunt flows and pressures in the mature fetal lamb. *Am J Physiol* **241**(1):H60–6, 1981.
11. Reuss ML, Rudolph AM. Distribution and recirculation of umbilical and systemic venous blood flow in fetal lambs during hypoxia. In *Journal of Developmental Physiology, Vol. 2* (ed. C.T. Jones), pp. 71–84. Oxford: Blackwell Scientific Publications, 1980.
12. Anderson DF, Faber JJ, Morton MJ, Parks CM, Pinson CW, Thornburg KL. Flow through the foramen ovale of the fetal and new-born lamb. *J Physiol (Lond)* **365**:29–40, 1985.
13. Nichols WW, O'Rourke MF. *McDonald's Blood Flow in Arteries: Theoretic, Experimental and Clinical Principles*, 3rd edn. Philadelphia: Lea & Febiger, 1990.
14. Langille BL, Adamson SL. Thoracic aortic pressure–flow relationships and vascular impedance in fetal sheep. *Am J Physiol* **263**:H824–32, 1992.
15. Meschia G, Cotter JR, Breathnach CS, Barron DH. The hemoglobin, oxygen, carbon dioxide and hydrogen ion concentrations in the umbilical bloods of sheep and goats as sampled via indwelling plastic catheters. *Quart J Exp Physiol* **50**:185–195, 1965.
16. Kirkpatrick SE, Friedman WF. Myocardial determinants of fetal cardiac output. In *Fetal and Newborn Cardiovascular Physiology, Vol. 1* (eds L.D. Longo & D.D. Reneau), pp. 369–389. New York: Garland STPM Press, 1978.
17. Anderson, PAW, Glick KI, Manring A, Crenshaw C, Jr. Developmental changes in cardiac contractility in fetal and postnatal sheep: *in vitro* and *in vivo*. *Am J Physiol* **247**:H371–9, 1984.
18. Jacobson S-L, Eicher AL, Paul MS, Giraud GD, Morton MJ, Thornburg KL. The sequential effects of estrogen administration and hypertension on cardiac function in ewes. *Am J Obstet Gynecol* **179**:610–619, 1998.
19. Rasanen J, Wood DC, Weiner S, Ludomirski A, Huhta JC. Role of the pulmonary circulation in the distribution of human fetal cardiac output during the second half of pregnancy. *Circulation* **94**:1068–1073, 1996.
20. Heymann MA, Creasy RK, Rudolph AM. Quantitation of blood flow patterns in the foetal lamb *in utero*. In: *Foetal and Neonatal Physiology* (eds K.S. Combline, K.W. Cross, G.S. Dawes & P.W. Nathanielsz) pp. 129–135. Cambridge: Cambridge University Press, 1973.
20a. Hoffmann JIE. Maximal coronary flow and the concept of coronary vascular reserve [review]. *Circulation* **70**(2):153–159, 1984.
21. Gilbert RD. Venous return and control of fetal cardiac output. In *Fetal and Newborn Cardiovascular Physiology, Vol. 1: Developmental Aspects* (eds L.D. Longo and D.D. Reneau), pp. 299–316. New York: Garland STPM Press, 1978.
22. Guyton AC, Lindsey AW, Abernathy JB, Richardson T. Venous return at various right atrial pressures and the normal venous return curve. *Am J Physiol* **189**:609–615, 1957.
23. Morin FC, Eagan EA. Pulmonary hemodynamics in fetal lambs during development at normal and increased oxygen tension. *J Appl Physiol* **73**:213–218, 1992.
24. Braunwald E, Ross Jr, J, Sonnenblick EH. *Mechanisms of Contraction of the Normal and Failing Heart*. Boston: Little, Brown, 1976.
25. Paterson SW, Starling EH. On mechanical factors which determine output of ventricles. *J Physiol (Lond)* **48**:357–379, 1914.
26. Friedman WF. The intrinsic physiologic properties of the developing heart. *Prog Cardiovasc Dis* **15**:87, 1972.
27. Maylie J, Thornburg KL, Faber JJ. E-C coupling in developing cat heart. *Biophys J* **24**:165 (Abstract), 1978.
28. Bishop VS, Stone HL, Guyton AC. Cardiac function curves in conscious dogs. *Am J Physiol* **207**:677–682, 1964.
29. Thornburg KL, Morton MJ. Filling and arterial pressures as determinants of RV stroke volume in the sheep fetus. *Am J Physiol* **244**(5):H656–63, 1983.
30. Thornburg KL, Morton MJ. Filling and arterial pressures as determinants of left ventricular stroke volume in fetal lambs. *Am J Physiol* **251**(5, Pt 2):H961–8, 1986.
31. Morton MJ, Pinson CW, Thornburg KL. *In utero* ventilation with oxygen augments left ventricular stroke volume in lambs. *J Physiol (Lond.)* **383**:413–424, 1987.
32. Reller MD, Morton MJ, Reid DL, Thornburg KL. Fetal lamb ventricles respond differently to filling and arterial pressures and to *in utero* ventilation. *Pediatr Res* **22**(6):621–626, 1987.
33. Pohlman AG. The course of the blood through the heart of the fetal mammal, with a note on the reptilian and amphibian circulations. *Anat Rec* **3**:75–109, 1909.
34. Cassin S, Dawes GS, Mott JC, Ross BB, Strang LB. The vascular resistance of the fetal and newly ventilated lung of the lamb. *J Physiol (Lond.)* **171**:61–79, 1964.
35. St John-Sutton MG, Gewitz MH, Shah B, Cohen A, Reichek N, Gabbe S, Huff DS. Quantitative assessment of growth and function in the cardiac chambers in the normal human fetus: a prospective longitudinal echocardiographic study. *Circulation* **69**:645–654, 1984.
36. Pinson CW, Morton MJ, Thornburg KL. An anatomic basis for fetal right ventricular dominance and arterial pressure sensitivity. *J Dev Physiol* **9**(3):253–269, 1987.
37. Pinson CW, Morton MJ, Thornburg KL. Mild pressure loading alters right ventricular function in fetal sheep. *Circ Res* **68**(4):947–957, 1991.
38. Fisher DJ, Heymann MA, Rudolph AM. Myocardial oxygen and carbohydrate consumption in fetal lambs and in adult sheep. *Am J Physiol* **238**:H399–405, 1980.
39. Fisher DJ, Heymann MA, Rudolph AM. Fetal myocardial oxygen and carbohydrate consumption during acutely induced hypoxemia. *Am J Physiol* **242**:H657–61, 1982.
40. Fisher DJ, Heymann MA, Rudolph AM. Regional myocardial blood flow and oxygen delivery in fetal, newborn, and adult sheep. *Am J Physiol* **243**:H729–31, 1982.
41. Reller MD, Morton MJ, Giraud GD, Wu DE, Thornburg KL. Maximal myocardial blood flow is enhanced by chronic hypoxemia in late gestation fetal sheep. *Am J Physiol* **263**(4, Pt 2):H1327–9, 1992.
42. Reller MD, Morton MJ, Giraud GD, Wu DE, Thornburg KL. Severe right ventricular pressure loading in fetal sheep augments global myocardial blood flow to submaximal levels. *Circulation* **86**(2):581–588, 1992.
43. Teitel DF. Circulatory adjustments of postnatal life. *Sem Perinatol* **12**:96–103, 1988.
44. Llanos AJ, Riquelme RA, Moraga FA, Cabello G, Parer JT. Cardiovascular responses to graded degrees of hypoxaemia in the llama fetus. *Progr Perinatal Physiol Reproduct Fertil Develop* **7**:247–250, 1995.
45. Nakazawa M, Miyagawa S, Ohno T, Miura S, Takao A. Developmental hemodynamic changes in rat embryos at 11 to 15 days of gestation: normal data of blood pressure and the effect of caffeine compared to data from chick embryo. *Ped Res* **23**(2):200–205, 1988.
46. Maylie JG. Excitation–contraction coupling in neonatal and adult myocardium of cat. *Am J Physiol* **242**(5):H834–43, 1982.
47. Cohn HE, Sacks EJ, Heyman MA, Rudolph AM. Cardiovascular responses to hypoxemia and academia in fetal lambs. *Am J Obstet Gynecol* **120**:817–824, 1974.
48. Longo LD, Wyatt JF, Hewitt CW, Gilbert RD. A comparison of circulatory responses to hypoxic hypoxia and carbon monoxide hypoxia in fetal blood flow and oxygenation. In: *Fetal and Newborn Cardiovascular Physiology* (eds L.D. Longo & D.D. Reneau), pp. 259–288. New York: Garland STPM Press, 1976.
49. Longo LD, Packianathan S. Hypoxia-ischaemia and the developing brain: hypotheses regarding the pathophysiology of fetal-neonatal brain damage. *Br J Obstet Gynaecol* **104**(6):652–662, 1997.
50. Peeters LLH, Sheldon RE, Jones MD Jr, Makowski EL, Meschia G. Blood flow to fetal organs as a function of arterial oxygen content. *Am J Obstet Gynecol* **135**:637–646, 1979.
51. Thornburg KL. Fetal response to intrauterine stress [review]. In: *Childhood Environment and Adult Disease* (eds G.R. Bock & J. Whelan), pp. 17–37. (Ciba Foundation Symposium 156) Chichester: John Wiley, 1991.
52. Thornburg KL, Morton MJ. Development of the cardiovascular system. In *Textbook of Fetal Physiology* (eds G.D. Thorburn, R. Harding), pp. 95–130. Oxford: Oxford University Press, 1994.
53. Versprille A, Jansen JRC, Harnick E, van Nie CJ, deNeef KJ. Functional interaction of both ventricles at birth and the changes during the neonatal period in relation to the changes of geometry. In *Fetal and Newborn Cardiovascular Physiology, Vol. 1* (eds L.D. Longo & D.D. Reneau), pp. 399–413. New York: Garland STPM Press, 1978.
54. Thornburg KL, Morton MJ, Pinson CW, Reller MD, Reid DL. Anatomic and functional distinctions between the fetal heart ventricles. In *Perinatal Development of the Heart and Lung* (eds J. Lipshitz, J. Maloney, C. Nimrod, & G. Carson), pp. 49–82. Ithaca, NY: Perinatology Press, 1991.
55. Thornburg KL, Morton MJ. Growth and development of the heart. In *Fetus and Neonate: Physiology and Clinical Applications, Vol. 1: The Circulation*, (eds M.A. Hanson, J.A.D. Spencer & C.H. Rodeck), pp. 137–159. Cambridge: Cambridge University Press, 1993.

Kidney and urinary tract

14

E. Marelyn Wintour, M. Dodic, H. Johnston, K. Moritz and A. Peers

Introduction

A knowledge of fetal renal development and function is essential for the understanding of the aetiology of certain disease states both in the fetus and in the adult. One of the most exciting areas of investigation currently is the role of factors operating before birth in the determination of the long-term health of the adult – the 'fetal origins of adult disease' hypothesis of David Barker and colleagues[1]. This hypothesis, based on a vast amount of epidemiological data linking weight at birth with increased incidence of hypertension, non-insulin-dependent diabetes mellitus and ischaemic heart disease in adult life, proposes that the first environment, the intrauterine one, may be crucial to long-term health. It has particular relevance to renal development. Babies who are growth-retarded have been found to have particularly low kidney weight, fewer nephrons, and higher levels of cord blood renin and angiotensin II[2–4]. As shown in Fig. 14.1, the potential exists for such small kidneys to begin to fail earlier in adult life, once subjected to a variety of risk factors, such as obesity, smoking, environmental pollutants or overuse of analgesics.

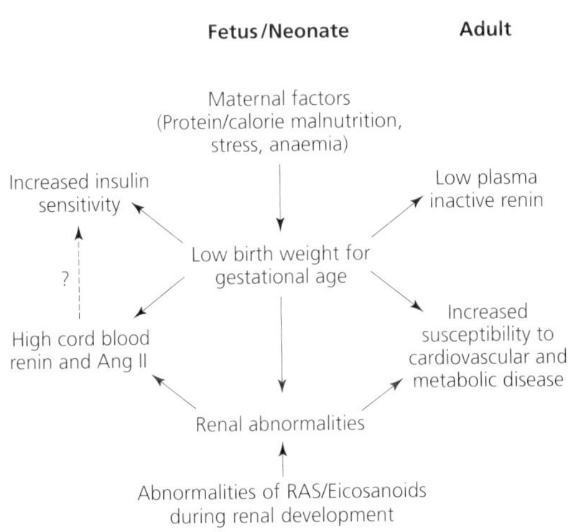

Fig. 14.1 Neonatal kidney failure.

Evidence is also accumulating that development of other organs, such as the adrenals and gonads, may be interrelated with the formation and regression of the temporary mesonephric kidney[5]. For that reason one section details the known data about the development and gene expression of the mesonephros.

The functions of the kidney, particularly relevant to fetal life, include the maintenance of blood pressure and the production of a large volume of dilute urine. The mechanisms by which a rather poorly perfused kidney, receiving only 3% of the cardiac output, manages to maintain a glomerular filtration rate which is at least half that of the adult kidney, on a body weight basis, are shown to involve the renin–angiotensin system. The production of a large volume of dilute urine by the fetal kidney is possible because of the relative insensitivities of both the release and the renal actions of arginine vasopressin (AVP). The roles of water channels, particularly that of aquaporin-1 (AQP_1) and aquaporin-2 (AQP_2) are quite important in this respect, and one section explores the most recent information on the water-channel genes, and the ontogeny and regulation of the expression of some relevant to fetal renal function. Urea transporters are crucial to the development of a medullary gradient, and these will be discussed, though little, as yet, is known of their ontogeny.

It is also important to realise that the normal development of the kidney may be affected adversely by drugs administered to the mother and crossing the placenta. There is evidence that two systems – the renin–angiotensin system and the prostaglandin–eicosanoid system – are particularly important in renal development and function and these are discussed in greater detail below.

Obstruction of the urinary tract, *in utero*, is detectable and potentially correctable before birth. However, the surgery is not without significant risk, and it is highly desirable to have some indication that the kidneys could function well, after such surgery, before exposing the patient to the risk and expense of such corrective procedures. Knowledge of normal fetal urine composition is essential for this diagnosis.

Some knowledge of renal development and function can be gained in the human by the examination of morphology and gene expression in fetal kidneys taken at pregnancy termination, and by ultrasound examination of both kidney size, and the volume and rate of filling/emptying of the bladder. Inferences about 'fetal' glomerular filtration rate (GFR) can be drawn from measurements of creatinine clearance in premature neonates. However, much of our knowledge of fetal renal function has come from experiments on the chronically cannulated sheep fetus. The morphological development time sequences of the human and ovine kidneys are remarkably similar, with the mesonephros being present over the period 10–40% of the total gestation period, metanephric formation starting at 12–18% of gestation, and metanephric nephrogenesis being complete before birth in both species[6]. Thus much of the physiology of the fetal kidney which will be discussed has been investigated in the sheep fetus.

Renal development

PRONEPHROS

The final, permanent metanephric kidney can only be formed normally if it is preceded by the development and subsequent regression of two more primitive forms – the pronephros and the mesonephros. The pronephros consists of one to three filtering units (the glomerulus) which filter(s) fluid into a body compartment – the nephrocoel. From here fluid is collected by the ciliated nephrostome and some reabsorption takes place into the surrounding blood sinus before excretion of the remainder into the cloaca. The pronephros has its origin in the nephrogenic ridge which forms on either side of the midline in the human embryo some 23–24 days after conception and the pronephros forms at the cranial end[6]. Whilst considered essential only in the provision of analgen of the Wolffian duct (which joins the cloaca by day 28 in the human fetus) in mammals, the pronephros does act as an embryonic kidney in some amphibia[7]. Interruption of pronephric function in the amphibian Amblystoma punctatum leads to oedema and death[8]. In the sheep no pronephros, as such, develops, but a 'giant glomerulus' is formed at the cranial end of the mesonephros[9]. The cranial and caudal nephrons of the mesonephros have been shown to vary in morphology and gene expression in the mouse, rat and chick[10,11], suggesting some differences in the two parts of the mesonephros in these species also. Mutant mice lacking expression of the genes *PAX-2* or *LIM1* do not form mesonephroi, while abnormal mesonephric development occurs with deletion of *WT1*[7]. The nephrostome of the pronephros persists in the mesonephros of the elephant fetus[12], suggesting an aquatic origin of this now terrestrial mammal.

MESONEPHROS

Development of the mesonephros is not so well studied, in terms of gene expression patterns, as the metanephros, but is thought to proceed along generally similar lines. Budding of the pronephric/Wolffian duct initiates condensation of mesenchyme and mesonephric tubule formation. The mesonephros does not form a loop of Henle and lacks the macula densa – a specialised segment of tubule between the top of the ascending limb of the loop of Henle and the distal tubule. There also appear to be two separate vascular poles, one each for the afferent and efferent arterioles and no juxtaglomerular apparatus[13]. The glomeruli of the mesonephros are much larger than those of the metanephros, and fewer in number (<100 compared to >500 000), as illustrated in Figs 14.2(A, B) and 14.3A. The mesonephros is a filtering kidney, producing a dilute urine[14], and is of special importance in ruminants which have a cotyledonary placenta, such as sheep and cow. The mesonephric urine enters the allantois from the bladder, via the urachus which runs in the umbilical cord. It is supposed that the expansion of the allantoic sac, as the mesonephric urine enters, allows apposition of the chorionic blood vessels to the predetermined sites on the uterus, caruncles, where the cotyledons of the placenta will form. A more detailed description of mesonephric/allantoic sac formation has been published recently[6].

The mesonephros is the permanent kidney of the fish, and the head kidney is the permanent site of erythropoiesis in fish[15,16]. As detailed later, the mesonephros is an important site of expression of the erythropoietin gene, which controls erythropoiesis.

Of potential importance to adrenal and gonadal deficiencies after birth are the recently explored roles of the mesonephros in development of these organs. By studying the expression of an early gene, steroidogenic factor 1 (*SF1*), it has been suggested that the steroidogenic cells of the adrenal cortex and gonad arise from a common pool[17]. If the *SF1* gene is 'knocked-out' mutant mice develop neither gonads

Fig. 14.2 Sagittal (A and B) and transverse (C and D) paraffin section of whole embryos demonstrating the development of the mesonephros. (A) In the pig embryo at 8 mm and (B) the sheep embryo at 27 days of gestation, the mesonephros is the most prominent organ in the future abdominal region. Large central mesonephric glomeruli are arranged segmentally and surrounded by mesonephric tubules. At later stages of development, both the mesonephros and metanephros can be identified (C) in the sheep embryo at 40 days of gestation and (D) in the human fetus at 8 weeks of gestation. The mesonephros has begun to regress and in the human embryo is less prominent in the abdominal cavity. MS, mesonephros; MT, metanephros. Magnification: A × 14; B × 12; C and D × 17. Reproduced with permission of Cambridge University Press[6].

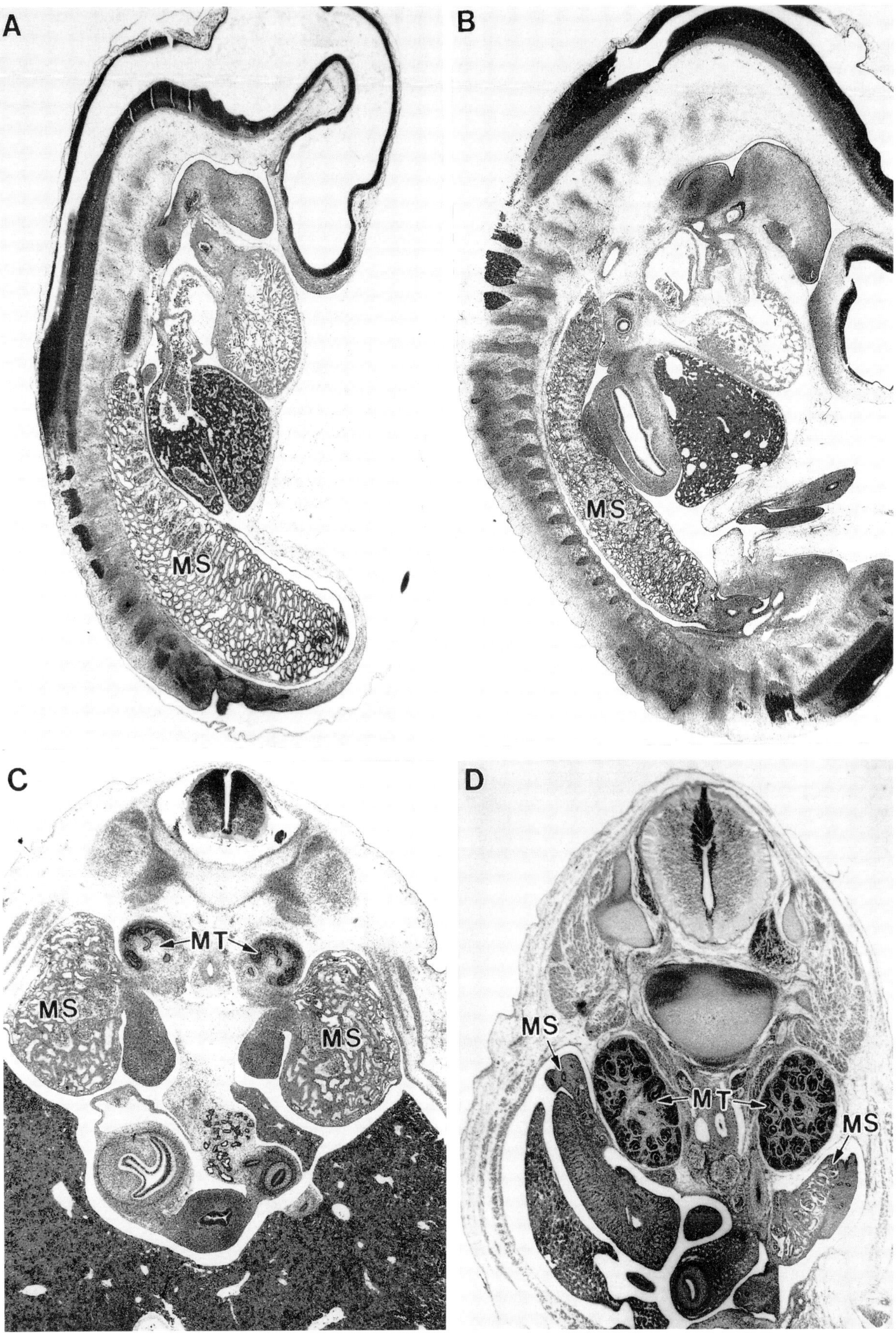
A
MS
B
MS
C
MT
MS
MS
D
MS
MT
MS

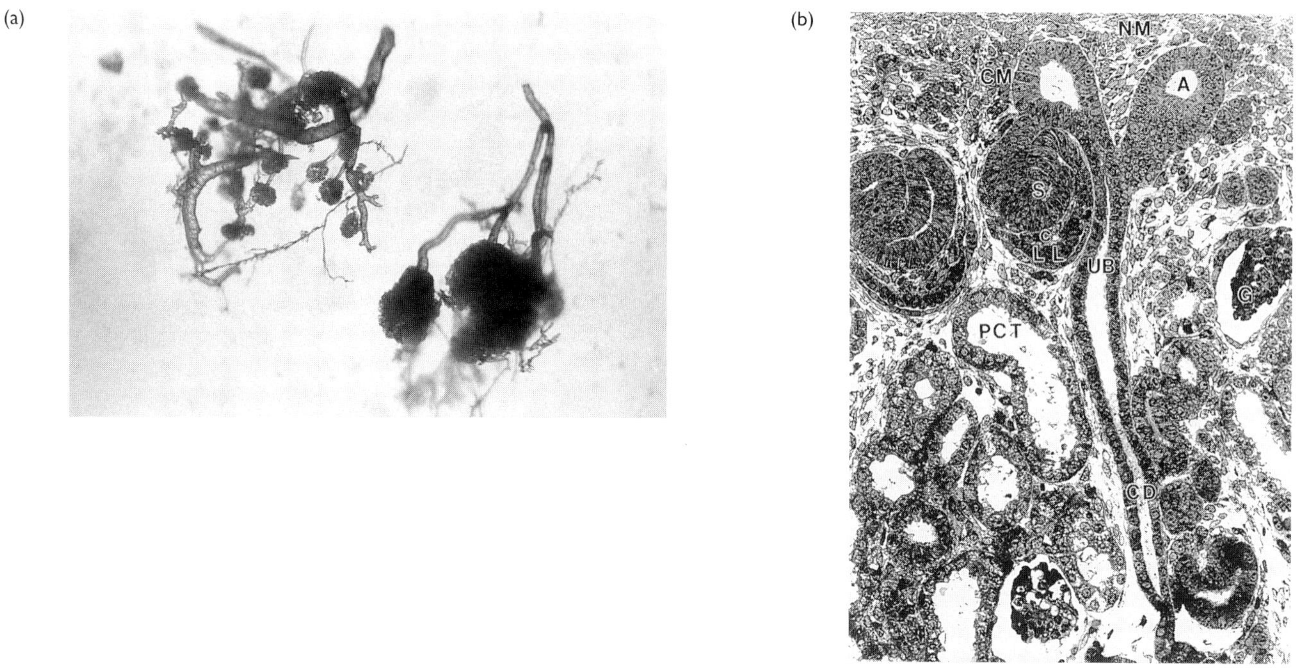

Fig. 14.3 (a) Acrylic vascular casts of glomeruli from the metanephros (upper) and mesonephros (lower) of one 50-day ovine fetus showing relative size of glomerulus. (b) A section of the developing metanephros from an ovine fetus at 50 days of gestation showing: A, ampulla of a branch of the ureteric bud (UB) – the UB is the future collecting duct; CM, condensing mesenchyme-metanephric blastema, close to an ampulla; G, primitive glomerulus, being invaded by capillaries c; NM, outer cortical nephrogenic zone of mesenchyme; PCT, proximal convoluted tubule of a more mature nephron in midcortex; S, S-shaped body. Magnification × 425. Reprinted with permission from Elsevier Science[199].

nor adrenals[18]. There have been claims on a morphological basis that mesonephric cells migrate into the developing adrenal[19]. With mice metanephroi, it has been possible to show the migration of genetically marked cells from the mesonephros to the developing testis, where they appear to form the endocrine Leydig cells[20]. Movement of mesonephric cells into the developing ovary of the sheep has also been proposed, though with less definitive proof[21]. It is certainly true that in all species examined, including human, the developing gonad can be seen physically attached to the mesonephros[5,6]. Earlier claims, however, that mesonephric development and limb bud development were linked, in the chick, have not been substantiated[22].

METANEPHROS

Metanephric development has been studied extensively at the morphological level, and the expression patterns of a large number of genes have been delineated[5,23–25]. There may well be redundancy in production of morphogenetic factors, because the expected phenotype does not always occur when a gene is deleted by homologous recombination[26]. The process of metanephrogenesis involves mutual induction. The ureteric bud arises from the caudal end of the Wolffian duct, on either side, and grows into the metanephric mesenchyme. Factors secreted by the metanephric mesenchyme stimulate the growth and division of the ureteric bud. At each division, one arm goes on to divide further, whilst the other forms an ampulla and secretes factors which induce condensation and ultimately epitheliarisation of the metanephric blastema (Fig. 14.3B). As the metanephric blastema epitheliarises, it first forms a comma shape, then S-shaped tubules. The lower limb of the S forms the glomerulus after invasion by capillaries, under the influence of vascular endothelial growth factor (VEGF) secreted by the developing epithelia, acting on Flk receptors in the mesenchymal derivatives. The S-shaped tubule, of mesenchymal origin, joins to the ureteric bud which forms the collecting duct. Progressive growth and differentiation occurs, so that proximal tubule, convoluted and straight, loop of Henle (descending thin limb and ascending thick limb, macula densa, and distal tubule) form. Nephrogenesis always occurs on the outermost rim of the developing kidney, and the 'oldest' glomeruli are pushed progressively to the innermost area of the cortex. The loops of these inner cortical nephrons grow into the inner medulla, whereas those of the last-formed outer glomeruli reach only as far as the outer stripe of the outer medulla. This area, then, is the last area of the kidney to mature.

Although the metanephros first develops caudal to the mesonephros, as it grows it ascends, posteriorly, to come to rest cranial to the regressing mesonephros so that in sections in which both mesonephric and metanephric kidneys can be seen (Fig. 14.2C,D) the mesonephros is the more caudal structure. As a percentage of body weight the metanephros is

TABLE 14.1
Growth of kidneys in Merino sheep fetuses

Gestation (days)	Body weight (g) (*n*)	Mesonephroi (2) weight (g)	Metanephroi (2) weight (g)	Body weight (metanephroi) (%)
40	5.0 ± 0.6 (18)	0.035 ± 0.008	0.034 ± 0.008	0.7
50	18.8 ± 3.6 (9)	0.027 ± 0.008	0.222 ± 0.051	1.2
60	63.8 ± 3.5 (6)	–	0.877 ± 0.112	1.4
80	254 ± 68 (18)	–	3.14 ± 0.53	1.2
90	394 ± 88 (8)	–	6.1 ± 1.3	1.6
100	918 ± 97 (5)	–	9.5 ± 1.4	1.0
110	1181 ± 202 (10)	–	12.1 ± 1.5	1.0
120	1817 ± 305 (7)	–	16.5 ± 2.0	0.9
130	2788 ± 356 (10)	–	21.2 ± 2.8	0.8
140	4185 ± 669 (10)	–	21.9 ± 3.1	0.5

Values are mean ± S.D. *n* = number of fetuses.

maximal (1.4–1.6%) between 60 and 90 days of gestation (term is 145–150 days) as shown in Table 14.1.

Functional development of the metanephros

The fetal metanephric kidney differs from the adult in that it has a low blood flow, only receiving 3% of cardiac output compared with 25% cardiac output in the adult, coinciding with a fetal kidney GFR approximately half that of the adult kidney[27,28]. Surprisingly, the fetal kidney can produce a large volume of hypotonic urine, averaging 10–15 ml/kg/h (equivalent to 25–35% bodyweight), which nevertheless contains 5% of the filtered sodium. At the time of birth, both GFR and sodium reabsorption rapidly increase[28]. In fetal kidney development this low GFR and high urine production appears to be maintained by the renin–angiotensin system within the ovine and human fetal kidney (see later). The equivalent urine production within an adult would result from deficiencies of secretion or lack of response to arginine vasopressin (AVP), such as that seen in patients suffering central or nephrogenic diabetes insipidus (NDI). Therefore the fetal kidney acts in a similar way to that of an adult with NDI, producing large amounts of dilute urine. Surprisingly, the already large urine flow rate can be increased in the fetal kidney with the introduction of hormones or stress that stimulates an increase in the GFR without decreasing the urine osmolality. An example of this is atrial natriuretic peptide (ANP) which is manufactured within adult hearts and has been detected in the human fetus at 10 weeks of gestation. Fetal levels of ANP are greater than maternal and can be increased by several factors such as atrial distension, isotonic and hypertonic saline loading and blood transfusion for anaemia within the human fetus[29,30]. Cortisol, angiotensin II and ANP all have a diuretic and natriuretic effect upon the immature fetal kidney partly due to an increase in GFR and also to a disruption of glomerulo-tubular balance[31,32].

Erythropoietin

Erythropoietin (Epo), a hormone required for red blood production, is predominantly produced in the kidney during adult life[34]. In the fetus, it was thought for many years that the liver was the site of Epo production and there was a gradual 'switching' to kidney production[34]. However, it has been demonstrated in the human fetal kidney that the *Epo* gene is expressed in interstitial cells close to proximal tubules from mid-gestation[35]. In the ovine fetus, the *Epo* gene is expressed at relatively high levels (compared to the liver) from early in gestation[36]. In fact expression of the *Epo* gene was highest at 60–100 days of gestation (term = 150 days) and declined thereafter. The mesonephros of the ovine fetus also expressed the *Epo* gene at 41 days of gestation, indicating the kidneys may contribute to plasma Epo levels from very early in gestation[37].

Plasma concentrations of Epo in the human fetus over weeks 20–40 have been reported to be low compared to the adult[38], whilst other studies have suggested an increase in concentrations towards term[39]. The method of fetal sampling may be important in interpreting these results[40]. In the unstressed ovine fetus, plasma levels are always lower than in the adult and are significantly lower at 140 days than at 100 days of gestation[41]. Although plasma Epo concentrations are low, erythropoiesis occurs at rapid rate such that the haematocrit is maintained during the rapid growth of the fetus. It may be during fetal development that Epo is more effective at stimulating erythropoiesis or alternatively, Epo synergizes with another factor[40]. Hepatocyte growth factor, thrombopoietin and the insulin-like growth factors have been suggested as possible candidates with which Epo may interact[40].

Epo gene expression in the ovine fetal kidney can be stimulated by haemorrhage from at least mid-gestation[42]. Recent studies have shown that glucocorticoids can influence *Epo* gene expression. Fetuses which had been treated with cortisol had markedly reduced *Epo* gene expression in their kidneys compared to controls, whilst fetuses which had been adrenalectomised increased gene expression fivefold[43]. This suggests that excess glucocorticoid, from the maternal circulation, may depress erythropoiesis in times of maternal stress. The plasma Epo response to haemorrhage after bilateral nephrectomy at 100 days of gestation was reduced significantly. The liver increased *Epo* gene expression only to the same extent as in the intact haemorrhaged fetus[42]. This indicates that the liver cannot compensate for the loss of kidney Epo production in times of erythropoietic stress, and that the kidney is a significant source, accounting for half the Epo hormone circulating in the fetus after haemorrhage.

Water channels

BACKGROUND

The water channels, known as aquaporins, are a family of intrinsic membrane proteins that span the phospholipid bilayer of cell membranes and serve as selective pores for the transfer of water. Even before the discovery of the aquaporins, their existence had always been suspected by the ratio of >1 for the osmotic permeability (P_f) to the diffusional permeability (P_d) which indicated that water passed across the epithelial membranes of the kidney at a rate greater than that possible by diffusion alone. Not all aquaporins are exclusive to water transport, with some showing varying degrees of permeability to either or both urea and glycerol (see Table 14.2).

The aquaporins range between 28 and 36 kDa in unglycosylated forms but generally most are found to exist in the glycosylated state. Based on freeze fracture and electron crystallography studies, the aquaporins consist of six membrane spanning domains connected by five loops, with a characteristic NPA (Asn-Pro-Ala) motif in each of the two most prominent loops[44–47].

At present, 10 mammalian aquaporins have been cloned, four highly expressed within the kidney and three at lower levels of expression[48–66]. Aquaporins 1, 2, 3, 4, 6, 8 and 9 are expressed in the kidney although the exact cellular localization for the recently discovered aquaporins 6, 8 and 9 is not yet known. Aquaporin-1 has been found to have a wide

TABLE 14.2
Synopsis of data on mammalian water channels

	Location	Permeability			Mercury sensitivity	Reference
		Water	Urea	Glycerol		
AQP_0 (MIP) (263)	Eye-lens	+	–	–	+	44
AQP_1 (CHIP28) (268–271)	PT and DTL of kidney, most organs, except brain	+	–	–	+	45, 46 47, 48
AQP_2 (AQP-CD) (271)	Kidney – cortical and medullary CD	+	–	–	+	49, 50
AQP_3 (GLIP) (279–292)	Lung, brain, colon, kidney – cortical and medullary CD	+	+	+	+	51, 52
AQP_4(MIWC) (301, 323)	Eye, lung, colon, salivary gland, lacrimal gland, skeletal muscle, ovary, brain. Medullary vasa recta, cortical and medullary CD	+	–	–	–	53, 54 55
AQP_5 (65–265)	Eye, salivary gland, lacrimal gland, lung	+	–	–	+	56, 57
AQP_6 (hKID) (282)	Kidney, ? location	+	–	–	+	58
AQP_7 (269)	Testis	+	+	+	–	59
AQP_8 (261, 263)	Testis, liver, pancreas, colon, salivary gland, placenta, heart, lung, spleen, submandibular gland, stomach, brain, diaphram Kidney cortex and medulla? location	+	+	–	+	60, 61 62
AQP_9 (342)	Adipose tissue, ? kidney	+	–	+	+	63

MIP = major intrinsic protein. CHIP28=channel-forming integral membrane protein of 28 kDa. AQP-CD=aquaporin of collecting duct. GLIP=glycerol intrinsic protein. MIWC=mercury-insensitive water channel. hKID=human kidney aquaporin. PT=proximal tubule. DTL=descending thin limb of loop of Henle. CD=collecting duct. Amino acid lengths are in parentheses.

distribution throughout the body but is strongly expressed in kidney in the apical and basolateral membranes of epithelial cells of proximal tubules and descending limb of loop of Henle[67,68]. Aquaporin-2, the vasopressin-regulated water channel, is found within cytoplasmic vesicles and the apical membrane of principal cells of cortical and medullary collecting ducts[50,69]. Aquaporin-3 is localized to basolateral membranes of these same cells[70,71]. Aquaporin-4 is expressed in medullary vasa recta and basolateral membrane of principal cells of cortical and medullary collecting ducts[72]. Aquaporin-6 and 8 exist in the kidney cortex and medulla but cellular localization is still unknown[58,62]. Aquaporin-9, almost exclusively expressed in human adipose tissue, was found by Northern blot analysis to have faint expression within the kidney but again exact location is yet to be determined[63]. The aquaporins are constitutive within the membranes with the exception of secretion-regulated AQP_1 insertion in cholangiocytes in the bile duct and AVP-regulated insertion of AQP_2 in collecting ducts[73,74].

A possible AQP_1 null phenotype exists in individuals that lack the Colton antigen who appear to have little (<1%) or no AQP_1 but surprisingly show no clinical manifestation[75]. AQP_1 knockout mice, while ostensively normal, appear to be unable to concentrate urine to more than two- to threefold plasma osmolality possibly due to the inability to develop the normal hypertonicity of the medulla[76].

Studies on AQP_2 gene expression have shown upregulation of AQP_2 to occur in cases of dehydration, cirrhosis and chronic heart failure[77,78], while downregulation occurred in chronic lithium-treated rats, persistent hypokalaemia, chronic ureteral obstruction and rats fed low protein diets[79–82].

The rare congenital disease nephrogenic diabetes insipidus (NDI) results from either the X-linked mutation of the AVP binding receptor (V_2) or with an autosomal recessive mutation in the gene for AQP_2[83].

Dehydration studies in otherwise phenotypically normal AQP_4 knock-out mice showed a defect in their ability to concentrate their urine normally[84].

ONTOGENY IN DEVELOPING KIDNEY

AQUAPORIN-1 (AQP_1)

With immunohistochemistry, AQP_1 was detected in developing proximal tubules at 14 weeks of gestation and strongly expressed in proximal tubules and developing loops of Henle at 17 weeks in the human fetal kidney. At birth, the AQP_1 protein concentration was only 47% of the adult value[85]. Expression within the developing rat kidney differed to the human in that AQP_1 was not significant until 3 days before birth, with a major induction at the time of birth[86]. The ovine fetus showed AQP_1 expression within the metanephros at 41 days gestation with increasing levels of expression over gestation[48,87]. However, adult levels were not reached until 6 weeks' postpartum. The variation of expression between the rat, sheep and the human is most likely due to the relative immaturity of the rat kidney at birth compared with the human and sheep kidney at birth.

Both dexamethasone and angiotensin II could increase AQP_1 expression at mid-to-late gestation, predominantly by increasing the length and maturity of the proximal straight tubules.

AQUAPORIN-2 (AQP_2)

Immunolocalization detected AQP_2 protein in apical membranes in rat embryonic day 18 (E18d) fetal kidneys; expression became strong at 4 weeks and reached a maximum at 2 months[88]. The ovine fetus exhibited low mRNA levels present at 40 days, with an increased expression at mid-gestation eventually reaching 41% of adult levels in the pre-term fetal kidney[89]. Steroid treatment did not affect AQP_2 expression but infusion of Ang I in late gestation did increase AQP_2 expression two- to threefold. This was not due to a direct effect of Ang II on collecting duct cells, as these contain no AT_1 or AT_2 receptors[90]. It was most likely an indirect effect due to factors secreted by the interstitial cells[91].

AQUAPORIN-3 (AQP_3)

Studies within the rat fetal kidney have found AQP_3 weakly detectable at E18d with expression becoming distinct at 1–2 weeks after birth and remaining constant throughout life[88]. AQP_3 is present in mid-gestation ovine fetal kidneys (unpublished observation).

Why fetal urine is hypotonic

AVP is an antidiuretic hormone present in most mammals, binding to V_2-type receptors present on the basolateral membranes of principal cells within the cortical and medullary collecting ducts. This initiates an increase in intracellular adenylate cyclase, stimulating a rise in cAMP which activates cAMP-dependent protein kinases that induce insertion of intracellular AQP_2 water-channel proteins into the apical membrane thereby increasing collecting duct water. The adult sheep kidney has a high sensitivity to AVP with doses as small as 0.003 μg/h inducing an antidiuretic effect[92]. This high sensitivity is not seen in the kidney of patients with hereditary NDI due to mutations in either the V_2 receptor gene, preventing AVP from binding, or within the gene coding for AQP_2 water channel preventing AVP insertion of active channels into the membrane[83]. AVP release in the fetus can result from stress such as hypoxia, haemorrhage, umbilical cord constriction, hypotension and increased plasma osmolality induced by dehydration[93]. However, a given osmotic stimulus releases less AVP in the fetus than in the adult[94]. Although the fetal response is qualitatively identical to that of the adult, resulting in reduced urine flow and increased urine osmolality, the level of AVP needed to induce this response is far greater and maximum osmolality achieved far less in the fetus than in the adult[95,96]. AVP is present within the fetus very early in gestation[97]. The decreased sensitivity within the fetus could be due to fewer functional V_2 receptors being present, decreased efficiency of the AVP-receptor second messenger system or the insufficient expression of AQP_2 water channels. Nephrogenesis is complete at birth within the human and the sheep but development of collecting ducts to maturity is not complete until just before birth, with substantial growth occurring in the last third of gestation. The density and affinity of V_2 receptors are similar in adult and fetal sheep kidneys, suggesting that AVP receptors are present and functional at that stage in gestation[98]. Recent studies within the ovine fetus have indicated that AQP_2 expression was only 17% of the adult at 100 days of gestation, increasing to 41% near term (145–150 days)[89]. This increase in functional AQP_2 expression coincided with the decreasing concentrations of AVP needed to induce a negative free-water clearance. In the human fetus AQP_2 protein was detectable at 12 weeks of gestation, increasing to 34% of adult value at mid-gestation[85]. AQP_2 was barely detectable in the rat fetus at birth, increasing to full adult expression levels at 4 weeks correlating with morphogenesis of the kidney[88,99]. These results indicate that the lower sensitivity observed in the early gestation kidney is related to the immaturity of collecting ducts, that are increasing in length and complexity at this time and therefore are gradually increasing expression of AQP_2 within the kidney. This is combined with normal low levels of AVP of ≈ 0.6 pmol/l[96], in the unstressed fetus.

Urea transporters

Although the kidney has many different functions, one of high importance is the ability to concentrate the urine. Due to the relative impermeability of the nephron and initial collecting duct system, urea collects along the kidney tubules in a progressive concentration gradient until reaching the terminal inner medullary collecting duct where it accounts for half of the urine osmolality. It is necessary for a hypertonic environment to exist in the deep medulla for the mechanism of water conservation to be effective. Urea specific channels, known as urea transporters, have been cloned from kidney and erythrocyte membranes in the human, rat and rabbit. The urea transporters, when expressed in *Xenopus* oocytes, increase urea permeability over fourfold with no change in water or small non-electrolyte permeability while exhibiting inhibition by urea homologues[100,101]. The erythrocyte urea transporter in humans (HUT 11) is proposed to protect erythrocytes from damage when passing through the renal medulla, allowing them to keep cell volume relatively constant[102]. Vasopressin-regulated urea transporters have been found within the kidney of the human, rat and rabbit. Two mRNA transcripts with distinct tissue distribution have been cloned each showing a high percentage homology between the human, rat and rabbit (>88% homology)[103]. A 2.9–3.0 kb transcript, later called UT2, is expressed within the descending limb of short loops of Henle and responded to hydration changes within the rat[104,105]. A 4.0-kb transcript, later called UT1, is expressed within the terminal inner medulla and responded to changes in the protein content of the diet[104,105]. Recently a third urea transporter, with a greater homology to HUT11, was cloned within the rat (UT3) and was found to be expressed in the medulla and epithelium of urinary tracts[106]. This location indicates the possible role of UT3 in countercurrent exchange important for maintaining hypertonicity in the medulla.

Clinical implications of urea transporters are seen within the Kidd blood group antigens whereby the null phenotype, JK(a–b–) have erythrocytes that appear lysis resistant in a concentrated urea solution compared with JK-positive cells and patients exhibit an inability to concentrate urine completely. Erythrocytes from JK(a–b–) patients exhibited a lack of carrier-mediated urea transport leading to suggestions the Kidd antigen is the red cell urea transporter[107]. While there are suggestions that the Kidd antigen and urea transporter are the same due to the same physical localization in a region on chromosome 18, the studies are still not conclusive[108]. There are no ontogony studies published to date.

Renin–angiotensin system (RAS)

During fetal development, the major action of the RAS appears to be on the kidney where it acts to maintain GFR and ensure a high rate of urine production[109]. Evidence is also accumulating to suggest that Ang II, the active product of this system, is necessary for normal morphological development of the metanephros[6]. As detailed below, all components of this system – renin, angiotensinogen, angiotensin converting enzyme and the angiotensin receptors – are produced in the fetal meso- and metanephros from very early in gestation allowing for local production and action. Information from the human is described where available and compared to experimental studies in the ovine fetus.

LOCALIZATION OF COMPONENTS

RENIN

It is possible to detect the mRNA for renin in the human mesonephros from as early as 28–30 days' post-conception[111]. There have been varying reports on when renin expression first appears in the metanephros. It is clearly evident at 56 days of gestation[110] but it may be present much earlier in just a very few cells[112]. By immunohistochemistry, renin was first observed in the walls of blood vessels outside the kidney and was subsequently seen in renal artery branches and arterioles[112]. Renin granules have also been observed in mesangial cells and in arterioles distant from the glomerulus[113] with the distribution of renin-containing cells in the fetal kidney being more widespread than in the adult. In the ovine fetus, renin-containing cells have been identified in the meso- and metanephros from 41 days of gestation[14]. In sheep, levels of mRNA and renal renin content increased from mid-gestation and were greater than in the adult at all stages[114].

Renin concentrations in human fetal cord blood between 16 and 24 weeks have been found to be high[115] and total renin content, measured in human fetuses from 12 to 25 weeks, were also greater than the adult[116].

ANGIOTENSINOGEN

The liver is the major site of angiotensinogen production in the adult but a small amount can be produced in the kidney[117]. The mRNA has been detected in human fetal mesonephroi at about day 25 and in the metanephros at day 56[111]. The protein is found in proximal tubule cells at this age which is also the site of mRNA for angiotensinogen in the ovine fetus[14]. In the sheep, the angiotensinogen can be identified at 41 days of gestation in both the meso- and metanephroi[14].

ANGIOTENSIN-CONVERTING ENZYME (ACE)

In human fetuses, ACE activity has been found in lung tissue from weeks 10 to 24 weeks and in the kidney the protein was detected from weeks 11 to 30[118]. Cells which labelled for ACE were in both proximal tubules and collecting ducts[111]. ACE gene expression could be detected in the ovine fetal meso- and metanephroi at 41 days using a polymerase chain reaction (PCR) method[14].

ANGIOTENSIN RECEPTORS

The angiotensin receptors (types 1 and 2) have been identified in the human fetus from day 23 to 25 of gestation in the mesonephros. The AT_1 receptor appears in presumptive mesangial cells of the developing glomerulus whilst the mRNA for the AT_2 receptor is seen in peripheral interstitial cells[111]. By 56 days, both receptors are observed in the metanephros where the AT_1 mRNA was again seen in glomeruli (in juxtaglomerular cells) and also in the proximal tubular epithelium. The AT_2 receptor mRNA and protein was present in the cortex surrounding the glomeruli and in the medullary rays. Some cells expressing the AT_2 receptor were at the vascular pole. In the ovine fetus, where expression of the receptors is similar to the human, hybridization histochemistry was used to localize the AT_2 receptor to cells of the macula densa during the period of active nephrogenesis[90].

FUNCTION OF THE RAS

It has been observed in clinical practice that women treated with ACE inhibitors during pregnancy often had oligohydramnios. This was associated with anuria and lung abnormalities after birth[119]. As these drugs cross the placenta, it is assumed that the fetal RAS was inhibited, at least to some degree, and this caused a decrease in fetal GFR and urine flow. Experimentally, giving ACE inhibitors to the late gestation ovine fetus causes a decrease in fetal GFR and an increase in renal vascular resistance[109]. As the fetal kidney only receives 3% of the cardiac output and is thus relatively underperfused compared to the adult, Ang II may be necessary to maintain kidney perfusion and fetal urine flow.

The idea that Ang II may be important for the normal morphological growth of the kidney has mainly come from studies in rodents. Rats treated with ACE inhibitors after birth (when most of nephrogenesis takes place in the rodent) caused changes in the morphology of the developing kidneys[120]. In mice in which the angiotensinogen has been 'knocked out', there are structurally deformed kidneys giving further support that Ang II is required for normal morphogenesis[121,122].

It is assumed that the effects mentioned above are due to Ang II acting on the AT_1 receptor, of which there are two forms (AT_{1A} and AT_{1B}) in the rodent. When both AT_{1A} and AT_{1B} genes are knocked out, some of the mutant mice show grossly abnormal kidneys, with marked medullary hypoplasia[123]. It is suggested that hypoplasia of the papilla may be secondary to hydronephrosis occurring because of aberrant ureter development.

What may be the actions via the AT_2 receptor? The AT_2 receptor is expressed at much higher levels in the fetus than in the adult, where it is not readily detectable. It is speculated that binding to the AT_2 receptor may trigger apoptosis[124] or have some growth-promoting effect[125]. This is currently an area of great interest. The use of specific angiotensin-receptor blockers may give clues as to the role(s) of this receptor during development in the kidney.

Kallikrein–kinin

The renal tubular dysplasia associated with the use of ACE inhibitors may be a consequence of induced hypotension which could result from accumulated bradykinin. Kininases, including ACE, degrade bradykinin[126], therefore ACE inhibitors – known to produce a drop in fetal mean arterial pressure[109] – are likely to potentiate the renal vasodilatory effects of bradykinin. A local tissue kallikrein–kinin system exists in both the adult and fetal kidney and comprises the low-molecular-weight (LMW) kininogen which is hydrolysed by kallikreins (serine proteases) to produce bradykinins (rat) or Lys-bradykinin (other species), kinin receptors, and kininases to inactivate the kinins[126]. All components have been found in the fetal rat kidney[127]. There is growing evidence that intrarenal kinins are not only important modulators of renal haemodynamics and sodium and water balance, but also have mitogenic properties. At least two bradykinin receptor isoforms are known to exist – the B_1 and B_2 receptors. The above effects appear to be mediated by the latter. B_2 is a seven transmembrane-spanning G-protein coupled receptor with only one gene in human and murine species. In the fetal rat, B_2 receptor mRNA is up to 30-fold that of the adult, the majority being intrarenally restricted to the differentiating distal tubule and collecting ducts. Late in weaning, receptor expression is seen mainly in outer medulla. A preliminary study using the B_2-receptor antagonist HOE-140 showed evidence of renal hypoplasia in the neonate and tubular dilatation and interstitial fibrosis in the fetus. Intrarenal kinin accumulates during rat renal development due to the upregulation and activity of kallikrein – which increases greatly in the neonate towards weaning – and downregulation and activity of kininase II[128]. Kallikrein enzyme activity has been measured in ovine fetal urine in the last third of gestation, and increased significantly after 120 days[129]. In the mouse, mRNA for the renal tissue kallikrein mGK6 is found at day E19d in the distal tubule[130]. In conclusion, the reported increase in kallikrein activity and upregulation of B_2-receptor mRNA probably reflects a kinin modulatory role in nephron maturation. ACE inhibitors may prematurely elevate fetal intrarenal bradykinin levels leading to abnormal tubules and premature differentiation of developing nephric structures.

Eicosanoids

Eicosanoids are derivatives of arachidonic acid which is synthesized via serial desaturation of the essential fatty acid, linoleic acid. The eicosanoid family include prostaglandins, thromboxane, leukotrienes, monohydroxylated eicosatetraenoic acids (HETES), and eoxides of arachidonic acid. All are synthesized in the adult kidney, though not all at elevated levels[131], and the distribution of various products varies over different cell types within the kidney. There are also species differences in the predominant type of product, though PGE_2 seems to be ubiquitously produced in the most liberal quantity[132]. However, in one study, in fetal sheep kidney, $PGF_{2\alpha}$ was the predominant renal product found, early in pregnancy[133]. Vasodilator prostaglandins are produced in large amounts by fetal kidneys, and the urinary excretion rate is higher in premature human neonates than in children or adults[134]. These prostaglandins are produced by the action of the enzyme, cyclooxygenase, which can be inhibited by compounds such as aspirin and indomethacin. Cyclooxygenase has two isoforms, constitutively expressed cyclooxygenase 1 (COX-1) and cyclooxygenase 2 (COX-2) which is expressed as part of the inflammatory response, but appears to be constitutively expressed in rat kidney[135]. Specific anti-COX-2 agents, such as flosulide have been recently developed to circumvent the gastric and, ironically, renal side effects of non-specific anti-inflammatory treatment. However, recent *COX-2*, but not *COX-1* gene knockout studies in mice have demonstrated renal defects of a developmental origin. Neonatal defects included retarded development of the mesenchyme, resulting in fewer mature nephrons, suggestive that COX-2 has a role in ureteric bud induction of the metanephric mesenchyme. Unlike humans, murine renal development continues postnatally, accentuating some renal defects due to the differing function of the kidney to meet the demands of extrauterine existence. In the COX-2 –/– mice, nephric cyst formation and dysplasia developed and blood urea nitrogen and serum creatinine were elevated[136]. In human fetal kidneys, temporal expression of the COX-2 isoform in the podocytes of post-vascularised glomeruli has been observed and is suggestive of a potential regulatory role in glomerular haemodynamics. The abundant expression of COX-1 during renal development suggests this isoform is more important in humans than in murine species, with renal impairment resulting from indomethacin treatment during pregnancy (see below) thought to relate more to inhibition of this isoform. It should be noted, however, that flosulide, the specific COX-2 inhibitor, has been clinically associated with renal impairment[135]. Thus caution is warranted until the potential renal effects of these specific anti-cyclooxygenase agents in the human fetus are studied further.

The role of prostaglandins in the fetal kidney has been explored predominantly by the inhibition of prostaglandin synthesis with indomethacin. When indomethacin has been administered directly to the chronically cannulated ovine fetus, the effect has depended on the dose, and the time of administration. Larger doses, or single bolus doses, tended to have no effect on fetal urine flow, or to increase it[137,138] whilst lower doses, given over longer periods, caused an approximate 50% reduction in flow, some increase in urine osmolality, and small to medium increases in plasma AVP levels[139,140]. When a blocker of the AVP-V_2 receptor was given in association with the indomethacin, the urinary changes were ablated[139]. This suggests that the normal effect of indomethacin, in decreasing urine flow rate, is not necessarily mediated by blockade of endogenous renal prostaglandin effects, but indirectly via a change in AVP release. Whatever the mechanism, indomethacin treatment has been previously associated with oligohydramnios[141] and in women with polyhydramnios has generally been effective in reducing amniotic fluid volume, and, when tested, it has been shown to decrease human fetal urine production[142–144]. Indeed, if indomethacin is continued until birth, some functional impairment of neonatal renal function may persist[145,146] and can lead to renal failure[141]. A recent retrospective study into indomethacin's effects upon the neonate after treatment for premature labour showed an association between raised serum creatinine and indomethacin administered prior to birth. In those women studied – whose babies were born less than 31 weeks' gestation – renal effects were greatest in those neonates born within 48 hours of treatment. All the women had also been treated with steroids and thyrotrophin releasing hormone at 24–32 weeks' gestation[141].

Renal agenesis and congenital urinary tract malformations

The increased use of ultrasound in pregnancy has resulted in an increase in the diagnosis of renal malformations of the fetus. Prenatal diagnosis is important and enables either special obstetric management, termination of pregnancy and the possibility of intrauterine intervention.

BILATERAL RENAL AGENESIS (POTTER'S SYNDROME)

Renal agenesis may be due to a defect either in the ureteric bud, or in the metanephric blastema resulting in a failure of the ureteric bud to induce development in the metanephric blastema, as described earlier. On inspection, the baby has widely spaced eyes, sweeping epicanthic folds, turned down tip of the nose, small jaw, and low-set misshapen ears[147]. The infant passes no urine and dies within hours of birth from a respiratory failure caused by pulmonary hypoplasia[148,149]. Pulmonary hypoplasia, characterized by a reduced number of lung cells, airways and alveoli[150], is at least in part due to the absence of amniotic fluid. Amniotic fluid surrounds the developing fetus and allows symmetrical growth[151]. The lack of amniotic fluid – oligohydramnios – causes compression of the fetus resulting in fetal deformations such as those seen in Potter's syndrome. Urine input is essential to normal amniotic fluid volume. Fetal urine, in the human, is excreted into the amniotic fluid compartment from at least 12 weeks of gestation, and although amniotic fluid differs significantly in composition from fetal urine, a steady input of dilute fetal urine is essential for normal amniotic fluid volume maintenance. If there are no kidneys or if there is ureteral or urethral obstruction, oligohydramnios results after mid-gestation. Oligohydramnios produced by urinary bladder obstruction in the ovine fetus in the first half of gestation results in pulmonary hypoplasia and renal dysplasia similar to that found in humans with congenital obstructive uropathy[152,153]. In addition, decompression reverses the effects of urinary bladder obstruction on lungs and kidneys, and postnatal outcome largely depends on the age of onset and the duration of obstruction[152,154,155].

ROLE OF THE FETAL KIDNEYS – WHAT WE HAVE LEARNT FROM EXPERIMENTAL BILATERAL NEPHRECTOMY

Roles of the fetal kidneys in growth, lung development, regulation of arterial pressure and erythropoietin production have been studied experimentally in nephrectomized fetuses. Removal of both fetal kidneys after mid-gestation results in decreases in fetal arterial pressure and in extracellular and blood volumes, alters composition of fetal plasma, and in some cases is accompanied by growth retardation.

EFFECT ON BLOOD PRESSURE AND FETAL FLUIDS

Fetal kidneys are important for the maintenance of the normal fetal arterial pressure and normal volume and composition of fetal body fluids. Bilateral nephrectomy in the ovine fetus, performed at 125 days of gestation, caused a significant reduction in basal mean arterial pressure[156]. The decrease in fetal arterial pressure was slower to develop than the drop in plasma renin concentration, and it was greater than that obtained when the angiotensin II blocker saralasin is given to fetal sheep with kidneys[109], suggesting the RAS is not solely responsible for maintaining normal fetal arterial pressure. In late-gestation ovine fetuses, bilateral nephrectomy for 5–8 days resulted in a significant decrease in extracellular fluid volume, as expressed in ml/kg body weight (from 496 ml ± 39 on day 0 to 458 ml ± 44 on day 3)[157]. There was also a decrease in plasma chloride, without a change in plasma sodium, and doubling of plasma creatinine, phosphate and magnesium[5]. In nephrectomized fetuses infused with a non-pressor dose of angiotensin II (1.5 μg/kg/h) for 3 days, the progressive decreases in extracellular volume and plasma chloride were prevented, but values were not restored to those of intact fetuses[158].

EFFECT ON FETAL GROWTH

One of the subsequent effects of decreased blood pressure after bilateral nephrectomy is a decrease in blood flow which leads to fetal tissue hypoxia. In addition, redistribution of fetal blood occurs with shunting to the brain, heart and adrenal glands. These effects of fetal nephrectomy could at least in part be responsible for the fetal growth retardation seen in some models of fetal bilateral nephrectomy[159]. Another possible mechanism that leads to fetal growth retardation is loss of kidney-related growth factors. The kidney is the major site of epidermal growth factor (EGF), synthesis of which directly stimulates synthesis of insulin-like growth factor-I (IGF-I) in the renal collecting duct[160,161]. Although fetal nephrectomy leads to a transient increase in the plasma concentration of IGF-I, reduced effectiveness may occur because of an increase in IGF-binding proteins[162–164]. In humans, circulating levels of IGF-I directly correlated with birth weight[165].

TAKING OUT THE FETAL KIDNEY IS NOT EQUAL TO TAKING OUT ALL THE URINE

Whilst urine output is essential for maintenance of fetal fluids (amniotic-human, amniotic and allantoic-sheep) drainage of urine to the exterior does not give the same changes in extracellular fluid volume and composition as does removal of the kidneys. Several studies in chronically cannulated ovine fetuses have demonstrated that, despite prolonged fetal urine loss, the fetus is able to maintain its growth and fluid and electrolyte homeostasis by obtaining water and electrolytes initially from the amniotic and allantoic fluids and subsequently from its mother[166,167]. The fetal fluid sacs are important sources of water and electrolytes in situations of maternal dehydration and hyperthermia[168].

CONGENITAL URINARY TRACT OBSTRUCTION

The common causes of congenital obstructive uropathies are pyeloureteric junction anomaly, vesicoureteric junction anomaly, ureteroceles and posterior urethral valves[169]. Severe obstruction to the urine flow in congenital urinary tract malformations initially leads to a renal interstitial fibrosis and hydronephrosis, associated with tubular dilatation and epithelial cell atrophy[170]. If it is not corrected during nephrogenesis, abnormalities in maturation or differentiation of renal structures – renal dysplasia – occur[153]. Experimental obstruction during fetal development in rabbits[171] and sheep[172,173] demonstrated that the extent of renal dysplasia and oligohydramnios is largely dependent on the timing and severity of the obstruction. Although pathogenesis of the renal dysplasia is not fully elucidated, recent studies in rats[174] demonstrated that neonatal unilateral ureteral obstruction leads to a profound activation of the ipsilateral intrarenal renin–angiotensin system leading to a profound renal dysplasia. In addition to its haemodynamic role, Angiotensin II may activate fibrinogenesis through stimulation of transforming growth factor (TGF-β1)[175]. In the ovine fetal model of bilateral urinary obstruction renal TGF-β1 immunoreactivity was increased in both hydronephrotic and dysplastic kidneys. More interestingly, urinary TGF-β1 concentration was elevated in hydronephrotic but not dysplastic kidneys, suggesting that TGF-β1 could be used as a biological marker of hydronephrosis[176].

ASSESSMENT OF THE FETAL RENAL FUNCTION IN OBSTRUCTIVE UROPATHY

Prenatal evaluation of the fetal kidney function largely depends on fetal ultrasound findings of amniotic fluid volume and renal parenchymal structure and biochemical analysis of fetal urine.

ULTRASOUND AS A TOOL IN ASSESSMENT OF FETAL RENAL FUNCTION

In addition to providing the diagnosis of the anatomical site of an obstructing lesion, a detailed study can focus specifically on amniotic fluid volume, renal size and parenchymal architecture, as well as bladder fullness and function. The two most significant prognostic findings that can be obtained from prenatal sonography include the presence or absence of oligohydramnios and renal cysts.

When severe obstructive uropathy results in oligohydramnios before 24 weeks of gestation, both renal and pulmonary dysplasia develop, which usually preclude fetal survival[177]. Studies in a fetal lamb model and in human fetuses, with bilateral hydronephrosis and oligohydramnios, without evidence of renal dysplasia, have shown that correction of the fetal urinary tract obstruction led to restoration of urine flow, amniotic fluid volume and pulmonary and renal development[178–181]. However, sonographic visualisation of the renal cortical cysts in fetal obstructive uropathy invariably indicates irreversible renal dysplasia that is unlikely to benefit from urinary tract decompression. Although sonographic visualisation of renal cysts is possible as early as 20 weeks of gestation, when renal cysts are not visible sonographically, it is not possible to predict accurately the absence of fetal kidney dysplasia[182]. Since fetal renal function cannot be accurately determined from ultrasound alone, it has to be further evaluated by biochemical analysis of fetal urine obtained by vesicocentesis.

BIOCHEMICAL ANALYSIS OF FETAL URINE

The healthy fetus produces hypotonic urine. At 16 weeks (0.4) of gestation, human fetal urine solutes (obtained by an ultrasound-guided needle inserted into the fetal bladder) showed the following concentrations (mmol/l): sodium 80–150, potassium 3, calcium 0.21, phosphate 0.91, creatinine 0.1 and urea 0.008[183]. When human fetal urine was analysed just before birth, there was a significant decrease in sodium (44 mmol/l) and an increase in urea and creatinine, being 4.7 and 5.0 mmol/l, respectively. The urinary concentrations of calcium and phosphate were not different. Similar gestational changes in fetal urine composition have been shown in chronically cannulated ovine fetuses, at 0.5 gestation and term[184,185].

Elevation in urinary sodium, chloride, calcium and osmolality are good indices of fetal renal injury and may suggest irreversible renal dysplasia. Some authors[186,187] proposed multiple fetal urine sampling (at least three times at 48- to 72-hour intervals) to improve diagnostic accuracy, instead of using a single urine sample (initial tap). They found that a combination of sodium <100 mmol/l, osmolality <200 mOsmol/kg water and total protein <20 mg/dl at tap 3 or 4 was always associated with normal renal function. However, fetal urine electrolyte parameters did not prove always reliable for the prediction of renal dysplasia. Nicolini and colleagues[183] found fetal urinary calcium as a most sensitive marker in predicting renal dysplasia, with a calcium <1.3 mmol/l suggesting normal renal function. Small gestational variations in urinary calcium concentrations may allow calcium to be a more sensitive predictor of renal function than the other urinary electrolytes.

Recently, β_2-microglobulin (molecular weight of 11 800 Da) and α_1-microglobulin (molecular weight of 33 000 Da) have been proposed as more sensitive indices of renal function[188]. As small proteins, they pass through the glomerular basement membrane and are almost entirely reabsorbed by proximal renal tubular cells, therefore elevated urinary levels are suggestive of proximal renal tubular dysfunction. Values of β_2-microglobulin $\geq$ 13 mg/l are almost invariably suggestive of poor outcome[189]. Mandelbrot and colleagues examined 15 biochemical parameters, including β_2-microglobulin, from aspirated urine in fetuses with bilateral obstruction and suggested that the combination of urinary sodium <70 mmol/l and β_2-microglobulin <4 mg/l are the best predictors for normal fetal renal function[190].

Elevation in urinary *N*-acetyl-β-D-glucosaminidase (lysosomal enzyme present throughout the entire length of the nephron) correlated well with renal cellular injury in both human and animal studies[191–194]. The enzyme proved to be a good marker for the evaluation of subsequent recovery since the removal of the source of urinary obstruction returned the urinary levels of the enzyme to normal values. Therefore this enzyme could be a useful marker, in both detection of renal cellular injury and for the evaluation of recovery.

The use of proton nuclear magnetic resonance spectroscopy to measure low-molecular-weight metabolites such as amino acids, amines and sugars may allow clear indentification of fetuses with impaired renal function[195]. In addition, medullary osmolytes, taurine, myo-inositol, and trimethylamide-*N*-oxide (TMAO) could be potentially used in evaluation of fetal renal function[196].

RECOMMENDATION

In conclusion, relief of the ureteric obstruction (fetal intervention) may protect or improve renal function, but when the kidneys become dysplastic and oligohydramnios persists, pulmonary hypoplasia cannot be prevented and prenatal intervention should not be considered[197]. The most recent study[198] testing the value of prognostic markers predicting perinatal death and evaluating the theoretical potential of postoperative decompression recovery suggested that after 20 weeks of gestation there is a good correlation between markers predicting poor prognosis and severity of renal lesions. However, the value of the markers before 20 weeks of gestation should be reconsidered.

Conclusion

In the adult, the kidneys are required to retain water and excrete waste products, predominantly urea, and thus excrete a hypertonic urine. In the fetus, the kidneys are required to produce a large volume of dilute urine for amniotic (and allantoic) fluid maintenance. The nephrogenic diabetes insipidus state in the fetus is maintained by the special role of angiotensin II in the fetus[199], to maintain GFR, by the resistance to release of AVP, and by the slow onset of AQP_2 gene expression, limiting the efficacy of the endogenous AVP. Inability to excrete the dilute fetal urine impacts most strongly on fetal lung development.

REFERENCES

1. Barker DJP. *Mothers, Babies and Diseases in Later Life*. London: BMJ Publishing Group, 1994.
2. Konje JC, Bell SC, Morton JJ, de Chazal R, Taylor DJ. Human fetal kidney morphometry during gestation and the relationship between weight, kidney morphometry and plasma active renin concentration at birth. *Clin Sci* **91**:169–175, 1991.
3. Hinchcliffe SA, Lynch MRJ, Sargent PH, Howard CV, van Velzen D. The effect of intrauterine growth retardation on the development of renal nephrons. *Br J Obstet Gynaecol* **99**:296–301, 1992.
4. Kingdom JCP, McQueen J, Connell JMC, Whittle MJ. Fetal angiotensin II levels and vascular (type I) angiotensin receptors in pregnancies complicated by intrauterine growth retardation. *Br J Obstet Gynaecol* **100**:476–482, 1993.
5. Moritz KM, Wintour EM. Functional development of the meso- and metanephros. *Pediatr Nephrol* (in press), 1999.
6. Wintour EM, Alcorn D, Rockell MD. Development and function of the fetal kidney. In *Fetus and Neonate: Physiology and Clinical Applications* (eds A.B. Brace, M.A. Hanson & C.H. Rodeck), pp. 3–56. Cambridge: Cambridge University Press, 1998.
7. Vize PD, Seufert DW, Carroll TJ, Wallingford JB. Model systems for the study of kidney development: use of the pronephros in the analysis of organ induction and patterning. *Dev Biol* **188**:189–204, 1997.
8. Howland RB. Experiments on the effect of removal of the pronephros of *Amblystoma punctatum*. *J Exp Zool* **32**:335–384, 1921.
9. Davies J. Nephric development in the sheep with reference to the problem of the ruminant pronephros. *J Anat* **85**:6–11, 1951.
10. Sainio K, Hellstedt P, Kreidberg JA, Saxen L, Sariola H. Differential regulation of two sets of mesonephric tubules by WT-1. *Development* **124**:1293–1299, 1997.
11. Friebova-Zemanova Z. Formation of the chick mesonephros. *Anat Embryol* **161**:341–354, 1981.
12. Gaeth AP, Short RV, Renfree MB. The development of the urogenital system of the African elephant. *Aust Soc Reprod Biol Proc 28th Annual Conf Canberra September 29–October 1 1997*; Abstract 62, 1997.
13. de Martino C, Zamboni L. A morphologic study of the mesonephros of the human embryo. *J Ultrastruct Res* **16**:399–427, 1966.
14. Wintour EM, Alcorn D, Butkus A, Congiu M, Earnest L, Pompolo S, Potcnik SJ. Ontogeny of hormonal and excretory function of the meso- and meta-nephros in the ovine fetus. *Kid Int* **50**:1624–1633, 1996.
15. Esteban MA, Meseguer J, Ayala AG, Agulleiro B. Erythropoiesis and thrombopoiesis in the head-kidney of the sea bass (*Dicentrarchus labrax* L.): an ultrastructural study. *Arch Histol Cytol* **52**:407–419, 1989.
16. Catton WT. Blood cell formation in certain teleost fishes. *Blood* **6**:39–60, 1951.
17. Hatano O, Takakusu A, Normura M, Morohashi K. Identical origin of adrenal cortex and gonad revealed by expression profiles of Ad4 BP/SF-1. *Genes to Cells* **1**:663–671, 1996.
18. Parker KL, Schimmer BP. Steroidogenic factor 1: A key determinant of endocrine development and function. *Endocr Rev* **18**:361–377, 1997.
19. Updhyay S, Zamboni L. Preliminary observations on the role of the mesonephros in the development of the adrenal cortex. *Anat Rec* **202**:105–111, 1982.
20. Buehr M, Gu S, McLaren A. Mesonephric contributions to testis differentiation in the fetal mouse. *Development* **117**:273–281, 1993.
21. Zamboni L, Bezard J, Mauleon P. The role of the mesonephros in the development of the sheep fetal ovary. *Ann Biol Anim Biochem Biophys* **19**:1153–1178, 1979.
22. Fernandez-Teran M, Piedra ME, Simandl BK, Fallon JF, Ros MA. Limb initiation and development is normal in the absence of the mesonephros. *Dev Biol* **52**:589–606, 1997.
23. Kanwar YS, Frank AC, Kumar A, Ota K, Wallner E. Role of extracellular matrix, growth factors and proto-oncogenes in metanephric development. *Kid Int* **52**:589–608, 1997.

24. Horster M, Huber S, Tschop J, Dittrich G, Braun G. Epithelial nephrogenesis. *Pflugers Arch (Eur J Physiol)* **434**:647–660, 1997.
25. Bard JBL, Davies JA, Karavanova I, Lehtonen E, Sariola H, Vainio S. Kidney development: the inductive interactions. *Sem Cell Dev Biol* **7**:195–202, 1996.
26. Sariola H. Does the kidney express redundant or important molecules during nephrogenesis? *Exp Nephrol* **4**:70–76, 1996.
27. Lumbers ER. Development of renal function in the fetus: a review. *Reprod Fertil Deve* **7**:415–426, 1995.
28. Robillard JE, Smith FG, Segar JL, Guillery EN, Jose PA. Mechanisms regulating renal sodium excretion during development. *Pediatr Nephrol* **6**:205–213, 1992.
29. Ross MG, Ervin MG, Lam RW, Castro L, Leake RD, Fisher DA. Plasma atrial natriuretic peptide response to volume expansion in the ovine fetus. *Am J Obstet Gynecol* **157**:1292–1297, 1987.
30. Robillard JE, Weiner C. Atrial natriuretic factor in the human fetus: effect of volume expansion. *J Pediatr* **113**:552–555, 1988.
31. Towstoless MK, McDougall JG, Wintour EM. Gestational changes in renal responsiveness to cortisol in the ovine fetus. *Pediatr Res* **26**:6–10, 1989.
32. Moritz KM, Wintour EM. Renal, hormonal, and cardiovascular responses to chronic angiotensin I infusion in the ovine fetus. *Am J Physiol* **272**:R1912–R1917, 1997.
33. Wintour EM, Butkus D. Ontogeny of hormonal and excretory function of the meso- and metanephros in the ovine fetus. *Kid Int* **50**:1624–1633, 1996.
34. Zanjani ED, Ascensao JL, McGlave PB, Banisadre M, Ash RC. Studies on the liver to kidney switch of erythropoietin production. *J Clin Invest* **67**:1183–1188, 1981.
35. Liapis H, Roby J, Birkland TP, Davila RM, Ritter D, Parks WC. *In situ* hybridization of human erythropoietin in pre- and postnatal kidneys. *Pediatr Pathol Lab Med* **15**:875–883, 1995.
36. Lim GB, Jeyaseelan K, Wintour EM. Ontogeny of erythropoietin gene expression in the sheep fetus: effect of dexamethasone at 60 days of gestation. *Blood* **84**:460–466, 1994.
37. Wintour EM, Butkus A, Earnest L, Pompolo S. The erythropoietin gene is expressed strongly in the mammalian mesonephros. *Blood* **88**:3349–3353, 1996.
38. Forestier F, Daffos F, Catherine N, Renard M, Andreux J. Developmental haematopoiesis in normal human fetal blood. *Blood* **77**:2360–2363, 1991.
39. Thomas RM, Canning CE, Cotes PM, Linch DC, Rodeck CH, Rossiter CE, Heuhns ER. Erythropoietin and cord blood haemoglobin in the regulation of human fetal erythropoiesis. *J Obstet Gynaecol* **90**:795–800, 1983.
40. Moritz KM, Lim GB, Wintour EM. Developmental regulation of erythropoietin and erythropoiesis. *Am J Physiol* **273**:R1829–R1844, 1997.
41. Wintour EM, Clemons GK, Butkus A, Horvath A, Moritz K, Towstoless MK. Immunoreactive erythropoietin concentration and haemoglobin type in the perinatal period in sheep of various haemoglobin genotypes. *J Dev Physiol* **14**:259–265, 1990.
42. Lim GB, Moritz K, Jeyaseelan K, Wintour EM. Effect of haemorrhage and nephrectomy on erythropoietin gene expression in the ovine fetus. *Mole Cell Endocrin* **117**:101–109, 1996.
43. Lim GB, Dodic M, Earnest L, Jeyaseelan K, Wintour EM. Regulation of erythropoietin gene expression in fetal sheep by glucocorticoids. *Endocrinology* **137**:1658–1663, 1996.
44. Gorin NB, Yancey SB, Cline J, Revel JP, Horwitz J. The major intrinsic protein (MIP) of the bovine lens fiber membrane. *Cell* **39**:49–59, 1984.
45. Preston GM, Agre P. Isolation of the cDNA for erythrocyte integral membrane protein of 28 kilodaltons: member of an ancient channel family. *Proc Natl Acad Sci USA* **88**:11110–11114, 1991.
46. Deen PMT, Dempster JA, Wieringa B, Van Os CH. Isolation of a cDNA for a rat CHIP28 water channel: high mRNA expression in kidney cortex and inner medulla. *Biochem Biophys Res Comm* **188**:1267–1273, 1992.
47. Patil RV, Yang X, Saito I, Coca-Prados M, Wax MB. Cloning of a novel cDNA homologous to CHIP28 water channel from ocular ciliary epithelium. *Biochem Biophys Res Comm* **204**: 861–866, 1994.
48. Wintour EM, Earnest L, Alcorn D, Butkus A, Shandley L, Jeyaseelan K. Ovine AQP_1: cDNA cloning, ontogeny and control of renal gene expression. *Pediatr Nephrol* **12**:545–553, 1998.
49. Fushimi K, Uchida S, Hara Y, Hirata Y, Marumo F, Sasaki S. Cloning and expression of apical membrane water channel of rat kidney collecting tubule. *Nature* **361**:549–552, 1993.
50. Sasaki S, Fushimi K, Saito F. *et al.* Cloning, characterization, and chromosomal mapping of human aquaporin of collecting duct. *J Clin Invest* **93**:1250–1256, 1994.
51. Ishibashi K, Sasaki S, Fushima K. *et al.* Molecular cloning and expression of a member of the aquaporin family with permeability to glycerol and urea in addition to water expressed at the basolateral membrane of kidney collecting duct cells. *Proc Natl Acad Sci USA* **91**:6269–6273, 1994.
52. Inase N, Fushimi K, ishibashi K, Uchida S, Ichioka M, Sasaki S, Marumo F. Isolation of human aquaporine 3 gene. *J Biol Chem* **270**:17913–17916, 1995.
53. Jung JS, Bhat RV, Preston GM, Guggino WB, Baraban JM, Agre P. Molecular characterization of an aquaporin cDNA from brain; candidate osmoreceptor and regulator of water balance. *Proc Natl Acad Sci USA* **91**:13052–13056, 1994.
54. Hasegawa H, Ma T, Skach W, Matthay MA, Verkman AS. Molecular cloning of a mercurial insensitive water channel expressed in selected water transporting tissues. *J Biol Chem* **269**:5497–5500, 1994.
55. Yang G, Ma T, Verkman AS. cDNA cloning, gene organization and chromosomal localization of a human mercurial insensitive water channel. *J Biol Chem* **270**:22907–22913, 1995.
56. Lee MD, Bhakta KY, Raina S. *et al.* The human aquaporin-5 gene. *J Biol Chem* **271**:8599–8604, 1996.
57. Raina S, Preston GM, Guggino WB, Agre P. Molecular cloning and characterization of an aquaporin cDNA from salivary, lacrimal, and respiratory tissues. *J Biol Chem* **270**:1908–1912, 1995.
58. Ma T, Yang B, Kuo W-L, Verkman AS. cDNA cloning and gene structure of a novel water channel expressed exclusively in human kidney: evidence for a gene cluster of aquaporins at chromosome locus 12q13. *Genomics* **35**:543–550, 1996.
59. Ishibashi K, Kuwahara M, Gu Y. *et al.* Cloning and functional expression of a new water channel abundantly expressed in the testis permeable to water, glycerol and urea. *J Biol Chem* **272**:20782–20786, 1997.
60. Ishibashi K, Kuwahara M, Kageyama Y, Toshaka A, Marumo F, Sasaki S. Cloning and functional expression of a second new aquaporin abundantly expressed in testis. *Biochem Biophys Res Comm* **237**:714–718, 1997.
61. Koyama Y, Yamamoto T, Kondo D. *et al.* Molecular cloning of a new aquaporin from rat pancreas and liver. *Biochemistry* **272**:30329–30333, 1997.
62. Ma T, Yang B, Verkman AS. Cloning of a novel water and urea-permeable aquaporin from mouse expressed strongly in colon, placenta, liver and heart. *Biochem Biophys Res Comm* **240**:324–328, 1997.
63. Kuriyama H, Kawamoto S, Ishida N. *et al.* Molecular cloning and expression of a novel human aquaporin from adipose tissue with glycerol permeability. *Biochem Biphys Res Comm* **241**:53–58, 1997.
64. Cheng A, Van Hoek AN, Yeager M, Verkman AS, Mitra AK. Three dimensional organization of a human water channel. *Nature* **387**:627–630, 1997.
65. Walz T, Hirai T, Murata K. *et al.* The three dimensional structure of aquaporin-1. *Nature* **387**:624–627, 1997.
66. Bai L, Fushimi K, Sasaki S, Marumo F. Structure of aquaporin-2 vasopressin water channel. *J Biol Chem* **271**:5171–5176, 1996.
67. Sabolic I, Valenti G, Verbavatz J, Van Hoek AN, Verkman AS, Ausiello DA, Brown D. Localisation of the CHIP28 water channel in rat kidney. *Am J Physiol* **263**:C1225–C1233, 1992.
68. Bondy C, Chin E, Smith BL, Preston GM, Agre P. Developmental gene expression and tissue distribution of the CHIP28 water-channel protein. *Proc Natl Acad Sci USA* **90**:4500–4504, 1993.
69. Sasaki S, Fushimi K, Saito H. *et al.* Cloning, characterization and chromosomal mapping of human aquaporin of collecting duct. *J Clin Invest* **361**:549–552, 1993.
70. Echevarria M, Windhager EE, Tate SS, Frindt G. Cloning and expression of AQP3, a water channel from the medullary collecting duct of rat kidney. *Proc Natl Acad Sci USA* **91**:10997–11001, 1994.
71. Ecelbarger CA, Terris J, Frindt G, Echevarria M, Marples D, Nielsen S,

Knepper MA. Aquaporin-3 water channel localization and regulation in rat kidney. *Am J Physiol* **269**:F663–F672, 1995.
72. Frigeri A, Gropper MA, Turck CW & Verkman AS. Immunolocalization of the mercurial-insensitive water channel and glycerol intrinsic protein in epithelial cell plasma membranes. *Proc Natl Acad Sci USA* **92**:4328–4331, 1998.
73. Marinelli RA, Pham L, Agre P, La Russo NF. Secretin promotes osmotic water transport in rat cholangiocytes by increasing aquaporin-1 water channels in plasma membrane. *J Biol Chem* **272**:12984–12988, 1997.
74. Knepper MA, Inoue T. Regulation of aquaporin-2 water channel trafficking by vasopressin. *Curr Opin Cell Biol* **9**:560–564, 1997.
75. Preston GM, Smith BL, Zeidel ML, Moulds JJ & Agre P. Mutation in aquaporin-1 in phenotypically normal humans without functional CHIP water channels. *Science* **265**:1585–1587, 1994.
76. Ma T, Yang B, Gillespie A, Carlson EJ, Epstein CJ, Verkman AS. Severely impaired urinary concentrating ability in transgenic mice lacking aquaporin-1 water channels. *J Biol Chem* **273**:4296–4299, 1998.
77. Asahina Y, Izumi N, Enomoto N, Sasaki S, Fushimi K, Marumo F, Sato C. Increased gene expression of water channel in cirrhotic rat kidneys. *Hepatology* **21**:169–173, 1995.
78. Xu D, Ohara P. Upregulation of aquaporin-2 water channel expression in chronic heart failure rat. *J Clin Invest* **99**:1500–1505, 1997.
79. Marples D, Christensen S, Christensen E, Ottosen PD, Nielsen S. Lithium-induced downregulation of aquaporin-2 water channel expression in rat kidney medulla. *J Clin Invest* **95**:1838–1845, 1995.
80. Marples D, Frøkiær J, Dorup J, Knepper MA, Nielsen S. Hypokalemia-induced downregulation of aquaporin-2 water channel expression in rat kidney medulla and cortex. *J Clin Invest* **97**:1960–1968, 1996.
81. Frøkiær J, Marples D, Knepper MA, Nielsen S. Bilateral ureteral obstruction downregulates expression of vasopressin-sensitive AQP-2 water channel in rat kidney. *Am J Physiol* **270**: F657–F668, 1996.
82. Sands JM, Naruse M, Jacobs JD, Wilcox JN, Klein JD. Changes in aquaporin-2 protein contribute to the urine concentrating defect in rats fed a low-protein diet. *J Clin Invest* **97**: 2807–2814, 1996.
83. Deen PMT, Verdijk MAJ, Knoers NVAM, Wieringa B, Monnens LAH, Van Os CH. van Oost, BA. Requirement of human renal water channel aquaporin-2 for vasopressin-dependent concentration of urine. *Science* **264**:92–95, 1994.
84. Ma T, Yang B, Gillespie A, Carlson EJ, Verkman AS. Generation and phenotype of a transgenic knockout mouse lacking the mercurial insensitive water channel aquaporin-4. *J Clin Invest* **100**:957–962, 1997.
85. Devuyst O, Burrow CR, Smith BL, Agre P, Knepper MA, Wilson PD. Expression of aquaporins-1 and -2 during nephrogenesis and in autosomal dominant polycystic kidney disease. *Am J Physiol* **40**:F169–F183, 1996.
86. Smith BL, Baumgarten R, Nielson S, Raben D, Zeidel ML, Agre P. Concurrent expression of erythroid and renal aquaporin CHIP and appearance of water channel activity in perinatal rats. *J Clin Invest* **92**:2035–2041, 1993.
87. Butkus A, Alcorn D, Earnest L, Moritz K, Giles M, Wintour EM. Expression of aquaporin-1 (AQP_1) in the adult and developing sheep kidney. *Biol Cell* **89**:313–320, 1997.
88. Yamamoto T, Sasaki S, Fushimi K. *et al.* Expression of AQP family in rat kidneys during development and maturation. *Am J Physiol* **41**:F198–F204, 1997.
89. Butkus A, Earnest L, Jeyaseelan K, Moritz K, Johnston H, Tenis N, Wintour EM. Ovine AQP_2–cDNA cloning, ontogeny and control of renal gene expression. *Pediatric Nephrology* (in press), 1999.
90. Butkus A, Albison A, Alcorn D. *et al.* Ontogeny of angiotensin II receptors, types 1 and 2, in ovine mesonephros and metanephros. *Kid Int* **51**:628–636, 1997.
91. Maric C, Aldred GP, Antoine AM *et al.* Effects of angiotensin II on cultured rat renomedullary interstitial cells are mediated by AT_{1A} receptors. *Am J Physiol* **271**:F1020–F1028, 1996.
92. Bell RJ, Laurence BM, Meehan PJ, Congiu M, Scoggings BA, Wintour EM. Regulation and function of arginine vasopressin in pregnant sheep. *Am J Physiol* **250**:F777–F780, 1986.
93. Ervin MG. Perinatal fluid and electrolyte regulation role of arginine vasopressin. *Semin Perinatol* **12**:134–142, 1988.
94. Bell RJ, Congiu M, Hardy KJ, Wintour EM. Gestation-dependent aspects of the response of the ovine fetus to the osmotic stress induced by maternal water deprivation. *Quart J Exp Physiol* **69**:187–195, 1984.
95. Wintour EM, Congiu M, Hardy KJ, Hennessy DP. Regulation of urine osmolality in fetal sheep. *Quart J Exp Physiol* **67**:427–435, 1982.
96. Horne RSC, MacIsaac RJ, Moritz KM, Tangalakis K, Wintour EM. Effect of arginine vasopressin and parathyroid hormone-related protein on renal function in the ovine foetus. *Clin Exper Pharmacol Physiol* **20**:569–577, 1993.
97. Levidiotis M, Oldfield B, Wintour EM. Corticotrophin-releasing factor and arginine vasopressin fibre projections to the median eminence of fetal sheep. *Neuroendocrinology* **46**:453–456, 1987.
98. Kullama LK, Ross MG, Lam R, Leake RD, Ervin MG, Fisher DA. Ovine maternal and fetal renal vasopressin receptor response to maternal dehydration. *Am J Obstet Gynecol* **167**:1717–1722, 1992.
99. Yasui M, Marples D, Belusa R, Eklof AC, Celsi G, Nielsen S, Aperia A. Development of urinary concentrating capacity: role of aquaporin 2 (AQP2). *Am J Physiol* **271**:F461–F468, 1996.
100. Hasegawa H, Verkman AS. Functional expression of cAMP-dependent and independent urea transporters in *Xenopus* oocytes. *Am J Physiol* **265**:C514–C520, 1993.
101. Marital S, Olives B, Abrami L. *et al.* Functional differentiation of the human red blood cell and kidney urea transporters. *Am J Physiol* **271**:F1264–F1268, 1996.
102. Macey RI, Yousef LW. Osmotic stability of red cells in renal circulation requires rapid urea transport. *Am J Physiol* **254**:C669–C674, 1988.
103. Olives B, Marital S, Mattei MG, Matassi G, Rousselet G, Ripoche P, Cartron JP, Bailly P. Molecular characterization of a new urea transporter in the human kidney. *FEBS Lett* **386**:156–160, 1996.
104. You G, Smith CP, Kanal Y, Lee W, Stelzner M, Hediger MA. Cloning and characterization of the vasopressin-regulated urea transporter. *Nature* **365**:844–847, 1993.
105. Smith CP, Lee WS, Marital S, Knepper MA, You G, Sands JM. Cloning and regulation of expression of the rat kidney urea transporter (rUT2). *J Clin Invest* **96**:1556–1563, 1995.
106. Tsukaguchi H, Shayakul C, Berger UV, Tokui T, Brown D, Hediger MA. Cloning and characterization of the urea transporter UT3: localization in rat kidney and testis. *J Clin Invest* **99**:1506–1515, 1997.
107. Gillin AG, Sands JM. Urea transport in the kidney. *Semin Nephrol* **13**:146–154, 1993.
108. Olives B, Mattei MG, Huet M, Neau P, Martial S, Cartron JP, Bailly P. Kidd blood group and urea transport function of human erythrocytes are carried by the same protein. *J Biol Chem* **270**:15607–15610, 1998.
109. Lumbers ER. Functions of the renin – angiotensin system during development. *Clin Exp Pharmacol Physiol* **22**:499–505, 1995.
110. Celio MR, Groscurth P, Inagami T. Ontogeny of renin immunoreactive cells in the human kidney. *Anat Embryol* **173**:149–155, 1985.
111. Schutz S, Le Moullec J-M, Corvol P, Gasc J-M. Early expression of all the components of the renin – angiotensin system in human development. *Am J Pathol* **149**:2067–2079, 1996.
112. Phat VN, Camilleri JP, Bariety J, Galtier M, Baviera E, Corvol P, Menard J. Immunohistochemical characterization of renin-containing cells in the human juxtaglomerular apparatus during embryonal and fetal development. *Lab Invest* **45**:387–390, 1981.
113. Graham PC, Kingdom JCP, Raweily EA, Gibson AAM, Llindop GBM. Distribution of renin-containing cells in the developing human kidney: an immunocytochemical study. *Br J Obstet Gynaecol* **99**:765–769, 1992.
114. Carbone GMR, Sheikh AU, Rogers S, Brewer G, Rose JC. Developmental changes in renin gene expression in ovine kidney cortex. *Am J Physiol* **264**:R591–R596, 1993.
115. Symonds EM, Craven DJ, Rodeck CH. Fetal plasma renin and renin substrate in mid-trimester pregnancy. *Br J Obstet Gynaecol* **92**:618–621, 1985.
116. Taylor GM, Peart WS, Porter KA, Zondek LH, Zondek T. Concentration and molecular forms of active and inactive renin in human and fetal kidney, amniotic fluid and adrenal gland: evidence for renin–angiotensin system hyperactivity in 2nd trimester of pregnancy. *J Hypertens* **4**:121–129, 1986.

117. Ohkubo H, Nakayama K, Tanaka T, Nakanishi S. Tissue distribution of rat angiotensinogen mRNA and structural analysis of its heterogeneity. *J Biol Chem* **261**:319–323, 1986.
118. Mounier F, Hinglais N, Sich M, Gros F, Lacoste M, Deris Y, Alhenc-Gelas F, Gubler M. Ontogenesis of angiotensin-1 converting enzyme in human kidney. *Kid Int* **32**:684–690, 1987.
119. Shotan A, Widerhorn J, Hurst A, Elkayam U. Risks of angiotensin-converting enzyme inhibition during pregnancy: experimental and clinical evidence, potential mechanisms, and recommendations for use. *Am J Med* **96**:451–456, 1994.
120. Alcorn D, McCausland JE, Maric C. Angiotensin receptors and development: the kidney. *Clin Exper Pharmacol Physiol* **23**:S88–S92, 1996.
121. Niimura F, Labosky PA *et al.* Gene targeting in mice reveals a requirement for angiotensin in the development and maintenance of kidney morphology and growth factor regulation. *J Clin Invest* **96**:2947–2954, 1995.
122. Kim H-S, Krege JH, Kluckman KD *et al.* Genetic control of blood pressure and the angiotensinogen locus. *Proc Natl Acad Sci USA* **92**:2735–2739, 1995.
123. Tsuchida S, Matsusaka T, Chen X *et al.* Murine double nullizygotes of the angiotensin type 1_A and 1_B receptor genes duplicate severe abnormal phenotypes of angiotensinogen nullizygotes. *J Clin Invest* **101**:755–760, 1998.
124. Kakuchi J, Ichiki T, Kiyama S, Hogan BLM, Fogo A, Inagami T, Ichikawa I. Developmental expression of renal angiotensin II receptor genes in the mouse. *Kid Int* **47**:140–147, 1995.
125. Stoll M, Meffert S, Stroth U, Unger T. Growth or antigrowth: angiotensin and the endothelium. *J Hypertens* **13**:1529–1534, 1995.
126. El-Dahr SS. Developmental biology of the renal kallikrein–kinin system. *Pediatr Nephrol* **8**:624–631, 1994.
127. El-Dahr SS, Chao S. Spatial and temporal expression of kallikrein and its mRNA during nephron maturation. *Am J Physiol* **262**:F705–F711, 1992.
128. El-Dahr SS, Figueroa CD, Gonzalez CB, Muller-Esterl W. Ontogeny of bradykinin B_2 receptors in the rat kidney: implications for segmental nephron maturation. *Kid Int* **51**:739–749, 1997.
129. Robillard JE, Lawton WJ, Weismann DN, Sessions C. Developmental aspects of the renal kallikrein-like activity in fetal and newborn lambs. *Kid Int* **22**:594–601, 1982.
130. Penschow JD, Coghlan JP. Sites of glandular kallikrein gene expression in fetal mice. *Mole Cell Endocrinol* **88**:23–30, 1992.
131. Schlondorff D, Ardaillou R. Prostaglandins and other arachidonic acid metabolites in the kidney. *Kid Int* **29**:108–119, 1986.
132. Mene P, Dunn MJ, Seldin DW, Giebish G. Vascular, glomerular, and tubular effects of angiotensin II, kinins, and prostaglandins. In *The Kidney: Physiology and Pathophysiology* 2nd edn. New York: Lippencott-Raven Press, 1992.
133. Pace-Asciak CR. Biosynthesis and catabolism of prostaglandins during animal development. *Adv Prost Thrombox Res* **1**:35–46, 1976.
134. Seikaly MG, Arant BS. Development of renal hemodynamics: glomerular filtration and renal blood flow. *Clin Perinatol* **19**:1–13, 1992.
135. Komhoff M, Hermann-Josef G, Thomas K, Hennsjoerg W, Seyberth HW, Nusing RM. Localization of cyclooxygenase-1 and 2 in adult and fetal human kidney: implications for renal function. *Am J Physiol* **272**:F460–F468, 1997.
136. Dinchuk JE, Car BD, Focht RJ *et al.* Renal abnormalities and an altered inflammatory response in mice lacking cyclooxygenase II. *Nature* **378**:406–409, 1995.
137. Stevenson KM, Lumbers ER. Effects of angiotensin II in fetal sheep and modification on its actions by indomethacin. *J Physiol (Lond)* **487**:147–158, 1995.
138. Walker MPR, Moore TR, Brace RA. Urinary and cardiovascular responses to indomethacin infusion in the ovine fetus. *Am J Obstet Gynecol* **167**:834–843, 1991.
139. Walker MPR, Moore TR, Brace RA. Indomethacin and arginine vasopressin interaction in the fetal kidney: a mechanism of oliguria. *Am J Obstet Gynecol* **171**:1234–1241, 1994.
140. Wlodek ME, Harding R, Thorburn GD. Effects of inhibition of prostaglandin synthesis on flow and composition of fetal urine, lung liquid, and swallowed fluid in fetal sheep. *Am J Obstet Gynecol* **170**:186–195, 1994.
141. Souter D, Harding J, McGowan L, O'Donnell C, McLeay E, Baxendale H. Antenatal indomethacin – adverse fetal effects confirmed. *Aust N Z J Obstet Gynaec* **38**:11–16, 1998.
142. Kirshon B, Mari G, Moise KJ. Indomethacin therapy in the treatment of symptomatic polyhydramnios. *Obstet Gynecol* **75**:202–205, 1990.
143. Kirshon B, Moise KJ, Wasserstrum N, Ou C, Huhta JC. Influence of short-term indomethacin therapy on fetal urine output. *Obstet Gynecol* **72**:51–53, 1988.
144. Mamopoulos M, Assimakopoulos E, Reece A, Andreou A, Zheng X, Mantalenakis S. Maternal indomethacin therapy in the treatment of polyhydramnios. *Am J Obstet Gynecol* **162**:1225–1229, 1990.
145. Heijden AJ, Provoost AP, Nauta J, Grose W, Oranje WA, Wolff ED, Sauer PJJ. Renal functional impairment in preterm neonates related to intrauterine indomethacin exposure. *Pediatr Res* **24**:644–648, 1988.
146. Van den Veyver IB, Moise KJ. Prostaglandin synthetase inhibitors in pregnancy. *Obstet Gynecol Surv* **48**:493–502, 1993.
147. Potter EL. Facial characteristics of infants with bilateral renal agenesis. *Am J Obstet Gynecol* **51**:885–890, 1946.
148. Bain AD, Scott JS. Renal agenesis and severe urinary tract dysplasia; a review of 50 cases with a particular reference to the associated abnormalities. *Br Med J* **i**:841–846, 1960.
149. Potter EL. Bilateral absence of ureters and kidneys. *Obstet Gynecol* **25**:3–12, 1965.
150. Hooper SB, Harding R. Fetal lung liquid: A major determinant of the growth and functional development of the fetal lung. *Clin Exper Pharmacol Physiol* **22**:235–247, 1995.
151. Brace RA. Physiology of amniotic fluid volume regulation. *Clin Obstet Gyn* **40**:280–289, 1997.
152. Peters CA, Docimo SG, Luetic T, Reid LM, Retik AB, Mandell J. Effect of *in utero* vesicostomy on pulmonary hypoplasia in the fetal lamb with bladder outlet obstruction and oligohydramnios: a morphometric analysis. *J Urol* **146**:1178–1183, 1991.
153. Peters CA, Carr MC, Lais A, Retik AB, Mandell J. The response of the fetal kidney to obstruction. *J Urol* **148**:503–509, 1992.
154. Harrison MR, Nakayama DL, Noall R, de Lorimier AA. Correction of congenital hydronephrosis *in utero*. II. Decompression reverses the effect of obstruction on the fetal lung and urinary tract. *J Pediatr Surg* **17**:965–974, 1982.
155. Glick PL, Harrison MR, Adzick NS, Noall R, Villa RL. Correction of congenital hydronephrosis *in utero*. IV. *In utero* decompression prevents renal dysplasia. *J Pediatr Surg* **19**:649–657, 1984.
156. Anderson DF, Barbera A, Faber JJ. Substantial reductions in blood pressure after bilateral nephrectomy in fetal sheep. *Am J Physiol* **266**:H17–H20, 1994.
157. Gibson KJ, Lumbers ER. The effects of bilateral nephrectomy on the volume and composition of fetal body fluids. *Proc Austral Soc Med Res* Abstract 032, 1993.
158. Gibson KJ. Personal communication, 1998.
159. Karnak I, Adrian F, Tanyel FC, Muftuoglu S, Cakar N, Buyukpamukcu N, Hicsonmez A. The effects of nephrectomy on the developing fetus. *Eur J Pediatr Surg* **6**:270–273, 1996.
160. Rogers SA, Miller SB, Hammerman MR. Growth hormone stimulates *IGF-I* gene expression in isolated rat renal collecting duct. *Am J Physiol* **259**:F474–F479, 1990.
161. Rogers SA, Miller SB, Hammerman MR. Enhanced renal IGF-I expression following partial kidney infarction. *Am J Physiol* **264**:F963–F967, 1993.
162. Blum WF, Ranke MB, Keitzmann K, Tonshoff B, Mehis O. Growth hormone resistance and inhibition of somatomedin activity by excess of insulin-like binding protein in uraemia. *Pediatr Nephrol* **5**:539–544, 1991.
163. Iwamoto HS, McConnell CJ. Effects of fetal nephrectomy on insulin-like growth factors and their binding proteins in sheep. *Biol Neonate* **71**:92–101, 1997.
164. Beanland C, Browne C, Young R, Owens J, Walton P, Thorburn G. Fetal plasma insulin-like growth factor-binding protein-3 concentrations are elevated following bilateral nephrectomy in fetal sheep. *Reprod Fertil Dev* **7**:345–349, 1995.
165. Fant M, Salafia C, Baxter RC, Schwander J, Vogel C, Pezzullo J, Moya FR. Circulating levels of IGFs and IGF binding proteins in human cord serum. Relationships to intra-uterine growth. *Regul Pept* **48**:29–39, 1993.

166. Wlodek ME, Harding R, Thorburn GD. Fetal–maternal fluid and electrolyte relationships during chronic urine loss in sheep. *Am J Physiol* **263**:F671–F679, 1992.
167. Gresham EL, Rankin JH, Makowski EL, Meschia G, Battaglia FC. An evaluation of fetal renal function in a chronic sheep preparation. *J Clin Invest* **51**:149–156, 1972.
168. Dickson KA, Harding R. Fetal and maternal fluid balance in sheep during hyperthermia with and without water deprivation. *Exp Physiol* **82**:777–789, 1997.
169. Mouriquand PDE, Wilcox D In *Fetus and Neonate: Physiology and Clinical Applications Volume 4: Body Fluids and Kidney Function* (eds R.A. Brace, M.A. Hanson & C.H. Rodeck), Chapter 7, pp. 177–206. Cambridge: Cambridge University Press, 1998.
170. Moeller JC, Skriver E, Olsen S, Maunsbauch AB. Ultrastructural analysis of human proximal tubules and cortical interstitium in chronic renal disease (hydronephrosis). *Virchows Arch Pathol Anat* **402**:209–237, 1984.
171. McVary KT, Maizels M. Urinary obstruction reduces glomerulogenesis in the developing kidney: a model in the rabbit. *J Urol* **142**:646–651, 1989.
172. Beck AD. The effect of intra-uterine urinary obstruction upon the development of the fetal kidney. *J Urol* **105**:784–789, 1971.
173. Glick PL, Harrison MR, Noall RA, Villa RL. Correction of congenital hydronephrosis *in utero*. III. Early mid-trimester ureteral obstruction produces renal dysplasia. *J Pediatr Surg* **18**:681–687, 1983.
174. Yoo KH, Norwood VF, El-Dahr SS, Yosipiv I, Chevalier RL. Regulation of angiotensin II AT_1 and AT_2 receptors in neonatal ureteral obstruction. *Am J Physiol* **273**:R503–R509, 1997.
175. Chung KH, Gomez RA, Chevalier RL. Regulation of renal growth factors and clusterin by angiotensin AT_1 receptors during neonatal ureteral obstruction. *Am J Physiol* **268**:F1117–F1123, 1995.
176. Medjebeur AA, Bussieres L, Gasser B, Gimonet V, Laborde K. Experimental bilateral urinary obstruction in fetal sheep: transforming growth factor-β1 expression. *Am J Physiol* **273**:F372–F379, 1997.
177. Crombleholme TM, Harrison MR, Golbus MS *et al*. Fetal intervention in obstructive uropathy: prognostic indicators and efficacy of intervention. *Am J Obstet Gynecol* **162**:1239–1244, 1990.
178. Harrison MR, Golbus MS, Filly RA. Fetal surgery for congenital hydronephrosis. *New Eng J Med* **306**:591–593, 1982.
179. Harrison MR, Golbus MS, Filly RA. Management of the fetus with congenital hydronephrosis. *J Pediatr Surg* **17**:728–742, 1982.
180. Harrison MR, Ross N, Noall R. Correction of congenital hydronephros *in utero*. I. The model: fetal urethral obstruction produces hydronephrosis and pulmonary hypoplasia in fetal lambs. *J Pediatr Surg* **18**:247–256, 1983.
181. Harrison MR, Golbus MS, Filly RA. Fetal hydronephrosis: selection and surgical repair. *J Pediatr Surg* **22**:556–558, 1987.
182. Mahony BS, Filly RA, Callen PW. Fetal renal dysplasia: sonographic evaluation. *Radiology* **152**:143–146, 1984.
183. Nicolini U, Fisk NM, Rodeck CH, Beacham J. Fetal urine biochemistry: an index of renal maturation and dysfunction. *Br J Obstet Gynaecol* **99**:46–50, 1992.
184. Wintour EM, Alcorn D, McFarlane A, Moritz K, Potocnik SJ, Tangalakis K. Effect of maternal glucocorticoid treatment on fetal fluids in sheep at 0.4 gestation. *Am J Physiol* **266**:R1174–R1181, 1994.
185. Lingwood B, Hardy KJ, Horacek I, McPhee ML, Scoggins BA, Wintour EM. The effects of antidiuretic hormone on urine flow and composition in the chronically-cannulated ovine fetus. *Quart J Exp Physiol* **63**:315–330, 1978.
186. Johnson MP, Corsi P, Bradfield W. Sequential urinalysis improves evaluation of fetal renal function in obstructive uropathy. *Am J Obstet Gynecol* **173**:59–65, 1995.
187. Evans M, Sacks AJ, Johnson MP. Sequential invasive assessment of fetal renal function and the intrauterine treatment of fetal obstructive uropathies. *Obstet Gynecol* **77**:545–550, 1991.
188. Konda R, Sakai K, Ota S, Takeda A, Orikasa S. Follow-up study of renal function in children with reflux nephropathy after resolution of vesicoureteral reflux. *J Urol* **157**:975–979, 1997.
189. Lipitz S, Ryan G, Samuell C *et al*. Fetal urine analysis for the assessment of renal function in obstructive uropathy. *Am J Obstet Gynecol* **168**:174–179, 1993.
190. Mandelbrot L, Dumez Y, Muller F. Prenatal prediction of renal function in fetal obstructive uropathies. *J Perinatal Med* **19**:283–287, 1991.
191. Huland H, Gonnermann D, Werner B, Possin U. A new test to predict reversibility of hydronephrotic atrophy after stable partial unilateral ureteral obstruction. *J Urol* **140**:1591–1594, 1988.
192. Carr MC, Peters CA, Retik AB, Mandell J. Urinary levels of renal tubular enzyme *N*-acetyl-β-D-glucosaminidase in relation to grade of vesicoureteral reflux. *J Urol* **146**:654–656, 1991.
193. Carr MC, Peters CA, Retik AB, Mandell J. Urinary levels of the renal tubular *N*-acetyl-β-D-glucosaminidase in unilateral uropathy. *J Urol* **151**:442–448, 1994.
194. Fung LCT, Atala A. Constant elevation in renal pelvic pressure induces an increase in urinary *N*-acetyl-β-D-glucosaminidase in a non-obstructive porcine model. *J Urol* **159**:212–216, 1997.
195. Foxall PJD, Bewley S, Neild GH, Rodeck CH, Nicholson JK. Analysis of fetal and neonatal urine using proton nuclear magnetic resonance spectroscopy. *Arch Dis Child* **73**:F153–157, 1995.
196. Sizeland PCB, Chambers ST, Lever M, Bason LM, Robson RA. Organic osmolytes in human and other mammalian kidneys. *Kid Int* **43**:448–454, 1993.
197. Coplen DE. Prenatal intervention for hydronephrosis. *J Urol* **157**:2270–2277, 1998.
198. Daikha Dahmane F, Dommergues M, Muller F, Nancy F, Lacoste M, Beziau A, Dumez Y, Guber M. Development of human fetal kidney in obstructive uropathy: correlations with ultrasonography and urine biochemistry. *Kid Int* **52**:21–32, 1997.
199. Wintour EM. The renin–angiotensin system and the development of the kidney. *Trends Endocrinol Metabol* **8**:199–207, 1997.

Amniotic and fetal fluids

15

R.A. Brace

Introduction

The fetal composition is unique in comparison with the adult. The fetal body is composed of 95% water at the beginning of the fetal period whereas the adult is composed of 55–60% water[1]. Although fetal body water content decreases progressively throughout gestation, the fetus at term still contains considerably more water than the adult and averages 72% water. In addition to the high fluid content, the fetus is unique in that fluid fluxes per unit body weight in the fetus are almost an order of magnitude greater than in the adult, including fetal cardiac output, urine production, swallowing, lymph flow and transcapillary filtration.

The fetus also differs from the adult by being surrounded by liquid (i.e. the amniotic fluid) rather than air as in later life. Since everything enclosed by the chorion and placenta is fetal tissue, the fetal compartment (i.e. the combined fetal–amniotic space) is 98–99% water early in gestation, and this decreases to 77% water at term. Similar to the rapid fluid fluxes within the fetal body, there are large and rapid fluid fluxes between the fetus and its surrounding amniotic fluid (AF) which occur over multiple pathways. This chapter summarizes what is known about the fetal–amniotic fluids and their interactions.

Fetal fluid volumes

At the transition from the embryonic to fetal period, the fetus weighs 5–10 g, 95% of which is water[1]. In contrast to the adult, most of this is extracellular fluid located within the interstitial space. Thus the fetus might be considered to be in a state of hydration analogous to whole-body oedema in the adult. These fetal–adult differences are due primarily to a smaller intracellular volume (relative to body weight) and to a larger interstitial volume in the fetus. The fetal interstitial space contains more ground substance and thus holds a large amount of interstitial fluid in the absence of oedema. The relative proportion of extracellular fluid decreases as gestation proceeds while the relative amount of intracellular fluid increases (Fig. 15.1A). That is, extracellular fluid decreases from approximately 70% of body weight at 16 weeks to 40% of body weight at term while intracellular fluid increases from 20 to 30% of body weight over the same time period. On an absolute scale, the amount of fluid in all fetal spaces increases with gestation due to fetal growth (Fig. 15.1B). Even though

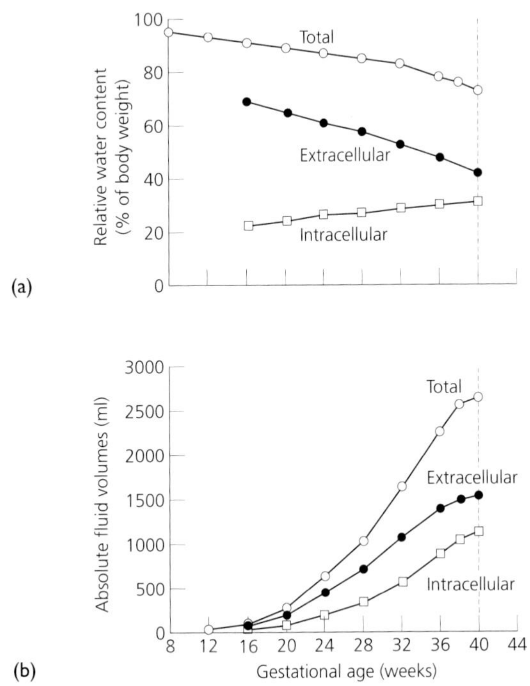

Fig. 15.1 Fluid spaces of the fetus during gestation. (a) Water content as a percentage of body weight. Data from Friis-Hansen[1]. (b) Total water content across gestation. Values calculated from relative water content (a) and average fetal body weights from Williams *et al.*[51]

the relative amount of extracellular fluid decreases with advancing gestation, the term fetus has roughly 50% more extracellular than intracellular fluid per unit weight and this is opposite to that in the adult which has roughly twice as much intracellular as extracellular fluid.

The fetal extracellular fluid is divided into three primary components: interstitial fluid, plasma and lung liquid. Interstitial volume is usually calculated as extracellular volume minus either plasma volume or minus the sum of plasma plus lung liquid volumes, depending on whether the extracellular marker (which was used to measure volume) penetrates the lung space. Animal data suggest that, although there is little liquid occupying the future airways during the first half of gestation, during the last third of gestation, lung liquid volume averages 3–4% of body weight or 30–40 ml/kg[2]. Thus, the sum of the plasma plus interstitial volumes is slightly less than the extracellular fluid volume indicated in Fig. 15.1(A) during the last trimester.

As for plasma volumes, the older literature had suggested that blood volume/kg fetus was considerably higher in younger than older fetuses, with individual early gestation values in excess of 350 ml/kg in fetal sheep[3] and over 200 ml/kg in human fetuses[4]. Since haematocrit is lower in younger fetuses, this implies that plasma volume/kg fetus is much higher in younger than older fetuses. However, these high blood volumes are now known to be overestimates since they were determined with indicator dilution techniques using dyes that are supposed to attach to plasma proteins. In fetuses, these dyes rapidly escape from the fetal circulation and thus overestimate plasma volume for two reasons. First, capillary permeability to plasma proteins in the near-term fetus is more than an order of magnitude greater than in the adult[5] and is most likely even higher in younger fetuses. Second, there may be a large fraction of unbound dye in young fetuses since the plasma protein concentration is low in early gestation and this would result in a decreased dye-binding capacity. Thus, the current interpretation of available data is that the circulating blood volume per unit fetal weight is constant across gestation and averages approximately 115 ml/kg[6]. Since fetal haematocrit increases slightly with advancing gestation, fetal plasma volume most likely decreases only slightly as gestation proceeds. Thus, the large decrease in the relative extracellular fluid volume shown in Fig. 15.1(A) is due primarily to a decrease in interstitial fluid volume per unit weight.

Amniotic fluid volume and composition

During embryonic development, the amnion forms and encloses the embryo in amniotic fluid. This in turn is surrounded by a thixotropic (jelly-like) coelomic fluid (i.e. the extraembryonic coelom). The coelomic fluid disappears early during the fetal period[7] while the amniotic fluid volume (AFV) expands progressively throughout the first two-thirds of pregnancy and mean changes in AFV across gestation are shown in Fig. 15.2. AFV reaches is peak at approximately 33 weeks gestation and averages 800 ml. There is little change in the mean AFV over 22 to 39 weeks gestation, with mean volumes ranging from 630 to 820 ml[8]. However, in post-term pregnancies, AFV can decrease, sometimes dramatically, and compromise the fetus due to cord compression.

As shown by the shaded area in Fig. 15.2, there is a wide range for normal AF volumes during the second half of gestation. For example, the 95% confidence interval for normal pregnancies at 33 weeks gestation ranges from 300 ml to 2150 ml. Figure 15.2 also shows that, during the first trimester, there is a much narrower range for normal AFV. At 12 weeks, the 95% confidence interval includes volumes from 25 to 173 ml. Because the data used to generate Fig. 15.2 have log-normal distributions and because the variances of the logs were uniform across gestation, the variability in AFV across gestation can be expressed in simple terms[8]. That is, the 95% confidence interval encompasses the range of 39 to 257% of the log mean volume for any gestational age[8]. In addition to the large range for normal AFV, there can be large day-to-day variations in AFV within any given pregnancy for both humans[9] and the most commonly studied experimental animal, i.e. sheep[10].

One of the unique aspects of amniotic fluid is that its composition is different from all other fetal fluids. Table 15.1 compares the osmolality and concentrations of the major solutes in amniotic fluid with other fluids that contribute to amniotic composition. To date, there has been little attempt to explain amniotic composition in terms of the flows into and out of the amniotic space. This lack of understanding of amniotic composition occurs because there is not enough known about the water and solute fluxes between amniotic fluid and fetus and this is discussed in more detail below.

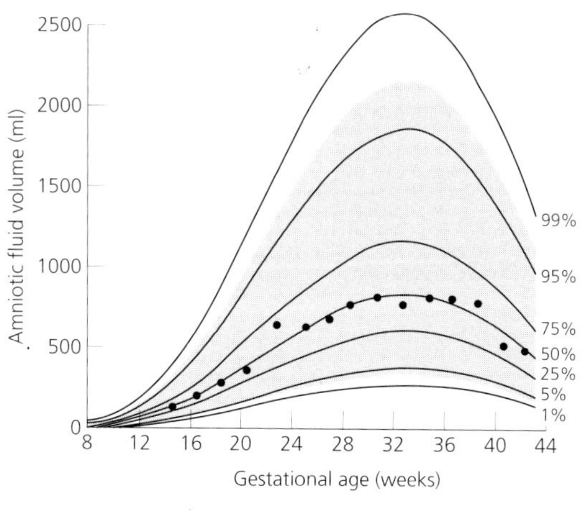

Fig. 15.2 Amniotic fluid volumes in human pregnancies with normal fetus. Shade area represents the 95% confidence interval as determined from 704 volumes. Reprinted with permission from Brace and Wolf[8].

TABLE 1
Comparison of compositions of fluids from late gestation fetal sheep*

Variable (units)	Amniotic fluid	Fetal plasma	Fetal Urine	Lung liquid	Swallowed liquid	Intramembranous flow
Osmolality (mOsm/kg)	278	298	150	298	280	?
Sodium (mmol/l)	116	142	40	143	118	?
Chloride (mmol/l)	97	108	40	147	102	?
Flow to/from amniotic fluid (ml/day)	–	–	950	165	–875	–240

*Data from Brace *et al.*[23,50] and Jang and Brace[25].

Interactions between fetus and amniotic fluid

There are five major pathways over which water and solutes move between the fetus and the amniotic fluid. These include the two primary sources of amniotic fluid during the second half of gestation, i.e. fetal urine and fetal lung liquid, and the two primary routes for reabsorption of amniotic fluid, i.e. fetal swallowing and absorption into fetal blood across the fetal surface of the placenta[11–15]. The latter is referred to as 'intramembranous' absorption[12]. The phrase 'intramembranous pathway' is used to describe not only reabsorption across the fetal surface of the placenta but also includes all direct exchange between fetal blood and amniotic fluid. Thus, intramembranous exchange includes water and solute exchange across the fetal skin prior to keratinization at 22–24 weeks gestation and exchange across the oral–nasal cavities (Fig. 15.3)[15]. The fifth pathway for fluid movement between fetus and amniotic fluid is the salivary glands and other oral–nasal secretions from the fetal head. Although the latter has yet to be studied in detail, preliminary estimates are that in the order of 8 ml/day/kg fetus are secreted by the oral–nasal cavities in late gestation[11]. Finally, transmembranous exchange between amniotic fluid and maternal blood within the wall of the uterus may also occur. These five fetal-amniotic and the transmembranous pathways are illustrated in Fig. 15.3.

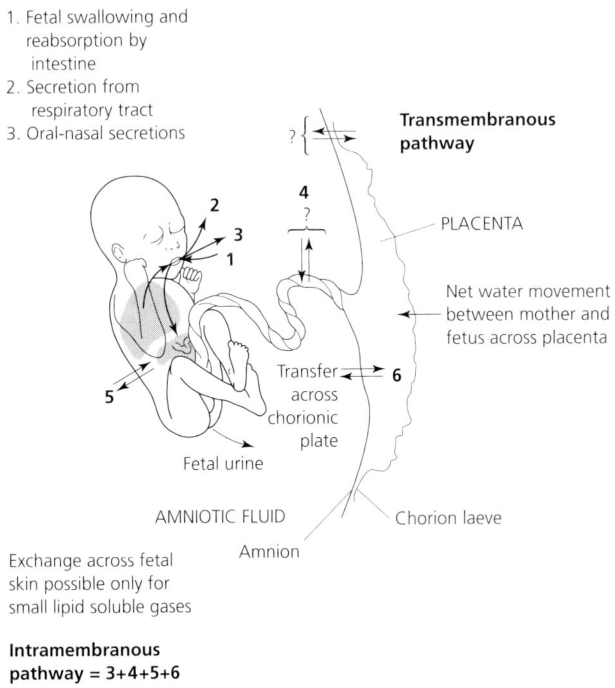

Fig. 15.3 Pathways for fluid movements between fetus and amniotic fluid. Figure redrawn from Seeds[52], with addition of intramembranous pathway, addition of fetal oral–nasal secretions, and inverting arrow to show fluid movement out of, rather than into fetal lungs.

Over the past decade, there has been steady progress in advancing our understanding not only of the fluxes between the fetus and amniotic fluid but also of the regulation of AFV and composition in that we know progressively more about the flow of water and solutes through each of the pathways depicted in Fig. 15.3. These flows are discussed next.

URINE FLOW

Fetal urine begins to enter the amniotic sac at the beginning of the fetal period. Urine is the primary source of amniotic fluid during the second half of gestation as renal agenesis or blockage of urine entry into the amniotic fluid almost invariably results in oligohydramnios. In spite of this important contribution of fetal urine to AF, normal urine flow rates in the human fetus have yet to be clearly defined. Early ultrasonographic work by Wladimiroff and Campbell[16] showed that urinary output progressively increased roughly in proportion to body weight during the latter half of gestation and averaged about 650 ml/day at term or 20% of fetal body weight/day. Although the latter study has been widely quoted, a more recent study suggested that the true human fetal urine flow rates are twice that reported by Wladimiroff and Campbell because more frequent sampling was needed in order to accurately determine flow rates[17]. This is equivalent to urine production at a rate of 40% of body weight per day. Even more recently, using carefully controlled conditions in human fetal cadavers, Hedriana and Moore[18] found that the formulation used for calculating urine production overestimated true rates by 40%, suggesting that human fetuses produce urine at a rate of approximately 25% of body weight/day. It is interesting to note that this is in close agreement with directly measured values most commonly found in the chronically catheterized fetal lamb over the past 20 years[19]. True daily ovine fetal urine flow may be closer to 30% of body weight/day as urine production displays a diurnal rhythm and is highest during the night whereas flow measurements are usually made close to midday when flows are lower[20].

In addition to its effects on AFV, fetal urine contributes importantly to amniotic fluid composition. This occurs because fetal urine normally has a dramatically different composition than fetal blood, with osmolality being approximately one-half, chloride concentration one-third, and sodium concentrations less than one-third of plasma values (see Table 15.1). In comparison, amniotic osmolality, sodium and chloride concentrations average only 10–20% less than those of plasma in fetal sheep (Table 15.1). These differences among fetal plasma, amniotic fluid and urine compositions have not been explained but are addressed below.

LUNG LIQUID

Over the past 20–25 years, there have been major changes in our understanding of the role played by the fetal lungs in determining AFV and composition. It is well established that the fetal lungs are not collapsed *in utero* as was once thought but are instead filled with liquid. In late gestation, the lung liquid volume is essentially the same as the air space in the newborn lung[2].

At fetal autopsy, a common finding has been that the amniotic fluid and associated material are found in the fetal lung liquid. Hence, it was accepted for many years that the fetal lungs normally absorb amniotic fluid. In contrast, it is now known that the fetal lungs secrete rather than absorb fluid under normal conditions and that absorption of fluid by the fetal lungs is a process that occurs only immediately prior to birth[21] or under severe stress or pathological conditions[2]. For over 20 years it has been clear that the fetal lungs normally secrete a volume of liquid equal to approximately 10% of fetal body weight/day[22].

While a small amount of this secreted fluid remains in the lungs for expansion with growth, over 99% of the secreted fluid exits the lungs via the trachea. Acute studies had suggested that essentially all of the lung liquid was swallowed as it exited the trachea. However, a recent study in near-term fetal sheep under physiological conditions suggest that only 50% of the lung liquid is swallowed as it exits the trachea and the other 50% enters the amniotic fluid[23]. Thus, fetal lung liquid is the source of the pulmonary surfactants within the AF.

With half of the fluid secreted by the lungs entering the AF, a volume of lung liquid equal to 5% of fetal body weight/day enters the amniotic space during late gestation. This volume is small compared to the urine entry of 25–30% of body weight/day noted above. Further, lung liquid osmolality and sodium concentration are similar to that of fetal plasma while chloride concentration is much higher that plasma, averaging 150 mmol/l compared to 110 mmol/l for plasma (Table 15.1).

INTRAMEMBRANOUS FLUXES

The most significant progress toward understanding AFV and composition as well as fetal–amniotic fluid interactions has been documentation of the fact that intramembranous fluxes not only exist[12] but may be large and thus contribute importantly to the regulation of amniotic fluid volume and composition[15]. In fact, intramembranous absorption has been termed the 'missing link' in understanding the regulation of AFV. For example, it is now well established that an average of 200–250 ml/day of water is absorbed from the amniotic sac directly into fetal blood via the intramembranous pathway in near-term fetal sheep under normal conditions[12,24,25]. Although estimates of normal absorption rates have yet to be experimentally determined in humans, there is a considerable body of older literature data from humans and primates[15] as well as new data from primates[26] which support the concept of extensive and rapid fluxes of water and solutes via the intramembranous pathway in primates including humans.

TRANSMEMBRANOUS FLUXES

Concomitant with the increased knowledge about fluxes through the intramembranous pathway, there has been an expansion of our understanding of transmembranous fluxes. Surprisingly, the data suggest that there is little if any transmembranous water or solute flux under normal conditions[15]. Even for low-molecular-weight substances such as urea and carbon dioxide which have high lipid solubilities, transmembranous fluxes are so low as to be undetectable[27,28,29]. Further, calculations by Anderson *et al.*[28] based on their earlier study suggest that transmembranous water fluxes may be in the order of 3.2 ml/day/kg fetal weight. However, this estimate may be greater than normal because the experimental data were collected after distending the amniotic space with 6 litres of saline and membrane stretching may have increased the permeability. The low flux through the membranes is surprising in view of the fact that isolated membranes have relatively high permeabilities *in vitro*[29–31]. Collectively, these data suggest that the uterine wall rather than the membranes may be the major barrier which limits transmembranous fluxes under normal conditions.

Integrated amniotic–fetal fluxes under normal conditions

In humans, there are insufficient data available to interpret or integrate basal fluxes between the AF and fetus. Currently, sufficient data are available only for fetal sheep, the most commonly studied chronic fetal preparation. Table 15.1 shows that, for late gestation fetal sheep, an average of 1115 ml/day of water flows into the amniotic sac and 1115 ml/day flows out. Perhaps an addition 5–10 ml/day enter the AF from fetal oral–nasal secretions and 5–10 ml/day exit the AF via the transmembranous pathway (discussed above) so that there is little net change in AFV.

Currently, our understanding of solute fluxes is far less clear than that for water. From the concentrations and flow rates of Table 15.1, it can be calculated that the two primary sources of AF, ie fetal urine and lung liquid, combined provide only 59.7% of the sodium which is removed from the AF by swallowing. Similarly, calculations from Table 15.1 show that only 69.8% of the chloride swallowed by the fetus is derived from fetal urine plus lung liquid. Presumably, the remaining 40.3% of the swallowed sodium and 30.2% of the swallowed chloride diffuses into the AF from fetal blood through the intramembranous pathway since the transmembranous pathway appears impermeable as discussed above. This possibility is supported by the fact that isolated membranes studied *in vitro* have sufficiently high permeabilities for such fluxes to occur. For example, with a near-term permeability of 2×10^{-5} cm/s[32,33], a concentration gradient from fetal plasma of 11 mmol/l (Table 15.1), and a total membrane surface area[34] of 5000 cm^2, 95 mmol/day of chloride would diffuse through the intramembranous pathway and enter the AF. This calculation is based on the fact that, in sheep and other related species, the fetal membranes are vascularized and perfused with fetal blood at high flow rates[34]. The calculated flux of 95 mmol/day is in excess of the 27 mmol/day deficit calculated from Table 15.1 and is consistent with the intramembranous fluxes playing an important role in determining AF composition[33]. Although measurement of *in vivo* fluxes are needed to further clarify intramembranous fluxes, it is clear that large fluxes of sodium and chloride must enter the AF each day by a route(s) other than the primary sources of water, i.e. fetal urine and lung liquid. It is interesting to note that, although fluxes of the primary AF solutes sodium and chloride through the intramembranous pathway are in the opposite direction to that of water, these fluxes are all down concentration gradients and thus appear to be passive.

Amniotic–fetal fluxes with fetal fluid loading

There have been several long-term animal studies in which fluids at varying rates and with varying amounts of solutes have been infused either into the ovine fetus circulation or into the ovine amniotic fluid over a period of days[10,35–38]. These provide several interesting observations and insights into amniotic–fetal fluid interactions: first, on a long-term basis during intravascular infusions of isotonic fluids, fetal urinary output increased by a volume slightly greater than the infusion rate[39]. There was a simultaneous increase in volume swallowed by the fetus. Further, although AFV increased during these long-term intravascular infusions, the increase was far less than expected from the infused volume or from the changes in urine flow plus fetal swallowing[39]. The same is true for direct intra-amniotic infusions[10,35]. That is, although fetal swallowing increased, there was an equal increase in fetal urine flow and AFV increased by only half the infused volume[35]. These differences between observed and expected changes in AFV were concluded to be due to absorption of fluid through the intramembranous pathway with subsequent transfer across the placenta to the mother.

During long-term intravascular infusions of hypertonic solutions, fetal urinary output increased without changes in urine osmolality so the entire solute load was excreted by the fetal kidney[37,38]. That is, the fetus appeared to acquire the free water necessary to dilute the hypertonic infusates and then excreted the resulting volume and solute load. Further, although urinary output increased by the same amount during equal molar infusions of hypertonic sodium chloride or hypertonic sodium lactate infusions, only the sodium lactate infusion was associated with sustained increases in AFV and thus polyhydramnios. The latter results suggest that sodium chloride but not sodium lactate can readily cross the intramembranous pathway and placenta[37,38]. The latter observation that sodium lactate causes extensive fluid acquisition by the fetus is strong support for the osmotic hypothesis of fluid acquisition across the placenta by the fetus[39–41] and further shows that amniotic acquisition/maintenance of fluid involves osmotic factors.

Collectively, these studies also show that, on a long-term basis, the fetal kidneys have a tremendously powerful ability to excrete fluid which may enter the fetus. In fact, sustained increases in fetal urinary output to as high as 10 ml/min have been observed during rapid intravascular infusions of isotonic fluids into ovine fetuses[42]. If the fetus maintained this extraordinary ability to excreted excess fluid under all conditions, then generalized hydrops fetalis would not be possible. A likely resolution of these conflicting ideas is that if antidiuretics, such as arginine vasopressin, are present during the fluid load then hydrops may result and without antidiuretics hydramnios occurs. More experimentation is needed to explore these possibilities.

Amniotic responses to oesophageal occlusion or atresia

The fetus excretes a large volume of urine into the AF and swallows a large volume of AF each day during the latter half of gestation. Hence polyhydramnios would be expected to develop if swallowing does not occur. In humans, polyhydramnios often but not always develops with oesophageal atresia or obstruction[43–45]. In monkeys, surgical ligation of the fetal oesophagus is followed by a transient polyhydramnios with AFV returning to normal over a period of several days[46].

In fetal sheep, ligation or obstruction of the oesophagus is followed by an increased AFV at 1–3 days[47], and normal AFVs at 5 days[12] and at 2–3 weeks[48]. Ovine fetal urinary output remains normal during the oesophageal obstruction/occlusion[47,49]. The combined volume of fluid from the fetal kidneys plus lungs would equal approximately 1000 ml/day (Table 15.1) which have to be absorbed from the amniotic compartment in order for AFV to remain within normal limits when swallowing does not occur. This appears to occur through an increased absorption via the intramembranous pathway since intramembranous absorption of both water and solutes is doubled after oesophageal ligation.[12,49] What mediates this large increase in the ability of the intramembranous pathway to absorb water and solutes has yet to be determined.

Summary

Over the past couple of decades there has been a tremendous increase in our understanding of the interactions between the fetus and its surrounding amniotic fluid. We now know more about what are normal and what are abnormal AFVs. The fetal lungs are now known to be a significant source rather than a sink of AF. Larger volumes of fetal urine appear to be excreted into the AF than was previously recognized, with daily volumes averaging in the order of 25–30% of fetal body weight. It is becoming increasingly clear that the transmembranous pathway may play little role in determining AFV or composition and this may be due to resistance within the uterine wall rather than in the membranes. Finally, it has become clear that there are rapid and large fluxes of water and solutes directly between amniotic fluid and fetal blood through the intramembranous pathway. Further, the capacity of the latter pathway to transfer water and solutes increases greatly under conditions such as impaired fetal swallowing. The next major step in understanding the regulation of fetal–amniotic fluid volumes and compositions will be the determination of permeability characteristics of the intramembranous pathway as functions of gestational age.

REFERENCES

1. Friis-Hansen B. Body water composition in children: changes during growth and related changes in body composition. *Pediatrics* **28**:169–178, 1961.
2. Harding R. Development of the respiratory system. In *Textbook of Fetal Physiology* (eds G.D. Thorburn & R. Harding) pp. 140–167. Oxford: Oxford University Press, 1994.
3. Barcroft J, Kennedy JA. The distribution of blood between the foetus and the placenta in sheep. *J Physiol* **95**:173–186, 1939.
4. Morris JA, Morgan CA, Gobuty A. Measurement of fetoplacental blood volume in the human previable fetus. *Am J Obstet Gynecol* **118**:927–931, 1974.
5. Gold PS, Brace RA. Fetal whole-body permeability–surface area product and reflection coefficient for plasma proteins. *Microvasc Res* **36**:262–274, 1988.
6. Brace RA. Regulation of blood volume *in utero*. In *Fetus and Neonate*. Volume 1. *The Circulation* (eds M.A. Hanson, J.A.D. Spencer & C.H. Rodeck), pp. 75–99. Cambridge Cambridge University Press, 1993.
7. Hamilton WJ, Mossman HW. *Human Embryology*, 4th edn. Baltimore, MD: Williams and Wilkins, 1972.
8. Brace RA, Wolf EJ. Normal amniotic fluid volume changes throughout pregnancy. *Am J Obstet Gynecol* **161**:382–388, 1989.
9. Queenan JT, Thompson W, Whitfield CR, Shah SI. Amniotic fluid volumes in normal pregnancies. *Am J Obstet Gynecol* **114**:34–38, 1972.
10. Tomoda S, Brace RA, Longo LD. Amniotic fluid volume regulation: basal volumes and responses to fluid infusion or withdrawal in sheep. *Am J Physiol* **252**:R380–R387, 1987.
11. Brace RA. Amniotic fluid volume and its relationship to fetal fluid balance: a review of experimental data. *Sem Perinatol* **10**:103–112, 1986.
12. Gilbert WM, Brace RA. The missing link in amniotic fluid volume regulation: intramembranous absorption. *Obstet Gynecol* **74**:748–754, 1989.
13. Gilbert WM, Moore TR, Brace RA. Amniotic fluid volume dynamics. *Fetal Med Rev* **3**:89–104, 1991.
14. Gilbert WM, Brace RA. Amniotic fluid volume and normal flows to and from the amniotic cavity. *Sem Perinatol* **17**:150–157, 1993.
15. Brace RA. Current topic: Progress toward understanding the regulation of amniotic fluid volume: water and solute fluxes in and through the fetal extraplacental membranes. *Placenta* **16**:1–18, 1995.
16. Wladimiroff JW, Campbell S. Fetal urine-production rates in normal and complicated pregnancy. *Lancet* **ii**:151–154, 1974.
17. Rabinowitz R, Peters MT, Vyas S, Campbell S, Nicolaides KH. Measurement of fetal urine production in normal pregnancy by real-time ultrasonography. *Am J Obstet Gynecol* **161**:1264–1266, 1989.
18. Hedriana HL, Moore TR. Accuracy limits of ultrasonographic estimation of human fetal urinary flow rate. *Am J Obstet Gynecol* **171**:989–992, 1994.
19. Gresham EL, Rankin JHG, Makowski EL, Meschia G, Battaglia FC. An evaluation of fetal renal function in a chronic sheep preparation. *J Clin Invest* **51**:149–155, 1972.
20. Brace RA, Moore TR. Diurnal rhythms in fetal urine flow, vascular pressures, and heart rate in sheep. *Am J Physiol* **261**:R1015–R1021, 1991.
21. Kitterman JA, Ballard PL, Clements JA, Mescher EJ, Tooley WH. Tracheal fluid in fetal lambs: spontaneous decrease prior to birth. *J Appl Physiol* **47**:985–989, 1979.
22. Mescher EJ, Platzker ACG, Ballard PL, Kitterman JA, Clements JA, Tooley WH. Ontogeny of tracheal fluid, pulmonary surfactant, and plasma corticoids in the fetal lamb. *J Appl Physiol* **39**:1017–1021, 1975.
23. Brace RA, Wlodek ME, Cock ML, Harding R. Swallowing of lung liquid and amniotic fluid by the ovine fetus under normoxic and hypoxic conditions. *Am J Obstet Gynecol* **171**:764–770, 1994.
24. Gilbert WM, Brace RA. Novel determination of filtration coefficient of ovine placenta and intramembranous pathway. *Am J Physiol* **259**:R1281–R1288, 1990.
25. Jang PR, Brace RA. Amniotic fluid composition changes during urine drainage and tracheoesophageal occlusion in fetal sheep. *Am J Obstet Gynecol* **167**:1732–1741, 1992.
26. Gilbert WM, Eby-Wilkins E, Tarantal AF. The missing link in primate amniotic fluid volume regulation: intramembranous absorption. *J Soc Gynecol Invest* **3**:272a, 1996.
27. Suzuki K, Plentl AA, Adamsons K. Exchange of carbon dioxide in the pregnant rhesus monkey: Multicompartmental analysis of carbon dioxide kinetics. *J Clin Invest* **48**:1967–1982, 1969.
28. Anderson DF, Faber JJ, Parks CM. Extraplacental transfer of water in the sheep. *J Physiol* **406**:75–84, 1988.
29. Abramovich DR, Page KR, Jandial L. Bulk flows through human fetal membranes. *Gynecol Invest* **7**:157–164, 1976.
30. Lingwood BE, Wintour EM. Permeability of ovine amnion and amniochorion to urea and water. *Obstet Gynecol* **61**:227–232, 1983.
31. Lingwood BE, Wintour M. Amniotic fluid volume and *in vivo* permeability of ovine fetal membranes. *Obstet Gynecol* **64**:368–372, 1984.

32. Battaglia FC, Meschia G, Makowski EL. Comparison of *in vitro* and *in vivo* placental permeability measurements. *Am J Physiol* **216**:1590–1594, 1969.
33. Wintour EM, Lingwood BE, MacIsaac RJ, Ryan GB, Towstoless MK. Role of fetal membranes in determining the composition of amniotic fluid. In *Human Fetal Membranes* (ed. B.F. Mitchell), pp. 199–211. Ithaca, New York: Perinatology Press, 1988.
34. Brace RA, Gilbert WM, Thornburg KL. Vascularization of the ovine amnion and chorion: a morphometric characterization of the surface area of the intramembranous pathway. *Am J Obstet Gynecol* **167**:1747–1755, 1992.
35. Gilbert WM, Brace RA. Increase in fetal hydration during long-term intra-amniotic isotonic saline infusion. *Am J Obstet Gynecol* **159**:1413–1417, 1988.
36. Brace RA. Fetal blood volume, urine flow, swallowing, and amniotic fluid volume responses to long-term intravascular infusions of saline. *Am J Obstet Gynecol* **161**:1049–1054, 1989.
37. Powell TL, Brace RA. Elevated fetal plasma lactate produces polyhydramnios in the sheep. *Am J Obstet Gynecol* **165**:1595–1607, 1991.
38. Powell TL, Brace RA. Fetal fluid responses to long-term 5 M NaCl infusion: where does all the salt go? *Am J Physiol* **261**:R412–R419, 1991.
39. Longo LD, Power GG. Long-term regulation of fetal cardiac output: a hypothesis on the role of carbon dioxide. *Gynec Invest* **4**:277–287, 1973.
40. Conrad EE, Faber JJ. Water and electrolyte acquisition across the placenta of the sheep. *Am J Physiol* **233**:H475–H487, 1977.
41. Wilbur WJ, Power GC, Longo LD. Water exchange in the placenta: a mathematical model. *Am J Physiol* **235**:R181–R199, 1978.
42. Brace RA, Moore TR. Transplacental, amniotic, urinary, and fetal fluid dynamics during very-large-volume fetal intravenous infusions. *Am J Obstet Gynecol* **164**:907–916, 1991.
43. Chamberlain PF, Manning FA, Morrison I, Harman CR, Lange IR. Ultrasound evaluation of amniotic fluid volume. II. The relationship of increased amniotic fluid volume to perinatal outcome. *Am J Obstet Gynecol* **150**:250–254, 1984.
44. Hill LM, Breckle R, Thomas ML, Fries JK. Polyhydramnios: ultrasonically detected prevalence and neonatal outcome. *Obstet Gynecol* **69**:21, 1987.
45. Kirshon B. Fetal urine output in hydramnios. *Obstet Gynecol* **73**:240–242, 1989.
46. Minei LJ, Suzuki K. Role of fetal deglutition and micturition in the production and turnover of amniotic fluid in the monkey. *Obstet Gynecol* **48**:177–181, 1976.
47. Fujino Y, Agnew CL, Schreyer P, Ervin MG, Sherman DJ, Ross MG. Amniotic fluid volume response to esophageal occlusion in fetal sheep. *Am J Obstet Gynecol* **165**:1620–1626, 1991.
48. Wintour EM, Barnes A, Brown EH, Hardy KJ, Horacek I, McDougall JG, Scoggins BA. Regulation of amniotic fluid volume and composition in the ovine fetus. *Obstet Gynecol* **52**:689–693, 1978.
49. Gilbert WM, Cheung CY, Brace RA. Rapid intramembranous absorption into the fetal circulation of arginine vasopressin injected intra-amniotically. *Am J Obstet Gynecol* **164**:1013–1020, 1991.
50. Brace RA, Wlodek ME, Graeme JM, Harding R. Swallowing and urine flow responses of ovine fetus to 24 h of hypoxia. *Am J Physiol* **266**:R1345–R1352, 1994.
51. Williams RL, Creasy RK, Cunningham GC, Hawes WE, Norris FD, Tashiro M. Fetal growth and perinatal viability in California. *Obstet Gynecol* **59**:624–632, 1982.
52. Seeds AE. Current concepts of amniotic fluid dynamics. *Am J Obstet Gynecol* **138**:575–586, 1980.

Lung development and maturation

16

R. Harding and S.B. Hooper

Introduction

At birth, when the umbilico-placental circulation is interrupted, the lungs of the newly born must take over from the placenta as the sole organ of gas exchange. In the majority of neonates, this transition is smooth and uneventful, which is remarkable given that prior to birth, the lungs had never performed this role. In this regard, the lung is somewhat unique amongst fetal organs, as most other organs have functioned before birth in a manner which is not dissimilar to their postnatal function. In the fetus, the lung is a liquid-filled, secretory organ that has a relatively modest blood supply (i.e. appropriate for its tissue mass, but inappropriate for gas exchange). In order for the lung to function effectively as an organ of gas exchange, its secretory activity must cease, the airways must be cleared of liquid and the vascular resistance of the lung must greatly decline, allowing it to receive the entire output of the right side of the heart; it must also be able to secrete surfactant which is necessary to prevent the collapse of the air-filled lung. During normal fetal development the lung becomes progressively prepared for these dramatic changes in function. This chapter will focus on the processes whereby the fetal lung grows and matures such that it is capable of functioning effectively as an organ of gas exchange immediately following term birth. Impaired lung growth or maturation *in utero* can lead to respiratory insufficiency in the newborn, and may contribute to the development of respiratory disorders in later life. Some of the more common respiratory complications in the neonate, and their fetal origins, will be discussed together with strategies for their treatment. Firstly, a brief overview of the major recognised stages of lung development is presented.

Stages in the development of the lungs

Detailed accounts of the structural development of the mammalian lung may be obtained in specialist reviews[1–6] and only a brief summary of major events will be given here. Although the emphasis will be on the human, similar stages of lung development can be recognised in all mammals; however, the stage of gestation at which they occur depends upon the length of gestation and the level of maturity of the fetus at birth. For example, in altricial species, such as mice and rats (and even more so in marsupials), the later stages of lung development may occur after birth. Pulmonary morphologists recognise five or six stages in lung development (Table 16.1).

EMBRYONIC STAGE (3–7 WEEKS)

During early embryonic development the lung first appears as an outgrowth of the primitive foregut (i.e. endodermal tissue) at 22–26 days' post-conception. This endodermal outpouching then divides to form buds on the left and right sides; these further divide to form the major units of the bronchial tree. By 34 days, each of the major bronchopulmonary segments has been formed. This early embryonic development results in 'airway' epithelial tissue being endodermal in origin, whereas the surrounding tissue into which the 'airways' grow is derived from splanchnic mesenchymal tissue. This mesenchymal tissue gives rise to the non-epithelial structures of the lung including blood and lymphatic vessels, airway cartilage and smooth muscle, fibrous tissue and other parenchymal components. The mature lungs contain more than 40 different cell types, all derived from embryonic endodermal and mesenchymal tissue.

TABLE 16.1
Stages of lung development in the human

Stage	Timing	Major events
Embryonic	4–7 weeks	Appearance of ventral bud in foregut. Epithelial tube branches and grows into surrounding mesenchyme. Vascular connections formed.
Pseudoglandular	5–17 weeks	Development of conductive airway tree, paralleled by formation of vascular tree. Lung periphery contains parenchymal precursors.
Canalicular	16–26 weeks	Addition of further generations of airways and of vascular tree. Differentiation of type I and type II epithelial cells. Formation of thin air–blood barrier. Start of surfactant production.
Saccular stage	25–40 weeks (term)	Formation of additional airway generations. Dilation of prospective gas-exchanging airspaces. Maturation of surfactant system.
Alveolar stage	36 weeks–18 months	Start of alveolar formation at 36 weeks. Formation of alveoli by outgrowth of secondary septa.
Microvascular maturation	Birth–3 years	Change from double- to single-capillary network. Reduction in interstitial tissue mass; fusion of capillaries; preferential growth of single-layered capillary network areas.

Reproduced in modified form, with permission, from Burri[5].

PSEUDOGLANDULAR STAGE (8–16 WEEKS)

During the pseudoglandular stage of lung development the lung resembles a typical secretory gland. The major bronchial airways and associated respiratory units of the lung (i.e. acini) are progressively formed. These developments are paralleled by the growth of pulmonary blood vessels, such that each major 'airway' is accompanied by a branch of the pulmonary artery. The formation of acini occurs as a result of repeated division of distal extremities of blind-ending tubes or 'airways' comprised of epithelial cells (Fig. 16.1a). The process of terminal branching, which is critical to the growth of new orders of 'airways', is stimulated by cellular interactions between cells of endodermal origin (airways) and the surrounding mesenchyme; this process probably depends upon mitogens acting in a paracrine manner. The developing airways are surrounded by mesenchymal tissue which, at this stage, has only a loose network of blood capillaries (Fig. 16.1a), thereby precluding, or at least greatly restricting, pulmonary gas exchange if the fetus were to be born at less than 16 weeks. Airway epithelial cells gradually differentiate (in a centrifugal direction) into ciliated cells (by 11–13 weeks), as well as goblet cells and mucous glands.

CANALICULAR STAGE (17–25 WEEKS)

The canalicular stage of lung development sees further growth and enlargement of airways (both widening and lengthening – i.e. canalisation) and the attenuation of mesenchymal tissue (Fig. 16.1b). This results in a substantial increase in the intraluminal volume (liquid-filled) relative to total lung volume. During the canalicular stage, the functional units of the lung (respiratory lobules) are formed, consisting of terminal bronchioles ending with enlargements that subsequently give rise to terminal sacs (the primitive alveoli). A network of blood capillaries becomes arranged around the lengthening and widening tubes of epithelial cells (terminal

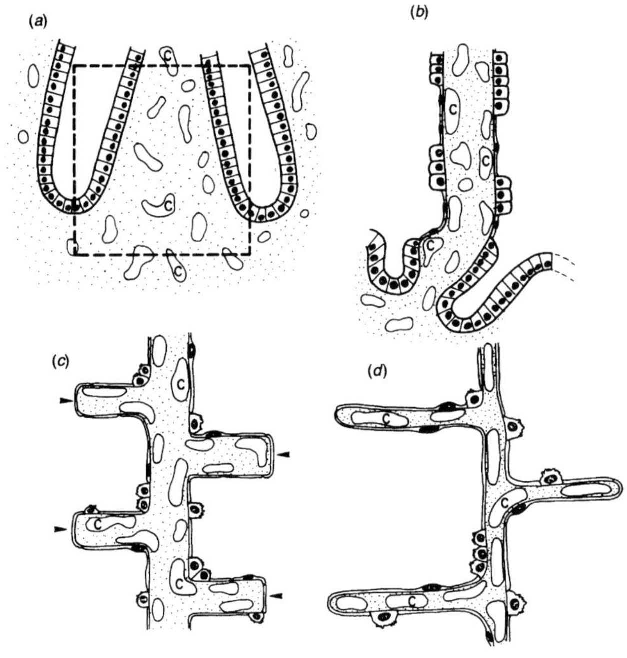

Fig. 16.1 Diagram showing development of lung parenchyma and its microvasculature. (a) Pseudoglandular stage, during which epithelial tubes lined by columnar epithelial cells invade the mesenchyme which contains a loose network of blood capillaries. (C=capillaries). (b)–(d) show further development of structures enclosed by the frame in (a). (b) Canalicular stage, showing differentiation of 'airspace' epithelium and expansion of airspaces resulting in attenuation of mesenchyme; capillaries are rearranged around the epithelial tubes so that walls between 'airspaces' contain a double layer of capillaries. A thin 'air'–blood interface develops and types I and II epithelial cells become apparent. (c) Terminal sac/alveolar stages, showing development of secondary septa (arrowheads) from primary septa; septa are primitive in that they contain a double capillary network and a central layer of connective tissue. (d) Mature lung, showing thin interalveolar walls containing a single capillary layer. Reproduced with permission from Burri[144].

airways). The increasing proximity of blood capillaries with the epithelial cell layer sees the beginnings of the air–blood interface that is required for effective gas exchange (Fig. 16.1b). Thus, the mid-late canalicular stage is the earliest that the lungs can potentially support independent life.

TERMINAL SAC STAGE (28–35 WEEKS)

This stage of lung development, sometimes called the saccular stage, sees a progressive enlargement of the peripheral 'airspaces'. This results from an attenuation of mesenchymal tissue and leads to an increase in luminal volume relative to total lung volume. During the terminal sac stage, the development of secondary septa (i.e. divisions between adjacent sacs) from primary septa occurs (Fig. 16.1c). These septa are considered primitive in that they are wider than in the mature lung and contain a double capillary network, rather than the single capillary layer of the mature lung. Elastic fibres are formed by cells within septa, providing the lung tissue with its elastic (recoil) properties. The epithelial layer becomes thinner and both type I and type II epithelial cells become recognisable. As a result of structural changes in the mesenchymal tissue and epithelial layer, the potential separation between luminal 'air' and capillary blood becomes smaller, thereby enhancing the ability of the lung to exchange respiratory gases should the need arise.

ALVEOLAR STAGE (36–40 WEEKS)

By the time of term birth in human infants, several million definitive pulmonary alveoli are present; estimates vary between 20 and 50 million. In the adult human lungs, some 300 million alveoli are present, indicating that most are formed postnatally. The alveolar stage of lung development continues for one or two years after birth. In species born at an earlier stage of development (e.g. rat) this stage occurs only after birth; at birth, gas exchange occurs across the simpler, more primitive terminal sacs.

During the alveolar stage, terminal sacs are further divided by the formation of secondary septa (Fig. 16.2), which leads to the development of alveoli. Initially, these alveoli resemble shallow cups, but they deepen due to elongation of the septa. Septal walls and epithelial cells lining the alveoli become thinner, leading to the formation of definitive alveoli. The mean alveolar diameter increases greatly, from ~30 μm at 30 weeks to ~150 μm at 40 weeks.

The final stage of alveolar maturation involves the restructuring of the capillary network, such that the more primitive double capillary system lining the terminal sacs/alveoli is replaced by a single layer of capillaries (Fig. 16.1d); this marks the existence of definitive alveoli.

Pulmonary circulation

STRUCTURAL DEVELOPMENT

Detailed accounts of the structural development of the pulmonary vasculature are provided in recent reviews[2,7,8]. The lung develops with two anatomically and functionally distinct vascular systems: the pulmonary system, later used in gas exchange, and the bronchial system, which perfuses the non-gas-exchanging regions of the lung. The arteries of the bronchial circulation follow the bronchi but generally do not reach the most peripheral parts of the bronchial tree; they give rise to capillaries which surround the walls of the bronchi and bronchioles; from these capillaries, blood enters the pulmonary veins. The arteries of the pulmonary circulation grow and branch along with the airways, all the main arteries being present by 14 weeks in the human. Although the pulmonary and bronchial circulations develop separately, there are known to be anastomoses[2]. The

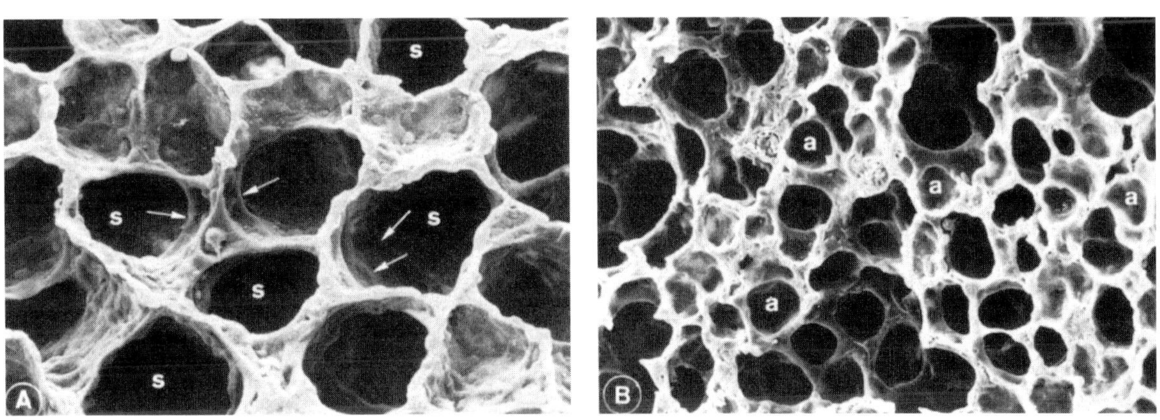

Fig. 16.2 Scanning electron micrographs showing formation of alveoli in the developing rat lung. Both are taken at the same magnification; scale bar = 20 μm. (A) Structure of rat lung at postnatal day 6 (terminal sac stage) showing smooth walled saccules (s) that gradually become partitioned by the formation of secondary septa (arrows). (B) Structure of the lung at postnatal day 17 (alveolar stage) showing increased height of secondary septa and subdivision of septa into alveoli (a). Reproduced with permission from Burri[145].

pulmonary arteries develop with a muscular wall, except near the periphery where the arteries are only partially muscularised. Pulmonary veins show a branching pattern similar to that of arteries, but do not follow the arteries and airways; rather they tend to run at right angles in the mesenchyme[2].

In the pulmonary circulation, arterioles are virtually absent; in the adult this results in pulmonary blood flow being determined largely by the resistance of the alveolar capillaries. In the fetus and newborn, however, the situation is different and resistance is apparently determined primarily by small pulmonary arteries. These vessels have thicker muscular walls, relative to their total diameter, than in the adult and this results in the pulmonary circulation of the fetus having a greater vascular resistance and greater vascular reactivity compared to that of the adult[9]. In the first few weeks after birth the arterial smooth muscle thins, leading to a reduction in wall thickness.

The creation of an effective air–liquid interface within the lung depends upon the development of a dense capillary bed in close proximity to the epithelium of the terminal sacs/alveoli. Early in development, blood capillaries form a loose network near the immature air spaces. During the canalicular stage, the number of capillaries increases greatly and they make contact with the primitive epithelial cells. By the terminal sac stage, the capillaries have formed a dense network around the terminal air spaces and, with attenuation of the septa between adjacent sacs, the separation between capillaries and the lumen becomes reduced.

FUNCTIONAL DEVELOPMENT

This topic has been dealt with in recent reviews[9–12]. During late fetal life, only 8–10% of total cardiac output flows through the pulmonary vascular bed; at mid-gestation this figure is only 3–4%[9]. In the fetus most of the right ventricular output is diverted away from the lungs to the descending aorta via the low resistance ductus arteriosus. Mean pulmonary arterial pressure in the near-term fetus is ~50 mmHg, which is slightly higher than mean aortic pressure. Although pulmonary vascular resistance declines progressively during fetal life, due to the formation of new arteries and an increase in total cross-sectional area, it remains much higher (up to eightfold) than after birth[9].

Pulmonary vascular resistance in the fetus is influenced by a range of factors, including the physical and oxygen environments of pulmonary vessels and the presence of vasoactive agents. Comprehensive reviews of this complex topic have been published recently[9,10] and only a brief outline will be provided here. Studies in fetal sheep have shown that there is a direct relation between lung liquid volume and pulmonary vascular resistance[13]. Increasing the volume, and hence pressure, of liquid in the terminal air-spaces may compress the small pulmonary arteries or capillaries, thereby increasing their resistance to flow[9]. The low P_{O_2} of blood perfusing the fetal lungs also contributes to their high vascular resistance; if the lungs of postnatal lambs are perfused with blood having a P_{O_2} similar to that of the fetus the normally low pulmonary vascular resistance is greatly increased[14]. Studies in fetal sheep have shown that lowering and raising the P_{O_2} of arterial blood (i.e. hypoxia and hyperoxia) induce, respectively, increases and decreases in pulmonary vascular resistance[9]. The mechanism by which oxygen tension influences the resistance of pulmonary blood vessels is unknown, but may involve the release of prostacyclin (PGI_2) and endothelium-derived nitric oxide (NO) both of which are known to affect vascular smooth muscle.

There is evidence that leukotrienes (LT) C_4 and D_4, both of which are potent vasoconstrictors in the pulmonary circulation, may be involved in maintaining the high pulmonary vascular resistance of the fetus. In fetal sheep, blockade of LT receptors or inhibition of LT synthesis leads to pulmonary blood flow increasing (by eightfold) to levels seen in the newborn[9]. Other vasoactive substances that may be involved in maintaining a high resistance in the pulmonary bed of the fetus include endothelin-1, a potential vasodilator released from endothelial cells, and thromboxane A_2, another product of arachidonic acid[9,10].

CHANGES AT BIRTH

With the clearance of liquid from the lungs and its replacement by air, and with the onset of continuous breathing and increase in arterial P_{O_2}, the resistance of the pulmonary vascular bed greatly diminishes; this allows pulmonary blood flow to increase by eight- to tenfold[9]. The increase in pulmonary blood flow and pulmonary venous return leads to an increase in left atrial pressure which results in closure of the foramen ovale. This, together with the closure of the ductus arteriosus, results in the effective separation of the pulmonary and systemic circulations soon after birth.

The mechanisms underlying the large fall in pulmonary vascular resistance at birth are complex and probably involve physical factors, the oxygen environment and alterations in the balance between vasodilator and vasoconstrictor substances in the pulmonary vascular bed. The creation at birth of an air–liquid interface in the alveoli, and the partial recoil of the lungs (see below), may alter the geometry of small pulmonary vessels such that they become dilated. Rhythmic expansion of the lungs at birth, and increased oxygenation, releases vasodilators such as PGI_2, possibly mediated by bradykinin (a potent vasodilator in the fetus) or angiotensin II. Nitric oxide (NO) is now thought to play a particularly important role in pulmonary vasodilation after birth. In sheep, the inhibition of NO synthesis prior to birth attenuates the birth-induced increase in pulmonary blood flow[15] and results in pulmonary hypertension in the newborn[9]. Clearly many factors are involved in the switch from tonic pulmonary vasoconstriction in the fetus to tonic vasodilation after birth.

Fetal breathing movements

It is now well established that breathing-like movements occur intermittently throughout much of gestation in healthy mammalian fetuses[16]. These movements, termed 'fetal breathing movements' (FBM), share important features with postnatal breathing and are thought to be an early expression of coordinated, rhythmical activity in brain regions responsible for the control of breathing throughout postnatal life. FBM involve rhythmic activation of the diaphragm and dilator muscles of the upper respiratory tract, particularly those of the larynx[17]. Expiratory muscles (e.g. intercostal muscles, upper airway constrictors) are not significantly active during unstimulated FBM[18]. Like postnatal breathing, FBM are stimulated by increased blood levels of carbon dioxide and by acidification of the blood or cerebrospinal fluid, probably via stimulation of centrally located chemoreceptors[19]. FBM are also influenced, like postnatal breathing, by behavioural states; that is, by different states of sleep and wakefulness. During late gestation, FBM are apparently inhibited (i.e. they are essentially absent or infrequent, depending on species) during the fetal state resembling quiet (slow wave or non-rapid-eye movement) sleep, and are common during the fetal state resembling rapid-eye movement (or active, or desynchronised) sleep[20]. Whether the fetus is ever in a state resembling wakefulness is controversial; however, those that believe that the awake state does exist in the fetus consider that FBM occur during this state. The suppression of FBM during the state of quiet (slow wave) sleep is of considerable interest, because this suppression must be overcome after birth when breathing must be continuous.

FBM differ from postnatal breathing in that the 'tidal volume' is very small, and each breath is essentially isometric and isovolumic; the reasons are complex, but are mainly attributable to the high viscosity (and inertia) of water relative to air, and the apparently high resistance of the fetal upper respiratory tract to the ingress of liquid[21]. In the ovine fetus, the 'tidal volume' is normally less than 1 ml[20,22], compared with 40–50 ml (8–10 ml/kg) of the newborn[23]; a similar difference exists in the human. That is, the change in lung luminal volume associated with individual FBM in a late-gestation ovine fetus is normally less than 1% of the resting (baseline) luminal volume. Thus, FBM resemble postnatal breathing with an obstructed upper airway; this presumably gives rise to the paradoxical nature of FBM; that is, during 'inspiration' the chest wall retracts and the abdominal wall moves out[24,25].

FBM can be readily detected ultrasonographically and are widely used in the assessment of fetal health; they have become an important part of the fetal biophysical profile[26]. The incidence of FBM is reduced in fetuses that are subjected to intra-uterine stresses such as the impaired delivery of primary nutrients (oxygen and glucose), to intra-uterine infection or to increased levels of prostaglandins[16,27]. FBM may be absent or impaired in fetuses with congenital abnormalities of the nervous system or skeletal muscle[28]. Maternal drug use can also abolish or attenuate FBM; for example alcohol[29], tobacco smoking[30] as well as common sedatives and narcotics[31,32] have been shown to inhibit FBM.

It is now recognised that the prolonged absence of FBM can lead to the development of lung hypoplasia; in this condition, the lungs are small, relative to body weight, and are structurally immature[33,34]. If severe, it can lead to death of the newly born, or may result in respiratory insufficiency. By resisting the tendency of the fetal lung to recoil, FBM play an important role in maintaining the fetal lungs in an expanded state. Lung expansion during late fetal life is known to be necessary for the normal growth and structural maturation of the lungs. The role of FBM in the maintenance of lung expansion and lung growth is discussed in more detail on page 188.

As well as being used in the assessment of fetal health, attempts have been made to use FBM to assess fetal lung development, in particular, the presence of lung hypoplasia. Given the role that FBM are known to play in maintaining fetal lung expansion and lung growth, it might be expected that their absence would be associated with lung hypoplasia. Some clinical studies have shown that, in patients in which there was a high risk of lung hypoplasia (i.e. in the presence of premature rupture of membranes and oligohydramnios), a strong association exists between the absence of FBM and evidence of lung hypoplasia in the newborn[35,36]. However, other studies found no association[37,38]. The different results could be due to the selection of different types of subjects or to differing definitions of FBM or lung hypoplasia.

Fetal lung liquid

LUNG LIQUID SECRETION

It is now well established that during fetal life the future airways of the lungs are filled with a liquid that is secreted by the pulmonary epithelium. Although it was once thought that this liquid was inhaled amniotic fluid, the findings that (i) liquid accumulates within the future airways when the trachea is obstructed[39,40] and that (ii) lung liquid has an ionic composition which is quite different to that of either amniotic fluid or plasma[41] (Table 16.2), indicate that lung liquid is neither inhaled amniotic fluid nor an ultrafiltrate of plasma. Indeed, measurements of unidirectional ion fluxes in fetal sheep lungs have indicated that lung liquid secretion results from the net movement of chloride ions across the pulmonary epithelium into the 'airway' lumen[42]. This generates an osmotic gradient across the epithelium which promotes the movement of water towards the lung lumen. The model proposed to describe the movement of chloride ions across the epithelium is based on that proposed for the shark rectal gland[43]. It is proposed that Na^+,K^+-ATPase, located on the basolateral surface of pulmonary epithelial cells, provides the electrochemical gradient

TABLE 16.2
Composition of fetal lung liquid in comparison to fetal arterial blood and amniotic fluid

Parameter	Arterial blood	Lung liquid	Amniotic fluid
Na^+ (mmol/l)	150 ± 0.7	150 ± 1.3	113 ± 6.5
K^+ (mmol/l)	4.8 ± 0.2	6.3 ± 0.7	7.6 ± 0.8
Cl^- (mmol/l)	107 ± 1.0	157.1 ± 4.1	87 ± 5
Ca^{2+} (mmol/l)	3.3 ± 0.1	0.8 ± 0.1	1.6 ± 0.1
HCO_3^- (mmol/l)	24 ± 1.2	2.8 ± 0.3	19 ± 3
Urea	291 ± 2	7.9 ± 2.7	10.5 ± 2.4
Osmolality (mOsm)	291 ± 2	294 ± 2	265 ± 2
Protein (mg/100 ml)	4090 ± 260	27 ± 2	100 ± 10
pH	7.34 ± 0.04	6.27 ± 0.5	7.02 ± 0.09

Values are derived from Adamson *et al.*[41].

for Na^+ to enter the cell coupled to Cl^-[43]. The Cl^- is then thought to exit the cell across its apical membrane and enter the lung lumen down its electrochemical gradient. Once secreted, fetal lung liquid leaves the lung by flowing out of the trachea into the pharynx, from where it is either swallowed or flows into the amniotic sac via the nose or mouth[44–47]. Consequently, the volume of liquid retained within the future airways must be controlled by a balance between the rate at which it is produced and the rate at which it leaves the lungs.

During the last third of gestation, before the onset of labour, healthy fetal sheep secrete lung liquid at a rate of 3–4 ml/kg/h (Fig. 16.3); for a given fetus, the rate of secretion is quite uniform throughout a 24-hour period. The rate of secretion of lung liquid is principally controlled by endocrine and metabolic factors, although recent studies indicate that physical factors may also play a role. Both adrenaline, acting via β-adrenergic receptors[48–50], and arginine vasopressin[51,52] are potent inhibitors of lung liquid secretion *in vivo*, possibly via activation of adenylate cyclase leading to an increase in intracellular cAMP concentrations[53]. Because the inhibitory effect of these hormones increases with gestational age in fetal sheep, it is generally considered that they play an important role in the reabsorption of lung liquid at birth (see below). Other hormones known to affect fetal lung liquid secretion include: epidermal growth factor (EGF) which inhibits secretion, although its effect may be mediated by an associated increase in fetal adrenaline release[54]; cortisol which increases lung liquid secretion *in vivo*[55,56] but inhibits it *in vitro*[57]; aldosterone which inhibits lung liquid secretion *in vitro*[57]; and prolactin which has been shown to stimulate lung liquid secretion when administered directly into lung liquid *in vivo*[58].

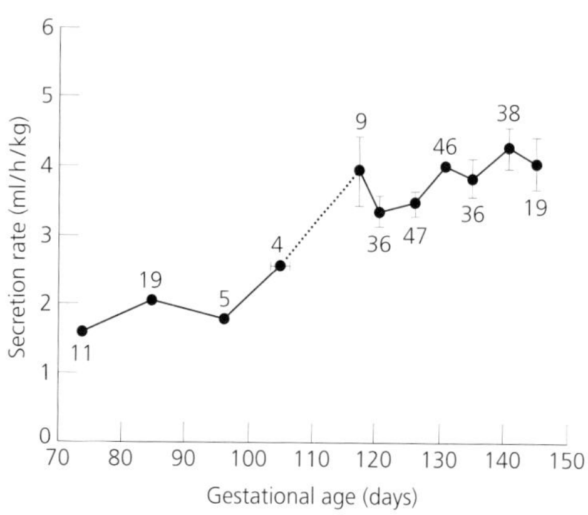

Fig. 16.3 The secretion rate of fetal lung liquid, measured by dye-dilution techniques, during the last half of gestation in fetal sheep. Numbers represent the number of measurements made at each gestational age. Values below 100 days of gestation were obtained from Olver *et al.*[146].

Hypoxaemia is also a potent inhibitor of fetal lung secretion[59,60]. Its effect is unlikely to be mediated by an associated stress-related increase in circulating adrenaline and vasopressin concentrations[50,61], but rather from a reduction in oxidative metabolism and/or associated changes in tissue pH[62]. Indeed, the lung liquid secretory process appears to be oxygen dependent[42,63] and acidaemia has been shown to enhance the inhibitory effect of hypoxaemia[62]. In this regard, it is of interest that acidaemia potentiates the reduction in pulmonary blood flow (and hence oxygen delivery) in fetal sheep that are exposed to hypoxaemia[64].

Physical factors also appear to influence the rate of secretion of fetal lung liquid. Experimental manipulations that lead to a reduction in fetal lung liquid volume, and hence a reduction in pulmonary luminal pressure, result in an increase in lung liquid secretion rates[65,66]; this also occurs following prolonged lung liquid drainage when the production rate of lung liquid is adjusted for the size of the lung[67]. On the other hand, manipulations that increase the volume of lung liquid, and hence increase luminal pressure, for example following tracheal occlusion, lead to an increase in intraluminal pressure and cause either a reduction[68] or complete cessation of fetal lung liquid secretion[67,69]. These alterations in secretion can be explained by alterations in intraluminal pressure. The driving force for the net movement of water across the epithelium must be governed by the sum of all forces affecting fluid movement. Under normal conditions, a small hydrostatic pressure exists across the lungs (lung lumen is 1–2 mmHg > amniotic sac pressure[70], which opposes the osmotic pressure resulting from the movement of chloride ions. Normally the osmotic pressure promoting liquid secretion must exceed the opposing hydrostatic pressure for liquid to cross the epithelium and enter the lung lumen. Thus, reductions or increases in the intraluminal pressure, resulting from alterations in lung liquid volume, would be expected to increase or reduce net production rates of lung liquid by altering the magnitude of the opposing hydrostatic pressure, i.e. without directly affecting the ionic mechanism of lung liquid secretion.

Although the presence of fetal lung liquid within the future airways is essential for normal fetal lung development (see below), this liquid must be cleared before birth so that the newborn can establish effective pulmonary gas exchange. Previous studies had suggested that, in fetal sheep, lung liquid clearance begins up to 10 days before the onset of labour[71]. However, this finding could not be confirmed in a recent study of healthy fetuses in normal pregnancies that proceeded to full term[72]; indeed large volumes of liquid (250–300 ml) remained within the future airways until the start of labour[72]. These results indicate that, in healthy fetuses, most of the liquid within the future airways must be cleared during labour itself. It is widely accepted that increased circulating concentrations of adrenaline and AVP in fetal plasma, which are released into the circulation in response to the stress of labour[49,73], play an important role in inhibiting secretion and inducing lung liquid reabsorption. These hormones are thought to induce lung liquid reabsorption via a cAMP-mediated activation of amiloride-blockable sodium channels on the luminal surface of pulmonary epithelial cells[53,73]. Activation of these channels is considered to cause an increase in Na^+ and Na^+-linked Cl^- flux away from the lung lumen to the interstitium, thereby reversing the osmotic gradient across the epithelium and leading to lung liquid reabsorption[73]. While this mechanism is likely to be very important for lung liquid clearance during labour, it is unlikely to be the only mechanism. For instance, in unstressed fetal sheep at term, we have observed that large amounts of lung liquid (~50%) leave the lungs during the early stages of labour before fetal circulating concentrations of adrenaline and AVP are elevated[72]. This reduction in lung liquid volume may be caused by compression of the lungs resulting from postural changes imposed on the fetus by the shortening of the uterine muscle during labour; it has been established that fetal trunk flexion causes substantial loss of lung liquid[74].

CONTROL OF LUNG LIQUID VOLUME

The volume of liquid retained within the future airways increases markedly over the last half of gestation in most species. In particular, over the last third of gestation in fetal sheep, lung liquid volumes increase from 25–30 ml/kg to 45–50 ml/kg near term (145–150 days) (Fig. 16.4). In contrast, the corresponding volume of the air-filled lung in newborn lambs (functional residual capacity; FRC) is approximately 20–25 ml/kg[75]. Thus, during late gestation, the fetal lung is hyperexpanded, compared with the air-filled newborn lung, and the lung partially collapses at birth (i.e. the volume approximately halves; see Fig. 16.4). The reasons why the fetal lung partially collapses at birth are self-evident. The clearance of lung liquid and the onset of air breathing not only removes lung liquid and the distending force that it in the fetus, but it also leads to the formation of an air–liquid interface, and hence surface forces, within the alveoli; the summation of these surface forces constitutes the major part of the postnatal lung's elastic recoil. Although the presence of surfactant greatly reduces these surface forces, it does not eliminate them and, as a consequence, the lung tends to collapse after birth. This partial recoil of the lung after birth results in the formation of a more sub-atmospheric pressure in the intrapleural space than existed in the fetus.

During fetal life, the volume of lung liquid is maintained at a relatively high level (approximately double the FRC after birth) primarily due to factors that control the efflux of liquid from the lungs. Lung liquid principally leaves the lungs via the trachea and its rate of efflux is principally controlled by the larynx and upper airway[21,44,76]. During 'non-breathing' periods (i.e. during fetal 'apnoea'), tonic activity in the laryngeal constrictor muscles imposes a resistance to lung liquid efflux[21,76], thereby opposing the tendency of the lungs to collapse as a result of their elastic recoil. This is analogous to constricting the neck of an inflated rubber balloon, and in the fetal lung results in the accumulation of liquid within the future spaces. However, during periods of FBM, the laryngeal dilator muscles are phasically active leading to widening of the glottis and a reduction in the resistance to lung liquid

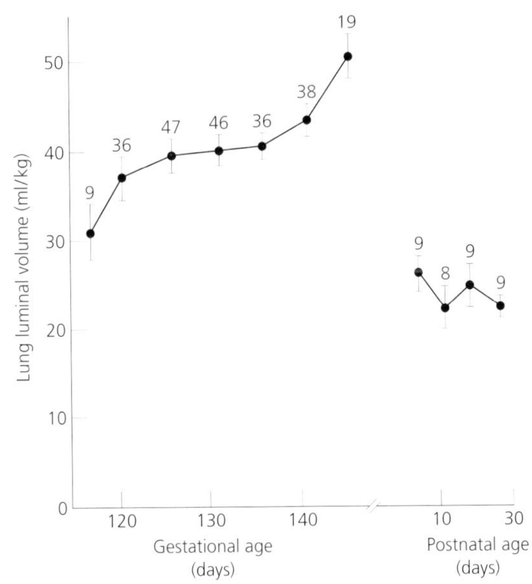

Fig. 16.4 The volume of fetal lung liquid, measured by a dye-dilution technique, during the last 40 days of gestation in fetal sheep. Measurements of functional residual capacity (FRC) in postnatal lambs, made using a He-dilution technique, have been included for comparison; these measurements were obtained from Jakubowska *et al.*[75]. Numbers represent the number of measurements made at each gestational or postnatal age.

efflux[21,76]. Consequently, due to the combined effect of the elastic recoil of lung tissue and the lowered resistance to lung liquid efflux, liquid loss from the lung accelerates and the lungs partially collapse during FBM episodes[21,46,76]. However, it is important to note that the loss of lung liquid during periods of FBM is apparently opposed by a simultaneous contraction of the diaphragm muscle[65,66,77]. That is, contraction of the diaphragm muscle during the inspiratory phase of FBM tends to oppose the elastic recoil of lung tissue, thereby limiting the loss of lung liquid. Thus, the high degree of lung expansion in the fetus is apparently due to (i) the low level of elastic recoil (owing to the absence of an air–liquid interface), (ii) the high resistance to lung liquid efflux offered by the larynx during non-breathing periods and (iii) the contractions of the diaphragm muscle during FBM episodes when the resistance to lung liquid efflux is reduced[77].

Processes in fetal lung growth

Most research to date indicates that mechanical influences, via alterations in the degree of stretch of lung tissue, play a critical role in normal fetal lung growth and development. Indeed, there is much evidence to indicate that most, if not all, of the many clinical conditions that result in inadequate lung growth (pulmonary hypoplasia) in human fetuses, result from a prolonged reduction in lung expansion. These include disorders that allow the fetal lung to collapse (e.g. diaphragmatic hernias), that reduce intrathoracic space (e.g. pleural fluid accumulation), that cause compression of the chest (e.g. oligohydramnios) and that impair skeletal muscle activity[77].

The physiological significance of fetal lung liquid first became apparent following experiments which showed that alterations in the volume of lung liquid caused marked changes in lung growth. In fetal sheep, prolonged drainage of lung liquid from the trachea, which causes the lungs to deflate, results in a total cessation of lung growth[67,78] which eventually results in severe lung hypoplasia[67,79]. On the other hand, increasing the volume of lung liquid, which can be readily accomplished by obstructing the fetal trachea, markedly increases fetal lung growth[40,79,80]. The lung growth response to tracheal obstruction is rapid and can cause an almost doubling in total lung cell number within 7 days[78]. Further research has shown that the acceleration in fetal lung growth, in terms of cell number, follows a specific time-course; it begins within 2 days and is complete within 7 days[69]. Thus, it would appear that the mechanisms by which increases in fetal lung expansion induce an acceleration in lung growth are only active within a relatively narrow window of time. The recent finding that the increase in lung cell number is very closely related to the increase in lung liquid volume ($r = 0.99$) following tracheal obstruction, but not to the increase in intraluminal pressure, provides an important clue as to how this response is regulated[69]. That is, the physical distortion of lung tissue, rather than an increase in intraluminal pressure *per se*, is most likely to be responsible for activating the growth response. Consequently, the reason for the acceleration in fetal lung growth ceasing within 7 days of obstructing the trachea is most probably the inability of the lung to continue to accumulate fluid after this time and undoubtedly results from the physical limitations imposed by the chest wall[69]. Thus, if the chest wall was not a limiting factor, for example if the diaphragm is herniated, it is likely that the lung would continue to expand and grow through the hernia into the abdomen. On the other hand, it is also possible that tracheal occlusion may not expand the lungs and stimulate lung growth in fetuses with hypoplastic lungs. For example, if the small lungs are so incompliant that the pressure required to expand them is greater than the osmotic pressure driving lung liquid secretion, the lungs may not expand.

STRETCH AND LUNG GROWTH: POTENTIAL MECHANISMS

The cellular and molecular mechanisms by which changes in fetal lung expansion affect lung growth are largely unknown, although the effect is specifically localised to expanded or deflated areas of the lung[80]. This response is not unique to the lung as mechanical forces are well known to affect DNA replication and/or the phenotypic expression, via the activation or repression of genes, of many different types of cells[81]. However, the mechanisms by which mechanical forces are translated into a cellular response are not known. We consider it likely that the distortion of lung tissue associated with a change in lung expansion is transmitted via the extracellular matrix and causes changes in cell shape and/or tension within the cytoskeleton. The translation of this stimulus into a cellular response may result from the direct activation of stretch sensitive ion channels and/or from the direct activation of second messenger systems (e.g. tyrosine kinases and phospholipases) associated with the proteins that interlink extracellular matrix receptors (e.g. integrins) with the cytoskeleton[82]. It is also possible that distortion of a cell may directly activate or inactivate genes and/or DNA replication enzymes via changes in tension or orientation of cytoskeletal and nuclear structural components[82]. Indeed, the recent finding of a specific stretch response element in the promoter region for α-actin indicates that stretch may be able to directly activate genes[83].

It is likely that alterations in the gene expression for a variety of growth factors play an important role in the growth response to changes in lung expansion, possibly by integrating and propagating the response. Indeed, alterations in fetal lung expansion induce corresponding changes in insulin like growth factor-II (IGF-II) gene expression[65,78]. IGF-II has potent mitogenic and differentiating activities and is thought to play an important role in fetal growth[84]. In addition, intermittent stretch of pulmonary epithelial cells in culture, designed to simulate FBM *in vivo*, is a potent stimulus for

DNA synthesis in those cells[85]. This physical stimulus also induces an increase in the gene expression for platelet-derived growth factor (PDGF) in cultured pulmonary epithelial cells[85]. The recent finding that the effect of phasic stretch on DNA synthesis in cultured pulmonary epithelial cells can be blocked by antisense oligonucleotides for PDGF, indicates that PDGF plays a crucial role in this response[86].

FETAL LUNG HYPOPLASIA

Fetal lung hypoplasia is commonly associated with an increased risk of neonatal morbidity and mortality. In humans, the fetal lung is classified as being hypoplastic if the lung to body weight ratio is <0.015 in fetuses younger than 28 weeks of gestation and <0.012 in fetuses older than 28 weeks[87]. Fetal lung hypoplasia occurs in ~1.1 babies per 1000 live births[88–90], although this value probably underestimates the true incidence due to the many neonates that survive following extensive postnatal treatment. However, of babies born after 35 weeks of gestation and who die in their first postnatal week, almost one-third have severe lung hypoplasia[89]. It is important to recognise that, in fetal lung hypoplasia, the lungs are not simply small, but are structurally immature. For example, hypoplastic lungs have been shown to contain reduced numbers of airways and alveoli[87,91–93], reduced elastin development[94], and narrower airways[95]. The proportion of airspace in the lung is also reduced[96]. The maturation of the respiratory epithelium is impaired, as evidenced by the persistence of cuboidal cells, particularly in the peripheral parts of the acinus[97,98]. This structural immaturity, which results in the reduced size and effectiveness of the gas-exchanging surface, contributes to the impaired gas exchange that results in neonatal respiratory compromise. However, the severity and range of pathological changes in the lungs will depend on the duration and degree of reduced lung expansion[99].

Fetal lung hypoplasia rarely occurs in isolation, but is usually associated with other types of developmental disorders. It is commonly associated with disorders of the central nervous system[28] and skeletal muscle[100] that affect the thorax, as well as disorders that reduce fetal intra-thoracic volume, for example pleural effusions and herniation of the diaphragm[101,102]. Oligohydramnios is also a common cause of fetal lung hypoplasia, whether the reduction in amniotic fluid results from premature rupture of the membranes or from renal or urinary tract abnormalities[100,103]. Although it appears that a diverse range of factors can cause fetal lung hypoplasia, it is likely that each of these factors leads to lung hypoplasia via a common final mechanism. It is now apparent that each of the factors thought to cause lung hypoplasia does so by causing a reduction in fetal lung expansion; thus, the associated lung hypoplasia most probably results from the absence of a growth stimulus (i.e. tissue stress), rather than from an active inhibition of growth.

Because fetal lung growth is so sensitive to alterations in lung expansion[78–80], it has been suggested that increasing the degree of fetal lung expansion may be used therapeutically to reverse lung growth deficits in human fetuses *in utero*. Indeed, obstruction of the fetal trachea, which results in intra-luminal fluid accumulation and increased lung tissue stress, has been shown experimentally to prevent the pulmonary hypoplasia caused by oligohydramnios[104,105] and congenital diaphragmatic hernias[106]. In addition, we have recently shown that as little as 6 days of tracheal obstruction in fetal sheep is sufficient to almost totally reverse an existing, severe deficit of lung growth, indicating that the period of tracheal occlusion need only be of short duration[67]. However, it has yet to be determined whether fetal lungs, subjected to accelerated growth by these procedures, are functionally normal after birth. The small amount of evidence that is presently available suggests that this procedure may be successful, although there are a number of unwanted side effects that need to be considered. For instance, tracheal obstruction alters the distribution of epithelial cell types in the terminal airways resulting in a reduced number of type II cells[79]. In addition, even short periods of increased lung expansion in the fetus greatly reduce surfactant protein-A, -B, and -C gene expression[107,108]. Thus, much more information is needed regarding the physiological consequences of altering the degree of fetal lung expansion to avoid complications that may result from this treatment.

Lung maturation

STRUCTURAL MATURATION

The unique architecture of the lung is largely dependent upon the components and organisation of its extracellular matrix (ECM) and on cell-to-cell and cell-substrate adhesion properties. Within the lung, the components of the ECM are synthesised by a variety of cell types and provide the structural support to which the lung cells attach[109]. Consequently, the ECM plays an integral role in lung development from the early stages of its growth *in utero* through to its ability to function as a gas-exchange organ during postnatal life. Indeed, different components of the ECM are considered to be critically involved with cell migration, branching morphogenesis, cellular proliferation and cyto-differentiation as well as determining tissue compliance[109]. The ECM of the lungs is primarily comprised of collagen (principally types I, III, V and VI), elastin, glycoproteins (e.g. fibronectin and laminin) and proteoglycans[109]. At the level of the peripheral airway units, these components form the epithelial and endothelial basement membranes and the structural fibres that course through the interstitium located at the interalveolar septa; these connect with axial fibres running in parallel with major conducting airways and blood vessels and are further braced by connective tissue elements projecting in from the pleura[110]. Thus, major alterations in lung architecture, such as those that occur during development, must involve remodelling of the ECM.

The increase in fetal plasma cortisol concentrations prior to parturition in most species is thought to play an important role in maturing the lung by either directly or indirectly influencing its structure, tissue compliance, the differentiation of epithelial cells and the synthesis of surfactant[111,112]. These changes lead to an increase in potential airspace volume, reduction in gas-diffusing distance and an increase in compliance of the air-filled lung. Indeed, over the last third of gestation in fetal sheep, there is a large increase in lung luminal volume (see Fig. 16.4) which is associated with increased alveolar surface area and reduced interalveolar tissue distances[113]. The findings that fetal infusions of corticosteroids accelerate these changes in lung architecture, whereas adrenalectomy (which removes the endogenous source of circulating corticosteroids in the fetus) retards them[55,56], indicates that corticosteroids are intimately involved in the structural modification of the lung during late gestation. Similarly, fetal hypophysectomy, which decreases circulating fetal plasma cortisol concentrations, has been shown to increase interalveolar wall thickness and to increase the volume density of septal tissue (i.e. it reduces the potential airspace volume)[114]. These structural features are characteristic of immature lungs and are reversed by the reinfusion of either cortisol or adrenocorticotrophin (ACTH)[114]. Collectively, these findings indicate that, at least in fetal sheep, over the last third of gestation a progressive increase in circulating concentrations of fetal corticosteroids plays an important role in promoting structural changes within the lung. This concept is consistent with numerous studies that have demonstrated that corticosteroid treatment greatly increases lung compliance[111,112,115] and ventilatory efficiency[116] in prematurely delivered fetuses. The relative involvement of thyroid hormones in the corticosteroid-induced changes in lung structure, however, is still unclear. It is interesting that sustained deflation of the lung during the last third of gestation in fetal sheep causes changes in lung structure that are very similar to those reported for corticosteroid withdrawal[79].

The mechanisms by which corticosteroids stimulate the structural maturation of the fetal lungs are not well understood, but most probably include remodelling of the ECM. Over the last third of gestation in fetal sheep, the content of collagen, particularly elastin, in lung parenchyma increases markedly, with most of the increase occurring over the final 25–30 days[117]. Similarly, it has been shown that elastin mRNA levels in ovine fetal lungs increase markedly over the last third of gestation and, in particular, tropoelastin (elastin precursor) production peaks just before the time of birth[118]. This period of gestation coincides with the exponential increase in circulating cortisol concentrations in the fetus and a large increase in the luminal volume of the fetal lungs[56,77]. Thus, because the components of the lung ECM are rapidly turned over, at least in culture[119,120], it is likely that endocrine factors like cortisol induce remodelling of the ECM by altering the expression of its specific components; corticosteroid-induced alterations in the rate of ECM turnover, occurring via alterations in the expression of metalloproteinases or their specific inhibitors, may also contribute to the remodelling[121]. Whatever the mechanisms, it is likely that endogenous glucocorticoids play an important role in regulating the ECM of the lung and, therefore, are able to influence its structural development and thus its ability to function as a gas exchange organ after birth. It is not known whether glucocorticoids act directly on specific cell types within the lung to effect these changes or whether their effects are mediated via numerous other endocrine factors that are also likely to be involved; these may include epidermal growth factor[122], transforming growth factor-β[123] and fibroblast–pneumonocyte factor[124]. It is possible that these growth factors act in a paracrine fashion to modulate the action of both glucocorticoids and physical influences, like alterations in lung expansion, which could explain the similarity in the effect of these stimuli on lung architecture and cellular differentiation.

EPITHELIAL CELL DIFFERENTIATION

The success of pulmonary gas exchange after birth depends on many factors. These include a sufficiently large surface area for gas exchange, an adequate blood flow in pulmonary capillaries, a thin barrier between air and blood, and a high degree of lung compliance. The last of these is highly dependent upon the maturation of pulmonary epithelial cells, without which postnatal respiratory function would be greatly impaired. During early stages of lung development, epithelial cells are either columnar (pseudoglandular stage) or cuboidal (canalicular stage) and are not suited to gas exchange; furthermore, they are not able to synthesise surfactant. These primitive epithelial cells characteristically contain abundant glycogen deposits. During the canalicular stage (by 22–24 weeks), epithelial cells begin to differentiate into thinner type I cells (which form the gas-exchange surface) and cuboidal type II cells (which are able to synthesise and release pulmonary surfactant).

The mechanisms which regulate the differentiation of pulmonary epithelial cell are largely unknown. However, these mechanisms have been the subject of considerable interest because appropriate epithelial cell differentiation is critical for respiratory function both in the neonate and adult. Indeed, type I epithelial cells make up >90% of the surface area of the lung and, therefore, are intimately involved in gas exchange. Type II cells, on the other hand, produce surfactant which is critical for lowering surface forces at the air-liquid interface (see Possmayer[125]).

Differentiation of the epithelial cells lining the peripheral airway units begins during the canalicular stage of lung development in sheep[113]. Initially, most epithelial cells within the terminal airways are undifferentiated[113] with approximately equal numbers of type I and type II epithelial cells[113,114]. As the structural development of the lung proceeds with gestation, the undifferentiated epithelial cells progressively differentiate and the density of type II cells decreases such that, by term, there are approximately twice as many type I as type II cells[114]. Although it is widely considered that both types of differentiated epithelial cells arise as daughter cells from proliferating type II stem cells[126], more recent data which identify the pattern of expression of cell-specific markers from very early in gestation indicate that this concept may not be accurate[127]. Indeed, in the sheep fetus, the presence of type I epithelial cells was detected at an earlier period in gestation than type II epithelial cells[113].

Whatever the mechanisms that control epithelial cell differentiation in the developing lungs, this process is influenced by both corticosteroids[114] and the degree of fetal lung expansion, or tissue stress[79]. Fetal hypophysectomy, which prevents the normal gestational age-related increase in fetal plasma cortisol concentrations and the onset of labour, prevents the gestational age-related decrease in type II cell density at the expected time of birth[114]. Replacement of glucocorticoids in hypophysectomised fetuses, by infusions of ACTH and cortisol, reduced the density of type II cells to control levels at the expected time of birth[114]. Similar changes in type II cell density can be observed following alterations in fetal lung expansion, indicating that there may be a common link between alterations in lung tissue stress and the action of corticosteroids. Studies in fetal sheep have shown that reduced tissue stress elicited by the continuous drainage of lung liquid increases the density of type II epithelial cells whereas increasing the degree of lung expansion and tissue stress reduces the density of type II epithelial cells[79].

Pulmonary surfactant

The presence of pulmonary surfactant at birth is essential for the lungs to function effectively; without adequate amounts of surfactant, the lungs are difficult to expand, the work of breathing is greatly increased, and gas exchange is impaired. Surfactant deficiency is common in preterm infants and can lead to the respiratory distress syndrome (RDS, or hyaline membrane disease); this is characterised by laboured breathing and progressive cyanosis due to ineffective respiratory gas exchange[128]. In preterm infants, the effects of surfactant deficiency may be exacerbated by structural immaturity of the lungs. Prenatal treatment with glucocorticoids can stimulate not only surfactant synthesis but, as outlined in the preceding section, can enhance structural maturation of the lungs[129]. Both of these effects are vital for effective lung function after birth.

COMPOSITION OF SURFACTANT

Pulmonary surfactant, which is a complex mixture of substances (approximately 90% lipid and 10% protein), is synthesised in the type II epithelial cells[130,131]. Once secreted, it leads to the formation of a monolayer of tightly packed lipid molecules at the interface between the liquid layer overlying alveolar epithelial cells and the air within the alveoli (Fig. 16.5), thereby greatly lowering surface tension, so that alveoli can be expanded more easily during inspiration, and effectively stabilising the alveoli so that they do not collapse during expiration.

Pulmonary surfactant is a complex mixture of phospholipids and protein[130,132]. Of the many recognised components of surfactant, the one with the greatest role in lowering surface tension is the principal lipid, dipalmitoyl phosphatidylcholine (DPPC); this is sometimes referred to as disaturated phosphatidylcholine (DSPC). It accounts for 45% of the weight of pulmonary surfactant obtained by broncho-alveolar lavage[133]. Other phospholipids that may be involved in the lowering of surface tension are phosphatidylglycerol and phosphatidylinositol.

In addition to lipids, four surfactant associated proteins (or apoproteins) have been identified; surfactant proteins (SP) A, B, C and D. SP-A, which is the largest and most abundant of the surfactant proteins, is a water-soluble glycoprotein with a molecular weight of 28–36 kDa and is made up of 18 subunits. *In vitro*, SP-A, together with SP-B and SP-C, accelerates the formation of a monolayer; without the presence of surfactant proteins, DPPC does not readily spread over a liquid surface[130]. SP-B is a smaller protein (8 kDa, 79 amino acids) which is lipophilic; SP-C is also a small lipophilic protein (5 kDa). Both of these are thought to play an important role in the formation of a surface layer of surfactant because, *in vitro*, they greatly accelerate this process. *In vivo*, mixtures of SP-B and phospholipids are able to increase lung compliance and alveolar stability in preterm animals[131]. SP-D is a hydrophilic

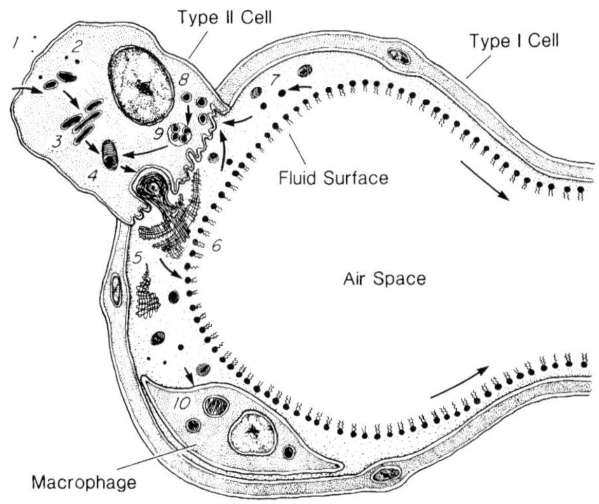

Fig. 16.5 Schematic diagram of a section through a single alveolus, showing the movement of surfactant components through the type II cell and alveolar liquid (not to scale). 1, surfactant precursors such as glucose, amino acids and fatty acids; 2, endoplasmic reticulum; 3, Golgi apparatus; 4, lamellar bodies; 5, tubular myelin; 6, surface film with adsorbed phospholipids; 7, vesicular and myelin forms of surfactant, possibly derived from material desorbed from the film; 8 and 9, endocytic compartments including multivesicular bodies; 10, alveolar macrophage. Reproduced with permission from Hawgood and Clements[147].

glycoprotein (43 kDa), but unlike other surfactant proteins, it does not appear to be involved in the formation of a surface layer or in the lowering of surface tension. SP-D bears some similarities to proteins that are involved in immunological responses and such a role has been postulated. *In vitro*, SP-D has been shown to bind to bacteria and to increase the formation of oxygen free radicals in alveolar macrophages. SP-D gene expression is associated with both type II cells and Clara cells of the distal bronchi[131].

It is now established that all of the lipid and protein components of surfactant are synthesised in alveolar type II cells[134]. Much of this material is recycled following its re-uptake by type II cells via endocytosis. Within the type II cells, the lipid and surfactant proteins (SP A–C) become components of lamellar bodies which are made up of concentrically arranged layers of phospholipids. Surfactant is released into the alveoli by a process of exocytosis following fusion of the lamellar body to the type II cell membrane (Fig. 16.5). Once outside the cell, the material from lamellar bodies forms a meshwork of tubular myelin made up of long tubules with intersecting lipid bilayer membranes containing SP-A and SP-B[135]. The phospholipids are then incorporated into the monolayer at the air–liquid interface.

ONTOGENY OF SURFACTANT SYNTHESIS AND RELEASE

In the human fetus, pulmonary concentrations of DPPC (mg/mg DNA) begin to increase after 20 weeks, when type II cells containing lamellar bodies are first detected[133]. By 24 weeks, concentrations have reached 35% of adult levels, although no surfactant is released from type II cells until about 30 weeks. Released surfactant can be first detected in amniotic fluid about this time. After 30 weeks, it is thought that the synthesis and release of surfactant from type II cells goes on increasing until term. The synthesis of DPPC is controlled by the enzyme fatty acid synthetase, the activity of which increases during late fetal life in parallel with increasing DPPC content of the lungs. Studies on the ontogeny of surfactant proteins show that levels increase during the latter half of gestation[133]. The presence of SP-A in amniotic fluid, like that of DPPC, is detected first around 30 weeks; after this, levels progressively increase. These changes are paralleled by increases in mRNA for the surfactant proteins in lung tissue.

The surfactant-producing status of fetal lungs can be assessed by measurements of components of surfactant in amniotic fluid. These components of surfactant are presumably transported into amniotic fluid by the on-going production of lung liquid (not all of which is swallowed by the fetus)[136]. Several tests are used for the assessment of fetal lung maturity[130]. The most widely used is the L/S ratio which is the ratio of the concentrations of lecithin (i.e. phosphatidylcholine) to sphingomyelin (a non-specific membrane lipid); this ratio increases markedly with increased surfactant release after 30 weeks of gestation. Other tests include measurements of phosphatidylcholine, phosphatidylglycerol and SP-A in amniotic fluid[130]. The 'shake test', in which the stability of bubbles produced by shaking samples of amniotic fluid is determined, can also be used to assess the amount of surfactant present.

GLUCOCORTICOID CONTROL OF SURFACTANT SYNTHESIS AND RELEASE

Endogenous fetal hormones are believed to play an important role in the maturation of the lungs; in particular, glucocorticoids appear to be necessary for the normal development of pulmonary surfactant production and its release[129,137,138]. The gestational age-related increase in circulating cortisol concentrations in fetal sheep is paralleled by an increase in pulmonary surfactant content and air-filled lung compliance[139]. Furthermore, a reduction in circulating glucocorticoid concentrations in fetal sheep, caused by hypophysectomy or adrenalectomy, inhibits surfactant production; replacement of cortisol or ACTH in treated fetuses leads to the stimulation of surfactant production[140]. Glucocorticoid receptors are present in the lung throughout most of gestation, and it is believed that these receptors mediate the actions of glucocorticoids in stimulating the synthesis of surfactant phospholipids and associated proteins.

It is now well established that the administration of exogenous glucocorticoids to the preterm fetus can accelerate the maturation of alveolar type II cells and surfactant synthesis[129,141]. The structural maturation of the lung is also accelerated, as indicated by an attenuation of mesenchymal tissue, an increase in the proportion of potential airspace, and an increase in the synthesis of elastin and collagen. Thus, the effect of cortisol in improving the lung distensibility of the preterm neonate is attributable to both enhanced structural maturation and increased surfactant synthesis[130].

ROLE OF THYROID HORMONES

Thyroid hormones appear to be important in lung development as fetal thyroidectomy impairs structural maturation as well reducing surfactant content in type II cells and lavage fluid[130]. *In vitro* and *in vivo* studies have shown that triiodothyronine (T_3), thyroxine (T_4) and TRH stimulate the synthesis of surfactant phospholipids[133,142]; T_3 appears to be more potent than T_4 in this regard. It has also been shown that the stimulatory effects of thyroid hormones are potentiated by glucocorticoids; that is, the effects of these hormones when administered together are greater than when given alone. This potentiation has formed the basis for recent clinical trials of the stimulation of lung maturation in cases of threatened preterm delivery[143]. In animal studies, a greater degree of potentiation was achieved when catecholamines were administered along with glucocorticoids and thyroid hormones. Catecholamines have been shown to stimulate the reabsorption of lung liquid and surfactant release from type II cells.

Studies in animals have indicated that lung maturation is dependent upon a number of key hormone systems, principally glucocorticoids, thyroid hormones and catecholamines, and it is likely that this also true in the human.

INTERVENTION IN LUNG IMMATURITY

Preterm birth is common worldwide and is the major cause of early postnatal respiratory disease and mortality. Of babies born at 30 weeks, approximately one-half will develop the respiratory distress syndrome (RDS). Antenatal therapy with glucocorticoids has greatly reduced the incidence of RDS in preterm infants, although, to be effective, they must be administered 1–2 days prior to birth[130]. In animal studies, glucocorticoids have been found to increase the activities of anti-oxidant enzymes in the lungs, as well as increasing surfactant synthesis.

Prenatal prevention of RDS with glucocorticoid alone is not always effective, and recent clinical trials have tested the combined administration of adding TRH[143]; however, the results of such trials have been conflicting, and further trials are needed. The treatment of RDS by the intrapulmonary administration of replacement surfactant has been successful, often in combination with prenatal glucocorticoid treatment (the latter also enhancing the structural maturation of the lungs). However, the earliest gestational age at which such treatments can be successful will be determined by the presence of the basic structural requirements for gas exchange (approximately 22–24 weeks, during the canalicular stage of lung development). Infants born earlier than this have been supported by ECMO (extracorporeal membrane oxygenation) until the lungs have developed sufficiently to support gas exchange.

REFERENCES

1. O'Rahilly R. The early prenatal development of the human respiratory system. In *Pulmonary Development* (ed. G.H. Nelson), p. 2. New York: Marcel Dekker, 1985.
2. Burri PH. Development and growth of the human lung. In *Handbook of Physiology* (eds A.P. Fishman, N.S. Cherniack, J.G. Widdicombe & S.R., Geiger), p. 1. Bethesda, MD: American Physiological Society, 1986.
3. Adamson IYR. Development of lung structure. In *The Lung: Scientific Foundations*, 2nd edn (eds R.G. Crystal, J.B. West, E.R. Weibel & P.J. Barnes), p. 993. Philadelphia: Lippincott-Raven, 1997.
4. Hodson WA. Normal and abnormal structural development of the lung. In *Fetal and Neonatal Physiology* (eds R.A. Polin & WW Fox), p. 771. Philadelphia: WB Saunders, 1992.
5. Burri PH. Structural development of the lung in the fetus and neonate. In: *Fetus and Neonate: Breathing* (eds M.A. Hanson, J.A.D. Spencer, C.H. Rodeck & D.V. Walters), p. 3. Cambridge: Cambridge University Press, 1994.
6. Thurlbeck WM. Pre- and postnatal organ development. In *Basic Mechanisms of Pediatric Respiratory Disease: Cellular and Integrative* (eds V. Chernick & R.B. Mellins), p. 23. Philadelphia: BC Decker, 1991.
7. de Mello DE, Reid LM. Pre- and postnatal development of the pulmonary circulation. In *Basic Mechanisms of Pediatric Respiratory Disease: Cellular and Integrative* (eds V. Chernick & R.B. Mellins), p. 36. Philadelphia: BC Decker, 1991.
8. Hoffman JIE, Heymann MA. Normal pulmonary circulation. In *Pulmonary Physiology: Fetus, Newborn, Child, Adolescent* (eds V. Chernick & R.B. Mellins), p. 233. Philadelphia: B.C. Decker, 1991.
9. Fineman JR, Soifer SJ, Heymann MA. Regulation of pulmonary vascular tone in the perinatal period. *Annu Rev Physiol* **57**:115–134, 1995.
10. Tod ML, Cassin S. Fetal and neonatal pulmonary circulation. In *The Lung: Scientific Foundations*, 2nd edn. (eds R.G. Crystal, J.B. West, E.R. Weibel & P.J. Barnes), p. 2129. Philadelphia: Lippincott-Raven, 1997.
11. Heymann MA. Regulation of the perinatal pulmonary circulation and the role of lipid mediators. In *Advances in Fetal Physiology: Reviews in Honor of G.C. Liggins* (eds P.D. Gluckman, B.M. Johnston & P.W. Nathanielsz), p. 55. Ithaca, NY: Perinatology Press, 1989.
12. Stenmark KR, Badesch DB, Durmowicz AG, Voelkel NF. Control of pulmonary vascular tone and cell proliferation. In *Basic Mechanisms of Pediatric Respiratory Disease: Cellular and Integrative* (eds V. Chernick & R.B. Mellins), p. 169. Philadelphia: B.C. Decker, 1991.
13. Walker AM, Ritchie BC, Adamson TM, Maloney JE. Effect of changing lung liquid volume on the pulmonary circulation of fetal lambs. *J Appl Physiol* **64**:61–67, 1988.
14. Rudolph AM. Fetal and neonatal pulmonary circulation. *Annu Rev Physiol* **41**:383–395, 1979.
15. Abman SH, Chatfield BA, Hall WG, McMurtry IF. Role of endothelium-derived relaxing factor during transition of pulmonary circulation at birth. *Am J Physiol* **259**:H1921–H1927, 1990.
16. Harding R. Fetal breathing movements. In *The Lung: Scientific Foundations*, 2nd edn. (eds R.G. Crystal, J.B. West, E.R. Weibel & P.J. Barnes), p. 2093. Philadelphia: Lippincott-Raven, 1997.
17. Harding R. The upper respiratory tract in perinatal life. In *Respiratory Control and Lung Development in the Fetus and Newborn* (eds B.M. Johnston & P.D. Gluckman), p. 331. Ithaca, NY: Perinatology Press, 1986.
18. Harding R, Johnson P, McClelland ME, McLeod CN, Whyte PL. Laryngeal function during breathing and swallowing in foetal and new-born lambs. *J Physiol* **272**:14P–15P, 1977.
19. Moore PJ, Hanson MA. Control of breathing: central influences. In *Fetus and Neonate: Breathing* (eds M.A. Hanson, J.A.D Spencer, C.H. Rodeck & D.P. Walters), p. 109. Cambridge: Cambridge University Press, 1994.
20. Dawes GS, Fox HE, Leduc BM, Liggins GC, Richards RT. Respiratory movements and rapid eye movement sleep in the foetal lamb. *J Physiol* **220**:119–143, 1972.
21. Harding R, Bocking AD, Sigger JN. Influence of upper respiratory tract on liquid flow to and from fetal lungs. *J Appl Physiol* **61**:68–74, 1986.
22. Maloney JE, Adamson TM, Brodecky V, Cranage S, Lambert TF, Ritchie BC. Diaphragmatic activity and lung liquid flow in the unanesthetized fetal sheep. *J Appl Physiol* **39**:423–428, 1975.
23. Jakubowska AE, Billings K, Johns DP, Hooper SB, Harding R. Respiratory function in lambs following prolonged oligohydramnios during late gestation. *Pediatr Res* **34**:611–617, 1993.
24. Patrick J, Natale R, Richardson B. Patterns of human fetal breathing activity at 34 to 35 weeks' gestational age. *Am J Obstet Gynecol* **132**:507–513, 1978.
25. Harding R, Liggins GC. Changes in thoracic dimensions induced by breathing movements in fetal sheep. *Reprod Fertil Dev* **8**:117–124, 1996.
26. Bocking AD, Gagnon R. Assessment of fetal health. In *Textbook of Fetal Physiology* (eds G.D. Thorburn & R. Harding), p. 186. Oxford: Oxford University Press, 1994.
27. Harding R. Fetal breathing: relation to postnatal breathing and lung development. In *Fetus and Neonate: Breathing* (eds M.A. Hanson, J.A.D. Spencer & C.H. Rodeck), p. 63. Cambridge: Cambridge University Press, 1994.
28. Dornan JC, Ritchie JWK, Meban C. Fetal breathing movements and lung maturation in the congenitally abnormal human fetus. *J Dev Physiol* **6**:367–375, 1984.

29. Smith GN, Patrick J, Sinervo KR, Brien JF. Effects of ethanol exposure on the embryo-fetus: experimental considerations, mechanisms, and the role of prostaglandins. *Can J Physiol Pharmacol* **69**:550–569, 1991.
30. Thaler I, Goodman JDS, Dawes GS. Effects of maternal cigarette smoking on fetal breathing and fetal movements. *Am J Obstet Gynecol* **138**:282–287, 1980.
31. Boddy K, Dawes GS, Fischer RL, Pinter S, Robinson JS. The effects of pentobarbitone and pethidine on foetal breathing movements in sheep. *Br J Pharmacol* **57**:311–317, 1976.
32. Piercy WN, Day MA, Neims AH, Williams RL. Alteration of ovine fetal respiratory-like activity by diazepam, caffeine and doxapram. *Am J Obstet Gynecol* **127**:43–49, 1977.
33. Wigglesworth JS, Desai R. Effects on lung growth of cervical cord section in the rabbit fetus. *Early Hum Dev* **3**:51–65, 1979.
34. Liggins GC, Vilos GA, Campos GA, Kitterman JA, Lee CH. The effect of spinal cord transection on lung development in fetal sheep. *J Dev Physiol* **3**:267–274, 1981.
35. Roberts AB, Mitchell J. Pulmonary hypoplasia and fetal breathing in preterm premature rupture of membranes. *Early Hum Dev* **41**:27–37, 1995.
36. Blott M, Greenough A. Neonatal outcome after prolonged rupture of the membranes starting in the second trimester. *Arch Dis Child* **63**:1146–1150, 1988.
37. Moessinger AC, Fox HE, Higgins A, Rey HR Haideri MA. Fetal breathing movements are not a reliable predictor of continued lung development in pregnancies complicated by oligohydramnios. *Lancet* **ii**:1297–1299, 1987.
38. Sival DA, Visser GH, Prechtl HF. Fetal breathing movements are not a good indicator of lung development after premature rupture of membranes and oligohydramnios – a preliminary study. *Early Hum Dev* **28**:133–143, 1992.
39. Jost A, Policard A. Contribution expérimentale a l'étude du développement prénatal du poumon chez le lapin. *Arch Anat Microscop* **37**:323–332, 1948.
40. Carmel JA, Friedman F, Adams FH. Fetal tracheal ligation and lung development. *Am J Dis Child* **109**:452–456, 1965.
41. Adamson TM, Boyd RDH, Platt HS, Strang LB. Composition of alveolar liquid in the foetal lamb. *J Physiol* **204**:159–168, 1969.
42. Olver RE, Strang LB. Ion fluxes across the pulmonary epithelium and the secretion of lung liquid in the foetal lamb. *J Physiol* **241**:327–357, 1974.
43. Silva P, Stoff J, Field M, Fine L, Forrest JN, Epstein FH. Mechanism of active chloride secretion by shark rectal gland: role of Na, K-ATPase in chloride transport. *Am J Physiol* **233**:F298–F306, 1977.
44. Harding R, Sigger JN, Wickham PJD Bocking AD. The regulation of flow of pulmonary fluid in fetal sheep. *Respir Physiol* **57**:47–59, 1984.
45. Harding R, Bocking AD, Sigger JN, Wickham PJD. Laryngeal resistance and lung liquid flow in relation to breathing activity in fetal sheep. In *The Physiological Development of the Fetus and Newborn* (eds C.T. Jones & P.W. Nathanielsz), p. 247. London: Academic Press, 1985.
46. Dickson KA, Maloney JE, Berger PJ. State-related changes in lung liquid secretion and tracheal flow rate in fetal lambs. *J Appl Physiol* **62**:34–38, 1987.
47. Brace RA, Wlodek ME, McCrabb GJ, Harding R. Swallowing and urine flow responses of the ovine fetus to 24 h of hypoxia. *Am J Physiol* **266**:R1345–R1352, 1994.
48. Walters DV, Olver RE. The role of catecholamines in lung liquid absorption at birth. *Pediatr Res* **12**:239–242, 1978.
49. Brown MJ, Olver RE, Ramsden CA, Strang LB, Walters DV. Effects of adrenaline and of spontaneous labour on the secretion and absorption of lung liquid in the fetal lamb. *J Physiol* **344**:137–152, 1983.
50. Hooper SB, Harding R. Effects of β-adrenergic blockade on lung liquid secretion during fetal asphyxia. *Am J Physiol* **257**:R705–R710, 1989.
51. Perks AM Cassin S. The effects of arginine vasopressin and other factors on the production of lung fluid in fetal goats. *Chest* **81S**:63S–65S, 1982.
52. Wallace MJ, Hooper SB, Harding R. Regulation of lung liquid secretion by arginine vasopressin in fetal sheep. *Am J Physiol* **258**:R104–R111, 1990.
53. Walters DV, Ramsden CA, Olver RE. Dibutyryl cAMP induces a gestation-dependent absorption of fetal lung liquid. *J Appl Physiol* **68**:2054–2059, 1990.
54. Kennedy KA, Wilton P, Mellander M, Rojas J, Sundell H. Effect of epidermal growth factor on lung liquid secretion in fetal sheep. *J Develop Physiol* **8**:421–433, 1986.
55. Wallace MJ, Hooper SB, Harding R. Effects of elevated fetal cortisol concentrations on the volume, secretion and reabsorption of lung liquid. *Am J Physiol* **269**:R881–R887, 1995.
56. Wallace MJ, Hooper SB, Harding R. Role of the adrenal glands in the maturation of lung liquid secretory mechanisms in fetal sheep. *Am J Physiol* **270**:R1–R8, 1996.
57. Kindler PM, Chuang DC, Perks AM. Fluid production by *in vitro* lungs from near-term fetal guinea pigs: effects of cortisol and aldosterone. *Acta Endocrinol* **129**:169–177, 1993.
58. Cassin S, Perks AM. Studies of factors which stimulate lung fluid secretion in fetal goats. *J Develop Physiol* **4**:311–325, 1982.
59. Hooper SB, Dickson KA, Harding R. Lung liquid secretion, flow and volume in response to moderate asphyxia in fetal sheep. *J Develop Physiol* **10**:473–485, 1988.
60. Hooper SB, Harding R. Changes in lung liquid dynamics induced by prolonged fetal hypoxemia. *J Appl Physiol* **69**:127–135, 1990.
61. Hooper SB, Wallace MJ, Harding R. Amiloride blocks the inhibition of fetal lung liquid secretion caused by AVP but not by asphyxia. *J Appl Physiol* **74**:111–115, 1993.
62. Wallace MJ, Hooper SB, McCrabb GJ, Harding R. Acidaemia enhances the inhibitory effect of hypoxia on fetal lung liquid secretion. *Reprod Fertil Dev* **8**:327–333, 1996.
63. Perks AM, Ruiz T, Chua B, Muhll IV, Kindler PM, Blair W. Reabsorption of lung liquid produced by 2,4-dinitrophenol in *in vitro* lungs from fetal guinea pigs. *Can J Physiol Pharmacol* **71**:1–11, 1993.
64. Rudolph AM, Yuan S. Responses of the pulmonary vasculature to hypoxia and H^+ ion concentration changes. *J Clin Invest* **45**:399–411, 1966.
65. Harding R, Hooper SB, Han VKM. Abolition of fetal breathing movements by spinal cord transection leads to reductions in fetal lung liquid volume, lung growth and *IGF-II* gene expression. *Pediatr Res* **34**:148–153, 1993.
66. Miller AA, Hooper SB, Harding R. Role of fetal breathing movements in control of fetal lung distension. *J Appl Physiol* **75**:2711–2717, 1993.
67. Nardo L, Hooper SB, Harding R. Fetal lung hypoplasia can be reversed by short-term obstruction of the fetal trachea in fetal sheep. *Pediatr Res* **38**:690–696, 1995.
68. Perks AM, Cassin S. The rate of production of lung liquid in fetal goats, and the effect of expansion of the lungs. *J Develop Physiol* **7**:149–160, 1985.
69. Nardo L, Hooper SB, Harding R. Stimulation of lung growth by tracheal obstruction in fetal sheep: relation to luminal pressure and lung liquid volumes. *Pediatr Res* **43**:184–190, 1998.
70. Vilos GA, Liggins GC. Intrathoracic pressures in fetal sheep. *J Develop Physiol* **4**:247–256, 1982.
71. Dickson KA, Maloney JE, Berger PJ. Decline in lung liquid volume before labor in fetal lambs. *J Appl Physiol* **61**:2266–2272, 1986.
72. Lines A, Hooper SB, Harding R. Lung liquid production rates and volumes do not decrease before labor in healthy fetal sheep. *J Appl Physiol* **82**:927–932, 1997.
73. Olver RE, Ramsden CA, Strang LB, Walters DV. The role of amiloride-blockable sodium transport in adrenaline-induced lung liquid reabsorption in the fetal lamb. *J Physiol* **376**:321–340, 1986.
74. Harding R, Hooper SB, Dickson KA. A mechanism leading to reduced lung expansion and lung hypoplasia in fetal sheep during oligohydramnios. *Am J Obstet Gynecol* **163**:1904–1913, 1990.
75. Jakubowski AE, Billings K, Johns DP, Hooper SB, Harding R. Respiratory function in lambs following prolonged oligohydramnios during late gestation. *Pediatr Res* **34**:611–617, 1993.
76. Harding R, Bocking AD, Sigger JN. Upper airway resistances in fetal sheep: the influence of breathing activity. *J Appl Physiol* **60**:160–165, 1986.
77. Hooper SB, Harding R. Fetal lung liquid: a major determinant of the growth and functional development of the fetal lung. *Clin Exp Pharmacol Physiol* **22**:235–247, 1995.

78. Hooper SB, Han VKM, Harding R. Changes in lung expansion alter pulmonary DNA synthesis and *IGF-II* gene expression in fetal sheep. *Am J Physiol* **265**:L403–L409, 1993.
79. Alcorn D, Adamson TM, Lambert TF, Maloney JE, Ritchie BC, Robinson PM. Morphological effects of chronic tracheal ligation and drainage in the fetal lamb lung. *J Anat* **123**:649–660, 1977.
80. Moessinger AC, Harding R, Adamson TM, Singh M, Kiu GT. Role of lung fluid volume in growth and maturation of the fetal sheep lung. *J Clin Invest* **86**:1270–1277, 1990.
81. Vandenburgh HH. Mechanical forces and their second messengers in stimulating cell growth *in vitro*. *Am J Physiol* **262**:R350–R355, 1992.
82. Ingber DE. The riddle of morphogenesis: a question of solution chemistry or molecular cell engineering – minireview. *Cell* **75**:1249–1252, 1993.
83. Carson JA, Yan Z, Booth FW, Coleman ME, Schwartz RJ, Stump CS. Regulation of skeletal α-actin promoter in young chickens during hypertrophy caused by stretch overload. *Am J Physiol* **268**:C918–C924, 1995.
84. D'Ercole AJ. The insulin-like growth factors and fetal growth. In *Modern Concepts of Insulin-like Growth Factors* (ed. E.M. Spencer), p. 9. New York: Elsevier, 1991.
85. Liu M, Xu J, Liu J, Kraw ME, Tanswell AK, Post M. Mechanical strain-enhanced fetal lung cell proliferation is mediated by phospholipases C and D and protein kinase C. *Am J Physiol* **268**:L729–L738, 1995.
86. Liu M, Liu J, Buch S, Tanswell AK, Post M. Antisense oligonucleotides against PDGF-B and its receptor inhibit mechanical strain-induced fetal lung cell growth. *Am J Physiol* **269**:L178–L184, 1995.
87. Askenazi SS, Perlman M. Pulmonary hypoplasia: lung weight and radial alveolar count as criteria of diagnosis. *Arch Dis Child* **54**:614–618, 1979.
88. Knox WF, Barson AJ. Pulmonary hypoplasia in a regional perinatal unit. *Early Hum Dev* **14**:33–42, 1986.
89. Moessinger AC, Santiago A, Paneth NS, Rey HR, Blanc WA, Driscoll JM, Jr. Time trends in necropsy prevalence and birth prevalence of lung hypoplasia. *Paediatr Perinat Epidermiol* **3**:421–431, 1989.
90. Husain AN, Hessel RG. Neonatal pulmonary hypoplasia: An autopsy study of 25 cases. *Pediatr Pathol* **13**:475–484, 1993.
91. Hislop A, Fairweather DVI, Blackwell RJ, Howard S. The effect of amniocentesis and drainage of amniotic fluid on lung development in *Macaca fascicularis*. *Br J Obstet Gynaecol* **91**:835–842, 1984.
92. Hislop A, Hey E, Reid L. The lungs in congenital bilateral renal agenesis and dysplasia. *Arch Dis Child* **54**:32–38, 1979.
93. Thibeault DW, Beatty EC, Hall RT, Bowen SK, O'Niell DH. Neonatal pulmonary hypoplasia with premature rupture of fetal membranes and oligohydramnios. *J Pediatr* **107**:273–277, 1985.
94. Haidar A, Ryder TA, Wigglesworth JS. Failure of elastin development in hypoplastic lungs associated with oligohydramnios: an electronmicroscopic study. *Histopathology* **18**:471–473, 1991.
95. Wigglesworth JS, Desai R. Is fetal respiratory function a major determinant of perinatal survival? *Lancet* **i**:264–267, 1982.
96. Gould SJ. Pulmonary hypoplasia, hyaline membrane disease and chronic lung disease. In *Fetus and Neonate: Breathing* (eds M.A. Hanson, J.A.D. Spencer, C.H. Rodeck & D. Walters), p. 214. Cambridge: Cambridge University Press, 1994.
97. Wigglesworth JS, Desai R, Guerrini P. Fetal lung hypoplasia: biochemical and structural variations and their possible significance. *Arch Dis Child* **56**:606–615, 1981.
98. Wigglesworth JS. Pathology of the lung in the fetus and neonate, with particular reference to problems of growth and maturation. *Histopathology* **11**:671–689, 1987.
99. Moessinger AC, Collins MH, Blanc WA, Rey HR, James LS. Oligohydramnios-induced lung hypoplasia: the influence of timing and duration in gestation. *Pediatr Res* **20**:951–954, 1986.
100. Page DV, Stocker JT. Anomalies associated with pulmonary hypoplasia. *Am Rev Respir Dis* **125**:216–221, 1982.
101. Adzick NS, Harrison MR, Glick PL, Nakayama DK, Manning FA, deLorimier AA. Diaphragmatic hernia in the fetus: prenatal diagnosis and outcome in 94 cases. *J Pediatr Surg* **20**:357–361, 1985.
102. Longaker MT, Laberge JM, Dansereau J, Langer JC, Crombleholme TM, Callen PW, Globus MS, Harrison MR. Primary fetal hydrothorax: natural history and management. *J Pediatr Surg* **24**:573–576, 1989.
103. Nimrod C, Varela-Gittings F, Machin G, Campbell D, Wesenberg R. The effect of very prolonged membrane rupture on fetal development. *Am J Obstet Gynecol* **148**:540–543, 1984.
104. Adzick NS, Harrison MR, Glick PL, Villa RL, Finkbeiner W. Experimental pulmonary hypoplasia and oligohydramnios: relative contributions of lung fluid and fetal breathing movements. *J Pediatr Surg* **19**:658–665, 1984.
105. Wilson JM, DiFiore JW, Peters CA. Experimental fetal tracheal ligation prevents the pulmonary hypoplasia associated with fetal nephrectomy: possible application for congenital diaphragmatic hernia. *J Pediatr Surg* **28**:1433–1440, 1993.
106. Hedrick MH, Estes JM, Sullivan KM, Bealer JF, Kitterman JA, Flake AW, Adzick NS, Harrison MR. Plug the lung until it grows (PLUG): A new method to treat congenital diaphragmatic hernia *in utero*. *J Pediatr Surg* **29**:612–617, 1994.
107. Lines A, Nardo L, Philips I *et al.* Alterations in lung expansion affect surfactant protein-A, -B and -C mRNA levels in fetal sheep. *Am J Physiol* **276**:L239–L245, 1999.
108. Piedboeuf B, Gamache M, Petrov P, Laberge JM, Chen MF. Fetal tracheal occlusion induce a dramatic change in lung cell population. *Am J Respir Crit Care Med* **153**:A553, 1997.
109. Schellenberg JC. The development of connective tissue and its role in pulmonary mechanics. In *Respiratory Control and Lung Development in the Fetus and Newborn* (eds B.M. Johnston & P.D. Gluckman), p. 3. Ithaca, NY: Perinatology Press, 1986.
110. Clark JG, Kuhn C, III, McDonald JA, Mecham RP. Lung connective tissue. *Int Rev Connect Tissue Res* **10**:249–331, 1983.
111. Liggins GC, Schellenberg J-C, Finberg K, Kitterman JA, Lee CH. The effects of ACTH1–24 or cortisol on pulmonary maturation in the adrenalectomized ovine fetus. *J Develop Physiol* **7**:105–111, 1985.
112. Mitzner W, Johnson JWC, Scott R, London WT, Palmer AE. Effect of betamethasone on pressure–volume relationship of fetal rhesus monkey lung. *J Appl Physiol* **47**:377–382, 1979.
113. Alcorn DG, Adamson TM, Maloney JE, Robinson PM. A morphologic and morphometric analysis of fetal lung development in the sheep. *Anat Rec* **201**:655–667, 1981.
114. Crone RK, Davies P, Liggins GC, Reid L. The effects of hypophysectomy, thyroidectomy, and postoperative infusion of cortisol or adrenocorticotrophin on the structure of the ovine fetal lung. *J Develop Physiol* **5**:281–288, 1983.
115. Jobe AH, Polk D, Ikegami M, Newnham J, Sly P, Kohen R, Kelly R. Lung responses to ultrasound-guided fetal treatments with corticosteroids in preterm lambs. *J Appl Physiol* **75**:2099–2105, 1993.
116. Polk DH, Ikegami M, Jobe AH, Newnham J, Sly P, Kohen R, Kelly R. Postnatal lung function in pretern lambs: effects of a single exposure to betamethasone and thyroid hormones. *Am J Obstet Gynecol* **172**:872–881, 1996.
117. Schellenberg J-C, Liggins GC. Elastin and collagen in the fetal sheep lung. I. Ontogenesis. *Pediatr Res* **22**:335–338, 1987.
118. Shibahara S, Davidson JM, Smith K, Crystal RG. Modulation of tropoelastin production and elastin messenger ribonucleic acid activity in developing sheep lung. *Biochemistry* **20**:6577–6584, 1981.
119. Rannels DE, Dunsmore SE, Grove RN. Extracellular matrix synthesis and turnover by type II pulmonary epithelial cells. *Am J Physiol* **262**:L582–L589, 1992.
120. Dunsmore SE, Rannels DE. Turnover of extracellular matrix by type II pulmonary epithelial cells. *Am J Physiol* **268**:L336–L346, 1996.
121. Minoo P, Penn R, deLemos DM, Coalson JL, DeLemos RA. Tissue inhibitor of metalloproteinase-1 mRNA is specifically induced in lung tissue after birth. *Pediatr Res* **34**:729–734, 1993.
122. Goetzman BW, Read LC, Plopper CG, Tarantal AF, Nascimento CG, Merritt TA, Whitsett JA, Styne D. Prenatal exposure to epidermal growth factor attenuates respiratory distress syndrome in rhesus infants. *Pediatr Res* **35**:30–36, 1994.
123. DiMari SJ, Howe AM, Haralson MA. Effects of transforming growth factor-β on collagen synthesis by fetal rat lung epithelial cells. *Am J Respir Cell Mol Biol* **4**:455–462, 1991.
124. Smith BT, Post M. Fibroblast–pneumonocyte factor. *Am J Physiol* **257**:L174–L178, 1989.
125. Possmayer F. The perinatal lung. In *The Biochemical Development of the Fetus and Neonate* (ed. C.T. Jones), p. 337. Amsterdam: Elsevier, 1982.
126. Adamson IYR, Bowden DH. Derivation of type I epithelium from type 2 cells in the developing rat lung. *Lab Invest* **32**:736–745, 1975.

dopaminergic system. Thus, dopamine agonist drugs inhibit prolactin secretion and are used in the treatment of hyperprolactinaemia. An increase in prolactin secretion is observed during pregnancy and lactation, but also in renal failure, during episodes of stress or hypoglycaemia and after breast stimulation, or the administration of dopamine antagonists, oestrogens, or thyrotropin-releasing hormone[34].

The raised fetal and maternal serum prolactin may be due to pregnancy-related stimulatory influences that are common to both the fetus and mother. However, the lack of significant association between fetal and maternal levels suggests the presence of independent control mechanisms. Experiments in rats have demonstrated that the fetal pituitary has a high sensitivity to prolactin releasing factors, such as TRH[35]. However, evidence from anencephalic fetuses suggests that it is unlikely that hypothalamic factors play a significant role in regulating prolactin secretion. Aubert *et al.* demonstrated that in anencephalic fetuses with no hypothalamus, the circulating concentrations of prolactin are normal[27]. Furthermore, several studies involving the administration of drugs to the mother, at timed intervals before delivery and measuring prolactin concentration in umbilical cord blood samples at birth, have demonstrated that fetal prolactin secretion is insensitive to TRH stimulation, and to both dopaminergic and H_2-receptor antagonism[36–41]. Although the precise role of prolactin in intrauterine life remains unclear, the finding of high serum concentrations suggests that it may have an important role in normal fetal development.

Posterior pituitary hormones

Three posterior pituitary hormones have been identified during fetal life, all are nonapeptides. Arginine vasopressin (AVP) and oxytocin are present from early gestation. Arginine vasotocin (AVT) is only found in fetal life. The posterior pituitary hormones are synthesised by enzymatic conversion of a precursor molecule to the nonapeptide hormone bound together with neurophysin, a carrier protein. AVP and oxytocin, together with their associated neurophysin, are found in granules in the cell bodies of the paraventricular, supraoptic and suprachiasmatic nuclei. The contents of the granules are released into the circulation after stimulation.

OXYTOCIN

Oxytocin appears in the pituitary in the second trimester. In a study of 38 human fetuses vasopressin and oxytocin were in all the studied glands and all the hypothalamic areas studied using microdissection and radioimmunoassay[42,43]. The concentration of oxytocin increases with advancing gestation. Labour stimulates a further rise in oxytocin levels, although the contribution of oxytocin from maternal sources is not clear and these also increase significantly during labour. The initially high ratio of AVP to oxytocin also decreases with gestation, reaching unity in the neonatal period. This ratio is maintained in adult life, while AVT is no longer present[43].

ARGININE VASOTOCIN

In the human fetus AVT is detectable from week 9 of gestation. Between weeks 12 and 19, the ratio of AVT to AVP decreases[39,40]. AVT is found not only in the pituitary, but *in vitro* studies have demonstrated it to be present in the pineal gland from weeks 8 to 17[44]. The role of AVT in the fetus is unclear, although it appears to have a osmoregulatory effect in animal models. In sheep and guinea pigs, AVT slows the transfer of water from the fetus to the mother[45,46].

ARGININE VASOPRESSIN

AVP is present from 12 weeks' gestation. AVP is an important vasoactive hormone, helping to maintain cardiovascular function under stress conditions. The fetal lamb has been extensively studied *in utero* and infusions of AVP elevate arterial pressure, decrease fetal heart rate and brings about a redistribution of cardiac output to the vital organs. At high doses AVP elevates venous pressure and decreases blood volume[47]. Conditions of stress such as fetal hypoxia and haemorrhage stimulate the release of AVP. AVP was assayed in amniotic fluid obtained from patients with rhesus isoimmunisation and compared with controls. It was concluded that amniotic AVP may act as a marker of fetal distress in rhesus isoimmunisation[48].

High concentrations of AVP have been found in the umbilical cord blood in situations which may non-specifically reflect increased levels of stress; for example, in growth-retarded fetuses, following documented fetal bradycardia or following the passage of meconium[49]. Although AVP concentrations are also considerably increased following vaginal delivery, studies in human neonates have found no correlation between AVP levels and fetal cord blood gases and therefore the role of AVP remains uncertain[50].

Fetal cardiovascular hormones

ATRIAL NATRIURETIC FACTOR

ANF is a hormone produced by the atrial cardiocytes in the heart and was discovered as recently as 1981. This hormone has powerful natriuretic and diuretic properties. Secretion of ANF appears to be regulated primarily by the prevailing pressure in the atria. In pharmacological doses, ANF rapidly elicits a natriuresis when administered to experimental animals or humans. In contrast infusions that increase plasma ANF by three- to fivefold tend to produce a slow diuresis[51]. It therefore appears to have a role in blood-volume regulation. In adults, plasma concentrations of ANF have been shown to rise in response to central volume expansion[52]. The principal action of ANF is in the kidney where it has a vasodilator effect on smooth muscle which mediates an increase in the glomerular filtration rate. In addition ANF has a direct action on the distal and collecting tubules.

In the human fetus, a functioning circulation is present from 4 weeks and by 8 weeks' gestation the four-chamber heart has developed. ANF has been demonstrated to be present in fetal atria from 10 weeks and is present in concentrations similar to those found in adult atria[53]. However, in contrast to the adult atria, ANF is present in the ventricles, but at low concentrations. The concentration in the right auricle is higher than in the left during fetal life, whereas that in the left is higher after birth. In the atria ANF remains present at a constant concentration throughout gestation, but in the ventricles the levels fall. In the fetal circulation the concentration of ANF is greater than that in the maternal circulation, and is not related the gestational age, sex or weight. Umbilical arterial concentrations are greater than in the venous circulation, suggesting that the placenta may act as a clearance site[54]. The higher concentrations of ANF observed in the fetus could be attributed to either an increase in secretion or reduced breakdown. The latter seems unlikely since the ovine fetus has been shown to have a rapid clearance rate of plasma ANF[55]. On the other hand, haemodynamic and endocrine conditions in the fetus favour increased ANF secretion as the fetal cardiac output is proportionately increased compared to that of adults. Furthermore, increased plasma concentrations of glucocorticoids, progesterone and aldosterone are present in the fetal circulation, and all of these factors are known to potentiate ANF secretion[51].

Fetal blood samples obtained at cordocentesis prior to fetal blood transfusion in fetuses at risk of rhesus haemolytic disease demonstrated that ANF is present in the fetal circulation as early as 19 weeks' gestation and its concentration rises in response to blood-volume expansion. This finding suggests the fetus is able to respond in an appropriate manner to adverse intrauterine stimuli. Fetuses with hydrops have elevated plasma ANF concentrations, but isoimmunized fetuses without hydrops have normal ANF levels. Fetuses with renal disorders such as renal agenesis and multicystic dysplastic kidneys have lower plasma ANF concentrations than normal fetuses. Plasma release of ANF in the fetus may play a role in fetal blood volume homeostasis[56,57] (Fig. 17.5).

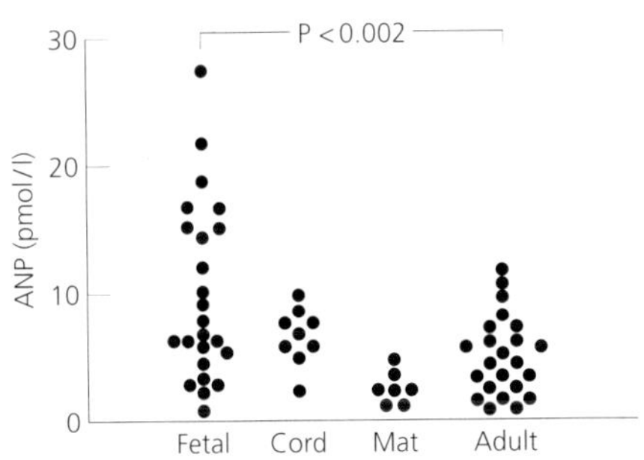

Fig. 17.5 Plasma atrial natriuretic peptide (ANP) concentration in fetal umbilical vein at 21–36 weeks' gestation (FETAL), umbilical cord vein at a full-term delivery of normal neonates (CORD), maternal plasma (MAT) and normal 18–32-year-old adults. Reproduced by permission of Panos *et al.*[56].

RENIN–ANGIOTENSIN–ALDOSTERONE SYSTEM

The role of the fetal renin–angiotensin system is poorly understood. In the adult it plays a crucial role in the regulation of blood pressure and vascular fluid volume, and helps to maintain sodium and potassium haemostasis. Renin is a carboxyl-peptidase enzyme that acts on a plasma α_2-globulin, to produce the biologically inactive decapeptide angiotensin I. A converting enzyme acts on angiotensin I to produce the octapeptide angiotensin II. Most of this conversion occurs during the passage of the blood through the lungs, but the converting enzyme is also found in the blood, kidney and during pregnancy in the placenta. Angiotensin II has a half-life of only 1–2 minutes, being inactivated by a group of enzymes collectively called the angiotensinases and forming the decapeptide angiotensin III. Angiotensin has two major actions, firstly it is the most potent vasoconstrictor known and secondly it has a stimulatory effect on aldosterone secretion from the adrenal gland. Angiotensin III has about 40% of the pressor activity of angiotensin II and is at least equal to it in aldosterone-stimulating activity.

Renin is produced by the kidney juxtaglomerular apparatus, located in the walls of the afferent arterioles as they enter the glomeruli. The human fetal kidney shows renin immunoreactivity from very early in gestation. At 5–6 weeks, renin containing cells are detectable in the wall of the arterioles of the mesonephros[58]. At 8 weeks, using transmission electron microscopy, renin granules are seen in juxtaglomerular epithelial cells of the metanephros[59]. In a study of 38 fetuses total kidney renin content increased between 12 and 25 weeks, although the renin activity decreased[60]. Despite this fall in activity the mean value of the specific fetal kidney renin activity was about 20 times greater than in the adult, suggesting it is chronically hyperactive *in utero*. Mirroring renal renin activity, fetal plasma renin concentration is highest in the third trimester and falls by the end of the third trimester. There are extrarenal sources of renin including the genital tract, umbilical cord vessels and the fetal lung. The contribution that these additional sources make may in part account for the high levels of plasma renin as compared to the adult, but in fetuses with renal agenesis plasma renin is absent suggesting that the kidneys are the critical site of renin production in the fetus. The stimuli for renin release appear the same in the fetus as in the adult. In the fetal sheep, a reduction in fetal blood volume of as little at 5% can induce plasma renin activity[61]. Situations associated with stress and a reduction in intravascular volume in the fetus have been demonstrated to increase plasma renin concentrations. Thus, in newborns whose umbilical blood pH and oxygen tension are decreased, plasma renin concentrations are elevated. The same response to hypoxaemia is observed in the human fetus with increased plasma renin activity, presumably mediated by stimulation of the renin–angiotensin system[62]. Growth retarded and non-immune hydropic fetuses have elevated plasma renin activity[63]. Newborns of hypertensive mothers may have elevated umbilical vessel plasma renin activity as compared to those of normotensive mothers[64,65], although no significant difference was described in an earlier study[66]. These findings have led some authors to conclude that the renin–angiotensin system is involved in the pathogenesis of pre-eclampsia[64].

In the fetus circulating angiotensin II concentrations are similar to those in the maternal circulation, but higher than in the non-pregnant adult. Following normal labour angiotensin II concentrations are higher in the umbilical vein than in the artery, suggesting that the placenta may be a site of conversion of angiotensin I to II. In addition, the concentrations in both the umbilical artery and vein are significantly greater than maternal values after vaginal delivery, but not following elective caesarean delivery[67].

Aldosterone is a mineralocorticoid produced by the zona glomerulosa of the adrenal cortex. It has a half-life of about 20 minutes. Its principal action is to act on the distal tubule and collecting duct to promote the reabsorption of sodium. It is present from the end of the first trimester, initially at low concentrations which increase with advancing gestation. In culture human adrenocortical cells secrete aldosterone in response to ACTH production[68]. The gradual increase in aldosterone production with advancing gestation suggests that the fetal adrenal gland matures during the second and third trimesters. Little other work has been undertaken in the human fetus, but in sheep aldosterone infusion decreases urinary sodium excretion and suppresses renin activity suggesting that *in utero* aldosterone has a negative feedback on renin release[69].

Pancreatic hormones and growth factors

Insulin is present in the fetal pancreas and circulation from 10 weeks' gestation. The maturation of the fetal pancreas is poorly understood, and it has been suggested that the insulin release by the pancreas is insensitive before 28 weeks' gestation[70]. Thus in term fetuses the maternal administration of glucose results in an increase of both glucose and insulin in fetal scalp blood in labour and cord at delivery[71,72], a study in fetuses at 15–20 weeks' gestation was unable to demonstrate an increase in insulin secretion following glucose infusion[73].

In a study of 68 fetuses between 17 and 38 weeks' gestation umbilical venous cord blood was obtained by cordocentesis without maternal fasting or sedation. This study showed that the fetal plasma insulin concentration and the fetal plasma insulin : glucose ratio increased exponentially with gestation[74]. The fetal glucose level correlated better with the maternal glucose concentration than with the level of fetal insulin, suggesting that the primary determinant of fetal glucose level is the maternal glucose concentration. This study seems to confirm that the maturation of the fetal glucose insulin relationship occurs in later gestation.

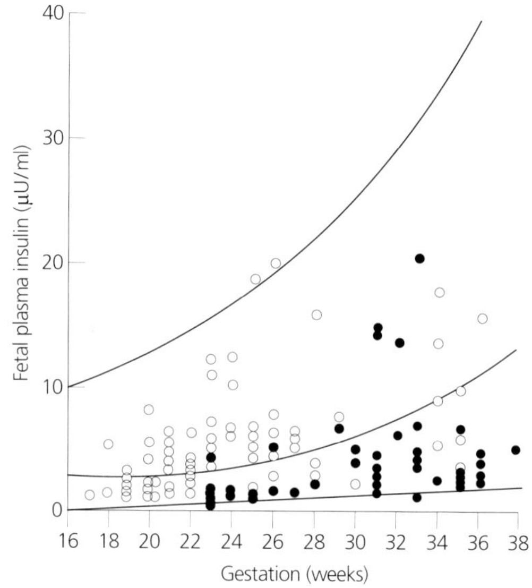

Fig. 17.6 Reference ranges for fetal insulin concentration with gestation (mean, 5th and 95th centiles). Individual values of appropriately grown (○) and small-for-gestational age (●) fetuses are also shown. Reproduced by permission of Economides *et al.*[74].

In normal fetuses, the mean umbilical venous blood glucose concentration is higher than in the umbilical artery, indicating that there is fetal glucose consumption[74,75]. In growth-retarded hypoxic fetuses, the insulin concentration falls further, the maternal glucose concentration is higher than the fetal and the levels in the two compartments are significantly correlated, indicating that the major source of fetal glucose is the mother (Fig. 17.6). The umbilical venous plasma insulin concentration and the fetal insulin to glucose ration increase exponentially with gestation[74]. These findings presumably reflect the progressive maturation of the endocrine activity of pancreatic β-cells. Pancreatic α-cell activity, as reflected in plasma glucagon concentration, does not change significantly with gestation[76].

Insulin-like growth factors I and II (IGF-I, IGF-II) increase with gestation especially after 33 weeks, and there are significant associations between fetal placental lactogen and IGF-I and II. These findings are consistent with the hypothesis that placental lactogen is involved in the regulation of IGF synthesis by human fetal liver[77]. Insulin and insulin-like growth factors may influence fetal growth through its action on nutrient uptake and utilisation.

Adrenal gland hormones

In animals, adrenal hormones are thought to play an important role both in maturation of fetal tissues and in the initiation of labour[15]. The target organ for the secreted ACTH, the adrenal gland, grows rapidly after week 10 of gestation. The fetal adrenal cortex doubles in size between 20 and 30 weeks and again between 30 weeks and term. This rapid growth is principally due to growth of the definitive outer zone, the part of the gland that will form the adult gland[78]. From 13 weeks' gestation the fetal adrenal gland synthesises cortisol, primarily in the definitive zone, while dehydroepiandrosterone sulphate (DHAS) is the main product of the inner fetal zone[79]. The ability of the adrenal gland to function after mid-gestation requires an intact fetal pituitary, as anencephalic fetuses have atrophic adrenals. However, in normal human fetuses there is no plasma cortisol surge before 36 weeks' gestation[13], by which time most fetal organs are mature. Although this evidence does not preclude a role for cortisol in human fetal organ maturation, it suggests that a late cortisol surge may not be necessary for this process.

Greenough *et al.* reported increased concentrations of plasma catecholamines in hypoxaemic growth-retarded fetuses[80]. Similarly, increased plasma noradrenaline concentration has been associated with low P_{O_2} and high P_{CO_2} in fetuses with non-immune hydrops and structural abnormalities[81]. These findings suggest that catecholamines are released in fetal blood when the fetus is exposed to intrauterine stress.

Thyroid gland

The thyroid gland produces thyroxine from 10–12 weeks' gestation[82,83]. The concentrations of fetal serum TSH, total and free thryoxine (T_4) and triiodothyronine (T_3) increase progressively during pregnancy[17,18] (Fig. 17.7 and 17.8). The increase in thyroid hormones presumably reflects the increasing maturation of the fetal thyroid gland. However, serum T_3 and free T_3 concentrations remain low throughout gestation and since the major source of T_3 is peripheral conversion of T_4, these findings suggest that in intrauterine life the processes required for this conversion are either immature or lack the necessary stimulus for their activation. An alternative explanation for the low T_3 could be rapid deiodination by the placenta.

The high fetal serum TSH concentration, even in the third trimester when adult concentrations of total and free T_4 are reached[18], suggest that the fetal pituitary is relatively insensitive to negative feedback from T_4. Alternatively, in the fetus circulating T_3 has a more important role in feedback than in the adult; since serum total and free T_3 concentrations are much lower in the fetus than in postnatal life, the threshold

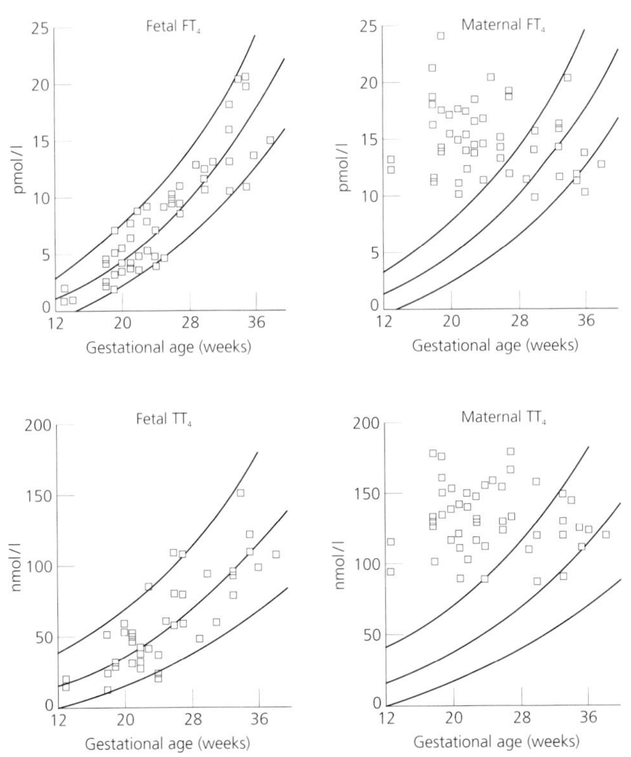

Fig. 17.7 Individual fetal (left) and maternal (right) serum total thyroxine (TT_4) and free serum thyroxine (FT_4) concentrations plotted on the fetal reference range for gestation (mean, 5th and 95th centiles). Reproduced by permission of Thorpe-Beeston *et al.*[18].

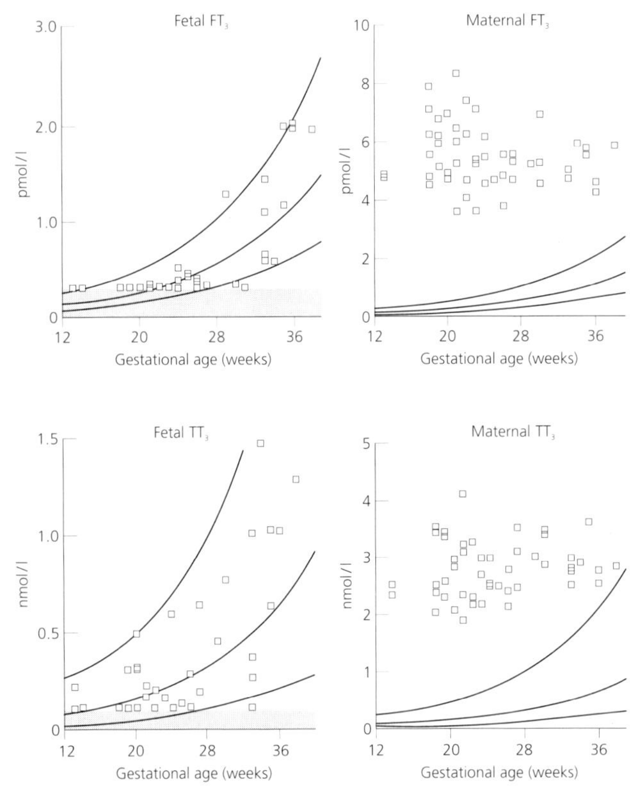

Fig. 17.8 Individual fetal (left) and maternal (right) serum total triiodothyronine (TT_3) and free serum thyroxine (FT_3) concentrations plotted on the fetal reference range for gestation (mean, 5th and 95th centiles). Reproduced by permission of Thorpe-Beeston *et al.*[18].

for negative feedback is never reached *in utero*. Growth-retarded fetuses exist in a state of relative hypothyroidism which may represent a beneficial adaptation to starvation, with a consequent decrease in metabolic rate and oxygen consumption[84]. The high concentration of TSH observed in growth retarded fetuses suggests that the low concentration of thyroid hormones does not constitute a purposeful adaptive mechanism in the face of a hostile intrauterine environment. Reduced synthesis of thyroid hormones may be due to (i) impaired placental perfusion and consequent reduction in the supply of oxygen and essential nutrients such as iodine, or (ii) developmental delay in the gestation related maturation of the thyroid gland, or (iii) underperfusion of the thyroid gland[85].

Irrespective of the underlying cause, the reduction in serum thyroid hormone concentration may affect the fetus adversely. Thus, the development of different regions in the brain follows a genetically determined time frame, and in thyroidectomized animals there is developmental delay and neurological deficits. Although these abnormalities may be corrected by subsequent administration of thyroxine, brain damage may become irreversible if hormone supplementation is not provided within certain critical periods of development[86]. Similarly in the human, untreated congenital hypothyroidism is associated with marked abnormalities in physical and neurological development[87].

Placental endocrine function

During the last 15 years our understanding of the role of the placenta in intrauterine life has changed dramatically. Initially, it was considered to solely have a role in gas exchange and the transfer of nutrients and waste. A growing number of studies have provided evidence that the fetal membranes and maternal decidua are capable of hormone production and metabolism. Intrauterine tissues are a source of brain, pituitary, gonadal, adrenocortical peptide and steroid hormone. The precise interaction between the intrauterine tissues and the fetus is poorly understood, but is believed to be modulated by paracrine and autocrine mechanisms within the intrauterine environment. Possible functional roles undertaken by these mediators include the local modulation of hormone release, the regulation of cell growth and differentiation and the regulation of uterine contractility. The autocrine, paracrine and endocrine mechanisms of the human placenta and membranes have recently been and extensively reviewed[88].

REFERENCES

1. Falin NI. The development of human hypophysis and differentiation of cells of its anterior lobe during embryonic life. *Acta Anat* **44**:188, 1961.
2. Mulchahey JJ, Jaffe RB. Detection of a potential progenitor cell in the human fetal pituitary that secretes both growth and prolactin. *J Clin Endocrinol Metab* **66**:24–32, 1988.
3. Siler-Khodr TM, Khodr GS. Studies in human fetal endocrinology. II: LH and FSH content and concentration in the pituitary. *Obstet Gynecol* **56**:176–181, 1980.
4. Siler-Khodr TM, Morgenstern LL, Greenwood FC. Hormone synthesis and release from the human fetal adenohypophysis *in vitro*. *J Clin Endocrinol Metab* **39**:891–905, 1974.
5. Goodyer CG, Hall CSG, Guyda H, Robert F, Giroud JP. Human fetal pituitary in culture: hormone secretion and response to somatostatin, luteinizing hormone releasing factor, thyrotropin-releasing factor and dibutyryl cyclic AMP. *J Clin Endocrinol Metab* **45**:73–85, 1977.
6. Kaplan SL, Grumbach MM, Aubert ML. The ontogenesis of pituitary hormones and hypothalamic factors in the human fetus: maturation of the central nervous system regulation of anterior pituitary function. *Rec Preg Horm Res* **32**:161–243, 1976.
7. Suganuma N, Seo H, Yamamoto N. *et al.* The ontogeny of growth hormone in the human pituitary. *Am J Obstet Gynecol* **160**:729–733, 1989.
8. Bugnon C, Fellman D, Bloch B. Immunocytochemical study of ontogenesis of the hypothalamic somatostatin-containing neurons in the human fetus. *Metabolism* **27**(suppl. 1):1161–1165, 1978.
9. Bresson JL, Clavequrin M-C, Fellman D, Bugnon C. Ontogeni of the neuroglandular system revealed with HPGRF44 antibodies in human hypothalamus. *Neuroendocrinology* **39**:68–73, 1984.
10. Roti E, Robuschi G, Alboni A. *et al.* Inhibition of fetal growth hormone (GH) and thyrotrophin (TSH) secretion after maternal administration of somatostatin. *Acta Endocrinol* **106**:393–399, 1984.
11. Gyevai A. Fine structure of, and ACTH production by, human fetal pituitaries taken at different periods of gestation. An *in-vitro* study. *Acta Biol Acad Sci Hung* **31**:107–120, 1980.
12. Allen JP, Cook DM, Kendall JW, McGilvra R. Maternal–fetal ACTH relationships in man. *J Clin Endocrinol Metab* **37**:230–234, 1973.
13. Economides DL, Nicolaides KH, Linton EA, Perry LA, Chard T. Plasma cortisol and ACTH in appropriate and small for gestational age fetuses. *Fetal Ther* **3**:158–164, 1988.
14. Robinson JS, Jones CT, Kingston EJ. Studies on experimental growth retardation in sheep. The effects of maternal hypoxaemia. *J Dev Physiol* **5**:89–100, 1983.
15. Liggins GC. Adrenocortical-related maturational events in the fetus. *Am J Obstet Gynecol* **126**:931–941, 1976.
16. Blumenfeld Z, Jaffe RB. Hypophysiotropic and neuro-modulatory regulation of ACTH secretion in the human fetal pituitary. *J Clin Invest* **78**:288–294, 1986.
17. Ballabio N, Nicolini U, Jowett T, Ruiz de Elvira MC, Ekins RP, Rodeck CH. Maturation of thyroid function in normal human foetuses. *Clin Endocrinol* **31**:565–571, 1989.
18. Thorpe-Beeston JG, Nicolaides KH, Felton CV, Butler J, McGregor AM. Maturation of the secretion of thyroid hormone and thyroid stimulating hormone in the fetus. *N Eng J Med* **324**:532–536, 1991.
19. Fisher DA, Dussault JH, Sack J, Chopra IJ. Ontogenesis of hypothalamic–pituitary–thyroid function and metabolism in man, sheep and rat. *Recent Prog Horm Res* **33**:59–116, 1977.
20. de Escobar GM, Obregon MJ, del Rey, FE. Fetal and maternal thyroid hormones. *Hormon Res* **26**:12–27, 1987.
21. Cooke NE, Coit D, Shine J. *et al.* Human prolactin. *J Biol Chem* **256**:4007–4016, 1981.
22. Wallis M. The molecular evolution of pituitary growth hormone, prolactin and placental lactogen: A protein family showing variable rates of evolution. *J Mol Evol* **17**:10–18, 1981.
23. Gluckman PD, Ballard PL, Kaplan SL, Liggins GC, Grumbach MM. Prolactin in umbilical cord blood and respiratory distress syndrome. *J Pediatr* **93**:1011–1014, 1978.
24. Hauth JC, Parker CR, MacDonald PC, Porter JC, Johnston JM. A role of fetal prolactin in lung maturation. *Obstet Gynecol* **51**:81–88, 1977.
25. Tyson JE. The evolutionary role of prolactin in mammalian osmoregulation: effects on fetoplacental hydromineral transport. *Sem Perinat* **6**:216–228, 1982.

26. Winters AJ, Colston C, MacDonald PC, Porter JC. Fetal plasma prolactin levels. *J Clin Endocrinol Metab* **41**:626–629, 1975.
27. Aubert ML, Grumbach MM, Kaplan SL. The ontogenesis of human fetal hormones. III. Prolactin. *J Clin Invest* **56**:155–164, 1975.
28. Schenker JG, Ben-David M, Polishk WZ. Prolactin in normal pregnancy: relationship of maternal, fetal and amniotic fluid levels. *Am J Obstet Gynecol* **123**:834–838, 1975.
29. Kaplan SL, Grumbach MM, Aubert ML. The ontogenesis of pituitary hormones and hypothalamic factors in the human fetus: maturation of central nervous system regulation of anterior pituitary function. *Recent Prog Horm Res* **23**:161–243, 1976.
30. Suganuma N, Seo H, Yamamoto N, Kikkawa F *et al.* Ontogenesis of pituitary prolactin in the human fetus. *J Clin Endocrinol Metab* **63**:156–161, 1986.
31. Thorpe-Beeston JG, Snijders RJM, Felton CV, Nicolaides KH. Serum prolactin concentration in normal and small-for-gestational age fetuses. *Br J Obstet Gynaecol* **99**:981–984, 1992.
32. Falin LI. The development of human hypophysis and differentiation of cells of its anterior lobe during embryonic life. *Acta Anat* **44**:188–205, 1961.
33. Pasteels JL, Gausset P, Danguy A, Ectors F, Nicoll CS, Varavudhi P. Morphology of the lactotropes and somatotropes of man and rhesus monkeys. *J Clin Endocrinol Metab* **34**:959–967, 1972.
34. Moran Campbell EJ, Dickinson CJ, Slater JDH, Edwards CRW, Sikora EK (eds). *Clinical Physiology*, p. 554. Oxford: Blackwell Scientific Publications, 1984.
35. Khorram O, Depalatis LR, McCann SM. Hypothalamic control of prolactin secretion during the perinatal period in the rat. *Endocrinology* **115**:1698–1704, 1984.
36. Roti E, Gardini E, Minelli R, Bianconi L, Alboni A, Braverman LE. Thyrotropin releasing hormone does not stimulate prolactin release in the preterm human fetus. *Acta Endocrinol* **122**:462–466, 1990.
37. Messinis IE, Lolis DE, Kanellopouos N, Dalkalitsis N, Kanaris C. TRH injection during labour: effect on maternal and fetal prolactin secretion. *Clin Endocrinol* **16**:193–198, 1982.
38. Messinis IE, Lolis DE, Dalkalitsis N, Kanaris C, Souvatzoglou A. Effect of metoclopramide on maternal and fetal prolactin secretion during labour. *Obstet Gynecol* **62**:686–688, 1982.
39. Messinis IE, Tsirkas N, Diamantis K, Vasakos S, Tsolas O, Lolis D. Effect of cimetidine on maternal and fetal prolactin secretion during labour. *J Endocrinol Invest* **11**:785–788, 1988.
40. Robuschi G, Emanuele d'Amato L, Salvi M *et al.* Effect of metoclopramide on maternal and fetal hyperprolactinemia. *J Endocrinol Invest* **6**:107–111, 1982.
41. Robuschi G, d'Amato L, Salvi M *et al.* Absent prolactin (PRL) response to thyrotropin releasing hormone (TRH) and somatostatin (SRIF) in at term fetus. *J Endocrinol Invest* **7**:521–524, 1984.
42. Khan-Dawood FS, Dawood MY. Oxytocin content of human fetal pituitary glands. *Am J Obstet Gynecol* **148**:420, 1984.
43. Schubert F, George JN, Rao, MB. Vasopressin and oxytocin content of human fetal brain at different stages of gestation. *Brain Res* **213**:111–117, 1981.
44. Legros JJ, Louis F, Demoulin A *et al.* Immunoreactive neurophysins and vasotocin in human foetal pineal glands. *J Endocrinol* **69**:289–290, 1976.
45. Vizsolyi E, Perks AM. The effects of arginine vasotocin on the isolated amniotic membrane of the guinea pig. *Can J Zool* **52**:371–386, 1974.
46. Leake RD, Palmer SM, Oakes GK, Artman HG, Morris AM, Fisher DA. Arginine vasotocin inhibits ovine fetal/maternal water transfer. *Pediatr Res* **15**:483, 1981.
47. Tomita H, Brace RA, Cheung CY, Longo LD. Vasopressin dose-response effects on fetal vascular pressures, heart rate, and blood volume. *Am J Physiol* (*Heart and Circulatory Physiology* 18) **249**:H974, 1985.
48. Stegner H, Fischer K, Pahnke VG, Kitschke HJ, Commentz JC. There is evidence that amniotic fluid vasopressin is a marker for foetal distress in Rhesus erythroblastosis. *Acta Endocrinol* **112**:267–270, 1986.
49. DeVane GW, Porter JC. An apparent stress-induced release of arginine vasopressin by human neonates. *J Clin Endocrinol Metab* **51**:1412–1416, 1980.
50. Pohjavuori M, Raivio KO. The effects of acute and chronic perinatal stress on plasma vasopressin concentration and renin activity at birth. *Biol Neonate* **47**:259–264, 1985.
51. Goertz KL. Physiology and pathophysiology of atrial peptides. *Am J Physiol* **254**:E1–15, 1988.
52. Anderson JV, Donckier J, McKenna WJ, Bloom SR. The plasma release of atrial natriuretic peptide in man. *Clin Sci* **71**:151–155, 1986.
53. Kikuchi K, Nakao K, Hayashi K. *et al.* Ontogeny of atrial natriuretic polypeptide in the human heart. *Acta Endocrinol (Copenh)* **115**:211–217, 1987.
54. Yamaji T, Hirai N, Ishibashi M, Takaku F, Yanaihara T, Nakayama T. Atrial natriuretic peptide in umbilical cord blood: evidence for a circulation hormone in the human fetus. *J Clin Endocrinol Metab* **63**:1414–1417, 1986.
55. Ervin MG, Ross MG, Lam RW *et al.* Atrial natriuretic peptide: ovine fetal cardiovascular reponses and arginine-vasopressin secretion. *Clin Res* **35**:233A, 1987.
56. Panos MZ, Nicolaides KH, Anderson JV, Economides DL, Rees L, Williams R. Plasma atrial natriuretic peptide in human fetus: response to intravascular blood transfusion. *Am J Obstet Gynecol* **161**:357–361, 1989.
57. Weiner CP, Robillard JE. Atrial natriuretic factor, digoxin-like immunoreactive substance, norepinephrine, epinephrine, and plasma renin activity in human fetuses and their alteration by fetal disease. *Am J Obstet Gynecol* **159**:1353–1360, 1988.
58. Ekblad H, Kero P, Arjamaa O, Erkkola R. Cord blood atrial natriuretic peptide (ANP) concentrations – lack of influence of labour stress. *Acta Paediatr Scand* **77**:312, 1988.
59. Celio MR, Groscurth P, Inagami T. Ontogeny of renin immunoreactive cells in the human kidney. *Anat Embryol* **173**:149–155, 1985.
60. Taylor GM, Peart WS, Porter KA, Zondek LH, Zondek T. Concentration and molecular forms of active and inactive renin in human fetal kidney, amniotic fluid and adrenal gland: evidence for renin–angiotensin system hyperactivity in 2nd trimester of pregnancy. *J Hypertens* **4**:121–129, 1986.
61. Hadeed A, Siegel SR. Plasma renin activity after birth and in the early newborn period. *Am J Perinatol* **1**:285–287, 1984.
62. Tannirandorn Y, Fisk NM, Shah V, Dillon MJ, Nicolini U, Rodeck CH. Plasma renin activity in fetal disease. *J Perinat Med* **18**:229–231, 1990.
63. Weiner CP, Robillard JE. Atrial natriuretic factor, digoxin-like immunoreactive substance, norepinephrine, epinephrine, and plasma renin activity in human fetuses and their alteration by fetal disease. *Am J Obstet Gynecol* **159**:1353, 1988.
64. Anat G, Raudrant D, Chappe J *et al.* Maternal and fetal plasma renin and dopamine-β-hydroxylase activities in toxemic pregnancy. *Obstet Gynecol* **52**:219–224, 1978.
65. Brar H, Kjos S, Dougherty W, Do Y, Tam H, Hsueh W. Increased fetoplacental active renin production in pregnancy induced hypertension. *Am J Obstet Gynecol* **157**:363–367, 1987.
66. Symonds E, Lamming G, Craven D. The fetal renin–angiotensin system in pregnancy-induced hypertension. *Br J Obstet Gynaecol* **91**:3–6, 1984.
67. Broughton Pipkin F, Symonds E. Factors affecting angiotensin II concentrations in the human infant at birth. *Clin Sci Molec Med* **52**:449, 1977.
68. Higashijima M, Nawata H, Kato K-I, Ibayashi H. Studies on lipoprotein and adrenal steroidogenesis. I: Roles of low density lipoprotein and high density lipoprotein–cholesterol in steroid production in cultured human adrenocortical cells. *Endocrinol Jpn* **34**:635–645, 1987.
69. Robillard JE, Nakamura KT, Lawton WJ. Effects of aldosterone on urinary kallikrein and sodium excretion during fetal life. *Pediatr Res* **19**:1048–1052, 1985.
70. Hill DJ, Milner RDG. The role of peptide growth factors and hormones in the control of fetal growth. *Recent Adv Perinatal Med* 79–102, 1987.
71. Milner RDG, Hales CN. Effect of intravenous glucose on concentration of insulin in maternal and umbilical cord plasma. *Br Med J* **1**:284–286, 1965.
72. Coltart RM, Beard RW, Turner RC, Oakley NW. Blood glucose and insulin relationships in the human mother and fetus before the onset of labour. *Br Med J* **4**:17–19, 1969.
73. Adam PAJ, Teramo K, Raiha N, Gitlin D, Schartz R. Human fetal insulin metabolism in early pregnancy. *Diabetes* **18**:409–416, 1969.
74. Economides DL, Proudler A, Nicolaides KH. Plasma insulin in appropriate and small for gestational age fetuses. *Am J Obstet Gynecol* **160**:1091–1094, 1989.

75. Nicolini U, Hubinont C, Santolaya J, Fisk NM, Coe A, Rodeck CH. Maternal–fetal glucose gradient in normal pregnancies and in pregnancies complicated by alloimmunisation and fetal growth retardation. *Am J Obstet Gynecol* **161**:924–927, 1989.
76. Hubinont C, Nicolini U, Fisk NM, Tanninrandorn Y, Rodeck CH. Endocrine pancreatic function in growth-retarded fetuses. *Obstet Gynecol* **77**:541–544, 1991.
77. Lassarre C, Hardouin S, Daffos F, Forestier F, Frankenne F, Binoux M. Serum insulin-like growth factors and insulin-like growth factor binding proteins in the human fetus. Relationship with growth in normal subjects and in subjects with intrauterine growth retardation. *Pediatr Res* **29**:219–225, 1991.
78. Johannison E. The foetal adrenal cortex in the human. *Acta Endocrinol* **58**(suppl. 130):7, 1968.
79. Seron-Ferre M, Lawrence CC, Siiteri PK, Jaffe RB. Steroid production by definitive and fetal zones of the human fetal adrenal gland. *J Clin Endocrinol Metab* **47**:603–609, 1978.
80. Greenough A, Nicolaides KH, Lagercrantz H. Human fetal sympathoadrenal responsiveness. *Early Hum Dev* **23**:9–13, 1990.
81. Okamura K, Watanabe T, Tanigawara S *et al.* Biochemical evaluation of fetus with hypoxia caused by severe pre-eclampsia using cordocentesis. *J Perinat Med* **18**:441–447, 1990.
82. Rosen F, Ezrin C. Embryology of the thyrotroph. *J Clin Endocrin Metabol* **26**:1343–1345, 1966.
83. Shepard TH. Onset of function in the human fetal thyroid: biochemical and radioautographic studies from organ culture. *J Clin Endocrin Metab* **27**:945–958, 1967.
84. Thorpe-Beeston JG, Nicolaides KH, Snijders RJM, Felton CV, McGregor AM. Thyroid function in small for gestational age fetues. *Obstet Gynecol* **77**:701–706, 1991.
85. Thorpe-Beeston JG, Nicolaides KH, Snijders RJM, Felton CV. Relationships between the fetal circulation and pituitary–thyroid function. *Br J Obstet Gynaecol* **98**:1163–1167, 1991.
86. Geloso JP, Hemon P, Legrand J, Legrand C, Jost A. Some aspects of thyroid physiology during the perinatal period. *Gen Comp Endocrinol* **10**:191–197, 1968.
87. McFaul R, Dorner S, Brett EM, Grant DB. Neurological abnormalities in patients treated for hypothyroidism from early life. *Arch Dis Child* **53**:611–619, 1978.
88. Petraglia F, Florio P, Nappi C, Geazzani AR. Peptide signalling in human placenta and membranes: autocrine, paracrine and endocrine mechanisms. *Endocrin Rev* **17**:156–186, 1996.

Blood and immune system 18

G. Brown and M.T. Drayson

Introduction

The haemopoietic (blood cell-forming) system is perhaps the most complex and certainly the most dynamic tissue in the adult organism. Development of blood cells starts in the first two months of intrauterine life and continues throughout life. At least eleven different types of blood cells are produced: platelets, erythrocytes, mast cells, basophils, eosinophils, neutrophils, monocytes, dendritic cells, natural killer cells, B-lymphocytes and T-lymphocytes. There are also sub-populations of cells within some of these well-defined cell types (see Table 18.1). The considerable functional diversity of leucocytes in total enables the selective clearance of effete or damaged tissues and of pathogens. Extracellular and intracellular bacteria, viruses, parasites and fungi are eliminated with minimal damage to self, as may be foreign tissue or tumour cells.

TABLE 18.1
Products of haemopoiesis: distribution of the 11 major types of blood cells between blood tissues

Marrow	Blood	Tissues
Megakaryoblast	Platelet	
Erythroblast	Erythrocyte	
Mast cell precursor	Mast cell	Mucosal and connective tissue mast cells
Myeloblast	Basophil Eosinophil Neutrophil	In sites of inflammation
Monoblast	Monocyte	Tissue/lymphoid tissue macrophages; Kupffer cell; osteoclast
Precursor?	Dendritic cell	Tissue dendritic cell/Langerhans cell; veiled cell; interdigitating cell
Precursor?	Natural killer cell	Lymphoid tissues; sites of inflammation
Pro-B cell (matures in marrow)	Type 1 and type 2 B cells in blood and secondary lymphoid tissues; plasma cells also in mucosal surfaces and bone marrow	
T-cell precursor (matures in thymus)	α/β and γ/δ T cells; $CD4^+$ and $CD8^+$ T cells; in blood, secondary lymphoid tissues and sites of inflammation	

Principles of haemopoiesis

Information on the population structure of the haemopoietic system has provided the foundation to understanding the development of blood cells. Early work focused on progressive stages of development within each cell lineage. This led to the concept of a tiered system of development and a 'generation structure' to haemopoiesis (see Fig. 18.1). It is generally accepted that all the blood cell types arise from a common

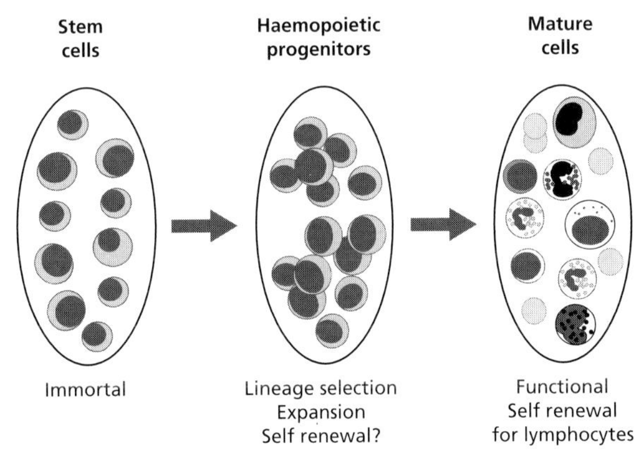

Fig. 18.1 Progressive stages in haemopoiesis. As cells progress from one cell compartment to the next, they lose and acquire cardinal properties.

stem cell, the haemopoietic stem cell (HSC). HSCs self-renew and their immortality and pluripotency are their hallmarks. As generations of cells are produced from the HSC they lose and gain cardinal properties. HSC progeny that are 'selected' for differentiation give rise to haemopoietic progenitor cells (HPCs). These cells are undergoing proliferative expansion and progressive commitment to a single differentiation option. Unipotent HPCs give rise to morphologically recognisable lineage precursors, for example, erythroblasts. HPCs together with recognisable lineage precursors are an amplifying and 'transit' generation. The 'end-generations' are functional cells (e.g. erythrocytes), which are expendable and have limited lifespans. Thus, haemopoiesis, in the fetus and the adult, entails: (i) the production and maintenance of HSCs, (ii) specification of HSC progeny to lineage fates, (iii) expansion of lineage-committed progenitor cells and (iv) maturation of unipotent progenitors to functional end cells. This sequence of events provides a rationale to the large numbers of mature cells that are produced.

Definition of cell lineages and the identification of committed HPCs allowed exploration of some of the questions that are most challenging to developmental biologists. For example, what are the precise origins of interrelated cell lineages? There are two components to this problem. The first is the issue of constructing a lineage map for the haemopoietic system. There is a long-standing map which has been challenged by more recent studies, but the exact relationships between haemopoietic cell lineages remains controversial. The second component is: What is the nature of the molecular mechanisms that are 'instructive' for lineage commitment? Levels of expression of transcription factors and cooperation between their activities appear to control haemopoiesis. Endeavours to understand haemopoiesis have focused on transcription factors that play roles in: (i) specification of ventral mesoderm to a haemopoietic fate, (ii) further lineage programming, (iii) maintenance and proliferation of committed progenitors and (iv) terminal maturation.

Beyond insight to the origin of the major haemopoietic lineages, there is the issue of the development, function and maintenance of innate and specific immunity. Specific immunity is enabled by antigen-specific receptors (ASR) on T and B lymphocytes. Early in lymphocyte ontogeny, genes for ASR are randomly rearranged with a potential for 10^{12} permutations. Once a successful rearrangement is made, it is retained for the life of that cell and of its progeny. Because the gene rearrangements are random, the ASR produced may be self-reactive. This necessitates mechanisms for the functional deletion of cells bearing self-reactive receptors. For a given foreign antigen the frequency of reactive lymphocytes is in the order of $1/10^5$. Development of a specific response to a target and memory of that developed response requires expansion and further differentiation of lymphocyte clones and maintenance of those changes over many years.

Innate immunity is engendered by neutrophils, macrophages and dendritic cells. In contrast to lymphocytes, either all or none of these cells recognise a given target. For each of these different cell types, recognition of a target and subsequent action is complex and diverse, but, in any given scenario, is identical and finite for all members of the population. Neutrophils, macrophages and dendritic cells are terminal effector cells with lifespans of days or weeks; replacement is almost entirely through further haemopoiesis.

Embryonic origins of haemopoietic stem cells

The generally accepted view is that the blood cell system in man derives solely from ventral mesoderm, but recent evidence suggests both ventral and dorsal contributions (see below). The first cells to appear, in developing mammals, are embryonic red cells, which are generated in the blood islands of the yolk sac. Vascular endothelium and haemopoietic cells appear at the same time within the yolk sac, which has led to the suggestion that these cells share a common precursor, termed a haemangioblast[1]. Evidence in favour of the existence of this cell has been obtained from studies of mice that are null for flk-1. Flk-1 is a receptor tyrosine kinase that responds to vascular endothelial growth factor (VEGF) and is an early marker for endothelial cell precursors[2]. There is a failure of blood island formation and defective vasculogenesis in flk-1 deficient mice[3]. This finding may reflect the importance of flk-1 expression in the hypothetical haemangioblast. Alternatively, loss of haemopoiesis may be secondary to a defect in vasculogenesis. In transforming growth factor-β (TGF-β) knock-out mice there is defective haemopoiesis and vasculogenesis, which can be interpreted in either of the above two ways[4].

What determines commitment of ventral mesoderm cells to a haemopoietic fate? A definite answer to this question is lacking. A candidate gene is that which encodes the basic helix–loop–helix transcription regulator SCL (also termed Tal-1). SCL is expressed in progenitors of haemopoietic and vascular cells during embryogenesis and in mature megakaryocytic, erythroid and mast cells[5,6]. Embryos lacking SCL fail to initiate yolk sac erythropoiesis and die at the yolk sac stage. Myeloid progenitors are also virtually absent within the yolk sac[7]. Furthermore, Orkin recently commented that preliminary studies have shown that SCL-null mouse embryonic stem cells are unable to generate definitive haemopoietic progenitors[8]. SCL may play a crucial role in progenitors of endothelial and haemopoietic cells and at early stages of haemopoietic cell development. In addition, SCL protein is present in the nucleus of erythroid cells as a complex with the LIM protein Rbtn2 (also termed LMO2)[9,10]. Rbtn2 null embryos also die at the yolk sac stage, due to an absence of erythropoiesis[11]; myeloid progenitors are also reduced. Interaction between SCL and Rbtn2 may thus be crucial to early haemopoietic cell development.

The temporal pattern of development of haemopoiesis

In developing mammals there are temporal waves of haemopoiesis. The first, termed primitive haemopoiesis, occurs in the islands of the yolk sac. At the second to the fifth month of intrauterine human life, definitive haemopoiesis occurs in the fetal liver and remains operative till around birth. Bone marrow haemopoiesis is apparent from the fifth month, and marrow becomes the major site of haemopoiesis shortly before birth. Thereafter, haemopoietic cells are normally produced in the bone marrow. As described later, the thymus is the site of T lymphopoiesis.

A long-standing concept in mammalian embryogenesis is that HSCs originate in the yolk sac and migrate to the fetal liver and from this site to the bone marrow (see Fig. 18.2, Model (a)). In birds and amphibians, yolk sac and analogues are responsible for primitive and transient haemopoiesis. Blood cells of the adult *Xenopus laevis*, that is, definitive haemopoietic cells, arise from stem-cell compartments that originated in the dorsal (paraortic) mesoderm[12], and recent studies in mice have revealed that two stem cell compartments may contribute differentially to primitive and definitive haemopoiesis. Investigators have identified a pool of stem cells in the aortic/gonad/mesonephros (AGM) or paraortic region of early embryos[13–15]. The source of these cells is uncertain. They arise before haemopoiesis in the liver, and unlike yolk sac cells, AGM region cells have stem cell-reconstituting activity in mice. It is therefore probable that the fetal liver of mice is seeded by a wave of stem cells from the yolk sac, and later by a second wave from the AGM region (see Fig. 18.2, Model (b)). This second wave of stem cells also populates the bone marrow. Hence, the principle of consecutive waves of ventral and dorsal stem cell compartments giving rise to primitive and to definitive (adult) haemopoiesis, respectively, may apply to all vertebrates.

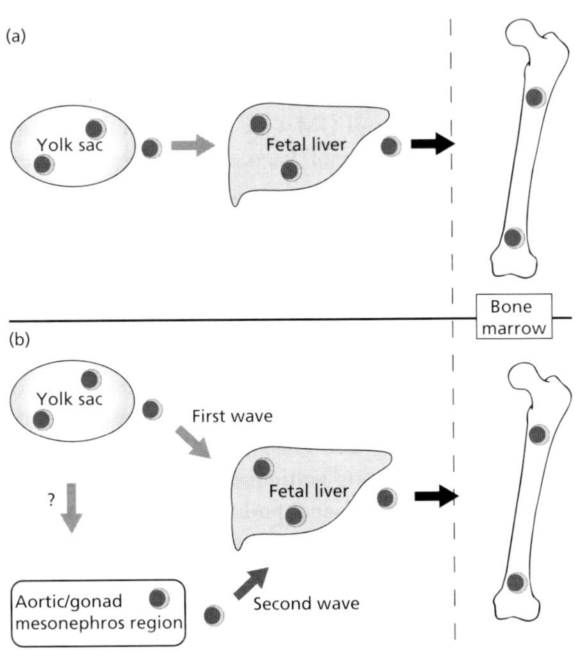

Fig. 18.2 Sites of haemopoiesis during embryogenesis. (a) A long-standing concept in mammalian embryogenesis, which is that yolk sac stem cells migrate to fetal liver and from this site to bone marrow. (b) Dual stem cells compartments may contribute to haemopoiesis.

Haemopoietic stem cell diversification

An understanding of what happens to HSCs to restrict them to development along pathways of maturation is central to describing the formation of the blood cell system. Recent work is focused on the mechanism of HSC diversification and has also led to a re-evaluation of the pathways of haemopoietic cell diversification.

THE CONVENTIONAL MODEL OF HAEMOPOIESIS

Researchers have inferred various connecting lines between HSCs and the blood cells they produce: a commonly depicted view is shown in Fig. 18.3. The central tenet of this model is that HSCs first give rise to two distinct progenitor cells. One of these, a lymphoid progenitor, gives rise to B and T lymphocytes and the other, a myeloid progenitor, generates all the remaining blood cell types. Myeloid progenitors are then further subdivided. It is customary to connect the neutrophil and monocyte lineages, since early studies of the growth of bone-marrow cells in semi-solid medium demonstrated the existence of a colony-forming cell (CFC) that can generate both neutrophils and monocytes (GM-CFC). There are unipotent progenitors for erythrocytes (BFU-E), eosinophils (Eo-CFC), megakaryocytes (Meg-CFC) and mast cells (Mast-CFC).

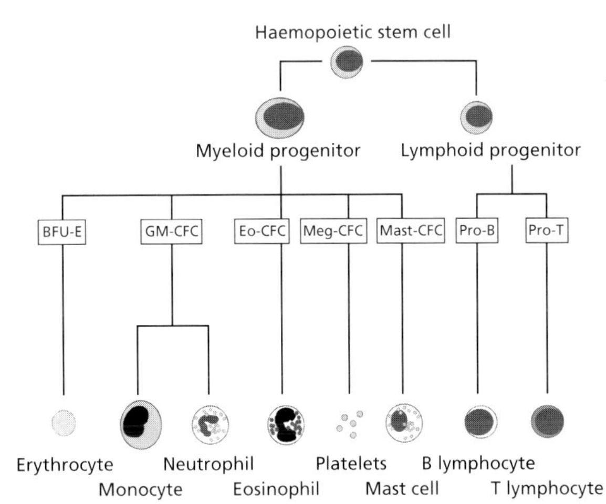

Fig. 18.3 Conventional model of haemopoiesis. The central tenet is that stem cells first give rise to myeloid and lymphoid progenitors.

allow sequential sampling of the various binary options. A cell is likely to be diverted along a particular pathway of differentiation whenever it simultaneously (i) encounters conditions conducive to a particular differentiated fate and (ii) samples one of the two binary options permissive to that fate.

The notion of a series of developmental options following one another originated from studies of the promyeloid cell line HL60, which can differentiate to neutrophils or monocytes, and of variants of this line that have restricted capacities for differentiation along one or both of these pathways. Analysis of the variant lines suggested that HL60 cells first acquire the capacity for neutrophil differentiation, as cells lose this capacity they acquire the potential for monocyte differentiation[35]. Dexter and colleagues had suggested previously that the sequence of development of committed progenitor cells during normal neutrophil and macrophage development is: G-CFC → GM-CFC → M-CFC[37].

The sequence of potential commitment stages, from megakaryocytes to T lymphocytes, takes into consideration the lineage potentials both of normal progenitor cells and of cell lines that are restricted to two differentiation potentials. For example, bipotent cells that differentiate to megakaryocytes and erythrocytes are present in bone-marrow cultures of human and murine cells[32]. The human cell line K562 can differentiate along both of these pathways[38,39]. McDonald and Sullivan have argued that the link between hypoxia stimulation of erythropoiesis and of thrombocytopenia in laboratory animals is competition between the two fates of a precursor cell for megakaryocytes and erythrocytes[40]. Collectively, these observations led to the notion that megakaryocytic and erythrocytic cells are closely related[40]. In 1985, the most controversial aspect of the sequential determination model was the postulate that monocytes and B lymphocytes might be closely related. It is now generally accepted that these lineages are linked. Further support for the pairings of differentiation pathways along the sequence is that the total ordering of potentials fits with the patterns of multiple lineage involvement seen in myelodysplastic and myeloproliferative disorders. Whenever two, three, four and five different lineages are involved in the disease process, they form a contiguous grouping within the sequence[41,42].

Pathways for mast cell, basophil and eosinophil differentiation were absent from the original model. Data that allow inclusion of these differentiation options in the sequence (see Fig. 18.5) and support for a model of this type emerged from analyses undertaken by Novak and Necas of the production rates of megakaryocytes, erythrocytes, mast cells, basophils, eosinophils, monocytes and neutrophils from murine bone marrow. These workers undertook a quantitative analysis of all of the published data on cell turnover in the normal steady state[43,44]. They concluded that production rates (fluxes) of all the lineages analyzed from bone marrow 'are fully consistent with a simple binary model of the sequential type, similar to that suggested by Brown and coworkers'.

The positions of progenitor states for dendritic cells and NK cells in the linear series of relationships shown in Fig. 18.5 are uncertain. In the thymus, T lymphocytes and dendritic cells develop simultaneously from a common precursor cell which can also give rise to monocytes and B lymphocytes[45]. So, the progenitor state for dendritic cells should fall in or next to the monocyte → B lymphocyte → T lymphocyte sector. NK cells are a type of lymphocyte and have functions similar to some T lymphocytes, so NK progenitors might be expected to fall in or next to the → B lymphocyte → T lymphocyte sector.

Finally, a sequence of successive restriction of differentiation potentials is a feature of the model proposed by Nicola and Johnson[46]. These workers interpreted their studies of committed HPCs to suggest that pluripotent HSCs progressively lose differentiation options until only the capacity to differentiate to erythrocytes remains. This model favours the concept of multipotent HSCs, which is argued against in the previous sequential determination model.

TRANSCRIPTION FACTOR UTILIZATION IN HAEMOPOIESIS

Studies of patterns of expression of transcription factors in various blood cell types and of the lineages that are ablated in knock-out experiments in mice have an important bearing on the fidelity of lineage maps. Recent reviews have highlighted the importance of the turning on and off of transcription factors to control of the availability of lineage options, the commitment of cells to a pathway and their maturation[8,47]. Analysis of knock-out mice can help elucidate the lineage map for haemopoietic cells by demonstrating that elimination of particular transcription factors causes the selective loss of certain groups of blood cell types.

Mice lacking the transcription factor ikarus fail to produce B and T lymphocytes[48]. Thus, ikarus is essential for the development of both these cell groups, which can be reconciled with both the conventional model (see Fig. 18.3) and the sequential determination model (see Fig. 18.5). The phenotype of ikarus knock-out mice does not exclude models in which progenitor cells are generated at random (see Fig. 18.4).

Mice carrying a mutation in the PU.1 locus (also termed Spi-1) show a particularly interesting pattern of blood cell development. They produce normal numbers of megakaryocyte and erythroid precursors, but have a multilineage defect in the generation of granulocytes, monocytes, B and T lymphocytes[49]. One interpretation of these findings is that the PU.1-dependent development of the latter cell types lies functionally down-stream of the PU.1-independent development of megakaryocytes and erythrocytes. This fits the sequential determination model, but is inconsistent with the conventional model. Observations in PU.1 null mice also further strengthen the opinion that cell differentiation options are not randomly associated.

The proto-oncogene product c-*myb* is expressed in immature erythroid, myeloid and lymphoid lineages, but c-*myb* expression is low or absent in mature cells. Loss of c-*myb* does not affect primitive haemopoiesis, and during definitive haematopoiesis megakaryopoiesis is spared[50]. Thus, c-*myb* expression may be necessary for HSCs to gain access to all the cell lineages that are downstream of the potential for megakaryocyte differentiation in the sequential model. When the ikarus, PU.1 and c-*myb* knock-out phenotypes are laid side by side, they define successively earlier 'breaks' in the backbone of a linear model of progenitor cell development (see Fig. 18.6).

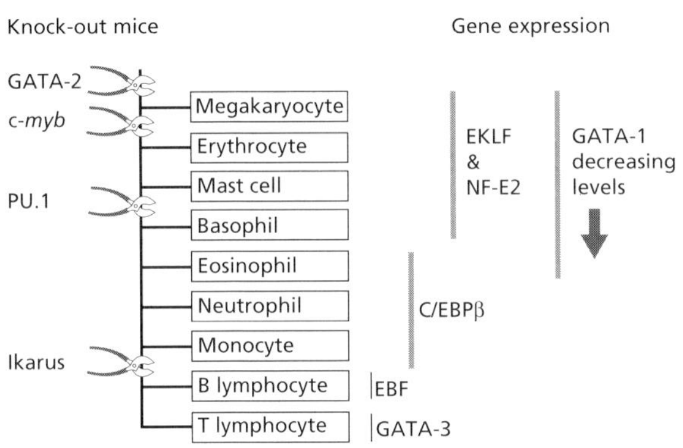

Fig. 18.6 Transcription factors and sequential determination. Lineages that are ablated in knock-out experiments in mice and patterns of expression of transcription factors are overlaid on the sequential determination model.

The extents to which expression of some transcription factors spread across several cell lineages may also point to certain close relationships. GATA-1 is expressed in megakaryocytes, erythroid cells, mast cells, basophils and eosinophils[51–54]. Expression of the Kruppel-like zinc-finger protein EKLF[55] and the basic leucine zipper protein NF-E2 (p45)[56] in megakaryocytes, erythroid cells, mast cells and basophils suggests that these cell types are closely related. The above two groups of cell types are all adjacent in the linear model (see Fig. 18.6). In a recent study, Kulessa and coworkers have investigated the effect of forced expression of GATA-1 in avian myelomonocytic cell lines and shown that GATA-1 can reprogram these cells into erythroblasts, thromboblasts and eosinophils[57]. Interestingly, when myeloblasts were transformed to either thromboblasts or eosinophils, a correlation was observed between the resultant phenotype and the level of GATA-1 expression. High levels were expressed by thromboblasts and lower levels by eosinophils, so the amount of GATA-1 may play an important role in lineage determination.

The transcription factor C/EBPβ is expressed in eosinophils, neutrophils and monocytes and their immediate precursors (Eo-CFC and GM-CFC)[58–60]. These progenitor cell compartments can be accounted for in the conventional model, in so much as Eo-CFC and GM-CFC are related. However, that GATA-1 is expressed by megakaryocytes, erythroid cells, mast cells and basophils, whereas C/EBPβ is expressed by eosinophils, neutrophils and monocytes is more in keeping with the sequential determination model.

It is clear that transcription factors are utilised in combination in haemopoietic cell differentiation[8,47]. In addition to the factors discussed previously, there are those that appear to play a role in HSC/HPC maintenance *per se*, for example GATA-2[8]. There are also factors that are apparently lineage-restricted, such as GATA-3 (T lymphocytes in mammals)[61], TCF-1 (T lymphocytes)[62] and EBF (early B cells)[63]. Transcription factors that are important in haemopoiesis are described in more detail in reviews by Ness and Engel[47] and by Orkin[8].

Whether the patterns of expression of transcription factors and of their combinatorial usage lead to margins that dictate a particular order to the development of HSCs is going to be a topic of considerable interest over the next few years. Levels of expression of transcription factors is also an important consideration, as illustrated by the studies of GATA-1 (see above). It is well established, from studies of the early stages of insect egg development, that gradients of transcription factors can switch on and off genes at various threshold levels to pattern the embryo. Hence, nuclei of cells can sense the available concentrations of transcription factors. Progressive increases and/or decreases in the levels of transcription factors in HSCs as they sample the various developmental options may allow cells to achieve a series of thresholds, with each relating to a possible differentiation fate. In this circumstance, each cell's career choices would be binary: an HSC would be moving from one threshold to the next, and at each threshold would lose one fate option but gain another.

AUTONOMY IN DIFFERENTIATIVE DECISIONS

In a recent editorial overview, Spiegelman and Watt suggest that cell autonomy in differentiative decisions is an increasingly important concept[64]. The best evidence for cell autonomy comes from studies of the development of the mouse gastrointestinal epithelium[65]. In these experiments, isografts of the gut endoderm (of 14-day-old embryos), that showed no morphologic variations, were implanted subcutaneously into adult mice and normal morphogenesis was observed. The capacity of cells to undergo differentiation along a particular pathway is seen as an intrinsic property in the random and sequential determination models of haemopoiesis. If this concept of cell autonomy is correct, then the processes that segregate developmental options need to be understood. One possibility is that cell cycling in the progenitor populations involves a cycling in the concentrations of key regulators, which might temporally separate differentiation options during a single cell cycle. Alternatively, cell division may result in an uneven distribution of key regulators.

Reaching maturity

Events that control differentiation of HPCs that are committed to a maturation pathway are outlined in regard to erythrocytes and lymphocytes. A description of erythropoiesis serves to highlight concepts relating to reaching maturity; lymphocytes are a special case as to their remarkable diversity. Furthermore, the production rate of lymphocytes is far in excess of the number recruited to the circulation. Elimination of 'unwanted' cells is a key feature of lymphopoiesis.

ERYTHROPOIESIS

Unipotent HPCs undergo expansion together with progressive maturation to give rise to morphologically recognisable precursors and mature cells. One of the most clearly defined pathways of cell differentiation is that which gives rise to erythrocytes[66]. There are two types of progenitors: burst-forming unit-erythroid (BFU-E) and colony-forming unit-erythroid (CFU-E). The less mature BFU-E give rise to diffuse colonies of 10 to 100 CFU-E, which in turn form a compact colony of 1000 to 10 000 mature erythrocytes. BFU-E and CFU-E are able to 'count' generations, in so much as there appears to be a fixed number of cell divisions. As CFU-E divide, they undergo inevitable changes in gene expression to alter their appearance and acquire functional activity.

The concept that unipotent HPCs undergo a fixed number of divisions leading to a loss of proliferative capacity has been challenged recently by the studies of avian erythroid differentiation by Beug and colleagues[66]. These workers have identified a self-renewing erythroid progenitor, which extends the property of self-renewal to cells immediately downstream of the pluripotent HSC. Long-term self-renewal of erythroid progenitors in culture requires the presence of TGF-α and estradiol; they also express *c-kit* and are termed stem cell factor (SCF)/TGF-α progenitors. SCF/TGF-α progenitors arise from a CFU-E-like progenitor, termed a SCF progenitor. These cells can undergo six to eight self-renewal divisions in the presence of SCF. The picture that is emerging is that the number of divisions during terminal differentiation is flexible. Furthermore, the division counting mechanism in HPCs and, in particular, their capacity to self-renew is affected by the presence of growth factors.

A second important concept from studies of erythroid differentiation is that of a 'master switch' that controls terminal maturation[66]. This 'master switch', in addition to eliciting a pattern of terminal gene expression, alters the control of cell cycle. This reprogramming is influenced by external signals in the following manner. Lack of exposure of SCF/TGF-α progenitors to TGF-α plus estradiol and of SCF progenitors to SCF, together with exposure of these cells to EPO and insulin, results in 'switch on' of the terminal programme and maturation to erythrocytes over five cell divisions. In these instances, external factors are affecting survival, self-renewal and cell-cycle control in cells that have already been recruited to erythroid differentiation. Of particular interest is whether a single, as yet unknown, transcription factor coordinates the entire pathway of erythropoiesis by turning on later gene regulators whose activity is influenced by surface receptor-mediated signalling pathways.

B LYMPHOPOIESIS

TYPES OF B LYMPHOCYTES

Studies of B lymphopoiesis, in mice in particular, indicate that two types of B lymphocytes are produced: B1 cells and B2 cells[67,68]. B1 cells are produced early in development, in the liver, and are the predominant type in the fetus. They persist throughout life in mice and are capable of self-renewal in the periphery[69]. The putative equivalent of B1 cells in man express the surface glycoprotein CD5 and decline as a proportion of total B cells in childhood. B lymphocytes that are produced in the bone marrow throughout life fall into the B2 category, hereafter termed B lymphocytes. A feature that distinguishes B1 cells from B lymphocytes is that they produce antibodies with broad reactivity[69]. Some of these antibodies bind to self-antigens, which has led to speculation that B1 cells may play a role in selection of the B-cell antibody repertoire[70,71]. However, the precise function of B1 cells remains unclear.

B lymphocytes are regarded as a single lineage that is further divided into cell types according to maturation status. There are three main types of B lymphocyte: newly produced virgin B lymphocytes, recirculating cells and those that reside in the marginal zone of secondary lymphoid organs. Virgin B lymphocytes give rise to recirculating cells and some of the recirculating cells mature to give rise to marginal zone cells. Around 20 million virgin B lymphocytes are produced in an adult mouse per day. Only 2–5% of these cells are recruited to the circulating pool of B lymphocytes. The failure of cells to enter the circulation is not merely deletion of B lymphocytes with reactivity to self-antigens, since when the recirculating pool is depleted a much greater proportion of newly produced virgin B lymphocytes survive to enter the recirculating pool to restore numbers.

SITES OF B LYMPHOPOIESIS

B lymphopoiesis originates in fetal liver at the end of the first trimester of pregnancy[72]. Later, production ceases at this site and B lymphocytes are produced in the splenic red pulp and the bone marrow. After birth, B lymphocytes are produced in the bone marrow.

STAGES OF B LYMPHOPOIESIS

The key process in B lymphopoiesis is rearrangement of immunoglobulin genes to generate cells with unique antigen

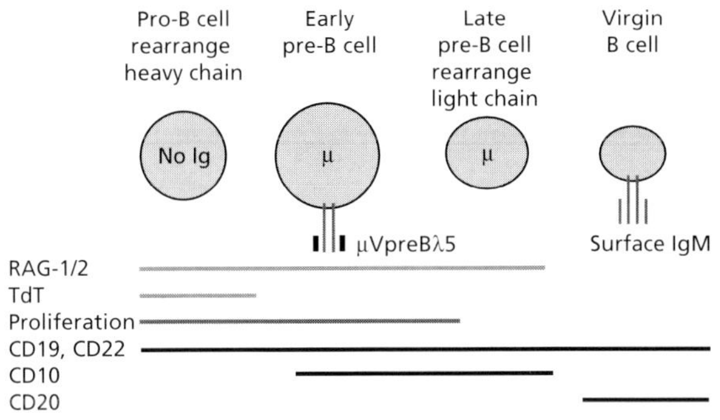

Fig. 18.7 B lymphopoiesis. Progressive stages of maturation are delineated in regard to rearrangement and expression of immunoglobulin genes and acquired expression of surface molecules.

receptors at their surface. Stages of B lymphocyte development are delineated with regard to steps in this process (see Fig. 18.7). Acquired expression of a number of surface molecules also typifies progressive stages of maturation[73]. The earliest markers of commitment of HSCs to the B-lymphocyte pathway are expression of CD19, CD22, CD24 and MHC class II molecules at the cell surface. A cell with this phenotype is termed a pro-B cell. This cell expresses the recombinase activating genes (Rag) 1 and 2. Rag-1 and -2 proteins are involved in rearrangement of the V-region of immunoglobulin genes and B lymphocyte maturation is arrested at the late pro-B stage in either Rag-1 or Rag-2 deficient mice[74,75].

There is a definite order to rearrangement of immunoglobulin genes[76,77]. The immunoglobulin heavy chain gene complex is located on chromosome 14 and the κ and λ complexes are located on chromosomes 2 and 22, respectively. The first rearrangements are of V-regions of the heavy chain. Three types of segments make up a complete variable region: V, D and J. D to J is attempted and completed, if possible, on both chromosomes[78,79]. The cell then rearranges DJ to a V segment on one of the chromosomes. Success results in transcription of VDJ together with the gene encoding the μ constant region. The enzyme terminal deoxynucleotidyl transferase (TdT) adds a random sequence of nucleotides at the V to DH and DH to J joints in heavy-chain gene rearrangement. This process greatly enhances the generation of diversity in the antigen-binding region. A cell with cytoplasmic μ heavy chain is termed a pre-B cell[72]. This cell must then express the μ heavy chain combined with a surrogate light chain (preBλ5) for further differentiation to occur[80]. If the first attempt to join DJ to V was not successful, then this rearrangement is attempted on the other chromosome 14. Failure a second time, and lack of expression of a μ heavy chain and surrogate light chain at the surface, results in death by apotosis.

Early pre-B lymphocytes are a proliferating population of cells and they receive a signal which allows them to come out of cell cycle to proceed to rearrange light chain genes. B lymphocytes express either a κ or a λ light chain, and, therefore, only transcribe one of their four light-chain gene complexes. First κ light chain genes are rearranged; failure to construct a functional κ gene leads to rearrangement of the λ light-chain genes[81]. In B lymphocytes producing a κ light chain, the λ genes remain in germline configuration[82]. A cell that expresses IgM at the cell surface is termed a newly-produced virgin B lymphocyte.

ELIMINATION OF SELF-REACTIVE VIRGIN B LYMPHOCYTES

Most autoreactive B lymphocytes are eliminated at the stage when they first express IgM at their surface though interaction with their specific antigen. Encounter with multivalent antigen, at this stage in the marrow, crosslinks the surface IgM, but fails to elicit full activation to effector function. Instead, the interaction results in apoptosis within the marrow or a state of anergy. B lymphocytes reactive to potential foreign antigens and those reactive to self-antigens not present in the marrow migrate to secondary lymphoid organs. Remaining autoreactive B lymphocytes are unlikely to survive and be activated to effector function, since this usually requires interaction with T lymphocytes specific for that self-antigen. Generally, these self-reactive T cells have been deleted in the thymus (see below). Newly produced B lymphocytes in the secondary lymphoid tissues express both IgM and IgD and most are not self-reactive. Nevertheless, they only survive for a few days unless one of two events occur. First, successful activation by antigen may occur in the context of T-cell help. Second, in the absence of specific antigen, cells receive an, as yet, unknown signal which allows entry to a longer lived (several weeks) pool of recirculating virgin B cells[83–85].

There is an extremely high death rate during B lymphopoiesis[86]. At the progenitor cell stage, there are those cells that produce non-productive V-region gene rearrangements. A cell may also produce light chains that fail to combine with heavy chains. A cell failing to express immunoglobulin at its surface dies by apoptosis. Autoreactive B lymphocytes are deleted at the newly produced virgin stage of B lymphopoiesis. Finally, there appear to be insufficient microenvironments in the periphery to support the survival of the very large number of virgin cells that enter the circulation. The overall viewpoint is that the body scrutinises and selects B lymphocytes as required in the circulation.

T LYMPHOPOIESIS

TYPES OF T LYMPHOCYTES

Two major types of T lymphocytes are produced by the thymus that differ in regard to the receptor molecules they express at their surface. Rearrangement of T-cell receptor (TCR) genes leads to cells that express either the γδ or αβ form of the TCR. These two populations share a common intrathymic precursor[87]. The first mature T lymphocytes to leave the thymus are of the γδ type. At later stages of human fetal development, 85–95% of cells leaving the thymus are of the αβ type. These are the predominant type of T lymphocytes that persists throughout life. αβ T lymphocytes have further diversified into two main subtypes. These are CD8-positive T lymphocytes, which recognise peptides in association with major histocompatibility complex (MHC) class I molecules, and CD4-positive T lymphocytes, which recognise peptides in association with MHC class II molecules. CD4 or CD8 are not expressed by many γδ T lymphocytes and the function of these cells in humans is uncertain.

SITES OF T LYMPHOPOIESIS

The thymus is essential to the development of the vast majority of T lymphocytes[88]. HSCs reaching the thymus undergo rearrangement of TCR genes. αβ T lymphocytes are subjected to rigorous positive and negative selection within thymic microenvironments. Positive selection allows cells that recognise foreign peptides in association with self MHC to mature to functional T cells. Negative selection removes T lymphocytes that recognise self peptides.

The nature of stromal cell types that develop in the thymus are important to the processes that govern selection of T lymphocytes. T lymphopoiesis proceeds in distinctive areas of cortical and medullary epithelium (see below). Early studies led to the suggestion that both ectoderm and endoderm contribute to thymic epithelium[89]. However, studies in birds have shown that pharyngeal endoderm minus ectoderm can result in complete thymic histogenesis, though the presence of neural crest derived mesenchyme cells is essential[90]. Interaction between mesenchyme and endoderm cells is necessary for morphogenesis of thymic epithelium[91]. As yet, the more precise origins of thymic epithelium cells are uncertain.

COLONIZATION OF THE THYMUS BY T-LINEAGE CELLS

HSCs arrive at the thymus via the bloodstream. An important question is: Are these cells already restricted to T cell development or do they have other differentiation potentials available to them? Eight- to nine-day-old murine yolk sac cells are able to colonize fetal thymus lobes *in vitro*[92,93]. Therefore, multipotent HSCs can colonize the thymus. However, multipotent HSCs and pro-thymocytes are present in murine fetal blood at day 15.5, which suggests that T-lineage commitment can precede thymus colonization[94]. In contrast, the presence of precursors of B cells, macrophages, dendritic cells and NK cells in the thymus[45,95,96] leads to the inference that multipotent HSCs enter the thymus and are then committed to T-cell differentiation. This need not be the case, since unipotent cells for other cell lineages may enter the thymus in addition to pro-thymocytes. As yet, the extents to which mutipotent HSCs and T-lineage committed cells enter the thymus, and the contribution of these cells to the development of αβ and γδ T cells are unclear.

Multipotent HSCs and/or T-lineage-committed progenitors colonize the thymic primordium prior to vascularization. Blood-borne progenitors leave pharyngeal vessels and traverse the surrounding mesenchyme. Mechanisms and chemoattractants that govern this migration to the thymus are unknown. Soon blood vessels, and associated mesoderm, invade the embryonic thymus. In addition, as lymphopoiesis proceeds, the epithelium becomes organized into an outer cortex region and an inner medulla. These regions have specialised types of stromal cells. For example, the outer cortex contains large epithelial cells termed 'nurse cells', which appear to have large numbers of lymphocytes lying within their cytoplasm. Dendritic cells are predominantly in the medulla. Macrophages are distributed throughout the cortex and medulla; the boundary of these regions is populated by cells termed sentinel macrophages The spatial distribution of dendritic cells and macrophages is probably important to their functional roles as mediators of negative selection and phagocytosis of apoptotic cells, respectively.

HSCs/T-lineage-committed progenitors proliferate in the thymus in the outer cortex. The proliferative potential of pro-thymocytes is extensive in that a single cell is able to populate an empty thymic lobe and generate the entire repertoire of T cells. Towards the end of this proliferative phase, TCR genes are rearranged in cells termed pre-thymocytes. Pre-thymocytes expressing a β chain/surrogate α-chain TCR (see below) undergo a second wave of proliferation that is probably driven by the pre-TCR. Pre-thymocytes traverse the cortex and then the medulla regions, and interact, via surface TCRs, with various stromal cells that express MHC molecules at their surface. This results in both positive and negative selection to generate an appropriate repertoire of T cells. The overall process of T-cell development is shown in Fig. 18.8.

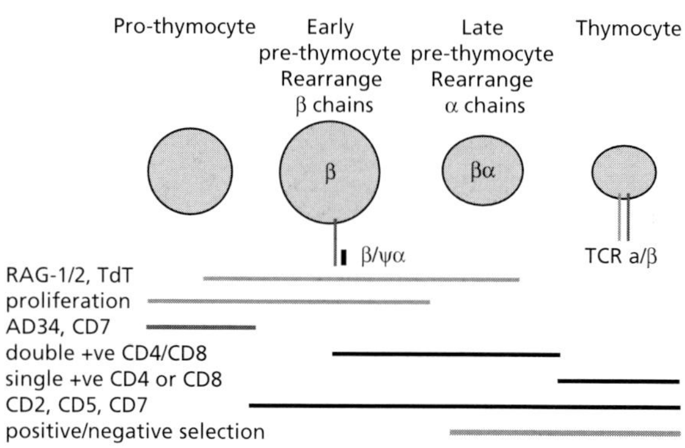

Fig. 18.8 T lymphopoiesis. The sequence of rearrangement of T-cell receptor genes and acquired expression of surface molecules are shown.

REARRANGEMENT OF T-CELL-RECEPTOR GENES

Expression of a definitive TCR complex consisting of an α and β chain is the starting point for the two processes of positive and negative selection of $\alpha\beta$ T cells. T-cell precursors express the Rag-1 and Rag-2 proteins and knock-out of these genes in mice results in a block in T-lymphocyte development[74,75]. Rearrangement of receptor genes occurs in a particular order in a manner analogous to rearrangement of immunoglobulin genes during B lymphocyte development. β-gene rearrangement occurs first. D is joined to J followed by V to DJ. This leads to a low level of expression of β chain, complexed with a surrogate α chain ($\psi\alpha$) and CD3, at the cell surface. At this stage, the cell starts to express low levels of both CD4 and CD8. Further β-gene rearrangement is halted and the CD4/CD8 double positive cell rearranges the α-chain genes. The processes of CD4/CD8 co-expression, arrest of β-chain rearrangement and initiation of α-chain rearrangement are, in part, mediated by signalling via the β-chain/surrogate α-chain/CD3 complex[97–99]. There are a large number of α-chain V and J gene segments. This allows developing T lymphocytes the possibility of multiple attempts at α chain gene rearrangement to produce an $\alpha\beta$ heterodimer that interacts with self MHC molecules. In addition, and unlike B lymphocytes, $\alpha\beta$ T cells do not show allelic exclusion of α-chain genes. Thirty percent of human peripheral T cells express two α chains and are, presumably, bispecific. Expression of an $\alpha\beta$ TCR, CD3 and both CD4 and CD8 allows T cells to progress to positive and negative selection.

SELECTION OF 'WANTED' CELLS AND ELIMINATION OF 'UNWANTED' CELLS

Positive and negative selection can operate at the same time on $CD4^+/CD8^+$ thymocytes[100,101]. There is also continued α-gene rearrangement. Thymocyte–stromal cell interactions that are crucial to selection of the T-cell receptor repertoire are described in detail in a recent review by Anderson and co-workers[102]. Thymic epithelial cells are essential for positive selection. Interaction with self MHC and positive selection leads to cessation of further α-gene rearrangement. Negative selection involves interaction of T-lymphocyte precursors with dendritic cells, though these cells may not be entirely responsible for this process. Cells that fail in their attempts to be positively selected and those that are negatively selected die by apoptosis. These cells are removed, in the thymus, by macrophages. Positively selected cells that also pass negative selection downregulate expression of either CD4 or CD8 and enter the circulation as $CD8^+$ and $CD4^+$ T lymphocytes.

As in the case of B lymphopoiesis, more than 95% of developing T lymphocytes, by virtue of failing either positive or negative selection, die by apoptosis. Rigorous screening of T lymphocytes during their development results in the generation of immunocompetent cells that are adapted to their role of looking at foreign peptides that are displayed at the surface of one's own cells.

Concluding remarks

Studies of the development of the blood cell system have revealed that there are multiple constraints at each and every stage which include renewal of HSCs, lineage commitment, expansion of HPCs, maturation of these cells and survival of end cells. The constraints are the inherent nature of developing cells together with the external signals they receive. Inherent nature is a matter of past history of cells, that is, their position in the process of development from specification to haemopoiesis *per se* to acquisition of a mature status. Past history and environmental signals combine to make various options available to cells. These include self-renewal, survival, proliferation and differentiation along one pathway versus another. Whether a cell is truly plastic in regard to all these options or that they arise as binary choices, such as apoptosis versus self-renewal and self-renewal versus differentiation, is uncertain.

Key control points in the process of haemopoiesis are those that are rate limiting. Availability of combinations of transcription factors appear to govern specification of HSCs to maturation pathways. Expression of transcription factors in developing HSCs may occur such that there is a definite order to the availability of lineage options. Alternatively, HSCs may be able to 'test out' many options simultaneously. However, the lesson from a number of developmental systems is one of limited and 'binary choices'. If choices are binary, then cells may follow an intrinsic course of action unless deviated by a specific signal.

Once HSCs become committed to a single differentiation option, the rate-limiting event may change. Survival of cells, and therefore their capacity to differentiate, is constrained by the availability of growth factors. Survival signals are crucial during the development of B and T lymphocytes. The high level of 'wastage' of cells is not entirely accountable by the process of selection of worthwhile and appropriate antigen specificities. It is possible that the generation of HPCs entails overproduction and competition for HGFs within appropriate microenvironments for survival. Thus, progenitor cells are inevitably present to meet demand; numbers are fine tuned by the prevailing circumstance in the body.

The antithesis of failure to survive and death, by apoptosis, is immortality. Immortality has long been regarded as a cardinal property of HSCs. The mortality status of HSCs is dependent on crucial interaction with stromal cells that provide a microenvironmental niche. The concept of cells undergoing self-renewal has now been extended to progenitor cells that are committed to differentiation options (for example, to erythrocytes). The mortality status of these progenitor cells is flexible, and clearly subject to the influence of HGFs. Finally, the repertoire of B- and T-lymphocyte reactivity evolves and is sustained throughout the lifespan of an individual. In this circumstance, there are immortal T- and B-lymphocyte clones generated by contact of lymphocytes with antigen and maintained by complex interactions within secondary lymphoid tissues.

The viewpoint that HSC produce a very diverse range of blood cell types in numbers as so required by the organism has led to the consideration that development of blood cells is a special case. This supply on demand pressure on HSCs and HPCs may require the system to be more plastic than any other developing tissue. There is plasticity in terms of the controls on self-renewal and survival of HSCs and HPCs; HGFs alter the levels of self-renewal and survival such that numbers of mature cells produced are in keeping with demand. However, ensuring that HSCs diversify in a certain manner may relate to an underlying degree of cell autonomy. Interplay between autonomy in differentiative decisions and permissive environmental signals would ensure that the system is tightly regulated and that there is an appropriate outcome. It is most likely that these rules, and others, gained from studies of the blood cell system are applicable to all systems in the body.

REFERENCES

1. Pardanaud L, Yassine F, Dieterlen-Lievre F. Relationship between vasculogenesis, angiogenesis, and haemopoiesis. *Development* **105**:473–485, 1989.
2. Yamaguchi TP, Dumont DJ, Conlon RA, Brietman ML, Rossant J. flk-1, an flt-related receptor tyrosine kinase is an early marker for endothelial cell precursors. *Development* **118**:489–498, 1993.
3. Shalaby F, Rossant J, Yamaguchi TP, Brietman ML, Schuh AC. Failure of blood island formation and vasculogenesis in flk-1 deficient mice. *Nature* **376**:62–66, 1995.
4. Dickson MC, Martin JS, Cousins FM, Kularni AB, Karlsson S, Akhurst RJ. Defective haematopoiesis and vasculogenesis in transforming growth factor-β_1 knock out mice. *Development* **121**:1845–1854, 1995.
5. Begley CG, Aplan PD, Denning SM, Haynes BF, Waldmann TA, Kirsch IR. The gene *SCL* is expressed during early hematopoiesis and encodes a differentiation-related DNA-binding motif. *Proc Natl Acad Sci USA* **86**:10128–10132, 1989.
6. Kallianpur AR, Jordan JE, Brant SJ. The *SCL/TAL-1* gene is expressed in progenitors of both the hematopoietic and vascular systems during embryogenesis. *Blood* **83**:1200–1208, 1994.
7. Schivasani R, Mayer E, Orkin SH. Absence of blood formation in mice lacking the T-cell leukemia oncoprotein tal-1/SCL. *Nature* **373**:432–434, 1995.
8. Orkin SH. Hematopoiesis: how does it happen? *Curr Opinion Cell Biol* **7**:870–877, 1995.
9. Valge-Archer VE, Osada H, Warren AJ, Forster A, Li J, Baer R, Rabbits TH. The LIM protein RBTN2 and the basic helix–loop–helix protein are present in a complex in erythroid cells. *Proc Natl Acad Sci USA* **91**:8617–8621, 1994.
10. Wadman I, Bash RO, Forster A, Osada H, Rabbits TH, Baer R. Specific *in vivo* association between the bHLH and LIM proteins implicated in human T cell leukemia. *EMBO J* **13**:4831–4839, 1994.
11. Warren AJ, Colledge WH, Carlton MBL, Evans MJ, Smith AJH, Rabbits TH. The oncogenic cysteine-rich LIM domain protein Rbtn2 is essential for erythroid development. *Cell* **78**:45–57, 1994.
12. Kau C-L, Turpen JB. Dual contribution of embryonic ventral blood island and dorsal plate mesoderm during ontogeny of hemopoietic cells in *Xenopus laevis*. *J Immunol* **131**:2262–2266, 1983.
13. Godin IE, Garcia-Porrero JA, Coutino A, Dieterlen-Lievre F, Marcos MAR. Para-aortic splanchnopleura from early mouse embryos contains B1a progenitors. *Nature* **364**:67–70, 1993.
14. Godin IE, Dieterlen-Lievre F, Cumano A. Emergence of multipotent hemopoietic cells in the yolk sac and paraaortic splanchnopleura in mouse embryos, beginning at 8.5 days post coitus. *Proc Natl Acad Sci USA* **92**:773–777, 1995.
15. Medvinsky L, Samoylina NL, Muller AM, Dzierzak EA. An early pre-liver intraembryonic source of CFU-S in the developing mouse. *Nature* **364**:64–66, 1993.
16. Cumano A, Paige CJ, Iscove NN, Brady G. Bipotent precursors of B cells and macrophages in murine fetal liver. *Nature* **356**:612–615, 1992.
17. Boyd AW, Schrader JW. Derivation of macrophage-like lines from the pre-B lymphoma ABLS8.1 using 5-azacytidine. *Nature* **297**:691–693, 1982.
18. Davidson WF, Pierce JH, Rudikoff S, Morse HC. Relationships between B cell and myeloid differentiation. Studies with a B lymphocyte progenitor line, HAFTL-1. *J Exp Med* **168**:389–407, 1988.
19. Wong AK-Y, Bunce CM, Lord JM, Salt J, Brown G. Evidence that precursor cells of monocytes and B-lymphocytes are closely related. *Exp Hematol* **17**:968–973, 1989.
20. Borzillo GY, Ashmun RA, Sherr CJ. Macrophage lineage switching of murine early pre-B lymphoid cells expressing transduced *fms* genes. *Mol Cell Biol* **10**:2703–2714, 1990.
21. Bunce CM, Lord JM, Wong AK-Y, Brown G. Near neighbour analysis of variant cell lines derived from the promyeloid cell line HL60. *Br J Cancer* **57**:559–563, 1988.
22. Klinken SP, Alexander WS, Adams JM. Haemopoietic lineage switch: v-*raf* oncogene converts Eμ-myc transgenic B cells into macrophages. *Cell* **53**:857–867, 1988.
23. Fisher AG, Burdet C, Bunce C, Merkenschlager M, Ceredig RH. Lymphoproliferative disorders in IL-7 transgenic mice: expansion of immature B cells which retain macrophage potential. *Int Immunol* **7**:415–423, 1995.
24. D'Andrea AD. Hematopoietic growth factors and the regulation of differentiative decisions. *Curr Opinion Cell Biol* **6**:804–808, 1994.
25. Nathan DG. Leukemia and the regulation of hematopoiesis. *Leukemia* **1**:683–696, 1987.
26. Liboi E, Carroli M, D'Andrea AD, Mathey-Prevot B. Erythropoietin receptor signals both proliferation and erythroid-specific differentiation. *Proc Natl Acad Sci USA* **90**:11351–11355, 1993.
27. Barber D, D'Andrea AD. Erythropoietin and IL-2 activate distinct JAK kinase family members. *Mol Cell Biol* **14**:2257–2265, 1994.
28. Linette GP, Korsmeyer SJ. Differentiation and cell death: lessons from the immune system. *Curr Opinion Cell Biol* **6**:809–815, 1994.
29. Till JE, McCullock EA, Siminovitch L. A stochastic model of stem cell proliferation based on the growth of spleen colony forming cells. *Proc Natl Acad Sci USA* **51**:29–36, 1964.
30. Gusella J, Geller R, Clark B, Weeks V, Housman D. Commitment to erythroid differentiation by Friend erythroleukaemia cells: a stochastic analysis. *Cell* **9**:221–229, 1976.
31. Nakahata T, Ogawa M. Clonal origin of murine hemopoietic colonies with apparent restriction to granulocyte–macrophage–megakaryocyte (GMM) differentiation. *J Cell Physiol* **111**:239–246, 1982.
32. Ogawa M, Porter PN, Nakahata T. Renewal and commitment to differentiation of hemopoietic stem cells [an interpretive review]. *Blood* **61**:823–829, 1983.
33. Suda T, Suda J, Ogawa M. Disparate differentiation in mouse hemopoietic colonies derived from paired progenitors. *Proc Natl Acad Sci USA* **81**:2520–2524, 1984.
34. Holtzer H. Stem cell concepts: comments and replies. *Differentiation* **14**:33–34, 1979.
35. Brown G, Bunce CM, Guy GR. Sequential determination of lineage potentials during haemopoiesis. *Br J Cancer* **52**:681–686, 1985.
36. Brown G, Bunce CM, Lord JM, McConnell FM. The development of cell lineages: A sequential model. *Differentiation* **39**:83–88, 1988.
37. Dexter TM, Garland J, Scott D, Scolnick E, Metcalf D. Growth of factor-dependent hemopoietic precursor cell lines. *J Exp Med* **152**:1036–1047, 1980.

38. Alitalo R. Induced differentiation of K562 leukemia cells: a model for studies of gene expression in early megakaryoblasts. *Leuk Res* **14**:501–514, 1990.
39. Rowley PT, Farley BA, LaBella S, Guiliano R, Leary JF. Single K562 human leukemia cells express and are inducible for both erythroid and megakaryocytic antigens. *Int J Cell Cloning* **10**:232–240, 1992.
40. McDonald TP, Sullivan PS. Megakaryocytic and erythrocytic cell lines share a common precursor cell. *Exp Hematol* **21**:1316–1320, 1993.
41. Brown G, Bunce CM, Rose PE, Howie AJ. Progenitor cells and classification of myelodysplastic and myeloproliferative disorders. *Lancet* (8460) 885, 1985.
42. Rose PE, Howie AJ, Galvin GP, Bunce CM, Brown G. Lineage determination during haemopoiesis and classification of myelodysplastic disorders. *Br J Haematol* **64**:626–628, 1986.
43. Novak JP. Proliferation–differentiation schema of murine haemopoietic lineages: a transient response. *Cell Prolif* **27**:635–642, 1994.
44. Novak JP, Necas E. Proliferation–differentiation pathways of murine haemopoiesis: correlation of lineage fluxes. *Cell Prolif* **27**:597–633, 1994.
45. Ardavin C, Wu L, Li C-L, Shortman K. Thymic dendritic cells and T cells develop simulataneously in the thymus from a common precursor population. *Nature* **362**:761–763, 1993.
46. Nicola NA, Johnson GR. The production of committed hemopoietic colony-forming cells from multipotent precursor cells *in vitro*. *Blood* **60**:1019–1029, 1982.
47. Ness SA, Engel JD. Vintage reds and whites: combinatorial transcription factor utilisation in hematopoietic differentiation. *Curr Opinion Genet Develop* **4**:718–724, 1994.
48. Georgopoulos K, Bigby M, Wang J-H *et al.* The ikarus gene is required for the development of all lymphoid lineages. *Cell* **79**:143–156, 1994.
49. Scott EW, Simon MC, Anastasi J, Singh H. Requirement of transcription factor PU.1 in the development of multiple hematopoietic lineages. *Science* **265**:1573–1577, 1994.
50. Mucenski ML, McLain K, Kier AB *et al.* A functional *c-myb* is required for normal murine fetal hepatic hematopoiesis. *Cell* **65**:677–689, 1991.
51. Evans T, Felsenfeld G. The erythroid-specific transcription factor Eryf1: a new finger protein. *Cell* **58**:877–885, 1989.
52. Tsai S, Martin DIK, Zon LI, D'Andrea AD, Wong GG, Orkin SH. Cloning of cDNA for the major DNA-binding protein of the erythroid lineage through expression in mammalian cells. *Nature* **339**:446–451, 1989.
53. Martin DIK, Zon LI, Mutter G, Orkin SH. Expression of an erythroid transcription factor in megakaryocytic and mast cell lineages. *Nature* **344**:444–447, 1990.
54. Romeo PH, Prandini MH, Joulin V *et al.* Megakaryocytic and erythrocytic lineages share specific transcription factors. *Nature* **344**:447–449, 1990.
55. Miller IJ, Bieker JJ. A novel, erythroid cell-specific murine transcription factor that binds to the CACCC element and is related to the Kruppel family of nuclear proteins. *Mol Cell Biol* **13**:2776–2786, 1993.
56. Andrews NC, Kotkow KJ, Ney PA, Erdjument-Bromage H, Tempst P, Orkin SH. The ubiquitous subunit of erythroid factor NF-E2 is a small basic-leucine zipper protein related to the v-*maf* oncogene. *Proc Natl Acad Sci USA* **90**:11488–11492, 1993.
57. Kulessa H, Frampton J, Graf T. GATA-1 reprograms avian myelomoncytic cell lines into eosinophils, thromboblasts, and erythroblasts. *Genes Develop* **9**:1250–1262, 1995.
58. Katz S, Kowenz-Leutz E, Muller C, Meese K, Ness SA, Leutz A. The NF-m transcription factor is related to C/EBPβ and plays a role in signal transduction, differentiation and leukemogenesis of avian myelomonocytic cells. *EMBO J* **12**:1321–1332, 1993.
59. Scott LM, Civin CI, Rorth P, Friedman AD. A novel temporal expression pattern of three C/EBP family members in differentiating myelomonocytic cells. *Blood* **80**:1725–1735, 1992.
60. Natsuka S, Akira S, Nishio Y *et al.* Macrophage differentiation-specific expression of NF-IL6, a transcription factor for interleukin-6. *Blood* **79**:460–466, 1992.
61. Ko LJ, Yamamoto M, Leonard MW, George KM, Ting P, Engel JD. Murine and human T-lymphocyte GATA-3 factors mediate transcription through a *cis*-regulatory element within the human T-cell receptor δ gene enhancer. *Mol Cell Biol* **11**:2778–2784, 1991.
62. Oosterwegel M, van de Wetering M, Timmerman J, Kruisbeek A, Destree O, Meijlink F, Clevers H. Differential expression of the HMG box factors TCF-1 and LEF-1 during murine embryogenesis. *Development* **118**:439–448, 1993.
63. Hagman J, Belanger C, Travis A, Turck CW, Grosschedl R. Cloning and functional characterisation of early B-cell factor, a regulator of lymphocyte-specific gene expression. *Genes Dev* **7**:760–773, 1993.
64. Spiegelman B, Watt FM. Cell differentiation: editorial overview. *Curr Biol* **6**:781–782, 1994.
65. Gordon JI, Hermiston ML. Differentiation and self-renewal in the mouse gastrointestinal epithelium. *Curr Opinion Cell Biol* **6**:795–803, 1994.
66. Beug H, Mullner EW, Hayman MJ. Insights into erythroid differentiation obtained from studies on avian erythroblastosis virus. *Curr Opinion Cell Biol* **6**:816–824, 1994.
67. Haughton G, Arnold LW, Whitmore AC, Clarke SH. B-1 cells are made, not born. *Immunol Today* **14**:84–87, 1993.
68. Herzenberg LA, Kantor AB. B-cell lineages exist in the mouse. *Immunol Today* **14**:79–83, 1993.
69. Kantor AB. The development and repertoire of B-1 cells (CD5 B cells). *Immunol Today* **12**:389–392, 1991.
70. Digheiro G, Lymberi P, Holmberg D, Lundquist I, Coutinho A, Avrameas S. High frequency of natural autoantibodies in normal newborn mice. *J Immunol* **134**:765–771, 1985.
71. Vakil M, Kearney JF. Regulatory influences of neonatal multispecific antibodies on the developing B cell repetoire. *Int Rev Immunol* **3**:117–131, 1988.
72. Owen JJT, Raff MC, Cooper MD. Studies on the generation of B lymphocytes in the mouse embryo. *Eur J Immunol* **5**:468–473, 1975.
73. Gordon J. Pathways of human B cell growth and differentiation. In *New Concepts in Immunodeficiency Diseases* (eds S Gupta, C Griscelli), pp. 27–44. New York: John Wiley, 1993.
74. Mombaerts P, Iacomini J, Johnson RS, Herrup K, Tonegawa S, Papaioannous VE. RAG-1-deficient mice have no mature B and T lymphocytes. *Cell* **68**:868–877, 1992.
75. Shinkai Y, Rathbun G, Lam K-P. *et al.* RAG-2 deficient mice lack mature lymphocytes owing to their inability to initiate V(D)J rearrangement. *Cell* **68**:855–867, 1992.
76. Schroeder HW. Jr, Perlmutter RM. Development of the human antibody repertoire. In *New Concepts in Immunodeficiency Diseases* (eds S Gupta, C. Griscelli), pp. 3–25, New York: John Wiley, 1993.
77. Melchers F, Hassner D, Grawunder U, Kalberer C, Karasuyama H, Winkler T, Rolnik AG. Role of IgH and L chains and of surrogate H and L chains in the development of cells of the B lymphocyte lineage. *Annu Rev Immunol* **12**:209–226, 1994.
78. Reth M, Alt FW. Novel immunoglobulin heavy chains are produced from DJH segment rearrangements in lymphoid cells. *Nature* **312**:418–423, 1984.
79. Gu H, Kitamura D, Rajewsky K. B cell development regulated by gene rearrangement: arrest of maturation by membrane bound Dμ protein and selection of DH element reading frames. *Cell* **65**:47–54, 1991.
80. Melchers F, Karasuyama H, Haasner D *et al.* The surrogate light chain in B-cell development. *Immunol Today* **14**:60–68, 1993.
81. Korsmeyer SJ, Hieter PA, Ravetch JV, Poplack DG, Waldmann TA, Leder P. Developmental hierarchy of immunoglobulin gene rearrangements in human leukemic pre-B-cells. *Proc Natl Acad Sci USA* **78**:7096–7100, 1981.
82. Hieter PA, Korsmeyer SJ, Waldmann TA, Leder P. Human immunoglobulin κ light-chain genes are deleted or rearranged in λ-producing B cells. *Nature* **290**:368–372, 1981.
83. MacLennan I, Chan E. The dynamic relationship between B-cell populations in adults. *Immunol Today* **14**:29–34, 1993.
84. Freitas AA, Rocha BB. Lymphocyte lifespans: homeostasis, selection and competition. *Immunol Today* **14**:25–29, 1993.
85. Coutinho A. Lymphocyte survival and V-region repertoire selection. *Immunol Today* **14**:38–39, 1993.
86. Osmond DG. The turnover of B-cell populations. *Immunol Today* **14**:34–37, 1993.
87. Dudley EC, Girardi M, Owen MJ, Hayday AC. αβ and γδ T cells share a late common precursor. *Curr Biol* **5**:659–669, 1995.

88. Miller JFAP, Osoba D. Current concepts of the immunological functions of the thymus. *Physiol Rev* **47**:437–520, 1967.
89. Cordier AC, Haumont SM. Development of thymus, parathyroids and ultimo-branchial bodies in NMRI and nude mice. *Am J Anat* **157**:227–263, 1980.
90. LeDourin N, Bussonnet C, Chaumont F. Etude des capacitiés de differenciation et due rôle morphogène de l'endoderme pharyngier chez l'embryon d'oisean. *Ann Embryol Morph* **1**:29–37, 1968.
91. Auerbach R. Morphogenetic interactions in the development of the mouse thymus gland. *Dev Biol* **2**:271–285, 1960.
92. Liu CP, Auerbach R. *In vitro* development of murine T cells from prethymic and preliver embryonic yolk-sac hematopoietic stem-cells. *Development* **113**:1315–1323, 1991.
93. Huang H, Auerbach R. Identification and characterisation of hematopoietic stem-cells from the yolk-sac of early mouse embryo. *Proc Natl Acad Sci USA* **90**:10110–10114, 1993.
94. Rodewald H-R, Kretzschmar K, Takeda S, Hohl C, Dressing M. Identification of pro-thymocytes in murine fetal blood: T cell lineage commitment can precede thymus colonisation. *EMBO J* **13**:4229–4240, 1994.
95. Rodwald H-R, Miongeon P, Lucich JL, Dosiou C, Lopez P, Reinherz EL. A population of early fetal thymocytes expressing Fcγ RI/II contains precursors of T lymphocytes and natural killer cells. *Cell* **69**:139–150, 1992.
96. Peault B, Khazaal I, Weissman IL. *In vitro* development of B cells and macrophages from early mouse fetal thymocytes. *Eur J Immunol* **24**:781–784, 1994.
97. Dudley EC, Petrie HT, Shah LM, Owen MJ, Hayday A. T cell receptor β chain gene rearrangement and selection during thymocyte development in adult mice. *Immunity* **1**:1–20, 1994.
98. Groettrup M, von Boehmer H. A role for a pre-T-cell receptor in T cell development. *Immunol Today* **14**:610–614, 1993.
99. Levelt CN, Ehrfeld A, Eichmann K. Regulation of thymocyte development through CD3. I. Timepoint of ligation of CD3ε determines clonal deletion or induction of development program. *J Exp Med* **177**:707–716, 1993.
100. Jameson SC, Hogquist KA, Bevan MJ. Positive selection of thymocytes. *Annu Rev Immunol* **13**:93–126, 1995.
101. Fowlkes BJ, Schweighhoffer E. Positive selection of T cells. *Curr Opinion Immunol* **7**:188–195, 1991.
102. Anderson G, Moore NC, Owen JJT, Jenkinson EJ. Cellular interactions in thymocyte development. *Ann Rev Immunol* **14**:73–99, 1996.

Myometrial physiology and parturition

19

S.J. Lye

Introduction

The control of myometrial contractile activity during pregnancy represents an extraordinary example of physiologic regulation in reproductive biology. Throughout the majority of pregnancy, this smooth muscle must be maintained in a quiescent and unresponsive state in order to allow the safe development of the embryo and fetus. Then, over a relatively short period, at the time of labour, the myometrium undergoes a remarkable transformation enabling it to develop the synchronous, intense contractions necessary for the effective expulsion of the fetus from the uterine cavity. For the most part, these events are subject to an exacting temporal control which results in this transformation of the myometrium at a time when the fetus is relatively mature. Unfortunately, in human pregnancy, these regulatory mechanisms can fail and lead to the premature birth of a baby whose physiologic organ systems have not matured to a degree when they are capable of sustaining life outside of the uterus. Preterm birth occurs in 5–10% of all pregnancies but is associated with 70% of all neonatal deaths and up to 75% of neonatal morbidity[1]. In the neonatal period, preterm infants are 40 times more likely to die than are term infants. They are also at increased risk of major complications including cerebral palsy, blindness, deafness, respiratory illness and complications of neonatal intensive care[2,3]. These complications result in tremendous costs to the health-care system. Perhaps even more disturbing are reports that significant numbers of children at school age who were born with low birth weights have neurological or developmental measures in the suspect or abnormal range requiring rehabilitation or early intervention services[4].

The poor prognosis for the very premature neonate has led to a myriad of treatments and protocols aimed at inhibiting or preventing myometrial contractions associated with preterm labour. In large part, this has involved the use of therapeutic agents adapted from other smooth-muscle systems (e.g. vascular and respiratory) with little consideration of the unique characteristics of the myometrium. In the past, the development of tocolytic regimes has been often empirical rather than being based on sound physiologic/pharmacologic principles. Clinical trials have sometimes lacked randomization or adequate controls and drug treatments are seldom compared against placebo raising concern over the significance of the results. Even with the widespread use of tocolytic drugs (estimated at >100 000 women per year) there has been no documented decrease in the incidence of preterm labour in the last two to three decades[5,6]. This is in part due to the failure to recognize the complexities and redundant pathways that are in place to ensure that labour and delivery occur. For example, it should not be surprising that blocking one stimulatory pathway (for example, with oxytocin receptor antagonists or with calcium-channel blockers) does not prevent preterm birth since other redundant pathways (for example, prostaglandins, or pathways activating intracellular calcium) remain active and can probably induce sufficient contractile activity to maintain effective labour. In this chapter we will describe the patterns of contractile activity that are present throughout pregnancy and during labour and discuss the physiologic, cellular and molecular mechanisms that control these patterns. A more detailed discussion of the control of myometrial activity can be found in other reviews[7,8].

Myometrial structure and function

TISSUE ARCHITECTURE

The myometrium is primarily composed of bundles of smooth-muscle cells embedded in an extracellular matrix together with blood vessels and nerves supplying or passing through this muscle. In most species, the myometrium is formed from an outer longitudinal muscle layer, running parallel to the long axis of the uterus, and in inner circular muscle layer, perpendicular to the long axis, though the human uterus has a much more complex structure with up to four layers of muscle. It is important to realize that the muscle layers arise from different embryologic origins which may account for the differences in activities and hormonal responses of the two layers[9–12]. This may in part explain the regionalization of uterine responses to uterotonic agonists and antagonists[13,14].

Internal to the myometrium is the endometrium (or decidua), and external is the serosal epithelium, which acts to protect the uterus and may act as a support on which the contracting muscle can develop tension. The myometrial cells are more or less spindle shaped and are 300–600 μm long by 5–10 μm in diameter. Their size and number are determined by the degree of distension and stage of pregnancy. While the myometrium receives adrenergic, cholinergic and peptidergic innervation, the role of this neural input is unresolved.

Surrounding all myocytes within the myometrium is a complex arrangement of extracellular matrix molecules including collagen and elastin. The myocytes are attached to the extracellular matrix at the site of the so-called dense bodies on the myometrial cell membrane. These 'spot welds' act in an analogous way to the tendons of skeletal muscle providing a support system which is critical to the myocytes being able to generate tension and shorten the myometrium. The matrix molecules are synthesized by the myocytes themselves, although the precise control of their production is not well understood.

INTRACELLULAR ORGANIZATION

Although little work has specifically examined intracellular structure of myometrial cells, it is believed to be similar to that of other types of smooth muscle. Extracellular calcium gains access to the contractile proteins though flask-shaped invaginations of the cell membrane called caveolae (analogous to T tubules of skeletal muscle). Closely associated with the caveolae is an extensive tubular network, the sarcoplasmic reticulum (SR), which acts as the intracellular calcium storage organelle. The SR membrane contains both calcium channels and Mg^{2+}-ATPase pumps for release and re-uptake of calcium during the contraction–relaxation cycle[15,16].

In additional to the contractile elements, actin and myosin, a network of fibrils connects electron-dense bodies within the cytoplasm to similar dense bands located on the inner surface of the cell membrane. This network is believed to form an internal 'scaffolding' providing support to the contractile elements during contraction. At the cell surface, this cytoskeleton forms complexes with intercellular membrane proteins forming the co-called focal adhesions. These focal adhesions not only enable tension development within the myometrium, but may also provide the means for the generated tension to be signalled to the cell through a cascade of protein kinases[17,18].

CELL–CELL COMMUNICATION

The optimum functioning of the myometrium during labour is due to its ability to develop well-coordinated synchronous contractions, which requires highly developed cell-to-cell coupling. Intercellular (or gap) junctions are formed as a result of interactions between intramembranous proteins within adjacent cell membranes. These proteins are organized into hexameric structures each of which forms a hemichannel. By mechanisms not understood, hemichannels in one cell membrane are able to align themselves with similar structures in the adjacent membrane to form a pore connecting the cytoplasm of the two cells. These pores provide sites for low-resistance electrical or ionic coupling between cells, as well as provide a pathway for transport of metabolites (<1–1.7 kDa) directly between cells. Hundreds or thousands of these individual channels arrange themselves into an organised plaque to form the gap junction.

The structural components of gap junctions are the 'connexins' (Cx), a highly related, multigene family of proteins, of which there are at least 16 distinct connexin proteins encoded by different genes. Connexins are classified according to their apparent molecular weights[19,20] and exhibit a complex cell type and temporal patterns of expression. Most cells express more than one connexin and there is evidence that the individual gap junction channels may be composed of more than one connexin protein. The connexins can also be expressed constitutively (e.g. Cx43 in the heart) or may be subject to distinct spatiotemporal changes in expression during various developmental and physiologic processes[21].

The myocytes of the myometrium express three connexin proteins (Cx43, Cx26 and Cx45) which exhibit distinct temporal patterns of expression[22,23]. Cx43 was the first connexin to be identified in the myometrium[24]. Messenger RNA and protein encoding Cx43 are expressed at low levels throughout pregnancy in all species so far examined; expression increases towards term with maximal levels being found during labour. The pattern of expression correlates with a decrease in electrical input resistance within the myometrium, a measure of electrical conductivity[25]. These electrophysiologic and expression data have led investigators to propose that Cx43 is responsible for the increased coupling within the myometrium that is essential for the development of effective labour contractions. The regulation of Cx43 expression during labour involves both hormonal and mechanical inputs (see below). In most species the major hormonal control is provided by progesterone (which negatively regulates expression) and oestrogen (a positive regulator)[26]. In a screen of connexins expressed in the myometrium, we identified Cx26 and Cx45 as other myocyte specific myometrial connexins[27]. Cx26 is expressed in the rat and human myometrium[22,28]. In the rat, Cx26 levels are low until day 17, rise to maximal levels on days 19–21, but fall to low levels prior to labour on day 23[22]. Data in the human suggest a similar expression profile[28]. The role of Cx26 is not known. In addition to its expression profile it exhibits different electrical properties to Cx43[29,30]. Moreover, in contrast to Cx43, progesterone appears to positively regulate Cx26 expression[22]. These data raise the possibility that Cx26 may contribute to the maintenance of pregnancy near term, possibly by inhibiting the development of a contractile phenotype. Cx45 is expressed at low levels in the myometrium throughout pregnancy[23,27]. Its expression does not seem to be regulated by steroid hormones, by the induction of preterm labour or when labour is blocked by progesterone administration[27].

In addition to transcription and translation of connexins, mechanisms must operate to control transport of the protein to the cell membrane, assembly into connexons, apposition of cell membranes, clustering of connexons into plaques and formation of functional channels. This complex process is poorly understood though, in the myometrium, the steroids oestrogen and progesterone are thought to play a role in at least some of these events (see below)[26,31,32]. In other tissues there is evidence to suggest that gap-junction formation may require the presence of cell adhesion molecules[33,34]. The mechanisms that regulate the opening and closing of gap junctions in the myometrium are poorly understood. Calcium ionophores[35], isoproterenol[36] and cAMP[36,37] reduce cell coupling, while they have opposing effects on uterine contractile activity. However, while calmodulin inhibitors reversed the effects of calcium ionophore in the rat, these compound actually reduced coupling in human myometrium[35]. Oxytocin has been reported to decrease coupling in the parturient rat myometrium consistent with the effect of elevated $[Ca^{2+}]_i$[38].

ION CHANNELS AND THE ELECTRICAL BASIS OF MYOMETRIAL CONTRACTILITY

The myometrium expresses a variety of ion-specific channels within the cell membrane that act to regulate the excitability of this smooth muscle. These channels include sodium, potassium, chloride and non-selective channels. Since these channels control the membrane potential of the myometrial cell, which, in turn, regulates the influx of calcium through voltage-dependent calcium channels, they are critically important to the control of myometrial contractility and may potentially be a target for tocolytic agents.

Voltage-gated sodium channels have been identified, electrophysiologically, in the myometrium of the rat[39,40] and human[41] and the number of cells expressing these receptors increases significantly towards term in the rat[42]. Tamkun and colleagues have identified transcripts encoding a novel class of sodium channels (bearing only around 50% sequence homology with previously cloned sodium channels) in the mouse and human uterus[43,44]. The expression of the mouse transcript increased significantly in late pregnancy and fell to low levels post-partum[43].

Calcium channels can be broadly divided into three major categories: (i) voltage-dependent channels (VDCC), (ii) receptor operated channels and (iii) calcium channels of organelles. An increase in the expression of VDCCs during late pregnancy in the rat has been demonstrated both electrophysiologically, biochemically and by the reverse transcription polymerase chain reaction (RT-PCR)[39,45,46]. Tezuka *et al.* also showed that the level of mRNA encoding the subunits of the VDCC, in the rat, was blocked by progesterone and could be increased by the progesterone antagonist, onapristone[46].

In addition to Na^+, K^+ ions play a major role in maintaining the resting membrane potential. Activation of K^+ channels inhibits pacemaker activity in myometrial cells[47], while blockade leads to depolarization and can thus increase contraction[48]. Several classes of K^+ currents have been reported in the myometrium, which play a role in neutralizing depolarization, inducing repolarization and inducing hyperpolarization[49]. These channels also exhibit differential hormonal regulation[50–52]. Of particular interest is the 'maxi' or large K^+ conductance that is activated by calcium since this channel is activated by myometrial relaxants such as β-agonists and relaxin[49].

While an examination of the electrophysiologic regulation of myometrial contractile activity is beyond the scope of the present review, the reader is referred to the reviews of Mironneau[40] and Sanborn[49]. It is important to state, however, that it is the state of polarization of the cell membrane that is the key in providing the means for the spread of electrical signals across the myometrium and for the influx of extracellular calcium that is critical for the generation of contractions. The resting membrane potential in myocytes is not static. It undergoes a regular cycling similar to the 'slow waves' of gastrointestinal smooth muscle. These slow waves cyclically hyperpolarize and depolarize the muscle and provide the basis for the phasic contractions typical of the myometrium. During the depolarization phase the membrane potential may reach the critical threshold at which calcium may enter the cell through the voltage-dependent calcium channels (VDCC) and induce a contraction. During the hyperpolarization phase the channels are closed and relaxation is more likely. Since the resting membrane potential is influenced by hormones (through activation or expression of ion channels), the potential for slow waves to lead to contractions can be reduced (for example, under progesterone domination) or increased (for example, during exposure to oestrogen).

CONTRACTILE ELEMENTS AND BIOCHEMICAL BASIS OF MYOCYTE CONTRACTION

The myosin molecule is a hexamer, approximately 160 nm in length, and is composed of two heavy chains (200 kDa each) and two pairs of light chains (one pair around 17 kDa and one around 20 kDa). The heavy-chain components form α-helices (130 nm in length). Towards the NH_2 terminal, these chains unfold to form two globular heads. Each globular head contains: (i) ATPase activity (localized only on the heavy-chain component); (ii) an actin-binding site; (iii) one light chain (20 kDa) that can bind Ca^{2+} and Mg^{2+} and can be phosphorylated, and another light chain (17 kDa) the functional role of which is unknown. The α-helical tail of the myosin molecule acts to transmit tension during shortening. The globular actin molecules (45 kDa) polymerize into long filaments, 6–9 nm in diameter. In smooth muscles, there are 11–15 thin filaments per myosin (thick) filament.

Interaction of actin and myosin occurs following the development of ATPase activity on the myosin head. This then allows the formation of crosslinks with the actin molecules. The myosin head then rotates as a result of conformational changes in the protein structure, leading to a pulling on the actin filament to create tension and produce a relative spatial displacement. The energy required for these changes is believed to result from the phosphorylation of the 20 kDa light chains of myosin (MLC20) by the enzyme myosin light chain kinase (MLCK). Other contractile proteins such as caldesmon, which interacts with myosin to increase the efficiency of actin–myosin coupling, may also play a role in regulating myometrial contraction.

MLCK can be considered a pivotal point in regulating smooth-muscle contraction. Most of our information on MLCK comes from enzyme isolated from the turkey gizzard although more recently we have gained information on MLCK from the sheep myometrium. These data can be summarised as follows. MLCK has an absolute requirement for calcium–calmodulin (Ca–CaM). In the presence of activating levels of calcium ($>10^{-6}$M) the Ca–CaM complex binds to a site on MLCK which in turn (presumably by some conformation change in MLCK) opens up the kinase site to enable the enzyme to phosphorylate MLC20 and hence initiate contraction.

Relaxation of smooth muscle as a result of reduction in the phosphorylation of MLC20, can occur due to a decrease in MLCK activity with the subsequent dephosphorylation of the light chains by MLC phosphatase. The reduction in MLCK activity can either be as a result of a fall in intracellular Ca^{2+} concentrations leading to a decrease in Ca–CaM levels or possibly due to phosphorylation of MLCK itself by a cAMP-dependent protein kinase (A-kinase). In this phosphorylated state the affinity of this regulatory protein for Ca–CaM is reduced. Thus the contractile state of the cell can, in large part, be represented as a balance between the actions of Ca^{2+} through calmodulin, and cAMP through A-kinase on the activity of the enzyme MLCK. Cyclic AMP can also affect contractility by reducing intracellular calcium levels either by increasing intracellular uptake of free calcium or increasing calcium efflux from the myocyte.

The resting intracellular Ca^{2+} concentration is 10^{-7}–10^{-8} and this must increase to at least 10^{-6} for MLCK to be activated and for contraction to occur. Under normal resting conditions, the extracellular calcium concentration is around 10^{-3} requiring the operation of active ATP-dependent (Ca^{2+}, Mg^{2+}-ATPase) and ATP-independent (Na^{+} exchange) cell-membrane Ca^{2+} pumps in order to maintain this electrical imbalance.

An increase in intracellular calcium to initiate contraction within the myometrial cell can occur through several mechanisms: (i) release of calcium from intracellular (sarcoplasmic reticulum, mitochondria, inner cell membrane bound) stores; (ii) inhibition of Ca^{2+} efflux; (iii) increase in calcium influx from extracellular sources. Depending on the stimulus, one or more of these events may occur during contraction. The entry of calcium from extracellular sources may occur via potential sensitive (during discharge of action potentials) or receptor-operated mechanisms. Mechanisms may also operate to link cell-membrane receptors to the intracellular calcium stores. Thus agonist–receptor activation of phospholipase C can lead to the hydrolysis of inositol phosphates leading to the release of inositol-1,4,5-triphosphate (IP_3). IP_3 in turn can cause the release of Ca^{2+} from intracellular stores. Diacylglycerol generated during inositol hydrolysis can also interact with intracellular signalling pathways as well as be a substrate for prostaglandin synthesis. Activation of these pathways by uterotonic agonists is described below. For a more detailed discussion of the biochemical mechanisms underlying smooth muscle contraction see Challis and Lye[7].

The myometrium during pregnancy

A requirement of the evolution of viviparity was that the products of conception be retained within the uterus where growth and development could occur in a protected environment to a stage at which the fetus is capable of surviving in the extrauterine environment. This requirement imposes two major challenges for the myometrium. Firstly, the growth and subsequent delivery of the fetus requires the cyclical growth and involution of the uterus with each pregnancy. Secondly, smooth-muscle cells are inherently spontaneously active and are stimulated by the mechanical stretch imposed by the growing fetus providing the additional challenge of developing mechanisms to inhibit this contractile activity.

MYOMETRIAL GROWTH DURING PREGNANCY

Depending upon the species, the uterus can exhibit a 500–1000-fold increase in volume and >15-fold increase in weight, representing one of the most spectacular examples of organ growth in mammalian biology. Then, within days of birth, remodelling and regression occur as the non-pregnant form is re-established. Despite the fundamental nature of these changes, there is little information as to the mechanisms that can produce such dramatic changes in uterine growth. The growth of the myometrium during pregnancy is believed to involve both hypertrophy and hyperplasia, though the precise contribution of each of these components remains controversial. It would appear the uterine growth during pregnancy is controlled by two pathways, one regulated by endocrine input and the other by mechanical inputs.

A number of growth factors and/or their receptors have been identified in the non-pregnant uterus including insulin-like growth factor-1 (IGF-1) mRNA and protein, IGF-1 receptor and IGF binding protein-1[53]; epidermal growth factor (EGF) receptor and EGF processing[54]; transforming growth factor-α (TGF-α) mRNA[55]; TGF-β_2[56]; TGF-β_1[57]; platelet-derived growth factor (PDGF) receptor[58], and beta fibroblast growth factor (β-FGF)[59]. All of these proteins are increased in the uterus following oestradiol treatment except IGF binding protein-1 (IGFBP-1) (which is decreased), TGF-β_1, TGF-β_2 and PDGF receptor (for which no information is available). TGF-β_2 mRNA is increased in the mouse uterus during pregnancy, peaking at d15 before falling to low levels prior to labour on d19[57]. β-FGF has been shown to increase DNA synthesis and cell proliferation in the rat and human myometrial cells[60]. The role of oestrogen and IGF-1 in promoting uterine growth was recently confirmed following the generation of mice carrying either a null mutation in the IGF-1 gene or overexpressing an IGF-1 binding protein (which reduces functional IGF-1 levels). These mice have very small uteri which showed no increase in growth in response to oestrogen. Oestrogen has also been reported, in other cell systems, to increase the activity of cyclin-dependent kinases which regulate the cell cycle and cell proliferation. However, studies of steroid treatment to non-pregnant animals suggests that hormonal mechanisms alone do not appear to be sufficient to account for the tremendous increase in uterine growth that occurs during pregnancy. While not abandoning the endocrine contribution to uterine growth, it is increasingly apparent that the primary factor regulating the growth of the uterus is the fetus itself. The fetus achieves this as a result of its growth producing a mechanical load on the uterine wall which in turn is transduced to induce hypertrophy and hyperplasia of the smooth muscle cells and remodelling of the extracellular matrix of the myometrium. It is quite clear that the pregnant myometrium is under increased mechanical tension during pregnancy as evidenced by amniotic pressure measurements[61]. Moreover, reports of mechanical distension of the uterus producing an increase in uterine weight go back many decades[62]. Several studies have shown that uterine distension during pregnancy is associated with increased smooth muscle RNA, DNA and protein concentrations[63,64] as well as collagen synthesis[65], although the mechanisms responsible are not known. Using data from other smooth muscles (e.g. vascular muscle) Vandenburgh[66] suggests two general mechanisms. In one, externally applied forces could directly influence nuclear events and cell growth as a result of anchoring of cells to the ECM through integrin – cytoskeletal network, possibly activating kinases at these focal adhesion sites. The second mechanism would involve stretch-induced alterations in plasma membrane associated molecules such as Na^+K^+-ATPase, ion channels, phospholipases, G proteins, and their associated second messengers including prostaglandins, cAMP, inositol phosphates, $[Ca^2]_i$, and protein kinase C. Interestingly, many of these mechanosensory-induced second messengers are also components of growth factor-receptor signalling pathways suggesting at the very least considerable overlap between these pathways which regulate cell growth. Interactions between these pathways could result from stretch induced increases expression of growth factors themselves or of their receptors, both of which have been reported in other cell systems[66]. The extent to which these mechanisms operate in the myometrium is not known, though data presented below suggest that stretch can have major effects on the expression of myometrial contraction-associated proteins such as connexin-43 and oxytocin receptors.

MYOMETRIAL QUIESCENCE DURING PREGNANCY

Throughout the majority of pregnancy the myometrium is inexcitable, relatively unresponsive to stimulation by uterotonic agonists (oxytocin, prostaglandins E and F) and the cells are poorly coordinated. However, the myometrium is not totally inactive. Low-frequency, low-amplitude contractions (termed 'contractures' see Harding *et al.*[67]) occur with a regular periodicity throughout pregnancy. Although contractures have no impact on cervical status, they do impact on physiologic and endocrine systems in the fetus[68,69]. Our own studies suggest that contractures are not the result of paracrine or endocrine stimulation but represent an inherent contractility of the myometrium possibly due to an underlying cyclicity of the resting membrane potential of these smooth-muscle cells[70–72]. The mechanisms that maintain the myometrium in a quiescent state have been reviewed in more detail elsewhere[7]. The relative quiescence of the uterus during most of gestation has been attributed, in large part, to progesterone[73]. In many species, progesterone-dominated uterine muscle is refractory to the stimulatory effects of oxytocin and prostaglandins[73]. Administration of exogenous progesterone to a number of species will decrease uterine activity[74] and delay parturition[26]. Progesterone may achieve these results through a number of mechanisms, including the uncoupling of excitation–contraction, inhibition of the synthesis of agonist receptors, gap junctions as well as the suppression of the production or formation of prostaglandins and inhibition of pituitary oxytocin release (see below and Challis and Lye[7]). While these effects on contractility are indirect in that they primarily involve modulating the expression of other proteins, there are some data which suggest that progesterone may directly inhibit myometrial contractile activity. However, for the most part this latter role has been attributed to other uterotonic inhibitors such as relaxin, prostacyclin, parathyroid hormone-related peptide (PTHrP) and β-adrenergic agonists.

Relaxin has been shown to inhibit spontaneous uterine activity in many species including sheep[75], humans[76] and rats[77]. The inhibition of myometrial activity in rats by relaxin is associated temporally with an increase in cyclic AMP levels and a decrease in MLCK activity[78]. The inhibitory effects of relaxin can be blocked by inhibitors of protein kinase A[79].

Relaxin affects MLCK by decreasing its affinity for calmodulin and myosin[78]. *In vitro* relaxin also blocks the action of stimulants such as oxytocin, carbachol and norepinephrine through mechanisms involving protein kinase A-mediated phosphorylation of phospholipase C-linked G-proteins. This in turn inhibits IP_3 turnover and the increase in $[Ca^{2+}]_i$[80,81]. A major action of relaxin has also been reported to be an activation of the calcium-activated 'maxi' K^+ channel which would induce hyperpolarization and relaxation[82].

Nitric oxide has been suggested to act as an endogenous inhibitor of uterine contractile activity; the uterine synthesis of nitric oxide is high during pregnancy and is reported to decrease during labour[83–85]. Data also suggest that generation of nitric oxide leads to the inhibition of myometrial contractile activity[85] and nitric oxide donors have been used clinically to relax the uterine muscle. Nitric oxide is believed to act by increasing the generation of cGMP within the myocytes, though the precise mechanisms by which cGMP produces an inhibition of the interaction of actin and myosin is not clear[86]. During labour, there is a decrease in the sensitivity of the myometrium to elevations in cGMP[87], thus it is questionable as to whether activation of the nitric oxide pathway in the labouring myometrium will prove to be an effective means of inhibiting preterm labour contractions. We have also found a decrease in the ability of the myometrium to generate cAMP during labour in response to agonist stimulation. It would appear, therefore, that a component of the increase in spontaneous myometrial activity during labour is due to a down-regulation of inhibitory systems in addition to the process of activation and stimulation described below.

Prostacyclin (PGI_2) inhibits ovine uterine contractility and electromyographic activity *in vivo*[88], and human myometrium *in vitro*[89]. PGI_2 is the major prostaglandin produced in the myometrium during pregnancy[90]. The production of a prostaglandin-like activity has been reported to be higher in areas of the myometrium over a conceptus than in other (unoccupied) areas[91]. However, the precise role of PGI_2 in the myometrium during pregnancy remains to be determined. PTHrP can also inhibit basal and oxytocin (but not $PGF_{2\alpha}$) stimulated myometrial contractions[92]. It is present in the myometrium in high levels during late pregnancy and its expression has been shown to be stimulated by the distension of the growing fetuses[93]. The action of PTHrP is enhanced by oestrogen[94]. While β-adrenergic agonists are potent pharmacological inhibitors of myometrial contractile activity *in vitro* and *in vivo* there is no evidence that they contribute to the maintenance of myometrial quiescence during pregnancy.

The myometrium during labour

The onset of labour is associated with a remarkable transformation in the pattern of contractile activity of the myometrium. With the approach of labour, the muscle demonstrates increased excitability (associated with a relative depolarization of the resting membrane potential)[72,95], it becomes highly responsive to uterotonic agents[96–98] and the smooth-muscle cells markedly increase their electrical coupling[36]. These changes act to increase the effectiveness of the uterotonic agents in generating high-frequency contractions and ensure that those contractions that are initiated rapidly spread to involve the entire uterus. We have termed this increase in the capability of the myometrium to develop contractions myometrial activation[99]. Once the myometrium is activated it can respond to the paracrine and endocrine stimulation resulting from the increased synthesis and release of uterotonic agonists (e.g. oxytocin, prostaglandins, endothelin-1). The combined effect of activation and stimulation is to enable the myometrium to generate the high-frequency, high-amplitude, intense contractions required to assist in the dilatation of the cervix and the delivery of the fetus. In most species this transformation takes place only during the onset of labour. However, in primate species, including humans, the myometrium exhibits a diurnal switch between the 'pregnant' and 'labour' state over several days leading up to labour and delivery, which may be related to the endogenous diurnal rhythm of oestrogen[100,101] as well as increases in oxytocin levels and myometrial responsiveness to this peptide[102]. For a more detailed review of the process of activation and stimulation the reader is referred to Challis and Lye[7] and Lye[103].

MYOMETRIAL ACTIVATION

We suggest that the activation state of the myometrium during pregnancy and at the time of labour reflects the profile of 'contraction-associated' proteins synthesized by the myometrium (e.g. ion channels, uterotonic agonist receptors, gap junctions, proteins involved in regulating $[Ca^{2+}]_i$ levels, etc). We also suggest that the expression of these 'contraction-associated proteins' (CAPs) is tightly regulated during pregnancy and that the steroids oestrogen and progesterone are intricately involved in the process. Substantial data suggest that oestrogen and progesterone, either directly or indirectly, regulate the synthesis of some or all of the 'contraction-associated proteins' described above and hence regulate the contractile state of the myometrium during pregnancy and labour. Receptors for both oestrogen and progesterone are present within the myometrium. There is clear evidence, in non-primate species, that receptor levels for these steroids are regulated throughout pregnancy and labour. In the human, the situation is much more complex, though a recent report suggests that an increase in mRNA encoding the oestrogen receptor (but not the progesterone receptor) may occur at the time of labour onset[104] within intrauterine tissues. There are also preliminary reports of elevated expression of the A isoform relative to the B isoform of the progesterone receptor in decidua from rhesus monkeys at term[105]. This may be of importance since transcriptional suppression by the full length B isoform can be blocked by the A isoform and hence induce a functional progesterone withdrawal.

REGULATION OF 'CONTRACTION-ASSOCIATED' PROTEINS DURING LABOUR

Our model of myometrial activation at labour suggests that there is a coordinated change in the expression of a series of myometrial proteins that together enable the muscle to increase its state of contractility. Using rodents as a model system, we and others have reported increased expression of the gap junction protein connexin-43[32], the oxytocin receptor[106], prostaglandin F receptor (but not EP subtypes)[107,108], the L-type calcium channel[46] and a component of the sodium channel near term and with the onset of labour[43].

This synchronous expression of CAPs at term suggests a coordinated mechanism (or switch) to regulate CAP expression. Clearly if the nature of this switch was known, it might be possible to develop novel strategies to prevent the activation of these *CAP* genes and thus prevent or inhibit myometrial activation in women in preterm labour. With this in mind we have extensively investigated the mechanisms that control expression of connexin-43. We found that mRNA and protein levels were low during pregnancy but increased markedly beginning some 48 hours prior to labour and reached maximal levels during labour[32]. Increased levels of connexin-43 mRNA were also found in sheep with the onset of labour[109]. In both species, this increase in connexin-43 mRNA and protein was related to an increase in the plasma oestrogen:progesterone ratio[32,109]. In subsequent studies of non-pregnant rats, we found that oestrogen acts to positively regulate connexin-43 mRNA and protein expression while progesterone has negative influence. The regulation of connexin-43 expression during pregnancy in the rat is closely regulated by progesterone. Thus, progesterone treatment at term blocks the increase in connexin-43 expression and the onset of labour, while removal of progesterone during pregnancy (either by administration of the receptor antagonist, RU486 or by ovariectomy) leads to preterm labour which can also be blocked by treatment with exogenous progesterone[110]. We have recently demonstrated that expression of the oxytocin receptor (OTR) and prostaglandin $F_{2\alpha}$ (FP) receptor are regulated in an identical manner to that of connexin-43, supporting our concept of synchronous control of myometrial CAP expression[106,107,111].

The precise mechanisms that regulate *CAP* gene expression remain to be determined. While there is some evidence that oestrogen increases transcriptional activity through effects on the connexin-43 promoter[112,113], other data suggest that this effect is indirect[110]. We have demonstrated a close relationship between the pattern of expression of Cx43 and the OTR in models of term and preterm labour and during post-term pregnancy in the rat and the expression of the transcription factor c-Fos[110]. This is important in that while the connexin-43 and OTR promoters have no palindromic oestrogen response element they each contain conserved AP-1 (Fos/Jun) binding sites[113–115]. It is possible, therefore, that the increased Fos expression during labour activates *CAP* genes through binding to the AP-1 site and contributes to myometrial activation and the onset of labour.

In addition to hormonal regulation of CAP expression, we have obtained data to suggest that mechanical stretch may be critical to the activation of *CAP* genes during labour. During pregnancy the growth of the fetus(es) results in an increase in myometrial wall tension (as indicated by increased amniotic fluid pressure[61]). In many systems, stretch is known to be a potent stimulant to muscle contractility. Previous data by Wathes and Porter[116] had demonstrated that myometrial stretch post-partum resulted in the maintenance of high levels of gap junctions compared to non-stretch control uteri; our data showed that this was due to a stretch-induced increase in connexin-43 expression. Moreover, preliminary data suggest that OTR expression is similarly increased by stretch[117].

During pregnancy, stretch produced minimal increases in connexin-43 and OTR (likely due to the effects of progesterone, since we found that progesterone administration to non-pregnant rats blocked the effects of myometrial stretch). It would appear that this pregnancy (progesterone) suppression of stretch-induced CAP expression is essential for the maintenance of pregnancy. In other studies in rats, we have shown that stretch plays a critical role in the increase in CAP gene expression during labour. These data indicate that in the absence of stretch but the presence of the normal endocrine changes associated with labour, myometrial CAP gene expression is not increased; however, when stretch is applied to the uterine horn (either by the presence of fetuses or of a polyvinyl tube) full CAP expression is achieved[118]. These studies suggest that mechanical stretch is an important contributor to the regulation of myometrial contractile activity during pregnancy. They also raise the possibility that the increased incidence of preterm birth in multifetal pregnancies may be due to premature activation of *CAP* genes due to the increased degree of mechanical stretch imposed on the myometrium.

The pattern of CAP expression is probably more complex in the human myometrium. Levels of connexin-43, OTR and FP receptor mRNA are already high in the myometrium prior to the onset of labour and it is not clear whether levels increase further with the onset of labour[111,119,120]. There are several possible explanations for these data. It may be that translational or post-translational events are more important in the human myometrium in generating functionally active CAP proteins. For example, the intracellular trafficking and assembly of gap junctions is subject to control by progesterone in the rat and it is possible that this is a major site of control in the human. It is also possible that data from the lower uterine segment (where virtually all samples are obtained in studies of human myometrium during labour) do not reflect changes in gene expression in the contractile fundal region of the uterus. This possibility is supported by our own preliminary data obtained[111] in which only the expression of putative inhibitory proteins (EP4 receptor and connexin-26) was found to increase in lower-segment myometrium during labour. In addition, there are a number of reports that have documented regional variation in contractile response to agonists that would promote fundal contractile and lower-segment relaxation[13,14].

In addition to being a useful model to understand the processes which are essential for the onset and establishment of labour, the concept of myometrial activation may have wider clinical significance. Most methods of tocolysis are aimed at suppression of the contractions themselves (e.g. β-adrenergic agonists, calcium-channel blockers) or reducing the effects of uterine stimulants (e.g. prostaglandin synthesis inhibitors, oxytocin antagonists). However, therapeutic strategies do not address the underlying changes that have occurred due to myometrial activation. It is not surprising therefore that these approaches are at best minimally effective in prolonging pregnancy. We suggest that new strategies should be directed towards reversing myometrial activation and switching the uterus back to its quiescent and unresponsive pregnancy state.

The concept of myometrial activation might also impact on approaches to electively induce labour. While the use of prostaglandins has proved quite effective as an inductive agent, the increased incidence of caesarian section associated with induction suggests that it is not optimal. We suggest that the state of myometrial activation is an important consideration, a view supported by observations that inductions are more successful if cervical ripening is advanced. It might be that once the process of myometrial activation is fully understood and can be controlled by hormonal or pharmacologic agents, optimal induction will involve strategies that induce myometrial activation and cervical ripening prior to administration of the uterotonic stimulants.

STIMULATION OF THE MYOMETRIUM

PRODUCTION OF UTEROTONIC AGONISTS

Once the myometrium is activated due to the increased expression of CAPs, it is in a state of preparedness for labour. However, labour is unlikely to precede until uterotonic stimulants are produced to drive this activated myometrium. Foremost amongst these uterotonic agonists are oxytocin and stimulatory prostaglandins, though there are many other agents that can stimulate myometrial contractions and which may play important roles. The mechanisms that induce the synthesis of these agents at term have been extensively reviewed elsewhere[7,121]; consequently only a brief overview will be provided here.

Prostaglandin $F_{2\alpha}$, thromboxane A_2 and in some situation PGE_2 are potent stimulators of uterine contractile activity in most species. While there is debate as to whether stimulatory prostaglandins are initiators of labour there is no doubt that these uterotonic agonists play a central role in the generation of labour contractions. Evidence clearly demonstrates that plasma and amniotic fluid prostaglandin levels increase during labour, inhibition of prostaglandin synthesis blocks term and preterm labour and administration of prostaglandins can induce labour[7,121]. The amnion (PGF_2) and decidua ($PGF_{2\alpha}$) are both major sites of prostaglandin production during labour. However, the chorion possesses a high capacity to metabolize prostaglandins (by activity of a prostaglandin dehydrogenase) and comparatively little prostaglandin can cross from the fetal to maternal compartment[122]. This suggests that decidual $PGF_{2\alpha}$ production may be critical to the generation of labour contractions.

Prostaglandins are formed from membrane phospholipids through the initial activity of phospholipase A_2 or C isozymes, forming unesterified arachidonic acid[123]. The arachidonic acid is further metabolized to the intermediate, PGH_2, by cyclooxygenase (COX) before being converted on to the primary prostaglandins. COX is present as two isoforms with molecular weights of 70–73 kDa and approximately 60% amino acid homology[121,124]. COX-1 is constitutively expressed and its gene has similar properties to other 'housekeeping' genes[125]; COX-2 is the inducible form of the enzyme and is characteristically upregulated by growth factors and cytokines[126–130]. Although null mutations in the *COX-1*[131] and *COX-2*[132] genes have been created in mice, the data are inconclusive as to which gene is critical for prostaglandin synthesis during labour in the mouse. In human pregnancy, major increases in COX-2 activity and mRNA occur in amnion and decidua, tissues that line the pregnant uterus in association with the increased production of prostaglandins in fetal and maternal compartments[133–136]. A major pathway in the metabolism of PGE_2 and $PGF_{2\alpha}$ is through the action of the type 1 15-hydroxyprostaglandin dehydrogenase (PGDH). Sangha and colleagues[137] have reported that PGDH expression and activity is decreased in the chorio-decidua during spontaneous and preterm labour, raising the possibility that reduced metabolism (as well as increased synthesis) of prostaglandins contributes to the considerable increase in prostaglandin levels at this time.

Our understanding of the physiologic role of oxytocin in the regulation of labour has been clarified in recent years. While there has been no question that oxytocin is a potent myometrial stimulant, few data could demonstrate increases in plasma oxytocin with the initiation of labour. This led some to propose that the major role of oxytocin was restricted to the second stages during passage of the fetus through the birth canal, when there is a reflex release of oxytocin from the posterior pituitary. However. the demonstration by Chibbar and colleagues[138] that human intrauterine tissues (excluding the placenta) can synthesize oxytocin and that there is a significant increase in oxytocin expression in the chorio-decidua with the onset of labour, has re-established oxytocin as a major physiologic regulator of labour contractions. While the mechanisms controlling oxytocin expression in intrauterine tissues is not fully established, expression can be increased by *in vitro* treatment with oestrogen[104]. For a complete discussion of the role and regulation of oxytocin in pregnancy the reader is referred to the recent publication edited by Ivell and Russell[139].

While a number of other hormonal agents (corticotrophin-releasing hormone [CRH], endothelin, bradykinin, platelet-activating factor) can stimulate myometrial activity under various circumstances, their precise role, if any, in the generation of labour contractions remains to be determined. In addition to their individual uterotonic actions, there is evidence to suggest that these myometrial stimulants might interact to regulate their expression and action. Oxytocin has been shown to stimulate the production of PGE_2 and $PGF_{2\alpha}$ from human and rat decidua[140,141], an effect blocked by oxytocin antagonists[142]. Inhibitors of prostaglandin synthesis or antagonists of prostaglandin action have been reported to block oxytocin-stimulated contractions of uterine strips in rabbits, although part of this effect may have been due to non-specific effects of the blockers used[143]. In rats, blockade of prostaglandin synthesis did not prevent oxytocin-stimulated myometrial contraction[140] nor was the number or affinity of oxytocin receptors affected by infusions of indomethacin or $PGF_{2\alpha}$[144]. Oxytocin may also interact with other uterine stimulants to regulate contractility. A synergistic effect of oxytocin and CRH to increase myometrial contractions in human myometrium has been reported[145], which may also act through effects on prostaglandins. In addition, oxytocin has been reported to stimulate endothelin-1 release from endometrial cells in culture[146].

ACTION OF UTEROTONIC AGONISTS

The mechanisms by which the uterotonic agonists induce contractile activity has been reviewed in detail elsewhere[7,8]. Essentially all agonists ultimately act to increase intracellular calcium levels and so activate the biochemical machinery that induces spatial reorganization of actin and myosin filaments (see above). An increase in intracellular calcium to initiate contraction within the myometrial cell can occur through several mechanisms: (i) release of calcium from intracellular (sarcoplasmic reticulum, mitochondria, inner cell-membrane bound) stores; (ii) inhibition of calcium efflux; (iii) increase in calcium influx from extracellular sources. Depending on the stimulus, one or more of these events may occur during contraction. The entry of calcium from extracellular sources may occur via potential sensitive (during discharge of action potentials) or receptor-operated mechanisms. Mechanisms may also operate to link cell-membrane receptors to the intracellular calcium stores. Thus agonist–receptor activation of phospholipase C can lead to the hydrolysis of inositol phosphates leading to the release of inositol-1,4,5-triphosphate (IP_3). IP_3 in turn can cause the release of Ca^{2+} from intracellular stores. While this spike in intracellular release of calcium is sufficient to initiate the contraction it is believed that it also induces an increase in calcium influx through L-type Ca^{2+} channels to produce the full contraction[147]. Diacylglycerol generated during inositol hydrolysis can also interact with intracellular signalling pathways as well as be a substrate for prostaglandin synthesis. α-Adrenergic agonists and oxytocin operate through the inositol phosphate pathway. Stimulatory prostaglandins act to increase the influx of calcium through cell-membrane channels, but this also probably involves an initial phospholipase C mediated IP_3-induced release of calcium from intracellular stores[148]. Oxytocin and prostaglandins have also been reported to inhibit calcium efflux and data also suggest that $PGF_{2\alpha}$ can stimulate the hydrolysis of arachidonic acid from phospholipids and that this arachidonic acid can act, in turn, as a mediator for the release of intracellular Ca^{2+}. Hence prostaglandins can have multiple actions to cause an elevation of intracellular Ca^{2+}.

Summary

The above discussion of elements of the structural, regulatory and functional characteristics of the uterine muscle, the myometrium, demonstrates the complex nature of this muscle. Its ability to develop contractile activity is dependent on structural elements within the myocytes and within the extracellular matrix within which the cells are embedded. The inherent spontaneous activity of the muscle is dependent upon a series of ion channels, pumps and cell–cell communication pathways. This spontaneous activity in turn is subjected to inhibitory and stimulatory influences from a plethora of endocrine, paracrine and autocrine signals during the menstrual cycle as well as during pregnancy and labour. Moreover, during pregnancy, it is now apparent that the growth of the fetus imposes a mechanical load on the myometrium that unchecked would likely lead to premature activation and preterm birth. It is not surprising, therefore, that attempts to impose pharmacologic regulation on this muscle by blocking individual elements of this organizational matrix have proven to be of limited value. However, we suggest that by considering the broader aspects by which the myometrium switches from its pregnancy state to that of labour, namely the mechanisms that control the process of myometrial activation and stimulation, it may be possible to provide a global control to the state of contractility of this muscle.

REFERENCES

1. Rush RW, Keirse MJNC, Howat P, Baum JD, Anderson ABM, Turnbull AC. Contribution of preterm delivery to perinatal mortality. *Br Med J* **ii**(6042):965–968, 1976.
2. Anonymous European Community collaborative study of outcome of pregnancy between 22 and 28 weeks' gestation. Working Group on the Very Low Birthweight Infant. [See comments.] *Lancet* **336**(8718):782–784, 1990.
3. McCormick MC. The contribution of low birth weight to infant

mortality and childhood morbidity. [Review.] *N Engl J Med* **312**(2):82–90, 1985.
4. Lipper EG, Ross GS, Auld PA, Glassman MB. Survival and outcome of infants weighing less than 800 grams at birth. [See comments.] *Am J Obstet Gynecol* **163**(1;Part 1):146–150, 1990.
5. Main DM. The epidemiology of preterm birth. *Clin Obstet Gynecol* **31**(3):521–532, 1988.
6. Iams JD. Current status of prematurity prevention. [Editorial.] *JAMA* **262**(2):265–266, 1989.
7. Challis JRG, Lye SI. Parturition. In *The Physiology of Reproduction*, 2nd edn. (eds E. Knobil & J. Neill). New York: Raven Press, 1994.
8. Monga M, Sanborn BM (eds). *Uterine Contractile Activity*. Philadelphia: W.B. Saunders, 1995.
9. Lambert FL, Pelletier G, Dufour M, Fortier MA. Specific properties of smooth muscle cells from different layers of rabbit myometrium. *Am J Physiol* **258**:C794–802, 1990.
10. Chow EH, Marshall JM. Effects of catecholamines on circular and longitudinal uterine muscle of the rat. *Eur J Pharmacol* **76**:157–165, 1981.
11. Hall S, Pennefather JN. Actions of forskolin and isoprenaline on the separated myometrial layers of the guinea-pig uterus: influences of ovarian steroids and pregnancy. *Eur J Pharmacol* **184**:33–42, 1990.
12. el Alj A, Bonoris E, Cynober E, Germain G. Heterogeneity of oxytocin receptors in the pregnant rat myometrium near parturition. *Eur J Pharmacol* **186**:231–238, 1990.
13. Wiqvist N, Bryman I, Lindblom B, Norstrom A, Wikland M. The role of prostaglandins for the coordination of myometrial forces during labour. *Acta Physiol Hung* **65**:313–322, 1985.
14. Wikland M, Lindblom B, Wiqvist N. Myometrial response to prostaglandins during labor. *Gynecol Obstet Invest* **17**:131–138, 1984.
15. Spencer GG, KI, Grover AK, Garfield RE. (eds) *Uterine Contractility. Calcium Regulation in Smooth Muscles*, **5**:pp. 53–68. Norwell, Massachusetts: Serono Symposia, 1990.
16. Sanborn BM, Anwer K, Garfield RE. (eds) *Uterine Contractility. Hormonal Regulation of Myometrial Intracellular Calcium*, **6**:pp. 69–84. Norwell, Massachusetts: Serono Symposia, 1990.
17. Eghbali B, Kessler JA, Reid LM, Roy C, Spray DC. Involvement of gap junctions in tumorigenesis: transfection of tumor cells with connexin 32 cDNA retards growth *in vivo*. *Proc Natl Acad Sci USA* **88**:10701–10705, 1991.
18. Otey CA. pp125FAK in the focal adhesion. *Int Rev Cytol* **167**:161–183, 1996.
19. Loewenstein WR. Junctional intercellular communication: the cell-to-cell membrane channel. *Physiol Rev* **61**:829–913, 1981.
20. Loewenstein WR. The cell-to-cell channel of gap junctions. *Cell* **48**:725–726, 1987.
21. Yancey SB, Biswal S, Revel JP. Spatial and temporal patterns of distribution of the gap junction protein connexin-43 during mouse gastrulation and organogenesis. *Development* **114**:203–212, 1992.
22. Orsino A, Taylor CV, Lye SJ. Connexin-26 and connexin-43 are differentially expressed and regulated in the rat myometrium throughout late pregnancy and with the onset of labor. *Endocrinology* **137**:1545–1553, 1996.
23. Albrecht JL, Atal NS, Tadros PN, Orsino A, Lye SJ, Sadovsky Y, Beyer EC. Uterine myometrium contains a second gap junction protein (connexin-45) with a differing temporal expression pattern from connexin-43. *Am J Obstet Gynecol* **175**:853–858, 1996.
24. Beyer EC, Kistler J, Paul DL, Goodenough DA. Antisera directed against connexin-43 peptides react with a 43-kDa protein localized to gap junctions in myocardium and other tissues. *J Cell Biol* **108**:595–605, 1989.
25. Sims SM, Daniel EE, Garfield RE. Improved electrical coupling in uterine smooth muscle is associated with increased numbers of gap junctions at parturition. *J Gen Physiol* **80**(3):353–375, 1982.
26. Petrocelli T, Lye SJ. Regulation of transcripts encoding the myometrial gap junction protein, connexin-43, by estrogen and progesterone. *Endocrinology* **133**(1):284–290, 1993.
27. Orsino A, Lye SJ. Differential expression of multiple connexins in the rodent myometrium during pregnancy and labour. Unpublished observations.
28. Teoh T, Orsino A, Lye SJ. Unpublished observations.
29. Rubin JB, Verselis VK, Bennett MV, Bargiello TA. Molecular analysis of voltage dependence of heterotypic gap junctions formed by connexins 26 and 32. *Biophys J* **62**:183–185, 1992.
30. Traub O, Eckert R, Lichtenberg-Frate H, Elfgang C, Bastide B, Scheidtmann KH, Hulser DF, Willecke K. Immunochemical and electrophysiological characterization of murine connexin-40 and -43 in mouse tissues and transfected human cells. *Eur J Cell Biol* **64**:101–112, 1994.
31. Garfield RE, McNellis D, Challis J, MacDonald P, Nathanielsz P, Roberts J (eds) Structural and functional studies of the control of myometrial contractility and labor. In *The Onset of Labor: Cellular & Integrative Mechanisms*, pp. 55–85. Ithaca, NY: Perinatology Press, 1988.
32. Lye SJ, Nicholson BJ, Mascarenhas M, MacKenzie L, Petrocelli T. Increased expression of connexin-43 in the rat myometrium during labor is associated with an increase in the plasma estrogen: progesterone ratio. *Endocrinology* **132**(6):2380–2386, 1993.
33. Mege RM, Matsuzaki F, Gallin WJ, Goldberg JI, Cunningham BA, Edelman GM. Construction of epithelioid sheets by transfection of mouse sarcoma cells with cDNAs for chicken cell adhesion molecules. *Proc Natl Acad Sci USA* **85**:7274–7278, 1988.
34. Meyer RA, Laird DW, Revel JP, Johnson RG. Inhibition of gap junction and adherens junction assembly by connexin and A-CAM antibodies. *J Cell Biol* **119**:79–89, 1992.
35. Cole WC, Garfield RE. Effects of calcium ionophore, A23187 and calmodulin inhibitors on intercellular communication in the rat myometrium. *Biol Reprod* **38**:55–62, 1988.
36. Sakai N, Tabb T, Garfield RE. Modulation of cell-to-cell coupling between myometrial cells of the human uterus during pregnancy. *Am J Obstet Gynecol* **167**(2):472–480, 1992.
37. Sakai N, Blennerhassett MG, Garfield RE. Intracellular cyclic AMP concentration modulates gap junction permeability in parturient rat myometrium. *Can J Physiol Pharmacol* **70**(3):358–364, 1992.
38. Blennerhassett MG, Garfield RE. Effect of gap junction number and permeability on intercellular coupling in rat myometrium. *Am J Physiol* **261**(6; Part 1):C1001–1009, 1991.
39. Ohya Y, Sperelakis N. Fast Na^+ and slow Ca^{2+} channels in single uterine muscle cells from pregnant rats. *Am J Physiol* **257**(2; Part 1):C408–412, 1989.
40. Martin C, Arnaudeau S, Jmari K, Rakotoarisoa L, Sayet I, Dacquet C, Mironneau C, Mironneau J. Identification and properties of voltage-sensitive sodium channels in smooth muscle cells from pregnant rat myometrium. *Mol Pharmacol* **38**:667–673, 1990.
41. Young RC, Herndon-Smith L. Characterization of sodium channels in cultured human uterine smooth muscle cells. *Am J Obstet Gynecol* **164**(1; Part 1):175–181, 1991.
42. Inoue Y, Sperelakis N. Gestational change in Na^+ and Ca^{2+} channel current densities in rat myometrial smooth muscle cells. *Am J Physiol* **260**(3; Part 1):C658–663, 1991.
43. Felipe A, Knittle TJ, Doyle KL, Tamkun MM. Primary structure and differential expression during development and pregnancy of a novel voltage-gated sodium channel in the mouse: *J Biol Chem* **269**:30125–30131, 1994.
44. George AL, Jr. Knittle TJ, Tamkun MM. Molecular cloning of an atypical voltage-gated sodium channel expressed in human heart and uterus: evidence for a distinct gene family. *Proc Natl Acad Sci USA* **89**:4893–4897, 1992.
45. Batra S. Characterization of [^{3}H]-nitrendipine binding to uterine smooth muscle plasma membrane and its relevance to inhibition of calcium entry. *Br J Pharmacol* **85**(4):767–774, 1985.
46. Tezuka N, Ali M, Chwalisz K, Garfield RE. Changes in transcripts encoding calcium channel subunits of rat myometrium during pregnancy. *Am J Physiol* **269**:C1008–1017, 1995.
47. Hollingsworth M, Amédée T, Edwards D, Mironneau J, Savineau JP, Small RC, Weston AH. The relaxant action of BRL 34915 in rat uterus. *Br J Pharmacol* **91**(4):803–813, 1987.
48. Sims SM, Singer JJ, Walsh JV Jr. Cholinergic agonists suppress a potassium current in freshly dissociated smooth muscle cells of the toad. *J Physiol (Lond)* **367**:503–529, 1985.
49. Sanborn BM. Ion channels and the control of myometrial electrical activity. *Semin Perinatol* **19**(1):31–40, 1995.
50. Toro L, Stefani E, Erulkar S. Hormonal regulation of potassium currents in single myometrial cells. *Proc Natl Acad Sci USA* **87**(8):2892–2895, 1990.
51. Boyle MB, Azhderian EM, MacLusky NJ, Naftolin F, Kaczmarek LK. *Xenopus* oocytes injected with rat uterine RNA express very slowly activating potassium currents. *Science* **235**:1221–1223, 1987.

52. Boyle MB, MacLusky NJ, Naftolin F, Kaczmarek LK. Hormonal regulation of K^+-channel messenger RNA in rat myometrium during oestrus cycle and in pregnancy. *Nature* **330**:373–375, 1987.
53. Murphy LJ, Ghahary A. Uterine insulin-like growth factor-1: regulation of expression and its role in estrogen-induced uterine proliferation. *Endocr Rev* **11**(3):443–453, 1990.
54. Hofmann GE, Rao CV, Barrows GH, Schultz GS, Sanfilippo JS. Binding sites for epidermal growth factor in human uterine tissues and leiomyomas. *J Clin Endocrinol Metab* **58**:880–884, 1984.
55. Borgundvaag B, Kudlow JE, Mueller SG, George SR. Dopamine receptor activation inhibits estrogen-stimulated transforming growth factor-alpha gene expression and growth in anterior pituitary, but not in uterus. *Endocrinology* **130**:3453–3458, 1992.
56. Altman DJ, Schneider SL, Thompson DA, Cheng H-L, Tomasi TB. A transforming growth factor-β_2 (TGF-β_2)-like immunosuppressive factor in amniotic fluid and localization of TGF-β_2 mRNA in the pregnant uterus. *J Exp Med* **172**(5):1391–1401, 1990.
57. Tamada H, McMaster MT, Flanders KC, Andrews GK, Dey SK. Cell type-specific expression of transforming growth factor-β_1 in the mouse uterus during the periimplantation period. *Mol Endocrinol* **4**(7):965–972, 1990.
58. Ronnstrand L, Beckmann MP, Faulders B, Ostman A, Ek B, Heldin CH. Purification of the receptor for platelet-derived growth factor from porcine uterus. *J Biol Chem* **262**:2929–2932, 1987.
59. Mangrulkar RS, Ono M, Ishikawa M, Takashima S, Klagsbrun M, Nowak RA. Isolation and characterization of heparin-binding growth factors in human leiomyomas and normal myometrium. *Biol Reprod* **53**:636–646, 1995.
60. Rauk PN, Surti U, Roberts JM, Michalopoulos G. Mitogenic effect of basic fibroblast growth factor and estradiol on cultured human myometrial and leiomyoma cells. *Am J Obstet Gynecol* **173**:571–577, 1995.
61. Fisk NM, Ronderos-Dumit D, Tannirandorn Y, Nicolini U, Talbert D, Rodeck CH. Normal amniotic pressure throughout gestation. *Br J Obstet Gynaecol* **99**(1):18–22, 1992.
62. Csapo A, Erdos T, De Mattos CR, Gramss E, Moscowitz C. Stretch-induced uterine growth, protein synthesis and function. *Nature* **207**:1378–1379, 1965.
63. Douglas AJ, Clarke EW, Goldspink DF. Influence of mechanical stretch on growth and protein turnover of rat uterus. *Am J Physiol* **254**(5; Part 1):E543–548, 1988.
64. Goldspink DF, Douglas AJ. Protein turnover in gravid and nongravid horns of uterus in pregnant rats. *Am J Physiol* **254**(5; Part 1), E549–554, 1988.
65. Woessner JF, JT, Brewer TH. Formation and breakdown of collagen and elastin in the human uterus during pregnancy and post-partum involution. *Biochem J* **89**:75–82, 1963.
66. Vandenburgh HH. Mechanical forces and their second messengers in stimulating cell growth *in vitro*. *Am J Physiol* **262**(3; Part 2):R350–355, 1992.
67. Harding R, Poore ER, Bailey A, Thorburn GD, Jansen CA, Nathanielsz PW. Electromyographic activity of the nonpregnant and pregnant sheep uterus. *Am J Obstet Gynecol* **142**(4):448–457, 1982.
68. Lye SJ, Wlodek ME, Challis JRG. Possible role of uterine contractions in the short-term fluctuations of plasma ACTH concentration in fetal sheep. *J Endocrinol* **106**(2):R9–R11, 1985.
69. Nathanielsz PW, Bailey A, Poore ER, Thorburn GD, Harding R. The relationship between myometrial activity and sleep state and breathing in fetal sheep throughout the last third of gestation. *Am J Obstet Gynecol* **138**:653–659, 1980.
70. Lye SJ, Freitag CL. An *in-vivo* model to examine the electromyographic activity of isolated myometrial tissue from pregnant sheep. *J Reprod Fertil* **82**(1):51–61, 1988.
71. Sigger JN, Harding R, Jenkin G. Relationship between electrical activity of the uterus and surgically isolated myometrium in the pregnant and nonpregnant ewe. *J Reprod Fertil* **70**(1):103–114, 1984.
72. Lye SJ. Evidence for an intrinsic control of myometrial contractile periodicity in sheep during pregnancy. *J Reprod Fertil* **96**:337–345, 1992.
73. Csapo AI. The 'see-saw' theory of parturition. *Ciba Found Symp* 159–210, 1977.
74. Lye SJ, Porter DG. Demonstration that progesterone 'blocks' uterine activity in the ewe *in vivo* by a direct action on the myometrium. *J Reprod Fertil* **52**:87–94, 1978.
75. Porter DG, Lye SJ, Bradshaw JM, Kendall JZ. Relaxin inhibits myometrial activity in the ovariectomized non-pregnant ewe. *J Reprod Fertil* **61**:409–414, 1981.
76. Szlachter N, O'Byrne E, Goldsmith L, Steinetz BG, Weiss G. Myometrial inhibiting activity of relaxin-containing extracts of human corpora lutea of pregnancy. *Am J Obstet Gynecol* **136**:584–586, 1980.
77. Porter DG, Downing SJ, Bradshaw JM. Relaxin inhibits spontaneous and prostaglandin-driven myometrial activity in anaesthetized rats. *J Endocrinol* **83**:183–192, 1979.
78. Hsu CJ, Sanborn BM. Relaxin treatment alters the kinetic properties of myosin light chain kinase activity in rat myometrial cells in culture. *Endocrinology* **118**:499–505, 1986.
79. Anwer K, Hovington JA, Sanborn BM. Involvement of protein kinase A in the regulation of intracellular free calcium and phosphoinositide turnover in rat myometrium. *Biol Reprod* **43**:851–859, 1990.
80. Anwer K, Hovington JA, Sanborn BM. Antagonism of contractants and relaxants at the level of intracellular calcium and phosphionositide turnover in the rat uterus. *Endocrinology* **124**:2995–3002, 1989.
81. Wen Y, Anwer K, Singh SP, Sanborn BM. Protein kinase-A inhibits phospholipase-C activity and alters protein phosphorylation in rat myometrial plasma membranes. *Endocrinology* **131**:1377–1382, 1992.
82. Meera P, Anwer K, Monga M, Oberti C, Stefani E, Toro L, Sanborn BM. Relaxin stimulates myometrial calcium-activated potassium channel activity via protein kinase A. *Am J Physiol* **269**:C312–317, 1995.
83. Sladek SM, Regenstein AC, Lykins D, Roberts JM. Nitric oxide synthase activity in pregnant rabbit uterus decreases on the last day of pregnancy. *Am J Obstet Gynecol* **169**:1285–1291, 1993.
84. Natuzzi ES, Ursell PC, Harrison M, Buscher C, Riemer RK. Nitric oxide synthase activity in the pregnant uterus decreases at parturition. *Biochem Biophys Res Commun* **194**:1–8, 1993.
85. Garfield RE, Ali M, Yallampalli C, Izumi H. Role of gap junctions and nitric oxide in control of myometrial contractility. *Semin Perinatol* **19**(1):41–51, 1995.
86. Izumi H, Garfield RE. Relaxant effects of nitric oxide and cyclic GMP on pregnant rat uterine longitudinal smooth muscle. *Eur J Obstet Gynecol Reprod Biol* **60**:171–180, 1995.
87. Izumi H, Yallampalli C, Garfield RE. Gestational changes in L-arginine-induced relaxation of pregnant rat and human myometrial smooth muscle. *Am J Obstet Gynecol* **169**:1327–1337, 1993.
88. Lye SJ, Challis JRG. Inhibition by PGI_2 of myometrial activity *in vivo* in non-pregnant ovariectomized sheep. *J Reprod Fertil* **66**(1):311–315, 1982.
89. Omini C, Folco GC, Pasargiklian R, Fano M, Berti F. Prostacyclin (PGI_2) in pregnant human uterus. *Prostaglandins* **17**(1):113–120, 1979.
90. Evans CA, Kennedy TG, Challis JR. Gestational changes in prostanoid concentrations in intrauterine tissues and fetal fluids from pregnant sheep, and the relation to prostanoid output *in vitro*. *Biol Reprod* **27**:1–11, 1982.
91. Kawano M, Mori N. The significance of prostacyclin produced by pregnant rat myometrium: the relationship between myometrial prostacyclin producing activity and passive stretch of myometrium by growing conceptus. *Prostaglandins* **35**(3):305–325, 1988.
92. Dalle M, Dauprat-Dalle P, Barlet JP. Parathyroid hormone-related peptide inhibits oxytocin-induced rat uterine contractions *in vitro*. *Arch Int Physiol Biochim Biophys* **100**:251–254, 1992.
93. Thiede MA, Daifotis AG, Weir EC *et al.* Intrauterine occupancy controls expression of the parathyroid hormone-related peptide gene in preterm rat myometrium. *Proc Natl Acad Sci USA* **87**:6969–6973, 1990.
94. Paspaliaris V, Vargas SJ, Gillespie MT *et al.* Oestrogen enhancement of the myometrial response to exogenous parathyroid hormone-related protein (PTHrP), and tissue localization of endogenous PTHrP and its mRNA in the virgin rat uterus. *J Endocrinol* **134**:415–425, 1992.
95. Marshall JM, Gatfield RE (eds) *Uterine Contractility. Relationship between Membrane Potential and Spontaneous Contraction of the Uterus*, **1**:pp. 3–8. Norwell, Massachusetts: Serono Symposia, 1990.
96. Lye SJ, Freitag CL. Local and systemic control of myometrial contractile activity during labour in the sheep. *J Reprod Fertil* **90**:483–492, 1990.

97. Crankshaw DJ, Gaspar V. Effects of prostanoids on the rat's myometrium *in vitro* during pregnancy. *Biol Reprod* **46**:392–400, 1992.
98. Fuchs A-R, Periyasamy S, Alexandrova M, Soloff MS. Correlation between oxytocin receptor concentration and responsiveness to oxytocin in pregnant rat myometrium: effects of ovarian steroids. *Endocrinology* **113**(2):742–749, 1983.
99. Challis JR, Lye SJ. Parturition. *Oxf Rev Reprod Biol* **8**:61–129, 1986.
100. Nathanielsz PW, Binienda Z, Wimsatt J *et al.* (eds) Patterns of myometrial activity and their regulation in the monkey. In *The Onset of Labour: Cellular and Integrative Mechanisms*, pp. 359–380. Ithaca, NY: Perinatology Press, 1988.
101. Figueroa JP, Honnebier MB, Binienda Z, Wimsatt J, Nathanielsz PW. Effect of a 48-hour intravenous delta 4-androstenedione infusion on the pregnant rhesus monkey in the last third of gestation: changes in maternal plasma estradiol concentrations and myometrial contractility. *Am J Obstet Gynecol* **161**:481–486, 1989.
102. Honnebier MB, Myers T, Figueroa JP, Nathanielsz PW. Variation in myometrial response to intravenous oxytocin administration at different times of the day in the pregnant rhesus monkey. *Endocrinology* **125**:1498–1503, 1989.
103. Lye S. The initiation and inhibition of labour: towards a molecular understanding. *Sem Reprod Endocrin* **12**(4):284–294, 1994.
104. Chibbar R, Wong S, Miller FD, Mitchell BF. Estrogen stimulates oxytocin gene expression in human chorio-decidua. *J Clin Endocrinol Metab* **80**:567–572, 1995.
105. Haluska GJ, Wells TR, Novy MJ. Progesterone receptor isoforms in gestational tissues from Rhesus monkeys. [Abstract] *J Soc Gynecol Invest* **3**(4):321A, 1996.
106. Chen Z, Qi S, Lye SJ. Myometrial expression and regulation of the rat oxytocin receptor during term and preterm labour. [Abstract] *J Soc Gynecol Invest* **3**(2):77A, 1996.
107. Chen Z, Qi S, Lye SJ. Myometrial expression of the prostaglandin FP receptor is increased during labour in the rat. [Abstract] *J Soc Gynecol Invest* **3**(2):325A, 1996.
108. Chen Z, Qi S, Lye SJ. Unpublished observations.
109. McNutt CM, Nicholson BJ, Lye SJ. ACTH-induced preterm labour in the ewe is associated with increased mRNA and protein levels of myometrial gap junction protein, connexin-43. *J Endocrinol* **141**(2):195–202, 1994.
110. Piersanti M, Lye SJ. Increase in messenger ribonucleic acid encoding the myometrial gap junction protein, connexin-43, requires protein synthesis and is associated with increased expression of the activator protein-1, c-fos. *Endocrinology* **136**(8):3571–3578, 1995.
111. Teoh T, Chen Z, Qi S, Lye SJ. Unpublished observations.
112. Yu W, Dahl G, Werner R. The connexin-43 gene is responsive to oestrogen. *Proc R Soc Lond B Biol Sci* **255**(1343):125–132, 1994.
113. Lefebvre DL, Piersanti M, Bai XH, Chen ZO, Lye SJ. Myometrial transcriptional regulation of the gap junction gene, connexin-43. *Reprod Fertil Dev* **7**:603–611, 1995.
114. Chen Z-O, Lefebvre D, Bai X-H, Reaume A, Rossant J, Lye SJ. Identification of two regulatory elements within the promoter region of the mouse connexin-43 gene. *J Biol Chem* **270**(8):3863–3868, 1995.
115. Rozen F, Russo C, Banville D, Zingg HH. Structure, characterization, and expression of the rat oxytocin receptor gene. *Proc Natl Acad Sci USA* **92**:200–204, 1995.
116. Wathes DC, Porter DG. Effect of uterine distension and oestrogen treatment on gap junction formation in the myometrium of the rat. *J Reprod Fertil* **65**(2):497–505, 1982.
117. Ou C, Lye SJ. Unpublished observations.
118. Ou C, Lye SJ. Unpublished observations.
119. Chow L, Lye SJ. Expression of the gap junction protein connexin-43 is increased in the human myometrium toward term and with the onset of labor. *Am J Obstet Gynecol* **170**:788–795, 1994.
120. Kimura T, Tanizawa O, Mori K, Brownstein MJ, Okayama H. Structure and expression of a human oxytocin receptor. *Nature* **356**(6369):526–529, 1992.
121. Olson DM, Mijovic JE, Sadowsky DW. Control of human parturition. *Semin Perinatol* **19**(1):52–63, 1995.
122. Nakla S, Skinner K, Mitchell BF, Challis JRG. Changes in prostaglandin transfer across human fetal membranes obtained after spontaneous labor. *Am J Obstet Gynecol* **155**(6):1337–1341, 1986.
123. Rice GE. Glycerophospholipid metabolism and human labour. *Reprod Fertil Dev* **7**:613–622, 1995.
124. Mitchell MD, Romero RJ, Edwin SS, Trautman MS. Prostaglandins and parturition. *Reprod Fertil Dev* **7**:623–632, 1995.
125. Wang L-H, Hajibeigi A, Xu X-M, Loose-Mitchell D, Wu KK. Characterization of the promoter of human prostaglandin H synthase-1 gene. *Biochem Biophys Res Commun* **190**(2):406–411, 1993.
126. Wong WYL, Richards JS. Evidence for two antigenically distinct molecular weight variants of prostaglandin H synthase in the rat ovary. *Mol Endocrinol* **5**(9):1269–1279, 1991.
127. Diaz A, Reginato AM, Jimenez SA. Alternative splicing of human prostaglandin G/H synthase mRNA and evidence of differential regulation of the resulting transcripts by transforming growth factor β_1, interleukin 1_β, and tumor necrosis factor-α. *J Biol Chem* **267**(15):10816–10822, 1992.
128. Xie W, Merrill JR, Bradshaw WS, Simmons DL. Structural determination and promoter analysis of the chicken mitogen-inducible prostaglandin G/H synthase gene and genetic mapping of the murine homolog. *Arch Biochem Biophys* **300**(1):247–252, 1993.
129. Zakar T, Hirst JJ, Mijovic JE, Olson DM. Glucocorticoids stimulate the expression of prostaglandin endoperoxide H synthase-2 in amnion cells. *Endocrinology* **136**(4):1610–1619, 1995.
130. Mitchell MD, Edwin SS, Lundin-Schiller S, Silver RM, Smotkin D, Trautman MS. Mechanism of interleukin-1 beta stimulation of human amnion prostaglandin biosynthesis: mediation via a novel inducible cyclooxygenase. *Placenta* **14**:615–625, 1993.
131. Langenbach R, Morham SG, Tiano HF *et al.* Prostaglandin synthase 1 gene disruption in mice reduces arachidonic acid-induced inflammation and indomethacin-induced gastric ulceration. *Cell* **83**(3):483–492, 1995.
132. Morham SG, Langenbach R, Loftin CD *et al.* Prostaglandin synthase 2 gene disruption causes severe renal pathology in the mouse. *Cell* **83**(3):473–482, 1995.
133. Rice GE, Freed KA, Aitken MA, Jacobs RA. Gestational- and labour-associated changes in the relative abundance of prostaglandin G/H synthase-1 and -2 mRNA in ovine placenta. *J Mol Endocrinol* **14**(2):237–245, 1995.
134. Hirst JJ, Teixeira FJ, Zakar T, Olson DM. Prostaglandin endoperoxide-H synthase-1 and -2 messenger ribonucleic acid levels in human amnion with spontaneous labour onset. *J Clin Endocrinol Metab* **80**(2):517–523, 1995.
135. Teixeira FJ, Zakar T, Hirst J, Guo F, Machin G, Olson DM. Prostaglandin endoperoxide H synthase (PGHS) activity increases with gestation and labour in human amnion. *J Lipid Mediat* **6**(1–3):515–523, 1993.
136. Hirst JJ, Teixeira FJ, Zakar T, Olson DM. Prostaglandin H synthase-2 expression increases in human gestational tissues with spontaneous labour onset. *Reprod Fertil Dev* **7**:633–637, 1995.
137. Sangha RK, Walton JC, Ensor CM, Tai HH, Challis JR. Immunohistochemical localization, messenger ribonucleic acid abundance, and activity of 15-hydroxyprostaglandin dehydrogenase in placenta and fetal membranes during term and preterm labor. *J Clin Endocrinol Metab* **78**:982–989, 1994.
138. Chibbar R, Miller FD, Mitchell BF. Synthesis of oxytocin in amnion, chorion, and decidua may influence the timing of human parturition. *J Clin Invest* **91**:185–192, 1993.
139. Ivell R, Russell JA. *Oxytocin: Cellular and Molecular Approaches in Medicine and Research.* New York: Plenum Press, 1995.
140. Riemer RK, Goldfien AC, Goldfien A, Roberts JM. Rabbit uterine oxytocin receptors and *in vitro* contractile response: abrupt changes at term and the role of eicosanoids. *Endocrinology* **119**(2):699–709, 1986.
141. Fuchs AR, Fuchs F, Husslein P, Soloff MS, Fernstrom MJ. Oxytocin receptors and human parturition: a dual role for oxytocin in the initiation of labor. *Science* **215**:1396–1398, 1982.
142. Chan WY, Powell AM, Hruby VJ. Antioxytocic and antiprostaglandin-releasing effects of oxytocin antagonists in pregnant rats and pregnant human myometrial strips. *Endocrinology* **111**(1):48–54, 1982.
143. Olson DM, Hertelendy F. Avian shell gland contractility: interaction of PGF2 alpha and arginine vasotocin with Ca^{2+}. *Am J Physiol* **244**:C150–7, 1983.
144. Engstrom T, Atke A, Vilhardt H. Oxytocin receptors and contractile response of the myometrium after long term infusion of prostaglandin

F2 alpha, indomethacin, oxytocin and an oxytocin antagonist in rats. *Regul Pept* **20**:65–72, 1988.

145. Quartero HW, Srivatsa G, Gillham B. Role for cyclic adenosine monophosphate in the synergistic interaction between oxytocin and corticotrophin-releasing factor in isolated human gestational myometrium. *Clin Endocrinol (Oxf)* **36**:141–145, 1992.

146. Peri A, Vannelli GB, Fantoni G, Giannini S, Barni T, Orlando C, Serio M, Maggi M. Endothelin in rabbit uterus during pregnancy. *Am J Physiol* **263**(1; Part 1):E158–167, 1992.

147. Zhuge R, Li S, Chen TH, Hsu WH. Oxytocin induced a biphasic increase in the intracellular Ca^{2+} concentration of porcine myometrial cells: participation of a pertussis toxin-insensitive G-protein, inositol 1,4,5-trisphosphate-sensitive Ca^{2+} pool, and Ca^{2+} channels. *Mol Reprod Dev* **41**:20–28, 1995.

148. Asboth G, Phaneuf S, Europe-Finner GN, Toth M, Bernal AL. Prostaglandin E_2 activates phospholipase C and elevates intracellular calcium in cultured myometrial cells: involvement of EP1 and EP3 receptor subtypes. *Endocrinology* **137**:2572–2579, 1996.

Maturation of the brain and behavioural states

20

J.G. Nijhuis

Introduction

The introduction of dynamic ultrasound techniques enabled both obstetricians and researchers to get a more direct approach into the developing human fetus and its central nervous system (CNS). And, although it is as yet not possible to assess the development of the fetal brain more invasively, the use of ultrasound has given a lot of information on the physiologic pathway that is followed during fetal (neuro-) development. One of the major points is that we have realised that we do not really investigate the fetal CNS, but rather the output of the CNS, which we call behaviour. Another major point is that we no longer regard the fetus as a 'living thing before birth' but that we do realise that the fetus, from its conception onward, follows a path with important milestones in which birth by itself is not the biggest issue, but rather just the change from fetal to neonatal life.

Initial fetal activity

The very first activity that can be observed is the beating fetal heart which can be detected from six menstrual weeks of gestation onward[1]. The initial rate of 100 beats per minute (bpm) increases to a mean rate of 167 bpm at nine weeks which will then be followed by a gradual decrease to 156 bpm. It is interesting to see that there is a close relationship between the heart rate and the crown–rump length (Fig. 20.1)[1]. From seven to eight weeks, the first fetal body movements can be observed, and very rapidly many different types of body movements can be distinguished[2]. At about seven to eight weeks of gestation one can observe the first 'vermicular' movements of the fetus which will then rapidly be followed by many other movements. De Vries *et al.* were the first to describe and classify the development of the different types of fetal movements in a longitudinal study of 12 fetuses of healthy nulliparous women. They described not only the first occurrence of each particular movement, but also how these movements were performed in terms of speed and amplitude. They emphasized also how important it is to be aware of the quality of movements, rather than the quantity of movements[2,3]. Their classification was based on a categorisation introduced by Prechtl in low-risk preterm and full-term infants[4,5]. Examples (with

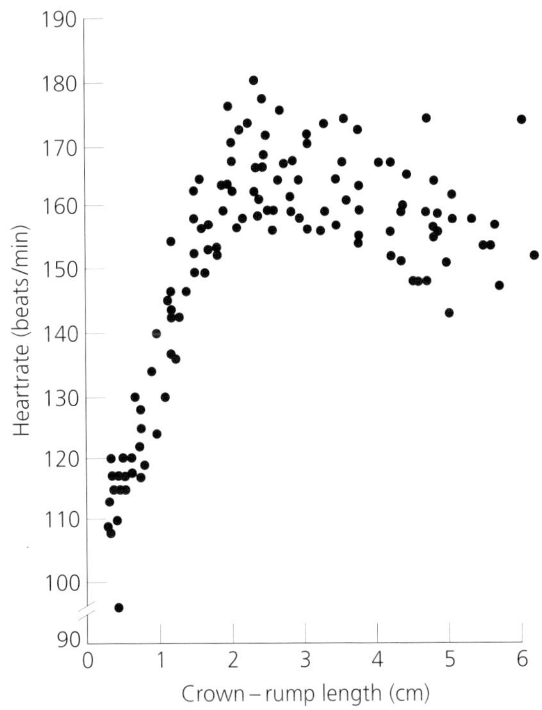

Fig. 20.1 Relationship between fetal heart rate and crown–rump length. The closest relationship can be seen before the peak frequency of heart rate has been reached. Reproduced with permission from Van Heeswijk *et al.*[1].

menstrual age of first occurrence in parentheses) are: 'just discernible movements' (7–8 weeks), startles and general movements (8–9 weeks), movements of arm or leg (9–10 weeks), breathing movements (10–11 weeks) and yawning, sucking and swallowing (12–13 weeks)[2]. In 1981, Birnholz showed that the first eye movements could be observed from 16 weeks of gestation[6]. Also in 1981, Bots *et al.* described how eye movements could be observed in the second half of pregnancy and they emphasized its importance for the study of fetal behaviour[7]. One of the striking differences during development is the increasing duration that movements can be absent: the longest period varies from about 12 min at 8 weeks to 5–6 min at 17 weeks[8]. In conclusion, during the first half of gestation the fetus already exhibits all movements that can also be observed after birth. Further maturation of the brain does not mean the introduction of new movements but rather a different organisation of (combinations of) movements.

Fetal behaviour in the second half of pregnancy

In the second half of pregnancy the observation of body movements can be combined with the recording of the fetal heart rate (FHR) using commercially available standard equipment (CTG). The combination of visible motility with the FHR is what is called 'fetal behaviour'. The developmental changes of fetal behaviour that can be observed are based on three aspects, i.e. change of cyclicity of individual variables, the development of specific combinations of movements (coincidence) and the occurrence of transitions from one situation into another.

CHANGING CYCLICITY OF INDIVIDUAL VARIABLES

We have already mentioned that in the first half of pregnancy, long periods of quiescence are scarce. In the second trimester, the cycles of absence and presence of movements change dramatically, meaning that the periods over which body movements can be absent increase significantly[9,10]. The same is true for the presence and absence of eye movements, for breathing movements[11], and also for the CTG that can be recorded. The periods of 'silent heart rate patterns' become increasingly longer[10,11].

SPECIFIC COMBINATIONS OF VARIABLES (COINCIDENCE)

During the second half of pregnancy specific combinations of variables become more frequent, e.g. when eye movements are in the 'off' condition, it is much more likely that body movements are also in the 'off' condition[9,12,13]. For fetal behavioural studies, it is the combination of fetal heart rate patterns (FHRP), eye movements and body movements that has gained the widest attention.

TRANSITIONS

Obviously, if the cycle duration increases, and specific combinations of variables are likely to occur, then the periods in between such situations will become short and can then be recognized as transitions. Figure 20.2 illustrates the combination of these three aspects nicely. Based on these aspects, it appeared possible to develop a concept of fetal behavioural states.

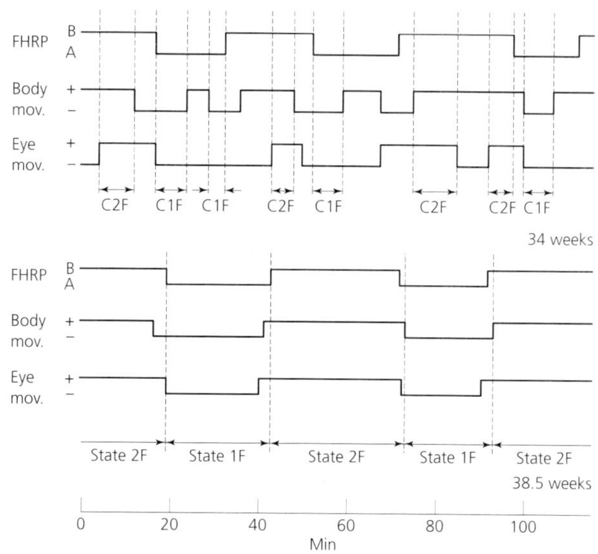

Fig. 20.2 Schematic representation of 114 min of the behaviour of a fetus at 34 weeks (upper part) and at 38.5 weeks of gestation (lower part). At 34 weeks, short periods of coincidence 2F (C2F) and coincidence 1F (C1F) can be seen, but clearly defined states are absent. At 38.5 weeks, states are present: there is coincidence of variables over a prolonged period with clear state transitions. FHRP, fetal heart rate pattern A or B; mov., movements; +, present; –, absent. Reproduced with permission from Nijhuis and Tas[53].

Fetal behavioural states

By 1979, Timor-Tritsch *et al.* had noted activity cycles of fetuses based on CTG recordings and fetal body movements[14]. Another big step forward followed in 1981 when it not only appeared possible to observe fetal eye movements with ultrasound, but also it became clear that these eye movements could be used as another state criterion[7]. In 1982, four behavioural states were defined by Nijhuis *et al.* and these definitions have now been widely accepted[10]. Fetal behavioural states are similar to the neonatal states described by Prechtl[15] and were therefore numbered 1F to 4F ('F' for fetal). The definitions are based on specific combinations of three variables, eye movements, body movements and the fetal heart rate patterns (FHRP) A to D. Eye movements and body movements are described in terms of 'absent' and 'present', and four separate heart rate patterns have been defined. State 1F is similar to state 1, quiet sleep or non-REM sleep in the neonate; state 2F is similar to state 2 or active or REM sleep; state 3F is similar to state 3 or quiet wakefulness and state 4F to state 4 or active wakefulness. A fetal behavioural state, similar to the neonatal state 5 – crying – has never been established.

The fetal behavioural states are defined as follows[10]:

State 1F: Quiescence, which can be regularly interrupted by brief gross body movements, mostly startles. Eye movements are absent. Fetal heart rate pattern (FHRP) A is a stable pattern with a small oscillation bandwidth and no accelerations, except in combination with a startle (Fig. 20.3).

State 2F: Frequent and periodic gross body movements – mainly stretches and retroflexions – and movements of the extremities. Eye movements are present. FHRP B has a wider oscillation bandwidth and frequent accelerations during movements (Fig. 20.3).

State 3F: Gross body movements absent. Eye movements present. FHRP C is stable but with a wider oscillation bandwidth than FHRP A and no accelerations (Fig. 20.3).

State 4F: Vigorous, continual activity including many trunk rotations. Eye movements are present. FHRP D is unstable, with large and long-lasting accelerations, often fused into a sustained tachycardia (Fig. 20.3).

It should be emphasized again that wakefulness *in utero* is not implied, only that behavioural states before and after birth are similar!

Following the description of fetal behavioural states in normal multigravidae, fetal behaviour was also studied in healthy primigravidae[16], in the intrauterine growth-retarded fetus[17,18], in mothers with diabetes[19–21], in mothers who used anti-epileptic drugs[22] or drugs such as cocaine[23], and in the fetus in post-term pregnancies[24]. All authors have confirmed the existence of fetal behavioural states, but the study of fetal behaviour in an individual fetus is still not sensitive enough to detect the fetus at risk. Recently, attention has also been focused on the value of the study of transitions[25]. Normally they last not more than three minutes in the near-term period, and the sequence of change of variables is also very consistent: in healthy fetuses, FHRP is the first to change during a transition from 1F to 2F, but the last to change in a transition from 2F to 1F[25]. This sequence is not present in the intrauterine growth-retarded fetus[26].

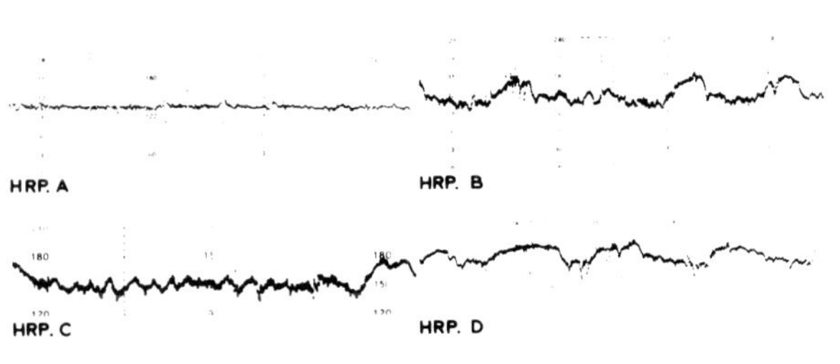

Fig. 20.3 Examples of the four heart-rate patterns (HRP) A to D, which are used for the definitions of fetal behavioural states, at a recording speed of 3 cm/min. For further definitions, see text.

Fetal behaviour and clinical testing

With the introduction of the concept of fetal behaviour and behavioural states it became apparent that fetal testing should be state-dependent. Good reviews have been published in recent years[27–29] and in this context we have to restrict ourselves to a few examples. Breathing movements are considered to indicate a good fetal condition. Breathing movements are therefore part of the fetal biophysical profile[30]. However, they are much more likely to be absent during state 1F than during state 2F[31]. Furthermore, they are more regular during state 1F[32]. Therefore, if we want to say something about fetal breathing, we should take fetal behavioural states into account.

Vibro-acoustic stimulation is another fetal test for fetal wellbeing. A fetal response, e.g. a transient fetal tachycardia, is considered to reflect a good fetal condition, both during pregnancy[33] and intrapartum[34]. The responsiveness of the fetus for this stimulus appears also to be state-dependent[35]. Because this test may induce prolonged periods of tachycardia, it has been asked whether this procedure is safe[36] and in many cases prolonged observation of the fetus without any intervention seems to be much more appropriate.

A possibly more sophisticated and more reasonable approach could be further research into the possibilities of an intrauterine neurologic investigation. Recently, Tas *et al.* have shown that the intercostal-to-phrenic-inhibitory reflex can be provoked, leading to arrest of breathing movements in the normal and growth-retarded fetus[37,38]. In this study, it appears that the effects in normal and growth-retarded fetuses are similar and it has, as yet, not been possible to detect a reliable test for the assessment of the integrity of the fetal CNS.

Yet another approach is to look at cardiovascular characteristics and fetal behaviour. Hitherto, in the human fetus, Doppler flow velocity measurements were very frequently used for this purpose, and also for the possible early detection of a deteriorating fetal condition[39,40]. The pulsatility index is significantly decreased in 2F as compared to 1F in the fetal descending aorta[41], and the fetal internal carotid artery[42], in the normal fetus but not in the growth-retarded fetus[43,44]. This difference is not observed in the umbilical artery, either in the normal[42,45], or in the growth-retarded fetus[44].

The recording of the fetal heart rate is probably the most frequently used technique for fetal surveillance. In general, the presence of accelerations is supposed to reflect a good fetal condition[46], while diminished variability and absence of accelerations is considered to be 'suspect'. Based on studies of fetal behaviour, it can be concluded that many suspect patterns are merely state-dependent and should be judged as FHRP A if they are 'silent'. Many 'sinusoidal-like' heart rate patterns can be produced by fetal sucking or mouthing movements[47,48]. Based on their observations, Nijhuis *et al.*[49] and Tas and Nijhuis[11] have established a differential diagnosis when a silent heart rate pattern is recorded. The first step is to extend the recording time to at least 50 min which is in agreement with other authors[29]. The use of drugs by the mother should be excluded, as should congenital anomalies and fetal brain death[49]. Finally, in the absence of decelerations, a cordocentesis can be considered a certain criterion to exclude fetal hypoxia or acidosis. In general, it is not the silent heart rate pattern that indicates fetal distress, but rather the presence of decelerations during or following a (Braxton–Hicks) contraction of the uterus. Visser *et al.* suggested a rank ordering in which several variables change in growth-retarded human fetuses with progressive deterioration of the fetal condition[50]. The first test to be abnormal is the umbilical artery waveform, followed by abnormal behavioural state development, qualitative movement changes, reduced amniotic fluid, heart rate decelerations, reduced heart rate variation, reduced general movements, reduced breathing movements, absence of movements, and, finally, a terminal heart rate pattern.

Conclusions

Although we used to judge the condition of a fetus without taking into account its age or behavioural state, it has now become clear that these facts must be taken into consideration if a proper assessment of the fetal condition is to be made. What may be normal for a fetus at 28 weeks can be very abnormal at 36 weeks. Furthermore, we must increasingly emphasize that the fetal environment is not as safe as has been previously assumed, and 'intrauterine accidents' with serious consequences may occur. The more we understand about the development of the fetal brain (reflected in fetal behaviour), the more we will realize that handicaps seldom arise from an accident during birth, but rather as a consequence of disturbances of development during pregnancy[51]. It is now clear that even in 1897, Freud understood this when he postulated that 'difficult birth in itself in certain cases is merely a symptom of deeper effects that influenced the development of the fetus'[52]. And this concept also helps us to understand why, despite intensive perinatal surveillance, the number of children born with a handicap does not really decrease. In the near future, we shall see how much progress can be made towards an early and adequate assessment of the fetal central nervous system, in order to come to better and more effective strategies to prevent, rather than to detect, pathology of the fetal CNS.

References

1. van Heeswijk M, Nijhuis JG & Hollanders HMG. Fetal heart rate in early pregnancy. *Early Human Develop.* **22**:151–156, 1990.
2. de Vries JIP, Visser GHA & Prechtl HFR. The emergence of fetal behaviour. I. Qualitative aspects. *Early Human Develop.* **7**:301–322, 1982.
3. de Vries JIP, Visser GHA & Prechtl HFR. The emergence of fetal behaviour. II. Quantitative aspects. *Early Human Develop.* **12**:99–120, 1985.
4. Prechtl HFR. The neurological examination of the full-term newborn infant. In *Clinics in Developmental Medicine*, Volume 63, London Heinemann, 1977.
5. Prechtl HFR & Fargel JW. Posture, motility and respiration in low-risk preterm infants. *Develop. Med. Child Neurol.* **21**:3–27, 1979.
6. Birnholz JC. The development of human fetal eye movement patterns. *Science* **213**:679–681, 1981.
7. Bots RSGM, Nijhuis JG, Martin Jr CB & Prechtl HFR. Human fetal eye movements: detection *in utero* by ultrasonography. *Early Human Develop.* **5**:87–94, 1981.
8. de Vries JIP. The first trimester. In *Fetal Behaviour. Developmental and Perinatal Aspects* (ed. J.G. Nijhuis), pp. 3–16. Oxford: Oxford University Press, 1992.
9. Drogtrop AP, Ubels R & Nijhuis JG. The association between fetal body movements, eye movements, and heart rate patterns between 25 and 30 weeks of gestation. *Early Human Develop.* **23**:67–73, 1990.
10. Nijhuis JG, Bots RSGM, Martin Jr CB & Prechtl HFR. Are there behavioural states in the human fetus? *Early Human Develop.* **6**:177–195, 1982.
11. Tas BAPJ & Nijhuis JG. Consequences for fetal monitoring. In *Fetal Behaviour, Developmental and Perinatal Aspects* (ed. J.G. Nijhuis), pp. 258–269. Oxford: Oxford University Press, 1992.
12. Nijhuis JG & van de Pas M. Behavioral states and their ontogeny: human studies. *Sem. Perinatol.* **16**:206–210, 1992.
13. DiPietro JA, Hodgson DM, Costigan KA, Hilton SC & Johnson TRB. Development of fetal movement – fetal heart rate coupling from 20 weeks through term. *Early Human Develop.* **44**:139–151, 1996.
14. Timor-Tritsch IE, Dierker LJ, Hertz RH, Deagan C & Rosen MG. Studies of antepartum behavioral states in the human fetus at term. *Am. J. Obstet. Gynecol.* **132**:524–528, 1979.
15. Prechtl HFR. The behavioural states of the newborn. [A review]. *Brain Res.* **76**:185–212, 1974.
16. van Vliet MAT, Martin Jr CB, Nijhuis JG & Prechtl HFR. Behavioural states in fetuses of nulliparous women. *Early Human Develop.* **12**:121–135, 1985.
17. van Vliet MAT, Martin Jr CB, Nijhuis JG & Prechtl HFR. Behavioural states in growth retarded human fetuses. *Early Human Develop.* **12**:183–197, 1985.
18. Arduini D, Rizzo G, Caforio L, Romanini C & Mancuso S. Behavioural state transitions in healthy and growth retarded fetuses. *Early Human Develop.* **19**:155–165, 1989.
19. Mulder EJH, Visser GHA, Bekedam DJ & Prechtl HFR. Emergence of behavioural states in fetuses of type-1 diabetic women. *Early Human Develop.* **15**:231–251, 1987.
20. Mulder EJH. Diabetic pregnancy. In *Fetal Behaviour. Developmental and Perinatal Aspects* (ed. J.G. Nijhuis), pp. 193–208. Oxford: Oxford University Press, 1992.
21. Gazzolo D, Scopesi R, Russo A, Camoriano R, Santi F, Di Renzo GC, Visser GHA & Bruschettini PL. Doppler velocimetry and behavioural state development in relation to perinatal outcome in pregnancies complicated by gestational diabetes. *Early Human Develop.* **41**:193–201, 1995.
22. van Geijn HP, Swartjes JM, van Woerden EE, Caron FJM, Brons JTJ & Arts NFT. Fetal behavioural states in epileptic pregnancies. *Eur. J. Obstet. Gynecol. Reprod. Biol.* **21**:309–314, 1986.
23. Hume Jr RF, O'Donnell KJ, Stanger CL, Killam AP & Gingras JL. *In utero* cocaine exposure: observations of fetal behavioral state may predict neonatal outcome. *Am. J. Obstet. Gynecol.* **161**:685–690, 1989.

24. van de Pas M, Nijhuis JG & Jongsma HW. Fetal behaviour in uncomplicated pregnancies after 41 weeks of gestation. *Early Human Develop.* **40**:29–38, 1994.
25. Arduini D, Rizzo G, Massacesi M, Boccolini MR, Romanini C & Mancuso S. Longitudinal assessment of behavioural transitions in healthy fetuses during the last trimester of pregnancy. *J. Perinat. Med.* **1**:67–72, 1991.
26. Arduini D, Rizzo G, Caforio L, Boccolini MR, Romanini C & Mancuso S. Behavioural state transitions in healthy and growth-retarded fetuses. *Early Human Develop.* **19**:155–162, 1989.
27. Groome LJ & Watson JE. Assessment of *in utero* neurobehavioral development. I. Fetal behavioral states. *J. Matern. Fetal Invest.* **2**:183–194, 1992.
28. Nijhuis JG (ed.) *Fetal Behaviour. Developmental and Perinatal Aspects.* Oxford: Oxford University Press, 1992.
29. Romanini C & Rizzo G. Fetal behaviour in normal and compromised fetuses. An overview. *Early Human Develop.* **43**:117–131, 1995.
30. Manning FA, Platt LD & Sipos L. Antepartum fetal evaluation: development of a fetal biophysical profile score. *Am. J. Obstet. Gynec.* **136**:787–795, 1980.
31. van Vliet MAT, Martin Jr CB, Nijhuis JG & Prechtl HFR. The relationship between fetal activity, and behavioural states and fetal breathing movements in normal and growth-retarded fetuses. *Am. J. Obstet. Gynec.* **153**:582–588, 1985.
32. Nijhuis JG, Martin Jr CB, Gommers S, Bouws P, Bots RSGM & Jongsma HW. The rhythmicity of fetal breathing varies with behavioural state in the human fetus. *Early Human Develop.* **9**:1–7, 1983.
33. Serafini P, Lindsay MBJ, Nagey DA, Pupkin MJ, Tseng P & Crenshaw C. Anterpartum fetal heart reponse to sound stimulation: the acoustic stimulation test. *Am. J. Obstet. Gynec.* **148**:41–45, 1984.
34. Edersheim TG, Hutson JM, Druzin ML & Kogut EA. Fetal heart rate response to vibratory acoustic stimulation predicts fetal pH in labor. *Am. J. Obstet. Gynec.* **157**:41–45, 1987.
35. Devoe LD, Murray C, Faircloth D & Ramos E. Vibroacoustic stimulation and fetal behavioural state in normal term human pregnancy. *Am. J. Obstet. Gynec.* **163**:1156–1161, 1990.
36. Visser GHA, Mulder HH, Wit HP, Mulder EJH & Prechtl HFR. Vibro-acoustic stimulation of the human fetus: effect on behavioural state organization. *Early Human Develop.* **19**:285–289, 1989.
37. Tas BAPJ, Nijhuis JG, Lucas AJ *et al.* The intercostal-to-phrenic inhibitory reflex in the human fetus near term. *Early Human Develop.* **22**:145–149, 1990.
38. Tas BAPJ, Nijhuis JG, Nelen W & Willems E. The intercostal-to-phrenic inhibitory reflex in normal and intra-uterine growth-retarded (IUGR) human fetuses from 26–40 weeks of gestation. *Early Human Develop.* **32**:177–182, 1993.
39. Almstrom H, Axelsson O, Cnattingius S, Ekman G, Maesel A, Ulmsten U, Arstrom K & Marsal K. Comparison of umbilical artery velocimetry and cardiotocography for surveillance of small for gestational age fetuses. *Lancet* **340**:936–940, 1992.
40. Doppler ultrasound in obstetrics. [Editorial.] *Lancet* **339**:1083–1084, 1992.
41. van Eyck J, Wladimiroff JW, Noordam MJ, Tonge HM & Prechtl HFR. The blood flow velocity waveform in the fetal descending aorta; its relationship to fetal behavioural states in normal pregnancy at 37–38 weeks. *Early Human Develop.* **12**:137–143, 1985.
42. van Eyck J, Wladimiroff JW, Noordam MJ, van den Wijngaard JAGW & Prechtl HFR. The blood flow velocity waveform in the fetal internal carotid and umbilical artery; its relationship to fetal behavioural states in normal pregnancy at 37–38 weeks of gestation. *Br. J. Obstet. Gynaecol.* **94**:736–741, 1987.
43. van Eyck J, Wladimiroff JW, Noordam MJ, Tonge HM & Prechtl HFR. The blood flow velocity waveform in the fetal descending aorta; its relationship to fetal behavioural states in the growth-retarded fetus at 37–38 weeks of gestation. *Early Human Develop.* **14**:99–107, 1986.
44. van Eyck J, Wladimiroff JW, Noordam MJ, van den Wijngaard JAGW & Prechtl HFR. The blood flow velocity waveform in the fetal internal carotid and umbilical artery; its relationship to fetal behavioural states in the growth retarded fetus at 37–38 weeks of gestation. *Br. J. Obstet. Gynaecol.* **95**:473–477, 1988.
45. Mulders LGM, Muysers GJJM, Jongsma HW, Nijhuis JG & Hein PR. The umbilical artery blood flow velocity waveform in relation to fetal breathing movements, fetal heart rate and fetal behavioural states in normal pregnancy at 37–39 weeks. *Early Human Develop* **11**:283–293, 1986.
46. Spencer JAD. Antepartum cardiotocography. In *Modern Antenatal Care of the Fetus* (ed. G. Chamberlain), pp. 163–188. Oxford: Blackwell Scientific Publications, 1990.
47. van Woerden EE & van Geijn HP. Heart-rate patterns and fetal movements. In *Fetal Behaviour. Developmental and Perinatal Aspects* (ed. J.G. Nijhuis), pp. 41–56. Oxford: Oxford University Press, 1992.
48. Nijhuis JG, Staisch KJ, Martin CB Jr & Prechtl HFR. A sinusoidal-like fetal heart-rate pattern in association with fetal sucking – report of 2 cases. *Eur. J. Obstet. Gynecol. Reprod. Biol.* **16**:353–358, 1984.
49. Nijhuis JG, Crevels AJ & van Dongen PWJ. Fetal brain death: the definition of a fetal heart rate pattern and its clinical consequences. *Obstet. Gynecol. Surv.* **46**:229–232, 1990.
50. Visser GHA, Ribbert LSM & Bekedam DJ. Sequential changes in Doppler waveform, fetal heart rate and movements patterns in IUGR fetuses. In *A Critical Appraisal of Fetal Surveillance* (eds H.P. Van Geijn & F.J.A. Copray), pp. 193–200. Amsterdam: Elsevier Science, 1994.
51. Nelson KB & Ellenberg JH. Intrapartum events and cerebral palsy. In *Prenatal Events and Brain Damage in Surviving Children* (ed. F.W. Kubli), pp. 139–148. Heidelberg: Springer-Verlag, 1988.
52. Freud S. Die infantile Cerebrallämung. In *Specielle Pathologie und Therapie* (ed. H. Nothnagel), pp. 1–327. Vienna: Holder, 1897.
53. Nijhuis JG & Tas BAPJ. Physiological and clinical aspects of the development of fetal behaviour. In *The Fetal and Neonatal Brainstem. Developmental and Clinical Issues* (ed. M.A. Hanson), pp. 268–281. Cambridge: Cambridge University Press, 1991.

The response of the fetal brain to asphyxia/ischaemia

21

A.J. Gunn and P.D. Gluckman

Introduction

The fetus is highly adapted to intrauterine conditions, which include low partial pressures of oxygen and relatively limited supply of other substrates compared with postnatal life. The compensatory mechanisms of the fetus may, however, be required to adapt to acutely compromised gas exchange or to chronic additional limitations of supply. It may be argued that every fetus is 'asphyxiated' in labour, in the formal sense that impaired uteroplacental gas exchange, with accumulation of metabolites and restriction of oxygen availability occurs. The response of the CNS helps determine whether this 'asphyxia' actually causes damage.

A seminal observation derived from *in vivo* and *in vitro* studies has been that although neurons may die during the actual ischaemic/asphyxial event (primary cell death), many neurons initially recover at least partially from the primary insult, only to die many hours, or even days later (secondary or delayed cell death). It was then shown *in vitro* that delayed cell death could be prevented by manipulation of the cell's biochemical environment, as discussed below. The effect of ischaemia on the supporting cells of the brain, the glia, has often been neglected. Although they are generally more resistant to ischaemia than neurons, they are still injured by many of the same factors, and with a relatively small increment in the severity of insults, infarction or pannecrosis, i.e. combined neuronal and glial death, may occur. Delayed glial death may also occur in a similar time course to neurons.

Recently, intensive research into the factors involved in cell death have made it clear that an acute event may activate both protective and damaging endogenous responses, many mediated by the glia. The acute response is modulated by the brain's maturity, metabolic status including temperature, and the severity, pattern and type of the insult[1]. Although the responses to hypoxia–ischaemia (which have been most closely studied) will be primarily discussed, similar principles apply to other acute metabolic derangements such as hypoglycaemia, and infections[2–8]. The response of the central nervous system (CNS) to chronic insults that do not cause any immediate damage, for example restriction of utero-placental blood flow[9], are poorly understood but may be quite different, and will be discussed separately.

PHASES OF CEREBRAL RESPONSE TO ISCHAEMIA/ASPHYXIA

There are two major types of hypoxic–ischaemic insult: transient (reversible) global insults and focal (usually permanent) insults[10]. After a reversible global insult several phases can be distinguished:

Primary phase. During the actual hypoxic–ischaemic insult itself.
Reperfusion phase. The immediate reperfusion – reoxygenation phase.
Latent phase. The interval between the reperfusion and secondary phases.
Delayed or secondary phase. The period of delayed cell death, often beginning between 6 and 12 hours after the insult, and lasting at least 72 hours.
Repair phase. After the acute perturbations resolve, healing and repair take place, with removal of cellular debris, remodelling and scar formation.

As will be discussed, the mechanisms involved in each of these phases are different, and are affected by the nature and severity of the injury. Naturally, the more severe the primary insult, the greater the proportion of cell death at this time[11]. Nevertheless, it is now clear that secondary damage accounts for a significant proportion of final cell loss even after very severe insults[12,13].

Biphasic CNS responses to transient hypoxia–ischaemia

Changes after varying periods of reversible global cerebral ischaemia and systemic asphyxia have been studied in the newborn piglet, fetal sheep and the rat. Magnetic resonance spectroscopy (MRS) has been used to measure cellular integrity. Although this technique cannot provide a continuous record of changes, it has provided direct evidence of secondary failure of energy metabolism (primarily mitochondrial function) in infants with moderate to severe encephalopathy. MRS was used to indirectly evaluate the relationship of ATP generation to consumption by measuring the ratio of phosphocreatine to inorganic orthophosphate (PCr/Pi)[14]. Thus, a relative fall in the amount of PCr suggests a failure of oxidative phosphorylation. Experimentally, in the newborn piglet subject to an hypoxic–ischaemic insult, the PCr/Pi ratio falls during the course of the hypoxia. After reoxygenation, the PCr/Pi ratio initially recovers, being normal at 8 h, only to fall again to very low levels by 24 h post-insult; the depth of the secondary fall correlates with apoptotic neuronal loss in the cingulate gyrus[14]. The same pattern of changes with time has been found in neonates with moderate-to-severe hypoxic–ischaemic encephalopathy (HIE); the PCr/Pi ratio after 24 h in infants is strongly correlated with the development of focal or generalised infarction, but also with neurodevelopmental outcome at one year of age[15], and four years.

Studies in the fetal sheep have emphasised continuous parasagittal parietal electroencephalographic (EEG) and impedance monitoring[12]. EEG intensity (power) reflects the amount of activity in large neurons (pyramidal cells) in the underlying cortex. Cortical impedance measurements, using a four-electrode technique, have been used to continuously estimate changes in extracellular space and intracellular volume. Since low-frequency currents are carried in the extracellular fluid, impedance rises during cytotoxic oedema, as fluid shifts from the extracellular to intracellular space reduce extracellular volume[16].

An example of the electrophysiological changes after a single 30-min episode of ischaemia is shown in Fig. 21.1. The EEG becomes isoelectric during the insult and remains suppressed for approximately 8 h after the insult, before there is a very abrupt increase in activity, corresponding with spike wave and poly-spike activity on the analogue EEG[11]. The seizures peak between 12 and 15 h and then resolve with no treatment, by approximately 36 h. Seizures rarely continue beyond 3 days. The EEG by 3 days is markedly suppressed compared with baseline but activity is returning, and between 3 and 5 days sleep state cycling can often be seen to be re-established, but at a severely reduced total intensity.

Corresponding with primary energy failure, there is an acute rise in cortical impedance, of approximately 100%, during the insult[12]. Even after the brain is reperfused, the impedance continues to rise for approximately 5 to 10 min, suggesting that it takes some time for the cells to re-establish membrane homeostasis, and also that there may be some ongoing injury[17]. The impedance then rapidly falls, and by 30-min post-insult has stabilised at only 10% higher than normal, and remains stable during the phase of suppression. A very large secondary rise, only slightly less in magnitude than that seen in the acute phase, begins hours after the onset of seizures, and also peaks much later, around 36 h post-insult, then gradually resolves by 3–4 days[12,18]. Microdialysis studies of amino acid neurotransmitter levels show a striking secondary rise in the excitotoxic index in parallel with the secondary rise in cortical impedance[19]. This suggests that post-ischaemic excitotoxicity is related primarily to membrane

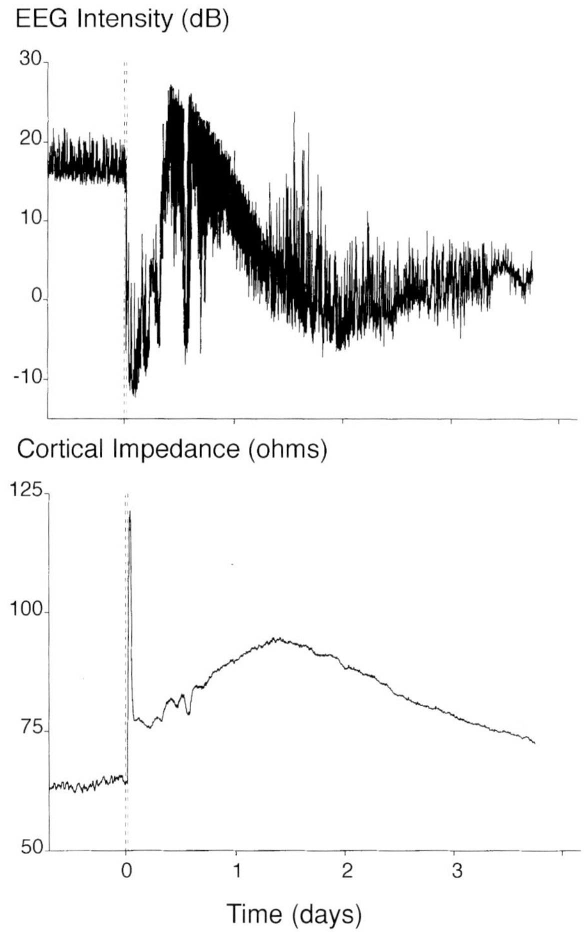

Fig. 21.1 An example of the changes in EEG intensity (top) and cortical impedance (bottom) after 30 min of cerebral ischaemia (vertical dashed lines), in fetal sheep[17,19]. Cortical impedance is a measure of cytotoxic or intracellular swelling. The two phases of injury are clearly seen: there is an initial rise in impedance during ischaemia which partially resolves during reperfusion. Then from ~ 9 h reperfusion there is a period of secondary EEG hyperactivity, which corresponds with tonic–clonic seizures, which peaks between 12 and 15 h. After the start of the delayed seizures, there is a secondary increase in impedance which peaks between 36 and 48 h before resolving.

dysfunction. Citrulline, a by-product of nitric oxide (NO) degradation, also increased after injury, consistent with increased production of NO during the secondary phase.

THE EFFECTS OF DURATION AND SEVERITY OF ISCHAEMIA ON CEREBRAL RESPONSES

Increasing duration of severe cerebral ischaemia in the fetal sheep leads to a stereotypic series of changes[11]. A minimal, 10-min insult leads to the acute changes in EEG and impedance discussed above. The EEG progressively recovers over about 6 h, with no secondary phase of hyperactivity; the impedance resolves fully with only minimal selective neuronal loss, mainly in the hippocampus and the parasagittal sulci. As the duration is increased, a progressively larger fraction of the fetuses demonstrate the pattern of delayed hyperactivity, and develop localised infarction in the parasagittal regions. After 40 min of ischaemia, the impedance remains substantially raised (>30% of baseline) shortly after the end of the acute insult. Although a secondary phase occurs, it is dramatically attenuated in amplitude compared with that seen after only 30 min of ischaemia. This suggests that over a critical threshold, much of the cerebral damage is occurring in the primary insult, with many fewer cells surviving to die in the secondary phase; global cortical infarction is seen after 3 days[11].

FOCAL INJURY

Focal hypoxic–ischaemic injury shows a different pattern of damage. Such insults, due to emboli, clots or other obstruction of a single artery (classically the middle cerebral artery) are usually not reversible. There is a dense ischaemic core in which primary cell death with pan-necrosis occurs. This core is surrounded by an ischaemic 'penumbra' which has some residual blood supply[20,21]. Damage tends to extend from the core out to the penumbra over a variable period of time[21]. The evolution of damage in the penumbra has been related to waves of depolarisation that may deplete cellular energetic reserves[22].

Mechanisms of injury after transient hypoxia–ischaemia

PRIMARY CELL LOSS

Cellular hypoxia leads to exhaustion of high-energy metabolites (primary energy failure) and depolarisation. *In vitro*, this can be tolerated for a remarkably long time[23,24], if the biochemical environment of the neurons is manipulated. Such studies suggest that three closely interrelated mechanisms are involved in the death of neurons during or following hypoxia–ischaemia.

Firstly, depolarisation due to hypoxia causes an influx of Na^+ and a lesser efflux of K^+ with passive Cl^- entry down the electrochemical gradient. This is turn favours further cation and water entry, leading to intracellular oedema. If sufficiently severe, this may cause immediate neuronal lysis[23]. Such swollen neurons can recover if the hypoxia is stopped or if the swelling is reduced by manipulating the osmotic environment[25].

Secondly, intracellular Ca^{2+} accumulation occurs due to both excessive entry of Ca^{2+}, due to activation of voltage-dependent and neurotransmitter-associated ion channels and also the failure during hypoxia of the energy-dependent processes of Ca^{2+} sequestration and removal by the Na^+–Ca^{2+} pump[24,26].

Thirdly, exposure to excitatory amino acids (EAAs), which are endogenous neurotransmitters, may cause both immediate swelling and lysis, by opening Na^+–K^+ channels[27], but also in lower concentrations increase calcium entry through specific NMDA (*N*-methyl-D-aspartate)-linked channels[24,28].

MEMBRANE INSTABILITY

Failure of energy-dependent Na^+ export, hypoxic depolarisation, and excitation of Na^+ conductances associated with non-NMDA receptors all lead to an increase in intracellular Na^+ and osmotic swelling. Associated with membrane lipid peroxidation due to free-radical production, this may lead to osmotic lysis. This appears to be a major component in severe primary injury. Agents such as GM_1 ganglioside and the lazaroids probably have their prime action by incorporating into the plasma membrane and thus providing stability/resistance to lipid peroxidation[29–32]. Thus they have not been consistently shown to be protective when used after the primary or reperfusion phases. GM_1 ganglioside is neuroprotective when given prior to or during hypoxic–ischaemic injury in the fetal sheep[33,34] but not when given more than 5 min post-insult in the adult rat[35].

REACTIVE CELL LOSS AND FREE RADICALS

Oxidative metabolism in the mitochondrial electron chain, as well as other oxidative–reductive reactions in the cytoplasm, normally produce oxygen free radicals (OFRs), i.e. an oxygen molecule that contains an uneven number of electrons in its outer orbit ($^{\cdot}O_2^-$). These species are highly reactive, and if not neutralised, can lead to degradation of cell membrane lipids (by peroxidation of the unsaturated fatty acids in the lipid bilayer). Part of the toxicity of excitatory amino acid release is mediated through OFR production, such that inhibition of lipid peroxidation also reduces glutamate toxicity[36]. The suggested sources of OFRs are shown in Fig. 21.2.

While the precise impact of OFRs remains controversial, there is increasing evidence that following hypoxia–ischaemia, they accumulate in excess of the metabolic capacity of endogenous scavenging systems[37–40], OFR exposure has been correlated with neuronal swelling[41] and impaired

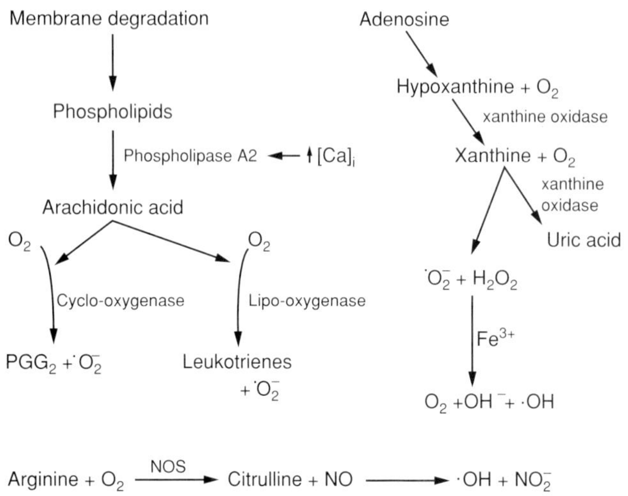

Fig. 21.2 Pathways leading to production of oxygen free radicals (OFRs). The metabolism of ATP during hypoxia leads to the accumulation of hypoxanthine. Activation of calpain by EAAs and calcium[333], favours conversion of the usual enzyme, xanthine dehydrogenase, to xanthine oxidase, which produces superoxide radicals as a byproduct of the metabolism of hypoxanthine to uric acid[334]. Thus inhibition of calpain activity may be protective for up to 6 h after reversible occlusion of the middle cerebral artery[68]. Similarly, the xanthine oxidase inhibitor, oxypurinol, reduces neuronal loss and nearly completely prevents OFR production during reperfusion[335]. Arachidonic acid, produced by EAA and calcium-mediated processes, is metabolised by cyclooxygenase to a variety of prostaglandins. The superoxide radicals produced by the cascade have been shown to promote lipid peroxidation, degrading the cell membrane[336]. Finally, activated neutrophils and macrophages produce large quantities of superoxide radicals and hydrogen peroxide following injury[336,337]. In particular, macrophages can produce nitric oxide (NO) in very concentrated bursts, that may mediate apoptosis[338,339].

cerebral metabolism[42,43]. Finally, OFR antagonists administered after hypoxia–ischaemia are neuroprotective both in immature[44,45] and adult brain[46,47].

CALCIUM

Increased intracellular Ca^{2+} levels, whether through specific neurotransmitter channels or just due to depolarisation and activation of voltage-dependent calcium channels, is an important mechanism mediating delayed cell death in neurons that recover from the acute swelling[24]. Under normal conditions, intracellular Ca^{2+} concentration is <0.1 μM, 10^{-4} times the extracellular Ca^{2+} concentration, with a variety of active mechanisms of Ca^{2+} removal which allow transient Ca^{2+} peaks to act as a signalling mechanism[48]. These mechanisms are disrupted by energy failure. *In vitro*, hypoxic neuronal death has been consistently shown to be greatly delayed by Ca^{2+} free media[24], while the intracellular injection of a calcium chelator reduced neuronal injury[49]. *In vivo*, microdialysis measurements have confirmed a fall in extracellular Ca^{2+} during hypoxia–ischaemia and a corresponding rise in cytosolic Ca^{2+} [50,51].

The contribution to pathological Ca^{2+} entry of excitatory neurotransmitter-linked channels relative to other sources such as the voltage-gated calcium channels[48], reverse operation of the Na^+–Ca^{2+} exchanger, Ca^{2+}-activated cation channels, stretch activated channels, intracellular endoplasmic reticulum release, simple membrane leaks, and failure of Ca^{2+} sequestration and removal[26], is unknown. While Ca^{2+} entry through neurotransmitter-associated channels is important[52], *in vitro*, where altered blood flow is not a factor, calcium antagonists, binding to receptors on the voltage-dependent channels, are protective against hypoxia[53–55], while calcium ionophores cause delayed neuronal death[56]. Furthermore, calcium-channel blockade has some anticonvulsant effects[57].

The excessive entry of Ca^{2+} is likely to continue until cellular homeostasis is restored[58]. Persisting elevation of resting intracellular Ca^{2+} levels after recovery from the acute insult has been linked to later delayed death[59]. The role of voltage-dependent Ca^{2+} entry however is probably mainly limited to the primary phase[60]. Voltage-dependent calcium-channel blockers such as flunarizine have been shown experimentally to confer some degree of neuroprotection. However while flunarizine clearly confers neuroprotection when given prior to hypoxic–ischaemic injury[61–64], it has no effect given immediately after injury[65] suggesting that calcium-channel activation is important in primary but not in secondary neuronal death. Other limitations to the use of such blockers include the cardiovascular compromise they generally induce, that may aggravate hypoperfusion during asphyxia[62].

Cytotoxins and calcium

A reciprocal relationship between oxygen free-radical production and calcium and excitatory amino acid production has been proposed. Oxygen free radicals increase glutamate release[66], while rising intracellular Ca^{2+} levels have been shown to uncouple mitochondrial electron transport, and so to promote free-radical production[67]. Calcium directly, or by inducing arachidonic acid production, induces a number of families of enzymes, such as protein kinase C, calpain, calmodulin regulated enzymes that may enhance excitatory synaptic efficiency, and circuit excitability[24]. Thus, for example, inhibition of calpain can reduce infarct volumes up to 6 h after reversible ischaemia in the rat[68]. Mechanisms of increased receptor stimulation include increased glutamate release[19], reduced reuptake by glial cells[19], increased postsynaptic response to depolarisation[69] and loss of inhibitory, mainly GABA, activity[70]. Perhaps more important than any change in receptor function may be impairment of glial regulation of ionic homeostasis[71]. Induction of the early response genes ('proto-oncogenes') has been proposed to promote this cascade[72].

EXCITOTOXINS

It has been strongly suggested that excitotoxins (the excitatory amino acid neurotransmitters, (EAAs)), particularly glutamate, play a key role in provoking this cascade of damaging events during hypoxia–ischaemia. *In vitro* and *in vivo*, glutamate and specific agonists to its receptors show dose-related toxicity[24]. Glutamate exposure is associated with extended neuronal depolarisation even after its removal *in vitro*, and reduced calmodulin binding, which tends to increase free intracellular calcium[73]. *In vitro*, mature cell cultures demonstrate trans-synaptic toxicity during hypoxia, which is blocked by antagonists to glutamate[74]. While the concentration of glutamate necessary to cause excitotoxic degeneration in immature cultures (in which synaptic connections have not yet been established) is very high (~1 mM)[75], the combination of excitotoxins with primary energy failure[76] dramatically potentiates glutamate toxicity such that only 10 μM is toxic. Such levels are consistently found during hypoxia–ischaemia *in vivo*, in adult animals[77–81]. The levels of EAAs begin to rise at a threshold of cerebral blood flow that is also associated with a fall in the amplitude of evoked potentials and of the EEG[82]. Finally, the protective effects of hypothermia are in some experimental paradigms closely correlated with reduced glutamate efflux[83].

The accumulation of excitotoxins cannot explain regional susceptibility, however, since similar rises are found throughout the brain, including regions spared from damage[84]. It has been suggested that susceptible neurons and regions have relatively high EAA afferents and receptors[23]. Thus, for example, the hippocampus is protected by lesioning of excitatory neural projections[85]. In the immature rat and human there is transient dense innervation of the basal ganglia with glutaminergic pathways[86], which correlates with increased damage due to exogenous excitotoxin exposure[87,88].

In any case, such a pivotal role for glutamate in the primary phase has not been established in the developing brain. No rise was found in the hippocampus of the neonatal rat[89], and modest rises, to levels much lower than seen in the adult brain, have been reported during systemic asphyxia[90] or cerebral ischaemia in the near-term fetal lamb[19]. This acute accumulation of excitotoxins was accompanied by a disproportionate rise in inhibitory neurotransmitters, as shown in Fig. 21.3[19]. In contrast, during the secondary phase there was a marked surge in excitatory transmitters which paralleled secondary cytotoxic oedema[19]. There is also some evidence to suggest greater injury of inhibitory neurons in the primary phase which may contribute to the loss of suppression of excitatory neurons in the secondary phase[91,92].

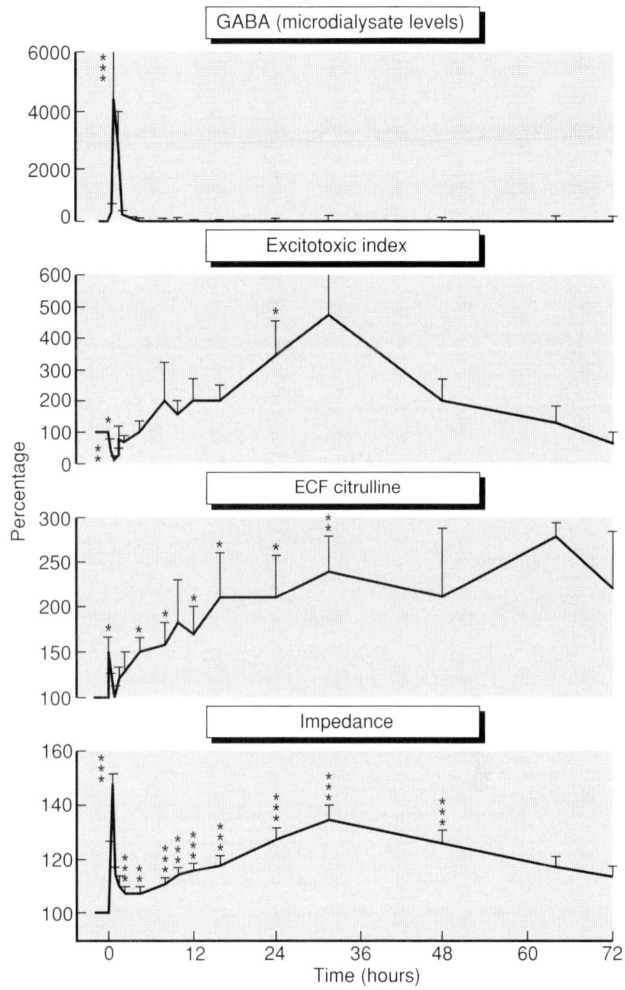

Fig. 21.3 The time course of changes in extracellular levels of amino acids within the parasagittal parietal cortex, measured by microdialysis, during and for 3 days after 30 min of cerebral ischaemia, in nine chronically instrumented near-term fetal sheep (119–133 days). Changes are related to changes in cortical impedance (bottom). Amino acid concentrations were measured using HPLC. During ischaemia, citrulline (byproduct of NO synthesis), glutamate, glycine, and gamma-aminobutyric acid (GABA) concentrations rose to 147 ± 18%, 180 ± 20%, 290 ± 50% and 4800 ± 1300% of baseline respectively (p <0.05). The excitotoxic index ([glutamate] × [glycine]/[GABA]) decreased to 15 ± 8%. Upon reperfusion, the cytotoxic oedema and amino acid accumulation largely resolved within 1 h, and the EEG was depressed. Citrulline began to rise again by 4 h (p <0.05), reaching a maximum (273 ± 21%) at 32 ± 2 h. Seizure activity developed at 7 ± 2 h, and impedance plus the excitotoxic index then rose progressively and peaked at 32 ± 2 h (480 ± 170%). At 72 h, there was severe neuronal loss and laminar necrosis within the parasagittal cortex. These data suggest that, several hours after a severe ischemic injury, NO synthesis increased, then seizures arose, and oedema developed concomitantly with the accumulation of excitotoxins. Data derived from Tan *et al.*[19].

SUBTYPES OF POSTSYNAPTIC GLUTAMATE RECEPTOR

Classically there were thought to be three types of glutamate receptor, each named for selective agonists. The NMDA receptor, which associated with a calcium channel, is involved in long-term potentiation and plasticity[93]. The two non-NMDA-mediated receptors, kainate and quisqualate, appear to mediate most of the fast synaptic transmission in the brain, through specific Na^+–K^+ channels[94]. Glutamate appears to exert neurotoxic effects via both NMDA and non-NMDA (particularly α-amino-3-hydroxy-5-methyl-3-isoxazole propionate (AMPA))-type receptors. Post-asphyxial seizures can be wholly blocked by the NMDA-receptor antagonist, MK-801[95]. While there is some neuroprotective effect of MK-801 when given after hypoxia–ischaemia[95–97], it is far less effective than when administered during the primary phase[98–101].

There are important developmental differences in the expression of the receptors[87,88]. In 7-day old rats, agonist responses follow the following hierarchy: NMDA ≥ quisqualic acid ≥ kainic acid. In adult rats the agonist responses follow a different pattern: kainic acid ≥ NMDA ≥ quisqualic acid[87]. Other investigators have emphasized however, that glutamate receptor expression does not become significant until relatively late in development, at the equivalent of 26 to 28 weeks' gestation in man. Thus, interventions designed to manipulate the glutamate receptor had no effect prior to this developmental stage[88,102].

NMDA RECEPTOR

Although activation of all three receptors can cause neuronal death during prolonged or sufficiently intense exposure, the NMDA receptor was originally suggested to have a singular role in causing Ca^{2+} entry and delayed neuronal death after even brief exposures *in vitro*[103]. This was supported by the protective effect of its selective antagonists, such as MK-801 *in vitro*, while *in vivo* NMDA agonists caused a pattern of selective neuronal loss that most closely matched that seen in ischaemia, sparing NADPH-diaphorase, somatostatin, vasointestinal peptide and cholecystokinin expressing inhibitory neurons[104,105]. Furthermore, MK-801, a highly potent and selective NMDA antagonist, appeared to reduce damage up to 24 h after brief ischaemia in the gerbil[106]. Recent experiments, however, have called these results into question. Studies of MK-801 in dense forebrain ischaemia, in adult species, have suggested that the protective effect seen in earlier studies was either wholly due to[107,108], or at least greatly augmented by hypothermia[109,110]. Indeed, selective non-NMDA antagonists may be more effective in this situation[111]. Moreover when regional protective effects were seen, the hippocampus appears to benefit less than the caudate nucleus[112], despite its high NMDA input.

Several factors may explain the discrepancy between the predominant NMDA and calcium-mediated role *in vitro*, and the relatively disappointing effects of selective NMDA antagonists in therapeutic trials. Some reported discrepancies are quite specific. NMDA antagonists appear to be relatively more efficacious in immature animals, in focal rather than global insults, or in incompletely ischaemic regions in global ischaemia, and in hypoglycaemia[113,114]. *In vitro*, NMDA activity is progressively impaired by acidosis with a progressive reduction in EAA neurotoxicity and hypoxia-mediated Ca^{2+} accumulation, and prolonged cell survival[115–117]. These data suggest that selective NMDA effects should be more important in regions of partial oxygenation and milder acidosis, such as is found in the penumbra of a stroke.

Non-NMDA glutamate receptors

Recently two novel features of the non-NMDA receptor system have been clarified (Fig. 21.2). Some subtypes of the kainic acid (KA) receptor have very high calcium conductance; this appears to be developmentally regulated in some regions, with greater expression in early life, possibly to modulate plasticity[118]. Quisqualate, on the other hand, acts on two separate receptors: the (fast) AMPA channel[74], and also via G-proteins to activate phospholipase C via the family of 'metabotrophic' receptors[27]. In high concentration, it may also activate NMDA receptors. Activation of the metabotrophic receptors increases hydrolysis of membrane phosphoinositides, producing diacylglycerol and inositol, and blocks glutamate excitatory synaptic transmission. This action, together with far greater expression in early development, suggests that they may be involved in long-term potentiation of glutamate synapses and synaptic plasticity. During ischaemia, however, excitation may be increased: the inositol may release intracellular Ca^{2+}, while the diacylglycerol acts as a primary substrate for the production of arachidonic acid. Arachidonic acid in turn promotes accumulation of glutamate by inhibiting re-uptake by astrocytes[119,120].

In vitro, intense or prolonged stimulation of each receptor can produce neuronal degeneration[74]. Immediate swelling is greatest with KA stimulation and least with AMPA and NMDA, but brief NMDA exposure caused the greatest late degeneration. The quinoxalines, such as CNQX (6 cyano-7-nitroquinoxaline-2,3-dione), show greater selectivity against the AMPA receptor, with lesser KA antagonism, but also some reduction of NMDA toxicity. Thus, post-insult protection in the rat with such agents, but not pure NMDA antagonists[111], does not rule out indirect NMDA-mediated effects. Further supporting evidence for specific role for excessive calcium entry comes from the marked augmentation of protection by NMDA antagonists following brief ischaemia provided by combination therapy with calcium-channel antagonists[121,122].

OTHER NEUROTRANSMITTER SYSTEMS

Other excitatory neurotransmitters have been implicated in the secondary phase. For example, there is a marked rise in the excitatory transmitter dopamine in the striatum during hypoxia–ischaemia[80], most of which is derived from the substantia nigra. Lesions of the substantia nigra reduce striatal injury following cerebral ischaemia[123]. These systems are of course, not isolated; there is evidence for glutaminergic stimulation of dopamine release[124], and for its inhibition by calcium antagonists *in vitro*[125]. Conversely, lesions of the inhibitory noradrenergic projections from the locus coeruleus increase damage in CA1 and the cortex[126].

SECONDARY CELL LOSS

MORPHOLOGY OF SECONDARY CELL DEATH

Microscopic studies demonstrated over a decade ago that some neurons surviving the primary phase apparently lose viability from 2 to even 72 h after the insult in adult[127,128] and immature animals[13,14], and for at least a week after cardiac arrest in man[129]. Two morphological patterns of cell death have been defined – necrosis and apoptosis[13,130]. Both may be precipitated by exposure to excitotoxins[131]. Necrosis is defined by loss of plasma membrane integrity associated with a random pattern of DNA degradation. Typically, there is swelling of the cytoplasm and organelles, with little change initially to the nucleus. Apoptosis is defined by shrinkage of the cell, 'karyorrhexis', associated with specific endonuclease mediated DNA degradation. Eventually the shrunken cell breaks into small fragments. Karyorrhexis is the classic microscopic picture of condensation of chromatin (i.e. a dark shrunken nucleus) with loss of the reticular formation in the cytoplasm (leading to eosinophilia on light microscopy). The active degradation of DNA by endonucleases which cleave the chromatin at internucleosomal points, leads to fragments of fixed size, with a characteristic laddering appearance on chromatography[132]. The terminal deoxynucleotidyl-transferase (TdT)-mediated dUTP-biotin nick end-labelling (TUNEL) technique has also been used to identify DNA cut by endonucleases *in situ*[133–135].

By analogy with the active process of developmental loss of excess cells, including neurons[130,136], it is suggested that an apoptotic morphology reflects active cell death, involving a cascade of 'suicide' processes[13,137–139]. In contrast, necrosis is suggested to reflect biophysical processes (cell-membrane instability, ion shifts, etc.), particularly lysis in the primary phase[13,140] Excitotoxic neuronal death, however, appears to be associated with a continuum of overlapping apoptotic and necrotic cell death, modulated by maturity and involvement of different glutamate-receptor subtypes[141]. There is, still controversial, evidence that apoptosis can be dependent on *de novo* protein synthesis or expression of inducible transcription factors[142–144], suggesting that it is due to a cell-death programme. Other studies however, suggest that apoptosis may occur or be prevented independent of RNA transcription[145,146]. Furthermore, *in vitro*, slowly evolving cell death triggered by excitotoxicity can occur by necrosis[147].

The concept remains an important one, since if neuronal and glial cell death is an active response, mediated by activation of second and third messenger events after an acute insult, (whether really due to a preset 'death programme' or to less specific pathways initiated by excess free Ca^{2+} and/or cytotoxins), then it should logically be possible to interrupt these events. This possibility of a 'therapeutic window' in time after an insult has driven much recent research. The balance of endogenous protective responses and cytotoxic events such as Ca^{2+} entry, oxygen free radicals and the excitotoxins, seizures, and cell swelling would then determine outcome.

APOPTOSIS VS. NECROSIS AFTER HYPOXIA–ISCHAEMIA

The balance of necrotic and apoptotic cell death has been studied using the modified 'Levine' model of carotid ligation, combined with a fixed period of hypoxia. In the immature rat, a mild insult (15 min of hypoxia) was associated with the progressive appearance of selective neuronal loss, in an apoptotic morphology, from 24 h[13]. In contrast, a severe insult (60 min of hypoxia) was associated with the massive death of neurons and glia with only a necrotic morphology (pannecrosis) between 10 and 24 h afterwards[13]. In the newborn piglet, a similar experimental approach results in moderate cortical selective death 48 h later, preponderantly with an apoptotic morphology[14]. The amount of apoptotic cell death correlated with the degree of energy failure as measured by MRS[14]. Interestingly, mild hypothermia after hypoxia is reported to reduce the number of apoptotic but not necrotic cells[148]. In adult rodent studies of focal injury, cell death in the penumbra of the infarct is reported to be predominantly apoptotic[134,149].

BIOCHEMISTRY OF APOPTOSIS

bcl-2 is one of a large family of genes that regulates homeostatic mechanisms during development and adult life[150]. In mammals, expression of the *bcl-2* gene can often inhibit apoptosis, whereas in the nematode *Caenorhabditis elegans* apoptosis is regulated by a mechanism controlled by the *ced-9* gene[151]. Since the human *bcl-2* gene can prevent cell deaths in *C. elegans*, this suggests that *bcl-2* and *ced-9* are homologous[151]. Thus, for example cells deprived of growth factor exhibit changes characteristic of apoptosis, such as DNA degradation; *bcl-2* expression protects these cells from factor withdrawal although not from cytotoxic T-cell killing. DNA degradation is therefore not specific to any one cell-death mechanism. Furthermore, *bcl-2* can protect cells from a wide variety of pathological, as well as physiological, events, suggesting that many triggers can activate the same suicide pathway, even some thought to cause necrosis, and not apoptosis. In contrast, other genes such as *bax* and *bcl-x* promote apoptosis[150]. The activation of a number of other immediate-early genes such as c-*myc* also appear to modulate the appearance of apoptosis[152]. The mechanism of action of these factors is unclear, however the bcl-2 protein acts in an antioxidant metabolic pathway, as well as modulating intracellular Ca^{2+} fluxes[150].

MICROGLIAL ACTIVATION

Activation of the microglia, the endogenous tissue scavenger cells, is closely related in time to apoptotic cell death after hypoxia–ischaemia, and have thus been proposed to contribute to cerebral damage[13,153]. Activated microglia express a number of cytotoxic cytokines such as tumour necrosis factor-α (TNFα) and also the cytotoxic radicals NO and H_2O_2; this response has probably evolved as a protective response to viral and bacterial infection at the cost of retaining a potential neurotoxic role[154]. Detailed studies *in vitro*, however, make it clear that activated microglia produce cell-survival factors as well as neurotoxins[155,156], although they may tend to promote astrocytic proliferation at the expense of neuronal survival[155]. Several of the putative inhibitors of microglial activation (e.g. transforming growth factor-β (TGFβ) may be neuroprotective or injurious depending on the extracellular levels[157,158].

Endogenous protective mechanisms

At least four potential endogenous protective systems exist, including neuromodulators/inhibitory neurotransmitters, cellular factors, neurotrophins and cerebral cooling. Additionally, as discussed separately, the cerebrovascular responses to asphyxia are clearly protective, since they tend to maintain preferential oxygen delivery to 'central' organs such as the brain and heart. As a strong illustration of the potential protective effects of endogenous responses, a single, subthreshold period of hypoxia or ischaemia or even heating, that does not cause damage, may markedly increase resistance to a subsequent more severe insult[159–161]. Both the intensity and, even more importantly, the timing of the preconditioning insult have to be quite precise – approximately 24 h – for this to occur, and after peaking the effect is rapidly attenuated by time. The mechanism is uncertain, but may be related to induction of anti-apoptotic genes such as *bcl*[162], growth factors such as fibroblast growth factor[163], free radical scavengers[164], adenosine or heat shock proteins[165].

NEUROMODULATORS

GABA

Inhibitory neuromodulators such as GABA and adenosine reduce cerebral metabolic demand by reducing neural activity and antagonise the excitotoxic responses[166]. Microdialysis experiments in the fetal lamb suggest although this response is very large during the primary phase, there is a rapid fall during the subsequent latent period, and no significant rise during the secondary phase[19]. This may be one factor determining the timing of the onset of the secondary phase of injury. Adult species such as the turtle that are very tolerant to hypoxia, show a similarly elevated GABA response to anoxia, which is suggested to reduce cerebral energy consumption[167]. Consistent with this, GABAergic agonists have been shown to have neuroprotective properties during ischaemia, both alone and in combination with NMDA antagonists[168,169].

ADENOSINE

The most clearly delineated inhibitory neurotransmitter system is that of adenosine, which is also massively increased after ischaemia[170]. Adenosine A1 (and A3) receptors on neurons are inhibitory and analogues binding to this site reduce glutamate release, while the A2 receptor primarily mediates local vasodilation[166,171]. In the late gestation fetal sheep, increased tissue adenosine levels were associated with improved cardiovascular adaptation to asphyxia, possibly due to improved cardiac perfusion[172]. Increased adenosine expression following asphyxia may cause some of the post asphyxia CNS depression seen in infants[173]. There is evidence that endogenous adenosine has a significant role in the brain after hypoxia–ischaemia, since theophylline, an adenosine antagonist, worsens delayed neuronal death when given post-insult[174]. Pretreatment with long-acting analogues of adenosine, or up-regulation of adenosine receptors has been reported to reduce neuronal loss, in some[174–176] but not all studies[166]. Rescue therapy was not effective[177].

ENDOGENOUS OPIOIDS

The κ-opioid system is one of the many subtypes of opiate receptors in the brain with diuretic, vasoconstrictor and neuromodulatory actions[178,179], which shows a large increase in activity after ischaemia[180]. Agents that selectively stimulate this system have been reported to reduce delayed neuronal death after brief ischaemia[179,181], but confusingly opiate antagonists have also been suggested to be protective[182–184]. Whether these contradictory effects are related to a reduction in acute neuronal swelling by osmotic effects or to a more direct receptor-mediated protection is not known. A non-specific opiate, dextromethorphan, that also has weak NMDA-antagonist actions[185], is also reported to be protective after ischaemia[186,187].

CELLULAR FACTORS

Biochemical responses within neurons may also help reduce damage after hypoxia–ischaemia. Increased expression of anti-apoptotic proteins such as *bcl-2* after subthreshold ischaemia may be important, as above[162]. A further potential modality is the transient increase in the expression of the calcium-binding protein calbindin D28k after ischaemia[188]. This response is postulated to buffer the increased free Ca^{2+} in neurons. A significant protective role for calbindin is supported by the differential expression of calbindin across different neuronal populations. Cell populations such as mature granule cells in the dentate gyrus of the hippocampus, and elsewhere, that are very resistant to ischaemic injury, express high levels of calbindin[189,190]. In their immature state, these cells do not express calbindin, and are as susceptible to ischaemia as other populations[189]; however, other groups have suggested that the developmental changes in selective neuronal death and of calbindin expression are distinct[191]. Finally, the neuroprotective actions of some neurotrophic factors have been related to induction of calbindin expression, supporting the concept that part of their action is mediated by stabilising calcium homeostasis[192–194].

NEUROTROPHIC FACTORS

While the observation that the brain enhances neurotrophic activity (defined by the ability to support neuronal survival *in vitro*) after injury is old[195], the neurotrophins involved have only recently been identified. Extensive studies have been performed in the 'Levine' model of unilateral hypoxic–ischaemic injury in the immature rat. These studies suggest that there are two phases of neurotrophin production after hypoxic–ischaemic injury. There is minimal induction, shortly after the end of hypoxia, of mRNAs coding for members of the early-immediate genes (*c-fos*, *c-jun*) and the nerve growth factor family (NGFβ, BDNF, NT3). Such induction is restricted to the hippocampus of the non-injured side and has been shown to be induced by post-asphyxial seizures rather than hypoxia itself[196].

Broader-spectrum growth factors, however, are induced intensely and for prolonged periods after hypoxia–ischaemia. Most attention has focused on insulin-like growth factor-1 (IGF-1) which has been shown to block developmental apoptosis for motoneurons *in vivo*[197], and experimental apoptosis in cerebellar granule cells *in vitro*[146]. After injury, IGF-1 mRNA is induced by injured glia in a dose-related manner, and reaches maximum levels 3–5 days after injury[198,199]. In an electrolytic damage model, enhanced IGF-1 release has been found in microdialysate several days after injury[200]. Two of the IGF-binding proteins (IGFBP), IGFBP-2 and IGFBP-3 are also induced early after injury[201]. In contrast, IGF-2 and IGFBP-5 are not induced until 3–10 days after injury, presumably as part of wound-repair mechanisms[202,203].

The implications of these data are unclear. The timing of IGF-1 expression would suggest that it and other neurotrophins with a broad spectrum of activity, are involved in the healing/repair phase rather than the earlier stages. The binding proteins may perhaps act to localise IGF-1 in the brain. In view of its potent anti-apoptotic effects, the effect of exogenous IGF-1 has been tested. In both the adult rat, and the fetal lamb, a single dose of intraventricular IGF-1 was associated with reduced secondary neuronal death[204,205]; in the rat, cortical infarction was reduced, while in the lamb partial cortical protection was obtained, with reduced seizure activity, and improved recovery of EEG activity. Interestingly, pretreatment with IGF-1 actually worsened damage[205], consistent with recent *in vitro* studies of other neurotrophins[206].

H^3-IGF-1 studies show that exogenous IGF-1 is rapidly transported via the perivascular space to the region where neurons are destined to die[207] – this specific localisation may be a result of early induction of IGFBP-2[201]. An analogue of IGF-1 with low affinity for the IGF-1 receptor is markedly less potent[208]: in the brain a protease cleaves IGF-1 at its N-terminal to produce a tripeptide glycine-proline-glutamate (GPE) and des(1–3)-IGF-1. Des(1–3)-IGF-1 is fully active at the IGF-1 receptor but has low affinity for IGFBPs. Des(1–3)-IGF-1 was protective at high dose only, confirming that protection is mediated by neuronal IGF-1 receptor activation[208]. However, at equimolar doses to IGF-1, GPE is also protective[209]. What receptor mediates the action of GPE is unclear – it may be a glutamate receptor subtype but the protective action was not mimicked by treatment with MK-801.

Basic fibroblast growth factor (bFGF) is also induced after injury but in a more limited manner and is reported to be neuroprotective in some[210–212], but not all studies[213]. There is one report suggesting its actions are mediated by IGF-1 induction[214]. Finally, TGFβ and activin are two members of a large evolutionarily related family of growth factors and are induced after injury[215–217]. $TGFβ_1$ also may reduce delayed neuronal death at appropriate doses[158], but it is not clear whether it is acting as a trophic factor or to inhibit microglial activation[157]. *In vitro* it directly antagonises excitotoxic injury[157].

HYPOTHERMIA

The protective effect of even a few degrees of hypothermia during hypoxia–ischaemia is well known[218]. Early studies of the effect of cerebral hypothermia after hypoxia–ischaemia had equivocal results, probably because of the focus on relatively brief early cooling. The key, interrelated factors that are now thought to determine the effectiveness or otherwise of rescue hypothermia, are the severity of the insult, the delay after reperfusion, the depth of hypothermia attained, and the duration of therapy. Even 1 to 2°C of cerebral hypo- or hyperthermia during or following the insult may modulate cerebral outcome[219–221]. Although 5 h of moderate hypothermia (32.5°C), initiated under anaesthesia in adult rats, is reported to reduce delayed neuronal death when started up to 12 h after brief ischaemia, the effectiveness of cooling declined markedly as the start of cooling was delayed beyond 2 h[222]. Similarly, after brief ischaemia in gerbils 12 h of moderate hypothermia reduced selective neuronal loss when started after 1 h[223,224] but not 3 h[223]. Critically, when the insult was made slightly more severe, the duration of hypothermia had to be extended from 12 h to 24 h to provide neuroprotection[224].

Although the exact period of cooling necessary is still unclear, the published data as a whole are consistent with the hypothesis that hypothermia is most effective when continued until the end of the phase of membrane instability – shorter periods of hypothermia may merely have the effect of delaying injury[225]. Thus, when (2–3°C) mild cerebral cooling, started immediately after injury, was continued through the entire secondary phase (3 days), this prevented the evolution of cortical infarction in the infant rat[226]. Cooling delayed until 6 h post-insult or 6 h of cooling started immediately were ineffective. Data have recently been presented suggesting that moderate cerebral hypothermia starting 90 min and continued for 72 h after severe cerebral hypoperfusion in the fetal sheep was able to abolish secondary cytotoxic oedema with a corresponding reduction in secondary neuronal loss[17].

HEAD TEMPERATURE AFTER BIRTH

These data, which highlight the importance of even small, clinically relevant changes in cerebral temperature, clearly suggest that the physiological cooling at birth (core temperature falls from ~37.5°C to 36.5–37°C after delivery) may be an important natural protective process. The effect of this normal change is increased in infants nursed in cots by a gradient between core temperature and that of the surface of the brain. This gradient increases cerebral cooling after birth[227]. This may be important, since infant-care practices such as nursing asphyxiated infants under an overhead heater may adversely affect the normal gradient between core temperature and the brain[228]. The major problem facing the therapeutic use of hypothermia, however, is to identify a sufficiently safe approach, as prolonged systemic hypothermia is associated with a number of potential adverse effects[229,230].

MECHANISMS OF HYPOTHERMIA

The mechanisms of hypothermic protection are still unclear. In principle, hypothermia might work by (i) reducing cellular metabolic demands, and so delaying neuronal depolarisation, (ii) reducing the excessive accumulation of excitotoxins such as glutamate, and so reducing intracellular Ca^{2+} accumulation or (iii) suppressing the toxic consequences of these events, such as activation of endonucleases or production of oxygen free radicals. Hypothermia produces a graded reduction in cerebral metabolic rate[231], of approximately 5.3% per 1°C, allowing high-energy metabolites to be maintained at blood flows significantly below the critical normothermic threshold for ischaemia[232]. Interestingly, however, direct comparison suggests that for similar reductions in metabolic rate, hypothermia delays neuronal depolarisation significantly more than general anaesthesia, suggesting that suppression of metabolism alone cannot explain all of its immediate cerebral effects[233].

The well-known rise in excitotoxins during ischaemia is consistently suppressed by mild-to-moderate hypothermia, both *in vitro*[234] and *in vivo*[77,83]. This mechanism, however, cannot account for all neuroprotective effects, since moderate hypothermia had no effect on the rise in excitotoxins after head injury in the rat[235], and yet markedly reduced subsequent damage. Consistent with this, *in vitro* hypothermia does not reduce glutamate receptor activity, or its toxic effects[234,236]. In contrast, prolonged hypothermia applied after the excitotoxins have been washed out of the culture media, is protective[234,237]. Furthermore, hypothermia during cardiac arrest in the rat prolongs anoxic depolarisation, despite having no effect on the acute transfer of Ca^{2+} from extracellular fluid into cells[51].

In summary, although it is likely that all of these effects of hypothermia are important, particularly in reducing damage in the primary phase, the effects of hypothermia in the secondary phase are likely to be mediated by a reduction in adverse changes in second or third messengers and in the production of other cytotoxic agents such as oxygen free radicals[83,238,239], rather than just reducing neurotransmitter release.

Responses of the whole brain to hypoxia–ischaemia

POST-ASPHYXIAL SEIZURES

Early studies of delayed neuronal death in the CA1 region following brief ischaemia suggested that this was associated with transient, delayed overactivity prior to the death of the neurons[240]. This was an attractive hypothesis, because it suggested that anticonvulsants in general and specific EAA antagonists in particular might be protective during this phase. However, while enhanced post-synaptic potentials have been reported which may mediate excessive calcium entry, there appears to be a progressive decrease in neuronal excitability[241]. Other recent studies of direct field potential recordings, both *in vivo*[242], and in hippocampal slices taken following brief ischaemia[243], found no phase of hyperexcitability. Instead, there was initial profound suppression followed by nearly complete recovery of function by 24 h, then an abrupt deterioration during the second day post-ischaemia, with nearly complete failure by day 3 or 4. Similarly, no cortical seizures were recorded after global ischaemia in the gerbil[244]. These studies suggest that early persistent depolarisation, which in hippocampal slices can be blocked by reducing Ca^{2+} levels in the media, may in fact be a better marker for later degeneration[245]. The period of post-asphyxial CNS depression (which may or may not precede seizures as below) is also, at least in part, related to the release of inhibitory neuromodulators such as serotonin[246] or adenosine[170].

Following more severe insults, however, post-asphyxial seizures often do occur in adult[247] and immature species[248]; such seizures are clinically associated with a poor outcome[249]. Status epilepticus *per se* may cause cerebral injury or death by causing an excessive increase in local metabolism despite adequate global oxygenation[250,251]. The benefits of treating delayed seizures due to hypoxia–ischaemia however remains equivocal. In the adult rat after severe ischaemia, diazepam reduced seizures and damage[247]. In the fetal sheep, low-dose therapy with a specific NMDA antagonist completely abolished delayed post-ischaemic seizures, with no change in the severe parasagittal cortical damage, but a reduction in hippocampal and temporal lobe damage[95]. These data suggest that the seizures were NMDA dependent and were primarily an effect of cortical damage rather than its cause. Barbiturates were amongst the first putative neuroprotective agents to be considered. Recent studies suggest that they may indeed be protective within 40 min following brief ischaemia in the gerbil[252,253], but that high doses exacerbate damage[252]. Finally, excessive suppression of seizures may impair functional recovery, as discussed below; the optimal balance remains unclear[254].

CEREBROVASCULAR CHANGES AFTER HYPOPERFUSION INJURY

The changes in cerebral blood flow after an insult are complex. Many investigators have noted that cerebral blood flow

(CBF) may be severely depressed after an ischaemic or asphyxial episode for many hours, and have postulated that this is in itself one cause of ongoing cerebral damage[255]. More recent data suggest that the reduction in CBF is coupled to depressed neuronal activity[256], and is not the cause of cerebral depression; reversing it with vasodilators has not been shown to be consistently beneficial[257,258]. In studies in adult rodents, the briefest period of ischaemia that causes neuronal depolarisation but no cell death at all is followed by transient hyperperfusion, and then by hypoperfusion[255,259]. As the duration of ischaemia is increased the hypoperfusion begins earlier but is usually not significantly more severe or longer; eventually, it begins nearly immediately after the insult. During this phase of hypoperfusion, which appears to correspond with the latent phase, as discussed above, the brain is more vulnerable to a second insult (see patterns of damage below)[260].

Recent cerebrovascular studies after cerebral ischaemia in fetal sheep suggest a similar pattern. Near infrared spectroscopy (NIRS) is a novel technique whereby changes in oxy- and deoxyhaemoglobin and the mitochondrial oxidative enzyme cytochrome a_3 may be followed in asphyxiated infants[261]. A rise in total haemoglobin suggests vasodilation. After severe cerebral ischaemia in the fetal lamb, NIRS measurements suggest that secondary vasodilation occurs, in parallel with cytotoxic oedema[18]. After resolution of seizures, there was an inverse relationship between total haemoglobin and neuronal damage, suggesting that greater damage was associated with reduced blood flow. Finally, these data suggested a fall in cytochrome a_3 during the secondary phase, consistent with mitochondrial failure at this time. Similar changes have been seen in small studies of infants with moderate to severe HIE[261,262].

The combination of secondary vasodilation, and hyperperfusion, with increased NO production in the secondary phase, suggested that perhaps this association was pathogenic. When the competitive antagonist of NO production, L-NNMA, was given, the secondary vasodilation was attenuated[263]. This effect was, however, associated with a trend to increased neuronal loss. It is not clear whether this was related to the perturbation in blood supply or to the local and microglial roles of NO.

Pathophysiological determinants of injury after systemic asphyxia

CARDIOVASCULAR AND CEREBROVASCULAR RESPONSES

Most of the above studies contributing to our understanding of the general and cellular responses of the brain were functional, i.e. they concentrated on producing cerebral injury, by either pure hypoperfusion, or the combination of inhalational hypoxia with partial hypoperfusion. Pathophysiological studies, however, have focused on reproducing the more realistic systemic asphyxia, to examine the mechanisms leading up to cerebral injury. As such, they are associated with greater or lesser cardiac compromise, and a greater mortality. Such studies have strongly suggested that the key factor precipitating cerebral damage is hypotension, and the consequent compromise of cerebral oxygen delivery[264–267].

The cardiovascular and cerebrovascular adaptations to relatively prolonged episodes of asphyxia in the normally grown fetus have been extensively studied; the mechanisms involved in adaptation to clinically relevant brief repeated asphyxia are likely to be similar but have not been adequately addressed. Initially, with mild-to-moderate asphyxia/hypoxia, there is usually a moderate transient bradycardia followed by a tachycardia. There is a rise in blood pressure and a redistribution of combined ventricular output which leads to an increase in blood flow to vital organs, the brain, heart and adrenals, at the expense of peripheral organs[268]. Oxygen consumption is little changed even if arterial oxygen content falls as low as 1 mmol/l thanks to compensating increases in cerebral blood flow (CBF) and oxygen extraction[269–271].

During acute severe asphyxia, the cardiovascular responses of the normal fetus are substantially different. Bradycardia is sustained and centralisation of the fetal circulation no longer occurs, although within the brain, blood flow is preferentially redirected to the brainstem to maintain autonomic function at the expense of such areas as the cerebrum[272]. When arterial oxygen content falls below 1 mmol/l, cerebral blood flow fails to rise due to a significant rise in cerebral vascular resistance. The fetus is unable to extract further oxygen and cerebral oxygen consumption falls[273]. During this insult, blood pressure initially increases markedly but this rise is not sustained and as asphyxia proceeds, the fetus becomes severely hypotensive, with a parallel fall in CBF[274].

The sustained bradycardia and increased peripheral resistance in the late gestation fetus are mediated by the carotid chemoreceptors; a logarithmic rise in catecholamine levels further augments the peripheral vasoconstriction[275]. The late hypotension is primarily related to impairment of myocardial contractility[276]. Studies of hypoxia in adult species have related this reduced contractility to depletion of high-energy metabolites such as ATP in mitochondria[277], but other factors such as profound acidosis[278] and depletion of myocardial glycogen stores are likely to contribute[279]. During a shorter episode, e.g. 5 min, of asphyxia, the fetus may not become hypotensive, but repeated 5-min episodes sensitise the heart to further insults, such that during each successive period of asphyxia the duration of hypotension increases; an example is shown in Fig. 21.4[280]. As cardiac function fails, the brain is also compromised; severe selective striatal damage occurs after repeated insults[280].

Very little is known about how fetal cardiovascular function alters in response to factors that cause growth retarda-

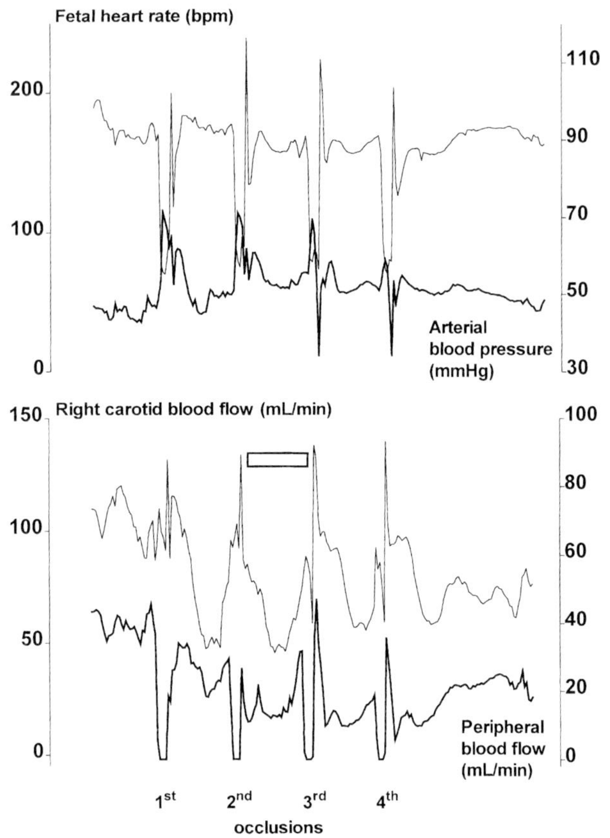

Fig. 21.4 An example of the cardiovascular and central adaptations to repeated severe asphyxia in a fetus subjected to 5 min of asphyxia, repeated four times at 30-min intervals[264]. The open box represents the interval between episodes of umbilical cord occlusion. Note the appearance of hypotension, and a fall in cerebral blood flow during the third and fourth occlusions. Despite this progressive fetal compromise, the bradycardic response to asphyxia remains similar in each episode.

tion, such as chronic hypoxia. It is known that the fetus can adapt to a compromised intrauterine environment: fetal heart rate, blood pressure, the incidence of fetal breathing and body movements may all return to normal in the absence of acidaemia despite continued hypoxia[281]. This may be a function of duration, as chronic hypoxia induced by placental embolisation from 0.7 gestation in the fetal sheep was associated with loss of fetal heart-rate variability[282]. These adaptations may detrimentally affect the way the fetus responds to further episodes of asphyxia/hypoxia. Experimentally, growth retarded fetuses exhibit sustained elevated plasma catecholamines and when challenged with hypoxia have a blunted rise in plasma catecholamines[283,284]. Human growth retarded fetuses have higher catecholamine levels in amniotic fluid[285]. Fetuses made chronically hypoxaemic exhibit altered and blunted cardiovascular responses to a further episode of hypoxia[275,286].

THE PATTERN OF ASPHYXIAL INSULTS

Recent large animal pathophysiologic studies have associated distinctive patterns of cerebral injury with clearly defined patterns of asphyxia. Such patterns of damage include selective damage to the striatum (basal ganglia), hippocampus, cerebellum, mixed striatal and cortical injury, and finally infarcts in the parasagittal cortex, thalamus and cerebellum. The mechanisms defining these different patterns have been only incompletely explored.

A single period of 10 min of total cord occlusion is associated with continuous bradycardia, with initial hypertension, then hypotension to well below the threshold of autoregulation. Histologically this insult produces selective neuronal loss particularly in the pyramidal cells of the hippocampus[266]. This pattern is similar to that produced by brief ischaemia in adult species, and as discussed above may be related to increased glutamate efflux.

Short insults that, individually, cause little or no damage, repeated before the neurons have fully recovered membrane function, may sensitise parts of the brain to damage. In the fetal sheep repeated short periods of subcritical ischaemia produced a disproportionate increase in striatal injury, compared with the cortex[287]. When the interval between insults was only 1 h, 3 × 10 min insults produced a similar degree of hippocampal and cortical injury to a single 30-min insult, but much greater striatal damage. When the interval was increased to 5 h, there was only minimal cortical damage, but striatal damage was still as great as that seen after the single 30-min insult. This sensitisation of the basal ganglia by many relatively short but severe insults is also seen after repeated episodes of 5 min of complete umbilical occlusion in the sheep[264,280]. Immunohistochemical studies suggested that the GABA-ergic medium sized neurons of the putamen were selectively lost[92]. In the adult rat, such repeated episodes of ischaemia do not produce greater release of glutamate, but are associated in some studies with enhanced ionic perturbations during successive insults[78].

Interestingly, enhanced striatal damage was also seen after a study of prolonged (1–4 h) partial asphyxia[265]. Here the major predictor of damage was the occurrence of discrete episodes of hypotension, rather than the degree of hypoxia or acidosis produced. Effectively then, prolonged partial asphyxia might be acting as several repeated insults, on a background of hypoxia, rather than as single continuous insult. The increased susceptibility of the striatum suggests a longer latency of recovery in the striatum at this age, which requires further investigation. In view of the often intermittent nature of asphyxia, with acute compromise during contractions, this mechanism may be a common precursor of status marmoratus; different spacing between insults would lead to variable associated cortical damage.

The above studies have focused on relatively prolonged episodes of asphyxia. Clinically, such severe and prolonged restrictions of fetal oxygenation are easily detected, and seldom present a therapeutic dilemma. Typical contractions, however, tend to be only 1 min or at most 2 min long. When uterine contractions compromise placental blood flow or compress the umbilical cord, a more likely pattern will be one of brief repetitive asphyxia, rather than prolonged periods of reduced placental gas exchange. Recent data in the fetal sheep suggest that if complete umbilical cord occlusions at a frequency of 1 min out of every 2.5 min are continued until severe hypotension (mean arterial blood pressure ≤ 20 mmHg for two successive occlusions) develops, they are associated with initial sustained hypertension for 30 min, followed by progressively worsening hypotension in a biphasic pattern during each occlusion[288]. Focal infarction in a watershed distribution was reported, with sparing of the hippocampus and striatum[289]. The cause of the vulnerability of the CA1 region to short, but intense insults[266], and its relative resistance in partial or brief repeated asphyxia[265,267,280], is unknown. Speculatively, it is possible that the greater (metabolic) acidosis seen with longer periods of asphyxia may have a protective effect, as suggested by *in vitro* studies[116,117].

DEVELOPMENTAL AGE

The resistance both of neurons to hypoxic depolarisation as well as the heart to hypoxia is greater earlier in gestation. Whereas 10 min of total cord occlusion results in severe hypotension and selective neuronal loss in the near term (0.9 gestation) fetal sheep, even 20 min of cord occlusion causes no cerebral damage, and only modest hypotension in the 0.65 gestation fetal sheep[290,291]. This reduced susceptibility to cerebral asphyxia with immaturity *in utero* is consistent with the long-established changes postnatally in a variety of species[292]. The relationships between developmental age, different insults and the different lesions seen at post-mortem or by modern imaging techniques, however, are still unclear. The lower limit of autoregulation of CBF is similar to resting arterial blood pressure in the fetal lamb, whereas it is significantly lower in the newborn lamb; thus the immature brain has a lesser margin of safety[293]. Total CBF increases with age, more so in the cortex than the hindbrain and the hypoxic increase in CBF increases with age[294], although the response to hypercapnia matures earlier[295]. Further, a preferential increase in CBF to the brainstem relative to the cortex is seen during hypoxic–ischaemic insults in all immature species studied compared to that seen in adults[296,297]. This differential perfusion may explain the pattern of parasagittal necrosis of the cortex and dorsal hippocampus seen in term infants[298]. This is clearly related to the watershed zone between the middle and anterior and posterior cerebral arteries, and is typical of pure hypotensive or ischaemic insults seen in adults and non-human primates[299].

Preterm infants appear to preferentially suffer lesions of the periventricular white matter although this may occur at term as well. This may be related to a watershed zone of superficial and deep blood arterial blood vessels, or to local tissue oedema[300]. Metabolic differences, due for example to rapid myelination, may explain some regional differences with age. Studies *in vitro* have highlighted the greater vulnerability of differentiating (as opposed to mature) oligodendrocytes to glutamate exposure[301]. This glutamate-induced oligodendroglia death was not due to a receptor mechanism, but was wholly due to glutamate uptake by the oligodendroglia. Glutamate was transported by high-affinity, sodium-dependent and by sodium-independent systems. This toxicity was closely coupled to oxygen free-radical production, due to glutathione depletion. This may have been due to the action of a glutamate–cystine exchange mechanism that results in cystine and glutathione depletion. The authors showed that depletion of glutathione levels occurred after glutamate exposure, and that this depletion preceded loss of cell viability. Since this selective damage could be prevented by exposure to free-radical scavengers such as vitamin E, this suggests a potential therapy for preterm infants at risk of white-matter damage.

Recovery

NEUROGLIAL RESPONSES TO INJURY IN THE CNS

Although neuronal proliferation does not occur in the mature CNS, a considerable amount of recovery can take place following injury and is probably greater in the immature brain. The redundancy of motoneuron innervation, for example, which is eliminated by normal neuronal death, allows much better recovery from a purely unilateral injury than from a more diffuse injury. Studies of adult survivors of stroke have shown that even the adult brain exhibits considerable functional plasticity. The main cellular events following cortical injury include dendritic stripping[302], then neurite growth followed by synaptogenesis in the neocortex, ipsilateral and contralateral to the injured area, in a pattern that corresponds with the timing of behavioural recovery[303,304]. Invading glial cells appear to separate the synapses during the first 5 days following injury in the hippocampus, with closely associated electrophysiologic changes[305]. The induction of growth factors during this phase may play a key role in re-establishing neuronal circuits[306]. Grafts of fetal tissue may improve recovery by their relatively exuberant growth factor production[307].

Much short-term recovery is, however, is not due to plasticity or 'remodelling', but rather to reversal of functional depression in undamaged structures that are interconnected with damaged regions. Both peptide growth factors and spontaneous electrical activity influence recovery, and are closely connected, as shown by the induction of nerve growth factor (NGF) by kindling[308], and conversely the delay in kindling after exposure to NGF antiserum[309]. Prolonged electrical suppression of neurons severely reduces their viability; this can be prevented by growth factors[310]. This action appears to be mediated by stabilising neuronal calcium homeostasis[311,312]. The role of neuronal electrical activity is complex; it may directly help maintain homeostasis in target neurons but also may stimulate the release of neurotrophic factors[313]. There is evidence that epileptiform activity may also help improve functional recovery[254]. Indeed stimulation with brief amphetamine therapy improved recovery from forebrain ablation in cats[314]. Conversely, suppression of EEG activity with GABA agonists or MK-801 may exacerbate or prevent secondary neuronal degeneration after cerebral lesions in adult rats[315,316]. These data suggest that the balance of excitatory and inhibitory inputs is crucial. The mechanism may be altered synaptogenesis during the early recovery phase: *in vitro*, suppression of neuronal activity suppresses synapse formation[317].

CHRONIC INSULTS

The fetal brain may be sensitised to asphyxial injury by chronic hypoxia or limitation of substrate leading to growth retardation[318], a conclusion supported by clinical observation[319]. Systemically, intrauterine growth retardation (IUGR) is likely to be compromised by reduced reserve capacity for cerebral oxygen delivery, reduced metabolic reserves and altered neurotransmitter activity. IUGR new-born piglets show reduced pressor and hyperglycaemic responses to acute hypoxia[284,320]. IUGR fetuses may show greater lipid peroxidation during hypoxia[321].

The major confounding variable, however, is that IUGR also affects cerebral development. Although cerebral oxidative metabolism is reported to be normal[322,323], retardation of the EEG spectra occurs with IUGR in the rat, with perturbations of neuromodulator and neurotransmitter expression[321,324,325]. Histologically, there may be reduced cerebral myelination[326–328], altered synaptogenesis[328], and smaller brain size[329]. Consistent with this, growth-retarded infants typically demonstrate delayed latency of evoked potentials, with an increased incidence of behavioural and developmental problems[330,331]. Paradoxically, IUGR has actually been associated with accelerated maturation of brainstem-evoked responses in some experimental paradigms[332], and in growth-retarded neonates whose mothers had gestational hypertension[330], illustrating the complexity of the multiple factors associated with growth retardation. Thus, it is often unclear how much of the long-term morbidity of IUGR is due to effects on neurodevelopment and how much may be related to acute prenatal events.

Conclusions

Over the last decade, complementary functional and pathophysiological studies have elucidated may of the key endogenous mechanisms determining outcome after an hypoxic–ischaemic insult. Such studies have continued to support a central role for excitotoxin exposure, and increased free cytoplasmic Ca^{2+}, but now highlight the overlapping roles of apoptosis, neurotrophic factor expression and glial cell dysfunction in the secondary phase of injury. Although much remains to be investigated, many of the mechanisms by which cerebral maturation, cooling and metabolic factors modulate cellular responses have been clarified. Finally, it is now clear that the temporal pattern of asphyxial insults is vital to understanding the spectrum of clinical asphyxial brain injury.

This improved understanding should promote more sophisticated fetal and neonatal monitoring, and has led to both innovative and better targeted proposals for therapeutic intervention, notably including exogenous growth factor therapy and cerebral cooling.

REFERENCES

1. de Haan HH, Gunn AJ, Gluckman PD. Experiments in perinatal brain injury: What have we learnt? *Prenatal Neonatal Med* **1**:16–25, 1996.
2. Auer RN, Siesjö BK. Hypoglycaemia: brain neurochemistry and neuropathology. *Baillière's Clin Endocrinol Metab* **7**:611–625, 1993.
3. Spar JA, Lewine JD, Orrison WW. Neonatal hypoglycemia: CT and MR findings. *Am J Neuroradiol* **15**:1477–1478, 1994.
4. Takashima S, Hirano S, Kamei S, Hasegawa M, Kimoto H. Cerebral hemodynamics on near-infrared spectroscopy in hypoxia and ischemia in young animal studies. *Brain Dev* **17**:312–316, 1995.
5. Geiger KD, Gurushanthaiah D, Howes EL, Lewandowski GA, Reed JC, Bloom FE, Sarvetnick NE. Cytokine-mediated survival from lethal herpes simplex virus infection: role of programmed neuronal death. *Proc Natl Acad Sci USA* **92**:3411–3415, 1995.
6. Thompson CB. Apoptosis in the pathogenesis and treatment of disease. *Science* **267**:1456–1462, 1995.
7. Pousset F. Cytokines as mediators in the central nervous system. *Biomed Pharmacother* **48**:425–431, 1994.
8. Rubinstein G. Schizophrenia, infection and temperature. An animal model for investigating their interrelationships. *Schizophr Res* **10**:95–102, 1993.
9. Salafia CM, Minior VK, Pezzullo JC, Popek EJ, Rosenkrantz TS, Vintzileos AM. Intrauterine growth restriction in infants of less than thirty-two weeks' gestation: Associated placental pathologic features. *Am J Obstet Gynecol* **173**:1049–1057, 1995.
10. Ginsberg MD, Busto R. Rodent models of cerebral ischemia. *Stroke* **20**:1627–1642, 1989.
11. Williams CE, Gunn AJ, Mallard EC, Gluckman PD. Outcome after ischemia in the developing sheep brain: An electroencephalographic and histological study. *Ann Neurol* **31**:14–21, 1992.
12. Williams CE, Gunn AJ, Gluckman PD. The time course of intracellular edema and epileptiform activity following prenatal cerebral ischemia in sheep. *Stroke* **22**:516–521, 1991.
13. Beilharz EJ, Williams CE, Dragunow M, Sirimanne ES, Gluckman PD. Mechanisms of delayed cell death following hypoxic–ischemic injury in the immature rat: evidence for apoptosis during selective neuronal loss. *Brain Res* **29**:1–14, 1995.
14. Mehmet H, Yue X, Squier MV *et al.* Increased apoptosis in the cingulate sulcus of newborn piglets following transient hypoxia–ischaemia is related to the degree of high energy phosphate depletion during the insult. *Neurosci Lett* **181**:121–125, 1994.
15. Roth SC, Edwards AD, Cady EB *et al.* Relation between cerebral oxidative metabolism following birth asphyxia, and neurodevelopmental outcome and brain growth at one year. *Dev Med Child Neurol* **34**:285–295, 1992.

16. Klein HC, Krop Van Gastel W, Go KG, Korf J. Prediction of specific damage or infarction from the measurement of tissue impedance following repetitive brain ischaemia in the rat. *Neuropathol Appl Neurobiol* **19**:57–65, 1993.
17. Gunn AJ, Gunn TR, de Haan HH, Williams CE, Gluckman PD. Dramatic neuronal rescue with prolonged selective head cooling after ischemia in fetal sheep. *J Clin Invest* **99**:248–256, 1997.
18. Marks KA, Mallard EC, Roberts I, Williams CE, Sirimanne ES, Johnston BM, Gluckman PD, Edwards AD. Delayed vasodilation and altered oxygenation following cerebral ischemia in fetal sheep. *Pediatr Res* **39**:48–54, 1996.
19. Tan WKM, Williams CE, During MJ, Mallard CE, Gunning MI, Gunn AJ, Gluckman PD. Accumulation of cytotoxins during the development of seizures and edema after hypoxic–ischemic injury in late gestation fetal sheep. *Pediatr Res* **39**:791–797, 1996.
20. Memezawa H, Minamisawa H, Smith ML, Siesjö BK. Ischemic penumbra in a model of reversible middle cerebral artery occlusion in the rat. *Exp Brain Res* **89**:67–78, 1992.
21. Folbergrova J, Memezawa H, Smith ML, Siesjo BK. Focal and perifocal changes in tissue energy state during middle cerebral artery occlusion in normo- and hyperglycemic rats. *J Cereb Blood Flow Metab* **12**:25–33, 1992.
22. Nedergaard M, Hansen AJ. Characterization of cortical depolarizations evoked in focal cerebral ischemia. *J Cereb Blood Flow Metab* **13**:568–574, 1993.
23. Rothman SM, Olney JW. Excitotoxicity and the NMDA receptor – still lethal after eight years. *Trends Neurosci* **18**:57–58, 1995.
24. Choi DW. Calcium: still center-stage in hypoxic–ischemic neuronal death. *Trends Neurosci* **18**:58–60, 1995.
25. Goldberg MP, Choi DW. Combined oxygen and glucose deprivation in cortical cell culture – calcium-dependent and calcium-independent mechanisms of neuronal injury. *J Neurosci* **13**:3510–3524, 1993.
26. Lipton P, Lobner D. Mechanisms of intracellular calcium accumulation in the CA1 region of rat hippocampus during anoxia in vitro. *Stroke* **21**:III60–III64, 1990.
27. Collingridge GL, Lester RA. Excitatory amino acid receptors in the vertebrate central nervous system. *Pharmacol Rev* **41**:143–210, 1989.
28. Connor J, Wadman W, Hockberger P, Wong R. Substained dendritic gradients of calcium induced by excitatory amino acids of CA1 hippocampal neurons. *Science* **240**:649–653, 1988.
29. Carolei A, Fieschi C, Bruno R, Toffano G. Monosialoganglioside GM1 in cerebral ischemia. *Cerebrovasc Brain Metab Rev* **3**:134–157, 1991.
30. Andrus PK, Taylor BM, Sun FF, Hall ED. Effects of the lipid peroxidation inhibitor tirilazad mesylate (U-74006F) on gerbil brain eicosanoid levels following ischemia and reperfusion. *Brain Res* **659**:126–132, 1994.
31. Park CK, Hall ED. Dose–response analysis of the effect of 21-aminosteroid tirilazad mesylate (U-74006F) upon neurological outcome and ischemic brain damage in permanent focal cerebral ischemia. *Brain Res* **645**:157–163, 1994.
32. Smith SL, Andrus PK, Zhang JR, Hall ED. Direct measurement of hydroxyl radicals, lipid peroxidation, and blood–brain barrier disruption following unilateral cortical impact head injury in the rat. *J Neurotrauma* **11**:393–404, 1994.
33. Tan WKM, Williams CE, Gunn AJ, Mallard EC, Gluckman PD. Pretreatment with monosialoganglioside GM1 protects the brain of fetal sheep against hypoxic–ischemic injury without causing systemic compromise. *Pediatr Res* **34**:18–22, 1993.
34. Tan WKM, Williams CE, Mallard CE, Gluckman PD. Monosialoganglioside GM(1) treatment after a hypoxic–ischemic episode reduces the vulnerability of the fetal sheep brain to subsequent injuries. *Am J Obstet Gynecol* **170**:663–670, 1994.
35. Simon RP, Chen J, Graham SH. GM1 ganglioside treatment of focal ischemia – a dose–response and microdialysis study. *J Pharmacol Exp Ther* **265**:24–29, 1993.
36. Monyer H, Hartley DM, Choi DW. 21-Aminosteroids attenuate excitotoxic neuronal injury in cortical cell cultures. *Neuron* **5**:121–126, 1990.
37. Bagenholm R, Nilsson UA, Gotborg CW, Kjellmer I. Free radicals are formed in the brain of fetal sheep during reperfusion after cerebral ischemia. *Pediatr Res* **43**:271–275, 1998.
38. Bagenholm R, Nilsson UA, Kjellmer I. Formation of free radicals in hypoxic ischemic brain damage in the neonatal rat, assessed by an endogenous spin trap and lipid peroxidation. *Brain Res* **773**:132–138, 1997.
39. Dorrepaal CA, Van Bel F, Moison RM, Shadid M, van de Bor M, Steendijk P, Berger HM. Oxidative stress during post-hypoxic–ischemic reperfusion in the newborn lamb: the effect of nitric oxide synthesis inhibition. *Pediatr Res* **41**:321–326, 1997.
40. Dorrepaal CA, Berger HM, Benders MJ, van Zoeren-Grobben D, van de Bor M, Van Bel F. Nonprotein-bound iron in postasphyxial reperfusion injury of the newborn. *Pediatrics* **98**:883–889, 1996.
41. Uenohara H, Imaizumi S, Yoshimoto T, Suzuki J. Correlation among lipid peroxidation, brain energy metabolism and brain oedema in cerebral ischaemia. *Neurol Res* **10**:194–199, 1988.
42. Rosenberg AA, Murdaugh E, White CW. The role of oxygen free radicals in postasphyxia cerebral hypoperfusion in newborn lambs. *Pediatr Res* **26**:215–219, 1989.
43. Dorrepaal CA, Shadid M, Steendijk P, Vandervelde ET, van de Bor M, Baan J, Van Bel F. Effect of post-hypoxic–ischemic inhibition of nitric oxide synthesis on cerebral blood flow, metabolism and electrocortical brain activity in newborn lambs. *Biol Neonate* **72**:216–226, 1997.
44. Palmer C, Roberts RL, Bero C. Deferrioxamine posttreatment reduces ischemic brain injury in neonatal rats. *Stroke* **25**:1039–1045, 1994.
45. Palmer C, Towfighi J, Roberts RL, Heitjan DF. Allopurinol administered after inducing hypoxia–ischemia reduces brain injury in 7-day-old rats. *Pediatr Res* **33**:405–411, 1993.
46. Toyoda T, Kassell NF, Lee KS. Attenuation of ischemia–reperfusion injury in the rat neocortex by the hydroxyl radical scavenger nicaraven. *Neurosurg* **40**:372–378, 1997.
47. Baker K, Marcus CB, Huffman K, Kruk H, Malfroy B, Doctrow SR. Synthetic combined superoxide dismutase catalase mimetics are protective as a delayed treatment in a rat stroke model – a key role for reactive oxygen species in ischemic brain injury. *J Pharmacol Exp Therap* **284**:215–221, 1998.
48. Siesjö BK. Calcium in the brain under physiological and pathological conditions. *Eur Neurol* **30**(Suppl 2):3–9, 1990.
49. Scharfman HE, Schwartzkroin PA. Protection of dentate hilar cells from prolonged stimulation by intracellular calcium chelation. *Science* **246**:257–260, 1989.
50. Uematsu D, Greenberg JH, Reivich M, Hickey WF. Direct evidence for calcium-induced ischemic and reperfusion injury. *Ann Neurol* **26**:280–283, 1989.
51. Kristian T, Katsura K, Siesjö BK. The influence of moderate hypothermia on cellular calcium uptake in complete ischaemia: implications for the excitotoxic hypothesis. *Acta Physiol Scand* **146**:531–532, 1992.
52. Benveniste H, Jorgensen MB, Diemer NH, Hansen A. Calcium accumulation by glutamate receptor activation is involved in hippocampal cell damage after ischemia. *Acta Neurol Scand* **78**:529–536, 1988.
53. Longo R, Sagratella S, Scotti de Carolis A. Effects of calcium antagonists on hypoxic and NMDA injury in rat hippocampal slices. *Life Sci* **55**:455–462, 1994.
54. Brooks KL, Kauppinen RA. Calcium-mediated damage following hypoxia in cerebral cortex *ex vivo* studied by NMR spectroscopy. Evidence for direct involvement of voltage-gated Ca^{2+}-channels. *Neurochem Int* **23**:441–450, 1993.
55. Louvel J, Abbes S, Godfraind JM, Pumain R. Effects of calcium channel blockers on neuronal calcium dependent processes. In: *Calcium Electrogenesis and Neuronal Functioning* (eds U Heinemann, M Klee, E Neker, W Singer), pp. 373–383 Berlin: Springer-Verlag, 1986.
56. Lehmann A. Neurotoxicity of calcium ionophore A23187 in immature rat cerebellar slices. *Neurosci Lett* **79**:263–266, 1987.
57. Palmer GC, Stagnitto ML, Ray RK, Knowles MA, Harvey R, Garske GE. Anticonvulsant properties of calcium channel blockers in mice: *N*-methyl-D, L-aspartate- and Bay K 8644-induced convulsions are potently blocked by the dihydropyridines. *Epilepsia* **34**:372–380, 1993.
58. Somjen GG, Aitken PG, Czeh G, Jing J, Young JN. Cellular physiology of hypoxia of the mammalian central nervous system. *Res Publ Assoc Res Nerv Ment Dis* **71**:51–65, 1993.
59. Limbrick DD, Churn SB, Sombati S, DeLorenzo RJ. Inability to restore resting intracellular calcium levels as an early indicator of delayed neuronal cell death. *Brain Res* **690**:145–156, 1995.

60. Rami A, Krieglstein J. Neuronal protective effects of calcium antagonists in cerebral ischemia. *Life Sci* **55**:2105–2113, 1994.
61. Xie Y, Zacharias E, Hoff P, Tegtmeier F. Ion channel involvement in anoxic depolarization induced by cardiac arrest in rat brain. *J Cereb Blood Flow Metab* **15**:587–594, 1995.
62. Gunn AJ, Williams CE, Mallard EC, Tan WKM, Gluckman PD. Flunarizine, a calcium channel antagonist, is partially prophylactically neuroprotective in hypoxic–ischemic encephalopathy in the fetal sheep. *Pediatr Res* **35**:657–663, 1994.
63. Lu HR, Van Reempts J, Haseldonckx M, Borgers M, Janssen PA. Cerebroprotective effects of flunarizine in an experimental rat model of cardiac arrest. *Am J Emerg Med* **8**:1–6, 1990.
64. Gunn AJ, Mydlar T, Bennet L, Faull R, Gorter S, Cook CJ, Johnston BM, Gluckman PD. The neuroprotective actions of a calcium channel antagonist, flunarizine, in the infant rat. *Pediatr Res* **25**:573–576, 1989.
65. Gunn AJ, Gluckman PD. Flunarizine, a calcium channel antagonist, is not neuroprotective when given after hypoxia-ischemia in the infant rat. *Dev Pharmacol Ther* **17**:205–209, 1991.
66. Pellegrini-Giampietro DE, Cherici G, Alesiani M, Carla V, Moroni F. Excitatory amino acid release and free radical formation may cooperate in the genesis of ischemia-induced neuronal damage. *J Neurosci* **10**:1035–1041, 1990.
67. Dugan LL, Sensi SL, Canzoniero LMT, Handran SD, Rothman SM, Lin TS, Goldberg MP, Choi DW. Mitochondrial production of reactive oxygen species in cortical neurons following exposure to *N*-methyl-D-aspartate. *J Neurosci* **15**:6377–6388, 1995.
68. Markgraf CG, Velayo NL, Johnson MP, McCarty DR, Medhi S, Koehl JR, Chmielewski PA, Linnik MD. Six-hour window of opportunity for calpain inhibition in focal cerebral ischemia in rats. *Stroke* **29**:152–158, 1998.
69. Collins DR, Davies SN. Potentiation of synaptic transmission in the rat hippocampal slice by exogenous L-glutamate and selective L-glutamate receptor subtype agonists. *Neuropharmacology* **33**:1055–1063, 1994.
70. Romijn HJ. Preferential loss of GABAergic neurons in hypoxia-exposed neocortex slab cultures is attenuated by the NMDA receptor blocker *d*-2-amino-7-phosphonoheptanoate. *Brain Res* **501**:100–104, 1989.
71. Largo C, Cuevas P, Somjen GG, Martin del Rio R, Herreras O. The effect of depressing glial function in rat brain *in situ* on ion homeostasis, synaptic transmission, and neuron survival. *J Neurosci* **16**:1219–1229, 1996.
72. Smeyne RJ, Vendrell M, Hayward M *et al.* Continuous c-*fos* expression precedes programmed cell death *in vivo*. *Nature* **363**:166–169, 1993.
73. Churn SB, Sombati S, Taft WC, DeLorenzo RJ. Excitotoxicity affects membrane potential and calmodulin kinase II activity in cultured rat cortical neurons. *Stroke* **24**:271–277, 1993.
74. Koh JY, Goldberg MP, Hartley DM, Choi DW. Non-NMDA receptor-mediated neurotoxicity in cortical culture. *J Neurosci* **10**:693–705, 1990.
75. Choi DW, Koh JY, Peters S. Pharmacology of glutamate neurotoxicity in cortical cell culture: attenuation by NMDA antagonists. *J Neurosci* **8**:185–196, 1988.
76. Novelli A, Reilly JA, Lysko PG, Henneberry RC. Glutamate becomes neurotoxic via the *N*-methyl-D-aspartate receptor when intracellular energy levels are reduced. *Brain Res* **451**:205–212, 1988.
77. Illievich UM, Zornow MH, Choi KT, Strnat MA, Scheller MS. Effects of hypothermia or anesthetics on hippocampal glutamate and glycine concentrations after repeated transient global cerebral ischemia. *Anesthesiology* **80**:177–186, 1994.
78. Ueda Y, Obrenovitch TP, Lok SY, Sarna GS, Symon L. Changes in extracellular glutamate concentration produced in the rat striatum by repeated ischemia. *Stroke* **23**:1125–1131, 1992.
79. Bullock R, Butcher SP, Chen M-H, Kendall L, McCulloch J. Correlation of the extracellular glutamate concentration with extent of blood flow reduction after subdural hematoma in the rat. *J Neurosurg* **74**:794–802, 1991.
80. Globus MY, Busto R, Dietrich WD, Martinez E, Valdes I, Ginsberg MD. Effect of ischemia on the *in vivo* release of striatal dopamine, glutamate and γ-aminobutyric acid studied by intracerebral microdialysis. *J Neurochem* **51**:1455–1464, 1988.
81. Benveniste H, Drejer J, Schousboe A, Diemer NH. Elevation of the extracellular concentrations of glutamate and aspartate in rat hippocampus during transient cerebral ischemia monitored by intracerebral microdialysis. *J Neurochem* **43**:1369–1374, 1984.
82. Penning DH, Goh JW, el Beheiry H, Brien JF. Effect of hypoxia on glutamate efflux and synaptic transmission in the guinea pig hippocampus. *Brain Res* **620**:301–304, 1993.
83. Busto R, Globus MY, Dietrich WD, Martinez E, Valdes I, Ginsberg MD. Effect of mild hypothermia on ischemia-induced release of neurotransmitters and free fatty acids in rat brain. *Stroke* **20**:904–910, 1989.
84. Globus MY, Busto R, Martinez E, Valdes I, Dietrich WD. Ischemia induces release of glutamate in regions spared from histopathologic damage in the rat. *Stroke* **21**:III43–III46, 1990.
85. Diemer NH, Johansen FF, Benveniste H, Bruhn T, Berg M, Valente E, Jorgensen MB. Ischemia as an excitotoxic lesion: protection against hippocampal nerve cell loss by denervation. *Acta Neurochir (Suppl) (Wien)* **57**:94–101, 1993.
86. Barks JD, Silverstein FS, Sims K, Greenamyre JT, Johnston MV. Glutamate recognition sites in human fetal brain. *Neurosci Lett* **84**:131–136, 1988.
87. McDonald JW, Silverstein FS, Johnston MV. Neurotoxicity of *N*-methyl-D-aspartate is markedly enhanced in developing rat central nervous system. *Brain Res* **459**:200–203, 1988.
88. Marret S, Gressens P, Gadisseux JF, Evrard P. Prevention by magnesium of excitotoxic neuronal death in the developing brain: an animal model for clinical intervention studies. *Dev Med Child Neurol* **37**:473–484, 1995.
89. Cherici G, Alesiani M, Pellegrini-Giampietro DE, Moroni F. Ischemia does not induce the release of excitotoxic amino acids from the hippocampus of newborn rats. *Dev Brain Res* **60**:235–240, 1991.
90. Kjellmer I, Andine P, Hagberg H, Thiringer K. Extracellular increase of hypoxanthine and xanthine in the cortex and basal ganglia of fetal lambs during hypoxia–ischemia. *Brain Res* **478**:241–247, 1989.
91. Shuaib A, Ijaz S, Miyashita H, Mainprize T, Kanthan R. Progressive decrease in extracellular GABA concentrations in the post-ischemic period in the striatum: a microdialysis study. *Brain Res* **666**:99–103, 1994.
92. Mallard EC, Waldvogel HJ, Williams CE, Faull RLM, Gluckman PD. Repeated asphyxia causes loss of striatal projection neurons in the fetal sheep brain. *Neuroscience* **65**:827–836, 1995.
93. Davis RE, Klinger PD. NMDA receptor antagonist MK-801 blocks learning of conditioned stimulus–unconditioned stimulus contiguity but not fear of conditioned stimulus in goldfish (*Carassius auratus* L.). *Behav Neurosci* **108**:935–940, 1994.
94. Mayer ML, Westbrook GL. The physiology of excitatory amino acids in the vertebrate central nervous system. *Progr Neurobiol* **28**:197–276, 1987.
95. Tan WKM, Williams CE, Gunn AJ, Mallard EC, Gluckman PD. Suppression of postischemic epileptiform activity with MK-801 improves neural outcome in fetal sheep. *Ann Neurol* **32**:677–682, 1992.
96. Dietrich WD, Lin B, Globus YT, Green EJ, Ginsberg MD, Busto R. Effect of delayed MK801 (dizocilpine) treatment with or without immediate postischemic hypothermia on chronic neuronal survival after global forebrain ischemia in rats. *J Cereb Blood Flow Metab* **15**:960–968, 1995.
97. Hagberg H, Gilland E, Diemer NH, Andine P. Hypoxia–ischemia in the neonatal rat brain: histopathology after post-treatment with NMDA and non-NMDA receptor antagonists. *Biol Neonate* **66**:205–213, 1994.
98. Lin B, Dietrich WD, Ginsberg MD, Globus MY, Busto R. MK-801 (dizocilpine) protects the brain from repeated normothermic global ischemic insults in the rat. *J Cereb Blood Flow Metab* **13**:925–932, 1993.
99. Murase K, Kato H, Kogure K. Limited but evident protective effects of MK-801 and pentobarbital on neuronal damage following forebrain ischemia in the gerbil under normothermic conditions. *Neurosci Lett* **149**:229–232, 1993.
100. von Lubitz DK, McKenzie RJ, Lin RC, Devlin TM, Skolnick P. MK-801 is neuroprotective but does not improve survival in severe forebrain ischemia. *Eur J Pharmacol* **233**:95–100, 1993.
101. Lyden PD, Hedges B. Protective effect of synaptic inhibition during cerebral ischemia in rats and rabbits. *Stroke* **23**:1463–1469, 1992.

102. Marret S, Mukendi R, Gadisseux JF, Gressens P, Evrard P. Effect of ibotenate on brain development: an excitotoxic mouse model of microgyria and posthypoxic-like lesions. *J Neuropathol Exp Neurol* **54**:358–370, 1995.
103. Siesjö BK, Bengtsson F. Calcium fluxes, calcium antagonists, and calcium-related pathology in brain ischemia, hypoglycemia, and spreading depression: a unifying hypothesis. *J Cereb Blood Flow Metab* **9**:127–140, 1989.
104. Ferriero DM, Simon RP. Neonatal striatal NADPH-diaphorase neurons are vulnerable to quisqualate and its analogue alpha-amino-3-hydroxy-5-methyl-4-isoxazole proprionate (AMPA). *Neurosci Lett* **126**:52–56, 1991.
105. Koh JY, Choi DW. Vulnerability of cultured cortical neurons to damage by excitotoxins: differential susceptibility of neurons containing NADPH-diaphorase. *J Neurosci* **8**:2153–2163, 1988.
106. Foster AC, Gill R, Woodruff GN. Neuroprotective effects of MK-801 *in vivo:* selectivity, and evidence for delayed degeneration mediated by NMDA receptor activation. *J Neurosci* **8**:4745–4754, 1988.
107. LeBlanc MH, Vig V, Smith B, Parker CC, Evans OB, Smith EE. MK-801 does not protect against hypoxic–ischemic brain injury in piglets. *Stroke* **22**:1270–1275, 1991.
108. Buchan A, Li H, Pulsinelli WA. The N-methyl-D-aspartate antagonist, MK-801, fails to protect against neuronal damage caused by transient, severe forebrain ischemia in adult rats. *J Neurosci* **11**:1049–1056, 1991.
109. Green EJ, Pazos AJ, Dietrich WD *et al.* Combined postischemic hypothermia and delayed MK-801 treatment attenuates neurobehavioral deficits associated with transient global ischemia in rats. *Brain Res* **702**:145–152, 1995.
110. Hayward NJ, McKnight AT, Woodruff GN. Brain temperature and the neuroprotective action of enadoline and dizocilpine in the gerbil model of global ischaemia. *Eur J Pharmacol* **236**:247–253, 1993.
111. Nellgard B, Wieloch T. Postischemic blockade of AMPA but not NMDA receptors mitigates neuronal damage in the rat brain following transient severe cerebral ischemia. *J Cereb Blood Flow Metab* **12**:2–11, 1992.
112. Warner MA, Neill KH, Nadler JV, Crain BJ. Regionally selective effects of NMDA receptor antagonists against ischemic brain damage in the gerbil. *J Cereb Blood Flow Metab* **11**:600–610, 1991.
113. Choi DW. Possible mechanisms limiting N-methyl-D-aspartate receptor overactivation and the therapeutic efficacy of N-methyl-D-aspartate antagonists. *Stroke* **21**:II20–II22, 1990.
114. Papagapiou MP, Auer RN. Regional neuroprotective effects of the NMDA receptor antagonist MK-801 (dizocilpine) in hypoglycemic brain damage. *J Cereb Blood Flow Metab* **10**:270–276, 1990.
115. Giffard RG, Weiss JH, Choi DW. Extracellular alkalinity exacerbates injury of cultured cortical neurons. *Stroke* **23**:1817–1821, 1992.
116. Giffard RG, Monyer H, Christine CW, Choi DW. Acidosis reduces NMDA receptor activation, glutamate neurotoxicity, and oxygen–glucose deprivation neuronal injury in cortical cultures. *Brain Res* **506**:339–342, 1990.
117. Tombaugh GC. Mild acidosis delays hypoxic spreading depression and improves neuronal recovery in hippocampal slices. *J Neurosci* **14**:5635–5643, 1994.
118. Miller RJ. The revenge of the kainate receptor. *Trends Neurosci* **14**(11):477–479, 1991.
119. Barbour B, Szatkowski M, Ingledew N, Attwell D. Arachidonic acid induces a prolonged inhibition of glutamate uptake into glial cells. *Nature* **342**:918–920, 1989.
120. Marin P, Stella N, Cordier J, Glowinski J, Premont J. Role of arachidonic acid and glutamate in the formation of inositol phosphates induced by noradrenaline in striatal astrocytes. *Mol Pharmacol* **44**:1176–1184, 1993.
121. Rod MR, Auer RN. Combination therapy with nimodipine and dizocilpine in a rat model of transient forebrain ischemia. *Stroke* **23**:725–732, 1992.
122. Hewitt K, Corbett D. Combined treatment with MK-801 and nicardipine reduces global ischemic damage in the gerbil. *Stroke* **23**:82–86, 1992.
123. Globus MY, Ginsberg MD, Dietrich WD, Busto R, Scheinberg P. Substantia nigra lesion protects against ischemic damage in the striatum. *Neurosci Lett* **80**:251–256, 1987.
124. Krebs MO, Desce JM, Kemel ML, Gauchy C, Godeheu G, Cheramy A, Glowinski J. Glutamatergic control of dopamine release in the rat striatum: evidence for presynaptic N-methyl-D-aspartate receptors on dopaminergic nerve terminals. *J Neurochem* **56**:81–85, 1991.
125. Epstein RP, Daly JW. Release of norepinephrine and dopamine from the brain vesicular preparations: effects of calcium antagonists. *Cell Mol Neurobiol* **2**:205–213, 1982.
126. Wieloch T, Lindrall O, Blomqvist P, Gage F. Evidence for amelioration of ischaemic neuronal damage in the hippocampal formation by lesions of the perforant pathway. *Neurol Res* **7**:24–26, 1985.
127. Kirino T, Sano K. Fine structural nature of delayed neuronal death following ischemia in the gerbil hippocampus. *Acta Neuropathol (Berlin)* **62**:209–218, 1984.
128. Andine P, Jacobson I, Hagberg H. Calcium uptake evoked by electrical stimulation is enhanced postischemically and precedes delayed neuronal death in CA1 of rat hippocampus: involvement of N-methyl-D-aspartate receptors. *J Cereb Blood Flow Metab* **8**:799–807, 1988.
129. Petito CK, Feldmann E, Pulsinelli W, Plum F. Delayed hippocampal damage in humans following cardiorespiratory arrest. *Neurology* **37**:1281–1286, 1987.
130. Lo AC, Houenou LJ, Oppenheim RW. Apoptosis in the nervous system: morphological features, methods, pathology, and prevention. *Arch Histol Cytol* **58**:139–149, 1995.
131. Ankarcrona M, Dypbukt JM, Bonfoco E, Zhivotovsky B, Orrenius S, Lipton SA, Nicotera P. Glutamate-induced neuronal death: a succession of necrosis or apoptosis depending on mitochondrial function. *Neuron* **15**:961–973, 1995.
132. Wyllie AH. Glucocorticoid-induced thymocyte apoptosis is associated with endogenous endonuclease activation. *Nature* **284**:555–556, 1980.
133. Krueger BK, Burne JF, Raff MC. Evidence for large-scale astrocyte death in the developing cerebellum. *J Neurosci* **15**:3366–3374, 1995.
134. Li Y, Chopp M, Jiang N, Zaloga C. *In situ* detection of DNA fragmentation after focal cerebral ischemia in mice. *Mol Brain Res* **28**:164–168, 1995.
135. Nitatori T, Sato N, Waguri S, Karasawa Y, Araki H, Shibanai K, Kominami E, Uchiyama Y. Delayed neuronal death in the CA1 pyramidal cell layer of the gerbil hippocampus following transient ischemia is apoptosis. *J Neurosci* **15**:1001–1011, 1995.
136. Raff MC. Social controls on cell survival and cell death. *Nature* **356**:397–400, 1992.
137. Yue X, Mehmet H, Penrice J *et al.* Apoptosis and necrosis in the newborn piglet brain following transient cerebral hypoxia–ischaemia. *Neuropathol Appl Neurobiol* **23**:16–25, 1997.
138. Dell'Anna E, Chen Y, Engidawork E, Andersson K, Lubec G, Luthman J, Herrera-Marschitz M. Delayed neuronal death following perinatal asphyxia in rat. *Exp Brain Res* **115**:105–115, 1997.
139. Edwards AD, Cox P, Hope PL, Azzopardi DV, Squier MV, Mehmet H. Apoptosis in the brains of infants suffering intrauterine cerebral injury. *Pediatr Res* **42**:684–689, 1997.
140. Scott RJ, Hegyi L. Cell death in perinatal hypoxic–ischaemic brain injury. *Neuropathol Appl Neurobiol* **23**:307–314, 1997.
141. Porteracailliau C, Price DL, Martin LJ. Excitotoxic neuronal death in the immature brain is an apoptosis–necrosis morphological continuum. *J Comp Neurol* **378**:70–87, 1997.
142. Goto K, Ishige A, Sekiguchi K *et al.* Effects of cycloheximide on delayed neuronal death in rat hippocampus. *Brain Res* **534**:299–302, 1990.
143. Shigeno T, Yamasaki Y, Kato G, Kusaka K, Mima T, Takakura K, Graham DI, Furukawa S. Reduction of delayed neuronal death by inhibition of protein synthesis. *Neurosci Lett* **120**:117–119, 1990.
144. Dragunow M, Preston K. The role of inducible transcription factors in apoptotic nerve cell death. *Brain Res Rev* **21**:1–28, 1995.
145. Deshpande J, Bergstedt K, Linden T, Kalimo H, Wieloch T. Ultrastructural changes in the hippocampal CA1-region following transient cerebral ischemia – evidence against programmed cell death. *Exp Brain Res* **88**:91–105, 1992.
146. Galli C, Meucci O, Scorziello A, Werge TM, Calissano P, Schettini G. Apoptosis in cerebellar granule cells in blocked by high KCl, forskolin, and IGF-1 through distinct mechanisms of action: the involvement of intracellular calcium and RNA synthesis. *J Neurosci* **15**:1172–1179, 1995.
147. Gwag BJ, Koh JY, Demaro JA, Ying HS, Jacquin M, Choi DW. Slowly triggered excitotoxicity occurs by necrosis in cortical cultures. *Neuroscience* **77**:393–401, 1997.

331. Kjellmer I, Liedholm M, Sultan B, Wennergren M, Gotborg CW, Thordstein M. Long-term effects of intrauterine growth retardation. *Acta Paediatr* **86**:83–84, 1997.
332. Cook CJ, Gluckman PD, Williams CE, Bennet L. Precocial neural function in the growth retarded fetal lamb. *Pediatr Res* **24**:600–605, 1988.
333. Robertslewis JM, Savage MJ, Marcy VR, Pinsker LR, Siman R. Immunolocalization of calpain I-mediated spectrin degradation to vulnerable neurons in the ischemic gerbil brain. *J Neurosci* **14**:3934–3944, 1994.
334. Saugstad O. Hypoxanthine as an indicator of hypoxia: its role in health and disease through free radical production. *Pediatr Res* **23**:143–150, 1988.
335. Phillis JW, Sen S. Oxypurinol attenuates hydroxyl radical production during ischemia/reperfusion injury of the rat cerebral cortex: an ESR study. *Brain Res* **628**:309–312, 1993.
336. Ikeda Y, Long D. The molecular basis of brain injury and brain edema: the role of oxygen free radicals. *Neurosurgery* **27**:1–11, 1990.
337. Matsuo Y, Onodera H, Shiga Y, Nakamura M, Ninomiya M, Kihara T, Kogure K. Correlation between myeloperoxidase-quantified neutrophil accumulation and ischemic brain injury in the rat – effects of neutrophil depletion. *Stroke* **25**:1469–1475, 1994.
338. Iadecola C, Xu XH, Zhang FY, Elfakahany EE, Ross ME. Marked induction of calcium-independent nitric oxide synthase activity after focal cerebral ischemia. *J Cereb Blood Flow Metab* **15**:52–59, 1995.
339. Albina JE, Cui SJ, Mateo RB, Reichner JS. Nitric oxide-mediated apoptosis in murine peritoneal macrophages. *J Immunol* **150**:5080–5085, 1993.

SECTION 3

Ethical issues

Ethical issues in maternal–fetal medicine

22

S. Bewley

Introduction

Discussions about ethics often seem irrelevant to practising doctors. Some are full of jargon and concepts that are alienating or cliquey. Others appear to be an attack on an aspect of medical practice. Why would one wish to submit oneself to the painful accusation or realisation of being unethical? Often they fail to provide answers to real and pressing clinical problems. As maternal–fetal medicine specialists, we know that ethics are relevant as we deal with precious and vulnerable lives, complex family decision making and future children and adults. We are questioned publicly about our ethics. In certain difficult cases we may also experience a visceral sinking or queasy feeling of 'Am I doing something wrong here?'

It is not possible in a small space to do justice to the depth and breadth of ethical issues in maternal–fetal medicine. A reading list at the end of the chapter points the interested reader to more detailed texts, books and journals. There are both great theoretical and elaborate individual problems. To illustrate this, Table 22.1 shows a list of contentious issues in this relatively new and rapidly developing medical field. Technological developments are bound to increase the list. Another approach starts with case-based scenarios which are also rich with complexity. A case study given below shows an example of an everyday case that poses ethical, as well as medical, problems for the participants. This chapter will attempt to draw a structure for discussions of all types of ethical issues in maternal–fetal medicine.

TABLE 22.1
Examples of current ethical issues in maternal–fetal medicine

Occurring at any time
Genetic knowledge – whose is it?
Property rights in genes, cells, etc.
Rights to know paternity
Requests for futile treatments
Iatrogenic creation of medical problems
Experimental treatments
Risk/benefit calculations for long-term or second generation harm
Informed consent
Research
Occurring pre-pregnancy
Contraception (coil, morning-after pill)
In vitro fertilisation
Embryo research
Surrogacy
Xenotransplantation
Artificial placenta
Cloning
Hybrids
Occurring first and second trimester
Abortion – rights and wrongs
Embryo reduction
Screening ('search and destroy'?)
Invasive testing risks
Selective reduction in multiple and discordant pregnancies
Fetal surgery
Occurring third trimester
Decisions re salvage or abandoning babies at edge of viability
Late karyotyping
Third-trimester termination and feticide
Monitoring during delivery
Enforced caesareans
Fetal and placental tissue donation
Occurring in neonatal life
Prematurity and sequelae
Withdrawal of intensive neonatal treatment
Value of the handicapped
Concept of the 'worthless life'
Infanticide

CASE STUDY

Jane, an illiterate 15-year-old single primigravida living in a mobile caravan with her mother on welfare is found to have a male fetus with megacystis and anhydramnios at 24 weeks' gestation. Apparently the 18-week anomaly scan was normal. The provisional diagnosis is posterior urethral valves and possible 'prune-belly'. There is severe hydronephrosis, and the kidney parenchyma is echogenic with a few cysts. Serial urine sampling shows relatively poor, but some, renal function. The previous week, the trainee talked optimistically about shunting without mentioning the poor long-term outlook and Jane is very keen to do everything possible to help the baby. However, even though the poor outlook has now been spelled out, she appears unrealistic about the possibility of neonatal death due to pulmonary hypoplasia or how she would manage long-term renal dialysis and childhood problems. She says 'I'm sure everything will be all right as the baby's moving OK'. Jane's mother understands about the low likelihood of survival and is pressing to terminate the pregnancy; 'Jane has always been slow and needed special schooling. It'll be me bringing this child up with my angina and arthritis. If it's ill we won't be able to manage. This child wasn't meant for this world and it'll be cruel to prolong its agony. I think you should end the pregnancy now, or at least leave it alone and let Nature decide'.

The case illustrates a number of problems. There is an *uncertain prognosis*, and procedures would be *invasive* with *risks of harm* to mother and baby. Is Jane *competent* to give *informed consent*? Who is the *patient* and to whom are *obligations* owed? How does one handle the *family dynamics*? If the doctor takes some or all of the *responsibility for decision making*, is this medical *paternalism* or appropriate? Would *late abortion* or early induction be wrong? Will *prematurity* add or *create harm*? How does one *alleviate suffering*? What are the *legal limits*?

Why should we consider ethics?

We all need to consider ethics for several reasons:

- To decide whether an action is right or wrong.
- To guide us in the future when a dilemma occurs.
- To know the extent of our professional obligations.
- For society to set boundaries of unacceptable behaviour through guidelines or laws.

An understanding of ethics may help doctors in a variety of ways. We may become aware of the underlying concepts guiding our everyday behaviour. We then have a basis for formulating questions about future actions and working out consistent and credible answers when asked to justify what we do or will do.

Ethics and law, although they have many parallels and connections, are not the same. An action may be legal but unethical: for example, walking past and ignoring an injured person in the street. An action may be ethical but not legal: for example, in the 'mercy-killing' debate, some argue that, although still illegal, it would be ethical to end the life of a terminally ill patient with intractable pain at their request. At the simplest level medical ethics is about the *highest* achievable standard of behaviour ('How can I be a good doctor?'), whereas law concerns itself with the *lowest* acceptable practice ('What is the lowest standard before redressing grievances or removing registration?'). Law is invoked to limit personal and professional judgements and freedoms when personal or professional ethics are not enough.

DESCRIPTIVE AND PRESCRIPTIVE ANALYSIS

An ethical analysis may have two parts:

1. *Descriptive. What is* the basis or foundation of the rules of behaviour? How does this or that group of doctors behave? Classically, we find different ethical cultures and laws in different countries, for example with regard to truth-telling and abortion.
2. *Prescriptive. What should be* the basis of the rules? For example, is abortion the taking of innocent life and absolutely wrong or a justifiable killing to prevent maternal harm? In an increasingly egalitarian world, should fathers have more rights to make decisions about their offspring when *in utero*?

These are similar to an individual's questions 'What *do* I do?' and 'What *should* I do?' If there is a discrepancy between what I do and what I should do, there is a pressure to change my belief or my behaviour. This is what makes the study of ethics so profoundly frightening. It may reveal inconsistencies in one's belief systems, or reveal that some pattern of behaviour is not right. This in turn may mean that we have previously been acting unethically or harming patients in our care. Patients can be harmed in a variety of ways; physically (for example, through disease, side-effects of treatment or negligent treatment), mentally (for example, through unsympathetic communication) and ethically. Patients are harmed ethically if they are treated without respect, treated against consent or treated as 'means' to an end rather than 'ends' in themselves (this last comes from Kant's categorical imperative[1]). Examples of patients being ethically harmed, without necessarily any physical or mental harm, would include being put into a research trial without their knowledge or being examined under anaesthetic without consent. Thus, being a good doctor is more than being good technically; it also includes communication and an ethically proper approach. If one has not been acting ethically, it must be better to face such a problem rather than carry on regardless.

Within 'What should I do?' are two further distinctions:

(i) distinction between an *intuition* and a *rational* argument;
(ii) distinction between *theory* and *practice*.

INTUITION AND RATIONAL ARGUMENT

For rationality: We have to overcome many gut reactions or instincts as doctors as they obstruct good medical practice. There is a social taboo about performing intimate examinations (for example a digital rectal examination, especially on a semi-stranger) but both the doctor and patient overcome the taboo by rational thought. We learn rituals to help both us and the patients overcome the instinctive upset and revulsion. We learn to hide our immediate dislike of certain individuals or groups as it is unprofessional and inappropriate. Our immediate intuition about the right course of action in a new and difficult ethical situation may equally be based on prejudice or ignorance that will give way on deeper thought and reflection. Philosophers are practitioners trained in the art and science of argument and can be extremely helpful in untangling and clarifying complex problems. However, they are theoreticians and may well belong to a particular school of thought or analysis, so doctors should not unthinkingly follow their prescriptions.

For intuition: Intuitions are worth some attention as they have evolved over many years and are often quicker than conscious thought processes, but they are fallible. Intuition may be related to caring when rationality can lead to cold, calculated and ultimately amoral behaviour. For example, if two people both require treatment and one is employed and the other unemployed, is it rational to treat only the first as the cost to society is more likely to be recouped? We may want more than mere calculations to guide our morality. If an intuition and rational argument do not match, one will have to give way, or both will have to be examined further to find the flaw.

THEORY AND PRACTICE

It is important to keep up a two-way dialogue between theory and practice. It is possible for health professionals to become bogged down in a morass of real-life complexity, or very involved with the feelings of the participants. They may then dismiss philosophy with 'well that's out of touch, ivory tower, academic nonsense'. Sometimes they can be so involved that they lose objectivity or the need for principles – not 'seeing the wood for the trees'. It is also possible for philosophers or medical ethicists to be insensitive to human life and concerns. They then miss out on field observations that enrich or enlighten theory. The best and most productive dialogue combines a mixture of both. Doctors should not be afraid to open their practice to scrutiny, as they may well have detailed information that empowers others to follow or defend their practice. Sometimes it must be tempting to ask someone else, maybe the ethics committee or board, to take away the awful responsibility for hurting patients, saying no to their demands for treatment or drawing boundaries for discussions or decisions. It would be comforting for someone else to be the expert or do the ethics. The only problem is that much of this is medicine, and doctors are expert at doctoring. They should not be so arrogant as to act alone, but nor should they be intimidated by ethical experts.

How can philosophers help?

Just as doctors look to scientific methods to support their understanding of disease and medicine, so we can look to moral philosophy and its methodology to help understand ethical problems. Philosophers are experts in argument and have available certain tools to help.

Firstly, philosophers *analyse words* and issues. They may draw our attention to the sloppiness of talking about 'euthanasia' for example. There may be many different topics under discussion; terminal care, relief of pain, the doctrine of double effect (acceptability of a good action, such as increasing pain relief, with the unintended but known side effect of shortening life), withdrawal of life support, active killing on request, or involuntary killing without consent. All the concepts (killing, intention, consent, etc.) are themselves divisible into parts and require much closer analysis.

Philosophers are used to *drawing distinctions*, or seeing morally relevant differences between situations. Consistency is a necessity in good arguments. If there is an appropriate ethical action for situation A, and situation B is essentially the same, so the ethical action should be the same. If, however, there is some discernible difference between A and B, then it might be justified to act differently. For example, one might consider that it is acceptable to induce labour for lethal anomalies. However, are there distinctions between types of lethal anomaly, and are they morally relevant? If there were three anomalies that were lethal at birth, one month or one year respectively, extra suffering might be caused to the baby if labour was induced (by adding prematurity to the problems of the newborn's short life). On the other hand, both maternal and neonatal suffering might be relieved by induction and death during or shortly after labour. The short life of suffering and inevitable death is lessened. Thus the type of anomaly might be a relevant distinction. A 'distinction without a difference' would be between two babies with different anomalies, say, but with exactly the same prognosis, when it is the prognosis that is weighed in the judgement about the right course of action.

Philosophers are also expert in the *use of logic* and pointing out that an argument does not flow logically when going from A to B to F and thus to conclusion G! They pin down the elements of an argument and find the jumps, leaps of faith or rhetoric that may be very emotionally persuasive or even comforting for doctors, but not necessarily logical.

Lastly, philosophers conduct '*thought experiments*'. These can seem ridiculous or trite, but are actually devices to separate several strands of an argument and examine them individually. Thought experiments are similar to controlled experiments in the laboratory where one variable is changed at a time to see its effect on the whole. It is to unpack our thoughts that they ask such unreal questions as 'What would you do if a prenatal diagnostic test for eye colour existed?' A thought experiment that tests the lengths to which we really sign up to 'informed consent' or 'beneficence' might be 'When would you refuse to do an amniocentesis?' Would it be at a 1 in 100 risk of aneuploidy, 1 in 1000, 1 in 10 000 or never (because it is the mother's informed choice)? 'What if a mother asked for a second (or third) amniocentesis when she already has a negative result?' Would you continue and do a completely unnecessary invasive procedure with a risk of fetal loss on maternal request because that is the mother's informed choice? Would you refuse, saying you know best and must not cause harm? Or, do you try and get out of the dilemma by suggesting the woman's choice does not have to be respected as it is not rational? In which case, are you really a believer in informed choices, or only those choices that agree with yours?

You can see from the above that what makes a good philosopher or medical ethicist is not someone who has *answers*, but someone who has *tools* to help ask the right questions. Someone who does not merely assert but justifies or explains. Good scientists are those who use sound and transparent methodology to test hypotheses, and whose results are consistent and reproducible. Philosophy can be seen as a scientific discipline in this way also. Good philosophers would not claim to be right or ethically superior, but would be rigorous, scientific and consistent. Like scientists, they are prepared to abandon a hypothesis if it proves to be flawed. This can be alarming for doctors when they find someone apparently passionately making an argument at one moment who says 'maybe I am totally wrong' and takes the opposite line in the next moment. As clinicians, our problem is that we must take decisions and actions that affect people's lives. We need a psychological certainty that it is ethical to do so (unless we are uncaring psychopaths!). This can create a conflict or tension when dealing with academic ethicists if they dissect our actions and ideology from what seems a safe and theoretical environment. If an action is questioned we may well feel defensive, uncomfortable, or even terrible and guilty.

It could be said that good philosophers pay more attention to the process than outcome. They would not just accuse doctors of being unethical or tell them how to behave. They would point out that, on the facts and arguments presented, a certain conclusion cannot be sustained and why it cannot. This may be discomforting, but allows for growth and learning. If doctors are to be responsible for their actions then we will have to go for the longer and harder route of understanding rather than 'I was only following orders'.

What is an ethical question?

What makes something an *ethical* issue? Ethics is the science of morals, the branch of philosophy that is concerned with human character and conduct. Thus any, and every, action within a doctor–patient relationship will have an ethical dimension. It is an inescapable fact of our everyday working life. Indeed, we take so much for granted that we stop noticing it. For example, there are systems of morals or rules of behaviour that have become ingrained. We have a duty of confidentiality and so would not tell our patients' stories to journalists. The obligation to obtain consent for examinations and procedures means we would not hold protesting patients down to do vaginal examinations or amniocenteses. We only appear to notice ethics when a conflict or an apparently insoluble problem arises, but ethics is always there.

What makes a conversation between a midwife and a pregnant woman about Down's screening an ethical issue whereas determining the decor in labour ward is not? We need to look at the three essential ingredients: an actor, an object and an act. The actor and object both have moral value. There has to be a relationship between them and something happens (including doing nothing if one could have done something). There are three main philosophical frameworks which all consider parts of this basic equation. They place major emphasis on one or other central tenet; the duties (crucially of the actor), the rights (crucially of the object) or the consequences (of the action). There are variations in views within each system, but they argue in different ways – that the ultimate 'good' is being good (duty-based), protecting the right-bearer (rights-based) or the maximising of good consequences (goal-based). We will consider who might be *actors* and *objects* of moral concern and then *special relationships* and lastly the *frameworks* of moral philosophy. The components of an issue of moral concern are thus:

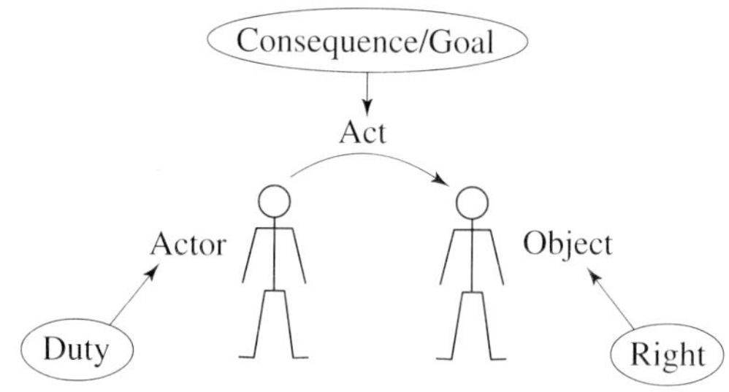

Table 22.2 gives examples of ethical issues and different views on the reasons that mothers should not smoke or doctors should maintain confidentiality or obtain consent.

The 'players' in maternal–fetal medicine

Table 22.3 contains examples of who or what might be an actor or object of moral concern. The 'objects' are divided into two lists: those that are autonomous and those that are non-autonomous. The meaning of autonomy is the power or right of self-government: the doctrine that the human will carries its guiding principle within itself[2]. The word 'autonomy' derives from the Greek for 'self-rule' and thus refers to beings that have self-awareness, can think and formulate actions.

We can see from the list that there will be many possible variations in the actor–object–act group, but that most actors and objects of moral concern are humans or groups of humans. Many appear on both lists. The only distinction between the lists is that it is a necessary, but not sufficient, condition to have a will or self-awareness or ability to formulate an action to appear on the 'actor' list. There are objects of moral concern without this that appear only on the objects list. Interestingly, some may appear temporarily on the object list, for example small children or unconscious patients, for

TABLE 22.2
Examples of ethical issues and components

Actor	Object	Act	Duty	Right	Goal
Mother	Fetus	Smoking	Mother's duty not to harm fetus	Either right to be born unharmed or no real 'right' as non-autonomous	Minimise number of damaged babies born
Doctor	Patient	Telling a secret	Doctor's duty of confidentiality	Patient's right to confidentiality	Confidentiality maintains trust in and efficacy of the medical profession
Surgeon	Patient	Operation	Touching is an assault unless prior consent	Right to bodily integrity. Consent can override	Must maximise health outcomes. Consent a device

TABLE 22.3
Possible actors and objects of moral concern

Actors (autonomous)	Objects (autonomous)	Objects (non-autonomous)
Doctor	Patient	Genes
Patient	Pregnant women	Gametes
Mother	Older child	Embryo
Father	Relative	Fetus
Donor	Mother	Neonate
Surrogate	Father	Young child
Relative	Doctor	Unconscious patient
Researcher	Researcher	Mentally incompetent
Government	Taxpayer	Animals
State	Donor	Future generations
Legal system	Surrogate	Precious commodities
Manager	Oppressed groups	
Taxpayer		
Pregnant women		
Pressure groups		
Interest groups		
Pharmaceutical companies		

whom others have to make decisions. However, at a later time, when they grow up or regain consciousness, they may also appear as actors. Others, such as the severely mentally disabled, may have to have some important decisions made on their behalf, although this should always be tested and not assumed. Some would dispute whether any moral value at all should be given to certain players on the object list (see later, 'What is the value or moral status of fetal life?'). What are the qualities that make something an agent or object of moral concern? Let us start with adult humans who have full moral worth.

What gives adult humans moral value?

We agree that adult human life is of value and adults should not be wantonly or unjustly killed. What are the qualities that make us worthy of moral consideration? There are a variety of reasons why adult human life may be of value:

1. '*We are part of God's creation and therefore sacred.*' This is also referred to as the 'sanctity of life' argument. The major problem with this argument is the absence of 'universalisability'. Any conclusions drawn from a religious view will not be generalisable or appeal to people of different or no religions. There is also still a debate about when God's creation started, or when the sanctity of life takes effect, although most religions hold that it starts at conception.
2. '*Humans are of value because we are human.*' Unfortunately this is not enough as it is a circular argument. What really matters is what distinguishes us from other animals, and does that hold for all human forms? Why would the possession of human DNA be particularly valuable? What happens when we get mixtures?
3. '*Our ability to feel pleasure, happiness, or form relationships is enough to justify protection.*' What then happens about humans who cannot have these feelings or animals who can?
4. '*We have the ability to suffer and feel pain.*' Conversely, it can be argued that it is the ability to suffer which creates a duty in others not to cause needless or unjustified suffering. This might be a reason to protect humans and higher-order animals from suffering, but would not necessarily create a duty to preserve life.
5. '*We are self-conscious and self-aware.*' These qualities make us very special and are what really make human life full and worth living. They are required to formulate intentions and motives, take responsibility and feel conscience. These may be the prerequisites for morality to avoid killing adult humans, either (a) because these are very special qualities or (b) because adults then themselves value their lives. These qualities may be used to justify moral status for the whole species (because most humans have self-consciousness the whole human race is of higher moral value). If it were used as a determinant of individual

moral worth then some humans at the extremes of life would not have worth. In addition, if an individual did not value his or her own life then the worth would diminish, or the duties to that individual would be lowered (e.g. voluntary euthanasia). Another higher function of adult humans is the *ability to form plans or express preferences* or aspirations. 'Utilitarians' say that the fulfilment of preferences, desires or aspirations is the greatest moral goal.

Then there may be a question of whether all humans are equal. Does one have more moral value than another because of a greater degree of intelligence, capability, sensitivity or strength of desire to be fulfilled? Generally, most philosophers sign up to equality of adults' moral value, although some consider that some humans lose it through incapacity (e.g. the embryo or mentally handicapped) or heinous behaviour (the criminal). It may be that the judgement about moral value is multilayered. Adult humans are important because they have all the qualities from (1) to (5). There may be moral responsibility, but lesser or different towards small animals because of (4) (the ability to suffer or feel pain).

What does 'moral value' confer? Most societies and religions agree that, at a minimum, (a) life should not be taken unjustly and (b) there is a general right not to be interfered with. There are many other protections and rights and they may follow a hierarchy. For example, although it is both wrong to kill and wrong to lie, it would be right to lie about someone hiding in your house to protect them from being killed by a murderous intruder. However, there are still very vigorous debates between people holding the same basic starting assumptions about the value of life, let alone different ones. These debates range from the rights and wrongs of capital punishment, to the ethics of 'a just war' to voluntary euthanasia.

If we could understand or analyse what gives adult human life value, we might be in a position to look at the smallest and earliest of human lives and their value. Do we value embryos or fetuses,

- for the same qualities as adults?
- for having those qualities in small amounts? – and therefore counting, but not as much as adults?
- for the potential to have adult qualities? – and does that mean they count now or not? or,
- for completely different reasons?

What is the value or moral status of fetal life?

With respect to comparison with adults there are only three possible answers to this question – full, some or none – although many reasons why it should be any of these answers.

Moral status	Example
Full	Adult human
Some	Animal
None	Inanimate object (e.g. chair)

Although some maternal–fetal medicine specialists, parents or ethicists may talk about the fetus as if it were of a certain value, it is important to be clear into which group they are categorising the fetus. For example, some argue for full moral status on the 'sanctity of life' argument which would entail doctors doing everything possible to increase, prolong or preserve fetal life. The moral status is intrinsic to the fetus and nothing makes killing or abortion right. Others would argue that the fetus has full moral status because the mother cares for it. The moral status thus derived extrinsically obliges doctors to do good ('beneficence'). The problem with this argument is that if a mother did not care then there would be no status and the doctor would be released from medical obligations. In this argument, the group 'fetus' actually has *no* intrinsic moral worth.

A doctor or mother may care for and value fetuses but still accept abortion for fetal abnormality. They must believe either (a) that abnormality diminishes moral status (from full status to some or none) or (b) that no fetus has full moral status and protection against being killed. Most Western democracies with abortion law appear to accord the fetus 'some' moral status, in that life cannot be taken during pregnancy wantonly but nor is it absolutely protected.

How does fetal moral worth change with time?

There is a time, most would agree, when there is no object of moral concern. The change from nothing to becoming an object of moral concern can only occur in one of three ways, suddenly, stepwise or gradually.

1. Suddenly

→ Full

→ None

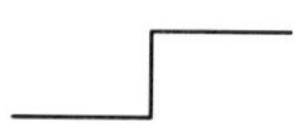

This sudden change might occur at conception (strict Catholic view), implantation, development of the neural tube (British Human Fertilisation and Embryology Act view for protection of human embryos against experimentation), viability ('fetus as a patient' view) or birth (woman's right to control her body view). Using a strict, sudden change allows a relatively simple analysis and resolution of problems in any dispute.

2. Stepwise

→ Full

→ None

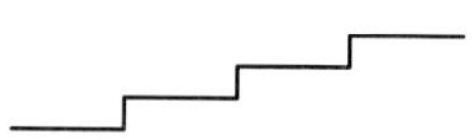

This view might correspond to the relationship of the mother to the developing fetus (e.g. status increasing in step with the pregnancy test and knowledge of pregnancy, quickening, first scan, birth and developmental milestones), or to a series of important physiological events (e.g.

implantation, formation of the neural tube, development of sensory cortical connections, viability, birth). Each step brings the fetus closer to adult status and ethical protection may increase stepwise also.

3. *Gradually*

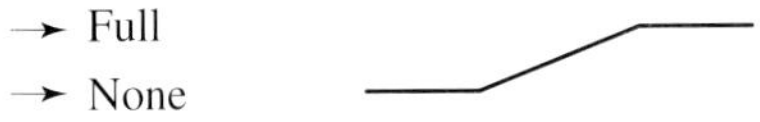

This might correspond to a developmental biological viewpoint, where status increases gradually with gestation, until a maximum is reached. The maximum could be being recognisably human, having the ability to sense pain or lay down memory, birth or self-awareness. This view means that each decision has to be individually weighed and balanced. What is acceptable ethically at 10 weeks might not be at 20 or 30 weeks. For example, with increasing gestation there will have to be a correspondingly greater justification for termination. Types (2) and (3), stepwise and gradually, are similar in that they require more complex judgements to be made.

Does birth make a difference?

Does birth make a difference to moral value? Intuitively it does, but is there a rational explanation? It is obvious that birth makes a difference to the mother as the fetus is now outside rather than inside her body. For example, if one is weighing countering claims of mother and fetus/child in situations where maternal behaviour is damaging or the mother is refusing beneficial intervention, removal of the child once born does not involve forcible incarceration or invasion of the mother. Thus after birth, any inhibition against violating her rights is removed. But does birth itself change the moral status of the fetus/child? We do know that the mother undergoes labour and delivery and puts work and effort into this. The baby undergoes a rapid and major adaptation to extrauterine life, becomes physically separate and breathes on his or her own, although is still extremely dependent. The baby enters the family and society and is given a name. Many powerful and important social events occur, but are any of these morally relevant? This is of particular interest to paediatricians who find it inexplicable, if not abhorrent, that they are involved in life-saving exercises for babies who are at such a low gestation that obstetricians may consider them previable. Thus at gestations around 24 weeks obstetricians may offer late termination, accept maternal refusal of caesarean section, decide not to monitor in labour, or deny classical caesarean section for fetal reasons.

What are the obligations of others and special relationships?

To whom do we owe a duty of care or responsibility? And what is its extent? The concept of 'special relationships' that bring extra and specific moral considerations into play is important. The most basic relationship is that of two strangers. What rights and responsibilities flow from a relationship of two strangers? How and why would the relationship of a mother to her child or two strangers be different? A stranger might be expected to keep a promise made to another, but not to buy all their clothes or wake repeatedly to feed every night, which would be expected of a mother for her child.

A doctor's duty to a patient is more than that of the stranger's. It may be characterised as doing one's best to increase life and decrease suffering. It may be characterised as respecting autonomy by fulfilling informed choices with regard to health outcomes, depending on the framework in which morality is being structured. However, being a doctor does not necessarily mean that one's duties to strangers or one's own children change or increase. Doctors may be concerned about the public health or be altruistic about global charity but do they actually have a moral duty to improving the health of others at some distance from themselves? This has implications when it comes to balancing conflicts of interests between patients. Doctors must have regard for all the patients in their clinic and have to ration their time. They have an equal duty of care to all the patients in a clinic. They may spend more or less time with each according to their medical problems but cannot spend two hours with the first one and always keep the rest waiting or shorten their appointments. Do doctors also have to ration their use of resources or costs, potentially depriving their patients of the best care, because other patients (not theirs) also have a claim to the limited resources? What does the implicit promise 'As your doctor, I will do my best for you' mean? There may be equal claims by patients on society, insurers or the state, or on doctors who manage budgets and priorities. Do doctors on the frontline fight for the needs of all 'their' individual patients or make decisions about competing needs? It may be that the same doctor sits in the morning on a committee allocating resources and in the afternoon with a patient denied that resource. Where does the responsibility lie? Or do we shift responsibility by using comfortable psychological devices so that we do not have to face unpalatable facts about limited resources?

Even if we agree that there is an ethical duty to care for a patient, the extent of this duty will be different for different individuals such as the doctor, nurse, relative, ward cleaner and passer-by. The standard, of doing one's best, might be the same, but that would entail different amounts from a generalist or a specialist, or a junior or senior doctor.

Frameworks for analysis

Normally, before communicating, discussing, arguing or negotiating with another person we make sure we speak the same language and work out whether we are starting from the same or different places. The reader must realise that in the fields of ethics and moral philosophy it is very easy to be mistaken that two people are speaking the same language or have the same concepts or assumptions. There are fundamental differences in approaches between individuals, philosophers and proponents of certain intellectual thoughts. They may use the same words differently or with different shades of meaning. For example, some may not include embryos on the 'moral worth' list at all. If embryos are included, one person might do so because they are intrinsically worthwhile themselves, but another might argue that embryos are worthwhile as someone else cares for them. One view is that embryos have intrinsic worth, which could be absolute, and the other is that they have extrinsic value, but maybe not as much as a living child. These differences will lead to very different views about the disposal of spare artificially created embryos even between two people agreeing they are of moral worth.

Not only are there differences about who or what appears on the moral agent and object lists and why, but then there are differences about how to analyse why some action is right or wrong. Most people agree that altruism and truth-telling are good and that murder and breaking promises are wrong, but they might give different reasons why. The answer to 'why?' may then lead to a difference of opinion, for example, regarding the next issue of payment for, or research on, human embryos.

The three main theoretical moral frameworks primarily examine the motives and intentions of the actor (duty-based), the object (rights-based) or the effects of the act (consequence or goal-based). There are variations within each philosophical system, but their underlying bases are fundamentally different. The ultimate 'good' is: being good (duty-based), protecting the right-bearer (rights-based) or the maximising of good consequences (goal-based). Careful listening or analysis can identify these different appeals.

In duty-based systems, conscience and motive are paramount. Originating from religion, and God judging the actor, there are also secular, humanist versions. We have duties and obligations to others and any 'rights' they possess flow from the duty. That is, the 'right to life' exists from the duty not to kill. Typically, fetuses may have a 'right to life' even though they have no self-expression. Doctors are not allowed to kill even if that is what the patient requests. The exception is when a doctor uses the Doctrine of Double Effect. That is when the doctor uses a drug such as morphine with a good intended effect (pain relief), but a known but non-intended side-effect (life-shortening). 'Rights' do not really have much force in duty-based systems although they are powerful rhetorically and politically. In a duty-based system abortion can only be acceptable if fetuses do not have full moral worth.

In rights-based systems, rights are inherently held by people, and duties flow secondarily from the right. They have largely been described in the twentieth century within political philosophy[3]. For example, if one has a right to vote, this makes a very powerful political claim on others to provide that right. These kinds of strong rights have the quality of being able to be waived. For example, one might have a 'right to vote' or a 'right of association' but not use either of them. Rights can only be held by those capable of making autonomous choices. In true rights-based systems, fetuses can have no rights as they cannot make choices or waive their rights. Thus they do not count at all. In obstetrics, women may claim certain rights (for example, to prenatal diagnosis or to choose the method of delivery). If one operates in a strong rights-based system, when rights exist doctors are obliged to provide the services. One might ask on what basis is there a right? For example, is there a right to reproduce, or a right to have a healthy child? Is there a fundamental right not to be interfered with, in which case clearly we should not stop women choosing to get pregnant or perform forcible abortion or sterilisation, but this is not the same as a right to get help.

In goal-based systems, an action is not inherently right or wrong as it depends on the outcome or consequence. This consequentialist or utilitarian approach was developed in the nineteenth century from the work of Mill and Bentham[1,4]. The ultimate purpose of morality is to increase the sum of happiness, or maximisation of pleasure or preferences. We should be acting for the maximisation of good outcomes. When it is impossible to work out all the possible consequences of an action, a rule might be invoked that generally has that effect. If there were a rule, such as 'do not kill', it is not that we should not kill as killing is inherently wrong, but that having such a rule means the world is a better place in which to live. Some killings will actually be judged as right (for example, of people who do not wish to live or dictators who cause harm). It is in utilitarianism that no-one has inherent value. Value is related to qualities possessed by the subject, such as sentience, preferences or ability to feel pain. A major criticism of utilitarianism is that of sacrificing one for the many, or overall benefit. Concepts of speciesism and replacement children belong here. Utilitarianism can be very attractive to doctors, as we spend our lives making harm/benefit calculations on the individual level and responding to parents' views of the worth of their fertility or offspring.

Spotting where an argument comes from, it can be weighed in its context. It is somewhat similar to giving one's vote to a politician. It helps to know which party they belong to and thus how their concept of freedom or equality of opportunity might be coloured.

'THE FETUS AS A PATIENT'

An example of identifying the philosophical framework being used is in the debate about 'the fetus as a patient'. There is a popular view in maternal–fetal medicine that 'the fetus is a patient'. Does this have any *ethical* meaning? Chervenak[5,6] and McCullough[7], in particular, have written a number of papers in the obstetric literature putting forward one particular model of maternal–fetal ethics. It is important to realise that, although this model dominates the American obstetric literature and claims to be 'ethically justified', it is not definitive and is far from being generally accepted in philosophical circles.[8]

The particular argument about fetuses (and counter-argument) runs thus:

- *Argument*: No-one can agree on the independent moral status of the fetus. There are diametrically opposed views. At one extreme, the 'sanctity of life', which is utterly opposed to abortion, at the other, notions of 'personhood' (which does not come until the child has interests, self-realisation or sentience, etc.). This latter is not the same argument as the ultra-feminist 'right to choose', but all those views that include 'personhood' accept abortion, as the fetus does not have it whilst *in utero*. Despite philosophers' best efforts there is no resolution nor any likelihood of resolution of this issue.
  Counterargument: Yes, there is disagreement about fundamental values. However, the existence of an impasse is not a justification for taking one side or the other. Does the concept of 'the fetus as a patient' end up being another version of one or other side of this impasse or is it a new view entirely that breaks the deadlock?
- *Argument*: We need to break the deadlock. So what do we agree upon? We all agree that the child is a patient to whom we have obligations. Therefore let us work backwards in time to identify our patients.
  Counterargument: We might well agree that we have obligations to treat children, but, as explained above, we might have different underlying reasons for our agreement. If we go further back in time, the reasons and agreement may become uncoupled. If we work back far enough, through child, baby, neonate, fetus, embryo and egg we may find that the thing we are dealing with has changed its nature and thus its moral status.
- *Argument*: Patients are those we can benefit, i.e. this starts at about 24 weeks when the fetus becomes viable.
  Counterargument: Firstly, is it agreed that 'patients are those we can benefit'? A more traditional definition is that 'patients are those under the care of a doctor' (whether we can benefit them or not). Otherwise we might find that we have unwilling and unwitting patients – those people who are unwell and can be benefited but who have not gone to see a doctor. Secondly, is it plausible that moral worth is determined by whether a doctor can benefit you? Does that mean that the size of a doctor's obligation relates to the amount he or she can do for you? And why should it? Another interesting possibility would be that the very sick and dying would not be patients or would count less than the remediably unwell. Are there obligations only to patients with treatable problems but not untreatable ones? We are always taught that it is reprehensible to walk past the beds of dying patients as they still require care even when cure is impossible. Is this only a symbolic need to care for the vulnerable? Thirdly, fetuses can be helped well before 24 weeks so there is no relevance of viability to 'the fetus as a patient' concept (excepting for the treatment of separation from the mother by delivery or enforced caesarean which can be justified only after viability). The ability to survive when separate from the mother is not the starting time when a fetus can be benefited. For example, cervical cerclage and blood transfusions for isoimmunisation can be administered much earlier. Particularly in the first trimester, when fetal vulnerability is greatest, teratogenic drugs can cause terrible harms well before 24 weeks. If a mother requested thalidomide for hyperemesis, should a doctor prescribe it under autonomy-based obligations to the mother at a time when she has not conferred status and the doctor has no beneficence-based obligations to the fetus? Doctors must have obligations not to cause harm at a time before the 'fetus as a patient' view starts.
- *Argument*: If the mother confers status and protection to her fetus beforehand, we will then also have beneficence-based obligations to fetus before 24 weeks.
  Counterargument: The mother can confer status. In other words, the status is granted by the mother as and when she sees fit. That is, the status is optional, and this means the fetus must actually be worth nothing intrinsically. There are only three views on *independent* moral status of the fetus (as described earlier): none, some or full. The 'sanctity of life' view gives fetuses full moral value. The 'personhood' view gives them none. There are views in between that take neither side of the impasse. What is the 'fetus as a patient' view? A view where value is *extrinsic* or *dependent* is actually one with a starting point of none (the default option) unless some property is identified. In this case the property that the fetus has that determines medical obligation is either the ability to be helped, or the mother conferring status (possibly as she has religious views or a sentimental attachment). Thus the concept of the 'fetus as a patient' does not break the deadlock of fundamental values. Any particular fetus may or may not have value depending on extrinsic facts. There is no intrinsic worth. The view merely shifts the starting point to 24 weeks (if and when a fetus can be helped).
- *Argument*: Various algorithms can then be devised to answer specific queries about the ethical permissibility of various treatments depending on gestation, and whether we have obligations to patients.
  Counterargument: If women do not do what

obstetricians consider as the best for their fetus, the 'fetus as a patient' argument can be used to enforce treatments in late pregnancy, on the basis of the mother's purported 'beneficence-based obligations' (that is, the obligations she has to help her fetus). The argument can be used to justify caesareans against consent. In reality, the 'fetus as a patient' (as already described and understood) is not a compromise view at all. It is a view that gives fetuses no intrinsic status and ends up conceptually being, in some senses, both anti-fetus and anti-mother. This is all a consequence of overstating the role of the doctor on whose judgement of benefit moral status turns. Superficially, the view is very appealing to doctors, who firstly are given intimations of omnipotence, and secondly, are given easy and comfortable solutions to difficult questions. The view should be rejected, even if, in part, it is our own fault for devising the medical slogan or concept of fetuses as patients. If the preceding steps are not accepted, no algorithm has to be followed.

CONCLUSION

Although apparently logical, the 'fetus as a patient' is actually an extraordinary and simplistic argument with many flaws[8]. It appears to have arisen from the medical language of the fetus as a patient, used by medical practitioners and fetal medicine pioneers themselves. It may have consolidated the emergent field of fetal medicine to point out to others that there are specific diseases and syndromes of fetuses. What is more, there are investigations and treatments specialists can apply. Fetal life and the importance of helping fetuses, because we can, have been drawn to public attention. However, to move from descriptions of medical advances to a redefinition of moral worth is a big leap.

Whatever the view on moral status during fetal life, one can argue that there is an obligation not to harm the child or adult who will eventually be born. However, there is an interesting difference in the obligations not to kill and not to harm when applied to adults and fetuses. In adult life, it is generally worse to kill than to harm because, even though damaged, the adult is still alive. However, during pregnancy it might logically be permissible to kill a fetus that has some moral worth if the argument is made that the abortion is of a lesser moral being and justified by some risk to the mother. However, at the same gestations it might not be permissible to harm it for the sake of the mother (for example, giving thalidomide for hyperemesis or induction of labour at 30 weeks owing to maternal discomfort) as it will later become a damaged greater moral being of full moral worth.

'HOW SHOULD I ACT?'

Having explained some of the concepts behind language, and some of the philosophical approaches, practitioners on the frontline still have to find an answer to 'what do I do *now*?' They have both ethical and legal obligations and the following section explains how these are described and then makes some simple practical recommendations.

Ethics – the highest ideal of behaviour

How might one work towards a high ideal of behaviour?

PROFESSIONAL ETHICS OR ETIQUETTE

The original description of a doctor's duty came from Hippocrates, and over the centuries this has become the *Hippocratic tradition*. In the eighteenth and nineteenth centuries, codes of etiquette were drawn up, that may have had more to do with professional demarcation than patient care. Many critics of medicine are particularly angry about the paternalism and authoritarianism that they feel is implicit in this tradition. One can try to act according to sets of rules devised by the profession. This might include professional codes of conduct (e.g. the GMC's *Duties of a doctor*[9]), international declarations (e.g. the Nuremberg Code[10] or the Declaration of Helsinki[11]) or specialty guidelines (e.g. RCOG guidelines on enforced treatment of pregnant women[12]). These might work most of the time but inevitably are general rather than specific and do not encourage independent thinking. The original Hippocratic Oath is now old-fashioned and inconsistent although there are attempts to update it. The value of professional rules is that they are drawn up by experts and can guide professionals who are too busy, tired or lazy to think. They also encourage consistency between practitioners and public accountability and transparency.

VIRTUE ETHICS

Virtue theorists consider that *virtues* should be inculcated and nourished in doctors and that this, rather than rules or intellect, will produce ethical doctors. Virtues might include motivation judgement and rapport[13], or self-effacement, self-sacrifice, compassion and integrity[14]. Other virtues might be knowledge, compassion, decisiveness, consistency, punctuality and responsibility. Vices might include being ideological, incompetent, prejudiced, irrational, inconsistent, irresponsible or weak. Unfortunately, merely being 'virtuous' is not enough as a guide. Are there better virtues to cultivate? How does one achieve them? How much self-sacrifice is the minimum, reasonable or supererogatory (more than is required, for the sake of greater perfection)? Are doctors who work tirelessly for their patients, never take holidays and neglect their own families commendable or not?

PRINCIPLES AND ALGORITHMS

In the late twentieth century, four principles, it is claimed, should guide and cover all ethical medical decision making[15,16]. These are *beneficence* (doing good), *non-maleficence* (avoiding harm), *respect for autonomy* and *justice*. Unfortunately, no guidance is given on which should give way when they clash, nor why doctors should follow them. If autonomy overrides all other considerations, this is significantly different from doctors' traditional duties to the vulnerable and non-autonomous. Should doctors be more concerned about justice because they are doctors, or should they be equally concerned just like other citizens? This matters when it comes to the distribution of scarce medical resources or rationing. Should a doctor fight for his or her individual patient (over the interests of the next doctor's patient) or should a doctor accept rationing (as a just way of delivering services) and accept what might be a second-best or 'good-enough' treatment or no treatment at all? It is not clear how far each of the principles goes in the individual special relationship. Algorithms have been devised[17,18] but either they merely describe all ethical dimensions to a problem or they are drawn up with ranking priorities in mind. For example, an algorithm will finally make beneficence give way to autonomy or vice versa.

DUTY, GOAL AND RIGHTS BASED PHILOSOPHIES

The frameworks as described are fundamentally mutually incompatible. This is not necessarily a counsel of despair as there may always be some fundamental underlying conflicts in human society that cannot be glossed over. The work of philosophers now is in assessing what is a good untangling, or an acceptable reason to veer in one direction or another. Whereas an algorithm may claim to give an answer to a problem, analytic philosophers can at least clarify what issues are at stake and who or what is being excluded or overridden in a decision.

Law – the lowest standard of behaviour

Enough of the theorising, the agonising, the introverted detailed analysis, the seeing all points of view, the 'on the one hand … and on the other …', what about real life and decision-making? A marvellous thing about medicine is that it is real and active. We have to make decisions and ignore certain information or interpretations, or order tests and treatments with good and harmful side-effects. But inevitably people get hurt and conflicts arise. Law is concerned with sorting out grievances and damage within a society. What does the law do?

- It sets limits by defining unacceptable behaviour.
- It criminalises the extremes.
- It is used to settle grievances or provide recompense for negligence.
- It may have a symbolic function in setting standards.

In maternal–fetal medicine, the most relevant criminal law usually relates to abortion and assault, though manslaughter may be relevant in maternal death. Negligence is usually a civil offence with financial recompense available. Law does not have to have the quality of 'generalisability' that is demanded of ethics. It varies greatly around the world. The main requirement of doctors is not to break local law. Law does not necessarily encourage ethical behaviour, nor lead to good medical practice, but sets a lowest common denominator below which the worst doctor should not fall. There is a view that excess concern about negligence claims leads to an overinvasive, non-holistic and expensive type of 'defensive' medical practice, that is not actually in the individual patient's interest (and therefore not ethical!). There is no evidence that defensive practice does actually keep claims down. If a claim is made, the defendant's lawyers are greatly helped by good documentation and standard practice. Thus, from a self-interested point of view, a doctor practising ethically and to a high medical standard is unlikely to fall foul of the lawyers. There are lawyers working on both sides, for the plaintiff and the defendant, and it is best not to get too worked up about them. All of us, as citizens, have to have the security of legal mechanisms to address grievances although it can be extremely personally upsetting to receive complaints.

When doctors are expected by the State to do something that is unethical, such as be involved in punishment of criminals, torture or labelling dissidents as mentally ill, they may find themselves in terrible personal conflict or danger. They have to heed a higher ethical calling and look for help and support from colleagues around the world. National medical organisations have been expelled from worldwide medical bodies for their toleration of persecution or abuse of doctors. Organisations such as Physicians for Human Rights or the World Medical Assembly may be helpful[19].

Real-life ethical trouble

When looking through notes of obstetric disasters, we often find a string of events, a series of small failures and many different people involved. It is rare to find that care was otherwise ideal and well documented but for one single mistake. Ethical crises are very similar. Many occur after miscommunication, muddled advice, poor medicine and in a muddied cultural context. If one starts at the beginning of the story and untangles it, the ethical component or dilemma is often much smaller than at first it appears. Thus, Table 22.4 shows advice about good medical practice that will also keep practitioners out of ethical trouble. The table contains examples of behaviour that gets doctors into trouble. Avoid such behaviour!

TABLE 22.4
How to get into ethical trouble in maternal–fetal medicine

Dealing with the patient
Do not read the referral letter
Assume you are a good communicator
Be rushed and too busy to pay full attention
Do not listen to the patient
Instead of the patient, find out what her husband or family want
Assume you and the patient share ethical and cultural values
Assume the patient is too stupid to understand concepts
Use medical jargon to ensure non-comprehension
Personality factors
Determine the patient's wishes by her clothes, educational level, income or demeanour
Assume everyone is monogamous, married or part of a happy family
Have fixed views about the world
Have strong and unyielding views about abortion, handicap, motherhood
Divide women into 'good' and 'bad'
Denigrate other doctors and health professionals
Be ignorant of the law (but certain you know it)
Have no idea about the effect of own personality on others
Respond excessively to gratitude
Be blissfully ignorant and complacent
Love media attention
Practical issues
Work on partial information
Stick to traditions and practices you learnt ten years ago
Do tests before working out the consequences of results you might obtain
Do large numbers of tests 'just in case'
Do not speak to colleagues (general practitioner, midwife, etc.)
Discuss cases loudly, especially in the hospital lift
Pay no attention to others' concerns
Assume you are the best (and only) doctor around
Get second opinions only from people who agree with you
Be pressurised to get answers *now*
When you do not know, guess!
Do new procedures 'for the sake of it' or because you need practice to help other patients
Confuse experimentation, research and audit
Special responsibilities of the Head of Department
Set a bad example and consider it leadership
Delegate the work to inexperienced juniors, and push people beyond their competence
Spend much time away and out of department
Pay no attention to facilities, equipment, servicing
Have no interest in protocols or procedures
Be ignorant of your department's numbers, workload, referral times, delays and complaints
Delegate complaints and policy to others
Blame everyone else when things go wrong

TABLE 22.5
Improving your own ethical expertise

Outside experts
Professional codes of conduct and guidelines
Specialty organisations (associations, colleges, unions)
Medical defence organisations
Ethics committees
University departments of philosophy, law, theology
Hospital religious advisers
Ethical education
Read ethics articles, books and journals
Attend ethics courses
Obtain an ethics, law or philosophy degree
Make friends: religious advisers, educationalists, philosophers, 'wise' men and women
Identify ethics within usual case discussions
Be proactive – set up regular multidisciplinary ethics meetings and seminars
Read and take part in informed public debate and outside opinion

How to get out of ethical trouble

Firstly, avoid getting into trouble (see above). Document your concerns closely and contemporaneously. If stuck, get second opinions (medical, legal, or refer to your ethics committee if you have one). It is important to recognise the morally 'queasy' feeling. You do not feel quite right, or are being pressurised to do something unusual or out of your depth. Although stopping is difficult, proceeding nevertheless gets you and the patient into deeper water. It is quite acceptable to say 'This is a difficult and complex problem and I would like to take advice about the best way to proceed. We will meet again on ...' If cornered, or feeling emotionally blackmailed, one can always say 'It would be unprofessional for me to carry on without reviewing the situation'. Often just taking stock or talking through a problem makes it vanish or at least manageable. Table 22.5 contains a variety of actions to improve your ethical expertise.

It is vitally important to *know your medicine* as many legal and ethical problems revolve around the medical facts. If there is a problem when offering a risky treatment, or rationing it, the problem may well become moot if the complication rate proves to be 5% rather than 95% or vice versa. No-one can make an individual ethical decision or judgement without medical knowledge. Indeed, it is this knowledge that is the justification for health professionals making ethical decisions in the first place. There is nobody else who can make medical ethical decisions *instead* of doctors, although there are several players who may make them *with* doctors (principally the patient). Indeed, it can be considered an abdication of one's responsibility to the patient to leave such decision making to committees at one remove!

When there is a conflict, identify;

- What are the *issues*?
- Who are the relevant *parties*?
- What are the vested *interests* or pressures?

Try to divide a problem into its medical, legal, social, psychological, communication and ethical components. You may need advice from several sources, each appropriate to their part. Get expert advice from relevant experts, not reflex opinions from your friends. Do not get specialist medical advice from a generalist. Do not ask for ethical advice from a lawyer nor infer religious beliefs from a distant relative.

Do not be pressured into acting beyond your level of competence. This means being self-reflective about skills and their maintenance, continuing your medical education and referring on to other specialists when it is in the patient's interests. Examine your own personal difficulties and beliefs and where they may interact differently from your colleagues. Just because you feel strongly that you are right does not mean you will be the best doctor for the patient. Be open, transparent and ready for criticism. If you want reflection about your practice, invite nurses, colleagues, juniors and visitors in to watch you and ask 'how could that have been improved?' If they do not make suggestions, challenge you or make you uncomfortable then you may not be creating the right or safe conditions for open discussion. Beware that you may have a powerful or fragile personality that does not look as if it is genuinely ready to receive advice or criticism. On the other hand, do not be disabled by self-reproach or guilt as these too can lead to decision paralysis.

When things go wrong, find the source and put the systems right for next time. Are risk assessment, counselling and support services available in your unit? Particularly when things go wrong, follow up the patients and make sure you have unhurried and uninterrupted time to discuss and listen.

Constantly ask 'what could I do better?'

Conclusions

- Every day is full of ethical decisions and practices.
- Doctors should not view ethics as an optional 'add-on' or something highly specialist.
- There are ethical skills that can be developed, honed and applied usefully to patient care.
- There are many sources of help for ethical difficulties including wise counsels, philosophers, lawyers, defence organisations, books, journals and patient organisations.
- An understanding of basic principles will enable doctors to examine their own practice critically and safely, defend such practice publicly and diminish their reliance on self-styled 'ethical experts'.
- Do not believe that there are easy solutions!!

REFERENCES

1. Norman R. Kant: Respect for persons. Chapter 6, pp. 94–123. *The Moral Philosophers: An Introduction to Ethics*. Oxford: Clarendon Press, 1990.

   An excellent introductory text ranging from Plato to modern Marxism and psychoanalysis.

2. Davidson GW, Seaton MA & Simpson J (eds) *The Wordsworth Concise English Dictionary*, p. 64. Edinburgh: Chambers, 1994.

3. Griffin J. *Well-being: Its Meaning, Measurement and Moral Importance*, pp. 224–253. Oxford: Oxford University Press, 1990.

   Difficult text on utilitarianism and rights-based morality.

4. Raphael DD. *Moral Philosophy*. Oxford: Oxford University Press, 1990.

   An excellent introduction to the wider field of moral philosophy.

5. Chervenak F & McCullough L. A practical method of analysis of the physician's ethical obligations to the fetus and pregnant woman in obstetric care. *Resid. Staff Physician* **35**(1):79–87, 1989.

   A model of conflicts between pregnant woman and physicians based on the autonomy/beneficence obligations of the physician to both and the mother to the fetus.

6. Chervenak FA & McCullough LB. The fetus as a patient: an essential ethical concept for maternal–fetal medicine. *J Mat–Fet Med* **5**:115–119, 1996.

   Expostulation of the concept of the fetus as patient to whom the obstetrician has beneficence-based obligations because he can do good.

7. McCullough LB & Chervenak FA. *Ethics in Obstetrics and Gynecology*. Oxford: Oxford University Press, 1994.

   Attempt to set out a framework for moral decision-making based on doctors' beneficence and autonomy-based obligations, and in particular a preventative approach by using informed consent.

8. Callahan JC. First steps in preventative ethics. *Hastings Centre Report* **26**(2):45–46, 1996.

   A strong critique of McCullough & Chervenak's book and 'the fetus as a patient' approach to obstetrics.

9. General Medical Council. *Duties of a Doctor*, 1995.

   British professional rules of conduct of the doctor–patient relationship.

10. Katz J. *Experimentation with Human Beings*, pp. 292–306. Russell Sage Foundation, 1972.

    Chilling indictments from the trial of Dr Karl Brandt and others before the Nuremberg Military Tribunals about war crimes and crimes against humanity involving medical experiments committed in concentration camps. Should be required reading by all researchers to know the extent of our history. Judgement contains the ten principles that became known as the Nuremberg Code.

11. World Health Organisation. Declaration of Helsinki (amended 1975 and 1983), 1964.

12. Royal College of Obstetricians and Gynaecologists. *RCOG Ethics Guidelines. No. 1. A consideration of the law and ethics in relation to court-authorised obstetric intervention*. April 1994 (supplement December 1996).

13. Brewin T. How much ethics is needed to make a good doctor? *Lancet* **341**:161–163, 1993.

    Argues that good doctors need the virtues of motivation, judgement and rapport but not academic ethics.

14. Chervenak FA, McCullough LB & Chez RA. Responding to the challenges posed by the business tools of managed care in the practice of obstetrics and gynecology. *Am J Obstet Gynecol* **175**:523–527, 1996.

    Four virtues to use proactively for conflicts of interest.

15. Beachamp TL & Childress JF. *Principles of Biomedical Ethics*. Oxford: Oxford University Press, 1979.

    Definitive work expostulating the four principles of beneficence, non-maleficence, respect for autonomy and justice.

16. Gillon R (ed.). *Principles of Health Care Ethics*. Chichester: John Wiley, 1994.

Multi-author and comprehensive text.

17. Seedhouse D & Lovett L. *Practical Medical Ethics*. Chichester: John Wiley, 1992.

A basic book with four-colour ethical grid and algorithms – useful for exploring practical problems.

18. Johnson AG. *Pathways in Medical Ethics*. London: Edward Arnold, 1990.

A simple text for medical students with a flow diagram on page 35 for breaking up all problems.

19. Anon. Health and human rights. *Lancet* **350**:586–587, 1997.

FURTHER READING

Journal articles

Berkowitz JM. How I was almost aborted: reflections on a prenatal brush with death. *J Med Eth* **17**:136–137, 1991.

A medical student finding out about the circumstances of his adoption contemplates his near non-existence and reflects on how he remains pro-choice.

Berkowitz RL. From twin to singleton. *Br Med J* **313**:373, 1996.

A good commentary on the present state of selective reduction.

Boss JA. First trimester prenatal diagnosis: earlier is not necessarily better. *J Med Eth* **20**:146–151, 1994.

Arguing against CVS both because of increased fetal loss and increased pressure on women to undergo testing in view of the social privacy and apparent ease of the test.

Chervenak FA & McCullough LB. An ethically justified, clinically comprehensive management strategy for third-trimester pregnancies complicated by fetal anomalies. *Obstet Gynecol* **75**:311–316, 1990.

Now argues for definite diagnosis of lethal disorder or no cognitive function, i.e. anencephaly and triploidy.

Chervenak FA & McCullough LB. Ethics, an emerging subdiscipline of obstetric ultrasound, and its relevance to the routine obstetric scan. *Ultrasound Obstet Gynecol* **1**:18–20, 1991.

Chervenak FA, McCullough LB & Wapner RJ. Selective termination to a singleton pregnancy is ethically justified. *Ultrasound Obstet Gynecol* **2**:84–87, 1992.

Chervenak FA & McCullough LB. An ethically justified algorithm for offering, recommending, and performing cesarean delivery and its application in managed care practice. *Obstet Gynecol* **87**:302–305, 1996.

Another algorithm, this time justifying caesarean on maternal request against medical advice.

Chervenak FA, Farley MA, Walters L, Hobbins JC & Mahoney MJ. When is termination of pregnancy during the third trimester morally justifiable? *N Engl J Med* **310**:501–504, 1984.

Argues for anencephaly only.

Cohen CB. 'Give me children or I shall die!' New reproductive technologies and harm to children. *Hastings Centre Report* **26**(2):19–27, 1996.

Argues for limits to IVF if children may have serious illness or disorders and against the Interest in Existing Argument (it is better to have been born with disabilities than not at all).

Consumers for Ethics in Research. *Spreading the word on research or patient information: how can we do it better?* 1993.

A very good leaflet about writing intelligible patient information (CERES, PO Box 1365, London N16 0BW).

Coverdale JH, Chervenak FA, McCullough LB & Bayer T. Ethically justified clinically comprehensive guidelines for the management of the depressed pregnant patient. *Am J Obstet Gynecol* **174**:169–173, 1996.

Draper H. Women, forced caesareans and antenatal responsibilities. *J Med Eth* **22**:327–333, 1996.

Argues that mothers have 'Good Samaritan' obligations towards their children, but that the existence of such an obligation does not mean others are at liberty or obliged to perform operations without consent.

Fisk NM, Fordham K & Abramsky L. Elective late fetal karyotyping. *Br J Obstet Gynaecol* **103**:468–470, 1996.

A controversial paper suggesting delaying karyotyping until the third trimester in the context of late feticide to avoid the risk of miscarriage.

Grundstein-Amado R. Teaching medical ethics. Values education: a new direction for medical education. *J Med Eth* **21**:174–178, 1995.

A description of values education and how students can fill in personal values diaries.

Heyd D. Prenatal diagnosis: whose right? *J Med Eth* **21**:292–297, 1995.

Examination of the rights to prenatal diagnosis from the parents', society's and fetus' points of view: all deficient.

Kallenberg K, Forslin L & Westerborn O. The disposal of the aborted fetus – new guidelines: ethical considerations in the debate in Sweden, *J Med Eth* **19**:32–36, 1993.

Discussion about the guidelines on the dignified treatment of late miscarriages and aborted fetuses > 12 weeks as objects of moral value despite possible upset to mothers.

Kennedy I. The law and ethics of informed consent and randomised controlled trials. In *Treat Me Right*, pp. 213–224. Oxford: Clarendon Press, 1988.

An interesting article suggesting that it is hard for RCTs to ever be ethical as equipoise does not really exist.

Nuffield Council on Bioethics. *Genetic Screening: Ethical Issues*. London: NCB, 1993.

Pinkerton JV & Finnerty JJ. Resolving the clinical and ethical dilemma involved in fetal–maternal conflicts. *Am J Obstet Gynecol* **175**:289–295, 1996.

An article supporting the use of ethics committees and court-orders but not the ultimate use of physical force to persuade women to undergo interventions on behalf of their fetuses.

Rodeck CH & Bewley S. Late abortion for fetal abnormality. In *Ethics in Obstetrics and Gynaecology* (eds S Bewley, RH Ward), pp. 262–267. London: RCOG Press, 1994.

Early observations of third trimester terminations in the United Kingdom following a relaxation of the law.

Swartz M. Pregnant woman vs. fetus: a dilemma for hospital ethics committees. *Cambridge Quart. Healthcare Ethics* **1**:51–62, 1992.

An analysis of the American law and a case study of a late diagnosis of hydrocephalus where the mother refused caesarean section and preferred cephalocentesis against recommendations of paediatric neurologist.

Thomasma DC, Muraskas J, Marshall PA, Myers T, Tomich P & O'Neill JA. The ethics of caring for conjoined twins: The Lakeberg twins. *Hastings Centre Report* **26**(4):4–12, 1996.

A very interesting case study of conjoined twins separated against medical advice in the midst of a media circus.

Thornton JG. Measuring patients' values in reproductive medicine. *Contemp Rev Obstet Gynaecol* **1**:5–12, 1988.

Interesting use of lotteries to find out women's values for different outcomes, e.g. amniocentesis vs. miscarriage, caesarean section vs. stillbirth to devise decision analysis.

Books

Bewley S & Ward RH. *Ethics in Obstetrics & Gynaecology*. London: RCOG Press, 1994.

Papers and discussions about a range of issues including rights, commerce, the doctor–patient relationship, beginning of life and problem pregnancies.

Boyd K, Callaghan B & Shotter E. *Life Before Birth. Consensus in Medical Ethics*. London: SPCK, 1986.

An ecumenical look at the ethics of abortion and the treatment of infertility primarily for church leaders and theological students.

Cohen M, Nagel T & Scanlon T (eds). *The Rights and Wrongs of Abortion. A Philosophy & Public Affairs Reader*. Princeton, NJ: Princeton University Press, 1974.

Good basic philosophy with Judith Jarvis Thomson's classic women's rights article 'A defence of abortion'.

Eyans D & Evans M. *A Decent Proposal. Ethical Review of Clinical Research*. Chichester: John Wiley, 1996.

A very detailed and practical book about the paternalistic responsibility of society and Research Ethics Committees to patients involved in research.

Gillon R. *Philosophical Medical Ethics*. New York: John Wiley, 1986.

Introduction to the four principles of biomedical ethics.

Harris J. *The Value of Life. An Introduction to Medical Ethics*. London: Routledge, 1989.

A comprehensive guide to medical ethics based on the values of worthwhile lives of persons. The utilitarian view well argued and written.

Heyd D. *Genethics: Moral Issues in the Creation of People*. Berkeley: University of California Press, 1992.

A book examining the implications of person-affecting versus impersonal theories of value in the sphere of procreation.

Kuhse H & Singer P. *Should the Baby Live? The Problem of Handicapped Infants*. Oxford: Oxford University Press, 1987.

Robust rational utilitarian arguments for withdrawal of treatment and euthanasia/infanticide of handicapped infants.

Mathieu D. *Preventing Prenatal Harm*. Dordrecht: Kluwer, 1991.

A book devoted to the question of state intervention in prenatal treatment finding the language of rights insufficient to cope with the complexity.

O'Hear A. *An Introduction to the Philosophy of Science*. Oxford: Clarendon Press, 1991.

Very good introduction of the philosophy of science for those wanting more intellectual stimulation.

Sutton A. *Prenatal diagnosis: Confronting the Ethical Issues*. London: The Linacre Centre, 1991.

A Catholic approach, against prenatal diagnosis of the purpose of selective abortion.

Journals

Bioethics. Journals Marketing, Blackwell Publishers, 108 Cowley Road, Oxford OX4 1JF or Blackwell Publishers, 238 Main Street, Cambridge, MA 02142 USA. E-Mail jnlsamples@cix.compulink.co.uk.

Bulletin of Medical Ethics. Publications Department, Royal Society of Medicine Press, 1 Wimpole Street, London W1M 8AE. Tel. 0171-290-2927/8, Fax 0171-290-2929.

Cambridge Quarterly of Healthcare Ethics. Cambridge University Press, The Edinburgh Building, Shaftesbury Road, Cambridge CB2 2RU or 40 West 20th Street, New York NY10011-4211, USA.

Hastings Centre Report. Hastings Centre, 255 Elm Road, Briarcliff Manor, New York 10510, USA. Tel. 914-762-8500.

Journal of Medical Ethics. BMJ Publishing Group, British Medical Journal, BMA House, Tavistock Square, London WC1H 9JR or British Medical Journal, PO Box 48, Franklin, MA 02038, USA. Website address: http://www.bmj.com/bmj/.

Philosophy & Public Affairs. The Johns Hopkins University Press, Journals Publishing Division, 2715 North Charles Street, Baltimore, MD21218–4319.

SECTION

4

Epidemiology

Primary prevention of neural tube defects

23

N.J. Wald and J. Noble

Introduction

Neural tube defects (NTDs) have been found in nearly all communities in which they have been sought. About half of all cases of NTDs are spina bifida alone and half have anencephaly with or without spina bifida. Historically, the birth prevalence of NTDs in different communities has ranged from about 0.5 in 1000 births to about 6 in 1000[1]. The approximately 12-fold variation in birth prevalence, together with the 10-fold increase among women who have had an affected child suggests both environmental and genetic causes.

In recent years, the range of variation in the birth prevalence of NTDs has widened, principally because some countries have introduced screening with the termination of affected pregnancies. Britain was among the countries that had the highest birth prevalence of NTDs and now largely through screening has one of the lowest. Figure 23.1 illustrates the decline in birth prevalence and Table 23.1 shows the numbers on which this is based.

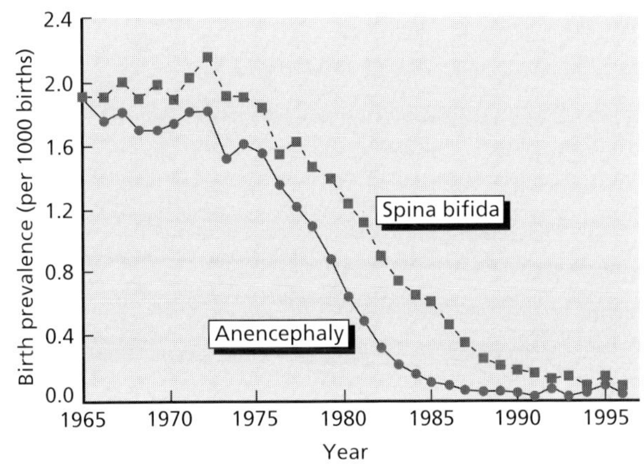

Fig. 23.1 Birth prevalence of anencephaly and spina bifida from 1965 to 1995.

TABLE 23.1
Number of births with anencephaly and spina bifida in England & Wales 1965–1996

Year	Anencephaly	Spina bifida	Total
1965	1346	1454	2800
1970	1137	1309	2446
1975	775	986	1761
1980	342	712	1054
1985	59	352	411
1990	25	116	141
1995	35	72	107
1996	24	57	81

Source: Office for National Statistics (ONS), *Congenital anomaly statistics notifications series* MB3, no. 10 (1994) and as a personal communication from Beverly Botting, ONS for 1995 and 1996.

Neural tube defects

PRIMARY PREVENTION

It has now been conclusively shown that about three-quarters of NTDs can be prevented by consuming sufficient folic acid immediately before pregnancy[2]. The possibility that folic acid might be involved was raised in 1965 when Hibbard and Smithells showed that a test indicating lack of folic acid or disturbed folic acid metabolism (the FIGLU test) was more often positive in a woman carrying a fetus with an NTD than in controls[3]. This finding precipitated a number of studies that investigated folic acid in relation to NTDs. It was the MRC Vitamin Study, an international multicentre randomised trial of vitamin supplementation[4], that showed that folic acid prevented NTDs. A supplement of 4 mg of folic acid taken around the time of conception reduced the risk of NTDs by 71%. There was no indication that other vitamins examined in this study were involved. Three other randomised studies addressed the issue and collectively this reduction was 76% (95% confidence interval 0.11–0.52)[5–7]. Table 23.2 summarises

TABLE 23.2
Studies of folic acid and neural tube defects

Type of study	Number of studies	Daily dose of folic acid (mg)	Number of neural tube defects	Relative risk	95% confidence interval
Randomised controlled trials					
Laurence *et al.* (1981)[5]		4	6	0.42	0.04–2.97
MRC Vitamin Study (1991)[4]		4	27	0.29	0.10–0.74
Kirke *et al.* (1992)[6]		0.4	1	0.00	*
Czeizel & Dudas (1992)[7]		0.8	6	0.00	0.00–0.85
All four	4	0.4–4	40	0.24	0.11–0.52
Non-randomised trials					
Smithells *et al.* (1983)[8]		0.4	27	0.14	0.03–0.47
Vergel *et al.* (1990)[9]		5	4	0.00	0.00–2.13
All four	2	0.4 or 5	31	0.12	0.04–0.41
Observational studies					
Vitamin supplements containing folic acid:					
Winship *et al.* (1984)[10]		about 0.4	561	0.14	0.003–1.11
Mulinaire *et al.* (1988)[11]		about 0.4	347	0.41	0.26–0.66
Mills *et al.* (1989)[15]		about 0.4	571	0.94	0.80–1.10
Milunsky *et al.* (1989)[12]		about 0.4	49	0.29	0.15–0.55
Werler *et al.* (1993)[13]		about 0.4	436	0.6	0.4–0.80
Bower & Stanley (1992)[14]		about 0.4	77	0.11	0.01–1.33
All, including Mills *et al.*	6	about 0.4	2041	0.47	0.29–0.76
All, excluding Mills *et al.*	5	about 0.4	1470	0.41	0.27–0.61
Dietary folate[a]	4	dietary	144		
Laurence *et al.* (1980)[17]		dietary	8	0.00	0–0.33
Yates *et al.* (1987)[16]		dietary	20	0.33	0.09–1.27
Bower & Stanley (1989)[18]		dietary	77	0.31[b]	0.10–0.97
		dietary		0.16[c]	0.06–0.49
Milunsky *et al.* (1989)[12]		dietary	39	0.42	0.16–1.15

[a]A combined risk for the dietary studies was not attempted as dietary folate intake was variable and difficult to standardise.
[b]Controls with congenital abnormalities other than neural tube defects.
[c]Normal controls.
*Insufficient data.

the results of the randomised trials plus other evidence based on non-randomised trials and observational studies[8–18].

GENETIC – ENVIRONMENTAL INTERACTION

Confirmation of the protective effect of folic acid supplementation encouraged research into how folic acid extended its preventive effect. A mutation in the 5,10-methylenetetrahydrofolate reductase (MTHFR) gene (*C677T*) was found to be associated with NTDs[19]. The mutation, associated with decreased MTHFR activity, low serum and red cell folate[20] and high plasma homocysteine[21–24] has been shown to be about four times as frequent in children affected with NTDs than in unaffected controls. Table 23.3 taken from Posey and colleagues[25] summarises the results of three case–control studies[19,26,27]. The *C677T* mutation is the first genetic cause of spina bifida to be identified; it is estimated to account for about 13% of NTDs. Folic acid supplementation overcomes the effects of this mutation. These findings are of great biological interest because they show how the interaction of an environmental factor (folic acid) with an abnormal gene can cause NTDs. They are of no practical consequence in the prevention of NTDs because only a small proportion of folic acid preventable cases are associated with the gene and all women stand to benefit by consuming more folic acid.

The environmental–genetic interaction has also been shown in an animal model. Administration of folic acid in pregnancy can suppress the development of acrania and meroanencephaly (a defect which corresponds to NTDs in humans) in the offspring of mice that are homozygous for a mutant gene that causes this defect[28].

Folic acid

DOSE

The randomised trials used a daily dose ranging from 0.4 to 4 mg of folic acid and most of the observational studies were based on taking 0.4 mg, all in the form of a supplement

TABLE 23.3

Pooled analysis of risk of neural tube defects according to thermolabile variant of MTHFR genotype. After Posey (1996)[25]

	Source	Heterozygous Percent (n)	Heterozygous OR (95% CI)	Heterozygous AP	Homozygous Percent (n)	Homozygous OR (95% CI)	Homozygous AP
Ou *et al.*[27]							
Cases (*n* = 14)	Fibroblast cultures	37% (15)	1.67 (0.69–4.01)	15%	22% (9)	7.2 (1.87–29.01)	19%
Controls (*n* = 109)	Convenience sample	33% (36)			5% (5)		
van der Put *et al.*[19]							
Cases (*n* = 55)	Live cases	47% (26)	1.52 (0.77–3.01)	16%	13% (7)	3.53 (1.07–11.56)	9%
Controls (*n* = 207)	Convenience sample	42% (86)			5% (10)		
Whitehead *et al.*[26]							
Cases (*n* = 82)	Live cases	39% (32)	1.06 (0.54–2.09)	2%	18% (15)	3.57 (1.15–11.56)	13%
Controls (*n* = 99)	Convenience sample	43% (43)			6% (16)		
Pooled analysis			1.35* (0.92–2.00)	11%		4.28* (2.26–8.10)	13%

AP = attributable proportions. OR = odds ratio. CI = confidence interval. *Mantel–Haenszel odds ratio.

(Table 23.2). The observational studies which used 0.4 mg of folic acid had an estimated risk reduction of about 50–60%, somewhat lower than the point estimate from the randomised trials which were in the main based upon a higher intake of supplemental folic acid.

The embryo obtains folate from the maternal plasma. Plasma folate levels reflect immediate intake of folates whereas red cell folate represents folate status over the previous months. A woman's risk of having a child with an NTD is associated with early pregnancy plasma folate and red cell levels in a continuous dose–response relationship[29]. When the data showing this are plotted on a log–log scale, a straight line is produced (see Figs 23.2(a) and (b)), which means that a specified percentage increase in plasma or red cell folate leads to a specified percentage decrease in the birth prevalence of NTDs. The quantitative relationship can be simply summarised: *a 10% increase in plasma folate results in a 7% reduction in the birth prevalence of NTDs* (Fig. 23.2(a) and Table 23.4). This is an important result because the quantitative relationship can be used to estimate the increase in folic acid consumption needed to achieve a specified reduction in NTDs. For an individual woman, the use of a plasma folate level is probably best because it reflects immediate folate status, but for monitoring population levels, red cell folate levels may be more appropriate because they represent folate levels over the previous months.

TABLE 23.4

Relative risk of having a NTD pregnancy according to maternal plasma folate level

Plasma folate arbitrary units	Relative NTD risk*
1.0	100
1.5	0.74
2.0	0.59
2.5	0.50
5.0	0.30
10	0.18

*log relative risk = – 0.7519 × [log relative plasma folate level]. From relationship in figure 23.2(a), taken from Daly *et al.*[29]

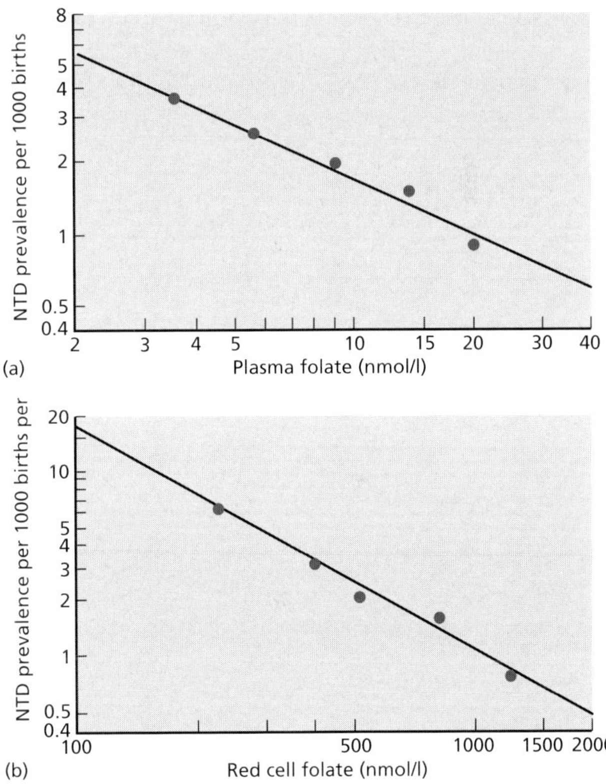

Fig. 23.2 (a) Birth prevalence of neural tube defects according to plasma folate. The equation for the line is NTD prevalence/1000 births expressed in $\log_{10}$ = 0.985 – (0.75 × $\log_{10}$ plasma folate). (b) Birth prevalence of neural tube defects according to red cell folate. The equation for the line is NTD prevalence/1000 births expressed in $\log_{10}$ = 3.62 – (1.19 × $\log_{10}$ red cell folate).

From a public health point of view the target level of extra folic acid needs to be specified. There is a consensus that an extra 0.4 mg per day is a reasonable target and this could be used at present and revised as necessary. The extent of fortification of flour to achieve a specified average blood level will vary according to changes in dietary folate intake but this could be reviewed by a monitoring authority and levels of fortification adjusted. In this way, fortification would be a flexible and rational means of implementing the prevention of NTDs.

FOLIC ACID AND FOLATE: TERMINOLOGY CONSIDERATIONS

The terms 'folic acid' and 'folate' are confusingly used as synonyms. They are not the same.

Folic acid is the name for pterylglutamic acid or 'PteGlu' (see Fig. 23.3). This consists of a double-ringed pteridine portion joined to *p*-aminobenzoic acid (PABA) and to glutamic acid. Folic acid is used in vitamin supplementation and food fortification and has four important features: (i) it is the oxidised form of folic acid and is therefore stable; (ii) it has only one glutamic acid 'residue'; (iii) it is synthetic and is not present in natural food; (iv) its bioavailability is about twice that of natural folate[30].

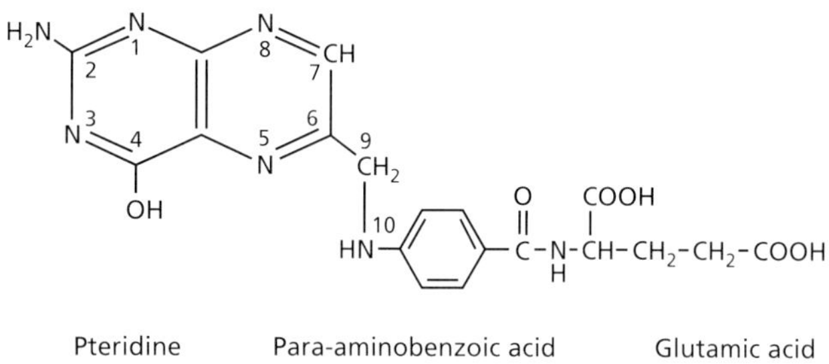

Fig. 23.3 Pterylglutamic acid (PteGlu).

Folate is a generic term that includes folic acid as well as other molecules that have the folic acid structure as their central element. Natural folates have two important features: (i) they exist in a reduced form by either having two extra hydrogen atoms on C5 and C6 (dihydrofolate, DHF or H_2PteGlu) or four extra hydrogen atoms on C5, C6, C7 and C8 (tetrahydrofolate, THF or H_4PteGlu); (ii) they have multiple glutamic acid residues designated, for example, $H_4PteGlu_n$, or if the number of glutamic acid residues is known, say 5, it is designated $H_4PteGlu_5$. Folates may carry a single C unit (formyl, CHO; methenyl, CH, methylene, CH_2; methyl, CH_3) and the position of attachment varies:

–CHO on N10
–CH_3 on N5
–CH and CH_2 as bridge compounds to both N5 and N10.

Oxidation of the reduced forms can lead to the molecule splitting at the 9–10 bond (see Fig. 23.3), destroying the molecule and its folic acid activity. Such oxidation readily occurs and is the reason that natural folate is unstable and can be destroyed by heat. The non-reduced synthetic folic acid is not subject to this effect and is therefore stable.

The enzyme dihydrofolate reductase converts folic acid,

$$\text{PteGlu} \rightarrow \text{H}_2\text{PteGlu} \rightarrow \text{H}_4\text{PteGlu}$$

on the mucosal surface of the gut. H_4PteGlu is then converted to 5-methylenetetrahydrofolate (5-MTHF) which enters the portal blood. 5-MTHF is the form of folate that enters cells. In order to be retained by cells it must be demethylated by methionine synthase and the resulting THF is conjugated to a variety of polyglutamates of which the long-chain forms such as pentaglutamates and hexaglutamates probably predominate. In this form, within a cell, it is biologically active and is involved in the intracellular synthesis of purines and pyrimidines which are required for the production of DNA and RNA. Figure 23.4 is a simplified scheme of the absorption, transport and cellular retention of folate in which the distinction between food folate and synthetic folate is shown. Dietary folate is subject to a variety of inhibitory conditions in the intestine that reduce its bioavailability to about half that of folic acid.

INCREASING FOLATE INTAKE

It has been shown that the consumption of extra folate as natural food is relatively ineffective in increasing red cell folate status but extra folic acid in the form of supplements or food fortification has a marked effect on increasing red cell folate, confirming that modest dietary alteration is not an effective means of providing sufficient extra folate to obtain the full potential effect in preventing NTDs[31].

On average, we consume about 0.2 mg of *folate* a day from our food, equivalent to 0.1 mg folic acid on the basis of a bioavailability of 0.5. To increase folic acid intake by the equivalent of 0.4 mg of folic acid (a threefold increase in folate or a fivefold increase in folic acid equivalents) by altering diet would involve an unrealistic change in diet. In folic acid equivalents, we would have to add about 20 glasses of orange juice, or 26 servings of broccoli or 10 servings of spinach or combinations of such foods to our regular daily diet to achieve this level (Table 23.5)[32]

The use of folic acid supplements is a practical and simple means of prevention but it means that women must be aware of the need to do this and do so before they become pregnant. The embryonic closure of the neural tube takes place about four weeks after conception, often before a woman is aware that she is pregnant. Probably about half of all pregnancies are unplanned, so this in itself will limit the efficacy of taking folic acid supplements.

The most effective option is to fortify a staple food with folic acid. The added folic acid, unlike folate, is stable. It is also inexpensive. There are no practical difficulties in fortifying

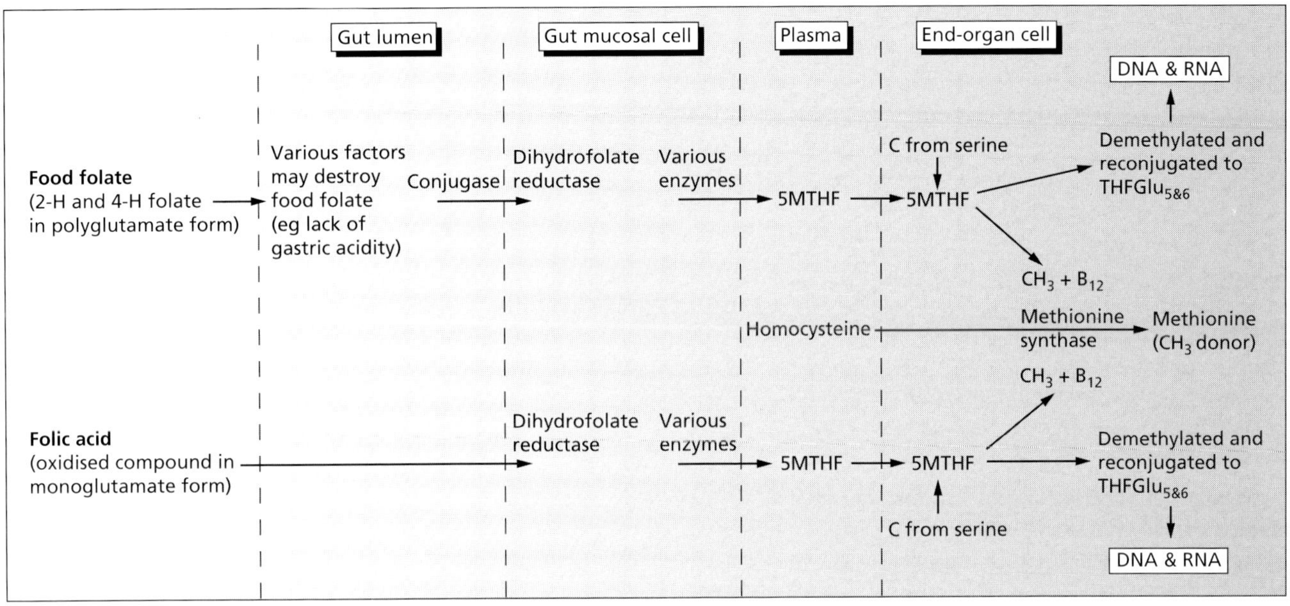

Fig. 23.4 A simplified schematic representation of the absorption, transport and cellular retention of folate showing the distinction between food folate and synthetic folate.

TABLE 23.5
Folate content of selected foods[32]

Food	Folate per serving (mg)	Folic acid equivalents per serving
Brussels sprouts	0.10	0.05
Spinach	0.08	0.04
Green beans	0.05	0.025
Potatoes	0.04	0.02
Orange juice	0.04	0.02
Broccoli	0.03	0.015
Cabbage	0.03	0.015
Carrots	0.01	0.005

food with folic acid and many breakfast cereals have been fortified for some time.

The Food and Drug Administration in the USA, part of the US Public Health Service, issued regulations that folic acid be added to flour at a level of 0.14 mg folic acid per 100 g flour which is equivalent to consuming about an extra 0.1 mg folic acid daily. While the level of fortification is too low to achieve the target intake, it is nonetheless an initiative that is a major public health advance. Other authorities, such as the UK Department of Health, are still considering the issue. In terms of effectiveness, economy and simplicity, fortifying flour with sufficient folic acid is the preferred public health strategy. It can ensure complete coverage of the population at risk and it avoids the need for people to consciously remember to take folic acid pills before becoming pregnant.

Figure 23.5 shows the distribution of dietary folate in folic acid equivalents (0.2 mg folate ≡ 0.1 mg folic acid) in Britain

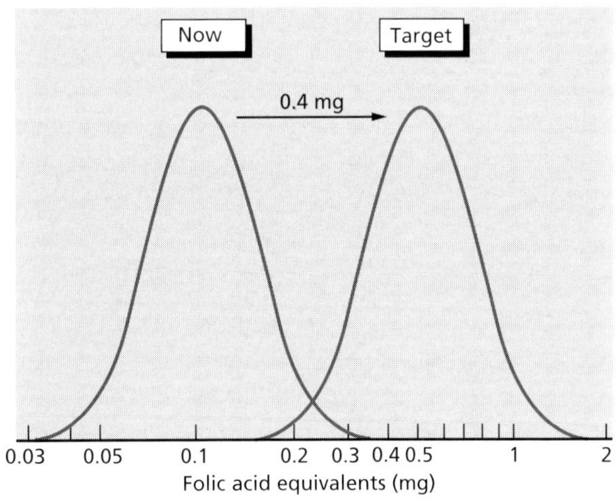

Fig. 23.5 Distribution of dietary folate in folic acid equivalents.

and how a 0.4 mg supplement will shift the distribution. The shift is large in relative terms but still represents a small absolute increase in folic acid intake.

OTHER HEALTH BENEFITS OF FOLIC ACID

A consensus is emerging that eating folic acid in the general diet will reduce the incidence of ischaemic heart disease. It does this by reducing the average levels of an amino acid, homocysteine, in the blood of men and women. There is persuasive evidence that homocysteine is causally associated with ischaemic heart disease and vascular disorders so increasing blood homocysteine will also reduce the incidence of cardiovascular disease. It is estimated that an extra 0.4 mg of folic acid daily would reduce the incidence of ischaemic heart disease by about 10%[33]. Folic acid supplementation *may* also reduce the risk of the congenital abnormalities cleft lip and cleft palate[34,35], but the position on this remains unresolved. There are also suggestions that it may reduce the risk of colon cancer[36–38].

FOLIC ACID IN MEDICAL PRACTICE

All women planning a pregnancy should be advised to take a daily 0.4 mg supplement of folic acid which is readily available from health food stores and pharmacists. Women who have previously had an affected pregnancy are advised to take a 4 or 5 mg folic acid supplement available on prescription. Women with epilepsy are at higher risk of having a pregnancy with a NTD and should be advised to have supplemental folic acid given at the higher dose. Those taking high doses of folic acid (≥ 5 mg) may be at an increased risk of having their anticonvulsant control destabilised. The risk may be more theoretical than real since studies have shown no increase in seizure activity in patients with drug-treated epilepsy taking 15–20 mg/day of folic acid and in epileptic patients on diphenylhydantoin given 3–5 mg/day of folic acid for 4–12 months[39]. Nonetheless, it would be prudent for physicians to monitor their anticonvulsant therapy closely.

The UK government, the UK Health Education Authority, and other authorities advise women to take folic acid supplements from the moment they plan to have a baby until the week 12 of pregnancy. This allows a measure of safety both before and after conception since the critical period of supplementation is likely to be around the time of the formation of the neural tube. Because of the risk of unintended pregnancy, the US Public Health Service recommends that all women of childbearing age take 0.4 mg folic acid per day regardless of whether they intend to become pregnant.

SAFETY OF FOLIC ACID

As a public health measure for prevention, the fortification of flour with folic acid is the method of choice. It has the potential to prevent up to three-quarters of cases of NTDs and a proportion of cases of cardiovascular disease. A concern over the safety has been raised; increased folic acid intake could 'mask' the anaemia of vitamin B_{12} deficiency and could possibly exacerbate the neurological features of the disorder.

The concern over this arose about fifty years ago when patients with pernicious anaemia were treated in error with folic acid. High-dose folic acid (> 5 mg/day) in a proportion of cases, treated the anaemia of the B_{12} deficiency but not the neurological lesions. In some cases, development of the disease was judged to have been more rapid with the use of folic acid than clinicians felt would have been the case had folic acid not been used. No objective evidence on this is available and it is recognised that the natural history of B_{12} deficiency can itself be highly variable[40]. What is agreed is that folic acid is not the cause of the diseases caused by B_{12} deficiency even though it may affect its presentation. It is also accepted that in current medical practice if B_{12} deficiency is suspected it can be diagnosed without the presence of an anaemia. There is therefore no reason to believe that any features of B_{12} deficiency are caused by folic acid. If there is a public health problem arising from B_{12} deficiency, this needs to be addressed as a separate issue and consideration given to fortifying a staple food with B_{12} as well as fortifying flour with folic acid.[41] This concern over safety is not supported by evidence and there is no doubt about the benefits of folic acid fortification and sound grounds for concluding that an increase in the daily intake of folic acid of 0.4 mg is completely safe.

The need for a population strategy for prevention

NTDs are a folate deficiency disorder. There is a reluctance to describe them as such on the grounds that they occur in Western populations who are not obviously malnourished. While it is recognised that extra folic acid reduces the risk of NTDs some argue that the problem is not a general one, but affects only one section of the population (women) at a particular stage in their lives (when having a baby), and then only in a minority (1–2 per 1000 pregnancies). However, without being able to predict who will have an affected pregnancy the problem is *de facto* a general nutritional one that is best solved using a general preventive strategy.

It is known that when a nutritional disorder is identified, not everyone who eats too much of the nutrient that causes the disorder or too little in the case of a deficiency, will suffer the disorder. Only a proportion may become affected because there are individual differences in metabolism and interactions with certain foods that can influence, for example, gastrointestinal absorption. There is a need to rectify a general dietary deficiency in a population that produces overt disease only in a few individuals.

The issue is well illustrated by using immunisation as an example'[42]:

> Immunisation programmes apply to all even though a small proportion of the population is likely to benefit. The prevention of rubella in pregnancy to avoid the congenital rubella syndrome originally focused on two target groups – teenage girls, who were vaccinated at school, and pregnant women who were screened and, if found to be susceptible, vaccinated after their pregnancy. This selective approach had only a partial effect. Aiming at vaccinating 10–14 year old girls kept a pool of infection among men and boys and younger girls. Vaccination against rubella is now offered to all, boys included. The population approach of collective action has been an essential part of most of the achievements in

public health. This is the strategy needed to prevent neural tube defects.

Historically, deficiency disorders have been of the type typified by scurvy or pellagra, but it is now recognised that while in Western populations disease can be caused by overnutrition (for example, the consumption of excess saturated fats) disease can also arise from a micronutrient deficiency in interaction with other factors. Indeed, as Western populations have become more sedentary and have reduced their daily calorie intake, they will necessarily have reduced their micronutrient intake. Without the fortification of foods with essential micronutrients, deficiencies relative to historic intakes of micronutrients in populations will necessarily occur. To avert this we should not, in principle, be averse to fortifying staple foods with micronutrients that have been shown to be effective in preventing disease and judged to be acceptably safe.

There is an urgent need to fortify flour with sufficient folic acid to overcome this deficiency in the population. Such a population strategy would be effective, economical and safe. The precise level of fortification needs to be assessed in relation to the consumption of flour-based products within a community and modified as the dietary intake of folate changes. No other public health measure would have as large an effect in the prevention of serious congenital abnormality.

Acknowledgements

We thank Rachel Jordan, Malcolm Law, Joan Morris and Christopher Schorah for their help and advice.

REFERENCES

1. Little J & Elwood M. Geographical variation. In *Epidemiology and Control of Neural Tube Defects* (eds MJ Elwood, J Little & JH Elwood). Oxford: Oxford University Press. pp. 96–145, 1992.
2. Wald NJ. Folic acid and neural tube defects: the current evidence and implications for prevention. *Ciba Foundation Symposium* **181**:192–211, Chichester: John Wiley, 1994.
3. Hibbard ED & Smithells RW. Folic acid metabolism and human embryopathy. *Lancet* **i**:1254, 1965.
4. MRC Vitamin Study Research Group Prevention of neural tube defects: results of the MRC Vitamin Study. *Lancet* **338**:132–137, 1991.
5. Laurence KM, James N, Miller MH, Tennant GB & Campbell H. Double-blind randomised controlled trial of folate treatment before conception to prevent recurrence of neural tube defects. *BMJ* **282**:1509–1511, 1981.
6. Kirke PN, Daly LE & Elwood JH. A randomised trial of low dose folic acid to prevent neural tube defects. *Arch. Dis. Child.* **67**:1442–1446, 1992.
7. Czeizel AE & Dudas I. Prevention of the first occurrence of neural-tube defects by periconceptional vitamin supplementation. *N. Engl. J. Med.* **327**:1832–1835, 1992.
8. Smithells RW, Seller MJ, Harris R *et al.* Further experience of vitamin supplementation for prevention of neural tube defect recurrences. *Lancet* **i**:1027–1031, 1983.
9. Vergel RG, Sanchez LR, Heredero BL, Rodriguez PL & Martinez AJ. Primary prevention of neural tube defects with folic acid supplementation: Cuban experience. *Prenat. Diag* **10**:149–152, 1990.
10. Winship KA, Cahal DA, Weber JCP & Griffin JP. Maternal drug histories and central nervous system anomalies. *Arch. Dis. Child.* **59**:1052–1060, 1984.
11. Mulinaire J, Cordero JF, Erickson D & Berry RJ. Periconceptional use of multivitamins and the occurrence of neural tube defects. *JAMA* **260**:3141–3145, 1988.
12. Milunsky A, Jick H, Jick SS *et al.* Multivitamin/folic acid supplementation in early pregnancy reduces the prevalence of neural tube defects. *JAMA* **262**:2847–2852, 1989.
13. Werler MM, Shapiro S & Mitchell AA. Periconceptional folic acid exposure and risk of occurrent neural tube defects. *JAMA* **269**:1257–1261, 1993.
14. Bower C & Stanley FJ. Periconceptional vitamin supplementation and neural tube defects; evidence from a case–control study in Western Australia and a review of recent publications. *J Epidemiol. Comm. Health* **46**:157–161, 1992.
15. Mills JL, Rhoads GG, Simpson JL *et al.* The absence of a relationship between the periconception use of vitamins and neural tube defects. *N. Engl. J. Med.* **321**:430–435, 1989.
16. Yates JRW, Ferguson-Smith MA, Shenkin A *et al.* Is disorder folate metabolism the basis for the genetic predisposition to neural tube defects? *Clin. Genet.* **31**:279–287, 1987.
17. Laurence KM, James N, Miller MH *et al.* Increased risk of recurrence of pregnancies complicated by fetal neural tube defects in mothers receiving poor diets, and possible benefits of dietary counselling. *BMJ* **281**:1592–1594, 1980.
18. Bower C & Stanley FJ. Dietary folate as a risk factor for neural tubes defects: evidence from a case–control study in Western Australia. *Med. J. Aust.* **150**:613–617, 1989.
19. van der Put NMJ, Steegers-Theunissen RPM, Frost P *et al.* Mutated methylenetetrahydrofolate reductase as a risk factor for spina bifida. *Lancet* **346**:1070–1071, 1995.
20. Molloy AM, Daly S, Mills JL, Kirke PN, Whitehead AS *et al.* Thermolabile variant of 5,10-methylenetetrahydrofolate reductase associated with low red-cell folates: implications for folate intake recommendations. *Lancet* **349**:1591–1593, 1997.
21. Frosst P, Blom HJ, Milos R *et al.* A candidate genetic risk factor for vascular disease: a common mutation in methylenetetrahydrofolate reductase. *Nat (Genet.)* **10**:111–113, 1995.
22. Kang SS, Passen EL, Ruggie N, Wong PWK & Sora H. Thermolabile defect of methylenetetrahydrofolate reductase in coronary heart disease. *Circulation* **88**:1463–1469, 1993.
23. Engbersen AMT, Franken DG, Boers GHJ *et al.* Thermolabile 5,10-methylenetetrahydrofolate reductase as a cause of hyperhomocysteinemia. *Am. J. Hum. Genet.* **56**:142–150, 1995.
24. Kluijtmans LAJ, van den Heuvel LPW, Boers GHJ *et al.* Molecular genetic analysis in mild hyperhomocysteinemia: a common mutation in the methylenetetrahydrofolate reductase gene is a genetic risk factor for cardiovascular disease. *Am. J. Hum. Genet.* **58**:35–41, 1996.
25. Posey DL, Khoury MJ, Mulinaire J *et al.* Is mutated MTHFR a risk factor for neural tube defects? *Lancet* **347**:686–687, 1996.
26. Whitehead AS, Gallagher P, Mills JL *et al.* A genetic defect in 5, 10-methylenetetrahydrofolate reductase in neural tube defects. *Q. J. Med.* **88**:763–766, 1995.
27. Ou CY, Stevenson RE, Brown VK *et al.* *V677T* homozygosity associated with 5,10-methylenetetrahydrofolate reductase as a risk factor for neural tube defects. *Am. J. Hum. Genet.* **57**: (Suppl), A223, 1995.
28. Zhao Q, Behringer RR & Crombrugghe B. Prenatal folic acid treatment suppresses acrania and meroanencephaly in mice mutant for the *Cart1* homeobox gene. *Nat (Genet.)* **13**:275–283, 1996.
29. Daly LE, Kirke PN, Molly A *et al.* Folate levels and neural tube defects. *JAMA* **274**:1698–1702, 1995.
30. Gregory III JF. The bioavailability of folate. In *Folate in Health and Disease* (ed. L.B. Bailey) New York: Marcel Dekker, pp. 195–235, 1995.

31. Cuskelly GJ, McNulty H & Scott J. Effect of increasing dietary folate on red-cell folate: implications for prevention of neural tube defects. *Lancet* **347**:657–659, 1996.
32. Expert Advisory Group. Folic acid and the prevention of neural tube defects. London: Department of Health, 1992.
33. Wald NJ, Watt HC, Law MR, Weir DG, McPartlin J & Scott JM. Homocysteine and ischaemic heart disease: results of a prospective study with implications on prevention. *Arch. Int. Med.* **158**:862–867, 1998.
34. Czeizel AE, Toth M & Rockenbauer M. Population-based case–control study of folic acid supplementation during pregnancy. *Teratology* **53**:345–351, 1996.
35. Shaw GM, Lammer EJ, Wasserman CR *et al.* Risks of orofacial clefts in children born to women using multivitamins containing folic acid preconceptionally. *Lancet* **346**:393–396, 1995.
36. Giovannucci E, Stampfer MJ, Colditz GA *et al.* Folate, methionine, and alcohol intake and risk of colorectal adenoma *J. Natl. Cancer Inst.* **85**:875–883, 1993.
37. Giovannucci E, Rimm EB, Ascherio A *et al.* Alcohol, low-methionine–low-folate diets, and risk of colon cancer in men. *J. Natl. Cancer Inst.* **87**:265–273, 1995.
38. Chen J, Giovannucci E, Kelsey K *et al.* A methylenetetrahydrofolate reductase polymorphism and the risk of colorectal cancer. *Cancer Res.* **56**:4862–4864, 1996.
39. Bailey LB. Folate requirements and dietary recommendations. In *Folate in Health and* Disease (ed. L.B. Bailey), p. 144. New York: Marcel Dekker. 1995.
40. Dickinson CJ. Does folic acid harm people with vitamin B_{12} deficiency? *Q. J. Med.* **88**:357–364, 1995.
41. Wald NJ & Bower C. Folic acid, pernicious anaemia, and prevention of neural tube defects. *Lancet* **343**:307, 1994.
42. Wald NJ & Bower C. Folic acid and the prevention of neural tube defects. *BMJ* **310**:1019–1020, 1995.

The application of epidemiology to fetal medicine

24

J.P. Neilson

Introduction

The science of epidemiology (the study of the distribution and causes of diseases in populations) has produced tools that are increasingly applied in the clinical arena, and there is an emerging specialism of 'clinical epidemiology'. This chapter will explore those tools and the concepts that underpin them, and will illustrate their application with reference to diagnostic and screening tests, and therapeutic interventions in fetal and perinatal medicine. Fetal medicine is itself, of course, a young specialism and its short history and rapid progress have perhaps inevitably resulted in some errors and blind alleys. It is incumbent on 'fetal physicians' of the future to try to ensure that lessons are learned from past mistakes and that future progress is based on sound scientific foundations to ensure that the application of fetal medicine contributes more good than harm. In the words of Murray Enkin[1]:

> In most fields of medical care, persons come to a doctor because they are ill and seek a cure or relief. In obstetrics, pregnant women come to us healthy but with an iatrogenic belief that obstetrical care will further improve the excellent outcomes that nature has already provided for them. The professionally engendered nature of our care increases our responsibility. The presence of the baby, who has no choice in the matter, doubles it.

Care during pregnancy and childbirth has been among the vanguard areas of clinical activity in moving towards 'evidence based' clinical practice. The basis of this process, the production of systematic reviews of scientifically rigorous studies, has been likened in scale and importance to the Human Genome Project[2]. Fetal medicine, with its obvious linkage to molecular genetics and its location within the field of pregnancy and childbirth, thus interlocks with the two most exciting thrusts in modern medicine – advances in molecular biology and in clinical epidemiology.

Routine datasets

Previous generations of perinatal epidemiologists have mostly concentrated on large datasets either collected routinely or derived for a specific research project. It is undeniable that important insights have been derived from such studies, although misleading evidence has also emerged from the 'data dredging' of such resources. In contrast, the modern perinatal epidemiologist is much more likely to try to address a specific hypothesis (or hypotheses) either through generating clinical experiments, notably randomised controlled trials, or by studying the results of a number of different clinical experiments to reach the most informative and least biased conclusion (through 'systematic reviews' and meta-analysis).

Previous studies of routinely collected data about maternal deaths and, more recently, perinatal deaths have been informative and may have contributed to lessening incidences of these disasters. Routine datasets continue to prove useful in a number of ways, e.g. generating hypotheses (some of which are best tackled definitively by a randomised controlled trial), identifying patterns of disease distribution in populations, and by identifying rare problems. Thus, the 'Barker hypothesis' linking undernutrition at critical stages of fetal life with adult diseases including coronary artery disease[3], and hypertension, has been generated by the study of routinely collected data on birthweights and placental weights and neonatal measurements, and linking these findings with health and disease in later adult life. The possibility of autosomal dominant or recessive inheritance of a genetic predisposition to develop pre-eclampsia has been investigated using carefully, and routinely, collected maternity records in Iceland between 1931 and 1947[4]. The possible link between chorion villus sampling and limb defects (if a true link, probably a very rare one) has been tested in a large routine dataset[5] – the potential for bias in this type of study has also, incidentally, been highlighted[6,7].

PERINATAL MORTALITY SURVEYS

The classification of perinatal mortality should have value in identifying both research and clinical service priorities in perinatal medicine. Different systems of classification have been used. It is highly unfortunate that the current British system still uses a modification of that first used by Sir Dugald Baird in the early 1950s that fails to differentiate between preterm low-birthweight babies and growth retarded low-birthweight babies[8]. This is not only uninformative to clinicians but is positively bizarre in the country that has spawned the epidemiological studies to produce the 'Barker hypothesis'. One system does recognise the importance of fetal growth restriction[9] and its application in a two-year regional audit identified this as potentially the largest avoidable group of deaths since those other causes that are responsible for a greater number of deaths are either difficult to modify, or were unpredictable[10] (Table 24.1).

TABLE 24.1
Classification of obstetric causes of extended fetal loss* in two-year regional study. After Neilson[10].

Fetal abnormality	75
Spontaneous preterm delivery	65
Intrauterine growth retardation	38
Unexplained intrauterine death	34
Antepartum haemorrhage	31
Hypertension	15
Intrapartum asphyxia	14
Infection	12
Others	9
Maternal disease	1
Trauma	0
Haemolytic disease	0
Total	294

*All stillborn babies from 20 weeks of pregnancy plus liveborn babies dying within 28 days plus ascertained deaths within the first year clearly attributable to perinatal causes.

The concept of 'avoidability' has been applied for many years in Britain to the scrutiny of maternal deaths in the triennial Confidential Enquiry reports[11]. This has, more recently, been applied to national studies of subsets of perinatal deaths as well[12], thus highlighting, in a study of intrapartum deaths, the problems of a lack of senior clinical involvement, and of failure to anticipate certain complications (including exaggerated response to oxytocic drugs, cord prolapse, shoulder dystocia and difficulties with delivery of the second twin).

Diagnostic tests

It is important to draw a clear distinction between screening tests, which are often relatively crude tests applicable to large populations to help identify clinically unsuspected disease, and diagnostic tests, which are usually much more precise and which are applied for specific clinical reasons.

The performance of tests can be assessed by calculating sensitivity, specificity and predictive values (Table 24.2). The *sensitivity* denotes the proportion of women with the condition who have a positive test result; the *specificity* denotes the proportion of women without the condition who have a negative test result. The optimal balance of sensitivity and specificity will depend on individual aims and circumstances. The ultrasound diagnosis of structural fetal defects, for example, should be highly specific to avert unwanted termination of pregnancies in which the fetuses are, in fact, normal; a screening test for fetal neural tube defects or chromosomal abnormalities can accommodate a lower level of specificity because final decisions about intervention are based on diagnostic tests (e.g. ultrasound or amniocentesis) that are triggered by the abnormal screening test result. The relationship between sensitivity and specificity can be displayed figuratively in *receiver operator curves (ROCs)*, the term being derived from radar technology during the Second World War. ROCs are useful in identifying the optimal trade-off between sensitivity and specificity for a given test so as to pinpoint the best cut-off value to differentiate 'normal' from 'abnormal' test results in a screening programme.

TABLE 24.2
Relationship between tests and disease (or other adverse outcome)

	Disease	
Test	Present	Absent
Positive	True postive [a]	False positive [b]
Negative	False negative [c]	True negative [d]

Sensitivity = a/a + c.
Specificity = d/b + d.
Positive predictive value = a/a + b.
Negative predictive value = d/c + d.

The *predictive value* of a test is influenced by the prevalence of the condition in question in the population being studied; thus, the positive predictive value of a raised maternal serum α-fetoprotein result will be greater in a Celtic population with a high incidence of neural tube defects. The more sensitive a test is, the better is the negative predictive value; the more specific a test is, the better is the positive predictive value.

Case studies

Case series or even single case reports can be useful in generating hypotheses that can be tested in experimental studies. Thus, a case report, describing an association between fetal nuchal translucency during the first trimester and chromosomal abnormality[13], has spawned further work of considerable current interest[14]. A potential problem with case studies is that these are sometimes seen as providing in themselves the basis for changing clinical practice. Such an example is the use of fetoscopically directed ablation of anastomostic vessels in twin–twin transfusion syndrome[15]; without an appropriately matched control group (as in that report), it is not possible to reach a firm conclusion about whether the manifest hazards of such an intervention are outweighed by improvement in outcome of these pregnancies (which undoubtedly have a relatively poor prognosis).

HISTORICAL CONTROL STUDIES

When a case series is collected outside the confines of a planned experimental study, a temptation exists to compare outcome with a control group identified with hindsight; one such model is the historical control group, i.e. a similar group of patients or pregnancies treated or observed before the intervention in question was introduced; another model would be a comparison group treated at a different hospital, or by a different doctor. Both models carry a major risk of bias and of misleading conclusions. In the case of historical controls, many changes may have occurred over the timescale of the observed period as to alter prognosis. Thus, one study that encouraged inappropriately optimistic expectations of the widespread use of electronic fetal heart rate monitoring during labour was a small, historical control study[16].

Experimental studies

CASE–CONTROL STUDIES

A major section of this chapter will be devoted to the methodology of the randomised controlled trial because this is the gold standard method of assessing the effectiveness of clinical interventions[17]. However, it must be recognised that not all important questions in fetal medicine can be addressed by the randomised controlled trial. Thus, the question of whether high-dose vitamin A is a teratogen cannot for ethical reasons be resolved by randomly allocating half of a group of women in early pregnancy to exposure to vitamin A. Here, the case–control study that has been widely used with benefit in human cancer studies may be helpful.

RANDOMISED CONTROLLED TRIALS

RANDOMISATION

The randomised controlled trial is a simple but powerful method of avoiding *systematic errors*, or *bias*, by ensuring that experimental (study) groups and control groups are comparable in all important respects other than in their exposure to the intervention being tested. By random allocation, the experimenter accounts not only for known confounding variables, but also for factors that are unknown but are also potentially important determinants of final outcome.

Random allocation depends on allocation solely on the basis of chance – metaphorically on the basis of the flip of a coin, but not on the actuality of the flip of the coin which can, of course, be flipped again if the doctor did not get the side he or she favoured. A potentially important trial of electronic fetal heart rate monitoring in a setting with significant risk of intrapartum death was weakened by the use of such a method[18]. The trial report describes markedly unbalanced overall numbers in the two groups (electronic monitoring: 746; intermittent auscultation: 682) as well as dramatic differences in the number of women having had labour induced (16% versus 7%) or augmented (52% versus 38%), suggesting the operation of *selection bias*.

The essence of secure randomisation requires that those involved in the study cannot know in advance to which group a particular woman will be allocated on entering a trial. Thus, the use of hospital case numbers or date of birth will not adequately conceal the direction of allocation and if a clinician has preconceptions about the effectiveness of the two treatment options, he or she may be influenced in whether or not that woman is actually recruited thus distorting the nature of two comparison groups. These methods are sometimes called 'quasi-random' and with current concepts of good trial methodology should not be used[19].

Even apparently robust methods of random allocation, such as the commonly employed sealed opaque envelope to be opened only after the woman has consented to entering the trial, have been known to be abused on occasion. The gold standard method, used now in most large trials, is telephone randomisation in which someone based at a remote site gives randomisation instructions only after basic descriptive data about the woman has been recorded on computer. This method was used for example in the CLASP trial of low-dose aspirin prophylaxis[20]. Electronic communication may be particularly difficult in parts of the developing world and randomised trials may be particularly important in such settings because of high rates of both maternal and fetal mortality may be high. The Collaborative Eclampsia Trial[21], which for the first time demonstrated the indisputable pre-eminence of magnesium sulphate as the anticonvulsant of choice for eclampsia, took place mainly in developing countries and used identical boxes containing either magnesium sulphate or diazepam or phenytoin with appropriate administration equipment to be opened when a woman had an eclamptic fit, and had a system to monitor the use of these numbered boxes.

EXPLANATORY VERSUS PRAGMATIC TRIALS

There are two types of randomised trial; both are valid and the appropriate trial design will depend on the question to be answered, but the differences between the two represent a common source of confusion. The *explanatory trial* assesses *efficacy* – the performance of the intervention under ideal circumstances; the *pragmatic trial* assesses *effectiveness* – performance under what may be less than optimal, but real life, circumstances. The European CVS Trial[22] was a pragmatic trial that compared the outcome of pregnancy after chorion villus sampling (CVS) compared to mid-pregnancy amniocentesis. Operators were required to meet certain minimum standards of experience of performing CVS, but many probably did not have very extensive experience. The trial showed a considerable disadvantage to women undergoing CVS – whether this reflects relative inexperience of operators or the nature of the technique could only be answered properly by a explanatory trial involving only those with great expertise and experience. Whatever that would show, there are clear messages for the generality of fetal medicine practice. The trial of early amniocentesis versus CVS in King's College Hospital, London[23] would approach the status of an explanatory trial, being performed in a busy tertiary referral centre of international repute, but the results might not be applicable to many other settings.

This raises the issue of *generalisability*. Ideally, important trials will provide guidance in many healthcare settings, but this is not always the case. The RADIUS trial[24] took place in the United States mainly in primary care settings and addressed the value of routine ultrasound examination of women who did not have one of a long list of factors that indicated a need for ultrasound in early pregnancy. There is no reason to believe that the sonographers involved in this pragmatic trial did not have the necessary skills to assess gestational age by accurate fetal measurement or to detect multiple pregnancies, but the detection rates of major fetal abnormalities was not only much lower than observational studies (e.g. Chitty *et al.*[25]) (which could potentially have been associated with biased reporting) but also the one other randomised controlled trial of routine ultrasound that seriously addressed the issue of screening for fetal abnormalities[26,27]. The generalisability of the findings of the RADIUS trial is therefore limited to similar primary care settings and not to secondary or tertiary maternity units where skilled anomaly scanning is practised.

POWER CALCULATIONS

Type I errors occur when the results of a trial suggest a difference when, in fact, none exists; *a type II* error occurs when the results do not suggest a difference although one does, in fact, exist. The principal protection against both types of error lies in adequate sample size in planning a trial and this should be calculated in advance of initiation. Fuller details can be accessed elsewhere[28].

DATA MONITORING

It is also a principle of good clinical trial design and execution to ensure that an independent panel of experts will have access to interim results to advise where or not a trial should continue. Advice may be given to abort a trial early if there is overwhelming evidence that either the treatment group or the control group are at significant advantage or disadvantage on the basis of treatment. What is not good practice is for the researchers themselves to continually monitor the results because of the possibility of stopping a trial once a 'statistically significant' result is obtained as this may well represent a type I error.

FACTORIAL DESIGN

It may be possible to answer two questions rather than one through factorial design. Thus, a trial of women with pre-eclampsia might comprise four groups with different patterns of administration of Drug A (an anticonvulsant) and Drug B (an antihypertensive): 1 (A + B), 2 (A/no B), 3 (no A/B), 4 (no A/no B). Comparison of the outcomes from groups 1 + 2 versus groups 3 + 4 addresses the value of Drug A; comparison of the outcomes from groups 1 + 3 versus groups 2 + 4 addresses the value of Drug B.

'INTENTION TO TREAT'

It is a feature of pragmatic trials (but not explanatory trials) that a woman may not receive the treatment or test to which she had been allocated. There are several reasons why this may happen – she might have delivered before the intervention could be implemented, she might have had second thoughts about involvement in the trial, or there may have been a mistake. Lack of appropriate treatment may, however, reflect the nature of the treatment. A course of drug treatment, for example, may have such unpleasant side effects that women stop taking medication. Since the fundamental aim of the pragmatic trial is to test the *policy* of allocating women to the treatment schedule in question, whether or not they actually receive the treatment in full, it is vital that analyses are based on 'intention to treat' to include *all* women allocated to the two groups.

The potential dangers of not including all randomised women in analyses can be illustrated by considering early trials of thyrotropin-releasing hormone (TRH) as a possible method of enhancing the effects of antenatal corticosteroids on fetal lung maturation before possible preterm delivery[29]. A meta-analysis (see below) included seven trials of TRH and demonstrated a statistically significant reduction in the incidence of respiratory distress among babies both exposed to prenatal TRH and 'optimally treated' (i.e. full course of treatment with delivery occurring > 24 hours and < 10 days post-treatment)[30]. However, only three of the trials[31–33] reported all babies included in an 'intention to treat' analysis and the pooled results from these showed no beneficial impact on the incidence of respiratory distress syndrome. Similar trends were also seen in perinatal deaths – these could only be explained if there were disadvantages from TRH treatment to babies who remained *in utero* for more than 10 days. One could, for example, envisage pregnancies in which there is uteroplacental insufficiency with associated fetal physiological compensation by circulatory readjustment and metabolic thrift, in which a sudden boost of TRH-stimulated increased metabolic rate may not best serve the long-term interests of the baby.

Systematic reviews

The importance of reviews to inform busy clinicians is obvious as we are now swamped by a huge primary medical literature and all of us struggle to keep up to date even with our special areas of clinical or scientific interest. Unfortunately, we are all too often ill served by conventional reviews whether published in books or in journals: they are frequently out of date at the time of publication if the topic is progressing rapidly; different 'experts' can reach entirely different conclusions after reviewing the same topic; as readers, we are usually not informed how the reviewer chose to select certain references and ignore others. As a consequence, we cannot be sure if the review can be trusted or not. The answer is the scientific or systematic review that, in contrast, is based on an explicit and rigorous process that includes:

- a clear description of the objectives
- explicit criteria for including studies
- an attempt to identify all relevant studies, whether published or not
- explicit description of why apparently relevant studies have not been considered
- extraction of data
- pooling of data from similar studies (meta-analysis)
- description of results
- drawing appropriate conclusions and discussing implications for clinical practice and future research.

META-ANALYSIS

In the perinatal field, large numbers of women or babies are usually needed to address important research questions about outcomes that may be rare, though important (e.g. fetal death). Such questions may be tackled by mounting very large studies or by pooling data from a number of different trials of similar structure and purpose – *meta-analysis*[34]. Meta-analysis is a component of systematic reviews, and there are now several examples of such analyses providing clear guidance about the value of interventions during pregnancy to try to optimise fetal outcome, e.g. corticosteroid treatment before likely preterm delivery[35,36], or the use of Doppler ultrasound to investigate umbilical artery waveforms in high risk pregnancies[37,38].

There are debates about whether large single trials are preferable to the meta-analysis of results from several smaller trials. Whatever may be better, clinically important differences, without explanation, are rare in the obstetric arena[39].

COCHRANE COLLABORATION

The Cochrane Collaboration is an international network of individuals and institutions committed to producing up-to-date systematic reviews of the effectiveness of health care measures[40]. The Collaboration is based on the principles of genuine collaboration, equity and inclusiveness, and it consists of four dimensions – review groups, centres, fields, and methodology and software development groups. The centres are scattered around the world and provide support for review groups based within their geographical area of responsibility; each centre also has responsibility for some strategic activity for the collaboration, e.g. trial registration, training of reviewers, software production. The 'fields' deal with large generic issues that transcend the interests of any one review group, e.g. children, the elderly, people living in developing countries. The collaborative review groups produce the systematic reviews and have expanded greatly in number since their genesis in the perinatal field; there are now, for example, productive review groups in the fields of stroke, tropical diseases, schizophrenia, and menstrual disorders and subfertility, and there are many others at an earlier stage in their development (e.g. fertility control). Each group has an administrative base, a coordinating editor, other editors, and (usually) a multidisciplinary, multinational panel of reviewers. The administrator coordinates electronic and hand searching of the relevant literature for randomised controlled trials (including identification of unpublished material and non-English language literature[41].

At present, the building blocks for Cochrane systematic reviews are exclusively randomised controlled trials both because of the scientific strength of this method of assessing clinical interventions, and because of the methodological difficulties of dealing with other types of scientific data (e.g. qualitative research data).

The main product of the Collaboration is the Cochrane Database of Systematic Reviews which is published in electronic form at three-monthly intervals within the 'Cochrane Library', together with databases of clinical trials, methodological papers, and abstracts of other systematic reviews.

Perinatal medicine provided prototype models for development of other Cochrane review groups. The first, pilot database produced was the Oxford Database of Perinatal Trials which followed the publication of the milestone book, *Effective Care in Pregnancy and Childbirth*[42]. The Oxford Database was developed by Iain Chalmers and colleagues at the National Perinatal Epidemiology Unit, Oxford, UK, and was successful in demonstrating that such a project was feasible and that it would attract, as reviewers, committed people from many different countries and several different professional backgrounds. With formation of the Cochrane Collaboration, the database metamorphosed into the Cochrane

Pregnancy and Childbirth Database, which continued to be published until the end of 1995, but has now temporarily ceased publication. At present, all reviews are published exclusively in the Cochrane Library.

Evidence-based medicine

Given the limited resources of all healthcare systems, there is increasing political pressure to deliver care according to clinical effectiveness. This should also, of course, be an imperative to all clinicians attempting to provide a high-quality service. As more and more interventions are scrutinised in robust clinical trials, and as more and more topics are reviewed systematically, it is now possible to identify treatments that are effective and which should be used widely; those that are ineffective or frankly harmful and which should be discarded; and those about which we are uncertain of effectiveness and which should be considered for future research agendas[43]. In these ways, clinical epidemiology is beginning to make a tangible impact on the way that healthcare is structured and delivered (Table 24.3).

TABLE 24.3
Synopsis of effectiveness of selected interventions related to fetal assessment or treatment. After Enkin *et al.*[43]

1. Beneficial forms of care (effectiveness demonstrated by clear evidence from controlled trials)
- Periconceptional folic acid supplementation to prevent neural tube defects.
- Iodine supplementation in populations with a high incidence of endemic cretinism.
- Doppler ultrasound of umbilical artery in pregnancies at high risk of fetal compromise.
- Tight as opposed to 'too strict' or 'moderate' control of blood glucose levels in diabetic women.
- Antibiotics during labour for women known to be colonised by β-haemolytic streptococci.
- Corticosteroids to promote fetal lung maturation before preterm delivery.
- Fetal acid–base balance assessment as an adjunct to fetal heart monitoring during labour.

2. Forms of care likely to be beneficial (the evidence in favour of these forms of care is not as firmly established as those in section 1)
- Advice to avoid excessive alcohol intake during pregnancy.
- Prepregnancy counselling for diabetic women.
- Selective use of ultrasound to answer specific questions about fetal size and structure.
- Ultrasound to facilitate intrauterine interventions.
- Transabdominal versus transcervical chorion villus sampling.
- Fundal height measurements.

3. Forms of care with a trade-off between beneficial and adverse effects
- Routine early ultrasound.
- Chorion villus sampling versus amniocentesis for diagnosis of chromosomal abnormalities.
- Routine fetal movement counting to improve fetal outcome.
- Corticosteroids to promote fetal lung maturation before preterm delivery in diabetic women.

4. Forms of care of unknown effectiveness (insufficient or inadequate quality data upon which to base a recommendation for practice)
- Placental grading by ultrasound to improve perinatal outcome.
- Fetal biophysical profile for fetal surveillance.
- Hospitalisation and bed rest for impaired fetal growth.

5. Forms of care unlikely to be beneficial (evidence against these forms of care not as firmly established as those in section 6 below)
- Routine use of ultrasound in late pregnancy.
- Routine use of Doppler ultrasound in all pregnancies.
- Screening for 'gestational diabetes'.

6. Forms of care likely to be ineffective or harmful (ineffectiveness or harm demonstrated by clear evidence)
- Non-stress cardiotocography to improve fetal outcome.
- Electronic fetal heart monitoring without access to fetal scalp sampling during labour.
- Prophylactic amnio-infusion for oligohydramnios.

REFERENCES

1. Enkin MW. The need for evidence-based obstetrics. *Evidence-Based Med.* **1**:132–133, 1996.
2. Naylor CD. Grey zones of clinical practice: some limits to evidence-based medicine. *Lancet* **345**:840–842, 1995.
3. Barker DJP. Fetal origins of coronary heart disease. *Br. Med. J.* **311**:171–174, 1995.
4. Arngrimsson R, Bjornsson S, Geirsson RT, Bjornsson H, Walker JJ & Snaedal G. Genetic and familial predisposition to eclampsia and pre-eclampsia in a defined population. *Br. J. Obstet. Gynaecol.* **97**:762–769, 1990.
5. Froster UG & Jackson L. Limb defects and chorion villus sampling: results from an international registry, 1992–4. *Lancet* **347**:489–494, 1996.

6. Firth H, Boyd PA, Chamberlain P, MacKenzie IZ & Huson SM. Limb defects and chorion villus sampling. *Lancet* **347**:1406, 1996.
7. Mastroiacova P & Botto LD. Limb defects and chorion villus sampling. *Lancet* **347**:1406–1407, 1996.
8. Baird D, Walker J & Thomson AM. The causes and prevention of stillbirths and first week deaths. *J. Obstet. Gynaecol. Br. Emp.* **61**:433–448, 1954.
9. Whitfield CR, Smith NC, Cockburn F & Gibson AAM. Perinatally related wastage – a proposed classification of primary obstetric factors. *Br. J. Obstet. Gynaecol.* **93**:694–703, 1986.
10. Neilson JP. Perinatal loss and appropriate fetal surveillance. In *A Critical Appraisal of Fetal Surveillance* (eds H.P. van Geijn & F.J.A. Copray), pp. 16–24. Amsterdam: Elsevier Science, 1994.
11. Lewis G, Drife JO *et al. Report on Confidential Enquiries into Maternal Deaths in the United Kingdom 1994–6.* London: HMSO, 1998.
12. Confidential Enquiry into Stillbirths and Deaths in Infancy. *Annual Report for 1 January–31 December 1993*, pp. 27–42. London: Department of Health, 1995.
13. Szabo J & Gellen J. Nuchal fluid accumulation in trisomy 21 detected by vaginosonography in first trimester. *Lancet* **336**:1133, 1990.
14. Snijders RJM, Noble J, Sebire N, Souka A & Nicolaides KH. UK multicentre project on assessment of risk of trisomy 21 by maternal age and fetal nuchal translucency thickness at 10–14 weeks of gestation. *Lancet* **352**:343–346, 1998.
15. De Lia JE, Kuhlmann RS, Harstad TW & Cruikshank DP. Fetoscopic laser ablation of placental vessels in severe previable twin–twin transfusion syndrome. *Am. J. Obstet. Gynecol.* **172**:1202–1211, 1995.
16. Edington PT, Sibanda J & Beard RW. Influence on clinical practice of routine intra-partum fetal monitoring. *Br. Med. J.* **3**:341–343, 1975.
17. Chalmers I. Evaluating the effects of care during pregnancy and childbirth. In *Effective Care in Pregnancy and Childbirth* (eds I. Chalmers, M. Enkin & M.J.N.C. Keirse), pp. 3–38. Oxford: Oxford University Press, 1989.
18. Vintzileos AM, Antsaklis A, Varvarigos I, Papas C, Sofatzis I & Montgomery JT. A randomized trial of intrapartum electronic fetal heart rate monitoring versus intermittent auscultation. *Obstet. Gynecol.* **81**:899–907, 1993.
19. Schulz KF, Chalmers I, Hayes RJ & Altman D. Empirical evidence of bias. *JAMA* **273**:408–412, 1995.
20. Collaborative Low Dose Aspirin Study in Pregnancy (CLASP trial) Collaborative Group. MRC Collaborative Low Dose Aspirin Study in Pregnancy (CLASP). *Lancet* **343**:619–629, 1994.
21. The Eclampsia Trial Collaborative Group. Which anticonvulsant for women with eclampsia? *Lancet* **345**:1455–1463, 1995.
22. MRC Working Party on the Evaluation of Chorion Villus Sampling. Medical Research Council trial of CVS. *Lancet* **337**:1491–1499, 1991.
23. Nicolaides KH, de Lourdes Brizot M, Patel F & Snijders R. Comparison of chorion villus sampling and amniocentesis for fetal karyotyping at 10–13 weeks' gestation. *Lancet* **344**:435–439, 1994.
24. Ewigman BG, Crane JP, Frigoletto FD, LeFevre ML, Bain RP & McNellis D, and the RADIUS study group. Effect of prenatal ultrasound screening on perinatal outcome. *N. Engl. J. Med.* **329**:821–827, 1993.
25. Chitty LS, Hunt GH, Moore J & Lobb MO. Effectiveness of routine ultrasonography in detecting fetal structural abnormalities in a low risk population. *Br. Med. J.* **303**:1165–1169, 1991.
26. Saari-Kemppainen A, Karjalainen O, Ylostalo P & Heinonen OP. Ultrasound screening and perinatal mortality: controlled trial of systematic one-stage screening in pregnancy. *Lancet* **336**:387–391, 1990.
27. Saari-Kemppainen A, Karjalainen O, Ylostalo P & Heinonen OP. Fetal anomalies in a controlled one-stage screening trial. A report from the Helsinki Ultrasound Group. *J. Perinat. Med.* **22**:279–289, 1994.
28. Grant A & Elbourne D. Clinical trials. In *Scientific Essentials of Reproductive Medicine* (eds S.G. Hillier, H.C. Kitchener & J.P. Neilson), pp. 555–565. London: W.B. Saunders, 1996.
29. Liggins GC, Schellenberg JC, Manzai M, Kitterman JA & Lee CC. Synergisms of cortisol and thyrotropin-releasing hormone in lung maturation in fetal sheep. *J. Appl. Physiol.* **65**:1880–1884, 1988.
30. Crowther CA & Alfirevic Z. Antenatal thyrotropin-releasing hormone (TRH) prior to preterm delivery. In *Pregnancy and Childbirth Module of The Cochrane Database of Systematic Reviews* (updated 4 March 1997) (eds J.P. Neilson, C.A. Crowther, E.D. Hodnett, G.J. Hofmeyr, M.J.N.C. Keirse) Issue 2. The Cochrane Collaboration. Oxford: Update Software. [Available in the Cochrane Library.]
31. Jikihara H, Sawada Y, Imai S *et al.* Maternal administration of thyrotropin-releasing hormone for prevention of neonatal respiratory distress syndrome. In *Proceedings of 6th Congress of the Federation of the Asia-Oceania Perinatal Societies, Perth, Western Australia* p. 87, 1990.
32. Knight DB, Liggins GC & Wealthall SE. A randomized controlled trial of antepartum thyrotropin-releasing hormone and betamethasone in the prevention of respiratory distress in preterm infants. *Am. J. Obstet. Gynecol.* **171**:11–16, 1994.
33. The Actobat Study Group. Australian Collaborative Trial of Betamethasone and Thyrotropin Releasing Hormone (ACTOBAT) for the prevention of neonatal respiratory disease. *Lancet* **345**:877–882, 1995.
34. Peto R. Why do we need systematic overviews of randomized trials? *Statistics Med.* **6**:233–240, 1987.
35. Crowley PA. Antenatal corticosteroid therapy: a meta-analysis of the randomized trials, 1972 to 1994. *Am. J. Obstet. Gynecol.* **173**:322–335, 1995.
36. Crowley P. Corticosteroids prior to preterm delivery. In *Pregnancy and Childbirth Module of The Cochrane Database of Systematic Reviews* (updated 4 March 1997) (eds J.P. Neilson, C.A. Crowther, E.D. Hodnett, G.J. Hofmeyr, M.J.N.C. Keirse) Issue 2. The Cochrane Collaboration. Oxford: Update Software. [Available in the Cochrane Library.]
37. Alfirevic Z & Neilson JP. Doppler ultrasonography in high-risk pregnancies: systematic review with meta-analysis. *Am. J. Obstet. Gynecol.* **172**:1379–1387, 1995.
38. Neilson JP & Alfirevic Z. Doppler ultrasound in high risk pregnancies. In *Pregnancy and Childbirth Module of The Cochrane Database of Systematic Reviews* (Updated 4 March 1997) (eds J.P. Neilson, C.A. Crowther, E.D. Hodnett, G.J. Hofmeyr, M.J.N.C. Keirse) Issue 2. The Cochrane Collaboration. Oxford: Update Software. [Available in the Cochrane Library.]
39. Cappelleri JC, Ioannidis JPA, Schmid CH, de Ferranti SD, Aubert M, Chalmers TC & Lau J. Large trials vs meta-analysis of smaller trials. How do their results compare? *JAMA* **276**:1332–1338, 1996.
40. Chalmers I, Dickersin K & Chalmers T. Getting to grips with Archie Cochrane's agenda. *Br. Med. J.* **305**:786–787, 1992.
41. Moher D, Fortin P, Jadad AR, Juni P, Klassen T, Le Lorier J, Liberati A, Linde K & Penna A. Completeness of reporting of trials in languages other than English: implications for conduct and reporting of systematic reviews. *Lancet* **347**:363–366, 1996.
42. Chalmers I, Enkin M & Keirse MJNC (eds) *Effective Care in Pregnancy and Childbirth.* Oxford: Oxford University Press 1979.
43. Enkin M, Keirse MJNC, Renfrew M & Neilson JP. *A Guide to Effective Care in Pregnancy and Childbirth.* Oxford: Oxford University Press, 1995.

Assessing the organisation and effect of perinatal care

25

J. Chapple

Background

More than 200 million women worldwide become pregnant each year[1]. The vast majority of these women receive no perinatal care and the price they pay is high. One very crude assessment of the effects of perinatal care is the number of mothers and babies dying. For 500 000 women each year, the complications of pregnancy are fatal and out of an estimated 8.1 million infants dying each year before their first birthday, half occur during the first month of life; 2.8 million babies each year die during the first week of life and for each of these deaths, another child is stillborn. The chief causes of this are poor maternal health, inadequate care during pregnancy, inappropriate management and poor hygiene during delivery and the critical few hours after birth, lack of care for newborn babies and care which discriminates between babies born with malformations or with the 'wrong' sex for a particular culture. All but 6000 of the 500 000 maternal deaths a year occur in developing countries. The introduction of community based healthcare systems can improve the outlook for mothers and babies dramatically. In the 1950s, most births in Sri Lanka (formerly Ceylon) took place at home with the assistance of untrained birth attendants and 555 out of every 100 000 women died. At the end of the 1980s, over 85% of all births were attended by trained people and maternal mortality had dropped to 95 per 100 000 with a fall of deaths due to sepsis from 25% to 10% of maternal deaths.

Provision of family planning and basic maternity care to women in developing countries is a human dilemma which has not yet been resolved, although the solutions to the problem are known. Access to care can also be problematic in countries such as the United States which do not have a system of universal healthcare nor a compulsory system of employment based health insurance. A study of ten countries with some form of national healthcare financing, prepaid prenatal and postnatal maternity leave and protective limits on the working circumstances of pregnant women showed they all had a lower infant mortality than the United States[2], although benefits cannot be inferred as the sole cause of these lower rates. This chapter focuses on care in developed countries with national systems of healthcare.

There has been a tradition of systematic programmes of maternity care in the United Kingdom, with the first Midwives Act 1902 laying down rules for midwifery training[3] and the second Act of 1918 making it compulsory for a midwife to summon medical help if a pregnancy or labour became abnormal[4]. It is illegal for a woman to deliver without arranging for the assistance of a trained midwife or qualified doctor in labour and there is a statutory duty for a midwife to provide care for at least ten days after delivery. This is a sharp contrast to all other areas of medicine, where an individual is free to choose whether to seek care and can choose anyone to provide it, with the proviso that the care provider does not pretend to be a qualified health professional if they are not.

Health service provision and improving social conditions have led to dramatic falls in deaths of both mothers and babies. In England & Wales, maternal mortality fell from 67.1 deaths per 100 000 births in 1955–57 to 6.1 in 1988–90[5] whilst stillbirths and first week deaths fell from 35 per 1000 births to 8.9 over the same period. Increasing medicalisation of maternity care has led to a system where over 97% of births in the UK now take place in hospital and no labour is regarded as normal except in retrospect. This has led to vigorous debate about the place of birth[6]. In North Thames (West) region, 67% of women will have an uncomplicated delivery by a midwife, only 6% of babies weigh < 2.5 kg and 5.8% of all singleton babies are admitted to a special care unit for more than 24 hours[7], yet the maternity and neonatal services are geared to the expectation that disaster will befall each woman with little detailed examination of the actual risks involved. There are tensions between women and their carers over the type of care provided and between clinicians over which specialty should have the lead role in care[8]. The introduction of the internal market in the National Health Service has also led to tensions between hospitals, especially between tertiary level specialist units and district general hospitals and competition to provide care.

Sophisticated and highly technical services are expensive. A study in Trent[9] estimated that in 1991 the cost of providing neonatal intensive care was up to £640 per baby per day. There is therefore an imperative to organise perinatal care so it is appropriate to the community in which it is based and to assess the outcome of increasingly complex technologies applied to the physiological process of pregnancy, delivery and adjustment to life outside the womb.

Care during pregnancy

Since the introduction of antenatal care in the UK in the 1920s, women have been taught that routine checks are important. They expect to be seen regularly and feel dissatisfied if they are not. However, the organisation of care grew in a haphazard way as a general screening programme with no stated aims and objectives and little monitoring for efficiency and effectiveness. Specialists were involved in care as a routine rather than when required.

Prediction and detection of obstetric problems is low in comparison with the resources and time of both health professionals and women invested in the visits. A retrospective analysis of the case records of 2186 women in Aberdeen[10] showed that the majority of antenatal admissions were for conditions which had arisen despite antenatal care and were not prevented or detected by it. Clinicians diagnosed fewer than half the cases of intrauterine growth retardation antenatally but for each case correctly predicted, there were 2.5 false-positive diagnoses and 1.3 false-positives for each correct diagnosis of pre-eclampsia or hypertension.

There are inititiatives to develop protocols for antenatal care, assess the woman's risk of developing complications of pregnancy, specify the objectives for each visit, reduce the overall number of visits and to assign each contact to the most appropriate carer (general practitioner, midwife or hospital obstetrician) and place (at home, community clinic or hospital). Observational data[11,12] and randomised controlled trials[13,14] suggest that new style care is as effective as traditional care in terms of variables related to pregnancy related hypertensive disorders, labour, and maternal and perinatal morbidity. Fewer visits to hospital also cut the number of ultrasound scans and day admissions for monitoring requested by obstetricians worried that they are missing growth retardation. This increased use of resources to allay obstetricians' fears is not associated with any measurable clinical effect, beneficial or otherwise[13,15].

People, whether professionals or patients, do not find change easy. A national programme in the UK[16] to give women more choice and control during pregnancy and childbirth and to improve continuity of care and carer has shown the tensions between these objectives when care is rationalised through evidence-based practice. One objective of the programme was to review of the total antenatal visits for women with uncomplicated pregnancies in the light of available evidence. In the study by Sikorski *et al.*[13], 26% of women eligible to enter into the trial of traditional versus new style reviewed care chose not to participate, mainly because they did not want to have fewer antenatal visits, even when the visits were more focused. Over half the women in the group receiving the new programme of care felt that some of the gaps between visits were too long. Most of these worries were about whether the baby was thriving and inability to cope postnatally and some of these feelings persisted into the postnatal period. Fewer different professionals were seen, so continuity of carer was improved in line with the *Changing Childbirth* initiative. Less conflicting advice was given, but women felt that staff did not remember them as well. Conservative approaches to care are therefore not confined to professionals[17]. Social support is important in pregnancy and antenatal care provides this, together with reassurance and information[18]. The answer may lie in allowing more time for talking rather than for testing during antenatal visits. As people are the most expensive resource in any healthcare system, focused antenatal care may not release large amounts of resources to be used elsewhere in maternity and other health services.

Care during labour

LOW-RISK PREGNANCIES

In recent years, there has been considerable controversy in the UK about the place of delivery and who should care for women in labour. The Select Committee on Midwives' registration reported that in 1890, 0.3% of births took place in workhouse infirmaries catering for women on poor relief and 1% in and charitable lying-hospitals[19]. Concern about conditions in people's homes during the First World War led to the introduction of maternity homes, built with gardens on the outskirts of town by local authorities and voluntary agencies. These ranged in size from 18 to 20 beds to larger homes with 25 to 50 beds in large towns. In 1927, when the General Register Office first tabulated births by place of delivery, 15% of births took place in institutions (hospitals, nursing homes, maternity homes and Poor Law institutions). A new technology of heavy sedation, scopolamine morphine narcosis or 'twilight sleep' led to a recommendation that hospitals with greatly increased nursing staff and a resident medical attendant were needed for its introduction[20]. This proportion of institutionalised births rose to 24% in 1932, 35% in 1937, 54% in 1946 and remained static at about 65% during the 1950s[21]. By 1992, 96.5% of all women delivering did so in NHS hospitals with consultant obstetric units, with 1.4% delivered in isolated general practitioner units, 0.7% in non-NHS hospitals and 1.3% at home.

Current UK practice on place of birth has developed from two assumptions. Firstly, that hospitals are the safest place to give birth and secondly, that the rapid decline in maternal, perinatal and neonatal mortality is a consequence of the move from home to hospital birth[21]. The debate centres around whether these assumptions are correct and whether mortality is the best outcome measure for maternity services. Numbers of deaths of both mother and baby are now so small that statistical comparisons are unreliable. Some stillbirths will occur before labour and are unlikely to be a consequence of place of delivery. Other deliveries to high-risk mothers who had always planned a hospital delivery to take advantage of specialist care will occur unexpectedly at home, but be counted as home deliveries. This is more likely to occur in rapid preterm labour with high-risk, low-birthweight babies.

International comparisons on safety are unreliable as there is considerable variation between countries in the way care is organised and between regulations on birth and death registration and the ways they are interpreted and applied[22,23]. However, the home-birth lobby frequently cites the example of maternity care in The Netherlands, where 31% of births took place at home in 1991, compared with 71% in 1971[24]. A study of 1692 low-risk women who had babies in Groningen in 1981 showed that women who chose a home birth experienced fewer problems during pregnancy, labour and the puerperium than those who gave birth in hospital, even when parity was taken into account[25]. These women initially had a free choice about a home or hospital birth, but were referred to hospital if any complications arose during pregnancy. In babies born without complications, morbidity leading to admission to a special care unit was lower for those born at home than in those born in hospital. Midwives in The Netherlands seem successful in selectively referring to obstetric care both primiparous and multiparous women who have problems diagnosed during pregnancy who initially booked with a midwife as they had no known risk factors[26].

HIGH-RISK PREGNANCIES

WHAT IS 'HIGH RISK'?

There is little debate about hospital delivery for women at high risk, but controversy about what constitutes risk. For example, 'elderly' primiparae and women with more than four previous births are often seen as high-risk patients who should be strongly advised not to have a home birth. The data on which this advice is based are collected through national record systems which produce cross-sectional data at one point in time, as birth registration records in the UK cannot be linked. Analysis in this way gives an erroneous view of the risks, as reproductive compensation may apply to women who have previously lost babies. Women who lose babies usually go on to have further pregnancies in order to achieve the size of famly they want. They are at high risk because of the previous poor outcome and are therefore of higher parity and of necessity, older. Higher age and parity in subsequent pregnancies may be the result of poor pregnancy outcome rather than the cause.

Cross-sectional studies show a U-shaped curve for distribution of perinatal mortality rates with maternal age and parity, with perinatal rates being high for first births and women under 20 years of age, dipping to lower levels and rising to fourth and subsequent births and for women over 35 years of age. Record linkage in Norway allowed cohort studies based on sibship size to be conducted between 1963 and 1973[27]. These showed that the mortality of fetuses over 16 weeks' gestation decreased with increasing maternal parity and as the rank in sibship size (birth order) increased. The fetal mortality increased with final family size, so that the mortality rate for the fourth child in a family was less than for a third, second or first child of any woman, but the mortality rate for the second child out of four was higher than that for the second child of a sibship of just two children. The decline of the perinatal mortality curve by parity is steeper the higher the maternal age at the time of first birth. If these data are looked at cross-sectionally, the traditional U-shaped association between parity and perinatal mortality rates is seen, and the self-selection bias towards trying for another pregnancy to achieve the wanted family size is not revealed. This research agreed with earlier work done in Aberdeen between 1949 and 1954 which concluded that the rate of unsuccessful pregnancies declined as birth order increased within cohorts of women having a given number of pregnancies[28]. A study of 3068 women doctors in England & Wales reported in 1978 that the risk of fetal loss (including miscarriage) at a given parity varied with the woman's gravidity, so that for each 'sibship' size the rate of fetal loss decreased with each successful pregnancy[29].

There is less debate about place of delivery for high-risk pregnancies where the mother has complications such as insulin-dependent diabetes, a multiple pregnancy or a breech presentation. Babies of insulin-dependent diabetic women have stillbirth and perinatal rates about five times higher than the population rate[30,31], as do babies from a multiple pregnancy. Breech delivery is also hazardous – a contentious report has suggested a perinatal mortality rate twenty times greater in women who deliver a term baby presenting by the breech vaginally than in those delivered by caesarean section[32,33]. These conditions are not common – in North Thames (West) in 1993, 0.4% of women had established diabetes at the start of pregnancy and 2.6% of deliveries were of multiple pregnancies[7].

The low prevalence of specific pregnancy complications raises the issue of specialisation and differing levels of healthcare for high-risk women and babies which will be a feature of the rest of this chapter. As more breech babies are delivered by caesarean section, expertise in vaginal breech delivery may diminish. In an overall maternity population of more than 41 000 women a year, fewer than five term babies presenting by the breech were delivered vaginally each week in the fifteen maternity units in North Thames (West) region. This is 3.5 deliveries per consultant per year. These numbers may be too small to train junior staff in vaginal breech delivery, so that expert help will be less accessible in the future for women who are anxious to deliver vaginally despite the breech presentation[7]. It also suggests that maintenance of expertise may become a problem – there may be too few cases available for each consultant to retain skills. The dilemmas of different levels of care for certain complications are: does practice make perfect and is big beautiful?

RELATIONSHIP BETWEEN VOLUME OF CASES AND QUALITY OF HEALTHCARE

> The organisation of medicine has become insufficient and ... fails to bring the advantages of medical knowledge to the people ... The general availability of medical services can only be effected by new and extended organisation ... This organisation is needed on the grounds of efficiency and cost, and is necessary alike in the interest of the public and of the medical profession.

Consultative Council on Medical and Allied Services (1920)

The Dawson Report[34] to the UK Parliament in 1920, from which the above quote was taken, was just one forerunner to current policy reviews on provision of care, not only for maternity and neonatal services, but for cancer, cardiac and surgical services. Cynics may say that concentration of hospital services on a few sites are finance driven, but there is considerable interest in whether improved health care outcomes can be gained from concentrating the hospital care of particular conditions or procedures. This may involve fewer clinicians or hospitals providing higher volumes of activity.

In an ideal world, organisation of services would be based on the best scientific evidence. The least biased way of making comparisons between similar groups of people receiving different forms of care is to do a randomised trial[35]. There are great difficulties in organising randomised controlled trials, especially when changes in technologies and patterns of care are already introduced before thorough evaluation by enthusiastic clinicians or are demanded by patients alerted to new developments in care by the media, as was suggested by George Bernard Shaw in 1906[36]:

> To advertise any remedy or operation, you have only to pick out all the most reassuring advances made by civilisation, and boldly present the two in relation of cause and effect; the public will swallow the fallacy without a wry face. It has no idea of the need for what is called a control experiment.

Also, mortality rates as a measure of outcome are now so low that the numbers of participants in trials needed to detect significant differences between types of care are prohibitively high to organise and finance.

VOLUME, OUTCOME AND CASE MIX

The NHS Centre for Reviews and Dissemination[37] has assessed over 200 mainly observational studies on the relationship between hospital or doctor volume[38], over 100 studies on volume and costs[39] and 47 papers on patient access[40]. Most reported a reduction in poor health outcomes (mainly hospital mortality) as volumes increased, but few made any assessment of difference in severity of illness. This is rather like comparing the quality of geriatric or terminal care to paediatric care using mortality rates – any unit which specialises in providing care for extremely ill, high-risk patients and has emergency and other referrals of 'difficult' cases from other non-specialist units will have a high overall mortality rate.

Case mix adjustment for mothers using maternity care is difficult. Concern about rapidly rising caesarean section rates led to the development of the 'standard primip' approach to interhospital comparisons. This takes a substantial group of low-risk women from each hospital population, omitting women who may have confounding factors for intervention. Variables for inclusion include parity (primiparous), ethnic group (Caucasian), age between 20 and 34 years, height of ≥155 c, singleton delivery, cephalic presentation, gestation of 37 weeks and over, delivering in the same unit in which the woman was booked (to exclude women referred for specialist care) and with no medical complications of pregnancy, such as diabetes and hypertensive disorders[41,42]. The 'standard primip' group does show lower levels of intervention, complications and better outcomes than 'non-standard' primips, suggesting that this methodology does define a low-risk group. However, there is still considerable variation in intervention and outcome between units, suggesting that factors due to staff, resources and organisation play an important role in quality of care in each unit.

VOLUME AND COSTS

It is often assumed that by concentrating hospital services into larger units, efficiency will be improved by economies of scale in which long-term average costs fall as the volume of activity rises. As the throughput increases, the average cost per case should fall, as the fixed costs of staff and equipment are spread over a larger number of cases. However, there is a critical volume beyond which average costs rise because of diseconomies of scale[43]. The issue of volume and cost has not been addressed for obstetrics, although there are recommendations for regionalisation of maternity and neonatal care which propose minimum numbers of deliveries each year for each of three levels of care[44]. These levels cover units which provide not only routine care for local patients but also intensive care for maternity and neonatal patients and special services for an entire region (level 3), standard units providing care for most complications (level 2) and services which exist only because of geographic necessity (level 1).

PATIENT ACCESS

Research in this area focuses almost entirely on the relationship between observed rates of utilisation and distance or travel time as a proxy for access. Most studies disregard other considerations affecting access, such as socio-economic group, language and personal mobility. Studies of accident & emergency self-referral, cervical cytology and mammography show that where perceptions of need and importance are low, there is a reduction in access with increasing distance from the facility providing it. However, when the illness (such as cancer) is perceived as serious, distance may not affect attendance[45]. This has implications for maternity care, which was not included in these studies. A number of studies have indicated women's preference for the more personal ambience and convenience of community-based clinics[46] and home delivery[47]. Women should feel convinced that there will be benefits for themselves and their baby in travelling to specialist centres for antenatal care or delivery or they may become defaulters and put themselves and their child at risk.

Care of the baby: neonatal intensive care (NIC)

WHY SHOULD NIC PROVISION BE REVIEWED?

In developed countries, small and sick babies are treated in neonatal intensive care units (NICUs). An interesting paradox has arisen with the provision of NIC. Professional advice from neonatologists suggests that NIC should be concentrated in a small number of well-resourced NICUs to produce the largest health gains in terms of mortality and morbidity[48]. However, data from monitoring North Thames (West) usage of NIC in fifteen maternity units between 1991 and 1993 (when the internal market had just been introduced in the NHS) shows an apparent decentralisation of care. Transfers to level 3 units dropped dramatically from 133 *in utero* transfers and 133 transfers after delivery in the 1991–92 financial year to 43 and 51 respectively in 1993–94. Level 2 units showed a decrease from 40 *in utero* and 44 *ex utero* transfers in 1991–92 to 13 and 12 in 1993–94. The total number of babies treated in level 2 and 3 units was 902 in 1991–92 and 858 in 1992–93 to 567 in 1993–94. This is a marked contrast to the situation which existed before the NHS internal market, when local paediatricians reported that they could not get babies transferred to specialist units either ante- or postnatally and an emergency bed service (EBS) was needed for the Thames regions to cut down on the time spent in arranging transfers. Since 1991, demand for transfers through the EBS has plummeted, and it is now extremely rare for there to be no cot available in a recognised specialist NICU. This change in activity was not seen in Trent region in over the same period of time[49,50]. Overall in England & Wales in this period, access to NIC improved while overall workload and transfers did not increase.

Requests from special care units in district general hospitals in North Thames (West) to be recognised for the provision of NIC suggest that many paediatricians are not referring preterm, low-birthweight (LBW) and ill babies to more specialist centres, but are looking after them in their own local units. All paediatricians are now trained in NIC and many believe that on consultant appointment to a district general hospital they can provide neonatal care, regardless of nursing and other resources available. Changes in purchasing services, with devolution to primary care, is felt to threaten the development of tertiary level services, which should be planned and purchased by groups responsible for larger populations than a single English health authority with a population of between 250 000 and 500 000[49,50].

Changes in care for ill babies which were introduced into general obstetric and paediatric practice the 1980s (giving steroids to mothers in preterm labour to prevent respiratory distress syndrome (RDS) and use of artificial surfactant to prevent and treat hyaline membrane disease (HMD)), together with changes brought by the internal market suggest that provision of NIC should be reviewed. A randomised controlled trial of extracorporeal membrane oxygenation (ECMO) is also underway nationally, which may promote the need for further review.

PROBLEMS IN REVIEWING NIC PROVISION

The main problems are those of defining what is being reviewed to avoid comparing apples with pears. These include the following.

DEFINITIONS OF POPULATIONS STUDIED

It is important to compare the outcome of NIC for entire populations rather than subgroups that did or did not get intensive care[51]. Many reports look at outcome only for those babies admitted to NICUs. Shann[48] has compiled a table (Table 25.1) of twelve papers covering different time periods between 1945 to 1984. These population studies have consistently shown a substantial improvement in perinatal mortality for babies treated in a NICU as compared with babies who were not. The exception is a study of all 206 054 births in New Zealand between 1978 and 1981[52]. This found that small rural maternity hospitals had lower mortality rates for babies > 1500 g, but higher mortality rates for babies < 1500 g – possibly because perinatal care in New Zealand is highly regionalised, with high-risk mothers being referred to larger hospitals before delivery. No volume threshold was found below which obstetric care was unsafe.

TABLE 25.1
Perinatal mortality and patient volumes

Reference	Years	Place	Number	Comments
Yankaner AMA, Allaway NC. An analysis of hospital neonatal mortality rates in New York State *J Dis. Child.* **95**:240–244, 1958.	1945–54	New York	1 489 175 (all births)	
Williams RL. Measuring the effectiveness of perinatal medical care. *Medical Care* **17**:95–110, 1979.	1960–73	California	3 441 448 (all births)	Found that a higher ratio of specialists to generalists was strongly associated with a lower observed to expected perinatal mortality ratio (10% increase in the proportion of specialists reduced mortality by 0.55 per 1000 births). Also lower mortality ratio of observed to expected deaths in larger delivery services, those with above average section rate, recording Apgar score, higher specialist to generalist ratios. Ratio significantly higher in mothers with Spanish sounding surnames and in private hospitals.
Horwood SP, Boyle MH, Torrance GW & Sinclair JC. Mortality and morbidity of 500 to 1499 g birth weight infants live born to residents of a defined geographic region before and after neonatal intensive care. *Pediatrics* **69**:613–620, 1982.	1964–69 and 1973–77	Ontario	638 births between 500–1499 g	The introduction of neonatal intensive care was associated with a significant reduction in mortality, but no significant change in morbidity.
Bakketeig LS, Hoffman HJ & Sternthal PM. Obstetric service and perinatal mortality in Norway. *Acta Obstet. Gynecol. Scand.* (suppl) **177**:1–19, 1978.	1967–73	Norway	454 358 births – all singleton births	Used an obstetric score based on personnel and equipment to divide country into three groups of counties, with low, medium and high obstetric scores. Significant differences in MRs (especially early NNMR) between counties with low obstetric scores and the 2 other groups.
Paneth N, Kiely JL, Wallenstein S, Marcus M *et al.* Newborn intensive care and neonatal mortality in low birth weight infants. *N. Engl. J Med.* **307**:149–155, 1982.	1976–78	New York City level 1–3 NICUs	13 560 singleton births between 501–2250 g	Looked at outcome by level 1–3 newborn intensive care units. Neonatal MR significantly lower for level 3 units (full NIC) – not explained by differences between groups in social/demographic status, prenatal care, medical complications of pregnancy.
Bowes WA. A review of perinatal mortality in Colorado, 1971–78 and its relationship to the regionalization of perinatal services. *Am. J. Obstet. Gynecol.* **141**:1045–1052, 1981.	1971–78	Colorado	319 040 live births	Neonatal MR halved in time period, no change in birth weight distribution. During this time, VLBW babies looked after more often in level 2 and 3 NICUs – greater survival rates of VLBW infants born in level 2 and 3 hospitals.
Rosenblatt RA, Reinken J, Shoemack P. Is obstetrics safe in small hospitals? Evidence from New Zealand's regionalised perinatal system. *Lancet* **ii**:429–432, 1985.	1978–81	New Zealand	206 054 all births in public maternity hospitals	Level 1 maternity units had lower birth weight specific PNMRs in all but the lowest body weight categories than the better equipped hospitals to which they refer. This may reflect cautious AN referral of problems and effective regionalisation. No evidence that satisfactory outcome depends on a minimum number of deliveries.
Saigal S, Rosenbaum P, Hattersley B & Milner R. Decreased disability rate among 3 year old survivors weighing 501–1000 g at birth and born to residents of a geographically defined region from 1982 to 1984 compared with 1977 to 1980. *J. Pediatr.* **114**:839–846, 1989.	1977–80 and 1982–84	Ontario	255 and 266 = 521 births between 501–1000 g	Use of tertiary care centre static between these time periods. Disabilities reduced over the time period, but infants delivered at community hospitals had higher prevalence of neurosensory impairments in the 2nd time period, compared with those delivering at level 3 unit.
Forbes JF, Larssen KE & Bakketeig LS. Access to intensive neonatal care and neonatal survival in low birthweight infants: a population study in Norway. *Paediatr. Perinat. Epidemiol.* **1**:33–42, 1987.	1979–81	Norway	4692 births below 2500 g	For infants weighing 1250–2499 g dose–response relationship between neonatal survival and level of immediate access to NIC. No similar pattern of survival for babies < 1250 g.
Victorian Infant Collaborative Study Group. Improvement of outcome for infants of birth weight under 1000 g. *Arch. Dis. Childh.* **66**:765–769, 1991.	1979–87	Victoria	911 births between 500–999 g	
Cooke RW. Referral to a regional centre improve outcome in extremely low birthweight infants. *Arch. Dis. Childh.* **62**:619–621, 1987.	1980–83	Liverpool	201 births below 1001 g	Referral of ELBW infants from district hospitals in a geographically defined area to a specialist regional centre significantly improved their chances of survival.
Verloove-Vanhorick SP, Verwey RA, Ebeling MCA, Brand R *et al.* Mortality in very preterm and low birth weight infants according to place of delivery and level of care. *Paediatrics* **81**:404–411, 1988.	1983	Holland	1338 births, 32 weeks or under 1500 g	All infants assigned to one of 3 levels of care according to hospital of birth. Uncorrected rates for all 3 levels were similar, but if adjusted for 4 and 22 potential confounding factors, mortality was significantly higher in level 1 and 2 hospitals.

From Shann, F. A review of the report 'The care of critically ill children' in *A Critical Appraisal of the Care of Critically Ill Children*. York: NHS Centre for Reviews and Dissemination, 1994.
MR = Mortality rate, NNMR = neonatal mortality rate, AN = antenatal

DEFINITIONS OF 'SPECIALIST UNITS'

Most papers use the terms 'level 1, 2 and 3' to denote increasingly specialist provision of NIC. Definitions of these levels vary from place to place. Experience from monitoring NIC usage in North Thames (West) suggests units find it very difficult to categorise the care received by individual babies, as the definitions of NIC produced by the British Association of Perinatal Medicine (BAPM) are complex. Units are often categorised by the resources that are available to them, rather than by workload cared for – a recent paper from Trent looking at survival and place of treatment after premature delivery[53] suggests that there are differences in outcome for babies born at < 28 weeks' completed gestation if a cut-off of 600 ventilator-days a year is used to differentiate levels of NIC.

DEFINITIONS OF BABIES TREATED IN NICUs

Some papers look at babies treated in terms of gestational age, usually, but by no means always, in terms of completed weeks of pregnancy. Gestational age can be difficult to assess accurately through clinical examination and comparison with ultrasound examination of the baby prenatally. Other papers categorise babies by birthweight, which often seems a more exact measure than gestational age, although scales may vary considerably. Babies are usually categorised as:

Low birth weight (LBW), <2500 g
Very low birthweight (VLBW), <1500 g
Extremely low birthweight (ELBW) babies, <1000 g

Epidemiological studies from Office of National Statistics (ONS) data suggest that the proportion of VLBW babies is static at about 1% of all births (although there is considerable local variation from district to district). This is probably because increasing survival of these babies, research on helping parents to cope with bereavement and changing parental attitudes encourages professionals to attempt to treat very small babies and acknowledge these infants as registrable births. Neither form of categorisation makes it possible to look at the outcome of NIC for a very vulnerable group – babies which are small-for-gestational age (SGA). The prevalence of SGA infants may vary considerably from one population to another.

TIME SCALES

All published studies cover different periods of time and none covers the recent period since 1990 when surfactant became widely available, more mothers were given steroids in preterm labour and more babies were treated locally. It is therefore difficult to know whether past studies in different countries are applicable to today's provision of care in the UK.

SHOULD CRITICALLY ILL BABIES RECEIVE NIC AT ALL?

There has been one randomised controlled trial of intensive care in neonates, performed in Melbourne, Australia, before the introduction of neonatal ventilation. Mortality was 18.3% in the intensive care group compared to 35% in the control group in the last two years of the four-year study ($p < 0.05$). There was no difference in mortality in the first two years of the study, suggesting experience of delivering intensive care is important in reaping benefits[54].

The twelve studies from several different populations and time periods referred to in Table 25.1 also show that perinatal mortality is reduced if babies receive NIC. However, mortality is not a good outcome measure for NIC, and there was concern during the late 1980s that as survival rates were increased, babies which previously would have died survived with severe handicaps. Concern on the outcome of NIC is now focusing on babies born at the extremes of prematurity and/or birthweight. Recent specific studies[55–59] show that the proportion of moderate-to-severe handicap in survivors remains constant. This means that, although the absolute numbers of children with disabilities caused by the complications of low birthweight may have increased slightly, they constitute a small minority of the overall number of children with disabilities requiring special educational and other services.

VOLUME AND OUTCOME

IS BIG BEAUTIFUL?

Field *et al.*[53] examined the short-term outcome (survival to discharge) in a one-year prospective study in Trent. Infants of ≤ 28 weeks' gestation who received all their perinatal care in one of five large centres (each providing more than 600 ventilator-days each year) showed significantly better survival rates than those infants electively treated throughout their entire course at one of the twelve smaller units (34 survivors from 65 infants (52%) compared with 8 survivors from 37 infants (22%)). These differences occurred despite the elective transfer of many of the sickest infants from the smaller units to the larger. Difference in survival between more mature infants were not significant. In her commentary on this paper, Mugford[60] highlights the problems of possible differentials in case mix between the two types of units.

CASE MIX

The problem of case mix is addressed in a paper from the International Neonatal Network[61] which used a neonatal scoring system which allocated scores for birthweight, gestational age, maximum and minimum fraction of inspired oxygen and maximum base excess during the first 12 hours and presence of congenital malformations to adjust mortality for factors other than birthweight. The score is known as the CRIB score – Clinical Risk Index for Babies[62]. All factors were recorded within 12 hours of birth. The study looked at 1300 infants in development and validation cohorts and 248 other infants of birthweight ≤ 1500 g or gestational age < 31 weeks treated at nine level 3 and four non-level 3 units in the UK. Without adjustment for initial risk, there was no clear difference in group mortality between the level 3 and non-level 3 units. Calculation of risk-adjusted mortality by means of the CRIB score showed that babies were twice as likely to die in non-level 3 units than level 3 units (odds ratio (O.R.) 2.12; 95% confidence intervals (C.I.) 1.39–3.24). Adjustment for birthweight alone also showed higher odds of death in non-level 3 units (O.R. 1.45; C.I. 1.01–2.11). No guidance is given in this paper as to the differences between level 3 units and non-level 3 units, other than the former were university teaching hospitals and the latter were district general hospitals.

In general, outcomes seem to be better in level 3 units and those with a workload of over 600 ventilator-days a year. However, it is impossible to define what constitutes a level 3 unit and to extrapolate what a minimum workload to define a level 3 unit might be. The study in Trent is supported by studies in the USA[63] and The Netherlands[64], but again, no definition of a level 3 unit is agreed.

TRANSPORT OF NEONATES

When there was a shortage of NIC cots, it was assumed that transfer between units, preferably antenatally, was important in improving survival through access to NIC. Advantages in transferring babies from level 2 units to level 3 have been shown[65,66]. However, a study in Auckland[67], New Zealand, of 40 infants born in a regional level 3 unit but transported to other level 3 units for NIC and 80 matched controls showed that transport appeared to affect respiratory status adversely but transiently. However, transported infants grew less well (32% were below third centile for weight at 36 weeks vs. 15% of controls), were more likely to suffer periventricular haemorrhage (40% vs. 21% of controls) and had a worse neurodevelopmental outcome (70% normal at follow-up vs. 83% of controls). The paper did not conclude whether the differences were due to the transport itself or the effects of possible differences in clinical practices in the different level 3 centres. All the other NICUs to which babies were transferred were smaller than those in Auckland itself, suggesting that size of unit may have an influence.

Another study in southern California[68] showed an improvement in outcome as a result of transport, but identified several variables which played a role in improving outcome. These included capacity at level 3 units.

COSTS OF NIC

There appear to be both clinical and financial advantages of treating sick babies in specialist units. A study in Trent[9] estimated the cost of providing NIC as £640 per baby per day in units providing 1000 occupied cot days at all levels of care (adjusted to 1991 prices) but £450 per day at units providing 5000 days per year – a difference of 20%. These costs include most of the costs of transporting babies to level 3 units, as staff from these units often collect babies.

CONCLUSIONS ON NEONATAL INTENSIVE CARE

Studies from around the world suggest there have been dramatic falls in mortality for small babies, largely because of the introduction of NIC, with the proportion of moderately to severely handicapped survivors remaining constant. This means that although the absolute numbers of children with disabilities caused by the complications of low birthweight may have increased slightly, they constitute a small minority of the overall number of children with disabilities requiring special educational and other services.

The literature strongly supports the hypothesis that big is beautiful and practice makes perfect, but does not define what is big and how much practice is needed before good outcomes are achieved. There is no evidence, apart from one paper from New Zealand[69], that small non-specialist units achieve comparable results in terms of mortality to larger specialist units and the results from this paper suggest that this may be due to good referral practice of high-risk cases to regional specialist centres. It is highly probable that there are considerable economies of scale in concentrating resources for NIC in a few high-volume centres. This advantage has to be balanced against access to local services and the maintenance of skills in resuscitation and emergency care in units without NICUs.

REFERENCES

1. World Health Organization. Maternal health and safe motherhood programme, Division of Family Health. Mother–baby package: Implementing safe motherhood in countries. Geneva: World Health Organization, 1994.
2. Miller CA. Maternal health and infant survival. Washington DC: National Center for Clinical Infant Programs. 1987.
3. Beard RW & Chapple J. An evaluation of maternity services. In *Reproductive Health Care for Women and Babies* (eds B. Sachs, R. Beard, E. Papiernik, C. Russell). Oxford: Oxford University Press 1995.
4. Chamberlain G. Organisation of antenatal care. *Br. Med. J.* **303**:647–650, 1991.
5. Department of Health *Report on confidential enquiries into maternal deaths in the United Kingdom 1991–1993*. London: HMSO, 1996.
6. Young GL. The place of birth. In *The Future of the Maternity Services* (eds G. Chamberlain & N. Patel). London: RCOG, 1994.
7. St Mary's Maternity Information system *North Thames (West) Region Annual Maternity Figures 1993*. London: North Thames Region, 1994.
8. Calder A. Contributions of the professions. In *The Future of the Maternity Services* (eds G. Chamberlain & N. Patel). London: RCOG, 1994.

9. Fordham R. Cost of neonatal care across a regional health authority. *J Public Health Med.* **14**:127–130, 1992.
10. Hall MH, Chng PK & MacGillivray I. Is routine antenatal care worthwhile? *Lancet* **ii**:78–80, 1980.
11. Kaminiski M, Blondel B & Breart G. Management of pregnancy and childbirth in England Wales and in France. *Paediatr. Perinatal Epidemiol.* **2**:13–24, 1988.
12. Hall M, MacIntyre S & Porter M. *Antenatal Care Assessed.* Aberdeen: Aberdeen University Press, 1985.
13. Sikorski J, Wilson J, Clement S, Das S & Smeeton N. A randomised trial comparing two schedules of antenatal visits: the antenatal care project. *Br. Med. J.* **312**:546–553, 1996.
14. Tucker JS, Hall MH, Howie PW, Reid ME, Barbour RS, du Florey C & McIlwaine G. Should obstetricians see women with normal pregnancies? A multicentre randomised controlled trial of routine antenatal care by general practitioners and midwives compared with shared care led by obstetricians. *Br. Med. J.* **312**:554–559, 1996.
15. Binstock MA & Wolde-Tsadik G. Alternative prenatal care: impact of reduced visit frequency, focused visits and continuity of care. *J. Reprod. Med.* **40**:507–512, 1995.
16. Department of Health. *Changing childbirth: a report of the expert maternity group.* London: HMSO, 1993.
17. Porter M & MacIntyre S. What is, must be best: a research note on conservative or deferential responses to antenatal care provision. *Soc. Sci. Med.* **19**:1197–1200, 1984.
18. Sikorski J, Wilson J & Clement S. Rituals in antenatal care: consider women's psychosocial needs. *Br. Med. J.* **307**:1064, 1993.
19. *Select Committee On Midwives Registration.* Report. Parliamentary papers 1892; IV.
20. Local Government Board. *Maternity and Child Welfare.* Report on the provision made by Local Authorities in England & Wales. London: HMSO, 1917.
21. Campbell R & Macfarlane A. *Where to be Born: The Debate and the Evidence*, 2nd edn. Oxford: National Perinatal Epidemiology Unit, 1994.
22. Macfarlane A & Mugford M. *Birth Counts: Statistics of Pregnancy and Childbirth.* London: HMSO, 1984.
23. Keirse MJNC. Perinatal mortality rates do not contain what they purport to contain. *Lancet* **i**:1164–1168, 1984.
24. Eske M & van Allen D. Review and Assessment of Maternity Services in The Netherlands. In *The Future of the Maternity Services* (eds G. Chamberlain & N. Patel). London: RCOG Press, 1994.
25. Damstra-Wijmenga SMI. Home confinement: the positive results in Holland. *J. Royal Coll. Gen. Practit.* **34**:425–430, 1984.
26. Van Alten D, Eskes M & Treffers P. Midwifery in The Netherlands. The Wormeveer study; selection, mode of delivery, perinatal mortality and infant morbidity. *Br. J. Obstet. Gynaecol.* **96**:656–662, 1989.
27. Bakketeig LS & Hoffman HJ. Perinatal mortality by birth order within cohorts based on sibship size. *Br. Med. J.* **2**:693–696, 1979.
28. Billewicz WZ. Some implications of self selection for pregnancy. *Br. J. Prev. Soc. Med.* **27**:49–52, 1973.
29. Roman E, Doyle P, Beral V *et al.* Fetal loss, gravidity and pregnancy order. *Early Human Develop.* **2**:131–138, 1978.
30. Casson IF, Clarke CA, Howard CV *et al.* Outcomes of pregnancy in insulin dependent diabetic women: results of a five year population cohort study. *Br. Med. J.* **315**:275–278, 1997.
31. Hawthorne G, Robson S, Ryall EA, Sen D, Roberts SH & Ward Platt MP. Prospective population based survey of outcome of pregnancy in diabetic women: results of the Northern Diabetic Pregnancy Audit, 1994. *Br. Med. J.* **315**:279–281, 1997.
32. Thorpe-Beeston JG, Banfield PJ & Saunders N StG. Outcome of breech delivery at term. *Br. Med. J.* **305**:746–747, 1992.
33. Multiple authors. Response to 'Outcome of breech delivery at term'. *Br. Med. J.* **305**:1090–1092, 1992.
34. Consultative Council on Medical and Allied Services. *Interim Report on the Future Provision of Medical and Allied Services.* London: HMSO, 1920.
35. Chalmers I. The implications of the current debate on obstetric practice. In *The Place of Birth* (eds S. Kitzinger & J.N. Davies). Oxford: Oxford University Press, 1978.
36. Shaw B. Preface to *The Doctor's Dilemma.* London: Constable, 1906.
37. NHS Centre for Reviews and Dissemination. *Effective Health Care: Hospital Volumes and Health Care Outcomes, Costs and Patient Access* 2; No. 8. Edinburgh: Churchill Livingstone, 1996.
38. NHS Centre for Reviews and Dissemination *Concentration and choice in the provision of hospital services: The relationship between hospital volume and quality of health outcomes.* CRD Report 8 (Part I). York: University of York, 1996.
39. NHS Centre for Reviews and Dissemination *Concentration and choice in the provision of hospital services: The relationship between volume and the scope of activity and hospital costs.* CRD Report 8 (Part II). York: University of York, 1996.
40. NHS Centre for Reviews and Dissemination *Concentration and choice in the provision of hospital services: The relationship between concentration, patient accessibility and utilisation of services.* CRD Report 8 (Part III). York: University of York, 1996.
41. Paterson CM, Chapple JC, Beard RW, Joffe M, Steer PJ & Wright CSW. Evaluating the quality of maternity services – a discussion paper. *Br. J. Obstet. Gynaecol.* **98**:1073–1078, 1991.
42. Cleary R, Beard RW, Chapple J, Coles J, Griffin M, Joffe M & Welch A. The standard primipara as a basis for inter-unit comparisons of maternity care. *Br. J. Obstet. Gynaecol.* **103**:223–229, 1996.
43. Shwartz M, Iezzoni LI, Moskowitz MA *et al.* The importance of comorbidities in explaining differences in patient costs. *Med. Care* **34**:767–782, 1996.
44. Ryan GM. Regional planning for maternal and perinatal health services. *Sem. Perinatol.* **1**:255–265, 1977.
45. Greenberg ER, Dain B, Freeman D, Yates J & Korson R. Referral of lung cancer patients to university hospital cancer centers. A population based study in two rural states. *Cancer* **62**:1647–1652, 1988.
46. Thomas J, Bowen-Simkins P, Stewart G *et al.* Survey of attitudes to testing for HIV infection in antenatal clinics in West Glamorgan. *Br. J. Obstet. Gynaecol.* **96**:1405–1409, 1989.
47. Ford C, Illiffe S & Franklin O. Outcome of planned home births in an inner city practice. *Br. Med. J.* **303**:1517–1519, 1991.
48. Shann F. A review of the report 'The Care of Critically Ill Children'. In *A Critical Appraisal of the Care of Critically Ill Children.* York: NHS Centre for Reviews and Dissemination, 1994.
49. Clinical Standards Advisory Group *Neonatal intensive care: access to and availability of specialist services.* Second report. London: Royal College of Paediatrics and Child Health, 1995.
50. Clinical Standards Advisory Group *Specialised services (1996).* London: The Stationery Office, 1996.
51. Mugford M. Commentary on paper by Field *et al.* on 'Survival and place of treatment after premature delivery'. *Arch. Dis. Childh.* **66**:410–411, 1991.
52. Rosenblatt RA, Reinken J & Shoemack P. Is obstetrics safe in small hospitals? – evidence from New Zealand's regionalised perinatal system. *Lancet* **ii**:429–432, 1985.
53. Field D, Hodges S, Mason E & Burton P. Survival and place of treatment after premature delivery. *Arch. Dis. Childh.* **66**:408–411, 1991.
54. Victorian Infant Collaborative Study Group. Improvement of outcome for infants of birth weight under 1000 g. *Develop. Med. Child Neurol.* **20**:605–618, 1978.
55. Coccia C, Pezzani M, Moro GE & Minoli I. Management of extremely low birthweight infants. *Acta Paediatr.* (Suppl.) **382**:10–12, 1992.
56. Whyte HE, Fitzhardinge PM, Shennan AT *et al.* Extreme immaturity: outcome of 568 pregnancies of 23–26 weeks gestation. *Obstet. Gynaecol.* **82**:1–7, 1993.
57. Roussounis SH, Hubley PA & Dear PR. Five year follow up of very low birthweight infants: neurological and psychological outcome. *Child: Care, Health Develop.* **19**:45–59, 1993.
58. Nishida H. Outcome of infants born preterm, with special emphasis on extremely low birthweight infants. *Baillière's Clin. Obstet. Gynaecol.* **7**:611–631, 1993.
59. Sutton L, Bajuk B, Duffey B *et al.* Short term outcome of mechanically ventilated infants weighing more than 2499 g at birth: a population based study. *J. Paed. Child Health* **29**:418–423, 1993.
60. Mugford M. Commentary on paper by Field *et al.* on 'Survival and place of treatment after premature delivery'. *Arch. Dis. Childh.* **66**:410–411, 1991.
61. International Neonatal Network. The CRIB (Clinical Risk Index for Babies) score: a tool for assessing initial neonatal risk and comparing performances of neonatal intensive care units. *Lancet* **342**:193–198, 1993.

62. Tarnow-Mordi W, Ogston S, Wilkinson AR, Reid E, Gregory J, Saeed M & Wilkie R. Predicting death from initial disease severity in very low birthweight infants: a method for comparing performance of neonatal units. *Br. Med. J.* **300**:1611–1614, 1990.
63. Paneth N, Kiely JL, Wallenstein S, Marcus M, Paktar J & Susser M. Newborn intensive care and neonatal mortality in low birthweight infants. *N. Engl. J. Med.* **307**:149–155, 1982.
64. Verloove-Vanhorick SP, Verwey RA *et al.* Mortality in very preterm and low birth weight infants according to place of delivery and level of care. *Pediatrics* **81**:404–411, 1988.
65. Delaney-Black V, Lubchenco I, Butterfield J, Goldson E, Koops BL & Lazotte DC. Outcome of very low birthweight infants: are populations of neonates inherently different after antenatal versus neonatal referral? *Am. J. Obstet. Gynaecol.* **160**:545–552, 1989.
66. Paneth N, Kiely JL & Susser M. Age at death used to assess the effect of interhospital transfer of newborns. *Pediatrics* **71**:854–861, 1984.
67. Harding JE & Morton SM. Adverse effects of neonatal transport between level III centres. *J. Paediatr. Child Health* **29**:146–149, 1993.
68. Chiu HSH, Vogt JF, Chan LS & Rother CE. Regionalization of infant transports: the southern California experience and its implications. I: Referral pattern. *J. Perinatol.* **8**:188–296, 1993.
69. Rosenblatt RA, Reinken J & Shoemack P. Is obstetrics safe in small hospitals? – evidence from New Zealand's regionalised perinatal system. *Lancet* **ii**:429–432, 1985.

The adult consequences of fetal disease

26

P.M. Clark, S.M.B. Morton and J.E. Harding

Introduction

'The child is father of the man.'
(William Wordsworth, 1770–1850)

The more we know, the clearer it becomes that the key to health and growth in childhood, and to adult health and disease, is to be found (at least in part) in fetal life. Outcomes examined in this chapter will include cerebral palsy, special senses and postnatal patterns of growth. These have long been recognised as possible outcomes of adverse events in the perinatal period. We will review the evidence that a number of adult diseases, including high blood pressure and non-insulin-dependent diabetes mellitus, are a product of a less than optimal fetal environment. We will examine some of the mechanisms that might link fetal experience with adult disease and, finally, we will look at the intergenerational effects of a woman's fetal experience on later reproduction.

Cerebral palsy

Cerebral palsy can be defined as a group of disorders of movements and posture owing to a defect or lesion of the brain. The lesion is by definition static, although the clinical picture evolves over time. The initial case histories of what we would now call cerebral palsy were published by Little in 1862[1]: 'On the influence of abnormal parturition, difficult labor, premature birth, and asphyxia neonatorum, on mental and physical conditions of the child, especially in relation to deformities.' Since then it has become increasingly clear that, where it is possible to diagnose the underlying cause of cerebral palsy, most cases are owing to pre- rather than perinatal causes.

PERINATAL ASPHYXIA

It appears that perinatal events are rarely the cause of cerebral palsy. Stanley and Watson analysed all cases of cerebral palsy in Western Australia born between 1968 and 1981[2]. Over this period, obstetric practice changed, with a greater use of fetal monitoring and of caesarean section. Perinatal mortality declined, but the number of cases of cerebral palsy changed little. This suggests that cerebral palsy is rarely due to perinatal factors, and further, that the route to prevention of cerebral palsy is unlikely to lie in increasingly invasive obstetric practice.

In a case–control study comparing children with cerebral palsy and a matched control group in Western Australia, clinical signs of birth asphyxia had been noted in 33.5% of children with cerebral palsy, and in 18% of neurologically normal children. The authors estimated that birth asphyxia was the cause of the cerebral palsy in ≤ 8% of the population[3]. Similarly, Nelson and Ellenberg studied some 54 000 deliveries, from which 189 children went on to develop cerebral palsy[4]. 'Birth asphyxia' had been described in some of the affected children, but the presence of a far higher incidence of major malformations in the children with cerebral palsy than in those without suggested a prenatal rather than perinatal cause in most cases.

PREMATURITY

There are several other recognised risk factors for cerebral palsy, including recurrent bleeding in pregnancy, having more than one fetus *in utero*, congenital infection, maternal pyrexia in labour and premature birth[5]. The risk of cerebral palsy increases as birthweight decreases, and within any birthweight category the risk of cerebral palsy increases as gestational age at birth decreases. As survival of very small babies increases, they may account for an increasing number of cases of cerebral palsy in the community. However, although the risk of a number of adverse outcomes is high in low-birthweight survivors, these children form only a small proportion of all children with these diagnoses[6,7] (Table 26.1).

TABLE 26.1
Estimated contribution of extremely low birthweight (ELBW) to childhood disability in England & Wales

	Survivors of:	
Disability	Normal birthweight *n* = 600 000	ELBW *n* = 1500
Cerebral palsy	1200 (0.2%)	150 (10%)
Blind	120 (0.02%)	30 (2%)
Deaf	1200 (0.2%)	15 (1%)
Low IQ	13800 (2.3%)	150 (10%)
Severe disability	10200 (1.7%)	105 (7%)

Extremely low birthweight babies (birthweight <1000 g) have a higher incidence of disability than do those of normal birthweight (>2500 g), but because of their low numbers, they contribute only a very small proportion of the total burden of disability in the country.

Figures are approximated from mortality statistics for England & Wales in 1995[6] and morbidity data from 1991–2, Victoria, Australia[7].

CONGENITAL INFECTION

The current contribution of congenital infection to cerebral palsy is hard to quantify. The most important infections are rubella and cytomegalovirus (CMV). Congenital rubella is a rare cause of cerebral palsy or other neurological problems in developed countries following the introduction of vaccination. However, up to half of pregnant women in developed countries are not immune to CMV, and congenital infection can also occur in women who are already antibody-positive. Thus the number of fetuses at risk and infected is large. Up to 5% of cerebral palsy in the UK could be due to congenital CMV infection[8].

Sensorineural hearing loss

Sensorineural hearing loss can develop years after congenital infection, and delayed sensorineural hearing loss is the main manifestation of congenital rubella infection in late gestation. Before the introduction of vaccination, some 16% of cases of moderate to severe deafness in England & Wales were due to congenital rubella[9]. As congenital rubella becomes less common, other causes, such as genetic disease, gain in relative importance. Congenital CMV now causes about 12% of congenital hearing loss in the UK[8], and sensorineural hearing loss is the most common manifestation of congenital CMV infection in people who are asymptomatic at birth[10]. Prematurity is also associated with deafness (Table 26.1). The proportion of sensorineural deafness due to infection, genetic causes and prematurity varies between countries, depending in part on immunisation strategies and levels of healthcare.

Visual impairment

Visual impairment of prenatal cause is often associated with other neurological problems. Prematurity accounts for a large proportion of childhood visual impairment and blindness in developed countries, and many of these children also have cerebral palsy (Table 26.1). Retinopathy of prematurity (ROP) was the single most common cause of childhood blindness in developed countries in the 1950s, but is now less common[11], although both retinopathy of prematurity and higher visual pathway damage continue to contribute to visual impairment in preterm survivors.

The contribution of infective and genetic causes of blindness varies between countries. For example, congenital rubella accounted for 22% of blindness in one school survey in Jamaica[12]. In contrast, in countries where consanguineous marriages are common and medical services good, up to 80% of cases of visual impairment may be genetic in origin[13]. Visual impairment following congenital toxoplasmosis has a low prevalence in most countries, but is a clear example of delayed effects of fetal disease.

Postnatal growth in small babies

Infants born small-for-gestation age (SGA) comprise a very heterogeneous group. They may be full term or premature, and their growth failure may be secondary to chromosomal disorder, intrauterine infection, maternal disease, placental dysfunction or multiple pregnancy. In most cases, however, the aetiology is not apparent. In spite of this heterogeneity, most children show a degree of catch-up growth in the first six months after birth. However, many still fail to reach the final adult height of their appropriate-for-dates peers. Catch-up growth is less likely in symmetrically small babies[14], in those born preterm, and in those with an earlier onset of fetal growth restriction[15]. An understanding of the determinants of adult height in these small babies is very relevant, as adult height has important social implications. Current studies suggest that it is possible to identify a subgroup of small babies as early as three months of age who will fail to exhibit catch-up growth and thus might benefit from interventions such as growth hormone therapy[16].

Breastfeeding has been shown to have beneficial effects on catch-up growth in SGA term babies. In particular, it has been associated with faster increases in weight, length and head circumference in the first 12 weeks of life, with the most pronounced effects being on head growth. These increases persist beyond the breastfeeding period and suggest that the first three months of postnatal life may be a critical period for catch up of body weight and brain growth in SGA babies[17].

Cardiovascular disease

Coronary heart disease and stroke may not be the most obvious consequences of adverse events in fetal life, but epidemiological studies and supporting animal work provide ever increasing evidence for such an association. The relationship was first examined in ecological studies. Barker and colleagues found a strong relationship between the standardised mortality ratios (SMR) for cardiovascular disease in men in local authority areas in England & Wales, and infant mortality in the years during which the men dying of heart disease would have been born[18]. Men born in areas with high infant[18] or neonatal[19] mortality rates were at increased risk of dying of ischaemic heart disease in adult life. As neonatal mortality increases with decreasing birthweight, it was postulated that reduced birthweight might be an indicator of factors important in determining adult susceptibility to cardiovascular disease.

Ledgers detailing the size at birth for men and women born in Hertfordshire from 1911 onwards allowed people to be traced and death certificates obtained. There was a strong inverse relationship between birthweight and the SMR for death from coronary heart disease and all cardiovascular disease[20]. Size at birth was not related to social class at the time of birth or death in this cohort. Thus it did not appear that size at birth was merely acting as a proxy for socio-economic conditions in childhood or adult life. The observation that reduced birthweight is associated with an increased rate of death from coronary heart disease has since been replicated in studies from a number of countries including the USA[21] and India[22].

SIZE AT BIRTH AND BLOOD PRESSURE

As hypertension is a recognised risk factor for coronary heart disease, it was proposed that hypertension might be a link between reduced size at birth and adult coronary heart disease. Reduced birthweight was indeed associated with raised blood pressure in the Hertfordshire cohort: systolic blood pressure decreased from a mean of 173 mmHg in those who weighed $\leq$ 5.5 lb at birth to 161 mmHg in those who weighed > 9.5 lb[23]. Rose has suggested that, if the population distribution of blood pressure were to be moved 2 mmHg to the left (i.e. if everyone's blood pressure were 2 mmHg lower), this would save as many lives as all the antihypertensive medication currently in use[24].

Birthweight is a relatively crude summary measure of growth *in utero*, while body proportions at birth reflect the *in utero* environment, and the timing of any adverse events[25]. Thin babies, as measured by low ponderal index at birth, were at increased risk of raised blood pressure in adult life[26]. In a Sheffield cohort, both systolic and diastolic blood pressures were higher in people of low birthweight, in those who had been short at birth, and in those who had had a small abdominal or head circumference at birth[27]. The relationships were independent of variables associated with adult lifestyle, including smoking, alcohol intake and obesity.

Placental weight is also important[26]. Adults who had a large placenta had raised systolic blood pressure. Adults who had been small at birth in relation to the size of the placenta tended to have the highest blood pressure[28]. Similar results have been reported for some[29,30], but not all[27,31] subsequent studies. This may reflect the complex relationships of maternal and fetal variables with placental growth.

STUDIES IN CHILDREN

The hypothesis that poor fetal growth can lead to hypertension in later life is strengthened by the demonstration of similar relationships between size at birth and current blood pressure in children. Allowing for current size, systolic blood pressure is inversely related to birthweight from about a year of age onwards, though the relationship is not found consistently in children studied between the ages of about 10 to 17 years, nor in all follow-up studies of children who were born prematurely (see Law and Sheil[32] for a review).

The relationship between size at birth and blood pressure occurs across the whole of the birthweight range, including weights usually considered to be normal or optimal. It is important to emphasise that later adult hypertension is not confined to SGA babies. This suggests that even babies of average or above average size may have suffered from adverse conditions *in utero*, and that they could have been larger if given an ideal fetal environment. It has also been possible to show that, in children as in adults, relatively raised blood pressure is associated with reduced size at birth independently of gestational age[29]. This suggests that it is not mild degrees of prematurity that predispose to higher blood pressure, but rather reduced fetal growth.

PROGRAMMING

The association of size at birth and later disease may be interpreted as evidence of programming. Programming is said to occur when an insult or stimulus, applied at a critical or sensitive period, causes long-lasting effects on the structure or function of an organism[33]. The timing of this sensitive period tends to be when the cells of the organ in question are dividing most rapidly.

Animal work has shown that maternal nutrition may be important in programming. Maternal undernutrition before and during pregnancy is associated with later hypertension in the offspring in rats[34]. An inverse, graded relationship between maternal protein intake in pregnancy and blood pressure of the offspring was evident. The effect was not mediated via changes in maternal blood pressure, and the association persisted throughout life[35].

Non-insulin-dependent diabetes mellitus

Epidemiological studies have linked size at birth with alterations in glucose and insulin metabolism. The proportion of Hertfordshire men with glucose intolerance or frank diabetes fell from 40% in those with birthweights of ≤ 5.5 lb (≤ 2.5 kg) to 14% in those with birthweights of ≥ 9.5 lb (≥ 4.3 kg)[23]. Reduced fetal growth was also associated with syndrome X, the combination of non-insulin-dependent diabetes mellitus, hypertension and hyperlipidaemia[36]. Syndrome X was associated with reduced birthweight in men from Hertfordshire and with both lightness and thinness at birth in men and women from Preston. These findings have now been replicated in Sweden[37]. The worst affected adults were those who were small at birth and currently most obese. Thus, fetal adaptations that may be beneficial *in utero* led to decompensation in the face of obesity, itself a recognised contributor to glucose intolerance.

Skeletal muscle is an important site of insulin action, and thin babies are born with decreased muscle mass. It follows that one mechanism linking thinness at birth and glucose intolerance could be insulin resistance at the level of skeletal muscle. Thinness at birth was associated with increased insulin resistance[38] and muscle metabolism was altered in subjects who were thin at birth[39].

Hypothalamo-pituitary–adrenal (HPA) axis

FETAL, PLACENTAL AND MATERNAL HPA AXIS

Programming of the HPA axis is an attractive hypothesis linking experiences in fetal life and later disease, as excess glucocorticoids can result in raised blood pressure, glucose intolerance, and central obesity; outcomes that are also related to reduced fetal growth. The fetus has low circulating levels of cortisol, and is protected from the far higher concentrations of maternal glucocorticoids by the placental enzyme 11β-hydroxysteroid dehydrogenase type 2 (11β-HSD2)[40]. This converts active cortisol to inactive cortisone. By protecting the fetus from maternal glucocorticoids, 11β-HSD2 could play an important role in maintaining the autonomy and perhaps even affecting the ontogeny of the developing fetal HPA axis.

ANIMAL MODELS

Exposure to maternal glucocorticoid could link reduced size at birth and later raised blood pressure. Placental 11β-HSD activity in rat placentas is inversely related to the birthweight of the offspring[41]. This suggests that more glucocorticoid could reach the developing fetus in rats with lower placental enzyme activity, resulting in the observed decrease in birthweight. Administration of dexamethasone to pregnant rats also resulted in moderately reduced birthweight and raised blood pressure in the offspring in later life[42]. Dexamethasone is not a substrate for 11β-HSD and thus crosses the placenta to reach the fetus. Pregnant rats treated with the 11β-HSD inhibitor carbenoxolone also gave birth to offspring with reduced birthweight. Moreover, such offspring grew up to have raised blood pressure[40].

EVIDENCE FROM HUMANS

Interpretable data on women given glucocorticoids during pregnancy are sparse. However, there is little evidence that exposure to exogenous glucocorticoids leads to reduced birthweight in humans[43] and the relationship of such exposure to later blood pressure has yet to be examined.

Limited human data link reduced fetal and infant size with evidence of altered activity of the HPA axis. Fetuses with estimated weights below the 10th centile for gestational age had raised cord venous cortisol and adrenocorticotrophic hormone (ACTH) concentrations when compared with heavier fetuses matched for gestational age[44]. At birth, cord venous and arterial corticotrophin-releasing hormone (CRH) levels were raised in babies with weights below the 10th centile for gestational age. Mean cortisol concentrations were also higher[45].

To date, the only study to examine the HPA axis in relation to size at birth in children found that reduced size at birth was associated with an increase in urinary glucocorticoid and adrenal androgen metabolite excretion[46]. Phillips and colleagues have recently reported that, in 370 men from Hertfordshire, fasting 9 a.m. cortisol was highest in those who had been lightest at birth[47]. Furthermore, fasting plasma cortisol concentrations were positively related to systolic blood pressure, and inversely related to measures of glucose tolerance, independent of body size.

Respiratory disease

Both prematurity and being small for gestational age are associated with chronic lung disease (CLD) and measurable differences in lung function in childhood[48]. CLD is more likely to occur in babies who are born small for gestational age[49] and those of extremely low birthweight[50]. The mechanisms underlying the association are likely to be complex, involving both prenatal and postnatal factors, as even low-birthweight babies without a history of ventilation had abnormal lung function tests in late childhood[48]. However, interruption of lung growth may be an important contributor, as even brief periods of undernutrition during the phase of rapid lung growth in animals results in markedly reduced lung size[51,52].

In adult men from the Hertfordshire cohort, low birthweight was associated with reduced forced expiratory volume in one second (FEV_1) but not with a reduction in forced vital capacity (FVC), findings similar to those in follow-up studies of small babies. The fall in FEV_1 with falling birthweight was marked, and was independent of adult height, age and smoking habits. It was found across the whole of the birthweight range. The relationship was also found within each social class[53]. In contrast, both FVC and FEV_1 were lower in Indian men and women who had been light at birth[54]. Both were reduced in Hertfordshire men who had been recorded by health visitors as having had whooping cough, bronchitis or pneumonia in infancy[53]. However, respiratory infection between the ages of one and four years was not associated with significant differences in these lung-function parameters.

Maternal smoking causes both a reduction in fetal growth and alterations in lung-function tests in infancy[48,50]. The significance of these early changes for later lung function and respiratory disease is still under investigation. A reduced FEV_1 in childhood or adult life may reflect adverse effects on airway growth *in utero*, while the association between respiratory infection in infancy and later reduction in both FEV_1 and FVC could indicate a sensitive period of lung and alveolar growth in infancy.

Effects on reproductive health

Size at birth and growth in infancy also affect the later reproductive health of women. Adrenarche[46,55] and menarche[56] may occur earlier in children who were light at birth. Menarche was also positively related to weight at seven years of age, the earliest menarche occurring in girls who were small at birth but had grown the most in childhood. In adult females, ovarian function was also related to neonatal events. Thin women with polycystic ovaries tended to have been born after 42 weeks of gestation. Obese hirsute women with this condition were more likely to have been heavy at birth and born to overweight women[57].

Age at menopause[58] and death from cancer of the ovary[59] are related to size in infancy, but not to size at birth. Women who were lighter at the age of one year had an earlier menopause and were more likely to have died of cancer of the ovary. These observations are compatible with a hypothesis that the hypothalamus is programmed *in utero*, with resulting effects on growth and reproductive hormones. Programming of the hypothalamus as a result of prolonged gestation could also explain the association between post-term births and later polycystic ovary disease.

INTERGENERATIONAL EFFECTS

Intergenerational effects are seen in the close correlation of mother and infant birthweight. Low-birthweight mothers (<2500 g) had a threefold increased risk of having a low-birthweight baby when compared with mothers who had weighed over 4 kg at birth[60]. In contrast, the risk of premature birth in mothers who were themselves born early appears very low[60,61].

The close relation between a mother's birthweight and that of her offspring has been interpreted by some[60,62] as an example of genetic inheritance. Observations of women conceived during the famine of the Dutch Hunger Winter of 1945 suggest otherwise. They show that fetal experiences that were not manifest in reduced size at birth can nevertheless affect the fetal growth of a woman's offspring. Women who were exposed to famine early in gestation were born with normal birthweights, but they tended to go on to have small babies[63,64]. The mechanisms underlying this intergenerational effect of famine *in utero* are not known. The development of the fetal uterus could be affected by maternal influences such as nutrition, and this in turn could perhaps affect placentation and placental function in later pregnancy. However, these, and other mechanisms such as programming of the hypothalamus, remain speculative. What is known, however, is that after 12 generations of malnutrition in rats, it takes several generations before birthweight returns to normal[65].

Summary

We have described a number of adult diseases that have fetal origins. Cerebral palsy, visual impairment and blindness, and hearing impairment have a number of prenatal causes, while intrauterine growth retardation can lead to shortness in later life and persisting abnormalities in lung function tests. There is also an expanding body of evidence linking fetal growth with a number of adult diseases. These associations span the whole of the birthweight range. The paradigm that coronary heart disease, and its risk factors of high blood pressure, obesity, and altered blood lipids, are programmed *in utero* suggests future avenues for prevention. Until then, the view of one newspaper may be right:

'Life in the womb will be written on your tomb.'
Sydney Morning Herald (October 1994)

REFERENCES

1. Little WJ. On the influence of abnormal parturition, difficult labor, premature birth, and asphyxia neonatorum, on mental and physical conditions of the child, especially in relation to deformities. *Trans. Obstet. Soc.* **3**:293–344, 1862.
2. Stanley FJ & Watson L. The cerebral palsies in Western Australia: trends, 1968 to 1981. *Am. J. Obstet. Gynecol.* **158**:89–93, 1988.
3. Blair E & Stanley FJ. Intrapartum asphyxia: a rare cause of cerebral palsy. *J. Pediatr.* **112**:515–519, 1988.
4. Nelson KB & Ellenberg JH. Antecedents of cerebral palsy. *N. Engl. J. Med.* **315**:81–86, 1986.
5. The Victorian Infant Collaborative Study Group. Improved outcome into the 1990s for infants weighing 500–999 g at birth. *Arch. Dis. Child.* **77**:F91–F94, 1997.
6. Office of National Statistics *Mortality Statistics 1995, Childhood, Infant and Perinatal, England and Wales* Series DH3, no.28. London: HMSO. 1998

7. Doyle LW. Outcome to five years of age of children born at 24–26 weeks' gestational age in Victoria. *Med. J. Aust.* **163**:11–14, 1995.
8. Peckham CS & Logan S. Congenital Infections. In *The Epidemiology of Childhood Disorders* (ed. I.B. Pless), pp. 153–172. Oxford: Oxford University Press. 1994.
9. Peckham CS. Congenital rubella in the United Kingdom before 1970: the prevaccine era. *Rev. Inf. Dis.* **7**:S11–S16, 1985.
10. Conboy TJ, Pass RF, Stagno, S *et al.* Intellectual development in school-aged children with asymptomatic congenital cytomegalovirus infection. *Pediatrics* **77**:801–806, 1986.
11. Ng YK, Fielder AR, Shaw DE & Levene MI. Epidemiology of retinopathy of prematurity. *Lancet* **ii**:1235–1238, 1988.
12. Moriarty BJ. Childhood blindness in Jamaica. *Br. J. Ophthalmol.* **72**:65–67, 1988.
13. Tabbara KF & Badr IA. Changing pattern of childhood blindness in Saudi Arabia. *Br. J. Ophthalmol.* **69**:312–315, 1985.
14. Fitzhardinge PM & Inwood S. Long-term growth in small-for-date children. *Acta. Paediatr. Scand.* (Suppl.) **349**:27–33, 1989.
15. Greisen G & Bloch Petersen M. Perinatal growth retardation in preterm infants. *Acta Paediatr. Scand.* (Suppl.) **360**:43–47, 1989.
16. Karlberg JPE, Albertsson-Wikland K, Kwan EYW, Lam BCC & Low LCK. The timing of early postnatal catch-up growth in normal, full-term infants born short for gestational age. *Horm. Res.* **48**:17–24, 1997.
17. Lucas A, Fewtrell MS, Davies PSW, Bishop NJ, Clough H & Cole TJ. Breastfeeding and catch-up growth in infants born small for gestational age. *Acta Paediatr.* **86**:564–569, 1997.
18. Barker DJP & Osmond C. Infant mortality, childhood nutrition, and ischaemic heart disease in England and Wales. *Lancet* **i**:1077–1081, 1986.
19. Barker DJP, Osmond C & Law CM. The intrauterine and early postnatal origins of cardiovascular disease and chronic bronchitis. *J. Epidemiol. Community Health* **43**:237–240, 1989.
20. Osmond C, Barker DJP, Winter PD, Fall CHD & Simmonds SJ. Early growth and death from cardiovascular disease in women. *BMJ* **307**:1519–1524, 1993.
21. Rich-Edwards J, Stampfer M, Manson J *et al.* Birthweight, breastfeeding, and the risk of coronary heart disease in the Nurses' Health Study. *Am. J. Epidemiol.* **141**:S78(Abstract), 1995.
22. Stein CE, Fall CHD, Kumaran K, Osmond C, Cox V & Barker DJP. Fetal growth and coronary heart disease in south India. *Lancet* **348**:1269–1273, 1996.
23. Hales CN, Barker DJP, Clark PMS *et al.* Fetal and infant growth and impaired glucose tolerance at age 64. *BMJ* **303**:1019–1022, 1991.
24. Rose G. Strategy of prevention: lessons from cardiovascular disease. *BMJ* **282**:1847–1851, 1981.
25. Barker DJP, Gluckman PD, Godfrey KM, Harding JE, Owens JA & Robinson JS. Fetal nutrition and cardiovascular disease in adult life. *Lancet* **341**:938–941, 1993.
26. Barker DJP, Godfrey KM, Osmond C & Bull A. The relation of fetal length, ponderal index and head circumference to blood pressure and risk of hypertension in adult life. *Paediatr. Perinat. Epidemiol.* **6**:35–44, 1992.
27. Martyn CN, Barker DJP, Jespersen S, Greenwald S, Osmond C & Berry C. Growth *in utero*, adult blood pressure, and arterial compliance. *Br. Heart J.* **73**:116–121, 1995.
28. Barker DJP, Bull AR, Osmond C & Simmonds SJ. Fetal and placental size and risk of hypertension in adult life. *BMJ* **301**:259–262, 1990.
29. Law CM, Barker DJP, Bull AR & Osmond C. Maternal and fetal influences on blood pressure. *Arch. Dis. Child.* **66**:1291–1295, 1991.
30. Moore VM, Miller AG, Boulton TJC *et al.* Placental weight, birth measurements, and blood pressure at age 8 years. *Arch. Dis. Child.* **74**:538–541, 1996.
31. Whincup P, Cook D, Papacosta O & Walker M. Birth weight and blood pressure: cross sectional and longitudinal relations in childhood. *BMJ* **311**:773–776, 1995.
32. Law CM & Sheill AW. Is blood pressure inversely related to birth weight? The strength of evidence from a systematic review of the literature. *J. Hypertension* **14**:935–941, 1996.
33. Lucas A. Role of nutritional programming in determining adult morbidity. *Arch. Dis. Child.* **71**:288–290, 1994.
34. Langley SC & Jackson AA. Increased systolic blood pressure in adult rats induced by fetal exposure to maternal low protein diets. *Clin. Sci.* **86**:217–222, 1994.
35. Langley-Evans SC, Phillips GJ & Jackson AA. *In utero* exposure to maternal low protein diets induces hypertension in weanling rats, independently of maternal blood pressure changes. *Clin. Nutrit.* **13**:319–324, 1994.
36. Barker DJP, Hales CN, Fall CHD, Osmond C, Phipps K & Clark PMS. Type 2 (non-insulin-dependent) diabetes mellitus, hypertension and hyperlipidaemia (syndrome X): relation to reduced fetal growth. *Diabetologia* **36**:62–67, 1993.
37. Lithell HO, McKeigue PM, Berglund L, Mohsen R, Lithell UB & Leon DA. Relation of size at birth to non-insulin dependent diabetes and insulin concentrations in men aged 50–60 years. *BMJ* **312**:406–410, 1996.
38. Phillips DIW, Barker DJP, Hales CN, Hirst S & Osmond C. Thinness at birth and insulin resistance in adult life. *Diabetologia* **37**:150–154, 1994.
39. Taylor DJ, Thompson CH, Kemp GJ *et al.* A relationship between impaired fetal growth and reduced muscle glycolysis revealed by ^{31}P magnetic resonance spectroscopy. *Diabetologia* **38**:1205–1212, 1995.
40. Lindsay RS, Lindsay RM, Edwards CRW & Seckl JR. Inhibition of 11-beta-hydroxysteroid dehydrogenase in pregnant rats and the programming of blood pressure in the offspring. *Hypertension* **27**:1200–1204, 1996.
41. Benediktsson R, Lindsay RS, Noble J, Seckl JR & Edwards CRW. Glucocorticoid exposure *in utero*: new model for adult hypertension. *Lancet* **341**:339–341, 1993.
42. Edwards CRW, Benediktsson R, Lindsay RS & Seckl JR. Dysfunction of placental glucocorticoid barrier: link between fetal environment and adult hypertension? *Lancet* **341**:355–357, 1993.
43. Crowley PA. Antenatal corticosteroid therapy: a meta-analysis of the randomized trials, 1972 to 1994. *Am. J. Obstet. Gynecol.* **173**:322–335, 1995.
44. Economides DL, Nicolaides KH, Linton EA, Perry LA & Chard T. Plasma cortisol and adrenocorticotropin in appropriate and small for gestational age fetuses. *Fetal Ther.* **3**:158–164, 1988.
45. Goland RS, Jozak S, Warren WB, Conwell IM, Stark RI & Tropper PJ. Elevated levels of umbilical cord plasma corticotropin-releasing hormone in growth-retarded fetuses. *J. Clin. Endocrinol. Metab.* **77**:1174–1179, 1993.
46. Clark PM, Hindmarsh PC, Shiell A, Law CM, Honour J & Barker DJP. Size at birth and adrenocortical function in childhood. *Clin. Endocrinol.* **45**:721–726, 1996.
47. Phillips DIW, Barker DJP, Fall CHD, Whorwood CB, Walker BR & Wood PJ. Low birthweight and raised plasma cortisol concentrations in adult life. *J. Endocrinol.* **152**:P2(Abstract), 1997.
48. Chan KN, Noble-Jamieson CM, Elliman A, Bryan EM & Silverman M. Lung function in children of low birth weight. *Arch. Dis. Child.* **64**:1284–1293, 1989.
49. Tyson JE, Kennedy K, Broyles S & Rosenfeld CR. The small for gestational age infant: accelerated or delayed pulmonary maturation? Increased or decreased survival? *Pediatrics* **95**:534–538, 1995.
50. Doyle LW, Ford GW, Olinsky A, Knoches AML & Callanan C. Bronchopulmonary dysplasia and very low birthweight: lung function at 11 years of age. *J. Paediatr. Child Health* **32**:339–343, 1996.
51. Harding JE. Periconceptual nutrition determines the fetal growth response to acute maternal undernutrition in fetal sheep of late gestation. *Prenat. Neonat. Med.* **2**:310–319, 1997.
52. Gaultier C. Malnutrition and lung growth. *Pediatr Pulmonol* **10**:278–286, 1991.
53. Barker DJP, Godfrey KM, Fall C, Osmond C, Winter PD & Shaheen SO. Relation of birth weight and childhood respiratory infection to adult lung function and death from chronic obstructive airways disease. *BMJ* **303**:671–675, 1991.
54. Stein CE, Kumaran K, Fall CHD, Shaheen SO, Osmond C & Barker DJP. Relation of fetal growth to adult lung function in south India. *Thorax* **52**:895–899, 1997.
55. Francois I & De Zegher F. Adrenarche and fetal growth. *Pediatr. Res.* **41**:440–442, 1997.
56. Cooper C, Kuh D, Egger P, Wadsworth M & Barker D. Childhood growth and age at menarche. *Br. J. Obstet. Gynaecol.* **103**:814–817, 1996.
57. Cresswell JL, Barker DJP, Osmond C, Egger P, Phillips DIW & Fraser RB. Fetal growth, length of gestation, and polycystic ovaries in adult life. *Lancet* **350**:1131–1135, 1997.
58. Cresswell JL, Egger P, Fall CHD, Osmond C, Fraser RB & Barker DJP. Is the age of menopause determined *in-utero*? *Early Hum. Dev.* **49**:143–148, 1997.

59. Barker DJP, Winter PD, Osmond C, Phillips DIW & Sultan HY. Weight gain in infancy and cancer of the ovary. *Lancet* **345**:1087–1088, 1995.
60. Magnus P, Bakketeig LS & Skjaerven R. Correlations of birth weight and gestational age across generations. *Ann. Hum. Biol.* **20**:231–238, 1993.
61. Tavares M, Rodrigues T, Cardoso F, Barros H & Leite LP. Independent effect of maternal birth weight on infant birth weight. *J. Perinat. Med.* **24**:391–396, 1996.
62. Magnus P, Bakketeig LS & Hoffman H. Birth weight of relatives by maternal tendency to repeat small-for-gestational-age (SGA) births in successive pregnancies. *Acta Obstet. Gynecol. Scand.* (Suppl.) **165**:35–38, 1997.
63. Lumey LH. Decreased birthweights in infants after maternal *in utero* exposure to the Dutch famine of 1944–1945. *Paediatr. Perinat. Epidemiol.* **6**:240–253, 1992.
64. Lumey LH, Stein AD, Ravelli ACJ. Timing of prenatal starvation in women and birth weight in their first and second born offspring: The Dutch Famine Birth Cohort Study. *Eur. J. Gynecol. Reprod. Biol.* **61**:23–30, 1995.
65. Stewart RJC, Sheppard H, Preece R & Waterlow JC. The effect of rehabilitation at different stages of development of rats marginally malnourished for ten to twelve generations. *Br. J. Nutr.* **43**:403–412, 1980.

Fetal malformation registers

27

M. Wyldes

Definition

A fetal malformation register is a systematic mechanism for the collection, storage and reporting of congenital malformations.

Introduction

Interest in fetal malformations is not new, the identification of 'monsters' antenatally being one of the stated aims of the organised programmes of antenatal care devised in the 1920s[1]. The structured collection of data and monitoring of congenital malformations in Birmingham England began during 1958[2]. A national surveillance system started in Hungary in 1962[3], and in Norway in 1967[4], with collaboration between the five Nordic countries from 1970 onwards[5]. A major early impetus for monitoring systems came from the thalidomide episode in the early 1960s, and prompted a national congenital monitoring system for England & Wales which continues to collect data and report suspected changes on a monthly basis to directors of public health[6].

The complexity of this task has, however, changed beyond all recognition since the widespread introduction and continued improvements of ultrasound imaging during pregnancy making precise prenatal diagnosis possible. Other chapters have detailed the timing and possible reasons for various fetal malformations occurring, usually during the period of embryogenesis, but the ability of healthcare services to modify the outcome of these pregnancies continues to change at a rapid rate. Certain types of malformation, such as neural tube defects, appear to have changed in incidence very markedly over relatively short periods of time, while others, such as congenital heart disease, remain relatively constant in different populations and time periods, and identifying the reasons for these changes is a challenge which requires accurate and complete data.

PHILOSOPHY

A fetal malformation registry is a mechanism which places itself at the heart of information relating to congenital anomalies. The precise focus will depend upon the individual circumstances of the register; there will be a substantial interest from specialists in public health, who will use the registry for broad questions of public health policy, and specific questions of cluster analysis or further investigation of specific incidents; obstetricians, sonographers and midwives who require information relating to prenatal diagnosis and follow-up of malformations; paediatric specialists requiring information relating to pregnancy and delivery as well as structured follow-up; clinical geneticists who span the spectrum of pre-pregnancy counselling through to diagnosis of difficult paediatric cases and sophisticated laboratory mechanisms for the screening and diagnosis of specific congenital malformations.

The task of bringing these groups together to collaborate effectively is difficult. Those not involved right at the beginning of the process may never feel a part of the structure, and the requirements of the different groups may at times be directly opposing. Links between these groups need to be encouraged, and the feedback of data is often the best way of achieving this.

A spirit of openness and easy access is important, with data being made available to those who request it. This needs to be balanced against the need to respect individual confidentiality, and although personal identifiers are important in validating and following up cases, these personal details should always be removed when any information is being released or reported.

AIMS

A fetal malformation register aims to provide basic data, with high levels of ascertainment for a particular population, and although there are widely different methods used throughout the world, the number of congenital anomaly registers in existence suggests that this is an area of work which has been seen as important in many different healthcare settings[7].

LINKS WITH FETAL MEDICINE

The purpose of a fetal malformation register is to allow accurate surveillance of birth defects, and linkage to possible causes of change, such as the possible adverse effects of environmental agents, or the possible beneficial effects of maternal health such as dietary supplementation. Without a fetal malformation register, there is little or no chance of measuring the effects of any intervention in the field of fetal medicine; even relatively specialised and uncommon events such as the outcome of intrauterine therapy cannot be properly interpreted without a knowledge of the natural history of conditions which may never be referred to fetal medicine specialists.

The task of a fetal malformation register therefore is to collect information on all possible cases which fit within the criteria, not just those which come through regional or national centres for fetal medicine. Although these centres of excellence are extremely important in providing accurate diagnosis in individual cases, they cannot provide the overview which is required for true progress to be made in the understanding of congenital malformations.

Fetal medicine is a new and fairly small subspecialty, with clear links to both obstetrics, paediatrics and genetics, and although the assessment and treatment of pregnancies affected by congenital malformations is not the whole specialty, most referral centres with specialists dedicated to this area will spend a large amount of time dealing with these patients. Clinical geneticists and some specialist paediatricians form the main structure of the clinical teams who will be involved in the management of these cases, alongside other professionals such as the laboratory specialists, specialist nurses and midwives. The fetal anomaly register is therefore an extremely important part of the work of these departments and is often the only means by which undiagnosed or unreferred cases can be identified.

Specialist centres for fetal medicine have high rates of diagnostic accuracy for the majority of structural congenital malformations, but within the vast majority of healthcare systems, even in the developed world, the overwhelming majority of pregnancies will not be assessed by experts in fetal medicine. The challenge for the healthcare service is therefore to put systems in place which offer the ability to identify fetal malformations. Other chapters present the details of screening programmes such as maternal serum alpha fetoprotein, serum screening for Down's syndrome and the various regimes for ultrasound assessment during pregnancy. These programmes are now widely used throughout the world, and a great deal of time and money is spent in this field, but the majority of these programmes have no formal audit structure, and their effectiveness in practice is therefore impossible to judge. The health economist can make predictions regarding the possible benefits of the introduction of a particular regime only when the information is available regarding the actual outcomes of the diseases being studied. The knowledge of how a condition, identified during pregnancy, is likely to effect the outcome of the pregnancy is fundamental to the whole basis on which these public health decisions are made.

Methodology

The most important basic requirement for a fetal malformation register is to ascertain as many cases as possible of the conditions which are of interest. This can be achieved in a number of ways.

A fetal malformation register must take data from multiple sources. A system which has only one data source is likely to miss cases[8], which threatens the validity of conclusions drawn from these data. The ascertainment levels can be estimated in a number of ways. The incidence of common fetal anomalies can be compared with published rates to give a crude estimate of likely underreporting, but to estimate accurately the number of missing cases an alternative data source is required. Comparisons with birth certificates in the New York State Congenital Malformation Registry yielded an overall additional 1.7% of cases of major malformation during 1983–1986[9], with the conclusion that the increased workload in routinely using this method was not justified for this relatively small additional number of cases. A case record study in Victoria, Australia, examined 500 cases of paediatric admissions with congenital malformations during 1992 and demonstrated improved ascertainment for the Victorian malformation register compared to 1986, with very high proportions of major structural malformations being registered[10].

Any professional who might come into contact with an affected fetus or child needs to be part of the reporting mechanism. The proportion of reports from different sources is presented for the West Midlands Congenital Anomaly Register for 1997 in Fig. 27.1. The majority of screening ultrasound scans in this region are performed by radiographers with additional specialist training, and these form the bulk of initial registrations in this survey. Antenatal clinic staff, delivery staff, especially midwives; neonatologists and nurse practitioners as well as specialists within paediatrics need to have the facility to report cases to the register. In the UK, a regional system for notification of perinatal death exists, with cases notified from 20 weeks' gestation up to one year of age, and the links which are required for the notification of these cases are extremely important in ensuring that cases of congenital malformation are not overlooked.

The mortality system, entitled CESDI (Confidential Enquiry into Stillbirth and Deaths in Infancy) will encompass those cases of congenital malformation which end in death. For deliveries during 1996, congenital malformations were the cause of death of 439/1317 (33%) of all cases regis-

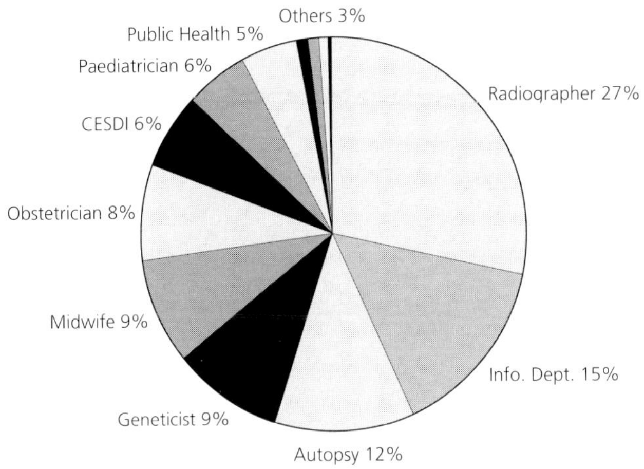

Fig. 27.1 Sources of notification of congenital anomalies 1995–1996.

tered between 20 weeks and one year of life, including terminations at any gestation for fetal malformation, and 124/740 (17%) of stillbirths and early neonatal deaths, in the West Midlands Region of England. Clearly this represents an extremely important area of overlap between the mortality and malformation surveillance programmes. This has led many congenital malformation registers in the UK to be intimately linked to the CESDI system, and in the West Midlands the two functions are so closely entwined that the same base dataset, computer software and largely the staff are shared between the mortality and congenital anomaly registration functions.

The introduction of prenatal screening programmes has led to an increasing number of cases of congenital malformation, which would previously have been registered as stillbirths or neonatal deaths, being terminated before the gestation at which birth notification is required. It is vital therefore that all cases of termination undertaken for suspected or confirmed fetal malformation should be collected within a fetal malformation register. This gives an opportunity to assess the impact of a screening programme on a population, and also highlights any false-positive diagnoses, which should be extremely rare, but are very important in the overall assessment of any programme. Validation of the number of cases terminated is difficult, and the precise post-termination diagnosis can be hard to verify if a structural malformation has been terminated surgically in early pregnancy. Karyotype abnormalities are easier to validate, although culture failures can occur using material from termination of pregnancy. If the number of cases undergoing termination of pregnancy is underestimated in comparison to other cases, the apparent effectiveness of any prenatal diagnosis programme will be reduced. Data relating to termination of pregnancy are some of the most potentially sensitive and the importance of adequate security to maintain individual confidentiality cannot be overstated.

A fetal malformation survey must also capture postnatal paediatric registrations. If the function of the register is, at least in part, to assess the ability of prenatal screening programmes to identify cases during pregnancy, it is fundamental to have an accurate method of collecting cases which were not identified. It seems clear that some of the conditions which are of interest will not be identified during pregnancy for many reasons, and it may therefore be more descriptive, and indeed more universally accepted, to use the term 'congenital malformation register' rather than to concentrate on fetal malformations. This does not deny the obvious fact that these conditions were present during fetal life, but recognises the paediatric diagnosis of conditions sometimes weeks, months or even years after the birth of the child.

INCLUSION AND EXCLUSION CRITERIA

A fetal malformation register should have strict inclusion and exclusion criteria. This is more a practical than a philosophical requirement. If infinite resources were available it may be very interesting to collect information on all suspected problems, but in the real world this tends to have a diluting effect on core data, and risks the register being swamped by large numbers of relatively minor problems. The boundaries are in practice difficult to draw. What a fetal medicine specialist may regard as of little consequence, such as a strawberry naevus, may be of great significance to the family and the dermatology specialists who will attempt to deal with the condition. Many other conditions which are relatively common at birth have been traditionally excluded from birth defect registers, and this does tend to reduce the ownership of the registry within the paediatric community, where the impact and importance of these conditions is seen. There is little point, however, in attempting to collect information on everything, even with the aim of making the registry more widely useful. The end result of this approach would be to have large amounts of poor quality data, which could never be properly analysed or even reported.

If a completely open-door policy were adopted to registration there would also be the temptation to extend the definition of congenital malformation to include cases outside a normal range of measurements. This might lead to the registration of all fetuses with a femur length shorter than the 3rd centile, or head circumference above the 97th centile, and although this might be very interesting and potentially important work, it would have the inevitable effect of overloading and potentially threatening the core function of a registry, to record suspected or confirmed *diagnoses* of congenital malformation.

The exclusion criteria for a congenital malformation register must be built into the foundations. If a decision is made to exclude a particular group of diagnoses at the outset it is extremely unlikely that these will ever be included. Although it is much easier to remove and edit data, using filters and sort criteria within a computer database package, the work which

TABLE 27.1
Alphabetical list of exclusions adapted from EUROCAT cases for exclusion

Accessory nipple	Heart murmur (unless referred to cardiologist)	Sacral dimple
Birth injuries	Hydrocoele	Skin tags
Birth marks (skin tags < 4 cm, naevae and haemangioma)	Hypospadias (if orifice distal to coronary sulcus)	Single umbilical artery
Cephalohaematoma	Inguinal hernia	Spina bifida occulta
Clicking hips (not dislocated)	Naevus (birth mark)	Talipes: positional
Chordee without hypospadias	Nipple accessory or ectopic	Testes undescended
Craniotabes (indentable cranial bones)	Phimosis	Toes minor webbing
Ectopic anus (if no other anomaly)	Pilonidal sinus	Toes overlapping
Ectopic nipple	Placental anomalies	Tongue tie
Facial palsy	Postural talipes	Two vessel umbilical cord
Haemangioma		Undescended testes
		Umbilical artery: single
		Umbilical hernia
		Vaginal skin tag
		Webbing of toes: minor

has been undertaken to gather these pieces of data will be largely wasted, and this must be considered when exclusion criteria are fixed. The EUROCAT collaboration has gathered information from a number of registries around Europe for many years. A list of conditions considered not suitable for inclusion in a malformation registry has been produced by this body, and this has been adopted by the majority of registries currently running in the Europe. This listing is by no means exhaustive, and tends to be based on the practicalities of reporting, rather than fundamental scientific or philosophical questions. See Table 27.1.

GENETICS

The inclusion criteria for chromosomal anomalies is a good example of a fundamentally grey area. Most registries would be very interested in aneuploidy, particularly trisomy 21 (Down's syndrome) for which prenatal screening and diagnosis has been evolving over many years, but other chromosomal rearrangements, even those appearing *de novo*, may be of little or no significance to the health of the individual, and with no easy way of grouping and collating these more subtle conditions together, this is much more an area of interest for clinical geneticists working case by case. If the fetal malformation registry is very much part of the clinical geneticist's domain, then these individual cases are best included, but in some registries there is little to be gained by adding this heterogeneous group, when they are most likely to be excluded from analysis for this very reason.

Single-gene defects present slightly different problems. They are present at conception and therefore fall with the group of diseases which potential could be diagnosed during pregnancy. However, when the effects of a disease process such as Huntington's chorea may not be apparent until middle life, there seems little in common with the other conditions which will be registered. Other single-gene defects such as cystic fibrosis seem to have much more relevance to the fetal malformation register and often will present with a 'structural' malformation such as echogenic bowel on ultrasound or immediate neonatal problems which would make these cases overlap with other causes of congenital gastrointestinal malformation. The place of cystic fibrosis, and other single-gene disorders, remains to be clarified, but our current practice is not to include these cases as they are already being grouped together and studied separately. Conversely, the inborn errors of metabolism, almost universally autosomal recessive conditions, have been classified within congenital malformations by the fetal and neonatal causes of death currently in use in CESDI in England & Wales[11]. These cases are important in fetal medicine because of their high recurrence risk and are frequently amenable to prenatal diagnosis. A condition should be included in a fetal malformation register if there is a high chance of the majority of cases being diagnosed in fetal or infant life.

GEOGRAPHICAL BOUNDARIES

A fetal malformation register must cover a particular geographical population. Ideally, the surrounding populations will also be covered by a similar system so that data can be exchanged with the aim of achieving full ascertainment of cases. If significant numbers of cases are delivered or managed in hospitals outside the area covered by the registry, a separate contact system may be needed to ensure information is not lost. This may be particularly important in cases of relatively rare conditions which may be transferred large distances for optimal management of their problem. The surgical correction of congenital heart disease is a field in which recent developments and published results have meant that children are frequently referred from great distances[12]. National centres for paediatrics, such as Great Ormond Street Hospital in London, will need to recognise their role in providing information for epidemiological studies, and the ever-present problems of communication between professionals may be partly alleviated by the improved used of information technology.

The analysis of data from a congenital anomaly register can only take place if the total population at potential risk of the condition is known (the denominator) and gives the opportunity to calculate the incidence of the condition, rather than reporting numbers of cases. Without this basic facility there is no useful information to be gained from the collection of information relating to congenital malformations, and the original design of any malformation register must take into account this fundamental requirement. The data which are available for the denominator population are likely to be the most important limiting factor in the analysis of data from a registry, and from this point of view, it may be justified to limit the data collection in the cases of malformation to that which is available for all births. In England & Wales the information recorded for each birth is limited, and although other sources, such as a computerised child health system and various hospital-based systems, are potentially available these are usually designed and funded with a particular purpose in mind and cannot easily be used as sources, even when those who own the data are keen to cooperate. The definition of the geographical area to be covered by the registry can cause some minor problems. We use the postcode of residence of the mother at the time of delivery, although for some postnatal registrations this can be difficult to ascertain and the postcode of the child at the time of paediatric attendance can be substituted in these cases with little loss of precision.

The size of the area to be covered by a registry is an important consideration. If the area is too small there will be relatively few cases reported, and therefore the statistical power with which it might be possible to say whether a particular malformation was becoming more or less common is very weak. Most individual hospital populations, even the very largest maternity hospitals will have too few deliveries to allow powerful analysis of an individual congenital malformation. If the area is too large it will become difficult to maintain contact with those who report cases, and the essential network for finding missing data will become fragile. The health regions in the UK, although recently reshaped, provide geographical areas covering between 40 000 and 80 000 births, which give the potential to maintain links with individuals within each reporting centre. This gives an important sense of ownership to a mechanism which is perceived as being local, although the success of this type of multihospital collaboration is to some extent dependent upon the goodwill of individuals rather than any sense of collective loyalty amongst hospital managers, who tend to have a competitive approach to the provision of healthcare. Competition and collaboration are tools which can be used together to establish and maintain an effective network.

COLLABORATION BETWEEN REGISTERS

When a congenital malformation registry has clearly defined geographical boundaries and a known denominator population, the data can be usefully pooled to examine trends over time, changes following healthcare interventions, and more wide-reaching geographical trends. This has been at the heart of the European Registration of Congenital Anomalies and Twins (EUROCAT) collaboration[13] which aims to bring together malformation registries in Europe. Very large collaborative ventures are required to examine trends in very rare conditions, but the most important results from these ventures are likely to be those which highlight particularly successful or unsuccessful strategies in healthcare. It seems that the current trend is towards grouping data together with increasing collaboration between registries[14]. This approach has a number of dangers, and there may be a tendency towards the very briefest of datasets, which have little valuable information for those working in the clinical setting. When two or more registries join together it is vital that the precise details of the information, and the way in which it is collected, checked and recorded, are examined. Any comparisons between registries in this type of collaboration are more likely to show difference between the registry methods than differences between the two populations. The potential power of a very large collaborative study, in statistical terms, is so great that the conclusions might be very hard to validate; the publication of data from the sources, especially those which compare one area with another, has the potential for misleading conclusions to be drawn by differences in methodology, coding, validation and recording.

DATASETS

The possible analysis from any source is defined by the actual dataset which is collected. The fundamental methods of collecting and storing information have been discussed. It is entirely useless to collect together a group of interesting case reports, because each will have a narrative which is applicable only to that case, and the ability to examine trends, common themes or differences will be lost. Case reports are very potent and powerful; a single interesting case published in a journal might be read by many thousands of professionals, and it is possible that those people will change their clinical practice on the basis of a small number of supporting case reports. For a case report to be interesting it must be unusual, and it may promote some novel association or idea which has not previously been stated. The association of a fetal malformation with some other factor in a particular case then raises the question of more general application. Fetal medicine contains many examples of potential links between ultrasound findings, biochemical results, history of drug ingestion, maternal infections and specific congenital malformations. Many have profoundly influenced medical practice and no doubt further fundamental discoveries will continue to enlighten clinical practice. The task of a fetal malformation register in this context is to attempt to answer a question, for which it was not originally designed. The answers which are possible depend upon the organisation or structure of the original data and in most circumstances the registry will only be the start of the trail.

The dataset contains information which is systematically collected on every case to allow analysis. This will contain fundamental details about the mother, the pregnancy, the delivery, the outcome and the baby as well as the actual diagnosis. The first methods of recording and retrieving information in a structured way relied upon asking questions with 'yes/no, true/false' answers which were recorded onto punchcard, with holes to represent the answers. Modern computer packages make it possible not only to record and search in a much more sophisticated way, but also to perform searches very rapidly through large sections of unstructured text, in order to find information within descriptive text. The fundamental of any registry is the dataset which it contains. This needs to be small enough to be completed accurately, but large enough to answer questions, some of which may not be predictable at the outset of the project. The task is made more difficult by the potential time span over which cases can be registered. For example, the dataset which may be required to answer questions relating to the identification of anencephaly on ultrasound at 12 weeks may be completely different to those which are needed to answer questions relating to the diagnosis of congenital heart disease within the first year of life. No standard exists, and the focus of different groups depends upon their own particular interests and biases.

The dataset which is collected by different registers will vary considerably, for justifiable reasons, depending upon their focus. Some will be primarily designed for fetal medicine, concentrating on questions of outcome following a particular diagnosis, while others may concentrate largely on paediatric issues. If too many registries are grouped together in an attempt to give greater power to the whole collaboration, there is a danger that the potential dataset will become so large that no case will be complete, and any particular piece of information within the dataset will be incomplete. This is a fundamental problem for all congenital malformation registries, but becomes more serious with increasing amalgamation of data from different sources.

CODING

The notification of a congenital malformation is usually made by a written description of the problem. The process of coding is to fit this text based description into a pre-existing disease classification, such that the case can take its place within a particular diagnostic group. The current International Classification of Diseases (revision 10) (ICD-10)[15] is generally recognised as a useful system for this purpose, with extensions giving additional focus provided by the Royal College of Paediatrics and Child Health. The conditions regarded as congenital malformations are grouped together with the suffix Q, which gives scope for the easy identification of cases using data collected for other purposes. This method is used in the West Midlands registry to identify paediatric admissions with a congenital malformation in the diagnostic code. The major purpose of coding the diagnoses in each case is to ensure clarity of definition. Allocating numbers to words has the additional benefit of allowing groups to be quickly and easily joined together during analysis. An illustration of the principles of the ICD-10 coding systems is presented in Table 27.2. The system used for data entry in the West Midlands includes a hypertext link to a computerised ICD-10 file which will identify the possible numerical codes which match any text entries. This allows coding to take place at the time of data entry for the majority of conditions, but relies on the data entry being undertaken by an experienced coder.

TABLE 27.2
International Classification of Diseases (ICD-10) coding system for congenital anomalies. Examples of groups and subgroups

Q 00 Anencephaly and similar malformations
Q 00.0 Anencephaly
Acephaly
Acrania
Amyelencephaly
Hemianencephaly
Hemicephaly
Q 00.1 Craniorachischisis
Q 00.2 Iniencephaly
Q 90 Down's syndrome
Q 90.0 Trisomy 21, meiotic nondisjunction
Q 90.1 Trisomy 21, Mosaicism (mitotic nondisjunction)
Q 90.2 Trisomy 21, Translocation
Q 90.9 Trisomy 21, unspecified

PRIMARY DIAGNOSIS

Summary analysis and presentation of data often require a single diagnosis for each case. This can cause problems when multiple diagnoses are recorded, for example a fetus with trisomy 18 might have many structural defects recorded within the dataset, and it may be important for some questions to examine how often a malformation, for example cleft lip, occurs in association with trisomy 18. For the purposes of reporting numbers of cases it is often valuable, however, to have a primary diagnosis. This means that when a well recognised syndrome or sequence occurs the primary malformation can describe the case, rather than relying on a particular constellation of problems, some of which may not be present in all cases.

The concept of a primary diagnosis does not fit every case – some will have two or more malformations without any obvious link – but for most cases it is useful for the purposes of analysis to assign a single primary diagnosis to one of the ICD-10 codes.

Computerisation and reporting by group

Data entry, efficient storage with back-up and flexible reporting are supported by modern information technology. The ability to validate data at the time of data entry reduces the numbers of errors which find their way into a system and can cause problems. The production of calculated fields to give the best estimate of gestation and other facilities are an integral part of the efficient use of computing software in this area.

Modern database design means that the facility exists to code any number of ICD-10 diagnoses, by having a 'one-to-many' database structure, with one table containing a single record of demographic details and one containing the ICD-10 codes and information specifically related to each diagnosis. Figure 27.2 illustrates how this can work, the computer terminology for this ability is a 'relational' database, and the complexity of the design is potentially infinite with pieces of information efficiently packaged into tables within which every field can be filled. Every table needs to contain the unique identifier which will allow linkage to all other tables,

Table 1
Fields which occur only once in each case

Unique ID	Mother's details	Field 1	Field 2
01234567	Smith	01/01/1962	Other data
01234568	Begum	06/06/1970	Other data

Table 2
Fields which could occur many times in each case

Unique ID	ICD-10 code	Date of diagnosis	Notifier	Notifying hospital
012345657	Q 37.0 Cleft palate	15.05.1997	Radiographer	Heartlands Hospital
012345657	Q 66.0 Talipes	10.06.1997	Labour ward midwife	Heartlands Hospital
012345657	Q 19.0 Trisomy 18	01.06.1997	Cytogenetic lab	Cytogenics lab
01234568	Q 01 Encephalocoele	02.06.1997	Radiographer	District general hospital
01234568	Q 01.2 Frontal encephalocoele	10.06.1997	Radiographer	Fetal medicine centre
01234568	Q 61.9 Cystic kidneys	10.06.1997	Radiographer	Fetal medicine centre
01234568	Q 61.9 Meckel–Gruber syndrome	21.06.1997	Pathologist	Post-mortem report

Fig. 27.2 Example of how two tables within a database can be linked to give complete flexibility and precision to each case.

giving great flexibility in analysis and reporting. Computerisation has been one of the major changes of recent decades, and has given powerful aids to those wishing to maintain and analyse data. The most important aspects of computerisation are the flexible nature of modern computer software, giving the ability to sort and report in many different formats, and the ability to produced data electronically which can then be amalgamated efficiently in collaborative studies. Computerisation allows complex multidiagnosis cases to be recorded in such a way that both the details of the case, and the broad systems involved, can be reported depending upon the precise requirements for each report.

OUTPUTS

A disease surveillance system such as a fetal malformation register will take a great deal of time and effort to establish, and the task of collecting, checking and entering data into a well constructed database can seem like an end in itself, but the only chance to achieve tangible results is when information comes out of the system. To some extent the method by which this happens is less important than the fact of it happening at all. There are very many examples of high-quality data being collected, but never reported. The annual report is a popular method, and this does ensure that regular output is maintained. There is a danger that a standard annual report is created and reproduced every year with little critical comment or analysis. Targeting particular topics is another method of reporting which allows the data to used to shed light on important areas of clinical practice, and often to be the focus for continued education and training for professionals working in clinical settings. The future of intervention programmes such as the maternal serum alpha-fetoprotein, serum screening for Down's syndrome and various regimes for ultrasound screening will need to be critically reviewed in future years, and it seems likely that the combined power of fetal anomaly registers working in different parts of the world will give relatively clean comparisons between different methods and should allow those with the responsibility to plan healthcare to commission the most effective programmes for their particular budget and population. A recent review of obstetric ultrasound policy highlights the relative paucity of information in this field and supports the concept of continued surveillence using population-based fetal malformation registers[16].

CLUSTER ANALYSIS

The reporting of rare events occurring together often generates a great deal of public anxiety and media interest. This can put the directors of public health for a certain area, the chief medical officer or health ministers in the position of having to quickly analyse and present known information relating to rare conditions, such as anophthalmia or limb reduction deformities. A well-organised system of fetal malformation registers gives the ability to provide data over a wide area for analysis, so that associations between the coastline or particular events of pollution can be rapidly examined. The most common result of previous cluster analysis has been to refute suggestions of any link, which might suggest causation. The thalidomide tragedy of the early 1960s, however, was an exception to this general trend that should lead us all to keep an open mind. This event has led doctors to be extremely cautious in the use of drugs during pregnancy and acted as a spur for a national congenital malformation monitoring system in England & Wales, and although this system still exists, it is not designed to identify fetal malformations before birth, does not link well with the system for registration of terminations of pregnancy for fetal malformation and is relatively inflexible with regard to postnatal registration.

COSTS

The current cost of maternity care in the UK is approximately £1500 per birth. This includes antenatal, intrapartum and postpartum care, with additional costs associated with paediatric care, when required. The surveillance of this whole area of healthcare has not been well funded and even a minimum maternity dataset has proved difficult to achieve in England & Wales[17]. There is little or no standardisation of the care which is recommended and a paucity of evidence on which to base judgements. Regions, districts, hospitals and individual clinicians have their own policies and practices. The cost of limited surveillance of some of the important outcomes of these episodes of care, including deaths and congenital malformation, is approximately 0.1% of the expenditure on the care itself and this would seem to be an extremely small amount, when the results will affect the future direction and therefore the future effectiveness of the entire system. It has been argued that competitive forces within a healthcare system will inevitable drive quality standards upwards, but if the very standards by which quality is judged have no valid foundation the whole system is brought into question. The fetal anomaly registry should be in a position to inform the process of healthcare commissioning, although the temptation to use the information to make comparisons between hospitals risks alienating those who are identified as being deficient.

Conclusion

Congenital anomaly registers have an important and probably growing place in the heart of pregnancy and child healthcare planning. The most efficient and effective policies for the majority of clinical screening and interventions are currently unknown, and without adequate disease surveillance will never be established. Additional research and development programmes are required to answer specific questions, but the fundamental outcomes of mortality and significant congenital defects will need to be recorded systematically. The development of congenital anomaly registers has relied in the past on local enthusiasm, but the future would seem to lie in collaboration of geographically based registries, offering a powerful and potentially flexible data source to address particular questions. The temptation to focus attention on the very rare and therefore most interesting cases must be resisted in favour of collecting high quality information on the relatively large number of common malformations occurring outside centres of fetal medicine expertise which form the bulk of the population of individuals who suffer from these diseases. The importance of the intrauterine environment should now be obvious and the importance of congenital malformation surveillance should be equally clear.

REFERENCES

1. Campbell J. *Protection of motherhood*. London: HMSO, 1927.
2. Knox EG & Lancashire R. *Epidemiology of Congenital Malformations*. London: HMSO, 1991.
3. Czeizel AE. First 25 years of the Hungarian Congenital Anomaly Registry. *Teratology* **55**:(5) 299–305, 1997.
4. Lie RT. Environmental epidemiology at the Medical Birth Registry of Norway; strengths and limitations. *Central Eur. J. Publ. Health* **5**:(2)57–59, 1997.
5. Bjerkedal T & Irgens LM. Medical birth registries: a gold mine for research. *Nordisk Med.* **108**:(8–9), 211–212, 218, 1993.
6. OPCS. *Congenital Malformation Statistics*. The OPCS Monitoring Scheme for Congenital Malformation. London: OPCS, 1995.
7. Van Cleave ML. Developing a birth defects registry for Tennessee. *J. Tennessee Med. Ass.* **87**(2):60–61, 1994.
8. Hemminki E, Merilainen J & Teperi J. Reporting of malformations in routine health registers. *Teratology* **48**(3):227–231, 1993.
9. Olsen CL, Polan AK & Cross PK. Case ascertainment for the state based birth defects registries: characteristics of unreported infants ascertained through birth certificates and their impact on registry statistics in New York State. *Paediatr. Perinatal Epidemiol.* **10**(2):161–174, 1996.
10. Kilkenny M, Riley M & Lumley J. Follow-up validation study of the Victorian Congenital Malformations Register. *J. Paediatr. Child Health* **31**(4):323–325, 1995.
11. Hey EN, Lloyd DJ & Wigglesworth JS. Classifying perinatal death: fetal and neonatal factors. *Br. J. Obstet. Gynaecol.* **93**:1213–1223, 1986.
12. Bullock FA, Stumper O, Jagtap R *et al.* Surgery for infants with a hypoplastic systemic ventricle and severe outflow obstruction; early results with a modified Norwood procedure. *Br. Heart J.* **73**:456–461, 1995.
13. EUROCAT. *European Registration of Congenital Anomalies*. Brussels: Department of Epidemiology, Catholic University of Louvain, 1990.
14. Lechat MF & Dolk H. Registries of congenital anomalies: EUROCAT. *Environ. Health Perspect.* **101**(Suppl.2):153–157, 1993.
15. World Health Organization. *International Classification of Diseases and related health care issues* 10th revision. Geneva: World Health Organization, 1992.
16. Royal College of Obstetricians & Gynaecologists. *Ultrasound screening for fetal abnormalities*. Report of the RCOG Working Party. London: RCOG, 1997.
17. MacFarlane A. At last – maternity statistics for England. *BMJ* **316**:RCOG 566–567, 1998.

SECTION

5

Prenatal screening and diagnosis

Genetic and post-pregnancy counselling

28

M. Mahoney

What is genetic counselling?

With varying emphases, genetic counselling is described as a communication process between healthcare personnel and counsellees that (1) describes fully a genetic disorder either present or having risk of occurrence in a family, (2) examines ways of responding to the risk of occurrence or recurrence, and (3) aids or guides the counsellee toward optimal adjustments to the disorder and/or choices about the risk of occurrence or recurrence[1]. In the context of fetal medicine, the disorders that are addressed are mostly those that affect the unborn, with conditions which become manifest either before or after birth, and the counsellees are usually a prospective mother, pregnant or considering pregnancy, and her partner. Disorders of the fetus that are not always or wholly genetic, especially anomalies due to teratogenic influences, usually fall within the purview of genetic counselling in obstetrics, alongside classic genetic disorders such as Down syndrome and cystic fibrosis.

Genetic counselling typically serves a twofold purpose: to educate and to counsel[2] (Table 28.1). Both are challenging. Prior knowledge about potential fetal disorders is often limited on the part of clients while the range of personal and family dynamics of client fears and hopes, of strengths and weaknesses, is huge. A counsellor or counselling team is often called upon to fill several roles – to be a teacher, psychologist, social worker and physician – in addition to being a counsellor. Sensitivity both to the general needs of every counsellee and the special needs of each individual counsellee is necessary for genetic counselling to achieve its goals and provide excellent service to patients.

TABLE 28.1
Elements of genetic counselling

- Accurate diagnosis of a genetic disorder or risk of genetic disorder in a family.
- Education of the family about the diagnosis.
- Information to the family of ways to respond to the risk of genetic disorders in their reproductive decisions.
- Assistance to the family in reaching personally satisfactory and meaningful decisions.

NON-DIRECTIVE COUNSELLING

A long-standing tenet of genetic counselling has been to be non-directive, to avoid heavily influencing or dictating a client's decision, to work to maintain a client's sense of autonomy and control over her life. The exercise of autonomy has high value for most persons and this is especially true in the realm of health and reproductive decisions. Yet it is self-evident that human communications like counselling can never be entirely value-neutral or opinion-neutral. Choice of words and subjects, verbal and non-verbal cues, selection of one example rather than another – all of these reveal thoughts, and perhaps biases, of the counsellor. It may be apparent that a client is overlooking an aspect of a decision, or is possibly too fearful to discuss it; she almost certainly will benefit from some level of direction[3]. Not infrequently, a patient will ask for a counsellor's opinion or even ask for direction. When genetic counsellors are observed, varying degrees of directiveness are found, but a recent study reported no association between perceived directiveness and a client's satisfaction with counselling[4].

Counsellors will continue to vary in their attempts at non-directive counselling and their beliefs about its value. They will derive styles of counselling that fit their own skills and often vary those styles in different client situations. It is likely that the genetic counselling profession will continue to debate and study the reality, value and nuances of nondirective counselling for some time. However the debate goes, it is suggested that it is paramount for a counsellor to do the following: to self-identify biases and make them explicitly known to the counsellee when they are relevant; to identify and explore a range of options and decisions with the counsellee; and, most importantly, as a health professional, to assist a counsellee in making a decision that is 'right' for that person or couple in their own terms, both when the decision is made and into the future.

QUANTITATIVE RISKS

Genetics has always been a field of probabilities, of chances, of risk figures. We are well into the Information Age and the language of probabilities and risks is being heard increasingly in other areas of medicine as well. This seems certain to increase in an era of population studies, clinical trials, and outcome measures. Quantitative statements do not come easily or naturally to a majority of our patients, however. They easily mistake the meaning of a 3% risk or a 1 in 250 chance, fail to recognize the equivalency of a 5% chance of a poor outcome versus a 95% chance of a good outcome, or do not readily translate a quantitative statement into a qualitative one that has personal meaning. Since we seem to be wed to quantitative risk figures, it behoves the counsellor to pay special attention to the understanding of risks by a counsellee and to use different ways of stating a probability, including qualitative terms.

Who receives genetic counselling?

Traditionally, those who deliver primary care have been urged to identify pregnancies in which there are or will be increased chances of a fetal disorder and to refer women and couples to genetics centres or prenatal diagnosis centres for information and counselling. Referral for genetic counselling should be as early in the pregnancy planning process as possible and should include both of the couple whenever possible. Ideally, referral should occur prior to conception in order to provide maximum information and options to the couple both about possibilities and methods of prenatal diagnosis, but also about considerations such as avoidance of pregnancy or the possibility of gamete donation. If preconception counselling cannot be accomplished, referral should occur early in a pregnancy. This will protect the availability of diagnostic approaches (e.g. chorionic villus sampling, early amniocentesis, or standard time amniocentesis) and secure required information to proceed legitimately with prenatal diagnosis. Such information often includes an accurately supported diagnosis in a proband or crucial gene or enzyme analyses in family members. Reasonable criteria for referral derive both from a careful, directed history from the couple concerning themselves and their families and from screening tests that are applied without regard to personal histories.

HISTORY-TAKING

Histories are meant to uncover circumstances that significantly increase the chance of serious fetal disorders, including ones that may be diagnosable, and perhaps even treatable, during fetal life and ones that might influence a decision of whether to undertake a pregnancy in the first place. Important factors are disorders, recognized or suspected to be genetic, and any other birth defects occurring in the prospective parents or in their first-degree (children, siblings, parents), second-degree (aunts, uncles, nephews, nieces, grandparents), or occasionally third-degree (cousins and others) relatives. Multiple miscarriages, unexplained fetal deaths or stillbirths, and neonatal deaths are often important. Consanguineous unions increase risks; so does the existence of rearranged or mosaic chromosomes in a prospective parent. Conditions characterized by mental retardation in a family member are included and even adult onset conditions will be important to some families (e.g. Huntington disease, myotonic dystrophy, polycystic kidney disease, hereditary cancer syndromes). Potential or actual exposure to teratogens (e.g. anticonvulsant medications) should be sought, including maternal disease states, like diabetes or phenylketonuria (PKU) that may be teratogenic. In general, a woman's medical history, past-pregnancy history and current pregnancy history should be scrutinized. It is instructive that a sizeable fraction of women referred for fetal chromosomal diagnosis because of advanced maternal age have other important prenatal diagnostic considerations after a careful history is taken[5].

SCREENING

Three methods of screening are potentially applied in all pregnancies to select women for referral to genetics or prenatal diagnosis services. Maternal age, because of its association with fetal aneuploidies, was the first to be used and today's routine practice generally uses the mid-thirties as a criterion for referral. Maternal serum screening programmes are also widely used and generate risk statements, during pregnancy, for Down syndrome, trisomy 18 and open neural tube defects. Increasingly, sonographic imaging, in first and second trimesters of pregnancy, is being used to identify fetuses with an increased chance of abnormalities. The trend is to combine the three modalities to give the most accurate assessment of fetal disease risks[6].

RECESSIVE GENE SCREENING

Another method of screening seeks to identify parents who are carriers of recessive genes that may result in recessive disease in a child. These screening efforts are aimed at persons without a significant family history of the disorder and thus are applicable to large segments of the population. Often, because of very different frequencies of a disorder in different ethnic groups, the ethnic background of prospective parents is used as a criterion for offering screening.

Several recessive disorders, with prenatal diagnosis being available, are currently the object of recessive gene screening. These include Tay–Sachs disease in the Jewish population (especially the Ashkenazim), for which there has been a long experience with screening. Very recently, screening for Canavan disease, Niemann–Pick disease type A and Gaucher disease has become available in that population. Screening for several severe haemoglobinopathies, the sickle-cell disorders and thalassaemias, has also been available for many years; peoples with increased risks include the populations (historic populations) of the Mediterranean region,. Africa, the Near East and West Asia, South Asia, Southeast Asia, and China. Emigrations have placed many of these peoples in the Americas, Australia and New Zealand in modern times.

Cystic fibrosis is a recent addition to population screening for recessive genes. The initial target population has been European origin peoples with more recent efforts aimed at better screening opportunities for Africans, Arabs, and some Asians. Recently in the United States, a government-convened consensus conference (convened by the National Institutes of Health) recommended the offering of carrier testing to all women and couples who are pregnant and to couples who are planning a pregnancy[7]. Experience with the logistics, successes, and problems of population screening for cystic fibrosis in a prenatal population are now being reported and, in general, are reassuring with regard to its acceptance[8,9] (Table 28.2).

TABLE 28.2
Traditional criteria for referral for genetic counselling

History
Medical and family histories of each prospective parent focused on genetic disorders and birth defects.
Miscarriages, fetal deaths, stillbirths, and neonatal deaths.
Teratogen exposures.
Screening
Maternal age (mid thirties).
Maternal serum screening results.
Sonographic imaging, first and second trimesters.
Recessive gene screening results.

Who delivers genetic counselling?

Genetic counselling is carried out in many health settings and by persons with different types of training. These include genetic counsellors, nurse geneticists, other nurse specialists, primary givers of obstetric care (nurse midwives, primary care obstetricians, family or general practitioners), perinatologists and medical geneticists. Availability of persons with different levels of training, consumer demands, differing organization of healthcare delivery systems, and economic considerations are all factors. The increasing complexity of fetal medicine and medical genetics increases the challenge for genetics specialists to inform and educate the young adult population and primary care-givers. Public education via multiple modalities must be emphasized. One mechanism that can be put to good use in some societies is the establishment of family registers to identify persons who have high personal risks of specific genetic disorders in their children[10]. These can serve to remind and educate concerned clients very early in the pregnancy planning process. Unfortunately, issues of privacy and of discrimination based on genetic identity can work against the utility of registers in other societies.

A major problem in delivering prenatal genetic services is that of sufficiently educating a pregnant woman and her partner about the consequences of having a screening test such as maternal serum screening or ultrasound imaging or a diagnostic test such as amniocentesis. These tests force information that is often ambiguous about the unborn baby to the forefront of a woman's consciousness. They may compel consideration of and decisions about invasive tests, with risks to the unborn baby, and about selective abortion of a fetus with disease. Many women and couples, in retrospect, wish they had never taken the first step down that path. The tests are generally offered by primary care-givers who may not have as much experience or sensitivity to issues of client decision-making, or time to devote to these issues, as has been the custom with genetic counsellors. Complicating the situation is the possibility that the test in question serves two purposes: (1) to address the prenatal diagnosis of a fetal disorder, which perhaps the woman does not wish to address; and (2) to give information about possible pregnancy risks that the obstetrician could use for better management decisions to the woman's and infant's benefit. This latter purpose had been suggested with the measurement of maternal serum alpha-fetoprotein in the second trimester, although clinical utility has been minimal, and now is again being suggested with late first-trimester ultrasound screening[11]. Whoever does genetic counselling, at any step along the way, will hopefully keep foremost in mind the necessity of engaging the patient in honest, informed decision-making that primarily serves her needs.

Critical issues in prenatal genetic counselling

Several recurring issues in prenatal genetic counselling deserve a special emphasis.

- Whenever possible, both members of a couple should be present during important counselling meetings. Information is often complex and suffers in translation when one member describes it to the other. Anxiety is invariably high and may inhibit the hearing or understanding of what is said. Joint decision-making about testing or about continuing or stopping a pregnancy usually provides better long-term outcomes for a couple, even if views conflict.

- Certain time considerations bring pressures to counsellees and these are best met by having information as early as feasible so as to allow adequate time for deliberation and decision. Whether to start a pregnancy, whether to have a prenatal test, whether to continue or stop a pregnancy – these are typical, high-anxiety questions. The last of them is the most problematic for there often are absolute deadlines for abortion procedures as a consequence of legal, social, or hospital policies. Abortion deadlines may also dictate when diagnostic tests can be done and which ones can be done if the information is being sought for abortion decision-making. People need time to gather information and opinions. They often find themselves weighing the burdens of one choice versus another and require time to try to understand the reality of each. On the other side, undue procrastination in making a decision can lead to increased distress and conceivably a counsellor could insist on an arbitrary deadline.
- Couples seek information about their unborn baby for many different reasons. The information may be used for fetal treatment decisions or to optimize the management of the pregnancy. It may be sought to direct abortion decisions. It may be sought to relieve anxiety about fetal disease or to have foreknowledge about the birth of an infant with a serious disorder or handicapping condition. Some prospective parents seem to delay the reality of the pregnancy or attachment to the unborn baby until diagnostic tests have been reported as normal[12]. The earlier information is available, the shorter this delay will be. Ultrasound images of a fetus are deemed desirable by most prospective parents, but not by all, especially if a decision about abortion is being considered. Asking patients about their wishes in this and similar matters is very important if one is striving to preserve patient autonomy and well-being.
- A common misconception holds that normal results from prenatal diagnosis equates with a normal, healthy baby. Optimism and a reluctance to focus too strongly on abnormal outcomes are natural to most people and 'good news' test results reinforce those feelings. Reality, of course, is somewhat different and counsellors should insist on accurate information about what a test does and does not accomplish. One hopes to minimize repercussions for both the family and for care-givers when the occasional bad outcome occurs. Equally difficult as trying to prevent unrealistic or unwarranted expectations is how to deal with ambiguity and uncertainty. A fetal diagnosis rarely predicts the severity of the condition or its treatability with high accuracy. Some findings, e.g. chromosomal mosaicism, have very low predictive value on the spectrum of normalcy to abnormalcy. These areas of uncertainty are very difficult for prospective parents and they will often need considerable assistance in accepting the uncertainty and making plans based on it[13] (Table 28.3).

TABLE 28.3
Critical issues in prenatal counselling

- Involve both prospective parents.
- Avoid or mitigate unrealistic time pressures placed on counsellees for decisions.
- Maximize participation and autonomy of counsellors.
- Avoid untrue or unrealistic expectations.
- Work to minimize uncertainty where possible.

Post-pregnancy counselling

Most women and their partners who interact with genetic services and counsellors during pregnancy are hoping desperately to have a normal child. Sometimes an abnormal fetus will die spontaneously in the womb, sometimes an infant will be born with unexpected abnormalities and sometimes a pregnancy will be electively terminated because of suspected or established fetal disease. All of these outcomes are unwanted and sad, in the sense of having lost the normal baby who was central to the parents' dreams, and all will trigger a grief reaction, surprisingly intense at times. Guilt, to some degree, about having conceived or otherwise caused an abnormal baby is extremely common, albeit often irrational. If elective abortion led to the death of the fetus, further mixed emotions, including guilt, will be present.

Recognition of these intense psychologic reactions has grown with the growth of prenatal diagnosis actitivity and interventions have been developed[14,15]. Central to them is the provision of full information and the concerted attempt to involve the parents in decisions and participation around the death of their baby. Parents differ considerably in how they wish to participate. Some will want to see or hold the baby, if the body is intact, and have someone explain any visible abnormalities. Some will want pictures, although perhaps not immediately; others will want a lock of hair, footprints or handprints. Some will choose ceremonies and private burials. Others will not want to participate in these ways but will want to talk about the loss and experiences they are going through. The important response for counsellors is to listen carefully to the parents, offer options and be flexible.

It is useful to warn the couple of the expected grief reaction. The depressive phase can last from a few days to a few weeks and be very inhibiting of usual activities. Most psychologically healthy persons move through their grief reaction with the support of family and friends and the interest and support of obstetric and genetics personnel they have known. A few require additional professional intervention. At times a woman and her partner are seriously out of concert with each other in their grieving process. Warning them about this possibility, encouraging communication, and helping them to progress can be very helpful. Support groups, made up of couples or individuals who have suffered similar losses, can also be of major benefit to some couples in their efforts at healing.

Another area in which a couple can be helped is with responses to and understanding of their children at home. The parents' distress cannot be hidden from their other children and open acknowledgment of it and sharing their sadness is almost always the appropriate behaviour. Children commonly think that they themselves may have somehow caused the death of the unborn baby or that they, too, may become sick and die. They need to be reassured about these matters and also reassured that their parents, although saddened, are still available to care for them (Table 28.4).

TABLE 28.4
Post-pregnancy counselling

- A grief reaction including a period of depression.
- Loss of the dreamed for 'normal' child.
- Non-parallel grieving by the couple.
- Support groups.
- Accurate diagnosis of a deceased fetus or infant.
- Future pregnancy planning including prenatal diagnosis options.

The quest for an answer of why did it happen, in a medical sense, is often achieved but it often cannot be. It is important to have good diagnostic facilities including autopsy, X-rays and photographs, and the capacity for molecular and biochemical analyses. Accurate interpretations will help ease guilt and are crucial for considerations of future pregnancies and possible prenatal diagnosis. In another sense, helping the parents to understand the imperfections and vagaries of biologic processes and how we can try to control them will be central to their healing.

REFERENCES

1. Royal College of Physicians of London. *Prenatal Diagnosis and Genetic Screening. Community and Service Implications.* London: RCOP, 1989.
2. Kessler S. Psychological aspects of genetic counseling. IX. Teaching and counseling *J. Genet. Counsel.* **6**:287–296, 1997.
3. White MT. 'Respect for autonomy' in genetic counseling: an analysis and a proposal. *J. Genet. Counsel.* **6**:297–313, 1997.
4. Michie S, Bron F, Bobrow M & Marteau TM. Nondirectiveness in genetic counseling: an empiric study. *Am. J. Hum. Genet.* **60**:40–47, 1997.
5. Rubin SP, Malin J & Maidman J. Genetic counseling before prenatal diagnosis for advanced maternal age: an important medical safeguard. *Obstet. Gynecol.* **62**:155–159, 1983.
6. Wald NJ & Hackshaw AK. Combining ultrasound and biochemistry in first-trimester screening for Down's syndrome. *Prenat. Diagn.* **17**:821–829, 1997.
7. NIH Consensus Statement. *Genetic Testing for Cystic Fibrosis* **15**(4):1–37, 1997.
8. Brock DJH. Prenatal screening for cystic fibrosis: 5 years' experience reviewed. *Lancet* **347**:148–150, 1996.
9. Rowley PT, Loader S & Levenkron JC. Cystic fibrosis carrier population screening: a review. *Genetic Testing* **1**:53–59, 1997.
10. Read AP, Kerzin-Storrar L, Mountford RC, Elles RG & Harris R. A register based system for gene tracking Duchenne muscular dystrophy. *J. Med. Genet.* **23**:581–586, 1986.
11. Souka AP & Nicolaides KH. Diagnosis of fetal abnormalities at the 10–14 week scan. *Ultrasound Obstet. Gynecol.* **10**:429–442, 1997.
12. Rothman BK. *The Tentative Pregnancy: Prenatal Diagnosis and the Future of Motherhood.* New York: Penguin, 1987.
13. Lippman-Hand A & Fraser FC. Genetic counseling: the postcounseling period: parents' perceptions of uncertainty. *Am. J. Med. Genet.* **4**:51–71, 1979.
14. White-Van Mourick M, Conner JM & Ferguson-Smith MA. The psychological sequelae of a second-trimester termination of pregnancy for fetal abnormality. *Prenat. Diagn.* **12**:189–204, 1992.
15. Elder S & Laurence K. The impact of supportive intervention after second trimester termination of pregnancy for fetal abnormality. *Prenat. Diagn.* **11**:47–54, 1991.

The stresses of prenatal screening and diagnosis

29

L. Abramsky

Introduction

Pregnancy has always been a time of uncertainty. In the fairly recent past the questions were: Would the baby be alive, normal and healthy when it was born? Would it be a boy or a girl? Would there be one baby or more? Would the mother live through the pregnancy, delivery and puerperium?

Now, in western countries, many of the questions about the baby are (or can be) answered prenatally, and the worry about the mother's well-being is greatly diminished. One might think that this would reduce the apprehension experienced by pregnant women, but these anxieties have been replaced by others which many find even more stressful. The fear of the unknown has now largely been replaced by the fear of what can be known, and by anxiety due to the degree of uncertainty that accompanies information obtained in some ways (screening tests)[1–5] and the risks to the pregnancy involved with obtaining more definite information[6–9]. The anxiety now is generated by the decisions which must be made – to know or not to know, to take the risks of invasive procedures or not to take them, to consider terminating a less than perfect pregnancy or to accept what God or nature provide, and even how to terminate if such a course of action is decided upon[10–12].

In addition to the anxiety engendered by having to make difficult decisions, the existence of prenatal screening and diagnostic tests has caused many couples to attempt to keep an emotional distance from the baby until it has been demonstrated to be 'normal'[13,14]. This phenomenon of the 'tentative pregnancy'[15] is becoming ever more common. Many couples do not tell their family, friends, or colleagues about the pregnancy until they have the results of prenatal tests. In addition to the emotional isolation this may cause, it has practical implications: for example, it is difficult to obtain time off work for antenatal clinic appointments or to be excused from certain physically difficult or even dangerous tasks if one's employer is unaware of a pregnancy. We do not know what, if any, effect this early denial of emotions has on the parents' ability to make a relationship with their child after birth.

We also do not know how many women having had some doubt raised during their pregnancy about the baby's condition retain that doubt after the birth, even if the baby appears to be entirely normal. I am reminded of the extreme case of Roberta. She had a chorionic villus sampling (CVS) for advanced maternal age. The direct chromosome result was normal male, but the culture did not grow. She was told that there was a possibility of missing subtle rearrangements on the direct, and she decided to have an amniocentesis. The result of the amniocentesis was normal except for one cell which was trisomic for chromosome 21. She was advised that this was likely to be a cultural artifact, but that low level mosaicism could not be ruled out. She went on to have a fetal blood sampling which revealed a normal karyotype. This, of course, still could not completely rule out low level mosaicism. After the birth of her son, Roberta was unable to relax and accept that he did not have Down Syndrome or some other abnormality. All the doctors said that he was normal, and he appeared to be normal, but she felt that there must be something wrong with him. In the face of this anxiety, he was, not surprisingly, a 'difficult' baby. She came to see me when deciding whether or not to embark on another pregnancy. She said that she felt unable to cope with her first child and thought she was a bad mother. She also said that she could not face going through prenatal tests in another pregnancy but that she felt unable to forgo having tests.

Joan's words expressed the same problem. She wrote in a personal communication '... if you live with a specific fear for many months, the stress cannot be switched off just like that. It has become a way of life. Even the reassuring sight of a healthy baby doesn't do it. It is just too difficult to believe, and there remains the fear of relaxing one's guard: something may still come to light, anything may still go wrong. There is even a reluctance to accept the doctor's opinion that all is as it should be.'

I will not discuss here the profound emotional reaction suffered by couples who undergo termination of pregnancy for fetal abnormality, as this issue is the subject of another chapter in this volume.

Screening tests

It is a fact that most people would rather have a 'normal' baby than one with some form of disability. For many people, but by no means all, the option of terminating the pregnancy if the fetus is abnormal is preferable to delivering a disabled baby. People who feel this way may welcome the chance to have screening tests in order to know more about their fetus before it is born. In so far as such tests are carried out with both expertise and humanity, and are carried out only on those who have given informed consent[16–20], it is to be hoped that the overall good done will outweigh the overall harm. Parental choice will have been increased; people will have more control over their own lives. However, there are many pitfalls to be overcome if these conditions are to prevail.

WHY DO WOMEN HAVE TESTS?

In western countries, a large proportion of pregnant women are offered an array of prenatal screening tests. The aim (as far as the carers are concerned) is to identify those pregnant women who may be carrying fetuses affected with congenital anomalies. The aim (as far as the women are concerned) is to be reassured that the babies are normal[21,22]. This difference in motivation is the cause of a great many problems. Many mothers have a screening test without being encouraged to consider the fact that the test could give a positive result and what that would mean in terms of future decision making[23]. Staff are faced with a dilemma: to insist that all women consider the possibility of a positive result means inducing stress in a large number of women who will, in the event, have a negative result; to collude with women who wish to think of the test as being a method of reassurance will result in some women having the test who later bitterly regret having to make the sorts of decisions with which they are then faced. All too often, we are faced with women who have received a positive serum screening result for Down Syndrome who are completely unprepared for dealing with it. One such woman wrote: 'I felt that if all it took was a simple blood sample to reassure myself that my child did not have spina bifida, Down Syndrome or anencephaly, then I would be a fool to turn it down. We weren't offered abnormality testing when I had my first baby four years ago. Surely this was progress?'[24]

The decision of whether or not to have a screening test (and if so which type(s)) may sometimes be more difficult for the better informed woman than for the less well informed. If she fully understands the nature and purpose of the screening test and what decisions she might have to make in the wake of the result, a woman is likely to be anxious. By contrast, the woman who has the test 'just to make sure the baby is all right' may be less anxious at the outset but extremely upset in the event of a positive result and extremely angry in the face of a false negative result.

I am reminded of Joyce who came to see me because she wanted to have serum screening for Down Syndrome. She was in her late thirties and had finally achieved a pregnancy as a consequence of her third *in vitro* fertilization (IVF) treatment. She had had a low risk result from her nuchal translucency scan and now wished to have serum screening. She was annoyed that I wanted to waste her time by discussing the test with her, and said that she had never had counselling before or after any of her IVF treatments and did not see why she should have any before a simple blood test. Joyce told me that under no circumstances would she have an amniocentesis, as the thought of causing herself to lose this long awaited pregnancy was far too terrible. When I asked why she wanted to have serum screening, she was unable to answer. She thought maybe it was for reassurance. I pointed out that a significant proportion of women her age did not get reassurance from the test, because they received a high risk result. After a lengthy discussion she said that she would rather not have serum screening because it might leave her very worried for the rest of her pregnancy. Joyce was made anxious by our discussion, and because she was not screened, I do not know whether, in her case, our session increased her anxiety unnecessarily or whether it saved her from an agonizing dilemma later.

WHEN DIFFERENT SCREENING TESTS GIVE CONFLICTING RESULTS

Screening tests, by definition, are not diagnostic, although some tests (such as ultrasound) can be screening tests for some conditions and diagnostic tests for others at the same time. Because screening tests will have false positives and false negatives, it is to be expected that many women having more than one type of test to screen for the same condition will be faced with contradictory results. For example, a 38-year-old woman is 'screen positive' for Down Syndrome using age as a screening test. If she then has the nuchal translucency test and the measurement is 1.5 mm, she will be informed that she is now 'screen negative' for Down Syndrome. If she proceeds to have serum screening and has a risk estimate of 1 in 140, she will be told she is 'screen positive' for Down Syndrome. If she waits and has an anomaly scan in which no abnormalities or markers for aneuploidy are found and the fetus is appropriately grown, she will be told she is 'screen negative' for Down Syndrome. What is she to think? What is she to do? Decision making is always stressful, even in the best circumstances; such contradictory information can hardly provide the best circumstances.

GESTATIONAL AGE AND SCREENING – WHEN SHOULD IT BE DONE?

There is a general feeling among both pregnant women and their carers that the earlier prenatal tests can be done and any subsequent terminations of pregnancy can be performed, the less stressful that will be for the woman[25–29]. This may well be true, although we have no proof of it. An ongoing study at the Centre for Family Research in Cambridge is addressing this issue. The benefits of a test being done early must be balanced against the fact that a large proportion of abnormal fetuses will miscarry naturally if given sufficient time[30–32]. The earlier we do prenatal tests, the more abnormal fetuses we will identify. This means that more women will be faced with that agonizing decision which they so often report as being the hardest thing about the pregnancy loss[33].

Anxiety generated and/or relieved by tests

Virtually all staff who counsel women either before or after screening tests will say that the tests generate a great deal of anxiety. However, it is also true that negative results relieve anxiety[34]. The question one must consider is the extent to which the anxiety relieved would have been there in the absence of the tests or whether the anxiety allayed by negative results was that which was first created by the test as some investigators argue[35]. Studies have been done to look at this issue[36–38] but they are hampered by the fact that women who are more anxious about fetal abnormality are more likely to have tests. Most studies measuring anxiety in tested and untested women are therefore not comparing like with like. A woman who desperately wants to have prenatal screening and/or diagnostic tests and is not able to have them will probably remain a good deal more anxious than a woman who never wanted to have the tests. We must incorporate in our thinking the fact that some of the anxiety caused by the tests is caused by their mere existence and the possibility of having them – even if they are not offered to a particular woman.

Routine anomaly scanning

Screening and diagnosis done on 'routine second trimester ultrasound' is almost always done without informed consent[39]. Carers rarely explain to the pregnant woman that the primary reason for the 'routine' anomaly scan is to look for abnormalities; nor do they ask whether she would want to know if the baby had an abnormality. Women are spared the anxiety such a discussion would generate, but the ordinary 'low risk' woman is totally unprepared if she is told after an anomaly scan that an abnormality or a marker for aneuploidy has been identified. Such a woman (and her partner) are then required to make decisions about whether or not to have invasive tests and/or whether or not to terminate the pregnancy.

Diagnostic tests (invasive procedures and non-routine ultrasound)

IN THE 'HIGH RISK' PREGNANCY

Diagnostic tests may be done because the pregnancy has been known to be high risk from the beginning. The couple are likely to be chronically anxious about the pregnancy even before it is conceived, and to be worried about having the test and about the results. They will not, however, be shocked at being offered a test. Such couples would, in the past, have suffered intense anxiety throughout the pregnancy, if they had the courage to embark on a pregnancy at all. Now, if they are lucky, the bulk of the worry can be limited to the early months of the pregnancy. Although they will be grateful for the existence of tests, they will still find such investigations highly stressful, and they should be offered support before, during and after the whole process.

IN THE 'LOW RISK' PREGNANCY

Couples who started the pregnancy as 'low risk' and were moved into the 'high risk' group because of something discovered about the pregnancy (such as a screening result) will suddenly be made acutely anxious[40]. For these couples, the existence of the tests has significantly damaged their enjoyment of the pregnancy. If the concerns eventually prove to be unjustified, there can be little doubt that in their cases the tests have done more harm than good. If, however, the concerns prove to be warranted, and the couple decide not to go ahead with an affected pregnancy, they may feel that the harm done to their experience of pregnancy was a price well worth paying.

ANXIETY LEVELS FOLLOWING INVASIVE DIAGNOSTIC TESTS

One of the benefits that people seek to obtain from having invasive diagnostic tests is reduction in the worry that they will have an affected baby, and they hope to experience a general reduction in anxiety. In other words, not only will the test ensure that they avoid the birth of a live baby with a specified abnormality but it will also give them peace of mind for the remainder of the pregnancy. While some studies demonstrate this 'peace of mind effect'[41], other do not; the latter have not found women with negative amniocentesis results to be less anxious than untested controls[42]. In the case of non-randomized studies, this must be at least partly due to self-selection (those who chose to have the invasive procedure were women with initially a higher level of anxiety than those who did not choose to have the test). Common sense tells us that a woman with a specific and reasonable worry about her baby having a chromosome abnormality will be more anxious if she remains untested than if she has a negative test result. This may not be true of a woman who is just generally anxious about the pregnancy; such a woman having ruled out a chromosome abnormality may just focus her worries on some other potential problem. It would appear that in large part, a woman's reaction to the process of prenatal diagnosis is determined by her reason for having it[43–45].

THE DECISION ABOUT WHETHER OR NOT TO HAVE INVASIVE TESTS

All women deciding whether to have an invasive test should consider whether they would wish to know antenatally if the baby had an abnormality and how they would use that information. They need to think about whether they want the information the investigation would provide enough to take the risks involved in having the test. The decision is likely to be influenced by such factors as: how great they perceive the risk of abnormality to be and how undesirable they think the abnormality in question would be, whether or not they have any other children, how difficult it was to achieve the pregnancy, whether they have suffered one or more pregnancy losses (particularly post-procedure losses), their age, and their perception of the likelihood of becoming pregnant again if they lost this pregnancy. It is also influenced by how the counselling is done and by whom[46,47].

When considering the above, women (and their partners) may feel under a great deal of pressure from family, friends, doctors, midwives and society in general to 'be responsible' and have tests which have been offered. The prevailing ethos in western society is that if something can be known, it should be known; and if it can be done, it should be done. It is a brave person who can say 'no'. No matter how non-directive carers try to be, the fact that people are offered testing to see if the baby has a particular condition implies that society (as represented by the carers) thinks that parents should prefer not to have children with that condition[48,49].

Getting the results of tests

Waiting for important news which will affect the rest of one's life is extremely stressful. Most of us have experienced the agony of dreading every time the phone rings because we are waiting to hear what might be very bad news. Similarly, the palpitations that can accompany every delivery from the postman are known to a number of us. It is inhumane to make people wait longer than necessary to obtain the results of tests. It is also unkind to spread out the anxiety. They should know, for example, if there will definitely not be a result for a specified period of time; this will at least make that period a bit less stressful.

People should never leave after having a prenatal screening or diagnostic test without knowing how, when and from whom they will be able to find out the result. If possible, they should be given some choice in the matter. For example, while many people prefer to be given the results over the phone, some find it more acceptable to make an appointment to come in to be given the results in person. This gives them a good deal of control about how, when, where and from whom they will hear. The practice of 'no news is good news', is extremely inhumane. How is a woman/couple to be sure that because the 'bad news' letter or phone call did not come today, it will not come tomorrow? When should she/they stop worrying? Anxiety levels in women who are not given their negative results stay high for longer and may remain higher for some time[50].

If the investigation in question provides an immediate result, such as happens with an ultrasound scan, provision needs to be made for the woman to be given the results at the time of the investigation. The woman needs to know from the beginning whether she will be 'talked through' the scan or whether the operator will be quiet for fairly long periods and explain later. An unexpected silence may be interpreted as a problem having been seen and may cause great apprehension even when that is unwarranted. It is unacceptable to send people off after a scan without a clear explanation of what is known and what is not known. If a sonographer sees or suspects he/she sees an abnormality, it is likely that this information will communicate itself to the woman in a number of ways, even if she is not told. A period of intense anxiety will ensue until an explanation is given. If the sonographer is not thought to be the best person to explain what has been seen on the scan, then another appropriate person needs to be available whenever scans are being done[51–53].

How parents interpret what is said to them

A forthcoming baby is incredibly important to a couple for a whole variety of reasons including: to love and be loved, to nurture, to cement their relationship, to let them into the 'parents' club', and to enhance their status due to the child being a desirable one. Because the baby remains somewhat of an enigma until it is born, the future parents are uncertain as to how well it will fulfil these roles. This uncertainty about something which is so important makes them extremely sensitive to real or imagined clues which they perceive. For example, a woman of advanced maternal age said to me that she was particularly worried about Down Syndrome because the sonographer had asked her if she was having screening for Down Syndrome the moment she saw the fetus on the screen. The woman took this to mean that something which the sonographer had seen had made her suspicious that the fetus had Down Syndrome. In fact, it was an 8-week dating scan, and nothing untoward had been seen. The timing of the question was unfortunate.

Non-verbal communication

It is also important to remember that we 'say' things in more ways than words: the expression on our faces, the tone of our voices, the way we stand or sit, the colleagues we do or do not call in, whether or not we offer a photo of a scan, and so on. All of these will be interpreted (perhaps incorrectly) by the woman or couple. A doctor who is rushed or who is feeling unwell and is consequently uncommunicative may be seen as a doctor who is hiding a piece of bad news. If care is not taken to ensure that people know what there is to know, we may be guilty of causing a great deal of unnecessary anxiety over a long period of time.

The offer of a termination of pregnancy

An offer of a termination of pregnancy for fetal abnormality is usually regarded as a suggestion that this would be a good idea and therefore an implication that the fetus is very severely affected. As one woman who was offered a termination for 47 XXX put it to me, 'I knew my baby must be severely abnormal, otherwise why would they have offered me a termination?' Such offers made with the intention of giving a couple the full range of choices can, in fact, be very hurtful and confusing. That particular woman, who decided to carry on with the pregnancy, commented that she wished she did not know the baby's karyotype and that it had completely spoiled her pregnancy.

This might be a good place to consider the difference (for the parents) between carers offering a termination of pregnancy and agreeing to that course of action if it is requested. There is a tendency to offer termination of pregnancy when certain fetal abnormalities are diagnosed even if those abnormalities would not be serious enough to justify doing the termination for an indication of '... a substantial risk that if the child were born it would suffer from such physical or mental abnormalities as to be seriously handicapped'. The thought is that it is the parents' right to know that termination is an option, and thus on both ethical and medico-legal grounds the offer should be made. However, the same argument could be used to offer termination to all pregnant women seen in the first trimester in countries allowing termination on social grounds. This is not, however, the usual practice. Normally, it is a question of agreeing to an explicit request or, in exceptional cases, of asking if the woman is considering termination. If it is felt to be appropriate to offer termination of a 'less than perfect' fetus in the absence of a request for it, parents might find it helpful to know if such a termination would be done because of 'a substantial risk of serious handicap' or because they would not wish to carry on with the pregnancy in the circumstances.

What does the word 'abnormal' mean?

We might also consider the different meanings which can be attached to the word abnormal. According the *Shorter Oxford Dictionary*, it means both 'unusual' and 'a monstrosity ... like a calf born with two heads'. If one includes both definitions, Einstein and Mozart are as abnormal as an anencephalic. The problem is that we sometimes use the word abnormal to mean 'differing from the norm', but the parents are apt to interpret it as meaning 'a monstrosity'. In addition to this, we may be referring to an unusual laboratory finding which is unlikely to have significant phenotypic expression, but the parents may again envision a severely 'abnormal' child (one with extremely undesirable characteristics). To say to parents that their child has an abnormality but is unlikely to be abnormal seems at best very confusing. Such parents will certainly feel they are being given mixed messages. If our intention is to convey the idea of a result being different from the norm but not 'bad', then we might make ourselves clearer by using words like 'unusual' or 'variant' rather than 'abnormal'.

When an abnormality is diagnosed – to terminate or to continue the pregnancy?

When a serious abnormality is diagnosed, the parents have to make what is likely to be the most difficult decision of their lives[54,55], and they may have to make it very quickly. As Caroline wrote in a poem to her baby, 'Please forgive me if I did wrong, I had to make choices and I didn't have too long'. The problem is, firstly, that there may be no acceptable option available. Most of us would not consider that we were being given much choice if we were offered only two alternatives – to have our child maimed or to have it killed. But we regularly have to ask couples to choose between two such unacceptable options.

Secondly, most couples having to decide between the two alternatives have never experienced either of them and can only imagine what they would be like. For example, most couples deciding whether or not to terminate a pregnancy in which the fetus has Down Syndrome have never looked after a Down Syndrome child and have never undergone a termination of pregnancy for fetal abnormality. The same can be said of most of the professionals who care for such couples.

As one woman, herself a doctor, wrote after she had a termination of pregnancy for fetal abnormality, 'A choice sounded better than not having a choice. Yet, the idea of choosing was overwhelming and confusing. We were devastated at the thought of either course of action ... For me, though, an earlier miscarriage paled in comparison with this. At least that was straightforward, and there was comfort in the fact that there was nothing I could have done to prevent it'[56]. Such a decision cannot be anything but highly stressful. However, there are many circumstances in which it becomes even more difficult:

- When the parents are ethically opposed to all termination of pregnancy for any reason but feel that in this case it is the best alternative. As Anita wrote in a letter to her terminated baby 10 years after the termination, 'I regret my decision very much. I feel guilty and I ask you to forgive me. I have done the worst possible thing a mother could do to a child ... I suffer up to this day and think I should be punished by God in the future'

- When the parents would wish to terminate but this would make them pariahs within the context of their church, family, or cultural group
- When one of them wishes to carry on with the pregnancy and the other thinks that termination would be a better course of action
- When they wish to carry on with the pregnancy but think that their carers and/or society will condemn them for this
- When they have a living child with the condition which the unborn child has. As John, the father of a William's Syndrome daughter, said, 'What would it say about our daughter if we terminated another pregnancy because of William's Syndrome?'
- When the diagnosis and/or prognosis is unclear and/or they are given conflicting information by different professionals

What to tell other people in the continuing pregnancy

Parents who decide to continue the pregnancy in which a diagnosis of fetal abnormality has been made have to decide what to tell other people. If the abnormality is incompatible with prolonged extrauterine life and they tell others, they risk many people making hurtful comments about what they perceive as the pointlessness in continuing the pregnancy. If they do not tell people, they have to, as Karen (a psychiatrist who continued to term with a baby suffering from renal agenesis) said, '... brave many kindly inquiries as to what we wanted and whether we were excited and how much I had knitted or bought in preparation[57].'

If the condition is compatible with extrauterine life and is not obvious to those who do not know laboratory results, there is the question of who to tell and when to tell them. There is also the question of how and when to tell the child him/herself. These issues are illustrated with antenatally detected sex-chromosome abnormalities. Parents fear, not without justification, that if others (such as the child's teachers) know, the child will be labelled as 'different'. Although there may be some benefits to others knowing, the benefits may well be outweighed by the disadvantages. The phenomenon of the self-fulfilling prophecy should not be ignored[58,59]. The question of how and when to tell a boy with Klinefelter syndrome, for example, that he will be infertile is one which causes much parental anxiety, and I have heard more than one mother say that she wished she did not know this information about her child. Parents should be told from the outset that they will be offered the chance to discuss these issues with appropriate professionals.

Conclusion

Prenatal screening/diagnosis is a two-edged sword. It enables us to give parents choices which were unheard of just a generation ago. It has the potential to alleviate much suffering. At the same time, it has the potential to cause great suffering (largely in the form of anxiety). The biggest challenge to all those involved in antenatal care today is to find a way of wielding this sword such that the benefits to most people outweigh the harm. This can be achieved only if women are enabled to give truly informed consent before all antenatal screening/diagnostic investigations, if the investigations are carried out as humanely as possible, the results given as quickly and sensitively as possible, and if high quality counselling is offered at all stages in the procedure.

REFERENCES

1. Berne-Fromell K, Uddenberg N, Kjessler B. Psychological reactions experienced by pregnant women with elevated S-AFP level. *J Psychosom Obstet Gynaecol* **2**:233, 1983.
2. Burton BK, Dillard RG, Clark EN. The psychological impact of positive elevations of maternal serum alpha-protein. *Am J Obstet Gynecol* **151**:77–82, 1985.
3. Burton BK, Dillard RG, Clark EN. Maternal serum alpha-fetoprotein screening: the effect of participation on anxiety and attitude toward pregnancy in women with normal results. *Am J Obstet Gynecol* **152**:540–543, 1985.
4. Roelofsen EEC, Kamerbeek LI, Tymstra TJ. Chances and choices. Psycho-social consequences of maternal serum screening. A report from the Netherlands. *J Reprod Inf Psychol* **11**:41–47, 1993.
5. Statham H, Green J. Serum screening for Down's syndrome; some women's experiences. *Br Med J* **307**:174–176, 1993.
6. Candian Medical Research Council. Diagnosis of genetic disease by amniocentesis during the second trimester of pregnancy (report no. 5). Ottawa: Minister of Supplies and Services, 1977.
7. NICHD National Registry for Amniocentesis Study Group. Mid-trimester amniocentesis for prenatal diagnosis: safety and accuracy. *JAMA* **236**:1471, 1976.
8. Canadian Collaborative CVS-Amniocentesis Clinical Trial Group. Multicentre randomized clinical trial of chorionic villus sampling and amniocentesis. *Lancet* **i**:1–6, 1989.
9. MRC Working Party on the Evaluation of chorion villus sampling. Medical Research Council European trial of chorion villus sampling. *Lancet* **337**:1491–1499, 1991.
10. Green JM. Calming or harming? A critical review of psychological effects of fetal diagnosis on pregnant women. London: Galton Institute Occasional Papers, Second Series, No. 2, 1990.
11. Abramsky L, Chapple J. *Prenatal Diagnosis: The Human Side*. London: Chapman and Hall, 1994
12. Davies BL. Decision making in prenatal genetic diagnosis. *Iss Health Care Women* **4**:69–76, 1983.
13. Caccia N, Johnson JM, Robinson GE, Barna T. Impact of prenatal testing on maternal-fetal bonding: chorionic villus sampling versus amniocentisis. *Am J Obstet Gynecol* **165**(4):1122–1125, 1991.

14. Sjogren B, Uddenberg N. Prenatal diagnosis and maternal attachment to the child-to-be. *J Psychosom Obstet Gynaecol* **9**:73–87, 1988.
15. Katz-Rothman B. *The Tentative Pregnancy: Prenatal Diagnosis and the Future of Motherhood.* New York: Viking, 1986.
16. Abramsky L. Counselling prior to prenatal testing. In *Prenatal Diagnosis: the Human Side* (eds L. Abramsky & J. Chapple). London: Chapman and Hall, 1994.
17. Davis AJ. Informed consent: how much information is enough? *Nurs Outl* **33**:40–42, 1985.
18. Donnai D. The management of the patient having fetal diagnosis. *Baill Clin Obstet Gynaecol* **1**:737–745, 1987.
19. Reid M. Consumer-oriented studies in relation to prenatal screening tests. *Eur J Obstet Gynecol Reprod Biol* **28** (Suppl):79–82, 1988.
20. Faulder C. *Whose Body Is It? The Troubling Issue of Informed Consent.* London: Virago, 1985.
21. Farrant W. Who's for amniocentesis? The politics of prenatal screening. In *The Sexual Politics of Reproduction* (ed. H. Homans). London: Gower, 1985.
22. Green J, Snowdon D, Statham H. Pregnant women's attitudes to abortion and prenatal screening. *J Reprod Inf Psychol* **11**:31–39, 1993.
23. Marteau TM, Slack J, Kidd J, Shaw RW. Presenting a routine screening test in antenatal care: practice observed. *Publ Health* **106**:131–141, 1992.
24. Radice S. Tested and found wanting. *The Guardian,* London, 3 January, 1995.
25. Bryce R, Bradley MT, McCormick SM. To what extent would women prefer chorionic villus sampling to amniocentesis for prenatal diagnosis? *Paed Perin Epidemiol* **3**:137–145, 1989.
26. Lippmann A, Perry TB, Mandel S *et al.* Chorionic villi sampling: women's attitudes. *J Med Genet* **22**:395–401, 1985.
27. McGovern MM, Goldberg JD, Desnick RJ. Acceptability of chorionic villi sampling for prenatal diagnosis. *Am J Obstet Gynecol* **155**:25–29, 1986.
28. Verp MS, Bombard AT, Simpson JL. Parental decision following prenatal diagnosis of fetal chromosome anomalies. *Am J Med Genet* **29**:613–622, 1988.
29. Turner L. Problems surrounding late prenatal diagnosis. In *Prenatal Diagnosis: the Human Side* (eds L. Abramsky & J. Chapple). London: Chapman and Hall, 1994.
30. Harper P. *Practical Genetic Counselling.* Bristol: John Wright, 1981.
31. Carr DH, Gedeon M. Population cytogenetics of human abortuses. In *Population Cytogenetics. Studies in Human Reproduction* (eds E.B. Hook & I.H. Porter). New York: Academic Press, 1977.
32. Hassold T, Chan N, Funkhouser J *et al.* A cytogenetic study of 1000 spontaneous abortions. *Ann Hum Genet* **44**:151–178, 1980.
33. Statham H. Parents' reactions to termination of pregnancy for fetal abnormality: from a mother's point of view. In *Prenatal Diagnosis: the Human Side* (eds L. Abramsky & J. Chapple). London: Chapman and Hall, 1994
34. Marteau T. Johnston M, Shaw R, Michie S, Kidd J, New M. The impact of prenatal screening and diagnostic testing upon the cognitions, emotions and behaviour of pregnant women. *J Psychosom Res* **33**:(1), 7–16, 1989.
35. Kolker A. Advances in prenatal diagnosis: social-psychological and policy issues. *Int J Technol Assess Health Care* **5**:601–617, 1989.
36. Marteau TM. Psychological aspects of prenatal testing for fetal abnormalities. *Irish J Psychol* **12**:121–132, 1991.
37. Statham H, Green J, Snowdon C. Psychological and social aspects of screening for fetal abnormality during routine antenatal care. In *Proceedings of Research and the Midwife*, November, 1992.
38. Lippman A. Prenatal genetic testing and screening: Constructing needs and reinforcing inequities. In *Genetic Counselling: Practice and Principles* (ed. A. Clarke). London: Routledge, 1994.
39. Chervenak FA, McCullough LB, Chervenak JL. Prenatal informed consent for sonogram. *Am J Obstet Gynecol* **161**:857–860, 1989.
40. Farrant S. Stress after amniocentesis for high serum alpha-fetoprotein concentrations, *Br Med J* **281**:452, 1980.
41. Beeson D, Golbus MS. Anxiety engendered by amniocentesis. *Birth Defects Orig Articl Ser* **15**:191–197, 1979.
42. Fava GA, Kellner R, Michelacci L *et al.* Psychological reactions to amniocentesis: a controlled study. *Am J Obstet Gynecol* **143**:509–513, 1982.
43. Tabor A, Jonsson MH. Psychological impact of amniocentesis in low risk women. *Prenat Diagn* **7**:443–449, 1987.
44. Evers-Kiebooms G, Swerts A, van den Berghe H. Psychological aspects of amniocentesis: anxiety feelings in three different risk groups. *Clin Genet* **33**:196–206, 1988.
45. Roghmann KJ, Doherty RA. Reassurance through prenatal diagnosis and willingness to bear children after age 35. *Am J Publ Health* **73**:760–762, 1983.
46. Marteau T, Drake H, Bobrow M. Counselling following diagnosis of a fetal abnormality: the differing approaches of obstetricians, clinical geneticists and genetic nurses. *J Med Genet* **31**:864–867, 1994.
47. Holmes-Siedle MN, Rynanen M, Lindenbaum RH. Parental decisions regarding termination of pregnancy following prenatal detection of sex chromosome abnormality. *Prenat Diagn* **7**:239–244, 1987.
48. Clarke A. Is non-directive genetic counselling possible? *Lancet* **338**:998–1001, 1991.
49. Sjogren B, Uddenberg N. Decision making during the prenatal diagnostic procedure. A questionnaire and interview study of 211 women participating in prenatal diagnosis. *Prenat Diagn* **8**:263–273, 1988.
50. Fearn J, Hibbard BM, Laurence KM, Roberts A, Robinson JO. Screening for neural-tube defects and maternal anxiety, *Br J Obstet Gynaecol* **89**:218–221, 1982.
51. Hollingsworth J. The sonographer's dilemma. In *Prenatal Diagnosis: the Human Side* (eds L. Abramsky & J. Chapple). London: Chapman and Hall, 1994.
52. *Support After Termination for Abnormality. Guidelines for Ultrasonographers.* Rugby: Support After Termination for Abnormality, 1992.
53. Cox DN, Wittmann BK, Hess M, Ross AG, Lind J, Lindahl S. The psychological impact of diagnostic ultrasound. *Obstet Gynecol* **70**:673–676, 1987.
54. White-van Mourik M. Looking in from the outside. In *Prenatal Diagnosis: the Human Side* (eds L. Abramsky & J. Chapple). London: Chapman and Hall, 1994.
55. White-van Mourik M. Termination of a second-trimester pregnancy for fetal anormality: psychosocial aspects. In *Genetic Counselling: Practice and Principles* (ed. A. Clarke). London: Routledge, 1994.
56. Brown J (pseudonym). A piece of my mind: the choice. *JAMA* **262**(19):2735, 1989.
57. Palmer K. Peace and pain. *Br Med J* **309**:279, 1994.
58. Garrett C, Carlton L. Difficult decisions in prenatal diagnosis. In *Prenatal Diagnosis: the Human Side* (eds L. Abramsky & J. Chapple). London: Chapman and Hall, 1994.
59. Puck MH. Some considerations bearing on the doctrine of self-fulfilling prophesy in sex chromosome aneuploidy. *Am J Med Genet* **9**:129–137, 1981.

Termination of pregnancy: methods, safety and recent developments

30

H. El-Refaey

Introduction

The introduction of new technologies to medicine throughout history has resulted in the development of better and safer procedures. Advances in technology have not always paralleled one another. Thus the advances in the diagnosis of major fetal anomalies that started with the introduction of ultrasound scanning in the 1960s were not matched by similar progress in the methods of abortion. Apart from the psychological distress associated with interrupting a wanted pregnancy, patients had to endure a variety of cumbersome abortion procedures. Most of these were not only invasive but were associated with protracted induction–abortion intervals, sometimes of several days. It is estimated, for example, that intra-amniotic hypertonic saline, when used alone, will terminate pregnancy within 24 hours in 20% of cases, in 48 hours in 85% and 72 hours in 97%[1]. The nature of these procedures was always a cause of major concern to patients, nursing staff and gynaecologists alike. Throughout the last two decades up to 30 different regimens have been proposed for second trimester abortion, indicating the extent of the problem.

The seriousness of psychological morbidity and lengthy induction–abortion interval is far outweighed by the physical morbidity associated with terminating pregnancies. Morbidity from abortion in general is known to increase with advancing gestational age. For example, a delay in abortion from 8 to 10 weeks increases the risk of major complication by 60%. Delay in abortion from 8 to 16 weeks' gestation increases the risk by 300–1300% depending on the abortion technique used[2].

Historically, methods of inducing abortion in the second trimester may be divided into two categories:

- Surgical, involving either uterine evacuation via the vaginal route (dilatation and evacuation) or uterine surgery such as hysterotomy or hysterectomy.
- Medical, predominantly involving intrauterine instillation of prostaglandins or hyperosmolar solutions. Intravenous oxytocin was frequently used as an adjuvant, particularly when the abortion process initiated by the intrauterine injection or instillation was slow.

Today, second trimester termination of advanced pregnancies due to anomalies or for social reasons is still an area that is surrounded by huge ethical and legal difficulties. Scientific communities worldwide therefore developed, often independently, their own regimens to handle this problem. Currently, practices vary widely from the complex life-threatening approach of the use of intra-amniotic infusion of hypertonic saline to the simple use of vaginal and oral misoprostol tablets.

It is not possible or beneficial to discuss all the different methods and regimens used to terminate pregnancies within the context of this chapter. However, two important developments have been the introduction of mifepristone, and subsequently misoprostol, to the field of abortion induction in general and to the second trimester in particular. The use of these two medications has simplified second trimester abortion considerably and it is now recognized that 50% of patients using the regimen detailed in Table 30.1 will abort in less than 6 h. The safety and simplicity of this approach will no doubt make other means of second trimster abortion obsolete. This chapter will therefore discuss in some depth the background of the use of mifepristone and misoprostol. Other methods for second trimester abortion will be discussed if they provide a background to changes in technology.

Surgical evacuation of the pregnant uterus

VACUUM ASPIRATION

Prior to 9 weeks' gestation, medical abortion is known to be acceptable to women and highly effective, with a success rate

TABLE 30.1
Clinical protocol for induction of abortion in second and third trimesters for fetal anomalies and antepartum fetal death

Stage 1.	Oral mifepristone (RU 486) 600 mg as soon as possible. Following administration, the woman is allowed home and asked to return to the labour ward 36–48 hours later.
Stage 2.	Induction of labour with misoprostol: First dosage: 800 μg vaginally Three hours later: 400 μg orally Every 3 h subsequently: 400 μg orally (maximum four dosages)

Patients with IUD or congenital anomaly might refuse to wait for 48 h prior to commencing misoprostol. In this case, administer RU 486 with the first misoprostol dose. However, if mifepristone (RU 486) is not available, Stage 2 may be carried out without prior treatment.

In cases of failure of the above regimen:

A	Repeat mifepristone (RU 486) with the last misoprostol dose
B	Repeat the misoprostol regimen as above

Remember complications can happen: ruptured uterus and infection are recognized complications.
High vaginal swabs, ultrasound scan (USS) and vaginal examination should be taken at this stage.

of around 95%[3]. However, the efficacy and patient acceptability of medical abortion are known to decrease with increasing gestational age[3,4] and therefore this method is only offered to women of less than 9 weeks' gestation. However, since only 20% of women in the UK undertake abortion prior to this gestation age, surgical abortion is likely to remain a widely performed operation[5]. Outside Europe, medical abortion is not an option: late presentation and the controversy surrounding the drug mifepristone mean that it will be a long time before medical abortion becomes available. In absolute numbers the majority of the 30 million terminations that are carried out every year are performed surgically and the safety of the operation is therefore a global public health issue.

The inherent risk associated with surgical abortion relates to the use of general anaesthesia and the invasive nature of the procedure. Induction of abortion under local anaesthesia is widely practised in the United States and is thought to increase the safety of the procedure. While this may be the case, in the UK, concerns about the acceptability of this approach has led to a situation in which the vast majority of cases are performed under general anaesthesia.

Techniques of dilating the cervix to pass an instrument into the uterus remained unchanged for more than two-and-a-half millennia until the middle of the nineteenth century. In 1874, Alfred Hegar demonstrated the operation of dilatation and curettage (D&C) which gained worldwide acceptance as a method of inducing abortion or treating incomplete abortions[6]. Vacuum curettage was first described by a Russian, Bykov, in 1927[7], and in the late 1950s Wu and Wu in the *Chinese Medical Journal of Obstetrics and Gynaecology* described electric vacuum suction curettage[8].

The safety of suction curettage became established after the Ljubljana study. This large comparative study established that in the first trimester, suction curettage was faster, and resulted in lower rates of perforation, haemorrhage and subsequent infection than sharp curettage[9]. Several retrospective studies have subsequently confirmed this and shown that the sharp curettage has a major complication rate 2.3 times higher than suction curettage[2,10,11].

The benefits of this change in technology had a wide effect on gynaecological practice. In the United Kingdom by 1985 more than 80% of all abortion cases were performed by suction curettage[12]. In the United States between 1972 and 1988 suction curettage had increased from 65% to 95% of first trimester abortions[13]. In Europe by 1990 it was estimated that 95% of all first trimester terminations were performed by suction curettage[14]. In developing countries, however, where most physicians are not trained in suction curettage and do not have the necessary equipment, sharp curettage is still widely practised.

DILATATION AND EVACUATION

Instrumental abortion in the second trimester is an invasive procedure that was made safer by changes in the technology and improvements in the atmosphere surrounding the abortion service. However, the skill of the operator is still one of the most important factors affecting the outcome of the procedure[2,15–17].

The problem of the protracted time required to achieve abortion by medical means led North American gynaecologists to rely on surgical abortion up to 20 weeks' gestation despite the distressing nature of the operation. Dilatation and evacuation (D&E), although an unpleasant operation to perform, is now the only surgical alternative to medical means for inducing second trimester abortions. Cervical priming is mandatory to allow easy dilatation of the cervix to 14 mm so that the relatively large fetal parts can be removed. The extracted fetal parts should be kept together to ensure that all fetal tissues, in particular the fetal spine and skull, have been removed[7]. The procedure is now being increasingly done under ultrasound scan guidance, allowing the surgeon to introduce the instruments safely, so minimizing the risk of perforation; it also allows removal of the placenta prior to the fetus.

Mechanical dilatation of the cervical canal with tapered metal cylinders of increasing diameters is essential to gain access to the uterine cavity. This integral part of the operation is associated with a variety of possible injuries, particularly with advanced gestational age. Cervical tears, uterine perforation and the creation of false passages in the cervix are recognized problems[2]. There is ample evidence that presurgical dilatation of the cervix by a variety of agents is effective in increasing the safety of the operation[16,17]. This important treatment effect has been recognized for a long time and there are reports to indicate that laminaria tents were used in traditional medicine[18].

Intracervical tents are hydrophilic agents that exert their effect by expanding within the cervical canal. The classical laminaria tent is an osmotic dilator made of seaweed sticks which expand to exert pressure on the cervical canal. Lamicel is a polyvinyl alcohol polymer sponge impregnated with magnesium sulphate and compressed to a tent. It expands to form a soft sponge but is not capable of exerting mechanical pressure on the cervical canal. Dilapan is a synthetic tent with an action similar to that of the natural laminaria tent, but seems to produce more rapid cervical dilatation. It is possible that laminaria and Dilapan tents exert their major effect on the cervix by applying a significant force per area for a relatively long time, whereas the Lamicel tents work mainly by taking up fluid from the cervix[19,20]. It is also possible that due to their effect on the cervix all tents may increase tissue production of prostaglandin and this may add to their clinical effect.

The transition from reliance on instillation procedures to curettage operations took almost a decade in the United States. In the early 1970s it was considered that curettage operations were too dangerous to perform after 12 weeks' gestation. It was customary to delay the abortion procedure to 16 weeks so that instillation techniques could be used[21]. Comparative studies in the early 1970s, however, have confirmed that vacuum curettage when performed by experienced surgeons between 13 and 16 weeks is safer than instillation procedures and that there is no observable difference in maternal mortality between the two methods after 16 weeks[15,22].

Although the safety of the operation is now beyond doubt, this may not be the main issue any more, since the medical approach has an equally established safety record. Medical pregnancy termination is preferable in the context of fetal medicine, since the gross fetal and placental anatomy can be examined post mortem and allows confirmation of the ultrasound diagnosis.

Medical abortion

PROSTAGLANDINS

Medical abortion was revolutionised by the introduction of prostaglandins. The efficacy of the procedure was increased considerably when uterine instillation (intra-amniotic or extra-amniotic) of prostaglandins was used in comparison to the use of intrauterine administration of hyperosmolar solutions. For example, when intrauterine hypertonic saline was used, only 20% of women aborted within 24 h[23]. By comparison, 50% of patients abort in less than 18 h when intra-amniotic prostaglandins are used[24].

The improved efficacy of prostaglandin regimens has led to a rapid increase in their usage in the UK. In 1968, prostaglandins were not used in the UK for second trimester abortion. By comparison, 38% of second trimester abortions in 1987 were performed using prostaglandins[25]. A variety of intra-amniotic and extra-amniotic prostaglandin agents were used such as the natural prostaglandin E and $F_2\alpha$ and several other analogues. Regimens have varied, involving single, intermittent or continuous infusion of prostaglandin agents. The extra-amniotic approach, however, has the advantage of being suitable throughout the second trimester, and less invasive than the intra-amniotic installation which is generally reserved for cases beyond 16 weeks' gestation and carries the risk of inadvertent systemic administration[1].

Since it was first introduced in 1968, extra-amniotic administration of prostaglandins has been used for more than 30 years. Although in general less invasive than other techniques, it is unpleasant and cumbersome. The procedure involved inserting a Foley's catheter through the cervix, with a small risk of introducing infection and/or the occasional rapid intake of prostaglandin from the choriodecidual space[26].

In 1989, Hill and MacKenzie provided a summary of the experience of the John Radcliffe Hospital in Oxford. They analysed and compared more than 1600 cases of second trimester termination of pregnancy and 700 cases of intra-amniotic PGE2 instillation. The mean induction–abortion interval of the two routes was similar (16 h). Morbidity rates were similar; vomiting occurred in more than 40% of cases, diarrhoea in 14% and a blood transfusion was required in less than 1% of cases.

The introduction of gemeprost, a prostaglandin E1 analogue, developed in the form of vaginal pessaries, has attracted special interest in this field. It is simple to administer and does not require skilled staff. In the first report examining its use in second trimester abortions, Sakamoto and others have pointed to the effectiveness of gemeprost 1 mg every 3 h being associated with a mean induction to abortion time of 16 h[27]. The use of gemeprost pessaries has also been compared in an open randomized trial with the extra-amniotic infusion of prostaglandin E2 for termination of pregnancy between 12–16 weeks' gestation. Abortion occurred within 24 hours in 77% in the gemeprost group and 79% in the extra-amniotic group. Side-effects were similar in both groups[28].

The administration of the prostaglandin analogues as vaginal pessaries was another important step in minimizing the morbidity of mid-trimester induction of abortion. For decades, research in the field of second trimester abortions has been concerned about the length of the induction–abortion interval. Even with prostaglandin agents such as gemeprost, this interval has been inappropriately long. A review of 900 cases of second trimester abortion has confirmed that the median induction–abortion interval is 16 h (range 1–120 h)[29]. The introduction of mifepristone to this field was important in reducing the induction–abortion interval and its implications will be discussed later.

MIFEPRISTONE (RU 486)

Mifepristone is a 19 nor-steroid which has a threefold greater affinity for the human progesterone receptor than progesterone and an affinity for the glucocorticoid receptor twice that of dexamethasone. It has a lesser affinity for the androgen receptor and does not seem to interact with the oestrogen or mineralocorticoid receptors[30]. It is a derivative of the synthetic progestin, norethindrone. Clinically, mifepristone has been used in trials of menstrual regulation, abortion, induction of labour, during treatment of breast cancer, ovarian cancer, meningiomas and adrenal disorders[31].

It is widely believed that progesterone helps to prevent premature labour by blocking myometrial contractility through an increase in calcium binding to the sarcoplasmic reticulum and myometrial cell membrane[32]. It is also believed that progesterone withdrawal is essential for the changes in uterine contractility normally observed during the secretory phase of the menstrual cycle, and that the inactivity of the early pregnant uterus is progesterone dependent[31].

Mifepristone also increases the uterine response to exogenous prostaglandins. In the uterus unprimed with mifepristone, prostaglandins increase the uterine tone. After priming with mifepristone this increase in tone is accompanied by coordinated contractions with increases in both frequency and amplitude[33,34]. The increase in uterine contractility consequent to mifepristone ingestion is maintained, however, in women in whom prostaglandin synthesis has been inhibited by indomethacin administration. This suggests that mechanisms other than prostaglandin must be involved in the increase in uterine contractility[35].

Clinically, the administration of mifepristone causes softening and dilatation of the cervix, the onset of regular uterine contractions and increased uterine sensitivity to prostaglandins but not to oxytocin or ergot alkaloids. These effects of mifepristone have resulted in the development of highly effective, non-surgical procedures to terminate early pregnancy based on the combined effects of mifepristone and prostaglandin analogues.

Mifepristone has been registered for medical abortion in France and China since September 1988, in Great Britain since July 1991 and in Sweden since September 1992. In France and China, mifepristone can be used for inducing abortion in pregnancies up to 7 weeks of amenorrhoea, while in Britain it is licensed up to 9 weeks[36]. In all four countries the recommended treatment is a single dose of 600 mg mifepristone followed 36–48 h later by a prostaglandin analogue such as sulprostone or gemeprost. It is now established that this combination is an effective and safe medical approach to induction of abortion. The WHO reported in 1991[37] and further in 1993 that a lower dose of 200 mg is equally effective[38].

MIFEPRISTONE AND MEDICAL ABORTION

FIRST TRIMESTER

When mifepristone is used without subsequent administration of prostaglandin in women who had amenorrhoea for less than 7 weeks the success rate ranges between 65–85%[39]. Mifepristone, followed 36–48 h later by the administration of a vaginal or intramuscular prostaglandin analogue, has become known as 'medical abortion'. A review of 16 369 women treated in France with mifepristone and gemeprost or sulprostone as the prostaglandin showed that the overall success rate was 95%[40]. The failures consisted of persisting pregnancies (1.2%), incomplete abortions (2.8%) and haemostatic surgical procedures in 0.7% of women. Blood transfusion was necessary in 0.1% of women and the median duration of bleeding following the procedure was 8 days.

In the UK the currently recommended regimen (for use up to 63 days of amenorrhoea) is mifepristone 600 mg followed 36–48 h later by 1 mg gemeprost vaginal pessary[36]. Several studies have established the safety and efficacy of medical termination of pregnancy. The method is increasingly acceptable to women and an increase in its use is anticipated[4,41,42]. Continuing pregnancies following attempts at medical induction of abortion is one of the major problems associated with the procedure. Prior to 64 days of amenorrhoea, less than 0.5% undergoing induction of abortion with mifepristone and gemeprost fail to respond and require vacuum aspiration due to persisting pregnancy[3,38].

Several large studies have established the safety of the combination of mifepristone and a prostaglandin analogue. Medical induction of abortion was shown to be well tolerated, acceptable and associated with very low rate of infectious complications[3,4,40,43].

A small number of serious side-effects are reported in the literature, however. After more than 60 000 cases of abortion induction with mifepristone, three myocardial infarctions were reported; one of them was fatal[44]. In all three cases the prostaglandin used was sulprostone. Noticeable cardiovascular events are also well documented in the literature. Three cases are known to have experienced severe hypotension that necessitated supportive therapy; all three patients recovered uneventfully. The three cases occurred within 1 h of administering the prostaglandin analogue. As a result, the question of possible potentiation of sulprostone by mifepristone was raised. No evidence, however, of such potentiality effects was obtained from animal studies[40]. It seems that these cardiovascular events are primarily related to the use of the prostaglandin component of the treatment. Animal studies have shown, for example, that sulprostone has a slight hypotensive effect[45]. There are also reported cases of serious cardiovascular events in association with sulprostone without prior administration of mifepristone[46].

The concern about potential cardiovascular complications like these prompted a revision of clinical guidelines to exclude women who are over the age of 35 years and more than light smokers[47]. As a further response to these cases Schering voluntarily withdrew sulprostone from the market[40].

Gemeprost, a prostaglandin E1, is therefore the preferred agent. It is administered vaginally and seems to avoid the risk of cardiovascular complications. Experience with gemeprost is less than that with sulprostone so definitive conclusions are not yet possible. There is a single report in the in the literature, however, that indicates that a cardiovascular event occurred subsequent to the sole administration of gemeprost[48]. Cardiac arrest requiring insertion of pacemaker occurred in a 19-year-old patient who received a total of 5 mg gemeprost (1 mg administered every 3 h) for second trimester abortion. The patient had uneventful recovery in this case. In addition the drug company have on record two reports of severe hypotension occurring during the course of treatment with gemeprost[49].

SECOND TRIMESTER

The introduction of mifepristone was an important advance in this area, particularly the reduced induction–abortion intervals. Pretreatment with mifepristone in the second trimester termination of pregnancy is advantageous for the patient and her attendant. It sensitizes the myometrium to prostaglandin agents, reducing the induction–abortion interval and the total prostaglandin dose required to achieve abortion[31,50–52]. In a study involving 49 patients, 20 of whom acted as controls, the mean induction–abortion interval was shown to be reduced from 12 h in the control group to 9 h in the mifepristone group. The extra-amniotic prostaglandin dose was also shown to be reduced from 18 mg to 11 mg respectively[51]. The second report has also confirmed these findings[50].

The benefits of mifepristone pretreatment are also evident when gemeprost is used. A double-blind placebo controlled trial has shown that when gemeprost is used, the median interval between the administration of gemeprost and abortion is significantly shorter in patients pretreated with mifepristone. The induction–abortion interval was 6.8 and 15.8 h for the mifepristone-pretreated group and the placebo group respectively. Similarly, the mean number of gemeprost pessaries was three (range 1–10) and five (range 2–10) in these groups[53].

In second trimester medical induction of abortion, a regimen consisting of mifepristone administration followed by the use of a prostaglandin agent has therefore evolved as the optimal procedure. In recent years, experience has been increasing with the prostaglandin agent gemeprost, due to the ease of its administration. Nevertheless, gemeprost requires specific conditions for storage and transfer[54]. It is also an expensive drug which, in second trimester abortions, requires multiple vaginal examinations for its insertion. Misoprostol seems to be the prostaglandin analogue that can be alternatively used in the field of medical induction of abortion. It was primarily developed for the management of gastroduodenal ulcer. The next section reviews its development, usage and safety.

MISOPROSTOL

MISOPROSTOL DEVELOPMENT AND UTEROTONICITY

Misoprostol is a potent, orally active prostaglandin E1 analogue, that possesses strong inhibitory effect on gastric acid secretion. It was developed by Searle Pharmaceutical for that purpose in the early 1970s. Misoprostol was released to international markets in 1986 and is now sold in more than 60 countries in the world. It is a safe and well-tolerated anti-ulcer treatment within the recommended dose of 800 μg per day. Higher total doses up to 1200 μg/day are also reported to be well tolerated for up to 3 months[55]. The safety of higher single or total doses of misoprostol is less well documented.

The uterotonic effects of misoprostol were not identified in animal studies[56]. The uterotonicity of misoprostol in pregnant women was described in 1987 and its use in pregnancy was therefore contraindicated.

Over-the-counter diagnosis and prescribing by pharmacy attendants, however, flourishes in many parts of the world. Many 'prescription only' drugs are freely available and many drugs are sold for indications that are not medically approved. A retrospective study conducted in one university hospital in Brazil had shown the growing misuse of misoprostol as abortifacient. It had shown that 12% of women admitted seeking emergency treatment for uterine bleeding reported using misoprostol as an abortion inducing agent in 1987. This figure has increased to 73% in 1990[57].

The misuse of misoprostol became an epidemiological fact in Latin America. Doses of 200–16 800 μg were reported. The drug was used orally in 65% and vaginally in 6% of women and both orally and vaginally simultaneously in 29% of women[58].

Concern about the teratogenicity of misoprostol started to increase in association with the apparent misuse of the drug in Latin America. Five newborns with unusual congenital malformation of the frontotemporal region were described from Brazil. The malformation consisted of a localized frontal and/or temporal defect with an asymmetrical, well-circumscribed defect of the cranium and overlying scalp, exposing dura matter through which the cerebrum could be seen[59]. It was debatable whether misoprostol was causal in such unusual malformation, especially as that the report was based on anecdotal testimony about ingesting misoprostol. However, the possible teratogenic potential of misoprostol was raised by this report despite the fact that animal studies have shown no evidence that it is teratogenic[60].

In 1991, Aubeny and Baulieu reported the first scientific study that examined the use of oral misoprostol and mifepristone for abortion induction[61]. This report was a landmark in the development of research in this field, and in a series of 100 patients the group reported a success rate close to 95% with minimal side-effects. The widespread phenomenon of self-administered misoprostol in Latin America also caught the attention of scientists there and reports about the efficacy of this drug in labour induction soon appeared[62–64]. Doses as low as 100 μg were shown to be superior to placebo and as effective as the prostaglandin E_2 dinoprostone when administered vaginally in inducing labour[64,65].

MISOPROSTOL AND SECOND TRIMESTER ABORTION

Misoprostol is an effective uterotonic agent that can be used reliably for second trimester induction of abortion in patients pretreated with mifepristone. Doses up to 2200 μg were investigated and were shown to be well tolerated. In women pre-treated with mifepristone, a prostaglandin regimen consisting entirely of misoprostol of up to 2200 μg has a success rate of 97% and a mean induction–abortion time of 6.4 h. This is comparable to regimens using mifepristone and prostaglandin agents[50,52,53,66]. When mifepristone and gemeprost are used it is reported that around 95% of patients abort within 24 h[53,66]. In comparison when mifepristone and an optimal misoprostol regimen is used 97% of patients abort within 14 h. Although comparison between different studies is difficult due to variations in sample size, management and gestational age it is clear that in patients pretreated with mifepristone an optimal misoprostol regimen is at least comparable to gemeprost.

Experience in the treatment of gastroduodenal ulcers has shown that 1200 μg of misoprostol in three divided doses over 24 h is a safe treatment that is associated with minimal side effects[67,68]. Dosages up to 2200 μg over 12 h are now reported to be well tolerated. Side-effects were largely gastrointestinal but these were mild in nature and no patient had to discontinue the treatment because of them. The need for anti-emetics, not associated with narcotic analgesia, occurred in only three cases. These findings become more pertinent when compared to the high incidence of gastrointestinal side-effects produced by orally administered prostaglandins for induction of labour. In the 1970s it was reported that 15% of patients had to discontinue such treatment because of side-effects[69].

Provided the first dose of misoprostol is administered vaginally, it appears there is no advantage in administering subsequent doses in this way. Thus the (vaginal/oral) regimen may offer advantages in relation to patient acceptability and risk of infection.

Retained placenta or incomplete abortion after medical abortion in the second trimester is a problem since it means that surgical intervention will be needed. Previous reports indicated that evacuation of the uterus was needed in more than 80% of cases[29,53] and that retained placentae occurred in more than half the cases[53]. This notion led many clinicians to adopt a policy of recommending routine D&C after medical abortion in the second trimester. The low incidence of incomplete abortion and retained placenta in some of the studies in this field highlights the effect of variation in practice in relation to this issue[70,71]. Ultrasound scan examination was not carried out unless there was a clinical indication. In the two studies described, out of 129 patients only 11 had retained placentae and D&C was performed because of persisting bleeding in five cases.

In the same series of patients, four women failed to abort in response to a regimen of mifepristone and a prostaglandin (misoprostol or gemeprost). It is of interest that three of those were multigravid. When gemeprost is used alone for abortion induction, 20% of patients fail to abort within 24 h. The introduction of mifepristone seems to decrease the incidence of this problem but does not abolish it. When mifepristone and gemeprost are used this incidence is close to 5%[53,66]. It remains to be seen whether the alteration of misoprostol regimens in future studies may bring an end to this problem.

Misoprostol without prior treatment with mifepristone can be of clinical value in the third and second trimester. Misoprostol was reported to be useful in the induction of labour in the third trimester. Intravaginal doses as low as 50 μg were successfully used for that purpose[62]. One report indicates that misoprostol without prior treatment with mifepristone is of clinical value in second trimester abortion induction. In a study involving 169 patients who requested abortion and were between 12–23 weeks' gestation, misoprostol in a single 800 μg dose was used to induce abortion. This dose was repeated 24 h later if abortion had not occurred or was not in progress. Five patients dropped out of the study. Out of the remaining 164 patients, abortion was successfully induced in 154 women (94%) with a mean induction interval of 14 h. The 10 failures required dilatation and evacuation to fulfil the procedure. Vacuum aspiration was carried out in all cases as a preventive measure[72]. This report confirmed that misoprostol has uterotonic features that can be of clinical value when used without prior treatment with mifepristone. The success rate and the induction–abortion interval is comparable to the sole use of gemeprost when used for second trimester induction of abortion[28]. Mifepristone pretreatment has been shown to sensitize the uterus to exogenous prostaglandins and reduce the induction–abortion time. The induction–abortion interval is almost half that reported when misoprostol is used without prior treatment with mifepristone.

SAFETY OF SECOND TRIMESTER ABORTION

Prostaglandin agents used for induced abortion are of established safety. Side-effects are usually of a minor nature. Rare life-threatening complications have been reported with different prostaglandin agents, however. These include uterine rupture[73], myocardial infarction[40] and cardiac arrest[48]. It is of interest that most reports occur during second trimester abortion, probably in relation to the high prostaglandin dose required to achieve abortion[48,74].

Genital tract trauma is rare but can be a serious complication of induced abortion. In a series of 900 patients undergoing medical abortion with gemeprost only one was reported to have developed a cervical tear[29]. Four cases of genital tract trauma was reported in a series of 2000 patients undergoing second trimester abortion with extra-amniotic or intra-amniotic instillation of prostaglandin. Three developed broad ligament haematomata and one was reported to have a cervical tear[24]. Uterine rupture after gemeprost administration has also been reported. A detailed case report depicts how such complications can develop. A 24-year-old multigravid woman undergoing medical induction of abortion at 16 weeks' gestation failed to abort after receiving five gemeprost pessaries. Oxytocin infusion was therefore commenced on the third day. By the fourth day she was pale, and abdominal examination revealed a large abdominal mass and rebound tenderness and guarding. Haemoglobin estimation revealed a haemoglobin drop to 6 g/dl. At laparotomy the findings were of a broad ligament haematoma, a ruptured uterus, and partially extruded fetus. Hysterectomy was performed and the patient did well subsequently[73]. One case of uterine rupture with misoprostol was reported from Brazil when the misoprostol was self-administered. The case illustrates that misoprostol, like other prostaglandin agents, can induce this problem[58].

The need for careful medical supervision is clear. Even though the self-administration of misoprostol dosages of 200–16 800 μg (sometimes over several days) has been reported from Brazil, resulting in less morbidity than other forms of illegal abortion, death was reported to have occurred in three cases (two sepsis, one ruptured uterus)[58]. Idiosyncratic reactions to misoprostol are possible as reported with a small vaginal dose of misoprostol[71].

Conclusion

Second trimester abortion is an important problem for women who have undergone prenatal diagnosis and have decided to terminate the pregnancy. Also, in the developing world, access to abortion services can be difficult and the skill and expertise for safe dilatation and evacuation may not always be available. The cost, specific storage conditions and the sophistication required in the transfer of the currently available prostaglandin agents hinder the wide use of medical abortion in these countries. Misoprostol is supplied in tablet forms and is cheap. It provides a suitable alternative of particular relevance to the developing world. The combination of mifepristone pretreatment with vaginally or orally administered misoprostol provides a simple, non-invasive and effective method for second trimester termination of pregnancy.

References

1. MacKenzie IZ. Prostaglandins and midtrimester abortion. In *Prostaglandins and the uterus* (eds J.O. Drife & A.A. Calder), pp. 119–133, 1992. London: Royal College of Obstetricians and Gynaecologists.
2. Grimes DA & Cates WC. Complications from legally-induced abortion. A review. *Obstet. Gynecol. Surv.* **34**, 177–191, 1979.
3. UK Multicentre Trial. The efficacy and tolerance of mifepristone and prostaglandin in first trimester termination of pregnancy. *Br. J. Obstet. Gynaecol.* **97**, 480–486, 1990.
4. Henshaw R, Naji SA, Russell IT & Templeton AA. Comparison of medical abortion with surgical vacuum aspiration: women's preferences and acceptability of treatment. *Br. Med. J.* **307**, 714–717, 1993.
5. Diggory P. Reducing late abortions. *Br. J. Obstet. Gynaecol.* **96**, 133–134, 1989.
6. David HP. Abortion in Europe, 1920–91: a public health perspective. *Stud. Fam. Plan.* **23**, 1–22, 1992.
7. Stubblefield PG. Surgical techniques of uterine evacuation in first and second trimester abortion. In *Termination of Pregnancy* (ed. J. Laferla), *Clin. Obstet. Gynaecol.* **13**(1), 53–70, 1986.
8. Population Reports. *Population and Birth Planning in the People's Republic of China.* Baltimore: Population Information Program, Johns Hopkins University, 1982.
9. Andolsek L. The Ljubljana abortion study, pp. 1–57. Maryland: National Institute of Health, Center for Population Research, 1974.
10. Edelman DA, Brener WE & Berger GS. The effectiveness and complications of abortion by dilatation and vacuum aspiration versus dilatation and rigid metal curettage. *Am. J. Obstet. Gynaecol.* **119**, 473, 1974.
11. Cates W, Grimes DA, Smith JC & Tyler CW. Legal abortion mortality in the United States. Epidemiologic surveillance, 1972–1974. *JAMA* **237**(5), 452–455, 1977.
12. Joint study of the Royal College of General Practitioners and the Royal College of Obstetricians and Gynaecologists. Induced abortion operations and their early sequelae. *J. R. Coll. Gen. Pract.* **35**, 175–185, 1985.
13. Council on Scientific Affairs A Induced termination of pregnancy before and after Roe v Wade. *JAMA* **268**, 3231–3239, 1992.
14. Henshaw SK. Induced abortion: a world review, 1990. *Fam. Plan. Perspect.* **22**, 76–89, 1990.
15. Grimes D, Schulz K, Cates W & Tyler C. Mid-trimester abortion by dilatation and evacuation. *N. Engl. J. Med.* **296**(20), 1141–1145, 1977.
16. Grimes DA, Schulz KF & Cates WJ. Prevention of uterine perforation during currettage abortion. *JAMA* **251**, 2108–2111, 1984.
17. Schulz KF, Grimes DA & Cates W. Measures to prevent cervical injury during suction curretage abortion. *Lancet* **i**, 1182–1184, 1983.
18. Newton BW. Laminaria tent: relic of the past or modern medical device? *Am. J. Obstet. Gynaecol.* **113**, 442–448, 1972.
19. Darney PD. Preparation of the cervix: Hydrophilic and prostaglandin dilators. In *Termination of Pregnancy* (ed. J. Laferla) *Clin. Obstet. Gynaecol.* **13**(1), 43–51, 1986.
20. Radestad A. Cervical softening in early pregnancy. In *Prostaglandins and the uterus* (eds J.O. Drife & A.A. Calder) (Royal College of Obstetricians and Gynaecologists Study Group Series), pp. 135–146, 1991. London: Springer-Verlag.
21. Cates W. Legal abortion: the public health record. *Science* **215**, 1586–1590, 1982.
22. Speroff L. Is there a best way to do mid-trimester abortion? *Contemp. Obstet. Gynecol.* **13**, 106–141, 1979.
23. Urquhart DR. Therapeutic abortion: methods used in second trimester. *Curr. Obstet. Gynaecol.* **3**, 17–22, 1993.
24. Hill NC & MacKenzie IZ. 2308 second trimester terminations using extra-amniotic or intra-amniotic prostaglandin E2: an analysis of efficacy and complications. *Br. J. Obstet. Gynaecol.* **96**, 1424–1431, 1989.
25. Munday D, Francome C & Savage W. Twenty one years of legal abortion. *Br. Med. J.* **298**, 1231–1234, 1989.
26. Keirse MJNC. Therapeutic uses of prostaglandins. In *Prostaglandins* (ed. M.G. Elder), pp. 787–808, 1992. London: Baillière.
27. Sakamoto S, Satoh K, Nishiya I *et al.* Abortifacient effect and uterine cervix-dilating action of 16, 16-dimethyl-trans- 2 PGE1 methylester (ONO 802) in the form of a vaginal suppository (a randomised, double blind, controlled study in the second trimester of pregnancy). *Prostagl. Leukotr.* **9**, 36–361, 1982.
28. Cameron IT & Baird DT. The use of 16,16-dimethyl-trans-prostaglandin E1 methyl ester (gemeprost) vaginal pessaries for the termination of pregnancy in the early second trimester. A comparison with extra-amniotic prostaglandin E2. *Br. J. Obstet. Gynaecol.* **91**, 1136–1140, 1984.
29. Thong KJ, Robertson AJ & Baird DT. Retrospective study of 932 second trimester terminations using gemeprost (16,16 dimethyl-trans PgE1 methyl ester). *Prostaglandins* **44**, 65–74, 1992.

30. Nieman LK & Loriaux DL. The use of anti-progesterones as a medical IUD. In *Anti-hormones in Clinical Gynaecology* (ed. D. Healy). *Baill. Clin. Obstet. Gynaecol.* **2**(3), 609–616, 1988.
31. Bygdeman M, Gemzell K, Gottlieb C & Swahn M. Uterine contractility and interaction between prostaglandins and antiprogestins. Clinical implications. *Ann. NY Acad. Sci.* **626**, 561–567, 1991.
32. Csapo AI. The see-saw theory of parturition. *Ciba Found. Sympos.* **47**, 159, 1977.
33. Smith SK & Kelly RW. The effect of the antiprogestins RU 486 and ZK 98734 on the synthesis and metabolism of prostaglandins F2a and E2 in separated cells from early human decidua. *J. Clin. Endocrinol. Metab.* **65**, 527–534, 1987.
34. Bygdeman M & Swahn ML. Progesterone receptor blockage. Effect on uterine contractility and early pregnancy. *Contraception* **32**, 45–51, 1985.
35. Norman JE, Wen Xuan W, Kelly RW, Glasier AF, McNeilly AS & Baird DT. Effects of mifepristone in vivo on decidual prostaglandin synthesis and metabolism. *Contraception* **44**, 89–97, 1990.
36. Editorial. UK approval for mifepristone. *Lancet* **338**, 111–112, 1991.
37. Anonymous. WHO suggests lower dose of mifepristone. *Br. Med. J.* **303**, 944, 1993.
38. World Health Organisation Task Force on Post-ovulatory Methods of Fertility Regulation. Termination of pregnancy with reduced doses of mifepristone. *Br. Med. J.* **307**, 532–537, 1993.
39. Baulieu EE. Contragestion and other clinical applications of RU 486, an antiprogesterone at the receptor. *Science* **245**, 1351–1357, 1989.
40. Ulmann A, Silvestre L, Chemama L *et al.* Medical termination of early pregnancy with mifepristone (RU 486) followed by a prostaglandin analogue. *Acta. Obstet. Gynaecol. Scand.* **71**, 278–283, 1992.
41. Heard M & Guillebaud J. Medical abortion safe, effective, and legal in Britain. *Br. Med. J.* **304**, 195–196, 1992.
42. Henshaw RC, Templeton AA, Naji SA & Russell IT. Medical abortion. *Br. Med. J.* **304**, 914, 1992.
43. World Health Organisation. Termination of pregnancy with reduced doses of mifepristone. *Br. Med. J.* **307**, 532–537, 1993.
44. Editorial. A death associated with mifepristone/sulprostone. *Lancet* **337**, 969–970, 1991.
45. Pons JC, Imbert MC, Elefant E, Roux C, Herschkorn P & Papiernick E. Development after exposure to mifepristone in early pregnancy. *Lancet* **338**, 763, 1991.
46. Fliers E, Duren DR & Van Zwieten A. A prostaglandin analogue as a probable cause of myocardial infarction in a young woman. *Br. Med. J.* **302**, 416, 1991.
47. Roussel Laboratories Limited. Mifegyne (mifepristone) tablets. Data sheet MF13, 1992.
48. Kalra PA, Litherland D, Sallomi DF, Critchley HOD, Falconer GF & Holmes AM. Cardiac standsill induced by prostaglandin pessaries. *Lancet* **333**, 1460–1461, 1989.
49. Personal communication with the drug company, 1994.
50. Urquhart DR & Templeton AA. The use of mifepristone prior to prostaglandin-induced mid-trimester abortion. *Hum. Reprod.* **5**, 883–886, 1990.
51. Urquhart DR, Bahzad C & Templeton AA. Efficacy of the antiprogestin mifepristone (RU 486) prior to prostaglandin termination of pregnancy. *Hum. Reprod.* **4**, 202–203, 1989.
52. Gottlieb C & Bygdeman M. The use of antiprogestin (RU 486) for termination of second trimester pregnancy. *Acta. Obstet. Gynaecol. Scand.* **70**, 199–203, 1991.
53. Rodger MW & Baird DT. Pretreatment with mifepristone (RU486) reduces interval between prostaglandin administration and expulsion in second trimester abortion. *Br. J. Obstet. Gynaecol.* **97**, 41–45, 1990.
54. Editorial. Misoprostol and legal medical abortion. *Lancet* **338**, 1241–1242, 1991.
55. Data sheet compendium. *ABPI Data Sheet Compendium*. London: Datapharm Publications, 1993.
56. Collins PW. Misoprostol: discovery, development and clinical applications. *Med. Res. Rev.* **10**, 149–172, 1990.
57. Schonhofer PS. Brazil: misuse of misoprostol as an abortifacient may induce malformations. *Lancet* **337**, 1534–1535, 1991.
58. Costa SH & Vessey MP. Misoprostol and illegal abortion in Rio de Janeiro, Brazil. *Lancet* **341**, 1258–1261, 1993.
59. Fonseca W, Alencar AJA, Mota FSB & Coelho HLL. Misoprostol and congenital malformations. *Lancet* **338**, 56, 1991.
60. Downie WW. Misuse of misoprostol. *Lancet* **338**, 247, 1991.
61. Aubeny E & Baulieu EE. Activite contragestivie de l'association au RU486 d'une prostaglandine active par voie'oral. *C.R. Acad. Sci. (III)* **312**, 539–546, 1991.
62. Marguilies M, Perez MC & Vato L. Misoprostol to induce labour. *Lancet* **339**, 64, 1992.
63. Sanchez-Ramos L, Kaunitz AM, Dell Valle GO, Delke I, Schroeder PA & Briones DK. Labour induction with prostaglandin E1 methyl analogue misoprostol versus oxytocin: a randomised trial. *Obstet. Gynecol.* **81**, 332–336, 1993.
64. Fletcher HM, Mitchell S, Simeon D, Frederick J & Brown D. Intravaginal misoprostol as a cervical ripening agent. *Br. J. Obstet. Gynaecol.* **100**, 641–644, 1993.
65. Fletcher H, Mitchell S, Frederick J, Simeon D & Brown D. Intraveginal misoprostol versus dinoprostone as a cervical ripening and labour inducing agents. *Obstet. Gynecol.* **83**, 244–247, 1994.
66. Thong KJ & Baird DT. Induction of second trimester abortion with mifepristone and gemeprost. *Br. J. Obstet. Gynaecol.* **100**, 758–761, 1993.
67. Collins PW. Misoprostol: discovery, development, and clinical applications. *Med. Res. Rev.* **10**, 149–172, 1990.
68. Herting RL & Nissen CH. Overview of misoprostol clinical experience. *Dig. Dis. Sci.* **31**, 47–54, 1986.
69. Gordon-Wright AP, Dutt TP & Elder MG. The routine use of oral prostaglandin E2 tablets for induction or augmentation of labour. *Acta. Obstet. Gynaecol. Scand.* **58**, 23–26, 1979.
70. El-Refaey H, Hinshaw K & Templeton A. The abortifacient effect of misoprostol in the second trimester. *Hum. Reprod.* **8**, 1744–1746, 1993.
71. El-Refaey H & Templeton A. Induction of abortion in the second trimester by a combination of misoprostol and mifepristone: a randomised comparison between two misoprostol regimens. *Hum. Reprod.* **10**(2), 475–478, 1995.
72. Bugalho A, Bique C, Almeida L & Faundes A. The effectiveness of intravaginal misoprostol (Cytotec) in inducing abortion after eleven weeks of pregnancy. *Stud. Fam. Plan.* **24**, 319–323, 1993.
73. Wiener JJ & Evans AS. Uterine rupture in midtrimester abortion. A complication of gemeprost vaginal pessaries and oxytocin. *Br. J. Obstet. Gynaecol.* **97**, 1061–1062, 1990.
74. Meyer WJ, Benton SL, Hoon TJ, Gauthier DW & Whiteman VE. Acute myocardial infarction associated with prostaglandin E2. *Am. J. Obstet. Gynaecol.* **165**, 359–360, 1991.

Bereavement and reaction to fetal loss

31

J. Lorenzen, J. Bitzer and W. Holzgreve

Introduction

The widely established possibilities of prenatal diagnosis influence the experience of pregnancy in the individual and within society as a whole. Most frequently prenatal diagnosis can remove anxieties from prospective parents, especially in those cases with an a priori increased risk. Having detected a fetal abnormality either by chance or due to a planned prenatal diagnosis, there are a few (though increasing number of) cases in which treatment is possible. Sometimes in cases of severe untreatable conditions, the parents have to decide whether they are going to continue or to terminate a possibly highly desired pregnancy. Parents always lose the hope for a 'healthy ideal baby', if a fetal malformation is diagnosed. This of course will change their experience of the further course of pregnancy. Some parents have to anticipate a possible miscarriage, stillbirth or neonatal death or have to cope with living with a handicapped child.

The members of obstetric teams are not usually adequately trained to help parents cope with these situations and the grief process following fetal loss. Bourne outlined the importance of the support of staff for the parents during a fetal loss: '... the danger lies not in the grief and distress; the danger is bypassing it, thereby promoting a variety of severe psychological complications. Moreover, the danger is not merely to the mother but also to her husband, her surviving children, and, worst of all, to the next baby'. 'Whereas grief is relatively understandable and obvious, these dangers are complex, their management and prevention are very hard'[1].

The main purpose of this chapter is to describe the internal processes of parents and families undergoing fetal loss and to give some advice for staff to facilitate grief and prevent pathological reactions in parents.

Neither the discussion of ethical issues, though necessary, can be included in this chapter (see section 3 of this book) nor the complex coping process of parents living with a handicapped child.

Development of bonding during pregnancy

The experience of pregnancy is influenced by several factors, including social and cultural circumstances, the individual setting, the pregnancy being planned or unplanned, physiological changes during pregnancy, medical factors (including prenatal diagnosis) and the psychic development and influence of the partnership. Looking at a possible fetal loss, the psychic development of bonding is the most interesting factor offering some guidelines on how to support parents' coping processes.

The term 'bonding' is used to characterize a special form of attachment. 'Attachment' is the arrangement one person wants with a preferred person, who is perceived as stronger, wiser and able to reduce anxiety or distress, and leads to a feeling of security. Mothers usually do not rely on their child as a source of security. The baby in utero becomes a preferred person for the pregnant woman by developing a wish for closeness and continuous contact with the child[2].

In terms of psychoanalytic theory and empirical studies, four phases describe prenatal bonding:

- In the first phase, before pregnancy, the wish for a child produces fantasies regarding motherhood and the future child-to-be
- In the second phase, during pregnancy, bodily sensations are perceived by proprioception. The baby is regarded as a separate object and is at the same time seen as part of the pregnant woman's body
- The third phase is characterized by the transformation of inner perceptions into fantasies regarding the evolving baby in the woman's body

- In the fourth phase the imaginations concerning the child-to-be evoke emotional response in the woman

The time and intensity of prenatal bonding varies widely from individual to individual depending on the personal capacities of anticipation, proprioception, imagination and emotional responses to pregnancy.

Quickening is a milestone in the development of bonding. Experiencing the ability of the child to act, the mother more easily perceives a person being separated from herself. With increasing prenatal activity of the child more personal characteristics are attributed to the baby[3].

The internal representation of the child and the experience of pregnancy will be influenced by the use of ultrasound (to confirm pregnancy, routine screening examinations to check for fetal development and fetal abnormalities)[4]. The experience of looking at the embryo reduces the fantasies about the baby and the possibility of normal ambivalence and denial in the first weeks of gestation. Therefore, these adaptive processes might be disturbed by the use of ultrasound. On the other hand, anxiety and stress due to possible fetal malformations might be reduced at an earlier stage of pregnancy. Watching the baby's growth with visual and proprioceptive information and knowing the gender of the baby seems to lead to earlier bonding during pregnancy[5].

Parents with an a priori increased risk for fetal abnormalities, or a previous history of child losses, often dare to plan another pregnancy only because of prenatal diagnosis. In order to protect themselves from disappointment and grief, they postpone bonding until the result of prenatal diagnosis indicates a healthy baby. It has been shown how weak this cognitive decision is, and that bonding develops nevertheless[6,7]. This topic should be addressed in preconception counselling.

Grief: loss of a significant object

Grief, mourning and bereavement apply to the psychological reactions of persons who experience the loss of a significant other. The phenomena of these reactions have been described by Lindemann[8], Parkes[9] and Bowlby[10] in a similar way. They distinguish several phases of grief with somatic, cognitive, emotional, behavioural, social and interpersonal characteristics.

According to Bowlby[10] the personal subjective experience of mourning goes through the following phases:

- Acute despair, numbness and protest. The first reaction on the death of a significant person may be denial, a sense of bewilderment and disbelief. Outbursts of anger and distress are common. Physical reactions include throat tightness, abdominal body sensations, crying and sighing. This state of shock may last some minutes to several weeks
- Intense yearning and searching for the deceased person. Once the searching proves to be ineffective, acute anguish, physical restlessness (including sleep disturbance) and an all-consuming preoccupation with thoughts and images of the deceased predominate for weeks or months. Feelings of guilt, self-accusation and aggression towards oneself, the deceased and all other people are common phenomena
- Disorganization. The reality of the loss begins to sink in. A sense of going through the emotions is dominant; the grieving person appears to be withdrawn, apathetic and listless. Many memories and dreams are activated. There may be an intense feeling of envy towards those who have not experienced such a loss
- Reorganization. Acceptance of the loss leads to a more balanced mood and less somatic symptoms. The bereaved is able to focus new goals, has integrated the experience of loss into the view of life and develops the capacity to become attached to someone else again

These phases may follow each other, but often they intermingle. In some bereaved, the phases occur several times before final progression is possible. Normal grief can thus be described as a biopsychosocial crisis challenging the coping capacity, passing through cyclic progression towards resolution and restitution of a new balance for the bereaved person.

Though the personality of the bereaved seems to be the strongest predictor of disordered mourning other factors are: the identity and personal meaning of the deceased person, social and personal circumstances of the bereaved and the circumstances of the loss[10].

Bowlby describes three different forms of disordered mourning:

- Chronic grief reaction. Long duration and very intense reaction without mourning but depression, anxiety, anger and self-reproach; prone to this reaction are those who show no reaction immediately after the loss
- Delayed grief reaction. Being very reserved, denying the meaning of the loss, withholding thoughts and feelings from meaningful others and compulsive care-giving for more than a week with no hint of mourning
- Euphoria. The bereaved denies that the loss has happened at all, feels the deceased is still around or denies the bonding

A review of the literature reveals that authors do not necessarily differentiate grief reactions from depression. Appetite, sleep and mood vary in response to the environment, with some capacity for transient pleasure in normal grief; they are consistently altered in depression. Bereaved persons experience sadness, while the depressed feel empty and 'dead inside'. Reality testing is intact in the bereaved (apart from hallucinations of baby kicking) and they feel worthy of the support of others and therefore do not isolate themselves from support like people tend to do in depression. Helplessness is common in grief, but usually some hope for the future is present, whereas depressed persons experience despair about the impossibility of change[11].

Reactions to fetal loss

Losing an embryo or fetus conveys different problems from those experienced if other, adult relationships are lost. The lost object is part of the body-self with a high degree of identification and difficulty on the part of the mother to separate herself from the embryo or fetus. The lost object is not visible and tangible but internally represented. Thus external mechanisms of mourning are reduced. The relationship is exclusive and not shared by others (except for the father). Therefore people other than the parents themselves are unlikely to perceive the loss as real. Even a highly desired pregnancy will be experienced with ambivalence in the beginning because every woman has to face disadvantages concerning her job, spare time, etc. Ambivalent relationships are more difficult to mourn[11].

In the case of abortion for fetal abnormality, the loss of the object is brought about actively by the decision of the parents. This process causes difficulties in coping with feelings of aggression and includes feelings of guilt and shame as well as grief. The latter are part of the mourning process in any loss.

In empirical studies, authors widely accept the loss of a child during pregnancy as a seriously distressing life event[12–16], leading to grief reactions in the majority of mothers for 6–9 months at least[11,17,18].

Pathological grief reaction following perinatal loss is estimated to affect from 13%[11] to 33%[13,16]. Because of the differences in definitions, times of assessment and instruments as well as kinds of losses, these results have to be interpreted with caution. In perinatal losses by abortion or stillbirth, the circumstances enhance pathological grief reactions. Usually the death is sudden and unexpected, and occurs within the mother; the relationship is exclusive and not supported by visual, acoustic or tactile sensations. In cases of known malformation or illness, the parents have to deal with feelings of insufficiency and have to restore their concept of themselves as having the capability to be a father or a mother. They have to deal with feelings of guilt, because they are not able to accept an ill or malformed baby. In some cases, they have decided to have their child killed, which can complicate the reactions to the loss.

If the death of the fetus has been diagnosed, midwives and doctors in many hospitals still stop using the term 'baby', try to hide the dead baby, and do not ask whether the parents want to bury the child. Their intention is to protect mothers from those difficult feelings of grief. Usually fathers are not encouraged to attend the abortion process. Parents being in a state of internal turmoil usually perceive their feelings as being 'wrong'. They doubt if they have the right to be sad. If there is no child but 'abortion material', they cannot start an adequate mourning process.

In western societies many rituals and ceremonies are lost which in former times facilitated coping with loss and the strong feelings within the community. Obstetric teams might accept the challenge to establish a helpful new way of dealing with losses to prevent long-term pathological effects on the parents, their partnership, the living and subsequent siblings and the potential subsequent pregnancies.

REACTIONS TO THE PRENATAL DIAGNOSIS OF A FETAL MALFORMATION

Diagnosis of a fetal malformation not only leads to the loss of the positive experience of being pregnant, but always to the loss of the illusion of a perfect child, sometimes to the loss of a child and the experience of parenthood. For both parents their self-esteem appears to be damaged[12,13,16,19–22].

It often takes several weeks from the first suspicion of a fetal malformation to the confirmation of the diagnosis. To reduce anxiety and stress, parents tend to deny their bonding, stop all preparations, sometimes hide the results from significant others because they are afraid to be reproached in case they decide to terminate the pregnancy. One can assume that parents have to deny that the child-to-be has a meaning for them in order to be able to judge on the life of the fetus (in the case of termination). It has been shown that parents stop the internal dialogue with the child[23].

Prenatal diagnosis usually includes several ultrasound examinations in which the parents can see an image of their child. This makes it more difficult for parents as they have to decide not only on 'interrupting a pregnancy' (a commonly used euphemism), but on the death of a nearly completely developed human baby. When a chromosomal anomaly was diagnosed by amniocentesis or chorion villus sampling (CVS) parents opted more often for termination of pregnancy if there was a visible malformation on ultrasound[24].

There is a need for detailed information about the prognosis of the child in any case of abnormality and parents need support during this stressful period. With severe malformations parents have to decide themselves on the course of the pregnancy, according to the legal conditions[25]. Ethical, religious and personal reasons, issues of the partnership and social circumstances might influence the process of decision on termination of pregnancy. Parents having decided to continue the pregnancy inspite of fetal malformation will usually be in need of support and encouragement[26,27]. They often expect social pressure if they give birth to a handicapped child after prenatal diagnosis[6].

Some authors describe chronic sorrow in parents of disabled children. Dealing repeatedly with lost expectations, daily frustrations, unattainable goals, and an uncertain future, some experience phases of acute grief over and over again, but for shorter duration[15,28].

REACTIONS TO MISCARRIAGE

The influence of the duration of pregnancy on the grief reaction has been the focus of several studies. Many authors found similar kinds of grief reactions in early pregnancy losses (first trimester) as in late pregnancy losses[29]. The duration of mourning seems to increase according to the length of pregnancy[30,31].

'For the majority of the women, around the 10th week of gestation, the embryo is psychologically represented in fantasies, dreams and concrete arrangements in reality'[32]. Early pregnancy losses are especially difficult to mourn, since they are usually not confirmed as personally significant events by significant others. Even the women themselves deny the importance of the loss. The lack of social support enhances delayed grief reactions[19,33,34].

There is much evidence that anxiety is high after several miscarriages. Tension has a negative psychological and physiological effect on the course of the following pregnancy[35]. Miscarriages due to complications of CVS or amniocentesis, though rare, seem to be similarly difficult to cope with as termination of pregnancy at the same time of gestation[36,37]. Even the decision to have used prenatal diagnosis seems to arouse feelings of guilt and sorrow.

REACTIONS TO TERMINATION OF PREGNANCY FOR FETAL ABNORMALITY

Many authors compare the intensity of grief reactions following termination of pregnancy for fetal abnormality in the second trimester of pregnancy with the reaction to perinatal death[22,38–43]. It is accepted that the loss is more difficult to cope with, if it is the result of a parental decision[17,23,36].

Frets et al.[44] studied the reactions of 41 couples undergoing second trimester termination of pregnancy. They found one-third experiencing strong emotions at two month follow-up, eight of whom needed long-term psychological help, one-third of the couples denying the emotional impact of the experience, and in the remaining couples the mourning process was in progress.

Parents are emotionally distressed by the conflict between their wish to continue the pregnancy and rational considerations to terminate[17,44]. If they have decided to abort the child, mourning seems to be inappropriate. To mourn would signify the child's importance and the relationship between parent and child, resulting in powerful feelings of guilt[23]. Lack of social support quite often complicates grieving as parents tend to hide the loss if it is due to a termination.

It has been shown that both women and men do mourn after a termination of pregnancy for fetal abnormality despite potentially strong feelings of guilt. The majority of mothers were convinced of the rightness of the decision, and they would again elect for termination in a similar situation in a following pregnancy[45–47]. But for a minority of mothers, feelings of guilt and doubts about the termination can be a serious problem[48].

Although a termination of pregnancy for fetal abnormality is widely accepted to be a seriously distressing life event, empirical data suggest most parents cope well. Only a minority will need psychiatric help[47,49]. All studies confirm that the facilitation of mourning by showing, holding and naming the dead baby is as well accepted after termination of pregnancy as it is after a spontaneous loss at the same time of pregnancy[23,38,40,44,46,47,50,51].

REACTIONS TO STILLBIRTH OR NEONATAL DEATH

According to the view[52] that the reaction of the parents is determined mostly by the reactions of staff, it seems to be easier to mourn after stillbirth or neonatal death. Neonatal death is much easier to mourn because there has been visible and tangible evidence that the child has existed that the loss is real[17]. 'Phantom crying' and the experience of kicking in the womb after the loss are common phenomena[14].

The physiological reactions of the postpartum period (e.g. milk coming in, afterpains, weight loss) are constant reminders that the body has prepared itself for a baby, but there is no baby to care for. Not only physical, but social problems arise as well.

Effects on partner and family

FATHERS

Quite often the obstetric team is in doubt whether and how to address the father during the abortion or delivery if a dead child is due to be born. With reference to the literature, the lack of interest in this subject is remarkable. Some studies have shown that there is a comparably strong paternal bonding to the fetus, though different in quality from the maternal bonding[3]. Kennell *et al.* described the paternal grief reaction being less strong but existent[13]. Empirical studies reveal the variation of grief reactions in fathers: some studies show lower scores and shorter duration of mourning, less anxiety, feelings of guilt and loneliness after all kinds of pregnancy losses in fathers than in mothers, while other authors found even more intensive paternal grief reactions[13,19,52,58–60].

There is evidence that the mother, the father and the partnership benefit if the father takes an active part in the abortion or delivery[30,52–54]. In more than 700 cases of miscarriage, stillbirth or neonatal death more than half of the fathers attended the birth, a quarter of them chose to hold their baby (the number of fathers increasing according to the duration of pregnancy) and one-fifth of fathers returned to follow-up appointments[54].

The quality of the marital relationship is a strong predictor for disturbed mourning in the mother. Lack of closeness, support and intimacy in the partnership and difficulties in communication can enhance pathological grief reactions[17,31]. As Costello *et al.* state: '... warning signs of a troubled relationship are over-involvement in work, church, or other groups, an increase in drinking or drug use, an affair, spending a large amount of time with parents, siblings or friends, doting on a surviving child, prolonged lack of sexual activity, and hearing themselves say "Yes we talk all the time but never get anything resolved" '[15]. Women feel misunderstood by their partners' helplessness, especially if partners try to avoid talking about the loss and cannot accept their wives' feelings of grief. Fathers usually try to hide their grief and look for distraction in vocational pursuits. Because of the increased risk of depression in the woman as well as the man, counselling seems to be helpful[16,55–57].

LIVING SIBLINGS

Parents usually avoid talking to their living children about the death of the sibling-to-be, as they do not want to burden them[16]. Even very small children experience changes in family life due to a pregnancy, and at the age of two years on, they develop an imagination of the sibling-to-be. They hope for a friend and are jealous at the same time. 'Magic thinking' easily leads to feelings of guilt at having killed the baby because of these ambivalent feelings.

Children's grief is different from adult reactions. Children act out and play the scene rather than talk about their feelings, are more active and sometimes aggressive[15,61,62]. If children are left alone with their fantasies they may try to replace the dead sibling-to-be to console the parents.

Children usually do not ask for explanation if they guess that parents are not willing to talk about the event. Therefore parents need advice to talk to their children and to avoid denial. Explanation should be given as soon as possible, in an honest way, without metaphor and adapted to the child's comprehensive capacity. It should be explained that the sibling is dead, nobody else in the family is in danger of dying, nobody is guilty of the death and that the parents are sad because they wanted the baby but are able to love several children[15,16,63]. Some authors suggest that the living children should be encouraged to see and touch the dead sibling as well[64,65]. Parents might find it helpful to re-establish their disrupted experience of being competent parents and therefore lift their self-esteem in enabling their living children to cope with the loss.

In twin pregnancies grief reaction is more complex if one fetus dies. The parents try to deny the importance of this loss to sustain the bonding to the surviving sibling[13,17,66,67].

SUBSEQUENT PREGNANCY AND CHILDREN

Clarification of risks for further pregnancies should be given soon. The immediate desire for another baby can usually be seen as an attempt to avoid grief and to extinguish the experience of the pregnancy loss. Many authors recommend an interval of 6–9 months before planning a new pregnancy. There may be an increased risk of a spontaneous abortion, probably due to endometrial insufficiency, and there seems to be a higher risk of pathological grief reaction, if a pregnancy occurs within 5 months of the loss[68]. The increased risk of miscarriage should be discussed if the subsequent pregnancy occurs sooner. Since this grief reaction will not be over before this time, it will be more complicated to engage in bonding to a new child-to-be.

Green and Solnit used the term 'replacement child syndrome' to describe the tendency of parents to attribute characteristics of the lost child to the next baby, to idealize the dead child and criticize the next baby. The inability to accept a new child in its own right is part of this syndrome. To minimize these risks counselling should focus on the choice of the name which should be a different one. If conception is planned, the date of delivery probably should not be in the month of anniversary of the lost pregnancy. The danger of a 'replacement child syndrome' is mentioned by several authors[11,48,68,69], though there is little empirical evidence[7].

Overall, 30% of all women become pregnant within 9 months after a fetal loss and 50–60% within 1–2 years[17,58,68,70]. Parents intentionally avoid pain in the following pregnancy by controlling their emotions towards the child-to-be. They often try not to show that they are pregnant, ignore signs of pregnancy, postpone preparations etc. Phipps[7] examined 15 women after pregnancy loss and found bonding processes in the subsequent pregnancy being undisturbed, though denied by the mothers[71]. Those women were more dependent on their gynaecologists. They needed more assurance that everything was all right, and needed more routine appointments. Nevertheless, anxiety was only be reduced for a short period of time[72,73].

Reaching the same stage in the subsequent pregnancy or anniversary dates can raise fears and tension. In many cases grief recurs when the next baby is born. Parents should be prepared for this normal reaction, as only then will they realize 'what' they have lost previously[7,19].

Coping with fetal loss

Many authors support the view[52] that the response of the social and medical environment is the strongest predictor for the grief reaction in perinatal loss. They therefore regret that the obstetric teams support the denial of the loss by using vague terms, by arranging the abortion process so that the dead child becomes invisible and avoiding the discussion of disposal of the body[12,16,17,74]. The state of information among medical staff about registration, autopsy, disposal, etc., was often poor[57,75–77]. Therefore a high percentage of women did not feel the obstetric team to be helpful[11,19,70]. The deficits and uncertainty in medical personnel in supporting parents' grief has led to many efforts to create a more favourable atmosphere which enhances the beginning of adequate grief reactions. The benefit of a better routine in dealing with bereaved parents is not only for the parents, but contributes as well to greater job satisfaction and improves coping with the tragedy of perinatal death in professionals[78].

In the meantime many programmes for grieving parents have been established, but are not yet standard in all hospitals. Bereavement counselling is emotionally draining and should be done within a team of professionals with specialized training and supervision[18].

FACILITATING GRIEF REACTIONS: BEREAVEMENT COUNSELLING

The primary tasks for the obstetric team in cases of fetal loss are:

- To help experience death as a reality
- To acknowledge parental feelings and assure parents that their feelings are normal
- To ensure that adequate grief reactions begin, including the father's and the siblings'
- To address feelings of guilt and anger explicitly
- To support the need for people to talk about the loss
- To prepare for negative reactions of the social environment
- To inform about contraception and subsequent pregnancies
- To meet the specific needs of individual patients[11,13,15,17]

Professionals often feel ill-prepared in knowing what to say if the death of the fetus is diagnosed. Initially, many words may not be as necessary as simply stating, 'I'm sorry this has happened', and remaining with the family. A quiet side room is much appreciated where the father and other family members and friends can attend.

It is difficult for the mother to cope with the reality of the death of the child and find the power to manage the delivery at the same time. If possible, women should have time to deal with the message of intrauterine death before labour is induced or a dilatation and evacuation is performed[74].

It is well established now that the offer to look at the dead child is the best help to facilitate an adequate grief process. Thereby parents can convince themselves that their child is real, that it is dead, and fantasies about anomalies can be corrected. In hospitals where parents were asked routinely if they wanted to see and hold their dead child after a perinatal loss, nearly 90% accepted this offer and no mother regretted this act later on[74,79]. Without exception all authors reported positive experiences of the parents, in spite of initial doubts whether to dare to look at the child. Parents appreciated having looked at their dead child, even in cases of maceration or obvious abnormalities. Mothers and fathers tend to focus on the familiar family characteristics. Their fantasies of the child, however, were often that of a monster. Even abnormalities which might look grotesque to the obstetric team are accepted by parents in this context and parents usually speak fondly of the experience. Quite often it seems to be easier for parents to accept the death if the cause is visible[11,17,47,76,79].

One should offer to show the dead child immediately after delivery, at the same time as a live baby would be presented. Abnormalities in colour or malformations should be explained in advance. Parents should be given the opportunity to see the baby naked. Many parents need encouragement to touch and hold the dead baby. A member of the staff should be present to answer questions, but should suggest that the parents might spend some time alone with the child as well.

In our study nearly all women wanted the option to see and hold the dead child 1–2 days after delivery[47]. Quite often women feel so exhausted by labour, under narcotics or overwhelmed by relief after delivery, that they refuse at first to look but develop the wish later on.

If possible, siblings or significant others should be invited to join. The offer to say goodbye should be made several times to encourage the parents. However, the parents have to decide, not members of staff, and their decision must be accepted and supported[15,63,74,80].

Not only the parents have to overcome disgust, horror and prejudices to be able to face the dead child. The staff are faced with the same kind of feelings and have to come to terms with their own emotions in order to offer genuine help to the parents. Otherwise, the parents will be easily discouraged by contradictory non-verbal or paralinguistic cues.

A photo should be taken. It can be kept in the files for some years, if the parents do not want to have it immediately. Quite often they change their mind and all kinds of mementoes (footprints, lock of hair, identity bracelet) are welcomed later on. An identity card including gender, length and weight, colour of hair and eyes should be written as well as the name if the parents choose one[11].

Without regard to legal conditions, parents should be encouraged to name their baby. Especially with living children, it is then less complicated to refer to the dead sibling. Many parents appreciate the option of having the baby baptized, anointed or blessed[15].

For the majority of parents the decision about autopsy is difficult. All questions should be answered carefully. Usually parents should be encouraged to agree to an autopsy even if there is only a small chance that their question, 'why it happened' will be answered by the results.

Parents often do not dare not to ask what is going to happen to the body. If the parents are not obliged to organize the disposal themselves, information should be given about the routine in case of miscarriage or intrauterine death. Staff should be able to give information how to organize a burial or cremation. The mother should be included in making decisions and plans, because this might help her to accept the reality of the death and enhance the grief process[15].

The majority of authors advise an immediate offer of bereavement counselling and at least two follow-up meetings

4–6 weeks and 2–4 months after the loss[15,13,70,81,82]. Emotional support can more easily be accepted if the offer includes help with practical issues like registration, autopsy or funeral arrangements. It has been shown[57] that 80% (n = 20 of 25) of parents after stillbirth or neonatal death accepted the offer of grief counselling in hospital and half of the group wanted one or two contacts after discharge (maximum eight meetings), including the fathers, who especially welcomed the offer. The study group showed less anxiety and depression and a higher status of general well-being after 6 months in comparison to the control group and no difference after 14 months. There was no difference in the rate of subsequent pregnancies. The number of women needing psychiatric help was slightly higher in the control group.

PSYCHOTHERAPEUTIC METHODS

The majority of bereaved persons recover without treatment. There has been much effort to predict who will need support because of disordered mourning, depression, somatization or post-traumatic stress syndrome. It is generally accepted that previous mental health treatment of the mother predisposes to pathological grief reactions[70,83]. Other predictors, e.g. age of the mother, living children, previous losses are controversial[11,14,15,19,31,52]. Zisook[84] adds the following risk factors as predictors for the need of formal psychotherapeutic interventions: past history of depression, loss through suicide or homicide, simultaneous losses or accidents in which the survivor was at fault, poor health, lack of social support, other distressing life events. The lack of social support in the bereaved seems to increase pathological grief reactions[11,57]. On the other hand, the interpersonal network might increase feelings of guilt and denial without intention[16].

After fetal loss a minority of parents might need professional help either in the form of specialized grief therapy or psychiatric help. The strategies of psychotherapeutic interventions are directed towards the different possible complications. They have to take into account the magnitude of the stressful life event of prenatal loss, the individual significance of this loss in the biography of the bereaved, pre-existing mental health disorders, the predominant defense mechanisms, the applied coping strategies, the lack or degree of social support or concomitant social stresses.

Zisook[84] describes four common features of the various approaches of grief therapy:

- Information about the grief process helps the bereaved to accept their confusing feelings, behaviours and somatic reactions
- Encouragement to express the full range of emotional reactions to the loss by using evocative techniques like role playing, writing to the deceased
- Clarification and definition of the relationship with the lost person. This can be obtained by exploring all aspects of the relationship and also by entering into an internal dialogue with the deceased
- Focusing the new identity of the bereaved person by trying to help with the integration of the traumatic experience into the self-concept of the bereaved and by discussing the changes regarding the general outlook on life and the view of the world

In cases of long duration of mourning, very strong grief reactions and delayed grief, Worden[85] has suggested a special kind of grief therapy in a group or single setting as a time-limited brief psychotherapy of 8–10 sessions. The focus of the grief therapy is to understand the present grief experience against the background of previous losses. To enable the development of a new relationship with the lost person, positive memories are collected and preserved. The 'tasks of mourning' are explained and gone through: accepting the reality of the loss, experiencing the painful feelings of grief together, adaptation to the surroundings without the lost child, dealing with questions of guilt and shame, engaging in other relationships, redefining the tasks of the couple and looking at possible conflicts and their resolution.

The aim is to restore or enhance the ego of the bereaved by accepting, not analysing defensive manoeuvres. The bereaved should be helped to develop better coping skills by teaching and advice. The therapist should be a coping model and a constantly reassuring figure on which the patient can rely.

Depending on the individual symptoms and complaints, further therapeutic interventions can be selected and adapted:

- With predominant emotional turmoil, feelings of guilt and persistent depression, the techniques of expressive and interpersonal psychotherapy[86,88] or cognitive therapy[89] may be helpful
- If the symptoms are mainly of post-traumatic stress syndrome, the techniques of Horowitz[89,90] can be used
- If interpersonal and marital conflicts are predominant, couple and marital or family therapy is indicated
- If depression becomes predominant, especially in the beginning of the grief reaction, antidepressant agents may be useful. Such medication does not prevent grieving
- Pharmacological treatment of anxiety and insomnia is controversial. We believe anxiolytic and hypnotic agents may be beneficial if they are used within a therapeutic alliance including counselling and psychotherapeutic interventions

Fetal loss is a major life event for most prospective parents. The majority of them will be able to cope with the loss, especially if they receive some support by professionals. But parents as well as obstetric staff are challenged by this unexpected confrontation with death.

REFERENCES

1. Bourne S. Stillbirths, grief and medical education. *Br Med J* **1**:1157, 1977.
2. Bowlby J. The nature of the child's tie to his mother. *Int J Psycho-Anal* **39**:350–371, 1950.
3. Condon JT. The parental-foetal relationship – a comparison of male and female expectant parents. *J Psychosom Obstet Gynecol* **4**:271–284, 1985.
4. Michelacci L, Fava GA, Grandi S, Bovicelli L, Orlandi C. Trombini G. Psychological reactions to ultrasound. *Psychother Psychosom* **50**:1–4, 1988.
5. Langer M, Ringler M, Reinhold E. Psychological effects of ultrasound examinations: changes of body perception and child image in pregnancy. *J Psychosom Obstet Gynecol* **8**:199–208, 1988.
6. Sjögren B, Uddenberg N. Prenatal diagnosis and maternal attachment to the child-to-be. *J Psychosom Obstet Gynecol* **9**:73–87, 1988.
7. Phipps S. The subsequent pregnancy after stillbirth: anticipatory parenthood in the face of uncertainty. *Int J Psychiat Med* **15**:243–264, 1985/86.
8. Lindemann E. Symptomatology and management of acute grief. *Am J Psychiat* **101**, 1944.
9. Parkes CM, Weiss RS. *Recovery from Bereavement*. New York: Basic Books, 1983.
10. Bowlby J. Processes of mourning. *Int J Psycho-Anal* **42**:317, 1961.
11. Condon JT. Prevention of emotional disability following stillbirth – the role of the obstetric team. *Aust NZJ Obstet Gynecol* **27**:323–329, 1987.
12. Giles PFH. Reactions of women to perinatal death. *Aust NZJ Obstet Gynecol* **10**:207–210, 1970.
13. Kennell JH, Slyter J, Klaus MH. The mourning response of parents to the death of a newborn infant. *N Engl J Med* **283**:344–349, 1970.
14. Kirkley-Best E, Kellner KR. The forgotten grief: A review of the psychology of stillbirth. *Am J Orthopsychiat* **52**:420–429, 1982.
15. Costello A, Gardner SL, Merenstein GB. Perinatal grief and loss. *J Perinatol* **8**:361–370, 1988.
16. Leon IG. The invisible loss: the impact of perinatal death on siblings. *J Psychosom Obstet Gynecol* **5**:1–14, 1986.
17. Stierman ED. Emotional aspects of perinatal death. *Clin Obstet Gynecol* **30**:352–361, 1987.
18. Morris D. Management of perinatal bereavement. *Arch Dis Child* **63**:870–872, 1988.
19. Peppers CG, Knapp RJ. *Motherhood and Mourning*. New York: Praeger, 1980.
20. Turco R. The treatment of unresolved grief following loss of an infant. *Am J Obstet Gynecol* **141**:503–507, 1981.
21. Lewis E. The management of stillbirth: coping with an unreality. *Lancet* **Sept. 18**:619–620, 1976.
22. Van Putte AW. Perinatal bereavement crisis: coping with negative outcomes from prenatal diagnosis. *J Perinat Neonat Nurs* **2**:12–22, 1988.
23. Ringler M. The influence of prenatal diagnosis on parent-fetus bonding. In *The Free Woman* (eds E. Van Hall & J.C. Everaerd). Carnforth: Parthenon, pp. 210–217, 1989.
24. Drugan A, Greb A, Johnson MP *et al*. Determinants of parental decisions to abort for chromosome abnormalities. *Prenat Diagn* **10**:483–490, 1990.
25. Holzgreve W, Miny P. Genetic counselling in prenatal diagnosis. *Eur J Obstet Gynecol Reprod Biol* **49**:125–129, 1993.
26. Spinnato JA, Cook VD, Cook CR, Voss DH. Aggressive intrapartum management of lethal fetal anomalies: beyond fetal beneficence. *Obstet Gynecol* **85**:89–92, 1995.
27. Julian-Reynier C, Aurran Y, Dumaret A, Maron A, Chabal F, Giraud F, Ayme S. Attitudes towards Down's syndrome: follow-up of a cohort of 280 cases. *J Med Genet* **32**:597–609, 1995.
28. Drotar D, Baskiewicz A, Irvin N, Kennell JH, Klaus MH. The adaptation of parents to the birth of an infant with a congenital malformation: a hypothetical model. *Pediatrics* **56**:710–717, 1975.
29. Zaccardi R, Abbott J, Koziol-McLain J. Loss and grief reactions after spontaneous miscarriage in the emergency department. *Ann Emerg Med* **22**:799–804, 1993.
30. Leppert HC, Pahlka BS. Grieving characteristics after spontaneous abortion: a management approach. *Obstet Gynecol* **64**:119–122, 1984.
31. Toedter LJ, Lasker JN, Alhadeff JM. The perinatal grief scale: development and initial validation. *Am J Orthopsychiat* **58**:435–449, 1988.
32. Beutel M, Deckard R, Schaudig K, Franke S, Zauner R. Trauer, Depressivität und Angst nach einem Spontanabort. *Psychother Psychosom Med Psychol* **42**:158–166, 1992.
33. Cecil R. 'I wouldn't have minded a wee one running about': miscarriage and the family. *Soc Sci Med* **38**:1415–1422, 1994.
34. Rajan L. Social isolation and support in pregnancy loss. *Health Visit* **67**:97–101, 1994.
35. Läpple M. Diagnostik, Beratung und Psychotherapie bei Spontanaborten und rezidivierenden Spontanaborten. *Z Klin Psychopath Psychother* **37**:277–290, 1989.
36. Beck Black R. A one and six month follow-up of prenatal diagnosis patients who lost pregnancies. *Prenat Diagn* **9**:795–804, 1989.
37. Beck Black R. Prenatal diagnosis and fetal loss: psychosocial consequences and professional responsibilities. *Am J Med Genet* **35**:586–587, 1990.
38. Elder SH, Laurence KM. The impact of supportive intervention after second trimester termination of pregnancy for fetal abnormality. *Prenat Diagn* **11**:47–54, 1991.
39. Von Gontard A. Psychische Folgen des Schwangerschaftsabbruchs aus kindlicher Indikation. *Monatsschr Kinderheil* **134**:150–157, 1986.
40. Jörgensen C, Uddenberg N, Ursing I. Ultrasound diagnosis of fetal malformation in the second trimester. The psychological reactions of the women. *J Psychosom Obstet Gynecol* **4**:31–40, 1985.
41. Kenyon SL, Hackett GA, Campbell S. Termination of pregnancy following diagnosis of fetal malformation: the need for improved follow-up services. *Clin Obstet Gynecol* **31**:97–100, 1988.
42. Langer M, Ringler M. Prospective counselling after prenatal diagnosis of fetal malformations: interventions and parental reactions. *Acta Obstet Gynecol Scand* **68**:323–329, 1989.
43. Lloyd J, Laurence KM. Sequelae and support after termination of pregnancy for fetal malformation. *Br Med J* **290**:907–909, 1985.
44. Frets PG, Los FJ, Sachs ES, Jahoda MGJ. Psychological counseling of couples experiencing a pregnancy termination after amniocentesis. *J Psychosom Obstet Gynecol* **11**:53–59, 1990.
45. Muth C, Exler U, Miny P, Holzgreve W. Die psychische Verarbeitung eines Schwangerschaftsabbruchs aus genetischer Indikation im zweiten Trimenon. *Z Geburtsh Perinat* **193**:96–99, 1989.
46. Leschot NJ, Verjaal M, Treffers PE. Therapeutic abortion on genetic indications. A detailed follow-up study of 20 patients. *J Psychosom Obstet Gynecol* **1**:47–56, 1982.
47. Lorenzen J, Holzgreve W. Helping parents to grieve after second trimester termination of pregnancy for fetopathic reasons. *Fetal Diagn Ther* **10**:147–156, 1995.
48. Dallaire L, Lortie G, Des Rochers M, Clermont R, Vachon C. Parental reaction and adaptability to the prenatal diagnosis of fetal defect or genetic disease leading to pregnancy interruption. *Prenat Diagn* **15**:249–259, 1995.
49. Jones OW, Penn NE, Shuchter S *et al*. Parental response to mid-trimester therapeutic abortion following amnicentesis. *Prenat Diagn* **4**:249–256, 1984.
50. Becker J, Glinski L, Laxova R. Long term emotional impact of 2nd trimester pregnancy termination after detection of fetal abnormality. *Am J Hum Genet* **36**:122, 1984.
51. White-van Mourik MC, Connor JM, Ferguson-Smith MA. Patient care before and after termination of pregnancy for neural tube defects. *Prenat Diagn* **10**:497–505, 1990.
52. Benfield DG, Leib SA, Vollman JH. Grief responses of parents to neonatal death and parent participation in deciding care. *Pediatrics* **62**:171–177, 1978.
53. Vance JC, Najman JM, Thearle MJ, Embelton G, Foster WJ, Boyle FM. Psychological changes in parents eight months after the loss of an infant from stillbirth, neonatal death or sudden infant death syndrome – a longitudinal study. *Pediatrics* **96**:933–938, 1995.
54. Revak-Lutz RJ, Kellner KR. Paternal involvement after perinatal death. *J Perinatol* **14**:442–445, 1994.
55. Beutel M. Verarbeitung von Spontanabort und Totgeburt in der Partnershaft. *Psychotherapeut* **40**:291–297, 1995.
56. Najmen JK, Vance JC, Boyle F, Embleton G, Foster B, Thearle J. The impact of child death on marital adjustment. *Soc Sci Med* **37**:1005–1010, 1993.
57. Forrest GC, Standish E, Baum JD. Support after perinatal death: a study

of support and counselling after perinatal bereavement. *Br Med J* **285**:1475–1479, 1982.
58. Theut SK, Zaslow MJ, Rabinovich BA, Bartko JJ, Morishisa JM. Resolution of parental bereavement after a perinatal loss. *J Am Acad Child Adolesc Psychiatry* **29**:521–525, 1990.
59. Stinson KM, Lasker JN, Lohman J, Toedter LJ. Parents' grief following pregnancy loss. A comparison of mothers and fathers. *Fam Relat* **41**:218–223, 1992.
60. Beutel M, Willner H, Deckardt M, von Rad M, Weiner H. Couples' grief after early pregnancy loss – results from a 12-months follow-up study. In *Advanced Research in Psychosomatic Obstetrics and Gynecology* (eds D. Richter & P. Nijs), pp. 49–46. Leuven/Belgium: Uitgeverij Peeters, 1995.
61. Cordell AS, Apolito R. Family support in infant death. *J Obstet Gynecol Nurs* **10**:281–285, 1981.
62. Hutton CJ, Bradley BS. Effects of sudden infant death on bereaved siblings: a comparative study. *J Child Psychol Psychiatry* **35**:723–732, 1994.
63. Furlong R, Hobbins J. Grief in the perinatal period. *Obstet Gynecol* **61**:497–500, 1983.
64. Goldmann-Posch U. *Wenn Mütter trauern*. München: Kindler, 1988.
65. Lothrop H. *Gute Hoffnung-jähes Ende*. München: Kösel, 1991.
66. Lewis E. Inhibition of mourning by pregnancy: psychopathology and management. *Br Med J* **ii**:27–28, 1979.
67. Bryan EM. The death of a twin. *Palliat Med* **9**:187–192, 1995.
68. Rowe J, Clyman R, Green C. Follow-up of families who experience a perinatal death. *Pediatrics* **62**:166–169, 1978.
69. Bourne S, Lewis E. Pregnancy after stillbirth or neonatal death: psychological risks and management. *Lancet* **i**:31–33, 1984.
70. Wolff JR, Nielson PE, Schiller P. The emotional reaction to a stillbirth. *Am J Obstet Gynecol* **108**:73–77, 1970.
71. Kemp VH, Page C. Maternal self-esteem and prenatal attachment in high-risk pregnancy. *Matern Child Nurs J* **16**:195–206, 1987.
72. Crowther ME. Perinatal death: worse obstetric and neonatal outcome in a subsequent pregnancy. *J R Army Med Corps* **141**:92–97, 1995.
73. Weeks JW, Asrat T, Morgan MA, Nageotte M, Thomas SJ, Freeman RK. Antepartum surveillance for a history of stillbirth: when to begin? *Am J Obstet Gynecol* **172**:486–492, 1995.
74. Kellner KR, Donnelly WH, Gould SD. Parental behavior after perinatal death: lack of predictive demographic and obstetric variables. *Obstet Gynecol* **63**:809–814, 1984.
75. Smialek Z. Observations on immediate reactions of families to sudden infant death. *Pediatrics* **62**:160–165, 1978.
76. Cohen L. Perinatal mortality: assisting parental affirmation. *Am J Orthopsychiatry* **48**:727–731, 1978.
77. Batcup G, Clarke JP, Purdie DW. Disposal arrangements for fetuses in the second trimester. *Br J Obstet Gynecol* **95**:547–550, 1988.
78. de Launiere MG, Boudreault A. Devant un deuil perinatal. *Can Nurse* **91**:41–46, 1995.
79. Kirk EP. Psychological effects and management of perinatal loss. *Am J Obstet Gynecol* **149**:46–51, 1984.
80. Jolly H. Family reactions to stillbirth. *Proc Roy Soc Med* **69**:835–837, 1976.
81. Lake M, Knuppel RA, Murphy J, Johnson TM. The role of a grief support team following stillbirth. *Am J Obstet Gynecol* **146**:877–881, 1983.
82. Schreiner RL, Gresham EL, Green M. Physician's responsibility to parents after death of an infant. *Am J Dis Child* **133**:723–726, 1979.
83. Hunfeld JA, Wladimiroff JW, Verhage F, Passchier J. Previous stress and acute psychological defence as predictors of perinatal grief – an exploratory study. *Soc Sci Med* **40**:829–835, 1995.
84. Zisook S. Death, dying and bereavement. In *Comprehensive Textbook of Psychiatry* 6th edn (eds H.J. Kaplan & B.J. Sadock). Baltimore: Williams and Wilkins, 1995.
85. Worden JW. *Grief Counselling and Grief Therapy*. New York: Springer, 1991.
86. Strupp H, Binder J. *Psychotherapy in a New Key*. New York: Basic Books, 1984.
87. Weisman M, Klerman GL (eds). *New Applications of Interpersonal Psychotherapy*. Washington: American Psychiatric Press, 1993.
88. Beck AT, Rush AJ, Shaw BF, Emery G. *Cognitive Therapy of Depression*. New York: Guilford Press, 1979.
89. Horowitz MJ, Marmar C, Krupnick J, Wilner N, Kaltreider N, Wallerstein R. *Personality Styles and Brief Psychotherapy*. New York: Basic Books, 1984.
90. Horowitz MJ. *Stress Response Syndromes*. New York: Aronson, 1986.

Screening for genetic disease in the community

32

B. Modell and M. Modell

Introduction

For the community to profit fully from developments in fetal medicine, couples at increased reproductive risk need to be identified and informed early enough to take advantage of prenatal diagnosis, and this depends largely on population screening. At present, screening for genetic reproductive risk is usually left until women reach the antenatal clinic. This is partly because the commonest preventable congenital malformations and chromosomal disorders arise sporadically at conception or in early embryonic development, and so can only be detected during pregnancy. In addition, pregnant women are a captive population, and there is a well-established system for collecting and analysing specimens already in place. However, antenatal screening as presently practised is not the ideal approach for preventing neural tube defects (and perhaps other congenital malformations), congenital infections, and inherited disorders, and is often done too late to permit first trimester prenatal diagnosis.

There is an increasingly strong case for promoting genetic screening and counselling in primary health care. The human genome project is rapidly increasing the possibilities for genetic testing, and once a test is available, carriers of inherited disorders can be detected and advised at any time of life. Couples 'at risk' for children with inherited disorders have a special need for timely counselling and the widest possible choice of options, because of their high (usually 25%) risk of an affected child, which recurs in every pregnancy. Detecting such at risk couples before pregnancy permits them to consider options other than prenatal diagnosis, and to choose early (first trimester) prenatal diagnosis in each pregnancy. In addition, close relatives of patients and carriers should be offered carrier testing ('cascade' testing), which is not feasible in the context of the antenatal clinic.

Fortunately, interest in genetic screening in primary health care is also increasing because of the likelihood that identifying people with a genetic predisposition to common disorders (including coronary heart disease and some cancers) will help to prevent or delay the onset of disease. On the other hand, most primary health care professionals were poorly trained in genetics while undergraduates, and as yet, few understand the growing relevance of genetics for primary care; therefore medical genetics hardly figures in continuing medical education for primary care workers.

In this chapter we demonstrate the inadequacy of antenatal screening for carriers of inherited disorders, and examine the desirability and practical feasibility of promoting pre- or very early pregnancy screening in primary care. If this is to be recommended as national policy, its advantages and disadvantages must be carefully compared with those of antenatal screening as presently practised. We therefore review the general principles of screening, examine the advantages and disadvantages of identifying genetic risk before pregnant women present at the antenatal clinic, and consider some community-based genetic screening programmes in Europe. We review the appropriateness of the UK primary care system as an infrastructure for supporting a wide range of genetic services including screening, preconception advice, and early identification of individuals (and families) at increased genetic risk, and consider the part that obstetricians, midwives and fetal medicine experts can play in promoting screening for reproductive risk in primary care. Many issues raised are relevant to other comprehensive community-based primary care systems (e.g. in the Netherlands), and to 'vertical' government programmes of preventive health care like the Maternal and Child Health programmes that are common in developing countries (e.g. in China) and the Hungarian 'optimal family planning programme' (A. Czeizel, personal communication).

General principles of genetic screening programmes

Before proceeding, it is necessary to define our interpretation of some key words and concepts in genetic screening.

Genetic screening

The aims are (a) to detect (or exclude) specific reproductive risks, or potential future inherited disease in people who consider themselves healthy, and (b) to inform people found to be at risk of the steps they can take to reduce or avoid the problem. The main clinical objective of counselling for reproductive risk is informed choice for the couples concerned, rather than a reduction in the number of affected births – though in practice the first usually leads to the second. This view leads us to emphasize the importance of providing full information at each stage of the programme.

Population screening

In epidemiological terms, a population is a selected group, such as all women seeking family planning advice, all pregnant women, all fetuses, all newborns, all people with learning disabilities, or all patients on a general practitioner's list. Population screening is an organized approach to screening *all* the selected population. Screening programmes often start with an identified cohort of the target population, e.g. newborns, or children attending school (e.g. rubella screening when there is no childhood immunization), so that with the passage of time ultimately the whole selected population will be tested.

Primary screening test

Most screening programmes start with a relatively simple *primary screening test* that is offered to as many of the selected population as possible – e.g. carrier screening for haemoglobin disorders is offered to people not of northern European origin*, and neonates are screened for phenylketonuria and hypothyroidism, and congenital dislocation of the hip. Usually the primary screen identifies a possible risk, and more complex tests are needed to reach a definitive diagnosis.

Genetic testing

Genetic testing is offered to selected individuals who are already known to be at high genetic risk because, for instance, they have a positive primary screening test, or a suggestive family history (e.g. first degree relative with familial hypercholesterolaemia or cystic fibrosis), or they suffer from a condition that may have a genetic origin (e.g. severe learning difficulty), or because a relative has been found to carry a genetic disorder by population screening.

Information and genetic counselling

It is important to discriminate between information and genetic counselling. In principle most health professionals (e.g. obstetricians, midwives, GPs, practice nurses) can provide basic information when offering screening, explain false positive screening results, and give preliminary information to people with true positive results. However, to do this they must themselves be informed, which is far from the case at present. Giving basic information need not be time consuming if the necessary tools (such as posters, leaflets, and information booklets to be handed to patients) are available, but they rarely are. Genetic counselling additionally involves helping patients to make the decision that is right for themselves, within recognized ethical principles (see below). It requires in-depth knowledge of the condition(s) involved, training in counselling techniques, time, and an appropriate personality. *Basic* genetic counselling for common reproductive risks is often provided by trained non-physician counsellors such as genetic associates, haemoglobinopathy counsellors or antenatal screening coordinators. For example, basic counselling for carriers (e.g. of a haemoglobin disorder or cystic fibrosis) detected by population screening must cover the implications for themselves, the desirability of testing their partner, and implications for their children and other relatives. Counselling at this level is also within the scope of trained primary care workers equipped with appropriate information materials. By contrast, people at risk for rare or complex disorders, and women at risk of having a child with a severe congenital or genetic disorder (especially if pregnant) require extensive *expert* genetic counselling by a specialist. Genetic counselling takes time, and so can be expensive.

IDENTIFYING GENETIC RISK: POPULATION SCREENING VERSUS THE GENETIC FAMILY HISTORY

The classical approach for identifying people at genetic risk is through family studies. When a clear genetic diagnosis is made in one family member, drawing up a pedigree allows a risk estimate for each relative (e.g. first degree relatives of a person who carries an abnormal gene have a 50% chance of also being carriers). Relatives often have to base important life decisions on such probabilistic information, but the new genetic technology is increasing their chance of finding out definitely if they are, or are not, a carrier.

Family studies have two important limitations.

- Preventing subsequent cases after the birth of the first affected child makes a relatively small difference to the

*In many countries this of course means the whole population. In Northern European countries it is increasingly difficult to identify those at risk by ethnic origin, because of population mixing, and universal antenatal and neonatal screening for haemoglobin disorders is becoming widespread.

birthrate of affected children in the population as a whole. For example, it is possible to offer prenatal diagnosis for a recessively inherited disorder in only 12% of all at risk pregnancies when final family size is small, and in less than 50% when it is large[1]

- Only a fraction of the carriers in the population who could benefit from knowledge of risk can be identified through family studies*. The maximum proportion of carriers of a recessively inherited disorder identifiable by family studies depends on carrier frequency. For example, in the UK no more than 6% of cystic fibrosis carriers (carrier frequency 4.5%) could be detected (Fig. 32.1).

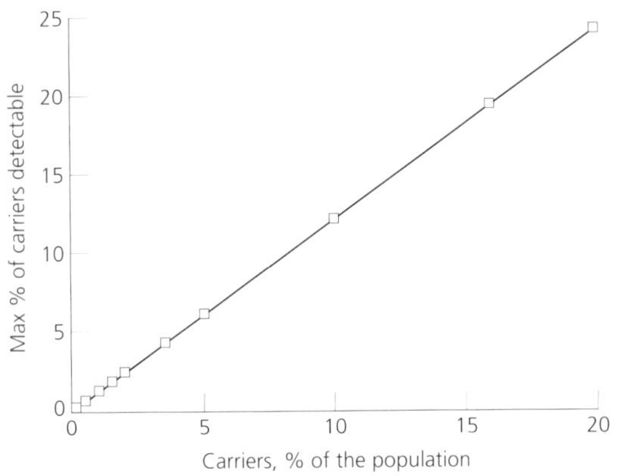

Fig. 32.1 Maximum percentage of carriers of a recessively inherited disorder detectable from family studies. The figure depends on mode of inheritance, carrier frequency, mean survival of affected people (which determines the number of index cases), and population characteristics such as average family size and whether 'random' partner choice or consanguineous marriage is preferred. The assumptions used here generate a maximum possible figure for a typical western population. They are: recessive inheritance, carrier frequency 4.5%, random mating, normal survival of index cases, and six carriers identified per index case.

By contrast, when a reliable carrier test is available it is possible to screen the whole population in order to identify as many at-risk couples as possible *before any* affected child is born into the family. In theory this approach could greatly reduce the number of affected cases: in practice the effect depends on the attitudes of the population being screened, and the efficiency of the service. The experience of carrier screening for haemoglobin disorders has provided a great deal of information on these aspects of genetic population screening over the past 20 years[2]. The results of more recent experience with carrier screening for cystic fibrosis closely reflect findings with the haemoglobin disorders[3].

*The proportion of carriers detectable varies with inheritance pattern. Calculations for recessively inherited disorders are relatively simple. The proportion of carriers of X-linked disorders (such as haemophilia, Duchenne muscular dystrophy and fragile X linked mental retardation) that can be detected by family studies does not exceed 50%, and varies with mutation rate and random factors such as inheritance in the female line. More carriers of dominant conditions can be detected, but the indications are complicated because of psychosocial implications.

Genetic population screening is a public health activity. It requires policy decisions, systematic planning, and support by the health authorities; it involves many aspects of the health service, needs an appropriate health infrastructure, and depends on outreach activities including training and information for health workers, information for the public, and regular audit. The reality, of course, is that in the initial phases of a screening programme there is no national policy, and screening is left to enthusiastic individuals in different parts of the country. They need to conduct well-designed pilot studies, and to analyse costs and benefits, to justify consideration of a national screening programme.

Family studies and genetic screening are complementary rather than alternatives. On the one hand, taking a basic genetic family history is a form of genetic screening for people who could benefit from referral to a specialist, and on the other, when population screening identifies a carrier their extended family should be offered carrier testing.

PRINCIPLES OF SCREENING

The general requirements for screening[4] summarized below apply for genetic screening. In this section, each requirement is discussed in turn.

- The primary screening test should be reasonably reliable
- The problem must be important
- There must be a well-mapped-out course of action following a positive test
- Facilities for information, testing and counselling should be generally available
- Tests must be acceptable to the target population
- The cost per test should be affordable

THE PRIMARY SCREENING TEST SHOULD BE REASONABLY RELIABLE

A primary screening test usually identifies a group that includes as many as possible of those who have the target condition (true positives), plus a variable number of people who do not (false positives). Definitive diagnosis then depends on further tests, each involving a smaller group of people. Table 32.1 lists types of primary genetic screening tests.

A basic *genetic family history* is already used in reproductive medicine to identify genetic risks that should not be missed (e.g. a parent or relative has a sickle cell disorder, achondroplasia, haemophilia or Duchenne muscular dystrophy). However, it is a very hit-and-miss affair in current practice. It needs to be put on a more formal basis, and practice should be standardized. Genetic screening using the family history is

TABLE 32.1
Types of primary screening tests

Test	Example
Family history	Previous affected child
Clinical examination	Deafness, CDH
Biochemical tests:	
– Non-specific (empirical) tests	msAFP, Down screen
– Specific test for secondary effects (e.g. metabolite)	PKU, CHT
– Specific test for primary product (usually protein)	Haemoglobin disorders
DNA tests	Cystic fibrosis

CDH = congenital dislocation of the hip
msAFP = maternal serum alphafetoprotein
PKU = phenylketonuria
CHT = congenital hypothyroidism

particularly appropriate in primary health care – if the doctors and nurses involved are adequately trained.

Clinical examination is in general less reliable than laboratory tests. For example screening for congenital dislocation of the hip calls for experience and judgement, but may be performed by relatively inexperienced doctors. Though this is unsatisfactory, a clinical screen for congenital dislocation of the hip is still recommended in the absence of more specific tests[5]. However, it could be replaced by ultrasound scanning in the future.

Many *biochemical tests* are quantitative, the number of false positives and negatives depending on the 'cutoff' value selected to distinguish a 'normal' from an 'abnormal' result. Meticulous laboratory practice and a quality-control system are necessary to obtain reliable results that can be reproduced at different centres.

- 'Non-specific' biochemical tests are related only indirectly to the underlying disorder (e.g. maternal serum AFP assay, maternal serum screening for Down Syndrome). There may be extensive overlap between the normal and abnormal ranges, and the number of false positives often greatly exceeds the number of true positives.
- Neonatal screening for PKU depends on measuring the level of a metabolite phenylalanine) that is normally processed by the enzyme under study (phenylalanine hydoxylase). This provides a much more specific test, with few false positives and almost no false negatives.
- Genetic tests that directly measure the affected protein (e.g. electrophoresis for abnormal haemoglobins) often give a qualitative yes/no result (when the mutation abolishes protein synthesis or produces an abnormal protein).
- *DNA tests* seem the most precise in principle, but in practice are often less precise than protein assay. Many genetic disorders (e.g. cystic fibrosis, thalassaemia) are caused by many different point mutations in the relevant gene, and it may only be cost-effective to screen for the commonest mutations. In the UK at present, carrier screening for cystic fibrosis is 100% specific (every positive is a true positive) but up to 15% of carriers are missed. DNA tests may prove highly effective for screening for conditions usually due to a specific mutation (e.g. achondroplasia) or to amplification of a repeating sequence (e.g. fragile X mental retardation, Friedreich's ataxia, myotonic dystrophy), or for simultaneous screening for multiple genetic risks.

Table 32.2 shows the proportions of *false positives* (unaffected people with a positive result) and *false negatives* (missed affected people) in some tests in current use. It should be kept in mind that a false positive result for a specific condition may have other clinical value – a pregnant woman with a raised serum AFP may have a non-viable pregnancy, or twins, and people with microcytosis may have iron-deficiency anaemia, or carry thalassaemia trait, or both. The figures show that primary screening tests for single gene disorders are among the most precise of the available tests.

THE PROBLEM MUST BE IMPORTANT

This could be because it is common, or because delay in diagnosis leads to severe disease, or both. Even when simple and precise tests are available, screening is not widely practised for disorders that do not usually lead to severe disease (e.g. G6PD deficiency, alpha-1-antitrypsin deficiency). On the other hand, the available screening tests for Down Syndrome fall far short of the ideal, but are widely implemented because the condition is common and severe.

The indication for genetic population screening also depends on the frequency of the mutation concerned, and the mode of inheritance. Table 32.3 lists some inherited disorders for which screening is already established, or could become so in the near future.

Most of the disorders that can (or could) appropriately be screened for are recessively inherited. In the UK, screening for haemoglobin disorders probably detects over 5000

TABLE 32.2
Proportions of false positives and false negatives in some current screening tests

Condition	Screening test	False positives	False negatives
Congenital dislocation of hip	Clinical	10:1	??
Neural tube defects	msAFP	3:1	<10%
Down syndrome	Maternal age >37	33:1	Approx. 60% of cases missed
Down syndrome	Triple test	33:1	>40% of cases missed
Phenylketonuria	Penylalanine assay	0.5:1	<1%
Congenital hypothyroidism	TSH assay	6:1	<1%
Abnormal haemoglobins	Hb electrophoresis	Almost 0	Almost 0
Thalassaemias	Red cell indices, Hb A_2 estimation	Very few	<2%
Cystic fibrosis (UK)	DNA for common mutations	0	15%

TABLE 32.3
Frequency of some conditions that are detected by population screening at present, or could be in the near future. Figures are given for the UK, with about 650 000 births/year at present

Condition	Carriers, % of population	Mode of inheritance	Affected births/ 1000	Pregnant carriers/year	At-risk pregnancies/ year	Potential affected births/year
Rhesus negativity	12	Recessive	2	78 000	9360	1300
Cystic fibrosis	4.5	Recessive	0.46	29 000	1200	300
Hb disorders[a]	0.88	Recessive	0.29	7120	869	217
Fragile X mental retardation	0.08	X-linked	0.02	520[b]	520	130
Phenylketonuria	1–2	Recessive	0.11	6500–13 000	300	75
Friedreich's ataxia	2–3	Recessive	0.1	13 000	260	65
Werdnig–Hoffman disease	2	Recessive	0.1	13 000	260	65

[a]Minimum figures[27,29]
[b]Carriers with the full fragile X mutation, i.e. at 25% risk of a severely affected son, plus a lower risk of a more mildly affected daughter

pregnant carriers per year. It could be worth the same effort to detect the far fewer carriers of fragile X mental retardation, since the affected birthrate is similar to that of the haemoglobin disorders.

THERE MUST BE A WELL-MAPPED-OUT COURSE OF ACTION FOLLOWING A POSITIVE TEST

Action may involve effective treatment, prenatal diagnosis with the option of selective abortion, or surveillance of people known to be at increased genetic risk for a serious disease. Screening for rhesus blood group is the oldest form of pregnancy-associated genetic screening. It addresses a common problem and provides a non-controversial and effective solution through routine administration of anti-D to rhesus negative women following delivery[6]. Screening for haemoglobin disorders is also well established, but was adopted more slowly because it took time for selective abortion to become recognized as an acceptable option. The appropriate action when genetic screening identifies individuals at increased risk of late onset disease can be problematic: lipid-lowering drugs lessen the risk of premature coronary heart disease for patients with familial hypercholesterolaemia, but it is uncertain whether enhanced surveillance, leading to early diagnosis, improves survival in inherited breast cancers.

FACILITIES FOR INFORMATION, TESTING AND COUNSELLING SHOULD BE GENERALLY AVAILABLE

It is a truism that appropriate pretest information is essential so that each person can make an informed choice of whether or not to be screened. Prescreening information should include:

- The target condition exists, and is inherited
- Carrier frequency
- The condition could affect *you*
- Risk can be detected reliably
- Consequences can be avoided

Carriers, once detected, require simple but complete information on the implications for their own health, and for their family.

Despite its crucial importance, information is often neglected in routine population screening in the context of a busy antenatal clinic or family medicine practice. Very little effort has so far been made to develop efficient and cost-effective approaches for patient information, and aids for counselling for common genetic risks. Unless the educational and financial resources for a national programme are provided centrally, standards will vary from one place to another. The ideal situation is likely to take years if not decades to establish, even in economically prosperous countries. Availability of information materials is therefore an appropriate concern for fetal medicine experts who wish to increase appropriate use of their service.

TESTS MUST BE ACCEPTABLE TO THE TARGET POPULATION

Primary screening tests should be as convenient and non-invasive as possible (e.g. a DNA sample may be obtained from a mouth wash rather than from blood) and culturally acceptable. For many members of some populations prenatal diagnosis may be unacceptable in the second trimester, but acceptable in the first trimester, for religious and cultural reasons[7].

COST PER TEST SHOULD BE AFFORDABLE

Economic analysis is important in evaluating pilot genetic screening studies[8]. However, it can be difficult to equate life-time costs for a family looking after a severely handicapped child, with the short-term expense of screening large numbers of mainly healthy people.

An increasing number of genetic tests meet the requirements discussed above: Table 32.3 includes some tests that could be considered in the near future. It is a truism that meticulously organized pilot projects are essential to decide which tests are suitable for introduction into national screening programmes, and that long-term follow-up and continuing evaluation are essential. However, there is often a long delay before a test that is demonstrably useful, acceptable and cost-effective is implemented on a large scale. For example, the safety, reliability, cost-effectiveness and acceptability of screening for haemoglobin disorders had been demonstrated by 1980[9], but screening was recommended nationally in the UK only in 1993[10]. Though similar data are now available for screening for cystic fibrosis, this is presently offered only where a highly motivated person persuades local health authorities of its value[11], or privately.

Delays in implementation may be partly attributed to the inertia of the health system, since considerable adaptations are needed to meet the following practical requirements for a genetic screening programme.

- Information for the people offered screening
- A network of diagnostic laboratories and a quality control system
- A system for collecting samples from the population and delivering them to the laboratory
- A system for recording results in an readily accessible way, both in the community and the laboratory
- Information and counselling for people with positive results, either by practice staff provided with the necessary information material, or other community-based counsellors
- Adequate expert centres for counselling at-risk couples and providing prenatal diagnosis
- Support for the woman or couple through any procedures they may undergo

Antenatal screening alone is inadequate

Once it has (finally) been decided that a genetic screening test is appropriate, the question needs to be addressed of where, when and to whom to offer it. Ideally it should be offered *routinely* at some point where the target group come into contact with the health system, and the above requirements can most easily be met. Genetic screening is still almost restricted to antenatal and neonatal screening because (in most communities) pregnant women routinely enter, and newborns routinely leave, obstetric care. Antenatal screening is efficient and cost-effective because the group most immediately at risk is targeted, patients and health workers perceive information on reproductive risk as highly relevant during pregnancy, other screening tests are done at this time, a system for specimen collection is already in place, and midwifery staff are experienced with screening.

However, it is easy to be complacent. Antenatal genetic screening as currently practised has important disadvantages, especially for couples at risk of inherited disorders. These couples naturally have a strong preference for the earliest possible diagnosis, because of the high level of anxiety caused by their high risk, and the distress associated with mid-trimester abortion. Fortunately first trimester diagnosis is possible for most diagnosable inherited diseases (by chorionic villus sampling followed by DNA, biochemical or chromosomal studies), and this makes a significant difference to the acceptability of prenatal diagnosis, especially for less predictable disorders. This difference has practical implications – only first trimester screening can have a major effect on the birth prevalence of these disorders – and is also an indicator of the unnecessary suffering caused by strategies that lead to mid-trimester abortion, when earlier diagnosis is possible.

Current antenatal booking policies, in the UK at least, are determined by factors other than the requirements of genetic screening, and differ widely by district. For example, in the former North East Thames Region in the UK, the proportion of women seen for the first time before 16 weeks' gestation ranges from 30% to over 90% at different hospitals (Fig. 32.2) because of variations in hospital policy.

When genetic screening is confined to the antenatal clinic but the majority of women are not booked in until after the first trimester, the following consequences are inevitably common.

- Many women or couples at risk are identified too late for prenatal diagnosis to be possible at all in the presenting pregnancy
- The majority of couples at risk are identified too late for first trimester diagnosis in the presenting pregnancy, especially when there are delays because family studies are needed to confirm a diagnosis of risk. Some couples who would request prenatal diagnosis in the first trimester, find second trimester testing unacceptably late
- Even when mid-trimester prenatal diagnosis is accepted, identification of a major genetic risk for the first time at this stage of the pregnancy is unnecessarily harrowing
- Some tests (e.g. carrier screening for Tay-Sachs disease) give less clear results during pregnancy
- Couples have only a short time to make the serious decisions needed, if a test turns out positive
- There is increased anxiety in pregnant carriers of a recessive disorder until the result of the partner's test is known
- Screening focused on women reinforces the false belief that only women have genetic problems
- 'Cascade' testing, though feasible in principle with the collaboration of family doctors, very rarely takes place in association with antenatal screening

These issues can all be illustrated from experience of antenatal screening for haemoglobin disorders. In the UK, antenatal screening for carriers of haemoglobin disorders is recommended practice[10]. Screening is required for clinical management as well as for genetic counselling: the differential diagnosis of iron deficiency and thalassaemia trait is important. Screening also detects women with sickle cell disorders, who are at increased risk of serious complications during or immediately after pregnancy and whose care needs specialist input from a haematologist. The 'haemoglobinopathy screen' consists of measuring the red cell indices, Hb A_2 estimation if there is microcytosis, and electrophoresis[12]. The methods are available in almost all haematology laboratories, and results are usually available in from 2 days to a week depending on the frequency with which electrophoresis and Hb A_2 estimation are carried out. New laboratory techniques (such as high performance liquid chromatography (HPLC)) increase the speed and accuracy, and reduce the expense of individual tests[13].

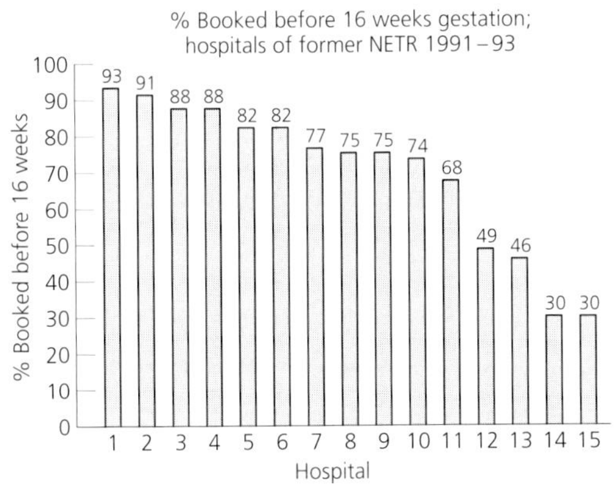

Fig. 32.2 Variation in gestation at antenatal booking at hospitals of the former North East Thames Regional Health Authority. The differences reflect differences in local policies. In many centres, it is clear that antenatal screening cannot lead to detection of carrier couples within the first trimester.

Screening for haemoglobin disorders usually follows a 'two-step' approach: the woman is tested at booking for antenatal care: the partner is offered testing if the woman is found to be a carrier. The stage at which risk is identified and counselling offered therefore depends on gestation at booking, and the pace of the subsequent process. First trimester diagnosis is possible in every case, and patients naturally have a very strong preference for it. Most couples at risk for thalassaemia major (a predictably highly burdensome disorder) choose to terminate affected pregnancies, even in the second trimester. The same is not true for sickle cell disorders, which are far less predictable. Here choice depends heavily on gestation at counselling: in the UK about 80% of referred couples at risk for a sickle cell disorder and counselled in the first trimester request prenatal diagnosis, compared to less than 50% of those seen later[7].

A recent national audit of the delivery of prenatal diagnosis for haemoglobin disorders in the UK has shown a wide gap between expectation (based on the observed choices of couples receiving expert counselling) and practice[14]. With an optimal service, it would be expected that over 50% of couples at risk for haemoglobin disorders would have a prenatal diagnosis, but in fact less than 20% do. This raises questions on the efficiency of screening (detection rate of at-risk couples), the adequacy of information for carriers, the timing of the steps in the screening process, and the nature of the counselling for at-risk couples – issues that are presently under investigation in the thalassaemia module of the National Confidential Enquiry into Genetic Counselling[15].

A study of the screening process for 30 at-risk couples detected in one year at a North London hospital[16] showed that though 50% of the women presented to their GP before the 11th week of pregnancy, only one was counselled in time for the offer of first trimester prenatal diagnosis. Twenty-seven were informed only in time for second trimester diagnosis, and three were informed too late for prenatal diagnosis to be an option. Only five women requested referral for discussion of prenatal diagnosis, three actually had a diagnosis, and one of nine affected pregnancies was terminated. The timing of counselling and referral was the same for women whose risk was detected for the first time in this pregnancy, and for those whose risk status had been detected previously, showing at-risk couples caught in an unproductive spiral of late referral and late counselling. The main reason for continuing late referral seemed to be because GPs assumed that everything would be dealt with in the antenatal clinic, but the antenatal routine progresses equally slowly for women with, and without a known risk. Only the five women who requested referral actually met the prenatal diagnosis (PND) team (a reassuring experience). According to regular practice at the centre, these couples were both informed of the possibility of early PND in subsequent pregnancies, and given clear written material including the centre's direct phone number, and told they could contact the PND service directly at first recognition of a subsequent pregnancy. The study was small, but it raises a multiplicity of questions, and points to a number of possibilities for improving the service. These call for increased involvement of primary care workers, but need not necessarily increase their workload.

Specific possibilities include the following:

- Encouraging carrier screening and basic counselling in primary care, both before and during pregnancy, e.g. opportunistic screening, screening of partners and relatives
- Promoting carrier screening as soon as a pregnancy is reported. This could be done either by the GP, or through an early hospital-based genetic counselling service for all pregnant women
- Promoting simultaneous screening of both partners when a pregnancy is first reported
- Encouraging GPs to refer at-risk couples directly for specialist counselling, instead of leaving this to the antenatal clinic

EXPERIENCE WITH COMMUNITY-BASED PROGRAMMES IN OTHER COUNTRIES

There is extensive experience in the Mediterranean region with community-based programmes for control of thalassaemia. Antenatal screening was rejected as the principal strategy in Italy, Greece and Cyprus, because it was felt that at-risk couples should have the choice of the full range of available options, including choosing not to marry another carrier, or avoiding pregnancy, or choosing early prenatal diagnosis. The strategies adopted in different areas all involve a government programme of intensive community education, including introducing specific teaching on the inheritance and meaning of thalassaemia in schools, publicizing the activities of support associations, and focusing on the issues involved in television programmes[17].

In Cyprus (where the potential birth rate of thalassaemia major is 7/1000) premarital carrier testing (in the government laboratory) is effectively mandatory, through a church ruling in the Greek community[18] and a government ruling in the Turkish community. Practically all at-risk couples are detected prior to marriage, and national statistics show that they use a variety of options: 3% choose not to marry, over 98% of those who do marry use prenatal diagnosis to obtain a healthy family, and on average at-risk couples have 20% fewer children than the national average, because many limit their family to two healthy children[19]. As a result, prevention is almost complete, though more recently, as the good results of present management are recognized, more couples are considering continuing affected pregnancies. There is also increasing pressure in the community for schoolchildren to be screened.

In Greece (potential affected births 2/1000) a programme of voluntary premarital testing has been established, based on a national network of dedicated screening centres, and a national education campaign[20]. However, the majority of couples who present for testing are already in early pregnancy, and there is a strong emphasis on integrating screening into obstetric practice. The government programme identifies about 50% of carriers, and the rest go to private laboratories. New affected births have fallen to 10–20% of expectation, but a plateau seems to have been reached, due largely to mistakes in carrier screening because of poor quality control in private laboratories.

The expert and well-supported Sardinian programme (potential affected births 3.5/1000) is based on community education, and outreach by mobile teams into the villages of this largely rural community[21]. The teams call village meetings, the aim being to motivate all people of reproductive age, and offer on-the-spot blood sampling. They return the next week to hand out sealed results, and hold a follow-up discussion, including the indications for testing relatives. This programme is also technically highly developed. Automated laboratory* and computer methods are used to achieve fast, cheap analysis and reliable records. Patients' results are recorded on magnetic 'smart' cards, which can be read on all screening centres' decoders. There are now very few affected births, and the main cause is still lack of information. The Regional Ministry of Health has provided a budget for a health education module in secondary schools, and in some schools optional carrier screening (with informed consent from the parents) is offered to pupils a few months later. However, screening in schools in limited because of differing attitudes among head teachers.

Surprisingly, there are now more living patients with haemoglobin disorders, and more affected births per year, in North-West than in Southern Europe. There are several reasons why it is particularly difficult to deliver carrier screening and counselling for haemoglobin disorders in Northern Europe: the disorders are considered as rare in the population

*Carrier screening is by haematological indices and automated HPLC analysis, which allows measurement of abnormal haemoglobins and Hb A_2 in a single step on all samples.

as a whole, though they are very common in minorities: the predominant problem is sickle cell disorder, for which genetic counselling is particularly difficult owing to its unpredictability: it is hard to deliver a specific service to diverse ethnic groups scattered in a large population not at risk: and a core of specially trained ethnic genetic counsellors is required because of cultural and linguistic diversity. The importance of the latter is clearly shown in the UK, where the choice to have prenatal diagnosis for sickle cell disorder has risen steadily in relation to the availability of trained counsellors of the relevant ethnic groups[22]. Perhaps the most important general lesson is the need to educate health workers in the principles of 'community genetics' to achieve successful community-based genetic screening.

SCREENING FOR CARRIERS OF CYSTIC FIBROSIS

Different approaches for information and carrier screening have been assessed for cystic fibrosis (CF). In primary care it has been concluded that the appropriate setting is during consultations relevant to reproduction, e.g. for family planning, or at first recognition of a pregnancy[23]. Antenatal screening has been studied in several settings. At present the preferred approach seems to be a form of couple testing, i.e. both partners are encouraged to give a sample simultaneously. There are then two options. One is to inform both partners of their result, and the implications for other family members. An alternative is to inform only couples where both partners are shown to be carriers that they are 'at risk': all other couples are considered 'screen negative' for that pregnancy, and informed accordingly. The main reason for choosing the latter approach is to limit costs, by avoiding counselling the numerous carriers identified – and indeed this may be the only way to initiate CF screening at present, in view of the financial restrictions affecting health services. The second approach also aims to reduce the anxiety caused when one partner is a carrier and the other tests negative, because of the residual (0.67%) risk that the negative partner is an undetected carrier, even though pilot programmes have not shown that this is a problem. On the other hand, the approach has the obvious disadvantage of excluding information and cascade screening for the majority of carriers detected. None of the current antenatal screening strategies focuses on achieving early detection of couples at risk.

Screening for genetic reproductive risk in primary care?

Though it is clearly not ideal, antenatal screening will always be needed as a back-up to any other approach for screening for reproductive risk. If genetic screening is to be extended into the community, new strategies will be needed. Table 32.4 summarizes the pros and cons of primary care systematic carrier screening for a condition such as cystic fibrosis, at different locations and times of life.

There have been a number of pilot projects to assess the feasibility and acceptability of genetic screening in general

TABLE 32.4
Primary care carrier screening

	Advantages	Disadvantages
When giving family planning or preconception advice	Often relevant, therefore the individual is unlikely to forget the result. Limited target population, and therefore more cost-effective. Before reproduction, allowing maximum reproductive choices	Requires genetic knowledge from health professionals who are often generalists, who find it difficult to explain genetic concepts in the context of a busy consultation. Specimen collection and processing system must be in place
Prepregnancy; adults of reproductive age	Before choice of partner and/or pregnancy, therefore allows maximum choices, including option of early PND. Cascade screening of relatives more likely. Both men and women can be offered testing	See above. Most costly option particularly if the percentage of carriers in the general population is low. Unlikely to be systematic, especially when there is no national primary care system. Individuals may forget result if there is a long time lag between test and reproduction
School-mid or late teens	Total population accessible. Before choice of partner or reproduction. Both sexes tested. Makes teaching of genetics and biology more personally relevant	Costly option. Hard to preserve confidentiality. Important to separate offer of test from teaching session. May damage 'healthy' self-image at a vulnerable time of life. Fear of stigmatization. Problem of informed consent. May forget result
Neonatal	Total population accessible. Blood spots already collected. Will also identify heterozygotes. Both sexes tested	Identifies less than half of carrier couples who may be offered PND in next pregnancy (a quarter of the first children will not be carriers, and a quarter will have the disease). Very long time lag before reproduction. No informed consent

practices and family planning clinics, and the following approaches have been tested.

- *Screening by invitation.* People are motivated to come for a specific test by writing to them, through media publicity, or through drives at community activities (e.g. through synagogues for Tay-Sachs disease, or ethnic community activities for haemoglobin disorders). This is considered a relatively inefficient approach, because even when there is an enthusiastic first response, it is not sustained and the general uptake rate is low[25]. However, such drives can be important in informing the community of the importance of testing.
- *Incidental or opportunistic screening.* People are offered screening when they attend a health professional for a reason related to reproduction, such as family planning or preconception advice, or on first reporting of a pregnancy[23,26]. Screening for genetic predisposition to common diseases could similarly be done in primary care when new patients register with a practice. Opportunistic screening is somewhat haphazard: it depends on variables such as individual health professional's level of interest, whether they remember to offer it at the appropriate moment, their training and ability to inform patients, and even on whether the patient or their employer pays (e.g. for a routine 'health check'). The general consensus is that in the initial stage, an opportunistic approach is the most feasible for all kinds of screening in primary care. This is then followed by a more systematic programme, with defined targets: an example is screening for cancer of the cervix[26].
- A community-based variant of antenatal screening, i.e. offering testing to women or couples *when a pregnancy is first reported to the primary care physician* (which is on average four weeks before the first hospital antenatal appointment)[23]. This greatly increases the chances that at-risk couples will be detected in time for first trimester prenatal diagnosis, and may be a very valuable strategy for primary care screening for reproductive risk.

Experience with the haemoglobin disorders indicates that there is no single 'best' approach for genetic screening, and population screening, cascade testing, antenatal and opportunistic screening all have their place in a community genetic counselling programme.

The percentage of carriers in the at-risk population is another important consideration in the cost-effectiveness equation of screening in primary care. Table 32.5 shows that screening for haemoglobin disorders should be offered opportunistically to Sub-Saharan Africans (25% of whom are carriers) whenever they enter the health care system. However, when the carrier frequency is lower there may be limited interest in offering screening to adolescents, or to all adults of reproductive age (unless there is some other health reason, as there may be with the haemoglobin disorders). It is likely to be felt that screening should be offered when individuals (and health professionals) perceive it as reproductively relevant, e.g. at consultations for family planning or as part of preconception advice, or when a pregnancy is first reported to the family doctor. This probably applies to cystic fibrosis in most North European communities.

The UK primary care system provides an infrastructure for genetic screening

Here we examine the UK primary care system, in relation to the requirements for systematic community involvement in genetic screening. Britain has a comprehensive system of community medical care with a long tradition of involvement in national screening programmes that, in principle, might be a very suitable vehicle for genetic screening. Over 95% of the population are registered with one of over 32 000 general practioners (GPs) or family doctors (half of all UK medical graduates). Access to hospital services is usually via referral from a GP, in contrast to the situation in most other countries where even when family physicians exist, people also have

TABLE 32.5
Percentage of carriers in at-risk populations

Population at risk	Carriers, % of population	Number of tests needed to detect one at-risk couple
Indians: Hb disorders	3	1144
North Europeans: CF	4	650
Pakistanis: Hb disorders	4.5	245[a]
Chinese: Hb disorders	8	268[b]
African Caribbeans: Hb disorders	12	78
Cypriots: Hb disorders	17	40
Sub-Saharan Africans: Hb disorders	25	20

[a]Calculation makes allowance for the high frequency of consanguineous marriage in this group
[b]Calculation makes allowance for the fact that two separate conditions, alpha and beta thalassaemia, are concerned

direct access to specialists. GPs are generalists, doctors of first contact who set no limits to the type of health (or social) problem a patient must suffer from before consulting, and their knowledge base must span the whole spectrum of medicine, albeit at a rather superficial level. It is unrealistic to expect GPs to introduce new treatments, or practice screening programmes, unless they are convinced (a) that these are relevant to *their* particular patients, and (b) that any new service can be easily incorporated into their working day.

Most GPs practise in groups of four or five, increasingly as members of a team of health professionals that usually also includes practice and community nurses (such as health visitors, who are responsible for health surveillance and support for young families). In contrast to hospital specialists, GPs are responsible for a defined list of patients from a restricted locality that usually (in urban areas) extends over a few square miles. An average practice includes a normal population of about 10 000 registered people, with the expected incidence and prevalence of diseases of that locality. GPs frequently look after several members of a family, who may live in the same house or neighbourhood for years, and they often develop a close relationship with their patients. From the population's perspective, it is the family doctor, not the hospital specialist, who provides personal and continuing care (though antenatal care is usually shared between GP and hospital). Individuals have lifelong personal practice-based records which follow them (when they move to a new area) to which ever practice they register with. In some practices the records of each family are filed together, because this helps the practice team relate illnesses in one family member with other family health and social problems. Family information is usually more accessible from general practice records than from hospital records.

British practices increasingly use computers for storing clinical data, and to facilitate surveillance of target groups (e.g. patients with asthma and diabetes). Availability of the computer during the consultation provides access to decision support programmes. This could be particularly helpful in genetic counselling, in helping to elicit and record the family history, and estimating specific risks and probabilities for individual patients as part of a baseline evaluation[27]. Electronic links to the outside world of computer software will give access to vast quantities of health information. For example, information leaflets tailored to the needs of individual patients are being produced, and could be a particularly effective way of informing health professionals as well as patients about genetic risks. Many information materials will become available on the Internet.

How can obstetricians and fetal medicine experts promote increased involvement of primary care workers?

Obstetricians and experts in fetal medicine have an important role to play in providing and disseminating information for community health workers. A general conclusion of studies of factors influencing GPs is that presenting them with patient-specific information relating directly to professional activity, in a user-friendly way, may change their clinical practice[28]. There is growing awareness of genetic screening in primary care, and some family doctors are already requesting tests, albeit in a haphazard and uncoordinated way. An initial baseline study (Fig. 32.3) showed that the number of haemoglobinopathy screening tests requested in 1994/5 by individual GPs served by the Whittington Hospital in North London varied from 0 to 120!

The authors have recently reported on a project based at this hospital, aiming to encourage local GPs to screen for haemoglobin disorders[27]. The objective is to promote opportunistic carrier screening, and encourage GPs to organize testing for partners rather than leaving this to the antenatal service. Early direct referral of couples at risk to expert counsellors is also encouraged. Twenty-six practices, randomized into study and control groups, took part in the study, and the main outcome measure was comparison of the number of requests for haemoglobinopathy screening from the practices.

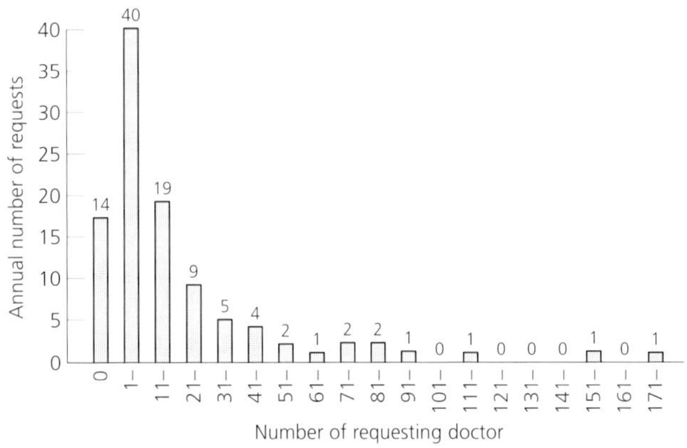

Fig. 32.3 Requests for a haemoglobinopathy screen from general practitioners using the Whittington Hospital haematology laboratory, January 1994 to June 1995.

RELEVANCE TO PRACTICE POPULATION; INFORMING STAFF AND PATIENTS

The area was chosen because a high percentage of births are in ethnic groups at risk for the haemoglobin disorders, and trained haemoglobinopathy counsellors are available. The demography of the area was discussed with the practice staff, to emphasize the relevance of screening for the practice population. A poster and leaflets informing people about haemoglobin disorders and the possibility of carrier testing, and a GP-oriented manual were produced for the practices.

HELPING PRACTITIONERS TO INTRODUCE A NEW SERVICE

A nurse facilitator was employed to liaise with and train the staff of the study practices. One of the first results of improved liaison was recognition that the laboratory lacked appropriate information leaflets for the carriers identified, to send to practices with the results. The research team and laboratory staff therefore produced a detailed, computerized set of information materials*. Whenever a carrier is identified, the laboratory now sends the practice a card plus a diagnosis-specific information leaflet to be given to the patient. The leaflet explains the implications of being a carrier for the person themselves, and for their relatives. The information is also incorporated into a letter to the GP, to be kept in the practice records and aid any counselling sessions. GPs also have the option of referring carriers they detect to the local haemoglobinopathy counsellors.

These steps led to an almost 100% increase in screening requests from study practices compared with controls. Closer examination of the data showed that most of the increase was due to a relatively small proportion of doctors, but the results show that carrier screening is feasible in primary care.

The future for genetic screening in primary care – increasing use of the family tree

The extension of population genetics beyond preconceptional and antenatal screening programmes, to the recognition of individuals, who would benefit from referral to a clinical geneticist and/or who are at genetic risk of prematurely developing specific serious diseases, has to be the task of physicians who look after families rather than just individuals.

The construction of a pedigree is the essential first step in the identification of individuals and families at increased genetic risk. In the UK, a person registering with a family doctor is expected to attend for an introductory consultation with the GP or nurse, during which brief details of the personal, past and family history are entered on a summary card that is placed at the front of the records and acts as an *aide-mémoire* at future consultations. This registration consultation, and other relevant consultations with a reproductive implication (family planning and preconception advice, or the first reporting of a pregnancy), present an ideal opportunity to construct a brief family tree, which will need to be updated every few years. In primary care the family tree is already extensively used as a shorthand method of highlighting events of both emotional and genetic significance, and to help in understanding the dynamics of the family. Progressing from taking this type of family history to constructing a simple pedigree is the key to increasing the involvement of the family doctor in community genetics. This pedigree will usually only need to include a limited number of relatives, unless genetic disease is suspected in a family member.

The aim of the genetic primary care family tree is to:

- Document the family pattern of illness with the objective of highlighting susceptibility to late-onset disease.
- Identify people with a family history that indicates that they may carry an X-linked or recessively inherited disease that confers a reproductive genetic risk.
- Identify people who would benefit from referral to a clinical geneticist.
- Identify relatives of patients with a known genetic disorder who may benefit from information and surveillance.

Conclusion

In this chapter we have presented the view that ideally there should be an integrated community/hospital approach to the identification of genetic risk[28]. At present the reality is that screening is mainly organized by the antenatal clinic. If carrier testing for common genetic diseases is to be offered before pregnancy by an outreach approach to the population, the practical screening requirements listed on p.364 will need modification as follows – additions in italics.

- *Informed and appropriately trained primary care workers. Though the infrastructure of UK family practice is steadily becoming more appropriate for community genetic screening, many tools for carrying out the task are not yet available. Posters, information leaflets, training for health workers in genetics and in counselling techniques, training videotapes, courses, books, reference materials and computer software are all still needed.*
- *Practitioners who have been persuaded that screening is relevant to the population they look after, and feasible in the context of a busy schedule of work. Primary care teams, as well as secondary care services, have to decide on their own screening policies, especially if there is no national guidance. Their decision will vary according to the proportion of likely carriers in the populations at risk (Table 32.5) and therefore the number of tests needed to detect one at-risk couple.*
- *Close collaboration between the referring doctor and the specialist, with a reliable system of reporting results and their interpretation to health professionals and people concerned.*
- Information for the population at risk – via national publicity, the media, school programmes for teaching genetics to teenagers, posters, leaflets, the internet, etc.
- A network of diagnostic laboratories and a quality control system.

*Information materials now available on the Internet at www.chime.ucl.ac.uk/APoGI

- A system for collecting samples from the population and delivering them to the laboratory.
- A system for recording results in a readily accessible way, both in the community and the laboratory.
- Information and counselling for people with positive results, either by practice staff provided with the necessary information material, or other community-based counsellors.
- Arrangements for testing the partner and other family members when necessary. Screening of partners and relatives will be a particularly important part of a community screening programme, though confidentiality dictates that these can only be approached via the index patient.
- Adequate expert centres for counselling at-risk couples and providing prenatal diagnosis.
- Support for the woman or couple through any procedures they may undergo.
- Discuss family planning and support in future pregnancies.

REFERENCES

1. Fraser GR. The short-term reduction in birth incidence of recessive diseases as a result of genetic counselling after the birth of an affected child. *Hum Hered* **22**:1–6, 1972.
2. WHO. Community control of hereditary anaemias: Memorandum from a WHO meeting. *Bull Wld Health Org* **61**:63–80, 1983.
3. Modell M. Screening for carriers of cystic fibrosis – a general practitioner's perspective. *BJ* **307**:849–852, 1993.
4. Wilson JMG, Jungner G. *Principles and Practice of Screening for Disease*. Geneva: WHO. Public Health Papers No. 34. 1968.
5. Hall DMB (ed). *Health for All Children*, 3rd edn. Oxford: Oxford University Press, 1996.
6. Clarke C. Prevention of Rh haemolytic disease by immunoglobulin anti-D. *Vox Sang* **44**:396–399, 1983.
7. Petrou M, Brugiatelli M, Ward RHT, Modell B. Factors affecting the uptake of prenatal diagnosis for sickle cell disease. *J Med Genet* **29**:820–823, 1992.
8. Beech R, Bekker H. Planning the development of cystic fibrosis gene carrier screening. *J Health Serv Res Pol* **1**(2):81–92, 1996.
9. Modell B, Ward RHT, Fairweather DVI. Effect of introducing antenatal diagnosis on the reproductive behaviour of families at risk for thalassaemia major. *BJ* **2**:737, 1980.
10. *Report of a Working Party of the Standing Medical Advisory Committee on Sickle Cell, Thalassaemia and other Haemoglobinopathies*. London: Her Majesty's Stationery Office, 1994.
11. Mennie ME, Gilfillan A, Compton M *et al*. Prenatal screening for cystic fibrosis. Lancet **340**:214–216, 1992.
12. British Society for Haematology. Guidelines for haemoglobinopathy screening. *Clin Lab Haemat* **10**:87–94, 1988.
13. Lorey F, Cunningham G, Shafer F, Lubin B, Vichinsky E. Universal screening for hemoglobinopathies using high-performance liquid chromatography: clinical results of 2.2 million screens. *Eur J Hum Genet* **2**:262–271, 1994.
14. Modell B, Petrou M, Layton M *et al*. Audit of prenatal diagnosis for haemoglobin disorders in the United Kingdom: the first 20 years. *Ann NY Acad Sci* **850**:420–422, 1996.
15. Harris R. How well do we manage families with genetic problems? A national confidential enquiry into counselling for genetic disorders should tell us. *BJ* **303**:1412–1413, 1991.
16. Neuenschwander H, Modell B. Audit of process of antenatal sickle cell screening at a north London hospital. *BMJ* **315**:784–785, 1997.
17. Kuliev AM. Thalassaemia can be prevented. *Wld Health For* **7**:286–290, 1986.
18. Angastiniotis MA, Hadjiminas MG. Prevention of thalassaemia in Cyprus. *Lancet* **1**:369–370, 1981.
19. Angastiniotis MA, Kyriakidou S, Hadjiminas M. How thalassaemia was controlled in Cyprus. *Wld Health For* **7**:291–297, 1986.
20. Loukopoulos D. Current status of thalassemia and the sickle cell syndromes in Greece. *Sem Hemat* **33**:76–86. 1996.
21. Cao A, Rosatelli. Screening and prenatal diagnosis of the haemoglobinopathies. *Bailliere's Clin Haemat* **6**:263–286, 1993.
22. Modell B. EC concerted action on developing patient registers as a tool for improving service delivery for haemoglobin disorders. In *Health Services Research* (eds G.N. Fracchia & M. Theophilatou). Amsterdam: IOS Press, 1993.
23. Bekker H, Modell M, Denniss G *et al*. Uptake of cystic fibrosis carrier testing in primary care: supply push or demand pull? *BMJ* **306**:1584–1587, 1993.
24. Harris HJ, Scotcher D, Craufurd D, Wallace A, Harris R. Cystic fibrosis carrier screening at first diagnosis of pregnancy in general practice. *Lancet* **339**:1539, 1992.
25. *General Practice in the National Health Service. The 1990 Contract*. Health Departments of Great Britain, August 1989.
26. Effective Health Care; Implementing Clinical Practice Guidelines 1994 No. 8.
27. Modell M, Wonke B, Anionwu E *et al*. Multidisciplinary approach for improving services in primary care: the example of screening for haemoglobin disorders. *BMJ* **317**:788–791, 1998.
28. Harris R, Harris H. Primary care for patients at genetic risk. *BJ* **311**:579–580, 1995.
29. Health Education Authority. Sickle Cell and Thalassaemia: Achieving Health Gain. Guidance for Commissioners and Providers. London: Health Education Authority, 1998.

Biochemical screening for neural tube defects and Down syndrome

33

J.E. Haddow and G.E. Palomaki

How prenatal screening began

The era of prenatal screening began in 1972, when Brock and Sutcliffe reported that alpha-fetoprotein (AFP) measurement was useful as a marker for detecting open neural tube defects (open spina bifida and anencephaly) in the fetus[1]. This initial discovery was limited to AFP levels in amniotic fluid, but it set the stage for the subsequent discovery of an association between fetal open neural tube defects and AFP levels in maternal serum[2,3]. Considerable overlap was found to exist between maternal serum AFP levels in affected and unaffected pregnancies, however. For that reason, maternal serum AFP measurement, while useful as a screening test, could not be used for diagnostic purposes. Pregnancies identified as being at high risk for open neural tube defects by virtue of elevated maternal serum AFP levels require diagnostic studies, such as AFP and acetylcholinesterase measurements in amniotic fluid and/or fetal scanning by an expert sonographer. A large-scale collaborative study was promptly organized in the United Kingdom to determine how to apply maternal serum AFP measurements most appropriately in population settings. The report of that study, in 1977, contained the scientific principles that continue to serve as guidelines for screening programmes[4].

Screening for open neural tube defects

WHY ALPHA-FETOPROTEIN IS USEFUL AS A MARKER FOR OPEN NEURAL TUBE DEFECTS

AFP was discovered in 1956 by Bergstrand and Czar. They observed an extra electrophoretic band in the α-1 region in fetal serum[5]. This extra α-1 band represented a protein not normally found in adults and was labelled alpha-1 fetoprotein. AFP is thought to be related evolutionarily to albumin. Genes for the two proteins are located on chromosome 4, and AFP has a similar molecular weight (69 000 daltons) and structure to albumin[6,7]. In spite of this structural similarity, antisera raised to AFP in a variety of animal species do not cross-react with albumin. AFP antisera can, therefore, be used successfully in laboratory assay systems for analysing AFP in body fluids that also contain albumin. The circulating use of AFP is approximately 4 days in the human adult.

AFP is synthesized in the fetal liver and yolk sac and is the dominant serum protein early in fetal life. It reaches a peak fetal serum concentration of approximately 300 mg/dl late in the first trimester. Thereafter, its concentration decreases steadily, but the fetal liver continues to produce AFP at a constant rate until approximately 30 weeks' gestation, after which production falls precipitously[8]. No functional role has been defined for AFP during fetal development. In three documented pregnancies, the fetuses produced minimal or no AFP, most probably as a result of a gene deletion similar to that seen with analbuminaemia[9]. All three pregnancies went to term and were associated with healthy newborns of normal weight.

HOW AFP REACHES AMNIOTIC FLUID

Fetal urine normally contains measurable concentrations of AFP, indicating that the fetal kidney has allowed small amounts to escape into the amniotic fluid. Peak amniotic fluid AFP concentration is found at around 12 weeks' gestation, after which levels steadily decrease, averaging 10% per gestational week during the second trimester[10]. This normally occurring background AFP makes it necessary to establish gestational age-specific reference ranges prior to measuring and interpreting AFP in amniotic fluid for diagnostic purposes (Fig. 33.1). Falsely elevated AFP levels can be present, when amniotic fluid is contaminated by fetal blood. This can make interpretation difficult, even when fetal blood contamination is recognized. Repeat atraumatic amniocentesis, carried out a minimum of 10 days later, will, as a rule, yield normal AFP levels in unaffected pregnancies[11].

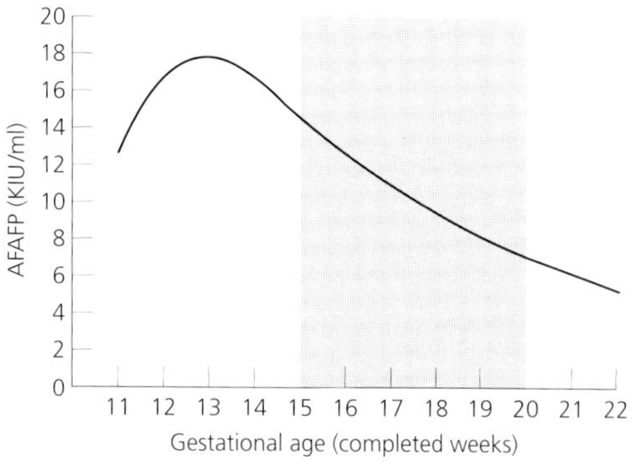

Fig. 33.1 Median amniotic fluid alpha-fetoprotein (AFAFP) levels between 11 and 21 weeks' gestation. The shaded area between 15 and 20 weeks' gestation indicates the appropriate time for interpreting AFP measurements for diagnostic purposes.

The exposed membrane and blood vessel surfaces found with open neural tube defects allow AFP to transudate into amniotic fluid, roughly in proportion to the size of the exposed areas[10,11]. The same is true for open ventral wall defects (omphalocele and gastroschisis). Gastroschisis always lacks a covering membrane, and nearly all cases are associated with AFP elevations[12]. Omphalocele is covered with a membrane and sometimes skin, as well; the AFP concentration in amniotic fluid is, therefore, more variable. Congenital nephrosis, a rare autosomal recessive condition, is characterized by high concentrations of amniotic fluid AFP[13]. About 20% of the cases of fetal spina bifida are classified as being closed, meaning that they are covered with skin or a thick membrane[14]. Such cases cannot be detected by AFP measurement but may be detected sonographically.

HOW AFP REACHES THE MATERNAL CIRCULATION

AFP normally reaches the maternal serum by two routes. About two-thirds reaches maternal serum by transplacental diffusion, and the remainder by transamnionic diffusion. When excess AFP resulting from fetal disorders is present in amniotic fluid, it reaches the maternal circulation by transamnionic diffusion. The restrictive amnionic membrane, in combination with a relatively high transplacental diffusion of normal background AFP, however, makes measurement of AFP in maternal serum both a less sensitive and a less specific test for the presence of open fetal malformations[4].

OTHER FACTORS INFLUENCING AFP LEVELS IN THE MATERNAL CIRCULATION

Taking into account the major variables that influence maternal serum AFP levels can considerably increase screening efficiency. Accurate gestational dating is critical, because maternal serum AFP levels normally increase steadily throughout the second trimester[4]. Race influences maternal serum AFP levels, as well. Maternal serum AFP levels average 10–15% higher in Black women than in Caucasian women at a comparable gestational week[15]. This can be taken into account either by establishing separate median values for both Black and non-Black populations or by establishing median values for either the Black or non-Black population, and then applying a conversion factor for the other[16,17].

A woman's weight also influences her maternal serum AFP level. Maternal weight was first identified as influencing the maternal serum AFP concentration in 1981, with lighter women having higher, and heavier women having lower, average concentrations[18]. Figure 33.2 demonstrates the relationship between maternal weight and AFP concentration in maternal serum. This relationship can be expressed mathematically as

$$\text{Expected MoM} = m \times (1/\text{maternal weight}) + b$$

where MoM stands for multiple of the median, and m and b are the slope and intercept of a log-linear regression analysis, respectively[19]. This allows maternal weight to be accounted for routinely when reporting the AFP MoM. Taking this into account leads to a reduction in falsely elevated maternal serum AFP measurements and a marginal improvement in detection[20]. Assay precision also affects the rate of falsely elevated maternal serum AFP measurements. When an assay's coefficient of variability is reduced from 15% to 4%, for example, about a third of the falsely elevated maternal serum AFP measurements may be eliminated. At present, nearly all assays are capable of yielding coefficients of variability below 10%. Twins give rise to maternal serum AFP levels that average twice as high as singletons, triplets three times, and quadruplets four times[21]. Identifying multiple gestations thus removes another source of falsely elevated maternal serum

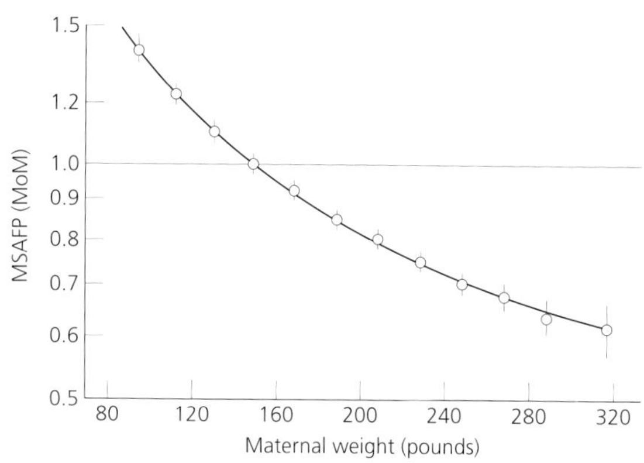

Fig. 33.2 The relationship between maternal serum alpha-fetoprotein (MSAFP) measurements and maternal weight. The MSAFP measurements are expressed as multiples of the median (MoM). The open circles indicate median MoM levels of MSAFP at the various maternal weight intervals. Vertical lines surrounding the circles are 95% confidence intervals.

AFP measurements. Unrecognized fetal death can cause maternal serum AFP levels to be elevated, as well. Ultrasound will immediately identify this source of falsely elevated AFP levels.

GESTATIONAL DATING AND MATERNAL SERUM AFP LEVELS

Once assay conditions have been optimized, gestational dating is the most important potential source of variability that can be taken into account for improving the screening performance of AFP measurement. If all pregnancy dates were to be verified by ultrasound prior to screening, the false positive rate would be approximately 40% lower than if only menstrual dates were available. The detection rate for open neural tube defects would also be slightly improved. A further improvement in detection would be gained if all of the ultrasound-derived dates were based only on biparietal diameter (BPD) measurements. This improvement is due to the BPD measurements of fetuses with open spina bifida being smaller, on average, than unaffected pregnancies[22]. This artifact makes the gestational age-adjusted maternal serum AFP measurements of these affected pregnancies appear higher and raises detection by approximately 10%.

UNEXPLAINED MATERNAL SERUM AFP ELEVATIONS AND PREGNANCY OUTCOME

Even when screening conditions have been optimized, there still remain falsely elevated maternal serum AFP measurements that cannot be explained. In such cases, the amniotic fluid AFP measurement is not elevated and/or no fetal defect is observed via ultrasound (i.e., the pregnancy is unaffected by a fetal malformation). This excess AFP in the maternal circulation is most probably transplacental in origin. One source is fetomaternal haemorrhage, sometimes associated with placental haematoma and/or infarcts. In one study, increased numbers of fetal red blood cells were demonstrated in the maternal circulation in a high proportion of women with maternal serum AFP elevations[23]. The integrity of the placental membrane interface might also be compromised by conditions such as fetal hydrops; this disorder has been found occasionally in association with maternal serum AFP elevation[24]. Placental lacunae have been described sonographically, as well, suggesting the possibility that excess AFP may somehow diffuse from these 'lakes' into the maternal circulation[25]. Most commonly, there is no explanation for falsely elevated maternal serum AFP measurements, but the high rate of low birthweight deliveries (three times as high as with normal maternal serum AFP measurements) and late fetal death (12 times as high as with normal maternal serum AFP measurements) indicates fetal or placental compromise[26]. Rarely, a malignant tumour in the pregnant woman may give rise to a maternal serum AFP elevation, sometimes reaching levels of several thousand nanograms per millilitre[27]. Maternal serum AFP elevation can also be found during the recovery phase from acute hepatitis[28].

Mathematical principles that underlie prenatal screening

An innovative system for normalizing and analysing data was developed as part of the first UK Collaborative Study[4]. That system continues to be used by prenatal screening laboratories, worldwide, for managing and interpreting AFP measurements, and, as well, other serum analyte measurements that will be discussed later in this chapter in relation to Down syndrome. The first component of the analytic system is the conversion of all laboratory measurements to multiples of the median (MoM). To accomplish this, a laboratory first performs maternal serum AFP measurements on about 100 pregnant women at each relevant gestational week (15–21 weeks' gestation)[29]. The measurements initially are expressed in traditional units (International Units or nanograms per millilitre). The laboratory then uses regression techniques to calculate median AFP levels for each gestational week. All AFP measurements are then converted into multiples of their week-specific median. This normalizing function serves several practical purposes:

- It immediately defines the population distribution of AFP measurements in unified terms
- It avoids the need for defining separate cutoffs for each gestational week (maternal serum AFP concentration normally rises by 10–15% per week)
- AFP values from the laboratory's own population can be reliably compared with published AFP distributions from neural tube defect pregnancies (this avoids the need for each laboratory to obtain its own measurements from affected pregnancies, before beginning to screen)
- Using MoM values as common currency, different laboratories can compare data, even when assays do not yield identical mass unit results
- Test results can be interpreted, based on a unified cutoff, and reported to physicians in more readily understandable terms
- The MoM value can be adjusted to take into account other variables, such as maternal weight or race, without disturbing the format used for test interpretation
- The population distribution of AFP measurements can be easily monitored by a laboratory on an ongoing basis and adjusted, as needed

The second component of the analytic system involves using published Gaussian distributions of AFP MoM values from unaffected pregnancies, pregnancies with open spina bifida, and pregnancies with anencephaly (Fig. 33.3)[4,30]. Each of these Gaussian distributions can be summarized by two

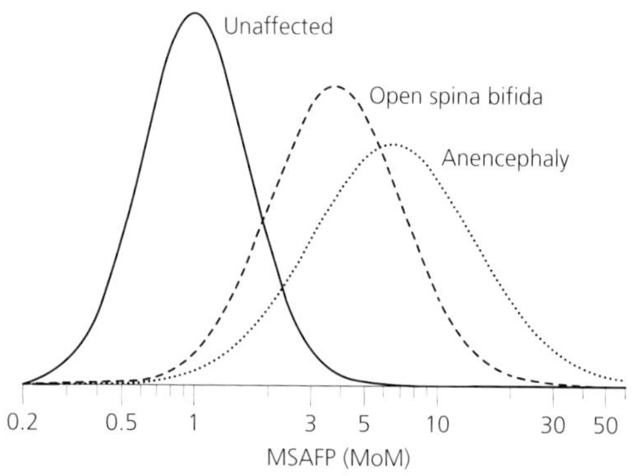

Fig. 33.3 The distribution of maternal serum alpha-fetoprotein (MSAFP) measurements in unaffected pregnancies and pregnancies with either open spina bifida or anencephaly. The median MSAFP value for unaffected pregnancies is by definition 1.0 MoM. For open spina bifida and anencephaly, median values are 3.7 MoM and 6.5 MoM, respectively.

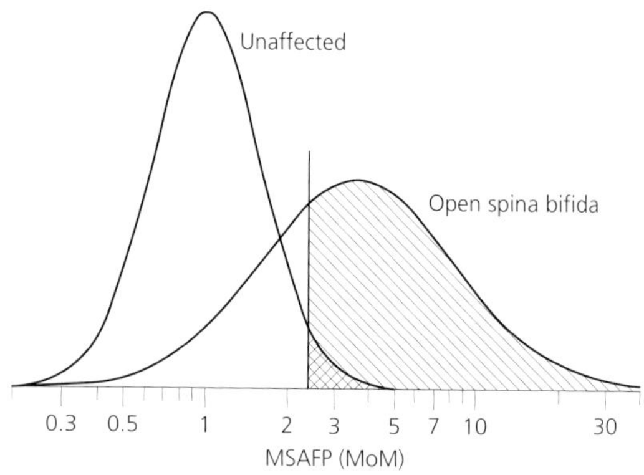

Fig. 33.4 The detection and false positive rate for open spina bifida in pregnancies with elevated maternal serum alpha-fetoprotein (MSAFP) measurements. A vertical line drawn from the baseline at 2.5 multiples of the median indicates the screening cutoff. The hatched area indicates the proportion of open spina bifida pregnancies above the cutoff (70%) and the cross-hatched area indicates the proportion of unaffected pregnancies above the cutoff (2%).

parameters; the log mean AFP MoM (equivalent to the log of the median) and the log standard deviation. These parameters describe the relationship between AFP measurements in the affected and unaffected populations. It is then possible to determine detection rates and false positive rates for the neural tube defects at various AFP MoM cutoff levels. A screening program can then select a cutoff that best suits its resources and population (most centres use AFP cutoff levels between 2.0 MoM and 2.5 MoM). As experience was gained in the 1980s with measuring maternal serum AFP for routine screening purposes, the AFP standard deviations for the affected and unaffected populations became smaller, for a variety of reasons. The net effect was to reduce the false positive rate at any given AFP MoM cutoff, with little or no effect on the detection rate.

A further analysis involves calculating the odds of being affected (with, for example, open spina bifida) given a positive result (OAPR). This calculation combines data derived from the overlapping Gaussian distributions with knowledge of how frequently open spina bifida occurs in the pregnancy population. The OAPR provides useful information for programmatic planning and is also helpful when AFP screening results are being explained to women with positive screening results. The OAPR can differ, depending upon factors such as geographic location, due to the differing prevalences of open spina bifida. A cumulative OAPR describes the overall odds in the group of women with positive screening tests. As an example, a screening programme's AFP cutoff is 2.5 MoM, the woman's AFP value is 2.8 MoM, and the frequency of open spina bifida in the population is 1:1000. Overall, 10 of the women will have an affected pregnancy and the remaining women (about 10 000) will have unaffected pregnancies. Seven of the 10 women with affected pregnancies will be screen positive (70% detection rate) along with about 200 unaffected pregnancies (2% false positive rate). The OAPR in this group of 208 women is 7:200, or about 1:30. The detection rate and false positive rate for the population of screen positive women as a whole can be shown visually by drawing a line vertically from the 2.5 MoM cutoff to intersect the overlapping distribution of affected and unaffected populations (Fig. 33.4). The proportions of affected and unaffected populations to the right of that line (the areas under the curves) represent the collective detection and false positive rates for all women with serum AFP values above that cutoff. More individualized odds for the woman with an AFP value of 2.8 MoM can be calculated by measuring the distance from the baseline at 2.8 MoM to the point of intersection with the respective curves (Fig. 33.5). At an AFP of 2.8 MoM, the distance to the intersection with the curve of affected

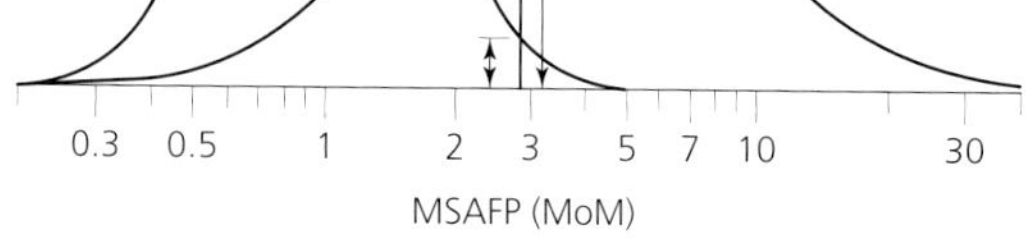

Fig. 33.5 The relative increase in an individual woman's open spina bifida risk when her serum alpha-fetoprotein level is 2.8 multiples of the median (MoM). The relative increase in risk (or likelihood ratio LR) can be estimated by measuring the distance from baseline to point of intersection with the curves of unaffected and affected pregnancies. In this example, the distance is seven times greater to the intersection with the curve from affected pregnancies.

pregnancies is seven times greater than the distance to the curve of unaffected pregnancies. This ratio, called the likelihood ratio, indicates that this woman is now seven times as likely as pregnant women in the general population to have an affected pregnancy. If the population background frequency is one per 1000, the woman's individual OAPR (or risk) is 7:1000 or about 1:140.

In addition to developing the mathematical principles of screening and presenting a rational system upon which to base screening policy decisions, the First UK Collaborative Study also defined the optimal time in gestation for screening (16–18 weeks) and the boundaries beyond which screening was either ineffective (<15 weeks) or not feasible (>21 or 22 weeks). The Collaborative Study also quantitatively defined risk for other pregnancy complications (low birthweight, fetal death) in relation to maternal serum AFP levels.

Diagnostic studies

The same mathematical principles that were developed for maternal serum AFP screening were subsequently applied to amniotic fluid AFP measurements in the Second UK Collaborative Study[10] and to amniotic fluid acetylcholinesterase measurements[31]. Performance characteristics of these diagnostic studies could then be described both separately and in combination, as defined once again by detection rates, false positive rates, and the odds of being affected, given a positive result. When acetylcholinesterase (AChE) measurements became available for diagnostic purposes, nearly all of the false positive amniotic fluid AFP measurements could be identified, with only minimal loss of detection.

Diagnostic ultrasound studies in the early 1980s initially were directed at visualizing the fetal spine defects, themselves[32]. This often proved difficult and was much less reliable than the amniotic fluid AFP and AChE measurements. The 1986 discovery of alternations in fetal head shape (the 'lemon' sign) and in cerebellum (the 'banana' sign) in the presence of open spina bifida markedly improved the ability of ultrasound to provide reliable diagnostic information[33]. Methods for combining information from ultrasound and biochemical diagnostic studies have been proposed for interpretive purposes[34]. Some centres now use ultrasound measurement almost exclusively.

The impact of screening on the birth prevalence of open neural tube defects

In the 20 years since AFP screening was first introduced, the birth prevalence of both anencephaly and open spina bifida has fallen sharply. This fall can be attributed in part to a lower prevalence of these disorders during early pregnancy in the UK and US, but prenatal screening is the major reason for this reduction.

The potential impact of folic acid supplementation on the incidence of open neural tube defects

Folic acid supplementation is now known to provide protection against the development of most open neural tube defects, when taken by women for the months before and immediately after becoming pregnant[35]. A daily supplement of 4 mg is recommended for women known to be at high risk because of a previous affected pregnancy. The greatest overall reduction in the rate of occurrence of those disorders would be achieved by supplementing the diets of all women in the childbearing years with 0.4 mg of folic acid, daily[36]. Efforts to introduce this supplement into the food supply have met with mixed success. In the United States, partial supplementation of grain products will begin in 1998[37]; in the United Kingdom no supplementation policy has yet been approved. In the absence of general folate supplementation of the food supply, the intake of folic acid supplements must rely on individual women's initiatives and on ongoing dissemination about the need for folic acid supplements by the health community.

Prenatal screening for Down syndrome

Presently available data indicate that the relationship between maternal age and Down syndrome risk is independent of geographic location and maternal race[38,39]. A consistent relationship has also been documented between the rate of occurrence of Down syndrome in the second trimester and at term. A recent analysis, combining data from several studies, demonstrates that 23% of all Down syndrome pregnancies end in spontaneous fetal loss between the early second trimester (16–18 weeks) and term[40]. For this reason, when pregnant women are provided with estimates for the odds of having an affected pregnancy, these odds will be higher if quoted for the second trimester. For example, a 35-year-old woman has a 1:380 risk at term for fetal Down syndrome but a 1:290 risk during the second trimester. When establishing screening policy for detecting Down syndrome prenatally, it is therefore necessary to adopt either the second trimester or term risk as the convention and then use that convention exclusively to avoid confusion.

Prenatal diagnosis for Down syndrome first became feasible in the 1970s, when amniocentesis was found to be relatively safe as a diagnostic procedure and the technique of chromosome analysis became refined. The first screening test for Down syndrome involved asking a pregnant woman her age and then offering amniocentesis and chromosome analysis as a diagnostic test, if her age at the estimated delivery date was 35 years or older. Down syndrome risk increases steadily but slowly in relation to a woman's age until her mid thirties, after which the risk increases at an accelerated pace (Fig. 33.6)[41]. The rationale for selecting age

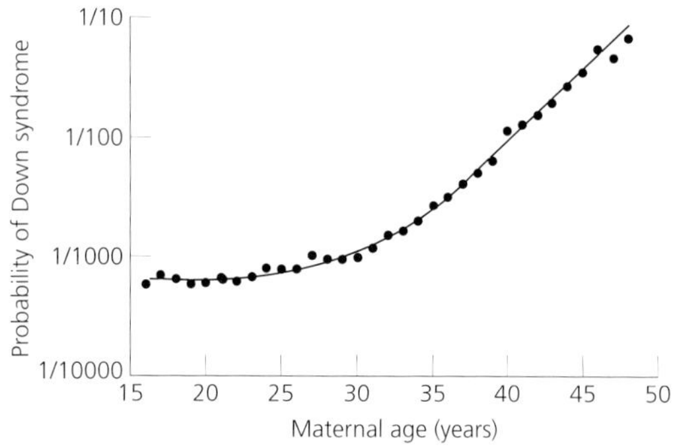

Fig. 33.6 The relationship between maternal age and the birth prevalence of Down syndrome. The filled circles indicate the probability of a Down syndrome birth occurring at each year of age between 16 and 48.

35 as the screening cutoff arose from an effort to balance the risk of having a pregnancy affected by a chromosome disorder with the risk of spontaneous fetal loss resulting from amniocentesis[42]. In the United Kingdom, the rationale for choosing any given age cutoff was often based upon the availability of regional resources for amniocentesis and chromosome culture.

In 1984 it was reported that maternal serum AFP levels averaged lower in pregnancies affected by Down syndrome than in unaffected pregnancies[43]. The extent of difference in AFP distributions between affected and unaffected pregnancies, although not great, was sufficient to be useful for screening purposes[44]. Serum AFP levels in affected and unaffected pregnancies were independent of maternal age, and this allowed the AFP measurements to be combined with maternal age to derive a risk, based on both pieces of information. Figures 33.7(a) and 33.7(b) compare the screening efficiency of using AFP measurements alone versus using maternal age alone, as a screening test for Down syndrome. In these examples, AFP values at or below 0.5 multiples of the unaffected population median (Fig. 33.7(a)) and women's ages at or above age 35 (Fig. 33.7(b)) are the defined cutoffs for identifying high risk women in the respective protocols. AFP screening identifies 20% of the Down syndrome pregnancies (detection rate) by classifying 5% of the pregnancy population as being at high risk (false positive rate).

Maternal age screening detects 31% of the Down syndrome pregnancies at a false positive rate of 7.5%. Given the independence between these two screening tests, overall screening efficiency ought to increase by combining them. Figure 33.7(c) displays the result achieved by merging the two screening tests and using the risk of a 35-year-old woman as a screening cutoff; a 33% detection rate is achieved by identifying 5.1% of the pregnancy population as being at high risk.

Combining these two screening tests involves, as a first step, deriving individual likelihood ratios for Down syndrome, based on the AFP measurement. Figure 33.8 shows that the midpoint of the distribution of AFP measurements in unaffected pregnancies is 1.0 multiples of the median (MoM), while the midpoint for pregnancies affected by Down syndrome is 0.72 MoM. Knowing these median AFP levels and the corresponding standard deviations allows individual likelihood ratios for Down syndrome to be calculated for any given AFP concentration, just as for neural tube defects, in the previous section. Three examples are contained in Fig. 33.9. At an AFP value of 0.35 MoM, the distance from the baseline to the intersection with the respective AFP curves is four times as great for affected as for unaffected pregnancies (likelihood ratio of 4). At an AFP value of 0.84 MoM (the point where the two curves cross), the likelihood ratio is 1. This means that the AFP measurement does not change the risk, based on age. At 2.20 MoM the likelihood ratio is 0.25 (or four times less likely than the population average for Down syndrome to be present).

The second step in combining information from the two screening tests can best be shown by using the following examples. In the first example the woman's age is 25 and her AFP measurement is 0.5 MoM. The overall term risk for

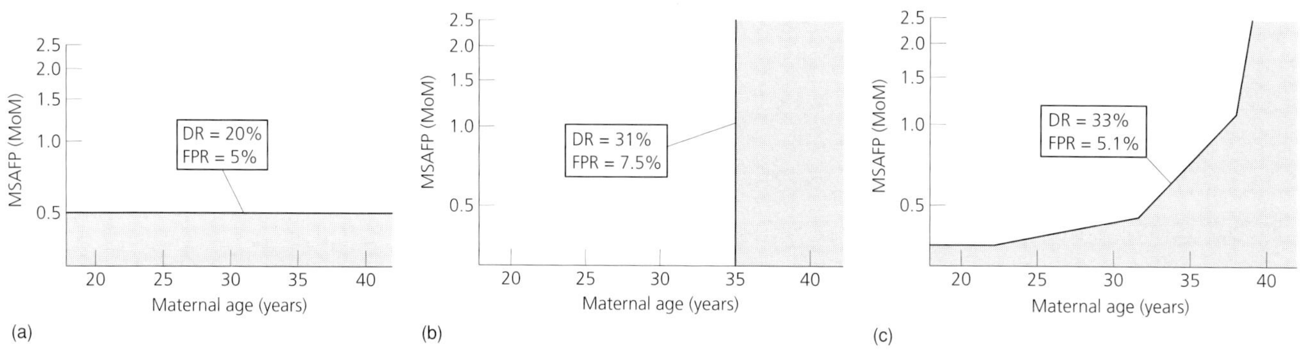

Fig. 33.7 Down syndrome screening performance using (a) maternal serum alpha-fetoprotein (MSAFP) measurements alone, (b) maternal age alone, and (c) a combination of maternal age and MSAFP measurements. Detection rates (DR) and false positive rates (FPR) are shown for the three screening methods. Combining the MSAFP measurements with risks based on maternal age yields the most efficient balance between DR and FPR.

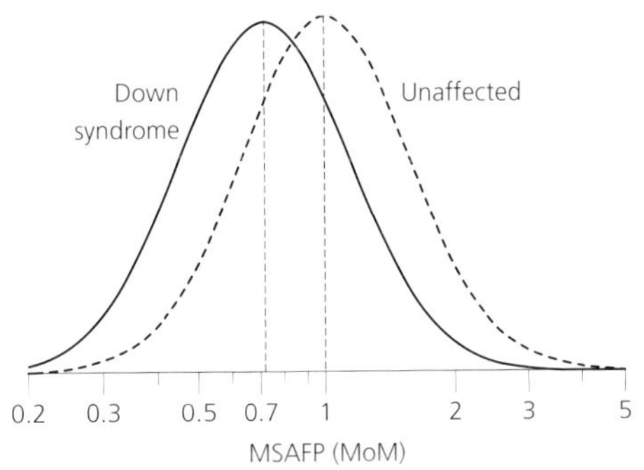

Fig. 33.8 The distribution of maternal serum alpha-fetoprotein (MSAFP) measurements in pregnancies with and without Down syndrome. The median MSAFP value in unaffected pregnancies is, by definition, 1.0 MoM. For pregnancies affected with Down syndrome the median value is 0.72 MoM. Considerable overlap is found for MSAFP values in the two groups.

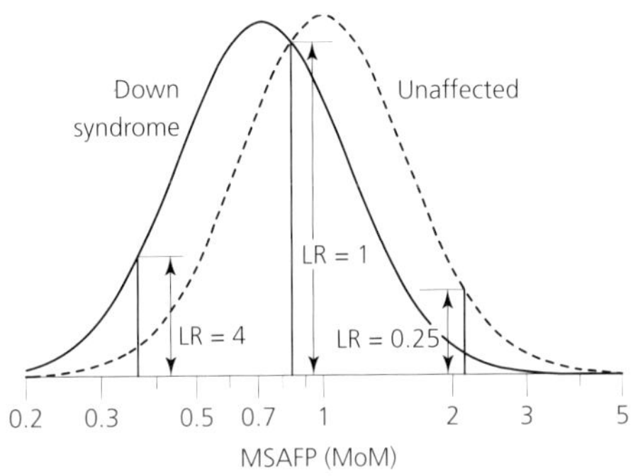

Fig. 33.9 The relative increase or decrease in Down syndrome risk at three different maternal serum alpha-fetoprotein (MSAFP) levels. At an MSAFP value of 0.35 MoM, the woman's individual risk for Down syndrome is four times that based on age alone. At 0.84 MoM, there is no change in age-based risk. An MSAFP value of 2.2 MoM lowers the risk fourfold.

Down syndrome in the pregnancy population is 1:830. Her likelihood ratio, based on her age, is 0.6; her AFP measurement yields a likelihood ratio of 4. Multiplying these two likelihood ratios together gives a combined likelihood ratio of 2.4, meaning that the woman is now 2.4 times as likely as the general pregnancy population (2.4:830, or 1:350) of having an affected pregnancy. In the second example the woman's age is 40 (likelihood ratio 7.4) and her AFP measurement is 2.2 MoM (likelihood ratio 0.25). Multiplied together (7.4 × 0.25 = 1.9), these likelihood ratios assign this pregnancy a risk of 1:440 (1.9:830) for being affected by Down syndrome. This system for deriving risk forms the basis of current population-based prenatal screening policies.

The AFP measurements available for the original Down syndrome case-control studies were originally performed as screening tests for open neural tube defects at between 15 and 21 weeks' gestation[43,44], the optimal time in gestation to perform such screening[4]. Screening for Down syndrome was initially viewed as an extension of the existing AFP screening for open neural tube defects, because both conditions could be screened for, using the same AFP measurement. For that reason, there was little interest in identifying whether AFP screening for Down syndrome might be effective earlier in gestation. Subsequently, however, evidence accumulated indicating that measurement of AFP in maternal serum can discriminate between Down syndrome and unaffected pregnancies as early as 9 to 11 weeks' gestation[45,46]. This will be discussed later.

DETERMINING RELIABLE EXPECTATIONS FOR PERFORMANCE OF AFP AS A SCREENING TEST FOR DOWN SYNDROME

As discussed earlier in this chapter, the three critical determinants that define any screening test's performance are: (a) the detection rate for the disorder being sought; (b) the false positive rate; and (c) the odds of being affected with the disorder, given a positive screening test result. It is possible to define these three determinants in relation to Down syndrome screening by knowing four pieces of information:

- The distribution of maternal serum AFP measurements in unaffected pregnancies
- The distribution of maternal serum AFP measurements in pregnancies affected by Down syndrome
- The second trimester (or term) prevalence of Down syndrome at each year of maternal age
- The maternal age distribution

Contrary to conventional wisdom, it is not always necessary to carry out large-scale clinical trials to obtain all of the necessary information for defining test performance. In fact, clinical trials are a relatively inefficient approach to gathering such data when the medical disorder being sought occurs at a low prevalence; clinical trials do, however, serve other useful purposes described later.

Knowledge of the distribution of serum AFP measurements in unaffected pregnancies was available at the time when the AFP–Down syndrome association was discovered. Similarly, as soon as outcomes of pregnancies with Down syndrome were identified from within the population of women having earlier been screened for open neural tube defects, AFP measurements from the Down syndrome pregnancies could be used to calculate the parameters for affected pregnancies. Knowledge of age-specific Down syndrome frequency was also available, both during the second trimester and among live births (23% of Down syndrome pregnancies are lost spontaneously between the second trimester and term)[40]. When applied to various hypothetical maternal age distributions, this collective information allowed reliable estimates to be calculated for all three of the critical screening determinants. These estimates, in turn, formed the basis for guiding policy development for the clinical trials which followed.

An intervention trial in New England was carried out during 1986 and 1987[47], restricted to women younger than age 35. Maternal serum AFP analysis and interpretation was limited to between 15 and 22 weeks' gestation. A second trimester Down syndrome risk cutoff of 1:270 (the approximate risk of a 35-year-old woman) was used to define the screen positive group. This 1:270 risk cutoff was estimated to give acceptable detection and false-positive rates of about 20% and 5%, respectively. All pregnancies dated by last menstrual period that were initially screen positive were then offered ultrasound to confirm gestational dates; low AFP measurements are strongly associated with incorrectly dated pregnancies. Since maternal serum AFP measurements normally increase by 15% per week during the second trimester, spuriously low AFP measurements will occur when a pregnancy is less far advanced than estimated from menstrual dates. When gestational dates are found by ultrasound to be within 8 days (or in some screening programmes 10 days) of menstrual dates, reinterpretation is not necessary. Otherwise, reinterpretation is performed in most centres. This often leads to the pregnancy being reclassified as screen negative, or it is determined that the sample was drawn prior to 15 weeks' gestation.

Figure 33.10 summarizes the findings of the trial[47]. Overall, 4.7% of the 77 273 enrolled women were initially placed in the high risk category (initial false positive rate). Subsequent reclassification by ultrasound dating removed 41% of those women from the high risk category, leaving 2.7% of the screened women to be offered amniocentesis (revised false positive rate or amniocentesis referral rate). Seventy-six percent of those women elected amniocentesis; one case of Down syndrome was identified for every 90 amniocenteses performed. Among those women choosing not to have amniocentesis, an additional four Down syndrome cases were identified at birth. The detection rate was estimated to be 25%.

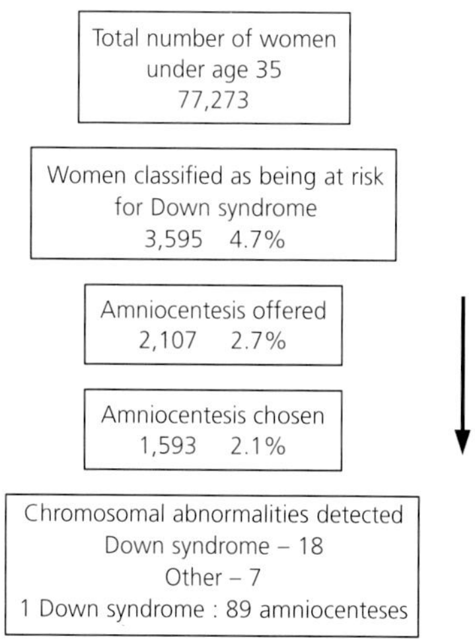

Fig. 33.10 Results of a multicentre intervention trial of combining maternal age and maternal serum alpha-fetoprotein levels to screen for Down syndrome in women under age 35.

The trial supported the feasibility of adding Down syndrome screening to AFP programme services. Using AFP screening, the cumulative OAPR was found to be more favourable for women younger than age 35 (1:89) than when amniocentesis was offered to all women in the 35 years or older category (1:150). Data from this trial were consistent with the estimates derived from modelling, based on findings from the earlier case-control study[44]. By 1988, AFP measurements in combination with maternal age were already widely used in the United States as a screening test for Down syndrome, with approximately 1 million pregnancies receiving such testing annually[48]. The relatively low detection rate, however, left considerable room for improvement.

HUMAN CHORIONIC GONADOTROPIN AND UNCONJUGATED ESTRIOL AS ADDITIONAL SCREENING TESTS

In 1987, human chorionic gonadotropin (hCG) measurements in maternal serum were discovered to average more than two times higher in the presence of Down syndrome during the second trimester[49]. Shortly thereafter, unconjugated estriol (uE3) levels in maternal serum were reported to average 25% lower in the presence of Down syndrome[50]. Both hCG and uE3 are better markers than AFP. Before either of the measurements could be incorporated into existing screening protocols, however, it was necessary once again to determine the extent to which information provided by these respective measurements was independent of information provided by AFP measurements and maternal age.

The biological basis for the association between AFP, uE3, and hCG levels and Down syndrome is less straightforward than that for AFP and open neural tube defects. Concentrations of AFP (a fetal product) and uE3 (a fetoplacental product) both are lower in the presence of Down syndrome, suggesting that either less is being produced, or more is being degraded. Concentrations of hCG (a placental product) are higher with Down syndrome, suggesting increased synthesis. Other placental and fetal products, as well, are now known to follow similar patterns. Levels of AFP, uE3, and hCG in maternal serum all change steadily as gestational age advances. Figure 33.11 displays median levels of these three analytes during the early second trimester. AFP and uE3 levels increase as gestational age increases, while hCG levels decrease.

In most instances, potential new screening tests are not discovered by analysing pre-existing laboratory measurements from large populations. The AFP data available for calculating Down syndrome screening performance are an exception. It is often possible, however, to set up case-control studies, using sera (or other biological materials) collected during pregnancy that are stored in a freezer bank and linked with pregnancy outcomes. This approach can provide information that allows calculation of reliable estimates for detection rates, false positive rates, and, finally, the OAPR. There are, however, several potential pitfalls to avoid:

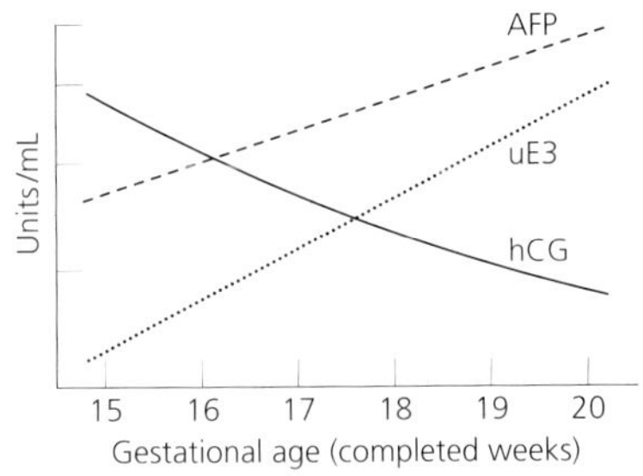

Fig. 33.11 The relationship between gestational age and maternal serum levels of alpha-fetoprotein (AFP), unconjugated estriol (uE3) and human chorionic gonadotropin (hCG). The lines for each of the three analytes represent median values at 15–20 weeks' gestation. AFP and uE3 values increase steadily, while hCG values decrease.

- There needs to be assurance that the 'cases' are representative of all cases. This means that they must be collected in a way that avoids their identification being related to levels of any marker being evaluated. One way to avoid this bias would be to identify all cases within a cohort
- Sufficient numbers of 'cases' (50 or more) need to be available to allow reliable distribution parameters (log mean and standard deviation) to be calculated for the marker
- Attention needs to be paid to appropriate matching of cases with controls (e.g. gestational age and time in freezer)
- Distributions of measurements, once determined, need to be adjusted to mimic the greater variability found in routine laboratory operation (otherwise the screening test's performance will be overestimated)
- The association between an analyte and a disorder, once observed, needs to be tested in a second, independent dataset, to confirm the association and robustness of the model, and to better define expectations under everyday conditions.

If analyses from case-control studies are carefully done, they will provide more reliable performance estimates for the critical determinants than clinical trials, in many instances. Clinical trials often require very large populations to be tested, in order to obtain sufficient numbers of cases, and complete ascertainment of missed cases can be difficult or impossible. As demonstrated by the clinical trial for AFP described earlier (Fig. 33.10), however, clinical trials can yield other useful information about screening performance, such as uptake rates, reclassification rates, and amniocentesis acceptance rates.

Following the initial observations about hCG and uE3 levels in Down syndrome pregnancies, a separate, larger case-control study was published in 1988 which simultaneously examined AFP, uE3, and hCG and determined that the three biochemical measurements were independent of maternal age and were largely (but not totally) independent of each other[51]. Figure 33.12 compares population distributions of these three analytes in unaffected and Down syndrome pregnancies. In this figure, detection rates are estimated at a constant false positive rate of 5%, and the measurements of all three analytes once again are expressed as multiples of the unaffected population median. AFP measurements yield the

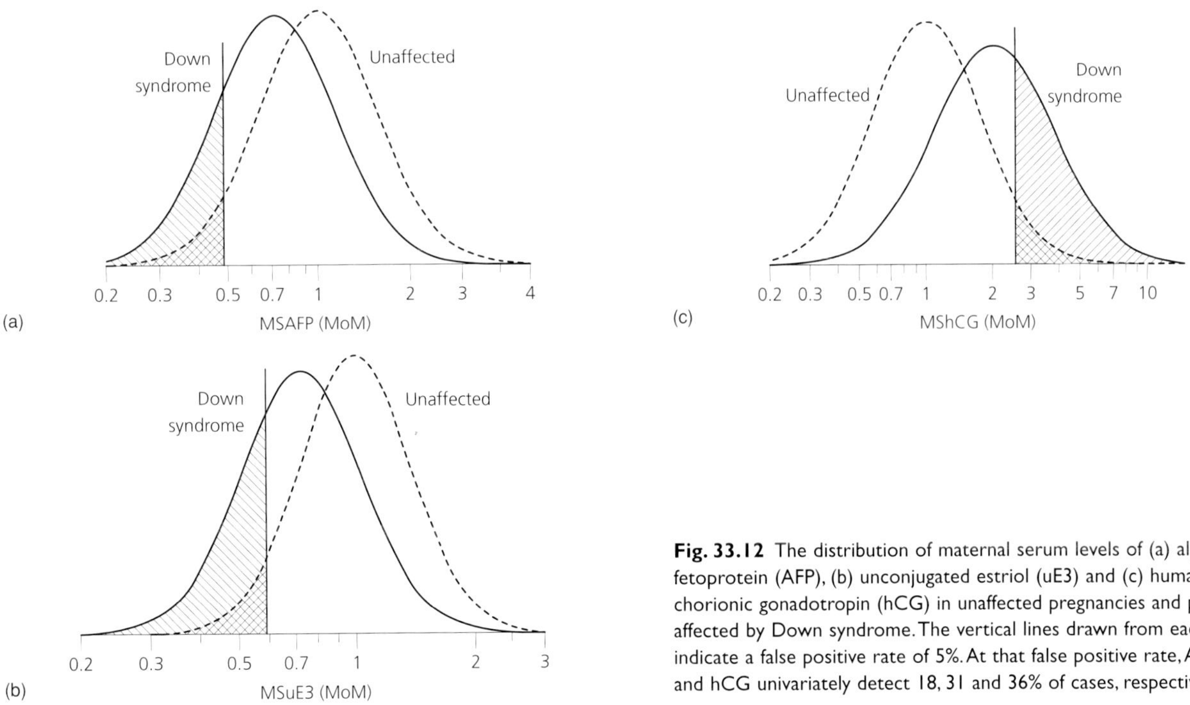

Fig. 33.12 The distribution of maternal serum levels of (a) alpha-fetoprotein (AFP), (b) unconjugated estriol (uE3) and (c) human chorionic gonadotropin (hCG) in unaffected pregnancies and pregnancies affected by Down syndrome. The vertical lines drawn from each baseline indicate a false positive rate of 5%. At that false positive rate, AFP, uE3, and hCG univariately detect 18, 31 and 36% of cases, respectively.

lowest detection rate (18%), uE3 measurements the next lowest (31%), and hCG the highest (36%). Case-control studies from many centres now provide extensive confirmation of the univariate differences between affected and unaffected pregnancies for the three analytes[52]. The collective median values all closely approximate those reported in the 1988 case-control study[51].

As a second step, the 1988 study provided an analysis of how the three measurements performed in combination. To display visually the extent to which combining the three biochemical measurements adds to the effectiveness of Down syndrome screening, it is first necessary to express the AFP, uE3, and hCG measurements for affected and unaffected populations in terms of risk (Fig. 33.13). The distribution of values for the population of Down syndrome pregnancies is now shifted to the right of the unaffected pregnancies for all three biochemical measurements. When the three biochemical markers and maternal age are used in combination (Fig. 33.13(d)), the separation between affected and unaffected populations is greatest (a 60% detection rate at a 5% false positive rate, using a term risk cutoff of 1:250).

Conceptually, calculating individual women's risks for fetal Down syndrome using all three biochemical markers requires first that individual likelihood ratios be defined for each of the measurements (along with maternal age) and then multiplied together. An additional factor needs to be inserted into the calculation, however, to take into account the extent of overlap in information (correlation) provided by the three biochemical measurements. Figure 33.14 displays likelihood ratios for three combinations of AFP, uE3, and hCG measurements in a hypothetical 27-year-old woman. In the first, the combination of low AFP, low uE3, and high hCG levels together with her age, raise her risk for Down syndrome from 1:830 to 1:160. The second combination of measurements yields a risk for Down syndrome equal to her age-related risk of 1:1200 (in this case, each of the measurements coincidentally is located at the point of intersection between the affected and unaffected curves). In the third example, relatively high AFP and uE3 measurements, in combination with a low hCG measurement, reduce the woman's risk of an affected pregnancy to less than 1:10 000.

AN INTERVENTION TRIAL TO FURTHER EVALUATE THE MULTIPLE MARKERS

Between 1989 and 1991 an intervention trial was carried out in two New England centres to evaluate the performance of the three biochemical markers in combination with maternal age[53]. One of the participating centres used a second trimester risk cutoff of 1:270 to define its high risk population. This

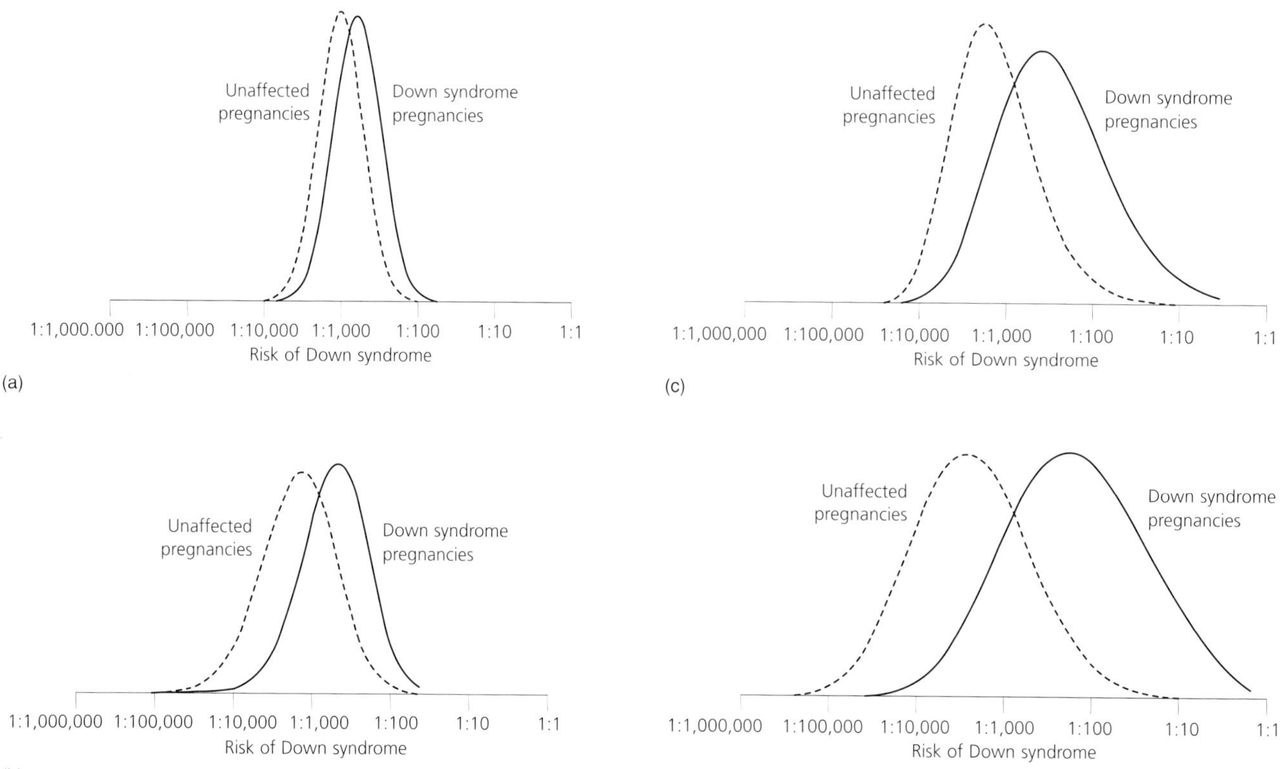

Fig. 33.13 The distribution of Down syndrome risk based on maternal serum levels of (a) alpha-fetoprotein, (b) unconjugated estriol and (c) human chorionic gonadotropin in unaffected and Down syndrome pregnancies; (d) the combination of maternal age and all the markers.

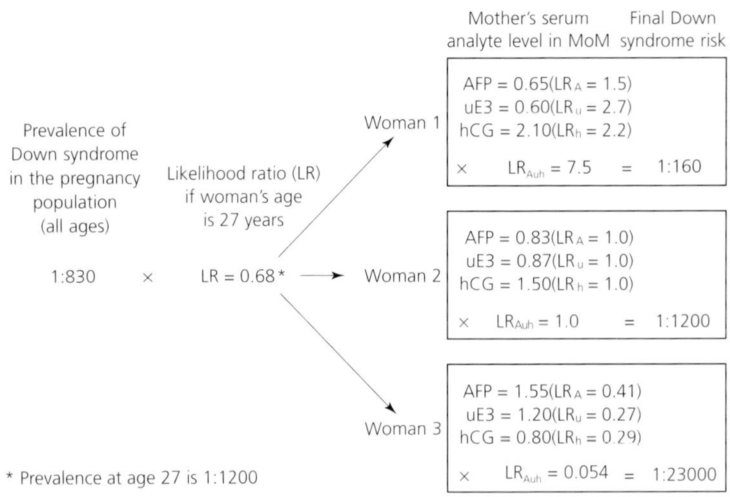

Fig. 33.14 The process of computing Down syndrome risk for three hypothetical 27-year-old women with different levels of maternal serum alpha-fetoprotein (AFP), unconjugated estriol (uE3) and human chorionic gonadotropin (hCG). The three examples provide some insight into how extensively the biochemical measurements can alter a pregnant woman's age-based risk for Down syndrome.

cutoff was estimated to yield an initial positive rate of 7–8%. The other centre selected a second trimester risk cutoff of 1:190 (estimated initial positive rate approximately 5%). Both centres converted AFP, uE3, and hCG measurements into risk estimates, using a published algorithm that was developed from data in the case-control study described on page 381[51]. Analysis and interpretation of serum samples was restricted to between 15 and 21 weeks' gestation, but samples were accepted from women aged 35 and older, as well as from younger women.

Figure 33.15 summarizes the findings of the study. Among the 25 207 enrolled women, 1661 (6.6%) were initially identified as having a second trimester Down syndrome risk of 1:190 or greater. Following confirmation of gestational dates by ultrasound and reinterpretation of risk, 962 (3.8%) remained in the high risk category. Amniocentesis was chosen by 760 of those 962 women (79%): 20 cases of Down syndrome and seven other chromosome disorders were identified within that group. With the possible exception of three cases of Turner syndrome, the other chromosome disorders were probably identified by chance. One additional case of Down syndrome was identified following delivery from among the 202 women who chose not to have amniocentesis.

Based upon the maternal age distribution of the study population, a total of 36 cases of Down syndrome were estimated to be present, in the second trimester. Follow-up of all cases identified at birth, combined with those identified via amniocentesis, revealed 35 cases. The detection rate was calculated at 58% (21/36), with a false positive rate of 3.8%. The OAPR in the group of women offered amniocentesis was 1:46 (21:962). Two additional Down syndrome cases were found in the women initially identified as being at high risk but were reclassified as being screen negative after ultrasound redating. As a result, the maximum detection rate was 64% in association with the initial positive rate of 6.6%. The detection and false positive rates associated with multiple marker screening for Down syndrome both increase steadily as maternal age advances. The estimated overall detection rate applies, therefore, to the population as a whole. This is in reasonable agreement with the earlier case-control study estimate of a 60% detection rate at a 5% false positive rate. The parameters computed from the case-control data[51] relied upon gestational dates estimated from the last menstrual period. Data were not available to assess the impact of revising risk estimates based on ultrasound-derived gestational dates. When compared with the earlier trial that involved AFP,

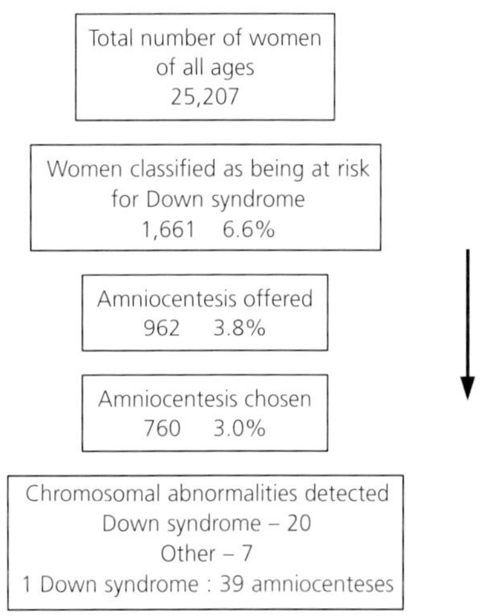

Fig. 33.15 Results of a multicentre intervention trial of combining maternal age with maternal serum alpha-fetoprotein, unconjugated estriol, and human chorionic gonadotropin measurements to screen for Down syndrome in women of all ages.

alone, the multiple marker protocol was associated with a slightly higher initial positive rate and revised false positive rate (women offered amniocentesis) but yielded a detection rate that was 2.3 times greater. This improved the ratio of Down syndrome cases detected to amniocenteses performed by a factor of two.

Several other intervention trials assessing the performance of the three serum marker have been published. A summary of their conclusions has also been published (Fig. 33.16)[54]. Their collective estimate of screening performance is once again consistent with predictions from the original case-control study. It is also apparent, however, that individual point estimates of Down syndrome detection from these intervention trials vary widely. This variability can be explained both by the relatively small numbers of Down syndrome cases occurring in most studies and by other factors, such as differing maternal age distributions, varying risk cut-off levels and variable use of ultrasound as the method of dating. In addition, several trials have examined the performance of two, rather than three, serum markers. Intact hCG and AFP were used in three studies; free β hCG in combination with AFP was used in two. Free β hCG is a breakdown product of the hCG molecule. Univariately, it appears to yield detection rates and false positive rates that are similar to, or slightly better than, the intact molecule. Figure 33.17 summarizes individual detection and false positive rates for the two marker studies, in comparison to the summary performance of the triple marker studies.

When the free β subunit of hCG (free β) was first introduced as a screening test for Down syndrome, some confusion existed as to how much benefit would be gained by substituting it for assays which measured the whole hCG molecule[55,56]. Free β is a breakdown product of the hCG molecule, and its circulating concentration is generally about one one-hundredth that of the intact molecule. The concentration of free β increases in vitro in a time- and temperature-dependent fashion[57]. The median free β level in Down syndrome pregnancies is 2.10 MoM, as opposed to 2.02 MoM for intact hCG. The greater separation between affected and unaffected pregnancies would provide a screening advantage, if all else were equal. This was found not to be the case, however. The distributions of free β measurements in unaffected and affected populations both were broader than found with the intact molecule. These broader distributions were associated with a relative increase in overlapping free β values between the two populations. The net effect is best shown by comparing estimated detection rates for the two measurements (in combination with maternal age, AFP and uE3 measurements) at a fixed false positive rate of 5% – intact hCG detected 58, and free β, 62%[58]. The two markers are thus very similar in screening performance. There may, however, be an advantage to using free β as a marker earlier in pregnancy; this will be discussed more fully later in this chapter.

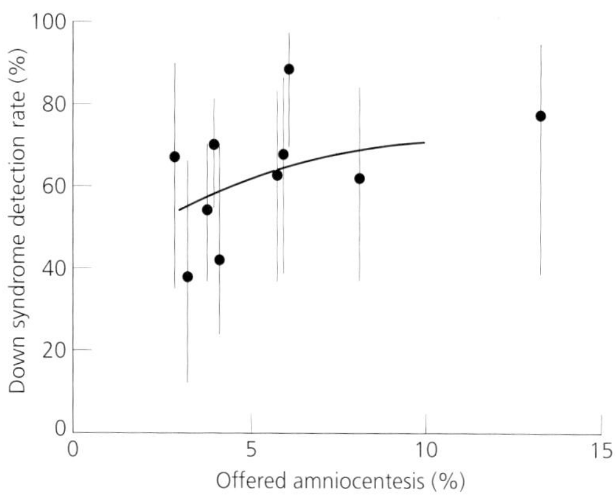

Fig. 33.16 A summary of the detection and false positive rates from 10 published triple marker intervention trials. The filled circles indicate detection rates and false positive rates found in the individual studies. The vertical lines attached to the circles represent 95% confidence intervals. The curve summarizes screening performance from the 10 studies.

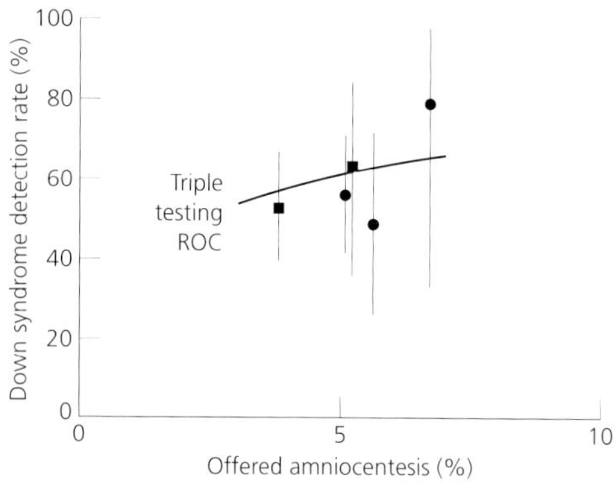

Fig. 33.17 A summary of the detection and false positive rates from five published double marker intervention trials. The curve shown here is taken from Fig. 33.16 and summarizes the collective estimates from 10 triple marker trials. The double marker trials are plotted individually, for comparison. Filled squares indicate free β/AFP combinations; filled circles indicate intact hCG/AFP combinations.

A fourth serum marker has recently been found suitable by a few laboratories as a screening test for Down syndrome during the second trimester. The free α subunit of hCG (free α) may have some advantage when combined with free β, AFP and uE3 measurements[59]. There has been some hesitation, however, on the part of most laboratories to add yet another marker to screening profiles, unless an important gain in detection (or reduction in false positives) is achieved. Such gain may be possible in the future by adding the measurement of dimeric inhibin[60]. Maternal serum levels of dimeric inhibin, a placental product, are higher, on average, when Down syndrome is present. These levels are largely independent of AFP, uE3, or hCG levels and, hence, can increase the detection rate for Down syndrome without raising the false positive rate. Many other fetoplacental markers have been investigated as possible candidates for screening. None has been found to add sufficient independent information to justify being incorporated into routine screening.

ADDITIONAL VARIABLES THAT INFLUENCE UE3 AND HCG MEASUREMENTS

Just as for AFP, other variables have been found to influence maternal serum levels of uE3 and hCG. These variables can be adjusted for, and the adjustments incorporated into the final expression of the values as multiples of the median. Adjusting AFP measurements for maternal weight is now routine. Levels of uE3 and hCG have also been discovered to be associated with maternal weight (Fig. 33.18), and these also can be adjusted to take maternal weight into account.

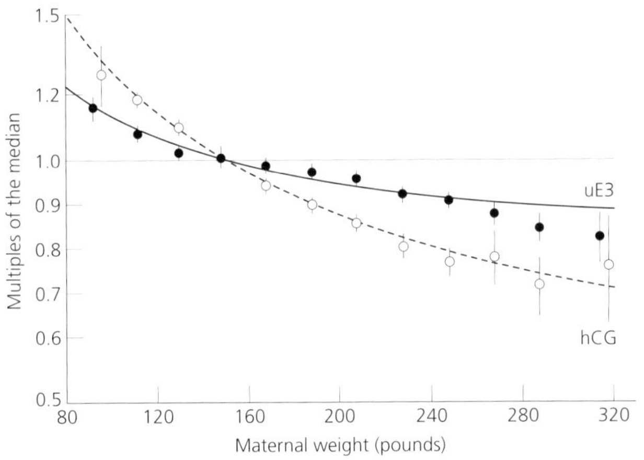

Fig. 33.18 The relationship between maternal weight, and maternal serum unconjugated estriol (uE3) and human chorionic gonadotropin (hCG) measurements. The open and filled circles indicate median values for hCG and uE3, respectively, at various maternal weight intervals. The vertical bars surrounding each circle represent 95% confidence intervals.

Insulin dependent diabetes in the pregnant woman is associated with maternal serum AFP levels that average 20% lower than the general pregnancy population[61]. The AFP value of a diabetic woman can be adjusted by dividing by 0.8. The influence of maternal insulin dependent diabetes on maternal serum levels of uE3 and hCG appears to be less than for AFP[62] but is still in the process of being defined. The influence of race upon maternal serum levels of uE3 and hCG is also in the process of being defined[63,64]. Cigarette smoking during pregnancy has a slight influence on maternal serum levels of AFP and uE3 when compared to levels in non-smokers. Serum levels of hCG, however, are 20–30% lower in the presence of cigarette smoking[65]. Adjusting for this effect is currently not recommended, in part due to the possible association between smoking and a lower Down syndrome prevalence[66].

Maternal age, in combination with AFP, uE3, and hCG as a screening test for trisomy 18

The standard multiple marker screening protocol for detecting Down syndrome does not serve as a screening test for trisomy 18. It has been discovered, however, that maternal serum levels of all three biochemical markers are depressed in the presence of trisomy 18[67]. This pattern is sufficiently distinctive that, when converted to a screening test, it detects one case of trisomy 18 for every 16 women with positive screening results. Furthermore, only four women per 1000 screened are identified as having this particular high risk profile. For that reason, it has been possible to insert this supplementary screening protocol into the Down syndrome screening sequence without appreciably altering the overall false positive rate[68]. The detection rate for trisomy 18, using this protocol, is estimated at about 60% with a false positive rate of 0.4 percent. More recently, a protocol based on assigning individualized risk for trisomy 18 has been developed[69]; no report of its prospective performance is yet available.

Prenatal screening for fetal disorders in the first trimester

The availability of chorion villus sampling and early amniocentesis as diagnostic sampling procedures in the first trimester led a number of investigators to study whether maternal serum screening for Down syndrome might be possible earlier in gestation[45,70–73]. The advantages of detecting fetal disorders such as Down syndrome in the first trimester might include greater assurance of privacy for women with affected pregnancies, less emotional stress, and less extensive surgery for those choosing termination. One disadvantage of first trimester screening would be the inability to detect fetal defects, such as open spina bifida. Maternal serum AFP measurement is not effective as a screening test for open spina bifida, prior to 15 weeks' gestation[4]. If serum screening for Down syndrome were to be performed in the first trimester, therefore, it would become necessary to carry out a second round of screening for open spina bifida in the second trimester. In addition to the extra screening procedures, this could lead to higher screening costs and more maternal anxiety. The pros and cons of separating screening tests for the two disorders are still being debated.

Beginning in 1986, a wide variety of fetoplacental products were studied, including not only familiar markers (i.e. AFP, uE3, hCG, free β, free α), but also a number of less familiar markers (pregnancy-associated plasma protein A [PAPP-A], CA-125, SP-1, dimeric inhibin-A, alpha inhibin, progesterone, and placental alkaline phosphatase). For many reasons, difficulties were encountered in achieving reliable appraisals of screening performance for these various analytes, either univariately or in combination. Maternal serum levels of some of the markers were near the lower sensitivity limits for existing assays (e.g. AFP, uE3, free β) and for others, reagents of reliable quality were difficult to obtain. For some of the markers, the relationship of serum levels in affected versus unaffected pregnancies differed, as gestation advanced from 9 to 14 weeks. Many of the studies included sera from relatively small numbers of affected pregnancies, and conclusions could not be confidently drawn. These studies have recently been summarized[74].

In spite of these difficulties, the studies collectively yielded data indicating that first trimester serum screening for Down syndrome might be feasible. Based on this, a collaborative study involving 22 centres from nine countries collected first trimester maternal sera from 77 cases of Down syndrome, each matched with five controls[75]. Measurements of AFP, uE3, total hCG, free β, free α, PAPP-A, and inhibin were then performed on all of the sera. Two markers in combination with maternal age were found to yield detection and false positive rates for Down syndrome screening that were comparable to those achievable in the second trimester. Serum levels of pregnancy-associated plasma protein A (PAPP-A), the first of these markers, averaged lower in the presence of Down syndrome (0.43 MoM); 42% of the PAPP-A values from affected pregnancies were at or below the fifth centile of unaffected pregnancies. Serum levels of free β-hCG, the second of these markers, averaged higher in the presence of Down syndrome (1.79 MoM); 18% of the free β-hCG values from affected pregnancies were at or above the 95th centile of unaffected pregnancies. The two markers were largely independent of each other, as judged by the low correlation coefficient (0.06), meaning that an advantage would be gained by using them in combination. When the two serum markers and maternal age were used together in a model, it was determined that 63% of the Down syndrome cases could be detected at a 5.5% false positive rate. It is likely that these markers will be incorporated into intervention trials and, if performance meets expectations, into routine practice.

Ultrasound measurement of nuchal translucency has also been found useful in first trimester screening, usually between 11 and 13 weeks' gestation[76]. In expert hands an 80% detection rate can be attained at a 5% false positive rate. If it were possible to achieve this level of screening performance as part of routine prenatal care, this measurement would be more effective than serum screening. Such is not presently the case, however[77]. As a next step, it may be possible to combine ultrasound and biochemical measurements to raise the detection rate for Down syndrome. Emphasis needs to be placed on training sonographers to perform nuchal translucency measurements properly[76], possibly in combination with software development. Ultimately, it may be possible to achieve a level of screening performance for ultrasound measurement that might allow it to be used independently. If that were to be the case, however, some type of independent, systematic quality assessment mechanism would need to be established[76], comparable to proficiency testing schemes already in place to monitor serum screening. Without such quality assessment, the reliability of ultrasound screening at the population level could not be assured.

REFERENCES

1. Brock DJH, Sutcliffe RG. Alpha-fetoprotein in the antenatal diagnosis of anencephaly and spina bifida. *Lancet* **2**:197–199, 1972.
2. Wald NJ, Brock DJ, Bonnar J. Prenatal diagnosis of spina bifida and anencephaly by maternal serum-alpha-fetoprotein. A controlled study. *Lancet* **1**:765–767, 1974.
3. Brock DJ, Bolton AE, Scrimgeour JB. Prenatal diagnosis of spina bifida and anencephaly through maternal plasma-alpha-fetoprotein measurement. *Lancet* **1**:767–769, 1974.
4. Wald NJ, Cuckle H, Brock DJ, Peto R, Polani PE, Woodford FP. Maternal serum-alpha-fetoprotein measurement in antenatal screening for anencephaly and spina bifida in early pregnancy. (Report of U.K. Collaborative Study on Alpha-Fetoprotein in Relation to Neural-Tube Defects.) *Lancet* **1**:1323–1332, 1977.
5. Bergstrand CG, Czar B. Demonstration of a new protein fraction in serum from the human fetus. *Scand J Clin Lab Invest* **8**:174, 1956.
6. Harper ME, Dugaiczyk A. Linkage of evolutionary-related serum albumin and alpha-fetoprotein genes within q11–22 of human chromosome 4. *Am J Hum Genet* **35**:565–572, 1983.
7. Ruoslahti E. Isolation and biochemical properties of alpha-fetoprotein. In *Prevention of Neural Tube Defects: the Role of Alpha-Fetoprotein* (ed. B.F. Crandall & M.A.B. Brazier), pp. 9–16. New York: Academic Press, 1978.
8. Tomasi TB. Structure and function of alpha-fetoprotein [Review]. *Ann Rev Med* **28**:453–465, 1977.
9. Greenberg F, Faucett WA, Rose E *et al.* Congenital deficiency of alpha-fetoprotein. *Am J Obstet Gynecol* **167**:509–511, 1992.
10. Amniotic-fluid alpha-fetoprotein measurement in antenatal diagnosis of anencephaly and open spina bifida in early pregnancy. (Second Report of the U.K. Collaborative Study on Alpha-Fetoprotein in Relation to Neural-tube Defects.) *Lancet* **2**:651–662, 1979.
11. Haddow JE, Miller WA. Prenatal diagnosis of open neural tube defects. In *Methods in Cell Biology. Prenatal Diagnosis: Cell Biological Approaches*, Vol. 26 (eds S.A. Latt & G.J. Darlington), pp. 68–93. New York: Academic Press, 1982.
12. Goldfine C, Haddow JE, Knight GJ, Palomaki GE. Amniotic fluid alpha-fetoprotein measurements in pregnancies associated with gastroschisis. *Prenat Diagn* **9**:697–700, 1989.
13. Ryynanen M, Seppala M, Kuusela P *et al.* Antenatal screening for congenital nephrosis in Finland by maternal serum alpha-fetoprotein. *Br J Obstet Gynæcol* **90**:437–442, 1983.
14. Althouse R, Wald NJ. Survival and handicap of infants with spina bifida. *Arch Dis Child* **55**:845–850, 1980.
15. Johnson AM. Racial Differences in Maternal Serum Alpha-fetoprotein Screening. In *Alpha-fetoprotein and Congenital Disorders* (eds G.J. Mizejewski & I.H. Porter), pp. 183–196. San Diego: Academic Press, 1985.
16. Crandall BF, Lebherz TB, Schroth PC, Matsumoto M. Alpha-fetoprotein concentrations in maternal serum: relation to race and body weight. *Clin Chem* **29**:531–533, 1983.
17. Baumgarten A. Racial difference and biological significance of maternal serum alpha-fetoprotein. *Lancet* **2**:573, 1986.
18. Haddow JE, Knight G, Kloza E, Smith DE. Relation between maternal weight and serum alpha-fetoprotein concentration during the second trimester. *Clin Chem* **27**:133–134, 1981.
19. Neveux LM, Palomaki GE, Larrivee DA, Knight GJ, Haddow JE. Refinements in managing maternal weight adjustment for interpreting prenatal screening results. *Prenat Diagn* **16**:1115–1119, 1996.
20. Johnson AM, Palomaki GE, Haddow JE. The effect of adjusting maternal serum alpha-fetoprotein levels for maternal weight in pregnancies with fetal open spina bifida: A United States collaborative study. *Am J Obstet Gynecol* **163**:9–11, 1990.
21. Wald NJ, Cuckle HS, Stirrat G. Maternal serum alpha-fetoprotein levels in triplet and quadruplet pregnancy. *Br J Obstet Gynæcol* **85**:124–126, 1978.
22. Wald NJ, Cuckle HS, Boreham J, Stirrat G. Small biparietal diameter of fetuses with spina bifida: implications for antenatal screening. *Br J Obstet Gynæcol* **87**:219–221, 1980.

23. Los FJ, de Wolf BT, Huisjes HJ. Raised maternal serum-alpha-fetoprotein levels and spontaneous fetomaternal transfusion. *Lancet* **2**:1210–1212, 1979.
24. Carrington D, Gilmore DH, Whittle MJ *et al.* Maternal serum alpha-fetoprotein – a marker of fetal aplastic crisis during intrauterine human parvovirus infection. *Lancet* **1**:433–435, 1987.
25. Perkes EA, Baim RS, Goodman KJ, Macri JN. Second-trimester placental changes associated with elevated maternal serum alpha-fetoprotein. *Am J Obstet Gynecol* **144**:935–938, 1982.
26. Haddow JE, Knight GJ, Kloza EM, Palomaki GE. Alpha-fetoprotein, vaginal bleeding, and pregnancy risk. *Br J Obstet Gynæcol* **93**:589–593, 1986.
27. Haddow JE, Thompson DK, Kloza EM. Maternal hepatoma detected during serum AFP screening. *Lancet* **2**:806–807, 1980.
28. Kew MC, Purves LR, Bersohn I. Serum alpha-fetoprotein levels in acute viral hepatitis. *Gut* **14**:939–942, 1973.
29. Haddow JE (ed.) *Prenatal Screening for Major Fetal Disorders. Vol. I: Fetal Disorders Associated with Elevated MSAFP Values.* Scarborough, ME: Foundation for Blood Research, 1990.
30. Wald NJ, Cuckle HS, Densem JW, Kennard A, Smith D. Maternal serum screening for Down's syndrome: the effect of routine ultrasound scan determination of gestational age and adjustment for maternal weight. *Br J Obstet Gynæcol* **99**:144–149, 1992.
31. Wald NJ, Cuckle HS, Nanchahal K. Amniotic fluid acetylcholinesterase measurement in the prenatal diagnosis of open neural tube defects. (Second Report of the Collaborative Acetylcholinesterase Study.) *Prenat Diagn* **9**:813–829, 1989.
32. Campbell S, Pryse-Davies J, Coltart TM, Seller MJ, Singer JD. Ultrasound in the diagnosis of spina bifida. *Lancet* **1**:1065–1068, 1975.
33. Nicolaides KH, Campbell S, Gabbe SG, Guidetti R. Ultrasound screening for spina bifida: cranial and cerebellar signs. *Lancet* **2**:72–74, 1986.
34. Wald NJ, Cuckle HS, Haddow JE, Doherty RA, Knight GJ, Palomaki GE. Sensitivity of ultrasound in detecting spina bifida. *N Engl J Med* **324**:769–771, 1991.
35. MRC Vitamin Study Research Group. Prevention of neural tube defects: results of the MRC Vitamin Study. *Lancet* **338**:132–137, 1991.
36. Centers for Disease Control and Prevention. Recommendations for the use of folic acid to reduce the number of cases of spina bifida and other neural tube defects. *MMWR Morb Mortal Wkly Rep* **41**(No.RR-14):1–7, 1992.
37. Food and Drug Administration. Food standards: amendment of standards of identity for enriched grain products require addition of folic acid. *Fed Regist* (March 5) **61**(44):8781–8797, 1996.
38. Hook EB: Down's syndrome, frequency in human populations and factors pertinent to variation in rates. In *Trisomy 21 Research Perspectives of NICHD* (ed. F. de la Cruz), p. 3. Mental Retardation Research Centers Series. Maryland: University Park Press, 1981.
39. Källen B, Knudsen LB. Effect of maternal age distribution and prenatal diagnosis on the population rates of Down syndrome – a comparative study of nineteen populations. *Hereditas* **110**:55–60, 1989.
40. Cuckle HS, Wald NJ. Screening for Down's syndrome. In *Prenatal Diagnosis and Prognosis* (ed. R.J. Lilford), p. 67. London: Butterworth, 1991.
41. Cuckle HS, Wald NJ, Thompson SG. Estimating a woman's risk of having a pregnancy associated with Down's syndrome using her age and serum alpha-fetoprotein level. *Br J Obstet Gynæcol* **94**:387–402, 1987.
42. Tabor A, Madsen M, Obel EB, Philip J, Bang J, Norgaard-Pedersen B. Randomised controlled trial of genetic amniocentesis in 4606 low-risk women. *Lancet* **i**:1287, 1986.
43. Merkatz IR, Nitowsky HM, Macri JN, Johnson WE. An association between low maternal serum alpha-fetoprotein and fetal chromosomal abnormalities. *Am J Obstet Gynecol* **148**:886–894, 1984.
44. Cuckle HS, Wald NJ, Lindenbaum RH. Maternal serum alpha-fetoprotein measurement: a screening test for Down syndrome. *Lancet* **1**:926–929, 1984.
45. Brambati B, Simoni G, Bonacchi I, Piceni L. Fetal chromosomal aneuploidies and maternal serum alpha-fetoprotein levels in first trimester. *Lancet* **2**:165–166, 1986.
46. Cuckle HS, Wald NJ, Barkai G *et al.* First trimester biochemical screening for Down's syndrome. *Lancet* **2**:851–852, 1988.
47. Combining maternal serum alpha-fetoprotein measurements and age to screen for Down syndrome in pregnant women under age 35. (New England Regional Genetics Group Prenatal Collaborative Study of Down Syndrome Screening.) *Am J Obstet Gynecol* **160**:575–581, 1989.
48. Palomaki GE, Knight GJ, Holman MS, Haddow JE. Maternal serum alpha-fetoprotein screening for fetal Down syndrome in the United States: results of a survey. *Am J Obstet Gynecol* **162**:317–321, 1990.
49. Bogart MH, Pandian MR, Jones OW. Abnormal maternal serum chorionic gonadotropin levels in pregnancies with fetal chromosome abnormalities. *Prenat Diagn* **7**:623–630, 1987.
50. Canick JA, Knight GJ, Palomaki GE, Haddow JE, Cuckle HS, Wald NJ. Low second trimester maternal serum unconjugated œstriol in pregnancies with Down's syndrome. *Br J Obstet Gynæcol* **95**:330–333, 1988.
51. Wald NJ, Cuckle HS, Densem JW *et al.* Maternal serum screening for Down's syndrome in early pregnancy. *BJ* **297**:883–887, 1988.
52. Haddow JE, Palomaki GE. Prenatal screening for Down syndrome. In *Essentials of Prenatal Diagnosis* (eds J.L. Simpson & S. Elias), pp 204–205. New York: Churchill Livingstone, 1993.
53. Haddow JE, Palomaki GE, Knight GJ *et al.* Prenatal screening for Down's syndrome with use of maternal serum markers. *N Engl J Med* **327**:588–593, 1992.
54. Palomaki GE, Neveux LM, Haddow JE. Can reliable Down's syndrome detection rates be determined from prenatal screening intervention trials? *J Med Screen* **3**:12–17, 1996.
55. Macri JN, Kasturi RV, Krantz DA, Copok EJ, Sunderji SG, Larsen JW. Maternal serum Down syndrome screening: Free β- protein is a more effective marker than human chorionic gonadotropin. *Am J Obstet Gynecol* **163**:1248–1253, 1990.
56. Spencer K. Evaluation of an assay of the free β-subunit of choriogonadotropin and its potential value in screening for Down's syndrome. *Clin Chem* **37**:809–811, 1991.
57. Sancken U, Bahner D. The effect of thermal instability of intact human chorionic gonadotropin (ihCG) on the application of its free β-subunit (free βhCG) as a serum marker in Down syndrome screening. *Prenat Diagn* **15**:731–738, 1995.
58. Wald NJ, Densem J, Stone R, Cheng R. The use of free beta-hCG in antenatal screening for Down's syndrome. *Br J Obstet Gynæcol* **100**:550–557.
59. Wald NJ, Densem JW, Smith D, Klee GG. Four marker serum screening for Down's syndrome. *Prenat Diagn* **14**:707–716, 1994.
60. Wald NJ, Densem JW, George L, Muttukrishna S, Knight PG. Prenatal screening for Down's syndrome using inhibin-A as a serum marker. *Prenat Diagn* **16**:143–153, 1996.
61. Wald NJ, Cuckle HS. Recent advances in screening for neural tube defects and Down's syndrome. In *Baillière's Clinical Obstetrics and Gynæcology. International Practice and Research. Vol. 1. Fetal Diagnosis of Genetic Defects* (ed. C. Rodeck), p. 649. London: Baillière Tindall, 1987.
62. Palomaki GE, Knight GJ, Haddow JE. Human chorionic gonadotropin and unconjugated estriol measurements in insulin- dependent diabetic pregnant women being screened for fetal Down syndrome. *Prenat Diagn* **14**:65–68, 1994.
63. Simpson JL, Elias S, Morgan CD, Shulman L, Umstot E, Andersen RN. Second trimester maternal serum human chorionic gonadotropin and unconjugated œstriol levels in blacks and whites. *Lancet* **335**:1459–1460, 1990.
64. Muller F, Boué A. A single chorionic gonadotropin assay for maternal serum screening for Down's syndrome. *Prenat Diagn* **10**:389, 1990.
65. Cuckle HS, Wald NJ, Densem JW *et al.* The effect of smoking in pregnancy on maternal serum alpha-fetoprotein, unconjugated œstriol, human chorionic gonadotrophin, progesterone and dehydroepiandrosterone sulphate levels. *Br J Obstet Gynæcol* **97**:272–274, 1990.
66. Palomaki GE, Knight GJ, Haddow JE, Canick JA, Wald NJ, Kennard A. Cigarette smoking and levels of maternal serum alpha-fetoprotein, unconjugated estriol, and hCG: Impact on Down syndrome screening. *Obstet Gynecol* **81**:675–678, 1993.
67. Canick JA, Palomaki GE, Osathanondh R. Prenatal screening for trisomy 18 in the second trimester. *Prenat Diagn* **10**:546–548, 1990.
68. Palomaki GE, Knight GJ, Haddow JE, Canick JA, Saller DN, Panizza DS: Prospective intervention trial of a screening protocol to identify fetal trisomy 18 using maternal serum alpha-fetoprotein, unconjugated œstriol and human chorionic gonadotropin. *Prenat Diagn* **12**:925–930, 1992.

69. Palomaki GE, Haddow JE, Knight GJ *et al.* Risk-based prenatal screening for trisomy 18 using alpha-fetoprotein, unconjugated œstriol and human chorionic gonadotropin. *Prenat Diagn* **15**:713–723, 1995.
70. Brambati B, Macintosh MCM, Teisner B *et al.* Low maternal serum levels of pregnancy associated plasma protein A (PAPP-A) in the first trimester in association with abnormal fetal karyotype. *Br J Obstet Gynæcol* **100**:324–326, 1993.
71. Spencer K, Aitken DA, Crossley JA *et al.* First trimester biochemical screening for trisomy 21: the role of free beta hCG, alpha fetoprotein and pregnancy associated plasma protein A. *Ann Clin Biochem* **31**:447–454, 1994.
72. Bersinger NA, Brizot ML, Johnson A, Snijders RJM, Abbott J, Schneider H, Nicolaides KH. First trimester maternal serum pregnancy-associated β1-glycoprotein in fetal trisomies. *Br J Obstet Gynæcol* **101**:970–974, 1994.
73. Brock DJH, Barron L, Holloway S, Liston WA, Miller SG, Seppala M. First trimester maternal serum biochemical indicators in Down's syndrome. *Prenat Diagn* **10**:245–251, 1990.
74. Wald NJ, Kennard A, Smith D. First trimester biochemical screening for Down's syndrome. *Ann Med* **26**:23–29, 1994.
75. Wald NJ, George L, Smith D, Densem JW, Petterson K. Serum screening for Down's syndrome between 8 and 14 weeks of pregnancy. *Br J Obstet Gynæcol* **103**:407–412, 1996.
76. Nicolaides KH, Sebire NJ, Snijders RJM, Johnson S. Down's syndrome screening in the U.K. *Lancet* **347**:906–907, 1996.
77. Haddow JE, Palomaki GE. Down's syndrome screening. *Lancet* **347**:1625, 1996.

Ultrasound screening for fetal abnormalities

34

L.S. Chitty

Introduction

Routine fetal anomaly scanning is widely practised throughout Europe. However, there is much controversy over the clinical effectiveness of this screening procedure for fetal abnormalities, and in the United States, the American College of Obstetricians and Gynecologists have concluded that large clinical trials are needed before implementing routine screening[1]. The recent publication of the results of a randomized controlled trial from America (the RADIUS study)[2,3] have supported the view that routine anomaly scanning is not effective, thus adding to the controversy. Furthermore, a meta-analysis reported in the *British Medical Journal* concluded that routine ultrasound scanning does not improve the outcome of pregnancy in terms of an increased number of live births or perinatal morbidity, although it may be useful as a screening test for malformations[4]. In this chapter, the effectiveness of routine fetal anomaly scanning will be reviewed and the benefits and burdens of such a policy discussed.

Review of routine screening programmes

The RADIUS study was a randomized study in which 15 530 women were allocated to ultrasound at 15–22 weeks and 31–35 weeks or to scanning on clinical indication only. There was no significant improvement in perinatal outcome in the routine screening cohort[2] and no significant effect on the frequency of abortion for fetal anomalies[3]. The meta-analysis included four randomized controlled trials which had evaluated the effect of routine ultrasound scanning on perinatal morbidity and mortality. The trials included a total of 15 935 pregnancies (7992 who underwent routine scanning and 7943 controls who were scanned on clinical indication only). This analysis demonstrated that the perinatal mortality was significantly lower in the ultrasound screened group, probably as a result of early detection of fetal abnormalities as reported in the Helsinki study and their subsequent therapeutic abortion[5]. The differences between these two studies can be largely attributed to the variation in the sensitivities of ultrasound in the detection of abnormalities reported, 40.9% in the Helsinki trial and 16.6% (before 24 weeks) in the RADIUS study. Any effect on perinatal mortality rates will depend both on the early detection of abnormalities, the approach to termination of pregnancy and the availability of effective treatments, either pre- or postnatally. In the Helsinki study the perinatal mortality rate was significantly lower in the women undergoing routine ultrasound screening (4.6/1000) compared with the control group (9.0/1000)[5]. Nearly half (49.2%) of this difference was due to termination of pregnancies because of serious fetal abnormalities, with 11/30 therapeutic abortions (total screened pregnancies 4691). Whereas in the RADIUS study[2] there were relatively few therapeutic abortions for fetal abnormalities (9/31, total screened pregnancies 76 859). Another recent randomized study reported from South Africa also failed to demonstrate any effect of routine ultrasound on perinatal outcome[6]. This, however, was a relatively small study comparing routine ultrasound performed between 18–24 weeks (n = 492) with a group of low risk women who were only scanned if there was a clinical indication (n = 492). Whilst more abnormalities were detected before 24 weeks in the study group (4 of 9) compared with control group (1 of 3), there was no difference in the number of therapeutic abortions, with one in each group.

These studies[2,4,6] all had different objectives and screening policies and only one included the detection of fetal malformations as a specific aim[5]. The meta-analysis includes only four studies, all with relatively small numbers (Table 34.1). Furthermore, these studies were performed 10 or more years ago when both understanding and technology was not as advanced as it is today. The study from South Africa also had relatively few women in each cohort and it is therefore

TABLE 34.1
Summary of studies included in the meta-analysis[4]

Study	Number	Period	Gestational age (weeks)	Scanning objectives
Helsinki[5]	9310	1986–1987	16–20	NF, GA, anatomy
Trondheim[8]	510	1979–1980	19–32	NF, GA, position growth
Stockholm[7]	4997	1985–1987	15 (13–19)	NF, GA
Missouri[9]	915	1984–1986	10–12 (up to 18)	NF, GA, (anatomy)

NF = number of fetuses
GA = gestational age

unlikely that any significant effect of detection of abnormalities could have been seen[6]. The RADIUS study was to be a randomized study of low risk pregnancies, but it would appear to be a study of highly selected low risk women as, of the 55 744 pregnancies registered, only 15 530 were randomized, with 32 317 being defined as ineligible or excluded and the remainder lost to follow-up or refusing to participate[2]. The detection rate of fetal abnormalities in the RADIUS study is low and compares unfavourably with most other descriptive studies of routine ultrasound programmes reported in the literature (Table 34.2). Although specificities of these programmes are very similar (99.8–100%), however, the sensitivities for the detection of fetal abnormalities vary considerably (21–85%), as was also found in those randomized studies which reported detection of abnormalities (16.6–76.9%). Reasons for such variation include the skill and experience of the sonographers, the gestational age at which screening is performed, the definition of abnormality and the degree of ascertainment of abnormalities postnatally.

SONOGRAPHER SKILL

The skill and experience of the sonographers who perform routine ultrasound screening is clearly an important factor in the detection of fetal abnormalities. Screening programmes in teaching hospitals report a higher detection rate (76.9% and 35%) than that reported in local hospitals (36% and 13%)[2,5] and it might be assumed that the level of expertise and under-

TABLE 34.2
Summary of studies reporting the detection of fetal abnormalities before 24 weeks using routine ultrasound

Study[a]	Period	Number of fetuses	Gestational age	Prevalence of abnormalities[b] (%)	Sensitivity (%)	Specificity (%)	TOP (%)	Sonographer[c]
Rosendahl and Kivinen[10]	1980–1988	9012	18	1.03	39.4	99.9	0.16	M, O
Saari-Kemppainen et al.[5]	1986–1987	4691	16–20	0.43	36–76.9	99.8	0.23	?
Chitty et al.[11]	1988–1989	8785	18–20	1.5	74.4	99.98	0.6	R
Levi et al.[12]	1984–1989	15 654	16–20	2.3	21	100	?	O,S,T
Shirley et al.[13]	1989–1990	6412	19	1.4	60.7	99.98	0.45	R
Luck[14]	1988–1991	8844	19	1.9	85	99.9	0.28	R
Ewigman et al.[2]	1987–1991	7617	15–22	2.46	16.6	—	0.11	O,T
Levi et al.[15]	1990–1992	9392	16–20	2.45	41	99.9	?	O, S, T
Geerts et al.[6]	1991–	496	18–24	1.8	44.4	—	1/496	O
Papp et al.[16]	1988–1990	?	18–20	2.26	63.1	100	?	O,S

[a]Data from Saari-Kemppainen, Ewigman and Geerts include ultrasound screened group only
[b]Ascertained postnatally
[c]M = midwife, O = obstetrician, R = radiographer, S = sonographer, T = technician, TOP = termination of pregnancy

standing was generally greater in the teaching hospitals. Training and increased experience was thought to account for the improvement in the proportion of abnormal fetuses detected in screening programmes in Hillingdon[13] and Belgium, where sensitivity increased from 21% to 41%[12,15]. Furthermore, a study in the southeast of England demonstrated that targeted training of sonographers in district general hospitals could significantly improve the detection of fetal cardiac abnormalities by attempting examination of the four-chamber view of the heart in all fetuses[17]. In this study in 1980–1988, before training the radiographers in 10 hospitals how to obtain and interpret a four-chamber view of the heart, eight cardiac abnormalities were identified prenatally. After training, in 1988–1990, 53 abnormalities were identified during routine second trimester ultrasound screening.

GESTATIONAL AGE

The gestational age at which routine ultrasound examination is performed is also a limiting factor in the detection of fetal abnormalities, as visualization of much of the fetal anatomy is more difficult at 15–17 weeks than at 18 weeks or later. It is for this reason that the RCOG recommendations suggest screening at 18–20 weeks[18]. Variation in the gestational age at which screening was performed may account in part for the differences in sensitivities reported (Table 34.2). In the Belgium and RADIUS studies[2,12,15] screening was performed at any time between 15 and 22 weeks, whereas in the UK studies[11,13,14] which report better detection rates (60–85%), screening was performed at 18–20 weeks. Examination of the four-chamber view of the heart has been reported by several authors to be easier after 18 weeks' gestation. Sharland and Allan[17] demonstrated that this view could only be obtained in 10% of fetuses under 18 weeks' gestation, but was visualized in 82% after 18 weeks. A Norwegian study confirmed this observation when it was shown that it was not possible to obtain a four-chamber in 9% of fetuses at 16 weeks, but by 21 weeks this figure fell to 2%[19].

FAILURE TO DEFINE PROTOCOL

A further confounding factor is that the studies vary in their definition of anomalies included. Some studies cannot define which pregnancies underwent ultrasound screening prior to 24 weeks[20,21] and others, whilst defining the screening policy clearly do not detail which abnormalities were detected as a result of the second trimester screening examination[22]. Such studies have therefore been excluded from further discussion. Some do not define their screening protocol, whilst others do not include examination of the face[14] examine the profile only[13], only include 'major' degrees of talipes[14] or do not include chromosomal abnormalities where there was no structural abnormality present sonographically or postnatally[11,14]. Adequate details regarding postnatal confirmation of abnormalities are often missing.[14] These discrepancies will contribute significantly towards the differences in reported detection rates, particularly in the Ascot[14] screening programme where 85% of abnormalities were detected but facial clefts and minor degrees of talipes were not included. These are two areas where the sensitivity of other programmes tends to be low (Tables 34.10 and 34.11), thus probably resulting in the unrealistically high sensitivity of the Ascot study. An obvious omission from nearly all studies is the absence of any prenatally detected cases of some minor abnormalities or chromosomal 'markers', for example choroid plexus cysts, echogenic bowel, mild ventriculomegaly, mild pyelectasis, etc. Inclusion of these findings (see below) would not affect the sensitivity but would clearly have a profound effect on the specificity of routine ultrasound in the detection of abnormalities.

VARIATION IN ASCERTAINMENT OF ABNORMALITIES POSTNATALLY

All the studies reported give the sensitivity of routine ultrasound in terms of abnormalities detected in the neonate. Virtually complete ascertainment of many major abnormalities and certainly those which are obvious on external examination (e.g. facial clefts, anterior abdominal defects, limb reduction defects, anencephaly and open neural tube defects) is likely. However, 'internal abnormalities', such as renal problems and cardiac abnormalities, may not be clinically evident and ascertainment of these will depend on the thoroughness of the neonatal/postmortem examination. Indeed, many renal abnormalities may be clinically silent until later in life and not evident on clinical examination alone. The incidence of cardiac abnormalities is probably a good indicator of the degree of ascertainment of less obvious abnormalities and this varied considerably in the studies (Table 34.5) from 1.4–12/1000 births. Overall, the incidence of all abnormalities varied from 0.43–2.46% (Table 34.2) and more complete ascertainment of less severe abnormalities must account in some degree for the apparently poor performance of the programmes reported from Belgium[12,15] and America (RADIUS)[2,3]. However, other factors, such as operator skill, must also have influenced the detection rates as all cases of spina bifida were detected in the British studies[11,13,14], none of whom used maternal serum alphafetoprotein measurement (MSAFP), compared with only 40% in the Belgium[12].

The majority of ultrasound programmes designed to detect fetal abnormalities involve scanning in the second trimester; however, other protocols are in use. Some units use an indication-based system where pregnancies are dated early in pregnancy and further scans are only performed if there is another indication, e.g. relevant past history, raised MSAFP. With advances in technology and the need to date pregnancies earlier to facilitate serum screening tests, there is a drive towards earlier scanning, and routine anomaly screening at the end of the first, or early second trimester is advocated by some. These various screening protocols will be discussed in turn.

Routine second trimester anomaly scanning

The sensitivity of routine second trimester ultrasound programmes for the detection of abnormalities varies considerably between systems (Table 34.3). There are many reasons why an abnormality may not be detected, including technical difficulties such as maternal obesity, fetal position or multiple pregnancies. In some cases, e.g. tracheo-oesophageal fistula, there is no sonographic sign associated with an abnormality. In others (bowel obstruction, hydrocephalus, microcephaly, etc.) the sonographic abnormality may not appear until the late second or third trimester and thus not be detected at the time of the routine scan.

CRANIOSPINAL ABNORMALITIES

Most recent studies report 100% detection of anencephaly with no false negatives, and many achieve rates approaching 100% for open spina bifida (Table 34.4). It is the recognition of the cranial signs associated with spina bifida and the Arnold–Chiari malformation which has resulted in significant improvement in the sensitivity of ultrasound for the detection of neural tube defects, such that it now compares favourably with MSAFP measurement which would identify about 80% of fetuses with open spina bifida[24]. The 'lemon' sign is a result of scalloping of the frontal bones, and the 'banana' sign refers to the abnormal shape of the cerebellum[25,26]. Using these cranial signs in high risk populations nearly all fetuses with open spina bifida can be successfully identified before 20 weeks[26–28]. A prospective evaluation in a low risk population has confirmed the value of the lemon and banana signs (J. Campbell, unpublished data). In this study of 11 778 pregnancies there were eight cases of spina bifida. All had an abnormal cerebellum (absent or banana-shaped) and seven had a lemon sign. The eight was scanned after 26 weeks' gestation and the skull was normal. The disappearance of the lemon sign as pregnancy progresses has been reported by others and it seems that this aid to the diagnosis of neural tube defects is only useful prior to 24 weeks[27,29].

Other intracranial abnormalities are detectable in the second trimester, but the sonographic signs associated with microcephaly and hydrocephaly may develop later in pregnancy, and these abnormalities are examples of those which

TABLE 34.3
Detection of fetal abnormalities (%) before 24 weeks using different screening protocols (from pooled data tables)

	Screening protocol		
	Second trimester	First trimester	Indication based
Anencephaly	99	100	94
Neural tube defects	88	–	77
Central nervous system	75	–	45
Thoracic	66	–	36
Cardiac	25 (2.5–82)	–	7
Anterior abdominal wall defects	85	–	100
Intestinal obstruction	35	–	8
Urinary tract	62	–	49
Musculoskeletal	39	–	8
Other	62	–	38
Chromosomal	26	70 (53–100)	52

TABLE 34.4
Detection of central nervous system abnormalities using routine second trimester ultrasound

Author	Anencephaly	Other NTD[a]	Hydrocephaly	Holoprosencephaly	Other
Chitty et al.[11]	6/6	7/7	3/3	2/3	2/2
Shirley et al.[13]	10/10	4/4	1/2	–	–
Levi et al.[12]	6/6	4/7	4/15	0/1	3/6
Luck[14]	7/7	3/3	–	1/1	–
Roberts et al.[23]	7/8	14/16	5/6	1/1	1/2
Crane et al.[3]	3/3	4/5	–	–	2/2
Papp et al.[16]	44/44	52/58	46/50	8/8	4/7
Overall	73/74	88/100	59/76	12/14	12/19
(%)	(99)	(88)	(78)	(86)	(63)

[a]NTD = Neural tube defect

may only be detected if a scan was initiated because of a clinical indication or if a third trimester scan were routinely offered. This is well illustrated in the study from Belgium[12] where only 4 of 20 cases of hydrocephalus were identified by scanning before 22 weeks' gestation with the remainder being identified later in pregnancy.

CARDIOVASCULAR ABNORMALITIES

Cardiac abnormalities occur in about one in every 120 births[30]. About half of these are likely to be life threatening and, of these, about 50% should be detectable prenatally by examining the four-chamber view of the heart[31]. At gestations of 18 weeks or greater a four-chamber view of the heart can be obtained in up to 98% of fetuses, and examining the fetal heart in this way has been shown to improve the detection of congenital cardiac abnormalities[17,32,33]. However, the sensitivity of routine ultrasound in the detection of cardiac abnormalities in most studies reported is low, with a mean of 39% (2.5–82%) (Table 34.5). Much of this variation must be accounted for by differences in postnatal ascertainment as there is a significant difference in the incidence of neonatal cardiac abnormalities reported in these studies. Other factors include a later gestational age at scanning, rescanning if the four-chamber view of the heart is not adequately identified on the first occasion and increased scanning time in some studies. The Norwegian study[32] probably gives the most realistic estimate of the efficacy of routine ultrasound in the detection of cardiac anomalies. When critical lesions (i.e. those which were likely to require surgery) were considered, 26% were detected by the routine scan. In 4% of cases the four-chamber view was not visualized due to practical difficulties and no arrangement was made for rescanning. Three critical lesions occurred in this group (many more than might have been expected). In the group classified as non-critical, none had required surgery and many small ventricular or atrial septal defects resolved spontaneously. It is possible that delay in closure in some cases is part of the spectrum of normality and therefore it is difficult to know whether or not to define them as congenital heart defects or not[34]. It may well be better to define detection rates in terms of clinically significant abnormalities although this may well be very difficult. However, many serious cardiac abnormalities will result in an normal four-chamber view of the heart at 18–20 weeks' gestation. If examination of the fetal heart is extended to include views of the great vessels, the number of cardiac defects detected are reported to increase from 48–78%[35].

Despite the differences in sensitivity reported, it seems clear that routine screening programmes are having some effect in as much as the referral pattern to tertiary centres for fetal echocardiography has changed significantly, with an increasing proportion being referred because of a suspicion on routine ultrasound rather than on the basis of a relevant family history[37]. Furthermore, there has been a significant fall in the number of neonates with hypoplastic left heart syndrome seen at a supraregional referral centre[38].

GASTROINTESTINAL ABNORMALITIES

The sensitivity of routine fetal anomaly scanning approaches 100% for the detection of anterior abdominal wall defects (Table 34.6) but intestinal obstruction or atresia is less amenable to diagnosis in the second trimester, because the classical signs of the dilated stomach or proximal loops of

TABLE 34.5
Detection of cardiac abnormalities with routine second trimester ultrasound

Author	Total population	Period of study	Cardiac abnormalities: Detected	Not detected	Not scanned	Incidence (/1000)	Sensitivity[a] (%)
Chitty et al.[11]	8733	1988–89	7	4	2	1.5	64
Shirley et al.[13]	6412	1989–90	5	4	–	1.4	56
Levi et al.[12]	16 370	1984–89	3	72	28	6.2	3
Vergani et al.[33]	9016	1985–89	35	14	–	5.4	71
		1985–86[b]	7	8	–	–	47
		1987–89[c]	28	6[c]	–	–	82
Achiron et al.[35]	5400	1988–90	11	12	–	4.3	48
Roberts et al.[23]	11 359	1988–89	4	23	–	2.4	15
Crane et al.[3]	7685	1987–91	5	33	–	4.9	13
Rustico et al.[36]	7024	1986–92	23	42	–	9.3	35
Tegnander et al.[32]	4435	1986–88[b]	3	46	–	11	6
	7459	1988–91[c]	6	90	–	12	7
Papp et al.[16]	63 794	1988–90	3	118	60	2.8	2.5
Overall			140	472	90	–	25

[a]Calculated including only those scanned before 24 weeks
[b]Prior to introducing four-chamber view
[c]Using four-chamber view

TABLE 34.6
Detection of gastrointestinal abnormalities with routine second trimester ultrasound

Author	TOF[b]	Omphalocele	Gastroschisis	Small bowel obstruction
Chitty et al.[11]	0/2	3/3	1/1	0/1
Shirley et al.[13]	–	1/1	1/1	0/1
Levi et al.[12]	1/7	2/2	2/2	0/1
Luck[14]	0/1	2/2	2/2	1/1
Roberts et al.[23]	0/1	0/2	3/3	0/4
Crane et al.[3]	0/3	1/1	–	1/1
Papp et al.[16]	2/5[a]	11/15	6/6	11/15
Overall (%)	3/19	20/26	15/15	12/24

[a]probably includes oesophageal atresias
[b]TOF = tracheo-oesophageal fistula

small bowel do not appear until later in pregnancy. Such abnormalities are often detected later in pregnancy when a scan is requested because of polyhydramnios. Isolated oesophageal atresia may be diagnosed at the time of routine second trimester screening if there is failure to visualize the stomach bubble on several occasions. However, in 95% of these cases there is a coexistent fistula to the trachea so that the stomach can fill via the trachea and thus the bubble will be visualized, although polyhydramnios may occur later in pregnancy. In the four studies which listed the types of intestinal atresia separately[2,11,14,23] none of the seven fetuses with tracheo-oesophageal atresia were identified in the second trimester. All anterior wall defects were identified and two of the four small bowel obstructions were diagnosed.

THORACIC ABNORMALITIES

Congenital diaphragmatic hernia is probably the most common abnormality of the respiratory system, occurring in about 1 in 2000 to 1 in 5000 births. This abnormality is amenable to diagnosis at a routine second trimester scan, but may often not be detected until later in pregnancy when scanning is performed because of polyhydramnios. Other pulmonary abnormalities include cystic lung lesions such as cystic adenomatoid malformation (CCAML) and pleural effusions. The majority of cases with cystic lung lesions are diagnosed at the time of the routine scan (Table 34.7) but there is often no confirmation of the prenatal diagnosis as the natural history of this condition is often for apparent resolution of the lesion in utero, such that the neonatal chest radiograph may appear normal. It is worth noting, however, that more detailed examination in some cases using computerized tomography or magnetic resonance imaging has revealed the presence of a significant abnormality in the lung despite a normal radiograph. Furthermore, postnatal ascertainment of lesions not detected prenatally may be difficult as most will be clinically asymptomatic.

URINARY TRACT ABNORMALITIES

Abnormalities of the renal tract account for about 15% of anomalies diagnosed prenatally. Evaluation of the efficacy of routine ultrasound screening for fetal urinary tract abnormalities is difficult, since, although neonates with severe, bilateral abnormalities of the renal tract (bilateral renal agenesis/dysplasia, urethral atresia) are likely to present with clinical problems in the newborn period, the majority of renal problems are clinically silent at birth. Accurate assessment of the sensi-

TABLE 34.7
Detection of thoracic abnormalities with routine second trimester ultrasound

Author	Diaphragmatic hernia	Cystic lung lesions[a]	Pleural effusion	Other
Chitty et al.[11]	2/2	4/4	1/3	–
Shirley et al.[13]	2/3	1/1	–	1/1
Levi et al.[12]	1/2	–	–	1/2
Luck[14]	2/5	1/1	–	–
Roberts et al.[23]	0/1	1/1	–	0/1
Crane et al.[3]	1/1	–	–	1/4
Papp et al.[16]	8/11	7/7	–	1/3
Overall	16/25	14/14	1/3	4/11

[a]Most will be asymptomatic at birth and thus poor postnatal ascertainment may bias these figures

tivity of any prenatal screening programme would require detailed, long-term follow-up of neonates in order to achieve more complete ascertainment. Even routine evaluation of the neonatal renal tract using ultrasound shortly after birth would be unlikely to determine the true incidence of problems as this has been shown to have a high false negative and false positive rate[39]. Review of routine screening programmes (Table 34.8) indicates that routine ultrasound varies in its effectiveness. It appears to be quite effective in detecting bilateral renal agenesis, but less good for the detection of renal dysplasia and obstructive uropathies. The potential impact of routine ultrasound screening is reflected by the results of the RADIUS study, where the incidence of hydronephrosis at birth in the ultrasound screened group (29/7685) was four times greater than the control group (7/7596)[2]. This observation also confirms the clinically silent nature of many renal abnormalities. In five of the routine screening studies[3,11–13,15] cases of mild hydronephrosis or mild pyelectasis were not included in the analysis. In the series reported from Ascot it would appear these were included, but details of the postnatal follow-up were not given and it is unlikely that all were pathological after birth[14]. Other studies in the literature describe improved detection rates of urinary tract abnormalities by scanning later in pregnancy[40,41]. This is also confirmed by some of the routine screening studies discussed above where only 29% of all cases with obstructive uropathy and bilateral renal agenesis and dysplasia were diagnosed before 24 weeks' gestation, with a further 57% being diagnosed later in pregnancy when scans were performed for other reasons (routine 32 week scan or other clinical indication) (Table 34.9). However, the true clinical significance of many of the prenatal findings, even when confirmed in the neonatal period, are unclear as the majority of neonates are clinically asymptomatic and many of the abnormalities detected in the newborn resolve spontaneously. The long-term significance of these prenatal findings must await further study.

MUSCULOSKELETAL ABNORMALITIES

Visualization of the fetal long bones and measurement of the femur is often incorporated as a routine part of the examination. Many of the lethal skeletal dysplasias have severe limb shortening which is evident by 18 weeks, making many amenable to detection with routine ultrasound, as demonstrated by the relatively good detection rates of skeletal dysplasias in the routine ultrasound screening programmes reported (Table 34.10). However, examination of the hands and feet may be more difficult and often, when performing a routine scan, there are time constraints which prevent detailed examination of the extremities. This results in relatively poor detection rates for abnormalities such as talipes and limb reduction defects.

TABLE 34.8
Detection of urinary tract abnormalities using routine second trimester ultrasound

Author	Obstructive uropathy	Renal dysplasia			Renal agenesis			Other
		Unilateral	Bilateral	All	Unilateral	Bilateral	All	
Chitty et al.[11]	10/10	3/5	2/3	5/8	1/1	4/4	5/5	1/2
Shirley et al.[13]	7/8	–	0/1	0/1	–	–	–	–
Levi et al.[12]	2/25	?	?	4/11	–	3/4	3/4	3/6
Luck[14]	11/11	4/4	–	4/4	–	–	2/2	–
Roberts et al.[23]	4/6	2/4	3/3	5/7	0/1	3/4	3/5	–
Crane et al.[3]	10/26	–	–	2/3	–	1/1	1/1	0/1
Papp et al.[16]	14/14	–	–	16/16	–	7/7	7/7	–
Overall	58/100	–	–	36/50	–	–	21/24	4/9

TABLE 34.9
Summary of papers detailing gestational age at diagnosis of renal abnormalities

	Gestation in weeks at time of detection								
	Obstructive uropathy			Bilateral renal agenesis			Bilateral renal dysplasia		
	<24	>24	ND	<24	>24	ND	<24	>24	ND
Levi et al.[12]	2	32	13	3	3	0	4	5	2
Crane et al.[3]	10	16	1	1	0	0	2	1	0
Chitty et al.[11]	7	0	0	4	0	0	2	1	0
Total (%)	19(21)	58(64)	14(15)	8(73)	3(27)	0(0)	8(47)	7(41)	2(12)

ND = not detected

TABLE 34.10
Detection of musculoskeletal abnormalities using routine second trimester ultrasound

Author	Abnormality				
	Limb reduction defect	Talipes	Spinal anomaly	Dwarfism	Other
Chitty et al.[11]	2/5	6/12	3/3	2/2	1/2
Shirley et al.[13]	1/1	0/6	–	1/1	–
Levi et al.[12]	0/1	3/14	0/2	0/2	1/4
Luck[14]	1/2	2/2	1/1	2/2	0/1
Roberts et al.[23]	2/2	0/4	0/1	6/7	–
Crane et al.[3]	1/5	1/20	0/1	–	–
Papp et al.[16]	4/13	N/C	N/C	11/14	N/C
Overall	11/29	12/58	4/8	22/28	2/7

N/C = No comment

OTHER ABNORMALITIES

Details of the detection of other anomalies are not clearly stated in most reports. Table 34.11 lists some other anomalies, as well as genetic and multiple malformation syndromes.

CHROMOSOMAL ABNORMALITIES

Many of the more commonly occurring chromosomal abnormalities are associated with structural abnormalities which are amenable to prenatal detection with ultrasound (Table 34.12). Studies from tertiary referral centres have found that nearly all fetuses with trisomy 13, 77–100% of fetuses with trisomy 18 and 33–50% of fetuses with Down syndrome have significant sonographic signs which may be detected by a second trimester scan[42–45]. It seems clear that the risk of chromosomal abnormality rises with increasing numbers of sonographic abnormalities in the fetus[46] and when multiple abnormalities are present the overall risk may be as high as 35%[47]. There is no prospective study in low risk patients, but in the two studies of routine second trimester ultrasound screening programmes where detection of chromosomal abnormalities was reported, 26% of fetuses (9 of 34) with an abnormal karyotype (4 of 24 cases of trisomy 21, all four fetuses with trisomy 18 and 1 of 2 with trisomy 13) were detected following the identification of a sonographic abnormality[11,13].

There are many minor sonographic appearances (markers) which may be present in normal fetuses, but which are reported to be associated with abnormal karyotypes (Table 34.12). Some, e.g. choroid plexus cysts, mild pyelectasis, nuchal oedema and mild ventriculomegaly, have potential for use in screening the low risk population for fetal karyotypic abnormalities because they can be relatively easily visualised at the time of a routine scan. Others such as clinodactyly, sandal gap, polydactyly, clenched fists, etc., are less readily seen as a routine, but are signs which should be sought in fetuses known to be at increased prior risk or where another sonographic abnormality has been found. One of the main problems with using these markers in the low risk population is that the majority of studies report data collected from selected populations and extrapolation of the associated risks to low risk pregnancies may be inappropriate. Furthermore, not all studies reach the same conclusions regarding the

TABLE 34.11
Detection of other malformations and syndromes using routine second trimester ultrasound

Author	Abnormality				
	Cystic hygroma	Facial cleft	Hydrops	Syndrome	MCA
Chitty et al.[11]	1/1	2/9	2/2	10/10	7/7
Shirley et al.[13]	2/2	3/9	0/1	–	–
Levi et al.[12]	5/5	0/11	2/6	1/5	–
Luck[14]	1/1	N/E	1/1	0/1	–
Roberts et al.[23]	–	0/4	–	–	–
Crane et al.[3]	1/1	1/8	0/2	–	–
Papp et al.[16]	6/6	N/C	31/32	8/8	10/20

MCA = multiple congenital anomalies
N/E = not examined
N/C = no comment

TABLE 34.12
Sonographic features associated with common chromosomal abnormalities

	Trisomy				
	21	18	13	45XO	Triploidy
Major abnormalities					
Holoprosencephaly	–	–	+	–	–
Microcephaly	–	+	+	–	–
Neural tube defect	–	+	–	–	–
Cystic hygroma	+	–	–	+	–
Cardiac abnormality	+	+	+	+	+
Diaphragmatic hernia	–	+	(+)	–	–
Exomphalos	–	+	(+)	–	–
Oesophageal atresia	–	+	–	–	–
Duodenal atresia	+	–	–	–	–
Renal abnormalities	(+)	+	+	+	–
Radial aplasia	–	+	(+)	–	–
Hydrops	+	–	–	+	–
IUGR	+	+	+	–	+
Minor abnormalities (markers)					
Mild ventriculomegaly	+	+	(+)	–	+
Choroid plexus cysts	(+)	+	–	–	–
Strawberry-shaped skull	–	+	–	–	–
Posterior fossa cyst	–	+	+	–	+
Facial cleft	–	uni	bi	–	–
Micrognathia	–	+	(+)	–	+
Macroglossia	+	–	–	–	–
Nuchal oedema ≥ 6 mm (2nd tm)	+	(+)	(+)	(+)	–
Nuchal translucency (1st tm)	+	+	+	+	+
Echogenic chordae tendenii	(+)	–	(+)	–	–
Mild pyelectasis	+	(+)	–	–	–
Echogenic bowel	+	+	–	–	–
Fisted hand	–	+	–	–	–
Talipes	–	+	(+)	–	–
Rocker bottom feet	–	+	(+)	–	–
Relatively short femur/humerus	+	+	–	+	+
Sandal gap	+	–	–	–	–
Clinodactyly	+	–	–	–	–

+ = common association; (+) = less common; – = rare
uni = unilateral; bi = bilateral/midline
tm = trimester

association with aneuploidy in the presence of various markers. A good example are choroid plexus cysts (CPCs) which were first identified in 1984 when they were described as a benign transient finding[48]. There have been many studies of CPCs published since then and estimates of risk for trisomy 18 in a fetus with isolated CPCs vary from 1:30 to 1:477[49] and if the data from unselected populations is pooled the risk lies around 1–2:100[50]. However, the vast majority of studies fail to take into consideration other risk factors such as raised maternal age or abnormal maternal serum biochemistry. If age is taken into consideration then the risk of aneuploidy can be modified[51,52]. Further evaluation of the efficacy of other minor markers in the detection of chromosomal abnormalities in low risk populations is needed and care should be taken before applying figures obtained from the high risk population to low risk pregnancies. The few studies which have considered maternal age as an independent risk factor have shown that risks are greater when a fetal abnormality is found in older women[51–54]. Some authors have suggested using multiple parameters by developing a index scoring system, whereby different markers are given different weightings (or scores) based on the sensitivity and specificity of an individual marker[43,55]. Using such a system Benacerraf et al.[43] claim a 73% sensitivity and 96% specificity for detecting Down syndrome in a high risk population, but there has been no evaluation in unselected pregnancies.

Screening for aneuploidy using second trimester aneuploidy is problematic. Minor sonographic markers are common and are found in a significant proportion of fetuses, at least 5%. Assignment of risk for aneuploidy following the identification of a marker in a low risk fetus is fraught with difficulty, as adequate data from low risk populations do not exist. The finding of a sonographic marker increases the risk of aneuploidy. Risks are higher when more than one marker or abnormality is found, and consideration of other factors such as serum screening results as well as age and past history may help in the assessment of risk. It is also important to remember that these minor findings may have other pathological associations, e.g. echogenic bowel with IUGR, cystic fibrosis and viral infections[56,57], mild pyelectasis with renal abnormalities[58].

First trimester fetal anomaly scanning

With improved technology, in particular the development of transvaginal ultrasound probes, it has become possible to examine the fetal anatomy in detail in the first trimester[59,60]. The advent of widespread maternal serum screening for Down syndrome means that there is a clinically driven need for early confirmation of gestational age. There is therefore a potential economic advantage in considering routine first trimester anomaly scanning, but there are relatively few reports of such programmes[61,62], although there are many papers looking in detail at high risk populations or specific abnormalities.

FETAL STRUCTURAL ABNORMALITIES

The optimum gestational age for early scanning will depend on several factors but one of the most important is the gestational age at which the majority of fetal structures can be visualized. This would appear to be around 12–13 weeks, whether using the vaginal or abdominal route (Table 34.13), although most authors report better overall visualization using the vaginal route[59,63,64]. The exception is one large study which reports the use of transabdominal ultrasound screening for anencephaly at 10–14 weeks' gestation[65]. Overall, 41 of 48 cases were identified. The study describes the effect of training sonographers to look specifically for this abnormality, and demonstrates that the detection rate can be improved to 100% following education. One of the studies describing the value of first trimester ultrasound in screening for all fetal malformations reported an overall incidence of congenital anomalies of 2.6% in fetuses examined between 9–16 weeks' gestation with transvaginal ultrasound[66]. However, they did not define their population, or give details of any false negative results, although they do comment that anomalies involving the obstruction of the passage of fluids may not be detected until later in pregnancy. Another study comparing transabdominal with transvaginal ultrasound[63] found an improved detection rate using transvaginal ultrasonography, but also reported a significant proportion of abnormalities which were not seen when scanned before 13 weeks but which were clearly visualized at a routine 18–20 week scan (Table 34.14).

As with second trimester screening there may be interpretational difficulties, for example the spontaneous resolution of cystic hygroma detected in the first trimester has been reported[67] and in the study from Israel 81 of the anomalies detected by transvaginal scanning between 9 and 16 weeks were transient, although there was a high rate of aneuploidy in the group (6.1%)[68]. Economides et al.[62] reported high incidences of choroid plexus cysts (3.6%) and hydronephrosis (3.2%) in fetuses scanned at 12–13 weeks. Other studies describing screening for urinary tract abnormalities also report high incidences (up to 4.5%) of transient dilatation of the upper urinary tract[69,70]. Megacystis has also been reported in fetuses scanned at 10–14 weeks of pregnancy[71]. This was observed to be transient in 7 of 15 cases, although in three

TABLE 34.13
Gestational age for visualization of fetal anatomy

	Gestational age (weeks) TA	Gestational age (weeks) TV	Reference
Cranium	11, 12–13	11–12	Braithwaite et al.[64], Timor-Tritsch et al.[60]
Spine	12–13	11	
Long bones	12–13	11	
Feet	?	13	
Four-chamber view	12–13	14	
Kidneys	12–13	11–12(80%) 13 (92–100%)	Bronshtein et al.[69], Rosati and Guariglia[70]
Bladder	12–13	13	
Anterior abdominal wall	12–13	12	Braithwaite et al.[64] Timor-Tritsch et al.[60]
Face	12–13	12	
Stomach	13	12	

TA = transabdominal
TV = transvaginal

TABLE 34.14
Results of first trimester ultrasound screening for fetal abnormalities

Author[a]	Population[b]	Period	Gestation	Detection of abnormalities[c]		Sensitivity (%)	
				TA	TV	TA	TV
Achiron and Tadmor[63]	?	1989–90	9–13	4/14	8/14	29	57
Bronshtein et al.[83]	M	?	12–16	–	42	–	?93
Bronshtein et al.[69]	M	?	10–16	–	35	–	–
Johnson et al.[65]	M	1992–96	10–13	39/47	–	83	–
		1992–95	10–13	23/31	–	74	–
		1995–96	10–13	16/16	–	100	–

[a]Johnson et al.[65] report anencephaly only; Bronshtein et al.[83] report skeletal abnormalities only
[b]M = mixed
[c]TA = transabdominal; TV = transvaginal

there was an underlying chromosomal abnormality and in four others there was progression to severe obstructive uropathy. These observations make it clear that the natural history of abnormalities (some of which may be physiological variants) must be more accurately defined before this technique can be considered for widespread application to the low-risk population and care must be taken in interpretation of findings. Furthermore, many of the false negative scans in second trimester screening are because the sonographic signs associated with many fetal malformations are not evident until after the time of the routine 18–20 week anomaly scan. This is likely to be a more important consideration in first trimester scanning and must in part account for the relatively high false negative rate reported in some studies.

In 1989, Bronshtein et al[68] reported the association of nuchal translucency, detected in the first trimester, and abnormal fetal karyotypes. Similar observations were made by Szabo and Gellen[72]. The value of this sign in screening for chromosomal abnormalities will be discussed below, but there is considerable evidence that an increased nuchal translucency may also be a marker for a wide variety of other underlying pathologies, some which may be definable in the first trimester (omphalocoele, anencephaly, limb anomalies, etc.), whereas the precise nature of others (e.g. urinary tract and cardiac anomalies) may not be clear until later in pregnancy. Table 34.15 summarizes the incidence of other pathologies in fetuses with an increased (≥3 mm) nuchal translucency. In particular, there appears to be an increased risk for cardiac abnormalities[73]. In one pathological study of fetuses terminated because of an increased NT and other abnormality, 19 of 21 cases had an abnormality of the heart or great vessels[74].

The majority of these studies report data from pregnancies scanned because of increased prior risk, usually for aneuploidy rather than other structural abnormalities. However, these data demonstrate that nuchal translucency measurement may be a useful screening tool, not just to identify fetuses at increased risk of aneuploidy, but also to identify those which would benefit from targeted second trimester anomaly and/or fetal cardiac scanning.

CHROMOSOMAL ABNORMALITIES

There are several sonographic markers which may be identified in the first trimester. These include nuchal translucency, fetal heart rate[75], a smaller than expected CRL, altered heart rate[75] and other major abnormalities such as exomphalos[53] cardiac anomalies[61] and urinary tract obstruction[71]. The sonographic finding of an abnormal collection of fluid at the

TABLE 34.15
Pathological findings in euploid fetuses with increased nuchal translucency (NT)

Author[a]	Population[b]	Gestational age	N[c]	Abnormality: Detected <14 weeks	Detected later	Detected postnatally
Cha'Ban et al.[92]	S	9–15	28	5	4	–
Trauffer et al.[93]	S	?	22	1	2	3
Pandya et al.[94]	S	10–13	177	8	13	1
Van Zalen-Sprock et al.[95]	U	10–16	15	0	4	1
Pandya et al.[73]	S	10–14	565	11	19	1

[a]In Pandya et al.[73] nuchal translucency ≥ 4 mm
[b]S = selected; U = unselected
[c]N = number in study

back of the fetal neck in the first trimester of pregnancy has been reported to have a strong association with fetal aneuploidy, and particularly fetal trisomy[62,68]. This sign has been variously defined as nuchal translucency[76], simple hygroma[77] and cystic hygroma[78] and has been the subject of considerable study over recent years as its application in the first trimester makes it an attractive option for population screening for Down syndrome[75]. However, much of the data have been collected in 'high risk' women already undergoing fetal karyotyping on the basis of advanced maternal age, parental anxiety or family history of chromosome abnormality (Table 34.16). Maternal age and nuchal translucency thickness have been combined as independent risk factors to improve the prediction of fetal trisomy[79]. The test has been well evaluated in selected populations, with most, but not all, studies reporting that an increased nuchal translucency measurement can identify around 77% (0–88%) of Down syndrome fetuses with a false positive rate of 6% (0.1–9.9%) (Table 34.16). However, there is little information on its utility in screening an unselected obstetric populations, although it appeared to have similar screening properties to the high risk population when introduced into two maternity units providing routine antenatal care[80]. There is considerable variation in the sensitivities reported both in selected and routinely screened populations (Table 34.16) and the overall detection rate is no greater that that reported for second trimester serum screening.

When considering implementation of first trimester screening, either for general structural or chromosomal abnormalities, consideration must be given to the fact that many pregnancies complicated with serious abnormalities will abort spontaneously in the first or early second trimester[81,82]. Whilst it may be helpful for parents to understand the reason for the pregnancy loss, this benefit must be carefully weighed against potential harm (which may last long beyond the perinatal period) which may be caused by making parents choose to terminate a wanted pregnancy which would have been lost spontaneously. Furthermore, for the majority of sporadic abnormalities, recurrence risks are based on data obtained at birth or later in pregnancy, and an increased recurrence risk for the future may be wrongly assigned.

Indication-based screening

An alternative screening policy employed in some units is to scan at booking in the first trimester (usually just to confirm the gestational age) and then only scan at 18–20 weeks if there is a clinical indication, positive family history, abnormal maternal serum screening, etc. However, this may still result in an unacceptably high false negative rate. In the study described above[63], the five abnormalities missed in the first trimester were hydrocephalus, agenesis of the corpus callosum, bilateral hydronephrosis and two major cardiac defects. None of these would have altered the serum biochemistry or would be likely to stimulate another clinical cause for a scan in the second trimester. Routine and indication-based (with-

TABLE 34.16
Summary of studies reporting the use of nuchal translucency measurement in screening for aneuploidy

	Gestational age (weeks)	NT (mm)	Number in study		Fetuses with ↑ NT and abnormal karyotypes		Sensitivity for the detection of aneuploidy		False positive rate (%)
			All(%)	↑NT	All(%)	Trisomy 21(%)	All(%)	Trisomy 21(%)	
Selected populations[a]									
Schulte-Valentin and Schinder[84]	10–14	4–7	917	9	75	7	7	70	0.1
Nicolaides et al.[79]	10–13	≥3	1273	88	33	21	72	84	4.4
Szabo et al.[85]	9–12	≥3	1380	69	34	23	92	88	2.6
Comas et al.[86]	9–13	≥3	481	51	9	4	37	57	9.9
Brambati et al.[87]	8–15	≥3	1819	70	13	?	30	?	3.2
Pandya et al.[88]	10–14	≥2.5	20 804	1548	127	66	77	77	6.9
Kornman et al.[89]	≥13	≥3	484	13	0	0	0	0	2.7
Total			27 158	1847	223(%)	121(%)	67	77[b]	6.0
Routine screening populations									
Szabo et al.[85]	9–12	≥3	2000	27	9	4	100	100	0.9
Hafner et al.[90]	10–13	≥2.5	1972	26	8	2	73	50	0.9
Kornman et al.[89]	≥13	≥3	439	23	2	2	67	67	4.8
Pandya et al.[80]	10–13	≥2.5	1763	63	4	3	76	75	3.4
Bower et al.[90]	8–13	≥3	2566	169	8	5	53	45	6.3
Total			6940	308	31	16	70	62	4.0

[a]Data from Comas *et al.*[86] includes nine cases of balanced translocations; data from Pandya *et al.*[80] are from a mixed population
[b]Excludes Brambati *et al.*[82]

out first trimester scanning) screening for fetal malformations has been compared[96]. More malformations were detected prior to 24 weeks by means of routine screening (18%) than by the indication-based (5%) screening (Table 34.17). This was not a randomized study, but a retrospective one comparing the different policies in operation at different times, indication-based screening in 1983–1984 and routine screening in 1990–1991. There are therefore several confounding factors which may have influenced these results, not least the fact that the technology had improved considerably between the two study periods. In a similar study, again retrospective but studying groups scanned over the same time period in a unit which used maternal serum alphafetoprotein measurement, 45% of abnormalities were detected in the fetuses scanned routinely at 16 weeks or later compared with only 30% in those scanned at booking only. The authors further refined the latter figure to 17% if only those booking scans done prior to 16 weeks were included[97].

Probably the best report of an indication-based screening programme is that by Chambers et al.[98]. In this study early scans were performed to date and establish the viability of the pregnancy combined with MSAFP estimation at 16 weeks. Thereafter, selective screening at 18–20 weeks was performed based on clinical indication (past history, raised MSAFP, etc). A total of 51% of abnormalities were diagnosed prenatally, 42% before 24 weeks' gestation. The overall sensitivity of this programme is less than that reported from other units in the UK[11,13,14], with the greatest shortfall in diagnosis occurring amongst cardiac and skeletal abnormalities and bowel obstruction (Tables 34.3, 34.17). This study was reported prior to the recognition of the association between increased nuchal translucency and cardiac abnormalities. It will be interesting to see whether the addition of NT measurement to an early dating scan can improve the sensitivity of indication-based screening programmes by including an increased NT as an indication for detailed second trimester ultrasound screening. Other screening policies should also be evaluated; for example, the addition of a routine late second or early third trimester scan to a dating scan (with or without NT measurement) may result both in the detection of many abnormalities not evident in first or second trimesters and in deviations from normal growth. Such a policy may result in the late detection of abnormalities but would still fulfil some of the potential benefits of ultrasound, such as allowing for the planning of delivery and postnatal treatment, and giving the parents time to prepare for the birth of a child with an abnormality. Detection rates for those abnormalities in which the sonographic signs develop later in pregnancy may also improve. However, for some it would remove the option of choosing to terminate a pregnancy if there was significant risk of a lethal or seriously handicapping abnormality, although in the UK there is no gestational age restriction for abortion in these circumstances.

Advantages and disadvantages of routine screening

The skill of the sonographer, gestational age at scanning and postnatal ascertainment of abnormalities all account for some of the variation in sensitivities of the studies reported, but is clear that if the staff are adequately trained and scanning is performed at 18–20 weeks' gestation, a significant proportion (around 70–80%) of lethal or severely disabling abnormalities (as well as many less serious ones) can be detected by a routine scan in low risk pregnancies. Prenatal detection of fetal

TABLE 34.17
Detection of fetal abnormalities before 24 weeks using an indication-based screening programme

System	Constantine[97]	Bernaschek[96]	Chambers[98]	Total (%)
Anencephaly	2/2	–	14/15	16/17 (94)
Other neural tube defect	4/4	–	16/22	20/26 (77)
Central nervous system	1/3	–	4/8	5/11 (45)
Thoracic abnormality	1/2	3/5	0/4	4/11 (36)
Cardiac abnormality	2/14	0/11	2/36	4/61 (7)
Anterior abdominal wall defect	1/1	–	7/7	8/8 (100)
Intestinal obstruction	0/1	–	1/12	1/13 (8)
Urinary tract abnormality	6/11	5/12	13/26	24/49 (49)
Skeletal abnormality	–	–	1/12	1/12 (8)
Facial cleft	–	–	1/20	1/20 (5)
Syndromes/MCA	1/3	–	2/6	3/9 (33)
Chromosomal	–	–	15/29[a]	15/29 (52)
Other	3/7	–	7/19	10/26 (38)
Total	18/46	38/92	83/196	112/272
Overall sensitivity < 24 weeks (%)	39	41	42	41

MCA = multiple congenital anomalies
[a]Includes cases karyotyped for other genetic indications

abnormalities would seem to be advantageous, but when screening the low risk population it is not without its problems.

EFFECTS ON PERINATAL MORBIDITY AND MORTALITY

There has been very little formal evaluation of the benefits of routine ultrasound screening for fetal malformations. The Helsinki study demonstrated a significant reduction in the perinatal mortality rate in their ultrasound screened cohort, much of which was due to the detection and subsequent termination of pregnancy in cases complicated by serious fetal malformations. Papp et al.[16], in their report of mid-trimester ultrasound screening in Hungary, conclude that prenatal detection and termination of pregnancies could significantly reduce the birth prevalence of severe abnormalities. Certainly giving parents the option to terminate a pregnancy where the fetus has been found to have a lethal or severely disabling abnormality is a potential advantage of a programme which screens for fetal abnormalities, albeit that the parents may be faced with difficult and unexpected decisions and not all parents will choose this option. In the latter case, forewarning of the adverse outcome of the pregnancy has been shown to be of value[99].

There is also potential for a reduction in perinatal morbidity in neonates requiring early neonatal surgical or paediatric interventions. The prior knowledge of the presence of a fetal abnormality allows both early implementation of therapy and for planning of the delivery in a unit with the appropriate facilities. Studies have shown that there is a reduction in morbidity in fetuses with gastroschisis, intestinal obstruction and cardiac abnormalities when the diagnosis has been made prenatally and delivery and postnatal treatment planned accordingly[100,101]. In the case of cardiac abnormalities, whilst there was no difference in the early survival rates between fetuses diagnosed in utero and those diagnosed postnatally, there was a significantly lower incidence of preoperative metabolic acidosis and no cardiac arrests in the group diagnosed prenatally. These factors may influence longer-term mortality and morbidity, but further study is needed before this benefit is proven[101]. Other investigators claim that the prenatal detection of renal abnormalities is beneficial and may reduce morbidity from reflux or infection. In one prospective study of 92 fetuses with a prenatally diagnosed urinary tract abnormality, 42 had the abnormality confirmed postnatally and the authors considered that in about half of these cases the baby had benefited from the prenatal diagnosis in that it allowed early treatment, either surgical or chemoprophylaxis[102]. Another study confirmed these observations and suggested that in their series benefit was conferred in about 75% of cases which would have otherwise remained clinically silent[103]. However, there has been no prospective study demonstrating a positive benefit. In addition, the high false positive rates reported (50 of the 92 abnormalities were not confirmed postnatally in one study), undoubtedly induced considerable unnecessary parental anxiety.

PARENTAL REASSURANCE

The majority of fetal abnormalities occur in pregnancies at low risk. Increasingly parents are aware that they all face a small but measurable risk of fetal abnormality in any pregnancy, and so possibly the greatest advantage of routine fetal anomaly scanning may be the reassurance it gives to most parents. The specificity reported for most ultrasound screening programmes is high (99.9–100%) and thus the majority of parents are correctly reassured. However, a few parents will be falsely reassured and their baby will have an unexpected abnormality. There have been no studies of the psychological consequences for parents when fetal anomalies have been missed, either following ultrasound or other screening tests for fetal anomalies, although parental anger in response to false reassurance has been reported. It is important that parents are aware of the possibility of a false negative (or false positive) diagnosis. In view of this the Royal College of Obstetricians and Gynaecologists[18] recommended that a written explanation of the reasons for and limitations of a scan should be given to women. Nevertheless, prescan counselling has been described as extremely poor in most British hospitals[104]. Smith and Marteau[105] found that fetal anomaly scanning was only discussed with 65% of women during general discussions regarding antenatal tests. The objectives of scanning were discussed in 37% of consultations, implications of abnormal findings in 15% and the possibility of false negative or false positive results were never discussed. In only 11% of cases was scanning presented as being optional. This study concluded that the lack of information given may make parents less able to make an informed choice should the need arise. Clearly, further study is needed to determine the optimum way of preparing parents for a scan in order to minimize any adverse psychological effects. Some may argue that detailed discussion of possible adverse consequences may deter parents from taking up the offer of a scan. This fear was not substantiated in a study reported from Sweden where midwives were trained to give detailed and uniform information to a group of women regarding anomaly scanning. Only 1% of women in this group declined detailed scanning, opting for a dating scan only, compared with none in a control group having standard antenatal care[106]. Anecdotal evidence would suggest that not all parents are aware of the implications of detailed fetal anomaly scanning and this issue must be addressed. Once an abnormality has been detected it is too late for such explanations.

PARENTAL PREPARATION FOR AN ABNORMALITY

It seems logical to suppose that in cases where the parents are faced with the unexpected finding of a fetal abnormality and the pregnancy continues, the prior knowledge may be helpful in allowing them to come to terms with the birth of a child with a congenital abnormality. There is no good evidence to support this view, but it is not uncommon to receive a request to scan a pregnancy at increased risk of an abnormality (for example a facial cleft), not because the parents would seek an abortion if the fetus were affected, but because they would like the forewarning. Prior knowledge of a fetal abnormality which will require surgery or other paediatric interventions also allows time for the parents to meet and discuss the postnatal management with the relevant health professionals, to see the neonatal intensive care unit if necessary and to adjust to the fact that their baby will have to spend some time in hospital after delivery. However, there is also evidence, again anecdotal, that for some parents the detection of an abnormality may cause so much concern that it impairs the parents' ability to cope with the child after birth[107].

FALSE POSITIVE DIAGNOSES

Most reports of routine ultrasound screening programmes give very low incidences of false positive results and none resulted in the termination of a normal fetus, although this is obviously a potential risk and has been described in reviews of pathological outcomes[108,109]. However, even the finding of a relatively minor abnormality, which is subsequently not confirmed, can cause considerably anxiety to the parents, the effects of which may last for some time after the birth of their child. For example, anomalies of the urinary tract are amongst those most frequently diagnosed prenatally, but where the incidence of false positive diagnoses can be high[102]. Furthermore, the majority of those with a postnatal abnormality will be asymptomatic with only mild to moderate degrees of upper tract dilatation of uncertain clinical significance. Further studies of the natural history of asymptomatic renal abnormalities in the neonate are required before the true significance in terms of postnatal renal function of many prenatal findings becomes clearer. Prenatal studies are also needed to try to define factors which may predict outcome more accurately and thus reduce the incidence of false positives. There are many other examples of these minor 'changes' (nuchal translucency, echogenic bowel, choroid plexus cysts, second trimester nuchal oedema, mild ventriculomegaly, etc.) which affect many fetuses. Most appear in fact be a variant of normal and there is an urgent need for large studies of low risk populations to accurately define the risks associated with these markers.

DIFFICULTY IN DEFINING PROGNOSIS

The unexpected discovery of an abnormality in a fetus is a source of great anxiety which is often compounded by an inability to give the parents accurate prognostic advice. In some cases the diagnosis may be clear but the pregnancy outcome very variable. In the case of a diaphragmatic hernia, for example, the mortality is high, but if the child survives surgery then the long-term prognosis is usually good. Other diagnoses may give rise to more difficult decisions. The finding of mild ventriculomegaly or agenesis of the corpus callosum are good examples of anomalies which occur with a higher frequency in developmentally delayed individuals, but may also be found as an incidental finding in otherwise normal people[110]. When detected prenatally both may be associated with an abnormal fetal karyotype, but once this has been excluded the prognosis is very variable. Review of the cases reported in the literature would suggest that the residual risk of handicap for both mild ventriculomegaly and agenesis of the corpus callosum[111] is of the order of 15%, much of which would be for significant degrees of developmental delay. However, these figures are derived from reports of selected cases, mainly reviewed retrospectively with very variable follow-up. Structured follow-up studies, looking both at the long-term paediatric outcome and the prenatal findings in more detail to try to elicit more reliable prognostic markers, are required in order to provide more accurate figures for counselling in these and other similar situations. When screening women who have a previously affected child the outcome in these situations is often clear, but there can be considerable difficulty in giving a confident prognosis in the low risk population.

Prediction of outcome of a recognizable abnormality may be difficult, but the prognosis for lesions not previously reported can be even more difficult to predict. This can only be overcome in time by accurate reporting in the literature of such cases.

SAFETY

As with most other aspects of routine ultrasound screening, there has been little formal evaluation of the safety of this procedure. The Norwegians performed two randomized controlled studies of ultrasound during 1979–1981. The screened group (1244 children) had been exposed to ultrasound at 16–22 weeks and most of the controls (1184 children) had not, although many (19%) were scanned later in pregnancy[8,112]. These cohorts of babies have recently been followed up to the age of 8–9 years. There was no difference in postnatal growth[113], reading and writing skills[114] or vision and hearing at the ages of 4 and 7[115] in the screened and control groups, although the data suggest a possible association between routine ultrasound exposure and subsequent non-righthandedness[116]. Whilst these studies did not produce any evidence to suggest that significant harm is done to the developing fetus, a recent paper from Australia found that fetuses (2834) exposed to repeated ultrasound and Doppler examinations tended to have slightly lower birthweights[117]. However, the difference between the group exposed to the frequent Doppler and those in the control group was small, and the authors concluded that further study looking specifically at this aspect was required. Furthermore, the exposure to ultrasound in this study was much greater and more frequent than that which would normally occur during routine ultrasound screening for fetal abnormalities. Further, by the age of 1 year there was no measurable difference in growth between the two groups in the Australian study[118].

Economic considerations

There has been no prospective cost–benefit analysis of routine ultrasound screening. Clearly costs will depend on a variety of factors including prevalence of abnormalities, skill of sonographers and rate of intervention following diagnosis of serious abnormalities. DeVore[118] examined the cost effectiveness of ultrasound in the centres participating in the RADIUS study[2]. He estimated that the cost per malformed fetus identified in tertiary centres (which had a significantly better detection rate) was around $30 000 compared with $115 000 in peripheral units. The only reasonable data from Europe come from an analysis of the screened group in the Helsinki ultrasound trial. They estimated a cost of $21 938 to avoid one perinatal death, and calculated that the cost of each ultrasound scan was $102, but that this resulted in a saving of $182 per woman due to fewer inpatient and outpatient visits and further investigations later in pregnancy[120].

Other issues

It must be remembered that fetal ultrasound is a screening test for fetal malformations. Whilst in some cases accurate diagnosis is possible prior to delivery, in many cases definitive diagnosis must await the results of other investigations. Expert perinatal pathology and radiology is often required to define the underlying pathology and can refine the ultrasound diagnosis in 35–46% of cases[108,121,122]. Accurate diagnosis is essential in order to define risks for future pregnancies and to decide which investigations may be appropriate. In one study, perinatal pathology increased the recurrence in 19% (25 of 133) cases, and decreased it 18% (24 of 133)[123]. It is worth noting that postmortem is sometimes refused and that in others, due to tissue autolysis, autopsy can provide less information than ultrasound[121].

Conclusions

In conclusion, further clinical cost–benefit evaluation of ultrasound screening programmes is needed before the true benefits and burdens of routine ultrasound screening for fetal malformations are clear. Long-term follow-up studies of the clinical significance of some sonographic markers in unselected pregnancies are needed. These will need to be multicentre, and probably multinational for some of the rarer conditions. Study of the psychological consequences of ultrasound is needed and consideration should be given to alternative screening protocols. Whilst the best way to evaluate routine screening is probably by randomized study, the time for this may well be past, since ultrasound is an accepted and indeed usually eagerly anticipated part of routine antenatal care (at least in Europe and the UK).

However, detailed descriptive evaluation must take place and every effort made to reduce any adverse sequelae. Lessons should be learnt from the failure to adequately evaluate this now widespread practice, and any potential advances must be formally evaluated in low risk populations before implementation. Screening programmes must be audited and the establishment of malformation registers, preferably those which access paediatric databases so that ascertainment of abnormalities goes beyond the newborn period, is an efficient mechanism for this. Finally, there must be a programme of structured training for all those who perform fetal anomaly scanning with accepted minimum standards of practice.

REFERENCES

1. Consensus Conference. The Use of Diagnostic Ultrasound Imaging During Pregnancy. *JAMA* **252**(5):669–72, 1984.
2. Ewigman BG, Crane JP, Frigoletto FD, LeFevre ML, Bain RP, McNellis D and the RADIUS Study Group. Effect of Prenatal Ultrasound Screening on Perinatal Outcome. *N. Engl. Med. J.* **329**(12): 821–827, 1993.
3. Crane JP, LeFevre ML, Winborn RC et al. and the RADIUS Study Group. A Randomized Trial of Prenatal Ultrasonographic Screening: Impact on the Detection, Management and Outcome of Anomalous Fetuses. *Am. J. Obstet. Gynecol.* **171**(2):392–399, 1994.
4. Bucher HC, Schmidt JG. Does routine ultrasound scanning improve outcome in pregnancy? Meta-analysis of various outcome measures. *Br. Med. J.* **307**:13–18, 1993.
5. Saari-Kemppainen A, Karjalainen O, Ylöstalo P, Heinonen OP. Ultrasound screening and perinatal mortality: controlled trial of systematic one-stage screening in pregnancy. *Lancet* **336**:387–391, 1990.
6. Geerts Lut TGM, Brand EJ, Theron GB. Routine obstetric ultrasound examinations in South Africa: cost and effect on perinatal outcome – a prospective randomised controlled trial. *Br. J. Obstet. Gynaecol.* **103**:501–507, 1996.
7. Waldenström U, Axelsson O, Nilsson S et al. Effects of routine one-stage ultrasound screening in pregnancy: a randomised controlled trial. *Lancet* **10**:585–588, 1988.
8. Bakketeig LS, Eik-Nes SH, Jacobsen G et al. Randomised controlled trial of ultrasonographic screening in pregnancy. *Lancet* **ii**:207–211, 1984.
9. Ewigman B, LeFevre M, Hesser J. A randomized trial of routine prenatal ultrasound. *Obstet. Gynecol.* **76**(2):189–194, 1990.
10. Rosendahl H, Kivinen S. Antenatal detection of congenital malformations by routine ultrasonography. *Obstet. Gynecol.* **73**(6):947–951, 1989.
11. Chitty LS, Hunt GH, Moore J, Lobb MO. Effectiveness of routine ultrasonography in detecting fetal structural abnormalities in a low risk population. *Br. Med. J.* **303**:1165–1169, 1991.
12. Levi S, Hyjazi Y, Schaaps JP, Defoort P, Coulon R, Buekens P. Sensitivity and specificity of routine antenatal screening for congenital anomalies by ultrasound: the belgian multicentric study. *Ultrasound Obstet. Gynecol.* **1**:102–110, 1991.

13. Shirley IM, Bottomley F, Robinson VP. Routine radiographer screening for fetal abnormalities by ultrasound in an unselected low risk population. *Br. J. Radiol.* **65**:565–569, 1991.
14. Luck C. Value of routine ultrasound scanning at 19 weeks: a four year study of 8849 deliveries. *Br. Med. J.* **304**:1474–1478, 1992.
15. Levi S, Schaaps JP, De Havay P, Defoort P. End-result of routine ultrasound screening for congenital anomalies: the Belgium multicentre study 1984–92. *Ultrasound Obstet. Gynecol.* **5**:366–371, 1995.
16. Papp Z, Toth-Pal E, Papp Cs et al. Impact of mid-trimester screening on the prevalence of fetal structural anomalies: a prospective epidemiological study. *Ultrasound Obstet. Gynecol.* 320–326, 1995.
17. Sharland GK, Allan LD. Screening for congenital heart disease prenatally. Results of a 2½ year study in the South East Thames Region. *Br. J. Obstet. Gynecol.* **99**:220–225, 1992.
18. Drife JO, Donnai D. *Antenatal Diagnosis of Fetal Abnormalities*, pp. 353–357. London: Springer-Verlag, 1991.
19. Tegander E, Eik-nes SH, Linker DT. Incorporating the 4-chamber view of the fetal heart into the second trimester routine fetal examination. *Ultrasound Obstet. Gynecol.* **4**:24–28, 1994.
20. Baronciani D, Scaglia C, Corchia C, Torcetta F, Mastroiacovos P. Ultrasonography in pregnancy and fetal abnormalities: screening or diagnostic test? IPIMC 1986–1990 register data. *Prenat. Diagn.* **15**:1101–1108, 1995.
21. Carrera JM, Torrents M, Mortera C, Cusi V, Munoz A. Routine prenatal ultrasound screening for fetal abnormalities: 22 years' experience. *Ultrasound Obstet. Gynecol.* **5**:174–179, 1995.
22. Stoll C, Dott B, Alembik Y, Roth MP. Evaluation of Routine Prenatal Diagnosis by a Registry of Congenital Anomalies. *Prenat. Diagn.* **15**:791–800, 1995.
23. Roberts AB, Hampton E, Wilson N. Ultrasound detection of fetal structural abnormalities in Auckland 1988–9. *New Engl. J. Med.* **106**:441–443, 1993.
24. Report of the UK Collaborative Study. *Lancet* **1**:1065–1080, 1975.
25. Nicolaides KH, Campbell S, Gabbe S, Guidett R. Ultrasound screening for spina bifida: cranial and cerebellar signs. *Lancet* **2**:72–73, 1986.
26. Thiagarajah S, Henke J, Hogge WA, Abbitt PL, Breeden N, Ferguson JE. Early diagnosis of spina bifida: the value of cranial ultrasound markers. *Obstet. Gynecol.* **76**:54–57, 1990.
27. Van den Hof MC, Nicolaides KH, Campbell J, Campbell S. Evaluation of the lemon and banana signs in 130 fetuses with open spina bifida. *Am. J. Obstet. Gynecol.* **162**:322–327, 1990.
28. Watson WJ, Chescheir NC, Katz VL, Seeds JW. The Role of ultrasound in evaluation of patients with elevated maternal serum alpha-fetoprotein: a review. *Obstet. Gynecol.* **78**:123–128, 1991.
29. Nyberg DA, Mack LA, Hirsch J, Mahony BS. Abnormalities of fetal cranial contour in sonographic detection of spina bifida: evaluation of the lemon sign. *Radiology* **167**:387–392, 1988.
30. Forfar JA, O'Neill GC. Demography, vital statistics in the pattern of disease in childhood. In *Textbooks of Paediatrics*, 2nd edn, p. 24. Edinburgh: Churchill Livingstone, 1978.
31. Allan LD, Crawford DC, Chita SK, Tynan MJ. Prenatal screening for congenital heart disease. *Br. Med. J.* **292**:1717–1719, 1986.
32. Tegnander E, Eik-Nes SH, Johansen OJ, Linker DT. Prenatal detection of heart defects at the routine fetal examination at 18 weeks in a non-selected population. *Ultrasound Obstet. Gynecol.* **5**:372–380, 1995.
33. Vergani P, Mariani S, Ghidini A et al. Screening for congenital heart disease with the four-chamber view of the fetal heart. *Am. J. Obstet. Gynecol.* **167** (4, pt 1):1000–1003, 1992.
34. Hirashi S, Agata Y, Nowatari M et al. Incidence and natural course of trabecular ventricular septal defect: two-dimensional echocardiography and color doppler flow imaging study. *J. Pediatr.* **120**(3):409–415, 1992.
35. Achiron A, Glaser J, Gelernter I, Hegesh J, Yagel S. Extended fetal echocardiographic examination for detecting cardiac malformations in low risk pregnancies. *Br. Med. J.* **304**:671–674, 1992.
36. Rustico MA, Benettoni A, D'Ottavio G et al. Fetal heart screening in low-risk pregnancies. *Ultrasound Obstet. Gynaecol.* **6**:313–319, 1995.
37. Allan LD. Diagnosis of fetal cardiac abnormalities. *Arch. Dis. Child.* **64**:964–968, 1989.
38. Allan LD, Cook A, Sullivan I, Sharland GK. Hypoplastic left heart syndrome: effects of fetal echocardiography on birth prevalence. *Lancet* **337**:959–961, 1991.
39. Dejter SW, Gibbons MD. The fate of infant kidneys with fetal hydronephrosis but initially normal postnatal sonography. *J. Urol.* **142**:661–662, 1989.
40. Helin I, Persson P. Prenatal diagnosis of urinary tract abnormalities by ultrasound. *Paediatrics* **78**:879–883, 1986.
41. Economou G, Eggington JA, Brookfield SK. The importance of late pregnancy scans for renal tract abnormalities. *Prenat. Diagn.* **14**:177–180, 1994.
42. Benacerraf BR, Miller WA, Frigoletta FD. Sonographic detection of fetuses with trisomies 13 and 18: accuracy and limitations. *Am. J. Obstet. Gynecol.* **158**:404–409, 1988.
43. Benacerraf BR, Nadel A, Bromley B. Identification of second-trimester fetuses with autosomal trisomy by use of a sonographic scoring index. *Radiology* **193**:135–140, 1994.
44. Nyberg DA, Resta RG, Luthy DA, Hickok DE, Mahony DS, Hirsch JH. Prenatal sonographic findings of Down syndrome: review of 94 cases. *Obstet. Gynecol.* **76**:370–377, 1990.
45. Benacerraf BR, Gelman R, Frigoletto FD. Sonographic identification of 2nd trimester fetuses with Down syndrome. *N. Engl. J. Med.* **317**:1371–1376, 1987.
46. Nicolaides KH, Snijders RJM, Gosen CM, Berry C, Campbell S. Ultrasonographically detectable markers of fetal chromosomal abnormalities. *Lancet* **340**:704–707, 1992.
47. Rizzo N, Pittalis MC, Pilu G, Orsini LF, Porolo A, Bovicelli L. Prenatal karyotype on malformed fetuses. *Prenat. Diagn.* **10**:17–23, 1990.
48. Chudleigh P, Pearce JM, Campbell S. Prenatal diagnosis of transient cysts of the choroid plexus. *Prenat. Diagn.* **4**:135–137, 1984.
49. Snijders RJ. Isolated choroid plexus cysts: should we offer karyotyping? *Ultrasound Obstet. Gynecol.* **8**:223–224, 1996.
50. Chitty LS. Choroid plexus cysts: the need for further studies. *Ultrasound Obstet. Gynecol.* **4**:444–445, 1994.
51. Snijders RJM, Shawa L, Nicolaides KH. Fetal choroid plexus cysts and trisomy 18: assessment of risk based on ultrasound findings and maternal age. *Prenat. Diagn.* **14**:1119–1127, 1994.
52. Chitty LS, Chudleigh P, Wright E, Campbell S, Pembrey ME. The significance of choroid plexus cysts in an unselected population: results of a multicentre study. *Ultrasound Obstet. Gynecol.* **12**:391–397, 1998.
53. Snijders RJM, Sebire NJ, Souka A, Santiago C, Nicolaides KH. Fetal exomphalos and chromosomal defects: relationship to maternal age and gestation. *Ultrasound Obstet. Gynecol.* **6**:250–255, 1995.
54. Drugan A, Johnson MP, Reichler A, Hume Jr, RF, Itskovicz-Eldor J, Evans MI. Second-trimester minor ultrasound anomalies: impact on the risk of aneuploidy associated with advanced maternal age. *Obstet. Gynecol.* **88**:203–206, 1996.
55. Vintzileos AM, Egan JFX. Adjusting the risk for trisomy 21 on the basis of second trimester ultrasonography. *Am. J. Obstet. Gynecol.* **172**:837–844, 1995.
56. Nyberg DA, Dubinsky T, Resta RG, Mahoney BS, Hickok DE, Luthy DA. Echogenic fetal bowel during the second trimester: clinical importance. *Radiology* **188**:527–531, 1993.
57. MacGregor SM, Tamura R, Sabbagha R, Brenhofer JK, Kambick MP, Pergament E. Isolated hyperechoic fetal bowel: significance and implications for management. *Am. J. Obstet. Gynecol.* **173**:1254–1258, 1995.
58. Corteville JE, Gray DL, Crane JP. Congenital hydronephrosis: correlation of fetal ultrasonographic findings with infant outcome. *Am. J. Obstet. Gynecol.* **165**:384–388, 1991.
59. Cullen MT, Green J, Whetham J, Salafia C, Gabrielli S, Hobbins JC. Transvaginal ultrasonographic detection of congenital anomalies in the first trimester. *Am. J. Obstet. Gynecol.* **163**:466–476, 1990.
60. Timor-Tritsch HE, Monteagudo A, Peisner DB. High-frequency transvaginal sonographic examination for the potential malformation assessment of the 9-week to 14-week fetus. *J. Clin. Ultrasound* **20**:231–238, 1992.
61. Bronshtein M, Blumenfeld Z, Drugan A et al. Detection of fetal cardiac malformations by transvaginal sonography in the first and early second trimester. *Ultrasound Obstet. Gynecol.* **1**(Supp. 1):85, 1991.
62. Economides DL, Braithwaite JM, Armstrong MA. First trimester fetal abnormality screening in a low risk population. In *Proceedings British Congress on Obstetrics and Gynaecology, Dublin, Abstracts* **455**, 1995.

63. Achiron R, Tadmor O. Screening for fetal abnormalities during the first trimester of pregnancy: transvaginal versus transabdominal sonography. *Ultrasound Obstet. Gyenecol.* **1**(3):186–191, 1991.
64. Braithwaite JM, Armstrong MA, Economides DL. Assessment of fetal anatomy at 12 to 13 weeks of gestation by transabdominal and transvaginal sonography. *Br. J. Obstet. Gynaecol.* **103**:82–85, 1996.
65. Johnson SP, Sebire NJ, Snijders RJM, Tunkel S, Nicolaides KH. Ultrasound screening for anencephaly at 10–14 weeks of gestation. *Ultrasound Obstet. Gynecol.* **9**:14–16, 1997.
66. Rottem S, Bronshtein M. Transvaginal sonographic diagnosis of congenital anomalies between 9 weeks and 16 weeks, menstrual age. *J. Clin. Ultrasound* **18**:307–314, 1990.
67. Cullen MT, Gabrielli S, Green JJ et al. Diagnosis and significance of cystic hygroma in the first trimester. *Prenat. Diagn.* **10**:643–651, 1990.
68. Bronshtein M, Rottem S, Yoffe N, Blumenfeld. First-trimester and early second-trimester diagnosis of nuchal cystic hygroma by transvaginal sonography: diverse prognosis of the septated from the nonseptated lesion. *Am. J. Obstet. Gynecol.* **161**(1):78–82, 1989.
69. Bronshtein M, Yoffe N, Brandes JM, Blumenfeld Z. First and early second-trimester diagnosis of fetal urinary tract anomalies using transvaginal sonography. *Prenat. Diagn.* **10**:653–666, 1990.
70. Rosati P, Guariglia L. Transvaginal sonographic assessment of the fetal urinary tract in early pregnancy. *Ultrasound Obstet. Gynecol.* **7**:95–100, 1996.
71. Sebire NJ, Von Kaisenberg C, Rubio C, Snijders RJM, Nicolaides KH. Fetal megacystis at 10–14 weeks of gestation. *Ultrasound Obstet. Gynecol.* **8**:387–390, 1996.
72. Szalo J, Gellen J. Nuchal fluid accumulation in trisomy 21 detected by vaginosonography in the first trimester. *Lancet* **ii**:1133, 1990.
73. Pandya PP, Kondylios A, Hilbert L, Snijders RJM, Nicolaides KH. Chromosomal defects and outcome in 1015 fetuses with increased nuchal translucency. *Ultrasound Obstet. Gynecol.* **5**:15–19, 1995.
74. Hyett J, Moscoso G, Papapanagiotou G, Perdu M, Nicolaides KH. Abnormalities of the heart and great arteries in chromosomally normal fetuses with increased nuchal translucency thickness at 11–13 weeks of gestation. *Ultrasound Obstet. Gynecol.* **7**:245–250, 1996.
75. Snijders RJM, Johnson S, Sebire NJ, Noble PL, Nicolaides KH. First-trimester ultrasound screening for chromosomal defects. *Ultrasound Obstet. Gynecol.* **7**:216–226, 1996.
76. Nicolaides KH, Azar G, Byrne D, Mansur C, Marx K. Fetal nuchal translucency: ultrasound screening for chromosomal defects in the 1st trimester of pregnancy. *Br. Med. J.* **304**:867–869, 1992.
77. Johnson MP, Johnson A, Holzgreve W et al. First-trimester smple hyroma: cause and outcome. *Am. J. Obstet. Gynecol.* **168**(1, pt 1):156–161, 1993.
78. Shulman LP, Emerson DS, Felker RE, Phillips OP, Simpson JL, Elias S. High frequency of cytogenic abnormalities in fetuses with cystic hygroma diagnosed in the first trimester. *Obstet. Gynecol.* **80**(1):80–82, 1992.
79. Nicolaides KH, Brizot ML, Snijders RJM. Fetal nuchal translucency: ultrasound screening for fetal trisomy in the first trimester of pregnancy. *Br. J. Obstet. Gynaecol.* **101**:782–786, 1994.
80. Pandya PP, Goldberg H, Walton B et al. The implementation of 1st trimester scanning at 10–13 weeks' gestation and the measurement of fetal nuchal translucency thickness in two maternity units, *Ultrasound Obstet. Gynecol.* **5**:20–25, 1995.
81. Macintosh MCM, Wald NJ, Chard T et al. The selective miscarriage of down's syndrome from 10 weeks of pregnancy. *Br. J. Obstet. Gynaecol.* **103**:1171–1172, 1996.
82. Hyett JA, Sebire NJ, Snijders RJM, Nicolaides KH. Intrauterine lethality of trisomy 21 fetuses with increased nuchal translucency thickness. *Ultrasound Obstet. Gynecol.* **7**:101–103, 1996.
83. Bronshtein M, Keret D, Deutsch M, Liberson A, Bar Chava I. Transvaginal sonographic detection of skeletal anomalies in the first and early second trimesters. *Prenat. Diagn.* **13**:597–601, 1993.
84. Schulte-Vallentin M, Schindler H. Non-echogenic nuchal oedema as a marker in trisomy 21 screening. *Lancet* **339**:1053, 1992.
85. Szabo J, Gellen J, Szemere G. First-trimester ultrasound screening for fetal aneuploidies in women over 35 and under 35 years of age. *Ultrasound Obstet. Gynecol.* **5**:161–163, 1995.
86. Comas C, Martinex JM, Ojuel J et al. First-trimester nuchal edema as a marker of aneuploidy. *Ultrasound Obstet. Gynecol.* **5**:26–29, 1995.
87. Brambati B, Cislaghi C, Tului L et al. First-trimester Down's syndrome screening using nuchal translucency: a prospective study in patients undergoing chorionic villus sampling. *Ultrasound Obstet. Gynecol.* **5**:9–14, 1995.
88. Pandya PP, Snijders RJM, Johnson SP, De Lourdes Brizot M, Nicolaides KH. Screening for fetal trisomies by maternal age and fetal nuchal translucency thickness at 10 to 14 weeks of gestation. *Br. J. Obstet. Gynaecol.* **102**:957–962, 1995.
89. Kornman LH, Morssink LP, Beekhuis JR, De Wolf BTHM, Heringa MP, Mantingh A. Nuchal translucency cannot be used as a screening test for chromosomal abnormalities in the first trimester of pregnancy in a routine ultrasound practice. *Prenat. Diagn.* **16**:797–805, 1996.
90. Hafner E, Schuchter K, Philipp K. Screening for chromosomal abnormalities in an unselected population by fetal nuchal translucency. *Ultrasound Obstet. Gynecol.* **6**:330–333, 1995.
91. Bower SJ, Chitty L, Bewley S et al. First trimester nuchal translucency screening of the general population: data from three centres. In *Proceedings British Congress Obstetrics and Gynaecology* Dublin:3, 1995.
92. Cha'Ban FK, van Splunder P, Los FJ, Wladimiroff JW. Fetal outcome in nuchal translucencyh emphasis on normal fetal karyotype. *Prenat. Diagn.* **16**:537–541, 1996.
93. Trauffer PML, Anderso CE, Johnson A, Heeger S, Morgan P, Wapner RJ. The natural history of euploid prenancies with first-trimester cystic hygromas. *Am. J. Obstet. Gynecol.* **170**(5 pt. 1):1279–1283, 1994.
94. Pandya PP, Brizot ML, Kuhn P, Snijders RJM, Nicolaides KH. First-trimster fetal nuchal translucency thickness and risk for trisomies. *Obstet. Gynaecol.* **84**(3):420–423, 1994.
95. van Zalen-Sprock RM, van Vugt JMG, van Geijn HP. First-trimester diagnosis of cystic hygroma – course and outcome. *Am. J. Obstet. Gynecol.* **167**(1):94–98, 1992.
96. Bernaschek G, Stuempflen, Deutinger J. The value of sonographic diagnosis of fetal malformations: different results between indication-based, screening-based investigations. *Prenat. Diagn.* **14**:807–812, 1994.
97. Constantine G, McCormack J. Comparative audit of booking and mid-trimester ultrasound scans in the prenatal diagnosis of congenital anomalies. *Prenat. Diagn.* **11**:905–914, 1991.
98. Chambers SE, Geirsson RT, Stewart RJ, Wannapirak C, Muir BB. Audit of a screening service for fetal abnormalities using early ultrasound scanning and maternal serum. *Ultrasound Obstet. Gynecol.* **5**:168–173, 1995.
99. Chitty LS, Barnes CA, Berry C. Continuation of the pregnancy following the diagnosis of a lethal abnormality: the experience of five couples and recommendations for management. *Br. Med. J.* **313**:478–480, 1995.
100. Romero R, Ghidini A, Costigan K, Touloukian R, Hobbins JC. Prenatal diagnosis of duodenal atresia: does it make any difference? *Obstet. Gynecol.* **71**:739–741, 1989.
101. Chang AC, Huhta JC, Yoon GY et al. Diagnosis, transport and outcome in fetuses with left ventricular outflow tract obstruction, *J. Thorac. Cardiovasc. Surg.* **102**:841–848, 1991.
102. Livera LN, Brookfields DSK, Egginton JA, Hawnaur JN. Antenatal ultrasonography to detect fetal renal abnormalities: a prospective screening programme. *Br. Med. J.* **198**:1421–1423, 1989.
103. Greig JD, Raine PAM, Young DG et al. Value of antenatal diagnosis of abnormalities of the urinary tract. *Br. Med. J.* **298**:1417–1419, 1989.
104. Morrall D. Should midwives carry out routine ultrasound scans? *Br. J. Midwif.* **2**(5):202–208, 1994.
105. Smith DK, Marteau TM. Detecting fetal abnormality: serum screening and fetal anomaly scans, *Br. J. Midwif.* **3**(3):133–136, 1995.
107. Griffiths DM, Gough MH. Dilemmas after ltrasonic diagnosis of fetal abnormality. *Lancet* **i**:623–624, 1985.
106. Crang-Svalenius E, Dykes AK, Joregensen C. Women's informed choice of prenatal diagnosis: Early ultrasound examination – routine ultrasound examination – age-independent amniocentesis. *Fetal Diagn. Ther.* **11**:20–25, 1996.
108. Medeira A, Norman A, Haslam J, Clayton-Smith J, Donnai D. Examination of fetuses after induced abortion for fetal abnormality – a follow-up study. *Prenat. Diagn.* **14**:381–385, 1994.
109. Grant HW, MacKinlay GA, Chambers SE, Keeling JW, Muir BB. Prenatal ultrasound diagnosis: a review of fetal outcome. *Pediatr Surg Int* **8**:469–471, 1993.
110. Jeret JS, Serur D, WWisniewski KE, Lubin RA. Clinicopathological findings associated with agenesis of the corpus callosum. *Brain Dev.* **9**(3):255–264, 1987.

111. Gupta JK, Lilford RJ. Assessment and management of fetal agenesis of the corpus callosum. *Prenat. Diagn.* **15**:301–312, 1995.
112. Eik-Nes SH, Okland O, Aure JC, Ulstein M. Ultrasound screening in pregnancy: a randomised controlled trial. *Lancet* **i**:1347–1349, 1984.
113. Salvesen KA, Jacobsen G, Vatten LJ, Eik-Nes SH, Bakketeig LS. Routine ultrasonography *in-utero* and subsequent growth during childhood. *Ultrasound Obstet. Gynecol.* **1**:6–10, 1993.
114. Salvesen KA, Bakketeig LS, Eik-Nes SH, Undheim JO, Okland O. Routine ultrasonography *in utero* and school performance at age 8–9 years. *Lancet* **339**:85–88, 1992.
115. Salvesen KA, Vatten LJ, Jacobsen G et al. Routine ultrasonography in utero and subsequent vision and hearing at primary school age. *Ultrasound Obstet. Gynecol.* **2**:243–247, 1992.
116. Salvesen KA, Vatten LJ, Eik-Nes SH, Hugdahl K, Bakketeig LS. Routine ultrasonography in utero and subsequent handedness and neurological development. *Br. Med. J.* **307**:159–164, 1993.
117. Newnham JP, Evans SF, Michael CA, Stanley FJ, Landau L. Effects of frequent ultrasound during pregnancy: a randomised controlled trial. *Lancet* **342**:887–891, 1993.
118. MacDonald W, Newham J, Gurrin L, Evans S. Effect of frequent prenatal ultrasound on birthweight: follow up at 1 year of age. *Lancet* **348**:482, 1996.
119. Devore GR. Opinion. Financial implications of routine screening ultrasound. *Ultrasound Obstet. Gynecol.* **7**:307–308, 1996.
120. Leivo T, Tuominen A, Saari-Kemppainen, Ylostalo P, Karjalainen O, Heinonen OP. Cost-effectiveness of one-stage ultrasound screening in pregnancy: a report from the helsinki ultrasound trial. *Ultrasound Obstet. Gynecol.* **7**:309–314, 1996.
121. Shen-Schwarz S, Neish C, Hill LM. Antenatal ultrasound for fetal anomalies: importance of perinatal autopsy, *Pediatr. Pathol.* **9**:1–9, 1989.
122. Brand IR, Kaminopetros P, Cave M, Irving HI, Lilford RJ. Specificity of antenatal ultrasound in the yorkshire region: a prospective study of 2261 ultrasound detected anomalies. *Br. J. Obstet. Gynaecol.* **101**:392–397, 1994.
123. Clayton-Smith J, Farndon PA, McKeown C, Donnai D. Examination of fetuses after induced abortion for fetal abnormality, *Br. Med. J.* **300**:295–300, 1990.

Fetal cells in the maternal circulation

35

J.L. Simpson and S. Elias

Introduction

The isolation and analysis of fetal cells in maternal blood for genetic diagnosis has not only been achieved, but may become sensitive enough to be competitive with other non-invasive techniques[1]. Attention is now being directed on choice of the best fetal cell type, selection of optimal method(s) of cell enrichment, consistency and reproducibility of cell recovery and analysis. This communication will update our previous reports on this topic[1–5].

Fetal karyotypes from maternal blood: historical overview (1969–1989)

Recovering fetal cells from maternal blood was first reported by Walknowska et al.[6], who found XY metaphases in maternal blood of pregnant women carrying male fetuses. In 1971, de Grouchy and Trubuchet also reported male metaphases from pregnant women carrying male fetuses[7], and other groups followed[3,8,9]. Y-chromatin-positive cells were also claimed by several groups[10–13]. Although relatively high proportions of fetal nucleated cells to maternal nucleated cells were reported (0.1–0.3%), not all individuals carrying male fetuses showed XY metaphases. This was explained on the basis of fetal cells being rare events in maternal blood; however, finding XY metaphases in some women carrying female fetuses was more disturbing. This was usually explained by clones of fetal cells having been established in the mother's bone marrow during prior pregnancies. Irrespective, the consensus arose that the 'fetal' XY metaphases could have represented cytogenetic misclassifications and the ostensible 'Y-chromatin' cells could have reflected autosomal fluorescence[14].

In the late 1970s, Herzenberg and colleagues applied flow sorting technology to enrich for fetal cells[15,16]. Their experimental design utilized HLA-A2 negative women whose spouse was HLA-A2 positive (heterozygote or homozygote). Any H2 positive cells recovered by flow sorting could thus be presumed to be fetal in origin, given the H2 antigen should have been present only as result of having been inherited from the father. In pregnancies where the fetus was male, Y-chromatin was used as an independent marker to verify that the cells were of fetal origin.

Later in the last decade, molecular techniques were applied. Using nested primer polymerase chain reaction (PCR) to amplify for Y sequences, Lo et al.[17,18] showed that fetal cells, or at least fetal DNA, indeed existed in maternal blood of women carrying a male fetus. The original work of Lo et al[17,18] was performed on unsorted nucleated cells. Later our own group[19] and many others confirmed these results with various separation schemes on sorted and non-sorted cells[20–23].

Clinical and biological questions

TIME OF APPEARANCE OF FETAL CELLS IN MATERNAL BLOOD

Using nested primer PCR for Y-specific DNA, signals can be detected early in pregnancy in the peripheral blood of pregnant women carrying male fetuses. Studies designed to identify the earliest time at which cells become detectable were pursued by Thomas et al[24], who followed five women who became pregnant by in vitro fertilization. In the two pregnancies with male fetuses, Y-specific signals were first detected at 33 and 40 days' gestation. In 18 pregnancies with male fetuses Thomas et al.[25] detected Y specific DNA sequences at the latest by 7 weeks. Liou et al.[26,27] sought ZFY and SRY sequences in blood of 19 women carrying male fetuses. Fetal cells were first detected at 6 weeks' gestation and consistently detected by 10 weeks. Hamada et al.[28] addressed this question with both fluorescence in situ hybridization (FISH) and nested PCR for Y sequences (Y 1.1, 1.2, 1.3, 1.4; Y 1.5, 1.6, 1.7 and 1.8). By 15 weeks' gestation, Y-signals were consistently observed in women carrying male fetuses.

The optimal time during pregnancy to analyse a maternal blood sample is uncertain. Our own data indicate that nucleated red cells are detectable in both the first and second trimester (10–18 weeks). The proportion of fetal cells in maternal blood relative to fetal mass could be higher in early pregnancy, yet fetal mass obviously increases as gestation increases. The absolute number in maternal blood could thus be sufficient to allow diagnosis in either trimester.

That Y DNA sequences are present by PCR provides no information about the type of cell present responsible for the PCR signal. Fetal cells present very early in gestation could be circulating only transiently, perhaps representing multinucleated syncytiotrophoblast buds that would not be readily amenable to diagnosis of aneuploidy by FISH with chromosome-specific probes.

FREQUENCY OF FETAL CELLS IN MATERNAL BLOOD

Estimates of the ratio of nucleated fetal cells to nucleated maternal cells have varied widely. The studies cited in the 1970s concerning ostensible presence of XY metaphases or Y-chromatin had suggested that the frequency was as high as 0.1–0.3%, but this now seems too high. Using an avidin-biotin-based immunoaffinity system, Hall and Williams[29] estimated the frequency of fetal nucleated cells to maternal nucleated cells was 1:4.75 × 10^6 to 1.6 × 10^7 but are unaware of these data being published in detail. Hamada et al.[28] attempted to provide precise estimates of the ratio of fetal nucleated cells to maternal nucleated cells by performing FISH on unsorted maternal blood using a probe for the repetitive Y DNA sequence DYZ1; the frequencies in successive trimesters were 0.27, 3.52 and 8.56 × 10^{-5}, respectively. A problem with the data of Hamada et al.[28] is that despite representing an enormous effort there is still concern about misclassification. The circumstance of only very rare cells showing three signals, admixed with many showing only two signals, raises the spectre of misclassification. Our own estimate is 1:1 × 10^7 to 1:1 × 10^8, based on flow cytometry data.

IS THE FREQUENCY OF FETAL CELLS AFFECTED BY KARYOTYPE?

The frequency of fetal cells in maternal blood may depend on fetal cytogenetic status. Higher percentages (10–15%) of sorted aneuploid cells have been observed by Gänshirt et al.[30] and by ourselves[2–4,31]. Only 1–2% of euploid (46, XY) fetal cells are recovered. Aneuploid cells might thus 'leak' into the maternal circulation, perhaps reflective of underlying placental pathology. Of course, this would be diagnostically salutary.

ENRICHMENT STRATEGIES

Given the frequencies noted, the detection of aneuploidies makes it necessary to enrich for rare fetal cells from maternal blood samples. To accomplish this one must first target a specific cell type (trophoblast, nucleated red blood cell, lymphocyte). One then generally utilizes density gradients or protein separation techniques, followed by either fluorescence activated cell sorting (FACS) or magnetic activated cell sorting (MACS) for selected characteristics. Only FACS has proved useful in our hands, but the technology is more expensive than MACS. The selection criteria we currently favour will be discussed below.

DO FETAL CELLS PERSIST AFTER DELIVERY?

A frequently voiced concern is that fetal cells from a prior pregnancy could persist in the maternal circulation and, hence, lead to diagnostic error. This fear would be especially relevant if aneuploid cells persist after a chromosomally abnormal live born offspring or a chromosomally abnormal spontaneous abortion. Fortunately, we believe this fear is unfounded given the selection criteria most commonly employed.

Hsieh et al.[32] followed 28 women delivered of a male fetus (Table 35.1). One week after gestation, 26 of 28 women delivered of males showed ZFY and SRY sequences in their blood. By 4 months, only 11 of the 28 showed Y-specific sequences, and by 8 months only two of 23. In 18 pregnancies with male infants followed by Thomas et al.[25], no Y-specific sequences were recognized after 8 weeks post partum. Our group recently studied 33 women delivered of males 14 months to 19 years ago but currently pregnant with a female. After FACS enrichment on the basis of CD71 or gamma globin and lack of CD45 expression, normal cells were identified in 32 of 33 cases, or 94 272 total cells scored in all 33 cases, only five[33]. These data indicate that persistence of fetal cells from prior pregnancies will be unlikely to compromise diagnostic accuracy. Indeed, Bianchi et al.[34] searched for antigens that would indicate presence of T cells, B cells and early haematopoietic cells. Women who delivered 6 months to 27 years ago were still likely to show fetal $CD34^+$ or $CD34^+$, $CD38^+$ cells from a prior pregnancy. This would be predicted with persistence of early haematopoietic cells. In conclusion, if fetal cells do persist from prior pregnancies,

TABLE 35.1
Postpartum persistence of fetal cells, based on detection of Y-specific DNA sequences (ZFY and SRY) by PCR. Data from Hsieh *et al.*[32]

Months after delivery	Cases showing ZFY and SRY
1/4	26/28
4	11/28
8	2/23

targeting the cell type for subsequent analysis should minimize the likelihood of error.

Diagnosis of fetal Mendelian traits by PCR for fetal DNA

FETAL SEX

Although obviously not the sole purpose of analysing fetal cells separated from maternal blood, fetal sex could be readily detected from either sorted or unsorted blood. Determination of fetal sex could be useful in couples at risk for X-linked recessive traits. Nested primer analysis for Y DNA sequences is the approach usually utilized, in fact by Lo et al.[17,18] to establish that fetal cells indeed exist in maternal blood. Other groups including our own have used this approach to verify experimentally the presence of fetal cells (male) in maternal blood, and new primers continue to be reported[35,36]. A caveat is that by PCR alone the fetal cell type being detected is not generally known.

DETECTION OF PATERNAL ALLELE NOT PRESENT IN THE PREGNANT FEMALE

Selected Mendelian traits can be detected by analysis of fetal cells in maternal blood. The general approach is to search for a mutant paternal gene, detection of whose DNA in the pregnant mother's blood indicates paternal transmission to the fetus. Camaschella et al.[37] were the first to do so, studying DNA obtained from maternal blood of three pregnancies at risk for β-thalassemia/haemoglobin Lepore$_{Boston}$. Haemoglobin Lepore$_{Boston}$ is a hybrid Δ-β globin gene that results from unequal crossing over between misaligned β and Δ genes, leading to a 7 kb deletion. Camaschella et al.[37] used PCR to amplify for haemoglobin Lepore$_{Boston}$-specific DNA in unsorted maternal blood of women whose male partners carried the Lepore$_{Boston}$ mutation. Paternal transmission was detected in two fetuses, and correctly excluded in a third. Although Camaschella et al.[37] did not enrich for any specific cell type, Hawes et al.[38] used a similar approach when they flow-sorted for trophoblasts and analysed for the presence of paternally transmitted β-thalassemia.

An attractive clinical application lies in rhesus isoimmunization. The affected mother is homozygous for absence of RhD (Rh negative), the genetic basis of which is most commonly gene deletion. If the father is homozygous for Rh(D), all fetuses must be heterozygous; every pregnancy would be at risk for Rh-isoimmunization. However, if the father is heterozygous, the likelihood is 50% that the fetus would inherit his Rh(D) gene and, hence, be affected. It could thus be very useful to know fetal Rh status early in gestation. Lo et al.[39] determined fetal Rh(D) status in Rh-negative-sensitized women where the father was heterozygous. Unsorted bloods from 21 RhD-negative women were subjected to PCR for Rh(D) DNA sequences. Of 11 women showing a positive PCR signal, seven had a RhD-positive fetus; of 10 not showing a PCR signal, only two had a RhD-positive fetus. Overall, eight of the 10 women carrying a RhD-fetus showed an Rh(D) signal. An improved set of primers was later recommended[40]. Geifman-Holtzman et al.[41] also studied Rh(D)-negative women. In seven of nine, Rh(D)-positive cells were identified, and in each of the seven fetal Rh status was confirmed. In the two other patients, no Rh(D) DNA was detected. In one of these two, the fetus was Rh-negative on the basis of amniotic fluid DNA testing; in the second, each of twin neonates was Rh-negative. This same group later determined fetal E/e status by PCR of maternal blood[42].

Another circumstance in which PCR could be used for detecting autosomal recessive traits exists when the father is heterozygous and the mother homozygously abnormal for an autosomal recessive trait. One can seek the normal allele that may or may not be transmitted by the heterozygous father. If blood from the homozygous mother shows amplification for DNA of the normal paternal allele when subjected to PCR, the fetus can be deduced to be heterozygous.

PCR-based diagnosis could also be applied if both parents are heterozygous for the same autosomal recessive mutant. However, one would need to search for a marker linked to the paternal mutant allele. This paternal marker should not be present in the mother.

Enriching for specific fetal cells types to detect fetal trisomy

PCR-based strategies can by themselves detect certain fetal genotypes. However, detection of fetal chromosome abnormalities ordinarily requires FISH with chromosome-specific probes. Given the low frequency of fetal cells in maternal blood (1:10^6), enrichment is necessary in order to allow efficient FISH analysis. As alluded to already, in order to enrich, a specific cell type must be targeted.

NUCLEATED FETAL RED CELLS (ERYTHROBLASTS)

The cell type that has led to the greatest success is the fetal nucleated red cell (erythroblast). This candidate cell is attractive because nucleated red blood cells (NRBCs) constitute about 10% of red cells in the 11-week fetus and 0.5% of the 19-week fetus. By contrast, NRBCs are rare in peripheral adult blood. Unlike lymphocytes, NRBCs do not persist longer than perhaps 5 days in the adult; thus, fetal NRBC persisting as clones in the maternal bone marrow seems less likely than for lymphocytes.

Bianchi et al.[20] were first to target this cell type, flow sorting on the basis of transferrin receptor (CD71) positivity and thereafter subjecting sorted cells to PCR for a Y sequence. Of eight samples showing a Y sequence, six were derived from pregnancies in which women were carrying male fetuses. Our initial experience failed to confirm the work of Bianchi et al.[20], but we were later successful when sorting not only for CD71 but also for cell size, cell granularity, transferrin receptor positivity and glycophorin-A positivity[2,4,19,43]. Using nested PCR primers for a Y sequence, we correctly identified male fetuses in 12 of 12 flow-sorted samples[19]. We identified female fetuses in five of six samples.

Using positive selection for glycopherin A and CD71, we became the first to detect fetal aneuploidy from analysis of maternal blood. In 1991 we detected trisomy 18 in blood taken prior to CVS[43] and one year later we detected trisomy 21[44]. Still in collaboration with Dr Katherine Klinger (Integrated Genetics, Framingham, MA), we had by 1993 studied 69 maternal blood samples (Table 35.2). Of eight aneuploidies, only one was not detected; however, diagnosis of a second case might have been arguable in a clinical setting because the percentages of cells with three signals was at 2.8%, relatively near the background at that time. We encountered no false-positive results in that series[4]. At least two other groups soon also detected trisomies using FISH. In 1992, Bianchi and Klinger[45] detected trisomy 21 in a maternal blood sample obtained and sorted after amniocentesis and Gänshirt-Ahlert et al.[46] detected five trisomy 18 and five trisomy 21 cases.

At present, various groups are attempting to optimize positive and negative selection criteria. For example, we abandoned positive selection for GlyA because the antibody often agglutinated non-nucleated RBCs, resulting in the latter falling into the same sorting gates as the desired fetal NRBCs[47,48]. In our experience Gly A monoclonal antibodies proved too variable and, hence, unreliable for use in large scale screening. Instead, we sought new enrichment schemes.

TABLE 35.2

The authors' initial experience encompassed analyses of maternal bloods, flow sorted from 69 women who carried chromosomally normal and abnormal fetuses. In 61 cases, the fetal karyotype was normal; trisomic cells were not found. In the eight cases detailed below a chromosomal abnormality existed in the fetus. In cases 3,4,6 and 8 blood samples were obtained before an invasive procedure (chorionic villus sampling); in cases 1,2,5 and 7 the sample was obtained after a procedure. Data from Simpson and Elias[4]

Case	Gestation (wks)	Fetal karyotype	Trisomic cells (FISH) among total cells scored
1	11	47,XX,+21	24/62 (38.7%)
2	19	47,XX,+21	21/113 (18.6%)
3	10	47,XX,+18	25/295 (8.5%)
4	11	47,XX,+21	3/104 (2.8%)
5	17	47,XX,+21	4/50 (8.0%)
6	10	47,XX,+21	74/100 (74.0%)
7	11	47,XXY	6/94 (6.4%)
8	11	47,XXY	0/93 (0.0%)

One attractive strategy was negative depletion which reduces the burden of isolating or enriching for cells that must be analysed by FISH. A useful negative selection marker proved to be CD45, an antigen present on lymphocytes and monocytes, but not NRBCs.

Another useful positive selection marker chosen has been γ-globin. The rationale is based on haemoglobin F constituting about 90% of haemoglobin in the 12–32 week fetus. Eventually haemoglobin A, which has two β-globin chains (α_2, β_2), replaces most of the haemoglobin F, which has two γ-globin chains (α_2, γ_2). The maternal circulation will contain a few NRBCs of maternal origin that express haemoglobin F, but most maternal cells will express haemoglobin A. Positive selection for γ-globin and negative selection for β-globin thus has a relatively higher likelihood of recovering fetal than maternal cells.

Recently we have been comparing between two methods of positive selection: $CD71^+$ or gamma globin[48]. In these studies we have used nuclear selection, phycoerthyrin-labelled CD45 after depletion ($CD45^-$), and positive selection by flow cytometry for either FITC-labelled anti-γ-globin or FITC-labelled CD71. In no trials was glyA selection attempted, and in all Ficoll separation was performed before sorting. FISH analysis used α-satellite centromere-specific probes for the X (biotin-labelled) and for the Y (digoxigenin-labelled) chromosomes.

The $CD71^+$ selection approach ($CD45^-$, $CD71^+$) detected male (fetal) cells in 10 of 18 pregnancies in which the fetus was 46,XY. The number of male (fetal) cells ranged from 0 to 7. The one trisomic case was successfully detected. Male cells were detected in none of five control pregnancies (46,XX fetuses). The anti-γ-globin approach ($CD45^-$, anti-γ-globin$^+$) detected male (fetal) cells in 12 of 14 pregnancies in which the fetus was 46,XY; the number of male cells ranged from 0 to 8. One additional trisomic case was successfully detected. Male cells were detected in one of the nine control pregnancies (46,XX fetuses).

At present we conclude that positive fetal cell selection for either CD71 or anti-γ-globin can be accomplished in 60–80% of samples. However, this detection efficiency cannot be achieved on a consistent basis.

TROPHOBLASTS

Trophoblasts are an obvious candidate cell, given their intimate relationship with the uterus. Indeed, it is widely accepted that syncytiotrophoblasts and cytotrophoblasts are present in relatively high numbers in the maternal circulation early in pregnancy, the inevitable result of uterine invasion to establish the fetal circulation. However, these cells become trapped and sequestered by the lung at their first passage[49]. Therefore, relatively few trophoblasts might be expected to be present in the peripheral venous circulation. Sequestration is consistent with data showing that trophoblasts were recovered readily from the inferior vena cava and uterine vein of women having eclampsia, whereas peripheral blood failed to show trophoblasts[50,51].

A persistent difficulty in recovering trophoblasts has been obtaining monoclonal antibodies specific for placental antigens. Generation of fetal specific antibodies has proved frustrating[52,53]. An aggressive effort was pursued in Adelaide, where Mueller et al.[21] generated 6000 monoclonal antibodies from placental tissue; five were believed specific for fetal tissue. Maternal blood from pregnant women was exposed to two of the five monocolonal antibodies, and presumptively isolated fetal cells subjected to PCR to detect the presence or absence of a Y DNA sequence. Fetal sex was correctly identified in each of seven males and in six of seven females. The same group[54] later applied immunohistochemical studies to demonstrate trophoblast fragments in maternal peripheral blood specific for certain placental monoclonal antibodies. Further evidence that trophoblasts were indeed being isolated from maternal blood by these antibodies came from analysis of a pregnancy at risk for β-thalassemia. Hawes and colleagues[38] sorted with a 'cocktail' of three different monocolonal antibodies, and used PCR to achieve a correct diagnosis of fetal status. We are unaware of recent data from this group.

Sbracia et al.[55] approached the problem differently, using antibodies against HLA-G. Fetal nucleated cells in maternal blood were separated using Ficoll Histo Paque density gradient, labelled with anti HLA-G monoclonal antibody conjugated to FITC, sorted by FACS, and then collected directly into Eppendorf tubes containing Ham's media. Standard cytogenetic techniques were then performed. Surprisingly, six of the 10 pregnant women studied had 46,XY fetuses and in all six 46,XY karyotypes were recovered. These fetal karyotypes are the first recovered by any modern technique and contrast with our own experience in failing to obtain fetal metaphases from flow-sorted lymphocytes[56,57].

A potential pitfall in analysis of fetal trophoblasts is that FISH analysis requires mononucleated cells. Multinucleated trophoblasts and anucleated cells would prove diagnostically difficult or impossible.

LYMPHOCYTES

It has been widely assumed that Herzenberg and colleagues[15,16] were seeking to isolate fetal lymphocytes. Recall that the strategy involved studying couples in which the father but not the mother was HLA-A2 positive. Cells separated by Ficoll Hypaque gradient were subjected to FACS for HLA-A2 positive cells. Among 12 pregnancies with male infants, five showed Y-chromatin cells (range 0.3% to 1.6% sorted cells); among the seven other mothers delivered of infants whose lymphocytes failed to react with HLA-A2 antiserum, none showed Y-chromatin cells.

Our group later tried to replicate this technique, using XY or trisomic fetal karyotypes as an end point for cell separation[56,57]. Unfortunately, we failed to detect a single fetal karyotype. Sargent et al.[14] used the same flow-sorting approach Y-specific DNA sequences in 48 couples in which the mother was HLA-A2 negative and the father HLA-A2 positive. Blood was obtained at 28- and 32-week gestations and DNA extracted without sorting. Paternal HLA-DR sequences were detected in maternal blood, indicating presence of fetal cells[14,58]. Actually, this work shows that DNA exists in maternal blood, but not necessarily of lymphocyte origin.

Lymphocytes may not be the ideal candidate cell for enrichment. First, paternal alleles must be known in order to devise an allele-specific strategy like that outlined. This would be expensive and complicated. Fetal cells could also persist from previous pregnancies as alluded to above. Bianchi et al.[34] flow sorted for antibodies that bind cell surface antigens present on B cells (CD19 and CD23), T lymphocytes (CD3, CD4, CD5) and haematopoietic stem cells (CD34 and CD38). Eight women delivered of male infants between six months and 27 years earlier were studied. In cells expressing B cell antigens no Y-specific amplification was detected; in cells expressing T cell antigens Y-specific amplification was detected in one of seven cases; however, Y-specific sequences for stem cell antigens were amplified in six of eight cases. The authors concluded that most postpartum women in fact are low grade mosaics for these fetal stem cells. On the other hand, our group has shown that sorting for $CD71^+$ $CD45^-$ yields no evidence for persistence[33].

Methods to facilitate fetal cells analysis after enrichment

Even after enrichment, fetal cells remain admixed among a great majority of maternal cells (1:10 to 1:100). Methods to identify the relatively few fetal cells would be greatly helpful for efficient analysis. Several general approaches appear feasible.

First, one might use micromanipulation techniques. Takabayashi et al.[59] identified nucleated red blood cells in maternal blood using Papenheim stain, and removed these cells from a slide with a micromanipulator. Nucleated fetal red cells were detected in 33 of 60 women between 8 and 23 weeks; 33 of 39 (85%) showed fetal cells. PCR of single cells for a Y sequence was performed in 11 cases; no signal was shown in the five cases with female fetuses, whereas five of six with male fetuses showed a signal. A disadvantage of this technique is its labour intensiveness.

Second, one could stain enriched cells for a gene product, like fetal haemoglobin ($\alpha_2\delta_2$). This should preferentially identify the fetal cells, which are far more likely to have haemoglobin F cells than the maternal cells, that contain haemoglobin A. This approach was employed by Zheng et al.[60] and Ferguson-Smith et al.[61], with confirmation by our own group[62]. We have, however, not found this technique sufficiently specific for fetal cells.

Third, one can identify fetal cells on the basis of their predominantly transcribing fetal haemoglobin. To identify transcribing cells, we use in situ primer extension with labelled uracil. Heavily labelled cells that are fetal in origin can be subjected to FISH analysis with chromosome-specific probes. In pregnancies with male fetuses, only the positively labelled cells show a signal for a Y-specific probe[63]. In pregnancies with female fetuses, the percentage of positively labelled (presumptively fetal cells) is similar to the percentage in male fetuses, offering promise that fetal XX cells can be distinguished from maternal XX cells.

Culturing the fetal cells circulating in maternal blood was the assumption underlying the early work of Walknowska et al.[6], who claimed recovery of fetal metaphases. In 1994, Alter[64] proposed that progenitor cells obtained from adult bone marrow could be cultured in vitro to erythroblasts by use of first stem cell factor and then erythropoietin. The 2–3 weeks theoretically required to culture fetal erythroblasts in maternal blood could be shortened because the fetal cells circulating in maternal blood are not progenitor cells but rather erythroid stem cells. Obtaining maternal blood (11–20 gestational weeks) from five women carrying male fetuses, Lo et al.[65] reported success by 'culture in erythropoietin-enriched medium'. In all five cases Y-positive cells were detectable (1/400 to 1/9500 female cells). This approach offers the exciting possibility of having fetal cells for analysis with no prior separation or sorting, as well as the possibility of obtaining metaphases for karyotyping.

Clinical evaluation

Since 1987, the US National Institute of Child Health and Development (NICHD) has sponsored collaborative investigations into the feasibility of isolating fetal cells from maternal blood for prenatal diagnosis. Phase I studies were first conducted by our group, then at the University of Tennessee, Memphis, and by colleagues at the University of California, San Francisco. Based upon encouraging preliminary results, NICHD moved in 1994 to Phase II clinical evaluation. Since 1996 clinical evaluation is underway in several centres: Baylor College of Medicine and University of Tennessee, Memphis; Jefferson Medical College; Tufts University/New England Medical Center; Wayne State University/Basel. Socioeconomic and demographic information are collected on all subjects, using standardized forms common to all centres and forwarded to a single data management team. Information on separation techniques, selection criteria, and FISH analysis are recorded. Subjects enrolled in this clinical trial are informed both verbally and by written informed consent that the results of the blood test will not be made available to them or their physicians. Determining sensitivity and specificity will require a study of at least 3000 women. Data relevant to the propriety of introducing this technology into clinical practice will probably be available in 1999. Until then traditional invasive techniques like chorionic villus sampling or amniocenteses should continue to be employed[66].

Acknowledgement

This work was sponsored in part by the National Institute of Child Health and Human Development (contract NOIHD43203), March of Dimes and US Agency for International Development.

REFERENCES

1. Simpson JL, Elias S. Isolating fetal cells in maternal circulation for prenatal diagnosis. *Prenat Diagn* **14**:1229–1242, 1994.
2. Elias S, Simpson JL. Prenatal diagnosis of aneuploidy using fetal cells isolated from maternal blood: University of Tennessee, Memphis experience. In *Fetal Cells in Maternal Blood: Prospects for Noninvasive Prenatal Diagnosis* (eds J.L. Simpson & S. Elias), pp. 80–91. New York: New York Academy of Science, 1994.
3. Elias S, Simpson JL. Prenatal diagnosis using fetal cells isolated from maternal blood. In *Screening for Down's Syndrome* (ed. J.G. Grudzinskas), vol. 13, pp. 193–210. London: Cambridge University Press, 1994.
4. Simpson JL, Elias S. Isolating fetal cells from maternal blood. *JAMA* **270**(19):2357–2361, 1993.
5. Simpson JL, Elias S. Isolating fetal cells in the maternal circulation. *Hum Reprod Update* **1**:409–418, 1995.
6. Walknowska J, Conte FA, Grumbach MM. Practical and theoretical implications of fetal/maternal lymphocyte transfer. *Lancet* **1**:1119–1122, 1969.
7. de Grouchy J, Trubuchet C. Transfusion foeto-maternelle de lymphocytes sanguins et detection du sexe du foetus. *Ann Genet* **14**:133–137, 1971.
8. Schindler AM, Graf E, Martin-Du-Pan R. Prenatal diagnosis of fetal lymphocytes in the maternal blood. *Obstet Gynecol* **40**:340–346, 1972.
9. Takahara H, Kadotani T, Kuzumi I, Makino S. Some critical aspects of prenatal diagnosis of sex in leukocyte cultures from pregnant women. *Proc Jap Acad* **48**:603–607, 1972.
10. Schroder J, de la Chapelle A. Fetal lymphocytes in the maternal circulation after delivery. *Blood* **39**:346–360, 1972.
11. Schroder J, Tiilikainen A, de la Chapelle A. Fetal leukocytes in the maternal circulation after delivery. *Transplant* **17**:346–360, 1974.
12. Grossett L, Barrelet V, Odartchenko N. Antenatal fetal sex determination from maternal blood during early pregnancy. *Am J Obstet Gynecol* **120**:60–63, 1974.
13. Zilliacus R, de la Chapelle A, Schroder J, Tiilikainen A, Kohne E, Kleihaue E. Transplacental passage of fetal blood cells. *Scand J Haemat* **15**:333–338, 1975.
14. Sargent IL, Choo YS, Redman CWG. Isolating and analyzing fetal leukocytes in maternal blood. In *Fetal Cells in Maternal Blood: Prospects for Noninvasive Diagnosis* (eds J.L. Simpson & S. Elias), pp. 147–153. New York: New York Academy of Science, 1994.
15. Herzenberg LA, Bianchi DW, Schroder J, Cann HM, Iverson GM. Fetal cells in the blood of pregnant women: Detection and enrichment by fluorescence-activated cell sorting. *Proc Natl Acad Sci* **76**:181–185, 1979.
16. Iverson GM, Bianchi DW, Cann HM, Herzenberg LA. Detection and isolation of fetal cells from maternal blood using the fluorescence-activated cell sorter (FACS). *Prenat Diagn* **1**:61–73, 1981.
17. Lo Y-MD, Wainscoat JS, Gilmer MDG, Patel P, Sampietro M, Fleming KA. Prenatal sex determination by DNA amplification from maternal peripheral blood. *Lancet* **2**:1363–1365, 1989.
18. Lo Y-MD, Pate P, Sampietro M, Gilmer MDG, Fleming KA, Wainscoat JD. Detection of single-copy fetal DNA sequence from maternal blood. *Lancet* **335**:1463–1464, 1990.
19. Wachtel SS, Elias S, Price J et al. Fetal cells in the maternal circulation: Isolation by multiparameter flow cytometry and confirmation by PCR. *Hum Reprod* **6**:1466–1469, 1991.

20. Bianchi DW, Flint AF, Pizzimenti MF, Knoll JHM, Latt SA. Isolation of fetal DNA from nucleated erythrocytes in maternal blood. *Proc Natl Acad Sci* **87**:3279–3283, 1990.
21. Mueller UW, Hawes CD, Wright AE et al. Isolation of fetal trophoblast cells from peripheral blood of pregnant women. *Lancet* **336**:197–200, 1990.
22. Kao SM, Tang GC, Hsieh TT, Young KC, Wang HC, Pao CC. Analysis of peripheral blood of pregnant women for the presence of fetal Y chromosome-specific ZFY gene deoxyribonucleic acid sequences. *Am J Obstet Gynecol* **166**:1013–1019, 1992.
23. Suzumori K, Adachi R, Okada S, Narukawa T, Yagami Y, Sonta S. Fetal cells in the maternal circulation: detection of Y-sequence by gene amplification. *Obstet Gynecol* **80**:150–154, 1992.
24. Thomas MR, Williamson R, Craft I, Yazhani N, Rodeck CH. Y Chromosome sequence DNA amplified from peripheral blood of women in early pregnancy. *Lancet* **343**:413–414, 1994.
25. Thomas MR, Tutschek B, Frost A et al. The time of appearance and disappearance of fetal DNA from the maternal circulation. *Prenat Diagn* **15**:641–646, 1995.
26. Liou J-D, Pao CC, Hor JJ, Kao S-M. Fetal cells in the maternal circulation during first trimester in pregnancies. *Hum Genet* **92**:309–311, 1993.
27. Liou J-D, Hsieh T-T, Pao CC. Persistence of cells of fetal origin in maternal circulation of pregnant women. In *Fetal Cells in Maternal Blood: Prospects for Noninvasive Prenatal Diagnosis*. (eds J.L. Simpson & S. Elias), pp. 237–241. New York: New York Academy of Science, 1994.
28. Hamada H, Arinami T, Kubo T, Hamaguchi H, Iwasaki H. Fetal nucleated cells in maternal peripheral blood: Frequency and relationship to gestational age. *Hum Genet* **91**:427–432, 1993.
29. Hall JM, Williams SJ. Isolation and purification of CD34++ fetal cells from maternal blood. *Am J Hum Genet* **51**:A257, 1992.
30. Gänshirt D, Börjesson-Stoll R, Burschyk M et al. Successful prenatal diagnosis from maternal blood with magnetic activated cell sorting. In *Fetal Cells in Maternal Blood: Prospects for Noninvasive Prenatal Diagnosis* (eds J.L. Simpson & S. Elias), pp. 103–114. New York: New York Academy of Science, 1994.
31. Elias S, Price J, Dockter M et al. Isolating fetal cells from maternal blood for prenatal diagnosis: University of Tennessee, Memphis experience. In *7th International Conference on Early Prenatal Diagnosis* (ed. H. Zakut), pp. 15–19. Bologna: Monduzzi Editor, 1994.
32. Hsieh TT, Pao CC, Hor JJ, Kao SM. Presence of fetal cells in maternal circulation after delivery. *Hum Genet* **92**:204–205, 1993.
33. Elias S, Lewis DE, Simpson JL et al. Isolation of fetal nucleated red blood cells from maternal blood: persistence of cells from prior pregnancy is unlikely to lead to false psoitive results. *J Soc Gynecol Invest* **3**:359A, 1996.
34. Bianchi DW, Zickwolf GK, Weil GJ, Sylvester S, DeMaria MA. Male fetal progenitor cells persist in maternal blood for as long as 27 years postpartum. *Proc Natl Acad Sci USA* **93**:705–708, 1996.
35. Adkinson LR, Andrews RH, Vowell NL, Koontz WL. Improved detection of fetal cells from maternal blood with polymerase chain reaction. *Am J Obstet Gynecol* **170**:952–955, 1994.
36. Lo Y-MD, Schmidtke J, Wainscoat JS et al. An improved PCR-based system for prenatal sex determination from maternal peripheral blood. In *Fetal Cells in Maternal Blood: Prospects for Noninvasive Prenatal Diagnosis* (eds J.L. Simpson & S. Elias), pp. 214–216. New York: New York Academy of Science, 1994.
37. Camaschella C, Alferno A, Gottardi E et al. Prenatal diagnosis of fetal haemoglobin $Lepore_{Boston}$ disease on maternal peripheral blood. *Blood* **75**:2102–2106, 1990.
38. Hawes CS, Suskin HA, Kalionis B et al. Detection of paternally inherited mutations for β-thalassemia in trophoblast isolated from peripheral maternal blood. In *Fetal Cells in Maternal Blood: Prospects for Noninvasive Prenatal Diagnosis* (eds J.L. Simpson & S. Elias), pp. 181–185. New York: New York Academy of Science, 1994.
39. Lo YD, Bowell PJ, Selinger M et al. Prenatal determination of fetal RhD status by analysis of peripheral blood of rhesus negative mothers [letter]. *Lancet* **342**:54–55, 1993.
40. Lo Y-MD, Bowell PJ, Selinger M et al. Prenatal determination of fetal rhesus D status by DNA amplification of peripheral blood of rhesus-negative mothers. In *Fetal Cells in Maternal Blood: Prospects for Noninvasive Prenatal Diagnosis* (eds J.L. Simpson & S. Elias), pp. 229–236. New York: New York Academy of Science, 1994.
41. Geifman-Holtzman O, Demaria M, Vadnaid TJ et al. Determination of fetal rhesus D Rh (D) type by PCR amplification of fetal cells in flow sorted Rh (D) negative maternal blood. In *7th International Conference on Early Prenatal Diagnosis* (ed. H. Zakut), pp. 41–45. Bologna: Monduzzi Editore, 1994.
42. Geifman-Holtzman O, Kaufman LM, Bernstein IM, Artal R. Rhesus E/e Genotyping of mother, father and fetal cells isolated from maternal blood. *J Soc Gynecol Invest* **3**:241A, 1996.
43. Price JO, Elias S, Wachtel SS et al. Prenatal diagnosis with fetal cells isolated from maternal blood by multiparameter flow cytometry. *Am J Obstet Gynecol* **165**:1731–1737, 1991.
44. Elias S, Price J, Dockter M, Wachtel S, Tharapel A, Simpson JL. First trimester prental diagnosis of trisomy 21 in fetal cells from maternal blood. *Lancet* **340**:1033, 1992.
45. Bianchi DW, Klinger KW. Prenatal diagnosis through the analysis of fetal cells in the maternal circulation. In *Genetic Disorders and the Fetus* (ed. A. Milunsky), pp. 759–770, 3rd edn. Baltimore: Johns Hopkins University Press, 1992.
46. Gänshirt-Ahlert D, Börjesson-Stoll R, Burschyk M et al. Detection of fetal trisomies 21 and 18 from maternal blood using triple gradient and magnetic cell sorting. *Am J Reprod Immunol* **30**:194–201, 1993.
47. Simpson JL, Lewis DE, Bischoff FZ, Elias S. Isolating fetal nucleated red blood cells from maternal blood: the Baylor experience. *Prenat Diagn* **15**:907–912, 1995.
48. Lewis DE, Schober W, Murrell S et al. Rare event selection of fetal nucleated erythrocytes in maternal blood by flow cytometry. *Cytometry* **23**:218–227, 1996.
49. Benirschke K. Anatomical relationship between fetus and mother. In *Fetal Cells in Maternal Blood: Prospects for Noninvasive Prenatal Diagnosis* (eds J.L. Simpson & S. Elias), pp. 9–20. New York: New York Academy of Science, 1994.
50. Douglas GW, Thomas L, Carr M, Cullen NM, Morris R. Trophoblast in the circulating blood during pregnancy. *Am J Obstet Gynecol* **78**:960–973, 1959.
51. Holzgreve W, Garritsen HSP, Gänshirt-Ahlert D. Fetal cells in the maternal circulation. *J Reprod Med* **37**:410–418, 1992.
52. Covone AE, Johnson PM, Latt SA, Adinolfi M. Trophoblast cells in peripheral blood from pregnant women. *Lancet* **75**:2102–2106, 1984.
53. Covone AE, Kozma R, Johnson PM, Latt SA, Adinolfi M. Analysis of peripheral maternal blood samples for the presence of placental-derived cells using Y-specific probes and McAb H315. *Prenat Diagn* **8**:591–607, 1988.
54. Hawes CS, Suskin HA, Petropoulos A, Latham SE, Mueller UW. A morphologic study of trophoblast isolated from peripheral blood of pregnant women. *Am J Obstet Gynecol* **170**:1297–1300, 1994.
55. Sbracia M, Scarpellini F, Lalwani S et al. Possible use of an unusual HLA antigen to select trophoblast cells from the maternal circulation to perform early prenatal diagnosis. In *Fetal Cells in Maternal Blood: Prospects for Noninvasive Diagnosis* (eds J.L. Simpson & S. Elias), pp. 170–174. New York: New York Academy of Science, 1994.
56. Tharapel AT, Jaswaney V, Dockter M et al. Can fetal cells in maternal blood be selected through cytogenetic means? *Am J Hum Genet* **45**(S):271, 1989.
57. Tharapel AT, Jaswaney VL, Dockter ME et al. Failure to detect fetal metaphases in lymphocytes flow sorted by maternal-fetal HLA differences. *Fetal Diagn Ther* **8**:95–101, 1993.
58. Yeoh SC, Sargent IL, Redman CWG, Wordsworth BP, Thein SL. Detection of fetal cells in maternal blood. *Prenat Diagn* **142**:50–53, 1991.
59. Takabayashi H, Kuwabara S, Ukita T et al. Fetal nucleated erythrocyte retrieval from maternal blood. In *7th International Conference on Early Prenatal Diagnosis* (ed. H. Zakut), pp. 45–52. Bologna: Monduzzi Editore, 1994.
60. Zheng Y-L, Carter MP, Price CM et al. Prenatal diagnosis from maternal blood: simultaneous immunophenotyping and FISH of fetal nucleated erythrocytes isolated by negative magnetic cell sorting. *J Med Genet* **30**:1051–1056, 1993.
61. Ferguson-Smith MA, Zheng YL, Carter NP. Simultaneous immunophenotyping and FISH on fetal cells from maternal blood. In *Fetal Cells in Maternal Blood: Prospects for Noninvasive Prenatal Diagnosis* (eds J.L. Simpson & S. Elias), pp. 73–79. New York: New York Academy of Science, 1994.

62. Park VM, Bravo RR, Price JO et al. A model system using fetal hemoglobin to distinguish fetal cells enriched from maternal blood. In *Fetal Cells in Maternal Blood: Prospects for Noninvasive Prenatal Diagnosis* (eds J.L. Simpson & S. Elias), pp. 133–135. New York: New York Academy of Sciences, 1994.
63. Bischoff FZ, Lewis DE, Nguyen DD et al. Greatly increased efficiency of analysis of fetal cells from maternal blood: identification of fetal cells based on CD71 expression, lack of beta globin expression and use of gamma globin mRNA to distinguish fetal (XX) from maternal (XX) cells. *J Soc Gynecol Invest* **3**:361A, 1996.
64. Alter BP. Biology of erythropoiesis. In *Fetal Cells in Maternal Blood: Prospects for Noninvasive Diagnosis* (eds J.L. Simpson & S. Elias), pp. 36–47. New York: New York Academy of Science, 1994.
65. Lo Y-MD, Morey AL, Wainscoat JS, Fleming KA. Culture of fetal erythroid cells from maternal peripheral blood. *Lancet* **344**:264–265, 1994.
66. de la Cruz F, Shifrin H, Elias S et al. Prenatal diagnosis by use of fetal cells isolated from maternal blood. (Letter.) *Am J Obstet Gynecol* **173**:1354–1355, 1995.

Invasive diagnostic methods

36

W. Holzgreve, S. Tercanli, D. Surbek and P. Miny

Introduction

Currently, prenatal diagnosis is characterized by the fact that a considerable variety of techniques for fetal diagnosis, especially karyotyping, is available throughout gestation including early chorionic villus sampling (CVS), early aminocentesis, conventional amniocentesis, placental biopsy (late CVS) as well as fetal blood sampling (FBS) and most recently endoscopy, with a general tendency to transfer invasive diagnostic methods to earlier stages of gestation. Some of these techniques (CVS, FBS) provide faster results than others (early amniocentesis). Therefore, there is an obligation now to select the appropriate technique based on an evaluation of the gestational age, the urgency to obtain a result, the risk of the procedures, and the *a priori* risk for a disorder in the fetus. The purpose of this review is to summarize the current experience with the various methods and to provide some guidelines for their choice. The selection of a specific invasive technique has to be based on the important data coming from large-scale randomized and multicentre studies but also on the individual familiarity of a prenatal diagnostic centre with the different techniques. Counselling about the various procedures has to take into account that the natural fetal loss rate decreases considerably with gestational age.

Even if prenatal karyotyping and the identification of children with non-lethal genetic or chromosomal disorders (e.g. cystic fibrosis or Down syndrome) *in utero* are considered to be valid aims, there are still two obvious reasons why invasive prenatal diagnosis should not be offered routinely to all pregnant women. Firstly, there is always a risk of damaging a pregnancy inherent to all *in utero* tissue samplings by needles or catheters, and secondly, there are costs involved which, if not covered privately, are also of public concern and have to be balanced against other needs in any healthcare system.

The different sampling techniques will be covered here more or less in the historic sequence of their introduction.

Conventional amniocentesis

During the last quarter of a century, amniocentesis in the second trimester of pregnancy has become the routine method to exclude chromosomal abnormalities and single-gene disorders of the fetus. Using ultrasound guidance 'classical' amniocentesis (in opposition to the so-called early amniocentesis, as covered later) is performed easily after 14 completed weeks of pregnancy and is accessible to patients in many regions of the world, because amniotic fluid has the additional advantage that it can be readily mailed to specialized laboratories.

HISTORICAL ASPECTS

The first reports about amniocentesis date back to 1881–82 when this technique was used for amniotic fluid drainage in cases of polyhydramnios in singleton and especially multiple pregnancies.[1,2] In the 1930s amniocentesis was used in France for abortion induction by introducing hypertonic saline.[3] The introduction of conventional amniocentesis is usually associated with a publication by Bevis in the *Lancet* (1952) who used it to evaluate Rhesus incompatibility. The development in cytogenetics then was a strong factor in bringing amniocentesis into the second trimester, and in the 1950s the X-chromatin was first identified in amniocytes.[4,5] Steele and Breg[6] were the first to report successful karyotyping after amniocentesis, and in 1968 the first cases of Down syndrome were diagnosed from amniotic fluid cells[7]. In the same year, Nadler also published the first successful prenatal diagnosis of an inborn error of metabolism, namely galactosemia. A first report of a larger series of some 150 amniocenteses in the second trimester appeared in 1970[8]. Recently, in addition to the established indications for amniocentesis, the polymerase chain reaction (PCR) technology has led to an increased list of indications for infectious disease workup by amniocentesis especially in toxoplasmosis[9,10], cytomegalovirus[11] and varicella infection[12], thus decreasing the overall risk incurred by cordocentesis which was previously necessary for a prenatal diagnosis of these diseases. Also, the new technology of fluorescence *in situ* hybridization (FISH) allows rapid exclusion of specific chromosomal abnormalities after amniocentesis with a speed comparable to karyotyping after direct chromosome preparation from chorionic villi or cordocentesis[13]. FISH analysis, however, does not provide a full karyotype.

The subsequent rapid development of prenatal diagnosis was triggered by the continuous improvement of ultrasound technology and, at the same time, by the increasing number of conditions diagnosable from amniotic fluid or its cellular components.

RISKS OF AMNIOCENTESIS

An NICHD trial in 1967 showed that the overall complication rate including spotting and amniotic fluid leakage was 2–3%. It has to be noted, however, that not all amniotic fluid leakages lead to spontaneous abortion[14]. Maternal complications are extremely rare, and only one maternal death due to sepsis in Germany is known to us. More frequent in the early stages of development of amniocentesis were fetal complications such as skin dimples (Fig. 36.1) (which, however, also occur in newborns without preceding amniocentesis). More serious complications such as cardiac tamponade[15], pneumothorax[16], arteriovenous fistula[17], gangrene of the leg[18], and eye injury[19] were rarely reported. The British Collaborative Amniocentesis Study[20] raised the suspicion that orthopaedic problems such as pes equinovarus or dislocation of the hip are more frequent in children after amniocentesis. These findings, however, were not confirmed by a US NICHD study nor by the Canadian Collaborative Study[21]. A British Working Party on amniocentesis, with 1342 children, also did not confirm any increased rate of birth defects. A recent population based study by Baird *et al.*[22] on 1631 children born after amniocentesis found only an increased rate of haemolytic disease due to isoimmunization, but no increase in other anomalies. Since older women have an increased rate of complications during pregnancy and an increased risk of fetal chromosomal abnormalities, only randomized studies can identify the true risk of an invasive procedure which is mainly performed for increased maternal age.

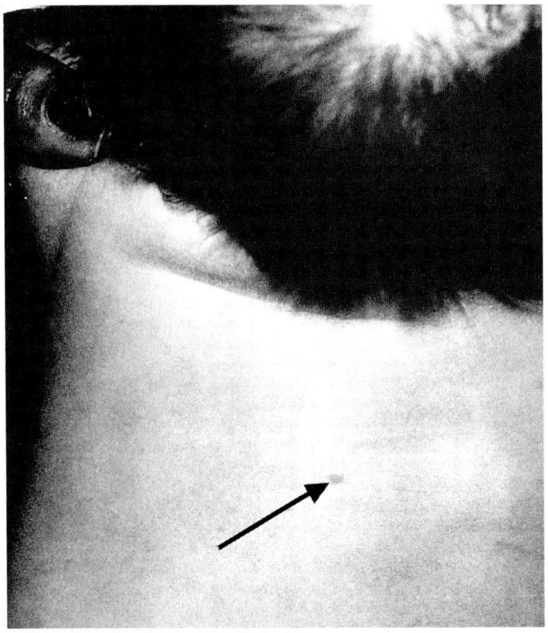

Fig. 36.1 Skin dimple on the back of a child born after amniocentesis in the second trimester of pregnancy.

In the British Collaborative Study[20], mentioned above, the spontaneous abortion rate after amniocentesis was 2.4% and in the control group 1.2%. In this case-controlled study, stillbirths occurred after amniocentesis in 1.2% and in the control group in 0.8%, neonatal deaths in 1.1 and 0.5% of the cases, respectively. To interpret these results, it is important to realize that in this cohort of patients 4% of the women were over 40 years old, and additionally, in this particular study the amniocenteses were performed in 10% of the cases for increased maternal serum alpha-fetoprotein (AFP) levels. The US Collaborative Study[23], mentioned above, evaluated the results of 1040 pregnancies after amniocentesis compared to 992 controls. In this study, there was a clear correlation between the number of needle insertions and the complication rate. The Canadian Collaborative Study in the same year found an increased risk when the needle diameter was larger than 19 gauge. In the Danish randomized study[24], which is probably still the best available to assess the risk of second-trimester amniocenteses, 4606 women between 25 and 34 years were evaluated and all procedures were performed with a 20-gauge needle by very experienced investigators. A spontaneous abortion rate of 1.7% after the procedure was significantly higher than that of the in the control group (0.7%, $p<0.01$). Orthopaedic problems were not increased in the amniocentesis group, but there was an increase of respiratory distress (relative risk = 2.1) and pneumonia (relative risk = 2.9). The most important studies comparing abortion rates after amniocentesis with control groups are summarized in Table 36.1.

TECHNICAL ASPECTS

Between weeks 15 and 17 of pregnancy, the total amount of amniotic fluid is about 200 ml and the uterus can be reached transabdominally without major risks of transversing the bladder or bowel. In the beginning the so-called 'free hand needle technique' was used which meant a puncture without continuous ultrasound guidance after preceding sonographical localization of the optimal puncture site, but nowadays continuous ultrasound surveillance during the puncture is the only acceptable method. An amniocentesis may be more difficult at the time of uterine contractions[25] and in cases where the needle is pushing a non-fused membrane into the uterus

TABLE 36.1
Risk of 'spontaneous' abortion after second-trimester amniocentesis compared to appropriate control groups

Multicenter studies	Post Amniocentesis	Control group	Difference
MRC (Canada)	3.3	2.3	1.0
NIH	3.6	2.5	1.1
MRC (UK)	5.7	2.6	3.1
DFG	2.4	1.3	1.1
Single studies			
Crandall (UCLA)	2.7	1.3	1.4
Porecco (UCSD)	2.8	2.1	0.7
PD Center (NY)	2.9	2.1	0.8
Leschot (Netherlands)	3.9	2.2	1.7
Tabor (Denmark)	1.7	0.7	1.0
			Total ≈ 1.0–1.2%

(so-called 'tenting'). When looking at the loss rates after transplacental, compared to non-transplacental amniocentesis, no difference between the two groups was found[26]. Although Golbus *et al.*[27] did not detect an increased rate of rhesus sensitization in 300 Rh-negative women not given anti-D after amniocentesis compared to 650 controls, most investigators have accepted an increased risk[28,29], so that usually the administration of 100–300 μg of anti-D is standard inmost countries after amniocentesis. Hanson *et al.*[30] have discussed that a lower dose might be sufficient before 20 weeks of gestation.

AMNIOCENTESIS IN MULTIPLE PREGNANCIES

A multicenter study in 1992[31] on 529 cases in 15 centers found a spontaneous abortion rate of 3.7% of which 2.3% occurred prior to 20 weeks of gestation. Anderson *et al.*[32] found a spontaneous abortion rate of 3.6% in 330 twin and 9 triplet pregnancies as compared to 0.6% in singleton pregnancies. In higher multiples, the experience is still too limited[33] for a proper risk assessment. With careful ultrasound guidance, needle entry into both sacs should be clearly demonstrated and the injection of dye should not be necessary. Methylene blue should certainly not be used for this purpose, because it increases the risk of fetal bowel atresia.[34] Jeanty *et al.*[33] and Sebire *et al.*[35] reported a single uterine entry technique for twin pregnancies and found the risk of fetal loss from this procedure to be similar to that in singleton pregnancies. If the absence of a septal lamda-sign has been demonstrated in the first trimester, indicating monochorionicity and therefore monozygosity, it is reasonable to puncture only one sac.

Early amniocentesis

During the last 15 years so-called early amniocentesis has been proposed as an alternative to CVS by a number of groups.[36–41] Usually the term early amniocentesis has been used for procedures before 15 completed weeks of gestation[42]. In an early series for example by Hanson *et al.*[30] out of 541 amniocenteses before week 16 of pregnancy, only 4 were performed during week 11 and 36 during week 12 of gestation, with 149 in week 13 and 352 in week 14 of pregnancy. In 8% of patients, more than two needle insertions were necessary and in 3.5% of the cases, no amniotic fluid could be obtained. Of all the pregnancies, 3.6% ended in spontaneous abortions, 0.7% in stillbirths and 0.3% in neonatal deaths. Also in the early series by Evans *et al.*[43] and Elejalde *et al.*[44] most procedures were done between weeks 13 and 14 of pregnancy. A more recent review by Byrne *et al.*[45] revealed that the vast majority of those procedures reported as early amniocentesis were performed at weeks 12 and 13 of gestation and only a very small number at or before 11 weeks. The safety of the procedure seems to vary significantly in relation to the gestational age before and after 13 weeks of gestation, e.g. 14.8% loss rate before and 1.8% between weeks 13 and 15 of pregnancy in the series reported by Stripparo *et al.*[46]. In 8 of the children in this series, orthopedic anomalies were found including four instances of club foot, one hyper-extended leg, a scoliosis as well as congenital dislocations of the knee and hip.

In a series by Hackett *et al.*[47] in 2 out of 106 cases of early amniocentesis between weeks 11 and 14 of pregnancy, the so-called tenting of the amniotic membrane was the most frequent reason for unsuccessful or repeated samplings. The average-failure rate to obtain a result in 15 series published until 1991 was about 2%[40]. The highest failure rate ('dry taps') of more than 20% was recorded in a series[48] where many procedures were performed before 10 weeks of gestation. Because the amniotic sac is still small in relation to the chorionic cavity in the first trimester of pregnancy (Fig. 36.2), there has been some concern about withdrawing amounts of amniotic fluid sufficient for a successful cell culture at that gestational age. In order to obtain a maximum number of cells

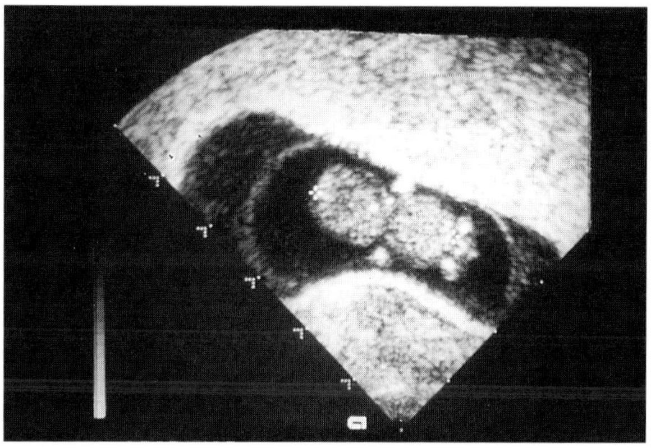

Fig. 36.2 Typical first-trimester sonogram showing that before a gestational age of 12 weeks the chorionic and the amniotic membrane are not fused yet.

amniofiltration systems have been proposed by different groups[49,50]. Recently, Sundberg *et al.*[51] published a study on 581 early amniocenteses compared to 579 CVS procedures, and although the abortion risk was similar in both groups, these authors found an association between early amniocentesis and talipes equinovarus. Another randomized trial[52–54] found an increase of respiratory problems (2.6% after early amniocentesis as compared to 1.6% in the mid-trimester amniocentesis controls). The effect of early amniocentesis on fetal and newborn lung development needs to be further evaluated. Crandall *et al.*[55] in their series on 693 consecutive early amniocentesis cases reported a spontaneous abortion rate of 1.5% as compared to 0.6% in the control group.

Regarding the cell culture success Djalali *et al.*[56] reported that long culture durations (more than 20 days) were more frequent after early amniocentesis. In the series by Eiben *et al.*[57], karyotyping was successful in 99.7% of the cases, but in 9.9% there was pseudomosaicism. Brumfield *et al.*[58] first described a significant rise in amniotic fluid AFP until 13 weeks of gestation and then a significant decline after 14 weeks. A large number of suspicious acetylcholinesterase (AchE) findings was reported by Eiben *et al.*[59], but a faint band of AchE was not associated with an increased number of fetal anomalies. In a comparative trial of early versus standard amniocentesis Brumfield *et al.*[60] found more post-procedure complications and a higher fetal loss rate within 30 days after amniocentesis in the early group. Also Eiben *et al.*[61] reported a 2% abortion rate up to 28 weeks after early amniocentesis as compared to 1.3% after standard amniocentesis. Nicolaides *et al.*[37,62] performed a comparison of chorionic villus sampling and early amniocentesis for karyotyping at 10 to 13 weeks, both by ultrasound guided techniques, and found a significantly higher loss rate after early amniocentesis compared to CVS. In a review of the currently available data on early amniocentesis versus CVS, Stranc *et al.*[63] concluded that: 'Ultimately the choice of prenatal diagnostic technique lies with the women herself, the choice being restricted mainly by the gestation at which she is referred for pre-test counselling and by the local availability of experienced practitioners.' More recently, the CEMAT trial, a randomized controlled study comparing early with second trimester-amniocentesis, has suggested higher loss rates and an increased incidence of talipes in the former, calling into question the continued use of early amniocentesis unless in special circumstances.

Early chorionic villi sampling (CVS)

The so-called 'direct' chromosome preparation from the cytotrophoblast and rapid culture techniques using the mesenchymal core of villi allow early and fast karyotyping in the first trimester of pregnancy. Exclusion of maternal age related aneuploidies is by far the most frequent indication for CVS followed by cases with a previous aneuploid child and cases at risk for monogenic disorders. The early gestational age may make CVS more acceptable as compared to conventional amniocentesis especially in high risk situations such as abnormal ultrasound findings, e.g. nuchal oedema, parental balanced structural chromosomal abnormalities or when a couple has already experienced a late termination of pregnancy due to aneuploidy. In addition to classic cytogenetic indications, villi can also be used for the diagnosis of chromosomal breakage syndromes and for rapid sexing in pregnancies at risk for X-linked diseases. Chorionic villi are an excellent source of DNA, supplying sufficient amounts for most molecular genetic techniques without prior culture. Therefore, CVS is the method of first choice in pregnancies at risk for monogenic disorders diagnosable by these techniques. The frequently high recurrence risks (25% with autosomal recessive diseases, 50% in male fetuses of carriers for X-linked conditions) are also in favour of an early diagnostic test, which allows a termination of pregnancy prior to 12 weeks, if so chosen by the parents. Due to the rapid progress in molecular genetics the number of diagnosable monogenic disorders is increasing steadily. In cases of doubt, a medical geneticist should be consulted as early as possible.

Biochemical testing after CVS is today possible for almost all metabolic diseases that can be diagnosed from amniotic fluid cells. As in other monogenic disorders CVS clearly appears advantageous, because of the high recurrence risks and the usually feasible use of fresh uncultured villi. A representative list of monogenic conditions diagnosed from chorionic villi by our own CVS programme is given in Table 36.2.

From the more than ten different techniques proposed for CVS in the first trimester, e.g. hysteroscopy (Fig. 36.3a) or metal biopsy forceps (Fig. 36.3b) only two have prevailed on a large scale, the transcervical (Fig. 36.4a) and transabdominal (Fig. 36.4b) sampling techniques. For transcervical sampling, most centres used the catheter originally designed by Ward *et al.*[64] although at his centre curved biopsy forceps are now used[65]. Some centres, including ours, use different kinds of catheters[66]. For the transcervical approach, a bendable polyethylene catheter with a metal obturator is introduced

TABLE 36.2
Monogenic conditions (n = 303) diagnosed from chorionic villi in the first 12 000 CVS procedures performed by our group in Basel and formerly in Münster

Indication	Result	*n*
Duchenne muscular dystrophy	X rec	62
Thalassemia/sickle-cell anemia	AR	59
Mucoviscidosis	AR	47
MPS I	AR	15
MPS II	X rec	9
MPS IV	AR	4
Haemophilia A/B	X rec	22
Acute granulomatous syndrome	AR	11
Others		74

*MPS = Mucopolysaccharidosis, X rec = X-linked recessive, AR = autosomal recessive.

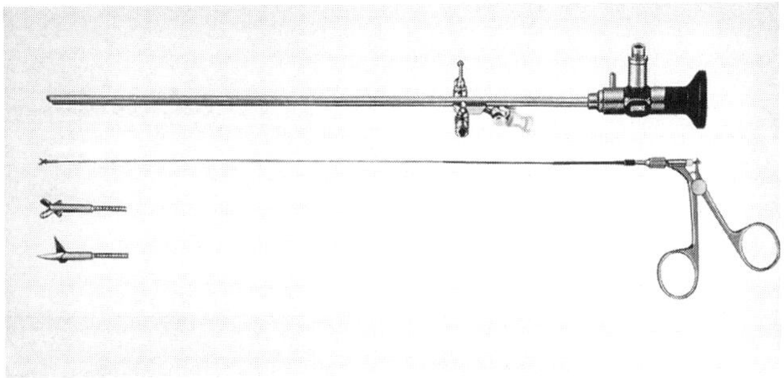

(a)

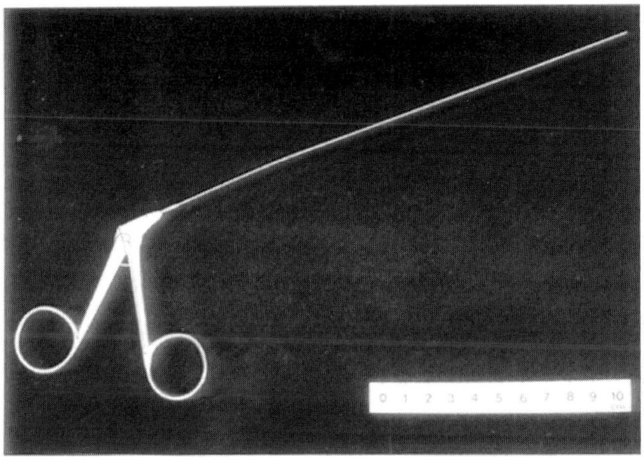

(b)

Fig. 36.3 Rarely used techniques for chorionic villi sampling (CVS): (a) with an endoscopic device; (b) with a metal biopsy forceps. Both are applied transcervically.

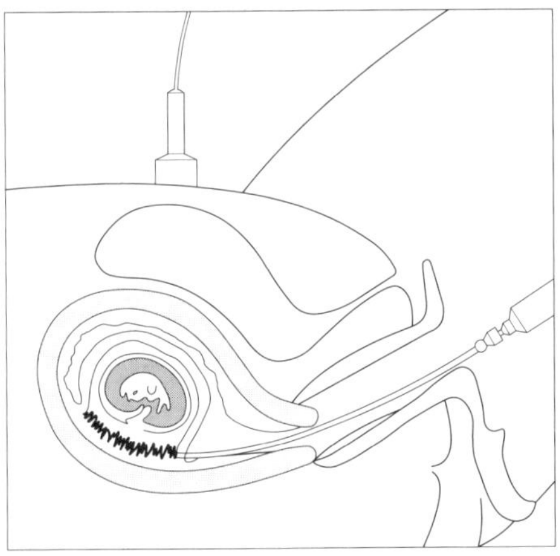

(a)

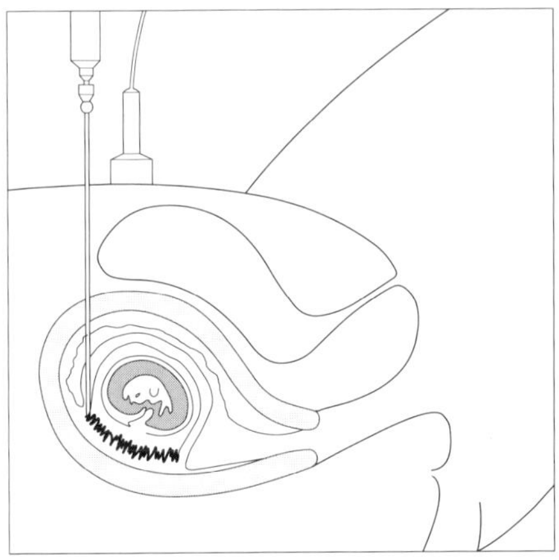

(b)

Fig. 36.4 Schematic depiction of the two frequently used CVS techniques: (a) transcervical catheter aspiration; (b) transabdominal puncture.

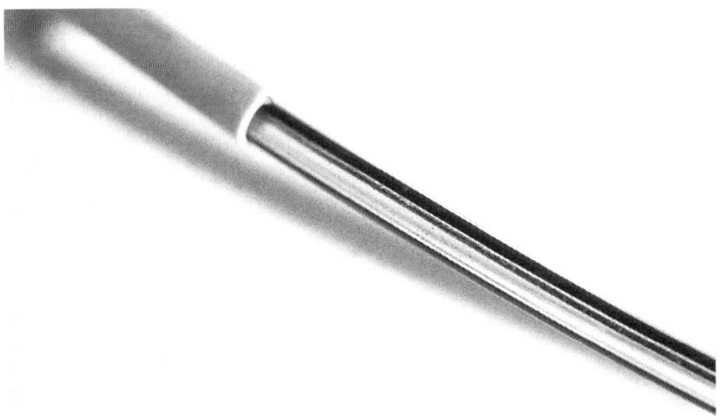

Fig. 36.5 Chorionic villus sampling catheter (developed by W. Holzgreve, Basel) with an echogenic bismuth stripe in its wall for enhanced echogenicity (Angiomed, Karlsruhe, Germany).

through the cervix and guided to the chorion frondosum under continuous ultrasound surveillance (Fig. 36.6a). With an attached syringe, which is partly filled with medium, a vacuum is applied and approximately 10–50 mg of tissue are aspirated and rinsed into a Petri dish.

The transabdominal technique was first developed in Denmark by Smid-Jensen and Hahnemann (1984)[67]. It can be applied either as a free-hand ultrasound-guided fine-needle aspiration or with a needle guide ultrasound transducer (Fig. 36.6b). A recent prospective comparative study on transabdominal chorionic villus sampling compared to amniocentesis performed at 10 to 13 weeks of gestation showed that the risk of fetal loss was higher and repeat testing was required more often after early amniocentesis than after CVS[68].

Regarding the medical risks of a pregnancy termination, which are considerably higher in later gestational ages[69], and

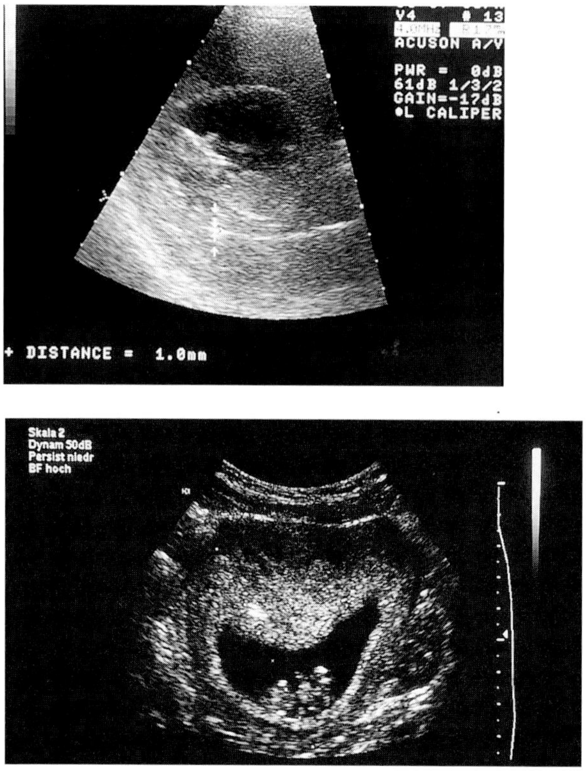

(a)

(b)

Fig. 36.6 Sonograms taken at the time of chorionic villus samplings: (a) transcervical technique; (b) transabdominal technique.

the psychological implication of waiting for a good or bad result and potentially facing a late termination, early diagnosis clearly seems to be advantageous[70]. Various studies[71,72] confirmed that women would prefer CVS to amniocentesis provided the risks of both procedures were equal. At Queen Charlotte's Hospital, women aged 35 years or over when asked after extensive counselling to choose between having no test, amniocentesis or joining the MRC trial[73] the majority chose to have some test and CVS was a more popular choice than amniocentesis[74]. A study reported by investigators at the Erasmus University, Rotterdam[38], revealed that only 29% of women who underwent amniocentesis had actually chosen this procedure, and 71% were too late for CVS.

There are currently two randomized trials[73,75] and one controlled[76] trial published, comparing the procedure-related risk rates of first-trimester CVS and conventional amniocentesis. Whereas the randomized Canadian[21] and the controlled US Collaborative[23] trials did not reveal a significant difference in the fetal loss rates, the MRC European trial[73] showed a significantly higher rate of liveborn infants who survived in the amniocentesis group. There were, however, 31 centres participating in the MRC trial contributing extremely variable numbers of cases and using different sampling and cytogenetic procedures. The number of repeat procedures was significantly higher in the CVS as compared to the amniocentesis group.

Later when CVS was more widely used clinically, concern was raised[77] that CVS might cause severe limb deficiencies (Fig. 36.7a) and the hypoglossia/hypodactyly syndrome (Fig. 36.7b), but reviewing the international experience and our own series with more than 3500 cases at that time, this could

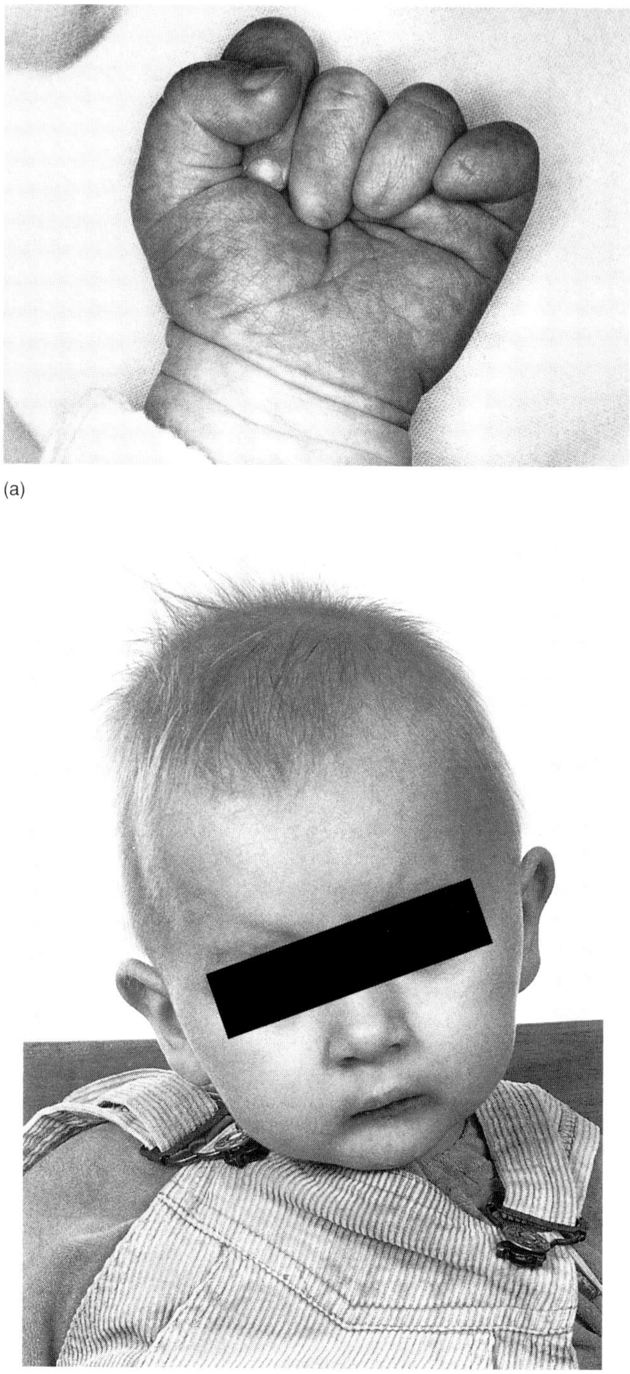

(a)

(b)

Fig. 36.7 Congenital malformations whose incidence was associated with early chorionic villus sampling. (a) Transverse terminal limb reduction defects (note missing fingernails). (b) Hypoglossia/hypodactyly syndrome (note retrognathia and thin lower lip).

not be confirmed[78]. Currently, the largest study on the issue of limb-reduction defects among infants exposed to CVS during pregnancy was published from the WHO International Registry[79]. Among 138 996 children born after CVS, 77 had limb-defects excluding syndromes, inherited disorders and defects occurring in previable fetuses. The percentage of transverse limb defects did not show any difference in the overall frequency compared to the background population including the pattern distribution of limb deficiencies. In a commentary in the same issue of *Lancet*[80] it was concluded that 'the decision whether or not to inform [a woman] of the potential increase, as yet unproven, in the risk of limb defects must remain with the conscience of the counsellors'. These studies, however, did not include early cases (6–8 weeks' gestation) as did the report of Firth *et al.*[77] and it is recommended that CVS not be performed before 10 weeks. A randomized clinical trial of transcervical versus transabdominal CVS by Brambati *et al.*[81] did not reveal a significant difference regarding safety and efficiency of both approaches, whereas Smidt-Jensen and Philip[82] found a higher risk in their transcervical CVS as compared to their transabdominal CVS and amniocentesis group. In accordance with data on the incidence and timing of pregnancy losses depending on maternal and gestational ages, Jahoda *et al.*[83] found that in older women the fetal loss rates after transcervical and transabdominal sampling was between 5.8 and 6.2%, whereas this rate dropped to 2.4% after 12 weeks. A single-centre comparison of results after 1000 CVS and the same number of amniocenteses revealed that the percentage of pregnancies with live-born infants was 95.8 and 95.7%, respectively[84].

Aspirated tissue needs to be separated carefully under a dissection microscope (Fig. 36.8) in order to exclude maternal cells (decidua, blood). Villi obtained by biopsy forceps are much clearer and easier for the laboratories to process[65]. This issue is especially critical in DNA diagnosis using amplification by PCR and in some biochemical examinations. In our series, the ability to obtain clean chorionic villi (Fig. 36.9) without maternal cell contamination was clearly related to the experience of the person separating the tissue microscopically. Clinical problems can be avoided by proper separation techniques and by additional cytogenetic analyses of chorionic villus cultures after direct preparation. There have been occasional diagnostic pitfalls due to erroneous interpretation of so-called confined placental mosaicism. The large-scale use of chorionic villi and placental cells for diagnostic purposes has greatly increased our understanding of early human development[85–87]. Today it is well established that aneuploidy (mosaic and rarely non-mosaic) may be confined to extraembryonic or extrafetal tissues, while the fetus proper has a normal chromosome count. A number of so-called false-positive (aneuploidy not confirmed in the fetus) and a few false-negative results (fetal aneuploidy not detected in chorionic or placental cells) have been reported after CVS or placental biopsy[88]. In larger series, true mosaicism was diagnosed in about 1% of samples. Most of these instances represent mosaicism which is confined to chorion or placenta. In these cases, confirmation of aneuploidy in the fetus by ultrasound, fetal blood sampling, or amniocentesis is mandatory before termination of pregnancy is considered. There is evidence now that confined placental mosaicism may lead to intrauterine growth retardation and an increased risk for spontaneous abortion. In some cases, uniparental disomy was confirmed in newborns after diagnosis of confined placental mosaicism[89,90] presumably originating from mitotic chromosomal loss in the early cleavages of a trisomic zygote, and even a prospective prenatal diagnosis of Prader–Willi syndrome due to maternal disomy for chromosome 15 following zygote rescue has been reported[87].

The so-called false-negative results after CVS or placental biopsy originate from mosaicism in fetus and/or placenta and were – with only very few exceptions – restricted to cases where direct preparations were performed exclusively. The simultaneous analysis of cultured cells reliably prevents diagnostic errors by raising the probability of detecting mosaicism present in placenta and fetus. As in any other tissue used for

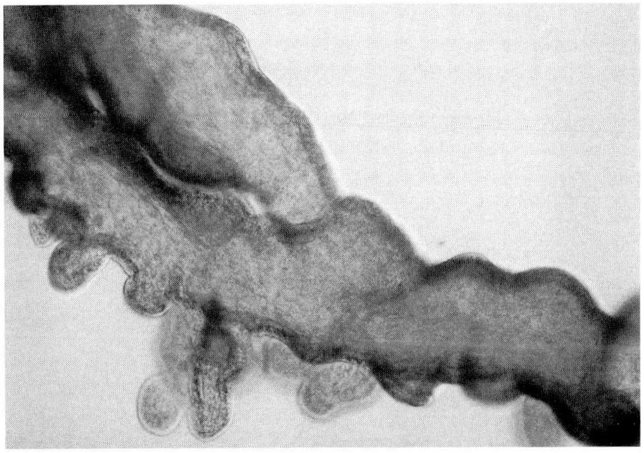

Fig. 36.9 Chorionic villus tissue among decidual contamination. Note Langhans cell layer on the edges of the villi.

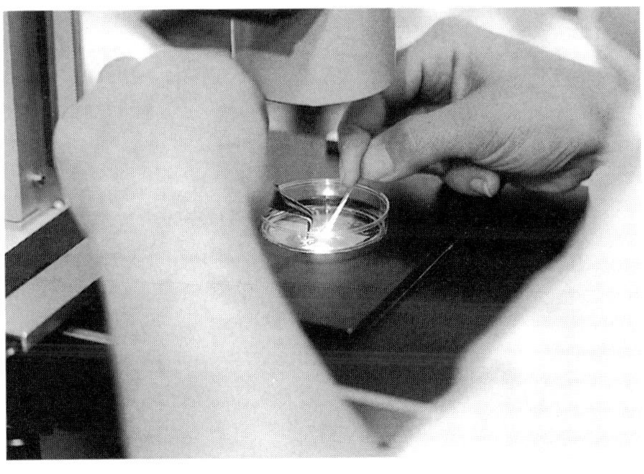

Fig. 36.8 Careful separation of chorionic villi after sampling under a dissecting microscope.

prenatal diagnosis of aneuploidy, it has to be kept in mind, however, that any realistic number of cells used for chromosome analysis represents an extreme selection and that low-grade mosaicism may remain undiagnosed.

Summarizing the present experience of larger centres including our own with CVS and placental biopsies, we conclude that CVS is as reliable as other diagnostic tools provided there is simultaneous use of direct preparation and cultured cells and a proper follow up of mosaicism. Karyotyping the placenta in some situations even provides valuable additional information not available by other means, e.g. amniocentesis or fetal blood sampling. The technique of transcervical retrieval of fetal cells by uterine lavage, endocervical lavage, cytobrush, and mucus aspiration which was developed by the group of Rodeck *et al.*[91] is covered in Chapter 40. Their preliminary assessment of the safety of mucus aspiration before transcervical chorionic villus sampling in continuing pregnancies found no difference in outcome compared to the control group of patients having only CVS. Cell yield and sample quality were estimated using monoclonal trophoblast specific antibodies, and there was a tendency for better samples obtained by lavage, although mucus aspiration samples showed improvement with increasing gestational age.

Placental biopsy in the second and third trimesters of pregnancy (late CVS)

Despite a probable reduction in mitotic index in the cytotrophoblast of the ageing placenta, rapid karyotyping after direct chromosome preparation is feasible in addition to culture techniques throughout gestation up to 40 weeks[92,93]. With this technique high rates of chromosomal abnormalities were found in patients with suspicious fetal ultrasound findings[94], but in some regions of the world this procedure is mainly used for the detection of single gene disorders, e.g. α-thalassemia in South-East Asia[95]. The most frequent indications in our programme for this so-called 'late CVS' were ultrasound findings suspicious of fetal aneuploidy followed by cases with late booking, e.g. due to failed amniotic fluid cell cultures or late maternal serum screening results. As compared to lymphocyte cultures after fetal blood sampling, direct chromosome preparation after placental biopsy can be faster if necessary (karyotyping on the same day). Furthermore, transabdominal placental biopsies (Fig. 36.10a,b) are easier to perform under certain circumstances, especially, poly-, oligo- or anhydramnios (Fig. 36.11). Karyotyping is indicated even in the third trimester of pregnancy in the presence of specific sonographic findings to optimize the pre- and perinatal management (e.g. avoidance of tocolysis or caesarean section with lethal aneuploidies in the fetus). Technical improvements of ultrasound machines and increasing experience of the investigators have already contributed to and will in the future further enhance the important role of sonography as a screening tool for the detection of pregnancies at risk for aneu-

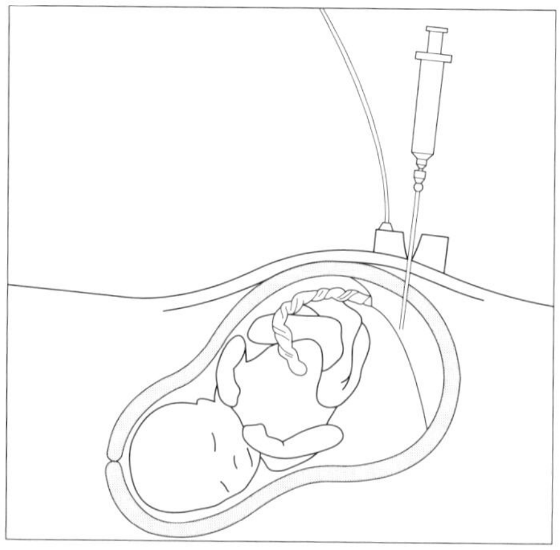

(a)

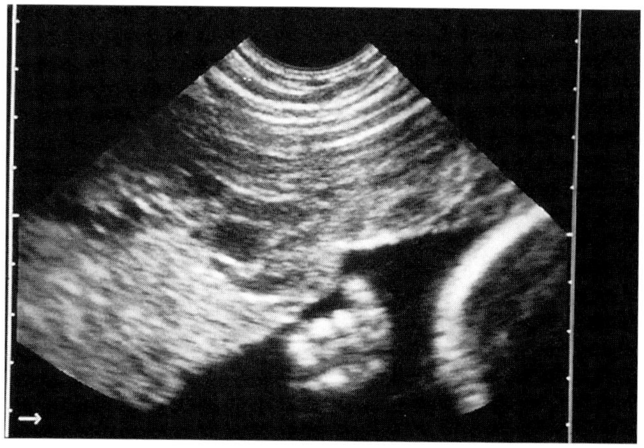

(b)

Fig. 36.10 Method of placental biopsy in the second and third trimester (late CVS) for rapid prenatal diagnosis. (a) Schematic depiction of the technique. (b) Sonogram showing an anterior placenta. The fetus points with the finger towards the placental edge which should not be the puncture site for late CVS, because maternal blood rather than chorionic villi is present in the marginal sinus of the placenta.

ploidy in an *a priori* low-risk population. Placental biopsy is currently the fastest option when a fetal karyotype is needed. For molecular genetic tests and also for some biochemical analyses, we also prefer placental biopsies as compared to amniocentesis even in the second trimester of pregnancy because fresh villi can be used. The molecular genetic confirmation of a suspected rubella infection in villi after placental biopsy or CVS saves a considerable number of women at risk the waiting time until fetal blood sampling for serological tests can be performed at around 23 weeks of gestation.

Placental biopsies in late gestation are only performed transabdominally using the same techniques as described above for the first trimester. The technique can be applied as late as 41 weeks of pregnancy when immediate perinatal decisions are required in the presence of suspicious ultrasound findings. Some investigators use a 'double needle' technique with a guide needle which is advanced through the uterine

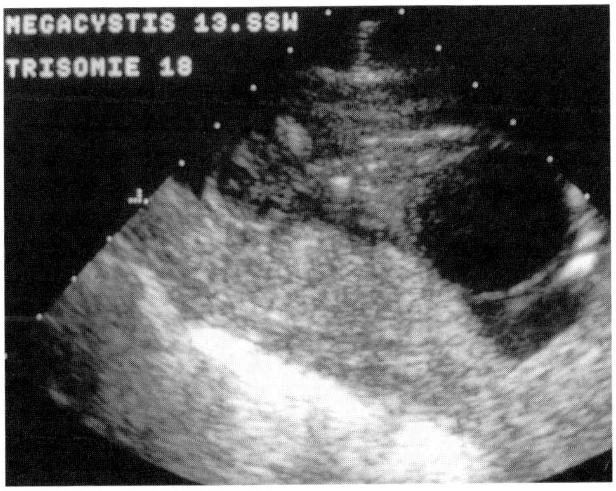

Fig. 36.11 Fetus with urethral obstruction and prominent occiput due to trisomy 18 at 13 weeks of gestation. Placental biopsy which revealed the karyotype within one day was easily performed despite the severe oligohydramnios.

wall and an inner needle for aspiration of villi, whereas others apply a 'single needle' approach usually with a 20 gauge spinal needle[93]. In a series of 335 cases published recently[96], it was found that the success rate in the study group increased from 90% in the first 60 procedures to 98.8% in the later cases.

The safety and reliability of late placental biopsies have been established in several individual series[97–99] as well as in a large international survey[93]. However, care should be taken to reduce the force of the procedure as transabdominal aspiration causes more fetomaternal haemorrhage (as judged by a rise in maternal AFP [MSAFP]) than does transcervical biopsy[100].

Classical fetoscopy

The term 'fetoscopy' was introduced in the 1970s by Scrimgeour[101] and is a combination of the Latin word for 'fetus' and the Greek word for 'viewing'. Fetoscopy originally was an endoscopic method for viewing the fetus and the placenta in the second trimester of pregnancy (Fig. 36.12a,b) and to sample blood skin and liver tissues from the fetus for prenatal diagnosis. First attempts at intrauterine endoscopic visualization of the fetus had been reported already by Westin[102]. He used a 10-mm hysteroscope transvaginally. Mandelbaum *et al.*[103] later used transabdominal fetoscopy to attempt to treat rhesus incompatibility by intraperitoneal transfusion. Valenti[104,105] reported the first successful fetoscopic blood aspiration with a modified paediatric cystoscope with a diameter of 6 mm in patients undergoing termination of pregnancy by hysterotomy. Hobbins and Mahoney (1974)[106] two years later introduced the 'Needlescope' (Dyonics, Woburn, Mass, USA) with a self-focusing rod lens and an outer diameter of 1.7 to 2.7 mm. This was the first clinically feasible percutaneous technique.

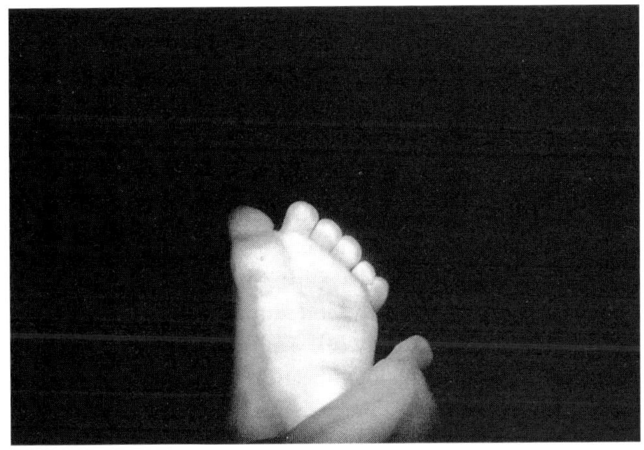

(a)

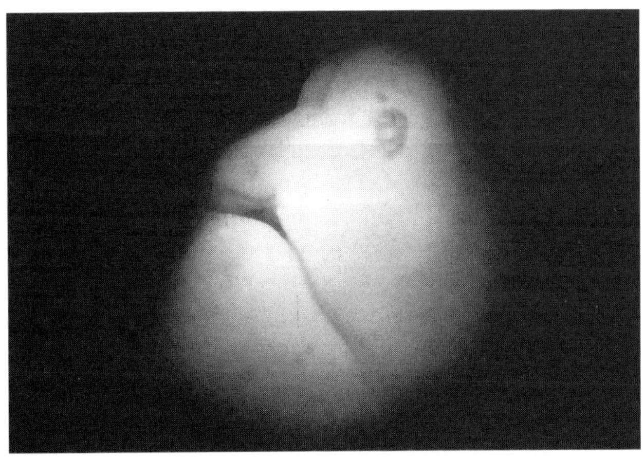

(b)

Fig. 36.12 Fetoscopic pictures obtained in the second trimester of pregnancy from a fetus with Ellis–van Crefeld syndrome, showing: (a) Polydactyly of the foot; (b) the typical cleft lip.

Before a classical fetoscopy between weeks 17 and 20 of gestation, an ultrasound assessment of the amniotic fluid volume and placental location was performed. The trochar was inserted after aseptic preparation and local anaesthesia. Rodeck and Campbell[107] found that even in cases of anterior placenta a 'window' for a safe entry could be found and a pure fetal blood sample could be obtained from the umbilical cord. Using this technique, Antsaklis[108] reported a spontaneous abortion rate below 5%. Second trimester fetoscopy for visualization has been replaced by ultrasound and fetoscopic cord sampling by ultrasound-guided cord puncture.

Embryoscopy

Over the last two decades, two important tendencies can be identified in prenatal medicine. Firstly, especially due to transvaginal sonography, there has been an ever increasing number of anomalies detectable in the first trimester. Secondly, the hope is growing that fetal therapy, e.g. by stem cell therapy,

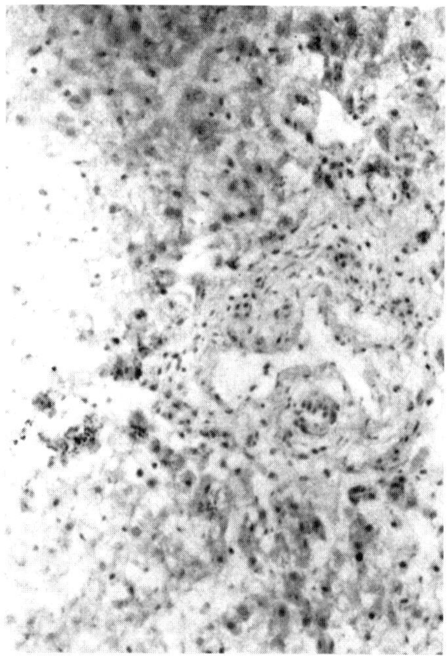
(a)

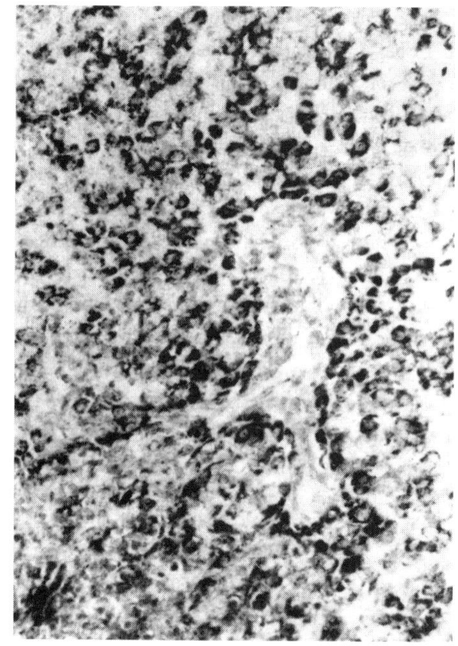
(b)

Fig. 36.16 Histochemical picture of fetal liver sections at 19 weeks of gestation obtained *in utero*. (a) Normal liver. (b) Liver of a fetus with ornithine transcarbamylase deficiency. Note the discrete lead depositions in the cytoplasm of the liver cells.

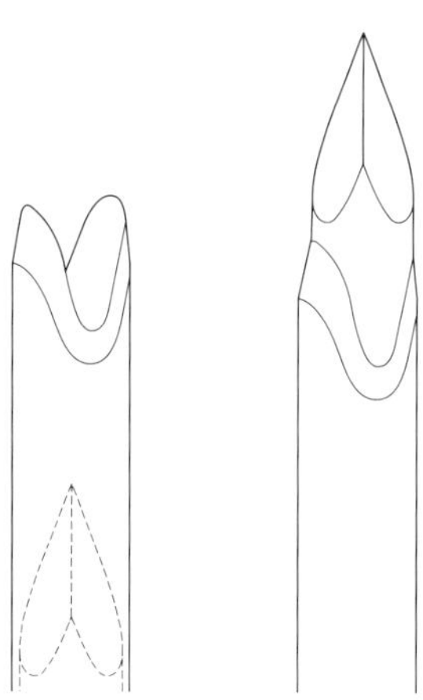
(a)

Fig. 36.17 Technique of ultrasound-guided fetal liver biopsy in the second trimester of pregnancy. (a) Schematic depiction of cut-biopsy needle (Squibb). (b) Biopsy cylinder obtained from fetal liver biopsy.

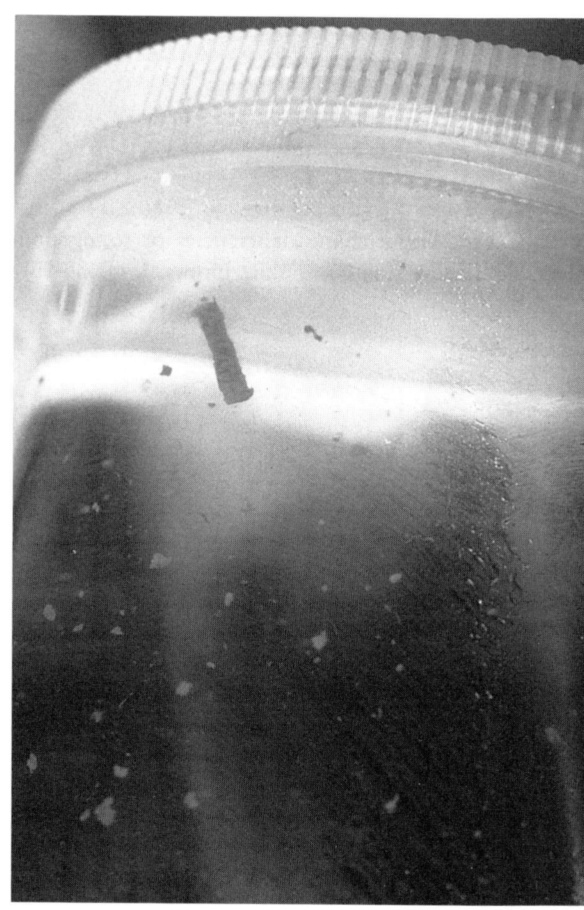
(b)

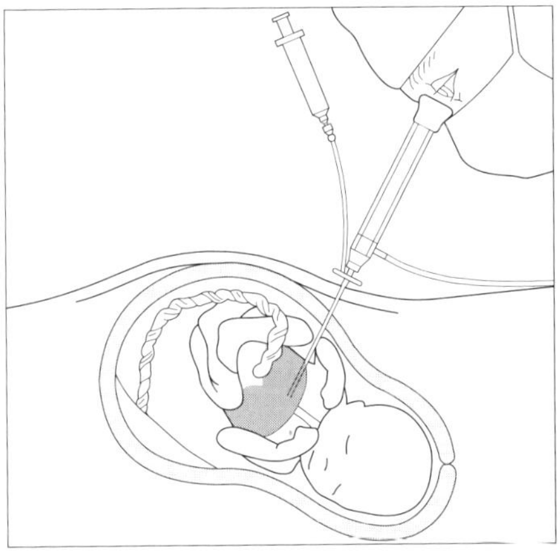

(a)

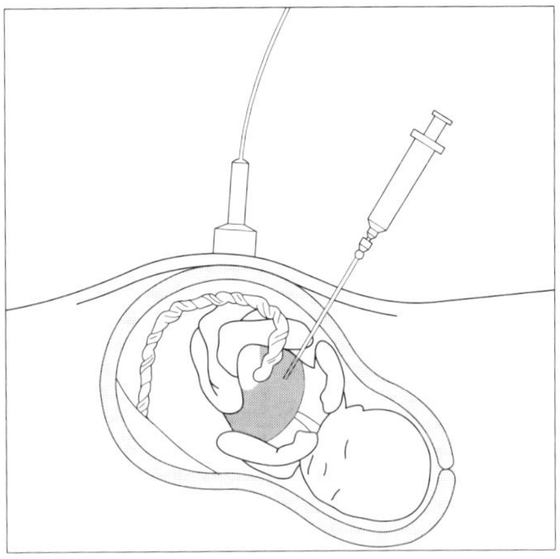

(b)

Fig. 36.18 The two methods of fetal liver biopsy. (a) Fetoscopic technique. (b) Ultrasound-guided technique.

of these non-invasive techniques for the assessment of fetal renal function, the importance of fetal kidney biopsies will be very limited.

Fetal blood sampling

Fetoscopic cord puncture[107] gave way to a direct ultrasound-guided approach[127] collection of pure fetal blood from the umbilical cord (Fig. 36.19 and Plates 36.2a and b). This paved the way for a considerable extension of the indications for prenatal diagnosis such as parvovirus B19 diagnosis and therapy, e.g. of infectious diseases (Fig. 36.20).

A fetal blood smear can even be a helpful diagnostic marker[128]. It must be verified that the prenatally obtained sample is pure fetal blood, because even a small trace of contamination with maternal blood or amniotic fluid can cause a false diagnosis, e.g. maternal IgM in cases of rubella or toxoplasmosis infections. The indications of our first 850 cases are summarized in Fig. 36.21. Daffos *et al.*[129] were the first to present large series for the exclusion of fetal infections and other diseases such as haemophilia or alloimmune thrombocytopenia. Other genetic diseases such as Wiskott–Aldrich syndrome[130], chronic granulomatous disease[131] or immunodeficiency disorders[132] which were previously diagnosed by fetoscopic blood sampling, can also be diagnosed by the ultrasound-guided technique.

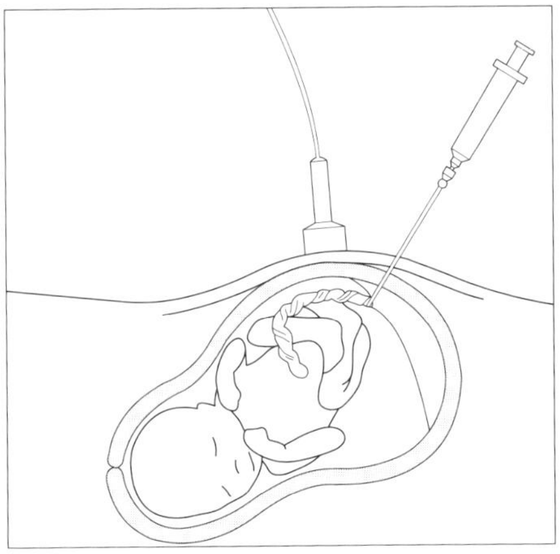

Fig. 36.19 Cordocentesis technique. Schematic depiction.

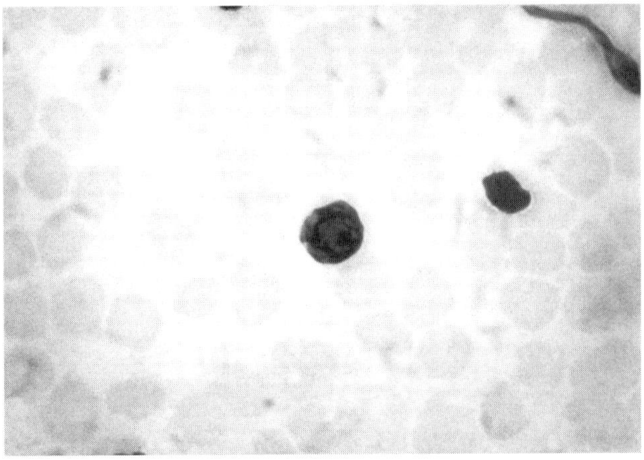

Fig. 36.20 Fetal blood obtained by cordocentesis in the second trimester of a case with maternal parvovirus B19 infection. Blood shows 'lantern' erythrocytes typical of fetal infection.

Cord puncture (or cordocentesis), like amniocentesis, can be performed either by the free-hand needle technique or with the help of a needle guide. Weiner and Okamura[133] found a total procedure-related loss rate of 0.2% and a higher loss rate with puncture of an umbilical artery as opposed to the umbilical vein. In a study of 1272 procedures, 861 before week 24 of gestation and 411 afterwards, a total procedure related loss rate of 2.3% was found with a 1.6% rate of intrauterine fetal death within 48 hours of the procedure and

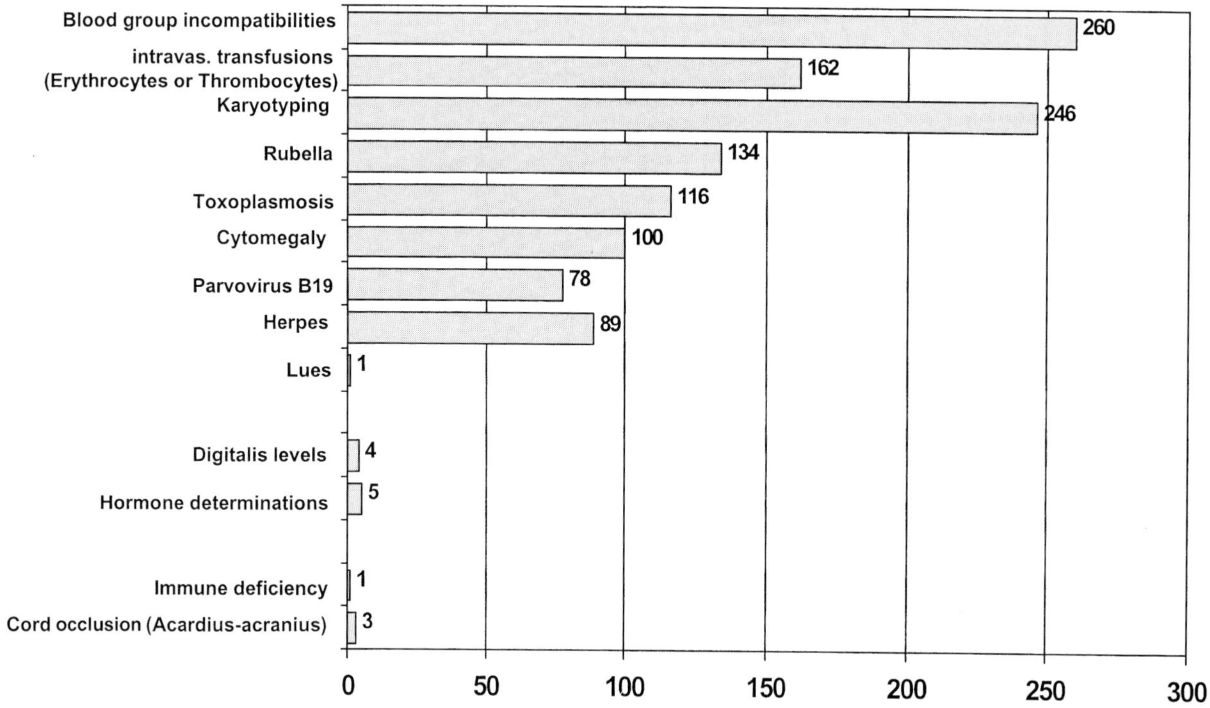

Fig. 36.21 Indications for cordocentesis.

0.7% spontaneous abortions in the 2 weeks following the procedure[134]. In centres for prenatal medicine, cordocentesis is now an established method of diagnosis which does not even require fetal anaesthesia, because there are no pain receptors in the umbilical cord.

However, fetal blood can also be obtained with a high degree of success and safety by puncture of the intrahepatic umbilical vein[123]. This has the advantage that there are no umbilical arteries in the vicinity, which are the main cause of complications with cord puncture.

Other factors that influence fetal loss rate after fetal blood sampling are gestational age and the indication for performing the procedure. The risk is higher before 20 weeks[135], and if the fetus has a life-threatening condition[136].

In recent years, fetal blood sampling has been declining in frequency for several reasons:

- the increasing use of molecular techniques for the prenatal diagnosis of genetic disorders and of fetal infections such as toxoplasmosis, and for fetal Rh and platelet genotyping;
- the development of molecular cytogenetics using fluorescent *in situ* hybridization (FISH) for chromosomal analysis;
- the increasing use of late CVS (placental biopsy) for fetal karyotyping; and
- improvement in the non-invasive assessment of Rh alloimmunization and intrauterine growth retardation.

REFERENCES

1. Lambl D. Ein seltener Fall von Hydramnios. *Zentralbl. Gynekol.* **5**:329, 1881.
2. Schatz F. Eine besondere Art von einseitiger Polyhydramnie mit anderstseitiger Oligohydramnie bei Zwillingen. *Arch. Gynecol.* **19**:329, 1882.
3. Aburel ME. Le déclenchement du travail par injections intraamniotique de serum sale hypertonique. *Gynaecol. Obstet.* **36**:398, 1937.
4. Fuchs F & Riis P. Antenatal sex determination. *Nature* **117**:330, 1956.
5. Makowski EL, Prem K & Kaiser IH. Detection of sex of fetuses by the incidence of sex chromatin in nuclei of cells in amniotic fluid. *Science* **123**:542, 1956.
6. Steele MW & Breg WR. Chromosome analysis of human amniotic fluid cells. *Lancet* **i**:383–385, 1966.
7. Nadler HL. Antenatal detection of hereditary disorders. *Pediatrics* **42**:912–918, 1968.
8. Nadler HL & Gerbie AB. Role of amniocentesis in the intrauterine detection of genetic disorders. *N. Engl. J. Med.* **282**:596–599, 1970.
9. Foulon W, Naessens A, de Catte L & Arny J-J. Detection of congenital toxoplasmosis by chorionic villus sampling and early amniocentesis. *Am. J. Obstet Gynecol.* **163**:1511–1513, 1990.

10. Hohlfeld P, Daffos F, Costa JM, Thulliez P, Forestier F & Vidaud M. Prenatal diagnosis of congenital toxoplasmosis with a polymerase chain reaction test on amniotic fluid. *N. Engl. J. Med.* **331**:695–699, 1994.
11. Lipitz S, Yagel S, Shalev E, Achiron R, Maschiach S & Schiff E. Prenatal diagnosis of fetal primary cytomegalovirus infection. *Obstet. Gynecol.* **89**:763, 1997.
12. Kustermann A, Zoppini C, Tassis B, Della Morte M, Colucci G & Nicolini U. Prenatal diagnosis of congenital varicella infection. *Prenat. Diagn.* **16**:71–74, 1996.
13. D'Alton ME, Malone FD, Chelmow D, Ward BE & Bianchi DW. Defining the role of fluorescence *in situ* hybridization on uncultured amniocytes for prenatal diagnosis of aneuploidies. *Am. J. Obstet. Gynecol.* **176**:769–776, 1997.
14. Simpson JL, Socol ML, Aladem S *et al.* Normal fetal growth despite persistent amniotic fluid leakage after genetic amniocentesis. *Prenat. Diagn.* **1**:277, 1981.
15. Berner HW, Seisler EP & Barlow J. Fetal cardiac tamponade. A complication of amniocentesis. *Obstet. Gynecol.* **40**:599, 1972.
16. Hyman CJ, Depp, R, Pahravan P *et al.* Pneumothorax complicating amniocentesis. *Obstet. Gynecol.* **41**:43, 1973.
17. Gottdiener JS, Ellison C & Lorenzo RC. Arteriovenous fistula after fetal penetration at amniocentesis. *N. Engl. J. Med.* **293**:1302, 1975.
18. Lamb MP. Gangrene of a fetal limb due to amniocentesis. *Br. J. Obstet. Gynaecol.* **82**:829, 1975.
19. Cross HE. Ocular trauma during amniocentesis. *Arch. Ophthalmol.* **90**:303, 1973.
20. Working Party on Amniocentesis An assessment of hazards of amniocentesis. *Br. J. Obstet. Gynaecol.* **85**(suppl. 2): 1, 1978.
21. Simpson NE, Dallaire L, Miller JR *et al.* Prenatal diagnosis of genetic disease in Canada: report of a collaborative study. *Can. Med. Ass. J.* **15**:739, 1976.
22. Baird, PA, Yee IM & Sadovnick AM. Population-based study of long-term outcomes after amniocentesis. *Lancet* **344**:1582, 1994.
23. NICHD-National Registry for Amniocentesis-Study Group. Mid-trimester amniocentesis for prenatal diagnosis. Safety and accuracy. *JAMA* **236**:1471, 1976.
24. Tabor A, Madsen M, Obel EB *et al.* Randomised controlled trial of genetic amniocentesis in 4606 low-risk women. *Lancet* **i**:1287, 1986.
25. Finberg HJ & Frigoletto FD. Sonographic demonstration of uterine contraction during amniocentesis. *Am. J. Obstet. Gynecol.* **139**:740, 1981.
26. Bombard AT, Powers JF, Carter S, Schwartz A & Nitowsky HM. Procedure-related fetal losses in transplacental versus nontransplacental genetic amniocentesis. *Am. J. Obstet. Gynecol.* **172**:868–872, 1995.
27. Golbus MS, Stephens JD, Cann HM *et al.* Rh-isoimmunization following genetic amniocentesis. *Prenat. Diagn.* **2**:149, 1982.
28. Murray JC, Karp LE, Williamson RA *et al.* Rh isoimmunization related to amniocentesis. *Am. J. Med. Genet.* **16**:527, 1983.
29. Miles JH & Kaback HD. Rh immune globulin after genetic amniocentesis. *Clin. Genet. Res.* **27**:103A, 1979.
30. Hanson FW, Zorn EM & Tennant FR. Amniocentesis before 15 weeks' gestation: Outcome, risks, and technical problems. *Am. J. Obstet. Gynecol.* **156**:1524, 1987.
31. Pruggmayer MRK, Jahoda MGJ, Van der Pol JG *et al.* Genetic amniocentesis in twin pregnancies: results of a multicenter study of 529 cases. *Ultrasound Obstet. Gynecol.* **315**:336, 1992.
32. Anderson RL, Goldberg JD & Golbus MS. Prenatal diagnosis in multiple gestation: 20 years' experience with amniocentesis. *Prenat. Diagn.* **11**:263, 1991.
33. Jeanty P, Shah D & Roussis P. Single-needle insertion in twin amniocentesis. *J. Ultrasound Med.* **9**:511, 1990.
34. Pruggmayer MRK, Jahoda MGJ, van der Pol JG *et al.* Genetic amniocentesis in twin pregnancies: results of a multicenter study of 529 cases. *Ultrasound Obstet. Gynecol.* **2**:6–10, 1992.
35. Sebire NJ, Noble PL, Odibo A, Malligiannis P & Nicolaides KH. Single uterine entry for genetic amniocentesis in twin pregnancies. *Ultrasound Obstet. Gynecol.* **7**:26–31, 1996.
36. Bravo RR, Shulman LP, Phillips OP, Grevengood, C & Martens PR. Transplacental needle passage in early amniocentesis and pregnancy loss. *Obstet. Gynecol.* **86**:437–440, 1995.
37. Nicolaides K, de Lourdes Brizot M, Patel F & Snijders R. Comparison of chrorion villus sampling and early amniocentesis for karyotyping in 1492 singleton pregnancies. *Fetal. Diagn. Ther.* **11**:9–15, 1996.
38. Brandenburg H, Jahoda MGJ, Pijpers L, Reuss A, Kleyer WJ & Wladimiroff JW. Fetal loss rate after chorionic villus sampling and subsequent amniocentesis. *Am. J. Med. Genet.* **35**:178–180, 1991.
39. Assel BG, Lewis SM, Dickerman LH, Park VM & Jassani MN. Single-operator comparison of early and mid-second-trimester amniocentesis. *Obstet. Gynecol.* **79**:940–944, 1992.
40. Lockwood DH & Neu RL. Cytogenetic analysis of 1375 amniotic fluid specimens from pregnancies with gestational age less than 14 weeks. *Prenat. Diagn.* **13**:801–805, 1993.
41. Daniel A, Ng A, Kuah KB, Reiha S & Malafiej P. A study of early amniocentesis for prenatal cytogenetic diagnosis. *Prenat. Diagn.* **18**:21–28, 1988.
42. Diaz Vega M, De La Cueva P, Leal C & Aisa F. Early amniocentesis at 10–12 weeks' gestation. *Prenat. Diagn.* **16**:307–312, 1996.
43. Evans MI, Drugan A, Koppitch III MS *et al.* Genetic diagnosis in the first trimester: The norm for the 1990s. *Am. J. Obstet. Gynecol.* **160**:1332, 1989.
44. Elejalde BR, de Elejalde MM & Acuna JM. Prospective study of amniocentesis performed between weeks 9 and 16 of gestation: Its feasibility, risks, complications and use in early genetic prenatal diagnosis. *Am. J. Med. Genet.* **35**:188, 1990.
45. Byrne D, Marks K, Azar G & Nicolaides KH. Randomized study of early amniocentesis versus chorionic villus sampling: a technical and cytogenic comparison of 650 patients. *Ultrasound Obstet. Gynecol.* **1**:235, 1991.
46. Stripparo L, Buscaglia M & Longatti L. Genetic amniocentesis: 505 cases performed before the sixteenth week of gestation. *Prenat. Diagn.* **10**:359, 1990.
47. Hackett GA, Smith JH, Rebello CTH *et al.* Early amniocentesis at 11–14 weeks gestation for the diagnosis of fetal chromosomal abnormality. A clinical evaluation. *Prenat. Diagn.* **11**:311, 1991.
48. Rooney DE, MacLachlan N, Smith J *et al.* Early amniocentesis: a cytological evaluation. *Br. Med. J.* **299**:25, 1989.
49. Sundberg K, Smidt-Jensen S & Philip J. Amniocentesis with increased cell yield, obtained by filtration and reinjection of the amniotic fluid. *Ultrasound Obstet. Gynecol.* **1**:91, 1991.
50. Byrne DL, Marks K, Braude PR & Nicolaides KH. Amniofiltration in the first trimester: feasibility, technical aspects and cytological outcome. *Ultrasound Obstet. Gynecol.* **1**:320, 1991.
51. Sundberg K, Bang J, Smidt-Jensen S, Brocks V, Lundsteen C, Parner J *et al.* Randomised study of risk of fetal loss related to early amniocentesis versus chorionic villus sampling. *Lancet* **350**:697–703, 1997.
52. Johnson JM, Wilson RD, Winsor EJT, Singer J, Dansereau J & Kalousek DK. The early amniocentesis study: A randomized clinical trial of early amniocentesis versus midtrimester amniocentesis. *Fetal Diagn. Ther.* **11**:85–93, 1996.
53. Wilson RD, Johnson JM, Windrim R *et al.* The early amniocentesis study: a randomized clinical trial of early amniocentesis and midtrimester amniocentesis. *Fetal Diagn. Ther.* **12**:97–101, 1997.
54. The Canadian Early and Mid-trimester Amniocentesis Trial (CEMAT) Group. Randomised trial to assess safety and fetal outcome of early and midtrimester amniocentesis. *Lancet* **351**:242–247, 1998.
55. Crandall BF, Kulch P & Tabsh K. Risk assessment of amniocentesis between 11 and 15 weeks: comparison to later amniocentesis controls. *Prenat. Diagn.* **14**:913–919, 1994.
56. Djalali M, Barbi G, Kennerknecht & Terinde R. Introduction of early amniocentesis to routine prenatal diagnosis. *Prenat. Diagn.* **12**:661–669, 1992.
57. Eiben B, Goebel R, Hansen S & Hammans W. Early amniocentesis – a cytogenetic evaluation of over 1500 cases. *Prenat. Diagn.* **14**:497–501, 1994.
58. Brumfield CG, Cloud GA, Davis RO, Finley SC, Hauth JC & Boots L. The relationship between maternal serum and amniotic fluid α-fetoprotein in women undergoing early amniocentesis. *Am. J. Obstet Gynecol.* **163**:903–906, 1990.
59. Eiben B, Goebel R, Hansen S & Hammans W. Alpha-fetoprotein and AChE in early amniocentesis. *Prenat. Diagn.* **16**:87–88, 1996.
60. Brumfield CG, Lin S, Conner W, Cosper P, Davis RO & Owen J. Pregnancy outcome following genetic amniocentesis at 11–14 versus 16–19 weeks' gestation. *Obstet. Gynecol.* **88**:114–118, 1996.

61. Eiben B, Hammans W, Hansen S *et al.* On the complication risk of early amniocentesis versus standard amniocentesis. *Fetal Diagn Ther.* **12**:140–144, 1997.
62. Nicolaides K, de Lourdes Brizot M, Patel F & Snijders R. Comparison of chorionic villus sampling and amniocentesis for fetal karyotyping at 10–13 weeks' gestation. *Lancet* **344**:435–439, 1994.
63. Stranc LC, Evans JA & Hamerton JL. Chorionic villus sampling and amniocentesis for prenatal diagnosis. *Lancet* **349**:711–714, 1997.
64. Ward RHT, Modell B, Petrou M *et al.* Method of sampling chorionic villi in first trimester of pregnancy under guidance of realtime ultrasound. *Br. Med. J.* **286**:1542, 1983.
65. Vaughan J & Rodeck CH. Interventional procedures. In *Clinical Ultrasound – A Comprehensive Text. Ultrasound in Obstetrics and Gynaecology* (eds K. Dewbury, H. Meire & D. Cosgrove), p. 463. Edinburgh: Churchill-Livingstone, 1992.
66. Holzgreve W & Miny P. Improved echogenicity of the catheter for chorionic villi sampling. In *First Trimester Fetal Diagnosis* (eds M. Fracare, G. Simoni & B. Brambati), p. 64. Berlin: Springer, 1985.
67. Smidt-Jensen S & Hahnemann N. Transabdominal fine needle biopsy from chorionic villi in the first trimester. *Prenat. Diagn.* **4**:163, 1984.
68. Cederholm M & Axelsson O. A prospective comparative study on transabdominal chorionic villus sampling and amniocentesis performed at 10–13 weeks' gestation. *Prenat. Diagn.* **17**:311–317, 1997.
69. Fletcher JC. Ethical issues in clinical trials of first trimester prenatal diagnosis. In *Chorionic Villus Sampling* (eds B. Brambati & G. Simoni), p. 2.
70. Perry TB, Vekemans MJJ, Lippmann A, Hamilton, EF & Fournier PJR. Chorionic villi sampling: clinical experience, immediate complications, and patients' attitudes. *Am. J. Obstet. Gynecol.* **151**:161–166, 1985.
71. Lippmann A, Perry TB, Mandel S & Cartier L. Chorionic villi sampling: women's attitudes. *Am. J. Med. Genet.* **22**:395–401, 1985.
72. McGovern MM, Goldberg JD & Desnick RJ. Acceptability of chorionic villi sampling for prenatal diagnosis. *Am. J. Obstet. Gynecol.* **155**:25–29, 1986.
73. MRC Working Party on the Evaluation of Chorion Villus Sampling. Medical Research Council European Trial of Chorion Villus Sampling. *Lancet* **337**:1491, 1991.
74. Abramsky L & Rodeck CH. Women's choices for fetal chromosome analysis. *Prenat. Diagn.* **11**:23, 1991.
75. Canadian Collaborative CVS Amniocentesis Clinical Trial Group. Multicentre randomised clinical trial of chorion villus sampling and amniocentesis. First report. *Lancet* **i**:1–6, 1989.
76. Rhoads GG, Jackson LG, Schlesselmann SE *et al.* The safety and efficacy of chorionic villus sampling for early prenatal diagnosis of cytogenetic abnormalities. *N. Engl. J. Med.* **320**:609, 1989.
77. Firth HV, Boyd PA, Chamberlain P *et al.* Limb abnormalities and chorion villus sampling. *Lancet* **ii**:51, 1991.
78. Schloo R, Miny P, Holzgreve W *et al.* Distal limb deficiency following chorionic villus sampling? *Am. J. Med. Genet.* **42**:404, 1992.
79. Froster UG & Jackson L. Limb defects and chorionic villus sampling: results from an international registry, 1992–94. *Lancet* **347**:489–494, 1996.
80. Evans JA & Hamerton JL. Limb defects and chorionic villus sampling. *Lancet* **347**:484–485, 1996.
81. Brambati B, Terzian E & Tognoni G. Randomized clinical trial of transabdominal versus transcervical chorionic villus sampling methods. *Prenat. Diagn.* **11**:285, 1991.
82. Smidt-Jensen S & Philip J. Comparison of transabdominal and transcervical CVS and amniocentesis: sampling success and risk. *Prenat. Diagn.* **11**:529, 1991.
83. Johada MGJ, Pijpers L, Reuss A & Sachs ES. Transabdominale Chorionzentese für die schnelle Diagnostik im zweiten Trimenon: Erfahrungen bei 147 Schwangeren. *Z. Geburtsh. Perinat.* **192**:101, 1988.
84. Young SR, Shipley CF, Wade RV *et al.* Single-center comparison of results of 1000 prenatal diagnoses with chorionic villus sampling and 1000 diagnoses with amniocentesis. *Am. J. Obstet. Gynecol.* **165**:255–263, 1991.
85. Kalousek DK, Barrett IJ & Gärtner AB. Spontaneous abortion and confined placental mosaicism. *Hum. Genet.* **88**:642–646, 1992.
86. Henderson KG, Shaw TE, Barrett IJ, Telenius AHP & Wilson RD. Distribution of mosaicism in human placentae. *Hum. Genet.* **97**:650–654, 1996.
87. Roberts E, Stevenson K, Cole T, Redford DHA & Davison EV. Prospective prenatal diagnosis of Prader–Willi syndrome due to maternal disomy for chromosome 15 following trisomic zygote rescue. *Prenat. Diagn.* **17**:780–783, 1997.
88. Miny P, Basaran S, Pawlowitzki IH *et al.* Validity of cytogenic analyses from trophoblast tissue throughout gestation. *Am. J. Med. Genet.* **33**:136, 1989.
89. Purvis-Smith SG, Saville T, Manass S, Yip MY, Lam-Po-Tang PR, Duffy B, Johnston H, Leigh D & McDonald B. Uniparental disomy 15 resulting from 'correction' of an initial trisomy 15. *Am. J. Hum. Genet.* **50**:1348, 1992.
90. Kalousek DK, Lang LS, Barrett I, Yam I, Wilson DR, Howarth-Pebles PN, Johnson MP & Giorgiutti E. Uniparental disomy for chromosome 16 in humans. *Am. J. Hum. Genet.* **52**:8, 1993.
91. Rodeck C, Tutschek B, Scherlock J & Kingdom J. Methods for the transcervical collection of fetal cells during the first trimester of pregnancy. *Prenat. Diagn.* **15**:933–942, 1995.
92. Nicolaides KH, Soothill PW, Rodeck GH, Warren RC & Gosden CM. Why confine chorionic villus (placental) biopsy to the first trimester? Lancet **i**:543–544, 1986.
93. Holzgreve W, Miny P, Gerlach B, Westendorp A, Ahlert D & Horst J. Benefits of placental biopsies for rapid karyotyping in the second and third trimester (late chorionic villus sampling) in high-risk pregnancies. *Am. J. Obstet. Gynecol.* **162**:1188–1192, 1990.
94. Podobnik M, Ciglar S, Singer Z, Podobnik-Sarkanji S, Duic Z & Skalak D. Transabdominal chorionic villus sampling in the second and third trimesters of high-risk pregnancies. *Prenat. Diagn.* **17**:125–133, 1997.
95. Ko T-M, Tseng L-H, Hwa H-L, Lee T-Y & Chuang S-M. Prenatal diagnosis by transabdominal chorionic villus sampling in the second and third trimesters. *Arch. Gynecol. Obstet.* **56**:193–197, 1995.
96. Borrell A, Costa D, Delgado, RD *et al.* Transcervical chorionic villus sampling beyond 12 weeks of gestation. *Ultrasound Obstet. Gynecol.* **7**:416–420, 1996.
97. Holzgreve W, Miny P, Basaran S, Fuhrmann W & Beller FK. Safety of placental biopsy in the second and third trimesters. *N. Engl. J. Med.* **317**:1159, 1987.
98. Hogdall CK, Doran TA, Shime J, Wilson S & Teshima I. Transabdominal chorionic villus sampling in the second trimester. *Am. J. Obstet. Gynecol.* **158**:345–349, 1988.
99. Chieri de PR & Aldini JR. Feasibility of placental biopsy in the second trimester for fetal diagnosis. *Am. J. Obstet. Gynecol.* **160**:581, 1989.
100. Rodeck CH, Sheldrake A, Beattie B & Whittle MJ. Maternal serum alpha-fetoprotein after placental damage in chorion villus sampling. *Lancet* **341**:500, 1993.
101. Scrimgeour JB. Other techniques for antenatal diagnosis. In *Antenatal Diagnosis of Genetic Disease* (ed. A.E.H. Emery), p. 40, 1973.
102. Westin B. Technique and estimation of oxygenation of the human fetus *in utero* by means of hysterophotography. *Acta Paediatr. Scand.* **46**:117, 1957.
103. Mandelbaum B, Pontarelli D & Brushenko A. Amnioscopy for prenatal transfusion. *Am. J. Obstet. Gynecol.* **98**:1140, 1967.
104. Valenti C. Endoamnioscopy and fetal biopsy: a new technique. *Am. J. Obstet. Gynecol.* **114**:561, 1972.
105. Valenti C. Antenatal detection of hemoglobinopathies. A preliminary report. *Am. J. Obstet. Gynecol.* **115**:851–853, 1973.
106. Hobbins JC & Mahoney MJ. *In utero* diagnosis of hemoglobinopathies: technique for obtaining fetal blood. *N. Engl. J. Med.* **290**:1065, 1974.
107. Rodeck C & Campbell S. Umbilical cord blood insertion as source of pure fetal blood for prenatal diagnosis. *Lancet* **i**:1244, 1979.
108. Antsaklis A. Fetoskopische Blutentnahmen zur pränatalen Diagnostik von Hämoglobinopathien. In *Pränatale Medizin* (ed. W. Holzgreve) p. 68. Berlin: Springer, 1987.
109. Hobbins JC. The future of first-trimester embryoscopy. *Ultrasound Obstet. Gynecol.* **8**:3–4, 1996.
110. Reece EA, Rotmensch S, Whetham J, Cullen MT & Hobbins JC. Embroyscopy: A closer look at first-trimester diagnosis and treatment. *Am. J. Obstet. Gynecol.* **166**:775–780, 1992.

111. Hobbins JC, Jones OW, Gottesfeld S & Persutte W. Transvaginal ultrasonography and transabdominal embryoscopy in the first-trimester diagnosis of Smith–Lemli–Opitz syndrome, type II. *Am. J. Obstet. Gynecol.* **171**:546–549, 1994.
112. Quintero RA, Abuhamad A, Hobbins JC, Mahoney MJ. Transabdominal thin gauge embryo fetoscopy: a technique for early prenatal diagnosis and its use in the diagnosis of a case of Meckel–Gruber syndrome. *Am. J. Obstet. Gynecol.* **168**:1552–1557, 1993.
113. Dommergues M, Lemerrer M, Couly G, Delezoides Al & Dumez Y. Prenatal diagnosis of cleft lip at 11 menstrual weeks using embryoscopy in the Van der Woude syndrome. *Prenat. Diagn.* **15**:378–381, 1995.
114. Cullen MT, Reece EA, Whetham J & Hobbins JC. Embryoscopy: Description and utility of a new technique. *Am. J. Obstet. Gynecol.* **162**:82–86, 1990.
115. Reece EA, Homko C, Goldstein I & Wiznitzer A. Toward fetal therapy using needle embryofetoscopy. *Ultrasound Obstet. Gynecol.* **5**:281–285, 1995.
116. Ville Y, Bernard JP, Doumerc S, Multori O, Fernandez H, Frydman R *et al.* Transabdominal fetoscopy in fetal anomalies diagnosed by ultrasound in the first trimester of pregnancy. *Ultrasound Obstet. Gynecol.* **8**:11–15, 1996.
117. Dumez Y. Embryoscopy and congenital malformations. *Proceedings of International Conference on Chorionic Villus Sampling and Early Prenatal Diagnosis* 28–29 May, 1990 Athens.
118. Holbrook, KA, Dale BA, Williams ML, Perry TB, Hoff MS, Hamilton EF, Fisher C & Senikas V. The expression of congenital ichthyosiform erythroderma in second trimester fetuses of the same family: morphologic and biochemical studies. *J. Invest. Dermatol.* **91**:521, 1988.
119. Rodeck CH, Eady RAJ & Gosden CM. Prenatal diagnosis of epidermolysis bullosa letalis. *Lancet* **i**:949, 1986.
120. Adzick NS & Longaker MT. Scarless fetal healing. Therapeutic implications. *Ann. Surg.* **215**:3, 1992.
121. Rodeck C, Patrick AD, Pembrey ME, Tzannatos C & Whitfield AE. Fetal liver biopsy for prenatal diagnosis of ornithine carbamyl transferase deficiency. *Lancet* **ii**:297, 1982.
122. Holzgreve W & Golbus MS. Prenatal diagnosis of ornithine transcarbamylase deficiency utilizing fetal liver biopsy. *Am. J. Hum. Genet.* **36**:320–328, 1984.
123. Evans MI, Greb A, Kunkel LM et al. In utero fetal muscle biopsy for the diagnosis of Duchenne muscular dystrophy. *Am. J. Obstet. Gynecol.* **165**:728, 1991.
124. Golbus MS, McGonigle KF, Goldberg JD, Filly RA, Callen PW & Anderson RL. Fetal tissue sampling: the San Francisco experience with 190 pregnancies. *West. J. Med.* **150**:423–430, 1989.
125. Lenz S, Lund-Hansen T, Bang J & Christensen E. A possible prenatal evaluation of renal function by amino acid analysis on fetal urine. *Prenat. Diagn.* **5**:259, 1985.
126. Holzgreve W, Lison A & Bulla M. SDS-PAGE as an additional test to determine fetal kidney function prior to intrauterine diversion of urinary tract obstruction. *Fetal Diagnosis and Therapy* **4**:93–96, 1989.
127. Daffos F, Capella-Pavlovsky M & Forestier F. A new procedure for fetal blood sampling *in utero:* preliminary results of 53 cases. *Am. J. Obstet. Gynecol.* **146**:985–987, 1983.
128. Forestier F, Hohlfeld P, Vial Y, Olin V, Andreux J-P & Tissot J-D. Blood smears and prenatal diagnosis. *Br. J Haematol* **95**:278–280, 1996.
129. Daffos F, Capella-Pavlovsky, M & Forestier F. Fetal blood sampling during pregnancy with use of a needle guided by ultrasound: a study of 606 consecutive cases. *Am. J. Obstet. Gynecol.* **153**:655, 1985.
130. Holmberg L, Gustavii B & Jonsson A. A prenatal study of fetal platelet count and size with application to fetus at risk for Wiskott–Aldrich syndrome. *J. Pediatr.* **102**:773, 1983.
131. Newburger PE, Cohen HJ, Rotchild SB *et al.* Prenatal diagnosis of chronic granulomatous disease. *N. Engl. J. Med.* **300**:178, 1979.
132. Linch DC, Beverly PC, Levinsky, RJ & Rodeck CH. Phenotypic analysis of fetal blood leucocytes: potential for prenatal diagnosis of immunodeficiency disorders. *Prenat. Diagn.* **2**:211, 1982.
133. Weiner C & Okamura K. Diagnostic fetal blood sampling—technique related losses. *Fetal Diagn. Ther.* **11**:169–175, 1996.
134. Buscaglia M, Ghisoni L, Bellotti M *et al.* Percutaneous umbilical blood sampling: indication changes and procedure loss rate in a nine years' experience. *Fetal Diagn. Ther.* **11**:106–113, 1996.
135. Orlandi F, Damiani G, Jakli C, Lauricello S, Bertolino O & Maggio A. The risk of early cordocentesis (12–21 weeks): analysis of 500 procedures. *Prenat. Diagn.* **10**:425–429, 1990.
136. Antsaklis A, Daskalakis G, Papantouiou N & Nicholas S. Fetal blood sampling indicating related losses. *Prenat. Diagn.* **18**:934–940, 1999.

Trends in cytogenetics

37

J. Philip and T. Bryndorf

Introduction

Human cytogenetics originated from the demonstration in 1956 that the human diploid chromosome number is 46[1]. Clinical cytogenetics is the study of chromosome structure and behaviour in relationship to clinical syndromes. Application of this knowledge for the diagnosis and screening of chromosome disease has been made possible by improvements in tissue culture, chromosome preparation and specific staining techniques to obtain banded chromosomes, in situ hybridization, computerized metaphase-finding and semi-automation of karyotyping. Chromosome analysis is performed on cells in metaphase after they undergo hypotonic treatment, fixation and staining. Originally, cytogenetic analysis was based on chromosome counting and categorization into seven groups. However, following the introduction of chromosome banding techniques, identification of each chromosome in the human complement, as well as a much more detailed analysis of structural abnormalities, became possible[2].

Chromosome banding can be produced by either fluorescent or non-fluorescent methods. For diagnoses of small abnormalities, e.g., microdeletions, elongated chromosomes in prometaphase are used. In situ hybridization techniques are also available for diagnosis of such abnormalities.

The normal human chromosome complement is illustrated in Fig. 37.1.

Chromosome abnormalities

NUMERICAL CHROMOSOME ABNORMALITIES (ANEUPLOIDIES)

Numerical chromosome abnormalities consist of monosomies (absence of one chromosome of a pair or of one sex chromosome), trisomies (three copies of a specific chromosome) and rarely, tetrasomy (four copies of a specific chromosome). In triploidy each chromosome in the complement is represented three times instead of two, the total chromosome number being 69.

Most monosomies and trisomies are lethal early in pregnancy. Trisomies 13, 18 (Fig. 37.2) and 21 and sex chromosome abnormalities are the most frequent chromosome aberrations present in newborns. Non-disjunction and anaphase lag are the two most frequent mechanisms responsible for numerical abnormalities.

STRUCTURAL CHROMOSOME ABNORMALITIES

A translocation involves transfer of genetic material between two chromosomes. As a consequence of translocation, genetic material may be lost or gained, or simply exchanged. Translocations may therefore be unbalanced or balanced.

- Unbalanced translocations cause partial trisomies or monosomies of the involved chromosomes. Balanced translocations frequently involve the acrocentric chromosomes, 13, 14, 15, 21, and 22 and are termed 'Robertsonian translocations'. Balanced translocations involving chromosomes other than the acrocentric chromosomes are termed 'reciprocal'
- Balanced translocations which may be familial do not appear to have obvious clinical consequences. There is, however, an increased risk of unbalanced translocations in the offspring. Distinguishing between balanced and unbalanced translocations is often difficult using conventional techniques. In situ hybridization (ISH) with probes that 'paint' entire chromosomes is often helpful in solving more complicated cases of structural rearrangements (Plates 37.1 and 37.2).

Although relatively rare, balanced de novo chromosome rearrangements and de novo marker chromosomes can arise during gametogenesis. Translocations which microscopically

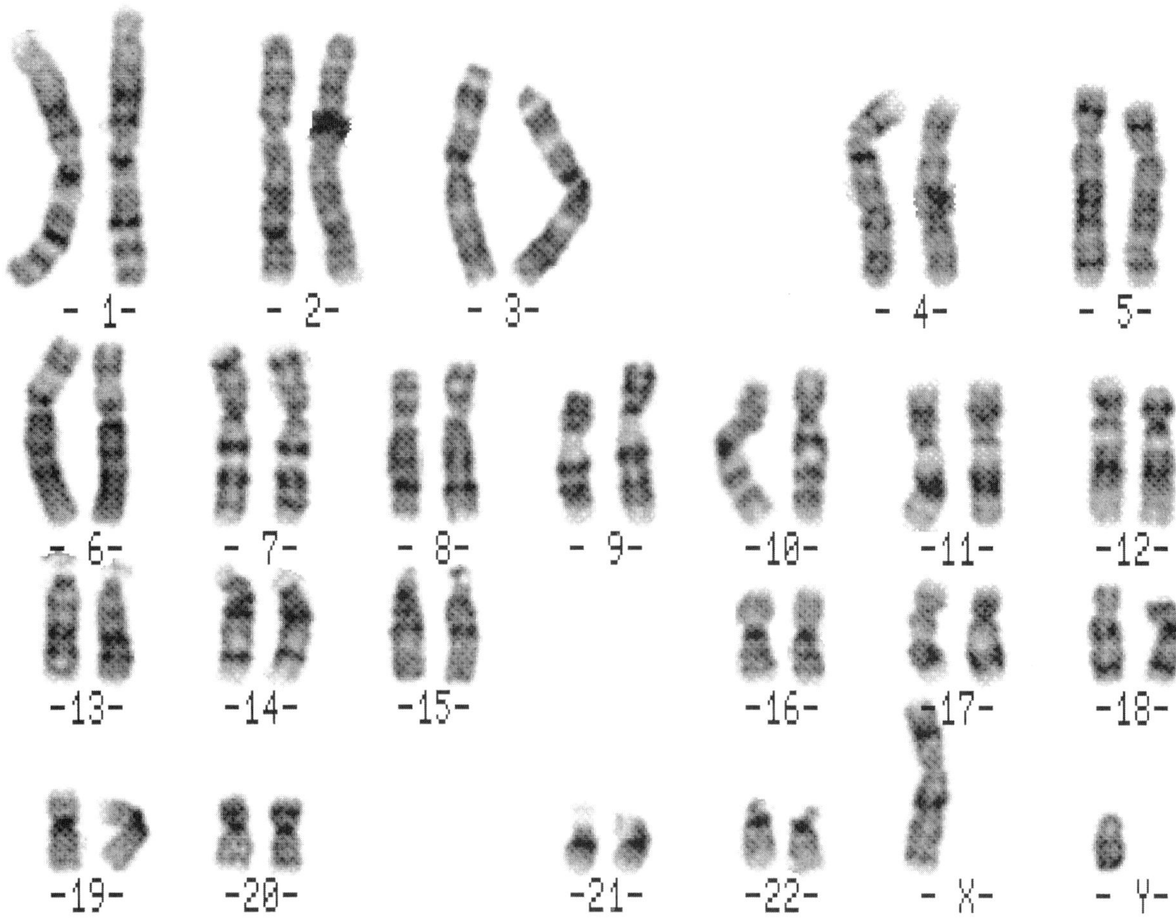

Fig. 37.1 G-banded chromosomes from a normal blood sample. The karyotype is 46, XY. For classical/conventional cytogenetic analysis the chromosome numbers in 10–15 metaphases are counted, and the structure and band pattern of the chromosomes is analysed. A karyotype is constructed by placing the chromosomes in pairs (homologues). The pairs are ordered according to size, centromere position and morphology (band pattern). Metaphase chromosomes have two chromatids, united at the centromere. The centromere is in the middle (metacentric) or to one side of the middle (submetacentric) or near the end (acrocentric). The short chromosome arm is designated the p arm, the long arm the q arm.

There are 22 pairs of autosomes (1–22) and two sex chromosomes (X and Y). Males have one X- and one Y-chromosome, while females have two X-chromosomes, one of them being partially inactivated[108].

Band patterns depend on the staining methods applied. The choice of staining method depends on the purpose. Routine staining is either by Giemsa (G-bands) or by fluorescent stains (Q-bands), which give similar patterns. Banding techniques which give opposite patterns to Giemsa are called R-band techniques.

Methods which stain telomeres (T-bands) or centromeres (C-bands) are used for specific purposes. Description of chromosome bands, including chromosome abnormalities, should be according to: An international system for human cytogenetic nomenclature (Mitelman F (ed); S Karger, Basel, 1995).

appear balanced may actually be submicroscopically unbalanced. In a similar fashion, small chromosome deletions, breaks within genes and other forms of rearrangement of genetic material may cause congenital malformations, but may not be detectable with current cytogenetic techniques.

De novo *balanced* translocations detected prenatally therefore represent a diagnostic dilemma. Little information is available regarding clinical prognoses in prenatally diagnosed translocations that appear balanced and in the case of supernumerary marker chromosomes of unknown origin[3]. Rather than depend on only risk figures for counselling about clinical prognosis, such newly developed ISH techniques as chromosome specific painting, reverse painting, and comparative genomic hybridization CGH (see below) may provide a specific diagnosis and the basis for decisions regarding continuation of a pregnancy.

A comprehensive study on the frequencies and clinical consequences of de novo balanced chromosome rearrangement and marker chromosomes was reported by Warburton[3]. The study was based on 377 357 pregnancies undergoing amniocenteses. One in 2000 pregnancies had a de novo reciprocal translocation, 1/9000 a de novo Robertsonian translocation, 1/10 000 a de novo inversion and 1/2500 a marker chromosome.

The indications for the amniocenteses were not described. Pregnancies in which abnormalities were diagnosed by ultra-

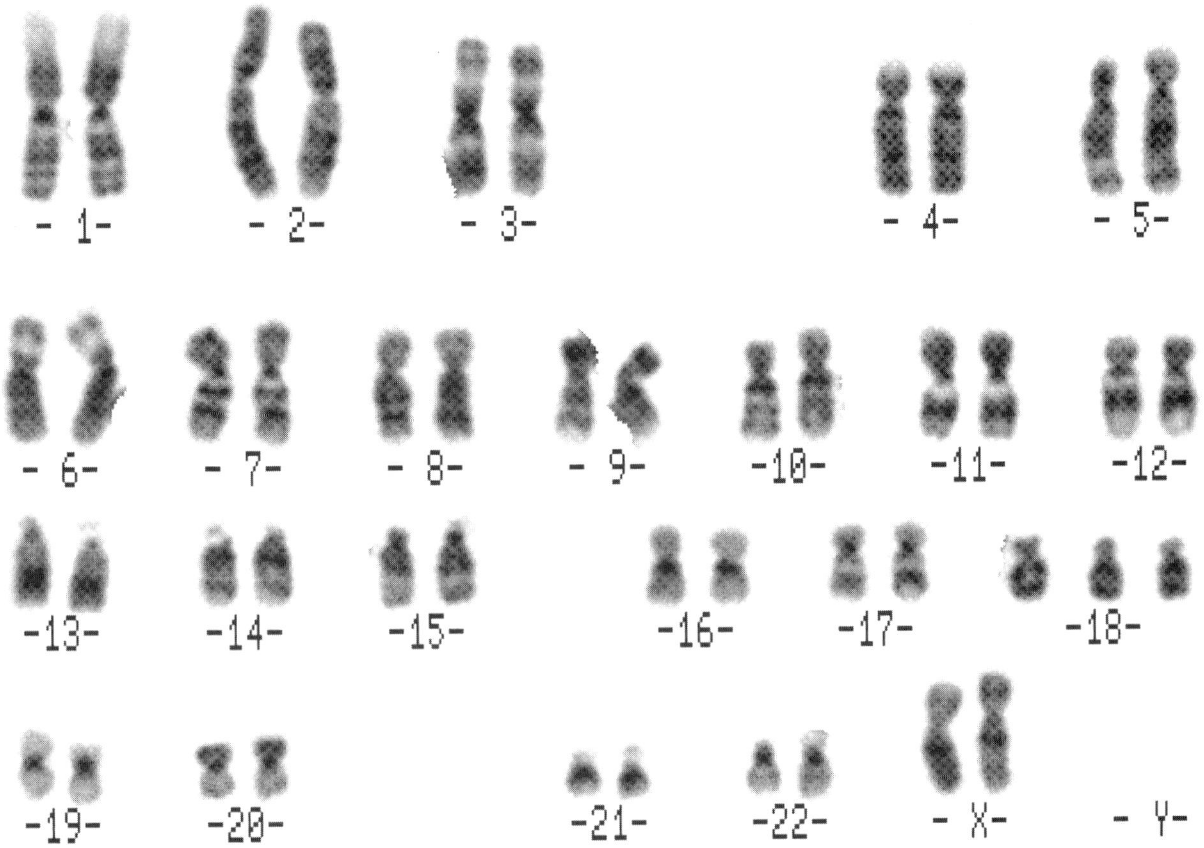

Fig. 37.2 G-banded chromosomes from a chorionic villus sample from a female with Edward's syndrome. The karyotype is 47, XX, +18.

sound before amniocentesis were excluded. Physical abnormalities associated with de novo structural abnormalities were as follows:

- Reciprocal translocations, 6.1%
- Robertsonian translocations, 3.7%
- Inversions, 9.4%

According to Warburton[3] the risk of a congenital abnormality in pregnancies with translocations and inversions was too small to correlate the chromosomal aberrations with congenital malformations. For marker chromosomes, the overall risk of somatic abnormalities was 13% (range 6.9–19.1%). This figure is definitely increased compared with the figures for the newborn. The nature of the material[3] did not allow systematic follow up. Clinical information about the somatic abnormalities was limited, and the frequencies of abnormalities may thus be misleading. The frequency of these chromosomal rearrangements at birth is estimated to be 0.067–0.07%.

Risk figures relevant in counselling pregnant women should be based on their occurrence in term pregnancies (and not at the time of amniocentesis).

The risk of *somatic abnormalities* associated with these rearrangements in the newborn may be slightly elevated but can be as high as 10%, compared with the average figure of 2–3% in the newborn.

The risk of *mental retardation* among carriers of de novo translocations is not known. However, among the mentally retarded, the frequency of de novo rearrangements is 0.24%. This is two to three times higher than among liveborn children[3].

Isochromosomes presumably arise by misdivision of the centromere and consist of two copies of one of the chromosome arms (duplication). At the same time, genetic material from the other arm is lacking (deletion). Duplications, insertions, and deletions of chromosomal material may also occur as a consequence of divisional errors during crossing over in meiosis, or be due to abnormal breaking and unification. Inversions within a chromosome results from two breaks, the segment between the breaks being rotated 180°.

Fragile sites represent apparent gaps between chromosome segments, giving the appearance of chromosome breakage. A fragile site at the end of the long arm of the X chromosome (Xq27.3) is associated with the Martin–Bell syndrome.

FRAGILE X SYNDROME

Fragile X syndrome is the most frequent familial cause of mental retardation in males and occurs with a frequency of 1:1000–1500. The molecular genetic findings (see later) explain to a large part the higher frequency of mental retardation in males compared with females. The estimated frequency of fragile X causing mild mental retardation in females is 1:2000–2500[4]. The syndrome is not only characterized by mental retardation but also by certain physical abnormalities such as macroorchidism, long face, and prominent ears. Fragile X was originally observed as a cytogenetic abnormality by Lubs[5]. Accurate diagnosis was difficult with conventional cytogenetic methods and the pattern of inheritance of the syndrome was also not well understood before its molecular basis was unravelled. The fragile site is located within the FMR-1 gene[6]. This gene is responsible for the transcription of a protein, which if absent causes the fragile X syndrome. At Xq 27.3 there is a repetitive DNA sequence consisting of triplets of nucleotides, cytidine, cytidine, and guanine, CCG repeats. The repeat is polymorphic. The function of the gene is disturbed by amplification of the CCG repeats. Carriers of the fragile X have an expanded number of CCG repeats ranging from 52 to 200; these are referred to as 'premutations'[7]. The risk of further expansion is correlated with the size of the amplified sequence and the sex of the carrier, i.e., in passing the amplified X chromosome on to the next generation the premutations may be further amplified, thus becoming a full mutation and resulting in the fragile X syndrome[8]. The risk for further amplification is greater in women than in men carrying the premutation. At >200 repeats the syndrome may become manifest. Phenotypic expression may also depend upon the degree of methylation. Diagnosis of the fragile X syndrome is now made by molecular analysis[9] and represents an example of the merging of cytogenetic and molecular genetics[10].

Frequency of chromosome abnormalities

The frequency of chromosome abnormalities does not seem to vary geographically. Surveys of the newborn period indicated that one in 156 (0.65%) of live births has a major chromosome abnormality (excluding mosaicism, fragile-X syndrome, and microdeletions)[11]. This included trisomy 21 in 0.12% of the newborn population. Trisomy 18 and 13 occurred in 0.013% and 0.004%, respectively, while in the cases of 47, XXY, 47, XYY and 47, XXX each occurred in 0.1%. Structural rearrangements occurred in 0.2%. These studies were based on analysis of unbanded chromosomes, but in a study of around 3600 newborns using banded chromosomes, similar frequencies were found[12].

In certain groups of patients chromosome abnormalities occur with relatively high but variable frequencies, e.g., early spontaneous abortions, stillborns, newborns with birth defects, mentally retarded, fetuses of mothers of advanced maternal age, etc. More than 50% of all conceptions are lost; in the case of clinically recognized pregnancies, more than 25% are lost. Chromosome aberrations are present in 50–60% of first trimester and about 20% of second trimester spontaneous abortions and approximately 5% of stillborn infants[13]. The risk of recurrence of abortions caused by chromosome abnormalities when the parents' chromosome complements are normal is estimated to be approximately 1%.

RISK OF CHROMOSOME ABNORMALITIES IN AMNIOTIC FLUID CELLS

The risk of chromosome abnormalities in *amniotic fluids* is correlated with maternal age and estimated to be 30% higher than the corresponding figures for *newborns* (see Table 37.1)[14]. This is primarily due to fetal loss of chromosomally abnormal fetuses after the 16th week of gestation, but underreporting of affected live births and selection of mothers with poor obstetric history have also been considered as reasons for the discrepancy. The risk figures derived in Table 37.1 were based upon 52 965 amniocenteses. The total frequency of chromosome abnormalities was 2.26% among women when the only indication for amniocentesis was maternal age ≥35 years.

RISK OF CHROMOSOME ABNORMALITIES IN CHORIONIC VILLUS BIOPSIES

Table 37.2 lists the risk of Down syndrome from the Danish Cytogenetic Central Register and demonstrates differences between amniocenteses and chorionic villus biopsies[15]. Frequencies of chromosome abnormalities in *chorionic villus biopsies* are higher than those in amniotic fluid specimens primarily because chorionic villus sampling (CVS) takes place earlier in pregnancy. Chromosomally abnormal fetuses, which would have been spontaneously aborted prior to amniocentesis, are diagnosed by CVS.

Chromosome abnormalities were present in 4.05% of CVS specimens obtained in 4122 pregnancies investigated because of advanced maternal age in 27 centres[16]. In the Canadian multicentre study of older pregnant women the frequency of cytogenetic abnormalities was significantly higher for CVS than for amniocentesis: 5.6% versus 3.4%[17]. The difference was mostly due to aneuploidies.

Mosaicism

Mosaicism continues to be a serious diagnostic dilemma in prenatal diagnosis. Mosaicism is defined as the presence of two or more cell lines with different chromosome constitutions (or other genetic differences) in an individual. Mosaicism is the result of abnormal cell division after conception. Such errors may be non-disjunction, anaphase lag or

TABLE 37.1

Crude maternal age specific rates (%) for chromosome abnormalities in pregnancies monitored because of maternal age ≥35 years

Maternal age	Number of pregnancies	Autosomal aberrations								Sex chromosome aberrations							Totals			
		+21	+18	+13	Extra marker	Mosaics etc.	Unbal.	Bal.	t13: 14	XXX	XXY	XYY	X	Mosaics etc.	Unbal.	Bal.	Abn.	Bal.	*De novo*	All aberrations
35	5409	0.35	0.07	0.05	0.04	0.04	0.02	0.26	0.07	0.07	0.09	0.05	0.05	–	0.05	0.05	0.91	0.39	0.02	1.29
36	6103	0.57	0.08	0.03	0.03	—	0.05	0.21	0.08	0.08	0.08	0.02	0.10	0.05	–	0.02	1.09	0.31	0.03	1.41
37	6956	0.68	0.09	0.03	0.07	0.07	0.04	0.18	0.03	0.07	0.04	0.03	0.06	0.06	–	0.03	1.24	0.26	0.04	1.50
38	7926	0.81	0.15	0.04	0.02	0.02	0.04	0.19	0.08	0.08	0.08	0.02	0.08	0.04	0.02	–	1.39	0.26	0.04	1.65
39	7682	1.09	0.19	0.06	0.05	0.03	0.05	0.16	0.03	0.12	0.16	0.04	0.03	0.04	0.01	0.04	1.87	0.22	0.05	2.10
40	7174	1.23	0.25	0.12	0.08	0.03	0.07	0.17	0.06	0.06	0.15	0.03	0.04	0.04	0.03	–	2.13	0.22	0.01	2.36
41	4763	1.47	0.36	0.17	0.06	0.04	0.02	0.17	0.02	0.15	0.29	0.04	–	0.04	–	–	2.64	0.19	0.02	2.83
42	3156	2.19	0.63	0.19	0.06	0.13	–	0.19	0.06	0.28	0.35	0.03	0.03	0.03	–	–	3.77	0.24	0.03	4.01
43	1912	3.24	0.78	0.05	0.10	0.10	0.05	–	0.05	0.31	0.31	–	–	–	0.05	–	5.02	0.05	–	5.07
44	1015	2.95	0.49	–	–	–	–	–	0.10	0.49	0.39	–	–	–	–	–	4.33	0.10	–	4.43
45	508	4.53	0.39	0.20	0.39	0.20	–	–	–	0.39	0.98	0.20	–	–	–	–	7.28	–	0.20	7.28
46	232	8.19	0.43	–	–	–	–	–	–	0.43	1.29	–	–	–	–	–	10.34	–	–	10.34
>46	129	2.33	0.77	–	–	–	–	–	–	1.55	1.55	0.77	–	–	–	–	6.98	–	–	6.98
≥35	52 965	1.16	0.23	0.07	0.06	0.04	0.04	0.18	0.05	0.12	0.16	0.03	0.04	0.04	0.02	0.02	2.01	0.25	0.03	2.26

+21, +18, +13 = autosomal trisomies

Unbal.=duplication-deficiencies resulting from structural rearrangements

Bal. =balanced structural rearrangements (translocations, inversions, excluding pericentric inversions of 9)

De novo=balanced or unbalanced rearrangements arising from new mutation

Abn.=all unbalanced aberrations

t 13:14 = translocation 13; 14

Source: Ferguson-Smith, M.A. Yatès, J.R.W. (1984) Maternal age specific rates for chromosome aberrations and factors influencing them: Report of a collaborative European study of 52 965 amniocenteses. *Prenat. Diagn.* **4**:5–44

TABLE 37.2

Risk figures for Down syndrome based on all cases registered from 1984 to 1993 in the Danish Cytogenetic Central Register[15]. Rates are divided according to sampling method and age of the pregnant women

	Total Prenatal Diagnoses		Trisomy 21			
Age	AC	CVS	AC	per 100 000 examinations AC	CVS	per 100 000 examination CVS
<20	466	56	0	0	0	0
20	413	52	0	0	0	0
21	626	99	1	159	0	0
22	961	151	1	104	0	0
23	1126	192	3	266	0	0
24	1481	336	2	135	2	595
20–24	4607	830	7	151	2	240
25	1775	398	3	169	0	0
26	1965	458	2	101	0	0
27	1983	542	3	151	2	369
28	2223	579	4	179	1	172
29	2166	584	5	230	4	684
25–29	10 112	2561	17	168	7	273
30	2322	591	5	215	2	338
31	2450	597	6	244	2	335
32	2424	675	8	330	0	0
33	2632	598	11	417	0	0
34	4068	1063	8	196	7	658
30–34	13 896	3524	38	273	11	312
35	7293	1979	25	342	9	454
36	6171	1718	33	534	14	814
37	4633	1367	25	539	14	1024
38	3522	1084	28	795	5	461
39	2370	768	24	1012	18	2343
35–39	23 989	6916	135	562	60	867
40	1561	547	15	960	8	1462
41	941	382	18	1912	7	1832
42	523	214	23	4397	10	4672
43	267	115	5	1872	7	6086
44	119	58	5	4201	3	5172
40–44	3411	1316	66	1934	35	2659
45+	83	43	3	3614	4	9302
Total	56 564	15 246	266	470	119	780

AC = amniocentesis; CVS = chorion villus sampling.

structural rearrangements. Ledbetter et al.[18] defined mosaicism in prenatal diagnosis as the presence of normal cells together with cells with an abnormal complement. A minimal demand is:

- Two or more identical, aberrant cells present in villi analysed by the direct (short term culture) method (CVS)
- At least one identical aberrant cell in each of two or more independent culture dishes (AC/CVS)
- At least one identical cell found both by the direct and the culture methods (CVS + AC)

In the direct method, spontaneous mitoses of the cytotrophoblast layer are studied. In the culture method, mitoses from cells which have proliferated in vitro are analysed.

Aberrant cells within only one culture vessel was considered to represent pseudomosaicism. Pseudomosaicism is an in vitro phenomenon; true mosaicism is an in vivo phenomenon. Mosaicism should not be confused with chimerism, in which the two cell lines (genotypes) originate from different individuals (zygotes).

Chromosome mosaicism may be present in cells *within* one tissue or *between* tissues from the same individual.

MOSAICISM AND PRENATAL DIAGNOSIS

Mosaicism presents a prognostic dilemma because it influences the postnatal phenotype of the individual in an unforeseeable manner. Extreme care must be exerted in counselling parents. An individual with 100% trisomic cells, for example, will express a phenotype characteristic for the trisomy in question. Having less than 100% trisomic cells may 'dilute' the phenotype, i.e., reduce frequency and/or severity of the chromosome syndrome. The degree of 'dilution' may depend upon the number of disomic (normal) and trisomic cells as well as which tissues are involved. It has also been found that the ratio of abnormal to normal cells may change over time. This is true in the fetus, as well as in the postnatal state.

Mosaicism is a recognized and established phenomenon in *amniotic cell cultures*. Hsu[19] collected US data from 62 279 amniocenteses from 59 participating centres and found an average of 0.25% of mosaicism with a range of 0% to 0.89%. Warburton[20], reviewing the literature regarding mosaicism in amniotic fluid cultures, found figures ranging from 0% to 20%. In her own experience the frequency was 9.1%. There are several reasons for these large differences, including sampling, culture methods, and others.

With the introduction of the technique of *chorionic villus biopsy* it became clear that cell lines with different chromosome complements could occur within the placenta. This phenomenon was termed 'confined chorionic mosaicism'[21]. The triple origin of the cells in the placenta from polar trophoectoderm, extraembryonic mesoderm and primitive embryonic streak, may predispose to this phenomenon.

Chromosome mosaicism present in placenta may or may not be present in amniocytes and/or fetal blood cells from the same pregnancy; one or both of these latter tissues may be chromosomally normal or abnormal. This phenomenon, different chromosome complements in different 'tissues', is frequently referred to as a discrepancy/discordancy rather than mosaicism. (For references see Kalousek and Dill[21]). Cells cultured from placenta or amniotic fluid may be chromosomally normal even if the fetus proper is in fact a mosaic containing abnormal and normal cells. Schneider et al.[22] failed to detect a mosaic trisomy 8 in two amniotic cell cultures from a fetus, later shown in blood cultures to have such a mosaic and features thereof. Smidt-Jensen[23] found mosaicism (discordancy) in 1.21% of 2483 CVS cases (30 cases) compared with 0.1% of 1074 amniocenteses, a tenfold difference. Only 12 of CVS mosaics were actually confirmed, mostly by amniocentesis. Among 11 855 CVS in the second European collaborative study, Vejerslev and Mikkelsen[24] found 1.2% mosaicism in CVS by direct (short term) analysis and in 0.6% after long term culture. In the US collaborative study on CVS[18] comprising 11 473 CVS procedures, (true) mosaicism was observed in 0.8% of all cases, while pseudomosaicism, including single trisomic cells, was found in 1.6%. Mosaicism present in placentas investigated only with the direct method was not confirmed as often (10%) as when cell culture was used (21%). Mosaicism present in the placenta investigated with both direct and long term culture was confirmed in 318 cases (37.5%)[18]. When the chromosome constitution of the placenta was investigated with both methods there was discordance in 0.5%. Pseudomosaicism was never confirmed.

It has become established that chromosome mosaicism must be confirmed in long term cell culture before any clinical action may be taken.

Prenatally diagnosed mosaicism is clinically significant for a number of reasons:

- Confirmation
- Fetal loss rate
- Adverse perinatal outcome
- Intrauterine growth retardation (IUGR)
- Congenital malformations.

Uniparental disomy (see later) is related to the occurrence of mosaicism. When chromosome mosaicism is found in prenatal diagnosis, there is an urgent need for *confirmation* or exclusion. It is generally accepted that cells from amniotic fluid are more likely to truly represent the fetus proper than placental cells. Fetal blood sampling allows the best estimate of the presence of mosaicism.

The confirmation or exclusion of mosaicism detected prenatally by CVS requires repeat sampling of fetal cells (amniotic fluid or fetal blood). Repeated sampling adds extra obstetrical risks and delays the final diagnosis. For women in whom CVS shows mosaicism, Sundberg et al.[25] introduced early amniocentesis with filter technique for the purpose of clarifying the fetal karyotype and reducing the waiting time for a karyotype. Forty-four pregnancies were examined. Mean gestational age for filter amniocentesis was 12.5 weeks (the 12th and 13th week of gestation) and the final karyotype was available at 13.9 weeks. Four pregnancies were interrupted because of confirmed abnormalities (9.1%).

Not all cases of mosaicism need further investigation; e.g., a mosaic cell line only present in the direct preparation of a placental biopsy and involving an abnormality unlikely to be present in the fetus does not warrant further examination[26]. The frequency of mosaicism will depend upon the material investigated, the number of cells counted and the care with which confirmation is sought. Once detected, mosaicism can never be definitively excluded.

Garber et al.[27] stressed the importance of combined cytogenetic and ultrasound examinations after a diagnosis of mosaicism in amniotic fluid cells. This is especially important in the cases of 45,X/46,XX mosaicism. Koeberl et al.[28] found a 'milder' phenotype among women with a prenatally diagnosed mosaicism of 45, X/46, XX, in comparison to a postnatally diagnosed group.

The higher risk of *fetal loss* associated with mosaicism may not be explained by any additional sampling required. Johnson et al.[29] found 6.7% pregnancy losses in confined placental mosaicism and 2.3% in the controls. Wapner et al.[26] had 8.6% fetal losses in cases of placental mosaicism, compared to 3.4% in the cytogenetically normal cases. Leschot et al.[30], however, did not find an increase in fetal loss in cases with chromosome mosaicism.

Some authors have reported an association between placental mosaicism and intrauterine growth retardation (IUGR)[21,29,31] (see later section on uniparental disomy); there is also a relative increase in the frequency of placental mosaicism in cases of IUGR. However, a number of publications have concluded that the association between IUGR and confined placental mosaicism is weak, if non-existent[26,32–34].

There are a number of factors that may influence the *clinical outcome* in the case of chromosome mosaicism[32]: the specific chromosome involved; the presence or absence of abnormal cells in the fetus proper; the parental origin of the chromosomes involved in the mosaic (uniparental disomy, see below); the distribution of trisomic cells in the placenta and the fetus; and the ratio of abnormal to normal cells found in the various parts of the placenta and the fetus. Some cells may have selective advantage under in vitro conditions, and the result of the chromosome analysis may not represent the in vivo condition. The importance of selective advantage is illustrated by the discrepancies between results of conventional cytogenetic analysis, which involves tissue culture, and interphase FISH, which does not involve tissue culture[35].

The concept of the vanishing twin as a possible explanation of placental mosaicism must also be considered[36].

When a prenatal diagnosis of placental mosaicism is made, postnatal cytogenetic analysis should be carried out if the pregnancy is not interrupted. Pletcher et al.[37] were able to confirm postnatally trisomy 16 mosaicism originally detected in two cases of amniotic fluid samples, despite the fact that a fetal blood sample taken during pregnancy was normal in one of the cases, as was ultrasound examination in both cases.

Technical problems other than mosaicism in prenatal diagnoses include: false positive or false negative results, failure of cell culture, difficulties in interpreting the cytogenetic findings, maternal cell contamination, and the need for obstetric, gynaecological, and paediatric follow-up.

In situ hybridization

The recent combination of chromosome banding techniques with the revolutionary technique of in situ hybridization contributes to the exact diagnosis of structural abnormalities not previously possible. In situ hybridization was first introduced using radiolabelling detection (see below)[38–40]; non-isotopic in situ hybridization (ISH) is now available[41]. ISH is quicker, simpler, cheaper and less polluting when compared to radiolabelling. The demonstration of the presence or absence of specific DNA/RNA sequences with sizes down to <1000 kilobasepairs (kb) in metaphase preparations or interphase nuclei, can be said to have removed the distinction between chromosomal and monogenic diseases.

PRINCIPLES OF IN SITU HYBRIDIZATION

ISH is a technique which allows the detection and localization of specific DNA (or RNA) sequences directly in interphase cells or metaphase chromosomes[42]. Labelled nucleic acid probe is annealed to complementary DNA sequences in cells or metaphase chromosomes that are fixed and located on a microscope slide. The binding of the probes to their homologous target nucleic acid sequences is visualized using fluorescent or absorbent dyes. The probes are labelled either with haptens, such as biotin, and detected using affinity reagents labelled with, e.g. fluorochromes, or the probes are labelled directly with fluorochromes. In this way the presence or absence of a specific DNA sequence can be determined in metaphase or interphase cells simply by observing whether a signal is present at the chromosome/in the nuclei or not. Since each chromosome has a defined spatial position in the interphase nucleus[43,44], the copy number of a specific chromosome may be determined by in situ hybridizing with a chromosome specific probe and simply counting the number of hybridization signals obtained in most interphase nuclei. NISH has been developed by a number of investigators (for references, see Adinolfi and Davies[45]).

PROBES

DNA probes may consist of satellite DNA (α-satellite or alphoid DNA), other repetitive DNA sequences, and unique DNA sequences. For practical purposes chromosome specific probes are categorized as 'repetitive' (centromeric) probes, 'painting' probes, and 'locus specific' probes according to their complementary location on the chromosomes. All three categories normally contain repetitive DNA elements; however, the latter two probe categories also contain unique sequences. When using probes containing unique DNA sequences (as well as repetitive non-specific sequences) suppression of the hybridization of the non-chromosome-specific repetitive DNA is accomplished by chromosome in situ suppression (CISS) using cohybridization with labelled probe and unlabelled repetitive sequences[46,47]. Arrays of alphoid repeats are located inter alia around the centromeres. Alphoid repeats are related, but divergent within and between chromosomes, which explains the chromosome specificity of the repetitive probes (for further elaboration, see review[48]). Centromeric repetitive probes are particularly useful in clinical studies, e.g., in the identification of chromosome markers[45]. Whole chromosomes may be recognized by fluorescence in situ hybridization (FISH) with chromosome specific painting probes[46,47] (Plates 37.1 and 37.2). Unique sequence probes (locus specific probes) can detect DNA sequences from 1 kb[49] to 1 Mb.

Several methods are available for obtaining probes for the identification of chromosomes. A painting probe specific for a whole chromosome may be obtained by isolation of a number of copies of that specific chromosome by flow cytometry, or from somatic cell hybrids only carrying this human chromosome. The chromosome in question may be amplified by degenerate oligonucleotide-primed polymerase chain reaction (DOP-PCR), and the resulting DNA used as the in situ hybridization probe[50].

A probe consisting of DNA from an abnormal chromosome, e.g. a marker chromosome or from a normal chromosome, may be obtained by microdissection of the same marker from a number of cells in metaphase, followed by amplification and labelling (DOP-PCR). By hybridization of the labelled DNA to normal metaphase preparations, the identity of the marker DNA can be determined[51]. This technique is called reverse chromosome painting.

Probes from several chromosomes may be used simultaneously in order to identify unknown markers or complicated structural abnormalities, on the condition that each probe is labelled by a specific colour (multicolour FISH[52,53]). Multicolour FISH is now being introduced using a specific combination of colours for each of the 24 different chromosomes[54].

COMPARATIVE GENOMIC HYBRIDIZATION

The principle of hybridization with differentially labelled DNA probes has been further developed in comparative genomic hybridization (CGH) for purposes of molecular cytogenetic analysis[55]. CGH was primarily applied for the cytogenetic analysis of solid tumours, but is also applicable to constitutive cytogenetics. Conventional cytogenetic analysis of solid tumours is hampered by the difficulties in obtaining satisfactory metaphases for study. However, DNA from tumours is in general easily obtained. The principle in CGH is to obtain genomic DNA from the tissue to be cytogenetically examined (test DNA) and genomic DNA from a normal individual (reference DNA). Test and reference DNAs are labelled with two different fluorescent colours, e.g. reference DNA with red fluorescence and test DNA with green fluorescence. Equal amounts of test and reference DNA are then hybridized to normal metaphases. The resulting hybridized metaphases are analysed by digital image microscopy and specific computer software, and the ratios between colour intensities along the chromosomes are measured. Where test and reference DNA are present in equal amounts, the colour will be the result of the equimolar mixture. Where test DNA is present in amplified amounts (duplications) green fluorescence will dominate and where it is missing (deletions), red fluorescence will dominate (Fig. 37.3, Plate 37.3).

Through CGH, the origin of larger amplifications and deletions in the tumour (test) DNA can be identified. Balanced translocations, however, cannot be identified. Another drawback of CGH is that most tumours are mixtures of clones with different chromosome complements and DNA from these various clones cannot be separated under normal circumstances. Nevertheless, CGH may provide important contributions to understanding malignant transformations. CGH may also be useful in diagnosing constitutive cytogenetic abnormalities responsible for congenital malformations and inherited diseases and therefore applicable in prenatal diagnosis[56].

CLINICAL CYTOGENETICS AND IN SITU HYBRIDIZATION

FISH is applicable to cells in metaphase as well as in interphase. FISH is useful for the analysis of intricate chromosome complements, e.g., complicated translocations, insertions and duplications, as well as for the diagnosis of microdeletions.

The following discussion emphasizes the use of interphase FISH for rapid detection of aneuploidies. NISH was introduced by Cremer et al.[57] in 1986. They demonstrated the use of a biotinylated probe of human repetitive DNA from chromosome 18 for the detection of trisomy 18 in interphase nuclei. The number of fluorescent signals in interphase nuclei could clearly distinguish trisomic cells (with three fluorescent signals) from disomic cells (with two fluorescent signals). Stringency conditions are important, since the probe consists of repetitive DNA having partial homology with DNA from other chromosomes. Lichter et al.[58] demonstrated that trisomy 21 could be diagnosed by counting signal numbers after in situ hybridization with chromosome 21 locus specific DNA in combination with chromosome in situ suppression hybridization (CISS). Rapid demonstration of numerical and structural abnormalities of chromosome 21 in both metaphase and interphase cells of lymphocytes, cultured chorionic villus cells and a tumour cell line was possible. Lichter et al.[59] found that not only the type of probes but also methods of cell preparation and hybridization were of utmost importance when signal numbers were to be quantitatively estimated. Single cosmid clones yielded the highest number of countable cells. Eighty to ninety percent of lymphocytes gave clear quantitative information, and 'the intranuclear signal was good enough to make it amenable to simple automated image analysis'[59]. They suggested that abnormalities of the five most common chromosomes showing aneuploides, 13, 18, 21, X, and Y, should be amenable to diagnosis in a single assay using in situ hybridization on interphase nuclei (Plate 37.4).

METHODOLOGICAL CONSIDERATIONS IN USING INTERPHASE IN SITU HYBRIDIZATION ON AMNIOCYTES

Julien et al.[60] claimed that FISH could be applied to uncultured amniocytes for prenatal diagnosis of Down syndrome.

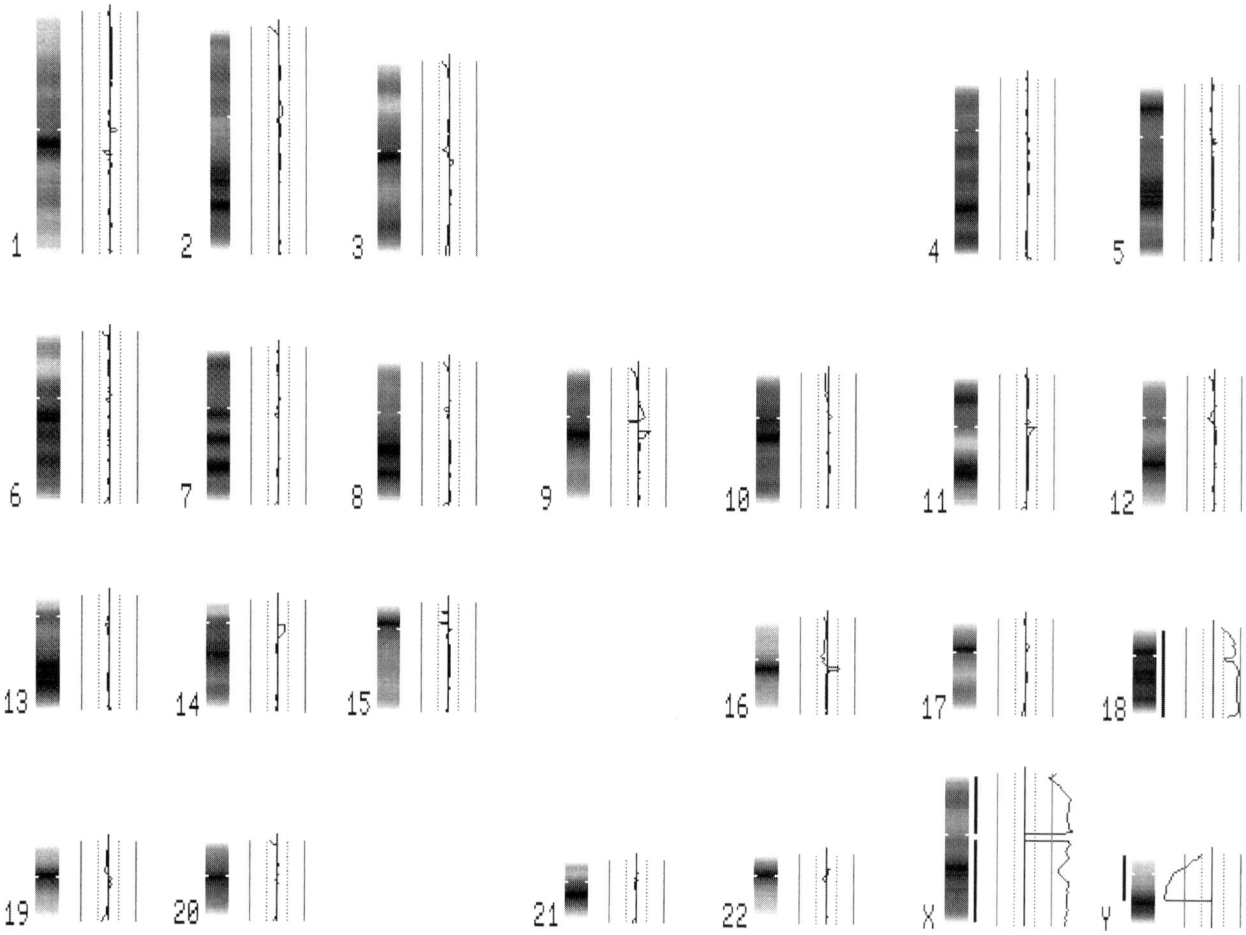

Fig. 37.3 Comparative genomic hybridization analysis of a chorionic villus sample. The ratios of green/red fluorescence are shown for each chromosome. Vertical lines represent ratios 0.5, 1.0 and 1.5 respectively. Ratios above or below the dotted line indicate gain or loss respectively of chromosomal material. All autosomes (1–22) except chromosome 18 show normal fluorescence ratios at 1.0. The fluorescence ratio for chromosome 18 is approximately 1.5, which indicates that this chromosome is trisomic in the chorionic villus sample. The chromosomal gain is illustrated as a black bar at the right side of chromosome 18. Since the chorionic villus sample is from a female and the normal DNA is from a male the fluorescence ratios of chromosome X and Y are different from 1.0.

The number of cases investigated in that study was not reported. We also demonstrated the possible use of in situ hybridization analysis of amniocytes[61–63]. We, and others, determined that cells from amniotic fluid present certain problems when used for prenatal, interphase FISH diagnosis: probes which give good results with other cell types such as lymphocytes, may present problems when applied to uncultured amniocytes. The hybridization efficiency of uncultured amniocytes is reduced with most of the available probes[64].

Kuo[65] found that painting probes specific for chromosomes 13, 18 and 21 produce intense, well localized and countable signals on *cultured* interphase amniocytes. Zheng et al.[66] compared painting probes and locus specific probes applied to *uncultured* amniotic fluid cells; they found that a locus specific probe developed by themselves was the only satisfactory probe for interphase analysis of chromosome 21.

In general, repetitive probes give clear, large, easily countable signals, while locus-specific probes give less intense signals. Repetitive (centomeric) probes are now available for chromosome 18, X and Y, and locus-specific probes for chromosomes 13 and 21 are available and useful also for uncultured amniocytes. A second problem in cytogenetic studies of amniocytes by interphase FISH is contamination by maternal leucocytes following amniocentesis. Contamination of fetal cells with maternal cells decreases the sensitivity, and increases the risk of a false negative diagnosis by FISH of trisomic cases[63]. The problem is significant. Ward et al. (to be published) found that 6.8% of clear 'straw coloured' amniotic fluids probably were contaminated by maternal cells. Out of over 10 000 samples, 3.2% had a mixture of male and female nuclei and 3.6% contained nuclei that were multilobulated and were likely polymorphonuclear cells of either maternal or fetal origin. Samples containing such cells have to be reported as uninformative by interphase-FISH analysis.

In contrast, maternal white blood cells are not a problem in *cultures* from amniotic fluid cells, since leucocytes will not grow in this type of tissue culture. Thus, conventional cytogenetic analysis is rarely hampered by maternal cell contaminations. However, when uncultured amniotic fluid cells undergo FISH, maternal leucocytes can be hybridized together with the fetal cells.

CLINICAL STUDY OF AMNIOTIC FLUID CELLS WITH FISH

Klinger et al.[71] reported the first major prospective study comparing results of classical cytogenetic analysis with interphase FISH on *uncultured* amniotic cells. They constructed chromosome specific DNA probes from loci on chromosomes 13, 18, 21, X, and Y in cosmids. These probes had high signal to noise ratios, acceptable spatial resolution of the fluorescent signals and high hybridization/detection efficiency. They analysed 526 samples. In 117 cases the number of cells present was suitable for all five chromosomes to be evaluated. Abnormalities tested for and present among the investigated samples were found. Two trisomy 21 cases had to be excluded because of maternal cell contamination.

Ward et al. (to be published) studied over 10 000 uncultured amniotic fluid samples with the probes previously described by Klinger et al.[71]. Results were obtained on 89.5% of the attempted FISH analyses. Detection rate was 78.2% for aneuploidies. There were 8961 normal samples and 283 showing aneuploidy. There was one false positive and seven false negative results (false negatives were only among the first 4500 samples)[72]. For informative samples, the sensitivity for the autosomal abnormalities was 97.1%; for sex chromosome abnormalities, 100%. Nineteen percent of all aneuploidies were uninformative, however.

The results of Klinger et al.[71] and Ward et al.[72] were confirmed in a smaller study by Spathas et al.,[73] in which a cosmid contig probe was used to correctly diagnose six cases of trisomy 21 in 500 uncultured amniotic fluid specimens. One false negative case involved an unbalanced 21/21 translocation. Modifying the protocol made it possible to diagnose this kind of abnormality as well. A retrospective study demonstrated that using multicolour FISH, it was possible to test for numerical abnormalities of chromosome 13, 18, 21, X, and Y in one hybridization procedure[74]. In both studies clear cutoff criteria for normal and abnormal cases were obtained[73,74].

Bryndorf et al.[75], using the same probes as Ward et al. in a study of 2000 *amniotic fluid* specimens, found that although abnormal samples were distinguishable from normal samples, the number of technically unsuccessfully hybridizations was too high for their practical use of the amnion interphase-FISH assay at the present time.

CLINICAL STUDY OF INTERPHASE FISH APPLIED ON CHORIONIC VILLUS CELLS

In the first large study of uncultured mesenchymal cells *from chorionic villus biopsies*, Bryndorf et al.[35] evaluated aneuploidy detection by interphase FISH using the probes of Klinger et al.[71] They blindly compared FISH with conventional chromosome analysis in 2709 samples and could easily distinguish normal and abnormal cases. There were 2567 karyotypically normal samples; 87 abnormal FISH results for chromosomes 13, 18, 21, X and Y were concordant with the conventional cytogenetic analysis. In disomies, an average of 0.3% (range 0–40%)* of nuclei showed three signals. Trisomies had 84% (range 52–96%) of cells exhibiting three signals. With regard to sex chromosomes (after a technical problem was corrected) female samples had 99% (range 44–100%) of their nuclei showing a two X-signal pattern. Male samples had 99% (range: 22–100%) of their nuclei showing one X-and one Y-signal. Samples with sex chromosome abnormalities had an abnormal signal pattern in 97% (range 94–100%) of their nuclei; this was concordant with the chromosome complement found by conventional cytogenetic analysis. Hybridization was successful in ≥94% of cases. Technical deviations from the protocol accounted for 43% of the unsuccessful hybridizations. One microdeletion of chromosome 18 was only identified by FISH and not by conventional cytogenetics. There were 11 mosaics as judged by conventional cytogenetics. In mosaic cases, however, there was no correlation between conventional cytogenetics and FISH analysis.

Using the diagnostic criterion defined by the study, four mosaic cases would be diagnosed as normal by FISH, four as uninformative, and three as abnormal. Detecting mosaicism will depend upon the criteria established, but in suspected cases amniocentesis is required. Maternal cell contamination was 0.3% (range 0–10%) and represented no problem for the FISH assay.

SUMMARIZING EXPERIENCE WITH PRENATAL FISH

FISH is an increasingly important tool in prenatal cytogenetics as well as in clinical cytogenetics in general. It allows:

- Rapid prenatal diagnosis of the major aneuploidies
- More complete prenatal diagnosis in clinically and cytogenetically difficult cases

FISH painting techniques, CGH, and the technique of chromosome microdissection and PCR amplification followed by in situ hybridization using the amplified DNA as a probe is useful not only for characterizing marker chromosomes of unknown origin but in excluding balanced states in familial translocation carriers[76,77]. FISH may be useful in the study of fixed (archival) material, and for screening for selected autosomal and sex chromosome abnormalities in chorionic villus biopsies.

---

* With the exclusion of a result from a hybridization that was allowed to hybridize for too long, an average of 0.3% (range 0–14%) three-signal nuclei were scored in karyotypically disomic samples.

INTERPHASE FISH IN PRENATAL DIAGNOSIS COMPARED WITH CONVENTIONAL CYTOGENETICS

The advantages of using interphase FISH compared with conventional chromosome analysis in prenatal diagnosis are that FISH is faster, may be more inexpensive, and fewer cells are required. Cell culture is not needed, and the FISH technique is less labour intensive than conventional cytogenetic analysis. FISH slide processing only takes hours and signal counting takes minutes. FISH reduces waiting time considerably and waiting for results is considered one of the important side-effects of prenatal diagnosis. When the risk of an abnormality is high, e.g., high maternal age, when ultrasound examination or low serum-AFP have raised suspicion of an abnormality of the fetus, or when prenatal diagnosis is performed late in the second trimester, a serious time constraint is present. FISH may be especially useful in such cases. Whiteman and Klinger[78] stated that FISH could identify up to 95% of clinically relevant abnormalities. Lebo et al.[79] stated that aneuploidies for 13, 18, 21, X, and Y represent 96% of the high risk chromosome abnormalities.

Mosaics, translocations and other relatively rare structural abnormalities are not detected by FISH. FISH without conventional cytogenetics limits anxiety, because diagnoses of a number of clinically insignificant abnormalities are avoided. However, this is not accepted everywhere.

Improvements in FISH are forthcoming all the time, e.g., dual colour (X and Y) FISH for evaluation of maternal blood contamination; and two fluorescent colours on the same probe for improvement of signal detection[80]. Multicolour FISH[81,82], applied to the 24 different human chromosome combined with automated analysis based on digital imaging microscopy is already being used in clinical cytogenetics[55].

Preimplantation cytogenetic diagnosis

Preimplantation cytogenetic diagnosis following in vitro fertilization has been carried out in several centres for sex-determination in order to exclude sex-linked disease and to exclude common chromosomal trisomies. Single gene disorders have also been diagnosed or excluded by preimplantation diagnosis[83]. (See Chapter 39.)

Embryonic sex may be determined by either PCR or in situ hybridization. Single cells may be removed from the embryo at the 6–10 cell stage (on the second–third day post-fertilization), and a diagnosis obtained by DNA amplification of specific sequences of the X and Y chromosomes or by in situ hybridization using chromosomes X and Y specific probes.

Misdiagnosis of embryonic sex has occurred with PCR[84]. PCR will give a positive result for the presence of an X chromosome in all possible complements including an X chromosome. Using PCR it is therefore not possible to distinguish between XX and abnormal X-complements such as X, XXX or XXXX.

The advantage of FISH compared with PCR can be summarized as follows: the risk of contamination by foreign DNA is excluded as a cause of false diagnosis; the nucleus can be visualized before and after the procedure; a clearly positive result is obtained (two X-signals for females or one X- and one Y-signal for males)[84].

There is now consensus that in situ hybridization is the method of choice for sex determination with the purpose of excluding sex-linked disease in preimplantation genetic diagnosis[85].

Conventional chromosome analysis is of interest in preimplantation genetics for purposes of excluding embryos with aneuploidy. Karyotypic analysis of early human embryos is, however, problematic[84] (cited from Coonen et al.[86]). Jamieson et al.[87] were only able to successfully karyotype 195 of 816 (23.9%) embryos available for study. Forty of the 195 embryos (22.5%) had an abnormal karyotype: 19.1% were aneuploids, 2.2% were mosaics, and 1.1% had structural anomalies. The difficulties in carrying out conventional cytogenetic analysis are low cell numbers, badly spread metaphases and poor banding quality. Chromosome analysis is also time consuming and cells in metaphase are not always available. Conventional cytogenetic analysis does not appear convenient for preimplantation diagnosis at this time.

Munné et al.[88] used FISH with probes for X, Y, 18, and 13/21 on 157 blastomeres from 30 human embryos. Seventy percent of abnormally developing, fragmented or arrested embryos and 70% of normally developing embryos from women with a mean maternal age of 40 years were chromosomally abnormal. Mosaicism, polyploidy, trisomy and monosomy were equally common in *abnormally and normally appearing embryos* (for review, see Zenses and Casper[89]).

Coonen et al.[86] investigated the occurrence of chromosome mosaicism in preimplantation embryos, using an improved spreading method combined with 'double target' chromosomes X and Y and 1 and 7 FISH, they had an extremely high hybridization efficiency (999/1000 on control leucocytes) which is necessary when using small numbers of cells. Forty-three cells from nine embryos (with two pronucleate) were readable and none was mosaic. However, Harper et al.[90] found mosaicism in normally developing embryos: 46% of 35 embryos showed autosomal abnormalities for chromosomes 1 and 17 including monosomy, trisomy and mosaicism. Such findings were in agreement with Munné et al.[91] It has been suggested that the majority of abnormal cells may be diverted to the trophectoderm and not to the embryo proper.

At the present time sex determination of preimplantation embryos using FISH with dual colour chromosomes X and Y specific probes appears reasonably safe and accurate. More than one cell should be biopsied for correct diagnosis[91]; however, survival of the embryo decreases when too many cells are removed[92].

It must also be understood that mosaicism may be unrecognized, that mosaicism is frequent, and that the biological significance of mosaicism in preimplantation embryos is unknown at present.

Genomic imprinting and uniparental disomy

Review of prenatal clinical cytogenetics is not possible now without referring to two related concepts: genomic imprinting and uniparental disomy. Genomic imprinting refers to the phenomenon that identical genetic material may have differential expression at the genomic, chromosomal, subchromosomal, or single locus level depending on parent of origin[93]. In short, genetic material on one homologue may be expressed, while the corresponding material on the other homologue is imprinted (inactivated).

Uniparental disomy means that the two homologous chromosomes are derived from only one parent[94]. The primary mechanism behind uniparental disomy is meiotic and mitotic non-disjunction. Uniparental disomy may arise from trisomy followed by loss of one of the 'extra' chromosomes ('trisomy rescue'). Monosomy duplication, somatic crossing over, gamete complementation are other possible mechanisms[95]. Uniparental disomy has been found in cases of placental mosaicism (diploid/aneuploid cell lines), together with a diploid fetus. Both homologous chromosomes of a diploid fetus may be of either paternal or maternal origin. The finding of complete trisomy or mosaicism in the placenta together with a karyotypically normal fetus may be explained by the loss of one of the three chromosomes in a trisomic embryo at the time of differentiation of the blastocyst into fetal and placental tissues[93,96]. The effect of the loss depends on the origin of the remaining two chromosomes (paternal or maternal) and on whether or not the paternal and maternal chromosome is imprinted (partially or totally inactivated).

When two chromosomes have their origin from the same parent, they may be identical, 'isodisomic', or different, 'heterodisomic'. The adverse effects that uniparental disomy may have on embryonic/fetal development are correlated with the isodisomic or heterodisomic state, and whether there is genomic imprinting of one or both chromosomes[96]. Uniparental disomy and imprinting may both affect outcome of pregnancy: abortion, preterm delivery, IUGR, and malformations. The effects of uniparental disomy and of imprinting may be difficult to distinguish from either the effects of chromosome mosaicism, or the possible expression of an autosomal recessive disease, manifest because of loss of heterozygosity[97].

There are now numerous examples in humans of uniparental disomy as a cause of both Prader–Willi and Angelman syndromes[98,99]. Both syndromes may be associated with a microdeletion in the proximal part of the long arm of chromosome 15 (the q11–13 region). However, in addition to microdeletion in the paternal chromosome 15, maternal uniparental disomy for chromosome 15 (no chromosome 15 from the father, two from the mother) can also cause Prader–Willi syndrome. A microdeletion in the maternal chromosome 15, or paternal uniparental disomy for chromosome 15 (no chromosome 15 from the mother, two from the father), can cause Angelman syndrome. Smith et al.[100] studied 87 patients with Prader–Willi syndrome and 49 with Angelman syndrome analysing for deletions (including single locus deletions) and uniparental disomy. The aetiology had to be revised in a number of suspected cases for both syndromes, because microdeletions were not found. Cases without microdeletions were shown by molecular techniques (homozygosity/loss of heterozygosity) to have uniparental disomy.

Chromosomes other than chromosomes 15 and 16 are also involved in uniparental disomy and/or imprinting: 11 pat, 7 mat and 14 mat are considered to have certain imprinting effects, while 16 mat, 14 pat, 6 pat, 2 mat, 20 pat and XX pat have possible effects[97].

For examples comparing clinical cases suspected of malformations resulting from uniparental disomy/genomic imprinting, see Table 37.3.

TABLE 37.3
References to literature suggesting association between congenital malformations (syndromes) and uniparental disomy/genomic imprinting

Chromosome	Abnormalities
7	Silver–Russell syndrome, growth retardation[109–111]
9[112]	
11	Wilm's tumour, embryonal rhabdomyosarcoma, neuroblastoma, Beckwith–Wiedemann's syndrome[113]
13[114]	
14	Short stature, precocious puberty. Further hydrocephalus, mental retardation, scoliosis etc.[113–117]
15[117–121]	
16	Growth retardation, congenital heart disease[122]
21[122–125]	Have all been found together with or suspected being involved in imprinting/mosaicism

It should be noted that the effect of chromosome abnormalities such as e.g. deletions, are influenced by the parental origin of the abnormal chromosome; Miller–Diecker syndrome (17q) (paternal); Di George syndrome 22q- (maternal); cri du chat 5q- (maternal)[93].

Prenatal aneuploidy detection in fetal cells isolated from maternal blood

Currently, prenatal genetic diagnosis of fetal cells has to be carried out on cells obtained through invasive procedures such as amniocentesis or chorionic villus biopsy, although endocervical or intrauterine lavage, which may be considered semi-invasive, has also been proposed[101].

Clinical and laboratory evidence that fetal cells are present in the peripheral circulation of the pregnant woman has been available for more than 100 years. As long as genetic analysis of fetal cells has been possible, there has been interest in isolating and investigating these fetal cells from maternal blood.

Adinolfi[102] recently reviewed the current status regarding the types of fetal cell present in maternal blood, including syncytiotrophoblasts, leucocytes, and erythroblasts and their availability and suitability for genetic analysis. The main obstacle to routine use of this non-invasive prenatal diagnostic approach is the small number of fetal cells present in maternal blood. Furthermore, syncytiotrophoblasts being multinucleated cells may not be suitable for interphase in situ hybridization; and fetal lymphocytes have not been studied in enough detail for this non-invasive approach. The most frequently studied cell type has been the fetal erythroblasts.

Although it has been claimed that mitotic chromosomes from male fetuses (46, XY) are present in maternal blood[103], sex determination and cytogenetic analysis of fetal cells has been carried out by PCR and in situ hybridization.

PCR on DNA from unsorted maternal peripheral blood has been applied to sex determination of fetuses[104]. The positive predictive value was 86%, 67%, and 87% in the first, second and third trimesters, respectively.

PCR OR ISH?

After cell sorting by flow cytometry, male sex was correctly identified in nucleated erythrocytes from 12 of 12 maternal blood samples in pregnancies with male fetuses[105]; female sex was correct in five of six samples of blood in pregnancies with female fetuses (for further references, see Price et al.[105] and Chapter 35).

Chromosome abnormalities have also been diagnosed by FISH on fetal cells isolated from the peripheral blood of pregnant women. Price et al.[105] found 38.7% cells with three signals after in situ hybridization with a chromosome 21 specific probe in a sorted sample of maternal blood. The blood sample that was taken after amniocentesis showed that the fetus had Down syndrome. In a fetus with trisomy 18, 8.5% of sorted cells (not further defined) showed three signals with a chromosome 18 specific probe; since no figures from normal fetuses regarding the chromosomes 18 and 21 specific probes were given, the results are difficult to interpret. The same group[106] published findings on trisomy 21 from a flow-sorted blood sample of a pregnant woman based on in situ hybridization with a chromosome 21 specific probe. Seventy-four percent of cells had three signals with the chromosome 21 specific probe. In five control samples with normal fetuses, 0 to 12.4% of the cells also had three signals with the chromosome 21 specific probe. Gänshirt-Ahlert et al.[107] studied maternal blood samples by in situ hybridization after cell sorting. In seven cases, blood sampling took place before any invasive procedure. Sampling was performed between gestational week 16 and 33. The number of nuclei with three signals in the 15 trisomic cases (9–17% three-signal nuclei) was different from the normal controls (0–7% three signals nuclei). However, these results have not been reproduced.

Further technical developments are required before genetic analyses based on fetal cells from the maternal circulation can be routinely applied to the prenatal diagnosis of chromosome abnormalities. Currently, there is considerable interest in this non-invasive approach because its implications include population-based prenatal genetic testing. If the isolation, identification and analysis of fetal cells in maternal blood proves to be successful, this technique may well revolutionize prenatal diagnosis in the future.

Acknowledgements

The figures were kindly provided by Maria Kirchhoff, M.Sci., The Chromosome Laboratory, Section of Clinical Genetics 4051.

Professor Eugene Pergament, Section of Reproductive Genetics, Northwestern University, Chicago, USA kindly revised the language.

REFERENCES

1. Tjio JH, Levan A. The chromosome number in man. *Hereditas* **42**:1–6, 1956.
2. Caspersson T, Lomakka G, Zech L. The 24 fluorescence patterns of human metaphase chromosomes distinguishing characters and variability. *Hereditas* **67**:89–102, 1971.
3. Warburton D. De novo balanced chromosome rearrangements and extra marker chromosomes identified at prenatal diagnosis: clinical significance and distribution of breakpoints. *Am J Hum Genet* **49**:995–1013, 1991.
4. Turner G, Robinson H, Laing S, Purvis-Smith S. Preventive screening for the fragile X syndrome. *N Engl J Med* **315**:607–609, 1986.
5. Lubs H. A marker X chromosome. *Am J Hum Genet* **21**:231–244, 1969.
6. Loesch DZ, Huggins R, Petrovic V, Slater H. Expansion of the CGG repeat in fragile X in the FMR 1 gene depends on the sex of the offspring. *Am J Hum Genet* **57**:1408–1413, 1995.
7. Kremer E, Pritchard M, Lynch S. et al. Mapping of DNA instability at the fragile X to a trinucleotide repeat sequence p (CCG) n. *Science* **252**:1711–1714, 1991.
8. Yu S, Mulley J, Loesch D. et al. Fragile-X syndrome: Unique genetics of the heritable unstable element. *Am J Hum Genet* **50**:968–980, 1992.
9. Rousseau F, Heitz D, Biancalana V. et al. Direct diagnosis by DNA analysis of the fragile X syndrome of mental retardation. *N Engl J Med* **325**:1673–1681, 1991.
10. Yu S, Pritchard M, Kremer E. et al. Fragile X genotype characterized by an unstable region of DNA. *Science* **257**:1179–1184, 1991.
11. Hsu LYF. Prenatal diagnosis of chromosomal abnormalities through amniocentesis. In *Genetic Disorders and the Fetus. Diagnosis, Prevention, and Treatment*, 3rd edn. (ed. A. Milunsky), pp. 155–210. Baltimore & London: The Johns Hopkins University Press, 1992.
12. Nielsen J, Wohlert M, Faaborg Andersen J. et al. Incidence of chromosome abnormalities in newborn children. Comparison between incidences in 1969–1974 and 1980–1982 in the same area. *Hum Genet* **61**:98–101, 1982.
13. Hook EB. Prevalence of chromosome abnormalities during human gestation and implications for studies of environmental mutagens. *Lancet* **2**:169–172, 1981.

14. Ferguson-Smith MA, Yates JRW. Maternal age specific rates for chromosome aberrations and factors influencing them: Report of a collaborative European study on 52 965 amniocenteses. *Prenat Diagn* **4**:5–44, 1984.
15. Danish Cytogenetic Register. Risk figures for Down's syndrome, based on all cases registered in Denmark (pre-and postnatal examinations 1984–1993). Personal communication from Jan Hansen, 1996.
16. Mikkelsen M, Aymé S. Chromosomal Findings in Chorionic Villi: a Collaborative Study. In *Human Genetics* (eds F. Vogel & K. Sperling), pp. 597–606. Springer Verlag, Berlin, 1987.
17. Lippman A, Tomkins DJ, Shime J, Hamerton JL. Canadian multicentre randomized clinical trial of chorion villus sampling and amniocentesis. Final report. *Prenat Diagn* **12**:385–408, 1992.
18. Ledbetter DH, Zachary JM, Simpson JL. et al. Cytogenetic results from the U.S. collaborative study on CVS. *Prenat Diagn* **12**:317–346, 1992.
19. Hsu LYF. United States survey on chromosome mosaicism and pseudomosaicism in prenatal diagnosis. *Prenat Diagn* **4**:97–130, 1984.
20. Warburton D, Yu CY, Kline J, Stein Z. Autosomal trisomy in cultures from spontaneous abortions. *Am J Hum Genet* **30**: 609–617, 1978.
21. Kalousek DK, Dill FJ. Chromosomal mosaicism confined to the placenta in human conceptions. *Science* **221**:665–667, 1983.
22. Schneider M, Klein-Vogler U, Tomiuk J. et al. Amniocentesis fails to detect mosaic trisomy 8 in a male newborn. *Prenat Diagn* **14**:651–652, 1994.
23. Smidt-Jensen S. Transabdominal chorionic villus sampling. Method, safety and accuracy. Thesis. *Danish Medical Bulletin* **45**:402–411, 1998.
24. Vejerslev LO, Mikkelsen M. The European collaborative study on mosaicism in chorionic villus sampling: Data from 1986 to 1987. *Prenat Diagn* **9**:575–588, 1989.
25. Sundberg K, Lundsteen C, Philip J. Early amniocentesis for further investigation of mosaicism diagnosed by chorion villus sampling. *Prenat Diagn* **16**:1121–1127, 1996.
26. Wapner RJ, Simpson JL, Golbus MS. et al. Chorionic mosaicism: Association with fetal loss but not with adverse perinatal outcome. *Prenat Diagn* **12**:347–355, 1992.
27. Garber A, Carlson D, Schreck R. et al. Prenatal diagnosis and dysmorphic findings in mosaic trisomy 16. *Prenat Diagn* **14**:257–266, 1994.
28. Koeberl DD, McGillivray B, Sybert VP. Prenatal diagnosis of 45, X/46, XX mosaicism and 45, X: Implications for postnatal outcome. *Am J Hum Genet* **57**:661–666, 1995.
29. Johnson A, Wapner RJ, Davis H, Jackson LG. Mosaicism in chorionic villus sampling: An association with poor perinatal outcome. *Obstet Gynecol* **75**:573–577, 1990.
30. Leschot NJ, Wolf H. Is placental mosaicism associated with poor perinatal outcome? *Prenat Diagn* **11**:403–404, 1991.
31. Kalousek DK, Howard-Peebles PN, Olson SB. et al. Confirmation of CVS mosaicism in term placentae and high frequency of intrauterine growth retardation association with confined placental mosaicism. *Prenat Diagn* **11**:743–750, 1991.
32. Wolstenholme J, Rooney DE, Davison EV. Confined placental mosaicism, IUGR, and adverse pregnancy outcome: a controlled retrospective U.K. collaborative survey. *Prenat Diagn* **14**:345–361, 1994.
33. Schwinger E, Seidl E, Klink F, Rehder H. Chromosome mosaicism of the placenta – a cause of developmental failure of the fetus. *Prenat Diagn* **9**:639–647, 1989.
34. Roland B, Lynch L, Berkowitz G, Zinberg R. Confined placental mosaicism in CVS and pregnancy outcome. *Prenat Diagn* **14**:589–593, 1994.
35. Bryndorf T, Christensen B, Vad M. et al. Prenatal detection of chromosome aneuploidies in uncultured chorionic villus samples by fluorescent in situ hybridization. *Am J Hum Genet* **59**:918–926, 1996.
36. Reddy KS, Petersen MB, Antonarakis SE, Blakemore KJ. The vanishing twin: An explanation for discordance between chorionic villus karyotype and fetal phenotype. *Prenat Diagn* **11**:679–684, 1991.
37. Pletcher BA, Sanz MM, Schlessel JS. et al. Postnatal confirmation of prenatally diagnosed trisomy 16 mosaicism in two phenotypically abnormal liveborns. *Prenat Diagn* **14**:933–940, 1994.
38. John HA, Birnstiel ML, Jones KW. RNA-DNA hybrids at the cytological level. *Nature* **223**:582–587, 1969.
39. Buongiorno-Nardelli M, Amaldi F. Autoradiographic detection of molecular hybrids between rRNA and DNA in tissue sections. *Nature* **225**:946–947, 1969.
40. Gall JG, Pardue ML. Formation and detection of RNA-DNA hybrid molecules in cytological preparations. *Proc Natl Acad Sci USA* **63**:378–381, 1969.
41. Manning JE, Hershey D, Brooker TR. A new method of in situ hybridization. *Chromosoma* **53**:107–117, 1975.
42. Hopman AHN, Raap AK, Landegent J, Wiegant J, Boerman RH, van der Ploeg M. Non-radioactive in situ hybridization. In *Molecular Neuroanatomy* (eds Van Leeuwen F, Buijs RM, Pool CW, Pach O), pp. 43–68. New York: Elsevier Science Publishers B.V. (Biomedical Division), 1988.
43. Manuelidis L. Individual interphase chromosome domains revealed by in situ hybridization. *Hum Genet* **71**:288–293, 1985.
44. Schardin M, Cremer T, Hager HD, Lang M. Specific staining of human chromosomes in Chinese hamster x man hybrid cell lines demonstrates interphase chromosome territories. *Hum Genet* **71**:281–287, 1985.
45. Adinolfi M, Davies AF. Non-isotopic in situ hybridization: Applications to clinical diagnosis and molecular genetics, p. 13. Austin, TX: R.G. Landers Company, 1994.
46. Pinkel D, Landegent J, Collins C. et al. Fluorescence in situ hybridization with human chromosome-specific libraries: Detection of trisomy 21 and translocations of chromosome 4. *Proc Natl Acad Sci USA* **85**:9138–9142, 1988.
47. Lichter P, Cremer T, Borden J, Manuelidis L, Ward DC. Delineation of individual human chromosomes in metaphase and interphase cells by in situ suppression hybridization using recombinant DNA libraries. *Hum Genet* **80**:224–234, 1988.
48. Griffin DK. Fluorescent in situ hybridization for the diagnosis of genetic disease at postnatal, prenatal, and preimplantation stages. *Int Rev Cytol* **153**:1–40, 1994.
49. Viegas-Péquignot E, Berrard S, Brice A, Apiou F, Mallet J. Localization of a 900-bp-long fragment of the human choline acetyltransferase gene to 10q11.2 by nonradioactive in situ hybridization. *Genomics* **9**:210–212, 1991.
50. Telenius H, Carter NP, Bebb CE, Nordenskjöld M, Ponder BAJ, Tunnacliffe A. Degenerate oligonucleotide-primed PCR: general amplification of target DNA by a single degenerate primer. *Genomics* **13**:718–725, 1992.
51. Meltzer PS, Guan XY, Burgess A, Trent JM. Rapid generation of region specific probes by microdissection and their application. *Nat Genet* **1**:24–28, 1992.
52. Nederlof PM, Robinson D, Abuknesha R. et al. Three-color fluorescence in situ hybridization for the simultaneous detection of multiple nucleic acid sequences. *Cytometry* **10**:20–27, 1989.
53. Wiegant J, Wiesmeijer CC, Hoovers JMN. et al. Multiple and sensitive fluorescence in situ hybridization with rhodamine-, fluorescein-, and coumarin-labeled DNAs. *Cytogenet Cell Genet* **63**:73–76, 1993.
54. Speicher MR, Ballard SG, Ward DC. Karyotyping human chromosomes by combinatorial multi-fluor FISH. *Nature Genet* **12**:368, 1996.
55. Kallioniemi A, Kallioniemi OP, Sudar D. et al. Comparative genomic hybridization for molecular cytogenetic analysis of solid tumors. *Science* **258**:818–821, 1992.
56. Bryndorf T, Kirchhoff M, Rose H. et al. Comparative genomic hybridization in clinical cytogenetics. *Am J Hum Genet* **57**:1211–1220, 1995.
57. Cremer T, Landegent J, Brückner A. et al. Detection of chromosome aberrations in the human interphase nucleus by visualization of specific target DNAs with radioactive and non-radioactive in situ hybridization techniques: diagnosis of trisomy 18 with probe L1. 84. *Hum Genet* **74**:346–352, 1986.
58. Lichter P, Cremer T, Tang CJ, Watkins PC, Manuelidis L, Ward DC. Rapid detection of human chromosome 21 aberrations by in situ hybridization. *Proc Natl Acad Sci USA* **85**:9664–9668, 1988.
59. Lichter P, Jauch A, Cremer T, Ward DC. Detection of Down's syndrome by in situ hybridization with chromosome specific DNA probes. *Progress in Clinical and Biological Research* **360**:69–78, 1990.
60. Julien C, Bazin A, Guyot B, Forester F, Daffos F. Rapid prenatal diagnosis of Down's syndrome with in-situ hybridisation of fluorescent DNA probes. *Lancet* **ii**:863–864, 1986.

61. Bryndorf T, Christensen B, Philip J, Hansen W, Yokobata K, Bui N, Gaizer C. New rapid test for prenatal detection of trisomy 21 (Down's syndrome), preliminary report. *Br Med J* **304**:1536–1539, 1992.
62. Christensen B, Bryndorf T, Philip J, Lundsteen C, Hansen W. Rapid prenatal diagnosis of trisomy 18 and triploidy in interphase nuclei of uncultered amniocytes by non radioactive in situ hybridization. *Prenat Diagn* **12**:241–250, 1992.
63. Christensen B, Bryndorf T, Philip J, Xiang Y, Hansen W. Prenatal diagnosis by in situ hybridization on uncultured amniocytes: reduced sensitivity and potential risk of misdiagnosis in blood-stained samples. *Prenat Diagn* **13**:581–587, 1993.
64. Bryndorf T. Development and clinical studies of in situ hybridization techniques in prenatal diagnosis. *Dan Med Bull* **45**:298–319, 1998.
65. Kuo WL, Tenjin H, Segraves R, Pinkel D, Golbus MS, Gray J. Detection of aneuploidy involving chromosomes 13, 18, or 21, by fluorescence in situ hybridization (FISH) to interphase and metaphase amniocytes. *Am J Hum Genet* **49**: 112–119, 1991.
66. Zheng YL, Ferguson-Smith MA, Warner JP, Ferguson-Smith ME, Sargent CA, Carter NP. Analysis of chromosome 21 copy number in uncultured amniocytes by fluorescence in situ hybridization using a cosmid contig. *Prenat Diagn* **12**:931–943, 1992.
67. Cacheux V, Tachdjian G, Druart L. et al. Evaluation of X, Y, 18, and 13/21 alpha satellite DNA probes for interphase cytogenetic analysis of uncultured amniocytes by fluorescence in situ hybridization. *Prenat Diagn* **14**:79–86, 1994.
68. Rao PN, Hayworth R, Cox K, Grass F, Pettenati MJ. Rapid detection of aneuploidy in uncultured chorionic villus cells using fluorescence in situ hybridization. *Prenat Diagn* **13**:233–238, 1993.
69. Pandya PP, Kuhn P, Brizot M, Cardy DL, Nicolaides KH. Rapid detection of chromosome aneuploidies in fetal blood and chorionic villi by fluorescence in situ hybridisation. *Br J Obstet Gynaecol* **101**:493–497, 1994.
70. Zahed L, Murer-Orlando M, Vekemans M. In situ hybridization studies for the detection of common aneuploidies in CVS. *Prenat Diagn* **12**:483–493, 1992.
71. Klinger K, Landes G, Shook D. et al. Rapid detection of chromosome aneuploidies in uncultured amniocytes by using fluorescence in situ hybridization (FISH). *Am J Hum Genet* **51**:55–65, 1992.
72. Ward BE, Gersen SL, Carelli MP. et al. Rapid Prenatal Diagnosis of Chromosomal Aneuploidies by Fluorescence In Situ Hybridization: Clinical Experience with 4, 500 Specimens. *Am J Hum Genet* **52**:854–865, 1993.
73. Spathas DH, Divane A, Maniatis GM, Ferguson-Smith ME, Ferguson-Smith MA. Prenatal detection of trisomy 21 in uncultured amniocytes by fluorescence in situ hybridization: a prospective study. *Prenat Diagn* **14**:1049–1054, 1994.
74. Divane A, Carter NP, Spathas DH, Ferguson-Smith MA. Rapid prenatal diagnosis of aneuploidy from uncultured amniotic fluid cells using five-colour fluorescence in situ hybridization. *Prenat Diagn* **14**:1061–1069, 1994.
75. Bryndorf T, Christensen B, Vad M. et al. Prenatal detection of chromosome aneuploidies by fluorscence in situ hybridization: Experience with 2000 uncultured amniotic fluid samples in a prospective preclinical trial. *Prenat Diagn* **17**:333–341, 1997.
76. Thangavelu M, Pergamen E, Espinosa R, Bohlander SK. Characterization of marker chromosomes by microdissection and fluorescence in situ hybridization. *Prenat Diagn* **14**:583–588, 1994.
77. Brandt CA, Lyngbye T, Pedersen S, Bolund L, Friedrich U. Value of chromosome painting in determining the chromosomal outcome in offspring of a 12;16 translocation carrier. *J Med Genet* **31**:234–237, 1994.
78. Whiteman DAH, Klinger K. Efficiency of rapid in situ hybridization methods for prenatal diagnosis of chromosome abnormalities causing birth defects. *Am J Hum Genet* **49** (suppl):A1279, 1991.
79. Lebo RV, Flandermeyer RR, Diukeman R, Lynch ED, Lepercq JA, Golbus MS. Prenatal diagnosis with repetitive in situ hybridization probes. *Am J Med Genet* **43**:848–854, 1992.
80. Davies AF, Barber L, Murer-Orlando M, Bobrow M, Adinolfi M. FISH detection of trisomy 21 in interphase by the simultaneous use of two differentially labelled cosmid contigs. *J Med Genet* **31**:679–685, 1994.
81. Nederlof PM, van der Flier S, Wiegant J. et al. Multiple fluorescence in situ hybridization. *Cytometry* **11**:126–131, 1990.
82. Ried T, Landes G, Dackowski W, Klinger K, Ward DC. Multi-color fluorescence in situ hybridization for the simultaneous detection of probe sets for chromosomes 13, 18, 21, X and Y in uncultured amniotic fluid cells. *Hum Mol Genet* **1**:307–313, 1992.
83. Harper J. Preimplantation diagnosis of inherited disease by embryo biopsy: An update of the world figures. *J Ass Reprod Genet* **13**:1–6, 1996.
84. Delhanty JDA, Griffin DK, Handyside AH. et al. Detection of aneuploidy and chromosomal mosaicism in human embryos during preimplantation sex determination by fluorescent in situ hybridization (FISH). *Hum Mol Genet* **2**:1183–1185, 1993.
85. Verlinsky Y. Preimplantation diagnosis of genetic and chromosomal disorders. *J Ass Reprod Genet* **11**:216–243, 1994.
86. Coonen E, Harper JC, Ramaekers FCS. et al. *Hum Genet* **94**:609–615, 1994.
87. Jamieson ME, Coutts JRT, Connor JM. The chromosome constitution of human preimplantation embryos fertilized in vitro. *Hum Reprod* **9**:709–715, 1994.
88. Munné S, Lee A, Rosenwaks Z, Grifo J, Cohen J. Diagnosis of major chromosome aneuploidies in human preimplantation embryos. *Hum Reprod* **8**:2185–2191, 1993.
89. Zenses MT, Casper RF. Cytogenetics of human oocytes, zygotes, and embryos after in vitro fertilization. *Hum Genet* **88**:367–375, 1992.
90. Harper JC, Coonen E, Handyside AH, Winston RM, Hopman AH, Delhanty JD. Mosaicism of autosomes and sex chromosomes in morphologically normal, monospermic preimplantation human embryos. *Prenat Diagn* **15**:41–49, 1995.
91. Munné S, Weier HUG, Grifo J, Cohen J. Chromosome mosaicism in human embryos. *Biol Reprod* **51**:373–379, 1994.
92. Tarin JJ, Conaghan J, Winston RM, Handyside AH. Human embryo biopsy on the 2nd day after insemination for preimplantation diagnosis: removal of a quarter of embryo retards cleavage. *Fertil Steril* **58**:970–976, 1992.
93. Hall JG. Genomic imprinting: Review and relevance to human diseases. *Am J Hum Genet* **46**:857–873, 1990.
94. Engel E, DeLozier-Blanche DD. Uniparental disomy, isodisomy, and imprinting: probable effects in man and strategies for their detection. *Am J Med Genet* **40**:432–439, 1991.
95. Engel E. Uniparental disomy revisited: the first twelve years. *Am J Med Genet* **46**:670–674, 1993.
96. Kalousek DG, Langlois S, Barrett J. et al. Uniparental disomy for chromosome 16 in humans. *Am J Hum Genet* **52**:8–16, 1993.
97. Ledbetter DH, Engel E. Uniparental disomy in humans: development of an imprinting map and its implications for prenatal diagnosis. *Hum Mol Genet* **4**:1757–1764, 1995.
98. Nicholls RD. Genomic imprinting and uniparental disomy in Angelman and Prader-Willi syndromes: a review. *Am J Med Genet* **46**:16–25, 1993.
99. Kokkonen H, Kahkonen M, Leisti J. A molecular and cytogenetic study in Finnish Prader-Willi patients. *Hum Genet* **95**:568–571, 1995.
100. Smith A, Prasad M, Deng ZM, Robson L, Woodage T, Trent RJ. Comparison of high resolution cytogenetics, fluorescence in situ hybridisation, and DNA studies to validate the diagnosis of Prader-Willi and Angelman's syndromes. *Arch Dis Child* **72**:397–402, 1995.
101. Rodeck C, Tutschek B, Sherlock J, Kingdom J. Methods for the transcervical collection of fetal cells during the first trimester of pregnancy. *Prenat Diagn* **15**:933–942, 1995.
102. Adinolfi M. Non- or minimally invasive prenatal diagnostic tests on maternal blood samples or transcervical cells. *Prenat Diagn* **15**:889–896, 1995.
103. Walknowska J, Conte FA, Brumbach MM. Practical and theoretical implications of fetal/maternal lymphocyte transfer. *Lancet* **1**:1119–1122, 1969.
104. Lo UD, Patel P, Baigent CN. et al. Prenatal sex determination from maternal peripheral blood using the polymerase chain reaction. *Hum Genet* **90**:483–488, 1993.
105. Price JO, Elias S, Wachtel SS. et al. Prenatal diagnosis with fetal cells isolated from maternal blood by multiparameter flow cytometry. *Am J Obstet Gyneol* **165**:1731–1737, 1991.
106. Elias S, Price J, Dockter M, Wachtel S, Tharapel A, Simpson JL. First trimester diagnosis of trisomy 21 in fetal cells from maternal blood. *Lancet* **340**:1033, 1992.

107. Gänshirt-Ahlert D, Börjesson-Stoll R, Burschyk M. et al. Detection of fetal trisomies 21 and 18 from maternal blood using triple gradient and magnetic sorting. *Am J Rep Immun* **30**:194–201, 1993.
108. Lyon MF. X-chromosome inactivation and the location and expression of X-linked genes. *Am J Hum Genet* **42**:8–16, 1988.
109. Kotzot D, Schmitt S, Bernasconi F. et al. Uniparental disomy 7 in Silver-Russell syndrome and primordial growth retardation. *Hum Mol Genet* **4**:583–587, 1995.
110. Hoglund P, Holmberg C, de la Chapelle A, Kere J. Paternal isodisomy for chromosome 7 is compatible with normal growth and development in a patient with congenital chloride diarrhea. *Am J Hum Genet* **55**:747–752, 1994.
111. Spotila LD, Sereda L, Prockop DJ. Partial isodisomy for maternal chromosome 7 and short stature in an individual with a mutation at the COL1A2 locus. *Am J Hum Genet* **51**:1396–1405, 1992.
112. Willatt LR, Davison BC, Goudie D. et al. A male with trisomy 9 mosaicism and maternal uniparental disomy for chromosome 9 in the euploid cell line. *J Med Genet* **29**:742–744, 1992.
113. Wada M, Seeger RC, Mizoguchi H, Koeffler HP. Maintenance of normal imprinting of H19 and IGF2 genes in neuroblastoma. *Cancer Res* **55**:3386–3388, 1995.
114. Slater H, Shaw JH, Dawson G, Bankier A, Forrest SM. Maternal uniparental disomy of chromosome 13 in a phenotypically normal child. *J Med Genet* **31**:644–646, 1994.
115. Bischoff FX, Feldman GL, McCaskill C, Subramanian S, Hughes MR, Shaffer LG. Single cell analysis demonstrating somatic mosaicism involving 11p in a patient with paternal isodisomy and Beckwith-Wiedemann syndrome. *Hum Mol Genet* **4**:395–399, 1995.
116. Slatter RE, Elliott M, Welham K, Carrera M, Schofield PN, Barton DE. Mosaic uniparental disomy in Beckwith-Wiedemann syndrome. *J Med Genet* **31**:749–753, 1994.
117. Healey S, Powell F, Battersby M, Chenevix-Trench G, McGill J. Distinct phenotype in maternal uniparental disomy of chromosome 14. *Am J Med Genet* **51**:147–149, 1994.
118. Sirchia SM, De-Andreis C, Pariani S, Grimoldi MG, Molinari A, Buscaglia M. Chromosome 14 maternal uniparental disomy in the euploid cell line of a fetus with mosaic 46, XX/47, XX, +14 karyotype. *Hum Genet* **94**:355–358, 1994.
119. Antonarakis SE, Blouin JL, Maher J, Avramopoulos D, Thomas G, Albot CCJ. Maternal uniparental disomy for human chromosome 14, due to loss of a chromosome 14 from somatic cells with t (13;14) trisomy 14. *Am J Hum Genet* **52**:1145–1152, 1993.
120. Temple IK, Cockwell A, Hassold T, Pettay D, Jacobs P. Maternal uniparental disomy for chromosome 14. *J Med Genet* **28**:511–514, 1991.
121. Woodage T, Deng ZM, Prasad M. et al. A variety of genetic mechanisms are associated with the Prader-Willi syndrome. *Am J Med Genet* **54**:219–226, 1994.
122. Vaughan J, Ali Z, Bower S, Bennett P, Chard T, Moore G. Human maternal uniparental disomy for chromosome 16 and fetal development. *Prenat Diagn* **14**:751–756, 1994.
123. Wilkins-Haug L. The emerging genetic theories of unstable DNA, uniparental disomy and imprinting. *Curr Opin Obstet Gynecol* **5**:179–185, 1993.
124. Mascari MJ, Gottlieb W, Rogan PK. et al. The frequency of uniparental disomy in Prader-Willi syndrome. Implications for molecular diagnosis. *N Engl J Med* **326**:1348–1350, 1992.
125. Whiteford ML, Coutts J, Al-Roomi L. et al. Uniparental isodisomy for chromosome 16 in a growth-retarded infant with congenital heart disease. *Prenat Diagn* **15**:579–584, 1995.

DNA analysis

38

D.E. Barton

Introduction

Advances in the technology available for the analysis of deoxyribonucleic acid (DNA) have formed the basis of the modern genetic 'revolution'. Drawing from advances in microbiology, virology, enzymology and gel electrophoresis, scientists working only some 20-odd years ago developed the core techniques which are today used in gene discovery and analysis, as well as in diagnostic and predictive testing. This chapter provides an introduction to the rudiments of DNA analysis, with particular emphasis on those techniques likely to be used in prenatal diagnosis. To understand the applications of this technology, some basic knowledge of DNA structure and behaviour is required.

DNA

Every cell that has a nucleus contains DNA in that nucleus. DNA is formed from two antiparallel strands of bases. The strands are held together by hydrogen bonds which form between the bases (Fig. 38.1A). The base adenine can only bond with thymidine, and guanosine only bonds with cytosine, so the base sequence on one strand must be complementary to that on the other for the double helix to form. This base pairing is fundamental to the way DNA behaves, both in vivo and in vitro. The hydrogen bonds holding the two strands together are fragile, and can be disrupted by raising the temperature or the pH, or by lowering the salt concentration of the DNA solution. This causes the double helix to separate or *denature* into single-stranded DNA. Under the appropriate conditions (high salt, low temperature, low pH), formation of double-stranded DNA is strongly favoured, and short single-stranded DNA molecules, or 'probes' will very rapidly find their complementary sequence, even in highly complex mixtures. This ability of DNA probes to locate and bind to their 'target' sequences is exploited throughout molecular genetics.

As DNA is the same substance whether it is viral, bacterial, plant or animal in origin, the enzymes produced by simple organisms to synthesize and maintain their DNA can be

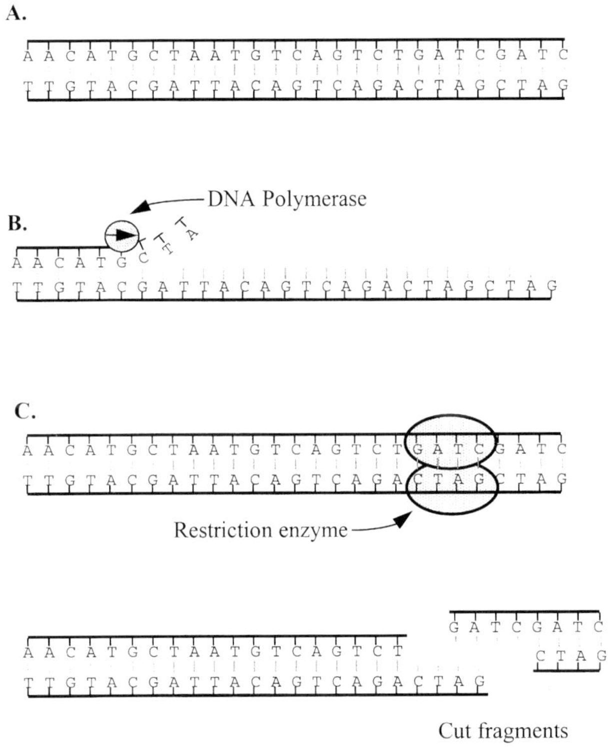

Fig. 38.1 (A) A stretch of double-stranded DNA showing the pairing of complementary bases, joined by hydrogen bonds. (B) DNA polymerase catalyses the addition of new bases to a short 'primer' strand, using the longer strand as a template. (C) A restriction enzyme first binds to its recognition sequence (GATC), then cuts both strands. Note the recognition sequence is the same on both strands.

isolated and used to manipulate human DNA in vitro. A wide range of such enzymes is commercially available, and they form part of the basic toolkit of the molecular geneticist.

DNA polymerase catalyses the synthesis of a complementary strand using a single-stranded template. All polymerases require at least a short *primer* sequence of double-stranded DNA (Fig. 38.1B). The primer is extended to match the template strand. DNA polymerases are used to amplify DNA in the polymerase chain reaction (see below) and to incorporate fluorescent, chemical or radioactive tracers or 'labels' into DNA to be used as 'probes'. The primer, by binding only to its precise complementary sequence on the template, determines what part of the template DNA gets replicated.

Restriction enzymes recognize specific four- to six-base sequences in double-stranded DNA, and cut the DNA strands within (or close to) their recognition sequence (Fig. 38.1C). Each restriction enzyme has a unique recognition sequence. These enzymes are produced by bacteria as a defence against viruses – they are called 'restriction' enzymes because they restrict the strains of bacteria which can be infected by the virus. Each enzyme is named for the strain of bacteria from which it is isolated. For example, EcoRI comes from *E. coli* strain R.

Mutations and polymorphisms

Each human cell contains six thousand million bases of DNA, and it would be extraordinary if this amount of information could be copied time after time without some changes creeping in. In fact, such changes, or *mutations* are the driving force of evolution. Most mutations involve the substitution of one base for another in the DNA code – the biological equivalent of a typographical error. Within a gene, such a substitution is likely to change or destroy the function of the protein encoded by that gene. There is an agreed nomenclature for such mutations[1,2], using the single letter code for the normal amino acid, followed by the position (amino acid number) in the protein, then the mutant amino acid; e.g. G551D is a common mutation in cystic fibrosis in which the glycine (G) at position 551 is changed to aspartic acid (D).

Mutations can also involve the removal (deletion) or insertion of one or more bases. If the insertion/deletion does not remove an integral number of coding units (three bases each), the reading frame of the gene is disrupted, and a nonsense protein produced. Such mutations are known as frameshifts. Less frequently, genes suffer much larger disruptions, such as deletion or duplication of all or most of the coding sequence, as is seen in Duchenne muscular dystrophy (see Ch. 44).

The DNA changes described above are identified as 'mutations' because they disrupt or eliminate the function of a gene. Many DNA variants, however, do not cause any change in a gene's function, but are passed through the generations as neutral 'polymorphisms'. These polymorphisms can be detected if the sequence change creates or destroys a recognition site for a restriction enzyme – so-called restriction fragment length polymorphisms (RFLPs). Like many forms of DNA variation, RFLPs were first recognized in humans in the β-globin gene[3] and their utility for diagnostic purposes was immediately recognized[3,4].

Other kinds of variation in DNA involve changes in stretches of short repeated sequences. Human DNA is liberally sprinkled with such sequences – a run of the bases cytosine and adenine repeated many times over is a common example, written (CA)n. The value of n can vary from one person to another, providing a further useful source of polymorphic markers for genetic analysis[5]. Such simple repeated sequences are variously referred to as di- (or tri- or tetra-) nucleotide repeats, microsatellites or short tandem repeats (STRs). In recent years, it has been recognized that triplet repeat stretches are occasionally important parts of genes or their regulatory regions, and that expansions in the size of these repeat stretches represent an important new type of disease-causing mutation, especially in inherited neurological disorders.

Both kinds of polymorphism – RFLPs and STRs – are used as genetic 'markers' in diagnostic testing when the mutation cannot be identified directly, in a technique known as linkage analysis (see below).

DNA analysis

The range of techniques now available for DNA analysis is very broad, and a review of all such techniques is beyond the scope of the present text. The techniques used in DNA-based prenatal diagnosis is much more limited, as one is invariably dealing with known mutations or polymorphic markers known to be informative in the family.

The purpose of taking prenatal samples from the fetus is to determine whether the fetus has inherited the disease-causing mutation(s) identified in the parent(s). There are several different techniques available to achieve this, most of which are based upon either the Southern blot or the polymerase chain reaction (PCR), but fundamental to almost all DNA analysis is the technique of gel electrophoresis.

GEL ELECTROPHORESIS

In electrophoresis, DNA fragments are separated according to size by forcing them through a porous matrix (gel) under the influence of an electric field. DNA is negatively charged in neutral or near-neutral pH solutions, and thus migrates from cathode to anode through the gel. The gel material is usually agarose or polyacrylamide. The smaller fragments move more rapidly through the gel than larger ones, so that the size of a fragment can be estimated by the distance it has travelled through the gel at a specific time, compared to a series of marker fragments of known size, a 'ladder'. DNA fragments are made visible after the gel run has finished, by staining with a fluorescent DNA-binding dye such as ethidium bromide, by staining with silver, or by autoradiography if the DNA has been made radioactive. Modern DNA analysers detect fluorescently labelled DNA fragments as they pass a fluorescence detector, producing 'traces' similar to an HPLC analyser (see Fig. 38.4). Most diagnostic tests are based on the presence, absence or change in size of a specific DNA fragment on an electrophoresis gel.

But how are such fragments produced and identified, when the human genome is so vast? Two very different approaches are taken to study specific DNA sequences from total human DNA.

SOUTHERN BLOTTING

The Southern blot was first described by Ed Southern in 1975[6], and remains an essential technique in the analysis of DNA from complex genomes. In essence, it allows us to identify a specific DNA fragment from a mixture of many millions of fragments, and to determine its size and even its relative abundance. In this technique, a mixture of DNA fragments – in the present context, a restriction digest of a patient's DNA – is first separated by size on an electrophoresis gel (Fig. 38.2). Such a digest typically contains over a million fragments, and it is of course impossible to determine the presence or absence of any particular fragment by inspection of the gel directly. In Southern's technique (Fig. 38.2), the DNA is chemically denatured in situ before being transferred by capillary action (blotting) onto a DNA-binding membrane. The membrane holds all the DNA from the gel in an exact image of the gel itself. The DNA on the membrane, being single stranded, is receptive to hybridization with a DNA 'probe' corresponding to the sequence of interest. This probe will have been generated from a portion of the gene or sequence under study cloned in bacteria, and will have been enzymatically modified to carry a 'label' which allows it to be detected visually. The probe is applied to the membrane under conditions conducive to the formation of double-stranded DNA, and the unbound probe is washed away. The probe is then detected by one of several techniques depending upon what label was used. The most common label is phosphorus 32, a strong emitter of beta radiation, which is detected by autoradiography. The size and intensity of the fragment(s) detected in the patient's DNA can be compared to appropriate control DNAs to detect abnormalities in the gene from which the probe is derived.

POLYMERASE CHAIN REACTION

The second key technique used to identify specific sequences from total human DNA is purely enzymatic, and, unlike Southern blotting, does not require prior digestion or electrophoresis of the patient's DNA. The polymerase chain reaction (PCR) makes it possible to amplify a specific sequence of DNA many millionfold, to the exclusion of all other sequences in the starting material. Invented in 1985[7], this rapid and powerful technique has replaced Southern blotting in many areas of molecular genetic diagnosis and research. The technique requires that the DNA sequences flanking the area of interest be known. Short, single-stranded synthetic DNA 'primers' corresponding to these sequences give the reaction its specificity. When bound to their matching sequences in the patient ('template') DNA, they can be extended enzymatically by a DNA polymerase to make a second copy of the area of interest (Fig. 38.3). Cycling this sequence of template DNA denaturation, primer binding and DNA synthesis allows the newly synthesized products from each round to act as templates in the next, giving rise to a logarithmic amplification of the sequences between the two primers. If total human DNA can be considered as a 24-volume encyclopaedia, PCR allows us to photocopy one word on one page of that encyclopaedia until we have enough of it to fill a room. Examining the products, we can concentrate on the word we have copied, and ignore the rest of the encyclopaedia. This technique can be used to detect any of the different kinds of mutations which cause inherited disorders, either by simple electrophoresis to detect, quantify or size the PCR products on a gel, or in combination with one of the mutation detection techniques described below.

Because of the power of PCR to amplify a template a millionfold in just 30 cycles, and potentially a million-millionfold in 45 cycles, it is essential to avoid contamination of the starting materials by products from previous reactions. Many laboratories now have physically separate areas, one for patient DNA preparation and PCR set-up, and one for PCR product analysis. Every set of PCR reactions should include a control tube which is identical to the others except that no template DNA is added. The presence of a PCR product in this tube indicates contaminated reagents and negates the results from the rest of the set. The risk from contamination is more acute when template DNA is limited and high cycle numbers are required, an extreme case being preimplantation diagnosis.

DELETION ANALYSIS AND DIRECT SIZING

Deletions can result in the absence of a fragment on Southern blot or absence of a PCR product. When investigated by PCR, steps need to be taken to distinguish the presence of a deletion from simple technical failure of the PCR reaction. Such deletion screens are often carried out in 'multiplex' reactions, in which many parts of a gene are amplified simultaneously in the same tube. Non-deleted fragments act as positive controls for the PCR reaction.

Triplet repeat expansions can be detected by Southern blot (Fig. 38.4) if they are very large (fragile X syndrome, myotonic dystrophy) or by PCR (Huntington's disease, dominant ataxias, Friedreich's ataxia, Fig. 38.5). As long as appropriate controls are included in the assay, this constitutes one of the most straightforward diagnostic approaches.

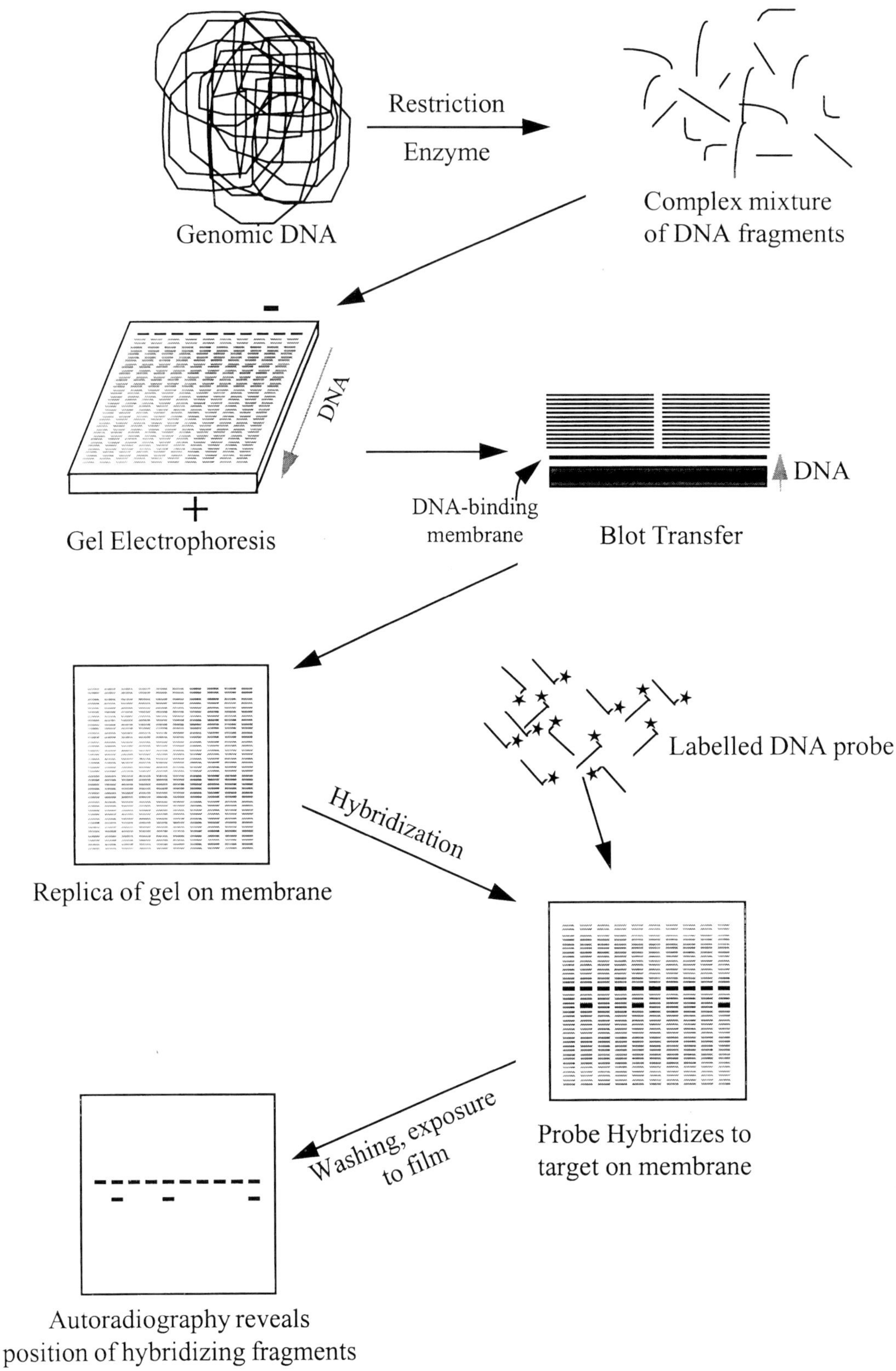

Fig. 38.2 Southern blotting of restriction-enzyme-digested human DNA. Typically, digesting human DNA with an enzyme with a six-base recognition sequence generates approximately one million different DNA fragments.

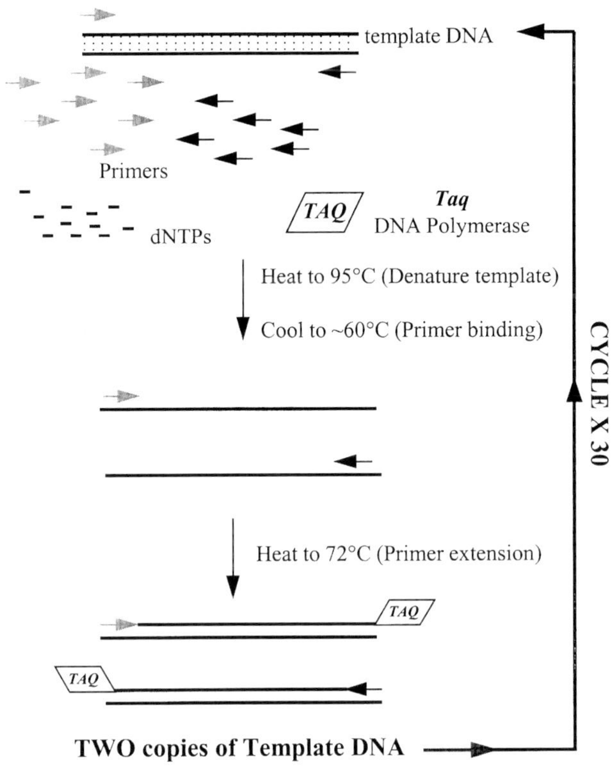

Fig. 38.3 The polymerase chain reaction. The ingredients are template DNA, short single-stranded 'primers', all four DNA building blocks (deoxyribonucleotide triphosphates, dNTPs) and *Taq* DNA polymerase.

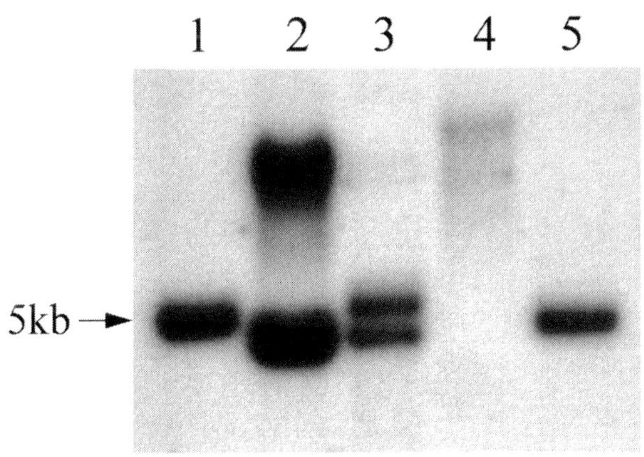

Fig. 38.4 Southern blot test for fragile X syndrome. An EcoRI digest of patient DNA is hybridized with probe Ox1.9, derived from the fragile X gene[20]. Triplet repeat expansions result in the appearance of fragments larger than normal. Lane 1, normal female; lane 2, affected female; lane 3, premutation carrier female; lane 4, affected male; lane 5, normal male. (*Source*: National Centre for Medical Genetics, Dublin, Ireland.)

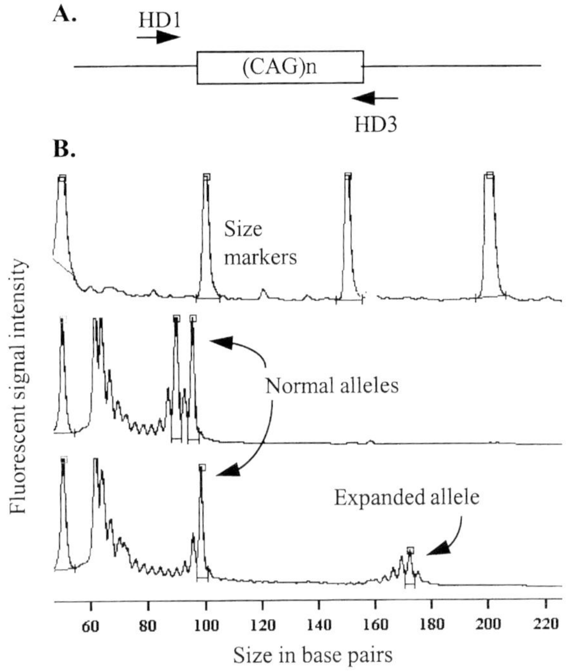

Fig. 38.5 Direct sizing of the (CAG)*n* repeat in the Huntington's disease gene by PCR. (A) Schematic showing positions of the PCR primers relative to the (CAG)*n* repeat[21]. (B) Fluorescently labelled PCR products are detected as they pass through a laser beam in the ALF™ DNA analyser (Amersham Pharmacia). The upper trace shows size standards; the middle trace shows an individual with two alleles in the normal range; the lower trace shows an affected individual, with one normal and one expanded allele. (*Source*: National Centre for Medical Genetics, Dublin, Ireland.)

RESTRICTION DIGESTION

Restriction enzymes, as described above, cut double-stranded DNA whenever they bind to a specific DNA sequence (Fig. 38.1C). Some disease-causing mutations will create or destroy one of these recognition sequences, and result in an altered fragment size. Restriction enzyme digestion is used in DNA diagnosis in conjunction with Southern blotting, when the patient's DNA is digested before electrophoresis and blotting, and in PCR, when the appropriate PCR products from the patient's DNA are tested by restriction digestion. Some caution must be exercised in interpreting the results of such tests. A change in *any* base of an enzyme's recognition sequence can result in a failure to cut, so it is preferable to use an assay where a new site is created rather than one where an existing site is eliminated. Even when testing for the creation of a new site, it is important to bear in mind that the creation of a restriction site elsewhere on the same PCR fragment by a naturally occurring polymorphism could yield a false positive result. This is a particular danger in mitochondrial DNA, which is known to be highly polymorphic[8].

ALLELE-SPECIFIC PCR

Mutations which do not cause changes in restriction enzyme recognition sites can still be detected by PCR. The DNA polymerases used for PCR are very sensitive to mismatches between the synthetic DNA primer and the template DNA, so that the PCR reaction will usually fail if one primer is not perfectly matched to the template. This characteristic can be exploited by designing a PCR reaction where one of the primers binds directly to the mutation site[9]. The PCR reaction will only produce a product if the mutation is present. A control reaction is carried out in which the test primer perfectly matches the normal sequence. With careful design of the PCR primers to give different product sizes, several mutations can be screened for at once in a multiplex reaction[10] (Fig. 38.6). This technique, known as allele-specific PCR or amplification refractory mutation system (ARMS™), forms the basis of a commercial kit for cystic fibrosis mutation screening.

ALLELE-SPECIFIC OLIGONUCLEOTIDE HYBRIDIZATION

Point mutations of all kinds can be detected without gel electrophoresis, by hybridization of the patient's PCR-amplified DNA with short synthetic DNA probes known as oligonucleotides. Early versions of this technique (Fig. 38.7A) involved spotting the target (patient) DNA onto a membrane (known as a dot-blot), and hybridizing it with labelled oligonucleotides corresponding to the mutant or the normal sequence, so-called allele-specific oligonucleotides (ASOs)[11]. If appropriate hybridization and washing conditions are used, single-base differences can be distinguished in this way. This approach is most useful when screening large numbers of samples for a single mutation. When one wants to screen smaller numbers of patients for many mutations simultaneously, it is more convenient to immobilize the ASO probes on the membrane and hybridize labelled, PCR-amplified patient DNA to them (reverse dot-blot, Fig. 38.7B)[12]. This technology is used in several commercially available DNA testing kits, for cystic fibrosis and for tissue typing, amongst other applications.

LINKAGE ANALYSIS

The preceding paragraphs have discussed diagnostic techniques in situations where the disease-causing mutation can be detected directly, but this is not always the case. Many disease genes have been mapped but not identified, meaning that we know which polymorphic markers are close (linked) to the gene, but we do not yet know the sequence of the gene itself. In other cases, finding the mutation can be impossible because the gene is too large and/or the pattern of mutations too variable. In these instances, linkage analysis is used to track the mutation through the family.

The polymorphic markers used can be any of the types of DNA variation described above, and a simple RFLP in the β-globin gene was used in the earliest reported DNA-based prenatal diagnosis[4]. However, microsatellites are now favoured, for their large numbers of alleles and high informativeness. To apply a linkage-based test, it is essential to have samples from several family members, usually including the index case and both parents (Fig. 38.8). The clinical status (affected or unaffected) of family members must be carefully assessed before linkage analysis is undertaken, and the diagnosis must be absolutely firm. The pattern of linked markers in these individuals is studied to determine if they are informative – that is, if the variants (alleles) present allow the mutated gene(s) to be followed through the family distinct from the normal copies. It is usual to test markers which lie on both sides of the disease gene (flanking markers), to guard against an incorrect result due to recombination (crossing over) between the marker used and the disease gene. The further a marker is away from the disease gene, the more likely it is that a crossover will be observed, so markers are selected to be as close to the disease gene as possible.

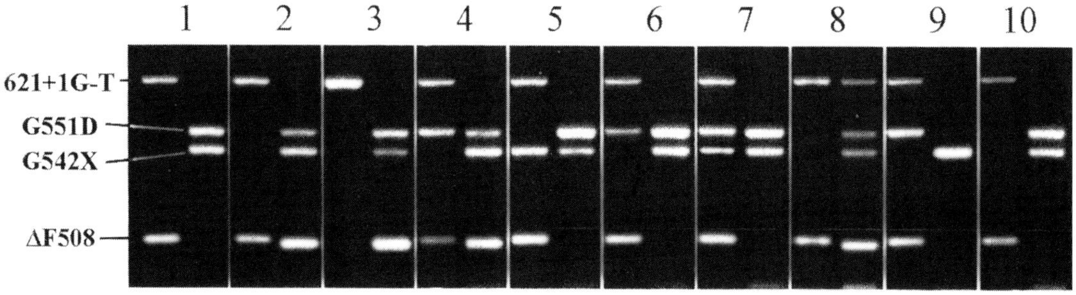

Fig. 38.6 Detection of mutations in the cystic fibrosis gene by allele-specific PCR or ARMS™. This multiplex reaction tests for four different mutations. Two lanes are run for each patient. Panel 1 shows the pattern from an normal sample, with two fragments present in each lane. When a mutation is present, the corresponding fragment shows up in the 'wrong' lane. Panel 2, ΔF508 carrier; panel 3, ΔF508/ΔF508; panel 4, G551D/ΔF508; panel 5, G542X carrier; panel 6, G551D carrier; panel 7, G551D/G542X; panel 8, 621+1G → T/ΔF508; panel 9, G551D/G551D; panel 10, normal. (*Source*: National Centre for Medical Genetics, Dublin, Ireland.)

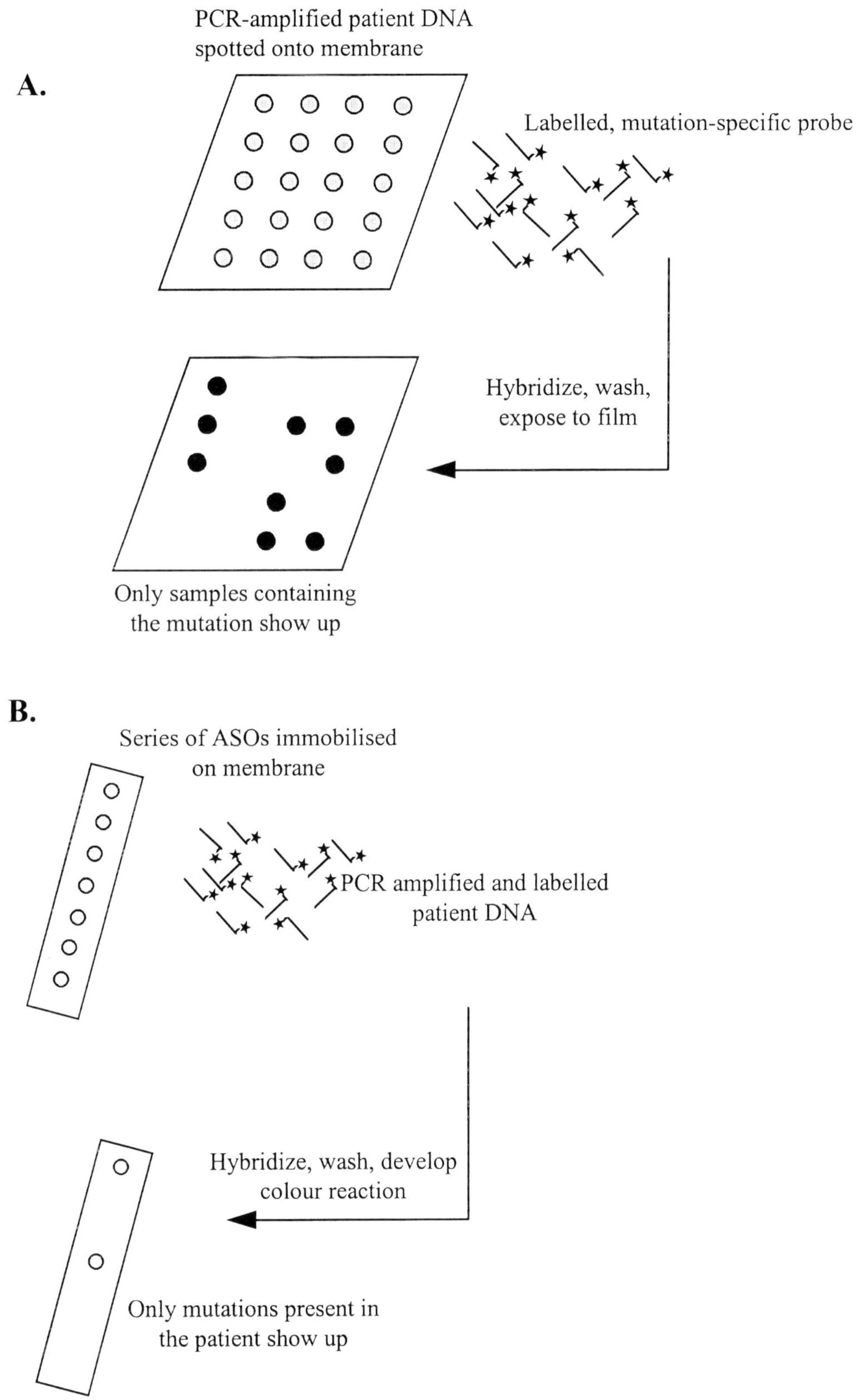

Fig. 38.7 Allele-specific oligonucleotide probe hybridization. Short synthetic probes can be used to detect single-base differences in patient samples. In the standard dot-blot (A) many patient samples are screened for a single mutation at once. In the reverse dot-blot (B) a single patient sample is screened for many mutations simultaneously.

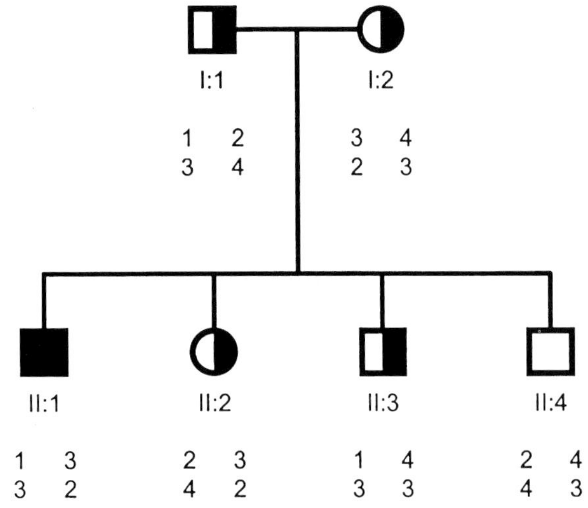

Fig. 38.8 An example of linkage-based diagnosis for an autosomal recessive disorder. The four children have inherited all possible combinations of alleles from the parents. Having determined which alleles segregate with the disease by testing the affected child, it is possible to determine that two of his siblings are carriers, while one has inherited two normal alleles.

Preparation of DNA

To analyse DNA from a patient sample, be it prenatal or otherwise, the DNA must first be released from the cells, and must often be further purified by removal of other cellular components. The cells are usually broken open using a non-ionic detergent such as sodium dodecyl sulphate, then the proteins are digested away using a fungal protease. The degraded proteins are removed by fractionation or precipitation before the DNA is precipitated out using alcohol. The precipitated DNA is redissolved in a buffer solution designed to prevent the action of DNA-degrading enzymes (nucleases), which are ubiquitous.

With prenatal samples, two concerns are overriding – the yield of DNA from the amount of sample (which is usually limiting), and the presence of contaminating maternal material.

Since the advent of PCR, DNA yield (and indeed purity) is less of a concern than heretofore, but some tests (notably fragile X syndrome and myotonic dystrophy) are still carried out using the Southern blot technique, which requires relatively large amounts of pure DNA. DNA yields are maximized by keeping the volume of solutions used as low as is practicable, and taking measures to minimize losses in tube-to-tube transfers.

MATERNAL CONTAMINATION

While the measures taken to combat losses during DNA preparation are the same for all three prenatal sample types (chorionic villus samples, amniocytes, and fetal blood), the measures taken to eliminate maternal contamination are specific to each sample type. Maternal 'decidua' must be assumed to be present in every chorionic villus biopsy, and are best removed by careful dissection under a microscope. The chorionic villus 'fronds' are clearly distinguishable (to the experienced eye) from the maternal decidua and can easily be dissected away. For PCR-based tests, many laboratories dissect out three individual fronds. Crude DNA is prepared from the three fronds and purified DNA from the rest of the sample, and the assay is performed in quadruplicate on these four DNA preparations. Any discrepancies in the results require further investigations to prove the sample is purely fetal in origin.

Similarly, maternal cells must be presumed to be present in all amniotic fluid samples when first taken. As no dissection is possible on these samples, the most effective way to eliminate the maternal contamination is by culturing the amniocytes exactly as for cytogenetic analysis. This is not always necessary, however, when maternal contamination would not confuse the results. For example, in determining fetal sex by PCR, the presence of maternal material will not mask the presence of a Y-chromosome, and in cases where the mother does not carry the mutation being tested for, unambiguous results can often be obtained from samples without dissection or tissue culture.

Even when the procedures outlined above are followed to minimize maternal cell contamination, it is advisable to use an independent method to assess the sample. The most reliable method is to use a highly polymorphic marker, and to verify the presence of both paternal and maternal alleles in the DNA prepared from the sample. This assay will also help to verify that the paternity of the sample is as expected, which is essential to the interpretation of the test results in many cases.

Preparing for a prenatal diagnosis

It is impossible to overemphasize the importance of investigating the family by molecular genetic testing *before* embarking upon a DNA-based prenatal diagnosis. The causative mutation must be identified in the index case or their parents wherever possible, and it is essential to determine which markers are informative before a linkage based prenatal test is initiated. There are two main reasons to test the family as early as possible – to save time and to confirm the diagnosis. Much DNA testing is sequential – laboratories will look for the most common mutations first, and only proceed to rarer mutations if this first test is negative – and the work-up of a family can take several weeks. Clearly, it is too late to start this when a consultand is already 10 or 12 weeks pregnant. Many genetic disorders are difficult to diagnose, or can be caused by mutations in different genes. Prenatal diagnosis is not possible in such cases unless the test to be applied has been verified to be applicable to the family in question. This will usually involve demonstration that a mutation is present in an affected member of the family. Preparation for linkage-based testing can involve the investigation of many different polymorphic markers before informative flanking markers are found. Patients considering prenatal diagnosis should be advised to seek genetic advice and testing *before the pregnancy has commenced*, as only then can they embark on the pregnancy in full knowledge of all the options available to them.

Future directions

The techniques described in this chapter have all been in use for molecular genetic diagnosis, including prenatal diagnosis, for many years. New techniques have been developed for screening for unknown mutations during that time, but these are rarely, if ever, used in prenatal diagnosis. However, several new technologies for the detection of specific mutations have also been described in recent times. Some of these have been designed with the express purpose of taking the gel electrophoresis out of the system, as gel electrophoresis is notoriously difficult to automate, and many of these developments are aimed at large scale, automated DNA testing rather than at prenatal diagnosis.

One way to get around the need for gel electrophoresis in DNA testing would be to develop probes whose characteristics change in some detectable way when they hybridize with their target. Two recently developed techniques have achieved this by using probes labelled with fluorophore–quencher pairs. These are pairs of molecules, one of which (the quencher) can absorb the fluorescence energy from the other (the fluorophore), so that no fluorescent signal is emitted. This quenching effect requires the quencher and fluorophore to be physically close together – the quenching efficiency decreases with the sixth power of the distance between the pair. Any assay which can effect a change in the probe to alter the distance between the fluorophore and quencher in the presence of perfectly matched target will have very high sensitivity.

MOLECULAR BEACONS

Tyagi and Kramer[13] described a type of short DNA probe with a fluorophore on one end and a quencher on the other. The two ends of the probe are complementary to each other, so that the probe forms a hairpin structure in the absence of its target sequence (Fig. 38.9). In this conformation, the fluorophore and quencher are brought close together, and the probe does not fluoresce. In the presence of perfectly matched target sequence, the hairpin unfolds as the central part of the probe hybridizes with the target, and the probe becomes fluorescent. The detection of this fluorescence confirms the presence of the target sequence in the sample without the need for electrophoresis.

TAQ-MAN

A slightly different way of using the fluorophore–quencher approach relies on the ability of *Taq* DNA polymerase to 'chew away' any DNA that it finds in its way when extending a primer. A probe is designed to bind to a PCR product when perfectly matched. The probe has a fluorophore–quencher pair attached at opposite ends, and fluorescence is quenched while both are attached to the same probe (Fig. 38.10). When the perfectly matched probe binds to the PCR product during amplification, *Taq* DNA polymerase degrades it, releasing the fluorophore into the solution, where it can fluoresce.

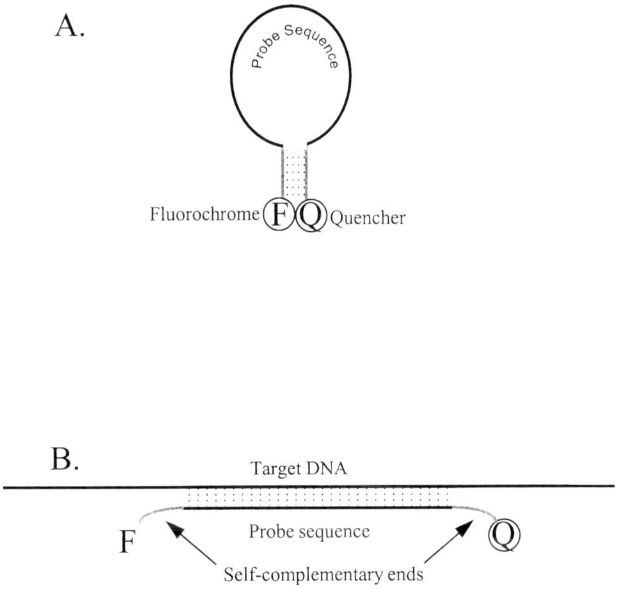

Fig. 38.9 Molecular beacons. When no target sequence is present, the probe folds into a hairpin structure, and the fluorescence energy is absorbed by the quencher (A). The probe unfolds in the presence of target sequence (B) and the fluorescence becomes visible.

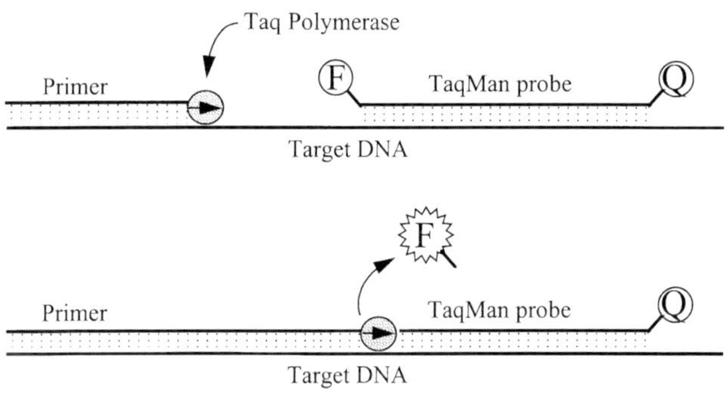

Fig. 38.10 '*Taq*-man' method for mutation detection. The probe, carrying a fluorophore–quencher pair, only binds to the PCR product if perfectly matched. If the probe binds, the *Taq* DNA polymerase cuts off the first nucleotide of the probe (with the fluorophore attached), releasing it into the solution, where it can fluoresce. The other half of the PCR reaction which generates the target has been omitted for clarity.

OLIGONUCLEOTIDE ARRAYS

The reverse dot-blot technique described above, in which amplified test (patient) DNA is hybridized to short probes immobilized on a surface, can be used to detect several mutations simultaneously. It has long been reasoned that if the number of probes was sufficiently great, any possible mutation could be detected. In effect, it even would be possible to determine the sequence of any stretch of DNA this way. The twin problems of synthesizing the very dense oligonucleotide arrays required and detecting the 'signals' from the hybridizing test DNA have now been largely overcome[14,15], and diagnostic tests based on DNA 'chips' are possible[16,17] (Fig. 38.11). This approach has the potential to replace many of the techniques currently in use in molecular genetics laboratories. Not only will it be possible, in a single assay, to screen for any possible mutation in an entire gene, but it will be possible to determine the pattern of expression of hundreds or thousands of genes simultaneously[18,19]. The introduction of such technology could in time also allow an individual (born or unborn) to be tested for variants or mutations in a large number of genes known to predispose to common disorders, and may be used to classify individuals into groups at higher risk of heart disease, diabetes, cancer etc. The technology will be there – it will be up to societies to decide if they wish to use it.

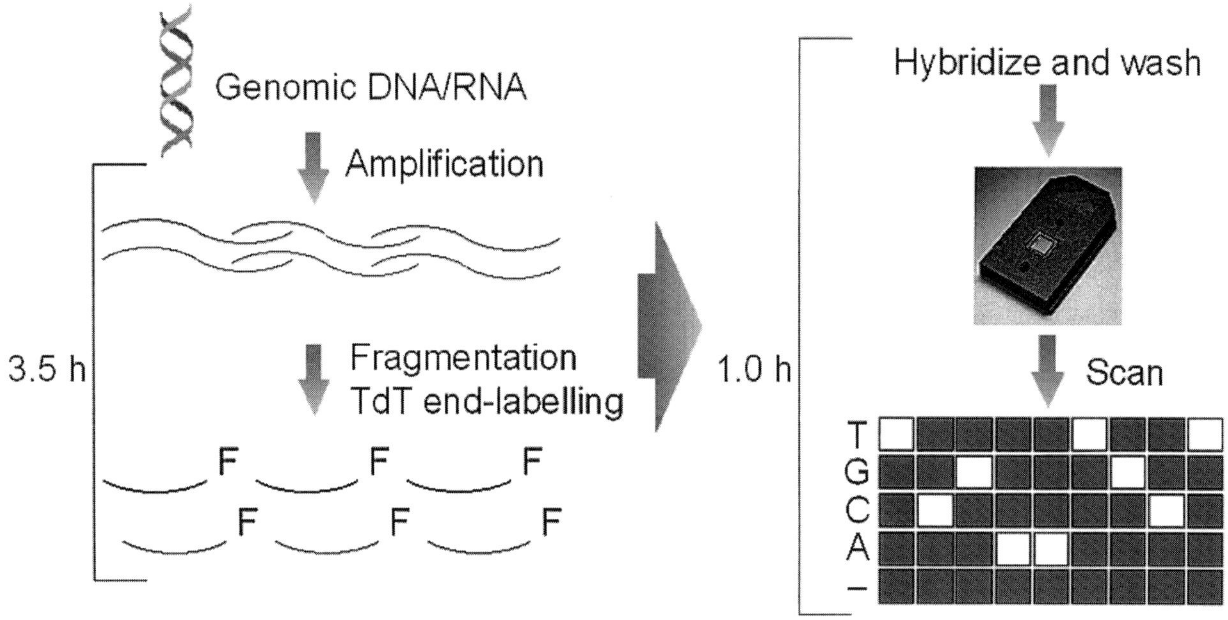

Fig. 38.11 Schematic of DNA analysis using an oligonucleotide array on a 'chip'. Patient DNA is amplified by PCR, fluorescently labelled and hybridized to the array in a specially designed cassette. Hybridization signals are detected in a purpose-designed apparatus using a confocal microscope. The output is a checkerboard pattern of hybridizing and non-hybridizing oligonucleotides. Attribution: Affymeltix Inc., Santa Clara, CA.

REFERENCES

1. Beaudet AL, Tsui LC. A suggested nomenclature for designating mutations. *Hum Mutat* **2**(4):245–248, 1993.
2. Beaudet AL, Antonarakis SE, Beutler E et al. Update on nomenclature for human gene-mutations. *Hum Mutat* **8**(3):197–202, 1996.
3. Kan Y, Dozy A. Polymorphism of DNA sequence adjacent to human beta-globin structural gene: relationship to sickle mutation. *Proc Natl Acad Sci USA* **75**(11):5631–5635, 1978.
4. Kan Y, Dozy A. Antenatal diagnosis of sickle-cell anaemia by DNA analysis of amniotic-fluid cells. *Proc Natl Acad Sci USA* **77**:6754–6758, 1978.
5. Weber JL, May PE. Abundant class of human DNA polymorphisms which can be typed using the polymerase chain-reaction. *Am J Hum Genet* **44**(3):388–396, 1989.
6. Southern E. Detection of specific sequences among DNA fragments separated by gel electrophoresis. *J Mol Biol* **98**(3):503–517, 1975.
7. Saiki RK, Scharf S, Faloona F et al. Enzymatic amplification of beta-globin genomic sequences and restriction site analysis for diagnosis of sickle-cell anemia. *Science* **230**(4732):1350–1354, 1985.
8. Torroni A, Wallace D. Mitochondrial DNA variation in human populations and implications for detection of mitochondrial DNA mutations of pathological significance. *J Bioenerg Biomemb* **26**(3):261–271, 1994.
9. Newton CR, Graham A, Heptinstall LE et al. Analysis of any point mutation in DNA – the Amplification Refractory Mutation System (ARMS). *Nucl Acids Res* **17**(7):2503–2516, 1989.
10. Ferrie RM, Schwarz MJ, Robertson NH et al. Development, multiplexing, and application of ARMS tests for common mutations in the CFTR gene. *Am J Hum Genet* **51**(2):251–262, 1992.
11. Conner BJ, Reyes AA, Morin C, Itakura K, Teplitz RL, Wallace RB. Detection of sickle-cell beta-s-globin allele by hybridization with synthetic oligonucleotides. *Proc Natl Acad Sci USA* **80**(1):278–282, 1983.
12. Saiki RK, Walsh PS, Levenson CH, Erlich HA. Genetic-analysis of amplified DNA with immobilized sequence-specific oligonucleotide probes. *Proc Natl Acad Sci USA* **86**(16):6230–6234, 1989.

13. Tyagi S, Kramer FR. Molecular beacons: probes that fluoresce upon hybridization. *Nature Biotechnology* **14**:303–308, 1996.
14. Chee M, Yang R, Hubbell E et al. Accessing genetic information with high-density DNA arrays. *Science* **274**(5287):610–614, 1996.
15. Fodor SPA. DNA sequencing – massively parallel genomics. *Science* **277**(5324):393, 1997.
16. Cronin MT, Fucini RV, Kim SM, Masino RS, Wespi RM, Miyada CG. Cystic-fibrosis mutation detection by hybridization to light-generated DNA-probe arrays. *Hum Mutat* **7**(3):244–255, 1996.
17. Hacia JG, Brody LC, Chee MS, Fodor SPA, Collins FS. Detection of heterozygous mutations in BRCA1 using high-density oligonucleotide arrays and 2-color fluorescence analysis. *Nature Genet* **14**(4):441–447, 1996.
18. Schena M, Shalon D, Davis RW, Brown PO. Quantitative monitoring of gene-expression patterns with a complementary-DNA microarray. *Science* **270**(5235):467–470, 1995.
19. Schena M. Genome analysis with gene-expression microarrays. *Bioessays* **18**(5):427–431, 1996.
20. Knight SJL, Hirst MC, Roche A et al. Molecular studies of the Fragile-X syndrome. *Am J Med Genet* **43**(1–2):217–223, 1992.
21. Warner JP, Barron LH, Brock DJH. A new polymerase chain-reaction (PCR) assay for the trinucleotide repeat that is unstable and expanded on Huntington's-disease chromosomes. *Mol Cell Probes* **7**(3):235–239, 1993.

Preimplantation genetic diagnosis

39

J. Harper and J. Delhanty

Introduction

The detection of genetic disease in the human embryo before implantation gives parents the chance of starting a pregnancy knowing that the baby will be free of the inherited disorder that is prevalent in their family. Pressure from several groups of patients for whom this approach held particular appeal led to the initiation of research towards this goal in the UK in the mid 1980s.

There are several groups of patients for whom preimplantation diagnosis is the preferred option. The first group includes couples at risk of passing on an X-linked disorder for which there is, as yet, no specific molecular diagnosis. The current treatment offered is fetal sex determination and selective abortion of all males, of which half will be unaffected.

Secondly, there are couples who have had to suffer repeated terminations of pregnancy, with or without a specific diagnosis. A third group consists of subfertile couples, possibly due to chromosomal translocation or gonadal mosaicism, who may resort to in vitro fertilization (IVF) treatment and wish to increase the chances of a normal zygote. This group would also include those needing IVF who are at risk of transmitting single gene disorders. Finally, there are those with moral or religious objections to pregnancy termination. This group would prefer selection to occur at the preimplantation stage, giving them a reasonable chance of starting with a normal pregnancy.

The approach to preimplantation diagnosis

The availability of IVF theoretically allows several approaches to genetic diagnosis at the preimplantation stage. These include first polar body analysis, or biopsy at the cleavage or blastocyst stage.

POLAR BODY ANALYSIS

Initially, first polar body analysis to detect genetic disease appears attractive[1]. It allows preconception diagnosis and it is non-invasive of the embryo, but overall, the disadvantages outweigh the advantages. In the case of a mother who is a carrier for a single-gene disorder, the assumption would be that if the first polar body is positive for the mutant gene then the oocyte itself will carry the normal chromosome. However, the frequent crossing-over between non-sister chromatids during first meiotic prophase in the human female leads to the situation where it is common to find the primary oocyte (and hence also the first polar body) carrying a chromosome that is heterozygous, with one chromatid bearing the mutation and the other normal. This situation is very difficult to detect technically, since there is a high probability that DNA from each chromatid will not amplify with equal efficiency during the polymerase chain reaction (PCR).

Polar body analysis has been applied clinically in two centres in the USA to avoid age-related aneuploidy in women aged 35 and above who are undergoing IVF treatment. The first, and/or in some cases the second polar body was removed, spread on a slide and analysed by fluorescent in situ hybridization (FISH) using DNA probes specific for chromosomes 18, 13/21 and X[2,3]. Early results from Verlinsky's group seem to show an improved ongoing pregnancy rate but there is as yet insufficient data for a full statistical comparison, as IVF rates are notoriously fickle. There are several difficulties with this approach. Firstly, having carried out an enormous amount of work in dissecting and analysing the first polar body, fewer than half of the analysed oocytes were normally fertilized and available for transfer. Since a substantial proportion of aneuploidy, particularly involving chromosome 18, arises at the second meiotic division, the attempt was made additionally to screen the second polar body. The success rate overall in first and second polar body analysis only amounted to 76%, meaning that one-quarter of the oocytes had to be discarded at the outset. The most frequent anomaly observed was the loss of a single chromatid from the first polar body; loss of a whole chromosome occurred with about one-tenth of the frequency[3]. This would be a most interesting finding if confirmed, but technical problems with the 13/21 probe in particular mean that at least some contribution from artefact must be expected, especially as the rate of chromatid loss far exceeded the rate of gain. On the grounds of cost alone this approach is unlikely to be applied in the UK, but if it were to be considered then improvements could be made by using an alternative probe set, including chromosome 16 and a locus-specific probe for chromosome 21. Although an improved ongoing pregnancy rate is claimed, the proportion ending in spontaneous abortion still amounted to 24%, which is not surprising, since chromosomes 13, 18 and 21 account for less than 20% of trisomies among miscarried pregnancies.

CLEAVAGE STAGE BIOPSY

The manipulation of embryos has been used in the bovine embryo transfer industry for many years. Adaptation of these techniques lead to the successful biopsy of mouse[4] and human[5] embryos (Plate 39.1a).

In the human, the cryopresevation of embryos in IVF treatment cycles is routine, and from frozen embryo replacement cycles up to 50% of blastomeres can be destroyed and the embryo is still capable of producing a viable fetus. No increase in fetal abnormalities have been reported following transfer of cryopreserved embryos in which some cells have been destroyed by freezing/thawing. Studies examining the effect of embryo biopsy have shown that at the eight-cell stage, removal of two cells was not detrimental to embryo metabolism or development[6] and is an efficient process with more than 90% of the embryos surviving. Biopsies performed at earlier stages (four cells) may alter the ratio of inner cell mass to trophectoderm cells which may be detrimental to embryo development[7]. Therefore, the main strategy used for embryo biopsy has been to biopsy embryos at the 6–10-cell stage, on day 3 post insemination. Removal of up to 25% of the embryo has been thought to be safe and not impair implantation or embryo development. To remove the blastomeres, acid Tyrodes solution is used to drill a hole in the zona pellucida and the blastomeres are aspirated (Plate 39.1b).

Two recent studies analysed the pregnancies obtained from biopsied embryos after preimplantation genetic diagnosis (PGD)[8,9]. Biochemical and ultrasound measurements showed that pregnancies did not show any significant developmental differences compared to controls, and deliveries, including birth weight and Apgar scores, were considered normal.

BLASTOCYST BIOPSY

Blastocyst biopsy was first tried in murine blastocysts where a small slit was made in the zona pellucida and as the blastomeres herniated through the slit, the cells were excised. Successful blastocyst biopsies have been performed in mice and primates with the delivery of healthy individuals[10,11]. In human, blastocyst biopsy can be performed on day 5 or 6 post insemination[12,13]. Dokras *et al.*[12] using the herniation technique examined human blastocyst viability by the production of hCG in vitro and found that the values for biopsied and non-biopsied controls was the same.

Development of this technique has been slow as more than 50% of cleavage stage human embryos arrest before the blastocyst stage[14]. One method which has been investigated has been the recovery of blastocysts by uterine lavage. Since the embryo floats freely in the uterine cavity before implantation, it is possible to flush the embryo from the uterus. Initially it was thought that this method could be used in conjunction with superovulation regimes, but since it seems impossible to be sure that all embryos have been flushed, the use of natural cycles has been employed (Simpson, personal communication).

Blastocyst biopsy has the advantage that a larger number of cells can be removed from the outer trophectoderm (TE) layer without affecting the inner cell mass (ICM) from which the fetus later develops. However, TE may have diverged genetically from the ICM as in at least 1% of conceptions, confined placental mosaicism (CPM) is observed, where the chromosome status of the embryo is different from the placenta. It may be a mechanism of early development that abnormal cells are preferentially allocated to the trophectoderm[15].

Chromosomal abnormalities in preimplantation embryos

Since the successful generation of human preimplantation embryos in vitro we have been able to examine chromosomes of early human embryos. As it is estimated that 60% of human conceptions are lost due to chromosome abnormalities, the possibility of examining preimplantation embryos may answer some of the questions of early human development and have important consequences for PGD.

Karyotypes of human preimplantation embryos are problematic, as it is difficult to arrest cells in metaphase, but using this technique mosaicism, aneuploidy and ploidy abnormalities have been observed[16–19] and mosaicism with normal and aneuploid or polyploid cell lines appears to be the most common abnormality[18,20]. Early studies showed the presence of a trisomy 1 embryo[21], but this work highlights the problem with karyotyping, since from the eight-cell embryo, metaphase spreads were only obtained for two cells and so the possibility of mosaicism could not be explored.

With the advent of interphase fluorescent in situ hybridization (FISH) we are able to examine the chromosome status of every cell within an embryo. The use of FISH using probes for chromosomes X and Y was developed to sex embryos for patients at risk of transmitting X-linked diseases[22,23]. Dual FISH gave the first indication of the frequency of chromosome mosaicism in diagnostic cleavage stage embryos[24].

FISH has been used for the analysis of chromosome patterns in human preimplantation embryos[25–27]. Studies on abnormally fertilized embryos (such as polyspermic embryos) has shown, as expected, that these embryos were highly abnormal[28], which is in agreement with the karyotype data obtained from such embryos[17].

Normally fertilized, normally developing embryos also show high levels of chromosomal abnormalities[27,29]. To try to categorize these abnormalities, the patterns have been divided into four groups[27,29].

- Uniformly diploid for the probes examined
- Uniformly abnormal, such as Down syndrome or Turner syndrome
- Mosaic, where usually both diploid cells and aneuploid, haploid or polyploid nuclei are present and can vary in proportion from mainly diploid to mainly abnormal
- Chaotic, where every nucleus shows a different chromosome complement

From the FISH data a higher rate of abnormalities has been observed than has previously been reported from karyotyping data. However, since mosaic and chaotic embryos are common, if only one or two cells are analysable from an embryo, then karyotyping would underestimate the level of chromosome abnormalities.

Normal, abnormal and mosaic embryos have all been observed in fetal development. The presence of two cell lines, as shown by mosaic embryos and in CPM, could arise due to abnormal chromosome segregation caused by a postzygotic event, or the chromosome loss from a trisomic embryo, which restores the diploid state (trisomic rescue). Several mechanisms indicate that these abnormal cells would most likely be found in the trophectoderm, and hence the placenta. First, only four cells from a blastocyst give rise to the embryo and so it would be unlikely that the abnormal cells would be found in the embryo; second, in most cases a fetus with abnormal chromosomes will not be compatible with life; or third, abnormal cells may be preferentially allocated to the trophectoderm[15].

Chaotic embryos have not been observed in later stages of embryonic development, probably because these embryos would arrest and fail to implant.

The accumulation of data on the chromosomal constitution of spare untransferred embryos from preimplantation diagnosis cycles has revealed that, despite the fact that these are embryos from women of proven fertility, the incidence of postzygotic chromosomal anomalies is similar to that in embryos from routine IVF patients[27]. This finding may provide one explanation for the apparently poor success rate of IVF procedures, i.e. that, at best, only one embryo transfer in five results in an ongoing pregnancy. A second significant finding is that the incidence of the most bizarre type of anomaly, chaotically dividing embryos, is strongly related to the particular patient. In repeated cycles, certain women regularly produced 'chaotic' embryos, while others did not, although the frequency of diploid mosaics was similar in both groups[27].

Diagnosis of single-gene defects and dominant disorders

Preimplantation diagnosis to avoid single-gene defects may be attempted either by the use of linked markers or, if the gene has been cloned, by the use of specific primers. For both approaches, a high efficiency of DNA amplification is required and nested PCR protocols are usual. The first clinical application was for couples at risk of transmitting cystic fibrosis (CF)[31,32]. Accurate detection of the common ΔF508 mutation is possible using nested PCR to amplify the affected exon from single cells followed by heteroduplex formation[33,34]. The birth of the first unaffected child following embryo selection using this method was reported in 1992[31]. A similar approach is possible for Tay–Sachs disease[35] but for diseases that are heterogeneous with respect to the mutation each family may require specific detection methods. This is true of β-thalassaemia which is caused by a variety of mutations within the β-globin gene. To overcome this, the approach of single-strand conformation polymorphism (SSCP) has been applied to detect mutations in a fragment of the β-globin gene at the single cell level[36]. The advantage of this method is that most mutations within the amplified fragment can be detected by altered mobility of the single stranded DNA or by the formation of heteroduplex bands.

PGD is frequently requested in families segregating for Duchenne muscular dystrophy. The simplest approach in this disorder is to sex the embryo and to transfer only females, but for a specific genetic diagnosis the problem of extreme heterogeneity again arises. However, since the mutations frequently involve large exonic deletions it is possible to test for the presence or absence of an intervening exon by simple gel electrophoresis[37]. Preimplantation diagnosis for the first autosomal dominant condition, Marfan's syndrome, has recently been achieved[38]. Dominant disorders pose particular problems in diagnosis at the single-cell level and to minimize these the authors incorporated primers for gender in a multiplex PCR reaction.

Potential sources of misdiagnosis in single-gene disorders are contamination by extraneous DNA (this could come from additional sperm that remain attached to the embryo) and analysis of sequences derived from a single chromosome only. This can be due to biopsy of a haploid cell, which may be found in about 15% of embryos or allele specific amplification failure so that DNA from the gene on one chromosome is not represented in the final reaction product. This is known as allele dropout (ADO) and is a particular problem when amplifying the genome from single cells. If both parents are carrying the same gene mutation in a recessive disorder ADO will not result in misdiagnosis of an affected embryo as unaffected, but problems can arise if the diagnosis relies on the detection of a common mutation, such as the three-base pair deletion causing CF, in one parent and a rare mutation in the other parent cannot be picked up. Here, the advantage of SSCP is apparent since each DNA strand may be visualized and the absence of one allele is immediately obvious.

ADO is a major problem when diagnosing dominant disorders as the failure of the mutant allele to amplify will lead to the diagnosis of a heterozygous (affected) embryo as homozygous normal. To overcome this problem primers for a closely linked genetic polymorphism may be included in the reaction, providing an independent system for analysis. Multiplex PCR may be used to achieve this, but is not always feasible. A development that provides an alternative approach is that of whole genome amplification by primer extension preamplification (PEP), which is a modified PCR using random primers to produce amplified fragments throughout the genome[39]. The advantage for preimplantation diagnosis is that samples of the PEP product can be used for secondary amplification of different sequences. This has recently been applied in the first diagnosis of a dominantly inherited cancer predisposition syndrome, familial adenomatous polyposis coli (FAPC) in the preimplantation embryo[40]. The use of the PEP product may also be appropriate in conditions where a specific gene diagnosis is not usually possible, such as the triplet repeat expansion disorders (e.g. Huntington's disease and fragile X syndrome) so that a combination of closely linked and intragenic markers could be used.

To eliminate the possibility of contamination by sperm released from the zona pellucida during the biopsy procedure, intracytoplasmic sperm injection (ICSI) should be used as the means of fertilization for the analysis of single-gene disorders. A high percentage of cystic fibrosis carrier males have congenital absence of the vas deferens and sperm aspiration techniques are required to obtain the sperm, followed by ICSI for efficient fertilization.

Embryo sexing to avoid X-linked disease

Sexing for X-linked disease is one of the major indications for PGD[41]. X-linked recessive diseases account for 6–7% of single-gene defects and include conditions such as Duchenne muscular dystrophy (DMD), haemophilia, and various mental retardation syndromes. The mother carries the mutation on one of her X chromosomes and so transmits the defective gene to half of her offspring. There are over 400 X-linked diseases. For some of these, the molecular nature of the mutation is known and a diagnosis of the disease is possible, either prenatally or postnatally. However, for many X-linked diseases, the location and mutation is unknown and so no genetic test is available. In these cases, all that can be offered prenatally is sexing of the fetus, with the option of terminating male pregnancies, knowing that there is only a 50% risk that the fetus will be affected. Therefore, for such X-linked diseases, PGD has an added benefit.

The first cycles of PGD performed used PCR to amplify a Y-chromosome repeat sequence to sex embryos for patients carrying X-linked disease[42]. Using this method, embryos showing no signal were assumed to be female and such embryos were considered for transfer. A diagnostic error occurred in one of the first seven pregnancies that resulted and the pregnancy was terminated as no specific molecular test was available for this disease. This misdiagnosis may have been due to amplification failure, ADO, an anucleate cell (or failure to put the cell in the tube) or mosaicism where an XO cell was biopsied from an XY embryo. Several groups have developed methods to control for amplification failure in the use of PCR for embryo sexing. These are basically of two types, those employing alphoid or other chromosome-specific repeat sequences from both X and Y in a multiplex PCR[43–45] or a combination of repeat and single-gene associated primers[46,47] and those relying on coamplification of related genes or pseudogenes with the same primers, such as amelogenin[48] steroid sulphatase[39] or ZFX/ZFY[43]. In the former, it is still possible that either sequence may independently fail to amplify, whilst the amplification of a fragment from a homologous X- and Y-linked gene avoids this[49].

In addition to amplification failure, there are two drawbacks that apply when amplifying DNA from single blastomeres in order to sex the embryo. The first applies to any reaction involving the PCR, that the risk of amplifying contaminating material is high. The second is that the presence of an amplified band only indicates that an X- or Y-chromosome is present and gives no information on copy number. In one series of five couples undergoing embryo sexing by FISH to avoid X-linked disease, no transfers took place for two of them despite the identification of X signals and no Y signals[24]. One embryo in this series was shown to be XO. Transfer of a potentially 45, X zygote could be disastrous when the aim is to avoid X-linked disease from the carrier mother, as the great majority of such embryos lack the paternal sex chromosome[50]. Since 45, X conceptuses are thought to occur with a frequency approaching 1% such a finding will not be rare when carrying out preimplantation diagnosis. An extra advantage of FISH is that the risk of contamination is minimal as the nucleus can be observed all at stages of the process.

The FISH procedure can be efficienly performed in 2 h using directly labelled DNA probes[26,51]. Most laboratories use three-colour FISH for PGD of sex with probes for chromosomes X, Y and an autosome, to provide additional information concerning aneuploidy and polyploidy (Plate 39.2).

The four groups of chromosome arrangements observed in human embryos have important implications for preimplantation diagnosis of sex. To date, there have been no reports of an XX nucleus in a male embryo, and so these abnormalities should not lead to a misdiagnosis of sex but care needs to be taken as cumulus cells could become attached to the slide and would be normal, female cells. However, XO nuclei have been observed in male embryos[29]. Therefore only an embryo where there are two X signals in the absence of a Y should be considered for transfer and an embryo with an XO nucleus should never be considered.

Detection of chromosome abnormalities

It has been estimated that 15% of all clinically recognized pregnancies spontaneously abort and of these 50% are chromosomally abnormal, the most common abnormality being aneuploidy. Some couples are at an even higher risk of transmitting a chromosome abnormality to their offspring as they carry a balanced translocation. Another group of patients that transmit such abnormalities are gonadal mosaics. Their blood karyotype is normal, but they repeatedly show the development of abnormal fetuses or offspring, such as Trisomy 21 (Down) fetuses.

Such patients may have severe problems trying to achieve a normal pregnancy. Their history often shows either failure to obtain a pregnancy, repeated spontaneous miscarriages, or an affected pregnancy after prenatal diagnosis which may lead to repeated induced abortions. Therefore, for such couples PGD may be the only way they can produce a normal pregnancy.

Two strategies have been used to examine embryos from such patients. One uses polar body analysis, where the first polar body is FISHed with chromosome paints to determine if the embryo is normal (Munné *et al.*, personal communication). The second uses cleavage stage embryo biopsy and interphase, multicolour FISH using combinations of alpha satellite and locus specific probes for the chromosomes in question[52–53]. To date, four couples have been treated in this way. One was a suspected gonadal mosaic for chromosome 21, and the remainder carried translocations for chromosomes 13/14, 6/21 and 13/21 respectively. The four couples underwent a total of eight cycles of IVF for PGD. In total over 70% of the embryos were chromosomally abnormal. In addition to frequent abnormal meiotic segregation, mosaicism was common but chaotically dividing embryos were observed only from two couples, both Robertsonian translocation carriers[54]. This perhaps provides some explanation for the unexpectedly poor reproductive history of these particular parents since such translocations are usually fairly benign in effect.

For the PGD of chromosome abnormalities, the frequent chromosome anomalies observed in preimplantation embryos (i.e. mosaicism and chaotic embryos) are problematic. In this situation, the biopsied cell may not be representative of the whole embryo. Trisomic cells in diploid embryos have been observed. In the case of a gonadal mosaic for chromosome 21, disomic cells have been seen in an otherwise trisomy 21 embryo. If a normal cell is biopsied, the embryo would be diagnosed as normal when it was affected. To reduce the chance of a misdiagnosis, for chromosome abnormalities only embryos where two nuclei are shown to be normal for the chromosomes analysed should be replaced.

The potential for misdiagnosis and implication of mosaicism

The last published world data for PGD (Table 39.1)[55] showed pregnancy rates of 28% per transfer which are comparable to those for routine IVF and confirm the initial in vitro data that embryo biopsy on day 3 does not affect preimplantation development[6]. Additionally the 34 babies born have no reported congenital malformations testifying to the pluripotent nature of the cells at that stage.

TABLE 39.1
Preimplantation genetic diagnosis world figures

	Cycles	Transfers	Pregnancy	Babies born
X-linked PCR	62	53	14	11
X-linked FISH	70	56	15	11
Single-gene defects	65	62	21	12
Total	197	171	50	34

Source: Harper[55]

Of more concern is that there were three misdiagnoses among the 50 pregnancies. The first misdiagnosis of sex was almost certainly the result of amplification failure. With the use of dual FISH there have been no further misdiagnoses of sex, nor with improved PCR methods. The two instances of CF misdiagnosis were both cases where only one parent carried the ΔF508 mutation and the mutation in the other parent was of a rarer type. Detection of the ΔF508 mutation in the embryo is essential in these cases, as such embryos could be affected if they also carried the alternative CF mutation. The reason for these misdiagnoses is presently unknown but it is recognized that failure to amplify both alleles can be a problem with DNA derived from blastomeres and the inadvertent incorporation of contaminating sperm is another possibility. A third possibility that now seems equally likely is chromosomal mosaicism in normally developing human embryos particularly of the diploid/haploid type.

For PGD to be successful, the biopsied cell should be representative of the whole embryo. In the investigation of mosaicism, we have not seen an XX nucleus in an otherwise XY embryo, leading us to believe that, providing we use dual FISH, mosaicism is unlikely to lead to misdiagnosis of sex. In the case of autosomal recessive disorders, where both parents are carriers for the same mutation, chromosomal mosaicism is unlikely to lead to misdiagnosis, since one or two extra or a missing copy of the relevant chromosome will not affect the detection of the mutation. Whereas for dominant conditions, autosomal or X-linked, absence of one homologue in the biopsied cell could lead to failure to diagnose an affected embryo (Table 39.2). Mosaicism is also an important consideration when attempting to diagnose trisomies or monosomies at the preimplantation stage; the effect will depend upon whether the embryo was initially trisomic or normally disomic for the chromosome in question (Table 39.3). For both of these situations, it would be advisable to analyse two independent blastomeres.

Future developments

Research currently is focused on methods of detecting chromosome imbalance in the preimplantation embryo and on improving the reliability of single gene diagnosis and extending the range of disorders amenable to specific diagnosis. In view of the frequency of chromosomal disorders in older women and in high risk couples, methods for diagnosing abnormal copy numbers with reliability are urgently needed. Multicolour FISH with centromeric probes for chromosomes 13/21, 18, X and Y has been used to screen IVF embryos prior to transfer in women of 40 and above[2,3] and polar body analysis is now being applied for the same purpose. However, it has yet to be demonstrated that screening with a limited set of probes will enhance the ongoing pregnancy rate.

The problem of gonadal trisomy mosaicism has been approached by developing locus specific probes for use in conjunction with the relevant centromere probe. Problems due to translocations are less easily solved because of the many possible types of unbalanced gamete, including 3:1 disjunctions, that one needs to detect. The approach of using a combination of centromere and locus specific probes that flank the breakpoint of one of the chromosomes has been applied[52]. It has become clear that for diagnostic purposes three is the maximum number of probes that can be reliably scored.

It is clear that what is needed is a whole genome screen for aneuploidy, both for high risk couples and older women having routine IVF treatment. Possible approaches that have been investigated include comparative genomic hybridization (CGH) by dual FISH of test and normal DNA onto normal metaphase chromosomes[57] following whole genome amplification from single blastomeres, and the use of fluorescent PCR primers for automated quantitative analysis of repeat sequences specific for the relevant chromosome region[58]. While CGH has given promising results[59], at the single cell level fluorescent PCR has proved to be an unreliable approach for the detection of chromosome imbalance[60]. Of the dominant single gene disorders, some of the most likely candidates for preimplantation diagnosis are the inherited cancer syndromes, such as retinoblastoma, Li Fraumeni syndrome and familial adenomatous polyposis coli. Couples who are reluctant to terminate an otherwise normal pregnancy may be more willing to consider selection at the preimplantation stage.

TABLE 39.2
The effect of monosomic or haploid chromosomal mosaicism on the single-cell diagnosis of dominant single-gene defects in the preimplantation embryo

Dominant inheritance	Embryo	Genotype	Minor cell line	Genotype
Autosomal	Disomic (chromosomally normal)	wt/m (affected)	Haploid or monosomic for chromosome carrying the gene	**wt** or m
X-linked	Disomy	wt/m (female affected) m (male affected)	X-chromosome monosomic X- or Y-chromosome monosomic	**wt** or m no result or m

wt: wild type (normal allele); m: mutant allele
wt: misdiagnosis of an affected embryo as unaffected

Source: Delhanty *et al.*[56]

TABLE 39.3
The effect of chromosomal mosaicism on the single-cell diagnosis of chromosome copy number in the preimplantation embryo

Embryo	FISH signals per nucleus	Minor cell line	FISH signals per nucleus
Disomic	●●	Monosomic or haploid, trisomic or triploid	● ●●●
Trisomic	●●●	Disomic or haploid	<u>●●</u> or ●
		Tetrasomic or tetraploid	●●●● or ●●●●●●

Inadvertent sampling of the minor cell line would always lead to misdiagnosis, but this would be serious only in the case of a trisomic embryo with a disomic (or haploid) cell line – <u>●●</u>

Source: Delhanty *et al.*[56]

References

1. Verlinsky Y, Ginsburg N, Lifchez A, Valle J, Moise J & Strom C. Analysis of the first polar body: preconception genetic diagnosis. *Hum. Reprod.* **5**, 826–829, 1990.
2. Munné S, Dailey T, Sultan KM, Grifo J & Cohen J. The use of first polar bodies for preimplantation diagnosis of aneuploidy. *Mol. Hum. Reprod.* **1**, 1014–1020, 1995.
3. Verlinsky Y, Strom C, Cieslak J, Kuliev A, Ivakhnenko V & Lifchez A. Birth of healthy children after preimplantation diagnosis of common aneuploidies by polar body fluorescent in situ hybridisation analysis. *Fertil. Steril.* **66**, 126–129, 1996.
4. Wilton LJ, Shaw JM & Trounsen AO. Successful single-cell biopsy, and cryopreservation of preimplantation mouse embryos. *Fertil. Steril.* **51**, 513–517, 1989.
5. Tarin JJ & Handyside AH. Embryo biopsy strategies for preimplantation diagnosis. *Fertil. Steril.* **59**, 943–952, 1993.
6. Hardy K, Martin KL, Leese HJ, Winston RML & Handyside AH. Human preimplantation development *in-vitro* is not adversely affected by biopsy at the 8-cell stage. *Hum. Reprod.* **5**, 708–714, 1990.
7. Tarin JJ, Conaghan J, Winston RML & Handyside AH. Human embryo biopsy on the 2nd day after insemination for preimplantation diagnosis: removal of a quarter of embryo retards cleavage. *Fertil. Steril.* **58**, 970–976, 1992.
8. Soussis I, Harper JC, Handyside AH & Winston RML. Obstetric outcome of pregnancies resulting from embryos biopsied for preimplantation diagnosis of inherited disease. *Br. J. Obstet. Gynaecol.* **103**, 784–788, 1996.
9. Soussis I, Harper JC, Kontogianni E *et al.* Pregnancies resulting from embryos biopsied for preimplantation diagnosis of genetic disease: Biochemical and ultrasonic studies in the first trimester of pregnancy. *J. Assist. Reprod. Genet.* **13**, 254–257, 1996.
10. Monk M, Muggleton Harris A, Rawlings E & Whittingham D. Preimplantation diagnosis of HPRT-deficient male and carrier female mouse embryos by trophectoderm biopsy. *Hum. Reprod.* **3**, 377–381, 1988.
11. Summers PM, Campbell JM & Miller MW. Normal in vivo development of marmoset monkey embryos after trophectoderm biopsy. *Hum. Reprod.* **1**, 89–94, 1988.
12. Dokras A, Sargent IL, Gardner RL & Barlow GH. Human trophectoderm biopsy and secretion of chorionic gonadotrophin. *Hum. Reprod.* **6**, 1453, 1991.
13. Muggleton Harris AL, Glazier A, Wall M & Pickering SJ. Genetic diagnosis using polymerase chain reaction and fluorescent in situ hybridisation analysis of biopsied cells from both the cleavage and blastocyst stages of individual cultured human preimplantation embryos. *Hum. Reprod.* **10**, 183–192, 1995.
14. Hardy K. Development of human blastocysts in vitro. In *Preimplantation Embryo Development* (ed. B. Bavister). Springer-Verlag, 1993.
15. James RM & West JD. A chimaeric animal model for confined placental mosaicism. *Hum. Genet.* **93**, 603–604, 1994.
16. Angell RR. Chromosome abnormalities in human preimplantation embryos. In *Development of Preimplantation Embryos and Their Environment*, pp. 181–187. New York: Alan R. Liss, 1989.
17. Plachot M, Mandelbaum J, Junca A-M, Grouchy J, de Salat-Baroux J & Cohen J. Cytogenetic analysis and developmental capacity of normal and abnormal embryos after IVF. *Hum. Reprod.* **4** (Suppl): 99–103, 1989.
18. Zenzes MT & Casper RF. Cytogenetics of human oocytes, zygotes and embryos after in vitro fertilisation, *Hum. Genet.* **88**, 367–375, 1992.
19. Jamieson ME, Coutts JRT & Connor JM. The chromosome constitution of human preimplantation embryos fertilised in vitro. *Hum. Reprod.* **9**, 709–715, 1994.
20. Zenzes MT, Wang P & Casper RF. Chromosome status of untransferred (spare) embryos and probability of pregnancy after in vitro fertilisation. *Lancet* **340**, 391–394, 1992.
21. Watt JL, Templeton AA, Messinis I, Bell L, Cunningham P & Duncan RO. Trisomy 1 in an eight cell human pre-embryo, *J. Med. Genet.* **24**, 60–64, 1987.
22. Griffin DK, Handyside AH, Harper JC *et al.* Clinical experience with preimplantation diagnosis of sex by dual fluorescent in-situ hybridisation. *J. Assist. Reprod. Genet.* **11**, 132–143, 1994.
23. Munné S, Tang YX, Grifo J, Rosenwaks Z & Cohen J. Sex determination of human embryos using the polymerase chain reaction and confirmation by fluorescence in situ hybridization. *Fertil. Steril.* **61**, 111–117, 1994.
24. Delhanty JDA, Griffin DK, Handyside AH *et al.* Detection of aneuploidy and chromosomal mosaicism in human embryos during preimplantation sex determination by fluorescent in-situ hybridisation. *Hum. Mol. Genet.* **2**, 1183–1185, 1993.
25. Munné S, Lee A, Rosenwaks Z, Grifo J & Cohen J. Diagnosis of major chromosome aneuploidies in human preimplantation embryos. *Hum. Reprod.* **8**, 2185–2191, 1993.
26. Harper JC, Coonen E, Ramaekers FCS *et al.* Identification of the sex of human preimplantation embryos in two hours using an improved spreading method and fluorescent in situ hybridisation using directly labelled probes. *Hum. Reprod.* **9**, 721–724, 1994.
27. Delhanty JDA, Harper JC, Ao A, Handyside AH & Winston RML. Multicolour FISH detects frequent chromosomal mosaicism and chaotic division in normal preimplantation embryos from fertile patients. *Hum. Genet.* **99**, 755–760, 1997.
28. Coonen E, Harper JC, Ramaekers FCS *et al.* Presence of chromosomal mosaicism in abnormal preimplantation embryos detected by fluorescent in situ hybridisation. *Hum. Genet.* **54**, 609–615, 1994.
29. Harper JC, Coonen E, Handyside AH, Winston RML, Hopman AHN & Delhanty JDA. Mosaicism of autosomes and sex chromosomes in morphologically normal, monospermic, preimplantation human embryos. *Prenat. Diagn.* **15**, 41–49, 1995.
30. Harper JC & Delhanty JDA. Detection of chromosomal abnormalities in human preimplantation embryos using FISH. *J. Assist. Reprod. Genet.* **13**(2), 137–139, 1996.
31. Handyside AH, Lesko JG, Tarin JJ, Winston RML & Hughes MR. Birth of a normal girl after in vitro fertilisation and preimplantation diagnostic testing for cystic fibrosis. *N. Engl. J. Med.* **327**, 905–909, 1992.
32. Ao A, Ray P, Harper JC, Lesko J *et al.* Clinical experience with preimplantation diagnosis of deltaF508 deletion in cystic fibrosis. *Prenat. Diagn.* **16**, 137–142, 1996.
33. Lesko J, Snabes M, Handyside AH & Hughes M. Amplification of the cystic fibrosis DF508 mutation from single cells: applications toward genetic diagnosis of the preimplantation embryo. *Am. J. Hum. Genet.* **49**(4), 223, 1991.
34. Liu J, Lissens W, Devroey P, Van Steirteghem A & Liebaers I. Efficiency and accuracy of polymerase-chain-reaction assay for cystic fibrosis allele delta F508 in single cell. *Lancet* **339**, 1190–1192, 1992.
35. Gibbons WE, Gitlin SA, Lanzendorf SE, Kaufmann RA, Slotnick RN & Hodgen GD. Preimplantation genetic diagnosis for Tay Sachs disease; successful pregnancy after pre-embryo biopsy and gene amplification by polymerase chain reaction. *Fertil. Steril.* **63**, 723–728, 1995.
36. El-Hashemite N, Wells D & Delhanty JDA. Preimplantation genetic diagnosis of β thalassaemia. *Lancet* **348**, 620–621, 1996.
37. Liu J, Lissens W, Van Broeckhoven C *et al.* Normal pregnancy after preimplantation DNA diagnosis of a dystrophin gene deletion. *Prenat. Diagn.* **15**, 351–358, 1995.
38. Harton GL, Tsipouras P, Sisson ME *et al.* Preimplantation genetic testing for Marfan syndrome. *Mol. Hum. Reprod.* **2**, 713–715, 1996.
39. Zhang L, Cui X, Schmitt K, Hubert R, Navidi W & Arnheim N. Whole genome amplification from a single cell: Implications for genetic analysis. *Proc. Natl. Acad. Sci. USA* **89**, 5847–5851, 1992.
40. Ao A, Wells D, Handyside AH, Winston RML & Delhanty JDA. Preimplantation genetic diagnosis of inherited cancer; familial adenomatous polyposis coli. *J. Assist. Reprod. Genet.* **15**, 140–144, 1998.
41. Verlinsky Y, Handyside AH, Grifo J *et al.* Preimplantation diagnosis of genetic and chromosomal disorders. *J. Assist. Reprod. Genet.* **11**, 236–243, 1994.
42. Handyside AH, Kontogianni EH, Hardy K & Winston RML. Pregnancies from biopsied human preimplantation embryos sexed by Y-specific DNA amplification. *Nature* **244**, 768–770, 1990.
43. Kontogianni EH, Hardy K & Handyside AH. Co-amplification of X- and Y-specific sequences for sexing preimplantation human embryos. In *Preimplantation Genetics* (eds Y. Verlinsky and C. Strom), pp. 139–145. New York: Plenum, 1991.
44. Grifo JA, Tang YX, Cohen J, Gilbert F, Sanyal MK & Rosenwaks Z. Pregnancy after embryo biopsy and co-amplification of DNA from X and Y chromosomes. *J. Am. Med. Ass.* **268**, 727–729, 1992.

45. Strom CM, Rechitsky S & Verlinsky Y. Reliability of gender determination using the polymerase chain reaction (PCR) for single cells. *J. I. V.F. E. T.* **8**, 225–229, 1991.
46. Levinson GL, Fields RA, Harton GL *et al.* Reliable gender screening for human preimplantation embryos, using multiple DNA target-sequences. *Hum. Reprod.* **7**, 1304–1313, 1992.
47. Bentley DR, Norwood FN, Holding C, Roberts RG & Bobrow M. Analysis of genetic variation in the single cell. In *Preconception and Preimplantation Diagnosis of Human Genetic Disease* (ed. R.G. Edwards), pp. 161–182. Cambridge: Cambridge University Press, 1993.
48. Nakahori Y, Hamanao K, Iwaya M & Nakagome Y. Sex identification by polymerase chain reaction using X-Y homologous primer. *Am. J. Med. Genet.* **39**, 472–473, 1991.
49. Chong SS, Kristjansson K, Cota J, Handyside AH & Hughes MR. Preimplantation prevention of X-linked disease: reliable and rapid sex determination of single human cells by restriction analysis of simultaneously amplified ZFX and ZFY sequences. *Hum. Mol. Genet.* **2** (8), 1187–1191, 1993.
50. Hassold T, Benham F & Leppert M. Cytogenetic and molecular analysis of sex chromosome monosomy. *Am. J. Hum. Genet.* **42**, 534–41, 1988.
51. Harper JC & Delhanty JDA. FISH in preimplantation diagnosis. In *Methods in Molecular Biology, Molecular Diagnosis of Genetic Disease* (ed. J. Walker), pp. 259–268. New Jersey, USA: Humana Press, 1996.
52. Conn CM, Harper JC, Winston RML & Delhanty JDA. Preimplantation diagnosis for trisomies 13, 14, 18 and 21 in translocation carriers using multicolour fluorescent in situ hybridisation. *Am. J. Hum. Genet.* **57** (Suppl. A), 1611, 1995.
53. Conn C, Harper JC, Winston RML & Delhanty JDA. Preimplantation diagnosis of autosomal aneuploidy using multicolour fluorescent in situ hybridisation (FISH). *Eur. J. Hum. Genet.* **4** (Suppl. 1), 125, 1996.
54. Conn C, Harper JC, Winston RML & Delhanty JDA. Infertile couples with Robertsonian translocations; preimplantation genetic analysis of embryos reveals chaotic cleavage divisions. *Hum. Genet.* **102**, 117–123, 1998.
55. Harper JC. Preimplantation diagnosis of inherited disease by embryo biopsy. An update of the world figures. *J. Assist. Reprod. Genet.* **13**(2), 90–94, 1996.
56. Delhanty JDA & Handyside AH. The origin of genetic defects in the human and their detection in the preimplantation embryo. *Hum. Reprod. Update.* **1**:201–215, 1995.
57. Kallioniemi A, Kallioniemi O-P, Suder D *et al.* Comparative genomic hybridization for molecular cytogenetic analysis of solid tumours. *Science* **258**, 818–821, 1992.
58. Pertl B, Yau SC, Sherlock J, Davies AF, Mathew CG & Adinolfi M. Rapid molecular method for prenatal detection of Down's syndrome. *Lancet* **343**, 1197, 1994.
59. Wells D & Delhanty J. Evaluating comparative genomic hybridisation (CGH) as a strategy for preimplantation diagnosis of unbalanced chromosome complements. *Eur. J. Hum. Genet.* **4** (Suppl. 1), 125, 1996.
60. Sherlock J, Cirigliano V, Pertl M, Tutschek B & Adinolfi M. Assessment of diagnostic quantitative fluorescent multiplex polymerase chain reaction assays performed on single cells. *Ann. Hum. Genet.* **62**:9–23, 1998.

Detection of fetal cells in transcervical samples in early pregnancy

40

M. Adinolfi and C.H. Rodeck

Introduction

The first report on the presence of fetal cells in the endocervical canal was published in 1971 by Shettles[1] who, intrigued by the fate of the cellular elements derived from the degenerating chorion villi, advanced the hypothesis that they were shed into the uterine cavity and could be used to assess the sex of the fetuses. Accordingly, he retrieved transcervical cells (TCCs) with cotton swabs and tested them for the presence of the Y chromosome using a fluorescent dye (quinacrine mustard). At the time of publishing his note, he had correctly diagnosed the sex of 10 fetuses out of 18 pregnancies investigated.

Using a similar approach Warren et al.[2] confirmed the detection of fetal cells in TCC samples obtained at various stages of gestation and diagnosed the sex of the fetuses in all 50 cases investigated. A few years later, Varner et al.[3] noticed the presence of multinucleated syncytial fragments in 60 out of 106 smears and successfully sexed the fetuses in 95% of these cases.

However, using the same procedure, other investigators observed a high proportion of false positive or negative diagnoses[4–8].

Based on the assumption that trophoblastic cells, shed from the placenta, would accumulate behind the cervical mucus plug, Rhine and collaborators[9–11] flushed the endocervical canal with sterile saline solution using a device referred to as 'antenatal cell extractor'. The collected cells were then cultured in vitro and analysed for the presence of metaphase chromosomes with staining patterns different from those detectable in maternal lymphocytes. This approach proved to be successful, since fetal cells in metaphase could be observed in 16 out of 34 TCC samples[10].

However, using the same procedures Goldberg et al.[12] detected only metaphases with a maternal banding pattern, although they had observed trophoblastic cellular elements in the original transcervical samples.

Following this last report and the discovery that chorion villus biopsies could provide fetal tissue for prenatal diagnostic tests, further attempts at performing non- or semi-invasive prenatal tests using TCCs were abandoned until 1992, when Griffith-Jones et al.[13] investigated the possibility of retrieving trophoblastic cells from the cervix and the endocervical canal with cotton swabs or lavage. Using the polymerase chain reaction (PCR) to detect chromosome Y-derived DNA sequences, the sex of nine male fetuses was correctly diagnosed, but false positive results were seen as well. However, doubts were raised about the diagnostic value of this approach by Morris and Williamson[14], who were not able to replicate these results, having observed too many false positive and negative results. Since, in both investigations, all TCC samples had been collected without asking the pregnant women to avoid sexual intercourse for at least a few days before the tests were performed, the false positive results could be attributed to PCR amplification of DNA sequences derived from contaminating sperm or seminal cells.

To avoid this possibility, fluorescent *in situ* hybridization (FISH) methods were employed to firmly establish whether trophoblastic cells could be found in TCC samples[15]. FISH tests with X and Y probes differentially labelled have the advantage that they can clearly identify diploid cells from sperm containing either the X or the Y chromosome. FISH can also assess the incidence of fetal cells in each sample and be used for the prenatal diagnosis of major chromosomal abnormalities. In the first study in which this procedure was employed, fetal sex was correctly diagnosed and a case of trisomy 18 was observed using TCC samples retrieved by lavage[15].

Subsequent investigations have confirmed the presence of fetal cells in the endocervical canal (Table 40.1)[16–25] and the possibility of performing *in vitro* cultures[19,26]. However, it has also emerged that the success of detecting trophoblastic cellular elements in TCC samples is strongly influenced by the method employed and the skill of the operator[16].

TABLE 40.1
Incidence of trophoblastic cells in TCC samples retrieved from mothers with male fetuses

Methods for collection		Test by FISH	Test by PCR	Authors
1	Transcervical swabs	—	9/9	Griffith-Jones et al.[13]
2	Endocervical lavage (10 ml)	7/7	6/6	Adinolfi et al.[15]
3	Endocervical lavage (10 ml)	5/6	6/6	Kingdom et al.[20]
4	Cytobrush	4/6	6/6	
5	Endocervical lavage (10 ml)	6/6	—	Adinolfi et al.[17]
6	Aspiration	1/1		
7	Aspiration[a]	2/5	7/14	Adinolfi et al.[18]
8	Endocervical lavage (5 ml)	1/1	2/2	
9	Aspiration	8/13	—	
	followed by lavage (5 ml)[b]	8/13	—	
10	Lavage (10 ml)	8/8[c]	—	Ishai et al.[19] (56% success in vitro cultures)
		21/21[d]	—	
11	Aspiration	12/13	12/13[e]	Briggs et al.[24]
12	Lavage (3 ml)[f]	—	7/7	Massari et al.[22]
13	Uterine lavage (20 ml)[a]	5/5	—	Chang et al.[23]
14	Lavage (10 ml)	13/13	—	Kawamura et al.[21]
15	Lavage (5–8 ml)	10/12	—	Daryani et al.[25]

[a]All samples were collected before TOP with the exceptions of samples in 7 and 13
[b]In total, 12 out of 13 samples were Y positive
[c]Double-colour FISH
[d]Single-colour FISH
[e]One false positive
[f]Out of 38 samples tested 17 contained fetal DNA

The main purpose of this review is to describe some of the papers dealing with this topic and to assess the feasibility of using this minimally invasive procedure for prenatal diagnostic tests of major chromosomal disorders and selected inherited diseases.

Methods for the collection of TCC samples

Shedding of fetal cells seems to occur mainly between 7 and 13 weeks of gestation, at a time when the decidua capsularis has not yet fused with the decidua parietalis and the uterine cavity is still present (Fig. 40.1).

Several techniques, with minor variations, have been employed for the collection of TCC samples: cotton swabs, endocervical or uterine lavage, mucus aspiration and cytobrush (Fig. 40.2 and Table 40.1). In most investigations, these procedures have been used to obtain samples before termination of pregnancy (TOP). The safety of using mucus aspiration before chorion villus sampling (CVS) has been assessed on a small group of women with continuing pregnancies (Table 40.2)[16].

It is now evident that cotton swabs cannot be used for collecting TCC samples, since the majority of the trophoblastic cells are shed in the endocervical canal and lower uterine cavity[16–18]. Lavage has been performed with different catheters and variable amounts of sterile saline

TABLE 40.2
Follow-up on 130 study cases (cervical mucus aspiration immediately before transcervical CVS) and 145 control cases (only transcervical CVS)

	Study group (n = 130)	Control group (n = 145)
Follow-up complete	113	121
Normal pregnancies	87	97
Miscarriages	2 (at 18 and 27 weeks)	7 (at 16, 16, and 15 weeks; 4 unknown)
Stillbirths	1 (at 40 weeks)	None
Terminations of affected pregnancies	23 (4 affected karyotypes, 8 blood disorders, 4 metabolic disorders, 7 others	17 (3 affected karyotypes, 8 blood disorders, 4 metabolic disorders, 2 others)

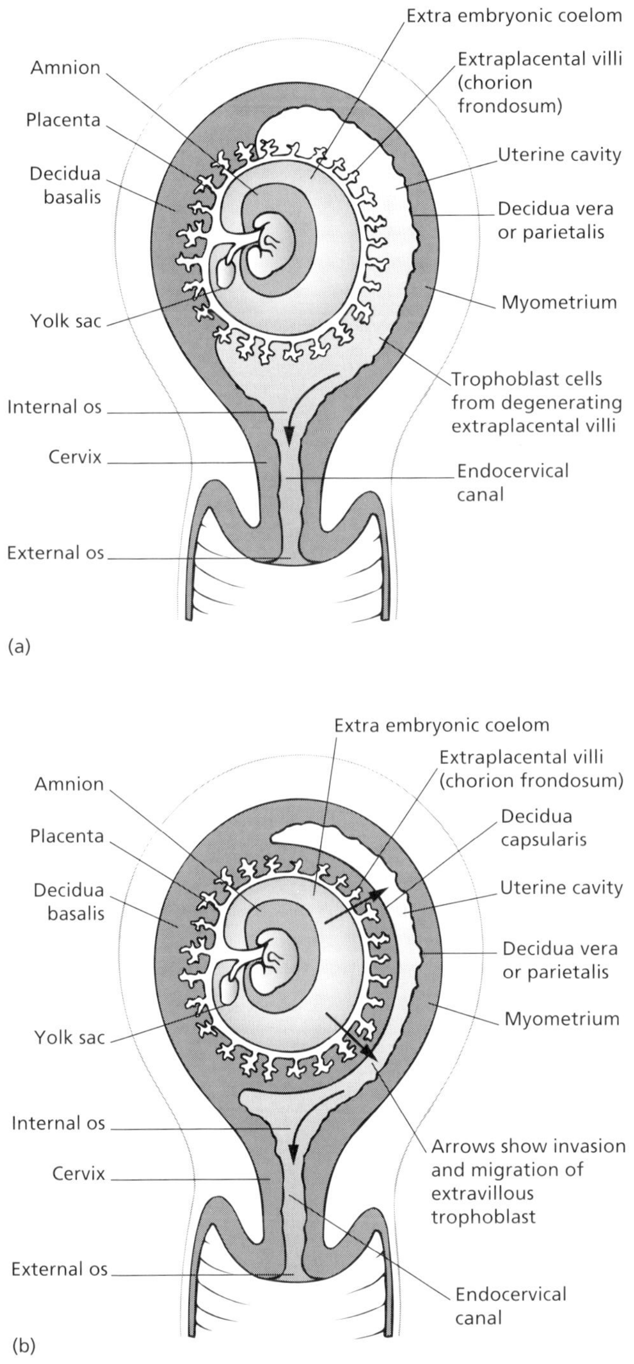

Fig. 40.1 (a) The earlier concept of how trophoblast cells appeared in the endocervical canal: by degeneration of and exfoliation from the extraplacental villi, in the process of the chorion frondosum becoming the chorion laeve. This ignores the fact that these villi cannot 'drop off' because they are covered by the decidua capsularis. (b) Our concept suggests that before the formation of the chorion laeve at 12–14 weeks, the invasive nature of the extravillous trophoblast in the decidua capsularis causes migration of some of these cells through into the uterine cavity (arrows). Since the decidua capsularis and parietalis do not fuse until about 12 weeks, these trophoblasts can collect in the uterine cavity.

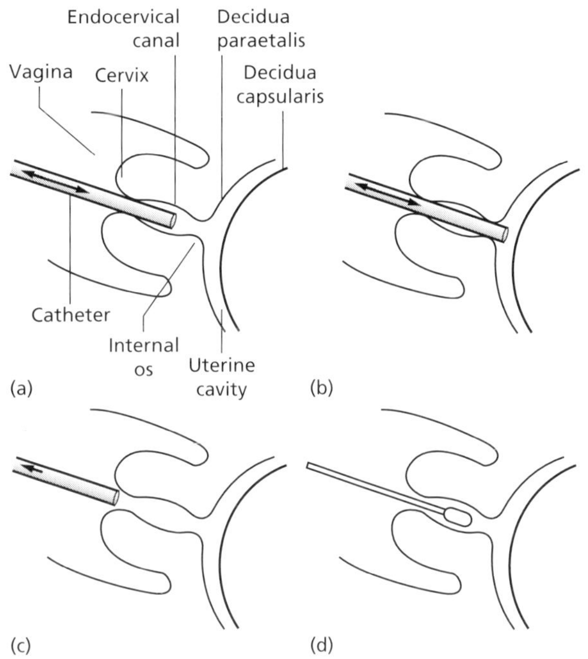

Fig. 40.2 Methods for collection of TCC samples: (a) endocervical lavage; (b) intrauterine lavage (arrows indicate instillation and aspiration of saline); (c) aspiration of cervical mucus; (d) cotton swab or cytobrush.

solution[9,10,13,15–18,20,22,24,27]. In our experience, good results can be obtained using a flexible plastic catheter 3 mm in diameter (Universal filling cannula, UN888/100, Universal Hospital Supplies Ltd., London, UK) attached to a syringe filled with 5 ml of sterile saline solution (*endocervical lavage*). Under visualization by transabdominal ultrasound the free end of the tube is passed 1 cm into the endocervical canal, the saline injected and immediately drawn back into the syringe[16–18]. For *intrauterine lavage*, the catheter is inserted through the cervical canal, the saline (10–20 ml) injected and then aspirated with gentle suction. Uterine lavage has been used on a large number of cases in Taiwan[27] but details about the procedure are lacking.

Aspiration of cervical mucus has been performed with a catheter attached to a 20–30 ml syringe containing 3–5 ml of saline. The catheter is inserted in the endocervical canal and the mucus retrieved in the syringe. As an alternative a small catheter with a piston (Pipelle) has been employed[28]. In a group of mothers, aspiration of mucus was followed by lavage with a small amount of saline; the purpose of this study was to establish whether TCCs were more frequently present in the cervical portion of the endocervical canal or in the uterine pole[16,17]. TCC samples have also been collected with a cytobrush (Sterling Winthrop, UK), placed in the lower part of the endocervical canal and rotated whilst being withdrawn to trap cells present in the mucus; the end of the brush was cut off, placed in a container with sterile saline solution and shaken to release the attached cells[20].

All procedures should be monitored by ultrasound scanning. They do not cause any discomfort to the pregnant women, last only a few minutes and can be performed without anaesthesia. At the time of the TCC sampling, a maternal peripheral blood sample is collected and a panel of clinical parameters recorded, including age of the mother, gestational age (by the last menstrual period and ultrasound scan), placental site and previous pregnancies, deliveries, miscarriages or abortions.

Soon after collection, TCC samples must be analysed under an inverted microscope and the cell content assessed (e.g. number of squamous cells, erythrocytes, clumps of presumed trophoblastic cellular elements, etc.). Aliquots of the specimen are then prepared for FISH, DNA extraction for PCR tests, isolation of cells or clumps and other tests. If large quantities of mucus are present, the samples must be treated with mucolytic agents[16].

Types of cells present in the endocervical canal

A variety of maternal and fetal cells are present in TCC samples. The type and number of cells vary greatly according to the method employed for their retrieval. Morphological examination using conventional staining reveals that endocervical lavage provides samples with maternal squamous and columnar epithelial cells, macrophages, leukocytes and red cells with variable frequency[16,29]. In these samples, multinucleated syncytial fragments have occasionally been detected often in association with groups of pleomorphic cells with a large hyperchromatic nucleus and abundant cytoplasm (Plate 40.1(a)) which have been identified as cytotrophoblast[29]. It seems that samples containing abundant cervical epithelial cells have low incidence of trophoblastic cellular elements and vice versa[29]. Endocervical and ectocervical cells are more abundant in TCC samples obtained by aspiration while the incidence of syncytial or trophoblastic fragments is low[29]. Samples collected with a cytobrush contain more debris and maternal cells than samples retrieved by aspiration or lavage; yet sufficient fetal cells are present, as judged by PCR assays[20].

In TCC samples examined with monoclonal antibodies (McAbs) raised against placental antigens, syncytial and trophoblastic cellular elements have been detected in a substantial number of specimens (Plate 40.1(b))[13,15,29].

In general, immunohistochemical stainings with McAbs are not as strong as those observed in control placental cells and often only a small proportion of cells in TCC samples are clearly stained[29]. Thus a lower incidence of fetal cells is observed in a sample tested with McAbs than in the same sample analysed by FISH. More accurate data should be obtained by using immunostaining with McAbs followed by FISH tests on single cells; with this approach TCCs derived from male fetuses should contain two fluorescent signals corresponding to the presence of a single X and one Y chromosome, while the membrane of the cell should show specific staining with the McAb. Trophoblastic cells from female fetuses should be immunostained and show two X chromosome signals. This technique is currently being investigated but the results are variable.

Incidence of fetal cells in TCC samples tested by FISH or PCR

PCR and FISH assays have been employed to study the frequency of trophoblastic cells in TCC samples collected with different methods (Table 40.1). In early studies, samples were analysed for the presence of chromosome Y-derived DNA sequences by PCR and/or single-colour FISH, but in subsequent investigations multicolour FISH, with probes for chromosomes X and Y and, in some cases, chromosomes 21, 18 and 13, was employed. The frequency of trophoblastic cells found in TCC samples obtained from pregnant women with male fetuses and tested with FISH or PCR techniques for the detection of Y specific DNA sequences is reported in Table 40.1. The great majority of these studies was performed on samples retrieved before TOP.

The observed variability is due to several factors, including the method employed for obtaining the TCC samples and the technique used for the identification of the fetal cells. As expected, the number of fetal (male) cells in each sample is also variable since, for example, it will be affected by the presence/absence of clumps of trophoblastic cells in the small aliquot of TCC sample tested by FISH. Table 40.3 shows the results of testing TCC samples retrieved by aspiration with a Pipelle before TOP[28]. PCR Y-derived signals could be seen in 68% of samples collected from mothers with male fetuses, while no false positive tests were seen in any of 31 TCC samples from mothers with female fetuses. It should be stressed that in this, as well as in other trials, the absence of Y-derived sequences in a TCC sample does not necessarily imply that the fetus is female, but that false positive results have not been observed.

In order to establish whether the lower incidence of fetal cells in TCC samples retrieved by aspiration – compared to that observed in specimens obtained by lavage – was due to a physiological difference between the frequency of trophoblastic cells in the cervical or the uterine pole of the endocervical canal, TCC samples have also been collected sequentially from the same subject, first by aspiration (cervical mucus) and then lavage[18]. When these samples were tested by double-colour FISH using probes for chromosomes X and Y, sexing was correctly diagnosed in eight out of 13 aspirated samples obtained from women with male fetuses. In nine out of nine cases with female fetuses all TCCs contained two chromosome X and no Y signals (Table 40.4). In TCC samples collected by lavage, no false positive Y signals were seen in nine samples retrieved from mothers with female fetuses, while the sex of the fetuses was correctly diagnosed in eight out of 13

TABLE 40.3
The presence of Y-derived and small tandem repeat (STR) sequences in placenta and TCC samples obtained by Pipelle

	Total	Placenta XY	TCC XY	Placenta XX	TCC XX[a]
PCR for X and Y	56	25	17 (68%)	31	31
	Total	STR fetal positive[b]	STR fetal negative	Possible[c]	Non-Informative
PCR for the STR markers	27	8 (29.6%)	5	2	12

[a] No TCC sample from female fetuses was found to be Y-positive
[b] There was full agreement between the results of testing placenta and TCC samples
[c] The fetal STR allele was observed in the TCC sample, but only at a very low level

TABLE 40.4
Double-colour FISH for X and Y chromosomes on TCC samples collected by sequential aspiration and lavage from 22 patients before TOP

Sample	Male (13)	Female (9)
Mucus aspirate	8	9
Lavage	8	9
Aspirate or lavage	12	9

samples obtained from mothers with male fetuses. Since, in some cases, fetal 'male' cells were seen in lavage but were absent in aspirated samples and *vice versa*, the combined analysis of all samples showed that a correct diagnosis of the sex of male fetuses was achieved in 12 out of 13 cases (Table 40.4).

Limited to a small group of samples, these results have not clarified whether fetal cells are more frequent in the cervical mucus or at the uterine pole of the endocervical canal; however, the general view is that trophoblastic cells are abundant in the uterine cavity between the decidua parietalis and capsularis until about 14 weeks of gestation (when this cavity disappears) and are shed in the endocervical canal from which the success of their collection depends on the method employed and the viscosity of the mucus.

The safety of performing aspiration of cervical mucus in continuing pregnancies has been assessed on a group of 130 women in whom the TCC samples were collected prior to an invasive CVS procedure. A control group of 145 women having transcervical CVS, but not TCC sampling, was included in the follow-up study (Table 40.2)[18]. The most important finding was the documentation that cervical mucus aspiration, performed before CVS, had no deleterious effects on the course of the pregnancies. In fact, the incidence of abortions was lower in the group of mothers tested for the presence of TCCs than in the control groups. It was particularly reassuring that infections were not observed in mothers belonging to the TCC aspiration group[16].

While false positive results have not or rarely been observed in all studies reported in Table 40.1, discordant results have been obtained by Overton et al.[30], who have often misdiagnosed the fetal sex. The high frequency of Y-derived DNA sequences noticed in samples retrieved from mothers with female fetuses was probably due to artefacts of the assay.

In several investigations TCC samples have also been tested by quantitative fluorescent PCR (QF-PCR) for the presence of chromosome specific small tandem repeats (STRs)[17,18,20,28]. These are highly polymorphic markers which characterize the phenotype of an individual and can be used to rapidly establish the presence of aneuploidies[31]. Most normal individuals will be heterozygous and produce two different STR products by QF-PCR. If a subject is trisomic for chromosome 21, three fluorescent STR markers or two products with a ratio 2:1 will be observed by QF-PCR analysis.

When this appoach is used to test a TCC sample, if the specimen contains only maternal cells, two PCR products similar to those present in the mother will be observed. Instead, if the TCC sample contains fetal cells as well, a third peak of fluorescent activity will be visible, corresponding to the PCR product of a gene inherited by the fetus from the father (Plate 40.2). This molecular approach is not as sensitive as the detection of Y-derived DNA sequences, but it provides evidence for the presence of fetal cells in TCC samples retrieved from mothers with female fetuses.

A new approach to the detection of fetal cells in TCC samples as well as maternal peripheral blood is based on the identification of a highly polymorphic pentanucleotide marker (X22) which maps on the pseudoautosomal region PAR 2 of the long arms of the X and Y chromosomes (Cirigliano *et al.* unpublished observation). Most normal individuals investigated by QF-PCR will be heterozygous for the marker and show two peaks of flourescent activities corresponding to the presence of different X22 alleles on the sex chromosomes. This STR can be employed for the rapid diagnosis of major aneuploidies affecting the X and Y chromosomes (Cirigliano *et al.* unpublished observation). When TCC samples are analysed with the X22 marker and QF-PCR, a paternal allele may be detected together with the two alleles present in maternal cells. This approach allows to identify cells derived from female fetuses and complements the detection of Y-derived sequences using amelogenin (AMXY) and QF-PCR.

In vitro cultures of transcervical cells

The first attempt at culturing TCCs was performed by Rhine et al.[9,10]. By flushing the mucus from the endocervical canal with physiological saline solution, cells could be collected that often had the morphological characteristics of trophoblastic cellular elements and could be cultured in vitro. In 17 out of 34 cultures, enough growth was obtained to perform comparative analyses between pairs of chromosome spreads prepared from the endocervical cells and the corresponding maternal lymphocytes. Using Q-banding staining, polymorphic differences were detected in 16 pairs of samples, suggesting that a proportion of the TCCs were of fetal origin[10]. In a subsequent paper, Rhine and Milunsky[11] confirmed the detection of trophoblastic cells in the endocervical samples on the evidence that some metaphases contained the Y chromosome.

However, Goldberg et al.[12] repeated these experiments, but failed to grow fetal cells despite having detected cytotrophoblastic cellular elements in the original samples.

A recent extensive study, aimed at culturing TCCs, has been carried out by Ishai et al.[19] who attempted short-term cultures of 28 TCC samples collected by lavage before TOP. In 19 cases, several metaphases could be obtained and karyotyped. Maternal contamination at a level near 10% proved to be less of a problem than anticipated. In six TCC samples, metaphases were detectable within 24 h following direct preparation. It has been claimed that in order to avoid contamination with maternal cells, TCC samples must be kept in culture for a brief period of time. Improvement of the in vitro cultures may provide, in a short period of time (48–72 h), clones of fetal cells suitable for the prenatal diagnosis of single-gene defects.

Detection of chromosomal and single-gene disorders

In the course of several investigations, chromosomal abnormalities have been detected by FISH analysis of TCC samples obtained by lavage or aspiration. A case of trisomy 18 was observed in the first small group of specimens retrieved by lavage[15]. In a recent study, two cases of trisomy 21 and several cases of sex chromosome aneuploidy were diagnosed in TCC samples collected before TOP and the results confirmed in placental tissues[32]. Other isolated cases of chromosome disorders have been reported by Massari et al.[22] and Briggs et al.[24].

While it is possible to diagnose major chromosomal abnormalities or the presence of the Y chromosome by testing TCC samples containing maternal cells, prenatal diagnosis of single-gene disorders, such as autosomal recessive or X-linked diseases, requires the isolation of fetal cells free of maternal contaminants[33,37]. Theoretically this could be achieved using McAbs raised against placental cells; however, this approach has not been yet successfully exploited.

Instead, the isolation of clumps of fetal cells from TCC samples (Plate 40.1(a)), has been attained by micromanipulation using an inverted microscope[34]. Clumps of cells, with the morphology of trophoblastic cellular elements, can then be removed, washed and then analysed by FISH or PCR amplification.

This method has been used to perform the first prenatal diagnoses of haemoglobinopathies on TCC samples in six couples, when both parents were carriers of thalassaemia or HbS[35]. The Hb mutations affecting each parent and the results of testing TCCs and CVS are shown in Table 40.5. Since clumps of trophoblastic cells may be contaminated with maternal cells, the only prenatal diagnoses that can be performed with certainty are those in cases where the clumps contain normal Hb genes (normal fetus) or a normal gene and the paternal mutation (heterozygous fetus). If parents carry the same mutation a correct diagnosis can also be achieved if clumps of cells show homozygosity for the mutated gene. However, tests can be extended to include chromosome specific polymorphic markers that can reveal the presence of paternal genes. An alternative is to test a series of single trophoblastic cellular elements.

As shown in Table 40.5, the diagnosis was correctly performed in four out of the six couples investigated, since the results of testing clumps of cells were in agreement with those obtained by CVS. Further evidence that prenatal diagnosis of haemoglobinopathies can be performed using TCC samples has been obtained by testing clumps of trophoblastic cells isolated from specimens retrieved at an early stage of gestation. In this study, one aliquot of the extracted DNA was tested for the presence of fetal DNA by STR and AMXY markers, and the other for the detection of the Hb mutations. This double test ensures that the clump of cells is not contaminated by maternal DNA (Cirigliano *et al.* unpublished observation).

Prenatal detection of fetal Rh(D) DNA sequences

In a pilot study, endocervical cells were retrieved from six mothers at about 10 weeks of gestation by aspiration of cervical mucus before CVS while, from another six women, TCC samples were obtained by lavage between 6 and 13 weeks before TOP[36]. All 12 mothers were serologically Rh(D)-negative. Two sets of primers specific for the 3′ untranslated region of Rh(D) and exon 4 of Rh(CD) were employed in a duplex PCR assay to analyse the samples together with maternal peripheral blood, chorionic villi or other fetal tissues; in four cases the fetal Rh phenotype was investigated serologically on cord blood samples collected at time of delivery.

TABLE 40.5
Results of testing clumps of cells from TCC samples for Hb mutations

	Mutations[a]		CVS	Clumps[b]							
Case	Mother	Father	result	1	2	3	4	5	6	7	Comments
1	+/110	+/110	+/+	**+/+**	**+/+**	+/110	—	—	—	—	Two normal clumps; fetus normal
2	+/5	+/C30	+/+	+/5	+/5	+/5	+/5	—	—	—	No paternal mutation in clumps
3	+/HbS	+/5	+/5	HbS/5	HbS/5	HbS/5	—	—	—	—	Compound heterozygote clumps. Maternal contamination
4	+/110	+/6	+/6	**+/6**	**+/6**	**+/6**	—	—	—	—	Three clumps with the paternal mutation, fetus heterozygous; non-affected
5	+/110	+/110	+/110	**+/110**	**+/110**	**+/110**	**+/110**	—	—	—	Heterozygous fetus?
6	+/del 1	+/del 2	del 1/del 2	**del 1/del 2**	**del 1/del 2**	**del 1/del 2**	**del 1/del 2**	+/del 1	+/del 1	+/del 1	Four clumps with maternal and paternal deletions

[a]Various mutations causing β-thalassaemia. Mutations 5, 6 and 110 occur in intron 1, and mutation C30 occurs in exon 1
In mother 3, the HbS mutation was in exon 1
In case 6 the maternal deletion (del 1) was four base pairs, and the paternal (del 2) was 619 base pairs
[b]Entries in bold are TCC clumps that agree with CVS result.

A good correlation was observed between the PCR results on TCC samples and those obtained on fetal tissues, with two exceptions when the TCC samples, retrieved by aspiration or lavage, appeared to be Rh(D)-negative, while the neonates or the placenta were Rh(D)-positive[36]. These discrepancies could be attributed to the absence of fetal cells or the low sensitivity of the test. Although promising, the Rh(D) detection by PCR on TCC samples requires technical improvements before it can be used for prenatal diagnosis.

Conclusions

Studies performed during the past 4 years have vindicated Shettles's claim that trophoblastic cells are present in the endocervical canal. Fetal cells are probably present in all TCC samples, at least judging from several studies in which specimens were collected by lavage. However, there is evidence that the successful retrieval of these cells depends on the technique employed (e.g. lavage, aspiration or cytobrush)[16]. Although lavage with 5 ml of saline solution, instilled before TOP, has provided satisfactory results, concern has been expressed about the use of this procedure in ongoing pregnancies in view of the possibility of introducing infections. In Taiwan, where uterine lavage has been used on a large scale, it was claimed that the success rate of sexing the fetus was over 90%. Unfortunately no data have been released on the safety of the procedure which was carried out in private clinics without ultrasound scanning and follow-up[27].

So far, aspiration of cervical mucus has been employed in small groups of pregnant women with a success rate between 50% and 70%. In a preliminary study, limited to about 130 ongoing pregnancies, when TCC samples were collected by aspiration before CVS, no major risks for the mothers or the fetuses were observed. This suggests that TCC samples retrieved by aspiration can be used for prenatal diagnosis of the most common chromosomal disorders. However, the failure to detect fetal cells in a high percentage of TCC samples collected by aspiration limits the diagnostic value of this approach. Improvement of the analysis of trophoblastic cells and their recovery may increase the rate of successes. Furthermore, a second specimen can be retrieved within a short period of time from the collection of the first sample[19].

Another important problem that remains to be solved is the isolation of trophoblastic cellular elements free from contaminating maternal cells. This is an essential step to perform prenatal diagnosis of autosomal recessive or X-linked disorders.

Isolation of clumps of trophoblastic cells from TCC samples has been attained by micromanipulation, but this is time consuming and is hampered by the possible contamination with maternal cells.

As briefly mentioned, a satisfactory technique for the isolation of trophoblastic cells using McAbs has not been reported as yet. However, it should be only a question of time before the right antibodies are produced for the detection and successful isolation of trophoblastic cells from TCC samples. Possibly, a preliminary enrichment by density gradients followed by the use of McAbs and magnetic beads could provide the best tools for the purification of fetal cells thus allowing the use of TCC samples for the prenatal diagnosis of the most common inherited disorders.

A final judgement on the possibility of exploiting the presence of trophoblastic cells in the endocervical canal requires further investigations and trials performed on ongoing pregnancies. At present, the TCC results obtained during the last 6 years should be evaluated in the light of other attempts at performing prenatal diagnoses by non or minimally invasive techniques, such as the detection of fetal nucleated cells in peripheral maternal blood samples which have been hampered by several difficulties, mostly associated with the extremely low incidence of these cells and their isolation from maternal contaminants[33,37].

Acknowledgement

We would like to thank The Dunhill Medical Trust and the Birth Defects Foundation for their financial support and many colleagues who have helped us in the course of our investigations.

REFERENCES

1. Shettles LB. Use of the Y chromosome in prenatal sex determination. *Nature* **230**:52, 1971.
2. Warren R, Sanchez L, Hammond D, McLeod A. Prenatal sex determination from exfoliated cells found in cervical mucus. *Am J Obstet Gynecol* **24**:22, 1972.
3. Varner RE, Younger JB, Finley SC. Fluorescent Y bodies from endocervical smears for prenatal sex detection. *Alabama J Med Sci* **14**:430, 1977.
4. Bobrow M, Lewis BV. Unreliability of fetal sexing using cervical material. *Lancet* **243**:539, 1971.
5. Tsuji K, Sasaki M. Absence of Y-body in the cervical mucus of pregnant women. *Nature* **243**:539, 1973.
6. Goldstein AI, Lukesh RC, Katchum M. Prenatal sex determination by fluorescent staining of the cervical smear for the presence of a Y chromosome: an evaluation. *Am J Obstet Gynecol* **115**:866, 1973.
7. Manuel M, Park IJ, Jones HW. Prenatal sex determination by fluorescent staining of cells for the presence of Y chromatin. *Am J Obstet Gynecol* **119**:853–854, 1974.
8. Amankwah KS and Bond EC. Unreliability of prenatal determination of fetal sex with the use of Y-body fluorescence in midcervical smears. *Am J Obstet Gynecol* **130**:300–301, 1978.
9. Rhine SA, Cain JL, Cleary RL, Palmer CG, Thompson JF. Prenatal sex detection with endocervical smears: successful results utilizing Y-body fluorescence. *Am J Obstet Gynecol* **122**:155–160, 1975.
10. Rhine SA, Palmer CG, Thompson JF. A simple alternative to amniocentesis for first trimester prenatal diagnosis. *Birth Def Orig Art Ser* **XII**:231–247, 1977.
11. Rhine SA, Milunsky A. Utilization of trophoblast for early prenatal diagnosis. In *Genetic Disorders and the Fetus: Diagnosis Prevention and Treatment* (ed. A. Milunsky), pp. 527–539. New York: Plenum Press, 1979.
12. Goldberg M, Chen TI, Ahu YW, Reidy JA. First trimester fetal chromosomal diagnosis using endocervical lavage: a negative evaluation. *Am J Obstet Gynecol* **138**:436–440, 1980.
13. Griffith-Jones MD, Miller D, Liford RJ, Scott J, Bulmer J. Detection of fetal DNA in transcervical swabs from the first trimester pregnancies by gene amplification: a new route to prenatal diagnosis? *Br J Obstet Gynaecol* **99**:508–511, 1992.
14. Morris N, Williamson R. Non-invasive first trimester antenatal diagnosis. *Br J Obstet Gynaecol* **99**:446–448, 1992.
15. Adinolfi M, Davies A, Sharif S, Soothill P, Rodeck C. Detection of trisomy 18 and Y-derived sequences in fetal nucleated cells obtained by transcervical flushing. *Lancet* **342**:403–404, 1993.
16. Rodeck CH, Tutschek B, Sherlock J, Kingdom J. Methods for the transcervical collection of fetal cells during the first trimester of pregnancy. *Prenat Diagn* **15**:933–942, 1995.
17. Adinolfi M, Sherlock J, Soothill P, Rodeck C. Molecular evidence of fetal-derived chromosome 21 markers (STRs) in transcervical samples. *Prenat Diagn* **15**:33–39, 1995.
18. Adinolfi M, Sherlock J, Tutschek B, Halder A, Delhanty J. Detection of fetal cells in transcervical samples and prenatal diagnosis of chromosomal abnormalities. *Prenat Diagn* **15**:943–949, 1995.
19. Ishai D, Amiel A, Diukman R et al. Uterine cavity lavage: adding FISH to conventional cytogentics for embryonic sexing and diagnosing common chromosomal abnormalities. *Prenat Diagn* **15**:961–965, 1995.
20. Kingdom J, Sherlock J, Rodeck C, Adinolfi M. Detection of trophoblast cells in transcervical samples by lavage or cytobrush. *Obstet Gynecol* **86**:283–288, 1995.
21. Kawamura M, Suzumori K, Yagami Y. Nucleated cells of fetal origin collected by uterine cavity flushing for prenatal diagnosis. *Nagoya Med J* **40**:41–50, 1995.
22. Massari A, Novelli G, Colosimo A et al. Non-invasive early prenatal molecular diagnosis using retrieved transcervical trophoblast cells. *Hum Genet* **97**:150–155, 1996.
23. Chang SD, Chang DJ, Chu KK, His DL. Rapid fetal chromosome fetal analysis using FISH on samples from uterine lavage. A preliminary experience in Taiwan. *Rec Adv Prenat Diagn Aneupl* (Abst) 132, 1996.
24. Briggs J, Miller D, Bulmer J, Griffith-Jones M, Rame V, Lilford R. Non-syncytial sources of fetal DNA in transcervically recovered cell populations. *Mol Hum Reprod* **10**:749–754, 1995.
25. Daryani YP, Penna LK, Patton MA. Detection of cells of fetal origin from transcervical irrigations. *Prenat Diagn* **17**:243–248, 1997.
26. Maggi F, Berdusco F, Liuti R, et al. First trimester chromosome diagnosis by lavage of the uterine cavity. *Prenat Diagn* **16**:823–827, 1996.
27. Hsi BL, Adinolfi M. Prenatal sexing of human fetuses and selective abortions. *Prenat Diagn* **17**:1–3, 1997.
28. Ruangvutilert P, Halder A, Jauniaux E, Ariengo M-P, Cirigliano V, Sherlock J. *Prenat Neonat Med* **3**:294–296, 1988.
29. Bulmer JN, Rodeck C, Adinolfi M. Immunohistochemical characterisation of cells retrieved by transcervical sampling in early pregnancy. *Prenat Diagn* **15**:1143–1153, 1995.
30. Overton TG, Lighten AD, Fisk NM, Bennett PR. Prenatal Diagnosis by minimally invasive first trimester transcervical sampling is unreliable. *Am J Obstet Gynecol* **175**:382–387, 1996.
31. Pertl B, Weitgasser U, Kapp S, Kroisel PM, Sherlock J, Adinolfi M. Rapid detection of trisomy 21 and 18 and sexing by quantitative fluorescent PCR. *Hum Genet* **98**:55–59, 1996.
32. Sherlock J, Halder A, Tutschek B, Delhanty JDA, Rodeck CH, Adinolfi M. Prenatal detection of fetal aneuploides using transcervical cell samples. *J Med Genet* **34**:302–305, 1997.
33. Adinolfi M, Breaking the blood barrier. *Nature Genet* **1**:316–318, 1995.
34. Tutschek B, Sherlock J, Halder A, Delhanty JDA, Rodeck CH, Adinolfi M. Isolation of fetal cells from transcervical samples by micromanipulation: molecular confirmation of their fetal origin and diagnosis of fetal aneuploidy. *Prenat Diagn* **15**:951–960, 1995.
35. Adinolfi M, El-Hashemite N, Sherlock J, Ward RHT, Petrou M, Rodeck CH. Prenatal detection of haemoglobin mutation using transcervical cells. *Prenat Diagn* **17**:539–543, 1997.
36. Adinolfi M, Sherlock J, Kemp T. et al. Prenatal detection of fetal RhD DNA sequences in transcervical samples. *Lancet* **345**:318–319, 1995.
37. Adinolfi M. Fetal nucleated cells in the maternal circulation. In *Prenatal Diagnosis and Screenings* (eds D.J.H. Brock, C.H. Rodeck, M. Ferguson-Smith), pp. 651–660. Edinburgh: Churchill Livingstone, 1992.

SECTION 6

Diagnosis of fetal genetic diseases

Haemoglobinopathies

J.M. Old

41

Introduction

The haemoglobinopathies are a diverse group of autosomal recessive disorders characterized by either the synthesis of a structurally abnormal globin (the haemoglobin variants) or the reduced synthesis of one or more of the globin chains (the thalassaemias)[1]. As a group they are the most common single gene disorder in the world and are found at high frequencies in many populations as a result of positive selection pressure due to falciparum malaria. Individuals with the carrier state are easily identifiable, permitting the control of the serious haemoglobinopathies by a programme of carrier screening, counselling and prenatal diagnosis. The most important disorders for which prenatal diagnosis is considered are α^0-thalassaemia, β-thalassaemia, sickle-cell anaemia and various compound heterozygous states which result in a clinically significant disease (Table 41.1).

The haemoglobinopathies are regionally specific and each local population has its own characteristic spectrum of haemoglobin variants and thalassaemia mutations. Therefore knowledge of the ethnic origin of a patient under study is often essential to enable the quick identification of the underlying molecular defects by the application of molecular biology techniques. This can be achieved in most cases as nearly all the globin gene mutations have now been identified and the particular mutations and their frequencies for most at-risk ethnic groups are known[2]. The majority of the molecular defects can be diagnosed using a variety of techniques involving the analysis of DNA amplified by the polymerase chain reaction (PCR). PCR-based techniques provide a quick and sensitive approach to fetal DNA diagnosis and normally enable a result to be obtained in 2–3 days.

The globin genes

Haemoglobin is a tetrameric protein made up of two α-like (α or ζ) and two β-like (ε, γ, δ or β) globin chains. Each globin chain is synthesized from its own globin gene located in two gene clusters, the α-like globin genes on chromosome 16 and the β-like genes on chromosome 11. The α-like globin cluster includes an embryonic gene (ζ2), two fetal/adult genes (α1 and α2), several pseudogenes (ψζ1, ψα1 and ψα2) and a gene of undetermined function (θ1) arranged in the order ζ2-ψζ1-ψα2-ψα1-α2-α1-θ. The β-globin cluster includes an embryonic gene (ε), two fetal genes (Gγ and Aγ), two adult genes (β and δ) and a pseudogene (ψβ) in the order ε-Gγ-Aγ-ψβ-δ-β. Throughout development there is a series of co-ordinated switches of the production of one type of haemoglobin to another. Embryonic haemoglobin ($\alpha_2\varepsilon_2$ – Hb Gower, $\zeta_2\varepsilon_2$ – Hb Gower 1 and $\zeta_2\gamma_2$ – Hb Portland) gives way to fetal haemoglobin ($\alpha_2\gamma_2$ – Hb F) which then switches to adult haemoglobin ($\alpha_2\beta_2$ – Hb A and $\alpha_2\delta_2$ – Hb A_2). The molecular mechanisms responsible for the switching on and off of the various globin genes have been the subject of intense research for many years because the clinical severity of β-thalassaemia or sickle-cell disease is ameliorated in individuals who have a naturally elevated level of Hb F. Several chemical agents such as hydroxyurea and butyrate induce the production of Hb F, and their effects in patients with sickle-cell disease and thalassaemia are being assessed in clinical trials[3]. Although the precise mechanism of action of these agents remains unknown, the most effective results obtained to date have been with hydroxyurea therapy in sickle-cell and sickle-β thalassaemia patients[4], in contrast to β-thalassaemia patients for which the results have been disappointing except in some patients with thalassaemia intermedia who are not transfusion-dependent[5].

TABLE 41.1
Phenotypes of thalassaemias, sickle-cell disease and various thalassaemia interactions

Type	Phenotype	DNA diagnosis
Homozygous state		
α^0-thalassaemia	Hb Bart's hydrops fetalis	S blot/PCR
α^+-thalassaemia	No clinical problems	S blot/PCR
β-thalassaemia:		
β^0 or severe β^+ mutation	Thalassaemia major	PCR
mild β^+ mutation	Thalassaemia intermedia	PCR
$\delta\beta^0$-thalassaemia	Thalassaemia intermedia	S blot/PCR
Hb Lepore	Variable: intermedia to major	PCR
Hb S	Sickle-cell disease	PCR
Hb C	No clinical problems	PCR
Hb D	No clinical problems	PCR
Hb E	No clinical problems	PCR
Compound heterozygous state		
α^0-thal/α^+-thal	Hb H disease	S blot/PCR
β^0/severe β^+	Thalassaemia major	PCR
Mild β^+/β^0 or severe β^+	Variable: intermedia to major	PCR
$\delta\beta^0/\beta^0$ or severe β^+	Variable: intermedia to major	S blot/PCR
$\delta\beta^0$/mild β^+	Mild thalassaemia intermedia	S blot/PCR
$\delta\beta^0$/Hb Lepore	Thalassaemia intermedia	S blot/PCR
$\alpha\alpha\alpha/\beta^0$ or severe β^+	Mild thalassaemia intermedia	S blot/PCR
Hb Lepore/β^0 or severe β^+	Thalassaemia major	PCR
Hb C/β^0 or severe β^+	Variable: β-thal trait to intermedia	PCR
Hb C/mild β^+	No clinical problems	PCR
Hb D/β^0 or severe β^+	No clinical problems	PCR
Hb E/β^0 or severe β^+	Variable: intermedia to major	PCR
Hb O Arab/β^0	Severe thalassaemia intermedia	PCR
Hb S/β^0 or severe β^+	Sickle-cell disease	PCR
Hb S/mild β^+	Usually mild sickle-cell disease	PCR
Hb S/Hb C	Sickle-cell disease, variable severity	PCR
Hb S/Hb D Punjab	Sickle-cell disease	PCR
Hb S/Hb O Arab	Sickle-cell disease	PCR

α-Thalassaemia

CLINICAL STATES

α-Thalassaemia is characterized by a deficiency of α-globin chain synthesis. Defective gene expression may occur in either one globin gene (called α-2 or α^+-thalassaemia) or in both (α-1 or α^0-thalassaemia) and thus there are four clinical states depending upon the number of functional α-globin genes (3, 2, 1 or 0).

The most severe form of α-thalassaemia is the homozygous state for α^0-thalassaemia, known as Hb Bart's hydrops fetalis syndrome. This condition results from a deletion of all four globin genes and an affected fetus cannot synthesize any α-globin to make Hb F or Hb A. Fetal blood contains only the abnormal haemoglobin Bart's (γ_4) and a small amount of Hb Portland. The resulting severe fetal anaemia leads to asphyxia, hydrops fetalis and stillbirth or neonatal death, and prenatal diagnosis is always indicated in order to avoid the severe toxaemic complications that occur frequently in pregnancy with hydropic fetuses.

Individuals with one functional α-gene have Hb H disease and are compound heterozygotes for α^+ and α^0-thalassaemia. They have a moderately severe hypochromic microcytic anaemia and produce large amounts of Hb H (β_4) as a result of the excess β-chains in the reticulocyte. Patients with deletional Hb H disease suffer from fatigue, general discomfort and splenomegaly, but they rarely require hospitalization and lead a relatively normal life. However, patients with non-deletional Hb H disease seem to exhibit more severe symptoms with a possible requirement of recurrent blood transfusions and splenectomy. In some situations couples at risk for the severe form of Hb H disease have opted for prenatal diagnosis and termination of an affected fetus[6].

Individuals with two functional α-globin genes are characterized by a normal Hb A_2 level and clearly reduced values for the red cell indices mean cell haemoglobin (MCH) and mean cell volume (MCV) and may be either homozygous for α^+-thalassaemia or heterozygous for α^0-thalassaemia. The two conditions have very similar phenotypes and can only be distinguished with certainty by DNA analysis. Finally, carriers of α^+-thalassaemia have three functional α-globin genes and exhibit slightly reduced red cell indices, but the overlap in these indices makes it impossible to distinguish carriers from normal individuals in many cases on the basis of MCV and MCH alone. The detection of Hb Bart's in neonates and the demonstration of occasional cells containing Hb H in adults also signify the presence of α-thalassaemia trait but again the tests do not clearly distinguish the various α-genotypes and do not detect all cases of α-thalassaemia trait.

MOLECULAR DEFECTS

Most α-thalassaemia mutations result from the deletion of gene sequences in the α-globin gene cluster[7]. The deletion of one of the two α-globin genes gives rise to the α^+-thalassaemia phenotype and although five different deletions have been identified, only two are commonly encountered in practice. These are the 3.7 kb deletion ($-\alpha^{3.7}$), which has reached high frequencies in the populations of Africa, the Mediterranean area, the Middle East, the Indian subcontinent and Melanesia, and the 4.2 kb deletion ($-\alpha^{4.2}$) which is commonly found in Southeast Asian and Pacific populations[2]. These deletions were created by unequal crossing over between homologous sequences in the α-globin gene cluster, resulting in a chromosome with only one α-gene (–α) and a chromosome with three α-genes (ααα). Further recombination events between the resulting chromosomes have given rise to quadruplicated α-genes (αααα). Various non-deletion defects have also been found to cause α^+-thalassaemia and a total of 17 mutations have been described to date, mostly in populations from the Mediterranean area, Africa and Southeast Asia[8]. All of the mutations except one are located in the dominant α2-globin gene and are denoted $\alpha^T\alpha$ in order to signify the affected gene. As there appears to be no associated change in expression of the remaining functional α1-globin gene (as occurs with the –α alleles) they give rise to a more severe reduction in α-chain synthesis than in deletion α^+-thalassaemia. The interaction of these non-deletional mutations with α^0-thalassaemia results in severe Hb H disease or, very rarely, Hb Bart's hydrops fetalis syndrome in infants with a very low level of α-globin chain synthesis[9].

α^0-Thalassaemia results from deletions which involve both α-globin genes and to date at least 14 different deletions have been described[8]. The deletions which have attained high gene frequencies are found in individuals from Southeast Asia and South China ($—^{SEA}$), the Philippine Islands ($—^{FIL}$), Thailand ($—^{THAI}$) and a few Mediterranean countries such as Greece and Cyprus ($—^{MED}$ and $-(\alpha)^{20.5}$). Although an α^0-thalassaemia mutation ($—^{SA}$) has been described in Asian Indians it is extremely uncommon and no α^0-thalassaemia deletions have been reported in individuals from sub-Saharan Africa. In Northern Europe α-thalassaemia occurs sporadically because of the lack of natural selection and several α^0-thalassaemia deletions have been reported in single British families. However, one particular molecular defect ($—^{BRIT}$) appears to turn up fairly regularly in DNA samples referred to my laboratory for α-thalassaemia investigations, especially from British individuals living in Cheshire and Lancashire.

MOLECULAR DIAGNOSIS

The two most common α^+-thalassaemia alleles, $-\alpha^{3.7}$ and $-\alpha^{4.2}$, together with three α^0-thalassaemia mutations, the $—^{MED}$, $-(\alpha)^{20.5}$ and the $—^{SEA}$ alleles, can now be diagnosed by a PCR-based technique, sometimes called GAP PCR, which uses two primers complementary to the sense and antisense strand in the DNA regions which flank the deletion[10–12]. Amplified product is obtained only from the deletion allele as the distance between the two primers is too great to amplify normal DNA. The normal allele (αα) is detected by amplifying DNA sequences spanning one of the breakpoints, using a primer complementary to the deleted sequence (Fig. 41.1). The non-deletion mutations may also be detected by PCR, by the technique of selective amplification of the α-2 gene and then analysis of the product for the particular mutations[13]. Several of the non-deletion mutations alter a restriction enzyme site and may be analysed by restriction enzyme analysis, in a similar manner to that reported for the mutation which gives rise to the abnormal Hb Constant Spring[6]. The amplification of the α-globin genes sequences is technically more difficult than that of other gene sequences such as the β-globin genes because of the high GC content of the α-globin gene cluster and requires more stringent conditions for success. For this and several other reasons, Southern blot analysis remains a useful and reliable approach to the molecular diagnosis of α-thalassaemia.

Southern blot analysis, using a combination of restriction enzyme digests and gene probes can be used to detect all the common deletions, including some not yet detectable by PCR and in addition, provides diagnostic information on triple and quadruple α-genes. A list of the characteristic abnormal restriction fragments used in my laboratory for diagnostic purposes is presented in Table 41.2. A *BamH* I digest hybridized to an α-globin gene probe is used to identify the single, double, triple and quadruple α-globin gene alleles and it also reveals the Mediterranean α^0-thalassaemia deletion $-(\alpha)^{20.5}$. A *BamH* I digest hybridized to a ζ-globin gene probe is used to detect the $—^{SEA}$ α^0-thalassaemia allele but the majority of the deletion mutations are identified by hybridization of a ζ-gene probe to a *Bgl* II digest (the $-\alpha^{3.7}$ and $-\alpha^{4.2}$ α^+-thalassaemia genes and the $—^{MED}$, $-(\alpha)^{20.5}$, $—^{SA}$, $—^{BRIT}$, and $—^{SEA}$ α^0 alleles as illustrated in Fig. 41.2), except for the $—^{THAI}$ and $—^{FIL}$ deletions, which require an Sst I digest hybridized to a DNA probe located downstream to the ζ-globin gene[14]. Although Southern blot analysis provides a comprehensive approach to the diagnosis of all the common α-gene deletions and rearrangements, the disadvantage of this approach is that the technique still takes 7–10 days to obtain a diagnostic result.

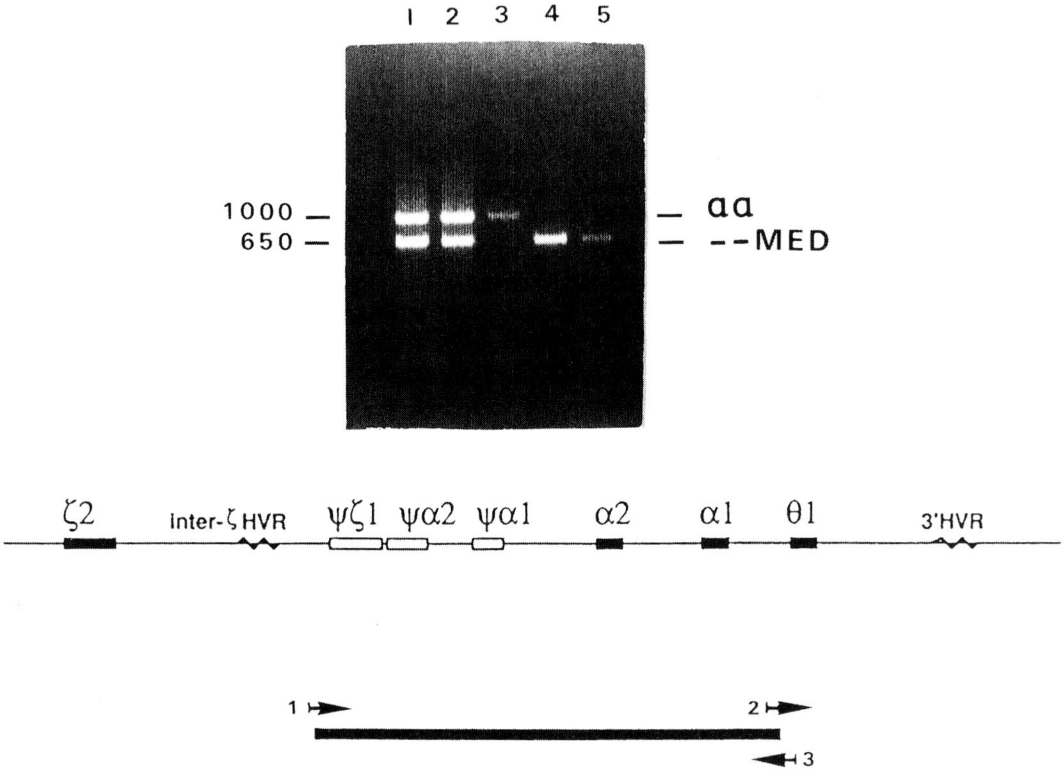

Fig. 41.1 Prenatal diagnosis for α^0-thalassaemia by GAP PCR. Lanes 1 and 2, maternal and paternal DNA heterozygous for the $—^{MED}$ deletion gene; Lane 3, normal DNA; Lanes 4 and 5, fetal DNA showing homozygosity for α^0-thalassaemia. A diagram shows the location of the $—^{MED}$ deletion within the α-globin gene cluster and the positions of primers 1 and 3 which amplify the mutant allele to give a 650 bp product and primers 2 and 3 which amplify only the normal allele to give a 1000 bp product.

TABLE 41.2
The diagnosis of α-thalassaemia and other alleles by Southern blotting

	Restriction enzyme/gene probe				
Allele	*BamH* I/α	*Bgl* II/α	*BamH* I/ζ	*Bgl* II/ζ	*Sst* I/LO
αα	14	12.6 7.4	10–11.3 5.9	12.6 or 5.2 10–11.3	5.0
ααα	18	12.6 7.4	10–11.3 5.9	12.6 or 16 10–11.3	5.0
αααα	22	12.6 7.4	10–11.3 5.9	12.6 or 20 10–11.3	5.0
$-\alpha^{3.7}$	10.3	16	10–11.3 5.9	16 10–11.3	5.0
$-\alpha^{4.2}$	9.8	8.0 7.4	10–11.3 5.9	10–11.3 8.0	5.0
$-(\alpha)^{20.5}$	4.0	10.8	5.9	10.8	5.0
$—^{MED}$	None	None	5.9	13.9	5.0
$—^{SEA}$	None	None	20 5.9	10.5	5.0
$—^{SA}$	None	None	5.9	7.0	5.0
$—^{BRIT}$	None	None	5.9	8.0	5.0
$—^{THAI}$	None	None	None	None	8.0
$—^{FIL}$	None	None	None	None	7.4

Fragment sizes are given in kilobase pairs. Characteristic abnormal fragments are underlined

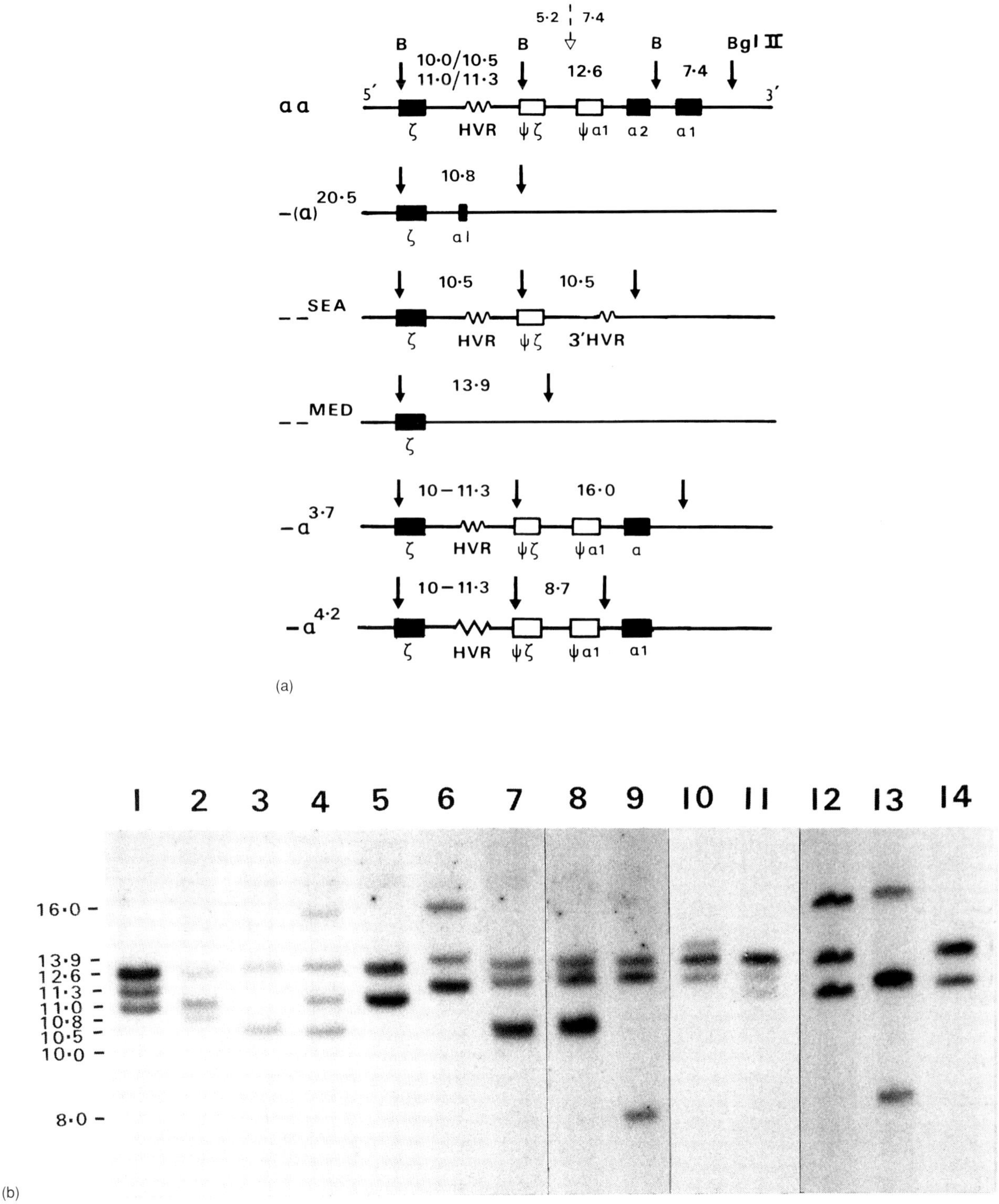

Fig. 41.2 (a) Diagram showing the positions of *Bgl* II sites in the normal α-globin gene cluster and five common α-thalassaemia deletion genes. A polymorphic *Bgl* II site is indicated by the dashed arrow. The hypervariable regions (inter-ζ HVR and 3′-HVR) are indicated by zig-zags. (b) Southern blot showing *Bgl* II digested DNA hybridized to a ζ-gene probe. The genotypes are: lane 1, αα/αα; lane 2, $-(\alpha)^{20.5}/\alpha\alpha$; lane 3, αα/αα; lane 4, $-\alpha^{3.7}/\alpha\alpha$; lane 5, αα/αα; lane 6, $-\alpha^{3.7}/\alpha\alpha$; lane 7, $—^{SEA}/\alpha\alpha$; lane 8, $—^{SEA}/\alpha\alpha$; lane 9, $—^{BRIT}/\alpha\alpha$; lane 10, $—^{MED}/\alpha\alpha$; lane 11, αα/αα; lane 12, $-\alpha^{3.7}/\alpha\alpha$; lane 13, $-\alpha^{3.7}/-\alpha^{4.2}$; lane 14, αα/αα.

β-Thalassaemia

CLINICAL STATES

β-Thalassaemia is characterized by a deficiency of β-globin chain synthesis. Individuals with β-thalassaemia trait are essentially healthy although they may have a slightly reduced Hb level and have typically low MCH and MCV values. In contrast to α-thalassaemia, the Hb A_2 concentration is elevated above the normal range to a level of 3.5–7.0% in all but a small minority of cases. β-Thalassaemia trait with a normal Hb A_2 level is due to either the coinheritance of δ-thalassaemia (12 different mutations are known to restrict the output of the δ-globin gene)[15] or to the inheritance of one of the six mild β-thalassaemia alleles known as silent β-thalassaemia mutations[16]. β-Thalassaemia trait with an unusually high level of Hb A_2 (above 7.0%) results from one of the larger deletions affecting the β-globin gene.

The majority of individuals homozygous for β-thalassaemia have the transfusion-dependent condition called β-thalassaemia major. This condition results from the homozygous state for a severe β-thalassaemia mutation or, more commonly, the compound heterozygous state for two different mutations. At birth, β-thalassaemia homozygotes are asymptomatic because of the high production of Hb F but as this declines, affected infants present with severe anaemia during the first or second year of life. Treatment is by frequent blood transfusion to maintain a haemoglobin level above 10 g/dl, coupled with iron chelation therapy to control iron overload, otherwise death results in the second or third decade from cardiac failure. This treatment does not cure β-thalassaemia major, although some patients have now reached the age of 40 in good health and have married and produçed children. With the prospects for gene therapy remaining as distant as ever, the only cure for β-thalassaemia for the foreseeable future is bone marrow transplantation. Although this form of treatment has proved successful when carried out in young children, it is limited by the requirement of an HLA matched sibling or relative.

Some individuals homozygous for β-thalassaemia have a milder clinical condition called thalassaemia intermedia. Such patients present later in life relative to those with thalassaemia major and are capable of maintaining a haemoglobin level above 6 g without transfusion. Thalassaemia intermedia is caused by a wide variety of genotypes and covers a broad clinical spectrum. Patients with a severe condition present between 2 and 6 years of age and although they are capable of surviving with an Hb level of 5–7 g/dl they will not develop normally and are treated with minimal blood transfusion. At the other end of the spectrum are patients who do not become symptomatic until they reach adult life and remain transfusion independent with Hb levels of 8–10 g/dl. However, even these milder patients tend to accumulate iron with age and many thalassaemia intermedia patients develop clinical problems relating to iron overload after the third decade.

MOLECULAR DEFECTS

β-Thalassaemia is caused by 13 large deletions of 44 nucleotides or greater and 170 point mutations or small insertions/deletions of DNA sequence in and around the β-globin gene[15]. The mutations either reduce the expression of the β-globin gene (β^+-type) or result in the complete absence of β-globin (β^0-type). Many of the mutations have attained high frequencies through a positive selection mechanism due to malaria and Table 41.3 lists the common β-thalassaemia mutations found in selected countries from the Mediterranean area, Asian India, Southeast Asia and Africa. For each region there are a small number of mutations which account for more than 90% of those found and the mutations are regionally specific, with each country within a region having its own characteristic spectrum of mutations.

A small number of β^+ mutations result in a milder phenotype than the majority of the β^+ and β^0 type mutations. These mutations include the transcription mutations located in the promoter region upstream of the β-globin gene, such as the mutations at nucleotide −88, −87, −30, −29 and −28 listed in Table 41.3, the CAP+1 site mutation, mutations between codon 24 and 27 such as the codon 24 mutation in Africans and the codon 26 mutation which creates Hb E, and the mutation at IVSI-6 mutation found in Mediterranean countries. The latter mutation, together with CAP+1 found in Indians, results in a Hb A_2 level of 3.5–4.0%, that is only just raised above the normal range and carriers of these mutations may be mistaken for having α-thalassaemia trait. However, these mutations do result in reduced MCV and MCH values, in contrast to three mutations observed in Italians, the promoter mutations, −101 (C→T) and −92 (C→T), and mutations IVSII-844 (G→C). Heterozygotes for these mutations exhibit completely normal MCV and MCH values in addition to a normal/borderline Hb A_2 value and cannot be detected by haematological screening tests, thus having a truly silent type of β-thalassaemia.

The mild β^+ mutations are characterized by having been identified in thalassaemia intermedia patients in either the homozygous or compound heterozygous state. However, predicting the phenotype of thalassaemia intermedia on the basis of a known genotype remains a problem. Homozygosity for a mild mutation nearly always results in intermedia but the combination of a mild and severe mutation results in thalassaemia major in some cases. In addition, the inheritance of ameliorating genetic factors such as α-thalassaemia, a high Hb F determinant, or other factors for which the molecular basis remains unclear[17] can result in a patient with a thalassaemia major genotype developing thalassaemia intermedia. Other causes of thalassaemia intermedia include the compound heterozygosity for a β-thalassaemia mutation and a triple or quadruple α-gene locus, and the heterozygous state for one of the rare β-thalassaemia mutations in exon 3 which cause inclusion-body haemolytic anaemia[18], sometimes called dominantly inherited β-thalassaemia.

TABLE 41.3
The distribution of the common β-thalassaemia mutations expressed as percentage gene frequencies of the total number of thalassaemia chromosomes studied

	Mediterranean			Indian		Chinese		African
Mutation	Italy	Greece	Turkey	Pakistan	India	China	Thailand	(US black)
−88 (C→T)					0.8			21.4
−87 (C→G)	0.4	1.8	1.2					
−30(T→A)			2.5					
−29(A→G)						1.9		60.3
−28 (A→G)						11.6	4.9	
CAP+1(A→C)					1.7			
CD5(−CT)		1.2	0.8					
CD6(−A)	0.4	2.9	0.6					0.8
CD8 (−AA)		0.6	7.4					
CD8/9(+G)				28.9	12.0			
CD15(G→A)				3.5	0.8			
CD16(−C)				1.3	1.7			
CD17(A→T)						10.5	24.7	
CD24(T→A)								7.9
CD39 (C→T)	40.1	17.4	3.5					
CD41/42(−TCTT)				7.9	13.7	38.6	46.4	
CD71/72(+A)						12.4	2.3	
IVSI-1 (G→A)	4.3	13.6	2.5					
IVSI-1 (G→T)				8.2	6.6			
IVSI-5 (G→C)				26.4	48.5	2.5	4.9	
IVSI-6(T→C)	16.3	7.4	17.5					
IVSI-110(G→A)	29.8	43.7	41.9					
IVSII-1(G→A)	1.1	2.1	9.7					
IVSII-654(C→T)						15.7	8.9	
IVSII-745(C→G)	3.5	7.1	2.7					
619 bp deletion				23.3	13.3			
Others	4.1	2.2	9.7	0.5	0.9	6.8	7.9	10.6

CD = codon; IVS = intervening sequence; bp = base pairs

MOLECULAR DIAGNOSIS

DNA sequences from the β-globin gene cluster are easily amplified under standard conditions and in theory all known mutations can be diagnosed by PCR techniques. Although a wide variety of techniques have been developed and new ones are still being published, most diagnostic laboratories use one or more of the techniques described below, following a strategy which depends upon knowing the most prevalent mutations likely to be encountered in the ethnic group of the individual being screened.

ALLELE SPECIFIC OLIGONUCLEOTIDES

The hybridization of allele specific oligonucleotide probes (ASOs) to amplified DNA bound to nylon membrane in the form of dots was the first method to be developed and is still widely used[19]. The method is based on the use of two oligonucleotide probes for each mutation, one complementary to the mutant DNA sequence and the other complementary to the normal β-gene sequence at that position. The probes can be labelled with either ^{32}P, biotin or horseradish peroxidase but the method is limited by the need for separate hybridizations to test for more than one mutation.

To overcome this problem the method of reverse dot blotting has been developed in which the roles of the oligonucleotide probe and target amplified DNA are reversed[20]. Probe pairs, complementary to mutant and normal DNA sequences, are bound to nylon membrane in the form of dots or slots and then the amplified DNA, labelled by either using end-labelled primers or the internal incorporation of biotinylated dUTP, is hybridized to the filter. This procedure allows multiple mutations to be tested for in one hybridization reaction. It has been applied recently to the detection of β-thalassaemia mutations in Mediterraneans[21], African-Americans[22] and Thais[23], using a two-step procedure with one strip for the common mutations and the other for the less common ones.

PRIMER SPECIFIC AMPLIFICATION

A number of different methods have been developed based on the principle of primer specific amplification, which is that a perfectly matched PCR primer is much more efficient in annealing and directing primer extension than one containing one or two mismatched bases. With the method known as the amplification refractory mutation system (ARMS)[24], the target DNA is amplified using a common primer and either of two allele specific primers, one complementary to the mutation to be detected (β-thalassaemia primer) and the other complementary to normal DNA at the same position (normal primer). A second pair of primers complementary to a different part of the β-globin gene are included in the PCR to amplify a fragment simultaneously in order to control the amplification step of the procedure. ARMS primers have been made to detect all the common β-thalassaemia mutations in the four major ethnic groups, namely the Mediterraneans, the Asian Indians, the Chinese and Africans[25] and are listed in Tables 41.4 and 41.5. The method provides a quick screening method which does not require any form of labelling as the amplified products are visualized simply by agarose gel electrophoresis and ethidium bromide staining (Figs 41.3 and 41.4). More than one mutation may be screened for at the same time in a single PCR reaction (multiplexing) provided the ARMS primers are coupled with the same common primer[26]. Fluorescent labelling of the common primer allows the sizing of the amplification products on an automated DNA fragment analyser[27].

If the normal and mutant ARMS primers for a specific mutation are coamplified in the same reaction they compete with each other to amplify the target sequence. This technique is called competitive oligonucleotide priming (COP) and requires the two ARMS primers to be labelled differently. Fluorescent labels permit a diagnosis to be made by means of a colour complementation assay[28]. A variation of this method is to simply use ARMS primers that differ in length and thus a diagnosis can be made by analysis of the different product sizes. This technique, called mutagenetically separated polymerase chain reaction (MS-PCR), has been applied to the prenatal diagnosis of β-thalassaemia in Taiwan[29].

TABLE 41.4
Primer sequences used for the detection of the common β-thalassaemia mutations by the allele-specific priming technique

Mutation	Oligonucleotide sequence	Second primer	Product size (bp)	Altered restriction site
–88(C→T)	TCACTTAGACCTCACCCTGTGGAGCCTCAT	A	684	+*Fok* I
–87(C→G)	CACTTAGACCTCACCCTGTGGAGCCACCCG	A	683	–*Avr* II
–30(T→A)	GCAGGGAGGGCAGGAGCCAGGGCTGGGGAA	A	626	
–29(A→G)	CAGGGAGGGCAGGAGCCAGGGCTGGGTATG	A	625	+*Nla* III
–28(A→G)	AGGGAGGGCAGGAGCCAGGGCTGGGCTTAG	A	624	
CAP+1(A→G)	ATAAGTCAGGGCAGAGCCATCTATTGGTTC	A	597	
CD5(–CT)	TCAAACAGACACCATGGTGCACCTGAGTCG	A	528	–*Dde* I
CD6(–A)	CCCACAGGGCAGTAACGGCAGACTTCTGCC	B	207	–*Dde* I
CD8(–AA)	ACACCATGGTGCACCTGACTCCTGAGCAGG	A	520	
CD8/9(+G)	CCTTGCCCCACAGGGCAGTAACGGCACACC	B	225	
CD15(G→A)	TGAGGAGAAGTCTGCCGTTACTGCCCAGTA	A	500	
CD16(–C)	TCACCACCAACTTCATCCACGTTCACGTTC	B	238	
CD17(A→T)	CTCACCACCAACTTCATCCACGTTCAGCTA	B	239	
CD24(T→A)	CTTGATACCAACCTGCCCAGGGCCTCTCCT	B	262	
CD39(C→T)	CAGATCCCCAAAGGACTCAAAGAACCTGTA	B	436	+*Mae* I
CD41/42(–TCTT)	GAGTGGACAGATCCCCAAAGGACTCAACCT	B	439	
CD71/72(+A)	CATGGCAAGAAAGTGCTCGGTGCCTTTAAG	C	241	
IVSI-1(G→A)	TTAAACCTGTCTTGTAACCTTGATACCGAT	B	281	–*BspM* I
IVSI-1(G→T)	TTAAACCTGTCTTGTAACCTTGATACCGAAA	B	281	–*BspM* I
IVSI-5(G→C)	CTCCTTAAACCTGTCTTGTAACCTTGTTAG	B	285	
IVSI-6(T→C)	TCTCCTTAAACCTGTCTTGTAACCTTCATG	B	286	+*SfaN* I
IVSI-110(G→A)	ACCAGCAGCCTAAGGGTGGGAAAATAGAGT	B	419	
IVSII-1(G→A)	AAGAAAACATCAAGGGTCCCATAGACTGAT	B	634	–*Hph* I
IVSII-654(C→T)	GAATAACAGTGATAATTTCTGGGTTAACGT*	D	829	
IVSII-745(C→G)	TCATATTGCTAATAGCAGCTACAATCGAGG*	D	738	+*Rsa* I
β^{S}CD6(A→T)	CCCACAGGGCAGTAACGGCAGACTTCTGCA	B	207	–*Dde* I
β^{C}CD6(G→A)	CCACAGGGCAGTAACGGCAGACTTCTCGTT	B	206	
β^{E}CD26(G→A)	TAACCTTGATACCAACCTGCCCAGGGCGTT	B	236	–*Mnl* I

The above primers are coupled as indicated with either primer A: CCCCTTCCTATGACATGAACTTAA; B: ACCTCACCCTGTGGAGCCAC; C: TTCGTCTGTTTCCCATTCTAAACT; or D: GAGTCAAGGCTGAGAGATGCAGGA. The control primers used were primers D plus E: CAATGTATCATGCCTCTTTGCACC (which yield an 861 bp product as shown in Fig. 41.1) for all the above mutation specific ARMS primers except the two marked '*'. Control primers used with these two are the $^{G}\gamma$-*Hind* III RFLP primers[25]

TABLE 41.5
Primer sequences used for the detection of the normal DNA sequence by the allele specific priming technique

Mutation	Oligonucleotide sequence	Second primer	Product size (kb)
–87 (C→G)	CACTTAGACCTCACCCTGTGGAGCCACCCC	A	683
CD5 (–CT)	CAAACAGACACCATGGTGCACCTGACTCCT	A	528
CD8 (–AA)	ACACCATGGTGCACCTGACTCCTGAGCAGA	A	520
CD8/9 (+G)	CCTTGCCCCACAGGGCAGTAACGGCACACT	B	225
CD15 (G→A)	TGAGGAGAAGTCTGCCGTTACTGCCCAGTA	A	500
CD39 (C→T)	TTAGGCTGCTGGTGGTCTACCCTTGGTCCC	A	299
CD41/42 (–TCTT)	GAGTGGACAGATCCCCAAAGGACTCAAAGA	B	439
IVSI-1 (G→A)	TTAAACCTGTCTTGTAACCTTGATACCCAC	B	281
IVSI-1 (G→T)	GATGAAGTTGGTGGTGAGGCCCTGGGTAGG	A	455
IVSI-5 (G→C)	CTCCTTAAACCTGTCTTGTAACCTTGTTAC	B	285
IVSI-6 (T→C)	AGTTGGTGGTGAGGCCCTGGGCAGGTTGGT	A	449
IVSI-110 (G→A)	ACCAGCAGCCTAAGGGTGGGAAAATACACC	B	419
IVSII-1 (G→A)	AAGAAAACATCAAGGGTCCCATAGACTGAC	B	634
IVSII-654 (C→T)	GAATAACAGTGATAATTTCTGGGTAACGC	D	829
IVSII-745 (C→G)	TCATATTGCTAATAGCAGCTACAATCGAGC	D	738
β^S CD6 (A→T)	AACAGACACCATGGTGCACCTGACTCGTGA	A	527
β^E CD26 (G→A)	TAACCTTGATACCAACCTGCCCAGGGCGTC	B	236

See Table 41.4 footnote for details of primers A–D and control primers

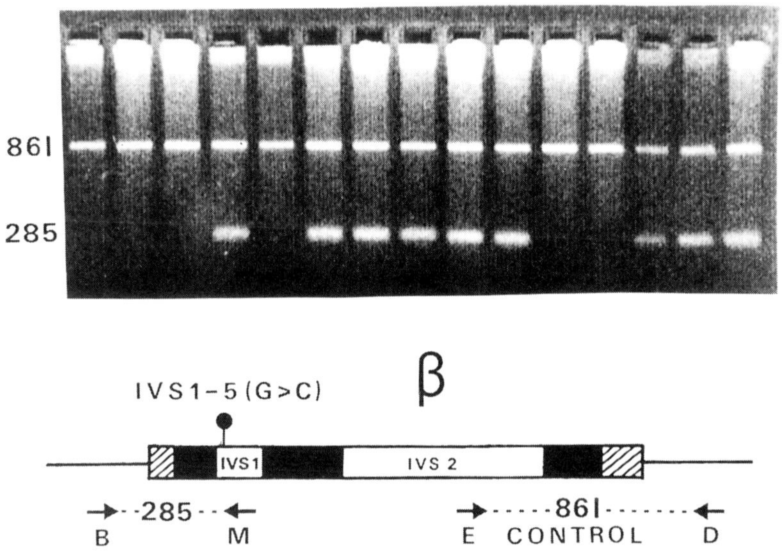

Fig. 41.3 Screening for the mutation IVS1-5 (G→C) by primer specific amplification. A diagram of the β globin gene shows the location of the mutation and its specific ARMS primer (M) plus the positions of the common primer (B) and two control primers (E and D) which generate an 861 bp product. Above, an ethidium bromide stained gel shows the results of screening a number of heterozygous β-thalassaemia individuals for IVS1-5 (G→C). The generation of the specific 285 bp product indicates an individual heterozygous for the mutation.

RESTRICTION ENZYME ANALYSIS

Approximately 40 β-thalassaemia mutations are known to create or abolish a restriction endonuclease site (Table 41.6). The majority of these can be detected simply and quickly by restriction endonuclease analysis of amplified DNA. The presence or absence of the enzyme site is determined from the pattern of digested fragments after agarose or polyacrylamide gel electrophoresis.

Mutations which do not naturally create or abolish restriction sites may be detected by the technique of amplification-created restriction sites (ACRS). This method uses primers that are designed to insert new bases adjacent to the mutation sequence and thus create a new restriction site allowing known mutants to be detected by restriction analysis of the PCR product[30].

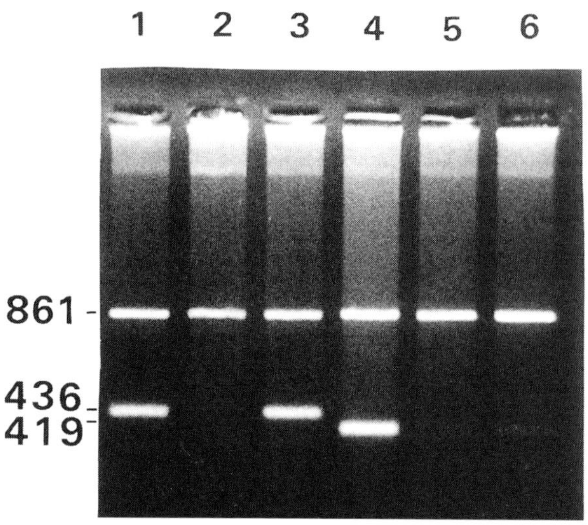

Fig. 41.4 Prenatal diagnosis for β-thalassaemia using ARMS primers to detect the mutations IVSI-110 (G→A) and codon 39 (C→T). Lanes 1 and 6 show fetal DNA, lanes 2 and 4 maternal DNA and lanes 3 and 5 paternal DNA. The first three lanes show the results with an ARMS primer for codon 39 and lanes 4–6 show the results with an ARMS primer for IVSI-110. The upper band is the 861 bp control product. The results show the fetus was heterozygous for codon 39.

GAP PCR

Deletion mutations in the β-globin gene sequence may be detected by PCR using two primers complementary to the sense and antisense strand in the DNA regions which flank the deletion. For large deletions, amplified product is obtained only from the deletion allele, as the distance between the two primers is too great to amplify normal DNA. In such cases the normal allele may be detected by amplifying a product spanning one of the breakpoints, using a primer complementary to the deleted sequence and one complementary to flanking DNA. As well as deletion β-thalassaemia, Hb Lepore and a number of δβ-thalassaemia and hereditary persistence of fetal haemoglobin (HPFH) deletion mutations can be diagnosed by this method[31].

UNKNOWN MUTATIONS

A number of techniques have been applied for the detection of β-thalassaemia mutations without prior knowledge of the molecular defect. The most widely used of these methods is denaturing gradient gel electrophoresis (DGGE), which allows the separation of DNA fragments differing by a single base change according to their melting properties[32]. Another approach is heteroduplex analysis by non-denaturing gel electrophoresis. Unique heteroduplex pattern can be generated for each mutation by annealing an amplified target DNA fragment with an amplified heteroduplex generator molecule, a synthetic oligonucleotide of about 130 bases in length containing deliberate sequence changes or identifiers at known mutations positions[33]. Other methods such as chemical mismatch cleavage (CMC), single-stranded conformational polymorphism analysis (SSCP), protein truncation test, are also good methods of detecting unknown mutations but they have not been applied to the haemoglobinopathies.

The above techniques simply pinpoint the presence of a mutation or DNA polymorphism in the amplified target sequence. Sequencing of the amplified product is then required to identify the localized mutation. This can now be done very efficiently using an automated DNA sequencing machine utilising fluorescence detection technology. The specialized equipment required for this technique is currently very expensive, but as the machines become more efficient the cost will come down and direct DNA sequencing will become the primary method of mutation detection.

δβ-Thalassaemia

CLINICAL STATES

δβ-Thalassaemia and the deletion types of hereditary persistence of fetal haemoglobin (HPFH) are characterized by the complete absence of Hb A and Hb A_2 in homozygotes and an elevated level of Hb F in heterozygotes. Both conditions are caused by large DNA deletions involving the β-globin gene cluster affecting the β and δ genes but leaving either one or both of the γ-globin genes intact. More than 50 different deletion mutations have been identified[34], and they can be classified into the $(\delta\beta)^0$- and $(^A\gamma\delta\beta)^0$-thalassaemias, HPFH conditions, fusion chain variants and $(\varepsilon\gamma\delta\beta)^0$-thalassaemia.

The $(\delta\beta)^0$-thalassaemias are characterized by the Hb F consisting of both $^G\gamma$- and $^A\gamma$-globin chains as both γ-globin genes remain intact in these conditions. Heterozygotes have normal levels of Hb A_2 and an Hb F level of 5–15% which, for the majority of mutations, is heterogeneously distributed in the red cells. There is a reduction of the non-α-globin chains compared to α-globin and the red cells are hypochromic and microcytic. Homozygotes for this condition have thalassaemia intermedia.

The $(^A\gamma\delta\beta)^0$-thalassaemias are characterized by the Hb F containing only $^G\gamma$-globin chains as the $^G\gamma$-globin gene has been deleted in these conditions. Apart from this distinction the phenotype of the heterozygous and homozygous states are identical to those for $(\delta\beta)^0$-thalassaemia.

The deletional HPFH conditions can be regarded as a type of δβ-thalassaemia in which the reduction in β-globin chain production is almost completely compensated for by the increased γ-globin chain production. Homozygous individuals have 100% F comprising both $^A\gamma$- and $^G\gamma$-globin chains but, in contrast to $(\delta\beta)^0$-thalassaemia homozygotes, are clinically normal. Heterozygotes have an elevated Hb F level of 17–35%, higher than that found in δβ-thalassaemia heterozygotes, and the Hb F is distributed uniformly (pancellular) in red cells with near normal MCH and MCV values.

TABLE 41.6
β-Thalassaemia mutations detectable by restriction enzyme digestion of amplified product

Position	Mutation	Ethnic group	Affected site
–88	C→T	African/Asian Indian	+*Fok* I
–87	C→G	Mediterranean	–*Avr* II
–87	C→T	Italian	–*Avr* II
–87	C→A	African/Yugoslavian	–*Avr* II
–86	C→G	Lebanese	–*Avr* II
–86	C→A	Italian	–*Avr* II
–29	A→G	African/Chinese	+*Nla* III
+43 to +40	(–AAAC)	Chinese	+*Dde* I
Initiation CD	T→C	Yugloslavian	–*Nco* I
Initiation CD	T→G	Chinese	–*Nco* I
Initiation CD	A→G	Japanese	–*Nco* I
CD5	(–CT)	Mediterranean	–*Dde* I
CD6	(–A)	Mediterranean	–*Dde* I
CD17	A→T	Chinese	+*Mae* I
CD26	G→T	Thai	–*Mnl* I
CD26	G→A	Southeast Asian (Hb E)	–*Mnl* I
CD27	G→T	Mediterranean (Hb Knossos)	–*Sau* 96I
CD29	C→T	Lebanese	–*BspM* I
CD30	G→C	Tunisian/African	–*BspM* I
CD30	G→A	Bulgarian	–*BspM* I
IVSI-I	G→A	Mediterranean	–*BspM* I
IVSI-I	G→T	Asian Indian/Chinese	–*BspM* I
IVSI-2	T→G	Tunisian	–*BspM* I
IVSI-2	T→C	African	–*BspM* I
IVSI-2	T→A	Algerian	–*BspM* I
IVSI-5	G→A	Mediterranean	+*EcoR* V
IVSI-6	T→C	Mediterranean	+*SfaN* I
IVSI-116	T→G	Mediterranean	+*Mae* I
IVSI-130	G→C	Turkish	–*Dde* I
IVSI-130	G→A	Egyptian	–*Dde* I
CD35	C→A	Thai	–*Acc* I
CD37	G→A	Saudi Arabian	–*Ava* II
CD38/39	(–C)	Czechoslovakian	–*Ava* II
CD37/8/9	(–GACCCAG)	Turkish	–*Ava* II
CD39	C→T	Mediterranean	+*Mae* I
CD43	G→T	Chinese	–*Hinf* I
CD47	(+A)	Surinamese	–*Xho* I
CD61	A→T	African	–*Hph* I
CD74/75	(–C)	Turkish	–*Hae* III
CD121	G→T	Polish, French, Japanese	–*EcoR* I
IVSII-I	G→A	Mediterranean	–*Hph* I
IVSII-4,5	(–AG)	Portuguese	–*Hph* I
IVSII-745	C→G	Mediterranean	+*Rsa* I

Two deletions in the β-globin gene cluster create an abnormal Hb chain as a result of unequal crossing over between globin genes. Hb Lepore is a hybrid globin chain comprising δ and β gene sequences and Hb Kenya comprises γ and β gene sequences. Hb Lepore homozygotes have a phenotype similar to thalassaemia major or severe thalassaemia intermedia. Hb Kenya has only been observed in the heterozygous state and is similar to heterozygous HPFH, with individuals having 5–10% HbF, normal red cell morphology and balanced globin chain synthesis.

The $(\varepsilon\gamma\delta\beta)^0$ thalassaemias are rare conditions that result from several different long deletions that start upstream of the ε-gene and remove all of the β-globin gene cluster, or in two cases the deletion ends between the δ- and β-genes, thus sparing the β-globin gene, but in both cases no β-globin synthesis occurs. This is because the deletions remove the β-globin gene cluster locus control region (LCR) located 50 kb upstream of the ε-gene. In adult life, heterozygotes for this condition have a similar haematological picture to β-thalassaemia trait with a normal Hb A_2 level. The homozygous condition is presumed to be incompatible with fetal survival.

Finally there is a group of conditions called non-deletion HPFH in which heterozygous individuals have normal red cells and no clinical abnormalities and an elevated Hb F level β-thalassaemia or sickle-cell disease can be identified prospectively by simple haematological tests and haemoglobin analysis, and informed of their risk of an affected child in each pregnancy and of the available options for prenatal diagnosis. Originally this was accomplished by sampling fetal blood at 18–20 weeks' gestation and measuring the relative amounts of globin chain synthesis, and although difficult the technique was established very successfully in more than 20 diagnostic laboratories worldwide. With the advent of DNA technology the fetal blood-sampling approach was replaced by the analysis of fetal DNA, first obtained from amniotic fluid and later by chorionic villus sampling. The original DNA methods were complex and expensive and prenatal diagnosis remained inaccessible for developing countries until the discovery of the polymerase chain reaction permitted the development of simple, rapid and less expensive non-radioactive methods of mutation detection.

CHORIONIC VILLUS DNA

Chorionic villus sampling is the method of choice for providing fetal DNA as it is carried out in the first trimester of pregnancy and provides a good yield of DNA. The average sample taken between 10 and 12 weeks' gestation by transcervical or transabdominal aspiration yields 35 μg of fetal DNA, sufficient for both PCR and Southern blot analysis of any known globin gene mutation. Villi collected by either method must be sorted to remove all traces of maternal tissue before DNA preparation. Sorted villi can then be transported to a DNA diagnosis laboratory in either tissue culture medium or, preferably, in a small volume of cell lysis buffer containing SDS and proteinase K, which lyses the villi in transit and provides a stable protective environment for the DNA for many days.

AMNIOTIC FLUID CELL DNA

Amniocentesis is often used for couples who present themselves too late for prenatal diagnosis by chorionic villus sampling. Less fetal DNA is obtained from an amniotic fluid sample than from chorionic villi; a 10 ml sample will yield between 1.5 and 5 μg of DNA. This is sufficient for most PCR-based diagnoses and usually just enough for one restriction enzyme digest in a Southern blot analysis. However, I have experienced the occasional failure to obtain DNA of good enough quality to amplify or produce bands on a Southern blot and thus a small portion of the amniotic fluid sample should always be set aside for culturing in case of failure. Cultured cells take 2 or 3 weeks to grow but will yield sufficient good quality DNA for all types of analysis.

DIAGNOSTIC STRATEGY

Since nearly all of the α- and β-thalassaemia mutations have been determined and most racial groups have only a few common mutations, it is now possible to offer prenatal diagnosis for couples at risk for thalassaemia who have not been previously studied by DNA analysis techniques. The strategy is to determine the mutations in the parents using a PCR based method such as ASO probe hybridization or ARMS primers and then to analyse the fetal DNA for their presence. Provided the ethnic origin of each partner is known, it is possible to identify the parental mutations and perform a fetal diagnosis in 3–4 days in more than 95% of couples at risk for β-thalassaemia. Obviously if the parental mutations are screened for before pregnancy the time taken to achieve a prenatal diagnosis result is even shorter and more importantly, one has the opportunity to identify a rare or new mutation in an individual by other DNA analysis methods.

DIAGNOSTIC PITFALLS

A problem with all PCR-based techniques used for fetal DNA diagnosis is the coamplification of maternal sequences. With chorionic villus samples this event can be avoided by the careful dissection of maternal decidua from the fetal trophoblast and by reducing the number of amplification cycles to 25, as shown by the experience of the Italian groups who have reported no misdiagnoses in 457 first-trimester fetal DNA analyses for β-thalassaemia[38]. Uncultured amniotic fluid samples are more of a problem, with a recent study finding the presence of maternal cell contamination in 21% of samples compared with 0.2% in cultured fluid[39], and all such cases in which the fetal diagnosis is identical to the maternal genotype should be retested using a back-up culture[40] or checked by DNA polymorphism analysis to avoid the possibility of misdiagnosis. The presence of coamplified maternal DNA sequences may be revealed by the amplification of informative polymorphic sequences such as the apolipoprotein B gene variable number tandem repeat sequence [41].

Another potential source of error is the failure to amplify one of the target DNA allele's. In my own experience this occurred once in a prenatal diagnosis of α^0-thalassaemia, for which the PCR-based result was different to that obtained by Southern blot analysis because of a failure of amplification of the fetal normal α-globin gene allele. Amplification failure may also result when the hybridization of a primer or probe is compromised by an unexpected change in the target DNA sequence[42].

Finally, because direct detection methods only detect the particular mutation screened for, a diagnostic error may occur if the fetus inherits an unsuspected mutation as a result of non-paternity, or as happened in two prenatal diagnoses for sickle-cell disease in my laboratory, when incorrect information was supplied about parental phenotypes and the partner in question was not available for testing at the time of the diagnosis. However, such instances are very uncommon and the overall diagnostic error rate in my laboratory for 1300 PCR-based fetal DNA diagnoses is 0.3%.

Summary

The visualization of amplified products by gel electrophoresis after ARMS analysis, gap PCR and restriction enzyme analysis provides a simple, quick and cheap approach to the direct detection of mutations, enabling developing countries such as India, Pakistan, Turkey and Iran to introduce prenatal diagnosis services for the haemoglobin disorders[43]. Dot blot analysis is popular for detecting small numbers of mutations, whereas reverse dot blotting offers the potential to screen large numbers of mutations simultaneously through the use of commercially developed kits of reagents. Fluorescence-based automatic DNA sequencing will become the method of choice for characterization of unknown mutations and possibly even for prenatal diagnosis as cheaper, second-generation machines are developed using capillary electrophoresis to separate amplified DNA fragments.

REFERENCES

1. Weatherall DJ & Clegg JB. *The Thalassemia Syndromes*, 3rd ed, p. 248. Oxford: Blackwell Scientific Publications, 1994.
2. Flint J, Harding RM, Boyce AJ & Clegg JB. The population genetics of the haemoglobinopathies. In *The Haemoglobinopathies* (eds D.R. Higgs & D.J., Weatherall), Baillière's Clinical Haematology, pp. 215–262. London: Baillière Tindall and W.B. Saunders, 1993.
3. Rodgers GP & Rachmilewitz EA. Novel treatment options in the severe β-globin disorders. *Br. J. Haematol.* **91**, 263–268, 1995.
4. Charache S, Terrin ML, Moore RD *et al.* Effect of hydroxyurea on the frequency of painful crises in sickle cell anemia. *N. Engl. J. Med.* **332**, 1317–1322, 1995.
5. Sher GD, Ginder GD, Little J *et al.* Extended therapy with intravenous arginine butyrate in partients with beta-hemoglobinopathies. *N. Engl. J. Med.* **332**, 1606–1610, 1995.
6. Ko TM, Tseng LH, Hsieh FJ & Lee TY. Prenatal diagnosis of HbH disease due to compound heterozygosity for south-east Asian deletion and Hb Constant Spring by polymerase chain reaction. *Prenat. Diagn.* **13**, 143, 1993.
7. Higgs DR, Vickers MA, Wilkie AOM *et al.* A review of the molecular genetics of the human α-globin gene cluster. *Blood* **73**, 1081–1104, 1989.
8. Higgs DR. α-thalassaemia. In *The Haemoglobinopathies*. (eds D.R., Higgs & D.J., Weatherall), Baillière's Clinical Haematology, pp. 117–150. London: Baillière Tindall, 1993.
9. Ko T, Hsieh FJ, Hsu PM & Lee TY. Molecular characterisation of severe α-thalassaemias causing hydrops fetalis in Taiwan. *Am. J. Med. Genet.* **39**, 317–320, 1991.
10. Dode C, Krishnamoorthy R, Lamb J & Rochette J. Rapid analysis of -$\alpha^{3.7}$ thalassaemia and $\alpha\alpha\alpha^{anti\ 3.7}$ triplication by enzymatic amplification analysis. *Br. J. Haematol.* **82**, 105, 1992.
11. Baysal E & Huisman THJ. Detection of common deletional α-thalassaemia-2 determinants by PCR. *Am. J. Hematol.* **46**, 208, 1994.
12. Bowden DK, Vickers MA & Higgs DR. A PCR-based strategy to detect the common severe determinants of α-thalassaemia. *Br. J. Haematol* **81**, 104–108, 1992.
13. Molchanova TP, Pobedimskaya DD & Postnikov YV. A simplified procedure for sequencing amplified DNA containing the α-2 or α-1 globin gene. *Hemoglobin* **18**, 251, 1994.
14. Fischel-Ghodsian N, Vickers MA, Seip M, Winichagoon P & Higgs DR. Characterization of two deletions that remove the entire human ξ-α globin gene complex ($—^{Thai}$ and $—^{Fil}$). *Br. J. Haematol.* **70**, 233–238, 1988.
15. Baysal E. The β-and δ-thalassemia repository. *Hemoglobin* **19**, 213–236, 1995.
16. Rosatelli MC, Faa V, Meloni A *et al.* A promoter mutation, C→T at position −92, leading to silent β thalassaemia. *Br. J. Haematol.* **90**, 483–485, 1995.
17. Camaschella C, Mazza U, Roetto A *et al.* Genetic interactions in thalassemia intermedia: analysis of beta-mutations, alpha-genotype, gamma-promoters, and beta-LCR hypersensitive sites 2 and 4 in Italian patients. *Am. J. Hematol.* **48**, 82–87, 1995.
18. Kazazian HH Jr, Dowling CE, Hurwitz RL *et al.* Dominant thalassemia-like phenotypes associated with mutations in exon 3 of the β-globin gene. *Blood* **79**, 3014–3018, 1992.
19. Ristaldi MS, Pirastu M, Rosatelli C & Cao A. Prenatal diagnosis of β-thalassaemia in Mediterranean populations by dot blot analysis with DNA amplification and allele specific oligonucleotide probes. *Prenat. Diagn.* **9**, 629–638, 1989.
20. Saiki RK, Walsh PS, Levenson CH & Erlich HA. Genetic analysis of amplified DNA with immobilized sequence-specific oligonucleotide probes. *Proc. Nat. Acad. Sci. USA* **86**, 6230–6234, 1989.
21. Maggio A, Giambona A, Cai SP, Wall J, Kan YW & Chehabb FF. Rapid and simultaneous typing of hemoglobin S, hemoglobin C and seven Mediterranean β-thalassaemia mutations by covalent reverse dot-blot analysis: application to prenatal diagnosis in Sicily. *Blood* **81**, 239–242, 1993.
22. Sutcharitchan P, Saiki R, Huisman THJ, Kutlar A, McKie V & Embury SH. Reverse dot-blot detection of the African-American β-thalassaemia mutations. *Blood* **86**, 1580, 1995.
23. Sutcharitchan P, Saiki R, Fucharoen S, Winichagoon P, Erlich H & Embury SH. Reverse dot-blot detection of Thai β-thalassaemia mutations. *Br. J. Haematol.* **90**, 809, 1995.
24. Newton CR, Graham A & Heptinstall LE. Analysis of any point mutation in DNA. The amplification refractory mutation system (ARMS). *Nucleic Acids Res.* **17**, 2503–2516, 1989.
25. Old JM. Haemoglobinopathies. Community clues to mutation detection. In *Methods in Molecular Medicine, Molecular Diagnosis of Genetic Diseases* (ed. R. Elles), pp. 169–184. Totowa, NJ: Humana Press, 1996.
26. Tan JAMA, Tay JSH, Lin LI *et al.* The amplification refractory mutation system (ARMS): a rapid and direct prenatal diagnostic techniques for β-thalassaemia in Singapore. *Prenat. Diagn.* **14**, 1077, 1994.
27. Zschocke J & Graham CA. A fluorescent multiplex ARMS method for rapid mutation analysis. *Mol. Cellular Probes* **9**, 447, 1995.
28. Chehab FF & Kan YW. Detection of specific DNA sequence by fluorescence amplification: a colour complementation assay. *Proc. Nat. Acad. Sci. USA* **86**, 9178, 1989.
29. Chang JG, Lu JM, Huang JM, Chen JT, Liu HJ & Chang CP. Rapid diagnosis of β-thalassaemia by mutagenically separated polymerase chain reaction (MS-PCR) and its application to prenatal diagnosis. *Br. J. Haematol.* **91**, 602, 1995.
30. Linderman R, Hu SP, Volpato F & Trent RJ. Polymerase chain reaction (PCR) mutagenesis enabling rapid non-radioactive detection of common β-thalassaemia mutations in Mediterraneans. *Br. J. Haematol.* **78**, 100, 1991.
31. Craig JE, Barnetson RA, Prior J, Raven JL & Thein SL. Rapid detection of deletions causing δβ thalassemia and hereditary persistence of fetal hemoglobin by enzymatic amplification. *Blood* **83**, 1673–1682, 1994.
32. Losekoot M, Fodde R, Harteveld CL, Van Heeren H, Giordano PC & Bernini LF. Denaturing gradient gel electrophoresis and direct sequencing of PCR amplified genomic DNA: a rapid and reliable diagnostic approach to beta thalassaemia. *Br. J. Haematol.* **76**, 269–274, 1991.
33. Savage DA, Wood NAP, Bidwell JL, Fitches A, Old JM & Hui KM. Detection of β-thalassaemia mutations using DNA heteroduplex generator molecules. *Br. J. Haematol.* **90**, 564, 1995.
34. Weatherall DJ, Clegg JB, Higgs DR & Wood WG. In *The Haemoglobinopathies in the Metabolic Basis of Inherited Disease* (eds C.R.

Scriver, A.L. Beaudet, W.S. Sly & D. Valle), pp. 2281–2339. New York: McGraw-Hill, 1989.

35. Kulozik AE, Wainscoat JS, Serjeant GR *et al.* Geographical survey of β^s-globin gene haplotypes: Evidence for an independent Asian origin of the sickle-cell mutation. *Am. J. Hum. Genet.* **39**, 239–244, 1986.
36. Powars DR. β^s-gene cluster haplotypes in sickle cell anemia. *Hematol./Oncol. Clin. N. Am.* **5**, 475–493, 1991.
37. Higgs DR, Aldridge BE, Lamb J *et al.* The interaction of alpha-thalassemia and homozygous sickle-cell disease. *N. Engl. J. Med.* **306**, 1441–1446, 1982.
38. Rosatelli MC, Tuveri T, Scalas MT *et al.* Molecular screening and fetal diagnosis of β-thalassaemia in the Italian population. *Hum. Genet.* **89**, 585, 1992.
39. Winsor EJT, Silver MP, Theve R, Wright M & Ward BE. Maternal cell contamination in uncultured amniotic fluid. *Prenat. Diagn.* **16**, 49, 1996.
40. Wang X, Seaman C, Paik M, Chen T, Bank A & Piomelli S. Experience with 500 prenatal diagnoses of sickle cell diseases: the effect of gestational age on affected pregnancy outcome. *Prenat. Diagn.* **14**, 851, 1994.
41. Decorte R, Cuppens H, Marynen P & Cassiman J-J. Rapid detection of hypervariable regions by the polymerase chain reaction technique. *DNA Cellular Biol.* **9**, 461–469, 1990.
42. Chan V, Chan TPT, Lau K, Todd D & Chan TK. False non-paternity in a family for prenatal diagnosis of β-thalassaemia. *Prenat. Diagn.* **13**, 977–982, 1993.
43. Petrou M & Modell B. Prenatal screening for haemoglobin disorders. *Prenat. Diagn.* **15**, 1275, 1995.

Prenatal diagnosis of haemophilia and allied haemostatic disorders

42

D.M. Layton and M.R.A. Lalloz

Introduction

The introduction in 1979 of fetoscopic[1,2] and subsequently ultrasound-guided[3] cordocentesis for prenatal diagnosis of haemophilia and allied haemostatic defects marked a turning point, providing families at risk with the possibility of specific fetal diagnosis in utero for the first time[4,5]. Prior to this the only option open to families with haemophilia seeking to avoid the birth of an affected child was to abort a fetus shown to be male by karyotypic analysis of amniocytes, an invidious choice given the equal likelihood of a normal or haemophilic fetus. Elucidation of the normal clotting factor profile during fetal life[6], coupled with the development of reliable fetal microassays for plasma clotting factors, permitted successful midgestation diagnosis of deficiencies of factor VIII (haemophilia A)[4,5,7,8], factor IX (haemophilia B)[5,9] and von Willebrand's disease[10,11], as well as several rarer inherited co-agulopathies (Table 42.1). While this approach yields a result within a few hours of cordocentesis, it suffers the detraction that fetal blood cannot be safely obtained before 20 weeks of pregnancy and carries the prospect of late termination of pregnancy, with its attendant psychological trauma[13]. This limitation has been circumvented to a large extent by progress in fetal medicine and molecular genetics. Many inherited defects of haemostasis are now amenable to first trimester prenatal diagnosis by chorionic villus DNA analysis. These advances have overtaken fetal blood bioassay for haemostatic disorders, which is reserved for cases in which genotypic analysis is precluded by late referral or lack of informativity and for confirmation of fetal normality predicted on the basis of an extragenic DNA polymorphism (see below). Fetal DNA diagnosis relies on the ability to track a genetic defect by association with polymorphism within (intragenic) or tightly-linked (extragenic) to the relevant gene or detection of the causative gene mutation. The facility with which each of these approaches can be applied differs among haemostatic disorders. The requirement for preliminary sometimes lengthy molecular analysis necessitates that genetic risk and the feasibility of prenatal diagnosis should, wherever possible, be assessed in affected families prior to invasive testing, preferably preconceptionally or in early pregnancy.

TABLE 42.1
Normal values for fetal blood coagulation factors at 18–22 weeks' gestation[a]

	Units	Range	Mean	*n*
Fibrinogen (factor I)	mg/dl	43–70	60	12
I:Ag	mg/dl	45–78	63	12
VC	%	45–76	56	50
VIIIC	u/dl	25–57	39	50
VWF:Ag	u/dl	51–79	58	12
Prothrombin (factor II)	%	15–20	17	12
II:Ag	%	15–20	17	12
VIIC	%	14–24	20	12
IXC	u/dl	5.9–11.8	9.1	50
IX:Ag	u/dl	1.7–8.2	4.3	12
XC	%	14–26	20	12
XIC	%	10–18	13	12
XIIC	%	13–25	21	12

Modified from Mibashan, Peake and Nicolaides[12] with permission

[a]Based on these values at King's College Hospital, London between 1979 and 1997, phenotypic diagnosis in vitro of haemophilia A and B, von Willebrand disease (type III), deficiencies of factors V, VII and X and afibrinogenaemia has been undertaken without error in over 400 consecutive pregnancies

Haemophilia

INHERITANCE

The X-linked recessive mode of inheritance of classical haemophilia has been recognized since antiquity[14]. It was not until 1947 that different forms of the disease were distinguished, when it was shown that the prolonged coagulation time of one patient could be corrected with plasma from another. The two types of haemophilia designated A and B are due to deficiency of factor VIII or factor IX (Christmas factor) respectively. Haemophilia A is the most important inherited bleeding disorder, affecting an estimated 1/5000 live male births. The incidence of haemophilia B is approximately five-fold less. In keeping with J.B.S. Haldane's prediction in 1935 that the gene frequency of an X-linked disorder associated with loss of reproductive fitness in affected males requires a high rate of spontaneous mutation[15], 30–40% of cases of haemophilia arise sporadically in the absence of any antecedent family history. By corollary, carriership cannot be assumed in the mother of a solitary affected male. This poses specific challenges for genetic counselling and prenatal diagnosis.

It is axiomatic that the phenotype of haemophilia breeds 'true' in individual families. Clinical severity correlates tightly with the level of residual plasma factor VIII or IX coagulant activity in hemizygous males. Based on United Kingdom national data, about 50% of cases are clinically severe (factor VIII:C or IX:C < 2 u/dl). Such cases, in the absence of factor replacement therapy, suffer frequent spontaneous haemorrhages. Factor levels are correspondingly higher in moderately severe (2–5 u/dl) or mild (5–30 u/dl) haemophilia. The less severe clinical course associated with these forms of haemophilia is reflected in the attitude to prenatal diagnosis among affected families, in whom uptake is low. Extremely rarely the development of inhibitory antibodies to factor VIII in a patient with mild or moderate haemophilia A results in conversion to a more severe clinical phenotype[16]. A variant of haemophilia B of particular interest has been identified in which the production of factor IX is enhanced significantly after puberty with concomitant clinical improvement[17]. This unusual phenotype has been shown to be due to mutation within the F9 gene promoter that disrupts transcription factor binding but spares steroid hormone response elements allowing recovery of factor IX level postpuberty[18]. These examples underscore the importance of careful clinical assessment as a prelude to genetic counselling in families at risk for haemophilia.

CARRIER ASSESSMENT

The possibility that a fetus might inherit haemophilia depends on whether the mother's carrier status is known with certainty or not. This may be evident from the family pedigree. Carriership is obligatory if she is the daughter of a haemophiliac or has more than one son (monozygotic twins excluded) or a son and relative(s) in the maternal line affected by haemophilia. With each conception the odds the defective gene will be transmitted by an obligate (or other proven) carrier are 1 in 2, the only exception being rare cases of somatic or gonadal mosaicism, in which the risk of haemophilia depends on the proportion of ova that carry the abnormal gene[19]. A woman may be excluded as a carrier if haemophilia segregates in the paternal line and her father is unaffected. In all other situations carrier probability must be estimated initially from analysis of the family pedigree, combined with discriminant analysis based on coagulation factor assays, age and blood group[20,21]. As a consequence of biological variation and Lyonization there is considerable (up to 15%) overlap in factor VIII or factor IX activity between carriers and non-carriers, which limits the predictive value of phenotypic methods. This inherent flaw may be overcome by genotypic analysis, which minimizes uncertainty in the majority of families.

MOLECULAR GENETICS OF HAEMOPHILIA A

Haemophilia A results from mutations in the gene coding for factor VIII (F8C) that lead to deficient or defective protein. Factor VIII is required for activation of factor X by factor IXa in the intrinsic coagulation pathway (Fig. 42.1). The F8C gene, one of the larger human genes, spans 186 kb of genomic DNA located at chromosome Xq28 close to the genes for red-green pigment defective in colour blindness and glucose-6-phosphate dehydrogenase[22,23]. The splice junctions between coding sequences contained in 26 exons ranging in size from 69 bp (exon 5) to 3106 bp (exon 14) conform to the GT/AG rule. The intron sequences range from 200 bp (intron 17) to greater than 32 kb (intron 22). The gene is transcribed into a 9 kb mRNA which in turn is translated into a single polypeptide chain with a 19-amino-acid hydrophobic leader sequence followed by 2332 amino acids. The precursor protein comprises three types of domain, A, B and C, and two short acidic regions, a_1 and a_2, in the order A1-a_1-A2-B-a_2-A3-C1-C2. Both A and C domains share homology with factor V and the triplicated A domains are homologous to those in the copper-binding protein ceruloplasmin. The function of the large B domain encoded by exon 14 is unknown.

Intracellular processing, which involves cleavage at sites within the B domain, generates two chains which associate in the presence of von Willebrand's factor (vWF) to produce the circulating form of factor VIII. The heavy chain extends at least 740 residues from the N-terminal Ala1, encompassing the A1 and A2 domains. The light chain begins at Glu1649, extending to the C-terminal Tyr2332. Heterodimers are non-covalently linked by divalent cations, e.g. Ca^{2+}, and further stabilized by binding to vWF. This pro-cofactor is activated by proteolytic cleavage by thrombin (factor IIa) and factor Xa at the carboxy terminal side of residues 372 and 1689. Cleavage at residue 336 by activated protein C inactivates factor VIII.

A large number of mutations responsible for factor VIII deficiency distributed throughout the F8C gene have been described[24]. These include nucleotide substitutions (183 missense/nonsense) which comprise 68% of all mutations, splice site mutants (15), small deletions (40), small insertions (11), large deletions (11), large insertions and duplications (3) and complex rearrangements including inversions (4). A mechanism of mutation unique to the F8C gene accounts for 40–50% of cases of severe haemophilia A (20–25% of all cases)[25]. Located within intron 22 of the factor VIII gene are

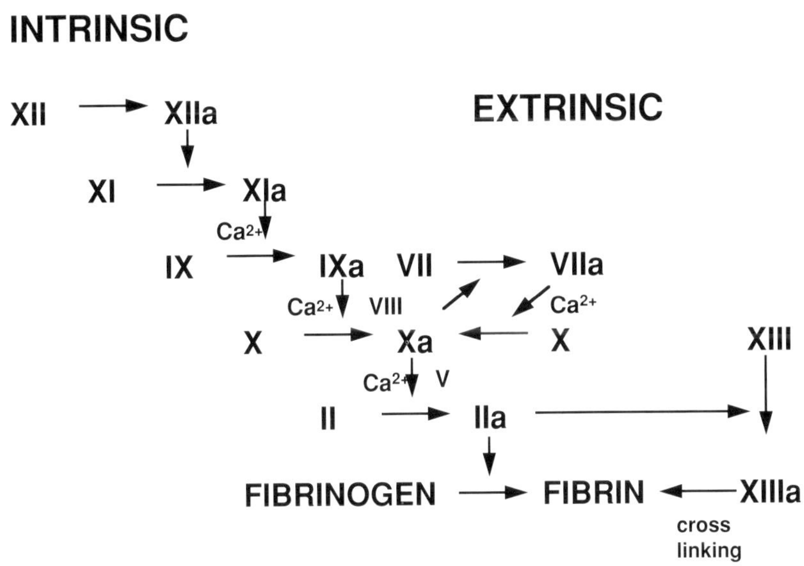

Fig. 42.1 The blood coagulation cascade

two open reading frames which encode protein products of unknown function. Two copies of one of these genes, F8A, lie 500 kb upstream of the F8C gene (telomeric). Homologous recombination between the intron 22 F8A gene and one of its two telomeric homologues divides the factor VIII gene placing exons 1–22 in opposite orientation to exons 23–26. The intron 22 inversion mutation originates predominantly during male gametogenesis[26] presumably because in females inter- rather than intrachromosomal recombination is favoured. This has important implications for genetic diagnosis of haemophilia A, since it follows that virtually all mothers of sporadic cases due to the intron 22 inversion will be carriers. This mutation may be readily detected by Southern blot analysis. Thus it is now possible by a single approach to offer carrier and prenatal diagnosis to nearly half of families with severe haemophilia.

For other families indirect analysis based on linkage to one of several DNA polymorphisms within or close to the F8C gene remains the mainstay of genetic diagnosis. The first genetic markers to be used for this purpose were restriction fragment length polymorphisms (RFLPs), single base variants which define the presence (denoted +) or absence (denoted –) of an endonuclease recognition site[27–33]. The frequency of heterozygosity in females for the most commonly used intragenic polymorphisms is shown in Table 42.2. In practice because of linkage disequilibrium, i.e. overlap in informativity only 70% of women are heterozygous for one or more intragenic RFLP. Differences in informativity for individual RFLPs exist among ethnic groups and should be taken into account in deciding the best diagnostic strategy[34]. The application of RFLP analysis to prenatal diagnosis of haemophilia A is illustrated in Fig. 42.2. Two additional extragenic polymorphisms reduce further to ≤3% the proportion of women who are homozygous, i.e. uninformative. Both are subject to risk of error due to recombination between the marker and gene during meiosis and this must be incorporated in prediction of carrier or fetal status based on their use. The chance of error is estimated from the recombination rate multiplied by the number of meioses distant from the proband. Since the maximum heterozygosity for any biallelic polymorphism is 50% it may be necessary to screen multiple RFLPs to establish informativity which can add unacceptable delay in the face of an established pregnancy. The use of simple sequence repeats (microsatellite polymorphisms) overcomes this problem. Two multiallelic dinucleotide repeats $(CA)_n$ have been identified within the F8C gene in introns 13 (10 alleles) and 22 (7 alleles)[35,36]. The combined informativity of these two polymorphisms which can be rapidly analysed singly or multiplexed by polymerase chain reaction (PCR) methods is over 80%.

Two outstanding obstacles which restrict the application of indirect genetic analysis are its dependence on the inclusion of key family members and limited utility in sporadic

TABLE 42.2
Factor VIII gene (F8C) polymorphisms

Polymorphism	Location	Allele frequency (%)
G/A	Intron 7	79/21
$13(CA)_n$	Intron 13	10 alleles
Bcl I	Intron 18	29/71
Hind III	Intron 19	70/30
Xba I	Intron 22	41/59
$22(CA)_n$	Intron 22	7 alleles
Bgl I	Intron 25	10/90
Msp I	3′ to exon 26	68/32
Bgl II (DX13)	3′ to exon 26	
Taq I (ST14)	5′ to exon 1	72/28

of cases seen during the past 10 years at our institution was carrier status known at the time of referral for consideration of prenatal diagnosis. Carrier testing in the face of an established pregnancy engenders additional psychological stress and introduces delay before a decision on prenatal diagnosis can be reached.

Whether undertaken preconceptionally or during pregnancy, carrier testing should be preceded by a balanced discussion of the nature and inheritance of haemophilia and its treatment. Account must be taken of phenotypic severity and the pregnant woman and family's individual, social, cultural and psychological perspective. For example, in families with adverse first-hand experience specific reassurance may be needed regarding the improved safety and outcome of modern replacement therapy. Conversely a woman who has a distantly affected male relative (and correspondingly low carrier risk) but little or no first-hand experience will be much less familiar with haemophilia and its consequences.

Advances in haemophilia care, notably the success of prophylactic factor replacement in prevention of chronic arthropathy and greater safety of modern factor concentrates that now include a recombinant form of factor VIII, have led to significant improvement in the outlook for haemophilia patients[52]. The life expectancy of patients with haemophilia is now close to that of the general population when deaths related to viral infection are excluded[53,54]. This is matched by improvement in quality of life. It should be borne in mind that the economic cost of progress in the treatment of haemophilia is prohibitive outside developed countries. In many parts of the world no infrastructure exists for treatment of haemophilia and the handicap it may cause[55]. It was estimated in 1990 that 80% of haemophiliacs worldwide (total 350 000) are without treatment. These factors influence the demand for prenatal diagnosis which is now greatest in developing countries.

PRENATAL DIAGNOSIS

The diagnosis of haemophilia A and B prenatally may involve early (chorionic villus sampling) or late (amniocentesis or cordocentesis) invasive or non-invasive (ultrasonographic assessment of fetal sex) approaches. As in other X-linked disorders determination of fetal sex which can be achieved reliably by ultrasonography from 16 weeks[7] gestation avoids the need for and risk incurred by invasive testing in 50% of pregnancies but suffers the disadvantage of delay in diagnosis of an affected pregnancy. This is compounded in the case of amniocentesis by the necessity to culture sufficient amniocytes for DNA analysis. This precludes the option of surgical abortion for some families.

Since 1979, over 500 prenatal diagnoses have been performed for haemophilia A or B in our institution. The proportions undertaken by different invasive procedures and gestational age at referral are shown in Fig. 42.4 and 42.5. These data suggest scope for improvement in the timeliness of referral of pregnant haemophilia carriers. This is supported by evidence that the primary indication for cordocentesis and phenotypic diagnosis of fetal haemophilia remains late referral rather than lack of informativity for genetic analysis. An idealized algorithm that addresses these issues and sets out the options open to families at risk for haemophilia is shown in Fig. 42.6.

Von Willebrand disease

CLASSIFICATION

Von Willebrand disease is the most common inherited disorder of haemostasis with a prevalence in population studies of up to 1%[56]. First described in 1926 by Erik von Willebrand in kindred in the Åland islands of Finland, it was distinguished

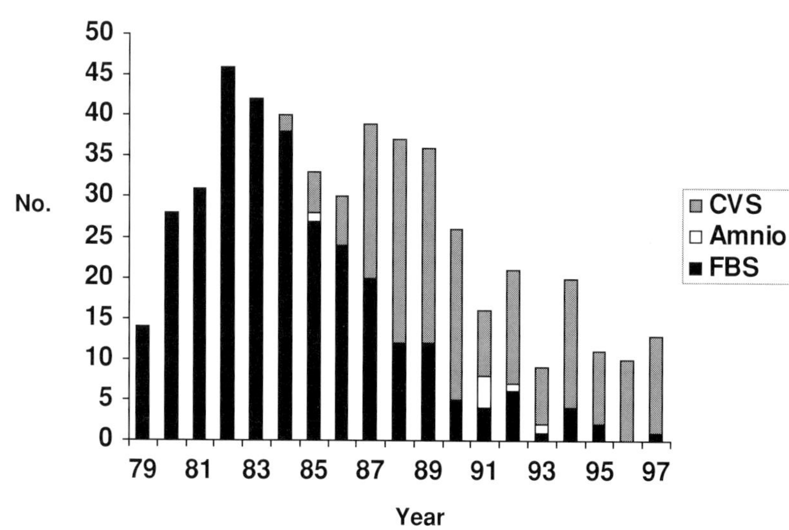

Fig. 42.4 Numbers of prenatal diagnoses of haemophilia undertaken at King's College Hospital, 1979–1997.

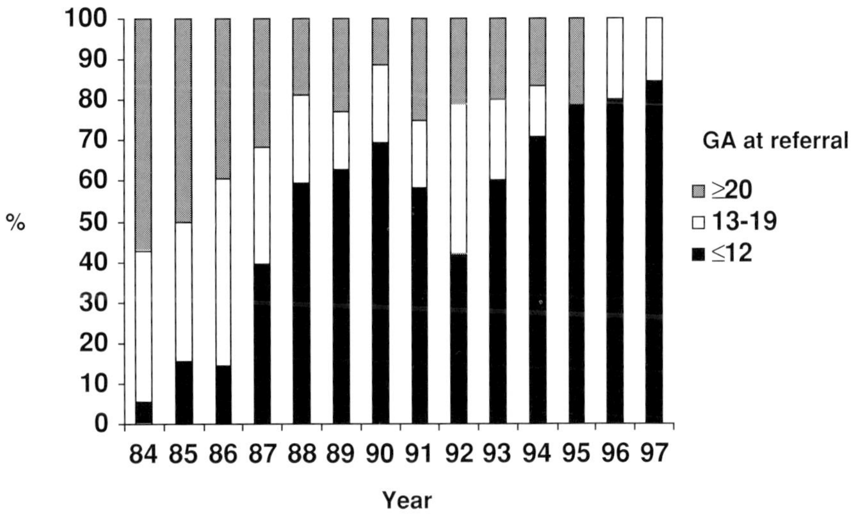

Fig. 42.5 Gestational age at referral showing that only 40% of families are seen in the first trimester.

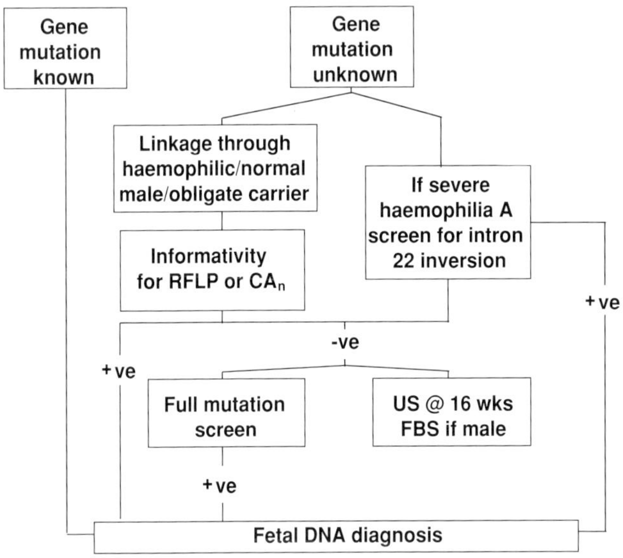

Fig. 42.6 Algorithm for carrier and prenatal diagnosis of haemophilia A.

from classical haemophilia by an autosomal dominant mode of inheritance predominance of mucocutaneous bleeding and prolonged bleeding time. These features may be reconciled with the function of vWF in plasma and platelets which serves both to promote platelet aggregation and formation of a platelet 'plug' at the site of vascular injury and as a carrier protein for circulating factor VIII. Deficiency of vWF thus affects both primary and secondary haemostasis.

Three major types of von Willebrand disease are recognized[57]. Types 1 and 2 reflect a partial quantitative deficiency or qualitative abnormality respectively. Both are usually inherited in an autosomal dominant manner, though penetrance is variable. Recent molecular studies in some forms of von Willebrand disease thought to be dominant, have revealed a recessive pattern of inheritance[58]. Type 3 von Willebrand disease results from recessive inheritance and is associated with severe quantitative deficiency with vWF antigen and activity levels typically below 5% of normal. The distinction of these types requires detailed assessment including blood cytometry, coagulation screening tests, assays for factor VIII coagulation activity (factor VIIIC), vWF antigen and vWF activity (ristocetin cofactor activity) and determination of the bleeding time. Thrombocytopenia is often present in type 2B von Willebrand disease due to increased binding of vWF to platelets and may worsen in pregnancy[57]. The different types of von Willebrand disease may also be differentiated on the basis of vWF multimer composition (see below) in plasma and platelets.

Prenatal diagnosis is seldom requested or warranted for a family history of type 1 or 2 von Willebrand disease. By contrast type 3 von Willebrand disease, a much rarer disorder with a prevalence of 0.5–5 per million, in which there are undetectable or trace amounts of vWF in the circulation, results in a bleeding disorder akin to haemophilia in severity. Patients with type 3 von Willebrand disease suffer from severe mucosal and cutaneous bleeding, persistent haemorrhage after minor trauma, menorrhagia and, in some cases, spontaneous haemarthrosis and tissue bleeds. Most prenatal diagnoses have been performed for type 3 von Willebrand disease.

MOLECULAR GENETICS

The vWF gene is located at chromosome 12p13[3]. It spans approximately 178 kb of genomic DNA and contains 52 exons ranging from 40 bp to 1379 bp and 51 introns from 97 bp to ~19.9 kb[59–63]. The signal peptide and propeptide are encoded by the first 17 exons and the mature subunit of von

Willebrand factor and the 3′-untranslated region by the remaining 35 exons of the gene. A partial unprocessed pseudogene which corresponds to exons 23 to 34 of the vWF gene is located on chromosome 22q11–q13. The presence of splice site and nonsense mutations indicates the pseudogene cannot yield a functional transcript.

The vWF gene is expressed in endothelial cells and megakaryocytes as a 9 kb mRNA. This is translated to a 2813-amino-acid polypeptide pre-pro-vWF which undergoes processing in the endoplasmic reticulum with removal of the signal peptide to generate pro-vWF. Pro-vWF dimerises by formation of a disulphide bond between the C-terminal ends of the subunits and is transported to the Golgi apparatus where further post-translational modification with cleavage of the propeptide occurs prior to assembly of mature vWF multimers. The mature protein is secreted into plasma or stored in endothelial cell Weibel–Palade bodies and platelet α-granules. In vitro, the synthesis of vWF in endothelial cells is stimulated by oestrogen. This may explain the characteristic rise in vWF (and factor VIII) level with gestation and why many pregnant women with types 1 and 2 von Willebrand disease suffer few bleeding problems during pregnancy.

Although mutations have now been defined in all types of von Willebrand disease[24] the size and complexity of the vWF gene and need to take account of possible homology with the partial unprocessed vWF pseudogene has hindered the wide application of mutation analysis in genetic diagnosis of von Willebrand disease. An exception in this respect is type 2 von Willebrand disease, in some forms of which clustering of mutations has been observed. Of particular interest are mutations identified in the vWF gene of patients with type 2N ('Normandy' variant) von Willebrand disease characterized by factor VIII deficiency due to defective factor VIII binding but otherwise normal vWF function (see above)[51]. Inherited in an autosomal recessive manner the 'Normandy' phenotype was originally ascribed to a missense mutation, ACG;Thr → ATG; Met, causing substitution of residue 28 of the mature WF subunit. Ten additional missense mutations at different codons within the WF gene have since been found in patients with type 2N von Willebrand disease. The resulting amino acid substitutions lie at the N-terminal region of the mature vWF subunit, within or near the major factor VIII binding domain.

A growing number of mutations of vWF gene have been identified in type 3 von Willebrand disease[24]. These include nonsense (6), missense (5) and insertion (2) mutations as well as several large deletions. A single cytosine deletion in exon 18 which causes premature translation termination is the predominant defect in Swedish type 3 patients. Type 3 von Willebrand disease arises either through homozygous (or compound heterozygous) inheritance of type 1 disease or true recessive inheritance of a variant that is phenotypically silent in the carrier state.

Approximately 20 RFLPs have been identified within or close to the vWF gene. The most informative polymorphism, however, is a tetranucleotide $(TCTA)_n$ repeat polymorphism in intron 40 of the vWF gene[65–69]. This multiallelic polymorphism is highly informative with a heterozygosity rate of up to 98%[70–72]. A dinucleotide repeat $(CA)_n$ within the vWF promoter with an observed heterozygosity of 77% has also been described[73].

PRENATAL DIAGNOSIS

Prenatal diagnosis was first performed for type 3 von Willebrand disease by fetal blood sampling[2,11]. Assay of plasma factor VIIIC in conjunction with vWF antigen and functional activity (ristocetin co-factor) has proved a reliable approach for the fetal diagnosis of severe forms of von Willebrand disease. Theoretically, due to defective primary haemostasis, there is a greater risk of haemorrhage or tamponade after cordocentesis in a fetus with type 3 von Willebrand disease.

Phenotypic diagnosis of von Willebrand disease in utero has been largely superseded by molecular diagnosis which allows diagnosis in the first trimester by chorionic villus sampling. Gene tracking using the highly polymorphic intron 40 variable number tandem repeat (VNTR) has been applied to the prenatal diagnosis of severe von Willebrand disease[67,74].

Prior to an invasive procedure consideration should be given to the need for replacement therapy with vWF or factor VIII concentrate in a pregnant woman with a family history of von Willebrand disease, particularly if she is symptomatically affected. Factor VIII and vWF levels should be carefully assessed. Elective abortion following the diagnosis of a severely affected fetus may also pose a risk of bleeding. Prolonged or excessive uterine bleeding after termination of pregnancy is most likely to be encountered in the early stages of pregnancy before the physiological rise in factor VIII and vWF levels has taken place. Treatment with DDAVP (1-diamino-8-D-arginine), a synthetic analogue of the antidiuretic hormone vasopressin which stimulates release of endogenous vWF and augments both vWF and factor VIII levels approximately threefold, or factor concentrates may be required. Not all patients with von Willebrand disease are equally responsive to DDAVP (desmopressin) and if its efficacy has not been established by a test dose prior to pregnancy replacement with factor concentrate is preferable. In ongoing pregnancies the presence of maternal von Willebrand disease is an important consideration in the context of obstetric care because of the risk of postpartum haemorrhage. This is greatest when vWF and factor VIII levels have fallen at around 4 to 5 days in the puerperum.

Hereditary deficiency of other coagulation factors

While haemophilia and von Willebrand disease account for the majority of inherited bleeding disorders, several haemostatic defects caused by deficiency of other coagulation factors exist. For the most part these show an autosomal recessive mode of inheritance and, with the exception of factor XI deficiency, which has a prevalence of 5% among Ashkenazi Jews, are rare. As in other recessive genetic disorders there may be a background of parental consanguinity. The nature and severity of the bleeding tendency varies widely among affected kindreds. Over the past 20 years families have been referred to our institution for prenatal diagnosis of afibrinogenaemia and congenital deficiencies of factors V, VII, X and XIII. In many cases this has been accomplished or is feasible by gene tracking or mutation analysis. There follows a brief review of some rarer haemostatic disorders for which prenatal diagnosis has been successfully performed.

DEFICIENCY OF VITAMIN K-DEPENDENT COAGULATION FACTORS

Congenital deficiencies of the serine proteases prothrombin (factor II), factor VII and factor X which, with factor IX, share dependence on vitamin K for biosynthesis in the liver are inherited in an autosomal recessive manner. These disorders are characterized clinically by a variable bleeding tendency which may, particularly in the case of factor VII or X deficiency, be of sufficient severity to justify prenatal diagnosis.

Prothrombin undergoes proteolytic activation on the surface of platelets to yield thrombin which cleaves the α and β chains of fibrinogen leading to the formation of a fibrin clot. Thrombin is also responsible for proteolytic activation of the procoagulant proteins factor V, factor VIII and factor XIII and the anticoagulant factor protein C. Prothrombin deficiency takes two forms, type I (hypoprothrombinaemia) and type II (dysprothrombinaemia) due respectively to reduced plasma levels and biological activity. Mutations of the prothrombin (F2) gene located at 11p11–q12 have been described in patients with prothrombin deficiency[24]. Several single nucleotide polymorphisms have been identified within the F2 gene[75–79]. These include a G→A nucleotide transition at position 20210 in the 3′ untranslated region which has been implicated as a risk factor for venous thrombosis[79]. To date prenatal diagnosis of prothrombin deficiency has not been reported.

Factor VII acts in the extrinsic coagulation pathway to convert factors IX and X to their active forms. Its function requires a cofactor, tissue factor, present in the vascular wall. Factor VII defiency may be associated with severe bleeding manifestations including intracranial haemorrhage, which occurs in up to 15% of homozygotes[80]. The risk appears greatest in the neonatal period and early infancy. There is poor correlation between the residual plasma factor VII level and bleeding symptoms. Although factor concentrates are available the short plasma halflife of factor VII (2–5 h) renders long-term replacement impractical.

A full-length human factor VII cDNA clone isolated from an expression library of poly(A)$^+$ mRNA allowed the amino acid sequence of the protein to be deduced[81]. Cytogenetic studies in a case of combined deficiency of factors VII and X localized both genes to the chromosome 13q34–qter segment[82]. The factor VII gene (F7) comprises nine exons (size range 25–1622 bp) and spans ~12.8 kb of genomic DNA situated only 2.8 kb 5′ to the factor X gene. F7 mRNA has multiple polyadenylated sites and can undergo alternative splicing[81].

Mutations responsible for factor VII deficiency that have been identified within the F7 gene include missense (26), nonsense (1), splice site (2), regulatory (1) and small deletions (4)[24]. Several polymorphisms have been identified in the F7 gene. These include a hypervariable region polymorphism which is the result of a variable number of tandem repeats in intron 7[83,84], a promoter decanucleotide (CCTATATCCT) insert at position –323 in the 5′-flanking region of the factor VII gene[85], and a G→A substitution (nucleotide 10976) at codon 353 in exon 8[86]. Arg353Gln affects factor VII levels by interfering with intracellular processing of the molecule and subjects homozygous for the A genotype (Glu 353) have levels of factor VII 20–30% lower than heterozygotes or homozygotes for the G genotype. An *Nla* III polymorphism silent at the amino acid level is located within exon 5 of the F7 gene[87]. These polymorphisms may be useful for genetic diagnosis of factor X deficiency as well as factor VII deficiency, since the factor X gene is closely linked to the factor VII locus.

Factor X acts at a key site at the point of conversion of the intrinsic and extrinsic coagulation pathways. After activation via the intrinsic pathway by factor IXa/factor VIIIa or the extrinsic pathway by factor VIIa/tissue factor complexes, factor Xa mediates the activation of prothrombin (see above). Factor X deficiency is a rare haemorrhagic disorder[88]. The bleeding tendency varies according to the severity of deficiency. At its most severe, factor X defiency may resemble severe haemophilia. Heterozygotes sometimes exhibit a lesser bleeding tendency. Factor X activity increases during pregnancy but this should be monitored prior to any invasive procedure to ensure a safe haemostatic level (≥40%) has been attained. If indicated replacement therapy may be given in the form of fresh frozen plasma or heat-treated intermediate purity factor IX concentrate (prothrombin complex concentrate) which contain significant amounts of factor X. Prothrombin complex concentrates carry a risk of thromboembolism and should be used with caution.

The factor X gene (F10) comprises eight exons which span >27 kb of genomic DNA located at chromosome 13q34 (see factor VII)[82]. The full-length cDNA sequence[89] comprises 5′ and 3′ untranslated sequences of 256 and 10 bp respectively, 120 bp coding for the 40-amino-acid pre-pro-leader sequence and 1344 bp that encodes the 448-amino-acid protein. Multiple missense mutations (18) and three deletions responsible for factor X deficiency have been identified within the F10 gene[24]. There are several reported RFLPs within or close to the F10 gene, of which *Taq* I, *Eco*R I, *Pst* I, *Hind* III and *Pvu* II can be analysed by Southern blotting[90–92] and a sixth (*Nla* IV) by the PCR method. Prenatal diagnosis of factor X deficiency has been performed by phenotypic analysis of cord blood.

Combined deficiency of vitamin-K-dependent coagulation factors associated with a bleeding disorder of variable severity may be due to an inborn error of vitamin K metabolism resulting in defective γ-carboxylation[94]. Skeletal abnormalities resembling warfarin embryopathy have been observed in some cases[95]. The molecular basis has not been elucidated but prenatal diagnosis could theoretically be undertaken by assay of multiple vitamin-K-dependent coagulation factors in fetal blood.

FACTOR V DEFICIENCY (PARAHAEMOPHILIA)

Factor V deficiency (parahaemophilia) is a rare autosomal recessive bleeding disorder with an estimated prevalence of one in one million[79]. Plasma factor V levels show little correlation with the bleeding tendency, which is dependent primarily on the amount of platelet surface-associated factor V. Heterozygotes are asymptomatic. Human factor V cDNA clones were isolated from a fetal cDNA library[96] and the gene (F5) mapped to chromosome 1 by Southern hybridization to somatic cell hybrid DNAs[97,98]. Detailed genetic mapping studies located the F5 gene to 1q23 and reveal tight linkage to the gene AT3 encoding antithrombin III[99]. The F5 gene comprises 25 exons (size range; 72–2820 bp) spanning 80 kb of DNA. The gene encodes a 28-amino-acid hydrophobic leader peptide and a protein of 2196 amino acids grouped on the basis of homologies both internal and with factor VIII (A and C domains; see factor VIII) and caeruloplasmin (A domains). Factor V is activated to factor Va by thrombin cleavage of the B domain (836 amino acids) generating a heavy chain (709 amino acids) and a light chain (651 amino acids) which are held together by calcium ions. Factor Va acts at the platelet surface as the receptor for the serine protease factor Xa, which in turn catalyses the conversion of prothrombin to the active clotting enzyme thrombin (see above).

Deficiency of a cofactor for activated protein C (APC), termed APC resistance, was identified in families with a tendency to thrombosis[100]. Further studies indicated the APC cofactor deficient in this disorder was factor V[101]. A guanine-to-adenine substitution at nucleotide 1691 in the F5 gene was subsequently identified as the basis of deficiency of the cofactor of activated protein C in APC resistance[102]. The codon 506(CGA; Arg → CAA; Glu) missense mutation commonly referred to as factor V Leiden is also known as FV Q506, R506Q and G1691A. Several studies have confirmed the increased risk of thrombosis in subjects homozygous or heterozygous for factor V Leiden[102–105]. Carrier frequencies have been estimated at 2–4% in Holland, 7% in Sweden[106] and 3.5% in England[107]. The high frequency of factor V Leiden may reflect positive selection, one suggested mechanism being that a mild prothrombotic tendency might favour embryo implantation[106]. A multiethnic survey of Americans found that Hispanics had the highest frequency of factor V Leiden (1.65%), while African Americans had the lowest frequency (0.87%)[108]. No instances of the mutation were found in Asian or Native Americans tested, indicating that factor V Leiden segregates in populations of Caucasian descent and is rare in other ethnic groups.

The size and complex structure of the factor V gene precludes rapid mutation detection. Only two mutations, a missense and a mRNA splice site mutation, have been reported in FV deficiency[24]. Few intronic RFLPs have been identified. A *Pst* I polymorphism by Southern blot analysis detected the 10.8 kb and 8.5 kb alleles to occur at a frequency of 0.74 and 0.26 respectively, in Caucasians[109]. Thirteen coding sequence polymorphisms have been identified[110–114]; 11 are within exon 13 which is the longest exon in the FV gene. Not all these neutral polymorphisms alter a restriction site. Two exon 13 polymorphisms which affect cleavage sites for *Taq* I (2391G/A) and *Eco*R I (2379A/G) were informative in kindreds with factor V Leiden[102]. In addition to these two, three other exon 13 RFLPs (2298C/T *Hinf* I; 2325T/C *Eco*R II; 2411G/A *Hinf* I) have been successfully used for prenatal diagnosis of severe factor V deficiency[115].

Combined deficiency of factor V and VIII, an autosomal recessive bleeding disorder, has recently been shown to be due to a mutation of a gene located at chromosome 18q21 that encodes a protein whose putative function involves intracellular transport between the endoplasmic reticulum and Golgi apparatus[116]. This rare disorder appears most prevalent in the Mediterranean basin.

HEREDITARY FIBRINOGEN DISORDERS

Fibrinogen plays a role in two essential processes in haemostasis, platelet aggregation (primary haemostasis) and clot formation (coagulation). The former activity is mediated through binding to surface glycoprotein IIb–IIIa on activated platelets and the latter by thrombin, which catalyses the conversion of fibrinogen to fibrin. Fibrinogen is a dimeric protein composed of six polypeptide chains ($\alpha_2\beta_2\gamma_2$). Mutations in the genes that encode these constituent chains lead to deficient (afibrinogenaemia or hypofibrinogenaemia; decreased production or assembly of fibrinogen) or defective (dysfibrinogenaemia; dysfunctional fibrinogen variants) protein.

Congenital deficiency of fibrinogen is rare. Afibrinogenaemia in which there is no detectable circulating fibrinogen results in a severe bleeding disorder whose characteristics include bleeding from the umbilical cord neonatally, mucosal haemorrhage, bruising, delayed wound healing and in affected females, recurrent abortion[117]. Death may occur from gastrointestinal or intracranial haemorrhage. Inheritance is autosomal recessive. Hypofibrinogenaemia is by contrast heterogeneous with respect both fibrinogen level and clinical severity. Some cases represent heterozygous forms of afibrinogenaemia. The clinical manifestations of dysfibrinogenaemia depend on the nature of the functional defect and include haemorrhage, recurrent abortion and thromboembolism. Most reported cases are heterozygous for mutation within one of the fibrinogen genes.

The α-fibrinogen gene (FGA) spans 8 kb of genomic DNA and consists of five exons. cDNA sequences comprise 5′ and 3′ non-coding regions of a minimum of 54 bp (due to ATG codons at −16 and −19) and either 217 or 234 bp respectively and 1875 bp that encodes the 625-amino-acid mature protein. Alternative processing of α-fibrinogen mRNA contains a sixth exon extending the length of the α-chain. The β-fibrinogen gene (FGB) spans 8 kb of DNA and consists of eight exons. The cDNA clone comprises 1383 bp encoding a 461-amino-acid protein and a 431 bp 3′-untranslated region. Since the ATG codon occurs at −16 and −27, the signal peptide is no more than 30 residues. Two mRNA species due to alternative transcription also exist for β-fibrinogen. The γ-fibrinogen gene (FGG) spans 10.5 kb of DNA and consists of 10 exons. The cDNA clone comprises 5′ and 3′ untranslated sequences of 71 and 207 bp and encodes a leader sequence of 26 amino acids and a 411-residue mature protein. The α- β- and γ-fibrinogen genes are located on the long arm of chromosome 4, forming a cluster at band q28. The genes lie within 55 kb of each other; α-fibrinogen is situated about 13 kb upstream of the β-gene and about 10 kb downstream of γ-fibrinogen (γ-α-β). The β-fibrinogen gene is transcribed in the opposite orientation to that of the α- and γ-fibrinogen genes, indicating the gene arose by duplication then transposition and inversion.

Mutations have been described in all three fibrinogen genes[24]. Polymorphisms of potential utility for genetic diagnosis have also been identified[118–125]. Prenatal diagnosis is possible by fetal blood bioassay.

REFERENCES

1. Hobbins JC, Mahoney MJ. In utero diagnosis of hemoglobinopathies: technique for obtaining fetal blood. *N. Engl. J. Med.* **290**:1065–1067, 1974.
2. Rodeck CH, Campbell S. Sampling pure fetal blood in the second trimester of pregnancy. *Br. Med. J.* **2**:728–730, 1978.
3. Daffos F, Capella-Pavlovsky M, Forestier F. A new procedure for fetal blood sampling in utero: preliminary results of fifty-three cases. *Am. J. Obstet. Gynecol.* **146**:985–987, 1983.
4. Firshein SI, Hoyer LW, Lazarchick J et al. Prenatal diagnosis of classic haemophilia. *N. Engl. J. Med.* **300**:937–941, 1979.
5. Mibashan RS, Rodeck CH, Thumpston JK et al. Plasma assay of fetal factors VIIIC and IXC for prenatal diagnosis of haemophilia. *Lancet* **i**:1309–1311, 1979.
6. Millar DS, Mibashan RS, Rodeck CH, Nocolaides KH. Coagulation in the normal human mid-trimester fetus. *Prenat. Diagn.* **5**:367–373.
7. Mibashan RS, Peak IR, Rodeck CH et al. Dual diagnosis of prenatal haemophilia A by measurement of fetal factor VIIIC and VIIIC antigen (VIIICAg). *Lancet* **ii**:994–997, 1980.
8. Hoyer LW, Carta CA, Golbus MS, Hobbins JC, Mahoney MJ. Prenatal diagnosis of classic hemophilia (hemophilia A) by immunoradiometric assays. *Blood* **65**:1312–1317, 1985.
9. Holmberg L, Gustavii B, Cordesius E et al. Prenatal diagnosis of hemophilia B by an immuno-radiometric assay of factor IX. *Blood* **56**:397–401, 1980.
10. Rodeck CH, Mibashan RS, Peak IR, Bloom AL. Prenatal diagnosis of severe von Willebrand's disease. *Lancet* **ii**:637–638, 1979.
11. Hoyer LW, Lindsten J, Blomback M et al. Prenatal evaluation of fetus at risk for severe von Willebrand's disease. *Lancet* **ii**:191–192, 1979.
12. Mibashan RS, Peake IR, Nicolaides KH. Prenatal diagnosis of hemostatic disorders. In *Methods in Haematology*, Vol 21. *Perinatal Hematology* (ed. BP Alter), pp. 64–107. Edinburgh: Churchill Livingstone, 1989.
13. Tedgård U, Ljung R, McNeil T, Tedgård E, Schwartz M. How do carriers of hemophilia experience prenatal diagnosis (PND)? Carrier's immediate and later reactions to amniocentesis and fetal blood sampling. *Acta Paediatr. Scand.* **78**:692–700, 1989.
14. Kazazian Jr. HH, Tuddenham EGD, Antonarakis SE. Hemophilia A and parahemophilia: deficiencies of coagulation factors VIII and V. In *The Metabolic and Molecular Bases of Inherited Disease*, Vol. 3 (eds C.H. Scriver, A.L. Beaudet, W.S. Sly, D. Valle), pp. 3241–3267. New York: McGraw Hill, 1995.
15. Haldane JBS. The rate of spontaneous mutation of a human gene. *J. Genet.* **31**:317–326, 1935.
16. Hay CRM, Ludlan CA, Colvin BT et al. Factor VIII inhibitors in mild and moderate severity haemophilia A. *Thromb. Haemost.* **79**:3, 1998.
17. Briet E, Bertina RM, Van Tilburg NH, Veltkamp JJ. Hemophilia B Leyden: A sex linked hereditary disorder that improves after puberty. *N. Engl. J. Med.* **306**:788–792, 1982.
18. Crossley M, Ludwig M, Stowell KM et al. Recovery from hemophilia B Leyden: An androgen responsive element in the factor IX promoter. *Science* **257**:377–379, 1992.
19. Sommer SS, Ketterling RP. The factor IX gene as a model for analysis of human germline mutations: an update. *Hum. Mol. Genet.* **5**:1505–1514, 1996.
20. Graham JB, Rizza CR, Chediak J et al. Carrier detection in haemophilia A: a cooperative international study. The carrier phenotype. *Blood* **67**:1554–1559, 1986.
21. Green PP, Mannucci PM, Briet E et al. Carrier detection in hemophilia A: a cooperative international study. II. The efficacy of a universal discriminant. *Blood* **67**:1560–1567, 1986.
22. Gitschier J, Wood WI, Goralka TM et al. Characterization of the human factor-VIII gene. *Nature* **312**:326–330, 1984.
23. Tantravahi U, Murty VVVS, Jhanwar SC et al. Physical mapping of the factor-VIII gene proximal to 2 polymorphic DNA probes in human-chromosome band Xq28 – implications for factor-VIII gene segregation analysis. *Cytogenet. Cell Genet.* **42**:75–79, 1986.
24. Cooper DN, Ball EV, Krawczak M. The human gene mutation database. *Nucleic. Acids. Res.* **26**:285–287, 1998.
25. Lakich D, Kazazian HH, Antonarakis SE, Gitschier JA. Inversions disrupting the factor VIII gene are a common cause of severe haemophilia A. *Nature Genet.* **5**:236–241, 1993.
26. Rossiter JP, Young M, Kimberland ML, et al. Factor VIII gene inversions causing severe hemophilia A originate almost exclusively in male germ cells. *Hum. Mol. Genet.* **3**:1035–1039, 1994.
27. Antonarakis SE, Waber PG, Kittur SD et al. Hemophilia-A- detection of molecular defects and of carriers by DNA analysis. *N. Engl. J. Med.* **313**:842–848, 1985.
28. Gitschier J, Drayna D, Tuddenham EGD et al. Genetic-mapping and diagnosis of hemophilia-A achieved through a BclI polymorphism in the factor-VIII gene. *Nature* **314**:738–740, 1985.
29. Wion KL, Tuddenham EGD, Lawn RM. A new polymorphism in the factor-VIII gene for prenatal-diagnosis of hemophilia-A. *Nucleic Acids Res.* **14**:4535–4542, 1986.
30. Ahrens, P, Kruse, TA, Schwartz, M et al. A new Hind-III restriction fragment length polymorphism in the hemophilia-A locus. *Hum. Genet.* **76**:127–128, 1987.
31. Youssoufian H, Phillips DG, Kazazian HH, Antonarkis SE. MspI polymorphism in the 3′ flanking region of the human factor-VIII gene. *Nucleic Acids Res.* **15**:6312, 1987.
32. Harper K, Pembrey ME, Davies KE, Winter RM, Hartley D, Tuddenham EGD. A clinically useful DNA probe closely linked to hemophilia-A. *Lancet* **ii**:6–8, 1984.
33. Oberle I, Camerino G, Heilig R et al. Genetic screening for hemophilia A (classic hemophilia) with a polymorphic DNA probe. *N. Engl. J. Med.* **312**:682–686, 1985.
34. Peake IR, Lillicrap DP, Boulyjenkov V et al. Haemophilia: strategies

for carrier detection and prenatal diagnosis. *Bull WHO* **71**:429–458, 1993.

35. Lalloz MRA, McVey JH, Pattinson JK, Tuddenham EGD. Haemophilia A diagnosis by analysis of a hypervariable dinucleotide repeat within the factor VIII gene. *Lancet* **338**:207–211, 1991.
36. Lalloz MRA, Schwaab R, McVey JH, Michaelides K, Tuddenham EGD. Haemophilia A diagnosis by simultaneous analysis of two variable dinucleotide tandem repeats within the factor VIII gene. *Br J Haematol* **86**:804–809, 1994.
37. Orita M, Iwahana H, Kanazawa H, Hayashi K, Sekiya T. Detection of polymorphisms of human DNA by gel electrophoresis as single-strand conformation polymorphisms. *Proc. Nat. Acad. Sci. USA* **86**:2766–2770, 1989.
38. Sheffield VC, Cox DR, Lerman LS, Myers RM. Attachment of a 40-base-pair G+C-rich sequence (GC-clamp) to genomic DNA fragments by the polymerase chain-reaction results in improved detection of single-base changes. *Proc. Nat. Acad. Sci.* USA **86**:232–236, 1989.
39. Cotton RGH, Rodrigues NR, Campbell RD. Reactivity of cytosine and thymine in single-base-pair mismatches with hydroxylamine and osmium-tetroxide and its application to the study of mutations. *Proc. Nat. Acad. Sci. USA* **85**:4397–4401, 1988.
40. Williams IJ, Abuzenadah A, Winship PR et al. Precise carrier diagnosis in families with haemophilia A: Use of conformation sensitive gel electrophoresis for mutation screening and polymorphism analysis. *Thromb. Haemost.* **79**:723–726, 1998.
41. Michaelides K, Schwaab R, Lalloz MRA, Schmidt W, Tuddenham EGD. Mutational analysis: new mutations. In *PCR II: A Practical Approach* (eds GR Taylor, MJ McPherson & BD Hames), pp. 255–288. Oxford: Oxford University Press, 1995.
42. Schwaab R, Oldenburg J, Lalloz MRA et al. Factor VIII gene mutations found by a comparative study of SSCP, DGGE and CMC and their analysis on a molecular model of factor VIII protein. *Hum. Genet.* **101**:323–332, 1997.
43. Naylor JA, Green PM, Montandon AJ, Rizza CR, Giannelli F. Detection of 3 novel mutations in 2 hemophilia-A patients by rapid screening of whole essential region of factor-VIII gene. *Lancet* **337**:635–639, 1991.
44. Yoshitake S, Schach BG, Foster DC, Davie EW, Kurachi K. Nucleotide-sequence of the gene for human factor-IX (antihemophilic factor-B). *Biochemistry* **24**:3736–3750, 1985.
45. Mattei MG, Baeteman MA, Heilig R et al. Localization by insitu hybridization of the coagulation factor-IX gene and of 2 polymorphic DNA probes with respect to the fragile-X site. *Hum. Genet.* **69**:327–331, 1985.
46. Thompson AR, Bajaj SP, Chen SH, MacGillivary RTA. 'Founder' effect in different families with haemophilia B mutation. *Lancet* **335**:418, 1990.
47. Saad S, Rowley G, Tagliavacca L et al. First report on UK database of haemophilia B mutations and pedigrees. *Thromb. Haemost.* **71**:563–569, 1995.
48. Winship PR, Anson DS, Rizza CR, Brownlee GG. Carrier detection in hemophilia-B using 2 further intragenic restriction fragment length polymorphisms. *Nucleic Acids Res.* **12**:8861–8872, 1984.
49. Hay CW, Robertson KA, Yong SL, Thompson AR, Growe GH, MacGillivray RTA. Use of a BamHI polymorphism in the factor-IX gene for the determination of hemophilia-B carrier status. *Blood* **67**:1508–1511, 1986.
50. Winship PR, Peake IR. A clinically useful RFLP in the 5′ flanking region of the factor IX gene. *Br. J. Haematol.* **80**:26a, 1992.
51. Mazurier C, Dieval J, Jorieux S, Delobel J, Goudemand M. A new vWF defect in a patient with FVIII deficiency but with normal level and multimeric patterns of both plasma and platelet vWF. Characterization of abnormal vWF/FVIII interaction. *Blood* **75**:20–26, 1990.
52. Lofqvist T, Nilsson IM, Berntorp E, Pettersson H. Haemophilia prophylaxis in young patients – a long-term follow up. *J Intern Med* **241**:395, 1997.
53. Triemstra M, Rosendall FR, Smit C et al. Mortality in patients with hemophilia – changes in a Dutch population from 1986 to 1992 and 1973 to 1986. *Ann. Inter. Med.* **123**:823–827, 1995.
54. Darby SC, Ewart DW, Giangrande PLF et al. Mortality before and after HIV infection in the complete UK population of haemophiliacs. *Nature* **377**:79–82, 1995.
55. Joint WHO/WFH meeting. Haemophilia care in the developing world. *Bull. WHO*, in press, 1997.
56. Sadler JE. Von Willebrand disease. In *The Metabolic and Molecular Bases of Inherited Disease*, Vol 3 (eds CH Scriver, AL Beaudet, WS Sly, D Valle). New York: McGraw Hill, 1995.
57. Sadler JE. A revised classification of von Willebrand disease. *Thromb. Haemost.* **71**:520–525, 1994.
58. Eikenboom JC, Reitsma PH, Peerlink KMJ, Briet E. Recessive inheritance of von Willebrand's disease type 1. *Lancet* **341**:982–986, 1993.
59. Sadler JE, Sheltoninloes BB, Sorace JM, Titani K. Cloning of CDNA and genomic DNA for human von Willebrand-factor. *Cold Spring Harbor Symp. Quant. Biol.* **51**:515–523, 1986.
60. Collins CJ, Underdahl JP, Levene RB et al. Molecular-cloning of the human-gene for von Willebrand-factor and identification of the transcription initiation site. *Proc. Nat. Acad. Sci. USA* **84**:4393–4397, 1987.
61. Bonthron D, Orkin SH. The human von Willebrand-factor gene – structure of the 5′ region. *Eur. J. Biochem.* **171**:51–57, 1988.
62. Assouline Z, Kerbiriounabias DM, Pietu G, Thomas N, Bahnak BR, Meyer D. The human-gene for von Willebrand-factor – identification of repetitive Alu sequences 5′ to the transcription initiation site. *Biochem. Biophys. Res. Commun.* **153**:1159–1166, 1988.
63. Mancuso DJ, Tuley EA, Westfield LA, et al. Structure of the gene for human von Willebrand-factor. *J. Biol. Chem.* **264**:19514–19527, 1989.
64. Zhang ZP, Blomback M, Egberg N et al. Characterization of the von-Willebrand factor gene (VWF) in Von-Willebrand disease type-III patients from 24 families of Swedish and Finnish origin. *Genomics* **21**:188–193, 1994.
65. Bignell P, Standen GR, Bowen DJ, Peake IR, Bloom AL. Rapid neonatal diagnosis of von Willebrands disease by use of the polymerase chain-reaction. *Lancet* **336**:638–639, 1990.
66. Standen GR, Bignell P, Bowen DJ, Peake IR, Bloom AL. Family studies in von Willebrands disease by analysis of restriction-fragment-length-polymorphisms and an intragenic variable number tandem repeat (VNTR) sequence. *Br. J. Haematol.* **76**:242–249, 1990.
67. Peake IR, Liddell MB, Moodie P et al. Severe type-III von Willebrands disease caused by deletion of exon 42 of the von Willebrand-factor gene – family studies that identify carriers of the condition and a compound heterozygous individual. *Blood* **75**:654–661, 1990.
68. Peake IR, Bowen D, Bignell P et al. Family studies and prenatal-diagnosis in severe von Willebrand disease by polymerase chain-reaction amplification of a variable number tandem repeat region of the von Willebrand-factor gene. *Blood* **76**:555–561, 1990.
69. Mannhalter C, Kyrle PA, Brenner B, Lechner K. Rapid neonatal diagnosis of type-IIb von Willebrand disease using the polymerase chain-reaction. *Blood* **77**:2539–2540, 1991.
70. Mercier B, Gaucher C, Mazurier C. Characterization of 98-alleles in 105 unrelated individuals in the F8vWF-gene. *Nucleic Acids Res.* **19**:4800, 1991.
71. Cumming AM, Armstrong JG, Pendry K, Burn MM, Wensley RT. Polymerase chain-reaction amplification of 2 polymorphic simple repeat sequences within the von Willebrand-factor gene – application to family studies in von Willebrand disease. *Hum. Genet.* **89**:194–198, 1992.
72. Haddad AP, Sparrow RL. Two novel alleles of the ATCT variable number tandem repeat locus VWF.VNTR I in intron 40 of the von Willebrand factor gene. *Br. J. Haematol.* **96**:298–300, 1997.
73. Zhang ZP, Deng LP, Blomback M, Anvret M. Dinucleotide repeat polymorphism in the promoter region of the human von Willebrand factor gene(vWF gene). *Hum. Mol. Genet.* **1**:780, 1992.
74. Mitchell M, Gaucher C, Jenkins E et al. Rapid genetic diagnosis of von Willebrand's disease. *Br. J. Haematol.* **84** (suppl 1):16, 1993.
75. Iwahana H, Yoshimoto K, Itakura M. Ncol RFLP in the human prothrombin (F2) gene. *Nucleic Acids Res.* **19**:4309, 1991.
76. Iwahana H, Mizusawa N, Yoshimoto K, Itakura M. Detection of a new polymorphism of the human prothrombin (F2) gene by combination of PASA and mutated primer-mediated PCR-RFLP. *Human Genet.* **90**:325–326, 1992.

77. Iwahana H, Yoshimoto K, Itakura M. Highly polymorphic region of the human prothrombin (F2) gene. *Human Genet.* **89**:123–124, 1992.
78. Poort SR, Rosendaal FR, Reitsma PH, Bertina RM. A common genetic-variation in the 3′-untranslated region of the prothrombin gene is associated with elevated plasma prothrombin levels and an increase in venous thrombosis. *Blood* **88**:3698–3703, 1996.
79. Kane WH, Davie EW. Blood-coagulation factor-V and factor-VIII – structural and functional similarities and their relationship to hemorrhagic and thrombotic disorders. *Blood* **71**:539–555, 1988.
80. Ragni MV, Lewis JH, Spero JA, Hasiba U. Factor VII deficiency. *Am. J. Haematol.* **10**:79–88, 1981.
81. Hagen FS, Gray CL, O'Hara P et al. Characterization of a cDNA coding for human factor VII. *Proc. Nat. Acad. Sci.* **83**:2412–2416, 1986.
82. Tariverdian G, Schroeder-Kurth T, Zimmermann R. Deficiency of coagulation factors VII and X in a girl with ring chromosome 13. In *Abstracts of the 1986 7th International Congress on Human Genetics*, Berlin, p. 76, 1986.
83. Ohara PJ, Grant FJ. The human factor-VII gene is polymorphic due to variation in repeat copy number in a minisatellite. *Gene.* **66**:147–158, 1988.
84. Marchetti G, Patracchini P, Gemmati D et al. Detection of two missense mutations and characterization of a repeat polymorphism in the factor VII gene (F7). *Hum. Genet.* **89**:497–502, 1992.
85. Marchetti G, Patracchini P, Papacchini M, Ferrati M, Ernardi F. A polymorphism in the 5′ region of coagulation-factor VII gene (F7) caused by an inserted decanucleotide. *Hum. Genet.* **90**:575–576, 1993.
86. Green F, Kelleher C, Wilkes H, Temple A, Meade T, Humphries S. A common genetic-polymorphism associated with lower coagulation factor-VII levels in healthy-individuals. *Arterioscler. Thromb.* **11**:540–546, 1991.
87. Chiang SH, Wallmark A, Berntorp E, High KA. A NlaIII polymorphism within the human factor-VII gene. *Hum. Genet.* **93**:722–723, 1994.
88. Perry DJ. Factor X and its deficiency states. *Haemophilia* **3**:159–172, 1997.
89. Leytus SP, Foster DC, Kurachi K, Davie EW. Gene for human factor X: a blood coagulation factor whose gene organization is essentially identical with that of factor IX and protein C. *Biochemistry* **25**:5098–5102, 1986.
90. Jaye M, Ricca G, Kaplan R et al. Polymorphism associated with the human coagulation factor-X (F10) gene. *Nucleic Acids Res.* **13**:8286, 1985.
91. Hay CW, Robertson KA, Fung MR, MacGillivray RTA. RFLPs for PstI and EcoRI in the human-blood clotting factor-X gene. *Nucleic Acids Res.* **14**:5118, 1986.
92. Hassan HJ, Guerriero R, Chelucci C. Multiple polymorphic sites in factor-X locus. *Blood* **71**:1353–1356, 1988.
93. Wallmark A, Ho C, Rose VL, Ljung R, High KA. A Nla IV polymorphism within the human FX gene. *Thromb. Haemost.* **65**:939, 1991.
94. McMillan CW, Roberts HR: Congenital combined deficiency of coagulation factors II, VII, IX and X. *N. Engl. J. Med.* **274**:1313–, 1966.
95. Pauli RM, Lian JB, Mosher DF, Suttie JW. Association of congenital deficiency of multiple vitamin K-dependent coagulation factors and the phenotype of the warfarin embriopathy: clues to the mechanism of teratogenicity of coumarin derivatives. *Am. J. Hum. Genet.* **41**:566–583, 1987.
96. Jenny RJ, Pittman DD, Toole JJ et al. Complete cDNA and derived amino acid sequence of human factor V. *Proc Nat Acad Sci* **84**:4846–4850, 1987.
97. Riddell DC, Wang H, Royle NJ et al. Regional assignment for the human genes encoding FII, FV, FXIII, ceruloplasmin and pseudoceruloplasmin. *Cytogenet. Cell Genet.* **46**:682, 1987.
98. Wang H, Riddell DC, Guinto ER, MacGillivray RTA, Hamerton JL. Localization of the gene encoding human factor V to chromosome 1q21–25. *Genomics* **2**:324–328, 1988.
99. McAlpine PJ, Coopland G, Guy C et al. Mapping the genes for erythrocytic alpha-spectrin 1 (SPTA1) and coagulation factor V (F5). *Cytogenet Cell Genet.* **51**:1042, 1989.
100. Dahlback B, Carlsson M, Svensson PJ. Familial thrombophilia due to a previously unrecognized mechanism characterized by poor anticoagulant response to activated protein C: prediction of a cofactor to activated protein C. *Proc Nat. Acad. Sci.* **90**:1004–1008, 1993.
101. Dahlback B, Hildebrand B. Inherited resistance to activated protein C is corrected by anticoagulant cofactor activity found to be a property of factor V. *Proc. Nat. Acad. Sci.* **91**:1396–1400, 1994.
102. Bertina RM, Koeleman BPC, Koster T, et al. Mutation in blood coagulation factor V associated with resistance to activated protein C. *Nature* **369**:64–67, 1994.
103. Greengard JS, Eichinger S, Griffin JH, Bauer KA. Variability of thrombosis among homozygous siblings with resistance to activated protein C due to an Arg-to-Gln mutation in the gene for factor V. *N. Engl. J. Med.* **331**:1559–1562, 1994.
104. Voorberg J, Roelse J, Koopman R et al. Association of idiopathic venous thromboembolism with single point-mutation at Arg506 of factor V. *Lancet* **343**:1535–1536, 1994.
105. Zoller B, Svensson PJ, He X, Dahlback B. Identification of the same factor V gene mutation in 47 out of 50 thrombosis-prone families with inherited resistance to activated protein C. *J. Clin. Invest.* **94**:2521–2524, 1994.
106. Majerus PW. Bad blood by mutation. *Nature* **369**:14–15, 1994.
107. Beauchamp NJ, Daly ME, Hampton KK, Cooper PC, Preston E & Peake IR. High prevalence of a mutation in the factor V gene within the U.K. population: relationship to activated protein C resistance and familial thrombosis. *Br. J. Haematol.* **88**:219–222, 1994.
108. Gregg JP, Yamane AJ, Grody WW. Prevalence of the factor V Leiden mutation in four distinct American ethnic populations. *Am. J. Med Genet* **73**:334–336, 1997.
109. McAlpine PJ, Dixon M, Guinto ER, Macgillivray RTA. A PstI polymorphism in the human coagulation factor-V (F5) gene. *Nucleic Acids Res.* **18**:7471, 1990.
110. Chang P, Alderman J, Caruso R, Aronson DL, Sanford S. Population parameters of factor-VIII, von-Willebrand-factor and factor-V in a heterogeneous population. *Blood* **82**(suppl 1):592, 1993.
111. Bayston TA, Ireland H, Olds RJ, Thein, SL, Lane DA. A polymorphism in the human coagulation-factor-V gene. *Hum. Molec. Genet.* **3**:2085, 1994.
112. Lunghi B, Iacoviello L, Gemmati D. Detection of new polymorphic markers in the factor-V gene-association with factor-V levels in plasma. *Thromb. Haemost.* **75**:45–48, 1996.
113. Ozawa T, Niiya K, Ejiri N, Sakuragawa N. A novel polymorphism in exon in of the factor V gene inducing an amino acid replacement of arginine to lysine at codon 485. *Thromb. Haemost.* **78**:1419–1420, 1997.
114. Lunghi B, Castoldi E, Mingozzi F, Bernardi F. A new factor V gene polymorphism (His 1254 Arg) present in subjects of African origin mimics the R2 polymorphism (His 1299 Arg). *Blood* **91**:364–365, 1998.
115. Lalloz MRA, Thompson LJ, Buggins AGS, Layton DM. Prenatal diagnosis of factor V deficiency by analysis of exon 13 restriction fragment length polymorphisms. *Br J Haematol* **89**:32, 1995.
116. Nichols WC, Seligsohn U, Zivelin A et al. Mutations in an endoplasmic reticulum-Golgi intermediate compartment protein cause combined deficiency of coagulation factors V and VIII. *Cell*, in press, 1998.
117. Chung DW, Ichinose A. Hereditary disorders of fibrinogen and factor XIII. In *The Metabolic and Molecular Bases of Inherited Disease*, Vol 3 (eds CH Scriver, AL Beaudet, WS Sly & D Valle), pp. 3223–3240. New York: McGraw Hill, 1995.
118. Humphries E, Imam AMA, Robbins TP et al. The identification of a DNA polymorphism of the α-fibrinogen gene, and the regional assignment of the human-fibrinogen genes to 4q26-qter. *Hum. Genet.* **68**:148–153, 1984.
119. Rixon MW, Chan WY, Davie EW, Chung DW. Characterization of a complementary deoxyribonucleic-acid coding for the alpha-chain of human-fibrinogen. *Biochemistry* **22**:3237–324, 1983.
120. Kant JA, Lord ST, Crabtree GR. Partial messenger-RNA sequences for human A-α, B-β, and γ-fibrinogen chains – evolutionary and functional implications. *Proc. Nat. Acad. Sci. USA Biol. Sci.* **80**:3953–3957, 1983.
121. Mills KA, Even D, Murray JC. Tetranucleotide repeat polymophism at the human alpha fibrinogen locus (FGA). *Hum. Mol. Genet.* **1**:779, 1992.

122. Murray JC, Buetow K, Chung D, Aschbacher A. Linkage disequilibrium of RFLPs at the β-fibrinogen (FGB) and γ-fibrinogen (FGG) loci on chromosome-4. *Cytogenet. Cell Genet.* **40**:707–708, 1985.
123. Ye S, Humphries S, Green F. Allele specific amplification by tetra primer PCR. *Nucleic Acids Res.* **20**:1152, 1992.
124. Humphries SE, Cook M, Dubowitz M, Stirling Y, Meade TW. Role of genetic-variation at the fibrinogen locus in determination of plasma-fibrinogen concentrations. *Lancet* **1**:1452–1455, 1987.
125. Thomas A, Lamlum H, Humphries S, Green F. Linkage disequilibrium across the fibrinogen locus as shown by 5 genetic polymorphisms, G/A(−455) (HaeIII), C/T(−148) (HindIII/AluI), T/G(+1689)(AvaII), and BclI (β-fibrinogen) and TaqI (α-fibrinogen), and their detection by PCR. *Hum. Mutat.* **3**:79–81, 1994.

Cystic fibrosis

43

D.J.H. Brock

Introduction

Cystic fibrosis (CF) is the most common life-shortening Mendelian disorder found in children and in young adults of Caucasian descent. It was first clearly described by Anderson[1] as 'cystic fibrosis of the pancreas', although the name was subsequently shortened to cystic fibrosis. An autosomal recessive mode of inheritance was suggested in the late 1940s[2] and is now universally accepted.

CF presents in a variety of ways, and although usually diagnosed within the first few years of life, may escape detection until the second or later decades. In early infancy a majority of patients present with a combination of respiratory symptoms, failure to thrive and steatorrhoea. Some 10–15% of newborns with CF have meconium ileus, and this is virtually diagnostic. A family history of the disorder should alert the paediatrician to search for more subtle presenting features. Isolation of *P. aeruginosa*, particularly in the mucoid form, from the lower respiratory tract of a child or young adult almost always signals CF[3].

Abnormally high concentrations of sodium and chloride ions in the sweat of CF patients were first noted by di Sant'Agnese et al.[4]. Although the sweat test is not without problems, a standard procedure in which sweating is stimulated by pilocarpine iontophoresis has become the primary laboratory test for CF. A sweat chloride concentration greater than 60 mEq/L, when found in association with other pulmonary manifestations, gastrointestinal symptoms, or history of CF in the immediate family, constitutes a certain diagnosis of the disorder.

The cloning of the CF gene[5–7] introduced a new laboratory method of diagnosis which can be absolutely definitive. However, as outlined below, there are a large number of mutant CF alleles, not all of which have been identified. The most prevalent of these, ΔF508, is found on 70–85% of CF chromosomes in populations of north European ancestry[8]. Homozygosity for this allele makes a diagnosis of CF inescapable. Homozygosity or compound heterozygosity for any other defined CF mutant allele (or alleles) is equally definitive. However, the inability to detect two copies of a defined mutant allele in an individual thought to have CF does not constitute a diagnostic exclusion.

For a genetic disorder, CF is unusually common in Caucasian populations. Epidemiological surveys show a birth prevalence ranging from about 1 in 1700 to about 1 in 6500[3], though many of these are bedevilled by incomplete ascertainment. Newborn screening using the serum immunoreactive trypsin (IRT) method is thought to have a sensitivity of 90–95% and has tended to show slightly higher birth prevalences[9]. There is now abundant evidence that the disease is caused by mutant alleles at a single genetic locus[10]. Thus if the birth prevalence is assumed to be 1 in 2500, the gene frequency is 0.02 and the heterozygote frequency 0.04 or 1 in 25. Data from completed trials of population screening suggest a heterozygote frequency between 1 in 22 and 1 in 23[11].

The prognosis for an individual born with CF is variable, ranging from death due to complications of meconium ileus in the neonatal period through to protracted survival to age 40 or 50. A survey made by the British Paediatric Association covering 1977 to 1985 suggested a median survival in the UK for boys of 21 years and for girls of 19 years[12]. Statistics from the Cystic Fibrosis Foundation indicate that in 1991 the median survival age in the USA was 30.6 years for males and 28.2 years for females[3]. An analysis of mortality data has projected that a child born with CF in the UK in 1990 may have a life expectancy of 40 years[13].

Molecular biology

The CF gene is localized on the long arm of chromosome 7. It spans some 230 kb of genomic DNA and contains 27 exons. The gene product, the cystic fibrosis transmembrane conductance regulator (CFTR), is expressed in those tissues primarily involved in the disease process, such as pancreas, nasal polyps, lung, colon, sweat glands, placenta, liver and parotid gland. It is a protein with a calculated molecular mass of 170 000, showing strong homology with a class of ATP-dependent membrane transport proteins[5–7]. Unfortunately, CFTR is not expressed in accessible tissues such as red or white red blood cells, and this means that tracking the CF gene through protein assays is impractical.

The predominant mutant allele at the CF locus is a 3 base-pair deletion in exon 10, which removes a phenylalanine residue at position 508 of the 1480 amino acid sequence of CFTR. This allele, known as ΔF508 (F is the single letter code for phenylalanine), makes up 50 to 90% of mutations in Caucasian populations (Table 43.1)[8,14]. It must be noted that these are the proportions of ΔF508 on single CF chromosomes, and that figures for homozygosity (i.e. affected individuals with both chromosomes carrying ΔF508) are obtained by squaring the ΔF508 proportions.

TABLE 43.1
Worldwide geographic distribution of the ΔF508 mutant allele[10,16]

Country	CF chromosomes	
	Total	ΔF508(%)
North America		
Caucasian, non-Ashkenazi	3193	2240 (70)
Black	169	60 (36)
Ashkenazi	95	30 (32)
Europe		
Denmark	586	511 (87)
Netherlands	1043	804 (77)
England	6085	4560 (75)
Belgium	982	734 (75)
Wales	341	245 (72)
Germany	3046	2166 (71)
France	5158	3595 (70)
Czechoslovakia	490	336 (69)
Scotland	836	571 (68)
Republic of Ireland	292	199 (68)
Switzerland	402	270 (67)
Northern Ireland	456	258 (57)
Bulgaria	202	112 (55)
Greece	326	173 (53)
Spain	1308	695 (53)
Italy	2331	1146 (49)

It is now known that CF is an extremely heterogeneous condition at the DNA level. Over 600 different mutant alleles have been described[15]. Many are extremely rare and have been found in one or a handful of patients. With the exception of ΔF508 only a few have been found at frequencies of more than 1% in the British population. Table 43.2 shows representative data for the United Kingdom[16].

TABLE 43.2
Percentage frequency of the more common CF alleles in the Scottish population[18]

Allele	Frequency (%)
ΔF508	74.2
G551D	5.9
G542X	3.7
R117H	1.2
1717-1G-A	1.0
A455E	0.6
N1303K	0.4
621 + 1G-T	0.4
ΔI507	0.4
R560T	0.2
W1282X	0.2
S549N	0.2

Diagnostic tests

It is possible to detect both normal and mutant CF alleles on any tissue which contains nucleated cells; in practice this means any tissue with the exception of mature red blood cells. Adequate amounts of DNA for the purpose of diagnosis can be extracted from 10 ml of whole blood, from 10 mg of a chorionic villus biopsy, or from a mouthwash sample, obtained by swilling out the mouth with 1 to 20 ml of isotonic saline, isotonic sucrose, distilled or even tap water. A mouthwash sample is in effect a self-administered buccal scrape and may sometimes fail; for this reason a spatula scrape gives more reliable material. DNA may also be amplified from dried blood spots or exfoliated cells in urine samples, and (if need be) from histological and archival specimens.

Laboratory detection of CF alleles is nearly always performed after prior amplification of the portion of the CF gene in which the relevant mutation lies. The standard technique used is the polymerase chain reaction (PCR), which employs a heat-stable DNA polymerase to produce between 10^7 and 10^9 copies of the target DNA sequence in a few hours. Commercial PCR-based kits for detection of the more common CF alleles (especially ΔF508) are now marketed. Not only is the PCR a quick and easy procedure, but it may also be applied to samples with an extremely low DNA content.

A disadvantage of the PCR is that it is most efficiently carried out when the target DNA sequence is comparatively small, ideally not more that 500 base-pairs. The CF gene, in common with most other genes in higher organisms, is made up of small exons separated by large intervening sequences (introns) which are spliced out during RNA processing and therefore not translated into the amino acids of the CFTR protein. Mutant CF alleles are scattered through the different exons and also at the beginning and ending of introns (where they interfere with correct RNA processing) in such a way that no single PCR amplification can cover all the points of mutation. In fact it is generally necessary to amplify each exon (and if necessary the adjacent intronic regions) in a separate PCR reaction, before searching for the presence or absence of a specific mutation.

Once the target DNA sequence has been amplified, the mutant CF allele may be detected by a number of procedures. In the case of the predominant ΔF508 allele (which encompasses a 3 base-pair deletion), the amplified material will be smaller than the normal allele by three nucleotides, and this difference can be directly visualized after electrophoresis and staining of products on an acrylamide gel[17–19]. There is a further advantage in this technique. Individuals who are ΔF508/normal heterozygotes not only show both ΔF508 and normal bands on the gel, but also a characteristic pair of heteroduplex bands which migrate more slowly (Fig. 43.1)[20].

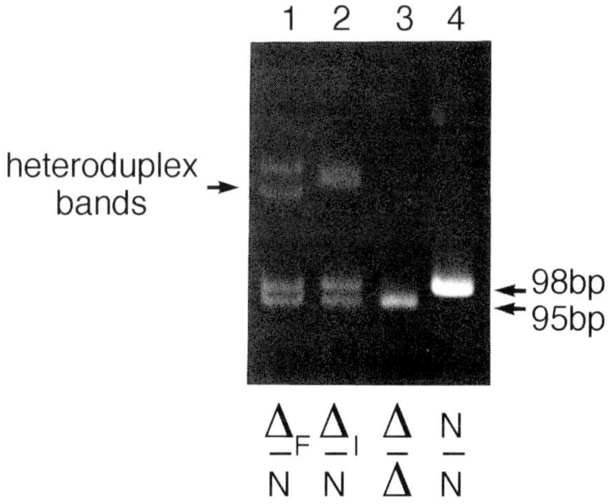

Fig. 43.1 Heteroduplex bands seen with ΔF508/normal (Δ_F/N) and ΔI507/normal (Δ_I/N) heterozygotes. (Courtesy of Dr Tony Shrimpton.)

These are non-covalent interactions between the different DNA fragments, with conformational changes resulting from incomplete annealing of the non-identical strands. A slightly different heteroduplex band is seen in the amplified DNA of an individual who is heterozygous for the ΔI507 and normal alleles[16]. Thus although it is not possible, by gel electrophoresis alone, to distinguish ΔF508/ΔF508 homozygotes from ΔI507/ΔI507 homozygotes or from ΔF508/ΔI507 compound heterozygotes, it is possible to distinguish ΔF508/normal and ΔI507/normal heterozygotes (Fig. 43.1).

A second procedure for detecting CF mutations employs the precise specificity of restriction enzyme digestion. If a mutation either destroys an existing restriction endonuclease recognition site, or alternatively creates a new one, it is possible to generate different size fragments from the normal and mutant alleles. An example is shown in Fig. 43.2 of detection of three specific mutations in exon 11[21]. The PCR amplification produces a product of 425 base pairs, which in normal

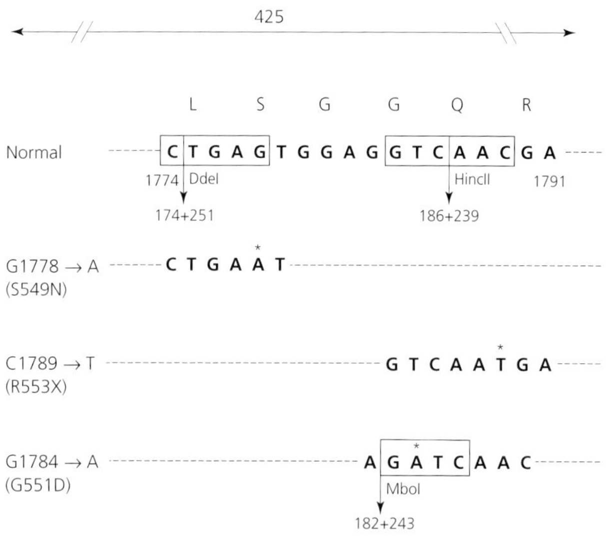

Fig. 43.2 Detection of three exon 11 mutations by differential restriction enzyme digestion. See text for details.

alleles can be cleaved by both *Dde*I and *Hinc*II. In the S549N mutation the *Dde*I restriction site is abolished by a G→A change at nucleotide 1778. In both R553X and G551D mutations the *Hinc*II restriction site is destroyed, the former by a C→T change at nucleotide 1789, and the latter by a G→A change at nucleotide 1784. However, in the latter the G→A change creates a novel *Mbo*I restriction site, which is not present in either the normal or the S549N and R553X alleles. Thus if exon 11 is amplified and the resulting sample digested with *Dde*I, *Hinc*II and *Mbo*I, the size of the fragments will reveal the presence or absence of these three mutant alleles.

A third method of detection uses hybridization to allele-specific oligonucleotides. For each specific mutation it is necessary to synthesize two short oligonucleotides, one exactly complementary to the region surrounding the mutation and the other exactly complementary to the equivalent region in the normal allele. Under conditions of high stringency (i.e. designed to permit hybridization when sequences are exactly complementary), the oligonucleotides will only anneal to their respective counterparts. Most individuals in a screened population will show a hybridization signal with the normal oligonucleotide, while heterozygotes for the specific mutation will produce signals with both oligonucleotides.

It is also possible to detect mutations by altering the specificity of the PCR in such a way that only the normal or only the mutant allele is amplified. This is referred to either as the amplification refractory mutation system (ARMS)[22] or as allele-specific amplification. The method requires synthesis of three amplification primers, one forward primer complementary to the normal allele, one forward primer complementary to the mutant allele, and one reverse primer complementary to both alleles (Fig. 43.3). Two separate amplifications are

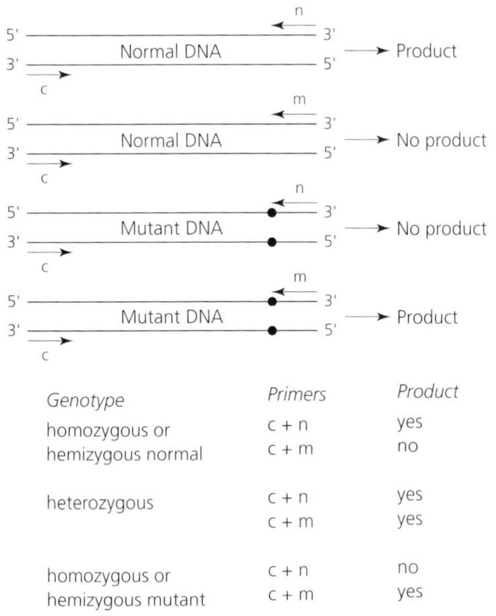

Fig. 43.3 Principle of the ARMS, or allele-specific amplification, technique.

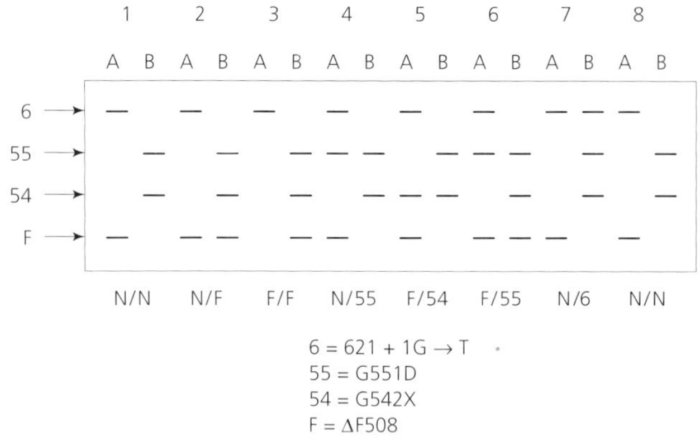

Fig. 43.4 Schematic representation of the use of multiplex ARMS to detect four common mutant CF alleles. Each sample is run in two reactions, A and B. In the absence of any mutation, the patterns shown in samples 1 and 8 are seen. The presence of G551D or G542X mutations is revealed by extra bands in reaction A and the presence of ΔF508 and 621+1G-T mutations by extra bands in reaction B. Note that in sample 3 the absence of a band in reaction A and an extra band in reaction B signals a homozygous ΔF508 mutation.

carried out, differing in the forward primer used, but each having the common reverse primer. DNA from normal homozygotes is only amplified in the reaction containing the complementary forward primer. The same is true for DNA from individuals homozygous for the mutation, although one would not expect to encounter these in screening a general population. DNA from individuals heterozygous for the specific mutation would be amplified in both reactions. Amplification products are inspected after electrophoresis on agarose gels and ethidium bromide staining.

It will be apparent from the above discussion that attempts to detect more than just the predominant ΔF508 allele are likely to become quite complicated. Two simplifying procedures are available. The first is to amplify several exons simultaneously (multiplexing) and then to sort out the products by electrophoresis, restriction enzyme digestion or allele-specific hybridization. The second is to concentrate on those CF alleles at highest frequency in the population being screened, and to design ARMS primers capable of selective amplification. The latter procedure – multiplex ARMS – has the virtue of being suitable for commercial kits. An example of a multiplex ARMS[23], designed to detect ΔF508, G551D, G542X and 621+1G→T, is shown in Fig. 43.4. It must be noted, however, that multiplex ARMS can only detect the specific mutations for which it is designed. In contrast exon multiplexing can in theory detect any mutation in the amplified exons.

Indirect testing for CF alleles

If defined CF mutations cannot be found in both members of an at-risk couple, the usual practice is to attempt to use linked DNA markers to carry out prenatal diagnosis. All evidence points to a single genetic locus for the disorder and thus the 'CF gene' may be regarded as single entity from the linkage point of view. The key to linkage-based diagnosis is the establishment of phase, i.e. determining which marker allele co-segregates with each parental CF allele. Establishing phase requires a sample from an index affected child or, if the index affected child is deceased, from appropriate stored tissues. The only problem is the small but finite possibility of recombination between the marker and CF locus during meiosis.

There are now a large number of closely linked DNA markers in use which render virtually all families fully informative. The most suitable of these are microsatellite repeats where there is such a high degree of heterozygosity that the two parental samples are likely to be different. One of the best systems is that originally described by Zielenski et al.[24], where the marker is a set of CA and TA repeats in intron 17b of the CFTR gene. There are at least 24 length variations for the TA repeat (7 to 56 units; see Fig. 43.5) and three for the CA repeat, giving a degree of heterozygosity of about 95%. Since the marker system is intragenic, the chance of recombination is essentially zero. Other intragenic microsatellites that have been reported are a TTGA repeat in intron 6a and the 5′ flanking region of exon 6b[25], and a GT repeat in intron 8[26].

Microvillar enzyme testing

Several years before the CF gene was cloned, it was noted that the activities of a number of microvillar enzymes were significantly depressed in amniotic fluid supernatant in the presence of a fetus with CF. These included γ-glutamyl-transpeptidase, aminopeptidase A[27], α-glucosidase and the

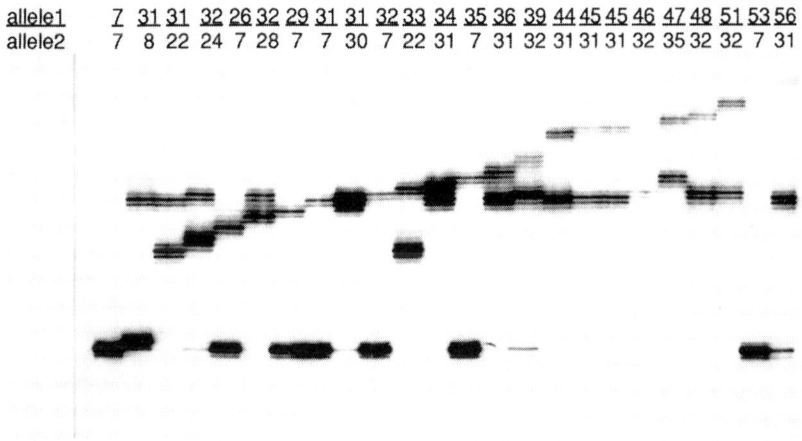

Fig. 43.5 Length variations of a TA repeat in intron 17b of the CF gene. The photograph shows 23 alleles on a sequencing type gel. (Courtesy of Dr L.C. Tsui and with permission of the University of Chicago Press and the *American Journal of Human Genetics*.)

intestinal isoenzyme of alkaline phosphatase[28]. The simplest explanation for this finding arose from the observation that these enzymes occurred at high levels in fetal meconium, and led to the belief that most CF fetuses at midtrimester have difficulty passing meconium. The blockage or partial blockage must be a transient phenomenon, for only about 15% of CF infants have an overt form of meconium ileus at birth.

Before the advent of DNA-based methods for detecting CF alleles or tracking the CF gene by linkage, microvillar enzyme testing was the only method for the prenatal diagnosis of the disorder. It was quite extensively used. Boue et al.[29] reported a series of 200 diagnoses on 1-in-4 risk pregnancies, with an admitted false positive rate of 0.7% and an admitted false negative rate of 3.4%. However, there were 53 terminations of pregnancy and 58 fetuses out of 200 (29.0%) were deemed to be or found affected, more than expected in a Mendelian recessive condition. Brock et al.[30] reported their experience on 258 pregnancies with a 1-in-4 risk, with an observed false positive rate of 2.3% and an observed false negative rate of 4.4%. Again, a higher than theoretical proportion of pregnancies (32.3%) were predicted or found to be affected.

It was thus obvious that microvillar enzyme testing was associated with considerable inaccuracy. The best available estimates for 'robust' figures suggest a false positive rate of 10% and a false negative rate of 5%. If these rates are applied to the calculation of predictabilities for both normal and abnormal test results, it can be seen that microvillar enzyme testing is inappropriate for anything other than a 1-in-4 risk pregnancy (Table 43.3). Given these data, it is not surprising that the system is now hardly ever used, and represents a 'last-gasp' approach to the prenatal diagnosis of CF.

TABLE 43.3
Predictabilities of microvillar enzyme testing using a sensitivity of 95% and a specificity of 90%

	Predictabilities	
Prior odds	Abnormal test	Normal test
1:4	3.2:1	1:54
1:9	1.2:1	1:144
1:16	1.1:6	1:270
1:50	1:5	1:980
1:100	1:10	1:1980
1:150	1:16	1:2980
1:200	1:21	1:3980

Systematic approach to prenatal diagnosis of CF

It will be apparent from the preceding sections that there is no method of prenatal diagnosis for CF that covers all possible situations. It is therefore necessary to use a stepwise approach, moving from direct testing for CF alleles, through indirect testing with linked DNA markers, and ending (if all else fails) with microvillar enzyme assay.

The ideal situation occurs when each parent carries a defined CF allele. In the United Kingdom, where some 85–90% of CF heterozygotes carry an allele detectable by routine tests, this situation occurs in 70–80% of pregnancies. In more heterogeneous populations, and particularly those with strong Jewish or Hispanic admixture, the proportion may be substantially lower. This problem can be overcome to some extent by increasing the range of detectable CF alleles in a laboratory's portfolio, and by tailoring the detection systems to the most prevalent mutations in the local population. But no laboratory is currently able to cover all the CF alleles it is likely to encounter, and there will always be a group of at-risk parents where one or perhaps both partners carry an undetectable mutation.

In this situation one would resort to indirect testing using one of the highly polymorphic intragenic marker systems described above. Given current awareness of the importance of keeping DNA samples from individuals with genetic diseases, it is now most unusual to encounter a pregnancy with a 1-in-4 risk of CF where there is no material from an index affected child. Thus the last resort method of microvillar enzyme testing is now almost a historical footnote.

REFERENCES

1. Anderson DH. Cystic fibrosis of the pancreas and its relation to celiac disease: clinical and pathological study. *Am. J. Dis. Child.* **56**:344–399, 1988.
2. Anderson DH & Hodges RGV. Genetics of cystic fibrosis of the pancreas with a consideration of etiology. *Am. J. Dis. Child.* **72**:62–68, 1946.
3. Welsh MJ, Tsui LP, Boat TF, Beaudet AL. Cystic fibrosis. In *The Metabolic and Molecular Bases of Inherited Disease*, 7th edn (eds CR Scriver, AL Beaudet, WS Sly & D Valle), pp. 3799–3877. New York: McGraw Hill, 1995.
4. Di Sant'Agnese PA, Darling RC, Perera GA & Shea E. Abnormal electrolyte composition of sweat in cystic fibrosis of the pancreas: clinical significance and relationship to disease. *Pediatrics* **12**:549–563, 1955.
5. Rommens JM, Iannuzzi MC, Kerem B et al. Identification of the cystic fibrosis gene; chromosome walking and jumping. *Science* **245**:1059–1065, 1989.
6. Riordan JR, Rommens JM, Kerem B et al. Identification of the cystic fibrosis gene: cloning and characterization of complementary DNA. *Science* **245**:1066–1073, 1989.
7. Kerem B, Rommens JM, Buchanan JA et al. Identification of the cystic fibrosis gene: genetic analysis. *Science* **245**:1073–1080, 1989.
8. The Cystic Fibrosis Genetic Analysis Consortium. Worldwide survey of the ΔF508 mutation. *Am. J. Hum. Genet.* **47**:354–359, 1990.
9. Brock DJH. Cystic Fibrosis. In *Prenatal Diagnosis and Screening* (eds DJH Brock, CH Rodeck & MA Ferguson-Smith), pp. 520–546. Edinburgh: Churchill-Livingstone, 1992.
10. Beaudet A, Bowcock A, Buchwald M et al. Linkage of cystic fibrosis to two tightly linked DNA markers: joint report from a collaborative study. *Am. J. Hum. Genet.* **39**:681–693, 1986.
11. Brock DJH. Prenatal screening for cystic fibrosis: five years experience reviewed. *Lancet* **347**:148–151, 1996.
12. British Paediatric Association Working Party on Cystic Fibrosis. Cystic fibrosis in the United Kingdom 1977–1985: an improving picture. *Br. Med. J.* **297**:1599–1602, 1988.
13. Elborn JS, Shale DJ, Britton JR. Cystic fibrosis: current survival and population estimates to the year 2000. *Thorax* **46**:881–885, 1991.
14. Schwarz MJ, Malone GM, Hayworth A et al. Cystic fibrosis mutation analysis: report from 22 UK regional genetics laboratories. *Hum. Mutat.* **6**:326–333, 1995.
15. Tsui LC, personal communication.
16. Shrimpton AE, McIntosh I, Brock DJH. The incidence of different cystic fibrosis mutations in the Scottish population: effects on prenatal diagnosis and genetic counselling. *J. Med. Genet.* **28**:317–321, 1991.
17. Taylor GR, Noble JS, Hall JL et al. Rapid screening for ΔF508 deletion in cystic fibrosis. *Lancet* **ii**:1345, 1989.
18. Scheffer H, Verlind E, Penninga T et al. Rapid screening for ΔF508 deletion in cystic fibrosis. *Lancet* **ii**:1345–1346, 1989.
19. Matthew CJ, Roberts RJ, Harris A, Bentley DR, Bobrow M. Rapid screening for ΔF508 deletion in cystic fibrosis. *Lancet* **ii**:1346, 1989.
20. Rommens JM, Kerem B, Grier W et al. Rapid non-radioactive detection of the major cystic fibrosis mutation. *Am. J. Hum. Genet.* **46**:395–396, 1990.
21. Cutting GR, Kasch LM, Rosenstein BJ et al. A cluster of cystic fibrosis mutations in the first nucleotide binding fold of the cystic fibrosis conductance regulator protein. *Nature* **340**:366–369, 1990.
22. Newton CR, Graham A, Heptonstall LE et al. Analysis of any point mutation in DNA. The amplification refractory mutation system. *Nucleic Acids Res.* **17**:2505–2516, 1989.
23. Ferrie RM, Schwarz MJ, Robertson NH et al. Development, multiplexing and amplification of ARMS tests for common mutations in the CFTR gene. *Am. J. Hum. Genet.* **51**:251–262, 1992.
24. Zielenski J, Markiewicz D, Rininsland F, Rommens JM, Tsui LC. A cluster of highly polymorphic dinucleotide repeats in intron 17b of the CFTR gene. *Am. J. Hum. Genet.* **49**:1256–1262, 1991.
25. Gasparini P, Dognini M, Bonizzatto A, Pignatti PF, Morral N, Estivill X. A tetranucleotide repeat polymorphism in the cystic fibrosis gene. *Hum. Genet.* **86**:625, 1991.
26. Morral N, Nunes V, Casals T, Estivill X. CA/GT microsatellite alleles within the CFTR gene are not generated by unequal crossing over. *Genomics* **10**:692–698, 1991.
27. Carbarns NJB, Gosden C, Brock DJH. Microvillar peptidase activity in amniotic fluid: possible use in prenatal diagnosis of cystic fibrosis. *Lancet* **i**:329–331, 1983.
28. Brock DJH. Amniotic fluid alkaline phosphatase isoenzymes in the prenatal diagnosis of cystic fibrosis. *Lancet* **ii**:941–943, 1983.
29. Boue A, Muller F, Nezelof C. Prenatal diagnosis in 200 pregnancies with 1 in 4 risk of cystic fibrosis. *Hum. Genet.* **74**:288–297, 1986.
30. Brock DJH, Clarke HAK, Barron L. Prenatal diagnosis of cystic fibrosis by microvillar enzyme assay on a sequence of 258 pregnancies. *Hum. Genet.* **78**:271–275, 1988.

Muscular dystrophies

44

M.I. Evans, E.L. Krivchenia, M. King and E.P. Hoffman

Introduction

The muscular dystrophies are often considered the paradigm of neuromuscular disorders, with Duchenne muscular dystrophy (DMD) being among the most common and devastating of all inherited diseases. They are categorized by progressive muscle wasting that is attributable primarily to muscular pathology. This is in distinction to neural pathology, which, for example, is commonly represented by amyotropic lateral sclerosis, also known in the United States as Lou Gehrig's disease.

DMD is the best studied of the muscular dystrophies, and is named after Geome Benjamin Amond Duchenne, who described this condition in publications in 1861 and 1868[1,2]. In retrospect, however, he was not the first person to have described the disorder. That distinction actually goes to Edward Maryon who had described the same pathology in 1852[3,4]. The predilection for males was recognized in the 19th century, but its official designation as an X-linked disorder took several more decades.

A milder form of muscular dystrophy, also X-linked, was first described by Dr Peter Becker in 1955, and is commonly now referred to as Becker's muscular dystrophy (BMD)[5]. Although there was controversy for a time, it is now understood that these two disorders are, in fact, allelic[6,7]. Gene-specific probes were first developed in 1985, and the protein product identified and named dystrophin by Hoffman in 1987[8–10].

The incidence of DMD has been documented in multiple studies to be approximately in 1 in 3 500 males, with a mutation rate of 1 in 10 000 genes per generation, which is the highest for any unifactorial disorder. Most newly ascertained cases are isolated, with many believed to represent spontaneous mutations[4].

DMD may occasionally present in the neonate as hypotonia, but is more likely to present later in life through the inability of a child to run properly, or a tendency to walk on toes. The most pathognomonic characteristics are difficulties in standing up caused by muscle weakness and inability to rise from the floor without pressing on their thighs – known as Gowers' sign. Muscles show progressive wasting, and boys are confined to wheelchairs by age 12. Contractures commonly develop, and scoliosis becomes a serious issue that can compromise respiratory function. Average lifespan has increased over the past several years, predominantly through secondary treatment of scoliosis and assisted ventilation.

In addition to the obvious striated muscle involvement, there is some evidence of smooth muscle involvement, as manifested by paralytic ileus, gastric dilatation, and bladder paralysis which are seen occasionally. Cardiac muscle is involved, leading to a particularly consistent finding of high R-waves on the right precordial leads on electrocardiography. Central nervous system involvement is also recognized, and the mean IQ of affected boys is approximately one standard deviation lower than unaffected siblings, with 20% having IQs less than 70.

The clinical diagnosis of DMD has traditionally been made on the basis of the pathognomonic hypertrophic calves, positive Gowers' sign, elevated serum creatinine kinase levels, abnormal electromyography, and findings on muscle biopsy (Fig. 44.1). Over the last decade, however, these have been generally usurped by molecular and immunohistochemical diagnoses of the dystrophin gene and product, which now serve as the gold standard for diagnosis (Figs 44.2, 44.3).

Dystrophin was shown to be the protein product of the Duchenne muscular dystrophy gene in 1987[8,9]. The gene is approximately 2.5 Mb in length, has 79 exons, and is transcribed into a 14 kb mRNA. The coding sequence is, therefore, less than 1% of the nucleotide composition of the locus. Approximately 70% of cases of DMD are associated with deletions of one or more exons of the gene, and 5–10% have duplications. Ninety percent of Beckers patients have deletions[4,11]. The remaining cases are secondary to point mutations, which can cause premature translational

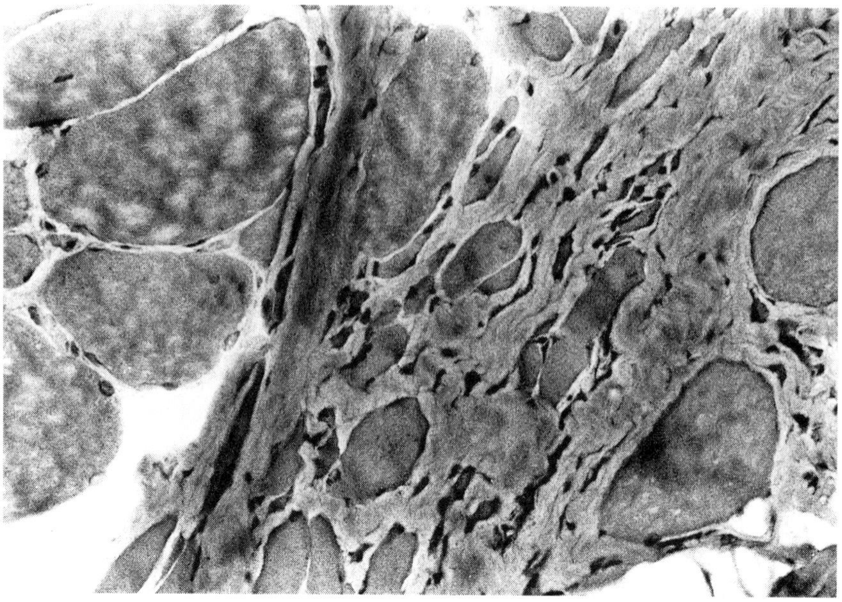

Fig. 44.1 Classic muscle wasting.

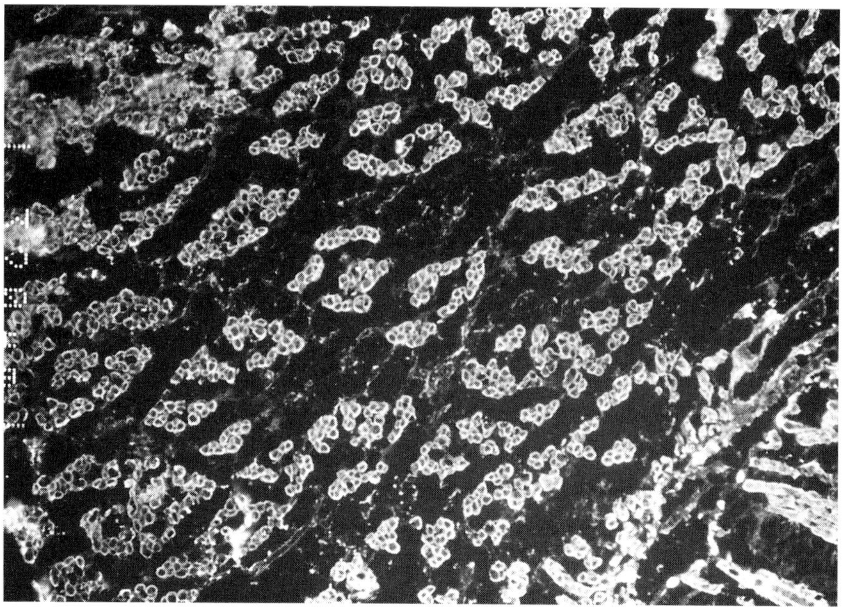

Fig. 44.2 Normal immunohistochemical muscle.

terminations, and result in deficiency of functional protein[12,13]. When deletions do occur, they are more likely to occur in two hot spots that occur in the first 20 exons, and at around 45–55.

The dystrophin protein has 3685 amino acids, and weighs 427 kDa. The rod-shaped protein has four domains: N-terminal, central rod, cystene rich, and C-terminal. Dystrophin is a cytoskeletal protein, localized to the muscle cell membranes via a dystrophin-associated protein complex. There are a number of isoforms of dystrophin, of which six have been clearly identified. Each has a different promoter that specifies the transcription of tissue specific dystrophins. The exact involvement of these isoforms of dystrophin in DMD is not certain. Mutations of the muscle promoter and first exon are sometimes associated with an the X-linked cardiomyopathy.

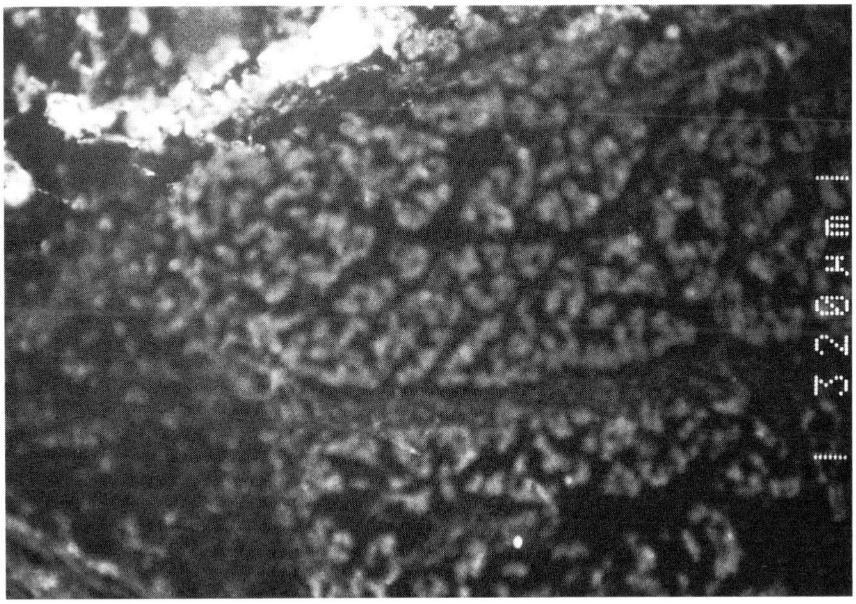

Fig. 44.3 DMD immunohistochemical muscle.

Genetic counselling and prenatal diagnosis

Patients presenting for genetic counselling about the possibility of prenatal diagnosis for DMD typically either have had an affected brother, or a previously affected child (Fig. 44.4). In our experience, most such couples are highly motivated to undergo prenatal diagnosis, and furthermore have a very high likelihood of choosing to terminate an affected fetus. For many years, prior to the isolation of the dystrophin protein and gene, the 'best' method for preventing the birth of a child with DMD or BMD was through the identification of fetal sex. Fifty percent of male fetuses would be expected to be affected with DMD, whereas 50% of females would be carriers, but clinically asymptomatic. Since the introduction of prenatal diagnostic techniques in the early 1970s through the late 1980s, termination of male fetuses 'at risk' for DMD was common under these circumstances. With the ability to predict with great certainty whether or not a male fetus is affected through DNA and protein studies, clinical decision making by sex selection alone has virtually disappeared.

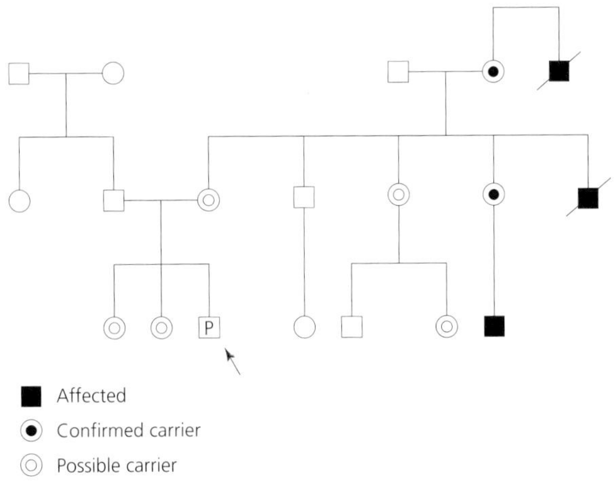

Fig. 44.4 DMD pedigree. (P = presenting patient.)

As with any molecular diagnosis, chorionic villus sampling is the preferred method because there is far more DNA in even the tiniest solid tissue specimen as compared to 20 cm^3 of amniotic fluid[14,15]. Thus, the diagnosis can be done in the first trimester, performed more quickly, and reported to the patient prior to her being seen to be clinically pregnant.

The isolation of the dystrophin gene[16] and identification of its normal protein product[8] have prompted the advent of what has been called 'molecular diagnosis' for this disorder[17].

However, in the 30% of families who do not have deletion mutations, both carrier detection and prenatal diagnosis are more difficult and less accurate. In such cases, restriction fragment length polymorphism analyses must be undertaken in an attempt to mark the affected X chromosome in the family. If only a single affected family member exists, it is often impossible to determine whether the mother of the affected boy is a carrier. This uncertainty has ramifications not only for future pregnancies of the mother but also for the carrier risks of other at-risk female relatives. With Bayesian analysis only, the probability of being a carrier can be generated. If the male fetus at risk of being affected with Duchenne muscular dystrophy inherits an X chromosome from his mother that is different from the previously affected male, then, with the exception of the small possibility of crossing over in meiosis, the diagnosis of Duchenne muscular dystrophy can be excluded[18]. However, if the male fetus inherits the *same* X chromosome as his previously affected sib, the risk that the fetus is affected is the same as the risk that the mother is, in fact, a carrier. Such uncertainty in risk assessment has been seen in other X-linked disorders, such as haemophilia[19].

In instances in which the genetic mutation in the DMD gene is known, the diagnosis by DNA methods is generally straightforward and relatively uncomplicated. The deletion or duplication mutation is identified in the affected male proband, then female relatives are assayed for carrier status based on presence or absence of the same deletion/duplication in their DNA. Prenatal diagnosis is done in carriers by testing for the same deletion or duplication. While it is technically difficult or impossible to identify non-deletion/duplication mutations (point mutations), carrier detection and prenatal diagnosis is still possible by genetic linkage analysis using polymorphic markers spaced throughout the Duchenne dystrophy gene.

There are four situations in which a mutation or detectable deletion may not be found, and DNA molecular diagnosis will generally be ambiguous. These situations include:

- A fetus whose mother has a normal creatinine kinase (CK) and a single affected son with no previous family history. If the fetus inherits the 'at risk' X chromosome, there is a 50% chance of being affected because of the possibilities of new mutations and gonadal mosaicism
- When the mother of a male fetus is at risk for being a carrier yet analysis of the polymorphisms proves uninformative (fails to show any differences between 2 maternal X chromosomes)
- When there has been a crossover event in meiosis between maternal X chromosomes such that it cannot be determined whether or not the DMD gene mutation was inherited
- There is a de novo X-autosomal translocation in a female fetus with breakpoints appearing to be within the DMD gene

Unfortunately, there are often complicating variables which limit the conclusiveness of genetic testing and counselling in DMD and BMD. First, affected male(s) in the pedigree may be deceased or unavailable for testing; this can make it more difficult to determine the causative mutation in a family. Second, the large size of the gene means that there is both a high mutation rate, and high recombination rate. Both of these variables can result in ambiguous risks being assigned to a male fetus. Under such circumstances, a fetal muscle biopsy may be the only, or best way to make a definitive diagnosis.

The clinical and laboratory techniques for fetal muscle biopsy have been developed within the past decade. The procedure is performed, under ultrasound guidance, with a coring biopsy gun inserted transabdominally into the uterine cavity, and inserted usually into the fetal buttock (Figs 44.5, 44.6). The coring biopsy chamber is then extended. When the trigger is pulled the core closes, entrapping a small amount of tissue. Identification of fetal muscle under a dissecting microscope is difficult under the best of circumstances and requires an experienced pathologist. The procedure must be performed with extreme care, making sure to go after the outer aspect of the buttock and thigh to minimize the potential for damage to nerves, vessels or scrotum. With such a procedure there is always the potential for damage despite the best efforts of all involved.

Over the past decade we, and others, have performed numerous procedures for patients whose indications were as listed above[20–25]. In general, these have been highly motivated patients who are willing to take risks to get a certain answer

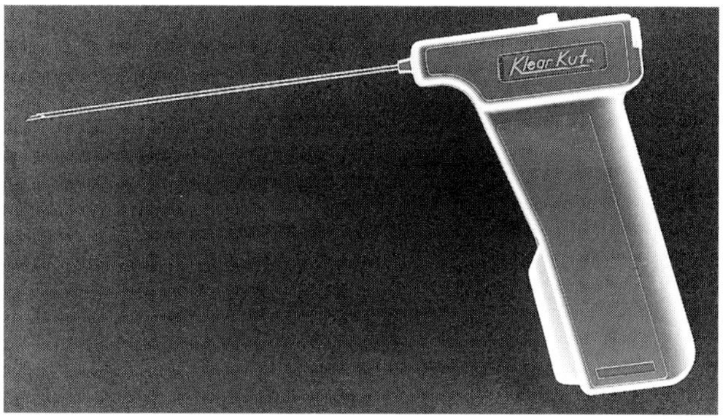

Fig. 44.5 Muscle biopsy gun.

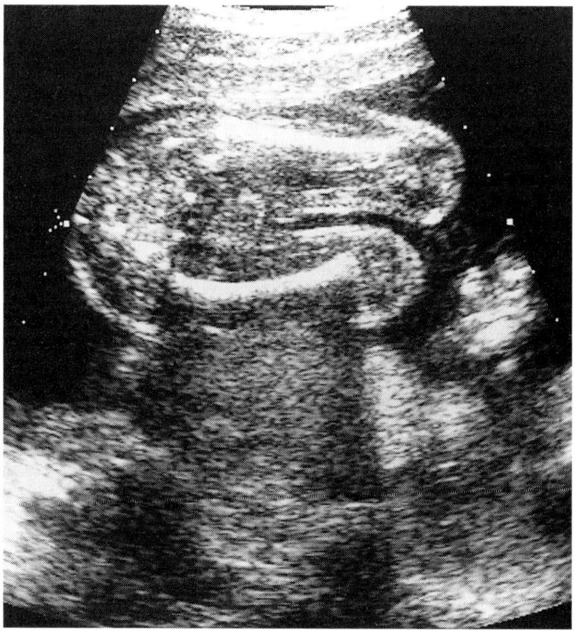

Fig. 44.6 Ultrasound of fetal muscle biopsy.

as to the status of their fetus when more controversial methods are insufficient to provide a definitive answer. In our experience we have found abnormalities in about 40% of cases, and all such couples have chosen to terminate.

A few cases of in utero muscle biopsy have been performed with endoscopic visualization in addition to ultrasound guidance. Our experience suggests that in the midtrimester, usually at 18 weeks or more, endoscopic assistance does not particularly improve the procedure[25]. As attempts are made to reduce the gestational age at which the procedure is done, however, endoscopic guidance will be essential (Fig. 44.7).

Initially, laboratory processing of the muscle biopsy specimen was done by immunoblotting. This technique requires a relatively large amount of muscle tissue, approximately 100 μg, which is beyond the normal amount available by the procedure. Immunohistochemical analysis by immunofluorescence has been the method used for most cases performed because it requires only a few fetal myofibres for an accurate analysis. Each fetal muscle biopsy specimen must be processed with both known, normal, and Duchenne specimens. At least two different dystrophin antibodies are used in separate experiments to make sure the results are unambiguous.

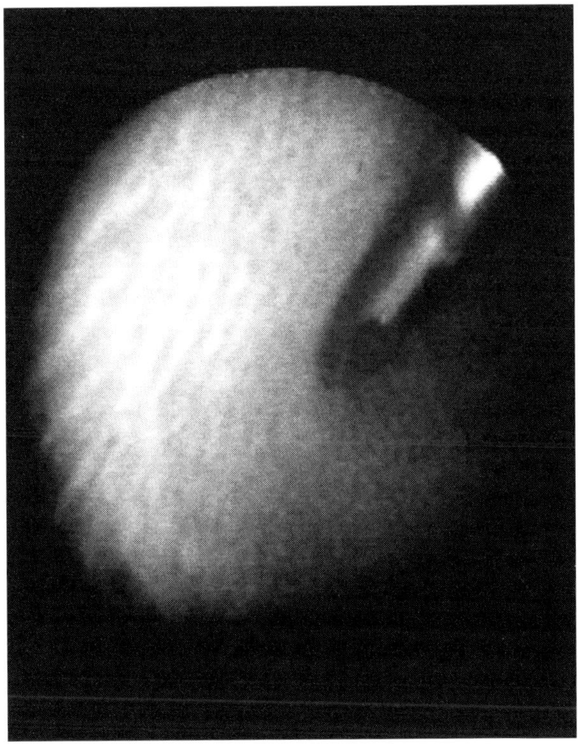

Fig. 44.7 Endoscopic visualization.

Potentials for gene therapy

Unfortunately, there are currently no 'cures' for Duchenne muscular dystrophy. Long-term use of steroids slows the progression of the disease somewhat, and palliative procedures (tendon lengthenings, spinal fusions, and respiratory support) can extend lifespan but will not abrogate the decline in muscle strength.

Considerable hope has been placed on strategies to overcome the primary biochemical defect, dystrophin deficiency. Efforts are underway to deliver the normal dystrophin gene via viral vectors (gene therapy), induce proteins that seem to share functional aspects with dystrophin (utrophin upregulation), or overcome the progressive deterioration of muscle through pharmacological approaches. The complete dystrophin protein has been successfully delivered to muscle cells using a recombinant adenovirus[26] and this approach shows great promise. However, significant hurdles remain before gene therapy can be expected to show efficacy in human patients. First, mature muscle is not infected by adenovirus. Thus, the dystrophin gene can only be delivered to neonatal or regenerating myofibres by this method. Second, intramuscular injection is the current method of delivering the recombinant virus to muscle, but the area of biochemical rescue is only on the order of a few millimetres. Thus, systemic delivery must be done to deliver the gene to muscle throughout the patient's body. Each of these barriers is being isolated and major research efforts are underway to overcome them.

REFERENCES

1. Duchenne GBA. *De l'electrisation localisee et son application a la pathologie et a la therapeutique*, 2nd edn. Paris, Baillière et Fils, 1861.
2. Duchenne GBA. Recherches sur la paralysie musculaire pseudohypertrophique ou paralysie myo-sclerosique. *Arch. Gen. Med.* **11**, 5–25, 179–209, 305–321, 421–443, 552–588, 1868.
3. Maryon E. On granular and fatty degeneration of the voluntary muscles. *Medico Chir. Trans.* (Lond.) **35**, 73–84, 1852.
4. Charrow J, Nadler HL & Evans MI. Prenatal diagnosis. In *Principles and Practice of Medical Genetics* (eds A.E.H. Emery & D.L. Rimoin), 2nd edn., pp. 1959–1994. New York: Churchill Livingstone, 1991.
5. Becker PE & Kiener F. Eine neue X-chromosomale Muskeldystrophie. *Arch. Psychiatr. Nervenkrankh.* **193**, 427–448, 1955.
6. Kingston HM, Thomas NST, Pearson PL *et al.* Genetic linkage between Becker muscular dystrophy and a polymorphic DNA sequence on the short arm of the X chromosome. *J. Med. Genet.* **20**, 255–258, 1983.
7. Kingston HM, Sarfarazi M, Thomas NST & Harper PS. Localisation of the Becker muscular dystrophy gene on the short arm of the X chromosome by linkage to cloned DNA sequences. *Hum. Genet.* **67**, 6–17, 1984.
8. Hoffman EP, Brown RH & Kunkel LM. Dystrophin. The protein product of the Duchenne muscular dystrophy locus. *Cell* **51**, 919–928, 1987.
9. Hoffman EP, Fishbeck KH & Brown RH *et al.* Dystrophin characterization in muscle biopsies from Duchenne and Becker muscular dystrophy patients. *N. Engl. J. Med.* **318**, 1363–1368, 1988.

10. Burmeister M, Monaco AP & Gillard EF *et al.* A 10-megabase physical map of human Xp21, including the Duchenne muscular dystrophy gene. *Genomics* **2**, 189–202, 1988.
11. Bushby KMD, Gardner-Medwin D & Nicholson LVB *et al.* The clinical, genetic and dystrophin characteristics of Becker muscular dystrophy. II. Correlation of phenotype with genetic and protein abnormalities. *J. Neurol.* **240**, 105–112, 1993.
12. Roberts RG, Barby TFM & Manners E *et al.* Direct detection of dystrophin gene rearrangements by analysis of dystrophin mRNA in peripheral blood lymphocytes. *Am. J. Hum. Genet.* **49**, 298–310, 1991.
13. Roberts RG, Bobrow M & Bentley DR. Point mutations in the dystrophin gene. *Proc. Natl. Acad. Sci. USA* **89**, 2331–2335, 1992.
14. Evans MI & Johnson MP. Chorionic Villus Sampling. In *Reproductive Risks and Prenatal Diagnosis* (ed. M.I. Evans), pp. 175–184. Norwalk, CT: Appleton & Lange, 1992.
15. Evans MI, Johnson MP, Bui TH, Holzgreve W & Wapner R. Prenatal Diagnosis. In *Principles and Practices of Medical Therapy in Pregnancy* (eds N. Gleisher, L. Buttino, U. Elkayam *et al.*) 3rd edn. pp. 178–192. Norwalk, CT: Appleton & Lange, 1998.
16. Koenig M, Hoffman EP & Bertelson CJ *et al.* Complete cloning of the Duchenne muscular dystrophy (DMD) cDNA and preliminary genomic organization of the DMD gene in normal and affected individuals. *Cell* **50**, 509–517, 1987.
17. Rowland LP. Clinical concepts of Duchenne muscular dystrophy. *Brain* **111**, 479–485, 1988.
18. Bieber FR, Hoffman EP & Amos J. Dystrophin analysis in Duchenne muscular dystrophy: use in fetal diagnosis and in genetic counseling. *Am. J. Hum. Genet.* **45**, 362–367, 1989.
19. Sarker G, Evans MI & Kogan S *et al.* Accurate prenatal diagnosis with novel polymerase chain reaction primers in a family with sporadic hemophilia A. *Obstet. Gynecol.* **71**, 414–417, 1989.
20. Evans MI, Greb A, Kazazian Jr HH *et al.* In utero fetal muscle biopsy for the diagnosis of Duchenne muscular dystrophy. *Am. J. Obstet. Gynecol.* **165**, 728–732, 1991.
21. Evans MI, Farrell SA, Greb A, Ray P, Johnson MP & Hoffman E. In utero fetal muscle biopsy for the diagnosis of Duchenne muscular dystrophy in a female fetus 'suddenly at risk'. *Am. J. Med. Genet.* **46**, 309–312, 1993.
22. Evans MI, Krivchenia EL, Johnson MP *et al.* In utero fetal muscle biopsy alters diagnosis and carrier risks in Duchenne and Becker muscular dystrophy. *Fetal Diagn. Ther.* **10**, 71–75, 1995.
23. Evans MI, Hoffman EP, Cadrin C, Johnson MP, Quintero RA & Golbus MS. Fetal muscle biopsy: collaborative experience with varied indications. *Obstet. Gynecol.* **84**, 913–917, 1994.
24. Kuller JA, Hoffman EP, Fries MH & Golbus MS. Prenatal diagnosis of Duchenne muscular dystrophy by fetal muscle biopsy. *Hum. Genet.* **90**, 34–40, 1992.
25. Evans MI, Quintero RA, King M, Qureshi F & Johnson MP. Endoscopically assisted, ultrasound guided fetal muscle biopsy. *Fetal. Diagn. Ther.* **10**, 168–173, 1995.
26. Chen HH, Mack LM, Kelly R, Ontell M, Kochanek S & Clemens PR. Persistence in muscle of an adenoviral vector that lacks all viral genes. *Proc. Natl. Acad. Sci. USA*, **94**, 1645–1650.

Inborn errors of metabolism

45

W.J. Kleijer

Introduction

More than 5000 human disorders are caused by single gene mutations[1]; they comprise conditions varying from slight deviations from the normal pattern to very severe disabling conditions and disorders which are practically incompatible with life. In most of these disorders metabolism must be affected in at least some stage of development, but only in a minority of the disorders (some 400) has the primary metabolic defect been established[1,2]. Mostly the defective gene product concerns an enzyme, but coenzymes, activators, hormones, transporter or receptor proteins and structural proteins are also involved. The specific diagnosis of these disorders is often complicated by the fact that most are quite rare and moreover clinically heterogeneous. Patients with the same enzyme deficiency or even the same mutations may present with different manifestations; conversely, similar patterns of symptoms may be caused by deficiencies of different but often related enzymes. This requires, in addition to clinical investigations, specialized studies of metabolites in blood and urine and of enzymes in leukocytes or cultured skin fibroblasts[2,3]. A precise diagnosis is needed as early as possible to allow adequate treatment, therapy and genetic counselling. Unfortunately, the possibilities for effective therapy are limited or absent for most severe metabolic diseases. Moreover, the available therapies often mean a considerable burden for patient and parents. Parents faced with the high 25% recurrency risk in subsequent pregnancies may therefore refrain from having further children unless the option of prenatal diagnosis is available with termination of the pregnancy if the fetus is affected. More than 100 inborn errors of metabolism can be diagnosed prenatally, mostly by testing the primary enzyme defect, sometimes by the demonstration of accumulating metabolites or storage material and increasingly also by the detection of the gene mutations.

Indications for prenatal diagnosis

The risk of a couple of having offspring with a metabolic disorder appears usually only after a first affected child has been born. The diagnosis of an autosomal recessive disorder establishes both parents as heterozygotes; in subsequent pregnancies their risk of recurrence is 25%. It is thus essential that the diagnosis is made as soon as possible to allow adequate counselling of the parents and prenatal diagnosis if wanted.

In general there are few possibilities to prevent a first affected child. Although it is possible to detect heterozygosity by enzyme or mutation analysis, this is inefficient in the absence of an indication of an increased risk. For some disorders with high incidence in certain populations screening for heterozygosity has been effective, e.g. for β-thalassaemia in Sardinia by mutation analysis and for Tay–Sachs disease in Ashkenazi Jewish populations in the USA and in Israel (Ch. 32). Also in families in which a metabolic disorder has been diagnosed in one or more patients, screening of their relatives together with their partners may be considered, especially in populations with a tradition of consanguineous marriage and in small closed communities.

For the much smaller, but important, group of X-linked recessive diseases the situation is quite different. The main indication for prenatal diagnosis of X-linked diseases is again the recurrence risk to mothers of patients. However, as soon as this mother is recognized as a (possible) carrier, all female relatives (e.g. sisters and daughters of the heterozygous mother) have a high risk of being heterozygote and thus that their sons will be affected. To some degree carrier detection is possible for X-linked disorders by biochemical methods, but it is unfortunately not possible to rule out heterozygosity with certainty. Therefore, prenatal diagnosis was, until recently, indicated for all close female relatives of a patient with a severe X-linked disease.

This policy is now changing due to the rapidly increasing possibilities of reliable carrier detection by mutation or linkage analysis (see section on DNA analysis). The main advantage of this approach is the ability to exclude heterozygosity in females at risk, so that unnecessary prenatal analyses can be avoided.

Prerequisites for prenatal diagnosis

Before prenatal diagnosis can be offered, the diagnosis in the proband – usually the affected child in the family – must be precisely established. A clinical diagnosis alone is not sufficient as there are many groups of disorders with similar or overlapping clinical manifestations, but based on different primary enzyme defects. On the other hand, extensive clinical heterogeneity occurs among patients with the same enzyme deficiency, but sometimes with different levels of residual activity; this should be known before prenatal diagnosis is undertaken. For many disorders demonstration of the primary enzyme defect is the preferred (or the only possible) approach for prenatal diagnosis. However, for several diseases abnormal and specific metabolite patterns in amniotic fluid have proven to be indicative for the affected status of the fetus[4]. Characteristic patterns of metabolite concentrations in urine and/or blood are associated with several disorders of, for example, amino and organic acid metabolism. A clearly abnormal metabolite pattern in urine is, however, no guarantee for similar abnormalities in amniotic fluid of an affected fetus. This can only be established by the demonstration of these abnormalities in affected pregnancies. However, irrespective of the method used for prenatal diagnosis, enzyme or metabolite analysis, it is essential that a precise diagnosis of the disorder or its possible variant type in the index patient has been established, not only by metabolite analysis, but if possible also by enzyme assay.

Although many enzyme deficiencies can be demonstrated primarily in blood cells, it is advantageous or necessary to have cultured fibroblasts available from the proband and often also from the parents for preparation for future prenatal analysis. Especially if the disease has an early fatal outcome, it is essential to take a skin biopsy at the earliest occasion and store the cultured fibroblasts in a cell bank.

A further requirement for prenatal diagnosis by enzyme assay is that the enzyme is expressed in the available fetal material and that its deficiency is evident in an affected fetus. Both requirements are not always met. Several enzymes are only active in liver, muscle, blood or other tissues which are much less accessible than chorionic villi or amniotic fluid (cells). Even if the enzyme is active, its deficiency may be obscured by isoenzymes or other interfering enzymes which specifically act in the fetal cells. Therefore at least one precedent, showing enzyme deficiency in an affected fetus, is needed before reliable prenatal diagnosis can be offered. Naturally, before undertaking prenatal diagnosis the laboratory must establish the normal ranges of metabolites in the fluid or enzyme activities in villi and cultured fetal cells[4,5]. Reliable and sensitive (micro)methods must have been developed which are not vulnerable and allow accurate measurements even at low metabolite concentrations or, as far as enzyme assay is concerned, in the usually small amount of material available.

All these requirements can only be fulfilled efficiently if the few requests for prenatal diagnosis for each of the rare metabolic diseases are handled by relatively few specialized laboratories per country or even per continent. This will enable these few centres to gain and maintain experience and organize their service in such a way that they are ready any moment to accept and handle any request immediately. Expertise on the technical level, although essential, is not the only prerequisite. The whole logistics of the many steps involved should ideally be arranged according to an established scenario with optimal mutual communication and cooperation in a small team coordinated by the clinical geneticist.

In many cases it will however be necessary to send material over long distances to the laboratory, which is, if arranged carefully, quite well possible.

Chorionic villi

The great advantages of chorionic villus sampling (CVS) are the early stage of sampling (10–12 weeks) and the immediate testing which provides definitive results within a day for many enzymes; for some metabolic tests and also for some DNA analyses several days to a week are necessary. This means that in case of an affected fetus the pregnancy can be terminated by aspiration as opposed to prostaglandin induction of labour, which is necessary at 13 weeks or later.

Cells can be cultured efficiently from the villi, which allows some metabolic tests which can only be performed on cultured cells, or if necessary, to confirm previous results of the direct assay on the villi. A disadvantage of the use of long-term CV cultures, however, is the occasional growth of maternal cells in these cultures. Although rare, this contamination may occur in 1–2% of the cultures[6,7].

The suitability of CV for direct prenatal analyses has in the past decade been demonstrated in large series, comprising a few thousand analyses for some 60 different metabolic disorders, with practically complete enzyme deficiencies in affected pregnancies[5,8–10]. This shows that pure fetal CV tissue can be reliably selected without admixture of maternal tissue. CV can easily be sent in sterile culture medium at room temperature over long distances for 24–48 h. It is essential, however, that adequate selection, cleaning and primary examination of the quality and quantity of the villi is done immediately at the site of sampling.

Amniocentesis

Amniocentesis allows analysis of both the amniotic fluid and of cultured amniocytes. Approximately 100 metabolic diseases have been diagnosed prenatally in this way. Compared to CVS the late stage of amniocentesis (16 weeks) and the 2–3 weeks needed to culture sufficient cells for biochemical analysis is a decisive disadvantage. For this reason amniocentesis has largely been replaced by CVS for the diagnosis of most metabolic disorders. However, amniocentesis remains indicated when the analysis of CV or cultured CV cells is not sufficiently reliable or when there is a need to confirm the initial results of the assay(s) on CV or CV cells. For some diseases the analysis of metabolites in amniotic fluid either or not in combination with enzyme assay in the cells is a more attractive choice.

Direct measurement of metabolites in the fluid allows a rapid diagnosis within 1 or 2 days after amniocentesis in the 15th to 16th week. The reliability of this approach has been demonstrated for a considerable number of diseases[4]. Recently a small number of centres has investigated the possibility of earlier amniocentesis in the 12th to 13th week[11]. This seems an advantage, especially for chemical analysis of the fluid, at least if this allows a definitive diagnosis without the need of further analysis of cultured amniocytes. In principle early amniocentesis and CVS could be performed simultaneously, to allow direct enzyme assay and metabolite measurement as well.

Fetal blood and other fluids and tissues

Fetal blood and tissues such as liver and skin offer the possibility to detect disorders which are not expressed in CV or amniotic fluid (cells) (Chapter 36). Fetal blood sampling has been practised for the diagnosis of haemoglobinopathies by globin chain analysis but the much earlier analysis of DNA from CV has replaced this approach. Fetal blood sampling may still be useful if the pregnancy is too advanced for amniocentesis and cell culture (e.g. late presentation, growth failure of amniocytes or ultrasound indication of abnormalities). However, in this situation placental biopsy may be a better choice.

Fetal liver biopsy has been carried out at 18–20 weeks of gestation for the assay of enzymes which are not expressed in CV or amniocytes. Thus diagnoses have been made for ornithine transcarbamylase deficiency, primary hyperoxaluria type I and glycogenosis I (Tables 45.4 and 45.6). As the genes involved in these disorders have been cloned, mutation or linkage analysis using DNA from CV is a better option if the mutations or informative markers in the family have been identified. Fetal skin biopsies have been used for the prenatal diagnosis of genodermatoses by light- or electronmicroscopy (Ch. 46).

Enzyme analysis

Prerequisites for enzyme assays used in prenatal diagnosis are that they are accurate, sensitive and relatively invulnerable. Usually the assays are performed directly in microlitre volumes of cell or tissue homogenates using appropriate fluorogenic, chromogenic or radioactive substrates[5]. Some activities may, however, be assessed indirectly in intact cells or CV by tracing radiolabelled precursors through their metabolic pathways. Examples are the assay of decarboxylases by measuring the release of $[^{14}C]CO_2$ and of reactions which may be followed by the incorporation of the radioactive products into high-molecular macromolecules (i.e. proteins, nucleic acids, phospholipids)[5]. To allow reliable interpretation of the results, the enzyme activities in the fetal cells or villi from the pregnancy at risk are always compared with a set of appropriate controls from stored or simultaneously sampled fetal material and also with the activities in cultured fibroblasts of the proband, parents and controls. For direct enzyme assays in cell homogenates, samples can be used which have been stored at −80°C. However, for metabolic tests using living cells or villi, also living controls are needed, which requires careful tuning of sampling in the hospital and analysis in the laboratory. In all samples a reference enzyme is tested simultaneously to check for possible loss of activity due to transport and further handling of the sample.

Most enzyme tests can be done equally well in CV and cultured amniotic fluid cells. Some enzymes have higher, others a lower activity in CV compared to amniocytes[5]. The latter is true for α-L-iduronidase, which is deficient in the Hurler syndrome; in this case heterozygote levels of activity in CV may approach the patients' range, which may occasionally necessitate further analysis of cultured CV cells or rarely even require amniocentesis.

Metabolite analysis

For a few dozens of metabolic diseases the (postnatal) diagnosis is indicated by elevated concentrations of specific metabolites in plasma and urine[3]. Similarly, prenatal diagnosis of several of these diseases has appeared possible by the demonstration of increased metabolite levels in amniotic fluid[4]. However, the possibility of postnatal diagnosis in urine cannot be extrapolated to the prenatal situation as is demonstrated by the normal levels of branched chain amino acids in amniotic fluid of fetuses affected with maple syrup urine disease. Also fetal metabolite patterns may be influenced by maternal diet or condition. Therefore the reliability of metabolite measurement for prenatal diagnosis must be established by the demonstration of abnormal concentrations in several affected pregnancies. This has now been accomplished for a considerable number of disorders which are listed below (Tables 45.1 to 45.7).

As the concentration of the relevant metabolites in amniotic fluid is often low their quantitation may require special methods using reference compounds labelled with stable isotopes and gas chromatography/mass spectrometry[4]. For most purposes rapid transport of the (sterile) centrifuged or unprocessed fluid at ambient temperature is adequate; for some the centrifuged (cell-free) fluid must be sent while frozen on dry ice.

DNA analysis

The development of the DNA technology has provided great diagnostic possibilities which are especially important for the numerous genetic disorders for which a primary protein defect or a secondary metabolic defect is not known or not easily detectable. These disorders and the techniques used to demonstrate mutations or to show linkage of certain markers with the disease-causing gene are discussed in other chapters (38, 41–44). In another category of disorders specific metabolic defects are known but they are either not expressed in the available fetal material or the available assays are not fully specific or technically vulnerable. Again DNA analysis, if reliable and practicable, will be desirable, as will be indicated in the tables and in the text below. For the majority of the metabolic disorders listed and discussed in this chapter rapid and reliable prenatal diagnosis is possible by enzyme or metabolic tests and the question may be raised: which role should DNA analysis play here? Most of the genes involved have been cloned and sequenced and for many of these disorders numerous mutations have been identified. For many metabolic diseases only rare or unique mutations have been found, whereas for some other diseases one or more relatively common mutations have been identified besides rare mutations. Until now the search for mutations has mainly been undertaken for research purposes. For diagnostic use the search for mutations in each newly diagnosed patient is at present time-consuming and expensive, but the technology is still rapidly developing towards higher speed and efficiency. The main potential use of mutation analysis is carrier detection, which is of great importance for females in families with X-linked diseases and for autosomal recessive disorders in affected families with consanguineous marriages or in populations with a high frequency of a specific mutation. In most other situations carrier screening (in high-risk relatives and their low-risk partners) seems rather inefficient, even if only a set of the most frequent mutations in the population is tested.

Diagnostic experience

The number of metabolic disorders which have been detected prenatally has expanded rapidly in the first two decades of prenatal diagnosis to more than a hundred. The discovery of primary enzyme (protein) defects has slowed down in the past 10 years; however, the number of other genetic disorders diagnosable by DNA analysis is now strongly increasing. The number of pregnancies tested varies strongly per disease depending on its incidence, severity, and probably the availability (and reliability) of pre- and postnatal diagnostic services for the disease concerned. For most of the rare diseases, with a recurrency risk as the major indication for prenatal diagnosis, the number of analyses per year may vary worldwide from none to several dozens. For a few disorders with higher incidence in some populations and for which prenatal diagnosis is offered as a result of carrier screening, the numbers tested are higher (e.g. Tay–Sachs disease by enzyme assay and cystic fibrosis and sickle cell anaemia by mutation analysis). The accuracy of prenatal diagnosis has been high for the majority of disorders. Pitfalls have been reported for some disorders, especially in the early stage of prenatal analysis, and for some the prenatal analysis is still in an experimental stage.

In Tables 45.1 to 45.7 disorders are listed for which prenatal diagnoses have been made by biochemical analysis in affected pregnancies or for which prenatal diagnosis seems quite feasible. For some of the metabolic disorders listed the preferential use of DNA technology is indicated; genetic disorders without a known metabolic defect but detectable by DNA analysis are not included. References to reports on the diseases are given in the tables and in the text; to restrict their number preference has been given to original first reports on the one hand and recent reports describing improved methods or larger series on the other. Additional references may be found in previous reviews[12,13].

Lysosomal storage diseases

A considerable proportion of prenatal analyses made for metabolic disorders concern lysosomal storage diseases (in our centre in Rotterdam 50%). This group comprises approximately 35 diseases with a defect in the degradation of complex cellular constituents or in the transport of some small metabolites leading to the accumulation of these products in the lysosomes. Although there is a wide clinical heterogeneity in each of these diseases, most of them include severe forms with progressive neurological and/or somatic anomalies which warrant prenatal diagnosis. Large numbers of prenatal diagnoses have been made for some disorders with a relatively high incidence such as Tay–Sachs disease (a few thousands[14]), Krabbe, Hurler, Hunter and Pompe disease (worldwide at least many hundreds for each); by contrast the numbers are very small for some extremely rare disorders such as Farber, Wolman, Schindler disease and β-mannosidosis.

LIPIDOSES (TABLE 45.1)

SPHINGOLIPIDOSES

Using adequate and practicable fluorogenic artificial substrates for the enzyme assays, the prenatal diagnosis for

TABLE 45.1
Lysosomal storage diseases – disorders of (sphingo)lipid metabolism

Disease	Defect	Sample[a]	Reference
Fabry disease	α-Galactosidase	CV	Kleijer *et al.*[15]
Farber disease	Ceramidase	(CV), AC	Fensom *et al.*[16]
Gaucher disease	β-Glucosidase	CV	Besley *et al.*[17]
GM1-gangliosidosis	β-Galactosidase	CV	Besley and Broadhead[18]
GM2-gangliosidosis (Sandhoff)	Hexosaminidase A+B	CV	Giles *et al.*[19]
GM2-gangliosidosis (Tay–Sachs)	Hexosaminidase A	CV	Grebner and Wenger[20]
Krabbe disease	Galactocerebrosidase	CV, VC, AC	Kleijer *et al.*[21]
Metachromatic leukodystrophy	Arylsulphatase A	CV	Fensom *et al.*[22]
Niemann–Pick type A (and B)	Sphingomyelinase	CV	Vanier *et al.*[23]
Niemann–Pick disease type C	Cholesterol transport	VC, AC, DNA	Vanier *et al.*[24]
Wolman disease/CESD	Acid lipase	CV	van Diggelen *et al.*[25]
Mucolipidosis:			
Type I (sialidosis)	Neuraminidase	AC	Sasagasako *et al.*[26]
Type II (I-cell disease)	Multiple lysosomal enzymes	AF, AC	Besley *et al.*[27]
Type IV	Accumulation of lipids	AC	Zeigler *et al.*[28]
Galactosialidosis	Protective protein/cathepsin A	(CV), AC	Kleijer *et al.*[29]

[a]CV = chorionic villi are indicated as the material of choice if suitable, additional samples are indicated only if they are occasionally needed or preferred; (CV) = possible on CV but positive cases not yet reported; VC = cultured chorionic villus cells; AF = amniotic fluid; AC = cultured amniocytes; FB = fetal blood; FL = fetal liver; DNA = analysis on DNA from chorionic villi.

GM1-gangliosidosis, Fabry, Gaucher, Sandhoff and Tay–Sachs disease is relatively uncomplicated: there is usually clear distinction between the enzyme deficiency which is characteristic for an affected fetus and the sometimes low levels of activity found in case of heterozygosity. For the X-linked Fabry disease, fetal sex determination is needed before a low α-galactosidase activity is interpreted to indicate an affected male rather than a female carrier[15]. A potential complication in carrier detection and prenatal diagnosis of Tay–Sachs disease is the occurrence of a mutation in the hexosaminidase A gene, which causes low enzyme activity but no disease[30]. A similar phenomenon called 'pseudodeficiency' (PD) is well-known and much more frequent in metachromatic leukodystrophy (in 10–15% of normal alleles[30,31]). If PD is suspected in one of the parents of a patient by the finding of very low arylsulphatase A activity it is necessary to test for PD mutation in this parent and in a subsequent prenatal analysis in this family. Special attention to the possible involvement of PD is needed in enzyme-based testing for heterozygosity in individuals with a low population risk. The chance may then be high that a reduced enzyme activity is due to a PD mutation rather than to a disease-causing mutation: this is certainly true for metachromatic leukodystrophy but also for Tay–Sachs, Krabbe and Pompe disease and the Hurler and Sly syndromes[14,30]. Another complication in metachromatic leukodystrophy has been the low arylsulphatase A activity in CV and the interference of much higher activities of the interfering enzymes arylsulphatase B and C. This problem was solved by a simple modification of the assay: at 0°C the interfering enzymes were completely inactive, while considerable activity of arylsulphatase A remained[22].

Although artificial substrates are also available and useful for the assay of the defective enzymes in Krabbe[32], Niemann–Pick A[33] and Wolman disease[25] the use of radiolabelled natural substrates is preferred. Many hundreds of prenatal diagnoses have successfully been made for Krabbe disease both on cultured amniocytes and fresh CV.

However, the activity of galactocerebrosidase in CV is relatively low, which may occasionally create a problem in distinguishing between a true enzyme deficiency and a low heterozygote level. In rare cases it may be necessary to exclude an affected fetus definitively by testing cultured villus cells or even amniocytes (in our centre this has been necessary in four out of 80 pregnancies at risk tested for Krabbe disease on CV).

The primary defect in Niemann–Pick disease type C is not precisely known but a cholesterol transport defect has been the basis of two successful prenatal tests: a cholesterol esterification test and a simple staining test using filipin to demonstrate accumulated cholesterol in the lysosomes[24]. The responsible gene has recently been identified and the first mutations have been demonstrated[34]. Farber disease has been diagnosed on amniocytes[16] and excluded on CV[35] using radiolabelled ceramide. Recently a new indirect assay using cultured cells has been described which may facilitate the (prenatal) diagnosis of this rare disease[36].

MUCOLIPIDOSES (TABLE 45.1)

Prenatal diagnosis of sialidosis (or mucolipidosis I) by analysis of amniocytes has been reported[26]. Fresh CV are less suitable because of the very low activity and the instability of neuraminidase[29]. Galactosialidosis may be detectable by a secondary β-galactosidase deficiency in CV like previously shown on amniocytes[37]; however, it seems recommendable to test also the primary defective protein, cathepsin A, which is known to protect and activate β-galactosidase and neuraminidase by forming a complex with them. An affected fetus was recently diagnosed by cathepsin A deficiency in cultured CV cells[38], but this should also be feasible by directly using fresh CV[29]. I-cell disease (or mucolipidosis II) has been diagnosed in CV by measuring the responsible defect of phosphorylation of lysosomal enzymes[39] but a more convenient and reliable approach is the demonstration of increased activities of several lysosomal enzymes in amniotic fluid (even at 10–12 weeks)[27,40] and of reduced activities of the same enzymes in cultured amniocytes (or CV cells).[27,40] The primary defect of mucolipidosis type IV is not known but prenatal diagnosis can be made by electron microscopy[28] and by phospholipid and ganglioside analysis of cultured amniocytes[28].

GLYCOPROTEINOSES (TABLE 45.2)

The glycoproteinoses listed in Table 45.2 are rare diseases, although higher incidences occur for aspartylglucosaminuria[41] and Salla disease[57] in Finland. All disorders, except Salla disease, can be diagnosed by convenient and sensitive enzyme assays using fluorogenic substrates[58]. Prenatal diagnosis for these disorders may seem rather uncomplicated. However, caution is needed with respect to residual enzyme activity in α-mannosidosis (K_M mutants)[43,59] and to strongly different levels of α-fucosidase activity in fibroblast-like and epithelial amniocytes (lower and higher activity respectively)[42] and CV (high activity)[5]. In fact the experience is very limited especially for fucosidosis (not diagnosed by CV), β-mannosidosis (only one heterozygote diagnosed by CV)[44] and Schindler disease[60] (not done).

Severe infantile sialic acid storage disease has been diagnosed by increased levels of free sialic acid in amniocytes and CV as detected by chemical assay and by electron-microscopy[45]. In Salla disease the lysosomal accumulation of free sialic acid is much less pronounced; the level in amniocytes seems too low for reliable diagnosis[57]. Haplotype or mutation analysis should be preferred for this disorder[57].

Various types of neuronal ceroid lipofuscinosis (CLN) may be diagnosed prenatally by electronmicroscopic study of CV tissue[46,47], but special care and expertise is needed. The identification of genes and mutations has improved the options for

TABLE 45.2
Lysosomal storage diseases – disorders of glyco(lipo)protein and mucopolysaccharide metabolism

Disease	Defect	Sample[a]	Reference
Glycoproteinoses:			
Aspartylglucosaminuria	Aspartylglucosaminidase	CV	Aula *et al.*[41]
Fucosidosis	α-Fucosidase	(CV), AC	Poenaru *et al.*[42]
α-Mannosidosis	α-Mannosidase	CV	Petushkova[43]
β-Mannosidosis	β-Mannosidase	(CV)	Kleijer *et al.*[44]
Salla/sialic acid storage disease	Sialic acid transport	CV	Lake *et al.*[45]
Schindler disease	α-*N*-acetylgalactosaminidase	(CV)	
Ceroid lipofuscinosis:	Accumulation of lipopigments		
Infantile (Santavuori)	Palmitoyl protein thioesterase	CV[b], DNA	Rapola *et al.*[46]
Juvenile (Batten)	CLN 3 protein	CV, DNA	Munroe *et al.*[47]
Mucopolysaccharidoses (MPS) type:			
I Hurler	α-L-iduronidase	CV, VC, AF	Young *et al.*[48]
II Hunter	Iduronate 2-sulphatase	CV	Kleijer *et al.*[49]
IIIA Sanfilippo A	Heparansulphamidase	CV	Kleijer *et al.*[50]
IIIB Sanfilippo B	*N*-acetylglucosaminidase	CV	Minelli *et al.*[51]
IIIC Sanfilippo C	Acetyl-CoA:α-glucosaminide *N*-acetyltransferase	CV	Di Natale *et al.*[52]
IIID Sanfilippo D	*N*-acetylglucosamine 6-S'ase	(CV, AF)	
IVA Morquio A	*N*-acetylgalactosamine 6-S'ase	CV[c], AF, AC	Zhao *et al.*[53]
IVB Morquio B	β-Galactosidase	(CV, AF, AC)	—
VI Maroteaux–Lamy	Arylsulphatase B	(CV), AF, AC	Kleijer *et al.*[54]
VII Sly	β-glucuronidase	CV	Chabas and Guardiola[55]
Mucosulphatidosis	Multiple sulphatases	CV, (AF, AC)	Patrick *et al.*[56]
Other:			
Glycogenosis II (Pompe) (see Table 45.4)			
Cystinosis (see Table 45.6)			
Hydrops fetalis, see text			

[a]See notes to Table I
[b]Done by PPT assay[64]
[c]Done on CV, unpublished

prenatal diagnosis, e.g. for the infantile type (Santavuori, CLN1)[61] and the juvenile type (Batten, CLN3)[62]. The infantile (CLN1) type as well as some juvenile (CLN1) variants are caused by a deficiency of PPT[61,63]. The feasibility of prenatal diagnosis by using a newly developed, convenient enzyme assay was recently demonstrated. In two affected pregnancies complete deficiency of palmitoyl protein thioesterase (PPT) activity was found in CV and in amniocytes respectively[64].

MUCOPOLYSACCHARIDOSES (TABLE 45.2)

A general approach for the diagnosis of all MPS types is the two-dimensional electrophoresis of glycosaminoglycans in amniotic fluid. The reliability of this method was shown by the study of a large series of fluids from pregnancies at risk (n = 72) by Mossman and Patrick in 1982[65] and the successful use has been described in many of the literature references given in this section, e.g. in reports from the author's laboratory on MPS IIIA[50], IIIB[66], IIIC[67], IVA[53] and VII[68]. This experience concerns largely pregnancies at 15–16 weeks of gestation; our experience in earlier pregnancy is limited to one clearly positive sample obtained after diagnosis of MPS II by CV and termination of pregnancy at 11 weeks. Another general method, which has been useful for the diagnosis of several MPS types (except MPS IV)[69] is the incorporation of ^{35}S-labelled sulphate in accumulating mucopolysaccharides in cultured amniocytes[70]. However, this method has become obsolete since enzyme assays on CV and GAG-electrophoresis of amniotic fluid have become more convenient and reliable and can be performed much earlier.

Artificial substrates are now available which allow convenient enzyme assays for the diagnosis of all MPS types[71], except type II which still requires a radiolabelled substrate. Some of these substrates have only recently been developed and applied for pre- and postnatal diagnosis of MPS IIIA[50], IIIC[67], IIID[72] and IVA[53]. The first-trimester diagnosis of the Hurler syndrome may occasionally be complicated as a result of the generally low activity of α-L-iduronidase in CV[48]. This hampers the distinction between affected fetuses and carriers with relatively or even very low activity due to a 'pseudodeficiency allele'[73]. Further investigation of cultured CV-cells or amniocentesis and GAG-electrophoresis may then be necessary[70]. In our experience this was necessary in 2 out of 51 pregnancies at risk for MPS I tested in the first trimester. Many mutations have been identified in the IDUA gene, some of which are rather common[74]. As the Hunter syndrome is X-linked only male fetuses are at risk; the iduronate sulphatase activity in males will be normal or deficient but not intermediate. Therefore the diagnosis of an affected fetus is only justified after establishing the male fetal sex. Very low activity may occur in amniocytes[75] or in CV[76] from a female fetus due to non-random X-chromosome inactivation or selection of one cell type. The chance that the female fetus would be affected seems extremely small but is not excluded[77] and therefore ascertainment may be wanted by electrophoresis of glycosaminoglycans in amniotic fluid. Many unique mutations have been identified in the IDUS gene but in 20% of the families this concerns a large deletion or a gross rearrangement which allows rapid carrier detection in female relatives in these families[78].

The occurrence of four types of Sanfilippo disease, each caused by a different enzyme defect, emphasizes the general requirement to confirm a clinical diagnosis by enzyme investigation. This has become much easier since convenient artificial substrates for all four enzymes became available. Relatively few prenatal diagnoses have been reported, although the incidence of Sanfilippo disease may be as high as Hurler and Hunter disease. The reason is probably that in the past, families were already completed before the diagnosis in the first affected child was made. The recent improvement of the enzyme assays should promote early postnatal diagnosis and prenatal diagnosis as well. First- and second-trimester diagnoses have been described for the types A[50], B[51,66,79] and C[52,67,80] but not yet for the extremely rare type D. For MPS IIIA at least one common mutation has been found[81].

Very few prenatal diagnoses have been made for the remaining MPS types and multiple sulphatase deficiency[56]. Diagnoses have been made for Morquio A[69] and Maroteaux–Lamy syndrome[54] in the second trimester but enzyme analysis of CV is possible as well[53,71]. MPS VII (Sly) has been diagnosed in several pregnancies affected with fetal hydrops[68,82]. β-Glucuronidase deficiency was demonstrated once in CV obtained at 17 weeks[55] and recently also in the 12th week[82]. The occurrence of pseudodeficiency alleles should be kept in mind and to anticipate complications in prenatal diagnosis, parental cells may be tested[83].

HYDROPS FETALIS

Fetal hydrops is associated with a large number of genetic and non-genetic conditions (see Ch. 56). Blood group incompatibilities, cardiovascular diseases, chromosome abnormalities and haematologic disorders (e.g. α-thalassaemia) are major causes but also lysosomal storage diseases should be kept in mind as a possible cause of fetal hydrops in fetuses or newborns. Cases of fetal hydrops have been described or briefly mentioned in a large number of reports which have been referred in reviews on hydrops fetalis in general[84,85] or in lysosomal diseases in particular[86]. The diseases are: Gaucher disease[84,85,87], GM_1-gangliosidosis[84,86], Farber disease[86], galactosialidosis[29,38,86], Niemann–Pick type C[86], mucolipidosis I[26,84,86] and II[84,86] sialic acid storage disease [64,88] and the mucopolysaccharidoses I[86], IVA[84,86] and especially VII[68,84–86].

The incidence of fetal hydrops due to lysosomal disorders may have been underestimated[84,85] because lysosomal enzymes have usually not been tested in cases indicated by echography and after miscarriage or (still)birth. In such cases it is essential that appropriate tissues, cells or fluids are sampled to allow routine screening for several lysosomal disorders after the major causes of fetal hydrops have been excluded[89]. Several of the prenatal diagnoses reported in the references in this section became possible only after finding the (lysosomal) cause of fetal hydrops in a previous pregnancy.

Peroxisomal disorders (Table 45.3)

Peroxisomal disorders are a group of diseases with often severe neurological involvement, caused by one or more of the peroxisomal functions such as the β-oxidation of very long chain fatty acids (VLCFA), ether-phospholipid biosynthesis, cholesterol biosynthesis, etc. In some disorders there is a generalized or multiple loss of peroxisomal functions due to the complete or partial deficiency of peroxisomal assembly respectively, whereas in others single peroxisomal enzymes are deficient. Clinical and biochemical aspects of some 20 peroxisomal disorders have recently been reviewed[94,95]. Many prenatal diagnoses have been made for the generalized severe Zellweger syndrome[90] (several hundreds) and to a much less extent for X-linked adrenoleukodystrophy (ALD) and some other disorders[91]. Several different methods may be used to demonstrate the metabolic abnormalities. For the Zellweger syndrome and for rhizomelic chondrodysplasia punctata the methods of choice, using fresh CV are dihydroxyacetonephosphate acyltransferase (DHAPAT) assay and immunoblot analysis of acyl-CoA oxidase or peroxisomal thiolase[95]. Other techniques such as the measurement of VLCFA levels and plasmologen biosynthesis are valuable alternatives using cultured CV cells or amniocytes[95]. In case of amniocentesis the measurement of bile acid intermediates is an important tool in the prenatal diagnosis of disorders in which bile acid biosynthesis is impaired[96]. For X-linked ALD and other peroxisomal β-oxidation defects cultured CV or AF cells are needed to measure VLCFA levels (C26:0/C22:0 ratio) and β-oxidation of VLCFA[95]. However, this approach has not always been successful. Therefore the use of DNA analysis may be considered. Intragenic and extragenic polymorphisms will allow segregation analysis in many families. Direct mutation analysis may be preferable both for prenatal diagnosis and carrier detection but this requires the search for a new mutation in practically each family[97]. The defective enzyme in hyperoxaluria type I (alanine: glyoxylate aminotransferase, AGT) is only expressed in liver. Prenatal diagnosis by fetal liver biopsy has been made but clearly the analysis of the AGT gene in DNA isolated from CV would be the method of choice whenever this is possible[92].

Mevalonic aciduria is caused by a defect in the first part of the cholesterol biosynthetic pathway which takes place in peroxisomes. Prenatal diagnosis of these disorders has been made by the demonstration of mevalonic acid in amniotic fluid[93], but should also be possible by direct or indirect enzyme assay in CV[98].

Disorders of carbohydrate metabolism (Table 45.4)

Only limited use is made of prenatal investigation for galactosaemia because this is a treatable disease. Unfortunately the long-term results of treatment appear not completely satisfactory[110]. Sometimes prenatal diagnosis is requested to decide whether maternal galactose restriction during pregnancy should be continued or not; however, it seems questionable whether maternal restriction is effective at all[111]. Prenatal diagnosis of galactosaemia is preferably done by enzyme assay in CV[99] or by galactitol measurement in amniotic fluid[99]; both methods provide a reliable diagnosis within 1 or 2 days after sampling. The presence of a common mutation in the GALT gene will allow carrier detection in many families[112].

TABLE 45.3
Peroxisomal disorders

Disease	Defect	Sample[a]	Reference
Zellweger syndrome	Generalized loss of peroxisomal functions	CV, AF, AC	Schutgens *et al.*[90]
Neonatal adrenoleukodystrophy		CV, AF, AC	
Infantile Refsum disease		CV, AF, AC	
Rhizomelic chondrodysplasia punctata	Partial loss of peroxisomal functions	CV, AC	
Zellweger-like syndrome		CV, AC	Wanders *et al.*[91]
X-linked adrenoleukodystrophy	Peroxisomal VLCFA-CoA synthetase	DNA, VC, AC	
Pseudo neonatal ALD	Acyl-CoA oxidase	CV, AC	
Pseudo Zellweger syndrome	Peroxisomal thiolase	CV, AF, AC	
Primary hyperoxaluria type I	Alanine:glyoxylate aminotransferase	DNA, FL	Danpure and Rumsby[92]
Mevalonic aciduria	Mevalonate kinase	(CV), AF, AC	Hoffmann *et al.*[93]

[a]See notes to Table 45.1

TABLE 45.4
Disorders of carbohydrate metabolism

Disease	Enzyme defect	Sample[a]	Reference
Galactosaemia	Galactose 1P-uridyltransferase	CV, AF, AC	Jakobs *et al.*[99]
Glycogenosis Ia	Glucose 6-P'ase	DNA, FL	Golbus *et al.*[100]
Glycogenosis II	Lysosomal α-glucosidase	CV	Kleijer *et al.*[101]
Glycogenosis III	Debranching enzyme	CV	Shin *et al.*[102]
Glycogenosis IV	Branching enzyme	(VC), AC	Brown and Brown[103]
Complex IV deficiency	Cytochrome C oxidase	CV	Ruitenbeek *et al.*[104]
PC deficiency	Pyruvate carboxylase	CV[b], AC	Marsac *et al.*[105]
PDH deficiency	Pyruvate dehydrogenase	DNA	Brown and Brown[106]
GK deficiency	Glycerolkinase	AF, AC, (CV)	Borresen *et al.*[107]
PK deficiency	Pyruvate kinase	DNA, (FB)	Rouger *et al.*[108]
GPI deficiency	Glucose phosphate isomerase	AC, (CV)	Whitelaw *et al.*[109]
CDG syndrome type Ia	Phosphomannomutase	(CV)[c]	
CDG syndrome type Ib	Phosphomannose isomerase	(CV)[c]	

[a]See notes to Table 45.1
[b]Made: Kleijer, unpublished
[c]Possible

The glycogen storage diseases (GSD) comprise more than 10 diseases but prenatal diagnosis seems only relevant for the types I to IV. Type II or Pompe's disease is a lysosomal storage disease caused by the deficiency of acid α-glucosidase (GAA). The incidence is relatively high and many hundreds of prenatal diagnoses have been made for the severe infantile form[101]. Direct enzyme analysis of CV is the method of choice not only because of the early result but also because of the high activity of GAA in CV compared to AF cells, which facilitates reliable diagnosis[101]. A few common mutations in the GAA gene are known, which is useful for carrier detection and for prenatal diagnosis in special cases[101].

As glucose 6-phosphatase is only expressed in liver, prenatal diagnosis by enzyme assay of GSD type I requires fetal liver biopsy[100]. Mutation analysis will thus be preferred if possible[113]. Direct enzyme analysis in CV has successfully been used for the diagnosis of GSD III[102,114] but for type IV prenatal diagnoses have so far only been made by investigating amniocytes[103].

Prenatal diagnosis for respiratory chain disorders, e.g. complex IV deficiency has been undertaken[104] but its general reliability remains to be established. The possibilities for prenatal diagnosis of defective mitochondrial function which are encoded by mtDNA are limited[115] as it is not clear whether CV or cultured cells are representative for other fetal tissues. Two disorders of pyruvate metabolism are also mitochondrial but nuclear DNA encoded. Pyruvate carboxylase (PC) deficiency has been demonstrated in AF cells[105] and in CV in the author's laboratory (unpublished). Pyruvate dehydrogenase (PDH) deficiency is usually demonstrated in muscle tissue; the activity in fibroblasts, amniocytes and CV is probably not sufficiently specific to allow reliable diagnosis[106]. The major form of PDH deficiency is X-linked; prenatal diagnosis will be possible in most families by DNA analysis[106].

Another X-linked disorder, glycerolkinase (GK) deficiency, has been diagnosed by the demonstration of accumulated glycerol in AF and of the enzyme deficiency in AF cells[107] but direct or indirect enzyme testing of CV also seems feasible. The prenatal diagnosis of the red cell pyruvate kinase (PK) deficiency, which causes non-spherocytic haemolytic anaemia, should preferably be attempted by DNA rather than by enzyme analysis. Polymorphisms and common mutations are known in different populations[116] and prenatal diagnosis has recently been reported[108]. Glucosephosphate isomerase (GPI) deficiency is another defect causing haemolytic anaemia and occasionally fetal hydrops. Prenatal diagnosis by enzyme analysis in AF cells has been reported[109] and should be possible in CV as well[117].

Finally Table 45.4 includes the carbohydrate-deficient glycoprotein (CDG) syndrome type I, which is caused by the primary deficiency of phosphomannomutase in most cases[118] or of phosphomannose isomerase in a minority of type I patients. Both enzymes are expressed in CV allowing early and rapid prenatal diagnosis.

Disorders of nucleotide metabolism and DNA repair (Table 45.5)

The diagnosis of the X-linked Lesch–Nyhan syndrome by direct enzyme analysis in CV has been reported[119,128] and is according to our experience with CV in 35 pregnancies tested with three affected fetuses rapid (1–2 days) and reliable. Complications have been reported, which only emphasize the need for proper selection of the CV sample, establishment of the fetal sex and of sufficient experience with the HPRT assay in CV. In case of any doubt (e.g. intermediate activity in a male fetus) cultured CV cells may be tested for confirmation. Linkage analysis or direct mutation analysis is especially

TABLE 45.5
Disorders of nucleotide metabolism and DNA repair

Disease	Defect	Sample[a]	Reference
Lesch–Nyhan syndrome	Hypoxanthine phosphoribosyltransferase	CV	Gibbs *et al.*[119]
ADA deficiency	Adenosine deaminase	CV	Dooley *et al.*[120]
PNP deficiency	Purine nucleoside phosphorylase	CV	Pérignon *et al.*[121]
Adenylosuccinase deficiency	Adenylosuccinase	(CV, DNA)[b]	
DHPDH deficiency	Dihydropyrimidine dehydrogenase	AF	Jakobs *et al.*[122]
Combined xanthine and sulphite oxidase deficiency	Molybdenum cofactor/ sulphite oxidase	CV, AF	Johnson *et al.*[123]
Xeroderma pigmentosum	DNA repair	VC, AC	Halley *et al.*[124]
Trichothiodystrophy	DNA repair	VC, AC	Sarasin *et al.*[125]
Cockayne syndrome	DNA repair/transcription	VC, AC	Lehmann *et al.*[126]
Ataxia telangiectasia	Radioresistant DNA synthesis	VC, AC	Kleijer *et al.*[127]

[a]See notes to Table 45.1
[b]Possible

important for carrier detection in female relatives[129]. This is illustrated in our own results: only seven affected fetuses were found in 77 pregnancies at risk. Probably more than half of these prenatal tests could have been prevented by timely exclusion of heterozygosity of the pregnant women.

Adenosine deaminase (ADA) and purine nucleoside phosphorylase (PNP) deficiencies have been demonstrated in CV[120,121] and in AF cells[130,131] from pregnancies at risk for these two rare immunodeficiencies. Molybdenum cofactor deficiency, which results in the combined deficiency of xanthine and sulphite oxidase, can be diagnosed by testing the latter enzyme in CV[123]; in case of amniocentesis enzyme assay in AF cells may be combined with S-sulphocysteine measurement in the fluid[132]. Dihydropyrimidine dehydrogenase (DHPDH) deficiency may not be detectable in CV but prenatal diagnosis has been made by measurement of increased levels of thymine and uracil in AF[122].

For the demonstration of the DNA repair defects xeroderma pigmentosum (XP), trichothiodystrophy (TTD), Cockayne syndrome (CS) and also of ataxia telangiectasia (AT) several methods are available which all require cultured CV (or AF) cells rather than fresh CV. Repair of DNA damage may be studied by direct measurement of repair DNA synthesis (XP[124,133], TTD[125]) or by studying the recovery of RNA or DNA synthesis after UV exposure (CS[126], XP[133], TTD[125]). AT is demonstrated by increased, so-called radioresistant DNA synthesis (RDS) after X-irradiation of cultured CV or AF cells[127], but the test is practised in very few places. The (major) gene responsible for this relatively frequent disease has been identified and many different mutations have been found[134]. This will probably lead to replacement of the RDS test by DNA analysis for prenatal diagnosis in many families. However, as for all metabolic disorders and especially in this group of DNA repair disorders, it is essential that the suspected biochemical defect is demonstrated in the proband in the family before prenatal diagnosis or even mutation analysis is considered.

Disorders of amino acid and organic acid metabolism (Table 45.6)

Many inborn errors of amino and organic acid metabolism appear in Table 45.6, but the list is not complete. Some disorders have already been listed in Table 45.3 and 45.4; other disorders have either been omitted or included but not discussed because prenatal diagnosis is seldom requested as they are rare or usually mild.

Phenylketonuria is a treatable disease for which prenatal diagnosis is in most countries rarely done. However, as the limitations of treatment are becoming clear and since DNA analysis of CV has become available, this option may be considered more often[159]. Similarly DNA analysis will be the method of choice for two of the urea cycle disorders (OTC and CPS deficiency) whenever this is possible[160]; the option of enzyme assay in fetal liver is clearly less favourable but its feasibility has been demonstrated[149,150,161]. DNA analysis will also be chosen for the prenatal diagnosis of Canavan disease if the mutations in the index patient can be found[162]; aspartoacylase activity in CV and AF cells is too low, but *N*-acetylaspartate measurement in AF at 16 weeks or later is probably reliable[137]. Tyrosinaemia type I can be diagnosed reliably in most but perhaps not all pregnancies at risk by increased succinylacetone in AF[163], probably even by early amniocentesis[138], but also fumarylacetoacetase assay in CV[138] and mutation analysis have been used[164].

The diagnosis of non-ketotic hyperglycinaemia can be made by the defective glycine cleavage system which can be detected in CV but not in cultured cells[139,165].

For several disorders, tests have been designed to study the relevant metabolic pathways in intact cultured cells or in uncultured CV; such tests are often more sensitive and more practicable than the direct enzyme assay in cell or tissue homogenates[5]. For example the lysosomal transport defect in cystinosis can be demonstrated by studying the uptake and

TABLE 45.6
Disorders of amino acid and organic acid metabolism

Disease	Enzyme defect	Sample[a]	Reference
Phenylketonuria	Phenylalaninehydroxylase	DNA	Lidsky *et al.*[135]
Phenylketonuria II	Dihydropteridine reductase	AC	Blau *et al.*[136]
Phenylketonuria III	6-pyruvoyl tetrahydropterin synthase	AF, FB	Blau *et al.*[136]
Canavan disease	Aspartoacylase	DNA, AF	Bennett *et al.*[137]
Tyrosinaemia I	Fumarylacetoacetase	DNA, CV, AF	Jakobs *et al.*[138]
Non-ketotic hyperglycinaemia	Glycine cleavage system	CV	Hayasaka *et al.*[139]
Cystinosis	Lysosomal cystine transport	CV	Patrick *et al.*[140]
Maple syrup urine disease	BCKA decarboxylase	CV	Kleijer *et al.*[141]
Isovaleric acidaemia	Isovaleryl CoA-dehydrogenase	CV, AF	Kleijer *et al.*[142]
3-MCC deficiency	3-methylcrotonyl CoA carboxylase	(CV, AF)	Jakobs *et al.*[4]
3-MGA deficiency	3-methylglutaconyl-CoA hydratase	(CV, AF)	Chitayat *et al.*[143]
3-HMG deficiency	3-hydroxy 3-methylglutaryl CoA lyase	CV, AF, AC	Chalmers *et al.*[144]
Multiple carboxylase deficiency	Holocarboxylase synthase	AF, AC	Packman *et al.*[145]
	biotinidase	(CV)	Chalmers *et al.*[146]
Citrullinaemia	Argininosuccinate synthetase	CV, AF	Kleijer *et al.*[147]
Argininosuccinic aciduria	Argininosuccinate lyase	CV, AF	Vimal *et al.*[148]
CPS deficiency	Carbamoyl phosphate synthetase	DNA, FL	Piceni Sereni *et al.*[149]
OTC deficiency	Ornithine carbamoyl transferase	DNA, FL	Rodeck *et al.*[150]
HHH syndrome	Ornithine transport	AC(CV)	Shih *et al.*[151]
Gyrate atrophy	Ornithine amino transferase	(CV, AC)	Shih *et al.*[151]
Propionic acidaemia	Propionyl CoA carboxylase	CV, AF	Rolland *et al.*[152]
Methylmalonic aciduria	Methylmalonyl CoA mutase	AF, AC, CV	Fowler *et al.*[153]
Glutaric aciduria I	Glutaryl CoA dehydrogenase	CV, VC, AF	Christensen[154]
Glutaric aciduria II	ETF or ETF dehydrogenase	AF, AC	Yamaguchi *et al.*[155]
MCAD deficiency	Medium chain acyl CoA dehydrogenase	DNA, AC	Bennett *et al.*[156]
VLCAD deficiency	Very long chain acyl CoA dehydrogenase	CV, AC, DNA	Nada *et al.*[157]
LCHAD deficiency	Long chain 3-hydroxyacyl CoA dehydrogenase	CV, DNA	Von Döbeln *et al.*[158]

[a]See notes to Table 45.1

accumulation of free ^{35}S-cystine in intact cells or CV[140,166]. Several disorders of leucine catabolism are amenable to prenatal diagnosis by direct or indirect enzyme assay or by measurement of specific metabolites. Increased metabolite levels have been demonstrated in amniotic fluid for isovaleric acidaemia[142] and 3-hydroxymethylglutaric aciduria[167] but not for maple syrup urine disease[4]. The latter disorder can be reliably diagnosed by measuring the decarboxylation of radiolabelled leucine in intact CV, providing results within a day. Since the first reported first-trimester diagnosis[141] we have successfully investigated CV from 45 pregnancies at risk, finding 12 affected fetuses, mostly after long-distance transport of the samples. Several prenatal diagnoses of isovaleric acidaemia have been made by showing strongly increased levels of isovalerylglycine in the amniotic fluid; recently a first diagnosis was made by the demonstration of defective incorporation of radiolabelled isovaleric acid in proteins in CV[142].

Incorporation tests using CV, as well as metabolite measurements in AF allow reliable prenatal diagnosis of two urea cycle disorders, citrullinaemia and argininosuccinic aciduria. A collaborative European report[161] of prenatal diagnosis of urea cycle disorders has summarized the results in 183 pregnancies at risk, with 47 affected fetuses, for the two disorders together. Some pitfalls in this large series and in other reports[148,168], were mainly related to the use of cultured AF and CV cells or may have been caused by maternal tissue in the CV sample; they should be avoidable.

Propionic acidaemia can be diagnosed reliably both by direct assay of propionyl CoA carboxylase in CV[152] and by measurement of methylcitrate in AF at 14–16 weeks as usual[169] or earlier[152]. The direct assay of the defective mutase in CV for methylmalonic acidaemia is possible[153] but not routinely available; fortunately measurement of methylmalonic acid in AF allows a reliable diagnosis[169]. Both types of glutaric aciduria, I and II, can be diagnosed by increased concentrations of glutaric acid in amniotic fluid[155,169,170], whereas type I has also been diagnosed in the first trimester by glutaryl CoA dehydrogenase deficiency in CV[154]. By far the most prevalent disorder of mitochondrial fatty acid oxidation is the medium chain acyl-CoA dehydrogenase deficiency. Early diagnosis of this often mild or even asymptomatic disorder is indicated in families at risk to anticipate severe complications. Prenatal diagnosis is possible by direct or indirect enzyme assay in cultured AF cells[156]. However, as a single highly prevalent mutation (A985G) is responsible for MCAD deficiency, prenatal or immediate neonatal screening for this mutation will be applicable in most families[171]. A common mutation is also present in LCHAD deficiency[172], but in contrast large mutational heterogeneity was reported for VLCAD deficiency[173]. Both disorders can however be diagnosed by direct enzyme assay[157,158,172,173] or by measurement of the production of the respective acylcarnitines[157].

Other disorders (Table 45.7)

Most of the disorders listed in Table 45.7 can be diagnosed prenatally by metabolic and by DNA methods; for several the DNA approach will be preferred if informative data are available. The first four disorders of the list are X-linked. This makes the option of DNA based carrier detection in females important for at least the two severe diseases, the Menkes[187] and Lowe[188] syndromes. Direct copper measurement in CV has provided many correct and early diagnoses for Menkes disease, but this method is susceptible to copper contamination[174,187]. Alternatively cultured amniocytes may be used for uptake studies with ^{64}Cu or with the more practical radioisotope ^{110m}Ag[189]. The primary enzyme defect in Lowe syndrome has recently been discovered but a practical enzyme assay is not (yet) available[188]. To anticipate complications at birth (delay of labour and failure of cervix dilatation) X-linked ichthyosis may easily be demonstrated in CV or placental biopsy material, but also the measurement of dihydroepiandrosterone sulphate in AF or specific steroid profiles in maternal urine and blood may be diagnostic[175]. For chronic granulomatous disease DNA analysis will be preferred for prenatal diagnosis as the available tests of enzyme activity in neutrophils require fetal blood[190]. Smith–Lemli–Opitz syndrome has been diagnosed by increased levels of 7-dehydrocholesterol in amniotic fluid[191] and in CV[184] but also direct assay of 7-DHC reductase in CV should allow first-trimester diagnosis[192].

References are given in Table 45.7 for prenatal diagnoses made by biochemical analysis. However, for most of these disorders the use of mutation or linkage analysis will be preferred, e.g. for the porphyrias[179], hypercholesterolaemia[193], leprechaunism[194], hypophosphatasia[182], and the collagen disorders[183]. Although DNA analysis is also the method of choice for prenatal diagnosis of cystic fibrosis, cases may remain where neither the mutations nor informative markers are available (Ch. 43). Microvillar enzyme testing in AF at 17–18 weeks then allows rapid prenatal diagnosis which may, in an experienced centre, reduce the risk from 25% to 1–2% ([195,196] and our personal updated experience in a series of 250 pregnancies at risk).

Past, present and future

The past decades have shown great progress in the prenatal diagnosis of inborn errors of metabolism in several respects. First, the number of disorders which can be diagnosed prenatally has increased rapidly to approximately 100 in the first two decades (1970–1990). In the past decade especially, DNA-based techniques have provided new possibilities to diagnose disorders for which the primary protein defect is not known or difficult to assess. Also for some of the disorders diagnosed thus far through their defective metabolic func-

TABLE 45.7
Other disorders

Disease	Defect	Sample[a]	Reference
Menkes syndrome	Copper transport (ATP'ase)	AC, CV	Tønnesen *et al.*[174]
Lowe syndrome	Phosphatidyl inositol 4,5biP5P'ase	DNA	
X-linked ichthyosis	Steroid sulphatase	CV, AF	Hähnel *et al.*[175]
Chronic granulomatous disease	NADPH-oxidase	DNA, FB	Huu *et al.*[176]
Congenital adrenohyperplasia	21-hydroxylase	DNA, AF	Raux-Demay *et al.*[177]
Acute intermittent porphyria	Porphobilinogen deaminase	AC, DNA	Sassa *et al.*[178]
Congenital erythropoietic porphyria	Uroporphyrin I	AF, DNA	Ged *et al.*[179]
Familial hypercholesterolaemia	LDL receptor	DNA, AC,	Brown *et al.*[180]
Leprechaunism	Insulin receptor	DNA, (CV), (AC)	Maassen *et al.*[181]
Hypophosphatasia	Alkaline phosphatase	CV, DNA	Brock and Barron[182]
Collagen disorders (E-D; OI)	Collagen	DNA, CV, VC	Raghunath *et al.*[183]
Smith–Lemli–Opitz syndrome	7-dehydrocholesterol reductase	CV, AF, AC	Mills *et al.*[184]
Sjogren–Larsson syndrome	Fatty aldehyde dehydrogenase	VC, AC	Rizzo *et al.*[185]
Cystic fibrosis	Cl transport (CFTR)	DNA, AF	Brock *et al.*[186]

[a]See notes to Table 45.1

tions, DNA analysis may provide more reliable or much earlier results (examples have been given in the Tables). However, for the majority of the disorders discussed in this chapter the metabolic tests are reliable, rapid and most importantly they are in principle applicable to all affected families. For these disorders DNA analysis seems neither necessary nor advantageous because this would either be applicable in only part (often a minority) of the families having common mutations or this would require a time-consuming and expensive search for rare mutations in each family.

Secondly, the introduction of CVS has allowed a much earlier and often almost immediate diagnosis. Potentially also amniocentesis may be moved forward by several weeks which would be useful especially for diseases diagnosed by metabolite measurement.

Thirdly, the reliability of prenatal diagnosis has increased by the expansion of available methods and of the experience acquired with them. The best combination can now be chosen from materials (CV, AF, cultured CV or AF cells) and methods (analysis at the DNA, protein or metabolite level) for each disorder and particular situation. More than one technique may occasionally be necessary to corroborate or clarify initial results.

Fourthly, DNA analysis has opened much better prospects for heterozygote detection. In cases of X-linked diseases this is especially important to avoid unnecessary prenatal diagnosis in female relatives of a patient, who appear not to be carrier. For autosomal recessive disorders the demonstration or exclusion of heterozygosity in relatives of a patient and their partners is possible and especially important in populations with one or more common mutations causing the disease concerned and in populations with a tradition of consanguineous marriage.

New, but still experimental, techniques to collect fetal cells from maternal blood (Ch. 35) or embryonal cells from blastomeres (Ch. 39) may in the future provide adequate material for prenatal diagnosis or preimplantation diagnosis by DNA analysis. Enzyme analysis would not only require the use of ultramicromethods, which are in principle available[197], but also depend on the consistent expression of metabolic functions in the fetal or embryonic cells and their deficiency in the affected case.

REFERENCES

1. McKusick VA. *Mendelian Inheritance in Man. A Catalog of Human Genes and Genetic Disorders*, 11th edn. Baltimore: The Johns Hopkins University Press, 1994.
2. Scriver CR, Beaudet AL, Sly WS & Valle D. *The Metabolic and Molecular Bases of Inherited Disease*, 7th edn. New York: McGraw-Hill, 1995.
3. Blau N, Duran M & Blaskovics M. *Physicians' Guide to the Laboratory Diagnosis of Inherited Metabolic Diseases*. London: Chapman and Hall, 1996.
4. Jakobs C, Ten Brink HJ & Stellaard F. Prenatal diagnosis of inherited metabolic disorders by quantitation of characteristic metabolites in amniotic fluid: facts and future. *Prenat. Diagn.* **10**, 265–271, 1990.
5. Kleijer WJ. First-trimester diagnosis of genetic metabolic disorders. *Contr. Gynecol. Obstet.* **15**, 80–89, 1986.
6. Roberts E, Duckett DP & Lang GD. Maternal cell contamination in chorionic villus samples assessed by direct preparations and three different culture methods. *Prenat. Diagn.* **8**, 635–640, 1988.
7. Ledbetter DH, Zachary JM, Simpson JL *et al.* Cytogenetic results from the U.S. collaborative study on CVS. *Prenat. Diagn.* **12**, 317–345, 1992.
8. Poenaru L. First trimester prenatal diagnosis of metabolic diseases: a survey in countries from the European community. *Prenat. Diagn.* **7**, 333–341, 1987.
9. Besley GTN, Young EP, Fensom AH & Cooper A. First trimester diagnosis of inherited metabolic disease: experience in the UK. *J. Inher. Metab. Dis.* **14**, 128–133, 1991.
10. Desnick RJ, Schuette JL, Golbus MS *et al.* First trimester biochemical and molecular diagnoses using chorionic villi: high accuracy in the U.S. collaborative study. *Prenat. Diagn.* **12**, 357–372, 1992.
11. Wilson RD. Early amniocentesis: a clinical review. *Prenat. Diagn.* **15**, 1259–1273, 1995.
12. Kleijer WJ & Galjaard H. Praenatale Diagnostik genetisch bedingter stoffwechselleiden. In *Murken Praenatale Diagnostik und Therapie*. pp. 100–132. Stuttgart: Enke, 1987.
13. Besley GTN. Enzyme analysis. In *Prenatal Diagnosis and Screening* (eds DJH Brock, CH Rodeck & MA Ferguson-Smith), pp. 127–145. Edinburgh: Churchill Livingstone, 1992.
14. Kaback M, Lim-Steele J, Dabholkar D, Brown D, Levy N & Zeiger K. Tay–Sachs disease – carrier screening, prenatal diagnosis, and the molecular era. An international perspective, 1970 to 1993. *J. Am. Med. Assoc.* **270**, 2307–2315, 1993.
15. Kleijer WJ, Hussaarts-Odijk LM, Sachs ES, Jahoda MGJ & Niermeijer MF. Prenatal diagnosis of Fabry's disease by direct analysis of chorionic villi. *Prenat. Diagn.* **7**, 283–287, 1987.
16. Fensom AH, Benson PF, Neville BRG, Moser HW, Moser AE & Dulaney JT. Prenatal diagnosis of Farber's disease. *Lancet* **ii**, 990–992, 1979.
17. Besley GTN, Ferguson-Smith ME, Frew C, Morris A & Gilmore DH. First trimester diagnosis of Gaucher disease in a fetus with trisomy 21. *Prenat. Diagn.* **8**, 471–474, 1988.
18. Besley GTN & Broadhead DM. Prenatal diagnosis of inherited metabolic disease by chorionic villus analysis: the Edinburgh experience. *J. Inher. Metab. Dis.* **12** (suppl 2), 263–266, 1989.
19. Giles L, Cooper A, Fowler B, Sardharwalla IB & Donnai P. First trimester prenatal diagnosis of Sandhoff's disease. *Prenat. Diagn.* **8**, 199–205, 1988.
20. Grebner EE & Wenger DA. Use of 4-methylumbelliferyl-6-sulpho-2-acetamido-2-deoxy-D-glucopyranoside for prenatal diagnosis of Tay–Sachs disease using chorionic villi. *Prenat. Diagn.* **7**, 419–423, 1987.
21. Kleijer WJ, Mancini GMS, Jahoda MGJ *et al.* First-trimester diagnosis of Krabbe's disease by direct enzyme analysis of chorionic villi. *N. Engl. J. Med.* **311**, 1257, 1984.
22. Fensom AH, Marsh J, Jackson M *et al.* First-trimester diagnosis of metachromatic leucodystrophy. *Clin. Genet.* **34**, 122–125, 1988.
23. Vanier MT, Boué J & Dumez Y. Niemann–Pick disease type B: first-trimester prenatal diagnosis on chorionic villi and biochemical study of a foetus at 12 weeks of development. *Clin. Genet.* **28**, 348–354, 1985.
24. Vanier MT, Rodriguez-Lafrasse C & Rousson R. Prenatal diagnosis of Niemann–Pick type C disease: current strategy from an experience of 37 pregnancies at risk. *Am. J. Hum. Genet.* **51**, 111–122, 1992.
25. Van Diggelen OP, Von Koskull H, Ämmälä P, Vredeveldt GTM, Janse HC & Kleijer WJ. First trimester diagnosis of Wolman's disease. *Prenat. Diagn.* **8**, 661–663, 1988.
26. Sasagasako N, Miyahara S, Saito N, Shinnoh N, Kobayashi T & Goto I. Prenatal diagnosis of congenital sialidosis. *Clin. Genet.* **44**, 8–11, 1993.
27. Besley GTN, Broadhead DM, Nevin NC, Nevin J & Dornan JC. Prenatal diagnosis of mucolipidosis II by early amniocentesis. *Lancet* **335**, 1164–1165, 1990.

28. Zeigler M, Bargal R, Suri V, Meidan B & Bach G. Mucolipidosis type IV: accumulation of phospholipids and gangliosides in cultured amniotic cells. A tool for prenatal diagnosis. *Prenat. Diagn.* **12**, 1037–1042, 1992.
29. Kleijer WJ, Geilen GC, Janse HC *et al.* Cathepsin A deficiency in Galactosialidosis: studies of patients and carriers in 16 families. *Pediatr. Res.* **39**, 1067–1071, 1996.
30. Thomas GH. 'Pseudodeficiencies' of lysosomal hydrolases. *Am. J. Hum. Genet.* **54**, 934–940, 1994.
31. Leistner S, Young E, Meaney C & Winchester B. Pseudodeficiency of arylsulphatase A: strategy for clarification of genotype in families of subjects with low ASA activity and neurological symptoms. *J. Inher. Metab. Dis.* **18**, 710–716, 1995.
32. Giles L, Cooper A, Fowler B, Sardharwalla IB & Donnai P. Krabbe's disease: first trimester diagnosis confirmed on cultured amniotic fluid cells and fetal tissues. *Prenat. Diagn.* **7**, 329–332, 1987.
33. Patrick AD, Young E, Kleijer WJ & Niermeijer MF. Prenatal diagnosis of Niemann-Pick desease type A using chromogenic substrate. *Lancet* **i**, 144, 1977.
34. Carstea ED, Morris JA, Coleman KG *et al.* Niemann-Pick C1 disease gene: Homology to mediators of cholesterol homeostasis. *Science* **277**, 228–231, 1997.
35. Akhunov VS, Gargaun SS & Krasnopolskaya XD. First-trimester enzyme exclusion of Farber disease using a micromethod with [^{3}H] ceramide. *J. Inher. Metab. Dis.* **18**, 616–619, 1995.
36. Levade T, Tempesta MC, Moser HW *et al.* Sulfatide and sphingomyelin loading of living cells as tools for the study of ceramide turnover by lysosomal ceramidase implications for the diagnosis of Farber disease. *Biochem. Mol. Med.* **54**, 117–125, 1995.
37. Kleijer WJ, Hoogeveen A, Verheijen FW *et al.* Prenatal diagnosis of sialidosis with combined neuraminidase and β-galactosidase deficiency. *Clin. Genet.* **16**, 60–61, 1979.
38. Itoh K, Miharu N, Ohama K, Mizoguchi N, Sakura N & Sakuraba H. Fetal diagnosis of galactosialidosis (protective protein/cathepsin A deficiency). *Clin. Chim. Acta.* **266**, 75–82, 1997.
39. Parvathy MR, Mitchell DA & Ben-Yoseph Y. Prenatal diagnosis of I-cell disease in the first and second trimesters. *Am. J. Med. Sci.* **297**, 361–364, 1989.
40. Poenaru L, Mezard C, Akli S, Oury JF, Dumez Y & Boue J. Prenatal diagnosis of mucolipidosis type II on first-trimester amniotic fluid. *Prenat. Diagn.* **10**, 231–235, 1990.
41. Aula P, Mattila K, Piiroinen O, Ämmälä P & Von Koskull H. First-trimester prenatal diagnosis of aspartylgucosaminuria. *Prenat. Diagn.* **9**, 617–620, 1989.
42. Poenaru L, Dreyfus J-C, Boué J, Nicolesco H, Ravise N & Bamberger J. Prenatal diagnosis of fucosidosis. *Clin. Genet.* **10**, 260–264, 1976.
43. Petushkova NA. First-trimester diagnosis of an unusual case of α-mannosidosis. *Prenat. Diagn.* **11**, 279–283, 1991.
44. Kleijer WJ, Geilen GC, Van Diggelen OP, Wevers RA & Los FJ. Prenatal analyses in a pregnancy at risk for β-mannosidosis. *Prenat. Diagn.* **12**, 841–843, 1992.
45. Lake BD, Young EP & Nicolaides K. Prenatal diagnosis of infantile sialic acid storage disease in a twin pregnancy. *J. Inher. Metab. Dis.* **12**, 152–156, 1989.
46. Rapola J, Salonen R, Ammäla P & Santavuori P. Prenatal diagnosis of infantile neuronal ceroid-lipofuscinosis, INCL: morphological aspects. *J. Inher. Metab. Dis.* **16**, 349–352, 1993.
47. Munroe PB, Rapola J, Mitchison HM *et al.* Prenatal diagnosis of Batten's disease. *Lancet* **347**, 1014–1015, 1996.
48. Young EP. Prenatal diagnosis of Hurler disease by analysis of α-iduronidase in chorionic villi. *J. Inher. Metab. Dis.* **15**, 224–230, 1992.
49. Kleijer WJ, Van Diggelen OP, Janse HC, Galjaard H, Dumez Y & Boue J. First trimester diagnosis of Hunter syndrome on chorionic villi. *Lancet* **ii**, 472, 1984.
50. Kleijer WJ, Karpova EA, Geilen GC *et al.* Prenatal diagnosis of Sanfilippo A syndrome: experience in 35 pregnancies at risk and the use of a new fluorogenic substrate for the heparin sulphamidase assay. *Prenat. Diagn.* **16**, 829–835, 1996.
51. Minelli A, Danesino C, Lo Curto F *et al.* First trimester prenatal diagnosis of Sanfilippo disease (MPSIII) type B. *Prenat. Diagn.* **8**, 47–52, 1988.
52. Di Natale P, Pannone N, D'Argenio G, Gatti R, Ricci R & Lombardo C. First-trimester prenatal diagnosis of Sanfilippo C disease. *Prenat. Diagn.* **7**, 603–605, 1987.
53. Zhao H, Van Diggelen OP, Thoomes R *et al.* Prenatal diagnosis of Morquio disease type A using a simple fluorometric enzyme assay. *Prenat. Diagn.* **10**, 85–91, 1990.
54. Kleijer WJ, Wolffers GM, Hoogeveen A & Niermeijer MF. Prenatal diagnosis of Maroteaux–Lamy syndrome. *Lancet* **ii**, 50, 1976.
55. Chabas A & Guardiola A. β-Glucuronidase deficiency: identification of an affected fetus with simultaneous sampling of chorionic villus and amniotic fluid. *Prenat. Diagn.* **13**, 429–433, 1993.
56. Patrick AD. Young E, Ellis C & Rodeck CH. Multiple sulphatase deficiency: prenatal diagnosis using chorionic villi. *Prenat. Diagn.* **8**, 303–306, 1988.
57. Schleutker J, Sistonen P & Aula P. Haplotype analysis in prenatal diagnosis and carrier identification of Salla disease. *J. Med. Genet.* **33**, 36–41, 1996.
58. Voznyi YaV, Keulemans JLM, Kleijer WJ, Aula P, Gray GR & Van Diggelen OP. Applications of a new fluorimetric enzyme assay for the diagnosis of aspartylglucosaminuria. *J. Inher. Metab. Dis.* **16**, 929–934, 1993.
59. Poenaru L, Girard S, Thepot F *et al.* Antenatal diagnosis in three pregnancies at risk for mannosidosis. *Clin. Genet.* **16**, 428–432, 1979.
60. Van Diggelen OP, Schindler D, Kleijer WJ *et al.* Lysosomal α-N-acetyl-galactosaminidase deficiency: a new inherited metabolic disease. *Lancet* **ii**, 804, 1987.
61. Vesa J, Hellsten E, Verkruyse LA *et al.* Mutations in the palmitoyl protein thioesterase gene causing infantile neuronal ceroid lipofuscinosis. *Nature* **376**, 584–587, 1995.
62. Munroe PB, Mitchison HM, O'Rawe AM *et al.* Spectrum of mutations in the Batten disease gene, CLN3. *Am. J. Hum. Genet.* **61**, 310–316, 1997.
63. Mitchison HM, Hofman SL & Becerra CHR. Mutations in the palmitoyl-protein thioesterase gene (PPT, CLN1) causing juvenile neuronal ceroid lipofuscinosis with granular osmiophilic deposits. *Hum. Mol. Genet.* **7**, 291–297, 1998.
64. De Vries BBA, Kleijer WJ, Taschner PEM *et al.* First-trimester diagnosis of infantile neuronal ceroid lipofuscinosis (INCL) using PPT enzyme assay and CLNI mutation analysis. *Prenat. Diagn.*, **19**, in press, 1999.
65. Mossman J & Patrick AD. Prenatal diagnosis of mucopolysaccharidosis by two-dimensional electrophoresis of amniotic fluid glycosaminoglycans. *Prenat. Diagn.* **2**, 169–176, 1982.
66. Kleijer WJ, Huijmans JGM, Blom W *et al.* Prenatal diagnosis of Sanfilippo disease type B. *Hum. Genet.* **66**, 287–288, 1984.
67. Wang He, Voznyi YaV, Huijmans JGM *et al.* Prenatal diagnosis of Sanfilippo disease type C using a simple fluorometric enzyme assay. *Prenat. Diagn.* **14**, 17–22, 1994.
68. Kagie MJ, Kleijer WJ, Huijmans JGM, Maaswinkel-Mooy P & Kanhai HHH. β-Glucuronidase deficiency as a cause of fetal hydrops. *Am. J. Med. Genet.* **42**, 693–695, 1992.
69. Von Figura K, Van De Kamp JJ & Niermeijer MF. Prenatal diagnosis of Morquio's disease type A (*N*-acetylgalactosamine 6-sulphate sulphatase deficiency). *Prenat. Diagn.* **2**, 67–69, 1982.
70. Kleijer WJ, Thompson EJ & Niermeijer MF. Prenatal diagnosis of the Hurler syndrome: report on 40 pregnancies at risk. *Prenat. Diagn.* **3**, 179–186, 1983.
71. Fensom AH & Benson PF. Recent advances in the prenatal diagnosis of the mucopolysaccharidoses. *Prenat. Diagn.* **14**, 1–12, 1994.
72. Wang He, Voznyi YaV, Boer AM, Kleijer WJ & Van Diggelen OP. A fluorimetric enzyme assay for the diagnosis of Sanfilippo disease type D (MPS IIID). *J. Inher. Metab. Dis.* **16**, 935–941, 1993.
73. Aronovicz EL, Pan D & Whitley CB. Molecular genetic defect underlying α-L-iduronidase pseudodeficiency. *Am. J. Hum. Genet.* **58**, 75–85, 1996.
74. Scott HS, Bunge S, Gal A, Clarke LA, Morris P & Hopwood JJ. Molecular genetics of mucopolysaccharidosis type I: diagnostic, clinical and biological implications. *Hum. Mutat.* **6**, 288–302, 1995.
75. Kleijer WJ, Mooy PD, Liebaers I, Van Der Kamp JJP, Niermeijer MF. Prenatal monitoring for the Hunter syndrome: The heterozygous female fetus. *Clin. Genet.* **15**, 113–117, 1979.
76. Cooper A, Thornley M & Wraith JE. First-trimester diagnosis of Hunter syndrome: very low iduronate sulphatase activity in chorionic

villi from a heterozygous female fetus. *Prenat. Diagn.* **11**, 731–735, 1991.

77. Sukegawa K, Song X-Q, Masuno M *et al.* Hunter disease in a girl caused by R468Q mutation in the iduronate-2-sulfatase gene and skewed inactivation of the X-chromosome carrying the normal allele. *Hum. Mutat.* **10**, 361–367, 1997.
78. Hopwood JJ, Bunge S, Morris CP *et al.* Molecular basis of mucopolysaccharidosis type II: mutations in the iduronate-2-sulphatase gene. *Hum. Mutat.* **2**, 435–442, 1993.
79. Mossman J, Young EP, Patrick AD *et al.* Prenatal tests for Sanfilippo disease type B in four pregnancies. *Prenat. Diagn.* **3**, 347–350, 1983.
80. Maire I, Epelbaum S, Piraud M, Mandon G, Dumoulin R & Mathieu M. Second trimester prenatal diagnosis of Sanfilippo syndrome type C. *J. Inher. Metab. Dis.* **16**, 584–586, 1993.
81. Weber B, Guo X-H, Wraith JE *et al.* Novel mutations in Sanfilippo A syndrome: implications for enzyme function. *Hum. Mol. Genet.* **6**, 1573–1579, 1997.
82. Van Eyndhoven HWF, Ter Brugge HG, Van Essen A & Kleijer WJ. β-Glucuronidase deficiency as cause of recurrent hydrops fetalis: The first early prenatal diagnosis by chorionic villus sampling. *Prenat. Diagn.* **18**, 959–962, 1998.
83. Vervoort R, Gitzelman R, Bosshard N, Maire I, Liebaers I & Lissens W. Low β-glucuronidase enzyme activity and mutations in the human β-glucuronidase gene in mild mucopolysaccharidosis type VII, pseudodeficiency and a heterozygote. *Hum. Genet.* **102**, 69–78, 1998.
84. Machin AG. Hydrops revisited: literature review of 1,414 cases published in the 1980s. *Am. J. Med. Genet.* **34**, 366–390, 1989.
85. Jauniaux E, Van Maldergem L, De Munter C, Moscoso G & Gillerot Y. Nonimmune hydrops fetalis associated with genetic abnormalities. *Obstet. Gynecol.* **75**, 568–572, 1990.
86. Kattner E, Schäfer A & Harzer K. Hydrops fetalis: manifestation in lysosomal storage diseases including Farber disease. *Eur. J. Pediat.* **156**, 292–295, 1997.
87. Tayebi N, Cushner SR, Kleijer WJ *et al.* Prenatal lethality of a homozygous null mutation in the human glucocerebrosidase gene. *Am. J. Med. Genet.* **73**, 41–47, 1997.
88. Poulain P, Odent S, Maire I *et al.* Fetal ascites and oligohydramnios: Prenatal diagnosis of a sialic acid storage disease (index case). *Prenat. Diagn.* **15**, 864–867, 1995.
89. Piraud M, Froissart R, Mandon G, Bernard A & Maire I. Amniotic fluid for screening of lysosomal storage diseases presenting in utero (mainly as non-immune hydrops fetalis). *Clin. Chim. Acta.* **248**, 143–155, 1996.
90. Schutgens RBH, Schrakamp G, Wanders RJA, Heymans HSA, Tager JM & Van Den Bosch H. Prenatal and perinatal diagnosis of peroxisomal disorders. *J. Inher. Metab. Dis.* **12**(suppl 1), 118–134, 1989.
91. Wanders RJA, Schutgens RBH, Van Den Bosch H, Tager JM & Kleijer WJ. Prenatal diagnosis of inborn errors in peroxisomal β-oxidation. *Prenat. Diagn.* **11**, 253–261, 1991.
92. Danpure CJ & Rumsby G. Strategies for the prenatal diagnosis of primary hyperoxaluria type 1. *Prenat. Diagn.* **16**, 587–598, 1996.
93. Hoffmann GF, Sweetmann L, Bremer HJ *et al.* Facts and artefacts in mevalonic aciduria: development of a stable isotope dilution GCMS assay for mevalonic acid and its application to physiological fluids, tissue samples, prenatal diagnosis and carrier detection. *Clin. Chim. Acta.* **198**, 209–228, 1991.
94. Fournier B, Smeitink JAM, Dorland L, Berger R, Saudubray JM & Poll-Thé BT. Peroxisomal disorders: A review. *J. Inher. Metab. Dis.* **17**, 470–486, 1994.
95 Wanders RJA, Barth PG, Schutgens RBH & Heymans HSA. Peroxisomal disorders: post-and prenatal diagnosis based on a new classification with flow charts. *Int. Pediat.* **11**, 203–214, 1995.
96. Stellaard F, Kleijer WJ, Wanders RJA, Schutgens RBH & Jakobs C. Bile acids in amniotic fluid: promising metabolites for the prenatal diagnosis of peroxisomal disorders. *J. Inher. Metab. Dis.* **14**, 353–356, 1991.
97. Imamura A, Suzuki Y, Song X-Q *et al.* Prenatal diagnosis of adrenoleukodystrophy by means of mutation analysis. *Prenat. Diagn.* **16**, 259–261, 1996.
98. Hoffmann GF, Brendel SU, Scharfschwerdt SR, Shin YS, Speidel IM & Gibson KM. Mevalonate kinase assay using DEAE-cellulose column chromatography for first trimester prenatal diagnosis and complementation analysis in mevalonic aciduria. *J. Inher. Metab. Dis.* **15**, 738–746, 1992.
99. Jakobs C, Kleijer WJ, Allen J & Holton JB. Prenatal diagnosis of galactosemia. *Eur. J. Pediatr.* **154** (suppl 2), S33–S36, 1995.
100. Golbus MS, Simpson TJ, Koresawa M, Appelman ZVI & Alpers CE. The prenatal determination of glucose-6-phosphatase activity by fetal liver biopsy. *Prenat. Diagn.* **8**, 401–404, 1988.
101. Kleijer WJ, Van Der Kraan M, Kroos MA *et al.* Prenatal diagnosis of glycogen storage disease type II: Enzyme assay or mutation analysis? *Pediatr. Res.* **38**, 103–106, 1995.
102. Shin YS, Rieth M, Tausenfreund J & Endres W. First trimester diagnosis of glycogen storage disease type II and type III. *J. Inher. Metab. Dis.* **12** (suppl 2), 289–291, 1989.
103. Brown BI & Brown DH. Branching enzyme activity of cultured amniocytes and chorionic villi: prenatal testing for type IV glycogen storage disease. *Am. J. Hum. Genet.* **44**, 378–381, 1989.
104. Ruitenbeek W, Sengers RCA, Trijbels JMF, Janssen AJM & Bakkeren JAJM. The use of chorionic villi in prenatal diagnosis of mitochondriopathies. *J. Inher. Metab. Dis.* **15**, 303–306, 1992.
105. Marsac C, Augereau CH, Feldman G, Wolf B, Hansen TL & Berger R. Prenatal diagnosis of pyruvate carboxylase deficiency. *Clin. Chim. Acta.* **119**, 121–127, 1982.
106. Brown RM & Brown GK. Prenatal diagnosis of pyruvate dehydrogenase E1*a* subunit deficiency. *Prenat. Diagn.* **14**, 435–442, 1994.
107. Børresen AL, Hellerud C, Møller P, Søvik O & Berg K. Prenatal diagnosis of glycerol-kinase deficiency associated with a DNA deletion on the short arm of the X-chromosome. *Clin. Genet.* **32**, 254–259, 1987.
108. Rouger H, Girodon E, Goossens M, Galacteros F, Cohen-Solal M & Mondor PK. Prenatal diagnosis of a frameshift mutation in the LR pyruvate kinase gene associated with severe hereditary non-spherocytic haemolytic anaemia. *Prenat. Diagn.* **16**, 97–104, 1996.
109. Whitelaw AGL, Rogers PA, Hopkinson DA *et al.* Congenital haemolytic anaemia resulting from glucose phosphate isomerase deficiency: genetics, clinical picture, and prenatal diagnosis. *J. Med. Genet.* **16**, 189–196, 1979.
110. Waggoner DD, Buist NRM & Donnell GN. Long-term prognosis in galactosaemia: Results of a survey of 350 cases. *J. Inher. Metab. Dis.* **13**, 802–818, 1990.
111. Jakobs C, Kleijer WJ, Bakker HD, Gennip AH, Przyrembel H & Niermeijer MF. Dietary restriction of maternal lactose intake does not prevent accumulation of galactitol in the amniotic fluid of fetuses affected with galactosaemia. *Prenat. Diagn.* **8**, 641–645, 1988.
112. Elsas LJ, Langley S & Steele E. Galactosemia: a strategy to identify new biochemical phenotypes and molecular genotypes. *Am. J. Hum. Genet.* **56**, 630–639, 1995.
113. Wong L-JC. Prenatal diagnosis of glycogen storage disease type 1a by direct mutation detection. *Prenat. Diagn.* **16**, 105–108, 1996.
114. Maire I, Mandon G & Mathieu M. First trimester prenatal diagnosis of glycogen storage disease type III. *J. Inher. Metab. Dis.* **12** (suppl 2), 292–294, 1989.
115. Poulton J & Marchington DR. Prospects for DNA-based prenatal diagnosis of mitochondrial disorders. *Prenat. Diagn.* **16**, 1247–1256, 1996.
116. Beutler E & Baronciani L. Mutations in pyruvate kinase. *Hum. Mutat.* **7**, 1–6, 1996.
117. Dallapiccola B, Novelli G, Ferranti G, Pachi A, Cristiani ML & Magnani M. First trimester monitoring of a pregnancy at risk for glucose phosphate isomerase deficiency. *Prenat. Diag.* **6**, 101–107, 1986.
118. Jaeken J, Artigas J, Barone R *et al.* Phosphomannomutase deficiency is the main cause of carbohydrate-deficient glycoprotein syndrome with type I isoelectrofocusing pattern of serum sialotransferrins. *J. Inher. Metab. Dis.* **20**, 447–449, 1997.
119. Gibbs DA, McFadyen IR & Crawford MD'A. First-trimester diagnosis of Lesch–Nyhan syndrome. *Lancet* **2**, 1180–1183, 1984.
120. Dooley T, Fairbanks LD & Simmonds HA. First trimester diagnosis of adenosine deaminase deficiency. *Prenat. Diagn.* **7**, 561–565, 1987.
121. Pérignon JL, Durandy A, Peter MO, Freycon F, Dumez Y & Griscelli C. Early prenatal diagnosis of inherited severe immunodeficiencies linked to enzyme deficiencies. *J. Pediatr.* **111**, 595–598, 1987.

122. Jakobs C, Stellaard F, Smit LME *et al.* The first prenatal diagnosis of dihydropyrimidine dehydrogenase deficiency. *Eur. J. Pediatr.* **150**, 291, 1991.
123. Johnson JL, Rajagopalan KV, Lanman JT *et al.* Prenatal diagnosis of molybdenum cofactor deficiency by assay of sulphite oxidase activity in chorionic villus samples. *J. Inher. Metab. Dis.* **14**, 932–937, 1991.
124. Halley DJ, Keijzer W, Jaspers NG *et al.* Prenatal diagnosis of xeroderma pigmentosum (group C) using assays of unscheduled DNA synthesis and postreplication repair. *Clin. Genet.* **16**, 137–146, 1979.
125. Sarasin A, Blanchet-Bardon C, Renault G, Lehmann A, Arlett C & Dumez Y. Prenatal diagnosis in a subset of trichothiodystrophy patients defective in DNA repair. *Br. J. Dermatol.* **127**, 485–491, 1992.
126. Lehmann AR, Francis AJ & Gianelli F. Prenatal diagnosis of Cockayne's syndrome. *Lancet* **i**, 486–487, 1985.
127. Kleijer WJ, Van Der Kraan M, Los FJ & Jaspers NGJ. Prenatal diagnosis of ataxia-telangiectasia and Nijmegen breakage syndrome by the assay of radioresistant DNA synthesis. *Int. J. Radiat. Biol.* **66**, S167–S174, 1994.
128. Graham GW, Aitken DA & Connor JM. Prenatal diagnosis by enzyme analysis in 15 pregnancies at risk for the Lesch–Nyhan syndrome. *Prenat. Diagn.* **16**, 647–651, 1996.
129. Marcus S, Steen AM, Andersson B, Lambert B, Kristoffersson U & Francke U. Mutation analysis and prenatal diagnosis in a Lesch–Nyhan family showing non-random X-inactivation interfering with carrier detection tests. *Hum. Genet.* **89**, 395–400, 1992.
130. Hirschhorn R, Beratis N, Rosen FS, Parkman R, Stern R & Polmar S. Adenosine deaminase deficiency in a child diagnosed prenatally. *Lancet* **1**, 73, 1975.
131. Kleijer WJ, Hussaarts-Odijk LM, Los FJ, Pijpers L, de Bree PK & Duran M. Prenatal diagnosis of purine nucleoside phosphorylase deficiency in the first and second trimesters of pregnancy. *Prenat. Diagn.* **9**, 401–407, 1989.
132. Ogier H, Wadman SK, Johnson JL *et al.* Antenatal diagnosis of combined xanthine and sulphite-oxidase deficiency. *Lancet* **2**, 1363–1364, 1983.
133. Cleaver JE, Volpe JPG, Charles WC & Thomas GH. Prenatal diagnosis of xeroderma pigmentosum and Cockayne syndrome. *Prenat. Diagn.* **14**, 921–928, 1994.
134. Savitsky K, Bar-Shira A, Gilad S *et al.* A single ataxia telangiectasia gene with a product similar to PI-3 kinase. *Science* **268**, 1749–1753, 1995.
135. Lidsky AS, Guttler F & Woo SLC. Prenatal diagnosis of classical phenylketonuria by DNA analysis. *Lancet* **1**, 549–551, 1985.
136. Blau N, Niederwieser A & Curtius HC. Prenatal diagnosis of atypical phenyketonuria. *J. Inher. Metab. Dis.* **12** (suppl 2), 295–298, 1989.
137. Bennett MJ, Gibson KM, Sherwood WG *et al.* Reliable prenatal diagnosis of Canavan disease (aspartoacylase deficiency): comparison of enzymatic and metabolite analysis. *J. Inher. Metab. Dis.* **16**, 831–836, 1993.
138. Jakobs C, Stellaard F, Kvittingen EA, Henderson M & Lilford R. First-trimester prenatal diagnosis of tyrosinemia type I by amniotic fluid succinylacetone determination. *Prenat. Diagn.* **10**, 133–139, 1990.
139. Hayasaka K, Tada K, Fueki N & Aikawa J. Prenatal diagnosis of nonketotic hyperglycinemia: enzymatic analysis of the glycine cleavage system in chorionic villi. *J. Pediatr.* **116**, 444–445, 1990.
140. Patrick AD, Young EP, Mossman J, Warren R, Kearney L, Rodeck CH. First trimester diagnosis of cystinosis using intact chorionic villi. *Prenat. Diagn.* **7**, 71–74, 1987.
141. Kleijer WJ, Horsman D, Mancini GMS, Fois A & Boue J. First-trimester diagnosis of maple syrup urine disease on intact chorionic villi. *New. Engl. J. Med.* **313**, 1608, 1985.
142. Kleijer WJ, van der Kraan M, Huijmans JGM, van den Heuvel CMM & Jakobs C. Prenatal diagnosis of isovaleric acidaemia by enzyme and metabolite assay in the first and second trimesters. *Prenat. Diagn.* **15**, 527–533, 1995.
143. Chitayat D, Chemke J, Gibson KM *et al.* 3-Methylglutaconic aciduria: a marker for as yet unspecified disorders and the relevance of prenatal diagnosis in a 'new' type ('type 4'). *J. Inher. Metab. Dis.* **15**, 204–212, 1992.
144. Chalmers RA, Tracey BM, Mistry J, Stacey TE & McFadyen IR. Prenatal diagnosis of 3-Hydroxy-3-Methyglutaric aciduria by GC-MS and enzymology on cultured amniocytes and chorionic villi. *J. Inher. Metab. Dis.* **12**, 286–292, 1989.
145. Packman S, Cowan MJ, Golbus MS *et al.* Prenatal treatment of biotin-responsive multiple carboxylase deficiency. *Lancet* **i**, 1435–1439, 1982.
146. Chalmers RA, Mistry J, Docherty PW & Stratton D. First trimester prenatal exclusion of biotinidase deficiency. *J. Inher. Metab. Dis.* **17**, 751–752, 1994.
147. Kleijer WJ, Thoomes R, Galjaard H, Wendel U & Fowler B. First-trimester (chorion biopsy) diagnosis of citrullinaemia and methylmalonicaciduria. *Lancet* **ii**, 1340, 1984.
148. Vimal CM, Fensom AH, Heaton D, Ward RHT, Garrod P & Penketh RJA. Prenatal diagnosis of argininosuccinicaciduria by analysis of cultured chorionic villi. *Lancet* **ii**, 521–522, 1984.
149. Piceni Sereni L, Bachmann C, Pfister U, Buscaglia M & Nicolini U. Prenatal diagnosis of carbamoylphosphate synthetase deficiency by fetal liver biopsy. *Prenat. Diagn.* **8**, 307–309, 1988.
150. Rodeck CH, Patrick AD, Pembrey ME, Tzannatos C & Whitfield AE. Fetal liver biopsy for prenatal diagnosis of ornithine carbamyl transferase deficiency. *Lancet* **ii**, 297–300, 1982.
151. Shih VE, Laframboise R, Mandell R & Pichette J. Neonatal form of the hyperornithinaemia, hyperammonaemia, and homocitrullinuria (HHH) syndrome and prenatal diagnosis. *Prenat. Diagn.* **12**, 717–723, 1992.
152. Rolland MO, Divry P, Mandon G *et al.* Early prenatal diagnosis of propionic acidaemia with simultaneous sampling of chorionic villus and amniotic fluid. *J. Inher. Metab. Dis.* **13**, 345–348, 1990.
153. Fowler B, Giles L, Sardharwalla IB, Donnai P & Clayton JK. First trimester of methylmalonic aciduria. *Prenat. Diagn.* **8**, 207–213, 1988.
154. Christensen E. Prenatal diagnosis of glutaryl-CoA dehydrogenase deficiency: experience using first trimester chorionic villus sampling. *Prenat. Diagn.* **14**, 333–336, 1994.
155. Yamaguchi S, Shimizu N, Orii *et al.* Prenatal diagnosis and neonatal monitoring of a fetus with glutaric aciduria type II due to electron transfer flavoprotein (β-subunit) deficiency. *Pediatr. Res.* **30**, 439–443, 1991.
156. Bennett MJ, Allison F, Pollitt RJ *et al.* Prenatal diagnosis of medium-chain acyl-CoA dehydrogenase deficiency in family with sudden infant death. *Lancet* **i**, 440–441, 1987.
157. Nada MA, Vianey-Saban C, Roe CR *et al.* Prenatal diagnosis of mitochondrial fatty acid oxidation defects. *Prenat. Diagn.* **16**, 117–124, 1996.
158. Von Döbeln U, Venizelos N, Westgren M & Hagenfeldt L. Long-chain 3-Hydroxyacyl-CoA dehydrogenase in chorionic villi, fetal liver and fibroblasts and prenatal diagnosis of 3-hydroxyacyl-CoA dehydrogenease deficiency. *J. Inher. Metab. Dis.* **17**, 185–188, 1994.
159. Scriver CR & Clow CL. Avoiding phenylketonuria: why parents seek prenatal diagnosis. *J. Pediatr.* **113**, 495–497, 1988.
160. Tuchman M, Morizono H, Reish O, Yuan X & Allewell NM. The molecular basis of ornithine transcarbamylase deficiency: modelling the human enzyme and the effects of mutations. *J. Med. Genet.* **32**, 680–688, 1995.
161. Kamoun P, Fensom AH, Shin YS *et al.* Prenatal diagnosis of the urea cycle diseases: a survey of the European cases. *Am. J. Med. Genet.* **55**, 247–250, 1995.
162. Shaag A, Anikster Y, Christensen E *et al.* The molecular basis of Canavan (apartoacylase deficiency) disease in European non-Jewish patients. *Am. J. Hum. Genet.* **57**, 572–580, 1995.
163. Grenier A, Cederbaum S, Laberge C, Gagné R, Jakobs C & Tanguay RM. A case of tyrosinaemia type 1 with normal level of succinylacetone in the amniotic fluid. *Prenat. Diagn.* **16**, 239–242, 1996.
164. Ploos van Amstel JK, Jansen RPM, Verjaal M, van den Berg IET & Berger R. Prenatal diagnosis of type I hereditary tyrosinaemia. *Lancet* **344**, 336, 1994.
165. Rolland O, Mandon G & Mathieu M. First-trimester prenatal diagnosis of non-ketotic hyperglycinaemia by a micro assay of glycine cleavage enzyme. *Prenat. Diagn.* **13**, 771–772, 1993.
166. Smith ML, Pellett OL, Cass MMJ *et al.* Prenatal diagnosis of cystinosis utilizing chorionic villus sampling. *Prenat. Diagn.* **7**, 23–26, 1987.
167. Mitchell GA, Jakobs C, Gibson KM *et al.* Molecular prenatal diagnosis of 3-hydroxy-3-methylglutaryl CoA lyase deficiency. *Prenat. Diagn.* **15**, 725–729, 1995.
168. Northrup H, Beaudet AL & O'Brien WE. Prenatal diagnosis of citrullinaemia: review of a 10-year experience including recent use of DNA analysis. *Prenat. Diagn.* **10**, 771–779, 1990.

169. Jakobs C. Prenatal diagnosis of inherited metabolic disorders by stable isotope dilution GC-MS analysis of metabolities in amniotic fluid: review of four years experience. *J. Inher. Metab. Dis.* **12**(suppl 2), 267–270, 1989.
170. Goodman SI, Gallegos DA, Pullin CJ *et al.* Antenatal diagnosis of glutaric acidemia. *Am. J. Hum. Genet.* **32**, 695–699, 1980.
171. Andresen BS, Bross P, Udvari S *et al.* The molecular basis of medium chain acyl-CoA dehydrogenase (MCAD) deficiency in compound heterozygous patients: is there a correlation between genotype and phenotype? *Hum. Mol. Genet.* **6**, 695–707, 1997.
172. IJlst L, Ruiter JPN, Hoovers JMN, Jakobs ME & Wanders RJA. Common missense mutation G1528C in long-chain 3 hydroxyacyl-CoA dehydrogenase deficiency. *J. Clin. Invest.* **4**, 1028–1033, 1996.
173. Andresen BS, Bross P, Vianey-Saban C *et al.* Cloning and characterization of human very-long-chain acyl-CoA dehydrogenase cDNA, chromosomal assignment of the gene and identification in four patients of nine different mutations within the VLCAD gene. *Hum. Mol. Genet.* **5**, 461–472, 1996.
174. Tønnesen T, Gerdes AM, Damsgaard E *et al.* First-trimester diagnosis of Menkes disease: intermediate copper values in chorionic villi from three affected male fetuses. *Prenat. Diag.* **9**, 159–165, 1989.
175. Hähnel R, Hähnel E, Wysocki SJ, Wilkinson SP & Hockey A. Prenatal diagnosis of X-linked ichthyosis. *Clin. Chim. Acta.* **120**, 143–152, 1982.
176. Huu TP, Dumez Y, Marquetty C, Durandy A, Boue J & Hakim J. Prenatal diagnosis of chronic granulomatous disease (CGD) in four high risk male fetuses. *Prenat. Diagn.* **7**, 253–260, 1987.
177. Raux-Demay M, Mornet E, Boue J *et al.* Early prenatal diagnosis of 21-hydroxylase deficiency using amniotic fluid 17-hydroxprogesterone determination and DNA probes. *Prenat. Diag.* **9**, 457–466, 1989.
178. Sassa S, Solish G, Levere RD & Kappas A. Studies in porphyria. IV. Expression of the gene defect of acute intermittent porphyria in cultured human skin fibroblasts and amniotic fluid cells: prenatal diagnosis of the porphyric trait. *J. Exp. Med.* **142**, 722–731, 1975.
179. Ged C, Moreau-Gaudry F, Taine L *et al.* Prenatal diagnosis in congenital erythropoietic porphyria by metabolic measurement and DNA mutation analysis. *Prenat. Diag.* **16**, 83–86, 1996.
180. Brown MS, Goldstein JL, Vandenberghe K *et al.* Prenatal diagnosis of homozygous familial hypercholesterolaemia. *Lancet* **i**, 526–529, 1978.
181. Maassen JA, Lindhout D, Reuss A & Kleijer WJ. Prenatal analysis of insulin receptor autophosphorylation in a family with leprechaunism. *Prenat. Diagn.* **10**, 13–16, 1990.
182. Brock DJH & Barron L. First-trimester prenatal diagnosis of hypophosphatasia: experience with 16 cases. *Prenat. Diagn.* **11**, 387–391, 1991.
183. Raghunath M, Steinmann B, Delozier-Blanchet C, Extermann P & Superti-Furga A. Prenatal diagnosis of collagen disorders by direct biochemical analysis of chorionic villus biopsies. *Pediatr. Res.* **36**, 441–448, 1994.
184. Mills K, Mandel H, Montemagno R, Soothill P, Gershoni-Baruch R & Clayton PT. First trimester prenatal diagnosis of Smith–Lemli–Opitz syndrome (7-dehydrocholesterol reductase deficiency). *Pediat. Res.* **39**, 816–819, 1996.
185. Rizzo WB, Craft DA & Kelson TL. Prenatal diagnosis of Sjögren–Larsson syndrome using enzymatic methods. *Prenat. Diagn.* **14**, 577–581, 1994.
186. Brock DJH, Clark HAK & Barron L. Prenatal diagnosis of cystic fibrosis by microvillar enzyme assay on a sequence of 258 pregnancies. *Hum. Genet.* **78**, 271–275, 1988.
187. Tümer Z & Horn N. Menkes disease: recent advances and new aspects. *J. Med. Genet.* **34**, 265–274, 1997.
188. Suchy SF, Olivos-Glander IM & Nussbaum RL. Lowe syndrome, a deficiency of a phosphatidyl-inositol 4,5-bisphosphate 5-phosphatase in the Golgi apparatus. *Hum. Mol. Genet.* **4**, 2245–2250, 1995.
189. Verheijen FW, Beerens CEMT, Havelaar AC, Kleijer WJ & Mancini GMS. Fibroblast silver loading for the diagnosis of Menkes disease. *J. Med. Genet.* **35**, 849–851, 1998.
190. De Boer M, Bolscher BGJM, Sijmons RH, Scheffer H, Weening RS & Roos D. Prenatal diagnosis in a family with X-linked chronic granulomatous disease with the use of the polymerase chain reaction. *Prenat. Diagn.* **12**, 773–777, 1992.
191. McGaughran JM, Clayton PT, Mills KA, Rimmer S, Moore L & Donnai D. Prenatal diagnosis of Smith–Lemli–Opitz syndrome. *Am. J. Med. Genet.* **56**, 269–271, 1995.
192. Honda A, Tint GS, Salen G, Batta AK, Chen TS & Shefer S. Defective conversion of 7-dehydrocholesterol to cholesterol in cultured skin fibroblasts from Smith–Lemli–Opitz syndrome homozygotes. *J. Lipid. Res.* **36**, 1595–1601, 1995.
193. Reshef A, Meiner V, Dann EJ, Granat M & Leitersdorf E. Prenatal diagnosis of familial hypercholesterolemia caused by the 'Lebanese' mutation at the low density lipoprotein receptor locus. *Hum. Genet.* **89**, 237–239, 1992.
194. Longo N, Langley SD, Still MJ & Elsas LJ. Prenatal analysis of the insulin receptor gene in a family with leprechaunism. *Prenat. Diagn.* **15**, 1070–1074, 1995.
195. Claass AHW, Kleijer WJ, van Diggelen OP, van der Veer E & Sips HJ. Prenatal detection of cystic fibrosis; comparative study of maltase and alkaline phosphatase activities in amniotic fluid. *Prenat. Diagn.* **6**, 419–427, 1986.
196. Baranov VS, Gorbunova VN, Ivaschenko TE *et al.* Five years' experience of prenatal diagnosis of cystic fibrosis in the former U.S.S.R. *Prenat. Diagn.* **12**, 575–586, 1992.
197. Galjaard H. Miniaturization of biochemical analysis of cultured (amniotic fluid) cells. In *Prenatal Diagnosis, Cell Biological Approaches* (eds SA Latt & GJ Darlington) *Meth. Cell. Biol.* **26**, 241–268, 1982.

Genodermatoses

46

R.A.J. Eady and J.A. McGrath

Introduction

The introduction of precise, reliable and generally safe methods for intrauterine fetal skin biopsy has been a significant development for the prenatal diagnosis of a number of hereditary skin disorders[1–7]. During the early 1980s accurate fetal tissue sampling depended to a large extent on direct visualization of the fetus using fetoscopy. More recently, with improvements in ultrasonography providing real-time high-resolution images, experienced operators have been successful in obtaining a variety of fetal tissue, including skin, without the need of a fetoscope. The past few years have seen the emergence of DNA-based methods for prenatal diagnosis of certain genodermatoses including major forms of epidermolysis bullosa, ichthyosis and oculocutaneous albinism. This chapter will briefly review the principal landmarks in prenatal diagnosis of genodermatoses based on analysis of fetal skin biopsy samples and cover some of the more recent developments using DNA technology.

Methods of prenatal diagnosis

FETAL SKIN BIOPSY

The skin samples, obtained at about 16–20 weeks of gestation, have to be collected and transported to the laboratory in special medium, and rapidly processed for microscopical analysis. This usually involves light microscopy (Fig. 46.1) and transmission electron microscopy[8], but immunohistochemistry (mainly indirect immunofluorescence microscopy) is now generally regarded as a valuable, if not essential, additional method of analysis, especially for junctional or recessive dystrophic forms of epidermolysis bullosa (Fig. 46.2)[9–13]. A range of highly specific monoclonal antibodies recognizing macromolecular components of the normal epidermal basement membrane zone (Fig. 46.3) has proved exceptionally helpful, not only for diagnosis, but also in the search for candidate proteins and genes in different forms of epidermolysis bullosa[14].

Results of prenatal diagnosis of inherited skin disease using fetal skin biopsy covering the period of 1979–1992 are summarized in the proceedings of a Workshop of the World Congress of Dermatology, held in New York in 1992[15]. Reporting centres were based in Seattle, Paris, London, Heidelberg, Tokyo and Nagoya. The total number of cases collectively was 468, of which 129 were affected and 337 unaffected. The major disorders being assessed in order of frequency were junctional epidermolysis bullosa[16,17], recessive dystrophic epidermolysis bullosa[18], non-bullous ichthyosiform erythroderma (or lamellar ichthyosis)[19,20] and harlequin ichthyosis[21]. Other categories included bullous congenital ichthyosiform erythroderma or epidermolytic hyperkeratosis[22–25], tyrosinase-negative oculocutaneous albinism[26,27], epidermolysis bullosa simplex[28], Sjögren–Larssen syndrome[29], X-linked hypohidrotic ectodermal dysplasia[30], restrictive dermopathy[31], and Chediak–Higashi syndrome[32].

In most centres carrying out fetal skin biopsy for prenatal diagnosis there is a close collaboration between the team undertaking the biopsy and the laboratory involved with the collection and analysis of samples. These centres have built up considerable experience over many years so the procedure has generally become reliable with a low rate of misdiagnosis and a similarly low incidence of complications leading to damage to the fetus from the skin biopsy procedure or loss of the pregnancy. Despite the impressive track record of fetal skin biopsy, as a midtrimester procedure, the introduction of DNA-based diagnosis has proved to be a welcome development.

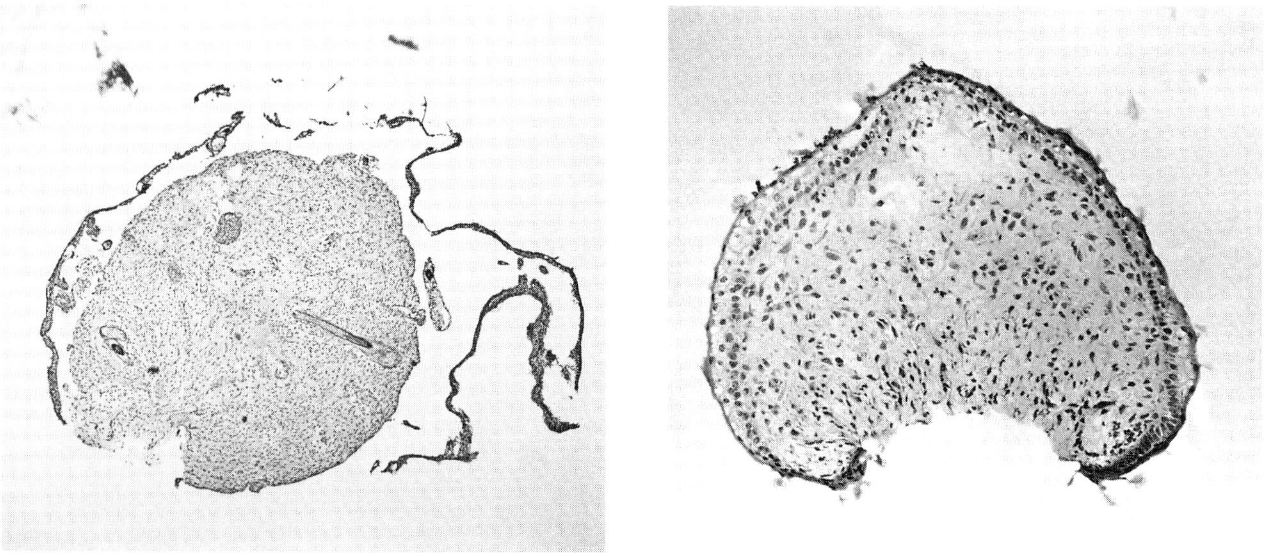

(a) (b)

Fig. 46.1 Light microscopy of semithin resin sections of fetal skin biopsy samples (16 weeks' gestation) used for the prenatal diagnosis of Herlitz (lethal) form of junctional epidermolysis bullosa. An extensive split is evident along the dermo-epidermal junction in (a) indicating that the fetus is affected. The control age-matched sample of normal fetal skin (b) is intact. (Magnification in (a) × 100 and (b) × 150.)

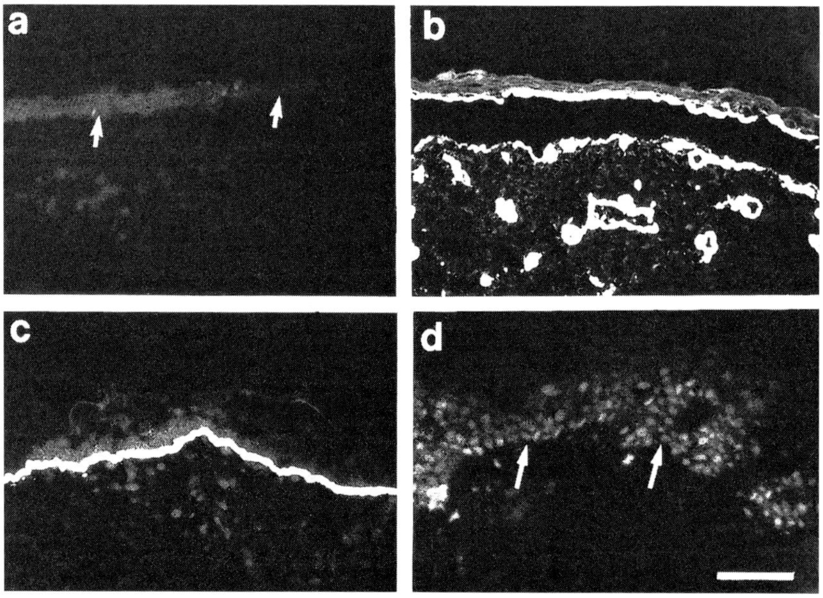

Fig. 46.2 Immunofluorescence micrographs illustrating use of monoclonal antibody GB3 (antilaminin 5) staining of 5 μm cryostat sections of fetal skin biopsy obtained at 17 weeks' gestation for the prenatal diagnosis of Herlitz junctional epidermolysis bullosa. (a) Virtual absence of GB3 staining at the dermo-epidermal junction (DEJ) (arrows) indicating fetus is affected. (b) Staining with antilaminin 1 antibody shows normal bright staining around dermal vessels. The DEJ shows extensive separation, as seen in this form of junctional EB. (c) Bright linear DEJ staining with GB3 in normal control fetal sample. (d) Absence of specific GB3 staining in control sample from another affected fetus. (Magnification bar = 50 μm.)

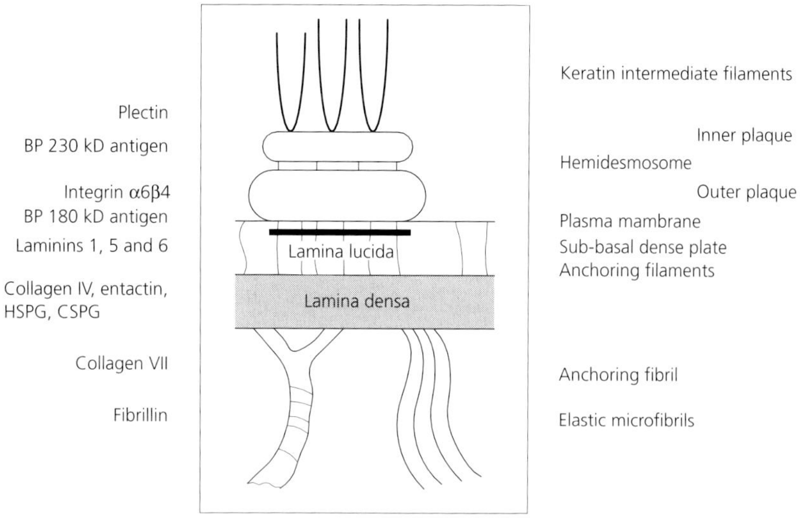

Fig. 46.3 Representation of the composition of the dermo-epidermal junction in the region of the hemidesmosome. Macromolecular components are shown on the left of the figure and ultrastructural components are listed on the right. HSPG = heparin sulphate proteoglycan, CSPG = chorioroitin sulphate proteoglycan.

DNA-BASED TECHNIQUES

JUNCTIONAL FORMS OF EPIDERMOLYSIS BULLOSA

The Herlitz type of junctional epidermolysis bullosa (EB) is autosomal recessive and involves mutations in the genes encoding the three chains of laminin 5 which is a component of the anchoring filament-hemidesmosome complex (Fig. 46.3). Mutations were first described in the *LAMC2* gene (encoding the γ2 chain)[33,34], and then in *LAMB3* (β3 chain)[35] and *LAMA3* (α3 chain)[36,37]. These are premature termination codon mutations causing a severe reduction or complete absence of one of the laminin 5 polypeptide chains and profound fragility of the skin and mucous membranes. The decreased protein synthesis at the dermal–epidermal junction would account for the reduced staining on skin sections with GB3 (antilaminin 5) monoclonal antibody antibody[10] (see Figure 46.2).

Because junctional EB is heterogeneous, DNA-based prenatal diagnosis in this disorder relies on mutational analysis rather than genetic linkage. In the first reported case in 1995[38], the fetus was predicted to be genotypically normal with respect to a homozygous 1 bp deletion in the *LAMB3* gene that had been detected previously in the index case. Other cases have involved mutational analysis of the *LAMA3* and *LAMB3* genes[39–41]. An example of DNA-based prenatal exclusion of junctional EB is shown in Fig. 46.4.

Further examples of the molecular heterogeneity of junctional EB are apparent. Mutations in the genes for the α6 and β4 integrin chains (*ITGA6* and *ITGB4*, respectively) have been found in the variant of junctional EB associated with pyloric atresia[42–46]. As in other forms of junctional EB, it is important first to discover the pathogenetic mutations in the index case or other affected family member, before proceeding to the DNA-based prenatal testing. Mutations in the gene for a different hemidesmosome-associated component, the 180 kDa bullous pemphigoid antigen (also known as BP-180, collagen XVII) may also give rise to non-lethal forms of junctional EB such as the 'generalized atrophic benign' variant[47]. Although the phenotypes resulting from mutations in the BP180 gene (*BPAG2*) tend to be less severe than other variants of junctional EB, several affected individuals have died in infancy[48], and therefore prenatal testing may be considered. A similar phenotype may result from mutations in the *LAMB3* gene[49]. Again, delineation of the pathogenetic mutations in each case will be necessary before embarking on DNA-based prenatal diagnosis.

DYSTROPHIC FORMS OF EPIDERMOLYSIS BULLOSA

In contrast to junctional EB both autosomal dominant and recessive forms of dystrophic EB are caused by mutations in a single gene (*COL7A1*) which encodes the anchoring fibril protein, type VII collagen (Fig. 46.3). *COL7A1* was originally identified by screening keratinocyte and fibroblast cDNA expression libraries with purified antisera from patients with the acquired autoimmune blistering skin disorder, EB acquisita, in which autoantibodies are directed against NC1 domain of type VII collagen[50–52]. The *COL7A1* gene was mapped to 3p21 and subsequent genetic linkage studies in both dominant and recessive dystrophic EB families confirmed *COL7A1* as the sole candidate gene for mutations in these forms of EB[53–56]. Several *COL7A1* mutations have now been described[57–63]. The most severe (Hallopeau–Siemens) type of recessive dystrophic EB is caused by premature termination codon mutations on both *COL7A1* alleles[57–60,63]. By contrast, dominant dystrophic EB is typically associated with

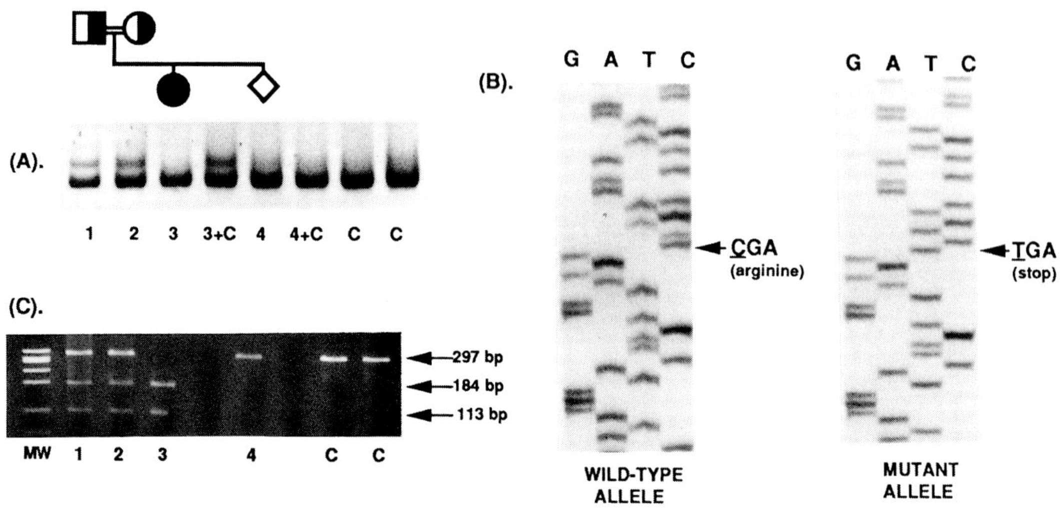

Fig. 46.4 Prenatal exclusion of junctional epidermolysis bullosa by LAMA3 mutation analysis. (A) Heteroduplex analysis of PCR products spanning part of the *LAMA3* gene reveals heteroduplex and homoduplex bandshifts (two bands) in the paternal and maternal DNA (lanes 1 and 2), but only a homoduplex bandshift (single lower band) in the index case (lane 3). However, when the affected child's amplified DNA is mixed with control DNA, a separate heteroduplex bandshift is seen (lane 3+C). Only a single homoduplex band is noted in the fetal DNA (lane 4), even with the addition of control DNA (lane 4+C). (B) Nucleotide sequencing of the affected child's DNA reveals a C-to-T transition that converts an arginine residue (CGA) to a stop codon (TGA). (C) Verification of the mutation by *Dde* I restriction endonuclease. The mutation results in a new cut site for *Dde* I. The index case is homozygous for a new restriction site, whilst the parents are heterozygous for the mutation. In contrast, the fetal DNA is not digested and is identical to the control DNA with no evidence for an additional *Dde* I site. This indicates that the fetus is genotypically normal with respect to this LAMA3 mutation and is predicted to be unaffected with junctional epidermolysis bullosa. (Previously published in McGrath, J.A., Kivirikko, S., Ciatti, S. et al. (1995) *Genomics* **29**, 282–284 and reproduced with permission.)

glycine substitution mutations within the helical region of the type VII collagen molecule[61,62].

Because only one gene appears to be involved in the pathogenesis of dystrophic EB, DNA-based prenatal diagnosis may be undertaken either by genetic linkage or by direct mutational analysis. Several intragenic and flanking *COL7A1* polymorphic markers suitable for linkage analysis have been reported[53–56,63]. The first full report of DNA-based prenatal diagnosis for the Hallopeau–Siemens form of dystrophic EB was in 1995[64]. Six pregnancies were assessed using fetal DNA extracted from chorionic villi or amniotic fluid cells with analysis by genetic linkage markers in four cases and by mutation detection in the other two cases. Several further examples have subsequently been reported[65–67]. The use of DNA markers for the exclusion of recessive dystrophic EB is illustrated in Fig. 46.5.

EPIDERMOLYSIS BULLOSA SIMPLEX

The more common forms of EB simplex are caused by point mutations in the keratin 5 or 14 genes, which are localized to the keratin gene clusters on chromosomes 12q and 17q respectively[68]. The Dowling–Meara form of EB is transmitted in an autosomal dominant manner, but most cases are sporadic. The disease can be very severe at birth, giving rise to widespread blistering and skin loss resulting in death of the affected infant. Prenatal assessment for the Dowling–Meara subtype has been achieved by direct sequencing and mutation analysis of either the K5 or K14 gene after the causative mutation had been identified in an affected parent[69]. A further, more recently identified form of EB simplex is associated with muscular dystrophy[70]. Unlike most other subtypes of EB simplex, this form is autosomal recessive and caused by mutations, in the *PLN* gene on chromosome 8q[71,72], which encodes a large multifunctional protein, plectin[73]. Plectin appears to be involved in the anchorage of the cytoskeleton to the plasma membrane in many cell types including epidermal keratinocytes, endothelial cells, Schwann cells and voluntary muscle cells[73]. Plectin was shown immunochemically to be deficient in skin and cultured cells from patients with EB simplex and muscular dystrophy[74]. Since mutations in *PLN* have been discovered in several unrelated families, DNA-based prenatal diagnosis should now be possible.

BULLOUS CONGENITAL ICHTHYOSIFORM ERYTHRODERMA (EPIDERMOLYTIC HYPERKERATOSIS)

This autosomal dominant disorder is caused by mutations in the genes encoding the suprabasal keratins 1 and 10[75,76]. It has been diagnosed in a fetus at risk by direct gene sequencing of keratin 10[77]. The fetal DNA was shown to contain the same mutant tyrosine residue within the highly conserved 1A-helical segment of keratin as seen in the affected father[77].

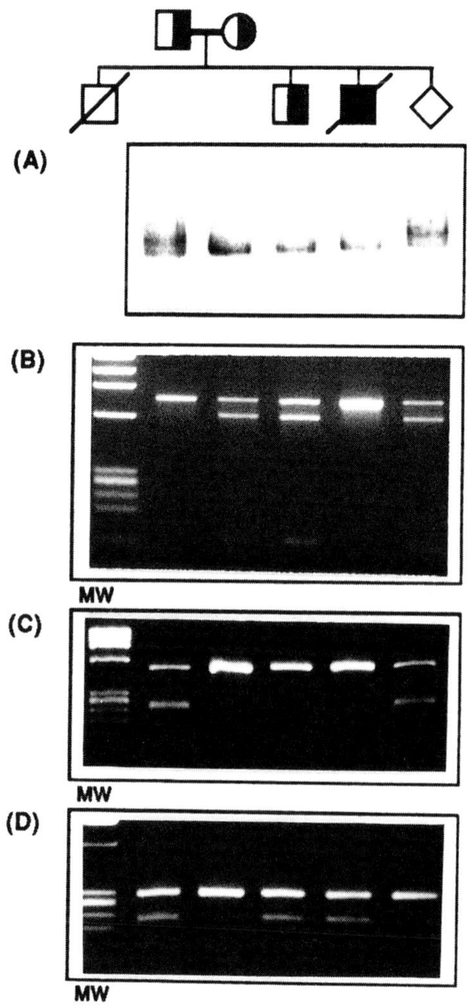

Fig. 46.5 Prenatal exclusion of dystrophic epidermolysis bullosa by linkage analysis. (A) Heteroduplex analysis to assess an intragenic COL7A1 gene polymorphism reveals heteroduplex and homoduplex bandshifts (two bands) in the paternal and fetal DNA, but only homoduplex bandshifts (single lower bands) in the other family members, including the index case. This indicates that the fetus has inherited the normal paternal COL7A1 allele. (B) *PvuII* restriction endonuclease digestion for an intragenic COL7A1 polymorphism shows a +/– haplotype in the maternal, fetal and unaffected child's DNA but a –/– haplotype in the paternal and previously affected child's DNA. This indicates that the fetus has inherited the normal maternal COL7A1 allele. Thus, by linkage analysis the fetus has inherited both normal COL7A1 alleles and is predicted to be unaffected with dystrophic epidermolysis bullosa. (C) *Msp* I restriction endonuclease digestion for a flanking polymorphism (D3S2) confirms the inheritance of the normal paternal COL7A1 allele in the fetal DNA. (D) Sex (X/Y) markers reveal single PCR digestion bands in the maternal and fetal DNA samples and an extra band in the other family members indicating that the fetus is female. (Previously published in McGrath, J.A., Dunnill, M.G.S., Christiano, A.M. et al. (1996) First trimester DNA-based exclusion of recessive dystrophic epidermolysis bullosa from chorionic villus sampling. *Br. J. Dermatol.* **134**, 734–739, reproduced with permission.)

LAMELLAR ICHTHYOSIS

Mutations in the keratinocyte transglutaminase gene may underlie lamellar ichthyosis in some families[78,79], and prenatal diagnosis has been achieved by direct mutational analysis of this gene[80,81]. However, because lamellar ichthyosis is heterogeneous[82], transglutaminase activity should first be assessed in the proband before undertaking DNA analysis.

OCULOCUTANEOUS ALBINISM

Genetic linkage to the tyrosinase gene locus at 11q14–q21 has been demonstrated in individuals with oculocutaneous albinism in whom tyrosinase enzyme activity is reduced or absent[83]. In albinos with normal tyrosinase activity, linkage has been shown to the P gene (equivalent of the mouse pink-eyed dilution gene) at 15q11.2.–q12[84,85]. Pathogenetic mutations in the corresponding patients have been delineated in either the tyrosinase gene[86,87] or the P gene[88]. The mutations in the P gene may also involve variable deletions of the long arm of chromosome 15 and, as a consequence, there is an association with the Prader–Willi and Angelman syndromes[89].

DNA-based prenatal diagnosis for oculocutaneous albinism associated with undetectable tyrosinase activity was described in 1994[90]. DNA was extracted from amniotic fluid cells at 14 weeks' gestation and assessed for tyrosinase gene mutations which had been previously characterized in an affected family member. The fetus was shown to be a heterozygous carrier of a mutant tyrosinase allele and a normal allele. The pregnancy continued with the birth of an unaffected child. A further example of DNA-based prenatal diagnosis for this disorder has been reported[91].

OTHER DISORDERS

Several other inherited disorders with skin manifestations have been tested for prenatally using DNA analysis. These conditions include xeroderma pigmentosum and PIBIDS syndrome[92,93], X-linked hypohidrotic ectodermal dysplasia[94,95], Wiskott–Aldrich syndrome[96].

The prenatal diagnosis of different types of porphyria should be feasible with recent progress in understanding the molecular basis of the porphyrias[97,98]. For example, congenital erythropoietic porphyria (Günther's disease) is an autosomal recessive disorder caused by mutations in the uroporphyrinogen cosynthesase III gene[99]. Identification of mutations causing Sjogren–Larsson syndrome[100] and Chediak–Higashi syndrome[101] should enable DNA-based prenatal diagnosis for these rare conditions.

Conclusion

The availability of prenatal diagnosis for a few potentially devastating genodermatoses has been a major step forward in attempts to eradicate or avoid these diseases and help couples at risk of having affected children to have normal offspring. During the early 1980s the use of fetal skin biopsy, with appropriate electron microscopical analysis, paved the way for DNA-based techniques. These newer methods were introduced some 10 years later and have since been found to be highly effective and reliable.

Acknowledgements

We thank DEBRA (Dystrophic Epidermolysis Bullosa Research Association) and the Special Trustees of St Thomas's Hospital for their support.

REFERENCES

1. Rodeck CH. Fetoscopy guided by real time ultrasound for pure fetal blood samples, fetal skin samples and examination of the fetus in utero. *Br. J. Obstet. Gynaecol.* **87**:449–456, 1980.
2. Anton-Lamprecht I. Prenatal diagnosis of genetic disorders of the skin by means of electron microscopy. *Hum. Genet.* **59**:392–405, 1981.
3. Eady RAJ, Rodeck CH. Prenatal diagnosis of disorders of the skin. In: *Prenatal Diagnosis.* Proceedings of the 11th Study Group, Royal College of Obstetrics and Gynaecologists. CH Rodeck and KH Nicolaides (eds), 147–158, 1984.
4. Elias S. Use of fetoscopy for prenatal diagnosis of hereditary skin disorders. *Curr. Probl. Dermatol.* **16**:1–13, 1987.
5. Eady RAJ. Genodermatoses. In *Prenatal Diagnosis and Screening* (eds DJH Brock, CH Rodeck & MA Ferguson-Smith), pp. 503–512. Edinburgh: Churchill Livingstone, 1992.
6. Sybert VP, Holbrook KA, Levy M. Prenatal diagnosis of severe dermatologic diseases. In *Advances in Dermatology*, Vol. 7 (eds JP Callen, MV Dahl, LE Golitz, HT Greenway & LA Schachner), pp. 179–209. St Louis: Mosby Yearbook, 1992.
7. Holbrook KA, Smith LA, Elias S. Prenatal diagnosis of genetic skin disease using fetal skin biopsy samples. *Arch. Dermatol.* **129**:1437–1454, 1993.
8. Eady RAJ, Gunner DB, Tidman MJ, Nicolaides KH, Rodeck CH. Rapid processing of fetal skin for prenatal diagnosis by light and electron microscopy. *J. Clin. Pathol.* **37**:633–638, 1984.
9. Heagerty AHM, Kennedy AR, Gunner DB, Eady RAJ. Rapid prenatal diagnosis and exclusion of epidermolysis bullosa using novel antibody probes. *J. Invest. Dermatol.* **86**:603–605, 1986.
10. Heagerty AH, Eady RAJ, Kennedy AR et al. Rapid prenatal diagnosis of epidermolysis bullosa letalis using GB3 monoclonal antibody. *Br. J. Dermatol.* **117**:271–275, 1987.
11. Fine JD, Eady RAJ, Levy ML et al. Prenatal diagnosis of dominant and recessive dystrophic epidermolysis bullosa: application and limitations in the use of KF-1 and LH7.2 monoclonal antibodies and immunofluorescence mapping technique. *J. Invest. Dermatol.* **91**:465–471, 1988.
12. Fine JD, Holbrook KA, Elias S, Anton Lamprecht I, Rauskolb R. Applicability of 19-DEJ-1 monoclonal antibody for the prenatal diagnosis or exclusion of junctional epidermolysis bullosa. *Prenat. Diagn.* **10**:219–229, 1990.
13. Shimizu H, Suzumori K, Hatta N, Nishikawa T. Absence of detectable α6 integrin in pyloric atresia-junctional epidermolysis bullosa syndrome: application for prenatal diagnosis in a family at risk for recurrence. *Arch. Dermatol.* **132**:919–925, 1996.
14. Eady RAJ, Dunnill MGS. Epidermolysis bullosa: hereditary skin fragility diseases as paradigms in cell biology. *Arch. Dermatol. Res.* **287**:2–9, 1994.
15. Eady RAJ, Holbrook KA, Blanchet-Bardon C, Anton-Lamprecht I. Prenatal diagnosis of skin diseases. In *Dermatology: Progress and Perspectives. The Proceedings of the 18th World Congress of Dermatology* (eds WHC Burgdorf & SI Katz), pp. 1159–1165. The Pantheon Publishing Group, 1993.
16. Rodeck CH, Eady RAJ, Gosden CM. Prenatal diagnosis of epidermolysis bullosa letalis. *Lancet* **1**:949–952, 1980.
17. Nazzaro V, Nicolini U, De Luca L, Berti E, Caputo R. Prenatal diagnosis of junctional epidermolysis bullosa associated with pyloric atresia. *J Med Genet* **27**:244–248, 1990.
18. Anton-Lamprecht I, Rauskolb B, Jovanovic V. Prenatal diagnosis of epidermolysis bullosa dystrophica Hallopeau–Siemens with electron microscopy of fetal skin. *Lancet* **2**:1077–1079, 1981.
19. Perry TB, Holbrook KA, Hoff MS. Prenatal diagnosis of congenital non-bullous ichthyosiform erythroderma (lamellar ichthyosis). *Prenat. Diagn.* **7**:145–155, 1987.
20. Arnold ML, Anton Lamprecht I. Problems in prenatal diagnosis of the ichthyosis congenita group. *Hum. Genet.* **71**:301–311, 1985.
21. Blanchet-Bardon C, Dumez Y. Prenatal diagnosis of harlequin fetus. *Semin. Dermatol.* **3**:225–228, 1984.
22. Golbus MS, Sagebiel RW, Filly RA, Gindhart TD, Hall JG. Prenatal diagnosis of congenital bullous ichthyosiform erythroderma (epidermolytic hyperkeratosis) by fetal skin biopsy. *N. Engl. J. Med.* **302**:93–95, 1980.
23. Holbrook KA, Dale BA, Sybert VP et al. Epidermolytic hyperkeratosis: ultrastructure and biochemistry of skin and amniotic fluid cells from two affected fetuses and a new born infant. *J. Invest. Dermatol.* **80**:222–227, 1983.
24. Holbrook KA. Progress in prenatal diagnosis of bullous congenital ichthyosiform erythroderma (epidermolytic hyperkeratosis). *Semin. Dermatol.* **3**:216–220, 1984.
25. Eady RAJ, Gunner DB, Lamblia Carbone L et al. Prenatal diagnosis of bullous ichthyosiform erythroderma: detection of tonofilament clumps in fetal epidermal and amniotic fluid cells. *J. Med. Genet.* **23**:46–51, 1986.
26. Eady RAJ, Gunner DB, Garner A, Rodeck CH. Prenatal diagnosis of oculocutaneous albinism by electron microscopy of fetal skin. *J. Invest. Dermatol.* **80**:210–212, 1983.
27. Shimizu H, Ishiko A, Kikuchi A, Akiyama M, Suzumori K, Nishikawa T. Prenatal diagnosis of tyrosinase-negative oculocutaneous albinism. *Lancet* **340**:739–740, 1992.
28. Holbrook KA, Wapner R, Jackson L, Zaeri N. Diagnosis and prenatal diagnosis of epidermolysis bullosa herpetiformis (Dowling–Meara) in a mother, two affected children, and an affected fetus. *Prenat. Diagn.* **12**:725–739, 1992.
29. Kousseff BG, Matsuoka LY, Stenn KS et al. Prenatal diagnosis of Sjogren–Larsson syndrome. *J. Pediatr.* **101**:998–1001, 1982.
30. Arnold M-L, Rauskolb R, Anton-Lamprecht I et al. Prenatal diagnosis of anhidrotic ectodermal dysplasia. *Prenat. Diagn.* **4**:85–98, 1984.
31. Happle R, Schuurmans Stekhoven JH, Hamel BCJ et al. Restrictive dermatopathy in two brothers. *Arch. Dermatol.* **128**:232–235, 1992.
32. Durandy A, Breton-Gorius J, Guy-Grand D, Dumez C, Griscelli C. Prenatal diagnosis of syndromes associating albinism and immune deficiencies (Chediak–Higashi syndrome and variant). *Prenat. Diagn.* **13**:13–20, 1993.
33. Aberdam D, Galliano MF, Vailly J et al. Herlitz's junctional epidermolysis bullosa is linked to mutations in the gene (LAMC2) for the γ2 subunit of nicein/kalinin (LAMININ-5). *Nat. Genet.* **6**:299–304, 1994.
34. Pulkkinen L, Christiano AM, Airenne T, Haakana H, Tryggvason K, Uitto J. Mutations in the γ2 chain gene (LAMC2) of kalinin/laminin 5 in the junctional forms of epidermolysis bullosa. *Nat. Genet.* **6**:293–297, 1994.
35. Pulkkinen L, Christiano AM, Gerecke D et al. A homozygous nonsense mutation in the β3 chain gene of laminin 5 (LAMB3) in Herlitz junctional epidermolysis bullosa. *Genomics* **24**:357–360, 1994.
36. Kivirikko S, McGrath JA, Baudoin C et al. A homozygous nonsense mutation in the α3 chain gene of laminin 5 (LAMA3) in lethal (Herlitz) junctional epidermolysis bullosa. *Hum. Mol. Genet.* **4**:959–962, 1995.
37. Vidal F, Baudoin C, Miquel C et al. Cloning of the laminin α3 chain gene (LAMA3) and identification of a homozygous deletion in a patient with Herlitz junctional epidermolysis bullosa. *Genomics* **30**:273–280, 1995.

38. Vailly J, Pulkkinen L, Miquel C et al. Identification of a homozygous one-base pair deletion in exon 14 of the LAMB3 gene in a patient with Herlitz junctional epidermolysis bullosa and prenatal diagnosis in a family at risk for recurrence. *J. Invest. Dermatol.* **104**:462–466, 1995.
39. McGrath JA, Kivirikko S, Ciatti S et al. A homozygous nonsense mutation in the α3 chain gene of laminin 5 (LAMA3) in Herlitz junctional epidermolysis bullosa: prenatal exclusion in a fetus at risk. *Genomics* **29**:282–284, 1995.
40. Christiano AM, McGrath JA, Uitto J. Prenatal exclusion of Herlitz junctional epidermolysis bullosa by mutation analysis in the LAMB3 gene in three families at risk for recurrence (abst). *J. Invest. Dermatol.* **105**:449, 1995.
41. Christiano AM, Pulkkinen L, McGrath JA, Uitto J. Mutation based prenatal diagnosis of Herlitz junctional epidermolysis bullosa. *Prenat. Diagn.* **17**:343–354, 1998.
42. Vidal F, Aberdam D, Miquel C et al. Integrin β4 mutations associated with junctional epidermolysis bullosa with pyloric atresia. *Nat. Genet.* **10**:229–234, 1995.
43. Pulkinnen L, Kurtz K, Xu Y et al. Genomic organization of the integrin β4 gene (ITGB4): a homozygous splice-site mutation in a patient with junctional epidermolysis bullosa associated with pyloric atresia. *Lab. Invest.* **76**:823–833, 1997.
44. Takizawa Y, Shimizu H, Nishikawa T et al. Novel ITGB4 mutations in a patient with junctional epidermolysis bullosa-pyloric atresia syndrome and altered basement membrane zone immunofluorescence for the α6β4 integrin. *J. Invest. Dermatol.* **108**:943–946, 1998.
45. Ruzzi L, Gagnoux-Palacios L, Pinola M et al. A homozygous mutation in the integrin α6 gene in junctional epidermolysis bullosa with pyloric atresia. *J. Clin. Invest.* **99**:2826–2831, 1997.
46. Pulkkinen L, Kimonis VE, Xu Y et al. Homozygous α6 integrin mutation in junctional epidermolysis bullosa with congenital duodenal atresia. *Hum. Mol. Genet.* **6**:669–674, 1997.
47. McGrath JA, Gatalica B, Li K, Owaribe K, McMillan JR, Eady RAJ, Uitto J. Mutations in the 180-kD bullous pemphigoid antigen (BPAG2), a hemidesmosomal transmembrane collagen (COL17A1), in generalized atrophic benign epidermolysis bullosa. *Nat. Genet.* **11**:83–86, 1995.
48. McGrath JA, Darling T, Gatalica B et al. A homozygous deletion mutation in the gene encoding the 180-kDa bullous pemphigoid antigen (BPAG2) in a family with generalized atrophic benign epidermolysis bullosa. *J. Invest. Dermatol.* **106**:771–774, 1996.
49. McGrath JA, Pulkkinen L, Christiano AM, Leigh IM, Eady RAJ, Uitto J. Altered laminin 5 expression due to mutations in the gene encoding the β3 chain (LAMB3) in generalized atrophic benign epidermolysis bullosa. *J. Invest. Dermatol.* **104**:467–474, 1995.
50. Parente MG, Chung LC, Ryynanen J et al. Human type VII collagen: cDNA cloning and chromosomal mapping of the gene. *Proc. Natl. Acad. Sci. USA.* **88**:6931–6935, 1991.
51. Christiano AM, Greenspan DS, Lee S, Uitto J. Cloning of human type VII collagen. Complete primary sequence of the α1(VII) chain and identification of intragenic polymorphisms. *J. Biol. Chem.* **269**:20256–20262, 1994.
52. Christiano AM, Hoffman GG, Chung-Honet LC et al. Structural organization of the human type VII collagen gene (COL7A1), comprised of more exons than any previously characterized gene. *Genomics* **21**:169–179, 1994.
53. Rynnanen M, Knowlton RG, Parente MG, Chung LC, Chu ML, Uitto J. Human type VII collagen: genetic linkage of the gene (COL7A1) on chromosome 3 to dominant dystrophic epidermolysis bullosa. *Am. J. Hum. Genet.* **49**:797–803, 1991.
54. Al-Imara L, Richards AJ, Eady RAJ, Leigh IM, Farrall M, Pope FM. Linkage of autosomal dominant dystrophic epidermolysis bullosa in three British families to the marker D3S2 close to the COL7A1. *J. Med. Genet.* **29**:381–382, 1992.
55. Hovnanian A, Duquesnoy P, Blanchet-Bardon C et al. Genetic linkage of recessive dystrophic epidermolysis bullosa to the type VII collagen gene. *J. Clin. Invest.* **90**:1032–1036, 1992.
56. Dunnill MG, Richards AJ, Milana G et al. Genetic linkage to the type VII collagen gene (COL7A1) in 26 families with generalised recessive dystrophic epidermolysis bullosa and anchoring fibril abnormalities. *J. Med. Genet.* **31**:745–748, 1994.
57. Hilal L, Rochat A, Duquesnoy P et al. A homozygous insertion-deletion in the type VII collagen gene (COL7A1) in Hallopeau-Siemens dystrophic epidermolysis bullosa. *Nat. Genet.* **5**:287–293, 1993.
58. Christiano AM, Anhalt G, Gibbons S, Bauer EA, Uitto J. Premature termination codons in the type VII collagen gene (COL7A1) underlie severe, mutilating recessive dystrophic epidermolysis bullosa. *Genomics* **21**:160–168, 1994.
59. Christiano AM, Uitto J. Molecular diagnosis of inherited skin diseases: the paradigm of dystrophic epidermolysis bullosa. *Adv. Dermatol.* **11**:199–213, 1996.
60. Dunnill MG, Richards AJ, Milana G, Mollica F, Eady RA, Pope FM. A novel homozygous point mutation in the collagen VII gene (COL7A1) in two cousins with recessive dystrophic epidermolysis bullosa. *Hum. Mol. Genet.* **3**:1693–1694, 1994.
61. Christiano AM, Ryynanen M, Uitto J. Dominant dystrophic epidermolysis bullosa: identification of a Gly→Ser substitution in the triple-helical domain of type VII collagen. *Proc. Natl. Acad. Sci. USA.* **91**:3549–3553, 1994.
62. Christiano AM, Uitto J. Molecular complexity of the cutaneous basement membrane zone. Revelations from the paradigms of epidermolysis bullosa. *Exp. Dermatol.* **5**:1–11, 1996.
63. Jarvikallio A, Pulkkinen L, Uitto J. Molecular basis of dystrophic epidermolysis bullosa: mutations in the type VII collagen gene (COL7A1). *Hum. Mutat.* **110**:179–182, 1997.
64. Hovnanian A, Hilal L, Blanchet Bardon C et al. DNA-based prenatal diagnosis of generalized recessive dystrophic epidermolysis bullosa in six pregnancies at risk for recurrence. *J. Invest. Dermatol.* **104**:456–461, 1995.
65. Dunnill MG, Richards AJ, Milana G, Mollica F, Eady RA, Pope FM. Use of type VII collagen gene (COL7A1) markers in prenatal diagnosis of recessive dystrophic epidermolysis bullosa. *J. Med. Genet.* **32**:749–750, 1995.
66. McGrath JA, Dunnill MG, Christiano AM et al. First trimester DNA-based exclusion of recessive dystrophic epidermolysis bullosa from chorionic villus sampling. *Br. J. Dermatol.* **134**:734–739, 1996.
67. Christiano AM, LaForgia S, Paller AS, McGuire J, Shimizu H, Uitto J. DNA-based prenatal diagnosis of recessive dystrophic epidermolysis bullosa in ten families at risk for recurrence. *Molec. Med.* **2**:59–76, 1996.
68. Leigh IM, Lane EB. Mutations in the genes for epidermal keratins in epidermolysis bullosa and epidermolytic hyperkeratosis. *Arch. Dermatol.* **129**:1571–1577, 1993.
69. Rugg EL, Shemanko CS, Magee GJ, Batty D, Boxer M, Lane EB. Taking epidermolysis bullosa simplex from mutation analysis to prenatal diagnosis. *J. Invest. Dermatol.* **108**:597(abstr), 1997.
70. Fine J-D, Bauer EA, Briggaman RA et al. Revised clinical and laboratory criteria for sub-types of inherited epidermolysis bullosa. *J. Amer. Acad. Dermatol.* **24**:119–135, 1991.
71. Smith FJD, Eady RAJ, Leigh IM et al. Plectin deficiency results in muscular dystrophy with epidermolysis bullosa. *Nat. Genet.* **13**:450–456, 1996.
72. McLean WHI, Smith FJD, Pulkkinen L et al. Loss of plectin causes epidermolysis bullosa with muscular dystrophy: cDNA cloning and genomic organization. *Genes. Dev.* **10**:1724–1735, 1996.
73. Wiche G. Plectin: general overview and its appraisal of its potential role as a subunit protein of the cytomatrix. *CRC Crit. Rev. Biochem. Mol. Biol.* **24**:41–67, 1989.
74. Gache Y, Chavanas S, Lacour JP et al. Defective expression of plectin/HD1 in epidermolysis bullosa simplex with muscular dystrophy. *J. Clin. Invest.* **97**:2289–2298, 1996.
75. Bonifas JM, Bare JW, Cheng MA et al. Linkage of epidermolytic hyperkeratosis phenotype and the region of type II keratin gene cluster on chromosome 12. *J. Invest. Dermatol.* **99**:524–527, 1992.
76. Cheng J, Syder AJ, Yu Q-C et al. The genetic basis of epidermolytic hyperkeratosis: a disorder of differentiation-specific epidermal keratin genes. *Cell* **70**:811–819, 1992.
77. Rothnagel JA, Longley NA, Holder RA, Kuster W, Roop DR. Prenatal diagnosis of epidermolytic hyperkeratosis by direct gene sequencing. *J. Invest. Dermatol.* **102**:13–16, 1994.
78. Huber M, Rettler I, Bernsasconi K et al. Mutations of keratinocyte transglutaminase in lamellar ichthyosis. *Science* **267**:525–528, 1995.
79. Russell LJ, Di Giovanna JJ, Rogers GR et al. Mutations in the gene for transglutaminase I in autosomal recessive lamellar ichthyosis. *Nat. Genet.* **9**:279–283, 1995.

80. Schorderet DF, Huber M, Laurini RN et al. Prenatal diagnosis of lamellar ichthyosis by direct mutational analysis of the keratinocyte transglutaminase gene. *Prenat. Diagn.* **17**:483–486, 1997.
81. Bichakjian CK, Nair RP, Wu WW, Goldberg S, Elder JT. Prenatal exclusion of lamellar ichthyosis based on identification of two new mutations in the TGM1 gene. *J. Invest. Dermatol.* **110**:179–182, 1998.
82. Huber M, Rettler I, Bernasconi K, Wyss M, Hohl D. Lamellar ichthyosis is genetically heterogeneous – cases with normal keratinocyte transglutaminase. *J. Invest. Dermatol.* **105**:653–654, 1995.
83. Barton DE, Kwon BS, Francke U. Human tyrosinase gene, mapped to chromosome 11 (q14–q21), defines second region of homology with mouse chromosome 7. *Genomics* **3**:17–24, 1988.
84. Ramsey M, Colman MA, Stevens G et al. The tyrosinase-positive oculocutaneous albinism locus maps to chromosome 15q 11.2–q12. *Am. J. Hum. Genet.* **51**:879–884, 1992.
85. Rinchik EM, Bultman SJ, Horsthemke B et al. A gene for the mouse pink-eyed dilution locus and for human type II oculocutaneous albinism. *Nature* **361**:72–76, 1993.
86. Tomita Y, Takeda A, Okinaga S, Tamagi H, Shibahara S. Human oculocutaneous albinism caused by single base insertion in the tyrosinase gene. *Biochem. Biophys. Res. Commun.* **164**:990–996, 1989.
87. Takeda A, Tomita Y, Matsunaga J, Tagami H, Shibahara S. Molecular basis of tyrosinase-negative oculocutaneous albinism. *J. Biol. Chem.* **265**:17792–17797, 1990.
88. Lee S-T, Nicholls RD, Bundey S, Laxova R, Musarella M, Spritz RA. Mutations of the P gene in oculocutaneous albinism, ocular albinism and Prader–Willi syndrome plus albinism. *N. Engl. J. Med.* **330**:529–534, 1994.
89. Magenis RE, Toth-Fejel S, Allen LJ et al. Comparison of the 15q deletions in Prader–Willi and Angelman syndromes; specific regions, extent of deletions, parental origins and clinical consequences. *Am. J. Med. Genet.* **35**:333–349, 1990.
90. Shimizu H, Niizeki H, Suzumori K et al. Prenatal diagnosis of oculocutaneous albinism by analysis of the fetal tyrosinase gene. *J. Invest. Dermatol.* **103**:104–106, 1994.
91. Borenstein TC, Holmes SA, Borochwitz et al. DNA-based carrier detection and prenatal diagnosis of tyrosinase-negative oculocutaneous albinism (OCA1A). *Prenat. Diagn.* **15**:345–349, 1995.
92. Savary JB, Vasseur F, Vinatier D, Manouvrier S, Thomas P, Deminatti MM. Prenatal diagnosis of PIBIDS. *Prenat. Diagn.* **11**:859–866, 1991.
93. Savary JB, Vasseur F, Deminatti MM. Routine autoradiographic analysis of DNA excision-repair. Report of prenatal and postnatal diagnosis in eleven families. *Ann. Genet.* **34**:76–81, 1991.
94. Zonana J, Jones M, Clarke A, Gault J, Muller B, Thomas NS. Detection of de novo mutations and analysis of their origin in families with x-linked hypohidrotic ectodermal dysplasia. *J. Med. Genet.* **31**:287–292, 1994.
95. Zonana J, Schnizel A, Upadhyaya M, Thomas NS, Anton-Lamprecht I, Harper DJ. Prenatal diagnosis of x-linked hypohidrotic ectodermal dysplasia by linkage analysis. *Am. J. Med. Genet.* **35**:132–135, 1990.
96. Schwartz M, Mibashan RS, Nicolaides KH et al. First-trimester diagnosis of Wiskott–Aldrich syndrome by DNA markers. *Lancet* **2**:1405, 1989.
97. Elder GH. Molecular genetics of haem biosynthesis. *J. Clin. Pathol.* **46**:977–981, 1993.
98. de Verneuil H, Ged C, Boulechfar S, Moreau-Gaudry F. Porphyrins: animal models and prospects for cellular and gene therapy. *J. Bioeng. Biomemb.* 239–248, 1995.
99. Bensidhoum M, Ged C, Hombrados I et al. Identification of two new mutations in congenital erythropoietic porphyria. *Eur. J. Hum. Genet.* **3**:102–107, 1995.
100. De Laurenzi V, Rogers GR, Hamrock DJ et al. Sjogren-Larsson syndrome is caused by mutations in the fatty aldehyde dehydrogenase gene. *Nat. Genet.* **12**:52–57, 1996.
101. Nagle DL, Karim MA, Woolf E et al. Identification and mutation analysis of the complete gene for Chediak–Higashi syndrome. *Nat. Genet.* **14**:307–311, 1996.

SECTION

7

Diagnosis and management of fetal malformations

Second-trimester sonographic features of aneuploidy

47

B.R. Benacerraf

Introduction

Until 10–15 years ago, amniocentesis was reserved for women ≥35 years of age. Over the past two decades, this group has formed approximately 5% of the pregnant population and produced 20% of the fetuses with Down syndrome[1,2]. More recently, the prenatal detection of fetuses with chromosomal abnormalities has progressed with the observation that a low maternal serum alpha fetoprotein (MSAFP) is associated with fetal chromosomal abnormalities – in particular, Down syndrome[3–5]. In 1984, two different laboratories (Cuckle et al.[3], Merkatz et al.[5]) found that a low MSAFP could be used to form the basis of a screening test for the detection of Down syndrome in women younger than age 35. This resulted in identifying 20–30% of pregnancies with Down syndrome fetuses among women <35 years old, while recommending amniocentesis for 5% of unaffected pregnancies. Since that time, there has been a multitude of studies evaluating the use of many serum markers, including human chorionic gonadotrophin (hCG) and unconjugated estriol (UE3) for detecting pregnancies complicated by chromosomal abnormalities.

While serum markers and maternal age are useful indirect parameters for evaluating the fetus, sonographic anatomic examination of the fetus is a more direct and potentially rewarding approach. During the evolution of these serum markers for the detection of Down syndrome, there has been a simultaneous effort to use ultrasound to identify anatomical markers in first- and second-trimester fetuses affected by chromosomal abnormalities (Table 47.1). The biochemical and sonographic areas of research have progressed largely independently but with the hope that, in the long term, a screening programme can be established that will use sonographic screening techniques as well as maternal age and biochemical screening for the best assessment of the risk that a fetus could be chromosomally abnormal.

Trisomy 18

Trisomy 18 or Edward syndrome (Table 47.1) is a rare chromosomal abnormality with an incidence of 1.4 per 10 000 births. The median life expectancy of newborn infants with trisomy 18 is 5 days, but it may range from birth to 18 months[6]. Fetuses with trisomy 18 have a multitude of malformations which are easily recognizable sonographically[7–16]. Some fetuses with trisomy 18 have a first-trimester nuchal translucency thickening which is thought to represent a cystic hygroma[17]. Most of the abnormalities associated with trisomy 18, however, are best seen in the second trimester, when visualization of the fetus is improved. Fetal malformations seen sonographically can be used to detect between 80% and 90% of second-trimester fetuses and up to 100% of third-trimester fetuses with trisomy 18[6,16,18].

Common abnormalities include major heart defects, cystic hygromata and nuchal thickening, omphalocele, diaphragmatic hernia, oesophageal atresia, large cisterna magna, strawberry-shaped skull, meningomyelocele and ventriculomegaly, micrognathia, renal anomaly, single umbilical artery, clubbed or rockerbottom feet, clenched hands, and severe intrauterine growth retardation (IUGR) associated with polyhydramnios (Figs 47.1–47.6)[7–20]. Choroid plexus cysts are also seen in approximately 30% of fetuses with trisomy 18 (Fig. 47.7). However, these cysts are also common among normal fetuses and, therefore, they are considered a marker rather than a true abnormality[21].

The most recognizable abnormality of fetuses with trisomy 18 seen on second-trimester ultrasound involves the fetal limbs[9,16,18,21]. The hands are almost always clenched in a characteristic configuration with an overlapping index finger (Fig. 47.6)[16,18,21]. The inability of most fetuses with trisomy 18 to open their hands is helpful in evaluating fetuses at risk for having trisomy 18; a picture of an open hand can be used to decrease the risk that a fetus has trisomy 18. Also, some fetuses

TABLE 47.1
Sonographic characteristics of fetuses with aneuploidy

Trisomy 18
Choroid plexus cysts
Strawberry-shaped cranium
Abnormal cerebellum/large cisterna magna
Cardiac defect
Omphalocele
Diaphragmatic hernia
Neural tube defect
Clubbed feet/rockerbottom feet
Clenched hands/overlapping fingers
Short radial ray
IUGR/polyhydramnios
Micrognathia
Cystic hygroma
Intrauterine growth retardation
Trisomy 13
Holoprosencephaly
Facial defects
Heart defects
Cystic kidneys
Polydactyly
Omphalocele
Cystic hygroma
Microcephaly
Triploidy
Early asymmetric growth retardation
Ventriculomegaly
Dandy–Walker malformations
Cardiac defects
Syndactyly
Oligohydramnios
Placental abnormalities
Neural tube defects
Cystic kidneys and hydronephrosis
Omphalocele
Facial defects
Turner syndrome (XO)
Cystic hygroma
Congenital lymphoedema
Hydrops
Cardiac defect (left heart lesions)
Short femur
Horseshoe kidney
Trisomy 9
Microcephaly
Facial cleft/micrognathia
Abnormal extremities
Cardiac defect
Kidney defects (cystic kidneys)
Cerebellar anomalies
Intrauterine growth retardation
Neural tube defect
Diaphragmatic hernia
Down syndrome (trisomy 21)
Nuchal fold ≥ 6 mm
Ventriculomegaly
Cardiac defects
Echogenic intracardiac focus
Hyperechogenic bowel
Pyelectasis
Short femur
Short humerus
Clinodactyly
Hypoplasia middle phalanx 5th digit
Sandal foot
Simian crease
Duodenal atresia

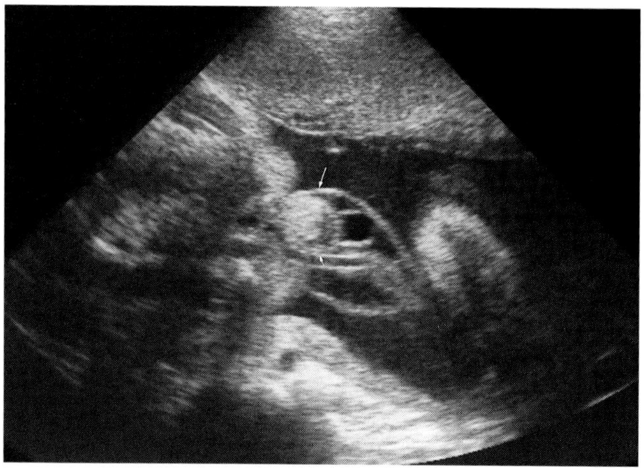

Fig. 47.1 Trisomy 18: transverse view through the fetal cord insertion in the third trimester, showing a small, bowel-containing omphalocele (arrows) within the umbilical sheath.

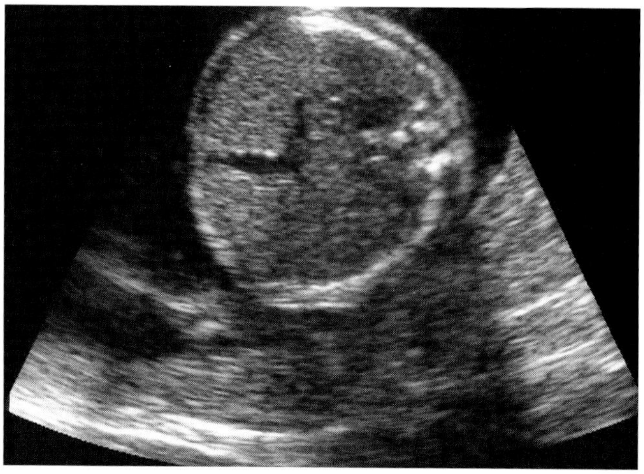

Fig. 47.2 Trisomy 18: transverse view through the fetal abdomen at the level of the portal vein, showing absence of the fetal stomach bubble.

with trisomy 18 have preaxial upper limb reduction, such as short radial rays and clubbed hands, as is often seen with Holt–Oram or Fanconi syndromes.

More than 90% of fetuses with trisomy 18 have heart defects, although these are difficult to diagnose in the first or very early second trimester. In a study by Nyberg et al., heart defects were identified in only 14% of fetuses with trisomy 18 between 14 and 24 weeks, as compared with 78% of those between 24 and 40 weeks[16].

Omphaloceles are present in approximately 20% fetuses with trisomy 18 (Fig. 47.1)[16]. Most of these omphaloceles, however, are small defects which contain only bowel (with no externalization of the fetal liver). Fetuses who have omphaloceles with an extracorporeal liver have a much lower incidence of chromosomal abnormalities.

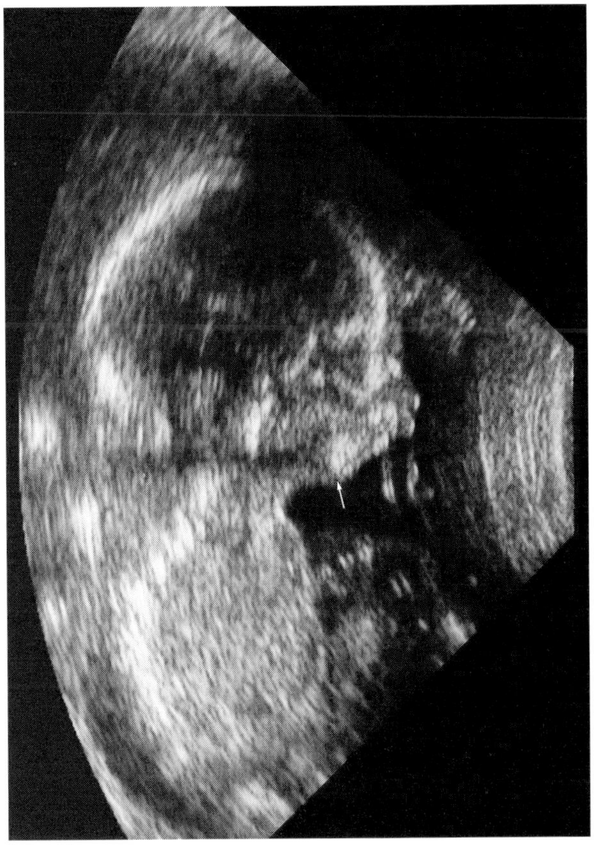

Fig. 47.3 Trisomy 18: longitudinal view of the fetal face, showing an abnormal fetal profile in the second trimester. Note the severe underdevelopment of the mandible, consistent with micrognathia (arrow).

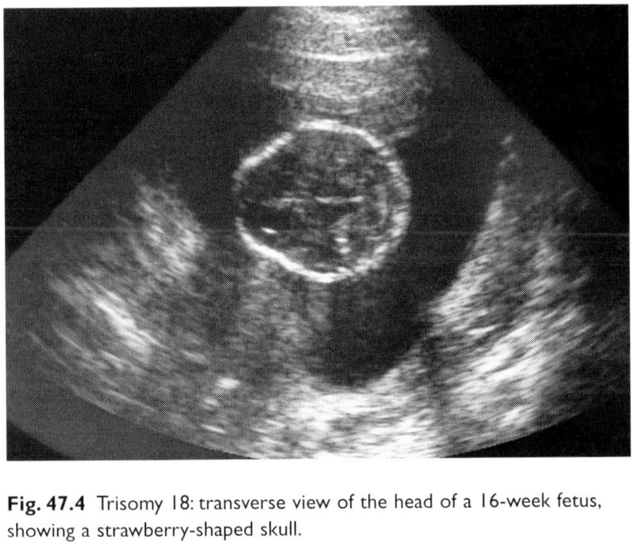

Fig. 47.4 Trisomy 18: transverse view of the head of a 16-week fetus, showing a strawberry-shaped skull.

The appearance of the head commonly seen in trisomy 18 includes a large cisterna magna with a small cerebellum as well as a strawberry-shaped skull (Fig. 47.4, 47.5)[7,8,11,12,16].

Fetal growth retardation is a very common feature of fetuses with trisomy 18[19,20]. This can develop early in

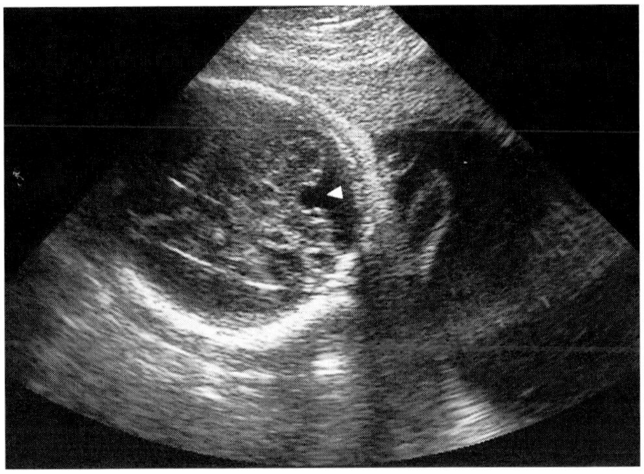

Fig. 47.5 Trisomy 18: abnormal development of the cerebellum, showing a Dandy–Walker malformation with absence of the cerebellar vermis and communication between the fourth ventricle and the cisterna magna (arrow head). Note the hypoplasia of the cerebellar hemispheres.

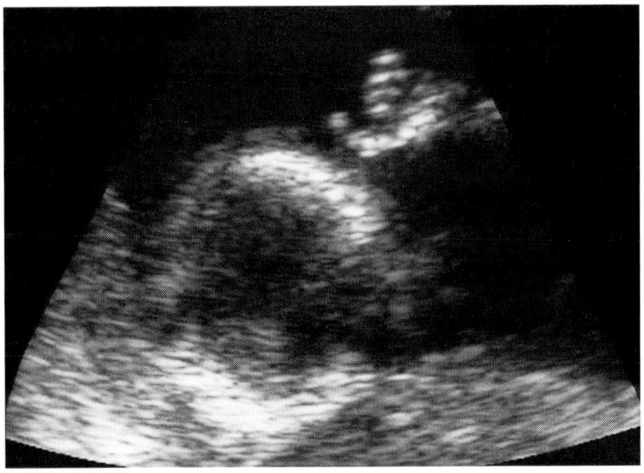

(a)

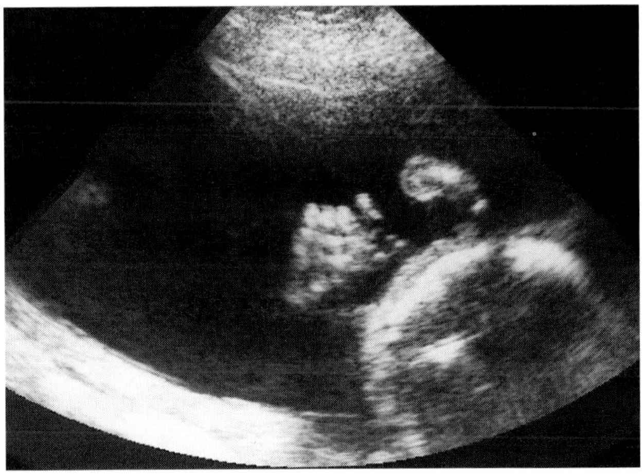

(b)

Fig. 47.6 Trisomy 18. (a) View of the fetal hand in the second trimester, showing clenched fist and overlapping index finger. (b) A different case showing a similar configuration of the fetal hand with a clenched fist and overlapping index finger.

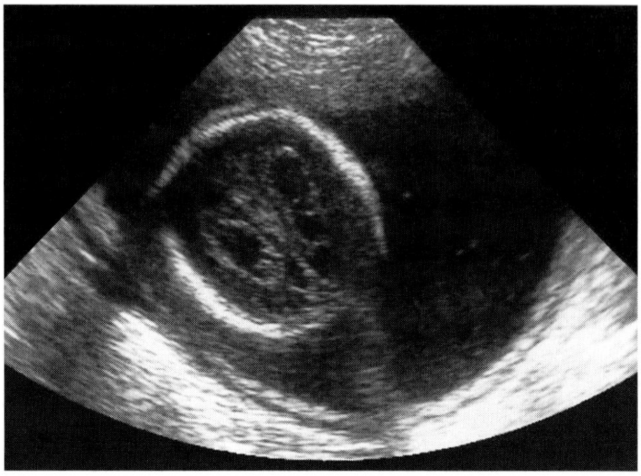

Fig. 47.7 Trisomy 18: transverse view of the fetal head showing large bilateral choroid plexus cysts.

pregnancy, although it is often not recognized until after the second trimester. Typically, fetuses with trisomy 18 have a combination of polyhydramnios and intrauterine growth retardation, with small abdominal circumferences. Evaluation of the umbilical cord may show a single umbilical artery as well as absent umbilical artery end diastolic flow in the third trimester. It is important to recognize that such anomalous fetuses do not have straightforward placental insufficiency but have a more serious aetiology for their severe intrauterine growth retardation. Umbilical cord cysts have also been documented in association with trisomy 18 and intrauterine growth restriction[22].

Choroid plexus cysts are transiently present in 1–2% of normal second-trimester fetuses and have been considered a normal variant for many years (Fig. 47.7)[21–28]. Thirty percent of second-trimester fetuses with trisomy 18 have choroid plexus cysts and, therefore, the risk of trisomy 18 is increased in fetuses who have these cysts[21]. Whether or not patients carrying fetuses with isolated choroid plexus should undergo amniocenteses remains controversial. It is widely acknowledged that trisomy 18 is a rare chromosomal abnormality which is easily recognizable sonographically by the presence of multiple congenital abnormalities. These include heart defects, limb abnormalities, facial malformations, and many other defects.

We reported that, in a hypothetical population, the chances that a second-trimester fetus with isolated choroid plexus cysts would have trisomy 18 is 1/477, thus suggesting that amniocentesis is not warranted unless an additional malformation is identified. However, the question of whether amniocentesis should be recommended to women carrying fetuses with isolated choroid plexus cysts remains highly controversial in what has become a large group of studies, most of which have less than 100 fetuses[21–44].

Different authors have varying success in detecting the major structural anomalies sonographically in fetuses affected with trisomy 18, thus resulting in conflicting recommendations. Table 47.2 summarizes most of the studies attempting to resolve this issue. Four studies stand out as containing the majority of fetuses with chromosomal abnormalities in fetuses with isolated choroid plexus cysts, indicating notable differences among ultrasound laboratories in detecting associated anatomical defects in chromosomally abnormal fetuses[35,36,38,40].

TABLE 47.2
Studies showing incidence of aneuploidy in fetuses with choroid plexus (CP) cysts

Study	Isolated CP cyst cases	Chromosomal anomalies
Achiron[29]	29	1
Benacerraf[26]	38	0
Gabrielli[32]	61	0
Chinn[30]	36	0
Clark[24]	5	0
Chan[23]	13	0
DeRoo[25]	17	0
Chitkara[31]	38	0
Hertzberg[33]	31	0
Ostlere[37]	96	0
Howard[34]	51	1
Nadel[18]	220	0
Nava[36]	193	4
Platt[39]	67	0
Porto[40]	59	2
Twining[41]	16	0
Thorpe-Beeston[43]	49	0
Walkinshaw[42]	152	4
Zerres[44]	14	0
Gross[28]	74	0
Perpignano[38]	86	5
Kupferminc[35]	98	4

Adapted from B. Benacerraf. The sonography of fetal syndromes. Harcourt Brace, 1998.

A recent study by Gross et al. summarizes the question of whether chromosomal studies are necessary in fetuses with isolated choroid plexus cysts, using a review and metanalysis of many of the larger studies in the literature concerning this issue[28]. Among 13 of the larger studies, Gross et al. demonstrate that the incidence of fetuses with trisomy 18 among fetuses with isolated choroid plexus cysts was only 0.27% or a risk of 1/374. This is lower than the usual accepted risk for suggesting amniocentesis. Gupta et al. also evaluated this issue, using a registry of fetal choroid plexus cysts over 3 years in the Yorkshire region and then analysing these together with 1361 cases from prospective studies reported in the English literature[27]. They showed that, when choroid plexus cysts were associated with any other abnormality, there was a high risk of chromosomal abnormality. In the absence of any other sonographic findings, however, the presence of choroid plexus cysts had a much lower predictive value for autosomal trisomy. Their recommendation was to regard choroid plexus cysts as an indication for detailed ultrasound assessment rather than invasive testing. Each centre, however, should develop its own data to determine its individual sensitivity for detecting fetuses with trisomy 18 sonographically, using other anatomical markers in fetuses with choroid plexus cysts.

Trisomy 13

Trisomy 13 is a rare autosomal trisomy, with a multitude of fetal malformations (Table 47.1) and a very poor outcome. The structural abnormalities include holoprosencephaly, major facial defects, heart abnormalities, cystic kidneys, anterior abdominal wall defects, polydactyly, and cystic hygromata (Figs 47.8–47.11)[6,45,46]. The ultrasound detection rate of these abnormalities is between 90% and 100%. Intrauterine growth retardation is also a feature of this syndrome – particularly in the third trimester.

The fetal facial malformations can be very severe, including median cleft lip and palate, severe hypotelorism, and cyclopia with a proboscis (Fig. 47.8)[46]. The prevalence of holoprosencephaly associated with trisomy 13 is around 40%, and enlargement of the cisterna magna with varying degrees of cerebellar abnormalities and Dandy–Walker variant have also been observed with trisomy 13 (Fig. 47.9)[45]. While cystic hygromata and nuchal oedema are features of trisomies 21 and 18, nuchal lucencies can occur also with trisomy 13. Hyperechogenic kidneys are present in 30% of fetuses with trisomy 13. The kidneys are enlarged and echogenic, making it difficult to distinguish trisomy 13 from other conditions such as Meckel–Gruber syndrome (Fig. 47.11).

Heart defects are present in more than 90% of fetuses with trisomy 13, although it is often difficult to diagnose heart defects in the early second trimester – such as ventriculo septal defect (VSD) and atrial septal defect (ASD). Sonography is not as successful in identifying fetuses with heart defects in the early second trimester as it is in the late second or third trimester. More recently, the presence of an echogenic intracardiac focus has been shown to be associated with trisomy 13, although this is also considered a normal variant and is present in 5% of all normal second-trimester fetuses[45,48]. Other abnormalities should be present, however, in the vast majority of fetuses with trisomy 13.

Polydactyly is a frequent feature of trisomy 13, involving both the hands and feet. Postaxial polydactyly is often an easy sonographic feature to detect and, when combined with holoprosencephaly, a diagnosis of trisomy 13 becomes highly probable (Fig. 47.10)[45,46].

When an omphalocele is present in a fetus with trisomy 13, it is likely to be a small, bowel-containing omphalocele, as larger, liver-containing omphaloceles are less often associated with chromosomal defects[45].

The outcome for trisomy 13 is extremely poor. Therefore, the knowledge of the karyotype, even in the third trimester, is crucial to facilitate decisions regarding the obstetrical management of affected fetuses. The severity of the anomalies is almost always fatal at birth, although some affected infants can live a few weeks or months.

Triploidy

Triploidy occurs in approximately 1% of conceptions, although most of these pregnancies are spontaneously aborted during the early first trimester[49]. Survival beyond 20 weeks for a fetus with triploidy is rare, and affected fetuses already have severe intrauterine growth restriction in the second trimester[49–53]. There is a lag in head growth, but even more severe delays in abdominal and skeletal growths, resulting in a very small fetus with severe head-to-body disproportion, with a body smaller than expected for head size. Affected fetuses also have multiple congenital abnormalities, affecting practically every organ system[49–55].

Congenital craniofacial abnormalities seen in triploidy include hydrocephalus, absence of the corpus callosum, holoprosencephaly, meningomyelocele, facial clefts, microphthalmia, and hypertelorism. Other abnormalities include heart defects, genitourinary malformations (including cystic kidneys and hydronephrosis), limb abnormalities (including syndactyly of the second and third digits), severe hypotonia, and omphalocele (Fig. 47.12–47.18)[49–55].

In addition, there are placental abnormalities associated with triploidy. Some placentae are large, cystic, and hydropic, consistent with a partial mole[52,56,57]. Such pregnancies are prone to early-onset preeclampsia and must be evacuated from the uterus due to maternal indications. Other placentae are small, calcified, and prematurely senescent, indicating early, poor placental function.

It is important to recognize triploidy, since the obvious associated intrauterine growth retardation would otherwise prompt early and operative delivery for a condition which is lethal and has no treatment. Detection of this entity can permit expectant management and non-interventional delivery of a stillborn.

Turner syndrome

Most conceptions with Turner syndrome abort spontaneously. The known incidence of X0 Turner syndrome is 1/5000 newborns; however, there are also many X0,XX mosaic individuals whose abnormality may not be detected in infancy.

Fetuses with Turner syndrome have a high incidence of congenital lymphoedema which is manifested by large, septated cystic hygromata around their necks (Fig. 47.19–47.21)[58–62]. The cystic hygromata can regress during gestation, as has been shown to happen with trisomies 21 and 18, resulting in a webbed neck deformity. When cystic hygromata are associated with generalized hydrops, the prognosis is poor. Most fetuses with Turner syndrome who develop hydrops die in utero.

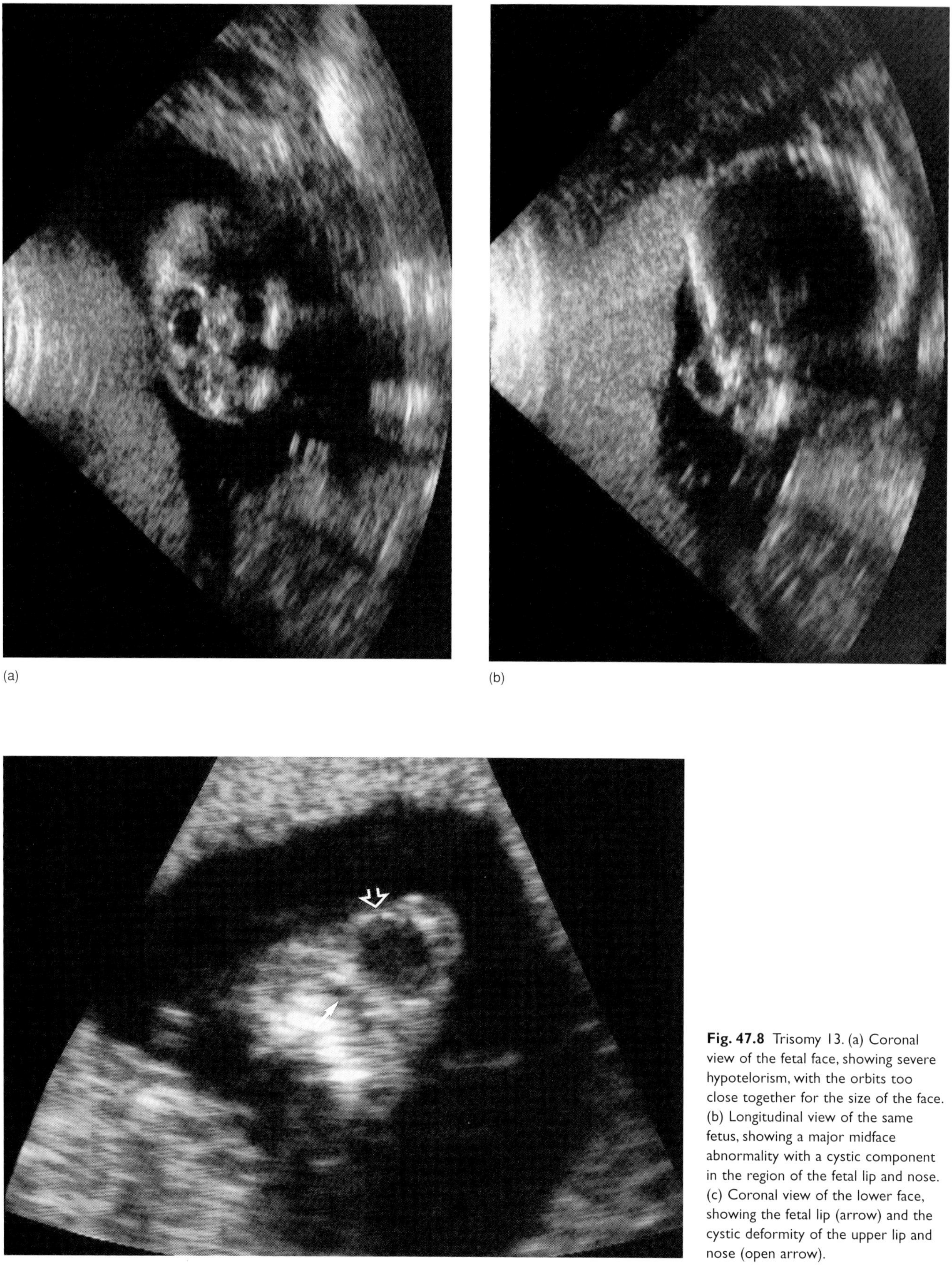

(a) (b) (c)

Fig. 47.8 Trisomy 13. (a) Coronal view of the fetal face, showing severe hypotelorism, with the orbits too close together for the size of the face. (b) Longitudinal view of the same fetus, showing a major midface abnormality with a cystic component in the region of the fetal lip and nose. (c) Coronal view of the lower face, showing the fetal lip (arrow) and the cystic deformity of the upper lip and nose (open arrow).

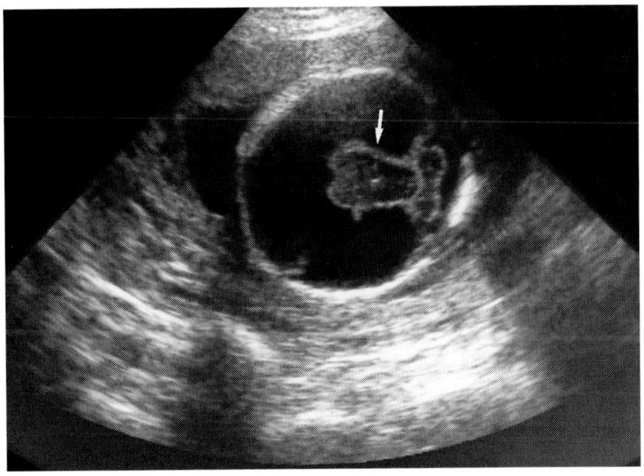

Fig. 47.9 Trisomy 13: coronal view of the head in the second trimester showing alobar holoprosencephaly. Note the abnormal thalami (arrow).

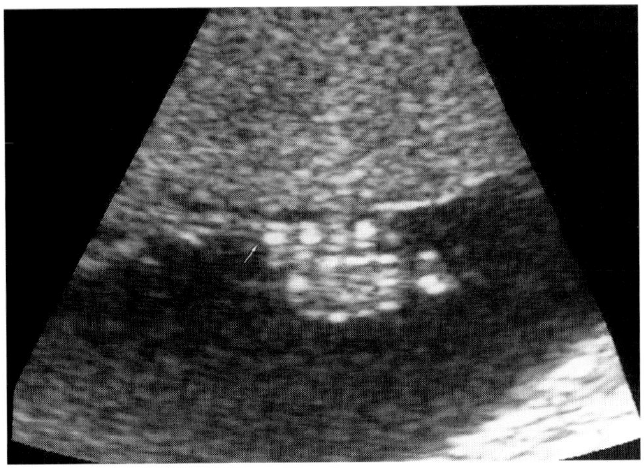

Fig. 47.10 Trisomy 13: view of a second-trimester fetal hand, showing polydactyly (arrow).

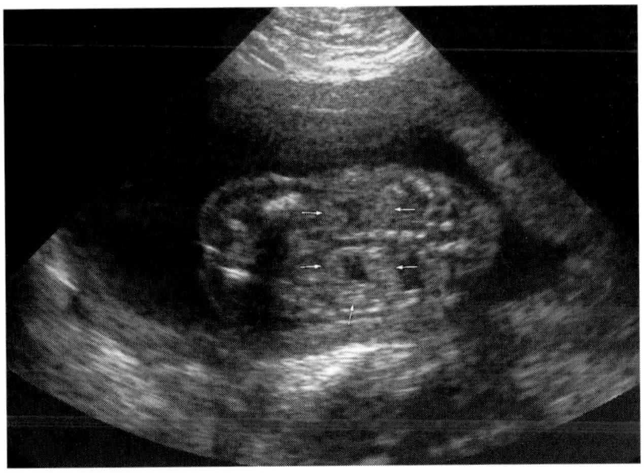

Fig. 47.11 Trisomy 13: coronal view of the fetal kidneys, showing hyperechogenicity of the renal parenchyma (arrows), consistent with cystic disease.

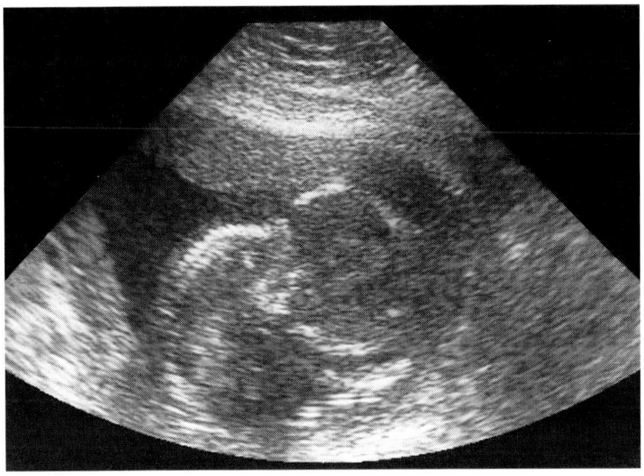

Fig. 47.12 Triploidy: transabdominal view of a 17-week fetus with oligohydramnios. Note that the fetus is curled, precluding a structural evaluation of the anatomy, and that the body is smaller than anticipated for the head.

Fetuses with Turner syndrome also tend to have slightly shorter femurs and, after birth, tend to be small in stature. Malformations include heart defects, which are usually localized on the left side of the heart. These include bicuspid aortic valve, coarctation of the aorta, and valvar aortic stenosis (Fig. 47.22). Sonographic examination can also reveal renal abnormalities, such as horseshoe kidneys[58].

In the absence of hydrops and generalized lymphoedema, the prognosis for survival of X0 Turner individuals is good.

Trisomy 9

Complete trisomy 9 is one of the rarest trisomies to give rise to a live fetus, and has a dismal prognosis with death at birth in practically all cases. Most of the reported cases of trisomy 9 are mosaic trisomy 9 and are exceedingly rare as live births. We previously reported two cases of complete trisomy 9 and have since had a third diagnosed by ultrasound with multiple congenital abnormalities[63]. In general, fetuses with trisomy 9 have abnormalities of most of the organ systems (Table 47.1), including microcephaly, cleft lip and palate, micrognathia, abnormal extremities (with flexion contractions of the fingers and toes), complex heart defects, renal malformations (such as multicystic kidneys), and neural tube defects (Figs 47.23–47.26)[63–66]. The phenotype of trisomy 9 by ultrasound can, at times, be similar to that of trisomies 18 and 13, and it is not possible to distinguish between them without a karyotype. While live births with trisomy 9 are very rare, this chromosomal abnormality should be considered when evaluating a fetus with multiple congenital abnormalities in a particular pattern which includes brain, heart, genitourinary tract, and limb anomalies as well as intrauterine growth restriction.

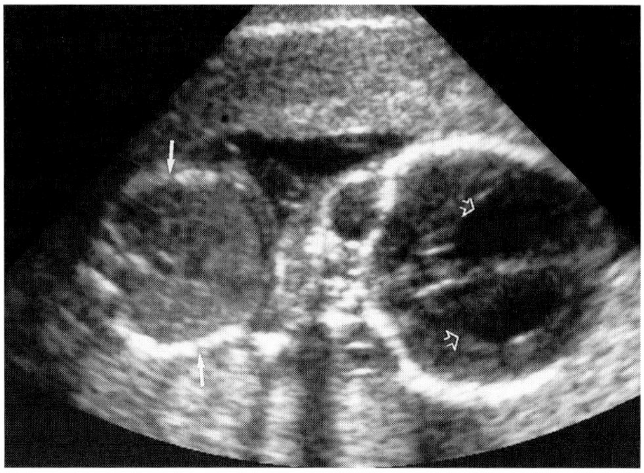

(a)

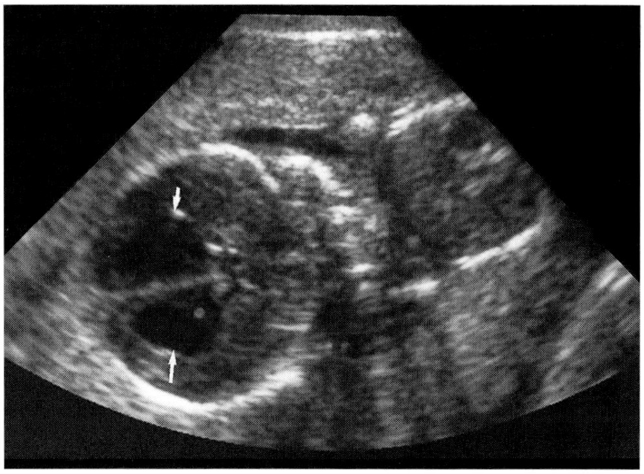

(b)

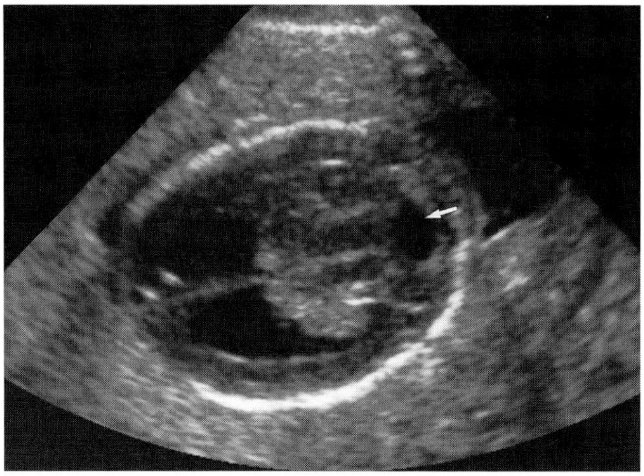

(c)

Fig. 47.13 Triploidy. (a) Transvaginal scan of a second-trimester fetus, showing that the cross-section of the abdomen (arrows) is small when compared with the size of the head. Also note ventriculomegaly (open arrows). This fetus was also noted to have hypertelorism. (b) Transvaginal view of the same fetus, showing the moderately severe ventriculomegaly (arrows) and the disproportionate size between the head and body. (c) Transverse view of the head of the same fetus, showing ventriculomegaly and a Dandy–Walker malformation with a cyst in the posterior fossa (arrow).

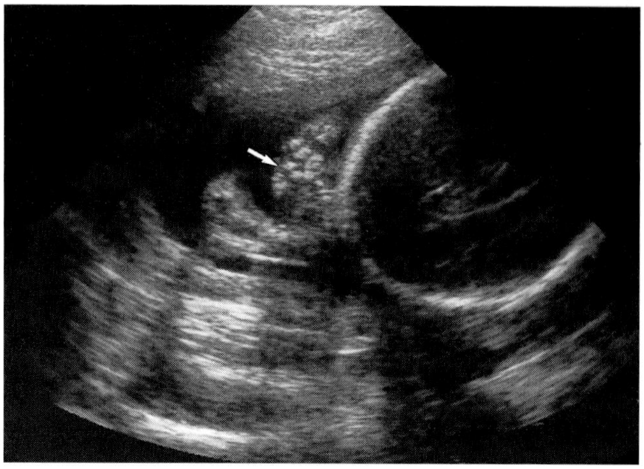

Fig. 47.14 Triploidy: view of the fetal hand, showing syndactyly of the third and fourth digits (arrow).

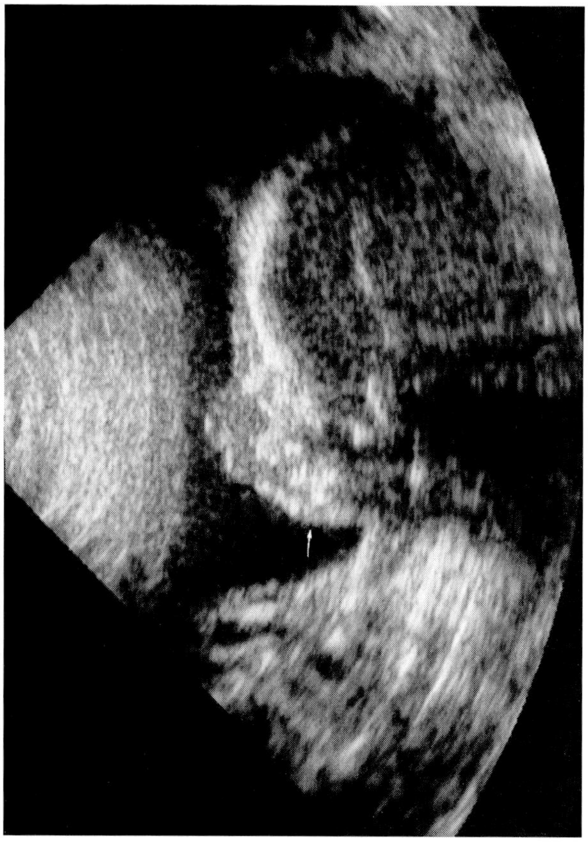

Fig. 47.15 Triploidy: longitudinal view of the fetal face, showing significant micrognathia (arrow).

Down syndrome

Trisomy 21 (Down syndrome) is the most common chromosomal abnormality giving rise to a live newborn[67,68]. Therefore, it is one of the most common causes of mental

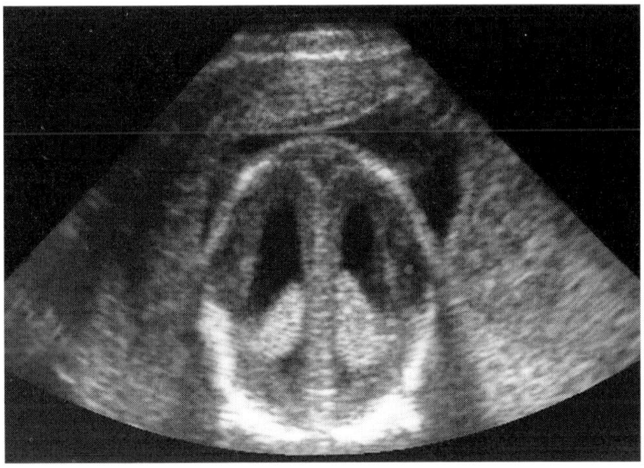

Fig. 47.16 Triploidy: transvaginal view of the head of a 15-week fetus, showing ventriculomegaly.

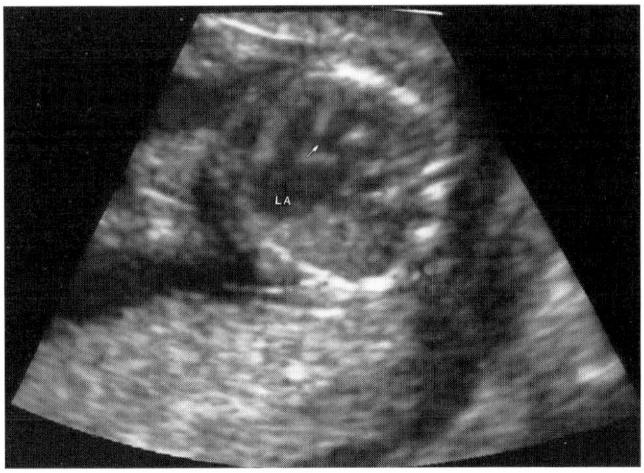

Fig. 47.17 Triploidy: transverse view of the fetal chest in the early second-trimester, showing cardiomegaly and an abnormal cardiac axis (almost 90° in its angle) within the chest. Note that there is dilatation of the left atrium (LA) as well as a ventriculoseptal defect. This fetus has a severe cardiac malformation.

retardation and infant morbidity, as well as mortality. Although advanced maternal age and serum screening have been used to identify women at increased risk of having a fetus with trisomy 21, the detailed anatomical evaluation of the fetus itself by ultrasound (Table 47.1) has yielded a high sensitivity and specificity for the detection of affected fetuses. Sonography enables us to identify the anatomical features of affected fetuses of women less than age 35 who may not have been candidates for amniocentesis based on maternal age. Also, second-trimester sonography may be used to reduce the risks of chromosomal abnormality for older women, at age-based risk for Down syndrome, whose second-trimester fetuses display none of the characteristic features. Thus, fewer of these older women would be subjected to unnecessary amniocentesis.

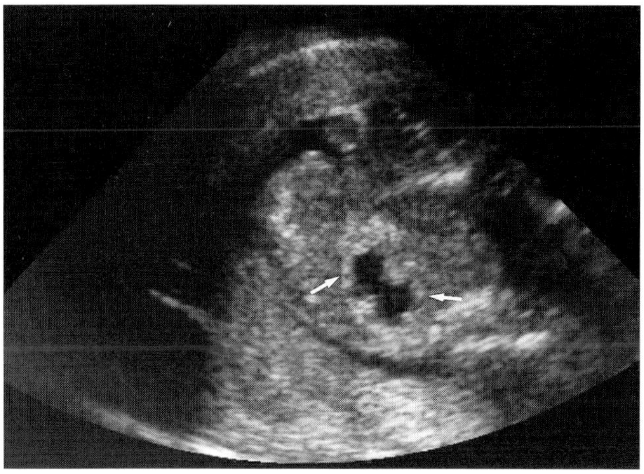

Fig. 47.18 Triploidy: longitudinal view of the fetal kidney, showing marked hydronephrosis and echogenic changes of the parenchyma (arrows).

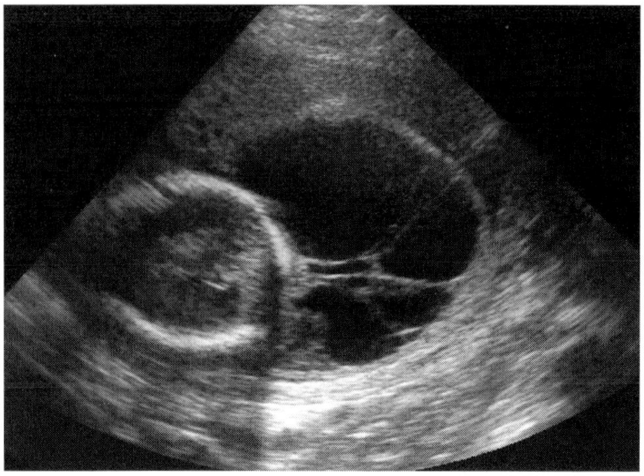

Fig. 47.19 Turner syndrome: transverse view of the fetal head, showing large, septated cystic hygromata which are larger than the head itself.

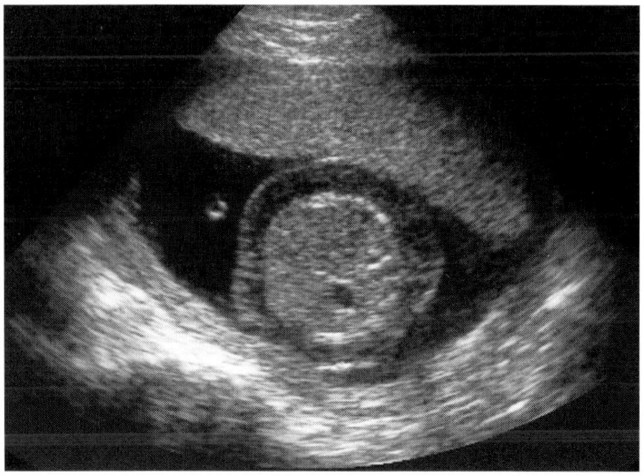

Fig. 47.20 Turner syndrome: transverse view of the fetal abdomen, showing severe lymphangiectasia with marked oedema of the soft tissues surrounding the abdomen.

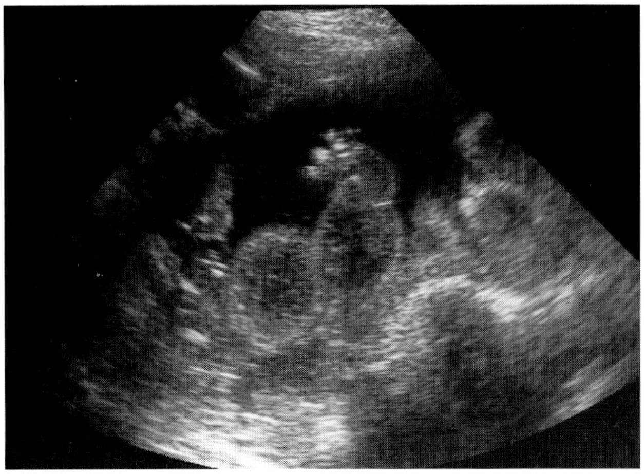

Fig. 47.21 Turner syndrome: view of the fetal upper extremity showing severe swelling of its soft tissues, consistent with lymphangiectasia.

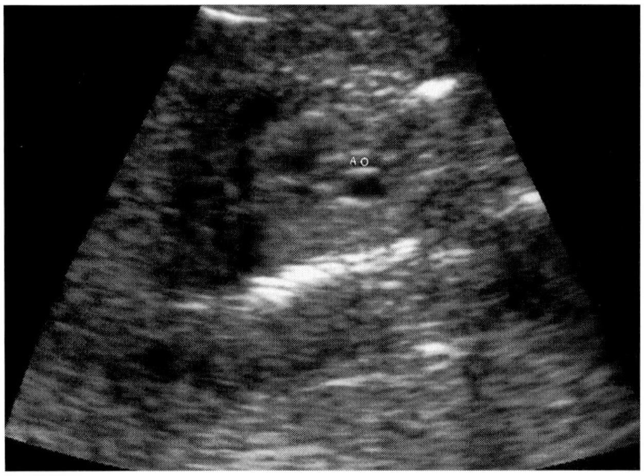

Fig. 47.22 Turner syndrome: long axis view of the heart, showing a very small aortic root (AO) when compared with the size of the other cardiac structures. This is consistent with coarctation of the aorta in a fetus with Turner syndrome.

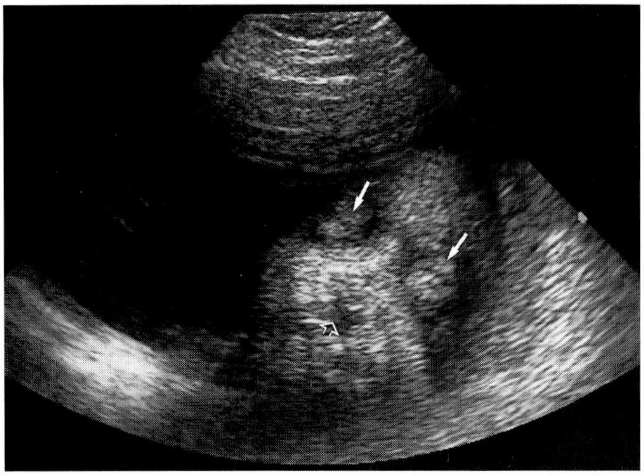

Fig. 47.23 Trisomy 9: coronal view of the fetal face, showing marked hypotelorism (eyes = arrows), with a large, midline, median cleft lip and palate (open arrow).

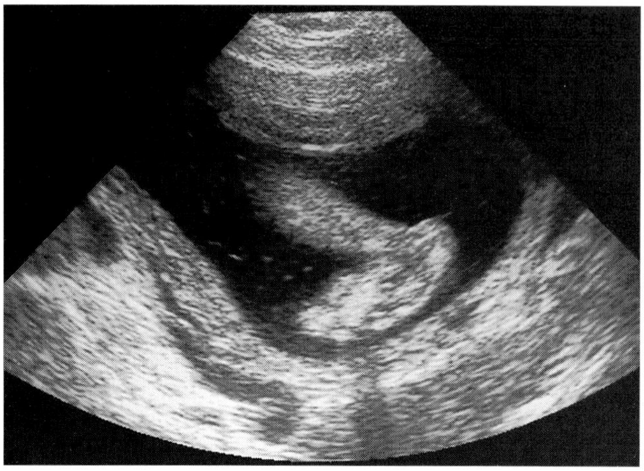

Fig. 47.24 Trisomy 9: longitudinal view of a rockerbottom foot associated with trisomy 9.

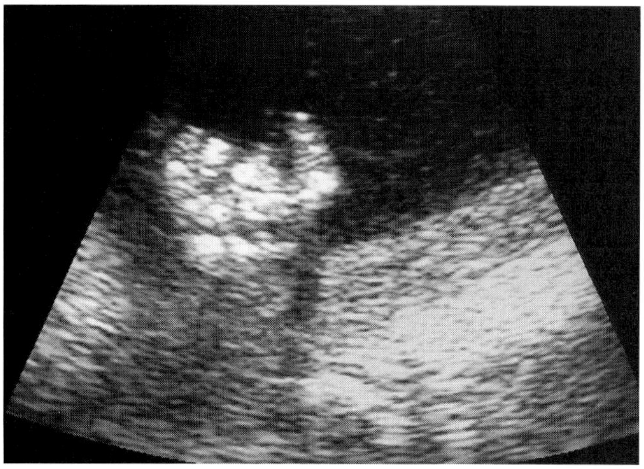

Fig. 47.25 Trisomy 9: magnified view of the fetal hand showing an unusually clenched fist with an overlapping index finger, similar to what is seen in trisomy 18.

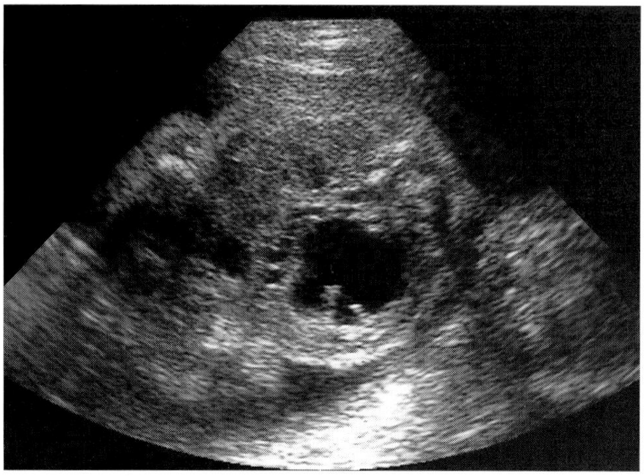

Fig. 47.26 Trisomy 9: coronal view of the fetal kidney, showing severe hydronephrosis with only a small amount of renal parenchyma present.

Fetuses with Down syndrome have an increased incidence of major structural defects, such as duodenal atresia, omphalocele, hydrothorax, ventriculomegaly, major heart defects such as endocardial cushion defect and ventriculoseptal defect (VSD), and abnormal facial profile[69–71]. However, Nyberg et al. and Benacerraf et al. found structural defects in only 30% of affected fetuses, and most of those anomalies were best seen after 24 weeks (Figs 47.27, 47.28)[71,72].

Traditionally, fetuses with Down syndrome have been identified due to the presence of a major congenital heart defect or duodenal atresia. However, only a small percentage of second-trimester fetuses with Down syndrome are identified in this way, since many of the heart defects are simple VSDs which are difficult to see sonographically in the second trimester and duodenal atresia is often not detectable until after 22 weeks. Although DeVore et al. have been able to detect small VSDs using colour Doppler ultrasound, thereby increasing the sensitivity for the detection of trisomy 21 by echocardiography, other investigators have not been able to duplicate these results, and the rate of identification of VSDs by early second-trimester ultrasound and colour Doppler remains low in most laboratories[73–75].

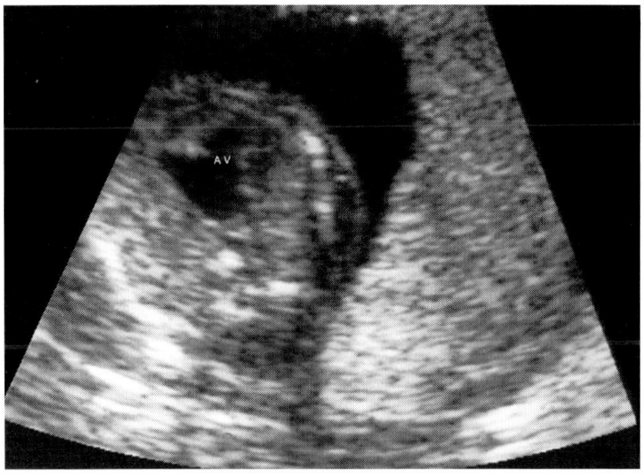

Fig. 47.28 Down syndrome: transverse view through the fetal chest in the second trimester, showing an atrial ventricular (AV) canal defect of the heart.

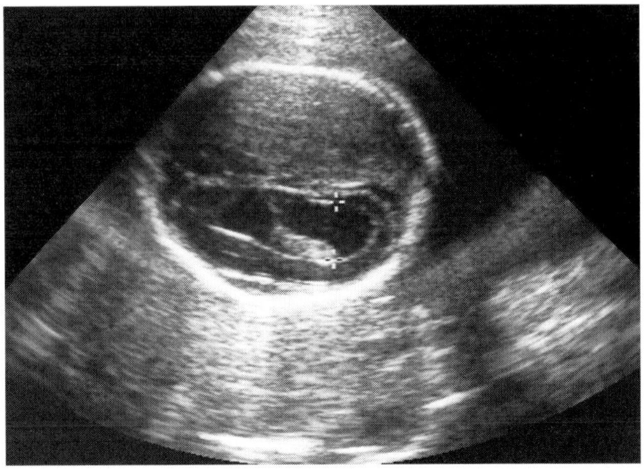

(a)

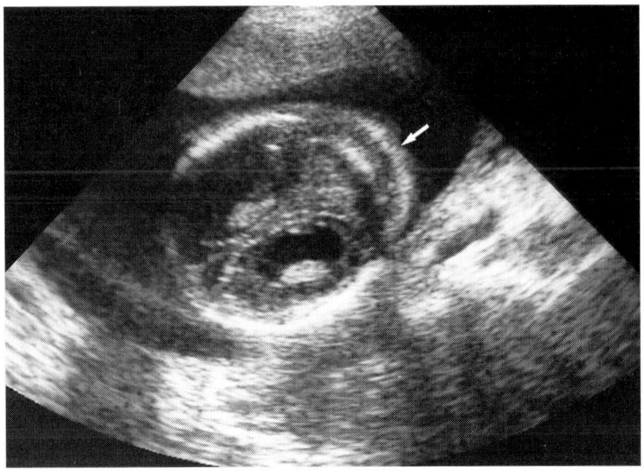

(b)

Fig. 47.27 Down syndrome (trisomy 21). (a) Transverse view through the head of a second-trimester fetus with Down syndrome, showing moderate ventriculomegaly. The lateral ventricular measurement is indicated by the calipers. (b) Modified coronal view of the fetal head and occiput showing displacement of the choroid plexes, associated with ventriculomegaly, as well as a thickened nuchal fold (arrow).

While karyotyping is necessary in fetuses with major congenital abnormalities, restricting amniocentesis to only those fetuses with structural anomalies identified in the early second trimester would leave 70% of fetuses with Down syndrome undetected.

THE NUCHAL FOLD

We first reported an association between a thickened nuchal fold (Fig. 47.29) and Down syndrome in 1985, when 5/11 fetuses with Down syndrome (45%) were found to have nuchal thickening of ≥6 mm[76,77]. Two of these patients had been undergoing sonography for dating, and an amniocentesis was prompted solely by the sonographic finding. Subsequently, an additional study from our laboratory showed that the nuchal fold was thickened in 4/10 fetuses with Down syndrome[78]. We further showed that the normal nuchal fold thickness gradually increases between 15 and 20 weeks' gestation, ranging from 1 mm to 5 mm. Most of the 5 mm measurements occurred after the 19th week. Among 303 normal fetuses, there were no nuchal folds of 6 mm between 15 and 20 weeks[79].

Other investigators confirmed the finding that a nuchal fold of ≥6 mm was associated with a markedly increased risk for Down syndrome, with a very low false-positive rate. Lynch et al. compared fetuses of twin pairs, only one of each pair having Down syndrome, and showed that the nuchal fold thickening identified 5/9 affected fetuses and was not present in

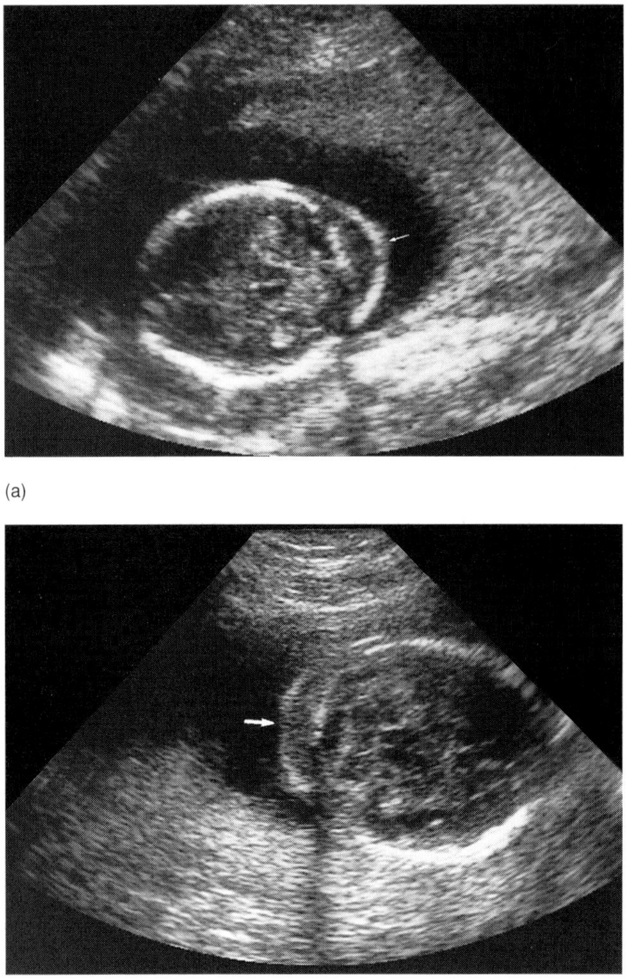

(a)

(b)

Fig. 47.29 Down syndrome. (a) Modified transverse view of the head of a fetus with Down syndrome the second trimester, showing a markedly thickened nuchal fold (arrow). (b) Second-trimester fetus with Down syndrome, also showing a thickened nuchal fold (arrow). Note that the nuchal fold is often measured at the same level at which the cerebellum can be visualized.

any of the normal cotwins[80]. Kirk et al. studied the nuchal fold between 15 and 20 weeks and found that among 7106 scans, 30 fetuses had nuchal thickening, 12 of whom had abnormal karyotypes[81]. Two of the fetuses with normal karyotypes and nuchal thickening, however, had other abnormalities, including Noonan syndrome and achondrogenesis. Seven of the 18 fetuses with normal karyotypes and abnormal nuchal thicknesses were beyond 20 weeks and were therefore at the upper limit of the gestational age range used for this measurement[81]. The investigators concluded that increased nuchal thickness identified 40% of fetuses with abnormal karyotypes, along with 0.4% of normal, second-trimester fetuses[81]. Watson et al. found a higher incidence of nuchal fold thickening in their general population of fetuses with normal karyotypes (2%); however, 8/14 fetuses with Down syndrome had abnormal ultrasound findings, four of which displayed an isolated thickened nuchal fold as the only sonographic abnormality[82]. Crane and Gray found the highest sensitivity for the detection of Down syndrome using the nuchal fold: 12/15 cases of fetuses with Down syndrome had abnormal nuchal folds of ≥6 mm in the second trimester (75%)[83]. Nuchal thickening was present in 1.4% of their general population. These reports suggested that the thickened nuchal fold is the single most sensitive and specific sonographic finding for the detection of trisomy 21. In another study, Gray and Crane suggested that the threshold for the nuchal fold measurement could be changed according to gestational ages, with a 5 mm limit from 14–18 weeks and a 6 mm limit for slightly older fetuses[84]. The use of the 5 mm limit improved the efficiency for detecting trisomy 21; whereas the positive predictive value was higher using the 6 mm limit, due to a lower false-positive rate.

Several investigators did not find as high a sensitivity and specificity for the detection of Down syndrome using the thickened nuchal fold measurement. Donnenfeld et al. found nuchal thickening in only 1/13 fetuses with Down syndrome[85]. Similarly, Toi et al. suggested that the nuchal fold had a low sensitivity and specificity for detecting Down syndrome, although their measurements were done retrospectively, on images that were most likely not taken for the purpose of evaluating nuchal soft tissue[86].

Other investigators evaluated the inter- and intraobserver variability of the measurement of the nuchal fold. Grandjean et al. reported a study in which 12 centres and 36 investigators measured the nuchal fold thicknesses of more than 33 000 fetuses[87]. They found abnormal thickening in 38% of the fetuses with Down syndrome. A false-positive rate below 5% was obtained by 81% of the investigators. Raising the cutoff of normalcy to 7 mm after 18 weeks resulted in a higher specificity. Donnenfeld et al. found that experienced sonologists were able to obtain second-trimester nuchal fold thicknesses within 1 mm of the estimated true value 95% of the time[88].

Most of the studies on the use of the nuchal fold for the detection of fetuses with Down syndrome were done within high-risk populations, composed of women ≥35 years of age or women with abnormal serum triple screening tests. Since the positive predictive value of such a sonographic feature would be different for a low-risk population, we evaluated the use of the nuchal fold in women *not* at risk for carrying fetuses with aneuploidy[89]. We studied 37 fetuses who were found to have thickened nuchal folds by prenatal sonography but who were not in the high-risk category defined by advanced maternal age or abnormal serum screening. Nine of 37 fetuses with thickened nuchal folds (24%) had abnormal karyotypes, indicating that this finding is a powerful tool for the detection of Down syndrome among low-risk patients.

FETAL RENAL PYELECTASIS

In 1990, our laboratory demonstrated an association between fetal pyelectasis and Down syndrome[90]. Among 7400 patients scanned during one year, 210 fetuses had pyelectasis – seven of whom had Down syndrome. The incidence of Down syndrome was 3.3% when pyelectasis was present in this non-selected population. Reviewed images of 44 fetuses with Down syndrome collected over a 5-year period revealed a 25% incidence of pyelectasis (Fig. 47.30). Crane and Gray also found pyelectasis in fetuses with Down syndrome[83]. Although they were evaluating the nuchal skin fold, they found that 3/16 fetuses with Down syndrome also had pyelectasis. Corteville et al. further studied the presence of pyelectasis in fetuses with Down syndrome and found that pyelectasis was observed in 17% of fetuses with Down syndrome versus only 2% of normal controls[91]. Although the positive predictive value of pyelectasis for the detection of Down syndrome was 1/90, most of the fetuses with Down syndrome had other sonographic abnormalities. When fetuses with other sonographic defects were excluded, the positive predictive value of isolated pyelectasis fell to 1/340 for the detection of Down syndrome.

While the finding of fetal pyelectasis is clearly associated with Down syndrome, it is also present in many normal fetuses. Therefore, most investigators suggest that an isolated finding of fetal pyelectasis, without any other sign of chromosomal abnormality, should prompt a careful and complete sonographic fetal survey but does not warrant karyotyping[83,90,91].

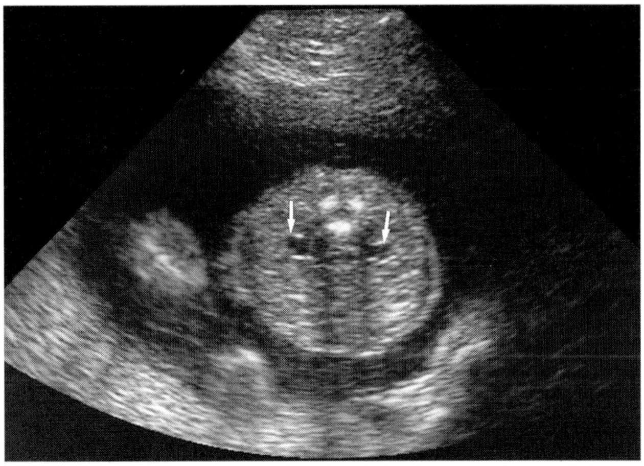

Fig. 47.30 Down syndrome: transverse view through the fetal back, showing mild pyelectasis (arrows), associated with an increased risk of Down syndrome.

HYPERECHOGENIC BOWEL

Nyberg et al. first reported that hyperechogenic bowel was a sonographic finding associated with Down syndrome[71]. In 1990, they found five fetuses with hyperechogenic bowel and Down syndrome and suggested that this was a new sonographic sign for the detection of this trisomy. Although hyperechogenicity of the lower abdomen had also been identified in case reports, Nyberg et al. were the first to look at hyperechogenic bowel as a specific sonographic sign for screening for fetuses with trisomy 21[92–94]. They found that hyperechogenic bowel was present in 0.8% of second-trimester fetuses but in 14% of second-trimester fetuses with trisomy 21. Fetuses with hyperechogenic bowel, therefore, carried a 17-fold greater risk for Down syndrome than those with normal bowel echogenicity. In a separate study at our laboratory, Bromley et al. confirmed the association between hyperechogenic bowel and Down syndrome in the second trimester and found that hyperechogenic bowel was present in 50/8680 fetuses (0.6%) in the general population of second-trimester fetuses (Fig. 47.31)[95]. Eight of the 50 fetuses (16%) with hyperechogenic bowel had chromosomal abnormalities, six of whom had Down syndrome. In addition, eight other fetuses with hyperechogenic bowel (16%) had severe intrauterine growth retardation. In our study, the risk of Down syndrome in fetuses with isolated hyperechogenic bowel was 1.4%, thus suggesting the need for karyotypic analysis in fetuses with this finding[95].

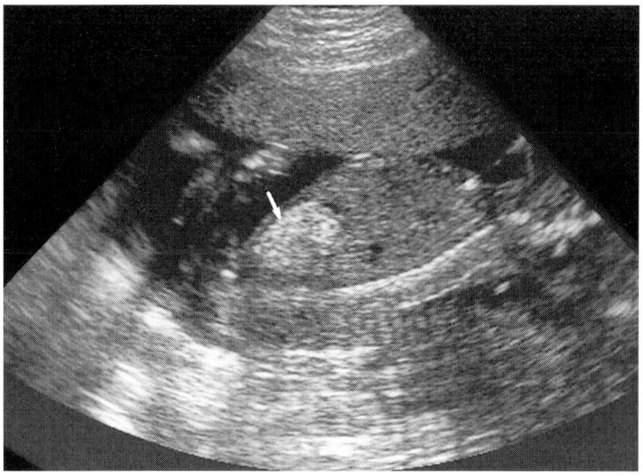

Fig. 47.31 Down syndrome: longitudinal view of the fetal abdomen, showing hyperechogenic bowel (arrow).

ECHOGENIC INTRACARDIAC FOCUS

Recently, several investigators have found an association between chromosomal abnormalities and an echogenic intracardiac focus in second-trimester fetuses[45,48,96,97]. This focus is thought to represent calcification in the papillary muscle and is usually found in the left ventricle (Fig. 47.32). The finding was first seen sonographically in association with aneuploidy by Lehman et al. who found an echogenic intracardiac focus in fetuses with trisomy 13[45]. Anecdotal case reports also suggested an association with Down syndrome[97]. The largest study, however, is in the pathology literature where the association between calcification of the papillary

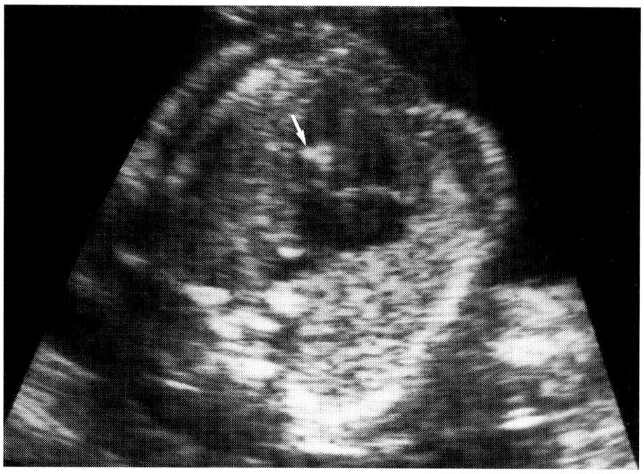

Fig. 47.32 Down syndrome: four-chambered view of the fetal heart, showing an echogenic intracardiac focus (arrow) in the left ventricle. This is associated with a fourfold increased risk of Down syndrome.

muscle of the heart and trisomies 13 and 21 is evident[96]. Recently, we evaluated this finding in vivo in second-trimester fetuses undergoing amniocentesis because of advanced maternal age or abnormal serum screening testing. We found that an echogenic intracardiac focus is present in 5% of normal fetuses and in 17% of fetuses with Down syndrome[48]. This resulted in a fourfold increase in the risk for Down syndrome among fetuses who have an intracardiac focus versus those who do not.

MISCELLANEOUS FINDINGS

Children with Down syndrome have many different, subtle findings which we have sought to identify sonographically in the second trimester. These anomalies include clinodactyly of the fifth digit of the hand as well as hypoplasia of the middle phalanx of that digit. Other findings include a gap between the first and second toes, reduced ear size, simian crease, brachycephaly and short frontal lobe dimensions, and unusual shape of the iliac crest.

Several studies have shown that clinodactyly of the fifth digit in fetuses with Down syndrome can be identified by ultrasound. Ultrasound is also successful in detecting hypoplasia of the middle phalanx of the fifth digit (Fig. 47.33)[98–100]. We demonstrated that a ratio of the length of the middle phalanx of the fifth digit over the length of the middle phalanx of the fourth digit can be helpful in detecting fetuses at risk for Down syndrome[99]. In our study of more than 1000 fetuses, the mean ratio was 0.85 for normal fetuses and 0.59 for fetuses with Down syndrome. By using a cutoff ratio of 0.70, the sensitivity and specificity for detecting fetuses with Down syndrome were 75% and 82%, respectively. Although this finding can be helpful in high-risk cases where other sonographic signs are evident, the high false-positive rate (18%) and the technically difficult measurement do not make this sonographic feature a candidate for general screening.

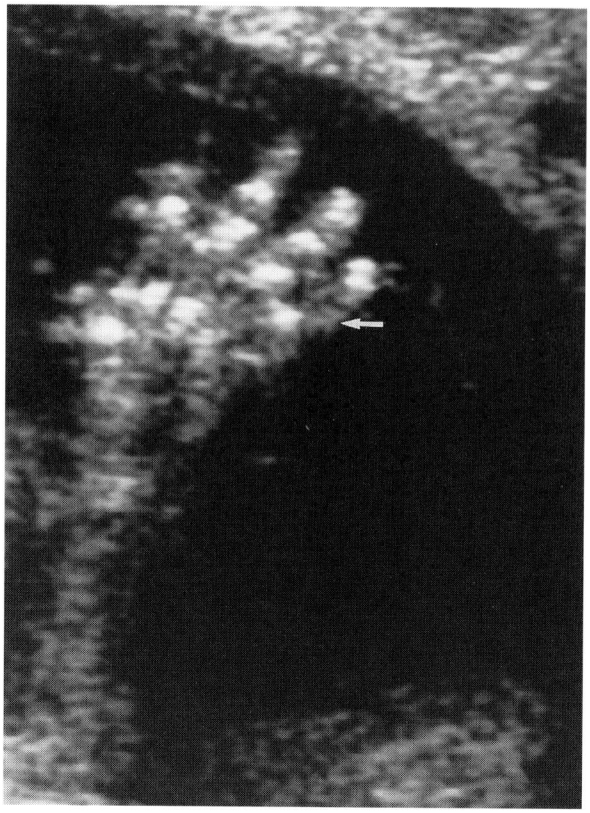

Fig. 47.33 Down syndrome: longitudinal view of the fetal hand in the second trimester, showing absence of the ossification of the middle phalanx of the fifth digit (arrow).

Jeanty demonstrated the ultrasound diagnosis of a simian crease in a fetus with Down syndrome[101]. Also, Wilkins described the separation of the great and second toes in fetuses with Down syndrome, in a double case report[102]. These findings, however, are impractical to apply to the general population as a screening protocol.

Other attempts to detect Down syndrome were made by using the transverse cerebellar diameter which, however, remained unaffected by Down syndrome[103]. The effect of the shortened frontal lobe and the brachycephalic head shape in fetuses with Down syndrome was also investigated. Although the frontal lobe dimension was found to be significantly shortened in fetuses with Down syndrome, the sensitivity was only 21%[104].

Measurement of the iliac length may be a helpful feature in the detection of Down syndrome, but it is not currently being used in most laboratories[105].

An attempt to use the fetal ear length was made by Gill et al. However, despite a statistically significant difference between normal ear size and that of trisomy 21 fetuses, the wide range of normal variation makes the ear length measurement impractical to utilize diagnostically[106].

More recently, fetal heart rate patterns appear to be abnormal in fetuses with trisomy 21, with abnormally low or high fetal heart rates in early pregnancy in affected fetuses[107]. More work is necessary to determine the use of this finding, although initial studies have shown that the detection rate of chromosomal abnormalities in high-risk populations was as high as 63%, with a positive predictive value of 17.9%.

LONG BONE BIOMETRY

Individuals with Down syndrome are known to be short in stature, so it is not surprising that they have slightly shorter femoral and humeral lengths when compared with their normal counterparts. Lockwood et al. were the first to demonstrate the slightly shorter femur length in affected fetuses[108]. Shortly thereafter, we showed that a ratio of measured-to-expected femur length (based on the biparietal diameter (BPD)) could be highly successful in detecting fetuses with Down syndrome[109,110]. Using a measured-to-expected femur length ratio cutoff of ≤0.91, we identified 40% of fetuses with Down syndrome and 5% of normal controls, for a positive predictive value of 3.1%[109]. Since eight of these 20 fetuses with Down syndrome also had thickened nuchal folds, these findings could be additive, thereby yielding a sensitivity of 45% and a positive predictive value of 4.3%. Other investigators confirmed our findings. Grist et al. used the measured-to-expected femur length and found a sensitivity and specificity of 46.2% and 94.1% respectively for the detection of all chromosomal abnormalities[111]. The sensitivity and specificity for Down syndrome in particular were 50% and 93.5%, resulting in a positive predictive value of 3% (Table 47.3).

Brumfield et al. used a BPD: femur length ratio and found that a ratio of ≥1.8 was 40% sensitive and 97.8% specific for predicting Down syndrome, with a false-positive rate of only 2.2%[112]. Hill et al. found that the BPD: femur length ratio had a sensitivity and specificity of 36.4% and 93.4% respectively[113]. Assuming a 1/1000 incidence of Down syndrome in the general population, the positive predictive value of a short femur would be 0.6%. Combining the femur length data with the nuchal fold thickening resulted in a sensitivity of 45% and a false-positive rate of 7%. Platt et al. found that the femur length:BPD ratio was particularly effective between 17 and 19 weeks for detecting fetuses with Down syndrome[114].

Several studies, on the contrary, did *not* find the femur length useful in detecting fetuses with Down syndrome[114–120]. Hadlock et al. found no difference between normal fetuses and those with Down syndrome[115]. Shah et al. report that the BPD:femur length ratio identified only 18% of fetuses with Down syndrome, with a 6% false-positive rate[116]. LaFollette et al. were unable to demonstrate a statistically significant difference between measured and predicted femur lengths in fetuses with Down syndrome[117]. Dicke found a sensitivity and false-positive rate of 29% and 4%, respectively, when comparing BPD:femur length ratios in fetuses with trisomies 21, 18, and 13 versus normal fetuses[118]. Nyberg et al. report a sensitivity and false-positive rate of 14% and 6%, respectively, for the measured-to-expected femur length ratio[119].

Lastly, Perrella et al. combined femur length shortening with the nuchal fold to detect fetuses with Down syndrome and found a sensitivity and specificity of 42% and 88%, respectively[121]. The relatively low specificity, however, may be a result of the retrospective nature of the study, making it difficult to obtain an accurate measurement of the nuchal fold.

Peters et al. attempted to explain the differing results of many of these studies when evaluating the femur length for the detection of Down syndrome. Although they demonstrated that the femur length was indeed shorter in fetuses with Down syndrome when compared with normal, the magnitude of this reduction in femur length may not be sufficient to permit this technique to be used in general screening[122]. Differences in patient populations, as well as in measurement techniques, may make it difficult for all laboratories to use the femur length for screening second-trimester fetuses for aneuploidy. Each ultrasound centre must decide what is useful in its own community.

Several centres have attempted to add the foot length, for a femur:foot length ratio in the detection of fetuses with Down syndrome[123,124]. Grandjean et al. found a sensitivity and false-positive rate of 35% and 4.6%, respectively, which was not an improvement over femur length alone[124]. Johnson et al. did a series of direct necropsy measurements of the leg:foot length ratio in autopsy specimens and found that they were able to identify 84% of fetuses with trisomy 21[123]. An ultrasonographic femur:foot length ratio of <0.9 had an 18 odds ratio risk for trisomy 21 in the high-risk population and correctly identified 71% of fetuses affected with trisomy 21.

FitzSimmons was the first to demonstrate that fetuses with Down syndrome had even shorter humerus lengths than femur lengths when compared with their normal counterparts[125]. Examining autopsy specimens, he showed that 9/32

TABLE 47.3
Studies using femur length to detect trisomy 21 in second trimester

Study	Sensitivity (%)	False-positive rate (%)
Benacerraf[110]	68	2
Ginsburg[136]	53	7
Lockwood[108]	51	7
Grist[111]	50	6.50
Benacerraf[109]	40	5
Brumfield[112]	40	2.20
Hill[113]	36	6.60
Perrella[121]	26	23
Hadlock[115]	25	20
Rotmensch[128]	19	9
Dicke[118]	18	4
Rodis[127]	18	5
Shah[116]	18	6
Nyberg[119]	14	6
LaFollette[117]	13	12

humeri fell below the normal regression for that bone, compared with only 3/37 femurs. Further evaluation, using ultrasound in vivo, showed that an abnormal measured-to-expected humeral length successfully identified 50% of fetuses with Down syndrome along with 6.25% of normals[126]. Adding the nuchal fold findings to the humeral length criteria resulted in identifying 75% of fetuses with Down syndrome in our laboratory. Rodis also found that an abnormal humeral length measurement had a sensitivity of 64% for the detection of fetuses with Down syndrome, compared with a sensitivity of 18% when using the femur length[127].

As with the femur, not everyone was successful in using the humeral length to detect second-trimester fetuses with Down syndrome[128]. Rotmensch only found a sensitivity of 28% and a specificity of 91% when using the humeral length to detect affected fetuses. It was clear that it would be the combination of the humeral and femoral lengths that would be most specific for detecting fetuses with trisomy 21. Several investigators found that the femur and humerus biometry can be combined for better results[129–131]. When both humerus and femur lengths were combined, a remarkable reduction of the false-positive rate occurred, resulting in a sensitivity and false-positive rate of 44.4% and 7.6% for the detection of fetuses with Down syndrome[130]. Nyberg found that fetuses with both short humeri and short femurs carried an 11-fold greater risk of Down syndrome than those with normal length long bones[131].

Further work on the use of the humeral and femoral lengths was done, looking for gender differences among second-trimester fetuses. Smulian studied 38 fetuses with Down syndrome and found that male fetuses with Down syndrome had a greater proportion of small humeral and femoral length measurements at given BPDs than did female fetuses[132]. Lockwood et al. also found that affected males had significantly smaller mean femoral and humeral lengths than euploid fetuses did; although, for both genders, the nuchal fold thickness of ≥5 mm was the single best sonographic predictor of Down syndrome[133]. We evaluated the impact of gender on the sonographic detection of Down syndrome and found that, although there were slightly more male than female fetuses with short femurs, the difference was not statistically significant[134]. Our data further showed that there was no statistically significant difference in the incidence of any of the sonographic findings, including nuchal fold, pyelectasis, heart defects, ventriculomegaly, and biometry when comparing male with female Down syndrome fetuses.

CHOROID PLEXUS CYSTS

Several investigators have suggested that choroid plexus cysts are not only associated with trisomy 18, but they also indicate an increased risk for trisomy 21[35,38,39]. We sought to determine whether the association between choroid plexus cysts and trisomy 21 was real or whether both findings in the same fetus could be coincidental. We established the prevalence of choroid plexus cysts among second-trimester fetuses in the general population of fetuses scanned in our department[135]. We found that 473 fetuses with choroid plexus cysts were identified from among 31 938 second-trimester fetuses (excluding those patients referred specifically for the evaluation of choroid plexus cysts). Sixteen were lost to follow-up, three had structural abnormalities and normal karyotypes, and 21 had abnormal karyotypes – most of whom had trisomy 18. Among them, however, were two fetuses with trisomy 21. The remaining 433 fetuses had normal karyotypes or were normal newborns. The prevalence of choroid plexus cysts in our general population, excluding chromosomal abnormalities, was 1.38%. During the study period, we saw 143 fetuses with trisomy 21 for amniocentesis in our laboratory, two of which (1.4%) had choroid plexus cysts. Both had other sonographic findings, indicating a high risk for trisomy 21. The difference in the incidence of choroid plexus cysts in fetuses with trisomy 21 and those with normal karyotypes was not significant. Therefore, we concluded that choroid plexus cysts occur with the same frequency in normal fetuses and fetuses with trisomy 21. The presence of choroid plexus cysts, therefore, should not be used to increase the patient's risk of carrying a fetus with trisomy 21[135].

COMBINATION OF FINDINGS AND SCORING SYSTEMS

Most of the investigating groups have come to the conclusion that the best approach to the prenatal detection of fetuses with trisomy 21, and perhaps even other trisomies, is to combine several of the sonographic findings[72,75,136–140]. Initially, long bone biometry and the thickened nuchal fold were used in combination by Ginsberg et al. who found that the sensitivity and specificity for the femur length ratio in detecting aneuploidy were 53% and 93%, while the thickened nuchal fold had a sensitivity and specificity of 44% and 100%[136]. The combined use of these sonographic measurements, however, resulted in an overall sensitivity of 81% and a specificity of 93% for trisomies 18 and 21[136].

We devised a scoring system where one point each was given to the following features: short femur, short humerus, pyelectasis, choroid plexus cysts, and hyperechogenic bowel[72,75]. Two points each were given to: thickened nuchal fold (≥6 mm) and any major structural malformation (Table 47.4). The initial study, using our scoring system, showed that, if a cutoff of 2 is utilized to indicate a risk of Down syndrome sufficiently high to warrant amniocentesis, 81% of fetuses with Down syndrome and 100% of those with trisomies 18 or 13 were identified, with an overall false-positive rate of 4.4%[72]. More recently, we performed a second study using the same criteria on a new data set, showing a sensitivity and a false-positive rate for detecting fetuses with Down syndrome of 73% and 4%, and an overall sensitivity for all three trisomies of 77%[75]. Vintzileos et al. devised a similar method

TABLE 47.4
Scoring index for detection of Down syndrome

Finding	Score	
Nuchal fold ≥ 6 mm	2	
Major anomaly	2	
Short femur[a]	1	
Short humerus[b]	1	
Pyelectasis[c]	1	
Hyperechogenic bowel	1	
Choroid plexus cysts	1	
Score of 2	**Sensitivity (%)**	**False-positive rate (%)**
Benacerraf[72]	81	4.40
Benacerraf[75]	73	4

[a]Exp. femur length = –9.3105 + 0.928 (BPD) Measured to exp. femur length ≤ 0.91
[b]Exp. humeral length = –7.9404 + 0.8492 (BPD) Measured to exp. humeral length ≤ 0.90
[c]PA diameter of renal pelvis ≥ 4 mm

using structural malformations, short humerus, short femur, nuchal fold, echogenic bowel, ear length, etc. and suggested an amniocentesis should be considered whenever second-trimester sonography reveals the presence of one or more of these features[138].

Until now, ultrasound has been used to detect Down syndrome in fetuses of women <35 years of age who would not be candidates for amniocentesis for other reasons. Recently, the question has arisen of whether women ≥35 years of age or those with a positive serum screen for Down syndrome could have their risks reduced by normal ultrasounds. We evaluated the risk of autosomal trisomy in women >35 years of age who had a normal sonogram, with a sonographic score of 0 based on the above scoring system. We found that, if a woman aged 35 has an age-based risk of a trisomy in midtrimester of 5.5/1000, a sonographic score of 0 decreases her risk to 0.9/1000[140]. A 42-year-old woman's probability of an autosomal trisomy when her sonographic score is 0 becomes equivalent to the age-based risk of a 35-year-old woman prior to the ultrasound. Our data demonstrated that sonography and maternal age can provide a more accurate estimate of the risk that a fetus has a trisomy than maternal age alone. This may help older women decide whether or not to pursue invasive antenatal testing.

A similar approach was used for women who tested positive for serum screen markers for Down syndrome. Bahado-Singh found that a normal nuchal thickness significantly reduces the risk of Down syndrome in patients who have abnormal triple screen results and may help to reduce the number of amniocenteses performed on normal fetuses[141]. Nyberg et al. found that abnormal sonographic findings increase the risk of Down syndrome among those with a positive maternal serum marker screen for Down syndrome[142]. However, normal findings were less predictive of normalcy. An abnormal ultrasound result increased the risk that a fetus had Down syndrome 5.6-fold, and a negative result reduced the risk by 45%.

Conclusion

Prenatal diagnosis for chromosomal abnormalities has evolved from simply using maternal age to detect pregnancies at increased risk for Down syndrome to using a combination of maternal age, several serum screening tests, as well as many ultrasound markers such as nuchal fold, biometry, pyelectasis, heart evaluation, structural malformations, etc. It is clear that a combination of these findings is most useful when trying to assess a patient's risk that she is carrying a fetus with a chromosomal abnormality. It also follows that a woman who does not display any of the sonographic features of Down syndrome and has a normal screening test probably has a markedly decreased risk of carrying a fetus with Down syndrome – even at age 35. The future of screening for chromosomally abnormal fetuses will most likely entail all of these tests together, to arrive at an assessment of each patient's *individual* risk that she is carrying a chromosomally abnormal fetus.

REFERENCES

1. Adams MM, Erickson JD, Layde PM, Oakley GP. Down's syndrome: recent trends in the United States. *JAMA* **246**(7):758–760, 1981.
2. Hook EB, Schreinemachers DM, Cross PK. Use of prenatal cytogenetic diagnosis in New York state. *N Engl J Med* **305**:1410–1413, 1981.
3. Cuckle S, Wald NJ, Lindenbaum RH. Maternal serum alpha-fetoprotein measurement: a screening test for Down syndrome. *Lancet* **1**:926–929, 1984.
4. DiMaio MS, Baumgarten A, Greenstein RM, Saai HM, Mahoney MJ. Screening for fetal Down's syndrome in pregnancy by measuring maternal serum alpha-fetoprotein levels. *N Engl J Med* **317**:342–346, 1987.
5. Merkatz IR, Nitowsky HM, Macri JN, Johnson WE. An association between low maternal serum alpha-fetoprotein and fetal chromosomal abnormalities. *Am J Obstet Gynecol* **148**:886–894, 1984.
6. Benacerraf B, Miller W, Frigoletto F. Sonographic detection of fetuses with trisomies 13 and 18: accuracy and limitations. *Am J Obstet Gynecol* **158**:404–409, 1988.
7. Thurmond AS, Nelson DW, Lowensohn RI, Young WP, Davis L. Enlarged cisterna magna in trisomy 18: prenatal ultrasonographic diagnosis. *Am J Obstet Gynecol* **161**:83–85, 1989.
8. Steiger RM, Porto M, Lagrew DC, Randall R. Biometry of the fetal cisterna magna: estimates of the ability to detect trisomy 18. *Ultrasound Obstet Gynecol* **5**:384–390, 1995.
9. Sepulveda W, Treadwell MC, Fisk NM. Prenatal detection of preaxial upper limb reduction in trisomy 18. *Obstet Gynecol* **85**:847–850, 1995.
10. Nyberg DA, Mahony BS, Hegge FN, Hickok D, Luthy DA, Kapur R. Enlarged cisterna magna and the Dandy–Walker malformation: factors associated with chromosome abnormalities. *Obstet Gynecol* **77**:436–442, 1991.

11. Nicolaides KH, Salvesen DR, Snijders RJM, Gosden CM. Strawberry-shaped skull in fetal trisomy 18. *Fetal Diagn Ther* **7**:132–137, 1992.
12. Hill LM, Marchese S, Peterson C, Fries J. The effect of trisomy 18 on transverse cerebellar diameter. *Am J Obstet Gynecol* **165**:72–75, 1991.
13. Hill LM, Macpherson T, Rivello D, Peterson C. The spontaneous resolution of cystic hygromas and early fetal growth delay in fetuses with trisomy 18. *Prenat Diagn* **11**:673–677, 1991.
14. Chervenak FA, Goldberg JD, Tsung-Hong C, Gilbert F, Berkowitz RL. The importance of karyotype determination in a fetus with ventriculomegaly and spina bifida discovered during the third trimester. *J Ultrasound Med* **5**:405–406, 1985.
15. Bundy AL, Saltzman DH, Pober B, Fine C, Emerson D, Doubilet PM. Antenatal sonographic findings in trisomy 18. *J Ultrasound Med* **5**:361–364, 1986.
16. Nyberg DA, Kramer D, Resta RG et al. Prenatal sonographic findings in trisomy 18: Review of 47 cases. *J Ultrasound Med* **2**:103–113, 1993.
17. Jackson S, Porter H, Vyas S. Trisomy 18: first-trimester nuchal translucency with pathological correlation. *Ultrasound Obstet Gynecol* **5**:55–56, 1995.
18. Nadel AS, Bromley BS, Frigoletto FD, Estroff JA, Benacerraf BR. Isolated choroid plexus cysts in the second-trimester fetus: is amniocentesis really indicated? *Radiology* **185**:545–548, 1992.
19. Droste S, FitzSimmons J, Pascoe-Mason J, Shepard TH. Growth of linear parameters in trisomy 18 fetuses. *Am J Obstet Gynecol* **163**:158–161, 1990.
20. Kurjak A, Kiekinen P. Ultrasonic growth pattern of fetuses with chromosomal abberations. *Acta Obstet Gynecol Scand* **61**:223–225, 1982.
21. Benacerraf BR, Harlow B, Frigoletto Jr FD. Are choroid plexus cysts an indication for second-trimester amniocentesis? *Am J Obstet Gynecol* **162**:1001–1006, 1990.
22. Ramirez P, Haberman S, Baxi L. Significance of prenatal diagnosis of umbilical cord cyst in a fetus with trisomy 18. *Am J Obstet Gynecol* **173**:955–957, 1995.
23. Chan L, Hixson JL, Laifer SA, Marchese SG, Martin JG, Hill LM. A sonographic and karyotypic study of second-trimester fetal choroid plexus cysts. *Obstet Gynecol* **73**:703–706, 1989.
24. Clark SL, DeVore GR, Sabey PL. Prenatal diagnosis of cysts of the fetal choroid plexus. *Obstet Gynecol* **72**:585–587, 1988.
25. DeRoo TR, Harris RD, Sargent SK, Denholm TA, Crow HC. Fetal choroid plexus cysts: prevalence, clinical significance, and sonographic appearance. *Am J Roentgenol* **151**:1179–1181, 1988.
26. Benacerraf BR, Laboda LA. Cyst of the fetal choroid plexus: a normal variant? *Am J Obstet Gynecol* **160**:319–321, 1989.
27. Gupta JK, Cave M, Lilford RF et al. Clinical significance of fetal choroid plexus cysts. *Lancet* **346**:724–729, 1995.
28. Gross SJ, Shulman LP, Tolley EA et al. Isolated fetal choroid plexus cysts and trisomy 18: a review and meta-analysis. *Am J Obstet Gynecol* **172**:83–87, 1995.
29. Achiron R, Barkai G, Katznelson B-M, Mashiach S. Fetal lateral ventricle choroid plexus cysts: the dilemma of amniocentesis. *Obstet Gynecol* **78**:815–818, 1991.
30. Chinn DH, Miller EI, Worthy LM, Towers CV. Sonographically detected fetal choroid plexus cysts: frequency and association with aneuploidy. *J Ultrasound Med* **10**:255–258, 1991.
31. Chitkara U, Cogswell C, Norton K, Wilkins IA, Mehalek K, Berkowitz RL. Choroid plexus cysts in the fetus: a benign anatomic variant or pathologic entity? Report of 41 cases and review of the literature. *Obstet Gynecol* **72**:185–189, 1988.
32. Gabrielli S, Reece A, Pilu G et al. The clinical significance of prenatally diagnosed choroid plexus cysts. *Am J Obstet Gynecol* **160**:1207–1210, 1989.
33. Hertzberg BS, Kay HH, Bowie JD. Fetal choroid plexus lesions: relationship of antenatal sonographic appearance to clinical outcome. *J Ultrasound Med* **8**:77–82, 1989.
34. Howard RJ, Tuck SM, Long J, Thomas VA. Short communication: the significance of choroid plexus cysts in fetuses at 18–20 weeks. An indication for amniocentesis? *Prenat Diagn* **12**:685–688, 1992.
35. Kupferminc MJ, Tamura RK, Sabbagha RE, Parilla BV, Cohen LS, Pergament E. Isolated choroid plexus cyst(s): an indication for amniocentesis. *Am J Obstet Gynecol* **171**:1068–1071, 1994.
36. Nava S, Godmilow L, Reeser S, Ludomirsky A, Donnenfeld AE. Significance of sonographically detected second-trimester choroid plexus cysts: a series of 211 cases and a review of the literature. *Ultrasound Obstet Gynecol* **4**:448–451, 1994.
37. Ostlere SJ, Irving HC, Lilford RJ. Fetal choroid plexus cysts: a report of 100 cases. *Radiology* **175**:753–755, 1990.
38. Perpignano MC, Cohen HL, Klein VR et al. Fetal choroid plexus cysts: beware the smaller cyst. *Radiology* **182**:715–717, 1992.
39. Platt LD, Carlson DE, Medearis AL, Walla CA. Fetal choroid plexus cysts in the second trimester of pregnancy: a cause for concern. *Am J Obstet Gynecol* **161**:1652–1656, 1991.
40. Porto M, Murata Y, Warneke LA, Keegan Jr KA. Fetal choroid plexus cysts: an independent risk factor for chromosomal anomalies. *J Clin Ultrasound* **21**:103–108, 1993.
41. Twining P, Zuccollo J, Clewes J, Swallow J. Fetal choroid plexus cysts: a prospective study and review of the literature. *Br J Radiol* **64**:98–102, 1991.
42. Walkinshaw S, Pilling D, Spriggs A. Isolated choroid plexus cysts – the need for routine offer of karyotyping. *Prenat Diagn* **14**:663–667, 1994.
43. Thorpe-Beeston JG, Gosden M, Nicolaides KH. Choroid plexus cysts and chromosomal defects. *Br J Radiol* **63**:783–786, 1990.
44. Zerres K, Schuler H, Gembruch U, Bald R, Hansmann M, Schwanitz G. Chromosomal findings in fetuses with prenatally diagnosed cysts of the choroid plexus. *Hum Genet* **89**:301–304, 1992.
45. Lehman CD, Nyberg DA, Winter III TC, Kapur RP, Resta RG, Luthy DA. Trisomy 13 syndrome: prenatal US findings in a review of 33 cases. *Radiology* **194**:217–222, 1995.
46. Benacerraf BR, Frigoletto Jr FD, Greene MF. Abnormal facial features and extremities in human trisomy syndromes: prenatal US appearance. *Radiology* **159**:243–246, 1986.
47. Rijhsinghani AG, Hruban RH, Stetten G. Fetal anomalies associated with an inversion duplication 13 chromosome. *Obstet Gynecol* **71**:991–994, 1988.
48. Bromley B, Lieberman E, Laboda LA, Benacerraf BR. Echogenic intracardiac focus, a sonographic sign for Down Syndrome? *Obstet Gynecol* **86**:998–1001, 1995.
49. Lockwood C, Scioscia A, Stiller R, Hobbins J. Sonograpphic features of the triploid fetus. *Am J Obstet Gynecol* **157**:285–287, 1987.
50. Edwards MT, Smith WL, Hanson J, Abu Yousef M. Prenatal sonographic diagnosis of triploidy. *J Ultrasound Med* **5**:279–281, 1986.
51. Crane JP, Beaver HA, Cheung SW. Antenatal ultrasound findings in fetal triploidy syndrome. *J Ultrasound Med* **4**:519–524, 1985.
52. Broekhuizen FF, Elejalde R, Hamilton PR. Early-onset preeclampsia, triploidy and fetal hydrops. *J Reprod Med* **28**(3):223–226, 1983.
53. Benacerraf BR. Intrauterine growth retardation in the first trimester associated with triploidy. *J Ultrasound Med* **7**:153–154, 1988.
54. Doshi N, Surti U, Szulman AE. Morphologic anomalies in triploid liveborn fetuses. *Hum Pathol* **14**:716–723, 1983.
55. Snijders RJM, Sherrod C, Gosden CM, Nicolaides KH. Fetal growth retardation: associated malformations and chromosomal abnormalities. *Am J Obstet Gynecol* **168**:547–555, 1993.
56. Rubenstein JB, Swayne LC, Dise CA, Gersen SL, Schwartz JR, Risk A. Placental changes in fetal triploidy syndrome. *J Ultrasound Med* **5**:545–550, 1986.
57. Pircon RA, Porto M, Towers CV, Drade M, Gocke SE. Ultrasound findings in pregnancies complicated by fetal triploidy. *J Ultrasound Med* **8**:507–511, 1989.
58. Smith DW. *Recognizable Patterns of Human Malformation*. Vol. VII in the series Major Problems in Clinical Pediatrics, pp. 11–23, 30–31, and 72–75. Philadelphia: WB Saunders Company, 1982.
59. Nadel A, Bromley BS, Benacerraf BR. Nuchal thickening or cystic hygromas in first- and early second-trimester fetuses: prognosis and outcome. *Obstet Gynecol* **82**:43–48, 1993.
60. Wax JR, Blakemore KJ, Baser I, Stetten G. Isolated fetal ascites detected by sonography: an unusual presentation of Turner syndrome. *Obstet Gynecol* **79**:862–863, 1992.
61. Garder AS, Benzie RJ, Miskin M, Gardner HA. Transactions of the forty-first annual meeting of the society of obstetricians and gynaecologists of Canada. *Am J Obstet Gynecol* **154**:221–225, 1986.
62. Chervenak FA, Isaacsoon G, Blakemore KJ et al. Fetal cystic hygroma: cause and natural history. *N Engl J Med* **309**:822–825, 1983.
63. Benacerraf BR, Pauker S, Quade BJ, Bieber FR. Prenatal sonography in trisomy 9. *Prenat Diagn* **12**:175–181, 1992.

64. Kurnick J, Atkins L, Feingold M, Hills J, Dvorak A. Trisomy 9: predominance of cardiovascular, liver, brain and skeletal anomalies in the first diagnosed case. *Hum Pathol* **5**:223–228, 1974.
65. Qazi HQ, Masakawa A, Madahar C, Ehrilich R. Trisomy 9 syndrome. *Clin Genet* **12**:221–226, 1977.
66. Schwartz S, Ashai S, Meijboom RJ, Schwartz MF, Sun CCJ, Cohen MM. Prenatal detection of trisomy 9 mosaicism. *Prenat Diagn* **9**:549–554, 1989.
67. Hook EB, Cross PK, Schreinemachers DM. Chromosomal abnormality rates at amniocentesis and in live-born infants. *J Am Med Assoc* **249**:2034–2038, 1983.
68. Cuckle H, Nanchahal K, Wald N. Birth prevalence of Down's syndrome in England and Wales. *Prenat Diagn* **11**:29–34, 1991.
69. Dicke JM, Crane JP. Sonographic recognition of major malformations and aberrant fetal growth in trisomic fetuses. *J Ultrasound Med* **10**:433–438, 1991.
70. Balcar I, Grant DC, Miller WA, Bieber F. Antenatal detection of Down syndrome by sonography. *Am J Roentgenol* **143**:29–30, 1984.
71. Nyberg DA, Resta RG, Luthy DA, Hickok DE, Mahony BS, Hirsch JH. Prenatal sonographic findings of Down syndrome: review of 94 cases. *Obstet Gynecol* **76**:370–377, 1990.
72. Benacerraf BR, Neuberg D, Bromley B, Frigoletto Jr FD. Sonographic scoring index for prenatal detection of chromosomal abnormalities. *J Ultrasound Med* **11**:449–458, 1992.
73. DeVore GR, Alfi O. The use of color Doppler ultrasound to identify fetuses at increased risk for trisomy 21, an alternative for high-risk patients who decline genetic amniocentesis. *Obstet Gynecol* **85**:378–386, 1995.
74. Bromley B, Estroff JA, Sanders S et al. Fetal echocardiography: accuracy and limitations in a population at high and low risk for heart defects. *Am J Obstet Gynecol* **166**:1473–1481, 1992.
75. Benacerraf BR, Nadel A, Bromley B. Identification of second trimester fetuses with autosomal trisomy by use of a sonographic scoring index. *Radiology* **193**:135–140, 1994.
76. Benacerraf BR, Frigoletto Jr FD, Laboda LA. Sonographic diagnosis of Down syndrome in the second trimester. *Am J Obstet Gynecol* **153**:49–52, 1985.
77. Benacerraf BR, Barss VA, Laboda LA. A sonographic sign for the detection in the second trimester of the fetus with Down's syndrome. *Am J Obstet Gynecol* **151**:1078–1079, 1995.
78. Benacerraf BR, Frigoletto Jr FD, Cramer DW. Down syndrome: sonographic sign for diagnosis in the second-trimester fetus. *Radiology* **163**:811–813, 1987.
79. Benacerraf BR, Frigoletto Jr FD. Soft tissue nuchal fold in the second trimester fetus: standards for normal measurements compared to the fetus with Down syndrome. *Am J Obstet Gynecol* **157**:1146–1149, 1987.
80. Lynch L, Berkowitz GS, Chitkara U, Wilkilns IA, Mehalet KE, Berkowitz RL. Ultrasound detection of Down syndrome: is it really possible? *Obstet Gynecol* **73**:267–270, 1989.
81. Kirk JS, Comstock CH, Fassnacht MA, Yang SS, Lee W. Routine measurement of nuchal thickness in the second trimester. *J Maternal-Fetal Med* **1**:82–86, 1992.
82. Watson WJ, Miller RC, Menard K et al. Ultrasonographic measurement of fetal nuchal skin to screen for chromosomal abnormalities. *Am J Obstet Gynecol* **170**:583–586, 1994.
83. Crane JP, Gray DL. Sonographically measured nuchal skinfold thickness as a screening tool for Down syndrome: results of a prospective clinical trial. *Obstet Gynecol* **77**:533–536, 1991.
84. Gray DL, Crane JP. Optimal nuchal skin-fold thresholds based on gestational age for prenatal detection of Down syndrome. *Am J Obstet Gynecol* **171**:1282–1286, 1994.
85. Donnenfeld AE, Carlson DE, Palomaki GE, Libruzzi RJ, Weiner S, Platt LD. Prospective multicenter study of second-trimester nuchal skinfold thickness in unaffected and Down syndrome pregnancies. *Obstet Gynecol* **84**:844–847, 1994.
86. Toi A, Simpson GF, Filley RA. Ultrasonically evident fetal nuchal skin thickening: is it specific for Down syndrome? *Am J Obstet Gynecol* **156**:150–153, 1987.
87. Grandjean H, Sarramon M, AFDPHE Study Group. Sonographic measurement of nuchal skinfold thickness or detection of Down syndrome in the second-trimester fetus: a multicenter prospective study. *Obstet Gynecol* **85**:103–106, 1995.
88. Donnenfeld AE, Meister D, Allison J, Brennan K, Ludomirsky A, Rightmire D. Interobserver variability of sonographically determined second-trimester nuchal skinfold thickness measurements. *Ultrasound Obstet Gynecol* **5**:119–122, 1995.
89. Benacerraf BR, Laboda LA, Frigoletto Jr FD. Thickened nuchal fold in fetuses not at risk for aneuploidy. *Radiology* **184**:239–242, 1992.
90. Benacerraf BR, Mandell J, Estroff JA, Harlow BL, Frigoletto Jr FD. Fetal pyelectasis, a possible association with Down syndrome. *Obstet Gynecol* **76**:58–60, 1990.
91. Corteville JE, Dicke JM, Crane JP. Fetal pylectasis and Down syndrome: is genetic amniocentesis warranted? *Obstet Gynecol* **79**:770–772, 1992.
92. Nyberg DA, Resta RG, Mahony BS et al. Fetal hyperechogenic bowel and Down's syndrome. *Ultrasound Obstet Gynecol* **3**:330–333, 1993.
93. Persutte WH. Second trimester hyperechogenicity in the lower abdomen of two fetuses with trisomy 21: is there a correlation? *J Clin Ultrasound* **18**:425–428, 1990.
94. Scioscia AL, Pretorius DH, Budorick NE, Cahill TC, Axelrod FT, Leopold GR. Second-trimester hyperechoic bowel and chromosomal abnormalities. *Am J Obstet Gynecol* **167**:889–894, 1992.
95. Bromley B, Doubilet P, Frigoletto Jr FD, Krauss C, Estroff JA, Benacerraf BR. Is fetal hyperechoic bowel on second trimester sonogram an indication for amniocentesis? *Obstet Gynecol* **83**:647–651, 1994.
96. Roberts DJ, Genest D. Cardiac histologic pathology characteristic of trisomies 13 and 21. *Hum Pathol* **23**(10):1130–1140, 1992.
97. Brown DL, Roberts DJ, Miller WA. Left ventricular echogenic focus in the fetal heart: pathologic correlation. *J Ultrasound Med* **13**:613–616, 1994.
98. Benacerraf BR, Osathanondh R, Frigoletto Jr FD. Sonographic demonstration of hypoplasia of the middle phalanx of the fifth digit, a finding associated with Down syndrome. *Am J Obstet Gynecol* **159**:181–183, 1988.
99. Benacerraf BR, Harlow B, Frigoletto Jr FD. Hypoplasia of the middle phalanx of the fifth digit, a feature of the second trimester fetus with Down syndrome. *J Ultrasound Med* **9**:389–394, 1990.
100. Goldstein I, Gomez K, Copel JA. Fifth digit measurement in normal pregnancies, a potential sonographic sign of Down's syndrome. *Ultrasound Obstet Gynecol* **5**:34–37, 1995.
101. Jeanty P. Prenatal detection of simian crease. *J Ultrasound Med* **9**:131–136, 1990.
102. Wilkins I. Separation of the great toe in fetuses with Down syndrome. *J Ultrasound Med* **13**:229–231, 1994.
103. Hill LM, Rivello D, Peterson C, Marchese S. The transverse cerebellar diameter in the second trimester is unaffected by Down syndrome. *Am J Obstet Gynecol* **164**:101–103, 1991.
104. Bahado-Singh RO, Wyse L, Dorr MA, Copel JA, O'Connor T, Hobbins JC. Fetuses with Down syndrome have disproportionately shortened frontal lobe dimensions on ultrasonographic examination. *Am J Obstet Gynecol* **167**:1009–1014, 1992.
105. Abuhamad AZ, Kolm P, Mari G, Slotnick N, Evans III AT. Ultrasonographic fetal iliac length measurement in the screening for Down syndrome. *Am J Obstet Gynecol* **171**:1063–1067, 1994.
106. Gill P, Vanhook J, FitzSimmons J, Pascoe-Mason J, Fantel A. Fetal ear measurements in the prenatal detection of trisomy 21. *Prenat Diagn* **14**:739–743, 1994.
107. Martinez JM, Comas C, Ojuel J, Borrell A, Puerto B, Fortuny A. Fetal heart rate patterns in pregnancies with chromosomal disorders of subsequent fetal loss. *Obstet Gynecol* **87**:118–121, 1996.
108. Lockwood C, Benacerraf B, Krinsky A et al. A sonographic screening method for Down syndrome. *Am J Obstet Gynecol* **157**:803–808, 1987.
109. Benacerraf BR, Cnaan A, Gelman R, Laboda LA, Frigoletto Jr FD. Can sonographers reliably identify anatomy features associated with Down syndrome? *Radiology* **173**:377–380, 1989.
110. Benacerraf BR, Gelman R, Frigoletto Jr FD. Sonographic identification of second trimester fetuses with Down syndrome. *N Engl J Med* **317**:1371–1376, 1987.
111. Grist TM, Fuller RW, Albiez KL, Bowie JD. Femur length in ultrasound prediction of trisomy 21 and other chromosome abnormalities. (Abstr.) *Radiology* **174**:837–839, 1990.
112. Brumfield CG, Hauth JC, Cloud GA, Davis RO, Henson BV, Cosper P. Sonographic measurements and ratios in fetuses with Down syndrome. *Obstet Gynecol* **73**:644–646, 1989.

113. Hill LM, Guzick D, Belfar RL, Hixson J, Rivello D, Rusnak J. The current role of sonography in the detection of Down syndrome. *Obstet Gynecol* **74**:620–623, 1989.
114. Platt LD, Medearis AL, Carlson DE et al. Screening for Down syndrome with the femur length/biparietal diameter ratio, a new twist of the data. *Am J Obstet Gynecol* **167**:124–128, 1992.
115. Hadlock FP, Harrist RB, Martinez-Poyer J. Fetal body ratios in second trimester, a useful tool for identifying chromosomal abnormalities? *J Ultrasound Med* **11**:81–85, 1992.
116. Shah YG, Eckl CJ, Stinson SK, Woods JR. Biparietal diameter/femur length ratio, cephalic index, and femur length measurements, not reliable screening techniques for Down syndrome. *Obstet Gynecol* **75**:186–188, 1990.
117. LaFollette L, Filly RA, Anderson R, Golbus MS. Fetal femur length to detect trisomy 21. *J Ultrasound Med* **8**:657–660, 1989.
118. Dicke JM, Gray DL, Songster GS, Crane JP. Fetal biometry as a screening tool for the detection of chromosomally abnormal pregnancies. *Obstet Gynecol* **74**:726–729, 1989.
119. Nyberg DA, Resta RG, Hickok DE, Hollenbach KA, Luthy DA, Mahony BS. Femur length shortening in the detection of Down syndrome: is prenatal screening feasible? *Am J Obstet Gynecol* **162**:1247–1252, 1990.
120. Marquette GP, Boucher M, Desrochers M, and Dallaire L. Screening for trisomy 21 with ultrasonographic determination of biparietal diameter/femur length ratio. *Am J Obstet Gynecol* **163**:1604–1605, 1990.
121. Perrella R, Duerinckx AJ, Grant EG, Tessler F, Tabsh K, Crandall BF. Second-trimester sonographic diagnosis of Down syndrome: role of femur-length shortening and nuchal-fold thickening. *Am J Radiol* **151**:981–985, 1988.
122. Peters MT, Lockwood CJ, Miller WA. The efficacy of fetal sonographic biometry in Down syndrome screening. *Am J Obstet Gynecol* **161**:297–300, 1989.
123. Johnson MP, Barr M, Treadwell MC et al. Fetal leg and femur/foot length ratio: a marker for trisomy 21. *Am J Obstet Gynecol* **169**:557–563, 1993.
124. Grandjean H, Sarramon M. Femur/foot length ratio for detection of Down syndrome, results of a multicenter prospective study. *Am Obstet Gynecol* **173**:16–19, 1995.
125. FitzSimmons J, Droste S, Shepard TH, Pascoe-Mason, J, Chinn A, Mack LA. Long-bone growth in fetuses with Down syndrome. *Am J Obstet Gynecol* **161**:1174–1177, 1989.
126. Benacerraf BR, Neuberg D, Frigoletto Jr FD. Humeral shortening in second-trimester fetuses with Down syndrome. *Obstet Gynecol* **77**:223–227, 1991.
127. Rodis JF, Vintzileos AM, Fleming AD et al. Comparison of humerus length with femur length in fetuses with Down syndrome. *Am J Obstet Gynecol* **165**:1051–1056, 1991.
128. Rotmensch S, Luo J, Liberati M, Belanger K, Mahoney MJ, Hobbins JC. Fetal humeral length to detect Down syndrome. *Am J Obstet Gynecol* **166**:1330–1334, 1992.
129. Johnson MP, Michaelson JE, Barr Jr M et al. Combining humerus and femur length for improved ultrasonographic identification of pregnancies at increased risk for trisomy 21. *Am J Obstet Gynecol* **172**:1229–1235, 1995.
130. Biagiotti R, Periti E, Cariati E. Humerus and femur length in fetuses with Down syndrome. *Prenat Diagn* **14**:429–434, 1994.
131. Nyberg DA, Resta RG, Luthy DA, Hickok DE, Williams MA. Humerus and femur length shortening in the detection of Down's syndrome. *Am J Obstet Gynecol* **168**:534–538, 1993.
132. Smulian JC, Vintzileos AM, Ciarleglio L, Rodis JF, Campbell WA. Gender-specific patterns of second trimester femur and humerus measurements in fetuses with Down's syndrome. *J Maternal-Fetal Med* **4**:225–230, 1995.
133. Lockwood, CJ, Lynch L, Ghidini A et al. The effect of fetal gender on the prediction of Down syndrome by means of maternal serum alpha-fetoprotein and ultrasonographic parameters. *Am J Obstet Gynecol* **169**:1190–1197, 1993.
134. Benacerraf BR, Miller WA, Nadel A, Pauker S, Bromley B. Does gender have an impact on the sonographic detection of second trimester fetuses with Down syndrome? *Ultrasound Obstet Gynecol* **5**:30–33, 1995.
135. Bromley B, Lieberman E, Benacerraf BR. Choroid plexus cysts: not associated with Down syndrome. *Ultrasound Obstet Gynecol* **8**:232–235, 1996.
136. Ginsburg N, Cadkin A, Pergament E, Verlinsky Y. Ultrasonographic detection of the second-trimester fetus with trisomy 18 and trisomy 21. *Am J Obstet Gynecol* **163**:1186–1190, 1990.
137. O'Brien WF, Knupper RA, Torres C, Sternlicht D. Potential prenatal predictions of Down syndrome, a statistical analysis. *Am J Obstet Gynecol* **163**:1796–1798, 1990.
138. Vintzileos AM, Egan, JFX. Adjusting the risk for trisomy 21 on the basis of second-trimester ultrasonography. *Am J Obstet Gynecol* **172**:837–844, 1995.
139. Seoud MA, Alley DC, Smith DL, Levy DL. Prenatal sonographic findings in trisomy 13, 18, 21 and 22. *J Reprod Med* **39**:781–787, 1994.
140. Nadel A, Bromley B, Frigoletto Jr FD, Benacerraf BR. Can the presumed risk of autosomal trisomy be decreased in fetuses of older women following following a normal sonogram? *J Ultrasound Med* **143**:297–302, 1995.
141. Bahado-Singh RO, Goldstein I, Uerpairojkit B, Copel JA, Mahoney MJ, and Baumgarten A. Normal nuchal thickness in the midtrimester indicates reduced risk of Down syndrome in pregnancies with abnormal triple-screen results. *Am J Obstet Gynecol* **173**:1106–1110, 1995.
142. Nyberg DA, Luthy DA, Cheng EY, Sheley RC, Resta RG, Williams MA. Role of prenatal ultrasonography in women with positive screen for Down syndrome on the basis of maternal serum markers. *Am J Obstet Gynecol* **173**:1030–1035, 1995.

Fetal nuchal translucency at 10–14 weeks of gestation

48

K.H. Nicolaides, A.P. Souka and P.L. Noble

Introduction

At 10–14 weeks of gestation there is a subcutaneous collection of fluid in the fetal nuchal region that can be visualized by ultrasonography as nuchal translucency (NT). During the last decade a series of studies have reported that increased NT is associated with chromosomal defects and a wide range of fetal abnormalities and genetic syndromes.

Nuchal translucency and chromosomal defects

OBSERVATIONAL STUDIES

In the early 1990s several reports involving high-risk pregnancies demonstrated a possible association between increased NT and chromosomal defects in the first trimester of pregnancy (Table 48.1). Although the mean prevalence of

TABLE 48.1
Summary of reported series on first trimester fetal NT providing data on gestational age in weeks, criteria for diagnosis of increased NT thickness and the presence of associated chromosomal defects

Reference	GA (wks)	NT (mm)	*N*	Chromosomal defects					
				Total	T21	T18	T13	45,X	Other
1	10–14	≥2.0	68	41 (60%)	16	9	2	9	5
2	10–14	≥2.0	29	12 (41%)	5	3	1	2	1
3	10–13	≥2.5	32	15 (47%)	4	4	3	4	—
4	10–13	≥3.0	88	33 (38%)	21	8	2	—	2
5	10–13	≥3.0	1015	193 (19%)	101	51	13	14	15
6	11–12	≥3.0	8	7 (88%)	7	—	—	—	—
7	8–11	≥3.0	14	3 (21%)	—	—	—	1	2
8	9–14	≥3.0	29	7 (28%)	4	3	1	—	—
9	10–14	≥3.0	43	21 (49%)	9	4	1	4	3
10	8–15	≥3.0	70	8 (19%)	?	?	?	?	?
11	9–13	≥3.0	51	13 (18%)	4	4	—	—	1
12	10–15	≥4.0	63	43 (68%)	15	15	1	10	2
13	9–12	≥4.0	24	19 (79%)	15	2	1	1	—
14	10–14	≥4.0	8	7 (88%)	7	—	—	—	—
15	10–14	≥4.0	18	5 (28%)	3	1	—	1	1
16	11–13	≥6.0	29	15 (52%)	6	2	—	4	3
17	8–14	≥10.0	13	8 (62%)	—	—	—	7	1
Total	8–15	2–10	1602	450 (28%)	217	106	26	67	36

GA = gestational age

chromosomal defects in 17 series on a total of 1602 patients was 28%, there were large differences between the studies with the prevalence ranging from 18% to 88%. This variation in results presumably reflects differences in the maternal age distributions of the populations examined and differences in the definition of minimum thickness of the abnormal NT, ranging from 2 mm to 10 mm.

SCREENING IN UNSELECTED POPULATIONS

In the last 4 years the results of a series of screening studies using fetal NT in unselected populations have been reported (Table 48.2). In the combined data from these studies on a total of 17 518 pregnancies the mean prevalence of trisomy 21 was 0.33%. In 74% of the trisomy 21 pregnancies the fetal NT was considered to be increased and the false positive rate was only 1.6%. The number of cases that were screened in each study was small and all but one of these studies ignored the gestational-age-related changes in fetal NT. Nevertheless, the overall results are remarkable and compare very favourably with the sensitivity of 60% and false positive rate of 5% achieved by a combination of maternal age and second trimester maternal serum biochemistry.

ASSESSMENT OF RISK BY COMBINING MATERNAL AGE AND FETAL NT

The risk for trisomy 21 increases with maternal age and decreases with gestation because there is preferential spontaneous fetal death for trisomy 21 compared to normal pregnancies.[24] In each pregnancy, the risk for trisomy 21 is calculated from this maternal age and gestational age-related prevalence which is then multiplied by the likelihood ratio from the NT measurement. The likelihood ratio is proportional to the degree of deviation in NT from normal; the greater the NT the higher is the risk for trisomy 21.[25–26] Since NT at 10–14 weeks of gestation normally increases with fetal crown–rump length (CRL), it is necessary to take into account the CRL measurement in calculating the likelihood ratio for a given NT. The median and 95th centile of NT at a CRL of 38 mm are 1.3 mm and 2.2 mm respectively and these increase linearly with gestation to 1.9 mm and 2.8 mm for CRL of 84 mm.

In an ongoing multicentre study the risk for trisomy 21 was estimated from a combination of maternal age and fetal NT at 10–14 weeks of gestation in 22 centres in the UK[28]. The ultrasound scans were carried out by 306 sonographers who had received the Fetal Medicine Foundation certificate of competence in the theory and practice of the 10–14 week scan. The sonographers had attended theoretical and practical courses and submitted images with measurements from 50 first trimester scans for approval before receiving the software for calculation of risks. To achieve uniformity of results from different operators the following criteria were used:

- A good sagittal section of the fetus was obtained
- The magnification was such that the fetus occupied at least 75% of the image
- Care was taken to distinguish between fetal skin and amnion
- The maximum thickness of the subcutaneous translucency between the skin and the soft tissue overlying the cervical spine was measured (Fig. 48.1)

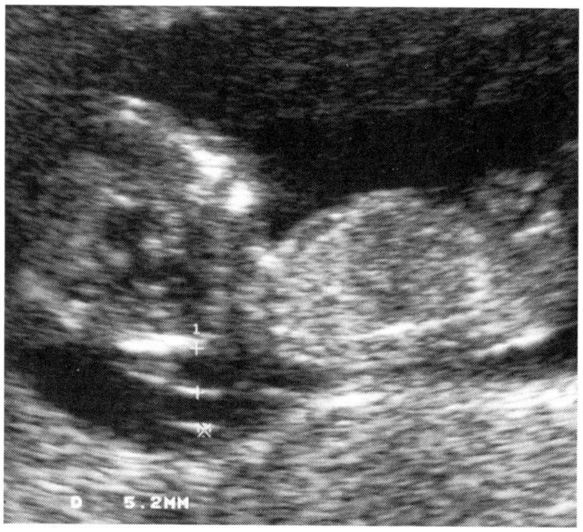

Fig. 48.1 Ultrasound picture of a 12-week fetus demonstrating increased nuchal translucency.

TABLE 48.2
Sensitivity and false-positive rate (FPR) of screening with fetal NT in unselected populations

Reference	Weeks	N	Prevalence of trisomy 21	NT cutoff	Sensitivity	FPR
18	9–12	3380	31 (0.92%)	NT ≥3.0 mm	28 (90.3%)	1.6%
19	8–14	1127	3 (0.27%)	NT ≥3.0 mm	1 (33.3%)	6.0%
20	8–13	537	4 (0.75%)	NT ≥3.0 mm	2 (50.0%)	6.3%
21	10–13	1302	6 (0.46%)	99th centile	5 (83.3%)	0.9%
22	10–14	6939	6 (0.09%)	NT ≥3.0 mm	4 (66.7%)	0.7%
23	10–13	4233	7 (0.17%)	NT ≥2.5 mm	3 (42.9%)	1.5%
Total		17 518	57 (0.33%)		43 (73.8%)	1.6%

The fetal NT and CRL were measured by transabdominal ultrasound examination unless visualization was poor, in which case vaginal sonography was carried out. The parents were counselled regarding the estimated risk for trisomy 21 and if they considered this risk to be high they were offered the option of an invasive diagnostic test – chorionic villus sampling or amniocentesis.

In the study population there were 326 pregnancies with trisomy 21 and 325 with other chromosomal abnormalities. The fetal NT was above the 95th centile of the normal range for CRL in 4209 (4.4%) of the normal pregnancies, in 234 (71.8%) of those with trisomy 21 (Fig. 48.2) and in 229 (70.5%) of those with other chromosomal defects (Table 48.3). The estimated risk for trisomy 21, based on maternal age and fetal NT, was ≥1 in 300 in 7907 (8.3%) of the normal pregnancies, in 268 (82.2%) of those with trisomy 21 and in 253 (77.8%) of those with other chromosomal defects. For a false positive rate of 5% the sensitivity was 77% (95% CI 72–82%).

The findings of this study demonstrate that assessment of risk for trisomy 21 can be carried out effectively during the first trimester of pregnancy using a combination of maternal age and fetal NT. Table 48.4 illustrates the observed prevalence of trisomy 21 according to the predicted risk based on maternal age and fetal NT. These results demonstrate the high degree of accuracy of the model. For the same rate of invasive testing (or screen positive rate) of 5%, the sensitivity of this method (about 80%) compares favourably with that of screening by maternal age alone (about 30%) or that of maternal age and serum biochemistry at 16 weeks (about 60%)[29]. However, as recommended by the RCOG Study Group on first trimester assessment of risk for trisomy 21, the implementation of this method should only be undertaken in centres with appropriately trained sonographers using high quality equipment, and results should be subject to an external agency for regular audit[30].

Assessment of risk for chromosomal defects in the first rather than the second trimester provides the option of earlier invasive diagnostic testing and consequently results in less trauma for those couples choosing termination of an affected pregnancy. A potential disadvantage is that earlier assessment of risk and prenatal diagnosis preferentially identifies those chromosomally abnormal pregnancies that are destined to miscarry. Approximately 40% of trisomy 21 fetuses die between 12 weeks of gestation and term[8]. This issue of intrauterine lethality of chromosomal defects is of course a potential criticism of all methods of antenatal screening, including second trimester maternal serum biochemistry; the

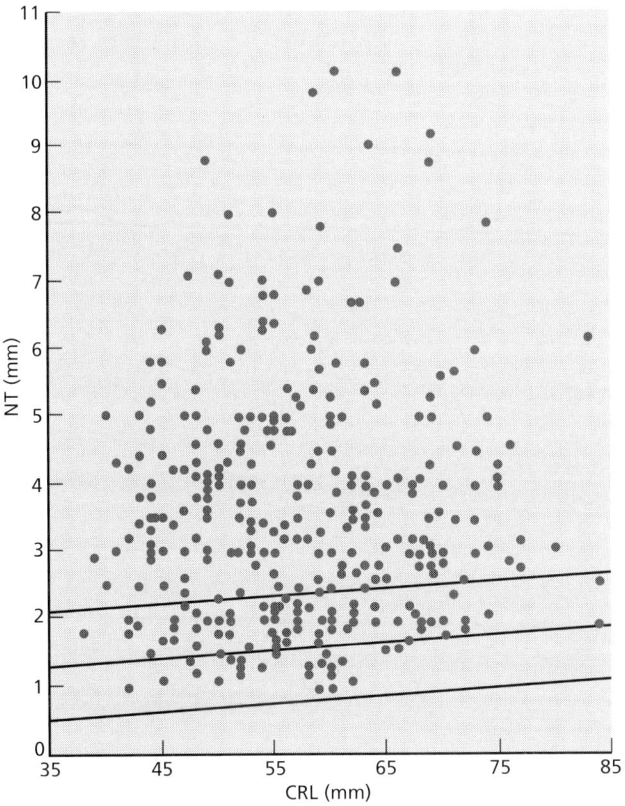

Fig. 48.2 Fetal nuchal translucency thickness (NT) in 326 trisomy 21 pregnancies plotted on the reference range with crown–rump length (CRL, median, 5th and 95th centiles).

TABLE 48.3
Number of pregnancies with NT thickness above the 95th centile and an estimated risk for trisomy 21 of ≥1 in 300

Fetal karyotype	*N*	NT >95th centile	Estimated risk ≥1 in 300
Normal	95 476	4209 (4.4%)	7907 (8.3%)
Trisomy 21	326	234 (71.8%)	268 (82.2%)
Trisomy 18	119	89 (74.8%)	97 (81.5%)
Trisomy 13	46	33 (71.7%)	37 (80.4%)
Turner syndrome	54	47 (87.0%)	48 (88.9%)
Triploidy	32	19 (59.4%)	20 (62.5%)
Other[a]	74	41 (55.4%)	51 (68.9%)
Total	96 127	4672 (4.9%)	8428 (8.8%)

[a]Deletions, partial trisomies, unbalanced translocations, sex chromosome aneuploidies

TABLE 48.4
Accuracy of estimated risk (range and median) for trisomy 21 by a combination of maternal age and fetal NT thickness

Estimated risk		Observed prevalence	
1 in 2 – 1 in 19	(1 in 7)	187 in 1305	(1 in 7)
1 in 20 – 1 in 99	(1 in 59)	49 in 2011	(1 in 41)
1 in 100 – 1 in 299	(1 in 198)	32 in 5096	(1 in 159)
1 in 300 – 1 in 999	(1 in 632)	31 in 18 279	(1 in 590)
1 in 1000 – 1 in 1999	(1 in 1504)	14 in 19 445	(1 in 1389)
1 in 2000 – 1 in 6000	(1 in 3702)	13 in 49 991	(1 in 3846)

estimated rate of intrauterine lethality between 16 weeks and term is about 30%[24].

In the multicentre study, trisomy 21 was diagnosed, either prenatally or postnatally, in 326 pregnancies. In the group with an estimated risk of >1 in 300, there were 268 cases of trisomy 21; in 250 cases the pregnancies were terminated but in 18 the parents chose not to have prenatal diagnosis or they decided to continue with the pregnancy despite the prenatal diagnosis of trisomy 21[28]. In the group with an estimated risk of <1 in 300, there were 35 live births with trisomy 21 and 23 other cases of trisomy 21 where the diagnosis was made prenatally and the pregnancies were terminated. On the basis of the maternal age distribution of the 96 127 pregnancies and the maternal-age-related prevalence of trisomy 21 in live births, it was estimated that 266 babies with trisomy 21 would have been liveborn had there not been any antenatal testing and selective termination of affected pregnancies[31]. On the extreme assumption that all intrauterine deaths are from the group with increased NT, then all 23 of the trisomy 21 pregnancies from the group with an estimated risk of <1 in 300 that were terminated would have resulted in live births. In such case, the number of trisomy 21 live births in this group would have been 58, or 22% of the total 266 potential live births with trisomy 21. Consequently, assessment of risk by a combination of maternal age and fetal NT, followed by invasive diagnostic testing for those with a risk of ≥1 in 300, and selective termination of affected fetuses would have reduced the potential live birth prevalence of trisomy 21 by 78%.

FETAL NT AND MATERNAL SERUM BIOCHEMISTRY

In trisomy 21, at 10–14 weeks of gestation the maternal serum concentration of free beta human chorionic gonadotrophin (free β-hCG) is higher, and pregnancy-associated plasma protein A (PAPP-A) is lower than in chromosomally normal pregnancies. In trisomy 21 pregnancies the deviation from normal in maternal serum PAPP-A and free-β hCG is independent of the increase in fetal NT[32–34]. It has been estimated that screening by a combination of maternal age, fetal NT and maternal biochemistry would identify about 90% of trisomy 21 pregnancies for a false positive rate of 5%.

Increased nuchal translucency with normal karyotype

REVIEW OF THE LITERATURE

In the literature there are 13 studies providing data on fetal defects in chromosomally normal pregnancies with increased NT thickness at 10–14 weeks of gestation and the data are summarized in Table 48.5. In the combined data on a total of 306 fetuses there were 49 (16%) with defects.

In addition to the above, a review of the literature for studies reporting the diagnosis of fetal abnormalities at the 10–14 week scan identified several conditions that were associated with increased NT thickness (Table 48.6).

TABLE 48.5
Studies reporting defects in chromosomally normal fetuses with increased NT thickness at 10–14 weeks of gestation

Reference	NT	N	Other defects	
1,9	>2.0	32	5	Megacystis (1), amnion rupture sequence (1), Noonan syndrome (1), unspecified syndrome (2)
35	≥2.5	32	1	Cystic hygromas (1)
23	≥2.5	72	7	Camptomelic dwarfism (1), cardiac defect (2), exomphalos (1), pentalogy of Cantrell (1), Ivemark syndrome (1), Toriello–Carey syndrome (1)
15	≥3.0	13	3	Megacystis (1), polycystic kidneys (1), Noonan syndrome (1)
2	≥3.0	10	1	Achondrogenesis
8	≥3.0	61	10	Facial cleft (1), cardiac defects (3), multicystic kidneys (1), exomphalos (1), FADS (2), unspecified syndrome (2)
36	≥3.0	5	2	Holoprosencephaly (1), cardiac defects (1)
37	≥3.0	35	3	Polycystic kidneys (1), Noonan syndrome (1), Joubert syndrome (1)
12	≥4.0	16	5	Facial cleft (1), cardiac defects (1), diaphragmatic hernia (1), exomphalos (1), FADS (1)
38	≥4.0	8	3	Cardiac defects (2), spina bifida (1)
39	≥4.0	18	7	Anencephaly (1), spina bifida (1), cardiac defects (3), Noonan syndrome (1), unspecified syndrome (1)
40	≥5.0	4	2	Cardiac defect (1), achondroplasia (1)

TABLE 48.6
Case reports and series of fetal abnormalities with increased NT thickness at 10–14 weeks of gestation

Abnormality	Gestation (weeks)	Increased NT	Reference
Major cardiac defect	10–14	17 of 21	41–44
Diaphragmatic hernia	10–14	7 of 19	45
Exomphalos	11–14	8 of 14	46
Megacystis	10–14	6 of 15	47
Body stalk anomaly	10–14	10 of 14	48
Achondrogenesis type II	11–12	2 of 2	49,50
Akinesia deformation sequence	10–14	2 of 2	51
Asphyxiating thoracic dystrophy	14	1 of 1	52
Frynn syndrome	12	2 of 2	53,54
Hydrolethalus syndrome	12	1 of 1	55
Jarcho–Levin syndrome	12	1 of 3	56
Robert syndrome	11	1 of 1	57
Smith–Lemli–Opitz syndrome	10–11	3 of 3	58–60

FETAL MEDICINE FOUNDATION STUDY

In the multicentre screening study for trisomy 21 by a combination of maternal age and fetal NT at 10–14 weeks of gestation involving about 100 000 pregnancies, there were 4116 singleton, chromosomally normal pregnancies with fetal NT above the 95th centile for CRL[61]. The patients were subdivided according to NT thickness into five groups; 95th centile to 3.4 mm, 3.5–4.4 mm, 4.5–5.4 mm, 5.5–6.4 and ≥6.5 mm. Nuchal translucency normally increases with CRL and the 95th centile is 2.2 mm for CRL of 38 mm and 2.8 mm for CRL of 84 mm; the 99th centile does not change significantly with CRL and is about 3.5 mm.

In the 4116 pregnancies, there were 3899 live births that survived the neonatal period, 38 neonatal deaths, 74 spontaneous abortions or intrauterine deaths and 77 terminations at the request of the parents because fetal abnormalities were detected by ultrasonography at 10–14 weeks or at follow-up scans; termination of pregnancy was also performed in 42 cases because of the uncertain prognosis since a repeat scan 2 weeks after presentation demonstrated persistence or increase in the large translucency (Table 48.7).

There was a wide range of structural defects and genetic syndromes and the prevalence of these increased with NT thickness (Table 48.8). The diagnosis of abnormalities was made by ultrasound examination in mid-pregnancy, or by pathological examination in terminations of pregnancy and intrauterine or neonatal deaths or by clinical examination and appropriate investigations in live births. In these calculations we did not include minor defects, such as choroid plexus cysts, pyelectasia, digital abnormalities or cardiac defects that would not require therapy.

These findings demonstrate that increased fetal NT thickness at 10–14 weeks of gestation is associated with a wide range of fetal abnormalities. The observed prevalence for some of the abnormalities, such as anencephaly, holoprosencephaly, microcephaly, facial cleft, gastroschisis, renal abnormalities, bowel obstruction and spina bifida, may not be different from that in the general population. However, the prevalence of major cardiac defects, diaphragmatic hernia, exomphalos, body stalk anomaly and fetal akinesia deformation sequence appears to be substantially higher than in the general population and it is therefore likely that there is an association between these abnormalities and increased NT thickness. Similarly, there may well be an association between increased NT and a wide range of rare skeletal dysplasias and genetic syndromes that are usually found in less than 1 in 10 000 pregnancies; however, the number of affected cases both in the present and previous series of fetuses with increased NT is too small for definite conclusions to be drawn.

In addition to the association between increased NT thickness and a wide range of fetal abnormalities, the data of this study demonstrate that the rates of miscarriage and perinatal death increase with fetal NT thickness. These data would be useful in counselling parents of affected pregnancies and in alerting sonographers to plan the appropriate follow up investigations for such pregnancies. However, it should be emphasized to the parents that increased NT thickness per se does not constitute a fetal abnormality and once chromosomal defects have been excluded about 90% of pregnancies with fetal NT below 4.5 mm would result in healthy live births; the rates for NT of 4.5–6.4 mm and 6.5 mm or more are about 80% and 45% respectively.

TABLE 48.7
Outcome in 4116 pregnancies with increased fetal NT in the Fetal Medicine Foundation study

Nuchal translucency	Total	Termination		Prenatal death	Postnatal death	Alive
		Total	Abnormal			
95th–3.4 mm	3423	49	36	47	29	3311 (96.8%)
3.5–4.4 mm	448	23	14	9	4	413 (92.2%)
4.5–5.4 mm	138	13	8	4	3	117 (84.8%)
5.5–6.4 mm	48	13	7	4	0	31 (64.6%)
≥6.5 mm	59	21	12	10	2	27 (45.8%)
Total	4116	119	77	74	38	3899 (94.7%)

TABLE 48.8
Fetal abnormalities and genetic syndromes identified in the 4116 pregnancies with increased fetal NT in the Fetal Medicine Foundation study

	Fetal NT thickness (mm)					Pregnancy outcome		
Fetal abnormality	<3.5	3.5–4.4	4.5–5.4	5.5–6.4	>6.5	TOP	Death	Alive
Anencephaly	4	1	—	—	—	5	—	—
Encephalocoele	3[a]	—	—	—	1	4	—	—
Ventriculomegaly	6	—	—	—	—	5	—	1
Dandy–Walker cyst	1	—	—	—	—	1	—	—
Holoprosencephaly	1	—	—	—	—	1	—	—
Microcephaly	1	—	—	—	—	—	—	1
Facial cleft	2	—	—	—	—	—	—	2
Microphthalmia	1[b]	—	—	—	—	—	—	1
Laryngeal cyst	1	—	—	—	—	—	—	1
Cystic hygroma	1	—	—	—	—	—	—	1
Major cardiac defect	12	12	6	3	10	19	9	15
Diaphragmatic hernia	4	1	3	—	—	1	5	2
Exomphalos	2[c]	3[de]	1[f]	1[g]	—	5	1	1
Gastroschisis	—	1	—	—	—	—	1	—
Bowel obstruction	2	—	—	—	—	—	—	2
Duodenal atresia	—	1	—	—	—	—	—	1
Hydronephrosis	2	2	1	—	—	1	—	4
Multicystic kidneys	4	—	—	—	—	3	—	1[b]
Polycystic kidneys	—	—	—	—	1	1	—	—
Renal agenesis	1	1	—	—	—	1	—	1[b]
Megacystis	7	1	—	—	—	2	2	4
Spina bifida	3	1	—	—	—	2	1	1
Kyphoscoliosis	—	—	—	1	—	1	—	—
Body stalk anomaly	1	3	1	1	4	10	—	—
Diastomatomella	1	—	—	—	—	—	—	1
Talipes	10	4	1	—	—	1	—	14
Akinesia deformation	2	—	—	1	3	6	—	—
Jarcho–Levin syndrome	1	—	1	—	—	1	1	—
Joubert syndrome	1	—	—	—	—	1	—	—
Nance–Sweeney syndrome	—	—	1	—	—	—	—	1
Noonan syndrome	—	—	—	—	1	—	—	1
Smith–Lemli–Opitz	1	—	1	1	—	2	1	—
Spinal muscular atrophy	1	—	—	—	—	—	1	—
Thanatophoric dysplasia	1	—	—	—	—	1	—	—
Trygonocephaly 'C'	1	—	—	—	—	—	—	1
Vacterl association	2	—	—	—	—	1	—	1
Unspecified syndrome	3	1	1	—	1	2	—	4

TOP = termination of pregnancy

[a]Encephalocele + AVSD; [b]Unilateral; [c]Spina bifida + cloacal exstrophy; [d] Beckwith–Wiedemann syndrome; [e]Extrocardia; [f]Spina bifida + anencephaly; [g]Spina bifida + coarctation

CARDIAC DEFECTS

Increased NT is of particular importance in its association with major abnormalities of the heart and great arteries. Cardiac defects are the most common congenital abnormalities with a birth prevalence of 3–8 per 1000; about half are classified as major because they are either lethal or require surgery and half are asymptomatic. Specialist echocardiography at around 20 weeks of gestation can identify most of the major cardiac defects, but the main challenge in prenatal diagnosis is to identify the high-risk group for referral to specialist centres. Currently, screening is based on examination of the four-chamber view of the heart at the 20-week scan, but this identifies only 26% of the major cardiac defects[62].

Studies involving pathological examination in both chromosomally abnormal and normal fetuses with increased NT at 10–14 weeks of gestation, have demonstrated a high prevalence of abnormalities of the heart and great arteries[63]. Additionally, there are several case reports or small series on the sonographic diagnosis of cardiac defects at 10–14 weeks of gestation; in a total of 21 fetuses with major cardiac defects, 17 (81%) had increased NT[41–44]. Furthermore, a study of 1389 chromosomally normal fetuses with increased NT at 10–14 weeks reported that the prevalence of major cardiac defects increased with translucency thickness[64].

In the Fetal Medicine Foundation study (Table 48.8), the prevalence of major abnormalities of the heart and great arteries was 10 per 1000 and increased exponentially with translucency thickness from about 4 per 1000 for NT of 95th–3.4 mm, 27 per 1000 for NT 3.5–4.4, 43 per 1000 for NT 4.5–5.4, 63 per 1000 for NT 5.5–6.4, and 169 per 1000 for NT of ≥6.5 mm. The clinical implication of these findings is that increased NT at 10–14 weeks constitutes an indication for specialist fetal echocardiography in later pregnancy. Furthermore, the findings suggest that measurement of NT thickness at 10–14 weeks is likely to prove to be a useful method of screening for abnormalities of the heart and great arteries in addition to its role in screening for chromosomal defects.

CONGENITAL INFECTION

In about 10% of 'unexplained' second or third-trimester fetal hydrops there is evidence of recent maternal infection and in these cases the fetus is also infected. In a study of 426 pregnancies with increased fetal NT and normal karyotype only 1.5% of the mothers had evidence of recent infection and none of the fetuses was infected[27].

In contrast to second- or third-trimester hydrops, in pregnancies with increased first-trimester NT the prevalence of maternal infection with the TORCH group of organisms is not higher than in the general population. Furthermore, in cases of maternal infection the presence of increased fetal NT does not signify the presence of fetal infection with these organisms. Therefore, increased NT in chromosomally normal fetuses need not stimulate the search for maternal infection unless the translucency evolves into second- or third-trimester nuchal oedema or generalized hydrops.

REFERENCES

1. Johnson MP, Johnson A, Holzgreve W *et al.* First-trimester simple hygroma: Cause and outcome. *Am. J. Obstet. Gynecol.* **168**, 156–161, 1993.
2. Hewitt B. Nuchal translucency in the first trimester. *Aust. NZ. J. Obstet. Gynaecol.* **33**, 389–391, 1993.
3. Shulman LP, Emerson D, Felker R, Phillips O, Simpson J & Elias S. High frequency of cytogenetic abnormalities with cystic hygroma diagnosed in the first trimester. *Obstet. Gynecol.* **80**, 80–82, 1992.
4. Nicolaides KH, Azar G, Byrne D, Mansur C & Marks K. Fetal nuchal translucency: ultrasound screening for chromosomal defects in first trimester of pregnancy. *Br. Med. J.* **304**, 867–869, 1992.
5. Pandya PP, Kondylios A, Hilbert L, Snijders RJM & Nicolaides KH. Chromosomal defects and outcome in 1,015 fetuses with increased nuchal translucency. *Ultrasound Obstet. Gynecol.* **5**, 15–19, 1995b.
6. Szabo J & Gellen J. Nuchal fluid accumulation in trisomy-21 detected by vaginal sonography in first trimester. *Lancet* **336**, 1133, 1990.
7. Wilson RD, Venir N & Faquharson DF. Fetal nuchal fluid–physiological or pathological? In pregnancies less than 17 menstrual weeks. *Prenat. Diagn.* **12**, 755–763, 1992.
8. Ville Y, Lalondrelle C, Doumerc S *et al.* First-trimester diagnosis of nuchal anomalies: significance and fetal outcome. *Ultrasound Obstet. Gynecol.* **2**, 314–316, 1992.
9. Trauffer ML, Anderson CE, Johnson A, Heeger S, Morgan P & Wapner RJ. The natural history of euploid pregnancies with first-trimester cystic hygromas. *Am. J. Obstet. Gynecol.* **170**, 1279–1284, 1994.
10. Brambati B, Cislaghi C, Tului L *et al.* First-trimester Down's syndrome screening using nuchal translucency: a prospective study. *Ultrasound Obstet. Gynecol.* **5**, 9–14, 1995.
11. Comas C, Martinez JM, Ojuel J *et al.* First-trimester nuchal edema as a marker of aneuploidy. *Ultrasound Obstet. Gynecol.* **5**, 26–29, 1995.
12. Nadel A, Bromley B & Benacerraf BR. Nuchal thickening or cystic hygromas in first- and early second-trimester fetuses: prognosis and outcome. *Obstet. Gynecol.* **82**, 43–48, 1993.
13. Savoldelli G, Binkert F, Achermann J & Schmid W. Ultrasound screening for chromosomal anomalies in the first trimester of pregnancy. *Prenat. Diagn.* **13**, 513–518, 1993.
14. Schulte-Valentin M & Schindler H. Non-echogenic nuchal oedema as a marker in trisomy 21 screening. *Lancet* **339**, 1053, 1992.
15. van Zalen-Sprock RM, van Vugt JMG & van Geijn HP. First-trimester diagnosis of cystic hygroma–course and outcome. *Am. J. Obstet. Gynecol.* **167**, 94–98, 1992.
16. Cullen MT, Gabrielli S, Green JJ *et al.* Diagnosis and significance of cystic hygroma in the first trimester. *Prenat. Diagn.* **10**, 643–651, 1990.
17. Suchet IB, Van der Westhuizen NG & Labatte MF. Fetal cystic hygromas: further insights into their natural history. *Can. Assoc. Radiol. J.* **6**, 420–424, 1992.
18. Szabo J, Gellen J & Szemere G. First-trimester ultrasound screening for fetal aneuploidies in women over 35 and under 35 years of age. *Ultrasound Obstet. Gynecol.* **5**, 161–163, 1995.
19. Bewley S, Roberts LJ, Mackinson M & Rodeck C. First trimester fetal nuchal translucency: problems with screening the general population II. *Br. J. Obstet. Gynaecol.* **102**, 386–388, 1995.
20. Komman LH, Morssink LP, Beekhuis JR, DeWolf BTHM, Heringa MP & Mantingh A. Nuchal translucency cannot be used as a screening test for chromosomal abnormalities in the first trimester of pregnancy in a routine ultrasound practice. *Prenat. Diagn.* **16**, 797–805, 1996.
21. Kadiz R & Economides DL. The effect of nuchal translucency measurement on second-trimester biochemical screening for Down's syndrome. *Ultrasound Obstet. Gynecol.* **9**, 244–247, 1997.
22. Taipale P, Hiilesmaa V, Salonen R & Ylostalo P. Increased nuchal translucency as a marker for fetal chromosomal defects. *N. Engl. J. Med.* **337**, 1654–1658, 1997.
23. Hafner E, Schuchter K, Liebhart E & Philipp K. Results of routine fetal nuchal translucency measurement at weeks 10–13 in 4,233 unselected pregnant women. *Prenat. Diagn.* **18**, 29–34, 1998.
24. Snijders RJM, Sebire NJ & Nicolaides KH. Maternal age and gestational age specific risk for chromosomal defects. *Fetal. Diag. Ther.* **10**, 356–367, 1995.
25. Nicolaides KH, Brizot ML & Snijders RJM. Fetal nuchal translucency thickness: ultrasound screening for fetal trisomy in the first trimester of pregnancy. *Br. J. Obstet. Gynaecol.* **101**, 782–786, 1994.
26. Pandya PP, Snijders RJM, Johnson SJ, Brizot M & Nicolaides KH. Screening for fetal trisomies by maternal age and fetal nuchal translucency thickness at 10 to 14 weeks of gestation. *Br. J. Obstet. Gynaecol.* **102**, 957–962, 1995a.
27. Sebire NJ, Bianco D, Snijders RJM, Zuckerman M & Nicolaides KH. Increased fetal nuchal translucency thickness at 10–14 weeks: is screening for maternal-fetal infection necessary? *Br. J. Obstet. Gynecol.* **104**, 212–215, 1997.
28. Snijders RJM, Sebire NJ, Noble PL, Souka AP & Nicolaides KH. UK Multicentre project on assessment of risk for trisomy 21 by maternal age and fetal nuchal translucency at 10–14 weeks of gestation. *Lancet* (in press), 1998.
29. Wald NJ, Cuckle HS, Densem JW *et al.* Maternal serum screening for Down's syndrome in early pregnancy. *Br. Med. J.* **297**, 883–887, 1988.
30. Recommendations of the 32nd Study Group of the Royal College of Obstetricians and Gynaecologists. In *Screening for Down Syndrome in the First Trimester* (eds JG Grudzinskas & RHT Ward), pp. 353–356. London: RCOG Press, 1997.

31. Hecht CA & Hook EB. The imprecision in rates of Down syndrome by 1-year maternal age intervals: a critical analysis of rates used in biochemical screening. *Prenat. Diagn.* **14**, 729–738, 1994.
32. Brizot ML, Snijders RJM, Bersinger NA, Kuhn P & Nicolaides KH. Maternal serum pregnancy associated placental protein A and fetal nuchal translucency thickness for the prediction of fetal trisomies in early pregnancy. *Obstet. Gynecol.* **84**, 918–922, 1994.
33. Brizot ML, Snijders RJM, Butler J, Bersinger NA & Nicolaides KH. Maternal serum hCG and fetal nuchal translucency thickness for the prediction of fetal trisomies in the first trimester of pregnancy. *Br. J. Obstet. Gynaecol.* **102**, 127–132, 1995.
34. Noble PL, Abraha HD, Snijders RJM, Sherwood R & Nicolaides KH. Screening for fetal trisomy 21 in the first trimester of pregnancy: maternal serum free β-hCG and fetal nuchal translucency thickness. *Ultrasound Obstet. Gynecol.* **6**, 390–395, 1996.
35. Shulman LP, Emerson DS, Grevengood C *et al.* Clinical course and outcome of fetuses with isolated cystic nuchal lesions and normal karyotypes detected in the first trimester. *Am. J. Obstet. Gynecol.* **171**, 1278–1281, 1994.
36. Salvesen DR & Goble O. Early amniocentesis and fetal nuchal translucency in women requesting karyotyping for advanced maternal age. *Prenat. Diagn.* **15**, 971–974, 1995.
37. Reynders CS, Pauker SP & Benacerraf BR. First trimester isolated fetal nuchal lucency: significance and outcome. *J. Ultrasound. Med.* **16**, 101–105, 1997.
38. Moselhi M & Thilaganathan B. Nuchal translucency: a marker for the antenatal diagnosis of aortic coarctation. *Br. J. Obstet. Gynaecol.* **103**, 1044–1045, 1996.
39. Thilaganathan B, Slack A & Wathen NC. Effect of first-trimester nuchal translucency on second-trimester maternal serum biochemical screening for Down's syndrome. *Ultrasound Obstet. Gynecol.* **10**, 261–264, 1997.
40. Fukada Y, Yasumizu T, Takizawa M, Amemiya A & Hoshi K. The prognosis of fetuses with transient nuchal translucency in the first and early second trimester. *Acta. Obstet. Gynecol. Scand.* **76**, 913–916, 1998.
41. Gembruch U, Knopfle G, Chatterjee M, Bald R & Hansmann M. First-trimester diagnosis of fetal congenital heart disease by transvaginal two-dimensional and Doppler echocardiography. *Obstet. Gynecol.* **75**, 496–498, 1990.
42. Gembruch U, Knopfle G, Bald R & Hansmann M. Early diagnosis of fetal congenital heart disease by transvaginal echocardiography. *Ultrasound Obstet. Gynecol.* **3**, 310–317, 1993.
43. Bronshtein M, Siegler E, Yoffe N & Zimmer EZ. Prenatal diagnosis of ventricular septal defect and overriding aorta at 14 weeks' gestation, using transvaginal sonography. *Prenat. Diagn.* **10**, 697–702, 1990.
44. Achiron R, Rotstein Z, Lipitz S, Mashiach S & Hegesh J. First-trimester diagnosis of fetal congenital heart disease by transvaginal ultrasonography. *Obstet. Gynecol.* **84**, 69–72, 1994.
45. Sebire NJ, Snijders RJM, Davenport M, Greenough A & Nicolaides KH. Fetal nuchal translucency thickness at 10–14 weeks gestation and congenital diaphragmatic hemia. *Obstet. Gynecol.* **90**, 943–946, 1997.
46. van Zalen-Sprock RM, van Vugt JMG & van Geijn HP. First-trimester sonography of physiological midgut herniation and early diagnosis of omphalocele. *Prenat. Diagn.* **17**, 511–518, 1997.
47. Sebire NJ, von Kaisenberg C, Rubio C, Snidjers RJM & Nicolaides KH. Fetal megacystis at 10–14 weeks of gestation. *Ultrasound Obstet. Gynecol.* **8**, 387–390, 1996.
48. Daskalakis G, Sebire NJ, Jurkovic D, Snidjers RJM & Nicolaides KH. Body stalk anomaly at 10 to 14 weeks of gestation. *Ultrasound Obstet. Gynecol.* **10**, 416–418, 1997.
49. Fisk NM, Vaughan J, Smidt M & Wigglesworth J. Transvaginal ultrasound recognition of nuchal oedema in the first-trimester diagnosis of achondrogenesis. *J. Clin. Ultrasound* **19**, 586–590, 1991.
50. Soothill PW, Vuthiwong C & Rees H. Achondrogenesis type 2 diagnosed by transvaginal ultrasound at 12 weeks of gestation. *Prenat. Diagn.* **13**, 523–528, 1993.
51. Hyett J, Noble P, Sebire NJ, Snidjers R & Nicolaides KH. Lethal congenital arthrogryposis presents with increased nuchal translucency at 10–14 weeks of gestation. *Ultrasound Obstet. Gynecol.* **9**: 310–313, 1997.
52. Ben Arni M, Perlitz Y, Haddad S & Matilsky M. Increased nuchal translucency is associated with asphyxiating thoracic dysplasia. *Ultrasound Obstet. Gynecol.* **10**, 297–298, 1997.
53. Bulas D, Saal H, Allen JF, Kapur S, Nies BM & Newman K. Cystic hygroma and congenital diaphragmatic hernia: early prenatal sonographic evaluation of Fryn's syndrome. *Prenat. Diagn.* **12**, 867–875, 1992.
54. Hosli IM, Tercanli S, Rehder H & Holzgreve W. Cystic hygroma as an early first-trimester ultrasound marker for recurrent Fryns' syndrome. *Ultrasound Obstet. Gynecol.* **10**, 422–424, 1997.
55. Ammala P & Salonen R. First-trimester diagnosis of hydrolethalus syndrome. *Ultrasound Obstet. Gynecol.* **5**, 60–62, 1995.
56. Eliyahu S, Weiner E, Lahav D & Shalev E. Early sonographic diagnosis of Jarcho–Levin syndrome: a prospective screening program in one family. *Ultrasound Obstet Gynecol.* **9**, 314–318, 1997.
57. Petrikovsky BM, Gross B, Bialer M, Solamanzadeh K & Simhaee E. Prenatal diagnosis of pseudothalidomide syndrome in consecutive pregnancies of a consanguineous couple. *Ultrasound Obstet. Gynecol.* **10**, 425–428, 1997.
58. Hobbins JC, Jones OW, Gottesfeld S & Persutte W. Transvaginal sonography and transabdominal embryoscopy in the first-trimester diagnosis of Smith–Lemli–Opitz syndrome, type 2. *Am. J. Obstet. Gynecol.* **171**, 546–549, 1994.
59. Hyett JA, Clayton PT, Moscoso G & Nicolaides KH. Increased first trimester nuchal translucency as a prenatal manifestation of Smith–Lemli–Opitz syndrome. *Am. J. Med. Genet.* **58**, 374–376, 1995.
60. Sharp P, Haant E, Fletcher JM, Khong TY & Carey WF. First-trimester diagnosis of Smith– Lemli–Opitz syndrome. *Prenat. Diagn.* **17**, 355–361, 1997.
61. Souka AP & Nicolaides KH. Diagnosis of fetal abnormalities at the 10–14-week scan. *Ultrasound Obstet. Gynecol.* **10**, 429–442, 1997.
62. Tegnander E, Eik-Nes SH, Johansen OJ & Linker DT. Prenatal detection of heart defects at the routine fetal examination at 18 weeks in a non-selected population. *Ultrasound Obstet. Gynecol.* **5**, 372–380, 1995.
63. Hyett JA, Moscoso G & Nicolaides KH. Abnormalities of the heart and great arteries in first trimester chromosomally abnormal fetuses. *Am. J. Med. Genet.* **69**, 207–216, 1997.
64. Hyett JA, Perdu M, Sharland GK, Snijders RSM & Nicolaides KH. Increased nuchal translucency at 10–14 weeks of gestation as a marker for major cardiac defects. *Ultrasound Obstet. Gynecol.* **10**, 242–246, 1997.

First-trimester diagnosis of fetal malformations

49

H.-G. Blaas and S.H. Eik-Nes

Ultrasound and the first trimester

More than 30 years ago ultrasound was introduced as a means to evaluate early pregnancy[1,2]. In the 1970s, measurements of the embryo and extra-embryonic structures were presented[3–5] initiating an avalanche of studies that described normal and abnormal early pregnancy. During the 1980s, with the introduction of real-time ultrasound, interest in the morphological development of the embryo increased. The developing conceptuses were studied by the transabdominal route and specific normal and abnormal first-trimester features could be described[6,7]. It was even possible to diagnose an omphalocele as early as at the end of the first trimester using a 4.5 MHz transducer[8].

During the 1990s transvaginal ultrasound has become established as the most important tool for the examination of early pregnancy. High-frequency transducers have improved the image quality to such an extent that a distinct description of the embryonic morphology has become possible[9]. The term sonoembryology[10] designates the description of the embryonic anatomy, the normal anatomic relations and the development of abnormalities as visualized by ultrasound. It has been possible to produce images of such a quality that sonoembryology has become a tool for basic research on the embryonic development[11–16].

An embryo of 10 postmenstrual weeks is less than half the length of an adult thumb, but already possesses several thousand named structures, practically any of which may be subject to developmental deviations[17]. Thus, the embryonic period proper is of particular importance because the majority of congenital anomalies make their appearance during that time.

In order to confirm the presence of normal anatomy or to make the diagnosis of an anomaly we need knowledge of the normal embryonic development, including the appearance of the normal embryo on the ultrasound screen. We must know when structural anomalies of various organs systems develop and what they can look like. This chapter provides a survey of this development along with examples of the anomalies that can be detected.

As documented in the classical embryological literature[17,18–23] the development of the human cyema displays dramatic morphological changes. The first-trimester embryo looks completely different from the second-trimester fetus and its appearance on the ultrasound screen changes from week to week; these changes have been shown in the sonoembryological studies[9–15,24,25]. Because of these drastic changes in embryonic development the standards for the assessment of the early conceptus must be quite different than the standard used for the second-trimester fetus, which is the usual object of routine scanning. An illustrative example is the central nervous system (CNS) development: during the first trimester, the embryonic brain dominates the appearance of the embryo; there are striking hypoechogenic areas that represent the wide ventricular system in the relatively large head[11,13–15,26]. This physiological phenomenon, if found in an 18-week fetus, would represent a serious CNS anomaly.

In the following overview of early development, all statements of time are based on last menstrual period, expressed in completed weeks and completed days, assuming a regular cycle with ovulation at 2 weeks 0 days. That applies also for the embryonic age, making the comparison of embryonic development with first-trimester ultrasound findings easy. For example, 'during week 8' means 8 completed weeks plus 0 to 6 days, and 'at the end of week 9' means 9 completed weeks plus 5 to 6 days.

Sonoembryological development

The developmental steps of the human embryo have been staged by the classical human embryologists[18,19,21–23,27]. The Carnegie staging system is based on the external form of the embryo and the analysis of its organ systems by light microscope where certain key features are determined[20]. The

Carnegie system is generally accepted for the dating and staging of human embryos. Twenty-three stages constitute the embryonic period from fertilization until about 10 weeks 1 day. The onset of marrow formation in the humerus was arbitrarily adopted as the conclusion of the embryonic period and the beginning of the fetal period of prenatal life[27]. In this presentation, the chronological development of the human embryo is described based on embryological literature[17,20,28,29] and on studies made with transvaginal sonography (TVS), using 6.5 MHz[10,25] and 7.5 MHz transducers[11–13,24].

GESTATIONAL AGE 4 WEEKS 0–6 DAYS

The major embryological event is the gastrulation of the embryonic disc, transforming the embryo into the trilaminar disc (ectoderm, mesoderm and endoderm). At the same stage, neurulation begins. This is a process which converts the neural plate via the neural folds into the hollow neural tube. The primitive heart tube appears at the end of week 4. At the middle of the week, the gestational sac with a diameter of about 2–3 mm becomes visible by *ultrasound*.

GESTATIONAL AGE 5 WEEKS 0–6 DAYS

With the closure of the caudal neuropore, the ventricular system of the CNS is created in week 5. The embryonic disc folds cephalocaudally and laterally, forming the three-dimensional body. The initially wide connection between the yolk sac and the embryo becomes the narrow vitteline duct (omphalomesenteric duct), keeping a continuous connection to the developing gut tube. At the end of the week the body stalk is established. The heart tube starts to beat at 5 weeks 1 day, showing peristaltic flow at stage 11 (5 weeks 3 days).

The yolk sac becomes *sonographically* visible at the beginning of the week. The embryonic pole can be identified at the second half of the week, the heart beats are identifiable at the end of week 5; the frequency is about 100 bpm.

GESTATIONAL AGE 6 WEEKS 0–6 DAYS, CROWN–RUMP LENGTH (CRL) 4–7 MM

At 6 weeks, the limb buds develop. The cerebral hemispheres develop as small evaginations from the telencephalon at about 6 weeks 4 days.

Sonographically the heart beats are always identifiable. The frequency increases from 105 to 130 bpm. At the end of the week the amniotic membrane may be seen. In the cranial pole of the embryo the rhombencephalic cavity appears as a tiny shallow hypoechogenic area. Sometimes the narrow mesencephalic cavity may be detected anteriorly[26].

GESTATIONAL AGE 7 WEEKS 0–6 DAYS, CRL 8–14 MM

At about 7½ weeks, the primary intestinal loop can be seen projecting further into the umbilical cord as the normal umbilical hernia. The metanephros (future kidney) is now reniform.

Sonographically the embryonic body appears like a triangle in the sagittal section. The sides consist of (1) the back, (2) the roof of the rhombencephalon, and (3) the frontal part of the head, the basis of the umbilical cord, and the embryonic tail. The limbs look like short hypoechogenic buds. All hypoechogenic brain cavities can be identified, including the separation of the cerebral hemispheres (Fig. 49.1). The rhombencephalic cavity on top of the embryonic body is the largest cavity. The future spine appears as two parallel lines. The heart is large and bright, the frequency increasing from 130 to 160 bpm. Details of the heart anatomy are not depictable, but the atrial and the ventricular compartments may be distinguished by the reciprocal movements of the walls[12]. The short umbilical cord shows a large coelomic cavity at its insertion, where the primary intestinal loop may be identified. The mean diameter of the amniotic cavity has a value which is approximately identical with the corresponding CRL. Blood flow can be seen in the grey-scale modus in the vitelline duct leading from the umbilical cord to the yolk sac.

GESTATIONAL AGE 8 WEEKS 0–6 DAYS, CRL 15–22 MM

The coalescence of the maxillary, medial and lateral nasal ridge-like swellings is completed. In the heart, the membranous part of the interventricular septum takes form. The septum secundum and the foramen ovale are starting to appear. The embryonic haematopoiesis shifts from the yolk sac to the liver. The cloacal membrane ruptures from urinary pressure in embryos of 16–17 mm CRL[30]; the anal membrane becomes defined. In most embryos the choroid plexuses are present in the rhombencephalon. Half of the diencephalon is covered by the hemispheres. The mesencephalon is on the top of the brain.

With transvaginal *ultrasound* the brain cavities are easily seen as large 'holes' in the embryonic head. The hemispheres enlarge, developing a crescent shape. The third ventricle is still rather wide, as is the mesencephalic cavity. Now, the mesencephalon lies on top of the head. The increased growth of the rostral brain structures and the deepening of the pontine flexure lead to the deflection of the brain. Slight movements of the body and some days later of the limbs are detectable. The arms and fingers are distinguishable at the end of the week. A kind of four-chamber view of the heart can be obtained, where the atrial compartment is wider than the ventricular part (Fig. 49.2)[12]. In some embryos the stomach becomes visible.

GESTATIONAL AGE 9 WEEKS 0–6 DAYS, CRL 23–31 MM

The chondrocranium and the skeletogenous layer of the head become recognizable. The falx cerebri starts to develop from

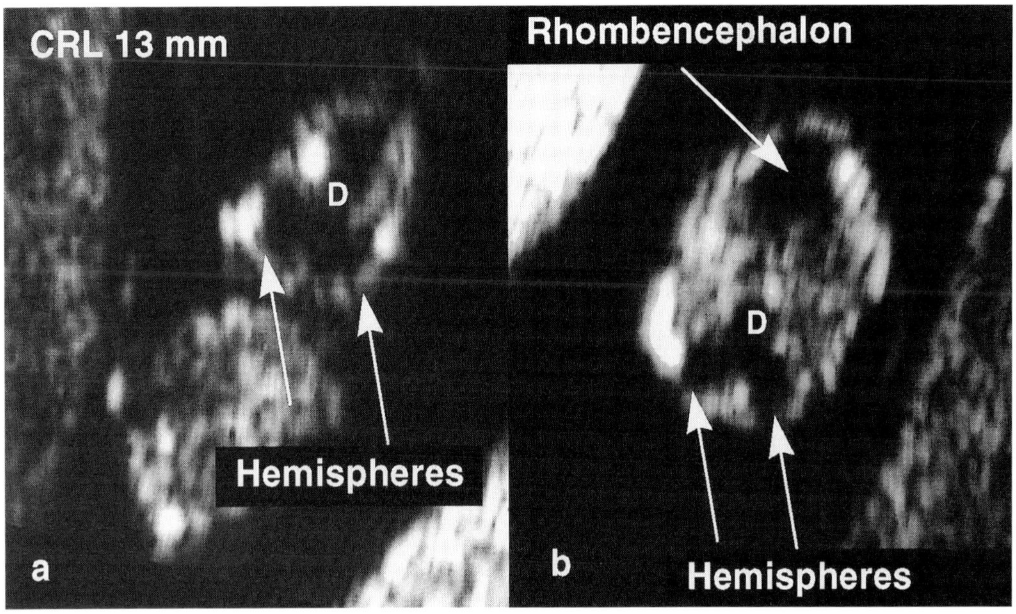

Fig. 49.1 Ultrasound images of a 7 week, 4-day-old embryo (CRL 13 mm). (a) The frontal section through the forebrain showing the hemispheres. The continuous connection between the lateral ventricles is called the telencephalon impar. (b) The oblique section through the rhombencephalic cavity and the cavities of the diencephalon (D) and hemispheres.

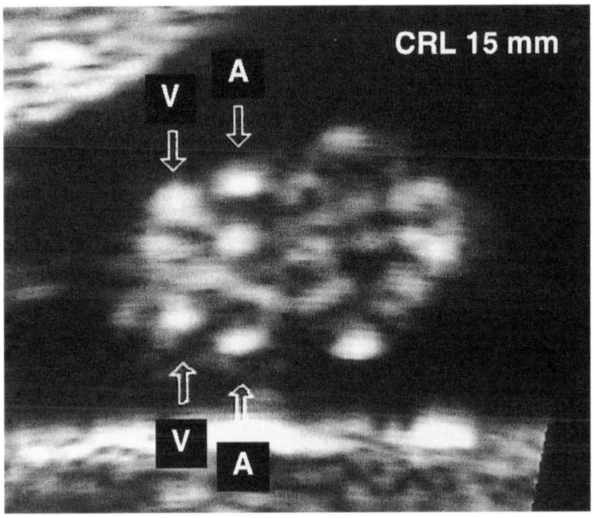

Fig. 49.2 Section through the embryonic thorax (CRL 15 mm); the spine is on the right side. The four chambers are depictable, the atria (A) are wider than the ventricles (V). In the real-time imaging there are reciprocal movements of the atrial walls versus the ventricular walls.

the skeletogenous layer. The thalami are thickening. The rhombic lips have developed into cerebellar hemispheres. The choroid plexuses of the fourth ventricle divide the roof into a pars membranacea superior and inferior. In the spinal column 33–34 cartilaginous vertebrae are present. The processi spinosi have not yet developed. The truncoconal swellings grow down onto the upper ridge of the ventricular septum and onto the inferior endocardial cushion, separating the right and left ventricles. The diaphragm is established dividing the pleuroperitoneal cavity. There is still a narrow pleuroperitoneal duct connecting the pleural and peritoneal cavities[31]. The anal membrane ruptures[30]. The kidneys ascend to level L 1–3. The genital tubercle represents the indifferent phallus in both sexes.

Fingers and toes are detectable with high frequency *ultrasound* transducers. The movements of the arms and legs increase. The embryos often 'clap their feet'. The toes become visible (Fig. 49.3). At the end of the week it is possible to obtain acceptable images of the profile, thus, it is possible to examine the mouth. The cerebellar hemispheres are easily detectable. The choroid plexuses of the fourth ventricle are bright landmarks dividing the ventricle into a rostral and caudal compartment. The border between the mesencephalic and diencephalic cavity becomes distinct by a narrow part of the walls. The width of the diencephalic cavity narrows gradually while the width of the mesencephalon remains wide. The hemispheres grow fast. The bright echogenic choroid plexuses fill the ventricles. The wall of the hemispheres is thin and smooth. The spine is still characterized by two echogenic parallel lines. The ventral body wall is well defined. The genital tubercle is relatively large (Fig. 49.4).

GESTATIONAL AGE 10 WEEKS 0–6 DAYS, CRL 32–41 MM, AND 11 WEEKS 0–6 DAYS, CRL 42–54 MM

EARLY POSTEMBRYONIC PHASE

The distinction between the embryonic period and the fetal period is arbitrarily put at the onset of marrow formation in

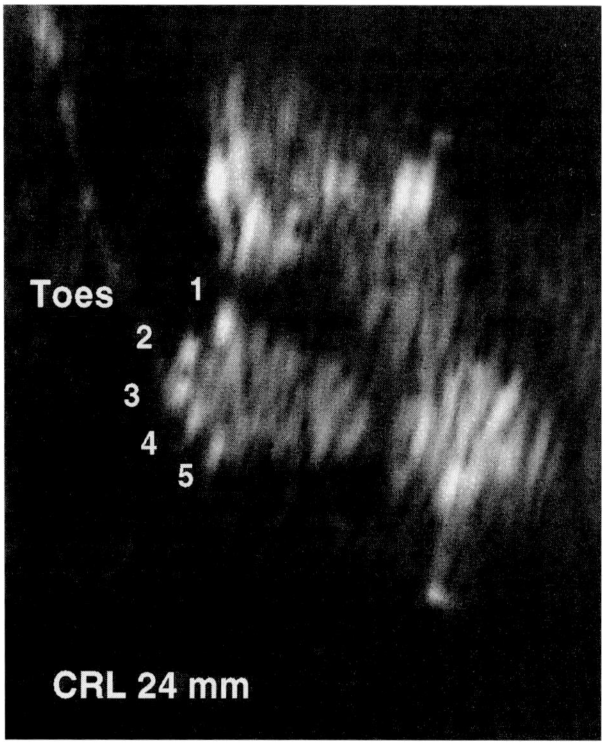

Fig. 49.3 Image of the foot in a 9-week-old embryo (CRL 24 mm). The toes are indicated by the numbers 1–5.

the humerus[27]. Among the most noticeable external changes of the brain are the union of the cerebellar hemispheres with the definition of the vermis and the increasing concealment of the diencephalon and mesencephalon by the cerebral hemispheres. The cerebellum enlarges, pulling the roof of the fourth ventricle beneath its caudal border. The development of the corpus callosum begins at about 12 to 13 weeks. The mesencephalic cavity is still wide. After a rotation of 270° the intestine returns into the abdominal cavity during week 11 (CRL approximately 45 mm)[32,33]. At the end of week 12 the physiological herniation is completed. The metanephros (kidneys) becomes functional. In fetuses longer than 50 mm (embryological measurement) it is safe to make an assessment of the external gender[20]. One must bear in mind that due to the fixation procedures, the length of embryos as measured in embryological studies may be about 1 to 5 mm less than equivalent in-vivo CRL measurements[34].

The human features of the fetus become clearer at the *ultrasound* examination. The head is still relatively large with a prominent forehead and a flat occiput. The limbs elongate further and the typical fetal posture appears. The future skull can be distinguished; ossification starts at about 11 weeks with the occipital bone[35]. The hemispheres occupy two-thirds of the head. The diencephalon lies between the hemispheres, and the mesencephalon gradually moves towards the centre

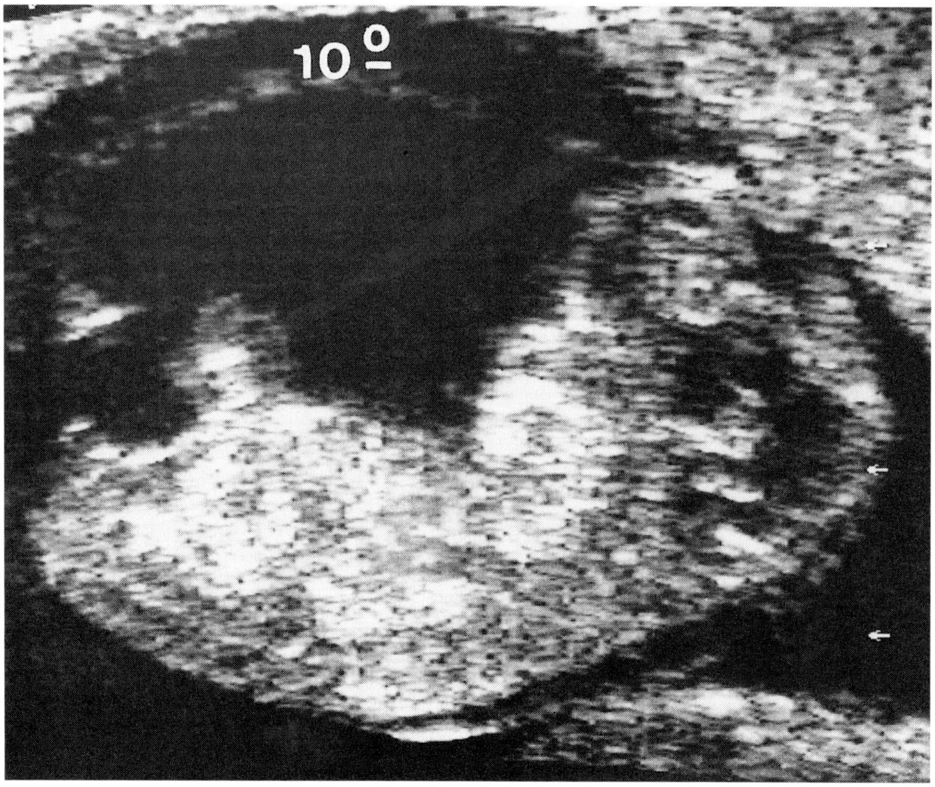

Fig. 49.4 Sagittal section through an embryo at the end of the embryonic period (CRL 32 mm). The ventral body wall is well established. The face is accessible for ultrasound evaluation. The bowel is visible in the coelom of the umbilical cord. The genital tubercle can be seen. It is not possible to identify the gender.

of the head. Due to the cerebellar growth, the choroid plexuses approach the caudal border of the cerebellum. Successively the ossification of the spine appears. The heart rate slows down to 165 bpm at the end of week 11. The ventricles, atria, septa, valves, veins and outflow tracts become identifiable. The midgut herniation has its maximal extent at the beginning of week 10; it returns into the abdominal cavity during weeks 10 to 11. The stomach is visible in most cases at the end of week 11. The kidneys are visible (Fig. 49.5); they are more echogenic than later in pregnancy.

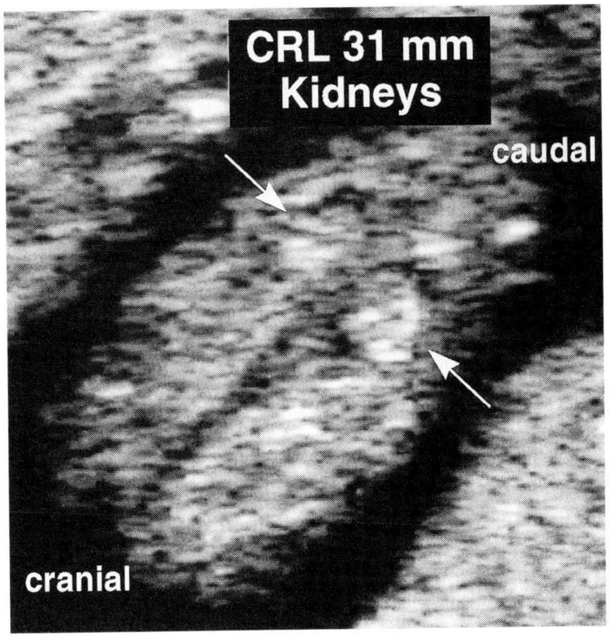

Fig. 49.5 Coronal section through the kidneys (arrows) at the end of the embryonic period (CRL 31 mm).

First-trimester anomalies

The uniform embryonic development as shown in embryological and sonoembryological studies constitutes the important basis for the evaluation of abnormal development. The balanced proportion between the embryo and its extra-embryonic structures is a guiding principle for normality. In imminent abortions, the measurement of extra-embryonic structures combined with the evaluation of the heart beats have often been used for clinical judgement. In early pregnancy, small dysmorphic structures instead of a normal embryo may be seen prior to spontaneous abortion. In some of such cases even heart beats can be detected (Fig. 49.6). Such findings represent a major structural defect of the embryo. There is a wide range between the uncharacteristic condition that later leads to an abortion and the development of a specific anomaly. One of the first fetal anomalies detected

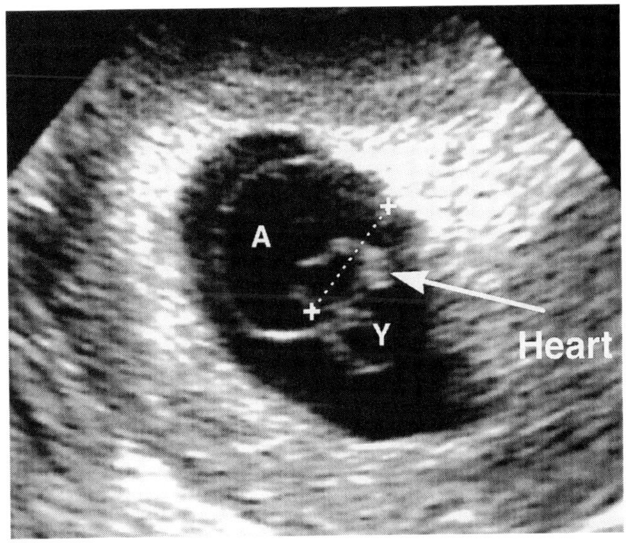

Fig. 49.6 Ultrasound image of an 8-week-old pregnancy, a few days prior to a spontaneous abortion. The amniotic cavity (A) and the yolk sac (Y) can be identified. The embryonic pole (calipers, dotted line) is too small compared to the amniotic cavity. The embryonic pole is dysmorphic with cystic structures; the beating heart was visible (arrow).

by ultrasound was an acrania at 31 weeks of gestation described by Sundén in 1964[2]. Twenty-five years later, in 1989, Rottem and co-workers reported the same diagnosis made by transvaginal ultrasound at 11 weeks of gestation[36], but they already suspected it during week 9. This was an important step towards a new challenge, namely the diagnosis of embryonic and early fetal anomalies.

Transient markers for embryonic and fetal maldevelopment

Compared with transabdominal ultrasound, transvaginal measurements of the *yolk sac* show less variability[37]. A high-frequency transvaginal transducer, combined with modern ultrasound equipment, gives accurate measurements in the range just below 1 mm. Under optimal conditions a 7.5 MHz probe may have an axial resolution of 0.4 mm and a lateral resolution of 0.8 mm. Recent studies with such sensitive measurements have shown the uniform slow growth of the yolk sac diameter until 9 to 10 weeks from mean 4.2 mm at 7 weeks to mean 5.4 mm at 10 weeks[24]. Significant deviation from this growth pattern before 10 weeks of gestation indicates an abnormal outcome[38,39]. In the presence of a living embryo such findings should initiate further evaluation of the anatomy and possibly later karyotyping (Fig. 49.7).

The mean diameter of the amniotic cavity and the mean CRL show a close correlation[24,40]. Embryologists have shown such a close relationship between the amniotic cavity volume and the fetal size[41]. Significant deviation from the normal size in a viable pregnancy before 11 weeks should cause further

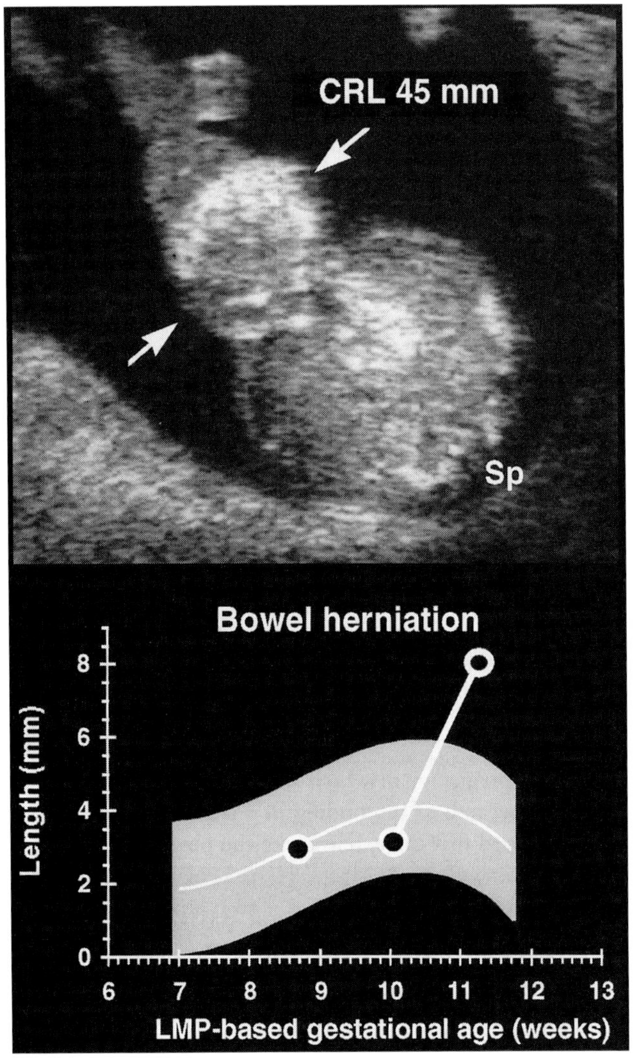

Fig. 49.17 Abnormal development of the bowel herniation in an embryo with a partial trisomy 13 (same case as in Fig. 49.7). The ultrasound image showed the increasing (instead of decreasing) size of the bowel herniation at 11½ weeks (CRL 45 mm). The diagram shows the development of the bowel herniation into a medial omphalocele in relation to the normal size of the physiological midgut herniation.

abnormalities and unidentifiable genitalia should make it possible to suspect this condition by ultrasound in the early postembryonic period[83].

COMPLEX DEFECTS

The complex body-wall defects include serious anomalies which present with gross alterations in the ultrasound image. A vascular disruption during 4–6 weeks of gestation is considered as the aetiology of the *LBWC*[84]. The amniotic membrane is always abnormal, continuing with the body wall to the placenta. In LBWC, persistence of the extraembryonic coelom may lead to the typical amniotic tags and adhesions[84]. Both in LBWC and in *ARS* the anomalous amniotic cavity should be detectable at 8–9 weeks. In LBWC no normal umbilical cord is found. Instead, two cord vessels should be found inside the amniotic membrane and continuing to the placenta. With a high-frequency transducer, further details such as abnormal limbs, kyphoscoliosis and bifid spine may be identifiable if present. In ARS, the seriousness of the abnormalities of the head and body wall depends on the onset of the amniotic rupture[85]. The early detectibility depends on the extension of the wall defect and possible associated anomalies such as reduction of the limbs (Plate 49.1(a)–(d)).

Gastrointestinal anomalies

There is a great variety of congenital gastrointestinal anomalies; most of them are obstructive conditions of the gastrointestinal tractus. Such anomalies are atresia, stenosis, and duplication of the gastrointestinal tract, cysts or tumours, and hepatic, splenic or pancreatic diseases. Alterations secondary to an anomaly such as polyhydramnios usually call the attention of the examiner and lead to the suspicion of the diagnosis. Oligohydramnios and polyhydramnios develop from imbalance of the amniotic fluid production due to disturbances of fetal urine production or resorption such as swallowing. During the first trimester, the volume of the amniotic fluid is related to the weight of the fetus[86]. Neither voiding nor swallowing start before the postembryonic period[87]. Therefore, alteration of the amniotic fluid amount due to possible imbalance of production and resorption by the fetal gastrointestinal and urinary system may not become significant until the second trimester. The fluid that can be found in the embryonic stomach as early as eight weeks probably originates from gastric secretion[12].

Obstruction of the oesophagus, the duodenum and the anus are the most common obstructive conditions of the alimentary tract[88]. *Oesophageal atresia* has been described histologically in embryos at stage 16 and later (8, 9, 18 and 19 mm CRL)[89]. An empty stomach in a second-trimester fetus leads to suspicion of oesophageal obstruction. We observed a grossly dilated stomach (diameter 6 mm) in a 10-week, 5-day-old triplet (pregnancy after in-vitro fertilization) (Fig. 49.18). After 12 weeks of gestation, the stomach was empty, and remained so for the rest of the pregnancy. This fetus proved to have an oesophageal atresia without fistula.

The question of epithelial plugging and/or vacuolation in the embryological development of the duodenum has been discussed. Some authors believe that non-recanalization of the completely plugged lumen at stage 19 is responsible for the duodenal atresia[88], while other authors doubt this hypothesis[90]. The diagnosis of oesophageal atresia associated with *duodenal stenosis* was described in a fetus of 12 to 13 weeks of gestation[91]. This fetus had no fistula from the upper oesophagus/trachea to the lower oesophagus. The lower oesophagus, the stomach and the duodenum were overdistended. Since swallowing can be excluded as a contribution to the gastric fluid in both cases, gastric secretion must be its origin.

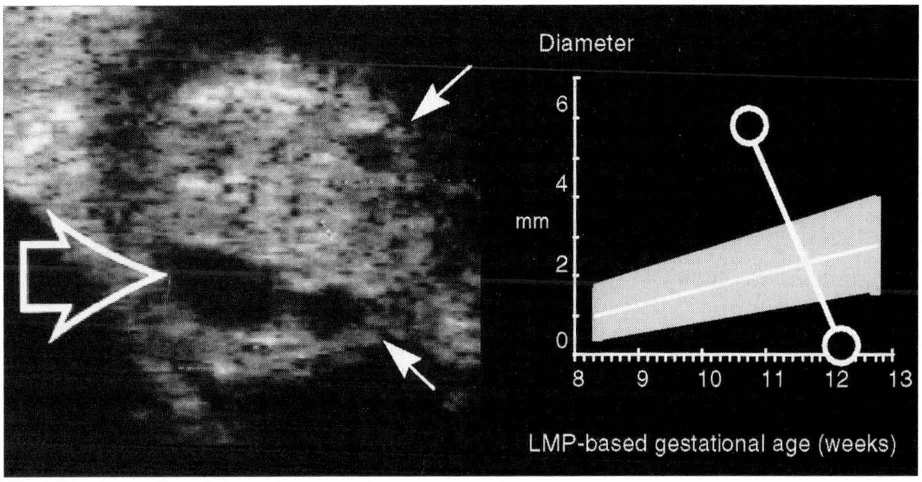

Fig. 49.18 Abnormal development of the stomach and bowel in a 10-week, 5-day-old fetus which proved to have oesophageal atresia. The ultrasound image showed the dilated stomach (open arrow) and dilated bowel loops (small arrows). The diagram shows the development of the stomach diameter in relation to the normal size: at 10 weeks, the stomach was dilated; at 12 weeks and later during the pregnancy, the stomach was empty.

So far, first-trimester diagnosis of gastrointestinal malformations are represented by a few case reports only. Intra-abdominal cysts or tumours, which usually are recognized in the second and third trimester, seem not to have a significant size for early recognition and, only exceptionally, intestinal obstructions seem to lead to dilation of the bowel.

Genitourinary anomalies

As with the gastrointestinal tract the development of the genitourinary tract is not complete before the postembryonic period. The outer genitalia differentiate so late that a safe ultrasound evaluation of the gender should not be made before 14 weeks, though an earlier definition is possible[20]. The gonads and the uterus have not yet been described by ultrasound during the first trimester. Anomalies of the amniotic fluid amount cannot be expected before the early second trimester. The kidneys can be imaged at 10 weeks (Fig. 49.5), the urinary bladder at 11 weeks. In a study of 537 singleton fetuses, the kidneys and the urinary bladder could be visualized in 92% at 13 weeks of gestation[92].

In *posterior valves syndrome* and in *urethral atresia* the dilation of the urinary bladder may become obvious at the early postembryonic period from 11 to 12 weeks. In a study group of 24 492 pregnancies between 10 and 14 weeks, 15 cases with megacystis were detected (1/1633)[93]. Three had chromosomal aberrations. In the chromosomally normal group, there were seven cases with spontaneous resolution. In four cases, a severe obstructive uropathy developed. The diameter of the bladder varied from 8 mm in a fetus of 44 mm CRL to 32 mm in a fetus of 69 mm CRL. In 300 control fetuses, the bladder was visualized in 92.7%; none of the normal bladders had a diameter of more than 6 mm.

Usually, early diagnoses of the urinary system are made at the end of the first trimester and at the beginning of the second trimester[94,95]. A *multicystic kidney* was described at 12 weeks 4 days[96]. In *renal agenesis* the relatively large hypoechogenic and discoid adrenal glands should not be mistaken for the kidneys, which are bright in the first trimester. Fluid may be found in the urinary bladder. This diagnosis was suspected as early as 12 weeks 5 days[94]. Failure in visualizing the fetal bladder at the end of the first trimester can be due to bladder exstrophy, or to cystic dysplastic conditions of the kidneys. An early variant of the *infantile polycystic kidney disease* (Potter I) has been diagnosed at 14 weeks[95]. Normal ultrasound appearance of the kidneys at the end of the first trimester in a high risk pregnancy does not exclude the diagnosis polycystic kidney disease, since the clinical course can vary considerably. *Tubular dysgenesis* is a disease where the clinical development during pregnancy ressembles that of Potter I[97].

Musculoskeletal anomalies

A large number of different disorders can cause local or general abnormal shape and size of the skeleton. The spectrum ranges from absence of a finger to the grotesque torsion of the fetal skeleton due to amniotic adhesions. There may be reduced growth of one limb due to vascular compromise, or general dwarfism caused by serious congenital dysplasia of the bone.

POLY- AND OLIGODACTYLY, LIMB DEFECTS

The early diagnosis of a musculoskeletal anomaly depends on the natural history and the scope of the disease. In gross anomalies such as ARS or LBWC the *reduction defects* of an extremity and the *kyphoscoliosis* may be easily detected at 9 weeks (Plate 49.1(d)) or even at the end of week 8. A signpost for the diagnosis is the abnormal shape of the amniotic cavity, which during 8 and 9 weeks usually looks like a well-demarcated balloon with the embryo in the inside. Small anomalies such as *polydactyly* can be made as demonstrated in an embryo of only 22 mm CRL with Meckel–Gruber syndrome (Fig. 49.10). Circumspection must be practised with the diagnosis of polydactyly, since reflections of the ultrasound beam from both sides of fingers and toes may give the false impression of hexadactyly. The difficulty of establishing the diagnosis of finger/hand abnormalities was illustrated in a case with split hand anomaly[98]. At the first ultrasound at 13 weeks, the hands did not open or close, and the fingers could not be seen separately. At 18 weeks, the split hand anomaly could be demonstrated by ultrasound. One might assume the hypothesis that it is easier to make this kind of diagnosis at 9–10 weeks when the fingers physiologically are not bent.

Arthrogryposis is a heterogeneous disease with diverse origins. Congenital arthrogryposis such as lethal multiple pterygium syndrome is characterized by the early onset of a general affection of the joints. Oedema or nuchal translucency may be an early sign of the disease[48,99]. Autosomal recessive and X-linked inheritance are described[100,101]. Two cases, which were diagnosed at 13 weeks, had nuchal translucency of 6.3 and 10.5 mm in addition to talipes and joint contractures[48]. We may assume that such serious alterations should be recognizable at least 1–2 weeks earlier in the early postembryonic period. Plate 49.4(a), (b) shows a case of lethal pterygium syndrome detected at 12 weeks, with extensive oedema, joint contractures and micrognathia. The postabortem photograph is from a fetus with the same condition from a previous pregnancy at the early second trimester.

Skeletal dysplasias are a heterogeneous group of rare bone maldevelopment resulting in abnormal growth and shape of the fetal skeleton. Recently, the normal embryonic and early fetal development of the skeleton has been described by ultrasound in a small study[35]. The diagnosis of a rare skeletal dysplasia that could lead to the termination of a pregnancy must be based on reliable and unambiguous images. The sizes of the measured objects in the embryos and young fetuses in this study were near the limits of resolution of the equipment. Thus, improvements of the image quality will be necessary before accurate measurements can be done[102]. In serious dysplasias such as *achondrogenesis* bone shortening may be obvious as early as 11 weeks[47]. The key for the diagnosis was not the measurement of the long bones, but the disproportion between body and limbs, the lack of limb movements, the lack of ossification in the limbs and vertebrae, and oedema. As described in lethal arthrogryposis nuchal translucency and oedema may be an early sign of such serious conditions. In other lethal conditions, as shown in *variant of thanatophoric dwarfism*[103], the appearance of the long bones was described as normal during the first trimester, before shortening was shown in the third trimester.

Embryofetoscopy

One of the most recent techniques for prenatal diagnosis and therapy is needle embryofetoscopy[104,105]. Today, there are flexible endoscopes of 0.5 mm and 0.7 mm in diameter which can fit through 20-gauge and 18-gauge needles. New solid optic endoscopes of diminutive diameter can provide images of remarkable clarity at a surprisingly wide field of view[106]. Early diagnoses of Meckel–Gruber syndrome at 10[107] and 11 weeks[108], neural tube defect at 11 weeks[108], Smith–Lemli–Opitz syndrome at 11 weeks[109], van der Woude syndrome at 11 weeks[110], encephalocele and club hand at 11 weeks, and a large median facial cleft at 12 weeks[111] were described. This list, which is not complete, shows the potential of this new technique. As this report has shown, however, most of the diagnoses made using embryofetoscopy have been made at even earlier stages using ultrasonographic examinations. Ultrasound is not invasive. The risk associated with endoscopy can never be zero and invasion of the intrauterine cavity at amniocentesis is not a harmless intervention[106]. Therefore, the indication for diagnostic embryofetoscopy should be carefully weighed against the potential risk involved, and against the possibility of transvaginal ultrasound diagnosis with high-frequency transducers. We believe that ultrasound techniques will improve to such an extent that there hardly will be any indication for invasive diagnostic imaging such as embryofetoscopy.

How to report an early anomaly?

The overview on the embryonic and early fetal development illustrates the high velocity of growth and of developmental changes. Many of the referred papers state the gestational age in weeks only. In order to get the correct aspect of the natural history of a malformation, the clinical data concerning the case have to be precise, e.g., the expression 'at the ninth week' may involve a period from 8 weeks 0 days to 9 weeks 6 days. During this long period, the embryo grows from 15 mm to 32 mm, and shows tremendous changes in the external appearance and in the developing organ systems. Further, there is obviously a difference in diagnosing an anomaly at the beginning of week 10 (CRL 32 mm), week 11 (CRL 42 mm) or week 12 (CRL 55 mm).

The correct description of a first-trimester anomaly should include the gestational age, if possible, in completed weeks and days based on the last menstrual period or the CRL. It is important to report measurements such as the precise CRL, and possibly biometric data including the BPD, the abdominal diameter or the femur length. The reader can only get the appropriate impression of the time aspect and of the dimension of the presented case if this information is included.

Future aspects

There is no reason to believe that the technological development of ultrasound has reached its endpoint. We will see ultrasound devices with even higher frequencies and improved resolution presented in the near future. Computer technology will be increasingly used to handle the pre- and postprocessing of the ultrasound imaging. Three-dimensional ultrasound has made its entry into the first trimester[112,113], giving us the possibility of analysing the recorded ultrasound volume offline in any plane including new sections through the embryo for a more precise diagnosis and the measurement of diameters and volumes of any structure of interest (Plate 49.5).

The overview of the normal embryological development gives an idea of the manifold dramatic processes which take place during the first trimester. The comparison with the sonoembryological development week by week shows the potential of ultrasound as a diagnostic tool. We do not know all about the natural history of the development of malformations. The classical embryologists were dependent on the accidental assignments of aborted malformed embryos and fetuses to study abnormal human development. Now, we can follow the development of the malformations longitudinally. Such examples are the description of an encephalocele originating from the roof of the mesencephalon in a case with cerebro-oculo-muscular syndrome (Fig. 49.11), or the description of club foot development in a case with early hydrocephaly[114]. This means that we are now able to study the human embryo longitudinally, and to describe step by step the development and possibly maldevelopment of organs. In the field of human embryology this implies a major development.

REFERENCES

1. MacVicar J, Donald I. Sonar in the diagnosis of early pregnancy and its complications. *J Obstet Gynæcol Br Cwlth* **70**:387, 1963.
2. Sundén B. On the diagnostic value of ultrasound in obstetrics and gynecology (Thesis). *Acta Obstet Gynecol Scand* **43**(suppl):121, 1964.
3. Robinson HP. Sonar measurement of fetal crown-rump length as means of assessing maturity in first trimester of pregnancy. *Br Med J* **4**:28–31, 1973.
4. Robinson HP. 'Gestation sac' volumes as determined by sonar in the first trimester of pregnancy. *Br J Obstet Gynaecol* **82**:100–107, 1975.
5. Robinson HP, Shaw-Dunn J. Fetal heart rates as determined by sonar in early pregnancy. *J Obstet Gynecol Br Cwlth* **80**:805–809, 1973.
6. Green JJ, Hobbins JC. Abdominal ultrasound examination of the first-trimester fetus. *Am J Obstet Gynecol* **159**:165–175, 1988.
7. Schmidt W, Yarkoni S, Crelin ES, Hobbins JC. Sonographic visualization of the physiologic anterior wall hernia in the first trimester. *Obstet Gynecol* **69**:911–915, 1987.
8. Curtis JA, Watson L. Sonographic diagnosis of omphalocele in the first trimester of fetal gestation. *J Ultrasound Med* **7**:97–100, 1988.
9. Timor-Tritsch IE, Warren WB, Peisner DB, Pirrone E. First trimester midgut herniation: a high frequency transvaginal sonographic study. *Am J Obstet Gynecol* **161**:466–476, 1989.
10. Timor-Tritsch IE, Peisner DB, Raju S. Sonoembryology: an organ-oriented approach using a high-frequency vaginal probe. *J Clin Ultrasound* **18**:286–298, 1990.
11. Blaas H-G, Eik-Nes SH, Kiserud T, Hellevik LR. Early development of the forebrain and midbrain: a longitudinal ultrasound study from 7 to 12 weeks of gestation. *Ultrasound Obstet Gynecol*, **4**:183–192, 1994.
12. Blaas H-G, Eik-Nes SH, Kiserud T, Hellevik LR. Early development of the abdominal wall, stomach and heart from 7 to 12 weeks of gestation: a longitudinal ultrasound study. *Ultrasound Obstet Gynecol*, **6**:240–249, 1995.
13. Blaas H-G, Eik-Nes SH, Kiserud T, Hellevik LR. Early development of the hindbrain: a longitudinal ultrasound study from 7 to 12 weeks of gestation. *Ultrasound Obstet Gynecol*, **5**:151–160, 1995.
14. Takeuchi H. Sonoembryology in the central nervous system. In *The fetus as a Patient. Advances in Diagnosis and Therapy* (ed. A Kurjak & FA Chervenak), pp. 141–150. New York–London: Parthenon Publishing, 1994.
15. Timor-Tritsch IE, Monteagudo A, Warren WB. Transvaginal ultrasonographic definition of the central nervous system in the first and early second trimesters. *Am J Obstet Gynecol* **164**:497–503, 1991.
16. Warren WB, Timor-Tritsch IE, Peisner DB, Raju S, Rosen MG. Dating the pregnancy by sequential appearance of embryonic structures. *Am J Obstet Gynecol* **161**:747–753, 1989.
17. O'Rahilly R, Müller F, Editors. *The Embryonic Human Brain. An Atlas of Developmental Stages*. New York: Wiley-Liss, 1994.
18. His W. *Anatomie menschlicher Embryonen*, vols 1–3. Leipzig: Vogel, 1880–1885.
19. Mall FP. On stages in the development of human embryos from 2 to 25 mm. long. *Anat Anz* **46**:78–84, 1914.
20. O'Rahilly R, Müller F. *Developmental Stages in Human Embryos*. Washington: Carnegie Institution Publications, 637, 1987.
21. Streeter GL. Developmental horizons in human embryos. *Contrib Embryol Carneg Inst* **30**:211–245, 1942.
22. Streeter GL. Development horizons in human embryos. *Contrib Embryol Carneg Inst* **199**:27–63, 1945.
23. Streeter GL. Developmental horizons in human embryos. *Contrib Embryol Carneg Inst* **211**:133–203, 1948.
24. Blaas H-G, Eik-Nes SH, Bremnes JB. Embryonic growth. A longitudinal biometric ultrasound study. *Ultrasound Obstet Gynecol*, **12**:346–354, 1998.
25. Timor-Tritsch IE, Farine D, Rosen MG. A close look at the embryonic development with the high frequency transvaginal transducer. *Am J Obstet Gynecol* **159**:678–681, 1988.
26. Blaas H-G, Eik-Nes SH. Ultrasound assessment of early brain development. In *Ultrasound and Early Pregnancy* (eds D Jurkovic & E Jauniaux), pp. 3–18. New York–London: The Parthenon Publishing Group, 1996.
27. Streeter G. Developmental horizons in human embryos (fourth issue). A review of the histogenesis of cartilage and bone. *Contrib Embryol Carneg Inst* **33**:133–203, 1949.
28. Hinrichsen KV. *Humanembryologie*. Berlin–Heidelberg–New York: Springer-Verlag, 1990.
29. Larsen WJ. *Human Embryology*. New York–Edinburgh–London–Melbourne–Tokyo: Churchill Livingstone, 1993.
30. Ludwig KS. Über die Beziehungen der Kloakenmembran zum Septum urorectale bei menschlichen Embryonen von 9 bis 33 mm SSL. *Z Anat Entwickl Gesch* **124**:401–413, 1965.
31. Kostovic I. Zentralnervensystem. In *Humanembryologie* (ed. KV Hinrichsen), pp. 381–448. Berlin–Heidelberg: Springer-Verlag, 1990.
32. Kiesselbach A. Der physiologische Nabelbruch. *Adv Anat Embryol Cell Biol* **34**:83–143, 1952.
33. Lauge-Hansen N. *Developmental Anatomy of the Human Gastro-intestinal Tract*. Aarhus: Munksgaard Aarhus Stiftsbogtrykkerie A/S. 1973.
34. Drumm JE, O'Rahilly R. The assessment of prenatal age from the crown-rump length determined ultrasonically. *Am J Anat* **148**:555–560, 1977.
35. Zalen-Sprock RMv, Brons JTJ, Vugt JMGv, Harten HJvd, Geijn HPv. Ultrasonographic and radiologic visualization of the developing embryonic skeleton. *Ultrasound Obstet Gynecol* **9**:392–397, 1997.
36. Rottem S, Bronshtein M, Thaler I, Brandes JM. First trimester transvaginal sonographic diagnosis of fetal anomalies. *Lancet* **I**:444–445, 1989.

37. Jauniaux E, Moscoso JG. Morphology and significance of the human yolk sac. In *The First Twelve Weeks of Gestation* (eds ER Barnea, J Hustin & E Jauniaux), p. 549. Berlin–Heidelberg–New York: Springer-Verlag, 1992.
38. Lindsay DJ, Lovett IS, Lyons EA et al. Yolk sac diameter and shape at endovaginal US: predictors of pregnancy outcome in the first trimester. *Radiology* **183**:115–118, 1992.
39. Stampone C, Nicotra M, Muttinelli C, Cosmi EV. Transvaginal sonography of the yolk sac in normal and abnormal pregnancy. *J Clin Ultrasound* **24**:3–9, 1996.
40. Grisiola G, Milano V, Pilu G et al. Biometry of early pregnancy with transvaginal sonography. *Ultrasound Obstet Gynecol* **3**:403–411, 1993.
41. Abramovich DR. The volume of amniotic fluid in early pregnancy. *J Obstet Gynaecol Br Cwlth*, **75**:728–731, 1968.
42. Thieme GA. Development malformations of the fetal ventral body wall. *Ultrasound Quarterly* **10**:225–265, 1992.
43. Nicolaides KH, Azar G, Byrne D, Mansur C, Marks K. Fetal nuchal translucency: ultrasound screening for chromosomal defect in first trimester of pregnancy. *Br Med J* **304**:869–869, 1992.
44. Hyett JA, Moscoso G, Nicolaides KH. First-trimester nuchal translucency and cardiac septal defects in fetuses with trisomy 21. *Am J Obstet Gynecol* **172**:1411–1413, 1995.
45. Nicolaides KH, Shawwa L, Brizot M, Snijders R. Ultrasonographically detectable markers of fetal chromosomal defects. *Ultrasound Obstet Gynecol* **3**:56–69, 1993.
46. Snijders RJM, Johnson S, Sebire NJ, Noble PL, Nicolaides KH. First-trimester ultrasound screening for chromosomal defects. *Ultrasound Obstet Gynecol* **7**:216–226, 1996.
47. Fisk N, Vaughan J, Smidt M, Wigglesworth J. Transvaginal ultrasound recognition of nuchal edema in the first-trimester diagnosis of achondrogenesis. *J Clin Ultrasound* **19**:586–590, 1991.
48. Hyett JA, Noble P, Sebire NJ, Snijders R, Nicolaides KH. Lethal congenital arthrogryposis presents with increased nuchal translucency at 10–14 weeks of gestation. *Ultrasound Obstet Gynecol* **9**:310–313, 1997.
49. Hyett JA, Clayton PT, Moscoso G, Nicolaides KH. Increased first trimester nuchal translucency as a prenatal manifestation of Smith–Lemli–Opitz syndrome. *Am J Genet* **58**:374–376, 1995.
50. Hyett JA, Perdu M, Sharland GK, Snijders RS, Nicolaides KH. Increased nuchal translucency at 10–14 weeks of gestation as a marker for major cardiac defects. *Ultrasound Obstet Gynecol* **10**:242–246, 1997.
51. Gillerot Y, Jauniaux E, Maldergem Lv, Fourneau C. Pathogenesis of human malformations. In *The First Twelve Weeks of Gestation* (eds ER Barnea, J Hustin & E Jauniaux) Berlin–Heidelberg–New York: Springer-Verlag, 1992.
52. Wood LR, Smith MT. Generation of anencephaly: 1. Aberrant neurulation and 2. conversion of exencephaly to anencephaly. *J Neuropathol Exp Neurol* **43**:620–633, 1984.
53. Nishi T, Nakano R. First-trimester diagnosis of exencephaly by transvaginal ultrasonography. *J Ultrasound Med* **13**:149–151, 1994.
54. Coerdt W, Ramsing M, Rehder H. Embryopathologische Untersuchungen an induzierten und spontanen Aborten im 1. Schwangerschaftstrimenon. *Pathologie* **15**:32–39, 1994.
55. Zalen-Sprock RMv, Vugt JMGv, Harten HJvd, Geijn HPv. Cephalocele and cystic hygroma: diagnosis and differentiation in the first trimester of pregnancy with transvaginal sonography. Report of two cases. *Ultrasound Obstet Gynecol* **2**:289–292, 1992.
56. Weinstein BJ, Benacerraf BR. Meckel syndrome, first trimester diagnosis. *Fetus* **4**(5):7598/4, 1994.
57. Zalen-Sprock RMv, Vugt JMGv, Geijn HPv. First-trimester sonographic detection of neurodevelopmental abnormalities in some single-gene disorders. *Prenat Diagn* **16**:199–202, 1996.
58. Achiron R, Achiron A, Lipitz S, Mashiach S, Goldman B. Holoprosencephaly: alobar. *Fetus* **4**:7422/9–12, 1994.
59. Nelson LH, King M. Early diagnosis of holoprosencephaly. *J Ultrasound Med* **11**:57, 1992.
60. Gardner E, O'Rahilly R, Prolo D. The Dandy–Walker and Arnold–Chiari malformations. *Arch Neurol* **32**:393–407, 1975.
61. Achiron R, Achiron A, Yagel S. First trimester transvaginal sonographic diagnosis of Dandy–Walker malformation. *J Clin Ultrasound* **21**:62–64, 1993.
62. Bronshtein M, Blumenfeld Z. Transvaginal sonography – detection of findings suggestive of fetal chromosomal anomalies in the first and early second trimester. *Prenat Diagn* **12**:587–593, 1992.
63. O'Rahilly R, Müller F. Ventricular system and choroid plexuses of the human brain during the embryonic period proper. *Am J Anat* **189**:285–302, 1990.
64. Blaas H-G, Eik-Nes SH, Kiserud T, Hagen CBvd, Smedvig E. Lissencephaly, type 1. *Fetus* **2**:7422/1–4, 1992.
65. Rustico MA, Benttoni A, D'Ottavio G et al. Fetal heart screening in low-risk pregnancies. *Ultrasound Obstet Gynecol* **6**:313–319, 1995.
66. Tegnander E, Eik-Nes SH, Linker DT. Prenatal detection of heart defects at the routine fetal examination at 18 weeks in a non-selected population. *Ultrasound Obstet Gynecol* **5**:372–380, 1995.
67. Dolkart LA, Reimers FT. Transvaginal fetal echocardiography in early pregnancy: Normative data. *Am J Obstet Gynecol* **165**:688–691, 1991.
68. Johnson P, Sharland G, Maxwell D, Allan L. The role of transvaginal sonography in the early detection of congenital heart disease. *Ultrasound Obstet Gynecol* **2**:248–251, 1992.
69. Achiron R, Rotstein Z, Lipitz S, Mashiach S, Hegesh J. First-trimester diagnosis of fetal congenital heart disease by transvaginal ultrasonography. *Obstet Gynecol* **84**:69–72, 1994.
70. Gembruch U, Knöpfle G, Bald R, Hansmann M. Early diagnosis of fetal congenital heart disease by transvaginal echocardiography. *Ultrasound Obstet Gynecol* **3**:310–317, 1993.
71. Cyr DR, Mack LA, Schoenecker SA, Pattern RM, Shephard TH, Shuman WP, Moss AA. Bowel migration in the normal fetus: Ultrasound detection. *Radiology* **161**:119–121, 1986.
72. Duhamel B. Embryology of exomphalos and allied malformations. *Arch Dis Child* **38**:142–147, 1963.
73. Zimmer E, Bronshtein M. Early diagnosis of fetal midline dysruption syndromes. *Prenat diagn* **16**:65–69, 1996.
74. Cantrell JR, Haller A, Ravitch MM. A syndrome of congenital defects involving the abdominal wall, sternum, diaphragm, pericardium, and heart. *Surg Gynecol Obstet* **107**:602–614, 1958.
75. Weissman A, Achiron R. Ultrasound diagnosis of congenital anomalies in early pregnancy. In *Ultrasound and Early Pregnancy* (eds D Jurkovic & E Jauniaux, trans. A Kurjak), pp. 95–119. New York–London: The Parthenon Publishing Group. 1996.
76. Brown DL, Emerson DS, Shulman LP, Carson SA. Sonographic diagnosis of omphalocele during 10th week of gestation. *Am J Roentgenol* **153**:825–826, 1989.
77. Nicolaides KH, Snijders RJM, Cheng HH, Gosden C. Fetal gastro-intestinal and abdominal wall defects: associated malformations and chromosomal abnormalities. *Fetal Diagn Ther* **7**:102–115, 1992.
78. Nyberg DA, Fitzsimmons J, Mack LA et al. Chromosomal abnormalities in fetuses with omphalocele. Significance of omphalocele contents. *J Ultrasound Med* **8**:299–308, 1989.
79. deVries PA. The pathogenesis of gastroschisis and omphalocele. *J Pediatr Surg* **15**:245–251, 1980.
80. Hoyme HE, Higginbottom MC, Jones KL. The vascular pathogenesis of gastroschisis: intrauterine interruption of the omphalomesenteric artery. *Pediatrics* **98**:228–231, 1981.
81. Bonilla-Musoles FM, Raga F, Ballester MJ, Serra V. Early detection of embryonic malformations by transvaginal and color Doppler sonography. *J Ultrasound Med* **13**:347–355, 1994.
82. Paidas MJ, Crombleholme TM, Robertson F. Prenatal diagnosis and management of the fetus with an abdominal wall defect. *Semin Perinatol* **18**:196–214, 1994.
83. Meizner I, Levy A, Barnard Y. Cloacal exstrophy sequence: An exceptional ultrasound diagnosis. *Obstet Gynecol* **86**:446–450, 1995.
84. Allen MIV, Curry C, Gallagher L. Limb body wall complex: I. Pathogenesis. *Am J Med Genet* **28**:529–548, 1987.
85. Higginbottom MC, Jones KL, Hall BD, Smith DW. The amniotic band disruption complex: Timing of amniotic rupture and variable spectra of consequent defects. *Pediatrics* **95**:544–549, 1979.
86. Lind T, Hytten FE. Relation of amniotic fluid volume to fetal weight in the first half of pregnancy. *Lancet* **1**:1147, 1970.
87. O'Rahilly R, Müller F. *Human Embryology and Teratology*. New York: Wiley-Liss, 1994.
88. Boyden EA, Cope JG, Bill AH. Anatomy and embryology of congenital intrinsic obstruction of the duodenum. *Am J Surg* **114**:190–202, 1967.
89. Smith EI. The early development of the trachea and esophagus in relation to atresia of the esphagus and tracheoesophageal fistula. *Contrib Embryol Carneg Inst* **36**:41–57, 1957.

90. Moutsouris C. The 'solid stage' and congenital intestinal atresia. *J Pediatr Surg* **1**:446–450, 1966.
91. Tsukerman GL, Krapiva GA, Kirillova IA. First-trimester diagnosis of duodenal stenosis associated with oesophageal atresia. *Prenat Diagn* **13**:371–376, 1993.
92. Rosati P, Guariglia L. Transvaginal sonographic assessment of the fetal urinary tract in early pregnancy. *Ultrasound Obstet Gynecol* **7**:95–100, 1996.
93. Sebire NJ, Kaisenberg CV, Rubio C, Snijders RJM, Nicolaides KH. Fetal megacystis at 10–14 weeks of gestation. *Ultrasound Obstet Gynecol* **8**:387–390, 1996.
94. Bronshtein M, Amit A, Achiron R, Noy I, Blumenfeld Z. The early prenatal sonographic diagnosis of renal agenesis: techniques and possible pitfalls. *Prenat Diagn* **14**:291–297, 1994.
95. Bronshtein M, Yoffe N, Brandes JM, Blumenfeld Z. First and early second trimester diagnosis of fetal urinary tract anomalies using transvaginal sonography. *Prenat Diagn* **10**:653–666, 1990.
96. Rottem S, Bronshtein M. Transvaginal sonographic diagnosis of congenital anomalies between 9 weeks and 16 weeks, menstrual age. *J Clin Ultrasound* **18**:307–314, 1990.
97. Allanson JE, Hunter AGW, Mettler GS, Jiminez C. Renal tubular dysgenesis: a not uncommon autosomal recessive syndrome: a review. *Am J Med Genet* **43**:811–814, 1992.
98. Haratz-Rubinstein N, Yeh M-N, Timor-Tritsch IE, Monteagudo A. Prenatal diagnosis of the split hand anomaly: how early is early? *Ultrasound Obstet Gynecol* **8**:57–61, 1996.
99. Kirkinen P, Herva R, Leisti J. Early prenatal diagnosis of a lethal syndrome of multiple congenital contractures. *Prenat Diagn* **7**:189–196, 1987.
100. Martin NJ, Hill JB, Cooper DH, O'Brien GD, Masel JP. Lethal multiple pterygium syndrome: Three consecutive cases in one family. *Am J Med Genet* **24**:295–304, 1986.
101. Tolmie JL, Patrick A, Yates JRW. A lethal multiple pterygium syndrome with apparent X-linked recessive inheritance. *Am J Med Genet* **27**:913–919, 1987.
102. Ashhurst DE. Assessing skeletal development. *Ultrasound Obstet Gynecol* **9**:373, 1997.
103. Macken MB, Grantmyre EB, Rimoin DL, Lachman RS. Normal sonographic appearance of a thanatophoric dwarf variant fetus at 13 weeks gestation. *Am J Roentgenol* **156**:149–150, 1991.
104. Reece EA, Goldstein I, Chatwani A, Brown R, Homko C, Wiznitzer A. Transabdominal needle embryofetoscopy: a new technique paving the way for early therapy. *Obstet Gynecol* **84**:634–636, 1994.
105. Reece EA, Rotmensch S, Whetham J, Cullen M, Hobbins JC. Embryoscopy: A closer look at first-trimester diagnosis and treatment. *Am J Obstet Gynecol* **166**:775–780, 1992.
106. Hobbins JC. The future of first-trimester embryoscopy. *Ultrasound Obstet Gynecol* **8**:3–4, 1996.
107. Dumez Y, Dommergues M, Gubler M-C, Bunduki V, Narcy F, Lemerrer M, Mandelbrot L, Berkowitz R. Meckel–Gruber Syndrome: Prenatal diagnosis at 10 menstrual weeks using embryoscopy. *Prenat Diagn* **14**:141–144, 1994.
108. Quintero RA, Abuhamad A, Hobbins JC, Mahoney MJ. Transabdominal thin-gauge embryofetoscopy: a technique for early prenatal diagnosis and its use in the diagnosis of a case of Meckel–Gruber syndrome. *Am J Obstet Gynecol* **168**:1551–1557, 1993.
109. Hobbins JC, Jones OW, Gottesfeld S, Persutte W. Transvaginal ultrasonography and transabdominal embryoscopy in the first trimester diagnosis of Smith–Lemli–Opitz syndrome type II. *Am J Obstet Gynecol* **171**:546–549, 1994.
110. Dommergues M, Lemerrer M, Couly G, Delezoide AL, Dumez Y. Prenatal diagnosis of cleft lip at 11 menstrual weeks using embryoscopy in the van der Woude syndrome. *Prenat Diagn* **15**:378–381, 1995.
111. Ville Y, Bernard JP, Doumerc S et al. Transabdominal fetoscopy in fetal anomalies diagnosed by ultrasound in the first trimester of pregnancy. *Ultrasound Obstet Gynecol* **8**:11–15, 1996.
112. Blaas H-G, Eik-Nes SH, Kiserud TW, Berg S, Angelsen B, Olstad B. Three-dimensional imaging of the brain cavities in human embryos. *Ultrasound Obstet Gynecol*, **5**:228–232, 1995.
113. Bonilla-Musoles FM, Raga F, Osborne N, Blanes J. The use of three-dimensional (3D) ultrasound for the study of normal and pathologic morphology of the human embryo and fetus: preliminary report. *J Ultrasound Med* **14**:757–765, 1995.
114. Bronshtein M, Liberson A, Lieberson S, Blumenfeld Z. Clubfeet associated with hydrocephalus: Evidence of gradual dynamic development in utero. *Obstet Gynecol* **79**:864–867, 1992.

Craniospinal and central nervous system defects

50

L.M. Hill

Introduction

Fetal central nervous system abnormalities are quite common. The improved resolution of both transabdominal and transvaginal sonography has allowed detailed imaging of normal central nervous system anatomy, and enhanced our understanding of development and pathology. The effect of specific central nervous system malformations upon fetal behavioural patterns has also become an area of intensive research. Prenatal and postnatal neurosonology, as well as computerized tomography (CT) and magnetic resonance imaging (MRI), all have a role to play in the evaluation of the fetal central nervous system and selected appropriate CT, and MRI images should provide the reader with a better visual understanding of specific nervous system malformations.

Supratentorial

DEVELOPMENTAL

AGENESIS OF THE CORPUS CALLOSUM

The corpus collosum makes up 11% of the supratentorial brain[1]. In the general population the incidence of agenesis of the corpus callosum (ACC) is estimated at 0.3% to 0.7%[2]. Since other non-callosal commissures may compensate for the absent interhemispheric pathways, 85% of individuals with isolated ACC are asymptomatic; other patients may have subtle neurological deficits[3,4]. The more severely affected patients with ACC have seizures, psychosis or varying degrees of mental retardation. However, patients in this latter group generally have associated central nervous system anomalies, rather than isolated ACC[5].

Although most cases of ACC are sporadic, there are some instances indicating autosomal recessive[6] or X-linked inheritance[7]. ACC is also associated with a 1 in 10 risk of chromosomal anomalies, specifically trisomies 13, 18 and 21 and mosaic trisomy[4,8–10]. Since fetuses with a karyotypic abnormality may have ACC as their only sonographic finding, karyotyping should be considered whenever ACC is detected. Fifty percent of cases with a lipoma of the corpus callosum will also have partial or complete callosal agenesis[11].

The corpus callosum functions as a conducting system between the two hemispheres of the brain. Development of the corpus callosum begins anteriorly at 8 weeks' menstrual age and proceeds caudally; formation is complete by 18–20 weeks' menstrual age. Hence, partial agenesis of the corpus callosum usually involves its posterior portion. When this occurs the frontal horns are normal and the cavum septum pellucidum is present, but there is occipital and temporal horn dilatation[7,12]. If there is partial absence of an anterior portion of the corpus callosum, it is due to a destructive process[13]. Complete absence of the corpus callosum results in an increased separation of the hemispheres with a prominent interhemispheric fissure (Fig. 50.1). When the anterior portion of the corpus callosum is absent, the third ventricle is elevated into the interhemispheric fissure (Fig. 50.2). With complete ACC the frontal horns of the lateral ventricle are widely separated and narrowed due to the overdevelopment of the lateral callosal bundles and medial cortex (Figs 50.1 and 50.2). The occipital horns of the lateral ventricles are generally mildly dilated. The severity of ventriculomegaly increases slightly with gestation[10]. Three percent of all fetuses with ventriculomegaly[14] and 10% of those fetuses with mild ventriculomegaly[15] have ACC.

Approximately 80% of cases with ACC have associated central nervous system anomalies that include hydrocephalus, porencephaly, microcephaly, encephalocele, holoprosencephaly, lissencephaly, Dandy–Walker malformation and spina bifida[9].

Non-nervous system malformations associated with ACC include micrognathia, hypertelorism, cleft lip or palate, malformed digits, horseshoe kidney, dysplastic kidney,

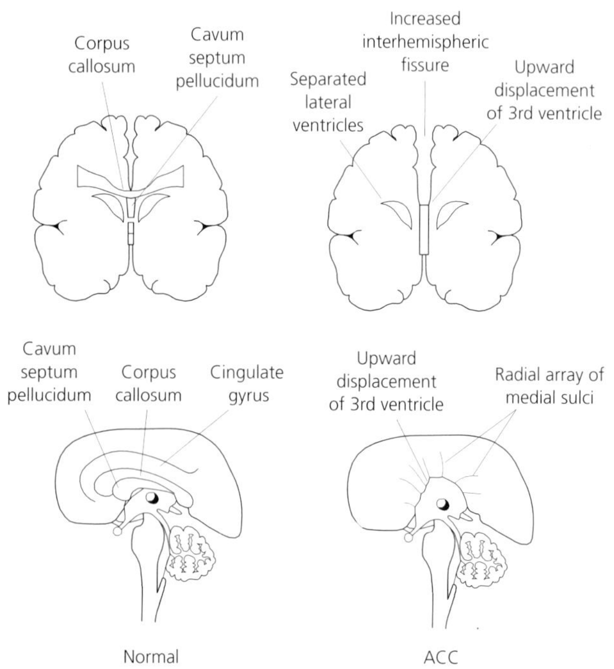

Fig. 50.1 Schematic representation of the findings associated with agenesis of the corpus callosum (ACC) that can be demonstrated with coronal and sagittal views of the brain. Coronal scans (upper drawings) are primarily useful for the direct demonstration of the absence of the corpus callosum–cavus septum pellucidum complex, but may also allow the visualization of a widening of the interhemisphereic fissure, of increased separation between the lateral ventricles and of upward displacement of the third ventricle. Sagittal views allow demonstration of the absence of the corpus callosum–cavum septum pellucidum complex and furthermore to appreciate a superiorly elongated third ventricle with a radial array of the medial gyri in the position normally occupied by the cingulate gyrus. (Pilu, G. et al. (1993) *Ultrasound Obstet. Gynecol.* **3**, 318. Used by permission.)

diaphragmatic hernia and congenital heart disease[16]. The frequency of associated malformations with ACC is outlined in Table 50.1.

A number of syndromes have agenesis of the corpus callosum as an associated finding (Table 50.2). The Aicardi syndrome is the most common syndrome with ACC and no other sonographically detectable findings. All of the reported

TABLE 50.1
Frequency of associated non-nervous system malformations with agenesis of the corpus callosum

Malformation	Percentage
Facial	34
Musculoskeletal	32
Cardiovascular	15
Genitourinary	11
Gastrointestinal	25
Respiratory	11

Modified from Parrish, M.L. et al. (1979) *Ann. Neural.* **6**, 349

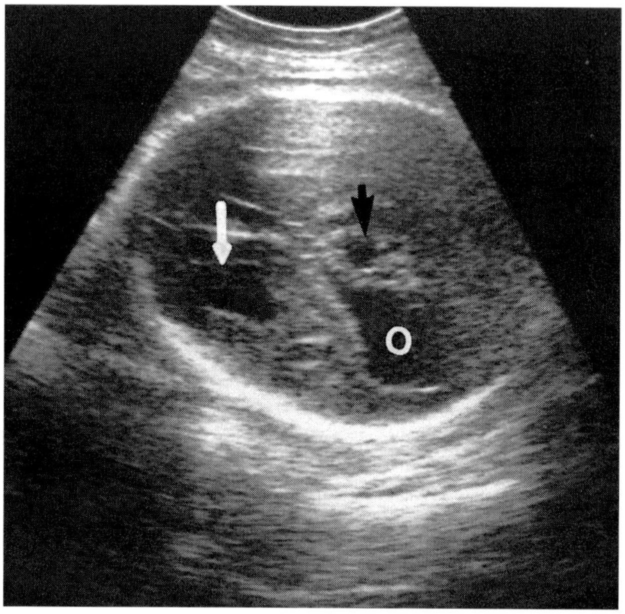

Fig. 50.2 In ACC, the medial wall of the anterior horn is displaced laterally (white arrow); the occipital horn of the lateral ventricle (O) is dilated (colpocephaly); and the third ventricle (dark arrow) is elevated and dilated.

cases have been in females. Since the Aicardi syndrome appears to result in early embryonic demise in males, the sonographic detection of a male fetus suggests that an isolated finding of ACC may not be associated with significant long-term morbidity[17]. Familial non-syndromic cases of ACC have been reported; the recurrence risk in this subset of patients is increased[18].

Sonographic findings

On a coronal scan the corpus callosum is visualized as a hypoechoic structure superior to the lateral ventricles. Since the corpus callosum forms the roof of the cavum septum pellucidum and the lateral ventricles, it is best imaged in a sagittal plane. Colour Doppler can be utilized to identify the pericallosal artery arcing over the corpus callosum (Fig. 50.3). Sonographic clues on a transaxial view include displacement and narrowing of the frontal horns of the lateral ventricles with simultaneous enlargement of the occipital horns. The third ventricle is also visualized at the level of the lateral ventricles, indicating its upward displacement. While the third ventricle is enlarged in all cases of ACC, it is not necessarily displaced[19]. Since the primary connecting fibres between the hemispheres are absent, there is an increased separation between the hemispheres and a prominent interhemispheric fissure (Fig. 50.4). On a sagittal view there is a radial array of the medial gyri in the position of the absent cingulate gyrus.

Sonographic findings associated with a good prognosis include an absence of upward displacement of the third ventricle and a normal interhemispheric fissure diameter. The

TABLE 50.2
Syndromes associated with agenesis of the corpus callosum

Syndrome	Inheritance pattern	Characteristics
Aicardi	X-linked dominant	Hemivertebrae Mental retardation Chorioretinitis Intractable seizures Lethal in males Infertility
Shaprio	Autosomal recessive	Spontaneous hypothermia
Ardermann	Autosomal recessive	Mental retardation Hypotonia
Walker–Warburg	Autosomal recessive	Hydrocephalus Cataracts Lissencephaly Encephalocele
Orofaciodigital	X-linked dominant	Cleft palate Asymmetric shortening of the digits Clinodactyly/syndactyly Lethal in males
Apert	Autosomal dominant	Craniosynostosis Syndactyly Frontal encephalocele
Fryn	Autosomal recessive	Holoprosencephaly Diaphragmatic hernia
Frontonasal dysplasia	Unknown	Cleft lip/palate Hypertelorism
Rubinstein–Taybi	Unknown	Microcephaly Congenital heart defects Mental retardation Scoliosis
Acrocallosal	Unknown	Polydactyly Duplication of big toes Hypertelorism Prominent forehead Mental retardation Cleft lip/palate

presence of a normal atrial diameter and cavum septum pellucidum along with normally positioned frontal horns excludes a diagnosis of complete ACC.

ARTERIOVENOUS MALFORMATIONS (AVM)

Intracerebral arteriovenous malformations usually involve the vein of Galen[20]. Knudsen and Alden[21] reported that 63% of symptomatic arteriovenous malformations in children less than 6 months of age involve the vein of Galen; cerebral (7.4%), superior sagittal sinus (6.2%) and carotid-jugular (2.6%) arteriovenous malformations were the next most common sites[21]. The number of sonographically detectable antenatal cases is too few to determine if the distribution of cerebral arteriovenous malformations is significantly different for the fetus. Since these are direct arteriovenous connections, blood flow through the brain is markedly increased.

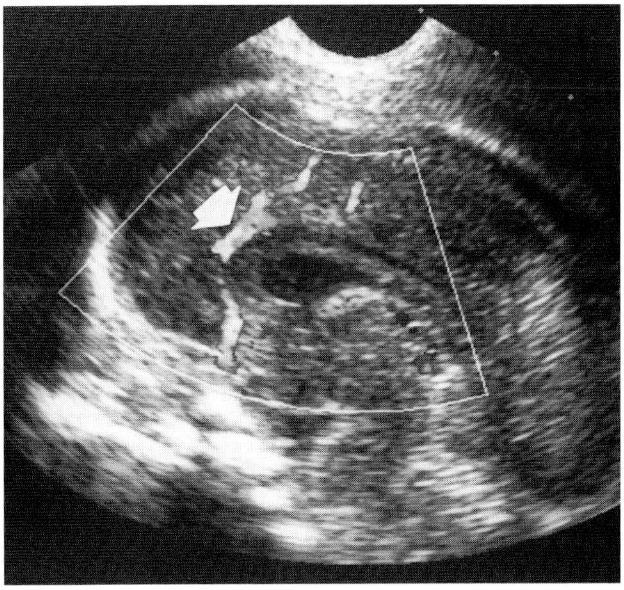

Fig. 50.3 Sagittal view of the corpus callosum at 27 weeks' gestation with colour Doppler (arrow); the pericallosal artery is visualized sweeping over the hypoechoic corpus callosum.

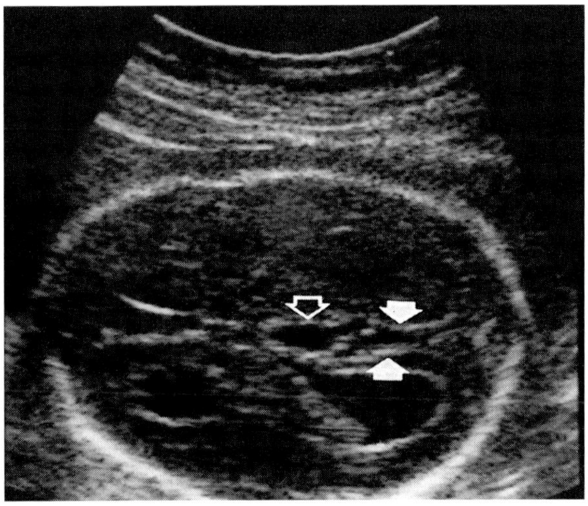

Fig. 50.4 With agenesis of the corpus callosum the hemispheres are separated with a prominent interhemispheric fissure (white arrows). A superiorly positioned third ventricle is demonstrated (hollow arrow).

Anatomically, the two internal cerebral veins enter into the vein of Galen, which then courses posteriorly into the straight sinus. Arteries that have been found to directly anastomose with the vein of Galen include the superior cerebellar artery, the anterior and middle cerebral arteries and the anterior and posterior choroidal arteries[22]. Because of the marked changes in blood flow that occur at the time of delivery, neonates frequently become symptomatic from an aneurysm of the vein of Galen. Loss of low resistance flow to the placenta results in an increase in vascular shunting to the arteriovenous malformation and subsequent cardiac decompensation. Infant mortality is characteristically secondary to central nervous system haemorrhage or congestive heart failure[23]. Operative management includes ligation or embolization of the feeder vessels or complete excision[24,25]. The reported mortality in symptomatic neonates is 90%[26]. While 25% of survivors are normal, the remaining infants have seizures, visual field defects, and intellectual impairment. In contrast to neonates, 74% of older children who are treated surgically for a symptomatic arteriovenous malformation are cured[27].

Sonographic findings

On prenatal sonography a vein of Galen aneurysm is a cystic non-pulsatile midline cerebral structure. If the straight sinus is also dilated, the characteristic circular vein of Galen aneurysm will have a linear or keyhole appearance[28]. Colour Doppler studies can be used to confirm the presence of flow within the apparent cyst (Plate 50.1)[25,29], as well as to detect feeding vessels around the periphery of the aneurysm. Serial ultrasound examinations indicate that a vein of Galen aneurysm usually does not develop until the third trimester[22]. Only three cases have been detected in the second trimester[30–32] with the earliest reported diagnosis at 23 weeks' gestation[30].

Hydrocephalus may result from compression of the ventricular system by an aneurysm of the vein of Galen. Subarachnoid haemorrhages and cerebral infarcts may also occur[29]. Heart failure is a common finding both in the third-trimester fetus and in the neonate[24,25,33]. Distension of the fetal neck veins is a pathognomonic finding (Fig. 50.5), indicating right heart failure[33]. Other sonographic signs associated with a poor prognosis include:(1) five or more feeding vessels; (2) retrograde aortic flow; (3) cardiomegaly[33A].

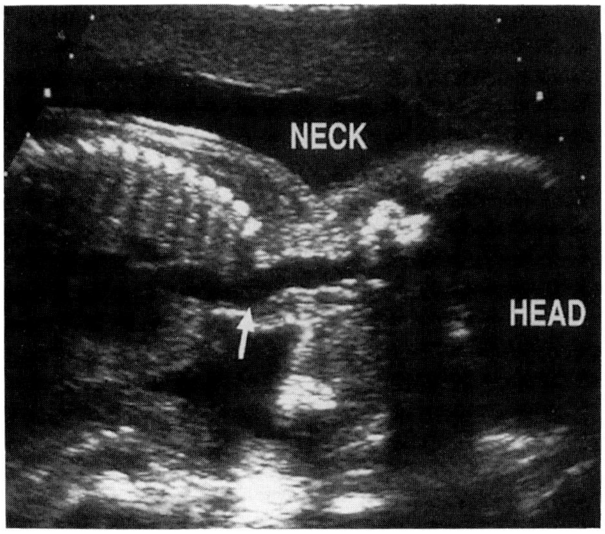

Fig. 50.5 Sagittal view of the fetus shows marked dilation of the neck vessels (arrow) which probably reflects increased right heart output. (Lee, W. et al. (1994) *J. Ultrasound Med.* **13**:645. Used with permission.)

Associated malformations with an aneurysm of the vein of Galen includes coarctation of the aorta and transposition of the great vessels[22].

ARACHNOID CYSTS

Arachnoid cysts represent approximately 1% of all intracranial masses[34]. They develop from congenitally malformed arachnoid tissue and may be either unilocular or multilocular. Haemorrhage into an arachnoid cyst may result from trauma. Cerebrospinal fluid becomes entrapped within the arachnoid loculations, resulting in secondary compression of adjoining structures[35]. Only rarely is the degree of compression by an arachnoid cyst sufficient to cause necrosis of surrounding cortical tissue.

Sonographic findings

When present above the tentorium, an arachnoid cyst may be confused with a porencephalic cyst. However, an arachnoid cyst displaces an intact cerebral cortex; with porencephaly there is an actual cortical defect that has passively filled with cerebrospinal fluid.

Intratentorial arachnoid cysts must be distinguished from a Dandy–Walker malformation. However, compression of the vermis by a large arachnoid cyst is difficult to distinguish from its congenital absence with a Dandy–Walker malformation[36]. A midline intrahemispheric arachnoid cyst may mimic agenesis corpus callosum (Fig. 50.6(a) and (b))[37]. If an arachnoid cyst obstructs the foramen of Monro or displaces the aqueduct, ventriculomegaly may result.

The primary treatment for an arachnoid cyst is shunting either into an adjoining ventricle or into the peritoneal cavity[38].

VENTRICULOMEGALY

Ventriculomegaly refers to an enlargement of the lateral ventricles, but does not imply a specific aetiology. Brain atrophy, brain destruction, or a failure of brain development can all result in ventriculomegaly. Hydrocephalus results from an excessive accumulation of cerebrospinal fluid within the brain due to either overproduction or more commonly an obstruction to normal outflow and absorption. Other causes of ventriculomegaly include: choroid plexus papilloma; intracranial haemorrhage; and congenital infection with cytomegalovirus or toxoplasmosis[39].

With hydrocephalus the level of obstruction will determine the sonographic signs associated with ventriculomegaly. Since cerebrospinal fluid flows through foramen of Monro to the third ventricle, obstruction at this level will result in ventriculomegaly with a normal third ventricle. Blockage of

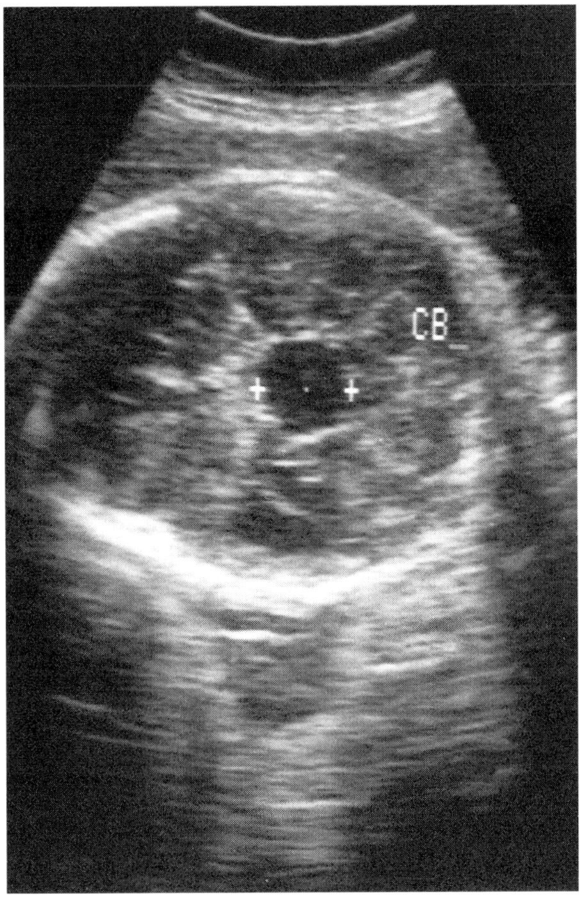

(a)

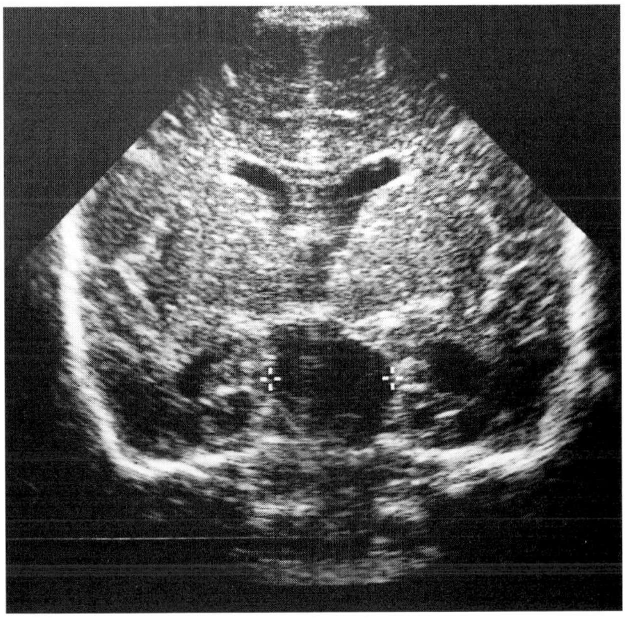

(b)

Fig. 50.6 (a) 1.9 cm arachnoid cyst (markers) is present in the midline between the third and fourth ventricle (CB = cerebellum). (b) Coronal neonatal image of the same arachnoid cyst between the markers.

either the left or right foramen of Monro results in unilateral hydrocephalus[40]. There are fewer associated central nervous system or extracentral nervous system anomalies with unilateral, in contrast to bilateral, hydrocephalus. The prognosis is also better with unilateral hydrocephalus[41]. The next passageway for cerebrospinal fluid is through the aqueduct of Sylvius to the fourth ventricle. If obstruction occurs at this level both lateral ventricles and the third ventricle are dilated (Fig. 50.7).

Uncomplicated hydrocephalus has a prevalence of 1/1000 births in the United States[42]. However, it is more typically part of a syndrome or associated with other congenital malformations (Table 50.3)[43–45]. Since approximately 30% of fetuses with hydrocephalus have an associated neural tube defect[44] a careful evaluation of the spine should always be performed after ventriculomegaly is diagnosed. Ventriculomegaly is also a marker for other underlying central nervous system abnormalities. Filly and co-workers[46] reported that 88% of fetuses with neural axis anomalies had lateral ventricular dilatation. Overall, 80% of fetuses with ventriculomegaly will have

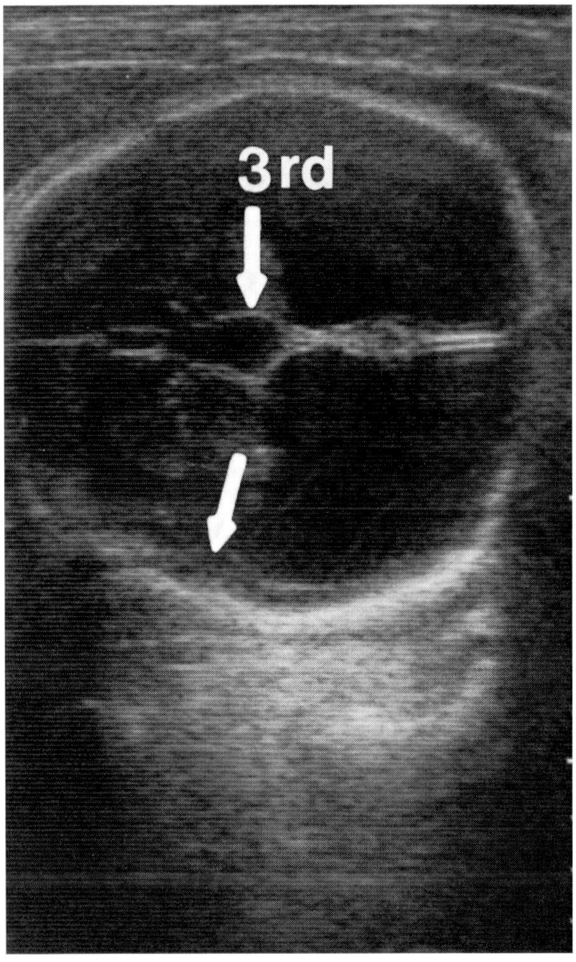

Fig. 50.7 Severe ventriculomegaly at 34 weeks' gestation. The dilated third ventricle (3rd) and rim of cortical tissue (arrow) anteriorly indicates hydrocephalus and not hydranencephaly.

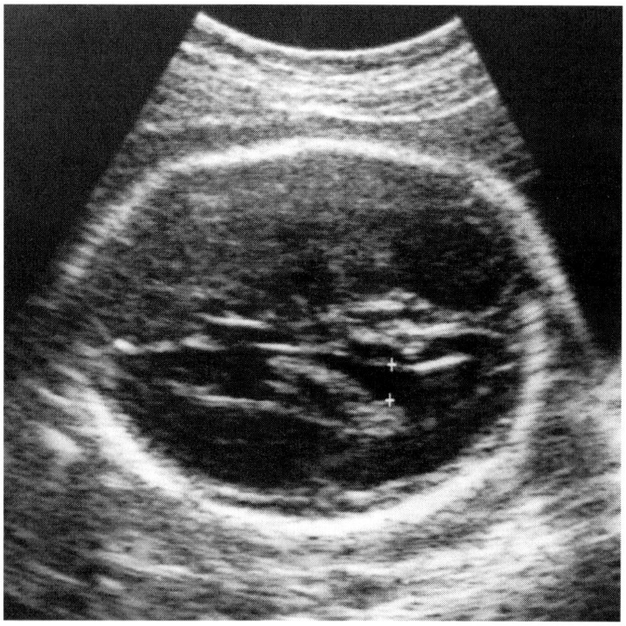

Fig. 50.10 Mild ventriculomegaly. There is a 6 mm gap between the medial border of the lateral ventricle and the choroid plexus (markers). The atrium of the lateral ventricles measures 12 mm.

routine second-trimester ultrasound examinations is 1 in 675[70]. When mild ventriculomegaly resolves on subsequent examinations and there are no other detectable malformations, the outcome is usually good[70A]. However, stable or progressive mild ventriculomegaly along with other congenital malformations is associated with a significant increase in perinatal morbidity and mortality[69]. Approximately 80% of fetuses with isolated mild ventriculomegaly develop normally, while 50% of fetuses with mild ventriculomegaly and other congenital defects are developmentally impaired[69]. Bloom et al.[70A] have reported a 36.4% prevalence of developmental delay at 2 years of age in children with antenatally detected mild ventriculomegaly. Mild ventriculomegaly has also been associated with karyotypic abnormalities, specifically trisomy 21 and trisomy 18[68]. Achiron and colleagues[70] have calculated that the risk of trisomy 21 in a fetus with mild isolated ventriculomegaly is 3.3%. It is of note that the maternal age of the eight cases reported by Achiron and co-workers[70] were between 23–32 years. In view of these findings mild ventriculomegaly should be considered an indication for genetic amniocentesis regardless of maternal age. Unfortunately, mild ventriculomegaly does not characteristically resolve until after 24 weeks' gestation.

HOLOPROSENCEPHALY

The forebrain (prosencephalon), midbrain (mesencephalon) and hindbrain (rhombencephalon) vesicles are formed during the fourth week after conception. In the following week the forebrain divides horizontally into the telencephalon (cerebral hemispheres and lateral ventricles) and diencephalon (thalami, neurohypophysis of the pituitary, and the third ventricle). Holoprosencephaly is due to an impairment in midline cleavage of the embryonic forebrain – the prosencephalon fails to divide sagittally into the cerebral hemispheres or horizontally into the telencephalon and diencephalon. Since the olfactory tracts are always absent, the term arhinencephaly was originally given to this brain malformation. In 1963, DeMeyer and Zeman[71] proposed the term holoprosencephaly, indicating that the prosencephalon had remained 'holistic'.

The incidence of all types of holoprosencephaly combined has been estimated at 1/16 000 births[72]. When embryos are studied, the incidence of holoprosencephaly is between 4.1 and 7.3 cases per 1000[73]. Hence, it is one of the more common embryonic malformations. The disparity in the liveborn and embryonic incidence of holoprosencephaly is due to the high attrition rate of fetuses with holoprosencephaly.

Holoprosencephaly is graded by severity as alobar, semilobar or lobar. In alobar holoprosencephaly there is an abnormally small brain with a monoventricle. A brain mantle of variable thickness surrounds the fluid collection. Since the brain consists of a single sphere, the corpus callosum and septum pellucidum are absent. The thalami are fused in the midline. The midbrain and cerebellum are structurally normal. However, compression by the superior dorsal sac and monoventricle may result in midbrain and cerebellar hypoplasia[74]. DeMeyer[75] subdivided alobar holoprosencephaly into 'pancake', 'cup' and 'ball' types, depending upon the amount of cortical tissue that is present (Figs 50.11–50.13).

In semilobar holoprosencephaly rudimentary cerebral lobes and an occipital interhemispheric fissure are present. There is less reduction in brain weight. A dorsal cyst is frequently present with lobar and semilobar holoprosencephaly. A ridge of cerebral tissue demarcates the dorsal cyst from the ventricles (Fig. 50.14). In lobar holoprosencephaly the two hemispheres are separated, except for fusion of the frontal lobes; the thalami are not fused.

There is a characteristic spectrum of facial abnormalities associated with holoprosencephaly (Figs 50.15–50.17, Table 50.4). The severity of facial anomalies generally reflects the severity of brain abnormalities[76]. However, there are exceptions to this rule – 17% of cases with alobar holoprosencephaly have normal facies and some cases of lobar holoprosencephaly are associated with severe facial dysmorphology[77,78].

The association between the facial and cerebral anomalies is due to the induction of the rostral neural ectoderm by the prechordal mesoderm. When the prechordal mesoderm is defective, the midline facial bones, as well as the division of the prosencephalon becomes arrested during development.

The entire spectrum of facial–brain anomalies with holoprosencephaly has been observed with trisomy 13. Indeed, holoprosencephaly to some degree is present in nearly every case of trisomy 13. Other chromosomal abnormalities associated with holoprosencephaly include 18p- and 13q-. Trisomy

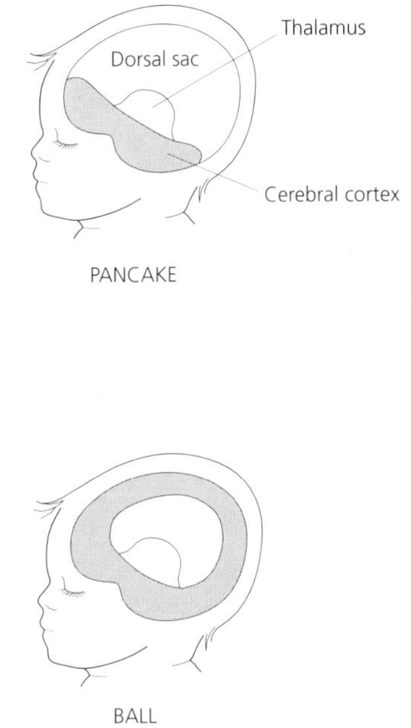

Fig. 50.11 Sagittal view of the 'pancake', 'cup' or 'ball' type of configuration with alobar holoprosencephaly. This concept is based on the amount of cerebral tissue that covers the monoventricular cavity; the residual tissue is similar in appearance to either a pancake, cup or ball. In both the pancake and cup forms, a dorsal sac protrudes from the monoventricular cavity. (From McGahan, J.P. & Porto, M. (1994) *Diagnostic Obstetrical Ultrasound*, p. 148. Phildelphia: J.B. Lippincott. Used by permission.)

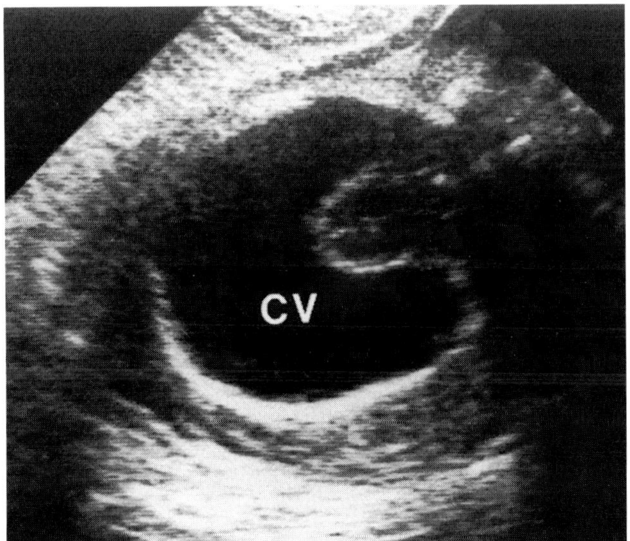

Fig. 50.12 Transverse scan of fetal head showing enlarged common ventricle (CV) with absence of midline echo. (From Chervenak, F.A. et al. (1985) *Obstet. Gynecol.* **66**, 322. Used with permission.)

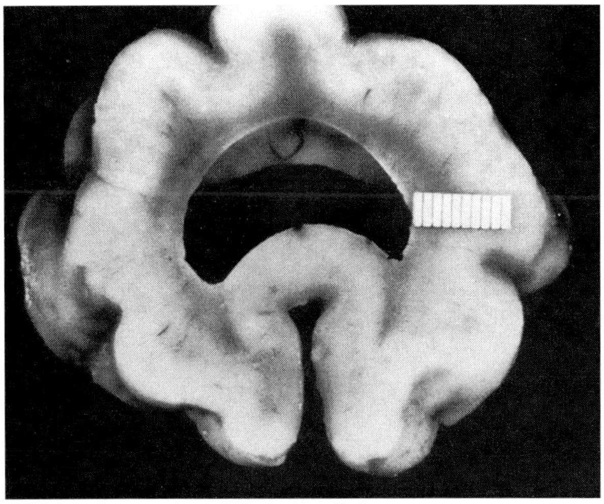

Fig. 50.13 An example of alobar holoprosencephaly with absent interhemispheric fissure and common ventricle. (From Chervenak, F.A. et al. (1985) *Obstet. Gynecol.* **66**, 322. Used with permission.)

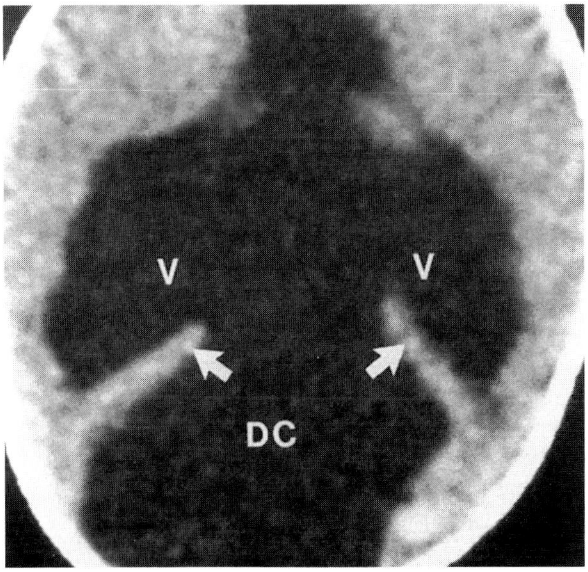

Fig. 50.14 Semilobar holoprosencephaly with a dorsal cyst. Computed tomography scan shows the relationship between the ventricles (V), dorsal cyst (DC) and ridge of cerebral tissue (arrows). (From Nyberg, D.A. et al. *AJNR* (1987) **8**, 871. Used with permission.)

18, trisomy 21 and triploidy are less frequently associated with holoprosencephaly[79]. An autosomal recessive, as well as an autosomal dominant, form of holoprosencephaly has been recognized; occurrence in families has also been reported[80]. About half of the neonates with holoprosencephaly are karyotypically normal and do not represent known monogenic syndromes[81,82]. When holoprosencephaly is the only malformation detected, a chromosomal anomaly is less likely[75]. The empirical recurrence risk for holoprosencephaly

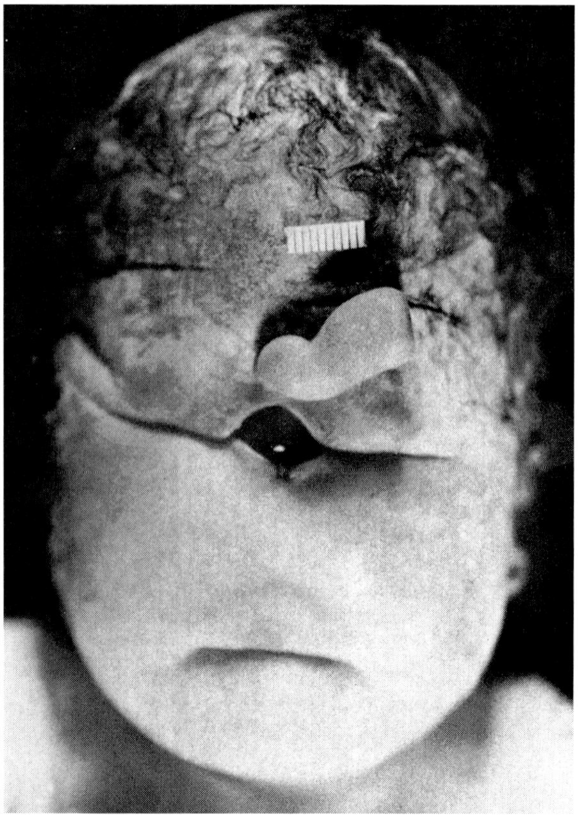

(a)

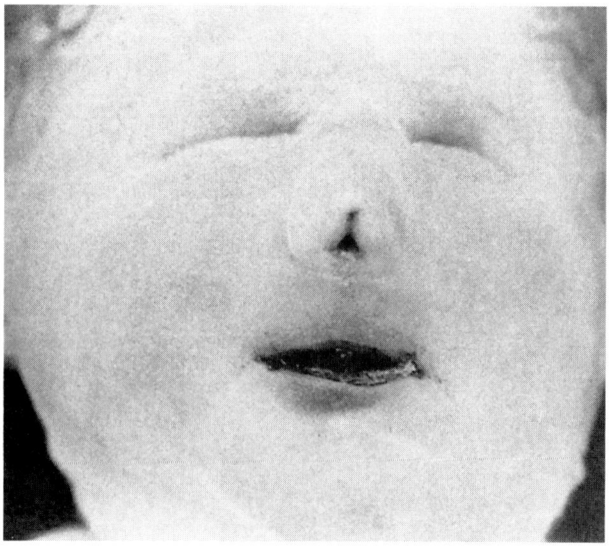

(b)

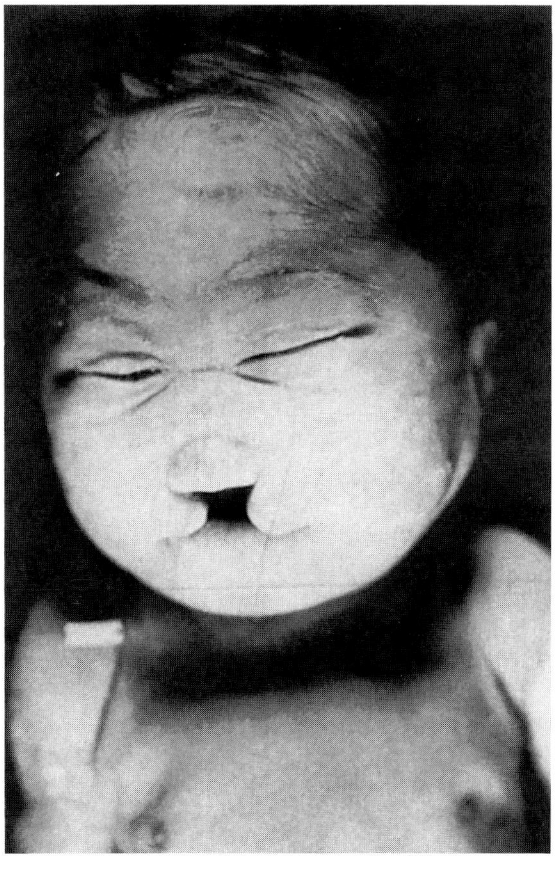

(c)

Fig. 50.15 Facial characteristics associated with holoprosencephaly. (a) Cyclopia with single fused orbit and proboscis above it. (b) Cebocephaly with hypotelorism and normally placed nose with a single nostril. (c) Median cleft lip and palate with hypotelorism. (From Chervenak, F.A. et al. (1984) *Obstet. Gynecol.* **63**, 115. Used with permission.)

with and without a karyotypic abnormality is 1% and 6%, respectively[71,79]. However, some couples will have a 25% recurrence risk associated with autosomal recessive inheritance. An increased incidence of holoprosencephaly has been reported in diabetic mothers[83]. Facial and cerebral anomalies occur as a unit, irrespective of karyotype.

Microcephaly is characteristic of alobar and semilobar holoprosencephaly. The head is of normal circumference in lobar holoprosencephaly; with severe ventriculomegaly, macrocephaly may occur. Holoprosencephaly represents approximately 16% of antenatally detected cases of 'hydrocephalus'[84]. Forty percent of cases with holoprosencephaly have hydrocephalus[85]; spina bifida and Dandy–Walker malformations may also occur.

Approximately 60% of holoprosencephalic fetuses have associated anomalies. The most common external anomalies noted with holoprosencephaly are polydactyly of the hands or feet. Major non-central nervous system structural defects include renal dysplasia, omphalocele, oesophageal atresia, bladder exstrophy and congenital heart defects[82]. Polyhydramnios[86] and intrauterine growth restriction are common associated findings with holoprosencephaly.

Neonates with alobar holoprosencephaly have only brain stem function. They invariably have seizures, are not conscious of their environment and do not appear to have useful vision or hearing. Neonates with alobar holoprosencephaly generally do not survive infancy. With semilobar holoprosencephaly, patients are severely retarded but may survive to

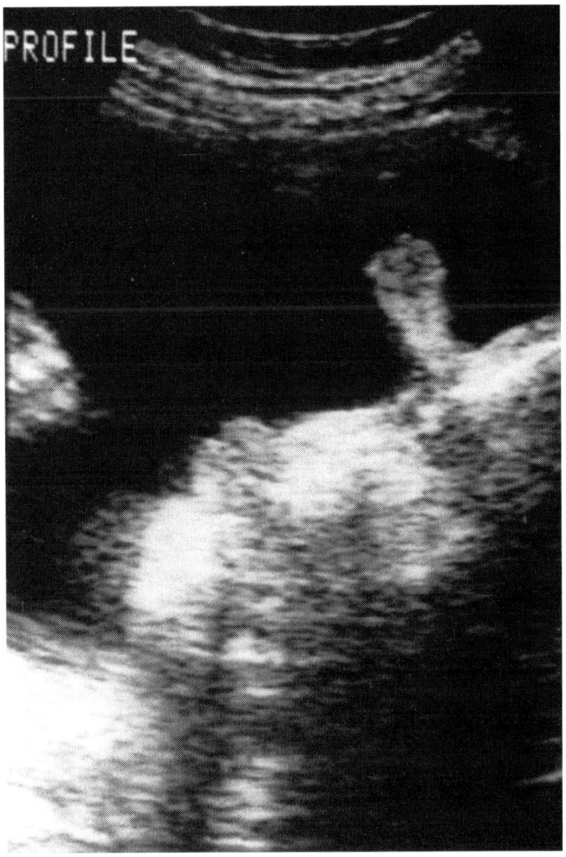

Fig. 50.16 Sagittal ultrasound view of a cyclops.

childhood. While most individuals with lobar holoprosencephaly are severely retarded, some are only mildly to moderately affected[71]. Visual abnormalities are common with lobar holoprosencephaly.

Sonographic findings

Nelson and King[87] utilized transvaginal sonography to diagnose holoprosencephaly at 10.5 weeks' menstrual age. In the latter part of the first trimester the posteriorly located normally developing rhombencephalon (Fig. 50.18) should not be confused with holoprosencephaly.

Pilu et al.[88] have described the characteristic sonographic findings with lobar holoprosencephaly. On a midcoronal scan the cavum septum pellucidum is absent, the frontal horns of the lateral ventricles are fused and communicate centrally with an enlarged third ventricle. The presence of a cavum septum pellucidum excludes a diagnosis of holoprosencephaly. The roofs of the frontal horns are typically squared (Fig. 50.19). Finally, the thalami are distinct rather than fused and rounded in shape. In the sagittal plane, the corpus callosum is present. Since the interhemisphere fissure is shallow and the falx cerebri is hypoplastic, the midline echo extends for a variable depth on a transaxial image.

Central nervous system malformations that have findings similar to lobar holoprosencephaly include severe hydrocephalus, Dandy–Walker malformations, agenesis of the corpus callosum and septooptic dysplasia. In mild to moderate hydrocephalus the frontal horns tend to be smaller than the

TABLE 50.4
Facial abnormalities associated with holoprosencephaly

Type of face	Facial features	Cranium and brain
I. Cyclopia	Single eye or partially divided eye in single orbit. Arhinia with proboscis	Microcephaly Alobar holoprosencephaly
II. Ethmocephaly	Extreme orbital hypotelorism but separate orbits. Arhinia with proboscis	Microcephaly Alobar holoprosencephaly
III. Cebocephaly	Orbital hypotelorism, proboscis-like nose but no median cleft of lip	Microcephaly. Usually has alobar holoprosencephaly
IV. With median cleft lip	Orbital hypotelorism, flat nose	Microcephaly and sometimes trigonocephaly. Usually has alobar holoprosencephaly
V. With median philtrum-premaxilla anlage	Orbital hypotelorism, bilateral lateral cleft of lip with median process representing philtrum-premaxillary anlage. Flat nose	Microcephaly and sometimes trigonocephaly. Semilobar or lobar holoprosencephaly

Source: DeMeyer, W. et al. (1964) *Pediatrics* 256–263

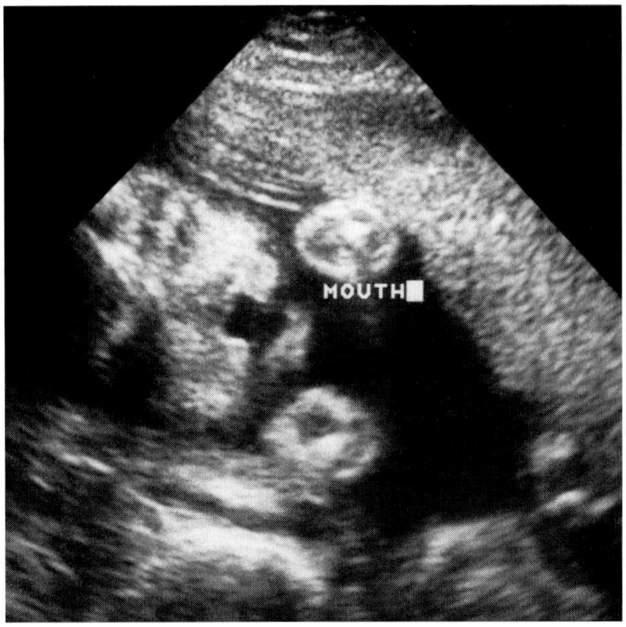

(a)

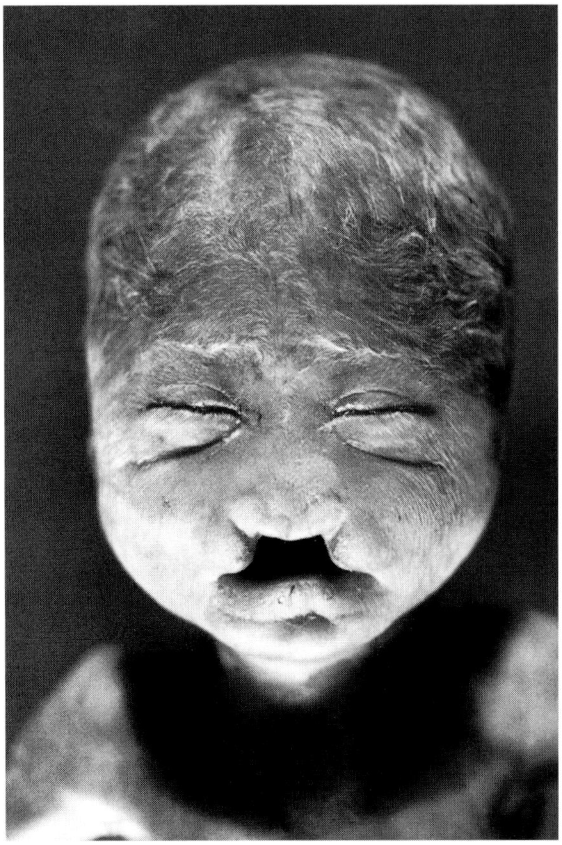

(b)

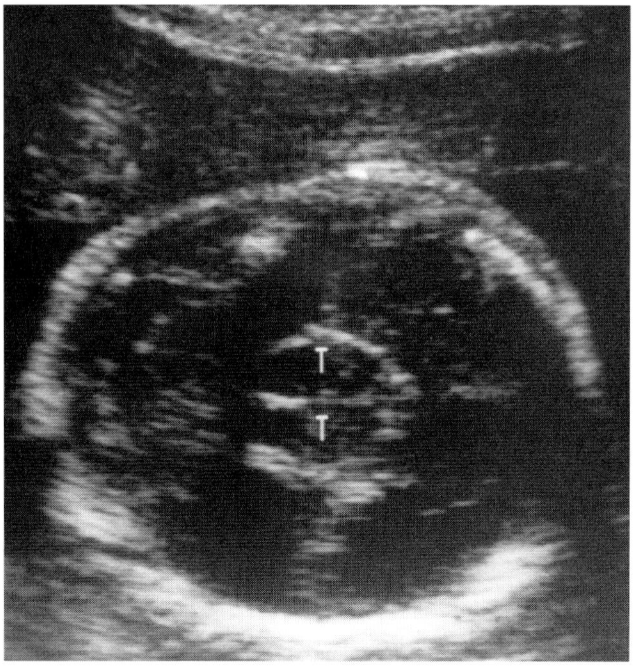

(c)

Fig. 50.17 Alobar holoprosencephaly. (a) midline cleft. (b) midline cleft at autopsy. (c) fused thalami (T) in a monoventricle.

occipital horns. However, with severe hydrocephalus the size of the frontal and occipital horns are of equivalent size. Compression atrophy of the falx cerebri, septum pellucidum and corpus callosum with severe hydrocephalus often makes the distinction between this congenital malformation and holoprosencephaly difficult. A large posterior fossa cyst associated with a Dandy–Walker malformation may simulate the dorsal sac of lobar holoprosencephaly. However, the walls of a dorsal sac are curved, while the margins of a posterior fossa cyst as it compresses the tentorium are straight. In addition, careful scanning will reveal the presence of an intact lateral ventricular system in cases of a Dandy–Walker malformation[74]. In agenesis of the corpus callosum, the entire corpus callosum rather than only the septum pellucidum is absent and the frontal horns are widely separated rather than fused. Unless the frontal horns can be well delineated, agenesis of the corpus callosum with an intrahemispheric cyst may be impossible to distinguish from lobar holoprosencephaly with a dorsal cyst[85]. Finally, there is usually a large third ventricle between the thalami in callosal agenesis, but not in lobar holoprosencephaly. Septooptic dysplasia consists of a triad of findings that includes absence of the septum pellucidum, aplasia of the optic discs, and hypopituitarism[89]. Since absence of the septum pellucidum is the only sonographically detectable abnormality with septooptic dysplasia, this anomaly and lobar holoprosencephaly may be difficult to differentiate[88].

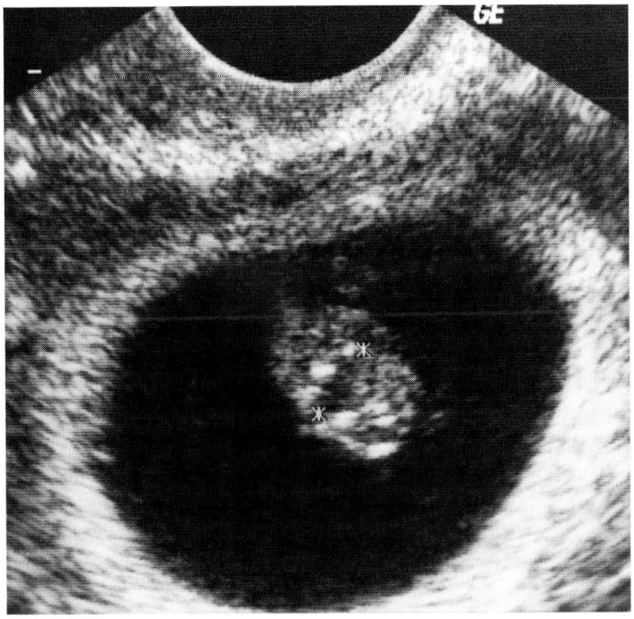

Fig. 50.18 Eight weeks' menstrual age. The normally developing rhombencephalon (markers) in the posterior aspect of the cranium.

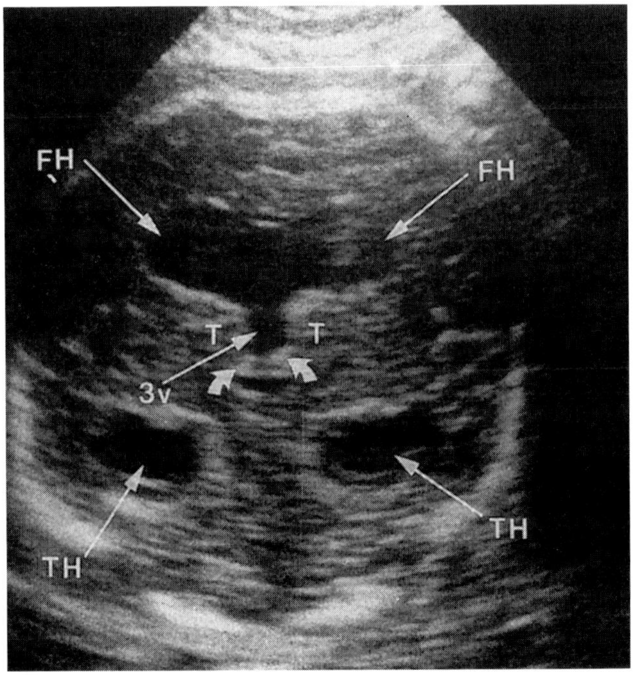

Fig. 50.19 Antenatal midcoronal scan in a 29-week fetus with lobar holoprosencephaly. The frontal horns (FH) are fused, have a square roof and communicate centrally with the inferior third ventricle (3 v). The choroid plexuses (curved arrowheads) are seen within the latter. The thalami (T) are rounded. The temporal horns (TH) are well formed and appear enlarged. Noise in the proximal field obscures the frontal cortex and does not allow the identification of the midline echo. (From Pilu, G. et al. (1992) *Ultrasound Obstet. Gynecol.* **2**, 88. Used with permission.)

LISSENCEPHALY (AGYRIA)

The term lissencephaly was initially used to describe the brain of lower mammalian species. In humans the term agyria, referring to an absence of convolutions, is more appropriate. Agyria is a disorder of cellular migration and differentiation that is determined before 7 weeks' gestation[90]. Agyria may involve either part or the entire brain. While reliable prevalence figures are not available, true agyria is quite rare. A few autosomal recessive syndromes[91] (Norman–Roberts, Neu–Laxova, Walker–Warburg, Zellweger) have agyria as a prominent finding. Partial deletion of the short arm of chromosome 17 (Miller–Dieker syndrome) results in agyria. Agyria may also occur in families[91]. The empirical recurrence risk for isolated agyria is <10%[92,93]. Neonates with agyria have profound mental and motor retardation. Approximately two-thirds of affected children die within the first year of life. Most patients with agyria are microcephalic[94]. The white matter is underdeveloped with a reverse of the normal grey to white matter ratios from 1:3 to 3:1. Secondary ventriculomegaly is due to a failure of white matter development. Additional central nervous system malformations with agyria include Dandy–Walker malformation, occipital encephalocele, hydranencephaly, and agenesis of the corpus callosum. Microophthalmia and cataracts are frequent findings. Reported associated malformations with agyria include congenital heart disease, polydactyly, duodenal obstruction, renal anomalies and polyhydramnios[95].

MICROCEPHALY

Microcephaly (Fig. 50.20) refers to a brain of subnormal size. A head circumference either two[96] or three[97] standard deviations below the mean for age and sex have been proposed as a definition for microcephaly. Since there is a stronger correlation between a head circumference three standard deviations below the mean and mental retardation, this definition is generally preferred. The reported incidence of microcephaly at birth using a head circumference of three standard deviations below the mean is approximately one in 6250[98]. Primary microcephaly is due to a disorder of neuronal proliferation and differentiation between the second and fifth month of gestation[99]. Secondary microcephaly may result from a prenatal infection (toxoplasmosis, rubella), hypoxia, or the fetal alcohol syndrome[100]. The offspring of untreated maternal phenylketonurics may have microcephaly, mental retardation and congenital heart disease[101,102]. Exposure to significant radiation prior to a gestational age of 15 weeks (e.g. survivors of the Hiroshima atomic bomb) can produce microcephaly[103]. Microcephaly is a characteristic of almost all malformed brains (holoprosencephaly, porencephaly). It is also a feature of a number of syndromes with mendelian inheritance. For example, Seckel syndrome[104] is an autosomal recessive disorder with microcephaly and severe intrauterine growth restriction.

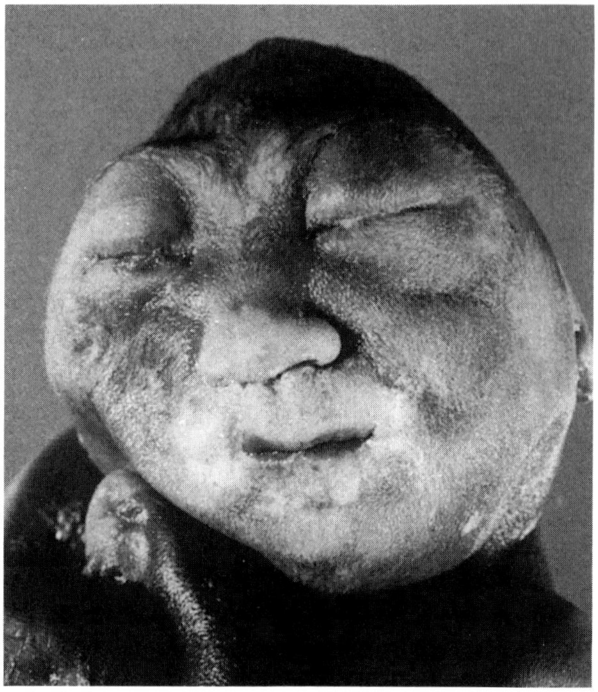

Fig. 50.20 Facial features of a 21-week fetus with atelencephalic microcephaly. (From Siebert, J.R. et al. (1986) *Teratology* **34**, 9. Used with permission.)

TABLE 50.5
Antenatal sonographic criteria for microcephaly[a]

Week no.	HC < –5 SD	H/A < –3 SD	F/HC > 3 SD
20	101	0.98	0.227
21	113	0.97	0.231
22	125	0.96	0.235
23	136	0.95	0.238
24	147	0.94	0.241
25	158	0.94	0.243
26	169	0.93	0.245
27	179	0.92	0.247
28	189	0.91	0.249
29	196	0.90	0.250
30	207	0.89	0.251
31	216	0.88	0.252
32	224	0.87	0.254
33	232	0.86	0.255
34	239	0.85	0.256
35	245	0.84	0.258
36	251	0.84	0.260
37	257	0.83	0.262
38	262	0.82	0.264
39	266	0.81	0.267
40	270	0.80	0.271
41	272	0.79	0.275
42	275	0.78	0.280

[a]A head circumference (HC) smaller than 5 SD below the mean; a head/abdomen ratio (H/A) smaller than 3 SD below the mean; and a femur/head circumference ratio (F/HC) greater than 3 SD

Modified from Chervenak F.A. et al. (1984) *Am. J. Obstet. Gynecol.* **149**, 512

TABLE 50.6
Antenatal sonographic criteria that exclude microcephaly[a]

Week no.	HC > –2 SD	H/A > –1 SD
20	145	1.16
21	157	1.15
22	169	1.14
23	180	1.13
24	191	1.12
25	202	1.11
26	213	1.1
27	223	1.1
28	233	1.09
29	242	1.08
30	251	1.07
31	260	1.06
32	268	1.05
33	276	1.04
34	283	1.03
35	289	1.02
36	295	1.01
37	301	1.00
38	306	1.00
39	310	0.99
40	314	0.98
41	316	0.97
42	319	0.96

[a]A head circumference (HC) larger than –2 SD and a head/abdomen ratio (H/A) larger than –1 SD

Modified from Chervenak, F.A. et al. (1984) *Am. J. Obstet. Gynecol.* **149**, 512

Microcephaly is also common with karyotypic abnormalities, such as trisomies 9, 13 and 18.

Any prediction of outcome with microcephaly must consider not only the head circumference, but also the aetiology of the reduction in brain size. Head circumference alone is a poor predictor of outcome in an individual case[105].

The forebrain or prosencephalon comprises two parts: the telencephalon and the diencephalon. The former includes the cerebral cortex and lateral ventricles. The diencephalon gives rise to the optic vesicles, the thalamus, the hypothalamus and the posterior or neurohypophysis. Secondary destruction of the telencephalic structures results in atelencephalic microcephaly[106]. Destruction of the entire prosencephalon is referred to as aprosencephaly[107]. Both conditions are rare causes of microcephaly.

Sonographic findings

Chervenak and co-workers[108,109] evaluated 24 cases of microcephaly and proposed the following criteria for in-utero diagnosis: (1) a head circumference 5 SD below the mean for gestational age; (2) a head circumference/abdominal circumference ratio of 3 SD below the mean; (3) a femur length/head circumference ratio of 3 SD above the mean (Table 50.5). When the head circumference was larger than –2 SD and the head circumference/abdominal circumference ratio was larger than –1 SD, fetal microcephaly could be excluded (Table 50.6). The use of multiple sonographic criteria optimized the diagnostic accuracy of predicting microcephaly.

Goldstein and co-workers[110] have reported a correlation between growth of the frontal lobe and gestational age. They measured the frontal lobe from the middle of the hyperechogenic frontal bone to the anterior edge of the medial wall of the frontal horn of the lateral ventricles (Fig. 50.21). Three cases of microcephaly confirmed after birth had a frontal lobe distance below 2 SD of the mean.

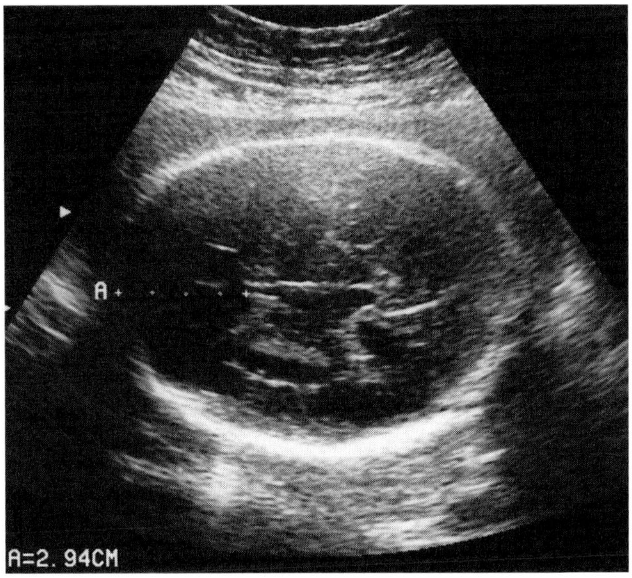

Fig. 50.21 Normal fetal frontal lobe distance at 27 weeks' gestation.

Serial examinations may be necessary in suspected cases of microcephaly. For example, Pescia and colleagues[111] diagnosed autosomal recessive microcephaly by a significant decrease in the biparietal growth rate between 18 and 23½ weeks' gestation. In cases of intrauterine growth restriction it must be determined if the head is disproportionately small. Hence the head/abdomen and femur length/abdominal circumference ratios, rather than the head circumference, should be used to make a diagnosis of microcephaly.

Microcephaly is generally due to a reduction in the size of the cerebral hemispheres; the cerebellum is less severely affected. Hence, the sonographic measurement of the frontal lobe has been proposed as another potentially more sensitive sonographic parameter for the detection of microcephaly[110].

The in-utero detection of a sloping forehead with redundant skin on a sagittal view of the face increases the likelihood that a small head circumference is due to microcephaly (Fig. 50.22).

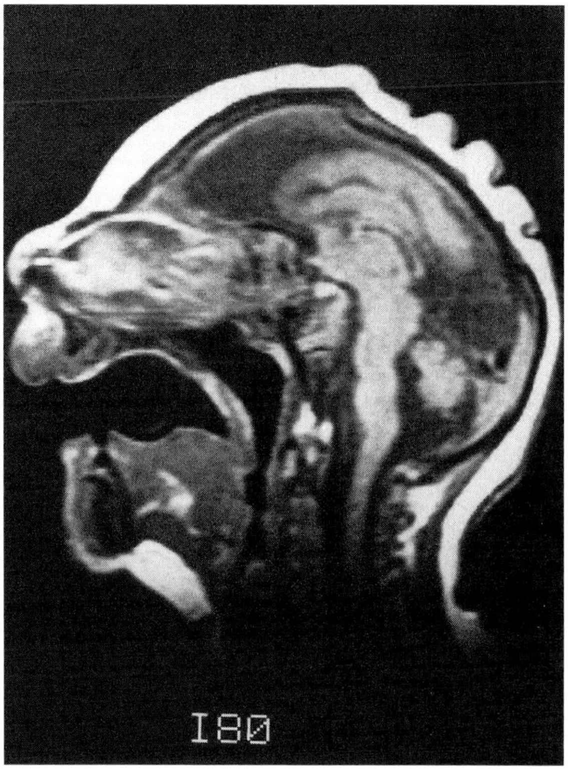

Fig. 50.22 Magnetic resonance image of neonate–midline sagittal cut. While midline structures are preserved, the cerebellum is very small with virtually no cerebrum. Note the sloping forehead and scalp skin folds. (From Persutte, W.R. et al. (1990) *Prenat. Diagn.* **10**, 631. Used with permission.)

MEGALENCEPHALY

Megalencephaly refers to a brain of unusually large size and weight. For newborns, brain weight averages 370 g and weights over 450 g are considered excessive[112].

Primary megalencephaly without associated findings is quite rare. Megalencephaly may be inherited as an autosomal recessive or as an autosomal dominant trait[113]. The male:female sex ratio with megalencephaly is 4:1[113]. While the enlargement of the brain with megalencephaly may involve the cerebellum and brain stem, usually only the cerebral hemispheres are involved[114]. Cortical thickness and the amount of white matter are usually increased. Unilateral megalencephaly with involvement of one cerebral hemisphere, usually the left, has been reported (Fig. 50.23)[114]. In some cases all parts of the brain on the same side, including the brain stem and cerebellum, are enlarged. Ipsilateral ventriculomegaly and asymmetry of the cranium are associated findings. Ramirez et al[115]. have diagnosed unilateral megalencephaly at 20 weeks' gestation with sonography and magnetic resonance imaging. In-utero megalencephaly is frequently present with Beckwith–Wiedemann syndrome and skeletal dysplasias (achondrodysplasia, thanatophoric dysplasia)[113]. With tuberous sclerosis and Tay–Sachs disease,

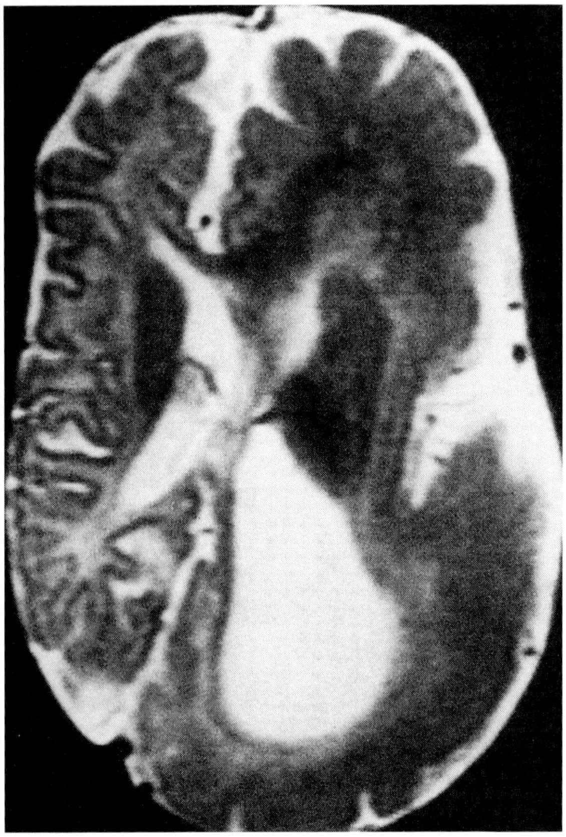

Fig. 50.23 Axial magnetic resonance image showing unilateral left hemispheric enlargement, ipsilateral ventricular enlargement, thickened cortex and poor differentiation of grey and white matter. (From Babyn, P. et al. (1992) *J. Ultrasound Med.* **11**, 563. Used with permission.)

megalencephaly may not occur until later in life. While megalencephaly has been associated with mental retardation, normal and even superior intelligence may occur.

DESTRUCTIVE

BRAIN TUMOURS

One percent of childhood brain tumours are categorized as congenital[116]. Teratomas, dermoids or choroid plexus papillomas make up 15% of the tumours; medulloblastomas account for 30%; and the remaining 55% are gliomas[117]. The prevalence of teratomas increases when only younger populations are evaluated. For example, at 2 months of age or less, 50% of cerebral neoplasms are teratomas[118].

Teratomas (Fig. 50.24) are derived from pluripotent cells and are composed of a wide variety of tissues. Most teratomas are supratentorial and are usually located either within the third ventricle, subtemporally or subfrontally. They may extend through the calvarium, or invade the oropharynx, nasopharynx or orbits[119,120]. Although long-term survival is possible, it is distinctly unusual; most neonates die within 9 months of birth[120,121].

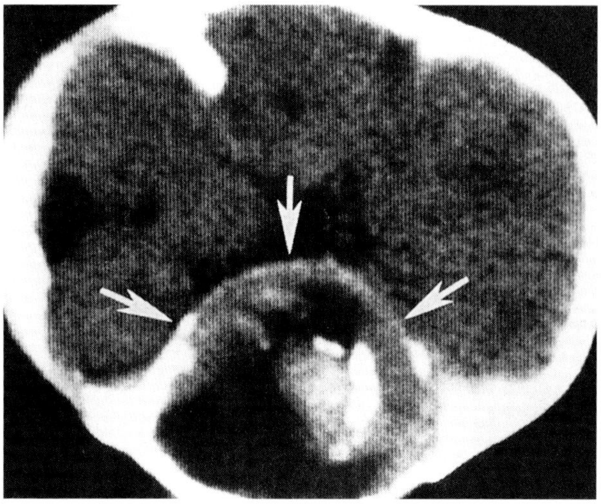

Fig. 50.24 Axial computed tomography scan of a neonate with a temporal intracranial teratoma (arrows) that enhances with contrast medium. (From Ulreich, S. et al. (1993) *J. Ultrasound Med.* **3**, 163. Used with permission.)

Gliomas constitute approximately 25% of fetal intracranial tumours. In contrast to teratomas, gliomas are echogenic tumours that occupy one hemisphere and shift the falx cerebri towards the contralateral side (Fig. 50.25). Intraventricular haemorrhage is an associated finding[122,122A].

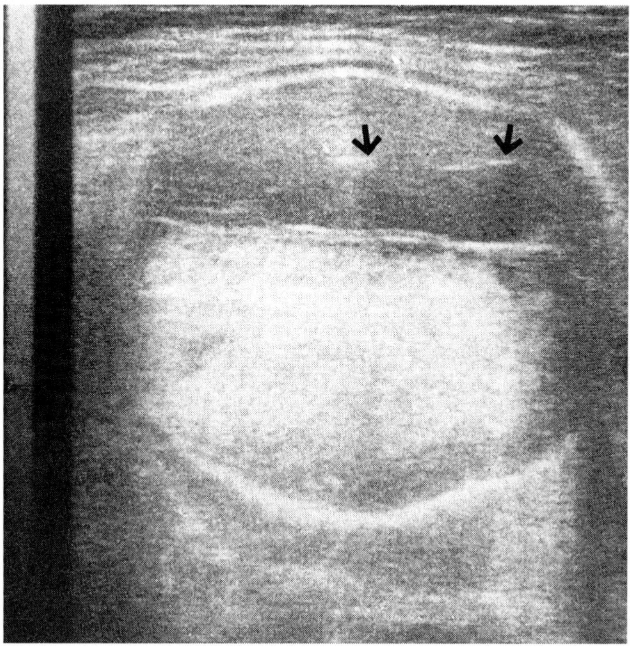

Fig. 50.25 Glioblastoma transverse section of the fetal head at 33 weeks demonstrating the enlarged right cerebral hemisphere almost completely replaced by tumour. The left internal ventricle is dilated (arrows) and the midline is shifted by the mass. (From Geraghty, A.V. et al. (1989) *Prenat. Diagn.* **9**, 613–616. John Wiley & Sons Ltd. Reproduced with permission.)

Choroid plexus papillomas usually arise in the lateral ventricles, but may also occur in the third and fourth ventricles. Sonographically, they are homogeneously echogenic (Fig. 50.26a and b)[123] with a loss of normal intracranial anatomy. If a choroid plexus papilloma is large enough, hydrocephalus can result from both overproduction of cerebrospinal fluid by the tumour and by obstruction[124]. Haemorrhage into a choroid plexus papilloma may occur. While calcifications are present microscopically, they are less frequently detected sonographically[119,125]. High-output cardiac failure due to arteriovenous shunting within the tumour and secondary polyhydramnios have also been described[119,126]. The rapid growth of these tumours occasionally results in labour dystocia[127,128]. Lipman and co-workers[119] reported a case with a normal 18-week ultrasound that by term had the entire brain replaced by tumour. Surgical removal of smaller tumours is generally associated with an excellent prognosis.

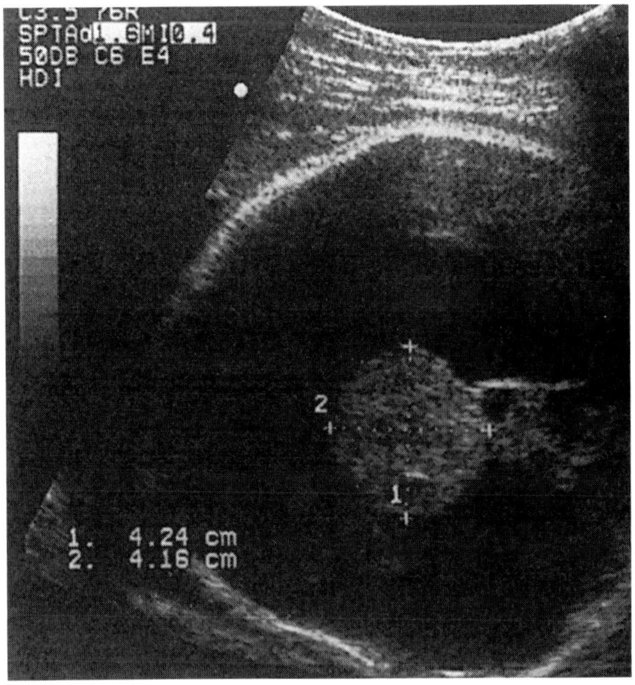

(a)

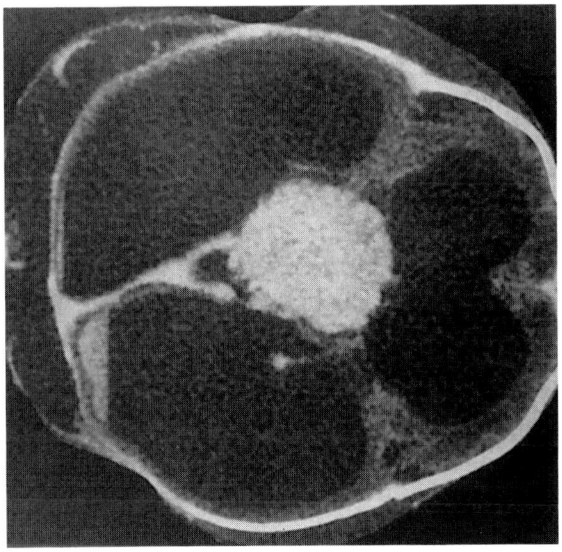

(b)

Fig. 50.26 Choroid plexus papilloma. (a) Sonogram of the fetal skull demonstrating a midline echogenic mass (4.24 cm × 4.16 cm) with massive hydrocephalus. (b) Neonatal computed tomography image of the brain at the same level showing identical findings. (From Adra, A.M. et al. (1994) *Prenat. Diagn.* **14**, 865–867. Used with permission.)

Lipomas of the choroid plexus have been detected antenatally. While they are also echogenic, their characteristic association with a lipoma of the corpus callosum helps to distinguish them from an isolated papilloma[129].

Craniopharyngiomas are benign tumours that produce damage by compressing adjoining normal brain. When they become sufficiently large, normal brain structures can no longer be identified. As with teratomas, craniopharyngiomas contain areas of calcifications[130]. Although craniopharyngiomas account for 5–10% of brain tumours in children, they are seldom diagnosed before 2 years of age.

Suresh and colleagues[116] have reported a case of cerebral neuroblastoma that was diagnosed prenatally by means of a fetal brain biopsy. The 6.0 cm heterogeneous mass had some areas of calcification.

Sonographic findings

A review of antenatally diagnosed brain tumours indicates that a definitive diagnosis must await histopathologic confirmation. However, from a prognostic standpoint failure to identify normal brain architecture in the presence of an intracranial tumour indicates that neonatal salvage will probably not be possible. The overall 5-year survival rate for congenital central nervous system tumours is approximately 20%[131]. Differentiation of an intracranial tumour from haemorrhage may not always be possible on a single ultrasound examination. Indeed, haemorrhage is an associated finding in 14% of brain tumours[132].

INTRACRANIAL HAEMORRHAGE

The aetiology of intracranial haemorrhage is not always apparent. Possible diagnoses include congenital vascular abnormalities, alloimmune thrombocytopenia, ingestion of drugs that affect platelet function (aspirin), maternal cocaine use, infection, trauma, and asphyxia[133,134]. Sims et al.[135] reported prelabour intracranial haemorrhage in 6% of stillbirths. The number of liveborn neonates who have had intracranial haemorrhage without subsequent sequelae remains unknown[136]. The pattern and distribution of central nervous system haemorrhages is similar to those found postnatally.

The extent of neurological damage depends on the location of the haemorrhage and the size of the infarction. If an intracerebral bleed perforates the ependyma, intraventricular haemorrhage will occur. The location of an intracranial haemorrhage may also suggest its arterial source. For example, a parietal haemorrhage is in the distribution of the right anterior cerebral artery, while a temporo-occipital lesion would be derived from the posterior cerebral artery[137].

Fetal manifestations of a significant intracranial haemorrhage are decreased fetal movements; an absence of fetal breathing movements; and a loss of beat-to-beat fetal heart rate variability.

Sonographic findings

On transabdominal (Fig. 50.27a) or transvaginal sonography, an intracranial haemorrhage initially appears as an irregular echodense mass that can significantly distort or obscure intracranial anatomy. Pulsed Doppler flow studies of the fetal middle cerebral and common carotid arteries indicate an increase in resistance after intracranial haemorrhage[138]. Over time the lysis of an intracerebral clot results in the formation of a fluid level within the lesion. Subsequent ultrasound examinations may detect cortical atrophy with secondary ventriculomegaly[133]. Periventricular haemorrhage is initially echodense; within 1–4 weeks periventricular cysts will appear[136]. An extensive intracerebral haemorrhage may ultimately result in hydranencephaly[139].

An intracranial haemorrhage may initially be confused with a neoplasm, most commonly a teratoma[140].

Vergani and co-workers[141A] have developed a prognostic

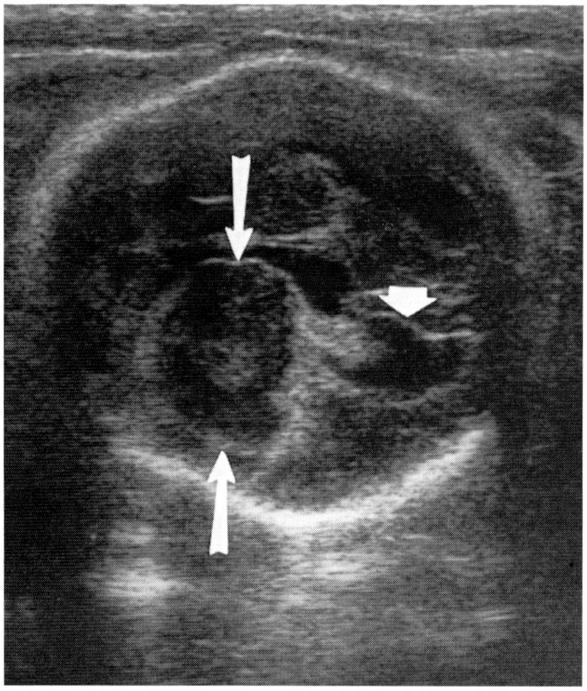

(a)

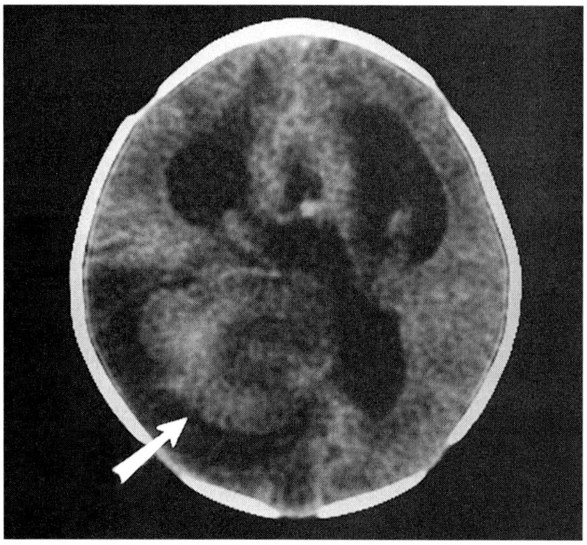

(b)

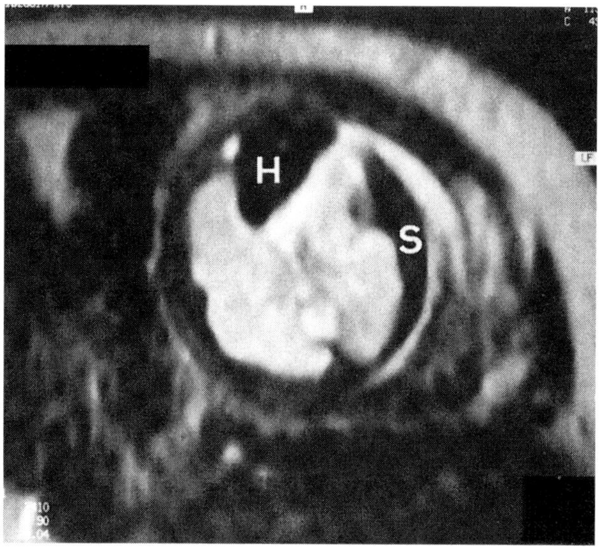

(c)

Fig. 50.27 Thirty-eight-week intrauterine gestation with an intracranial haemorrhage. (a) A 4 cm mass of mixed echogenicity in the left frontoparietal region (arrow) with medial displacement of the lateral ventricle. There is mild ventriculomegaly (arrowhead). (b) CT after delivery of 4 cm left frontoparietal haemorrhage (arrow). (c) T_2-weighted axial magnetic resonance image of the fetal head in the 34th gestational week showing a low-intensity mass (H) located frontally and protruding between the cerebral hemispheres. A sickle-shaped mass (S) is located around the right cerebral mantle, imaged together with the skull bone. The findings were caused by a recent subdural haemorrhage. (From Kirkinen, P. et al. (1997) *J. Reprod. Med.* **42**, 467. Used with permission.)

scoring system for intraventricular haemorrhage based on the prenatal ultrasound findings. They found that the prognosis was poor in 90% of cases with either parenchymal or subdural haemorrhage; fetuses with an intraventricular haemorrhage had a poor prognosis in 45% of cases.

Magnetic resonance imaging can be used to further evaluate and date a fetal intracranial haemorrhage (Fig. 50.27c)[141B].

Percutaneous umbilical blood sampling should be considered, not only to narrow the differential diagnosis with a suspected intracranial haemorrhage, but also for possible intrauterine treatment should an anaemia be detected[141].

HYDRANENCEPHALY

Hydranencephaly is characterized by an absence of the cerebral hemispheres with intact meninges and a skull of normal appearance (Fig. 50.28). An intact falx separates the two cystic hemispheres of hydranencephaly. The membrane forming its wall is thin and translucent. In addition to an absence of cerebral tissue, there is no evidence of the lateral ventricles.

Hydranencephaly results from the secondary destruction of a normal or abnormally developed brain enclosed within its meninges and skull[142]. Cerebrospinal fluid subsequently replaces the absent cerebral hemispheres. Parts of the temporal and/or occipital lobes, as well as the choroid plexi, may be preserved. The cerebellum has been reported as normal, small, or absent[142,143]. Reduction of the hemispheres to a single unilocular cavity has been reported. Unilateral hydranencephaly has also been described[144].

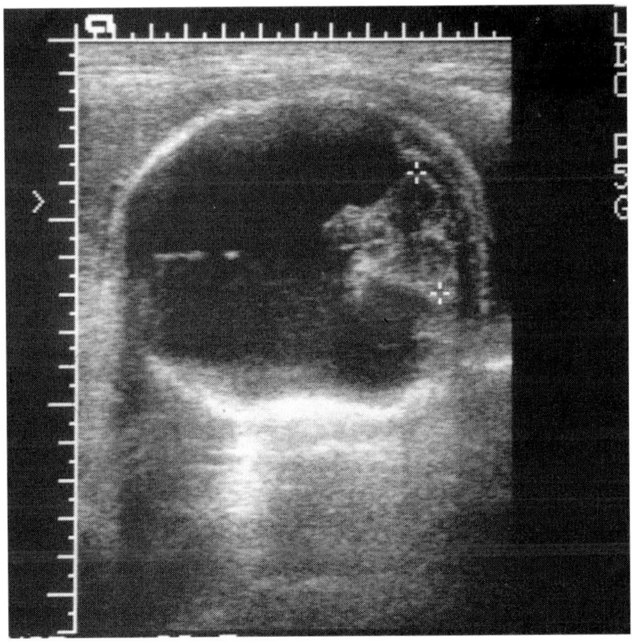

Fig. 50.28 Fetus with hydranencephaly. The cerebral hemispheres are absent; the cerebellum (markers) is intact.

The loss of cerebral tissue with hydranencephaly corresponds to the distribution of the carotid arteries or the anterior and middle cerebral arteries. Characteristically, the arteries that supply the absent parts of the brain are small. Animal studies have confirmed that interference with carotid blood flow early in pregnancy can result in hydranencephaly[145]. It has been suggested that transient vascular occlusion leads to cerebral necrosis. When the circulation is re-established, haemorrhagic destruction of the remaining brain occurs[146]. Cytomegalovirus and toxoplasmosis may cause hydranencephaly by either destroying periventricular tissue or by a disseminated intravascular coagulation resulting in cerebral hypoxia and microinfarcts[147,148]. Trauma to the developing brain may also cause hydranencephaly.

Neonates with hydranencephaly are usually stillborn or die soon after birth. However, survival for several months to a year has been reported. The length of survival is determined by the amount of residual brain. While there tends to be a complete absence of supratentorial structures in those infants that die soon after birth, neonates who survive have residual basal ganglia and a cerebellum[143]. In 1951 Johnson and co-workers[149] reported 16 cases of hydranencephaly – three lived longer than 1 year. The vast majority of survivors are physically and mentally severely handicapped.

Sonographic findings

Green and colleagues[146] have sonographically documented the presence of a normal appearing brain that was subsequently destroyed (Fig. 50.29a and b). At delivery the child had hydranencephaly with preservation of the inferior aspects of the temporal lobes, the basal nuclei, cerebellum and brain stem. Hydranencephaly has been documented sonographically as early as 12 weeks' menstrual age[150].

Differentiation between severe hydrocephalus, alobar holoprosencephaly and hydranencephaly is frequently difficult. A 'pancake' or 'horseshoe' frontal cortex, fused thalami and facial abnormalities are characteristic of holoprosencephaly. In hydranencephaly there may be islands of cerebral cortical tissue that have persisted due to collateral circulations. For example, residual occipital cerebral cortex is supplied by the vertebrobasilar circulation. A dilated third ventricle would suggest a diagnoses of severe hydrocephalus rather than hydranencephaly.

Russell and co-workers[148] have reported three cases of hydranencephaly with microcephaly and overlapping sutures. They hypothesized that partial destruction of the brain during the second or third trimester resulted in a diminution in intracranial hydrostatic pressure and subsequent collapse of the skull. In the usual case of hydranencephaly, the size of the cranium is normal due to a balance between brain destruction and cerebrospinal fluid production. In cases of hydranencephaly with microcephaly, cerebrospinal fluid production is diminished.

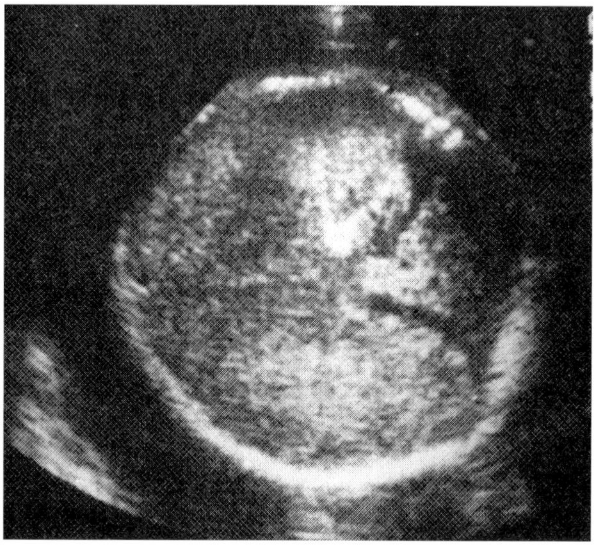

(a)

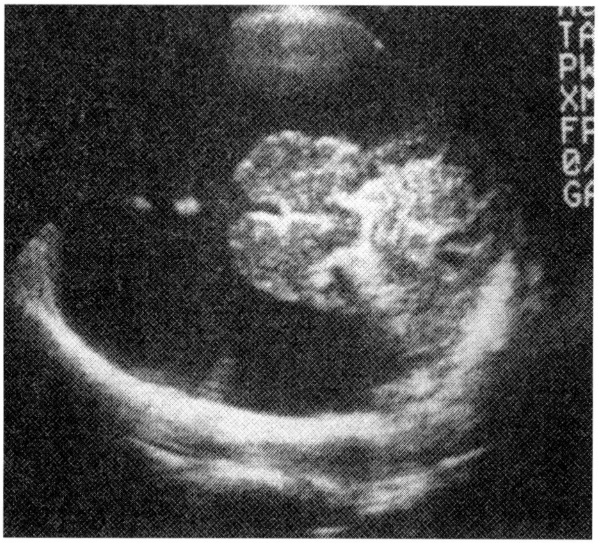

(b)

Fig. 50.29 Evolving hydranencephaly. (a) Coronal sonogram of a fetal head at 27 weeks' gestation showing bright homogeneous material filling the entire supratentorial region without any recognizable brain matter or lateral ventricles. (b) Transaxial sonogram of the fetal head 3 weeks after (a), showing a marked change in echogenicity; the entire lateral hemispheres are filled with low-level echoes. There is no recognizable cerebral tissue. (From Green, M.F. et al. (1985) *Radiology* **156**, 779. Used with permission.)

PORENCEPHALY

Porencephaly refers to fluid-filled cavities within the brain that connect with the subarachnoid space (external), ventricles (internal), neither (central), or both. Porencephalic cysts that do not connect with either the lateral ventricles or the subarachnoid space are also referred to as false or pseudoporencephalic cysts. Porencephaly is due to destruction of part of the fetal brain. The subsequent 'cyst' replaces the white and grey matter that has necrosed. The cyst wall consists of remaining white matter. A porencephalic cyst does not produce a mass effect. Ipsilateral hydrocephalus is due to the loss of cortical tissue rather than to obstruction.

A circulatory origin for porencephaly is consistent with its characteristic location within the distribution pattern of the carotid arteries[151]. Maternal trauma as well as fetal infection have also been implicated[152]. The destructive process involves the entire thickness of the brain. The white matter lining of a porencephalic cyst may be seen on a neonatal magnetic resonance image[153]. The brain stem and cerebellum are usually unaffected. The disturbances in the brain's gyrial pattern, as well as other associated central nervous system malformations, indicates that porencephaly generally occurs around 20 weeks' gestation[154]. While patients with porencephaly may be asymptomatic, mental and neurological sequelae are common. Most neonates do not learn to walk or speak.

Vintzileos and colleagues[155] have reported the prenatal sonographic findings with porencephaly.

SCHIZENCEPHALY

Schizencephaly is a developmental anomaly that results in grey-matter-lined clefts within the substance of the brain. These clefts may be extremely narrow with actual fusion of the cleft walls to very wide clefts due to the absence of large portions of the brain (Fig. 50.30)[156,157]. Barkovich and

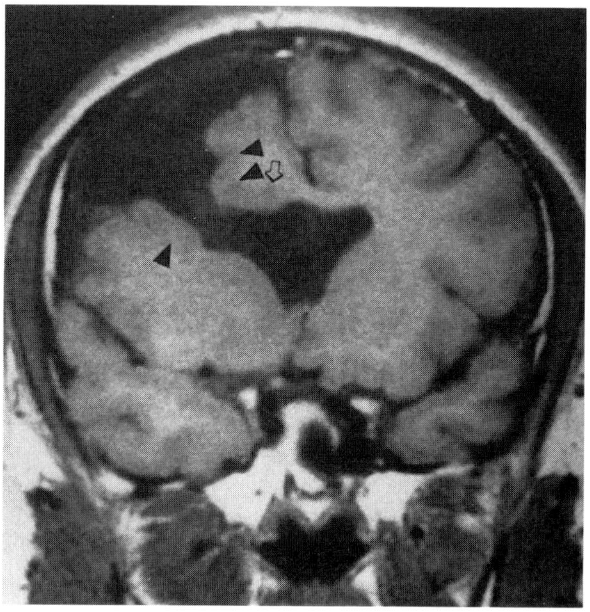

Fig. 50.30 Schizencephaly. Coronal magnetic resonance image showing a large cleft in continuity with the lateral ventricle. Continuity of grey matter through the cleft is clearly shown (arrowheads) as is a focus of heterotopic grey matter along the roof of the right lateral ventricle (open arrow). There is absence of the septum pellucidum. (From Barkovich, A.J. and Norman, D. (1988) *Am. J. Radiol.* **150**, 1391. Used with permission.)

Norman[158] have hypothesized that the aetiology of this congenital malformation is an ischaemic episode during the seventh week of gestation. Hence, the severity of ischaemia would determine the size of the cleft. Unilateral, as well as bilateral, clefts have been described. Only cases of schizencephaly with extensive clefts have been detected prenatally (Fig. 50.31)[156,159]. Ventriculomegaly, agenesis of the corpus callosum and microcephaly are associated findings with schizencephaly.

Neurological impairment is dependent upon the degree of cerebral mantle involvement. Some patients with unilateral fused clefts have normal intelligence. However, patients with large bilateral clefts invariably have developmental delay[160]. Seizures are a common finding in all patients with schizencephaly[158,161].

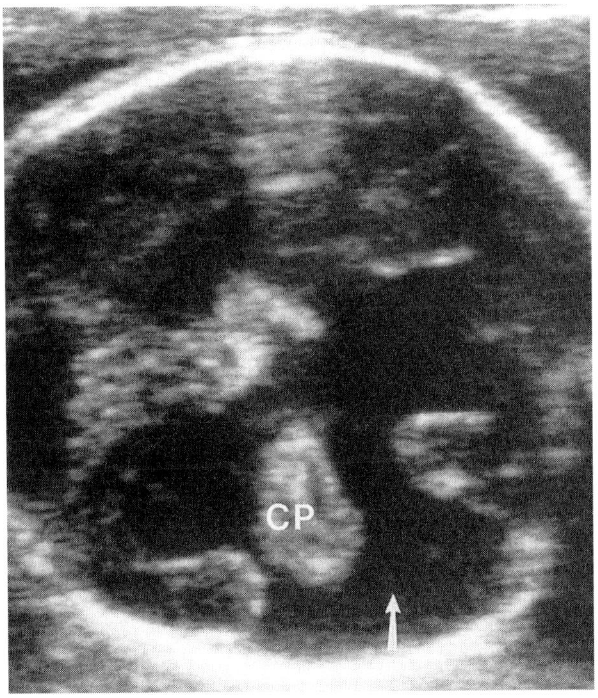

Fig. 50.31 Axial sonogram at 37 weeks' gestation demonstrating cerebral cleft consistent with schizencephaly (arrow) (CP, choroid plexus). (From Komarniski, C.A. et al. (1990) *J. Ultrasound Med.* **9**, 305. Used with permission.)

Infratentorial

DANDY–WALKER MALFORMATION

A careful assessment of the posterior fossa should be performed during every second- and third-trimester obstetrical ultrasound examination[162]. The cerebellar hemispheres, vermis and cisterna magna can be visualized in the same transaxial image. The depth of the normal cisterna magna is 5 ± 3 mm from 15 to 40 weeks' gestation; a depth of <2 mm or >10 mm is considered abnormal[163,164]. An axial view of the posterior fossa slightly caudal to the transcerebellar view will demonstrate the square-shaped fourth ventricle (Fig. 50.32) between the cerebral peduncles anteriorly and the echogenic inferior cerebellar vermis. Sonographic continuity between the fourth ventricle and the cisterna magna is required before a diagnosis of a Dandy–Walker variant should be entertained. A pseudo-Dandy–Walker variant can be easily created by obliquely imaging the cisterna magna[165].

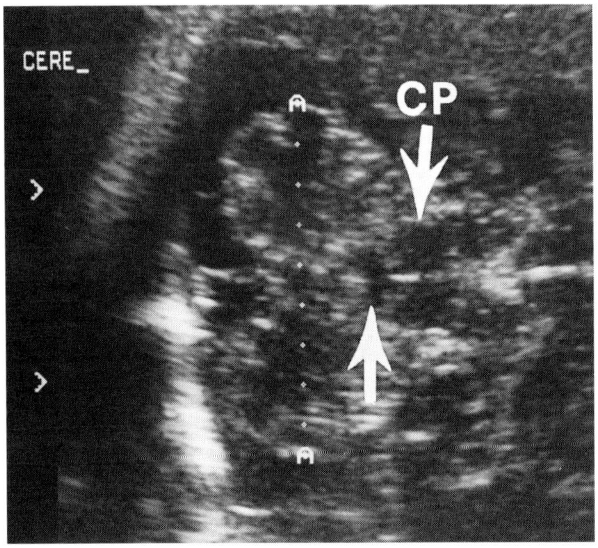

Fig. 50.32 Transaxial view of the normal fourth ventricle (arrow) between the cerebral peduncles (CP) and the echogenic inferior cerebellar varmis. The markers outline the transverse cerebellar diameter.

The characteristic triad identified as the Dandy–Walker malformation includes: (1) cystic dilatation of the fourth ventricle; (2) an enlarged posterior fossa with upward displacement of the tentorium; (3) the cerebellar vermis is either absent (25% of cases) (Fig. 50.33) or small and abnormally developed. When there is partial absence of the cerebellar vermis, it is the inferior portion that is missing. The midline foramen of Magendie and the laterally positioned foramina of Lushka are either narrowed or atretic.

There is a significant difference in the reported incidence of ventriculomegaly between neonatal and antenatal series of Dandy–Walker malformations. Hirsch et al.[166] reported a 20% incidence of ventriculomegaly with Dandy–Walker malformations at birth. However, the incidence of ventriculomegaly in antenatal series of Dandy–Walker malformations varies between 50% and 70%[167–169]. This suggests that the fetal loss rate with severe Dandy–Walker malformations is substantial. There is no correlation between the size of the posterior fossa cyst and the degree of ventriculomegaly[170]. The Dandy–Walker malformation accounts for between 2% and 4% of neonatal hydrocephalus[166].

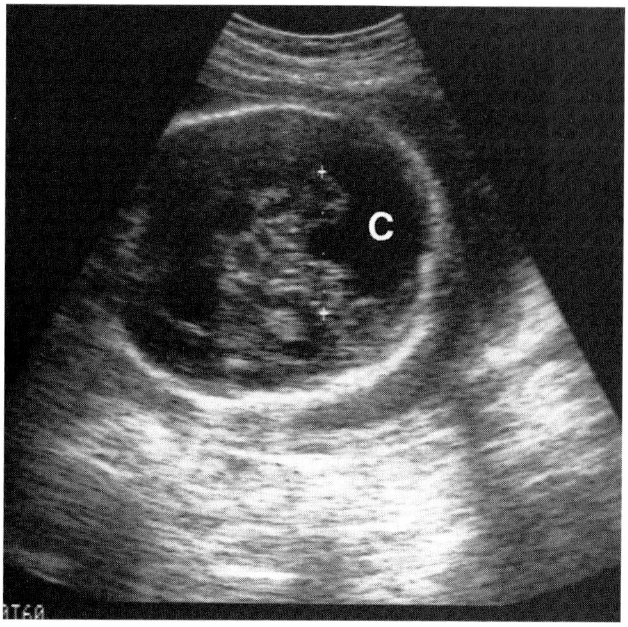

Fig. 50.33 Dandy–Walker malformation at 22 weeks' gestation. The cerebellar hemispheres (markers) are hypoplastic; the vermis is absent; and there is a large posterior fossa cyst (C).

The pathogenesis of the Dandy–Walker malformation is an arrest in hindbrain development with persistence rather than atrophy of the membranous roof of the fourth ventricle[170–171]. The cerebellum develops from symmetrical centres in the rhombencephalon. Fusion of the cerebellar hemispheres begins anteriorly at approximately 9 weeks' menstrual age and is completed by 17 weeks. Hence, a definitive diagnosis of a Dandy–Walker variant cannot be made until after a gestational age of 18 weeks. The overproduction of cerebrospinal fluid by the fourth ventricle results in herniation of the rhombencephalic roof and eventually cerebellar hypoplasia. The association of facial anomalies and polydactylism with Dandy–Walker malformations places the timing of the latter malformation prior to 8 weeks' menstrual age[166,170,171].

Dandy–Walker malformations have been described with single-gene disorders, chromosomal aberrations, after congenital infections (cytomegalovirus) or as an isolated defect[172]. Chromosomal abnormalities associated with Dandy–Walker malformation include not only trisomies 13,18 and 21[166,168], but also duplication malformations (i.e. 5P, 8P and 8q)[172]. The risk of a chromosomal abnormality increases with extra-CNS anomalies[172]. The incidence of Dandy–Walker malformation is between 1 in 25 000 to 1 in 35 000 births. Familial cases of Dandy–Walker malformation have been reported[166]. The recurrence risk for isolated Dandy–Walker malformation is 1% to 5%[172]. With transvaginal sonography the diagnosis of a Dandy–Walker malformation has been made as early as 11[173] and 14 weeks' menstrual age[174]. However, Dandy–Walker malformation may not always be apparent even in the latter part of the second trimester. Russ and co-workers[167] have reported a case of a Dandy–Walker malformation with a normal posterior fossa (7 mm) at 24 weeks' gestation; 10 weeks later the posterior fossa was enlarged and the cerebellar hemispheres were hypoplastic.

With Dandy–Walker malformations, associated central nervous system malformations occur in 68% of patients and include encephalocele, microcephaly, aqueductal stenosis, and lipomas[170]. Agenesis of the corpus callosum is present in 7%[166] to 17%[175] of cases. Hypoplasia of the brain stem is an associated finding in a significant number of cases.

The frequency of non-central nervous system anomalies with the Dandy–Walker malformation is between 25% to 73% of cases. Facial angiomas, cleft lip/palate, congenital heart disease, renal anomalies and skeletal malformations have all been reported[167,170,171,176]. Congenital heart defects associated with a Dandy–Walker malformation include ventricular septal defects, coarctation of the aorta, pulmonary stenosis, tetralogy of Fallot and hypoplastic right ventricle[167].

A Dandy–Walker malformation is compatible with a normal life[163]. Overall mortality rates of 12% to 50% have been reported[163]. The presence of additional malformations adversely affects the survival rate[164]. Additional concurrent CNS malformations also play an important part in subsequent long-term outcome.

The differential diagnosis of a posterior fossa cyst includes a Dandy–Walker variant, a prominant cisterna magna, an arachnoid cyst and semilobar holoprosencephaly. A mega cisterna magna (≥1.0 cm) accounts for 54% of cystic posterior fossa malformations[177]. Unlike a Dandy–Walker malformation, an enlarged cisterna magna is not associated with a vermian defect or other cerebellar abnormalities. Although it was initially considered a benign condition[163] a mega cisterna magna may also be associated with karyotypic abnormalities, specifically trisomy 18[178,179]. In cases of trisomy 18, the cisterna magna is prominent due to cerebellar hypoplasia. Since tables are available for the transverse cerebellar diameter at a given gestational age[180], a physiological enlargement of the cisterna magna can now be distinguished from a large cisterna magna secondary to cerebellar hypoplasia. The Dandy–Walker variant accounts for up to one-third of posterior fossa lesions[177]. The variation in the severity of the defects between a Dandy–Walker malformation, a Dandy–Walker variant, and a mega cisterna magna may relate to the timing and severity of the initial central nervous system insult[177]. The postnatal outcome for fetuses with a Dandy–Walker variant is similar to the outcome with a true Dandy–Walker malformation and ranges from normal development to severe disability or death. The prevalence of karyotypic abnormalities, as well as central nervous system and non-central nervous system anomalies is similar with the Dandy–Walker malformation and Dandy–Walker variant[181].

In order to differentiate a posterior fossa arachnoid cyst

from a Dandy–Walker malformation, the symmetry of the cerebellar hemispheres should be evaluated. While a Dandy–Walker malformation has laterally displaced symmetrical cerebellar hemispheres, an arachnoid cyst is either positioned off the midline, or if centrally located, expands asymmetrically. In addition, a Dandy–Walker cyst has a triangular shape, while an arachnoid cyst tends to be rounded[167,175]. A posterior arachnoid cyst may displace the cerebellum, but the cerebellar hemispheres are not separated and the vermis is intact. An arachnoid cyst may produce ventriculomegaly by compression. Since agenesis of the corpus callosum is an associated finding of the Dandy–Walker malformation, ventriculomegaly secondary to compression by the posterior fossa cyst or colpocephaly (occipital horn dilatation) secondary to agenesis of the corpus callosum may be observed.

Characteristics of semilobar holoprosencephaly that distinguish it from a Dandy–Walker malformation include a supratentorial cyst that communicates with a single ventricle, fused thalami and complete or partial absence of the midline falx[168].

Aplasia of the vermis with occipital encephalocele (tectocerebellar dysraphia) is a rare sporadic malformation. In addition to absence of the vermis, these infants have an occipital encephalocele that contains cerebellar cortex. Additional central nervous system malformations are characteristically present[182].

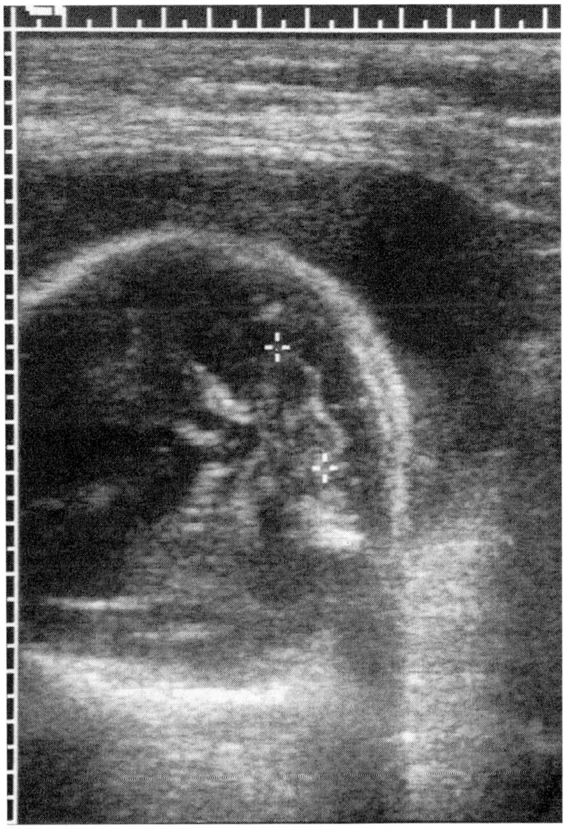

Fig. 50.34 Cerebellar hypoplasia at 28 weeks' gestation with a cerebellum (between markers) consistent with a 24-week intrauterine pregnancy.

CEREBELLAR ABNORMALITIES

Cerebellar abnormalities are frequently associated with chromosomal anomalies. In the infant with Down syndrome, cerebellar weight is decreased by 34%[183]. However, in the second trimester the transverse cerebellar diameter is within the normal range[184]. This suggests that either the transcerebellar diameter is not sensitive enough to detect the reduction in cerebellar weight, or that with trisomy 21 cerebellar hypoplasia does not occur until after the second trimester. With trisomy 18, 57.9% of second trimester transcerebellar diameter measurements are greater than 2 SD below the mean[185]. Other causes of cerebellar hypoplasia include infection[186], exposure to teratogens[187] and hypotensive brain stem necrosis[188] (Figs 50.34, 50.35).

Cerebellar agenesis may be complete or incomplete[189]. Joubert syndrome is an autosomal recessive disorder with agenesis of the cerebellar varmis. The cerebellar hemispheres, rather than being separated, are immediately adjacent to one another. Hence, the fourth ventricle is not enlarged. Additional subtle central nervous system malformations may account for the symptoms of Joubert syndrome, namely hyperpnoea, ataxia, abnormal eye movements, and mental retardation[190,191]. Agenesis of the cerebellar vermis is also compatible with a normal life[192]. Daffos et al.[193] have described a case of atrophy of the left cerebellar lobe with secondary cisternal dilatation.

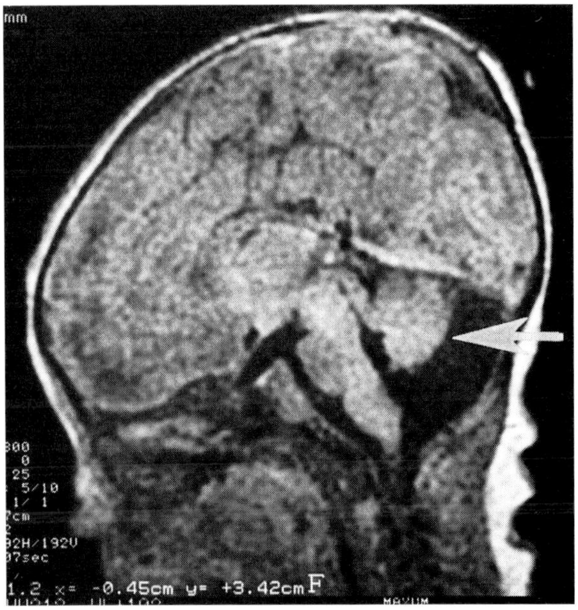

Fig. 50.35 Parasagittal magnetic resonance image of cerebellar hypoplasia (arrow) and an enlarged cisterna magna in a neonate.

Spinal column

ANENCEPHALY

Embryologically the neural plate forms at 18 days postovulation. Closure of the rostral and caudal aspects of the neuropore occurs on postovulatory day 24 and day 26, respectively (Table 50.7). The spinal cord distal to S-2 forms by secondary neurulation (postovulation day 28–56), i.e. neural crest cells migrate into the dorsal midline of the mesoderm, form a canal, and eventually fuse with the distal end of the spinal cord.

Anencephaly was the first fetal anomaly diagnosed with antenatal sonography[194]. Anencephaly is due to a failure of rostral neural tube closure at 3–4 weeks after conception. Since the developing brain is not initially affected, exencephaly is the first stage in the development of anencephaly[195]. The time period during which the cerebral tissue atrophies is highly variable.

In 1925, Nañangas[196] classified anencephaly into five types based upon cranial morphology (Fig. 50.36). This classification extends from the classic anencephalic (Type I) with minimal or no area cerebrovasculosa; to anencephaly with craniorachischisis (Type II); to meroanencephaly with a prominent area cerebrovasculosa (Type III); to iniencephaly (Type IV); and exencephaly (Type V).

The reported incidence of anencephaly in the United States is approximately 0.3 per 1000 births[197]. However, this rate is dependent upon race, sex, and geographic location. Anencephaly is more common in whites than blacks and orientals. There is a clear female predominance with a female-to-male ratio of between 2:1 and 4:1. Multiple gestations have a higher incidence of anencephaly[198].

Anencephaly is generally considered multifactorial in origin, i.e. the result of the interaction between genetic predisposition and presumed environmental factors. Byrne and Warburton[199] have shown that 9.3% of all karyotypically abnormal spontaneous abortuses have a neural tube defect. In addition, from 12% to 20% of neural tube defects have conditions that are aetiologically distinct from an isolated neural tube defect[200].

Approximately 65% of anencephalics die in-utero; most liveborn anencephalics die soon after birth. Brackbill[201] described one anencephalic infant who survived for 5½ months. The widespread use of second-trimester maternal serum alpha fetoprotein testing and antenatal sonography in the US has had a significant impact on the incidence of liveborn anencephalics. In Massachusetts between 1972 and 1975, 47% of anencephalics were liveborn; in 1986–87 only 3% were liveborn[202].

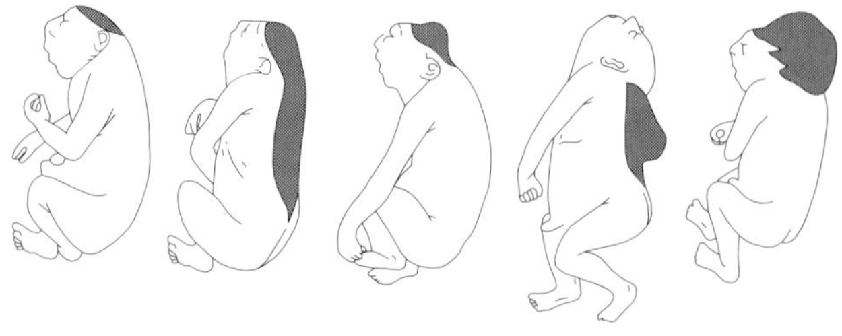

Fig. 50.36 Classification of the different types of anencephaly according to Nanagas. (I) Anencephalic acrania. (II) Anencephalic craniorachischisis. (III) Microcephalic acrania (merocrania). (IV) Iniencephaly (microcephalic craniorachischisis). (V) Exencephalic acrania. (From Salamanca, A. et al. (1992) *US Obstet. Gynecol.* **2**, 95. Partridge: Parthenon Publishing used with permission.)

Although movement patterns are observed in anencephalic fetuses, their motor behaviour is distinctly abnormal – most movements are jerky in character and of large amplitude, indicating lower motor neuron reflex activity[203]. The upper extremities of anencephalic fetuses tend to be abnormally long when compared to the lower extremities[196].

Lung hypoplasia is commonly present with anencephaly and may be present as early 16 weeks' menstrual age. Since both breathing movements and normal amniotic fluid are present with anencephaly, the aetiology for pulmonary hypoplasia has yet to be elucidated[203].

Sonographic findings

First-trimester fetuses seen as apparently normal by transabdominal sonography have subsequently been found to have anencephaly. In these instances the contour of the exposed brain was considered the calvarium (Figs. 50.37a and b)[204]. Transvaginal sonography has made it possible to reliably

TABLE 50.7
Timing of neurulation defects

Defect	Event	Menstrual age (weeks)	Crown–rump length (mm)
Craniorachischisis	Non-fusion of neural folds	4.4–5.3	1.0–3.5
Anencephaly	Non-closure of anterior neuropore	5.3–5.8	2.5–4.5
Meningomyelocele	Non-closure of posterior neuropore	5.8–6.3	3.0–5.0

Modified from Lemire, R.J. (1983) *Clin. Neurosurg* **30**, 165

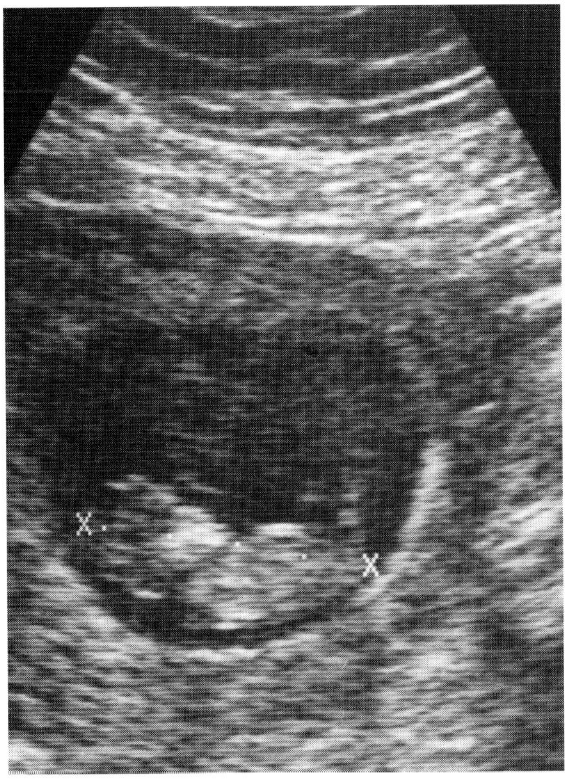

(a)

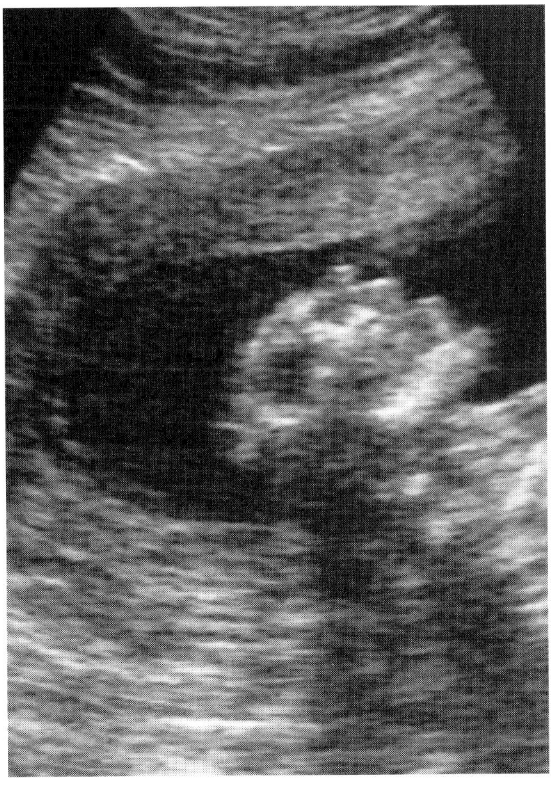

(b)

Fig. 50.37 Anencephaly. (a) Transabdominal image of the crown–rump length (between markers) at 11.2 weeks' gestation. (b) Profile of the same fetus as in (a) with anencephaly at 16 weeks' gestation.

exclude a diagnosis of anencephaly by 10–11 weeks' menstrual age[204]. The brain is eventually replaced by a discoid mass of tissue, the area cerbrovasculosa. Microscopically, the area cerbrovasculosa consists of fibrous tissue, randomly dispersed neurons and choroid plexus. Although the area cerbrovasculosa is quite disorganized, it may sonographically appear 'brain-like'. The brain stem and cerebellum are less severely involved[205]. Since the orbits are shallow, the eyes protrude from their sockets.

Fifty percent of anencephalic fetuses have a spinal defect. The common embryological origin of anencephaly and spina bifida (i.e., non-closure of the rostral and caudal aspects of the neural tube, respectively) explains the high association of these two defects. Polyhydramnios is present with 50% of third-trimester anencephalics[205].

Anencephaly can usually be distinguished from the cranial defects associated with the amniotic band syndrome. With the latter malformation, the cranial defects are characteristically asymmetric and do not follow established anatomic divisions. In addition, there may be limb or body-wall deformities. Amniotic bands are not necessarily visualized sonographically within the amniotic cavity.

EXENCEPHALY

In exencephaly a large portion of the brain is present despite the absence of the calvarium (see classification of anencephaly). Although exencephaly characteristically progresses to anencephaly, cases with sonographically detectable third-trimester exencephaly have been reported[206,207]. Transvaginal sonography has diagnosed exencephaly as early as 10½ menstrual weeks[208]. In the second and third trimester, differentiation from a large cephalocele should be possible by identifying the skull through which the encephalocele protrudes. As with the other classifications of anencephaly, the amniotic band syndrome should be ruled out. Concurrent anomalies that are associated with the amniotic band syndrome or the identification of bands attached to the fetus will enable the examiner to distinguish between this anomaly and isolated exencephaly. Although the remaining brain in exencephaly may have convolutions (Figs 50.38, 50.39), normal brain anatomy is not present.

The presence of limb, abdominal wall and spinal deformities in association with exencephaly should suggest the limb–body-wall complex[209].

INIENCEPHALY

Iniencephaly (Figs 50.40–50.42) describes a group of malformations that consist of: (1) a bony defect in the occipital region of the skull; (2) partial or total absence of the cervical and thoracic vertebra; (3) spina bifida or rachischisis of the cervical and thoracic spine; (4) fixed retroflexion of the head. Two types of iniencephaly have been described, with (apertus) and without (clausus) an accompanying encephalocele.

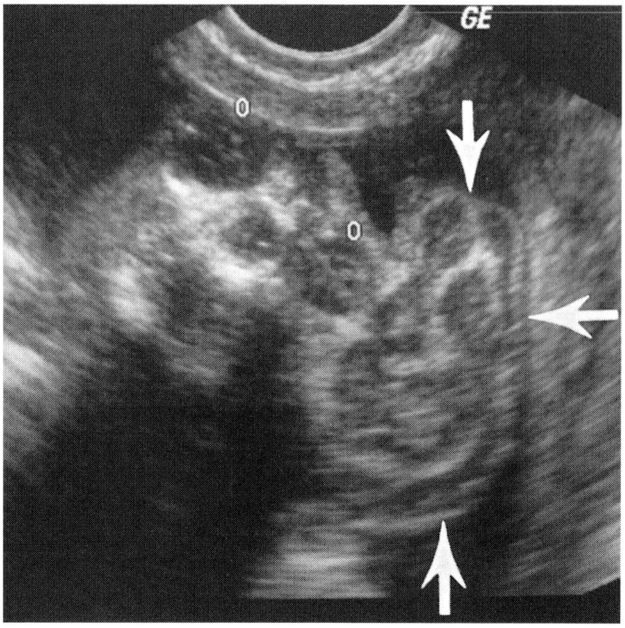

Fig. 50.38 Exencephaly (arrows) at 18 weeks' gestation (O = orbits).

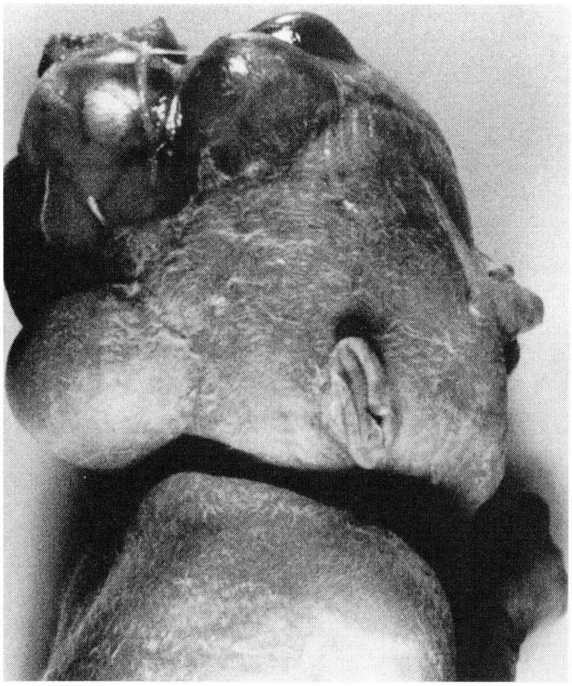

Fig. 50.39 Gross appearance of an exencephalic fetus. (From Hendricks, S.K. et al. (1988) *Obstet. Gynecol.* **72**, 898. Used with permission.)

The reported incidence of iniencephaly is one in every 1000 to 2000 births[210]. Some authors consider the incidence to be substantially higher due to underreporting. Central nervous system malformations that have been associated with iniencephaly include: microcephaly, hydrocephalus, and holoprosencephaly. Non-central nervous system malformations that occur more frequently with iniencephaly include congenital heart defects, diaphragmatic hernia, encephalocele, genitourinary malformations, single umbilical artery and clubfoot[210]. Polyhydramnios is characteristically present in the latter part of the second and in the third trimester. A correct prenatal diagnosis is critical since iniencephaly is inevitably fatal in the neonatal period[211].

ENCEPHALOCELE

Encephaloceles refer to a protrusion of intracranial contents through a bony defect of the skull. They arise from a failure in closure of the rostral end of the neural tube during the fourth week after conception. A simultaneous disruption of the neural tube at its caudal end results in a concurrent spinal defect, a lesion that occurs with 7–15% of cephaloceles[212,213].

Jeanty and co-workers[214] have listed four types of encephaloceles (Fig. 50.43): (1) cranial meningocele, consisting of membranes and cerebellar spinal fluid; (2) cranial meningomyelocele, when a small amount of neural tissue is present within the herniated sac; (3) encephalomeningocele, if the herniated neural tissue is contiguous with the brain; (4) encephalocystomeningocele when a portion of the lateral ventricles, as well as brain tissue, are present within the herniated sac (Fig. 50.44–50.46). Encephaloceles usually connect to one hemisphere and cause disfiguration of adjoining brain[215]. The involved hemisphere is usually smaller than the contralateral hemisphere. As a result, the normal hemisphere may extend beyond the midline. While large amounts of brain within a herniated sac are easily detected sonographically, cranial meningomyeloceles may be mistaken for cranial meningoceles.

Encephaloceles characteristically arise in the midline. Seventy-five percent of encephaloceles in the western world are occipital in location; frontal (13%) (Figs 50.47, 50.48) and parietal (12%) encephaloceles may also occur. The incidence of anterior encephaloceles is estimated at 1/40 000 births in the western world and 1/5000 births in Asia[216,217]. The rarest form of encephalocele occurs through the base of the skull and presents as a pharyngeal mass[219]. When an encephalocele is not in the midline, it is usually associated with the amniotic band syndrome[216].

Encephaloceles may appear as an isolated lesion or as part of a genetic or non-genetic syndrome (Table 50.8)[219]. Roberts syndrome and frontonasal dysplasia may have a frontal enceophalocele. Karyotypic abnormalities associated with an encephalocele include trisomy 13, trisomy 18, triploidy, Turner syndrome, mosaic trisomy 20 and unbalanced translocations[219,220].

Other central nervous system anomalies associated with encephaloceles include the Dandy–Walker syndrome, agenesis of the corpus callosum and microcephaly. The impairment in the flow of cerebrospinal fluid by large encephaloceles results in ventriculomegaly[213,221,222]. The recurrence risk for an isolated encephalocele is approximately 2%[223].

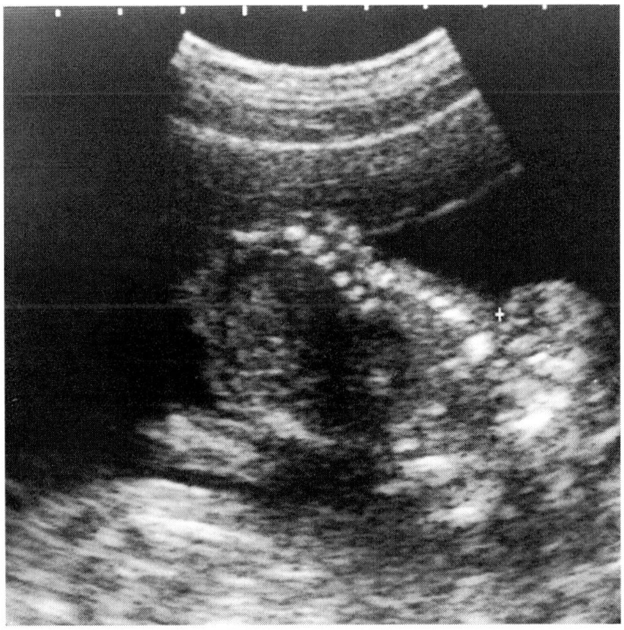

(a)

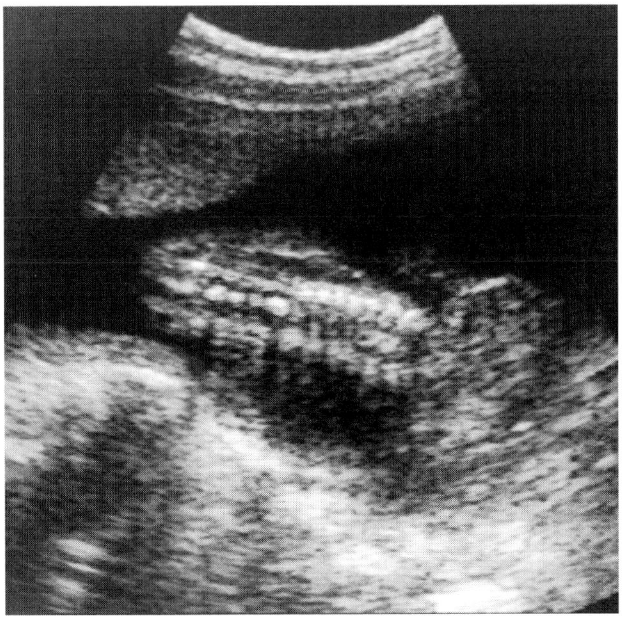

(b)

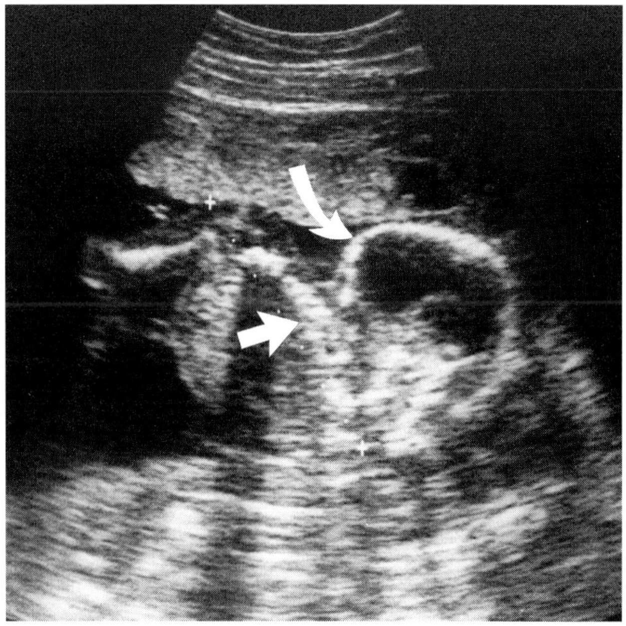

(c)

Fig. 50.40 Iniencephaly at 18 weeks' gestation. (a) An occipital encephalocele is between the markers. There is marked kyphoscoliosis of the spine. (b) Rachischisis of the spine. (c) Fixed retroflexion of the head. (Straight arrow = spine; curved arrow = occiput.)

The factors that correlate with neonatal outcome are:

- Site of the lesion
- Size of the lesion
- Content of the lesion
- Microcephaly
- Associated abnormalities
- Operability of the lesion

The presence of microcephaly, associated congenital malformations or a cephalocele as part of certain genetic syndromes are poor prognostic signs. In general, 50% of patients

TABLE 50.8
Syndromes associated with encephaloceles

Inheritance	Additional sonographic characteristics
Autosomal recessive	
Meckel–Gruber	Polycystic kidneys
	Polodactyly
	Microcephaly
	Cleft lip and palate
	Clubfoot
Roberts	Tetra phocomelia
	Bilateral cleft (lip/palate)
	Microcephaly
	Growth restriction
Orofaciodigital	Micrognathia
	Polysyndactyly
	Dandy–Walker malformation
	Renal agenesis
Walker–Warburg	Retinal detachment
	Hydrocephalus
	Microphthalmia
Chemke	Hydrocephalus
	Cataracts
Knobloch	Meningocele
	Retinal detachment
Uncertain	
Frontonasal dysplasia	Median cleft palate
	Hypertelorism
Hemifacial microsmia	Facial asymmetry
	Hypoplasia of mandible
	Microtia
	Absence of orbit

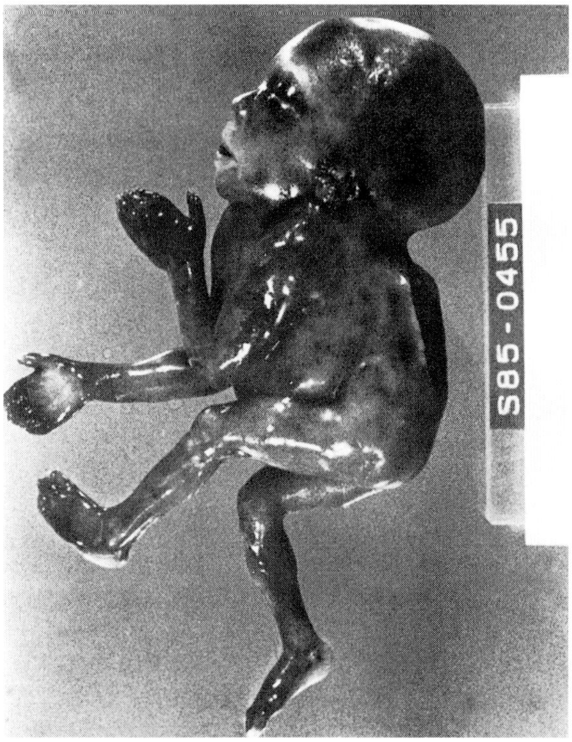

Fig. 50.41 A side view of a fetus with iniencephaly. There is a short neck with hyperextension of the head and fusion of the occiput to the cervical and upper thoracic spine. A large open neural tube defect (T9–sacrum) begins below the point of fusion of occiput and spine. (From Fuderero, A.E. et al. (1987) *J. Clin. Ultrasound* **15**, 550. Used with permission.)

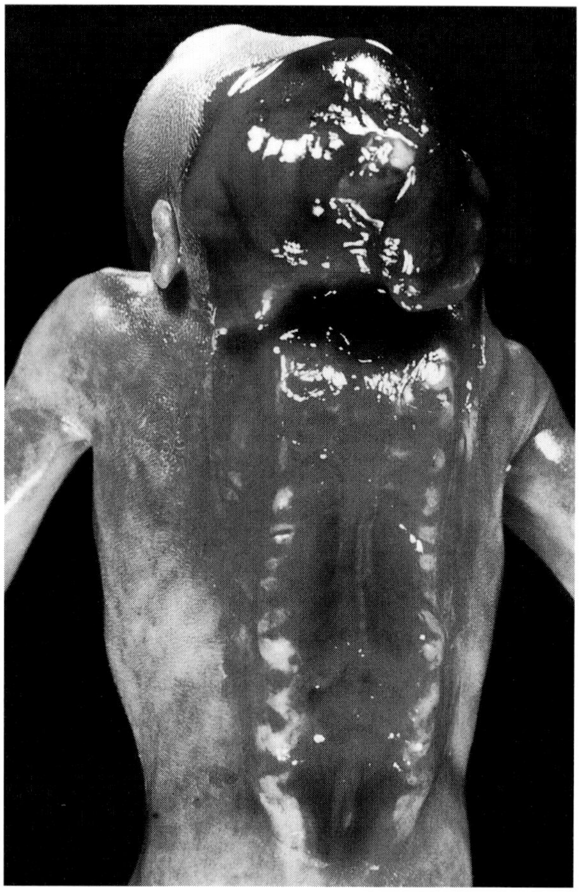

Fig. 50.42 Iniencephaly. There is rachischisis of the spine and retroflexion of the head.

born with an encephalocele survive and 74% of survivors are mentally retarded[213]. In the subset of patients with an isolated meningocele, 60% of cases have normal intelligence after surgical repair. Externalized brain is generally abnormal and therefore, resected at the time of encephalocele repair. When cerebral tissue is removed most survivors have significant mental deficiencies, as well as developmental delay[222,224].

In addition to having a better prognosis, frontal enceophaloceles are generally not inherited and do not recur in families[212,219].

Non-central nervous system anomalies that have been associated with cephaloceles include facial clefts, cystic renal disease, short limbs and congenital heart disease[219].

Sonographic findings

The bony defect of an encephalocele may only be a few millimetres in diameter and therefore, difficult to visualize sonographically. Hanley et al.[225] reported a case of an apparent cranial meningomyelocele that regressed to a cranial meningocele between 26–31 weeks' menstrual age. The tissue visualized within the encephalocele may have been dura and arachnoid rather than brain. Bronshtein and Zimmer[226] detected an 8 mm occipital meningocele with transvaginal sonography at 13 weeks' gestation. The meningocele changed

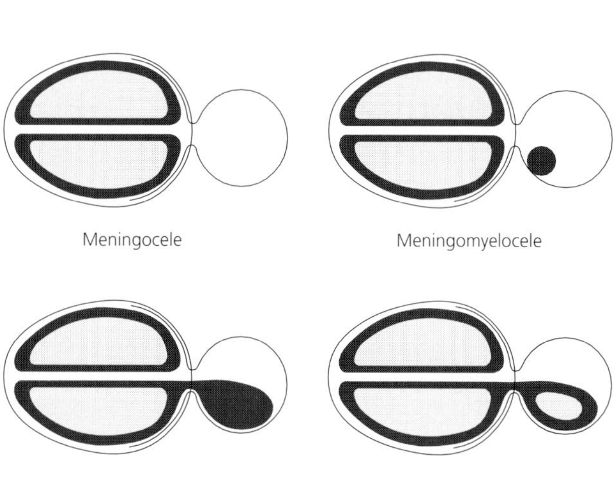

Fig. 50.43 Schematic representation of the types of cephaloceles. (From Jeanty, P. et al. (1991) *Am. J. Perinatol.* **8**, 144. Used with permission.)

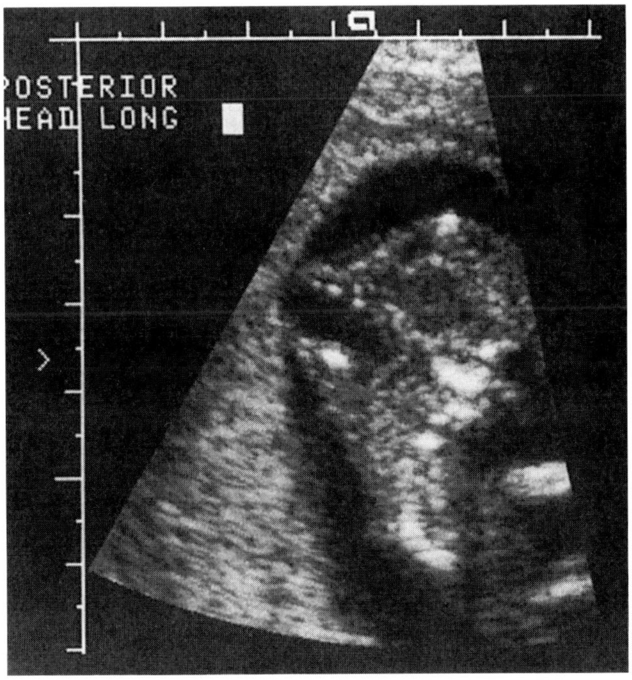

Fig. 50.44 Familial recurrence of Meckel–Gruber syndromes diagnosed at 12 weeks' gestation. A posterior encephalocele is identified. (From Wininger, S.J. & Donnenfeld, A.E. (1994) *Prenat. Diagn.* **14**, 839. Copyright John Wiley & Son Ltd. Reproduced with permission.)

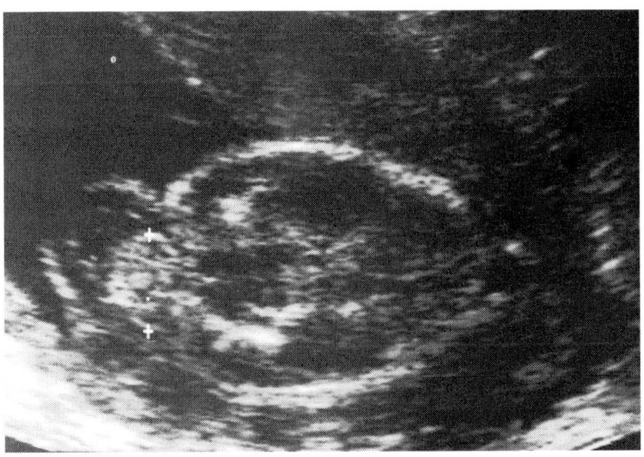

Fig. 50.45 Occipital encephalomeningocele (markers) at 23 weeks' gestation. The markers delineate the brain tissue within the meningocele sac.

to an encephalomingocele in 1 week, completely disappeared at 16 weeks, and was detected again at 19 weeks' menstrual age. Hence, the changing appearance of encephaloceles indicates that prognosis cannot always be accurately predicted antenatally[219].

The 'lemon sign' characteristically associated with spina bifida occurs in approximately 25% of cases with an encephalocele. A beaked tectal plate (Fig. 50.49) and flattening of the occiput may also occur[222]. An encephalocele may

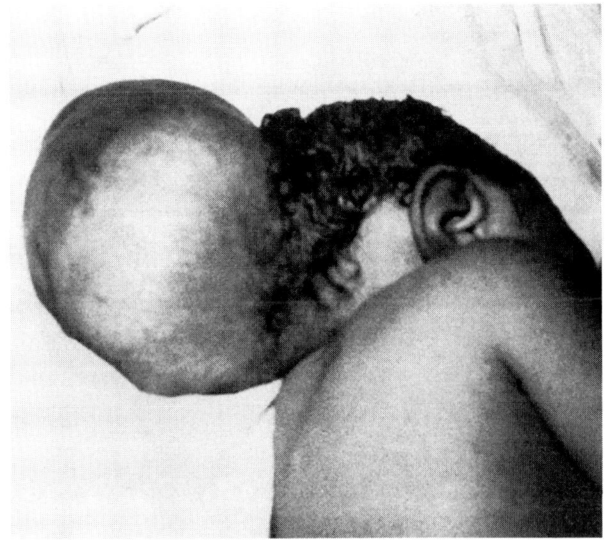

Fig. 50.46 Neonate with occipital encephalocele (From Chatterjee, M.S. et al. (1985) *Am. J. Obstet. Gynecol.* **153**, 646. Used with permission.)

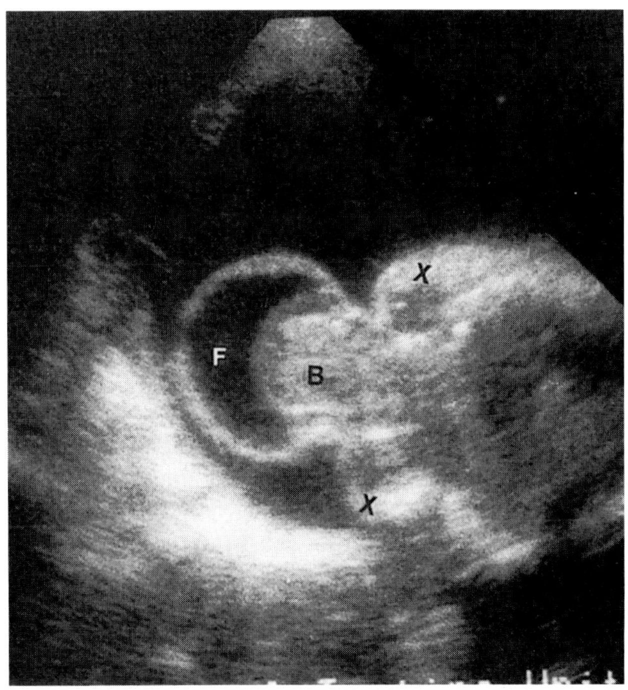

Fig. 50.47 Prenatal sonogram at 33 weeks' gestation of fetus with frontoethmoidal meningoencephalocele (F). Herniated brain tissue (B) and outer orbital margins (X) are marked. (From Donnenfeld, A.E. et al. (1988) *Am. J. Perinatol.* **5**, 51. Used with permission.)

present as a cyst within a cyst and therefore resemble a myelocystocele[222].

With current high-resolution sonographic equipment, there are few lesions that should be mistaken for an occipital encephalocele. While a cystic hygroma is located in the posterior occipital region, a cranial defect is not present and the

157. Yakovlev PI & Wadsworth RC. Schizencephalies. A study of the congenital clefts in the cerebral mantle. II Clefts with hydrocephalus and lips separated. *J. Neuropthol. Exp. Neurol.* **5**:169–206, 1946.
158. Barkovich AJ & Norman D. MR imaging of schizencephaly. *Am. J. Roentgenol.* **150**:1391–1396, 1988.
159. Lituania M, Passamonti U, Cordone S, Magnano GM & Toma P. Schizencephaly: prenatal diagnosis by computed sonography and magnetic resonance imaging. *Prenat. Diagn.* **9**:649–655, 1989.
160. Miller GM, Stears JC, Guggenheim MA & Wilkening GN. Schizencephaly: a clinical and CT study. *Neurology* **34**:997–1001, 1984.
161. Komarniski C, Cyr DR, Mack LA & Weinberger E. Prenatal diagnosis of schizencephaly. *J. Ultrasound Med.* **9**:305–307, 1990.

Dandy–Walker malformation

162. Hill LM, Martin JG, Fries J & Hixson J. The role of the transcerebellar view in the detection of fetal central nervous system anomaly. *Am. J. Obstet. Gynecol.* **164**:1220–1224, 1991.
163. Mahony BS, Callen PW, Filly RA & Hoddick WK. The fetal cisterna magna. *Radiology* **153**:773–776, 1984.
164. Pretorius DH, Kallman C, Grafe MR, Budorick NE & Stamm ER. Linear echoes in the fetal cisterna magna. *J. Ultrasound Med.* **11**:125–128, 1992.
165. Laing FC, Frates MC, Brown DL, Benson CB, DiSalvo DN & Doubilet PM. Sonography of the fetal posterior fossa: false appearance of mega-cisterna magna and Dandy–Walker variant. *Radiology* **192**:247–251, 1994.
166. Hirsch J-F, Pierre-Kahn A, Renier D, Sainte-Rose C & Hoppe-Hirsch E. The Dandy–Walker malformation. A review of 40 cases. *J. Neurosurg.* **61**:515–522, 1984.
167. Russ PD, Pretorius DH & Johnson MJ. Dandy–Walker syndrome: a review of fifteen cases evaluated by prenatal sonography. *Am. J. Obstet. Gynecol.* **161**:401–406, 1989.
168. Nyberg DA, Cyr DR, Mack LA, Fitzsimmons J, Hickok D & Mahony BS. The Dandy–Walker malformation prenatal sonographic diagnosis and its clinical significance. *J. Ultrasound Med.* **7**:65–71, 1988.
169. Pilu G, Romero R, DePalma L et al. Antenatal diagnosis and obstetric management of Dandy–Walker syndrome. *J. Reprod. Med.* **31**:1017–1022, 1986.
170. Hart MN, Malamud N & Ellis WG. The Dandy–Walker syndrome. *Neurol.* **22**:771–780, 1972.
171. Gardner E, O'Rahilly R & Prolo D. The Dandy–Walker and Arnold–Chiari malformations. Clinical, developmental and teratological considerations. *Arch. Neurol.* **32**:393–407, 1975.
172. Murray JC, Johnson JA & Bird TD. Dandy–Walker malformation: etiologic heterogeneity and empiric recurrence risks. *Clin. Genet.* **28**:272–283, 1985.
173. Achiron R & Tadmor O. Screening for fetal anomalies during the first trimester of pregnancy: transvaginal versus transabdominal sonography. *Ultrasound Obstet. Gynecol.* **1**:186–191, 1991.
174. Achiron R & Achiron A. Transvaginal ultrasonic assessment of the early fetal brain. *Ultrasound Obstet. Gynecol.* **1**:336–344, 1991.
175. Sawaya R & McLaurin RL. Dandy–Walker syndrome. Clinical analysis of 23 cases. *J. Neurosurg.* **55**:89–98, 1981.
176. Nyberg DA, Mahony BS, Hegge FN, Hickok D, Luthy DA & Kapur R. Enlarged cisterna magna and the Dandy–Walker malformation: factors associated with chromosome abnormalities. *Obstet. Gynecol.* **77**:436–442, 1991.
177. Altman NR, Naidich TP & Braffman BH. Posterior fossa malformations. *AJNR* **13**:691–724, 1992.
178. Thurmond AS, Nelson DW, Lowensohn RI, Young WP & Davis L. Enlarged cisterna magna in trisomy 18: prenatal ultrasonographic diagnosis. *Am. J. Obstet. Gynecol.* **161**:83–85, 1989.
179. Hill LM, Marchese S, Peterson CS & Fries J. The effect of trisomy 18 on transverse cerebellar diameter. *Am. J. Obstet. Gynecol.* **165**:72–75, 1991.
180. Hill LM, Guzick D, Fries J, Hixson J & Rivello D. The transverse cerebellar diameter in estimating gestational age in the large for gestational age fetus. *Obstet. Gynecol.* **75**:981–985, 1990.
181. Estroff JA, Scott MR & Benacerraf BR. Dandy–Walker variant: Prenatal sonographic features and clinical outcome. *Radiology* **185**:755–758, 1992.
182. Friede RL. Uncommon syndromes of cerebellar vermian aplasia. II. Tecto-cerebellar dysraphia with occipital encephalocele. *Dev. Med. Child Neurol.* **20**:764–772, 1978.

Cerebellar abnormalities

183. Crome L, Cowie V & Slater E. A statistical note on cerebellar and brain-stem weight in mongolism. *J. Met. Defic. Res.* **10**:69–72, 1966.
184. Hill LM, Martin JG, Fries J & Hixson J. The role of the transcerebellar view in the detection of fetal central nervous system anomaly. *Am. J. Obstet. Gynecol.* **164**:1220–1224, 1991.
185. Hill LM, Marchese S, Peterson C & Fries J. The effect of trisomy 18 on transverse cerebellar diameter. *Am. J. Obstet. Gynecol.* **165**:72–75, 1991.
186. Ceballus R, Ch'ien LT, Whitley RJ & Brans YW. Cerebellar hypoplasia in an infant with congenital cytomegalovirus infection. *Pediatrics* **57**:155–157, 1976.
187. Fischer DS & Jonas HM. Cerebellar hypoplasia resulting from cytosine arabinoside treatment in the neonatal hamster. *Clin. Res.* **13**:540, 1965.
188. Gessaga EC, Herrick MK & Urich H. Necrosis of the fetal brain stem with cerebellar hypoplasia. *Acta Neuropathol.* (Berl.) **69**:326–331, 1986.
189. Mendelsohn DB, Hertzanu Y, Glass RBJ & Spino F. Unilateral cerebellar hypoplasia. *J. Comput. Assist. Tomogr.* **7**:1077–1078, 1983.
190. Joubert M, Eisenring J-J, Robb JP & Andermann F. Familial agenesis of the cerebellar vermis. *Neurology* **19**:813–825, 1969.
191. Kendall B, Kingsley D, Lambert SR, Taylor D & Finn P. Joubert syndrome: a clinico-radiological study. *Neuroradiology* **31**:502–506, 1990.
192. Michaud J, Mizrahi EM & Urich H. Agenesis of the vermis with fusion of the cerebellar hemispheres, septo-optic dysplasia and associated anomalies. *Acta. Neuropathol.* (Berl.) **56**:161–166, 1982.
193. Daffos F, Forestier F, Mac Aleese J et al. Fetal curarization for prenatal magnetic resonance imaging. *Prenat. Diagn.* **8**:311–314, 1988.

Anencephaly

194. Campbell S, Johnstone FD, Holt EM & May P. Anencephaly: early ultrasonic diagnosis and active management. *Lancet* **2**:122–126, 1972.
195. Wilkins-Haug L & Freedman W. Progressions of exencephaly to anencephaly in the human fetus – an ultrasound perspective. *Prenat. Diagn.* **11**:227–233, 1991.
196. Nañangas JC. A comparison of the growth of the body dimensions of anencephalic human fetuses with normal growth as determined by graphic analysis: an empirical formula. *Am. J. Anat.* **35**:455–494, 1925.
197. Kurtzke JF, Goldberg ID & Kurland LT. The distribution of deaths from congenital malformations of the nervous system. *Neurology* **23**:483–496, 1973.
198. Medical Task Force on Anencephaly. The infant with anencephaly. *N. Engl. J. Med.* **332**:669–674, 1990.
199. Byrne J & Warburton D. Neural tube defects in spontaneous abortions. *Am. J. Med. Genet.* **25**:327–333, 1986.
200. Khoury MJ, Erickson JD & James LM. Etiologic heterogeneity of neural tube defects: clues from epidemiology. *Am. J. Epidemiol.* **115**:538–548, 1982.
201. Brackbill Y. The role of the cortex in orienting: orienting reflex in an anencephalic infant. *Devel. Psychol.* **5**:195–201, 1971.
202. Medearis DN Jr & Holmes LB. Anencephalic infants as organ donors: two unaddressed issues. *Am. J. Hum. Genet.* **45**(suppl):A54 abstract, 1989.
203. Visser GHA, Laurini RN, de Vries JIP, Bekedam DJ & Prechtl HFR. Abnormal motor behavior in anencephalic fetuses. *Early Hum. Devel.* **12**:173–182, 1985.
204. Goldstein RB, Filly RA & Callen PW. Sonography of anencephaly: pitfalls in early diagnosis. *J. Clin. Ultrasound* **17**:397–402, 1989.
205. Goldstein RB & Filly RA. Prenatal diagnosis of anencephaly: spectrum of sonographic appearances and distinctions from the amniotic band syndrome. *Am. J. Roentgenol.* **151**:547–550, 1988.

Exencephaly

206. Cox GG, Rosenthal SJ & Holsapple JW. Exencephaly: sonographic findings and radiologic-pathologic correlation. *Radiology* **155**:755–756, 1985.
207. Hendricks SK, Cyr DR, Nyberg DA, Raabe R & Mack LA. Exencephaly – clinical and ultrasonic correlation to anencephaly. *Obstet. Gynecol.* **72**:898–901, 1988.
208. Kennedy KA, Flick KJ & Thurmond AS. First-trimester diagnosis of exencephaly. *Am. J. Obstet. Gynecol.* **162**:461–463, 1990.
209. Patten RM, Van Allen M, Mack LA et al. Limb–body wall complex: In utero sonographic diagnosis of a complicated fetal malformation. *Am. J. Radiol.* **146**:1019–1024, 1986.

Iniencephaly

210. Mórocz I, Szeifert GT, Molnár P, Tóth Z, Csécsei K & Papp Z. Prenatal diagnosis and pathoanatomy of iniencephaly. *Clin. Genet.* **30**:81–86, 1986.
211. Meizner I, Levi A, Katz M & Maor E. Iniencephaly. A case report. *J. Reprod. Med.* **37**:885–888, 1992.

Encephaloceles

212. Mealey J, Ozenitis AJ & Hockley AA. The prognosis of encephaloceles. *J. Neurosurg.* **32**:209–218, 1970.
213. Lorber J & Schofield JC. The prognosis of occipital encephalocele. *Z. Kinderchir.* **28**:347–351, 1979.
214. Jeanty P, Shah D, Zaleski W, Ulm J & Fleischer A. Prenatal diagnosis of fetal cephalocele: a sonographic spectrum. *Am. J. Perinatol.* **8**:144–149, 1991.
215. Karach SB & Urich H. Occipital encephalocele: a morphological study. *J. Neurol. Sci.* **15**:89–112, 1972.
216. Suwanwela C & Suwanwela N. A morphological classification of sincipital encephalomeningoceles. *J. Neurosurg.* **36**:201–211, 1972.
217. Thu A & Kyu H. Epidemiology of frontoethmoidal encephalomeningocele in Burma. *J. Epidemiol. Commun. Health* **38**:89–98, 1984.
218. Pollock JA, Newton TH & Hoyt WF. Transphenoidal and transethmoidal encephaloceles. A review of clinical and roentgen features of 8 cases. *Radiology* **90**:442–453, 1968.
219. Goldstein RB, LaPidus AS & Filly RA. Fetal cephaloceles: diagnosis with ultrasound. *Radiology* **180**:803–808, 1991.
220. Winninger SJ & Donnenfeld AE. Syndromes identified in fetuses with prenatally diagnosed cephaloceles. *Prenat. Diagn.* **14**:839–843, 1994.
221. Brown MS & Sheridan-Pereira M. Outlook for the child with a cephalocele. *Pediatrics* **90**:914–919, 1992.
222. Budorick NE, Pretorius DH, McGahan JP, Grafe MR, James HE & Slivka J. Cephalocele detection in utero: sonographic and clinical features. *Ultrasound Obstet. Gynecol.* **5**:77–85, 1995.
223. Holmes LB, Driscoll SG & Atkins L. Etiologic heterogeneity of neural tube defects. *N. Engl. J. Med.* **294**:365–369, 1976.
224. Date I, Yagyu Y, Asari S & Ohmoto T. Long-term outcome in surgically treated encephalocele. *Surg. Neurol.* **40**:125–130, 1993.
225. Hanley ML, Guzman ER, Vintzileos AM, Leiman S, Doyle A & Shen-Schwarz S. Prenatal ultrasonographic detection of regression of an encephalocele. *J. Ultrasound Med.* **15**:71–74, 1996.
226. Bronshtein M & Zimmer EZ. Transvaginal sonographic follow-up on the formation of fetal encephalocele at 13–19 weeks' gestation. *Obstet. Gynecol.* **78**:28–30, 1991.
227. Bronshtein M, Bar-Hava I & Blumenfeld Z. Early second-trimester sonographic appearance of occipital haemangioma simulating encephalocele. *Prenat. Diagn.* **12**:695–698, 1992.
228. Ferriman EL & McCormack J. An epidermal scalp cyst simulating an encephalocele. [Letter to the editor]. *Prenat. Diagn.* **15**:981–984, 1995.

Spina bifida

229. McLone DG & Knepper PA. The cause of Chiari II malformation: a unified theory. *Pediatr. Neurosci.* **15**:1–12, 1989.
230. Laurence KM & Tew BJ. The natural history of spina bifida cystica and cranium bifidum cysticum: the central nervous system malformations in South Wales Part IV. *Arch. Dis. Child.* **467**:127–138, 1971.
231. Pang D. Surgical complications of open spinal dysraphism. *Neurosurg Clin. N. Am.* **6**:243–257, 1995.
232. Hahn YS. Open myelomeningocele. *Neurosurg Clin. N. Am.* **6**:231–241, 1995.
233. Lorber J & Ward AM. Spina bifida – vanishing nightmare? *Arch. Dis. Child.* **60**:1086–1091, 1985.
234. Creasy MR & Alberman ED. Congenital malformations of the central nervous system in spontaneous abortions. *J. Med. Genet.* **13**:9–16, 1976.
235. Greenberg F, James LM & Oakley GP. Estimates of birth prevalence rates of spina bifida in the United States from computer-generated maps. *Am. J. Obstet. Gynecol.* **145**:570–573, 1983.
236. Davis CF & Young DG. The changing incidence of neural tube defects in Scotland. *J. Pediatr. Surg.* **26**:516–518, 1991.
237. Timson J. The sex ratio in spina bifida. *Genetica* **40**:427–433, 1969.
238. Main DM & Mennut MT. Neural tube defects: issues in prenatal diagnosis and counselling. *Obstet. Gynecol.* **67**:1–16, 1986.
239. Khoury MJ, Erickson JD & James LM. Etiologic heterogeneity of neural tube defects: clues from epidemiology. *Am. J. Epidemiol.* **115**:538–548, 1982.
240. Lammer EJ, Sever LE & Oakley GP Jr. Teratogen update: Valproic acid. *Teratology* **35**:465–473, 1987.
241. Rosa FW. Spina bifida in infants of women treated with carbamazine during pregnancy. *N. Engl. J. Med.* **324**:674–677, 1991.
242. Nyberg DA, Shepard T, Mack LA, Hirsch J, Luthy D & Fitzsimmons J. Significance of a single umbilical artery in fetuses with CNS malformations. *J. Ultrasound Med.* **7**:265–273, 1988.
243. Harmon JP, Hiett AK, Palmer CG & Golichowski AM. Prenatal ultrasound detection of isolated neural tube defects: Is cytogenetic evaluation warranted? *Obstet. Gynecol.* **86**:595–599, 1995.
244. Kalousek DK, Fetch N & Paradice BA. *Pathology of the Human Embryo and Previable Fetus: an Atlas*, p. 188. New York: Springer-Verlag; 1990.
245. Kalousek DK, Fetch N & Paradice BA. *Pathology of the Human Embryo and Previable Fetus: an Atlas*, p. 190. New York: Springer-Verlag; 1990.
246. Dimmick JE & Kalousek DG. *Development Pathology of the Embryo and Fetus*, p. 102. Phildelphia: J.B. Lippincott Co, 1992.
247. Nyberg DA, Kramer D, Resta RG et al. Prenatal sonographic findings of trisomy 18: Review of 47 cases. *J. Ultrasound Med.* **2**:103–113, 1993.
248. Benacerraf BR, Miller WA & Frigoletto FD. Sonographic detection of fetuses with trisomies 13 and 18: accuracy and limitations. *Am. J. Obstet. Gynecol.* **158**:404–409, 1988.
249. Nyberg DA, Resta RG, Luthy DA, Hickok DE, Mahony BS & Hirsch JH. Prenatal sonographic findings of Down syndrome: review of 94 cases. *Obstet. Gynecol.* **76**:370–377, 1990.
250. Babcook CJ, Goldstein RB & Filly RA. Prenatally detected fetal meylomeningocele: is karyotype analysis warranted? *Radiology* **194**:491–494, 1995.
251. Drugan A, Johnson MP, Dvorin E et al. Aneuploidy with neural tube defects: another reason for complete evaluation in patients with suspected ultrasound anomalies or elevated maternal serum alpha-fetoprotein. *Fetal Ther* **4**:88–92, 1989.
252. Holmes LB, Driscoll SG & Atkins L. Etiologic heterogeneity of neural-tube defects. *N. Engl. J. Med.* **294**:365–369, 1976.
253. Yen S & MacMahon B. Genetics of anencephaly and spina bifida? *Lancet* **2**:623–626, 1968.
254. Smithells RW, Nevin NC, Seller MJ et al. Further experience of vitamin supplementation for prevention of neural tube defect recurrences. *Lancet* **1**:1027–1031, 1983.
255. Mills JL, McPartlin JM, Kirk PN et al. Homocysteine metabolism in pregnancies complicated by neural-tube defects. *Lancet* **345**:149–151, 1995.
256. Seeds JW & Jones D. Lipomyelomeningocele. Prenatal diagnosis and management. *Obstet. Gynecol.* (suppl) **67**:34–37, 1986.
257. Cameron AH. The spinal cord lesion in spina bifida cystica. *Lancet* **2**:171–174, 1956.
258. Emery JZ & Lendon RG. The local cord lesion in neurospinal dysraphism (meningomyelocele). *J. Pathol.* **110**:83–96, 1973.

259. Williams RA & Barth RA. In utero sonographic recognition of diastematomyelia. *Am. J. Roentgenol* **144**:87–88, 1985.
260. Silverman FN. *Caffey's Pediatric X-ray Diagnosis: an integrated teaching approach*, pp. 295–300. Chicago: Year Book Medical Publishers, 1985.
261. Cleland J. Contribution to the study of spina bifida, encephalocele and anencephalus. *J. Anat. Physiol.* **17**:257–292, 1883.
262. Chiari H. Über Veränderungen des Kleinhirns infolge von Hydrocephalie des Grosshirns. *Dtsch. Med. Wochenschr.* **17**:1172–1175, 1891.
263. Chiari H. Veränderungen des Kleinhirns, des Pons und der Medulla oblongata in Folge von congenitaler Hydrocephalie des Grosshirns. *Den. Kschrift. Akad. Wiss. Wien* **63**:71–116, 1896.
264. Arnold J. Myelocyste, Transposition von Gewebskeimen und sympodie. *Beitr. Pathol. Anat.* **16**:1–28, 1894.
265. Russel DS & Donald C. The mechanism of internal hydrocephalus in spina bifida. *Brain* **58**:203–215, 1935.
266. Garceau GJ. The film terminale syndrome (the cord-traction syndrome). *J. Bone Joint Surg.* **35-A**:711–716, 1993.
267. Müller F & O'Rahilly R. The human chondrocranium at the end of the embryonic period, proper, with particular reference to the nervous system. *Am. J. Anat.* **159**:33–58, 1980.
268. Barry A, Patten BM & Stewart BH. Possible factors in the development of the Arnold–Chiari malformation. *J. Neurosurg.* **14**:285–301, 1957.
269. Variend S & Emery JL. The weight of the cerebellum of children with myelomengingocele. *Dev. Med. Child Neurol.* **15** (suppl 29):77–83, 1973.
270. Van Gool JD, Bruinese HW & Kriek R. Early fetal movements in myelomeningocele. (Letter.) *Lancet* **1**:917–918, 1986.
271. Epstein F, Marlin A, Hochwald G & Ransohoff J. Myelomeningocele: a progressive intrauterine disease. *Dev. Med. Child Neurol.* **18** (suppl 37):12–15, 1976.
272. Leonard CO & Freeman JM. Spina bifida: a new disease. *Pediatrics* **68**:136–137, 1981.
273. Warsof SL, Abramowicz JS, Sayegh SK & Levy DL. Lower limb movements and urologic function in fetuses with neural tube and other central nervous system defects. *Fetal Ther.* **3**:129–134, 1988.
274. McLone DG, Czyzewski D, Raimondi AJ & Sommens RC. Central nervous system infections as a limiting factor in the intelligence of children with myelomeningocele. *Pediatrics* **70**:338–342, 1982.
275. McLaughlin JF & Shurtleff DB. Management of the fetus and newborn with neural tube defects. *J. Perinatol.* **4**:3–12, 1984.
276. Roberts CJ, Hibbard BM, Roberts EE, Evans KT, Laurence KM & Robertson IB. Diagnositic effectiveness of ultrasound in detection of neural tube defect. The South Wales Experience of 2509 scans (1977–1982) in high-risk mothers. *Lancet* **2**:1068–1069, 1983.
277. Roberts AB & Campbell S. Fetal head measurements in spina bifida. *Br. J. Obstet. Gynaecol.* **87**:927–928, 1980.
278. Nicolaides K, Campbell S, Gabbe S & Guidelti R. Ultrasound screening for spina bifida: cranial and cerebellar signs. *Lancet* **2**:71–74, 1986.
279. Van dem Hof MC, Nicolaides KH, Campbell J & Campbell S. Evaluation of the lemon and banana signs in one hundred thirty fetuses with open spina bifida. *Am. J. Obstet. Gynecol.* **162**:322–327, 1990.
280. Williams B. Cerebrospinal fluid pressure gradients in spina bifida cystica, with special reference to the Arnold–Chiari malformation and aqueductal stenosis. *Dev. Med. Child Neurol.* **17** (suppl 35):138–150, 1975.
281. Campbell J, Gilbert WM, Nicolaides KH & Campbell S. Ultrasound screening for spina bifida; cranial and cerebellar signs in a high-risk population. *Obstet. Gynecol.* **70**:247–250, 1987.
282. Goldstein RB, Podrasky AE, Filly RA & Callen PW. Effacement of the fetal cisterna magna in association with myelomeningocele. *Radiology* **172**:409–413, 1989.
283. Babcook C, Golstein RB, Barton RA, Damato NM, Callen PW & Filly RA. Prevalence of ventriculomegaly in association with myelomeningocele: correlation with gestational age and severity of posterior fossa deformity. *Radiology* **190**:703–707, 1994.
284. Laurence KM, Dew JO, Dyer C & Downey KH. Amniocentesis carried out for neural tube indications in South Wales 1973–1981: outcomes of pregnancies and findings in the malformed abortuses. *Prenat. Diagn.* **3**:187–201, 1983.
285. Watson WJ, Chescheir NC, Katz VL & Seeds JW. The role of ultrasound in evaluation of patients with elevated maternal serum alpha-fetoprotein: a review. *Obstet. Gynecol.* **78**:123–128, 1991.
286. Dennis MA, Drose JA, Pretorius DH & Marco-Johnson ML. Normal fetal sacrum simulating spina bifida: 'pseudodysraphism'. *Radiology* **155**:751–754, 1985.
287. Rottem S & Bronshtein M. Transvaginal sonographic diagnosis of congenital anomalies between 9 weeks and 16 weeks, menstrual age. *J. Clin. Ultrasound* **18**:307–314, 1990.
288. Blumenfeld Z, Siegler E & Bronshtein M. The early diagnosis of neural tube defects. *Prenat. Diagn.* **13**:863–871, 1993.
289. Morrow RJ, McNay MB & Whittle MJ. Ultrasound detection of neural tube defects in patients with elevated maternal serum alphafetoprotein. *Obstet. Gynecol.* **78**:1055–1057, 1991.
290. Nadel AS, Green JK, Holmes LB, Frigoletto FD JR & Benacerraf BR. Absence of need for amniocentesis in patients with elevated levels of maternal serum alpha-fetoprotein and normal ultrasonographic examinations. *N. Engl. J. Med.* **323**:557–561, 1990.
291. Robbin M, Filly RA, Fell S et al. Elevated levels of amniotic fluid alpha-fetoprotein: sonographic evaluation. *Radiology* **188**:165–169, 1993.
292. Kollias SS, Goldstein RB, Cogen PH & Filly RA. Prenatally detected myelomeningoceles: sonographic accuracy in estimation of the spinal level. *Radiology* **185**:109–112, 1992.
293. Thornton JG, Lilford RJ & Newcombe RG. Tables for estimation of individual risks of fetal neural tube and ventral wall defects, incorporating prior probability, maternal serum alpha fetoprotein levels, and ultrasonographic examination results. *Am. J. Obstet. Gynecol.* **164**:154–160, 1991.

Conclusion

294. *Guidelines for Performance of the Antepartum Obstetrical Ultrasound Examination.* American Institue of Ultrasound in Medicine, 1994.

Diagnosis and management of fetal heart disease

51

J.A. Copel, C.S. Kleinman and A. Friedman

Introduction

The diagnosis and management of fetal cardiac disease has evolved into a distinct cross-disciplinary subspeciality over the past 15 years. In many ways, this has foreshadowed much of perinatal medicine. From the beginning of fetal cardiac assessment it has been obvious that neither of the specialities most actively involved, the general fetal imagers and the pediatric cardiologists, had sufficient breadth of training and experience to work independently. Full appreciation of the breadth of fetal cardiac diseases that can be present, as well as the many associated extracardiac anomalies that can also occur[1], requires a collaborative approach, as does the rational antepartum and intrapartum management of affected pregnancies. Finally, appropriate prenatal counselling requires a complete familiarity with up-to-date postnatal management of pediatric patients with cardiac disease, all further necessitating close teamwork in the diagnosis and management of affected pregnancies.

The first step: referral for prenatal diagnosis

Most patients referred for fetal cardiac evaluation are sent because of historical risk factors placing them at increased risk of carrying a fetus with congenital heart disease. Most of these risks are established from epidemiological studies. Reliance on small antenatal or postnatal case series is insufficient to determine risks accurately for rare events.

The background risk of congenital heart disease in large neonatal screening studies from unselected populations is generally estimated to be approximately 8/1000 births, although the true number may be somewhat higher[2,3]. It is possible that neonatal case ascertainment underestimates the true incidence of cardiac anomalies, since some children will not manifest congenital heart disease until after closure of the ductus arteriosus and/or the postnatal decrease in pulmonary vascular resistance, which may occur several days postpartum. Additionally, some children with ventricular septal defects may not develop clinically noticeable murmurs until weeks or months after birth, and some mild lesions such as bicuspid aortic valve may not become apparent for months or years[2,4]. The incidence of congenital heart disease may be even higher in fetuses, especially if case detection is sought in the midtrimester, as early spontaneous loss of severely anomalous fetuses may also remove these fetuses from postnatal series.

Actuarial studies suggest that families having a previous child with congenital heart disease in the absence of a recognized genetic syndrome have a 2–3% risk of recurrence with subsequent pregnancies, although there may be some variation with different lesions[2,5,6]. If the previous child had a cardiac anomaly as part of a syndrome, then the recurrence risk is the same as that for the syndrome (e.g. autosomal dominant, autosomal recessive). With advances in our understanding of the genetic basis of fetal anomalies, including congenital heart disease, our counselling regarding recurrence risks is evolving.

Mothers with congenital heart disease have an increased risk of delivering a child with a cardiac anomaly. This risk has been calculated to range from 5–10%[5–9]. As with previously affected children, the subsequently affected family member may have more severe or less severe disease, or may in many cases have an apparently different type of disease (e.g. first affected family member coarctation of the aorta, next family member tetralogy of Fallot). Recurrence risks for affected fathers have not been established.

Many patients are referred for fetal echocardiography because of more distant family histories of congenital heart disease. The recurrence risks for second- and third-degree relatives must begin to approach those of the general population, but in practice many of these families have been emotionally traumatized by the loss of a child, and the reassurance provided by a normal prenatal echocardiogram is significantly reassuring.

Whether screening based on historical risk factors is 'cost effective' in the current era of cost cutting in the United States depends on many factors, but perhaps none is as important as the perspective of the person making the decision. If we assume a conservative $500 cost for a Level II ultrasound and fetal echocardiogram, for those families with a previously affected child imparting a 2% recurrence risk, the cost of finding another affected child in the same family would be approximately $25 000. This is not a large amount of money, but certainly cannot be expected to be offset simply by cost-savings in the care of the correctly identified child. More important than simple dollar-and-cents arguments, we believe, is the peace of mind provided to the 98% of families who are given reassuring news. This cannot be cost-accounted in a simple fashion.

Many drugs[10,11] have been identified as potential cardiac teratogens, e.g.:

- Vitamin A analogues
  - Isotretinoin[12] (topical preparations not a risk[13])
  - Nutritional supplements[14]
- Antiseizure medications
  - Phenytoin[15,16]
  - Carbamazepine[17]
  - Valproic acid[18]
  - Trimethadione[19]
- Alcohol[10]
- Lithium carbonate[10]

Many of the risks available in the literature are derived from retrospective studies, or from voluntary report registries, either of which might exaggerate the true risks. For any medically indicated medication, such as antiseizure drugs, the risks to the patient of not taking the drug must be balanced against the potential risks to the fetus[10]. For more elective medications, such as isotretinoin (Accutane™), or vitamin A nutritional supplements[12–14], discontinuing the medication well before attempting conception appears to be judicious. The teratogenicity of the antiseizure medications[15–19] may be attenuated with folate supplementation[20].

Maternal metabolic derangements may be teratogenic, and both diseases in this category include the fetal heart among their target organs. Diabetes mellitus carries a higher risk of congenital heart disease in the offspring of affected women, with the risk for cardiac and other abnormalities inversely proportional to the degree of metabolic control achieved during embryogenesis[21–24]. Phenylketonuria carries similar risks[25,26]. Preconceptional metabolic control is the mainstay of preventive treatment in both diseases.

The preceding referral indications have been historical in nature; those remaining are intrinsic to the fetus, and therefore can be expected to impart substantially higher risks. We have made it a practice to perform fetal echocardiography on virtually all fetuses identified to have structural abnormalities. It is beyond the scope of this chapter to review all of the associations between extracardiac and cardiac anomalies in fetuses and neonates[27]. It is important to note that syndrome identification is dependent on complete ascertainment of all effects in the fetus. For those families choosing to terminate a pregnancy with multiple fetal anomalies, the combination of ultrasound, and perhaps autopsy, will be relied upon to make a full diagnosis. Accurate counselling regarding recurrence risks is dependent on a correct diagnosis. For those families continuing pregnancies with a fetus with multiple anomalies, preparation for postnatal management can be planned based on the information available from prenatal studies.

Fetuses with polyhydramnios have a high rate of congenital anomalies, especially when the amniotic fluid index exceeds 24 cm[28]. We have also found that a great many fetuses with non-immune hydrops have either structural cardiac anomalies or fetal arrhythmias as the underlying cause[29,30].

While Chapter 61 addresses the management of fetal arrhythmias, it is important to emphasize here the association between fetal bradycardia and structural heart disease. About half of fetuses with complete heart block have complex cardiac anomalies as the underlying cause[29–32]. These are usually either abnormalities of situs (the heterotaxy syndromes including polysplenia), or other lesions resulting in absence of the normal electrical connection between the atria and ventricles. Fetal tachycardia is rarely associated with structural heart disease.

In 1987 we reported our experience with the four-chamber view as part of a formal fetal echocardiogram[33]. In that retrospective study, we found that 94% of fetuses with congenital heart disease had an identifiable abnormality on the four-chamber view of the heart. That study was imperfect as an evaluation of the four-chamber view as a screening test for several important reasons. It was not a prospective study in a low-risk population, rather the study was retrospective in a population referred for their risks of having a fetus with congenital heart disease. The diagnoses were also known to us at the time the contribution of the four-chamber view to the recognition of cardiac abnormalities was recorded. Nevertheless, the point of the report was to stimulate examination of the four-chamber view in a more general population.

This has now been the subject of numerous other reports[34–42], with the sensitivity in low-risk populations ranging from as low as 0%[40] to as high as 81%[37]. The final sensitivity numbers are, in part, dependent on the postnatal case ascertainment method, as without careful follow-up on all fetuses examined, there might be an inflation of the sensitivity, should failures to appreciate pathology not be reported back to the study centre. The wide variation in sensitivity makes interpretation of the literature difficult; however, we believe that the final consensus will fall at about 50% sensitivity. Far from indicating a lack of value to the four-chamber view, we believe that this portion of the population with congenital heart disease represents the most severe cases, those most likely to benefit from prenatal diagnosis, and that finding half the affected fetuses is better than finding none. Whether the addition of outflow tract views will enhance sensitivity to heart defects remains preliminary[43], but common sense suggests that the more of the fetus we scrutinize as part of our routine examination the more we will find.

Conversely, the referral of fetuses with abnormal four-chamber views remains a major contributor to the pool of prenatal diagnoses of congenital heart disease. We have found that 50–60% of fetuses referred for this indication do, in fact, have cardiac abnormalities (unpublished data).

Fetal cardiovascular physiology

Understanding the appearance of the normal and the abnormal fetal heart first requires an appreciation of the physiology of the heart in utero[44]. More detail is found in Ch. 13, but it is relevant to review a few facts here. There are several major differences between the fetal heart and the neonatal heart. The fetal ventricles work in parallel with each other rather than serially, with right ventricular output being slightly greater than left. Because of the physiological shunts that are present in the fetus, the foramen ovale between the atria and the ductus arteriosus between the pulmonary artery and the aorta, the pressures generated in the ventricles are very nearly equal, and the ventricles therefore are approximately equal in size. When discussing cardiac output, the operative consideration is the combined ventricular output. Hypoplasia of one ventricle may be compensated for by increased flow through the other ventricle with no net effect on combined output.

The intracardiac shunt between the atria serves the important function of directing oxygenated blood returning from the placenta to the left ventricle. The umbilical venous return enters the inferior vena cava through the ductus venosus near the inferior vena cava's insertion into the right atrium. The ductus venosus is quite narrow, and blood flows through it at high velocities. There is pronounced streaming of blood from different sources in the inferior vena cava, with little mixing of the ductus venosus flow with flow from the lower body.

The highly oxygenated stream in the inferior vena cava remains in the dorsal and leftward portion of the vessel, and is directed across the foramen ovale by the crista dividens. The remaining inferior venal caval flow, as well as superior venal caval blood, crosses the tricuspid valve into the right ventricle. The most oxygenated blood has thus been separated by flow into the left atrium, where it mixes with the relatively minor pulmonary venous return contribution before entering the left ventricle. Its major distribution is to the coronaries, the brain and the upper limbs. Only about a third of this blood crosses the aortic isthmus to enter the descending aorta.

The deoxygenated blood in the right ventricle is ejected into the main pulmonary trunk, where most flows into the ductus arteriosus and from there perfuses the lower trunk, the viscera, the lower limbs and, most importantly, the placenta where it can be reoxygenated. The right ventricle can be thought of as always perfusing the organ of respiration, the placenta before birth and the lungs after.

Fetal echo technique

The evaluation of the fetal heart requires the sonographer or sonologist to be flexible in order to accommodate the many varying positions of the fetus. The acquisition of the necessary images for a complete diagnostic evaluation cannot always be performed in a rigid sequence, but all must be achieved[45].

The first order of business is to establish fetal position, and abdominal situs. The fetal head and spine must be located, which should immediately orient the fetus in terms of the right and left sides of the fetal body. The stomach must be seen on the fetal left, and the umbilical vein should be seen as it curves to the fetal right. Tilting cephalad while maintaining the same relationship to the axial plane of the fetus should bring the four-chamber view into the image.

The apex of the fetal heart should be seen on the left side of the body, concordant with the stomach. The right and left atria should be approximately equal in size, with the left atrium closest to the spine. The superior and inferior vena cavae should be seen entering the right atrium, while the left atrium should have the flap valve of the foramen ovale visible within it. The pulmonary veins can also be seen to enter the left atrium. The foramen ovale can be seen in the midportion of the atrial septum and should be the only communication between the atria. It occupies about a third of the length of the atrial septum.

In the fetal four-chamber view both ventricles should appear approximately equal in size, although typically the right ventricle is slightly larger than the left, due to the slightly greater stroke volume of the fetal right ventricle. Neither ventricle should dominate the cardiac apex, however. The chamber closest to the anterior chest wall should be the right ventricle, notable for its trabeculated walls and the presence of the moderator band near its apex. The left ventricle has a smoother appearance, and the papillary muscles can be seen within it.

The interventricular septum is best examined when the orientation of the heart places the septum horizontally on the screen, allowing the sonologist to use the axial resolution of the image. When the septum is vertical on the screen, one is relying on lateral resolution to see the thinnest portion of the wall, and the artefactual appearance of septal defects may be observed at the thinnest portion of the septum, just below the atrioventricular valves.

Examination of the atrioventricular valves should also be a part of the four-chamber view. The tricuspid valve should be seen to insert into the interventricular septum slightly closer to the cardiac apex than does the mitral valve. Failure to observe this relationship, or the visualization of both valves inserting linearly into the septum, should raise the question of an atrioventricular septal defect, also known as an endocardial cushion defect or an atrioventricular canal defect. Free movement of both valves should be present. The valves can be assessed with the orientation of the septum either horizontal or vertical on the screen.

The axis of the interventricular septum should be approximately 45° ± 15°[46,47]. Deviation toward the right suggests mesocardia, which may be seen with the heterotaxy syndromes, atrioventricular septal defects, or right lung hypoplasia. Deviation to the left can be seen with double outlet right ventricle, and other outflow tract abnormalities. While elaborate measurement techniques have been described, simply examining the four-chamber view generally suffices in our experience. Inclusion of this new criterion as part of the four-chamber view may improve the sensitivity of this screening approach.

Slight rotation of the transducer brings the long axis view of the left ventricle (Fig. 51.1). This view is useful to assess the relationship between the interventricular septum and the ascending aorta. Fetuses with a discontinuity between the septum and the aorta may have an anterior displacement of the aorta, as can be seen with double outlet right ventricle and with tetralogy of Fallot (Fig. 51.2)[48]. It is also important to confirm that the posterior wall of the aorta is contiguous with the mitral valve. The mitral valve can be seen to move freely in this view, although the tricuspid valve is not seen. Movement of the aortic valve can also be seen within the aorta. Often an area of sonolucency is seen above the aortic valve in this orientation. This is an artefact of azimuthal resolution from the pulmonary artery as it crosses anteriorly to the aorta. Posterior displacement of the outflow septum may be found in association with complex left ventricular outflow obstruction.

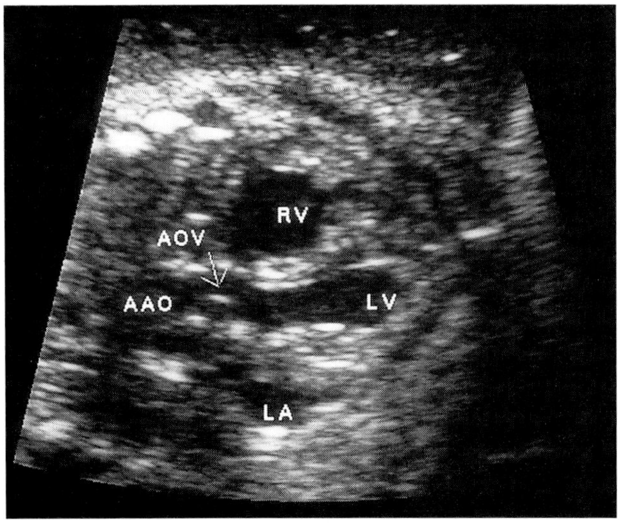

Fig. 51.1 Normal long axis view of the left ventricle at 32 weeks' gestation. The aorta (AAO) can be seen exiting the left ventricle (LV). The intact interventricular septum separates the LV from the right ventricle (RV), extending up to the level of the aortic valve (AOV). (LA = left atrium.)

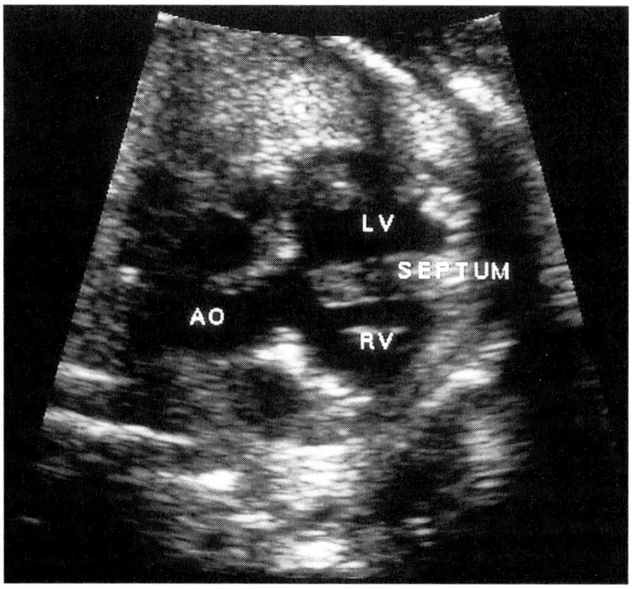

Fig. 51.2 Long axis view of left ventricle in a 32-week fetus with tetralogy of Fallot. The aorta (AO) is seen above the top of the septum. The aortic valve is visible just to the right of the defect. (RV = right ventricle, LV = left ventricle.)

SHORT AXIS VIEW OF THE GREAT VESSELS

The short axis view of the great vessels is useful to confirm that the vessel leaving the anterior ventricle is, in fact, the pulmonary artery. The atria can be seen with the foramenal flap in the left atrium, and the right ventricle and pulmonary artery wrap from the right atrium around the aortic root. With favourable resolution and fetal positioning the aortic valve cusps can be seen. The identification of the pulmonary artery is confirmed by its bifurcation. In the short axis view the right pulmonary artery is seen passing behind the aorta and the initial segment of the ductus arteriosus is the second prong of the fork.

AORTIC AND DUCTAL ARCHES

The correct identification of the great arteries as they leave the heart is an essential component of the fetal echocardiogram. The aorta leaves the posterior ventricle and moves slightly to the right as it ascends in the thorax, while the pulmonary artery leaves the anterior ventricle and is directed to the left before the ductus arteriosus courses posteriorly to enter the descending aorta. The aortic arch view can be achieved by scanning in a sagittal plane from just to the left of the fetal spine with the transducer directed anteriorly and to the right in the fetus. Alternatively the transducer can be placed in a position to look sagittally from the right of the fetal sternum toward the left side of the fetal spine. The arch resembles the handle of an umbrella, taking a full 180° turn in its direction from an initial orientation toward the head to a caudal direction. At the top of the arch, three vessels can be seen leaving the cephalic side of the curve, the innominate, left carotid, and left subclavian arteries.

The course of the ductal arch describes more of a 90° turn as it enters the descending aorta, as a consequence of its more anterior origin just beneath the sternum, and a more horizontal path.

VENOUS CONNECTIONS

The venous connections to the heart are also important to evaluate. The superior and inferior vena cavae can be seen in sagittal views of the chest. The most common cause of anomalies of the inferior vena cava are the situs abnormalities (heterotaxy syndromes). With left atrial isomerism there will be interruption of the inferior vena cava above the renal veins, with continuation of lower body venous return to the heart through the azygous vein and the superior vena cava.

Pulmonary venous return to the heart can be evaluated by examination of the left atrial walls. The right and left pulmonary veins can be seen in realtime sonography as irregularities of the atrial wall with sonolucencies extending into the pulmonary parenchyma. Colour Doppler or power Doppler can be used to confirm the flow pattern into the atrium.

Making diagnoses

It is impossible to review the full spectrum of diagnoses that can be established by fetal echocardiography, and it is sufficient to say that the entire breadth of postnatally established diagnoses have been and will be seen in the fetus. The most common diagnoses tend to be those that clearly distort the four-chamber anatomy, since that is the view most commonly obtained by prenatal sonographers. Thus, the two most common diagnoses in our experience have been atrioventricular septal defect (Fig. 51.3 and Plate 51.1), and hypoplastic left ventricle (Fig. 51.4 and Plates 51.2, 51.3), both of which result in easily detected changes in four-chamber anatomy[29,30].

Any discordance in the size of the atrial or ventricular chambers requires careful evaluation. Although the right ventricle is usually slightly larger than the left, major differences in size mandate full assessment (Fig. 51.5). Tables of chamber diameters have been reported, suggesting that simply determining whether one chamber is too small or the other too big will provide diagnostic information. These size differences should be evaluated by pulsed and colour Doppler assessment of flow into and out of each chamber to identify any obstructions to flow that may be present. We have seen pulmonic stenosis in association with both enlarged and small right ventricles, the former seen with later onset moderate disease with tricuspid regurgitation, and the latter seen with early onset severe disease of long standing with intact tricuspid valve function.

The interatrial septum should contain the normal foramen ovale, occupying the middle third of the wall. A small foramen ovale may be seen in fetuses with coarctation of the aorta as well as hypoplastic left ventricle reflecting diminished right to left transforamenal flow[49,50]. Any other defect in the septum will generally be seen in the lower third, due to defective formation of the septum secundum.

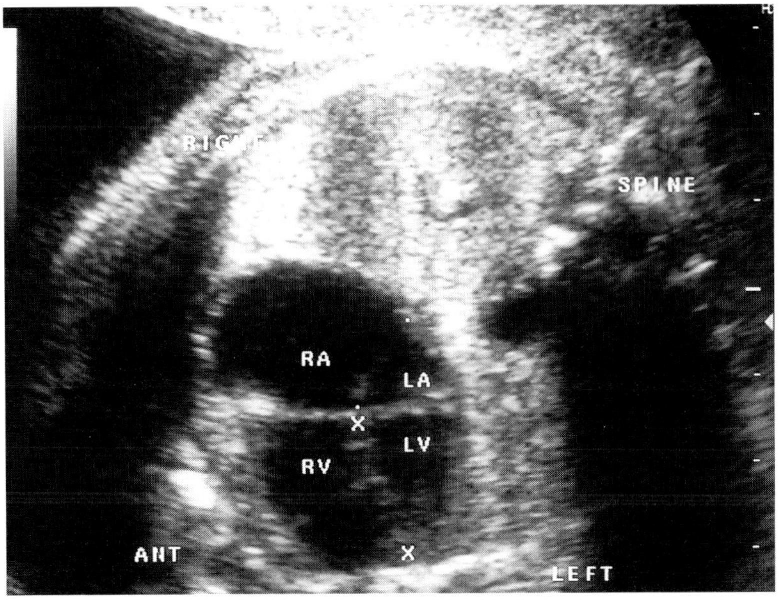

Fig. 51.3 Four-chamber view of fetus with complete atrioventricular septal defect. Note linear appearance of atrioventricular valves, lacking the usual apical displacement of the tricuspid valve.

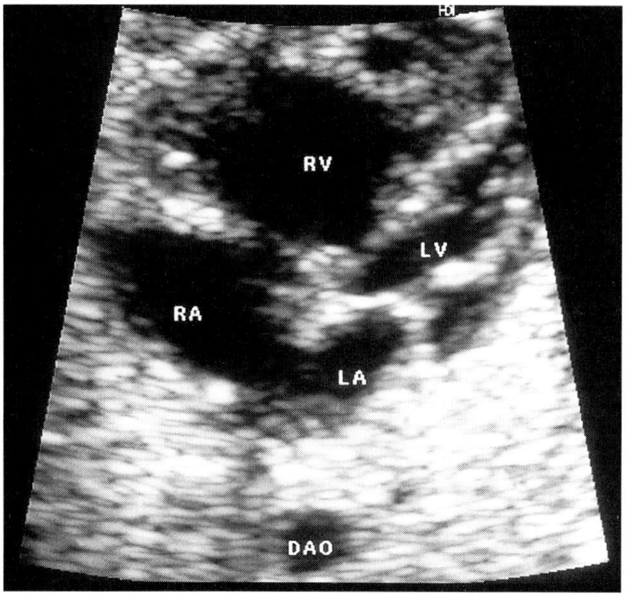

Fig. 51.4 Four-chamber view of fetus with hypoplastic left heart syndrome secondary to Turner syndrome (45, X). The left atrium (LA) and ventricle (LV) are much smaller than the right atrium (RA) and ventricle (RV). (DAO = descending aorta.)

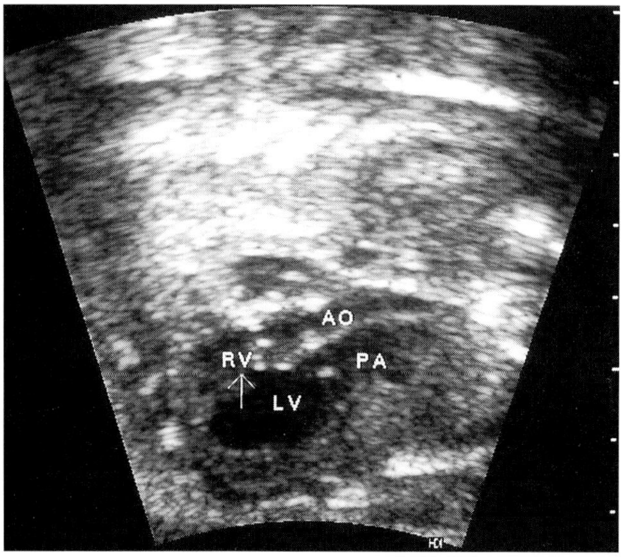

Fig. 51.5 Outflow tracts of fetus with transposition of great arteries and hypoplastic right ventricle. Note smaller size of right than left ventricle (RV, LV), and of aorta (AO) than pulmonary artery (PA).

The ventricular septum may be more difficult to evaluate, because it must be seen in at least two planes, the four-chamber view and the long axis view. Even then, small defects may be hard to appreciate in the fetus, although the smaller septal defects are unlikely to be haemodynamically of clinical significance. In fact, many close spontaneously and the remainder rarely require surgical intervention. Examination of the portion of the ventricular septum just beneath the atrioventricular valves is especially tricky. Any defect suspected from an apical orientation must be confirmed with a long axis four-chamber view.

The presence of echogenic foci in the ventricles has recently been reported to be associated with fetal trisomy 21[51–54]. Although we have not systematically reviewed our own data, the association has not been a prominent pediatric finding. Full understanding of the implications for prenatal diagnosis and counselling will require prospective confirmation from other investigators.

Whenever a fetal abnormality is detected, it must be assumed that other abnormalities are also present[27,55,56]. A thorough search for associated anomalies is a requirement of any fetal cardiac examination, in our opinion, but especially when a cardiac anomaly is present. Along with the (ultrasonic) physical examination of the fetus, a relevant history is also necessary, including family history, maternal medication intake, and pregnancy complications. Using all the information together can result in a more thorough diagnosis and specific syndromes can be discussed with the family.

There is a common association between congenital heart disease and fetal chromosome abnormalities, with abnormal karyotypes being detected in up to 30% of affected fetuses[57,58]. The distribution of karyotypes encountered is different from that seen in unselected populations[29]. We see an equal number of trisomy 21 and trisomy 18 fetuses, while the former is 10 times more common than the latter in midtrimester amniocenteses. The next most common karyotype seen is Turner syndrome (45, X). The high frequency of these relatively uncommon aneuploidies is due to the method of case ascertainment, since congenital heart disease is common with both trisomy 18 and Turner syndrome. Fetuses with multiple anomalies, in the case of trisomy 18, and non-immune hydrops, in the case of Turner syndrome, are also more likely to come to the attention of the sonographer.

It has become our practice to offer a karyotype whenever fetal cardiac defects are detected. When severe chromosome abnormalities such as trisomy 18 or 13 are found, the families are counselled that surgery is not indicated, because of the poor prognosis that is present with these neonates even in the absence of cardiac abnormalities. When trisomy 21 is present, some families decide to terminate the pregnancy, and others to continue, although surgery is not withheld in these cases. For some families who may live a significant distance from the nearest tertiary care centre that can perform neonatal cardiac surgery, knowing that surgery will not be an option for the neonate will allow them to avoid unnecessary travel and to deliver at their local hospital as originally planned.

Recently new genetic microdeletions have been described in fetuses with conotruncal abnormalities[59,60]. These have been seen in fetuses and children with DiGeorge syndrome, as well as the velo-cardial-facial syndrome, and localized to the long arm of chromosome 22 (22q11). The diagnosis of DiGeorge syndrome is important because the thyroid and parathyroid abnormalities may have important metabolic consequences for the neonate. The thymic abnormalities that are also seen in DiGeorge syndrome may compromise the child's immune function, as well.

Antenatal and intrapartum management

Although we have previously reported a 5% incidence of stillbirth among fetuses with congenital heart disease, the deaths we have seen in utero have been limited to fetuses with karyotype abnormalities and/or non-immune hydrops[29]. Antepartum fetal heart rate testing is not necessary for the fetus with a cardiac anomaly, unless some other standard indication for such testing is present (e.g. maternal diabetes, hypertension).

The intrapartum management of affected fetuses is not different from obstetrical norms. Intrapartum fetal heart rate monitoring should be performed as per standards. The only exception to this is the fetus with complete heart block due to structural abnormalities. In these cases the ventricular rate will be fixed and not respond to hypoxia with the usual expected decelerations. Internal electronic fetal heart rate monitoring measures R–R intervals, and will only reflect the ventricular rate, so it will not be useful. On occasion the atrial rate can be monitored externally, and will be useful[61]. Otherwise caesarean delivery is indicated until other techniques for fetal assessment, such as continuous transcutaneous PO_2 monitoring, become widely available.

One of the most commonly asked questions by parents on being informed of fetal cardiac abnormalities is whether caesarean delivery offers advantages to the neonate. To the contrary, the normal physiological fetal chest compression that occurs during passage through the bony pelvis may be beneficial. We do not offer elective caesarean delivery for these patients. We do use labour induction liberally, however, because many patients referred to a regional centre for diagnosis and treatment will live significant distances from the hospital. Timed delivery offers the patient reassurance that a rushed trip to the hospital over a long distance can be avoided.

We do routinely recommend that delivery be planned for a tertiary centre so that any necessary paediatric intervention can be initiated with a minimum of delay by the team that will provide definitive care. The only exceptions to this approach have been non-viable fetuses, and those with lesions with anticipated haemodynamic consequences such that cardiology intervention can reasonably be anticipated to be deferred until days or weeks after delivery, such as small, isolated ventricular septal defects.

The wide availability of prostaglandin E_1 to maintain ductal patency has reduced the urgency of many neonatal transfers for congenital heart disease. Keeping the ductus open permits a more leisurely assessment of the fetus with either right or left heart obstruction. Even with prostaglandin available at the referring hospital, we believe that there are advantages to having both parents and the baby in the same hospital rather than the mother in one hospital, the baby in another, and the father shuttling between the two.

Postnatal management

The management of fetuses with congenital heart disease is the subject of entire texts, and it would be impossible to cover the breadth of the field even in an entire chapter. A few general principles bear reviewing for the fetal diagnostician.

Fetuses with either right or left heart obstruction may benefit from prostaglandin E_1 to maintain patency of the ductus arteriosus. Mild and moderate pulmonic stenosis may improve somewhat after delivery as pulmonary vascular resistance drops, but the fetus with severe pulmonic stenosis, pulmonic atresia or tricuspid stenosis will have poor pulmonic blood flow if the ductus closes. Similarly the fetus with left heart obstruction will develop shock from inadequate systemic perfusion if the ductus is allowed to close. Fetuses with severe coarctation of the aorta also will benefit from prostaglandin E_1.

Another group that may become significantly ill in the newborn period includes those with transposition of the great arteries. Unless a ventricular septal defect is present to allow mixing of oxygenated and deoxygenated blood, severe hypoxaemia will ensue. Neonatal balloon atrial septostomy can be lifesaving for these fetuses, with an arterial switch procedure performed in an unhurried fashion over the next several days.

In the absence of obstruction, the major remaining group of prenatally diagnosed fetuses have septal defects. These neonates do well initially, and develop pulmonary congestion over the first few postnatal weeks, as pulmonary vascular resistance drops. This can be managed initially with digoxin and diuretics, with later performance of cardiac surgery.

Conclusions

The prognosis for fetuses with congenital heart disease has improved since initial reports of our ability to make intrauterine diagnoses. This is clearly due to improvements in neonatal and surgical care. Improvements in ultrasound technology have resulted in earlier and more precise prenatal diagnoses. This has allowed greater experience with the evolution of fetal cardiac anomalies, and time to counsel parents about expected outcomes.

The optimal approach to the fetus with heart disease includes a multidisciplinary team involving obstetricians, paediatric cardiologists, and geneticists. Additional personnel to complete the team include sonographers and nurses. Using a collaborative approach, the family can receive care in a continuous manner both before and after birth, easing their transition through a stressful birth and neonatal course.

REFERENCES

1. Copel JA, Pilu G & Kleinman CS. Congenital heart disease and extracardiac anomalies: associations and indications for fetal echocardiography. *Am. J. Obstet. Gynecol.* **154**, 1121–1132, 1986.
2. Moller JH. Incidence of cardiac malformations. In *Fetal, Neonatal, and Infant Cardiac Disease* (eds J.H. Moller & W.A. Neal), pp. 361–369. Norwalk, CT: Appleton & Lange, 1990.
3. Hoffman JIE & Christianson R. Congenital heart disease in a cohort of 19,502 births with long-term follow-up. *Am. J. Cardiol.* **42**, 641–647, 1978.
4. Feldt RH, Avasthey P, Yoshimasu F, Kurland LT & Titus JL. Incidence of congenital heart disease in children born to residents of Olmsted County, Minnesota, 1950–1969. *Mayo Clin. Proc.* **46**, 794–799, 1971.
5. Nora JJ & Nora AH. The genetic contribution to congenital heart diseases. In *Congenital Heart Disease: Causes and Processes* (eds J.J. Nora & A. Takao), pp. 3–13. Mt. Kisco, NY: Futura, 1984.
6. Boughman JA, Berg KA, Astemborski JA *et al.* Familial risks of congenital heart defect in a population-based epidemiologic study. *Am. J. Med. Genet.* **26**, 839–849, 1987.
7. Whittemore R, Hobbins JC & Engle MA. Pregnancy and its outcome in women with and without surgical treatment of congenital heart disease. *Am. J. Cardiol.* **50**, 641–651, 1982.
8. Rose V, Gold RJM, Lindsay G & Allen M. A possible increase in the incidence of congenital heart defects among offspring of affected parents. *J. Am. Coll. Cardiol.* **6**, 376–382, 1985.
9. Allan LD, Crawford DC, Chita SK, Anderson RH & Tynan MJ. Familial recurrence of congenital heart disease in a prospective series of mothers referred for fetal echocardiography. *Am. J. Cardiol.* **58**, 334–337, 1986.
10. Zierler S. Maternal drugs and congenital heart disease. *Obstet Gynecol.* **65**, 155–165, 1985.
11. Zierler S & Rothman KJ. Congenital heart disease in relation to maternal use of Bendectin and other drugs in early pregnancy. *N. Engl. J. Med.* **313**, 347–352, 1985.
12. Lammer EJ, Chen DT, Hoar RM *et al.* Retinoic acid embryopathy. *N. Engl. J. Med.* **313**, 837–841, 1985.
13. Jick SS, Terris BZ & Jick H. First trimester topical tretinoin and congenital disorders. *Lancet* **341**, 1181–1182, 1993.
14. Rothman KJ, Moore LL, Singer MR, Nguyen UDT, Mannino S & Milunsky A. Teratogenicity of high vitamin A intake. *N. Engl. J. Med.* **333**, 1369–1373, 1995.
15. Hanson JW, Myrianthopoulos NC, Harvey MAS & Smith DW. Risks to the offspring of women treated with hydantoin anticonvulsants, with emphasis on the fetal hydantoin syndrome. *J. Pediatr.* **89**, 662–668, 1976.
16. Monson RR, Rosenberg L, Hartz SC, Shapiro S, Heinonen OP & Slone D. Diphenylhydantoin and selected congenital malformations. *N. Engl. J. Med.* **289**, 1049–1052, 1973.
17. Jones KL, Lacro RV, Johnson KA & Adams J. Pattern of malformations in the children of women treated with carbamazepine during pregnancy. *N. Engl. J. Med.* **320**, 1661–1666, 1989.
18. Ardinger HH, Atkin JF, Blackston RD *et al.* Verification of the fetal valproate syndrome phenotype. *Am. J. Med. Genet.* **29**, 171–185, 1988.
19. Zackai EH, Mellman WJ, Neiderer B & Hanson JW. The fetal trimethadione syndrome. *J. Pediatr.* **87**, 280–284, 1975.
20. Dansky LV, Andermann E, Rosenblatt D, Sherwin AL & Andermann F. Anticonvulsants, folate levels, and pregnancy outcome: a prospective study. *Ann Neurol* **21**, 176–182, 1987.
21. Miller E, Hare JW, Cloherty JP *et al.* Elevated maternal hemoglobin A_{1c} in early pregnancy and major congenital anomalies in infants of diabetic mothers. *N. Engl. J. Med.* **302**, 1331–1334, 1981.
22. Becerra JE, Khoury MJ, Cordero JF & Erickson JD. Diabetes mellitus during pregnancy and the risks for specific birth defects: a population-based case-control study. *Pediatrics* **85**, 1–9, 1990.
23. Ferencz C, Rubin JD, McCarter RJ & Clark EB. Maternal diabetes and cardiovascular malformations: predominance of double outlet right ventricle and truncus arteriosus. *Teratology* **41**, 319–326, 1990.
24. Shields LE, Gan EA, Murphy HF, Sahn DJ & Moore TR. The prognostic value of hemoglobin A1c in predicting fetal heart disease in diabetic pregnancies. *Obstet. Gynecol.* **81**, 954–957, 1993.
25. Lenke RR & Levy HL. Maternal phenylketonuria and hyperphenylalaninemia: an international survey of the outcome of untreated and treated pregnancies. *N. Engl. J. Med.* **303**, 1202–1208, 1980.
26. Platt LD, Koch R, Azen C *et al.* Maternal phenylketonuria collaborative study, obstetric aspects and outcome: the first 6 years. *Am. J. Obstet. Gynecol.* **166**, 1150–1160, 1992.
27. Copel JA, Pilu G & Kleinman CS. Extracardiac anomalies and congenital heart disease. *Semin. Perinatol.* **17**, 89–105, 1993.
28. Carlson DE, Platt LD, Medearis AL & Horenstein J. Quantifiable polyhydramnios: diagnosis and management. *Obstet. Gynecol.* **75**, 989–993, 1990.
29. Smythe JF, Copel JA & Kleinman CS. Outcome of prenatally detected cardiac malformations. *Am. J. Cardiol.* **69**, 1471–1474, 1992.
30. Baumann P, Copel JA & Kleinman CS. Management of the fetus with cardiac disease. *Ultrasound Quart.* **10**, 57–58, 1992.
31. Kleinman CS, Copel JA & Hobbins JC. Combined echocardiographic and Doppler assessment of fetal congenital atrioventricular block. *Br. J. Obstet. Gynaecol.* **94**, 967–974, 1987.
32. Schmidt KG, Ulmer HE, Silverman NH, Kleinman CS & Copel JA. Perinatal outcome of fetal complete atrioventricular block: a multicenter experience. *J. Am. Coll. Cardiol.* **91**, 1360–1366, 1991.
33. Copel JA, Pilu G, Green J, Hobbins JC & Kleinman CS. Fetal echocardiographic screening for congenital heart disease: the importance of the four chamber view. *Am. J. Obstet. Gynecol.* **157**, 648–655, 1987.
34. Fermont L, DeGeeter B, Aubry J *et al.* A close collaboration between obstetricians and pediatric cardiologists allows antenatal detection of severe cardiac malformations by 2D echocardiography. In *Pediatric Cardiology: Proceedings of the Second World Congress* (eds E.F. Doyle, M.E. Engle, W.M. Gersony *et al.*), pp. 34–37. New York: Springer-Verlag, 1986.
35. Hegge FN, Lees MH & Watson PT. Utility of a screening examination of the fetal cardiac position and four chambers during obstetric sonography. *J. Reprod. Med.* **32**, 353–358, 1987.
36. Eik-Nes SH. Presentation to International Perinatal Doppler Society, Malmo, Sweden, September, 1991.
37. Vergani P, Mariani S, Ghidini A *et al.* Screening for congenital heart disease with the four chamber view of the fetal heart. *Am. J. Obstet. Gynecol.* **167**, 1000–1003, 1992.
38. Luck CA. Value of routine ultrasound scanning at 19 weeks: a four year study of 8849 deliveries. *Br. Med. J.* **304**, 1474–1478, 1992.
39. Shirley IM, Bottomley F & Robinson VP. Routine radiographer screening for fetal abnormalities by ultrasound in an unselected low risk population. *Br. J. Radiol.* **65**, 564–569, 1992.
40. Ewigman BG, Crane JP, Frigoletto FD *et al.* A randomized trial of prenatal ultrasound screening in a low risk population: impact on perinatal outcome. *N. Engl. J. Med.* **329**, 821–827, 1993.
41. Wyllie J, Wren C & Hunter S. Screening for fetal cardiac malformations. *Br. Heart J.* **71**(suppl), 20–27, 1994.
42. Rustico MA, Benettoni A, D'Ottavio G *et al.* Fetal heart screening in low-risk pregnancies. *Ultrasound Obstet. Gynecol.* **6**, 1–7, 1995.
43. Kirk JS, Riggs TW, Comstock CH, Lee W, Yang SS & Weinhouse E. Prenatal screening for cardiac anomalies: the value of routine addition of the aortic root to the four-chamber view. *Obstet. Gynecol.* **84**, 427–431, 1994.
44. Rudolph AM. *Congenital Diseases of the Heart.* Chicago: Yearbook, 1974.
45. McCurdy CM & Jr Reed KL. Basic technique of fetal echocardiography. *Semin. Ultrasound.* CT MRI **14**, 267–276, 1993.
46. Smith RS, Comstock CH, Kirk JS & Lee W. Ultrasonographic left cardiac axis deviation: a marker for fetal anomalies. *Obstet. Gynecol.* **85**, 187–191, 1995.
47. Shipp TD, Bromley B, Hornberger LK, Nadel A & Benacerraf BR. Levorotation of the fetal cardiac axis: a clue for the presence of congenital heart disease. *Obstet. Gynecol.* **85**, 97–102, 1995.
48. Lee W, Smith RS, Comstock CH, Kirk JS, Riggs T & Weinhouse E. Tetralogy of Fallot: prenatal diagnosis and postnatal survival. *Obstet. Gynecol.* **86**, 583–588, 1995.
49. Feit LR, Copel JA & Kleinman CS. Foramen ovale size in the normal and abnormal human fetal heart: an indicator of transatrial flow physiology. *Ultrasound Obstet. Gynecol.* **1**, 313–319, 1991.
50. Phillipos EZ, Robertson MA & Still KD. The echocardiographic assessment of the human fetal foramen ovale. *J. Am. Soc. Echocardiogr.* **7**, 257–263, 1994.

51. Brown DL, Roberts DJ & Miller WA. Left ventricular echogenic focus in the fetal heart: pathologic correlation. *J. Ultrasound Med.* **13**, 613–616, 1994.
52. Bromley B, Lieberman E, Laboda L & Benacerraf B. Echogenic intracardiac focus: a sonographic sign for fetal Down syndrome. *Obstet. Gynecol.* **86**, 998–1001, 1995.
53. Petrikovsky BM, Challenger M & Wyse LJ. Natural history of echogenic foci within ventricles of the fetal heart. *Ultrasound Obstet. Gynecol.* **5**, 92–94, 1995.
54. Sepulveda W, Cullen S, Nicolaides P, Hollingsworth J & Fisk NM. Echogenic foci in the fetal heart: a marker of chromosomal abnormality. *Br. J. Obstet. Gynaecol.* **102**, 490–492, 1995.
55. Copel JA, Pilu G & Kleinman CS. Congenital heart disease and extracardiac anomalies: associations and indications for fetal echocardiography. *Am. J. Obstet. Gynecol.* **154**, 1121–1132, 1986.
56. Fogel M, Copel JA, Cullen MT, Hobbins JC & Kleinman CS. Congenital heart disease and fetal thoracoabdominal anomalies: association in utero and the importance of cytogenetic analysis. *Am. J. Perinatol.* **8**, 411–416, 1991.
57. Copel JA, Cullen M, Green JJ, Mahoney MJ, Hobbins JC & Kleinman CS. The frequency of aneuploidy in prenatally diagnosed congenital heart disease: an indication for fetal karyotyping. *Am. J. Obstet. Gynecol.* **158**, 409–413, 1988.
58. Berg KA, Clark EB, Astemborski JA & Boughman JA. Prenatal detection of cardiovascular malformations by echocardiography: an indication for cytogenetic evaluation. *Am. J. Obstet. Gynecol.* **159**, 477–481, 1988.
59. Wilson DI, Goodship JA, Burn J, Cross IE & Scambler PJ. Deletions within chromosome 22q11 in familial congenital heart disease. *Lancet* **340**, 573–575, 1992.
60. Driscoll DA, Salvin J, Sellinger B *et al.* Prevalence of 22q11 microdeletions in DiGeorge and velocardiofacial syndromes: implications for genetic counselling and prenatal diagnosis. *J. Med. Genet.* **30**, 813–817, 1993.
61. Kleinman CS, Copel JA & Hobbins JC. Combined echocardiographic and Doppler assessment of fetal congenital atrioventricular block. *Br. J. Obstet. Gynaecol.* **94**, 967–974, 1987.

Thoracic malformations

52

P. Johnson

Introduction

Congenital intrathoracic lesions are of importance in that any space occupying lesion present in the fetal chest may restrict normal lung growth with the possibility of resultant pulmonary hypoplasia (PH). Hydrops fetalis may occur if venous cardiac return is embarrassed, with associated poor prognosis. However, in fetal life, the presence of even a very large lesion may not be accompanied by any adverse consequences as the lungs are not required to function in gas exchange. Prenatal diagnosis of such abnormalities permits relevant further investigation and, in some circumstances, the potential for intrauterine therapy.

As with many other congenital anomalies, the behaviour of intrathoracic lesions is dynamic, with marked changes occurring during gestation, including complete resolution. This dynamic nature requires serial assessments for appreciation of the natural history and in order to be able to offer an accurate prognosis.

Embryology of the thorax

The trachea has a common endodermal origin with the foregut of the embryo, arising from the laryngotracheal groove in the pharyngeal floor around week 4 of development. The groove fuses to form a tube which grows caudally into the splanchnic mesoderm. The caudal end of the tube becomes the trachea. Lung buds develop from this and are thus surrounded by mesoderm. The buds grow laterally into the pleural coelom, with the right bud dividing into three and the left two lobes, corresponding to the lobes of the postnatal lung. The trachea divides into two main bronchi which then branch in a dichotomous fashion until the terminal bronchioles and alveoli are formed. This process continues after birth.

Each lung receives a covering of visceral and parietal pleura from the splanchnic and somatic mesoderm respectively. The mesenchyme which surrounds the endodermal bronchial tree develops into connective tissue, cartilage, muscle, pulmonary and bronchial blood vessels.

Pleural effusions

AETIOLOGY

In fetal life, pleural effusions are non-specific collections of fluid within the pleural cavity which can be identified by ultrasound. Whilst the commonest cause of pleural effusions in the neonate is accumulation of chyle or lymph[1], the aetiology of such effusions in the fetus remains unclear. When chylothorax is confirmed postnatally, the aetiology is thought to be related to a possible fistula or atresia of the thoracic duct[2,3]. Pleural effusions may occur in isolation, or in association with other thoracic lesions such as pulmonary sequestration[4]. Other possible causes include fetal goitre[5] and infection[6]. There are reports of familial congenital pleural effusions[7,8]. In such cases, the aetiology may be of a different nature and includes interlobular septal lymphatic hypoplasia. Congenital pulmonary lymphagiectasis (CPL) has also been described as a cause of pleural effusions[9,10]. Such pathogenesis is usually sporadic but may present in siblings. CPL may also be the mechanism underlying the development of pleural effusions in Down and Noonan syndromes.

However, the majority of cases of congenital pleural effusion do not require postnatal surgery, and tissue for histological study will thus not be available from the survivors. Thus, for many cases, the cause remains speculative.

NATURAL HISTORY

The natural history of fetal pleural effusions remains unclear. The literature is plentiful in case reports, but few large series have been published. The timing of diagnosis can vary from late first trimester to term, but this will depend on the indication for the ultrasound scan. With the practice of routine scanning being more widely adopted, early diagnosis is becoming more common. However, in those fetuses where a previous anomaly scan has been reported as normal, late presentation may be by way of investigation for polyhydramnios which complicates approximately 42% of pregnancies complicated by pleural effusions[11] or premature labour.

Spontaneous resolution does occur[12] and has been reported in up to 10% of cases[11,13,14] with one series[15] reporting resolution in six of 11 cases (55%). In addition, resolution has been seen followed by recurrence[16]. Such changes are associated with a good prognosis.

Isolated pleural effusions may also demonstrate progression to fetal hydrops, which can occur over a relatively narrow timespan[17]. This necessitates regular follow-up with ultrasound after the initial diagnosis. Survival varies with the gestational age at presentation, uni- or bilateral effusions, the coexistence of associated anomalies and the presence of hydrops. Early diagnosis with hydrops is associated with a poor prognosis, with a mortality rate of at least 50%[13]. However, outcome in isolated effusions may not be very much better, with estimates of mortality as high as 36%[11] and 47%[18].

The presentation of pleural effusions may be delayed until after delivery. In this group of neonates, chylothorax is the commonest cause. The neonates will usually present with respiratory distress or embarrassment immediately or within 24 h of birth[19]. Treatment consists of drainage, usually followed by spontaneous resolution, although in persistent cases, pleurectomy or thoracic duct ligation may be necessary. Provided that immediate treatment is successful, the outlook is good, with the majority of affected infants having a normal clinical examination at the end of the first year of life.

DIAGNOSIS

Pleural effusions appear as an echo-free area lying between the chest wall, diaphragm and lung. They may be unilateral or bilateral, and of varying size, with large bilateral effusions giving the lungs the appearance of butterfly wings (Fig. 52.1). They may be isolated or associated with generalized hydrops fetalis which may be related to mediastinal shift. Polyhydramnios is a common finding.

The diagnosis of pleural effusions may be made during the investigation of obstetric problems, for example, polyhydramnios, but now most frequently occurs during routine ultrasound examination of the fetus. The first reports of prenatal diagnosis of this condition were in the late 1970s[20,21].

When a pleural effusion is diagnosed, it is essential that a detailed and careful examination of the fetus is undertaken to establish the presence of associated anomalies and any underlying pathology. In some cases, the presence of other anomalies may point to the aetiology of the effusion, e.g. congenital

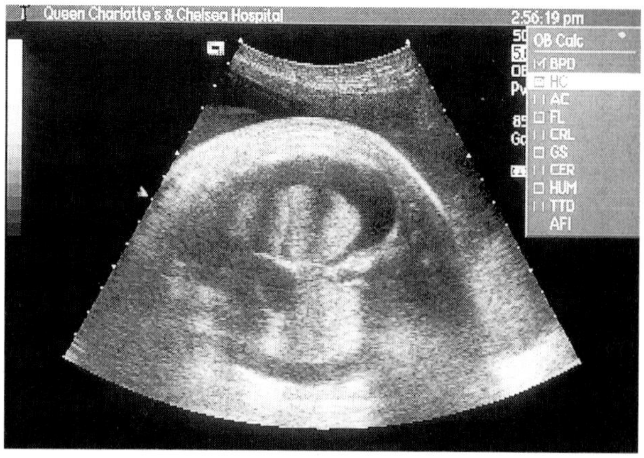

Fig. 52.1 Ultrasound picture of pleural effusion.

diaphragmatic hernia[22,23]. Many congenital anomalies are also associated with pleural effusions including tracheo-oesophageal fistula, Noonan syndrome and other multiple malformation syndromes. There is a well-recognized association between pleural effusions and aneuploidy, particularly trisomy 21[22,24] and Turner syndrome[1] and thus fetal karyotyping is of value in assessing the aetiology and prognosis. In some series, the risk of aneuploidy in association with pleural effusion is as high as 33%.

In cases of hydrops fetalis, it may not be possible to assess whether the effusion is a cause of the hydrops, or secondary to fetal heart failure. A thorough investigation for the underlying cause must be made in these cases. The prognosis in the presence of hydrops is very poor, with the associated mortality rate being of the order of 75–95%[25,26] with pulmonary hypoplasia being the most common cause of postnatal loss irrespective of the underlying aetiology of the effusions.

INVESTIGATIONS

Detailed ultrasound examination of the fetus is the mainstay of diagnosis of pleural effusions and associated anomalies. However, additional investigations will often assist in the assessment, e.g. by confirming or excluding the presence of aneuploidy. At the time of diagnosis, a careful search for other structural anomalies must be carried out, including fetal echocardiography to exclude structural heart disease and cardiac dysrhythmias. Other investigations may then be indicated which may be maternal or fetal.

MATERNAL

In many cases, maternal blood will be taken for full blood count, blood group and antibodies, Kleihauer–Betke test, syphilis serology, viral screen including parvovirus and screening for diabetes. Additional investigations which may be indicated include haemoglobin electrophoresis and antiphospholipid screen. Many of these tests are performed routinely during antenatal care.

FETAL

Further investigations of the fetus require invasive procedures such as amniocentesis, chorion villus sampling and fetal blood sampling. The nature of test performed will depend upon gestational age and the possible aetiologies. For example, if anaemia is suspected, only fetal blood sampling will permit assessment of the haematological status whereas karyotyping can be performed on liquor, villi or blood. Each case needs to be assessed individually and decisions made to choose the test which will maximize benefit with the minimum risk. It must be recognized that invasive testing in the presence of hydrops increases the risk of pregnancy loss[27].

Aspiration of the effusion may assist in visualization of the intrathoracic structures. In addition, examination of the aspirate has been thought to have potential value in the differentiation between chylothorax and other types of pleural effusion by the colour of the fluid[11] or the lymphocyte count[28–32]. Whilst such investigation is diagnostic after alimentation has commenced postnatally, it is of less value prenatally. The fluid aspirated from a pleural effusion may be suitable for cytogenetic examination[33].

MANAGEMENT

Once all the diagnostic information is available, management options will include termination of pregnancy, drainage of the effusion or a conservative approach.

TERMINATION OF PREGNANCY

This option may be considered in the presence of aneuploidy, additional structural abnormalities or hydrops, depending upon gestational age and the local law governing termination of pregnancy. Whilst it is difficult to provide accurate information regarding prognosis in isolated pleural effusions, the chances of intact survival are markedly reduced by the presence of other abnormalities, particularly hydrops.

ASPIRATION OF EFFUSION

Aspiration of an effusion by ultrasound guidance permits further assessment of intrathoracic anatomy and may lead to resolution. It has been suggested that expansion of the lung after aspiration is a good prognostic indicator, implying that the lung tissue has not undergone irreversible damage. Reaccumulation of the effusion after aspiration may lead to further aspiration or shunting to permit continued drainage. The speed of reaccumulation varies from 1 h to 10 days[34,35]. However, aspiration just before delivery may assist in the resuscitation of the neonate[36–38].

THORACOCENTESIS AND SHUNTING

Aspiration under ultrasound guidance has become an accepted procedure in the management of pleural effusions complicated by ascites and hydrops fetalis. Although one of the aims of in-utero drainage is to allow lung growth to prevent respiratory embarrassment at birth, this is only relevant if the fetus does not succumb in utero from hydrops, or die from prematurity due to polyhydramnios. Thus a more immediate aim is restoration of normal haemodynamics and swallowing[39]. The role of intervention in isolated hydrothorax is less clear with up to 50% resolution occurring spontaneously[15]. The drainage of bilateral effusions may be achieved by a single needle insertion[40]. Insertion of a double pigtail catheter (Rocket of London, London UK) into the pleural space either uni- or bilaterally permits continued drainage of the effusion into the amniotic cavity (Fig. 52.2 and 52.3). Other approaches include the insertion of an epidural catheter into the pleural effusion through the maternal abdominal wall and draining into a sterile bag[41]. Drainage may

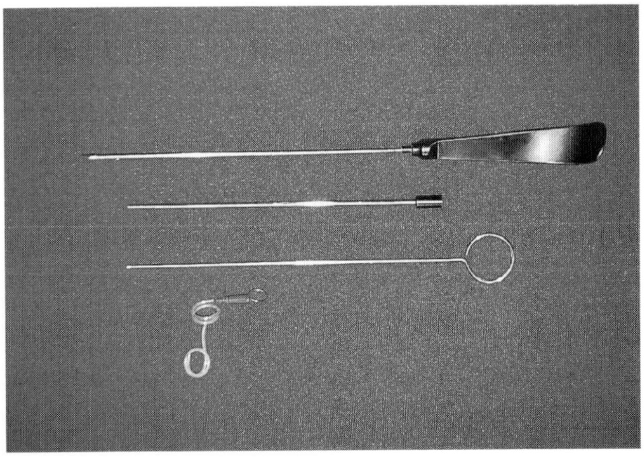

Fig. 52.2 Double pigtail catheter and introducer.

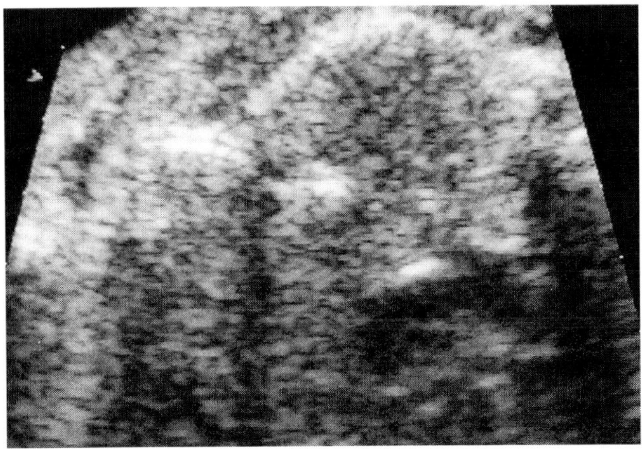

Fig. 52.3 Ultrasound picture of shunt in situ.

be attempted in both isolated effusions[42] and those with an identifiable cause such as extralobar pulmonary sequestration[43].

The primary aim of drainage by whatever means is to permit re-expansion of the lungs and thus minimize the risk of PH. The efficacy of the procedure in permitting lung growth is shown in follow-up studies of babies who underwent shunting in utero[44]. In severe cases, drainage of the effusions by aspiration[45] or thoracoamniotic shunting[22] may lead to the resolution of hydrops (Figs 52.4 and 52.5). When bilateral effusions are accompanied by hydrops, drainage of only one side may lead to partial resolution[46].

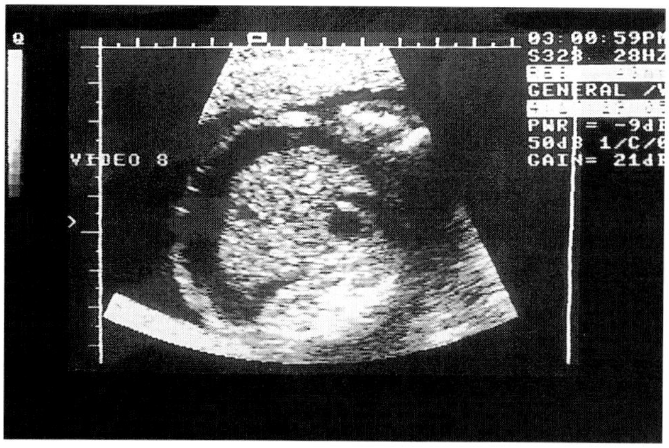

Fig. 52.4 Ultrasound picture of ascites related to pleural effusion.

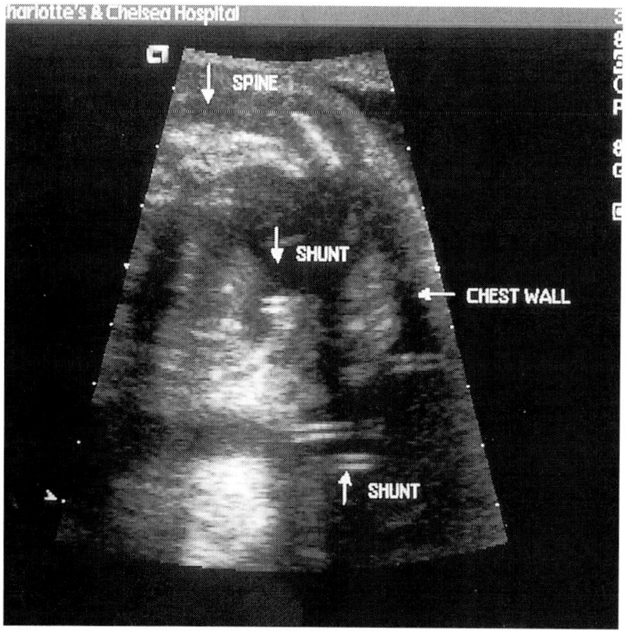

Fig. 52.5 Fetus after insertion of thoracoamniotic shunt.

The insertion of a thoracoamniotic shunt is a procedure which carries procedure-related risks which may lead to abortion or intrauterine death. The shunt may block after insertion, become displaced or even be pulled out by the fetus. In one series of seven euploid cases of pleural effusion accompanied by hydrops treated by bilateral shunting, the gestational age varied between 22 and 33 weeks (mean 28) and the overall survival rate was 29%[47]. However, in selected cases, insertion of a shunt has been associated with a much higher survival (10 of 11)[11]. Nicolaides and colleagues have reported on a series of 74 cases, with 47 survivors and five pregnancies terminated following the confirmation of aneuploidy in the fetus. The survival rate in the non-hydropic fetuses was 100% (n = 28) whereas only 46% of those with hydrops survived (19 of 41)[48]. Mussat et al.[49] reported a series of 25 fetuses with pleural effusions complicated by hydrops. Twenty underwent the insertion of a pigtail catheter and five had aspiration of the effusions. Three pregnancies were terminated (two for aneuploidy, one for failure of improvement of hydrops after shunting). Of the 22 remaining fetuses, 16 were liveborn with three postnatal deaths. Thus, with an active policy of drainage of effusions with accompanying hydrops, a survival rate of 13 of 25 (52%) was achieved.

If a shunt has been inserted, it is important that it is clamped immediately after delivery and then removed to reduce the risk of pneumothorax. An alternative approach is to electively intubate and ventilate the neonate. The shunt can then be used for postnatal drainage of the pleural space.

CONCLUSION

The ideal management of fetal pleural effusions remains unclear. Detailed investigation including karyotype and fetal echocardiography is recommended. The indications for aspiration and shunt insertion remain unclear. In the presence of hydrops thought to be secondary to the effusion, mediastinal shift or cardiac embarrassment, drainage of the effusion may lead to resolution and improvement in outcome. Conservative management is appropriate in the presence of a unilateral effusion with no associated problems. Drainage immediately before delivery may improve resuscitation and perinatal outcome.

Congenital cystic adenomatoid malformation

AETIOLOGY

Congential cystic adenomatoid malformation (CCAM) is a rare malformation of the lung which can be diagnosed prenatally by ultrasound. It is caused by an overgrowth of the terminal bronchioles at the expense of the saccular tissue. It appears to arise at the point of connection of the conducting airways, which are derived from endoderm, and the respiratory component of the lung which arises from mesoderm. The embryological origin is likely to be at approximately 7 weeks of menstrual age, and may be caused by a maturation defect in lung embryogenesis[50] or localized bronchial atresia[51]. The exact nature of this defect remains unclear, but there appears to be an abnormality of paracrine growth[52].

NATURAL HISTORY

The lesion is usually unilateral, although bilateral cases have been reported. It will generally affect one lobe of the lung, but the size of the lesion may lead to compression of the other lobe and the other side of the lung. Stocker[53] proposed a classification of CCAM into three groups according to the size of the cysts. Type 1 has large cysts present, whereas type 2 has multiple small cysts up to 1.2 cm in diameter. Type 3 has a non-cystic appearance on ultrasound. An alternative classification has been proposed of macrocystic (that is with cysts greater than 5 mm) and microcystic (with cysts of up to 5 mm in diameter). This second classification essentially puts types 1 and 2 into the macrocystic group and type 3 into the microcystic group.

CCAM may undergo spontaneous resolution, although without confirmatory histology, such disappearing lesions cannot be proven to be of this type[54–56].

DIAGNOSIS

This is generally made by ultrasound examination in the second and third trimesters of pregnancy (Fig. 52.6). Although the lesion must exist in the first trimester, diagnosis at this time has not been reported. The majority of cases are diagnosed on routine ultrasonography at between 16 and 22 weeks' gestation. However, some cases will be diagnosed in the third trimester, generally as part of an investigation of complications such as polyhydramnios. The differential diagnosis includes congenital diaphragmatic hernia, bronchogenic cysts, lung sequestrations, pulmonary lobar hypoplasia, laryngeal and bronchial atresia[57]. Ultrasound appearances depend upon the type of CCAM. The macrocystic lesions appear as multiple cysts occupying one side of the chest. It is often extremely difficult to identify normal lung tissue on the same side of the chest. There is frequently mediastinal shift and compression of the contralateral lung. The microcystic lesions appear on ultrasound to have a uniform echogenic appearance. Fetal lung biopsy has been utilized in assisting with the diagnosis of such lesions[58].

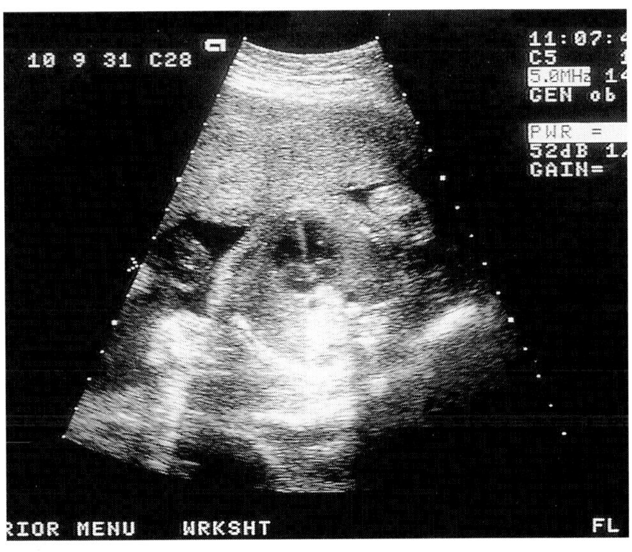

Fig. 52.6 Ultrasound picture of CCAM type III.

Associated anomalies are rare, but have been reported to include renal anomalies, cardiac anomalies and aneuploidy. The foregut origin of CCAM means that other anomalies of the same embryological origin may occur[59]. Type 2 CCAM is more commonly associated with other abnormalities[60]. Polyhydramnios frequently complicates pregnancies where the fetus has CCAM. It is thought that the thoracic lesion interferes with fetal swallowing, thus leading to an increase in amniotic fluid volume. Compression of venous return may lead to the development of hydrops, which is a bad prognostic sign.

In general terms, CCAM has been associated with a poor prognosis, particularly the microcystic or type 3. However, more recent reviews have shown that the survival rate can be as high as 86%[60] or 90%[61]. The factors most frequently associated with poor prognosis are large size of lesion, severe mediastinal shift, the presence of hydrops and other abnormalities[62]. Some authors have described poor outcome in type 3[63]. However, Adzick[64] and Bromley et al.[60] have demonstrated that the prognosis depends primarily on size. If the lesion affects only part of the lung there is an up to an 86% survival, but if the lesion affects the entire lung there is only a 36% survival rate.

INVESTIGATIONS

Once diagnosis has been made, a careful search for other abnormalities should be carried out and consideration given to checking the karyotype. Counselling with the aid of a paediatric surgeon experienced in the postnatal management of this condition is extremely useful.

Subsequent follow-up scans should be performed, particularly as the natural history of CCAM is unclear. Some lesions do resolve, with eight of a series of 15 becoming smaller during the pregnancy[60]. Follow-up scans also permit the identification of hydrops if it develops. In the presence of large cysts and hydrops, consideration can be given to drainage of the cysts, either by thoracocentesis or the insertion of a shunt. There have been reported successes of intrauterine surgery for excision of lesions of this nature[64,65]. However, the majority of cases can be managed conservatively.

MANAGEMENT

As many of these lesions (up to 30%) resolve[61], ultrasound follow-up is essential. It is also important to be aware of the possibility of the development of hydrops as this carries such a poor prognosis. Fetal surgery (see above) and drainage of large cysts[66,67] have been successfully performed, and relief of associated polyhydramnios by serial amniocentesis has also been shown to be of value[68]. Outcome is optimized if the babies are delivered in a centre where neonatal facilities are available, particularly as difficulties with respiration may be evident in the first few days of life. The neonate should be examined by chest X-ray and magnetic resonance imaging, and surgery may be necessary to remove the affected tissue.

ACCURACY OF PRENATAL DIAGNOSIS

Following histological examination of the affected lesions, it has become evident that the ability to correctly assess these lesions by prenatal ultrasound is limited. In one series of 13 consecutive cases, McCullagh et al.[69] demonstrated that five lesions were confirmed and two were almost certainly present postnatally, although no histological diagnosis was available. Two fetuses were completely normal on postnatal examination, with another two having pulmonary sequestration. One baby had primary pulmonary lobar hypoplasia and another had bronchial atresia. In a different series[70] eight of 14 were correctly identified by prenatal diagnosis. Five out of 10 fetuses thought to have type 1 were confirmed after delivery, with three having type 2 on histology. Two fetuses did not have CCAM confirmed. Only one fetus thought to have type 3 was confirmed to have this, the other having type 2. With these inaccuracies in mind, it is extremely important to assess all the information available when counselling patients regarding the prognosis. The size of lesion, mediastinal shifts, hydrops and polyhydramnios are the most important prognostic indicators.

Lung sequestration

AETIOLOGY

These lesions are normally developed lung tissue which is not in contact with the bronchial tree. They are perfused by blood from the systemic circulation rather than the pulmonary vessels. The embryological origin is probably a separate outgrowth from the primitive foregut or a segment of normally developing lung which has lost its connection with the bronchial tree. Sequestered lobes may appear above or below the diaphragm[43] and must be considered in the differential diagnosis of echogenic lesions in the abdomen.

Pulmonary sequestration is also associated with CCAM, with both histological diagnoses being present simultaneously in some cases[71,72].

DIAGNOSIS

The differentiation between pulmonary sequestration and CCAM, particularly type 3, is very difficult as the ultrasonic echogenicity may be the same. A sequestered lobe often has a pyramidal appearance on ultrasound examination. Identification of a vessel supplying the lesion arising from the systemic circulation using colour Doppler will confirm the diagnosis, but this is not easy, and frequently the correct diagnosis can only be confirmed by histological study. CCAM and pulmonary sequestration can coexist and in these cases, histological examination is the only method of diagnosis. Ultrasound guided needle biopsy has been employed postnatally in the diagnosis[73] and could be applied prenatally.

NATURAL HISTORY

As with CCAM, if the lesion is large and causes mediastinal shift, there may be associated hydrops[74] which leads to a poor outcome. In addition, heart failure in the neonate may develop if the anomalous blood supply leads to the development of a left–right shunt. However, in the absence of hydrops, the outlook for the pregnancy is usually good.

Lesions which have the ultrasonographic appearances of pulmonary sequestration may disappear, as with other echogenic lesions in the fetal chest. Whilst this may represent true resolution, the possibility of obstruction of a bronchus by a mucous plug has been proposed as a possible explanation[75].

INVESTIGATIONS

The investigation of a pregnancy where the fetus is thought to have a sequestered lobe is as for CCAM. The embryological origin of the condition, however, means that associated anomalies are more common, particularly those related to the foregut, heart and diaphragm, including diaphragmatic hernia.

MANAGEMENT

Fetal surveillance should be instigated by serial ultrasound examinations once the diagnosis has been made and other anomalies excluded. There is a possibility of neonatal respiratory embarassment, so neonatal care facilities should be available at the place of delivery. Postnatal investigation by chest X-ray and other imaging modalities will help elucidate the exact nature of any lesion.

BRONCHOGENIC CYSTS

Bronchogenic cysts are rare lesions which probably have their origins in abnormal outgrowths from the laryngeal tube and primitive foregut. They appear on ultrasound as isolated cystic lesions which may arise from the mediastinum or be located within the lung tissue. Occasionally, the cysts may separate from the site of origin and thus be present in the neck ot the subpleural space. They may be associated with other anomalies of the foregut such as lung sequestration.

The presence of an isolated cyst does not require any intervention, but as for the lesions described above, enlargement leading to mediastinal shift or hydrops may be an indication for drainage.

Congenital diaphragmatic hernia

AETIOLOGY

The diaphragm is formed from the septum transversum, pleuroperitoneal membranes and the oesophageal mesentery. It forms between the 8th and 10th week, and fusion is normally complete before the intestines return to the abdominal cavity. The septum transversum is a mass of mesoderm which forms from the fusion of the third, fourth and fifth myotomes. It thus has its motor nerve supply from the third, fourth and fifth cervical nerves (the phrenic nerve). Migration caudally occurs with the descent of the heart into the thorax. The pleuroperitoneal membrane grows medially on each side from the body wall to fuse with the septum transversum anteriorly and the oesophageal mesentery posteriorly. Mesoderm from the septum transversum migrates into the other parts of the diaphragm and forms the entire muscle.

The two main hypotheses to account for the origin of diaphragmatic hernias are (a) failure of fusion and (b) a primary defect.

Congenital diaphragmatic hernias (CDH) are classified according to the site of the defect, which in turn is reflected in the embryological origins. The commonest defect is posterolateral (Bochdalek) where the hernia is through the pleuroperitoneal canal (85–90%) and may be uni- or bilateral. Left sided lesions are commonest (80%), probably related to the later fusion on the left side than the right. Bilateral defects are least common (5%). Morgagni hernias, which are rare, accounting for 1–2% of all CDH, occur in the anterior portion, between the costal and sternal origins of the diaphragm. Septum transversum defects are midline and arise from a defect in the central tendon of the diaphragm. Hiatus hernias are clinically of less importance, as the large oesophageal orifice does not usually permit the egress of abdominal viscera into the thoracic cavity.

The incidence of CDH varies depending upon whether data are pre- or postnatal or from surgical series. This relates to the losses from termination of pregnancy, associated defects and immediate neonatal mortality. The neonatal incidence is about 1:3000 to 1:5000, with a prenatal incidence of 1:2000. There is a high association with other anomalies, including aneuploidy, and some genetic syndromes.

NATURAL HISTORY

Time of diagnosis is related to outcome, and there are well-documented cases of normal midtrimester prenatal sonography and a diaphragmatic hernia diagnosed at birth or on late scan[76,77]. It has been noted that the survival of cases diagnosed at birth or in the third trimester is better than those diagnosed early[78], although when compared to cases in which the diagnosis was not made prenatally, cases identified by prenatal ultrasound had a similar outcome[79]. However, why the herniation appears to occur later in some cases than others has no satisfactory explanation in embryological terms. Most cases are sporadic, although familial CDH has been described[80].

Pregnancies in which the fetus has a diaphragmatic hernia may be complicated by polyhydramnios, which predisposes to premature labour and delivery. Survival is dictated by the presence of other abnormalities, including aneuploidy and the degree of pulmonary hypoplasia.

ASSOCIATED ANOMALIES

The presence of other anomalies with CDH is common, occurring in between 30 and 70%[81–83] of those identified prenatally and 40% in liveborn infants[84]. Karyotype anomalies include the major trisomies and other complex abnormalities including translocations[83,85], and may occur in up to 34%[83,86] particularly in the presence of other anomalies[78]. Additional structural anomalies occur in up to 73% of cases of CDH diagnosed prenatally[81] and include cardiac in 20%[83,84] skeletal, genitourinary and neurological systems. The presence of associated anomalies markedly adversely affects survival[77] and therefore a careful search for such must be made at the time of initial diagnosis.

PRENATAL DIAGNOSIS

Diaphragmatic hernia can be diagnosed by ultrasound, usually at the time of the routine anomaly scan at 18 to 20 weeks. The ultrasound appearances vary and include the presence of the stomach on the same view as the four-chamber view of the heart, mediastinal shift, presence of bowel in the thorax, paradoxical movement of organs during fetal respiratory movements and absence of the normal integrity of the diaphragm seen in longitudinal views. It is well documented that ultrasound diagnosis may occur later in pregnancy following a normal midtrimester anomaly scan[76]. Many series report a false negative rate of detection of the order of 50%[79,87], more common in the case of a right-sided defect.

Once the diagnosis has been made, a careful examination of the fetus for associated anomalies and investigation of karyotype should be performed. At the time of diagnosis, the side of the lesion and the nature of herniated abdominal organs should be identified if possible. In addition, an attempt should be made to assess the degree of mediastinal shift, cardiac compression, and lung volume. Many methods of assessing lung volume have been described[77,88,89] and assessment of fetal breathing characteristics has also been investigated as a possible predictor of outcome[90]. However, the ability to predict outcome from ultrasound findings prenatally in the presence of an isolated defect is limited with most studies showing very disappointing results[77,83] although in some the presence of polyhydramnios is associated with a poor outcome[78,91]. The addition of magnetic resonance imaging to ultrasound examination prenatally enhances the ability to detect liver herniation[92], the absence of which is associated with a better survival[77].

POSTNATAL SURVIVAL

Predicting the prognosis of CDH is extremely difficult when a prenatal diagnosis is made. Advances in neonatology and paediatric surgery have led to improvements in survival, with some centres now reporting excellent figures up to 100% in the presence of an isolated lesion with diagnosis after 25 weeks[76,77]. However, comparison of data from different centres is difficult, as some use only those cases in which prenatal diagnosis had been made, and others use postnatal presentation regardless of prenatal diagnosis. Table 52.1 demonstrates the variety of survival figures from the literature.

Modern methods of postnatal management appear to have variable effect. Extracorporeal membranous oxygenation (ECMO) and high-frequency oscillatory ventilation (HFOV) have had disappointing results, with no improvement in survival[96,97] although HFOV with conventional ventilation has been shown to give similar results to ECMO[93]. ECMO may also be associated with long-term developmental problems and requires careful follow-up[98]. Partial liquid ventilation, however, shows promise in improving pulmonary function in babies with CDH[99]. Delaying surgery until the neonate has been stabilized does appear to be associated with improved postsurgical outcome, but this may relate to the presurgery deaths in the worst affected infants.

The principal causes of death in babies with CDH are pulmonary hypoplasia and hypertension In an attempt to reduce the risks of these problems, Harrison and his team have performed fetal surgery[94,95]. The results of this have generally been disappointing, although related to overall survival figures rather than those derived from postnatal series, the survival is similar. Fetal surgery has remained controversial[100] and alternative methods involving tracheal ligation have been explored[101]. Whilst the theory of this approach is promising, further studies must be performed before the potential can be assessed. Fetal surgery carries the risk of significant morbidity for the mother, and therefore the improvements in survival adopting such an approach must outweigh the risks.

Pulmonary hypoplasia

AETIOLOGY

Pulmonary hypoplasia (PH) is the main cause of death in neonates affected by space-occupying lesions within the thorax. It is also a common complication of pregnancies affected by reduced or absent liquor such as obstructive uropathies or very early rupture of membranes. The three prerequisites for normal fetal lung growth are:

- Adequate intrathoracic space
- Normal fetal breathing movement
- Presence of adequate amniotic fluid

If one or more of these are deficient during the canalicular phase of lung development (between 17–26 weeks) PH is likely to occur[102]. Some conditions which predispose to PH are not relevant to the neonate (ruptured membranes), or are

TABLE 52.1
Survival in congenital diaphragmatic hernia

Author	No. of patients	Percentage survival	Prenatal diagnosis	Isolated lesion survival (%)
Azarow et al.[93]	223	54.7		
Bollmann et al.[81]	44	18	Yes in 33	43.7
Bronshtein et al.[76]	15	40	Yes	75
Chan et al.[91]	19	21	Yes in 16	
Dommergues et al.[82]	135	22	Yes	33
Guibaud et al.[88]	43	43 (excl. TOP)	Yes in 40	
Harrison et al.[94,95]	52	40	Yes <25/40	40
Howe et al.[83]	48	27	Yes	50
Lewis et al.[79]	136	53 or 77	Yes in 61	
Manni et al.[78]	28	14	Yes	30
Metkus et al.[77]	55	65	Yes	
Shaw et al.[87]	36	64		89 (if survived to surgery)
Wilson et al.[96]	196	53		56

TOP = termination of pregnancy

amenable to postnatal correction (obstructive uropathies, diaphragmatic hernia). In these, prevention of PH should improve the chances of survival after delivery. However, in conditions which are lethal, e.g. bilateral renal agenesis, there is no role for prenatal interventions to prevent PH.

Antenatal intervention is thus focused on three areas:

- Relief of lung compression from intrathoracic space-occupying lesions, e.g. pleural effusions
- Correction of oligohydramnios in fetuses with functioning renal tissue; e.g. bladder outflow obstruction
- Restoration of amniotic fluid volume following amniorrhexis

Animal studies have demonstrated that compression of the developing lung by intrathoracic space-occupying lesions produces PH, whereas its relief is associated with continued lung growth. Harrison et al.[103] showed in controlled experiments in fetal sheep (canalicular period 80–125 days) that inflating an intrathoracic balloon between 100–140 days' gestation resulted in PH and fatal respiratory insufficiency at birth; deflating the balloon at 120 days permitted improved lung growth and allowed survival at birth. Similarly, in the same animal model, repair of experimentally created diaphragmatic herniae in utero before the end of the canalicular period improves lung size and morphometry, and survival.

There is a strong causal relationship between PH and oligohydramnios, although the underlying mechanism of oligohydramnios-related PH remains controversial[104]. It is known that loss of lung liquid occurs in oligohydramnios-related PH[105]. Chest compression, at least in the resting state[106], and/or a reduction in fetal breathing movements do not seem to be involved[107,108]. In addition, follow-up studies confirm that, in premature preterm rupture of membranes, PH is not inevitable[109]. Our poor understanding of the method of pathogenesis makes the development of therapeutic options very difficult, apart from the simple intervention of restoration of amniotic fluid volume by amnioinfusion.

Animal models of bladder outflow obstruction have facilitated study of the effects of amnioinfusion and diversion of urine flow at the appropriate gestational age (before the end of the canalicular phase). Such interventions have significant beneficial effects on lung and enhance postnatal survival[110,111].

The importance of normal liquor volume has been shown in cases of twins, with renal agenesis in one of monamniotic twins failing to develop PH[112]. Clinical experience of oligohydramnios suggests that the likelihood of PH depends on three variables: the gestation at onset, the duration and the severity of oligohydramnios[113–117]. PH secondary to amniorrhexis is unlikely when membrane rupture occurs after 25 weeks' gestation or if the resultant oligohydramnios lasts ≤5 weeks[114]. The relative risk of PH following amniorrhexis is highly gestation dependent[118] and declines from 50% at 19 weeks to 15% at 24 weeks[116]. PH is also 10 times more likely to occur after severe rather than mild to moderate oligohydramnios (60% vs 6%)[115].

DIAGNOSIS

Various parameters of lung size assessed by ultrasound have been proposed for the prediction of risk of PH. These include thoracic circumference, thoracic area, thoracic area minus heart area, lung area, thoracic circumference/abdominal circumference ratio, thoracic area/heart area ratio, thoracic area minus heart area/thoracic area ratio and lung area/thoracic area ratio[119,120]. Pulmonary blood flow has also been investigated[121]. These methods show promise, although many doubts have been raised concerning the reproducibility of the measurements. However, longitudinal studies suggest that in PH, progressive lag in other biophysical parameters does not occur ≥24 weeks (i.e. the end of the canalicular phase[122–124]. Thus, these parameters may only be of value in detecting established PH, rather than selecting those suitable for intervention.

The role of fetal breathing movements has also been investigated, with significantly fewer breathing movements being detected in fetuses which developed PH when compared with those that did not[125,126]. It is thought that the mechanical stretch caused by fetal breathing movements is needed for normal lung growth[127].

PREVENTATIVE INTERVENTIONS

In survivors of PH, catch-up lung growth occurs[128] and thus preventative strategies need to be concentrated on those at risk of lethal PH. Antenatal interventions to promote lung growth may be considered before the end of the canalicular period in those fetuses at risk of lethal PH, where the primary aetiological condition is non-lethal. Possible interventions include ultrasound-guided needling for aspiration or drainage of pleural effusions, drainage for obstructive uropathies or open fetal surgery. Prior to any of these, associated anomalies and aneuploidy should be excluded. To maximize expertise and chances of success, these procedures should only be performed in centres which have experience and the multidisciplinary back-up necessary.

RELIEF OF LUNG COMPRESSION

The drainage of pleural effusions and cystic lesions has been described above.

Resection of pulmonary lesions by open fetal surgery has been performed. Although the natural history of echogenic lung lesions is still being elucidated, large microcystic adenomatoid malformations carry a poor prognosis when associated with hydrops[129–131]. Based on experience with fetal surgery for diaphragmatic herniae, macrocystic lesions have been excised by open fetal surgery with some success[64,132].

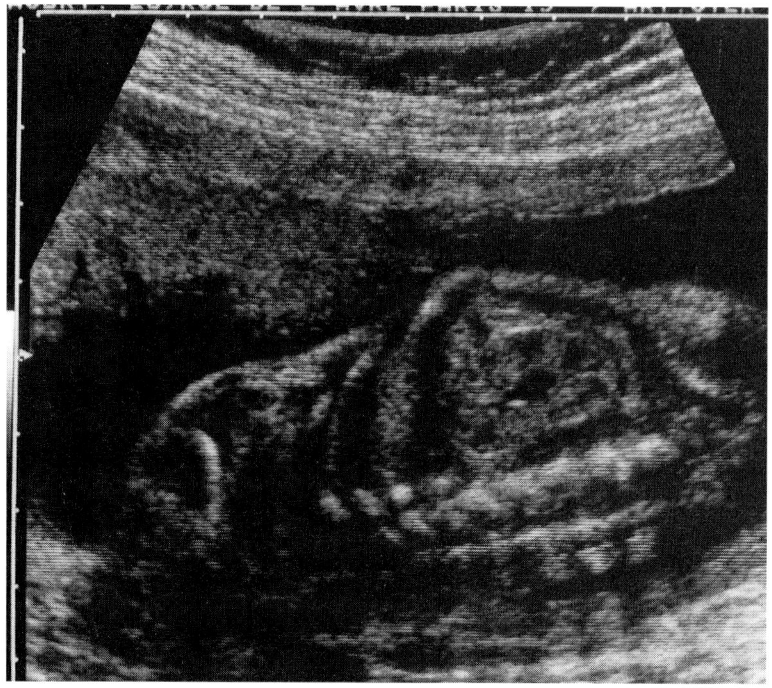

Fig. 53.4 Frontal cross-section of a normal fetal kidney at 21 weeks showing the corticomedullary differentiation.

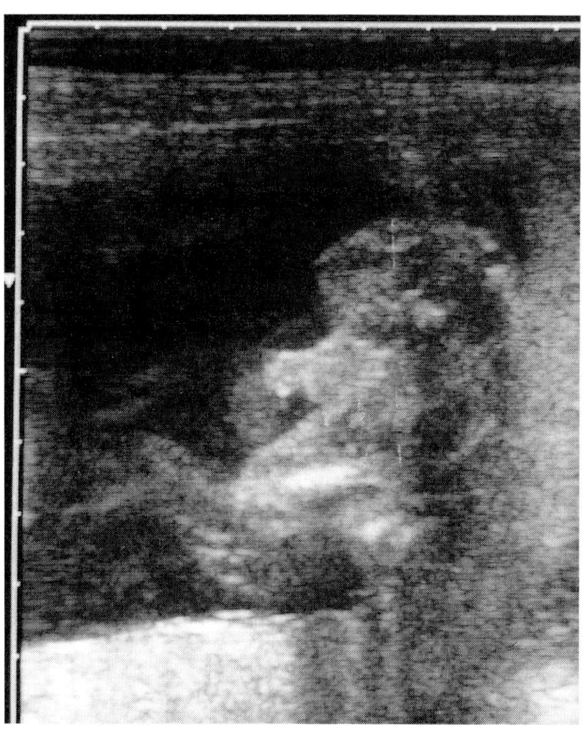

Fig. 53.5 Fetal penis and scrotum at 20 weeks.

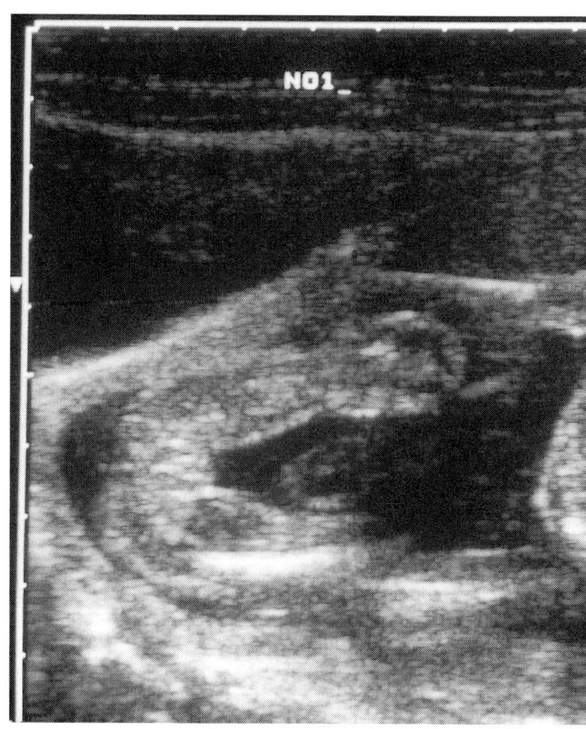

Fig. 53.6 Female external genitalia at 20 weeks.

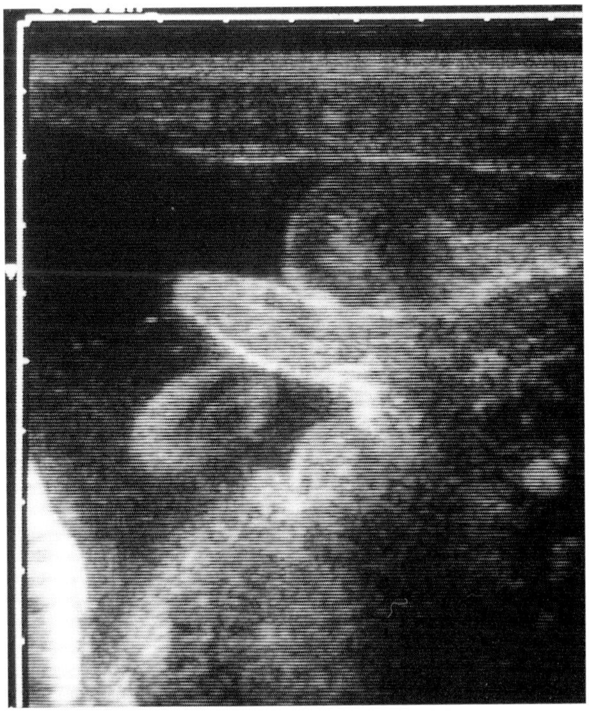

Fig. 53.7 Urethral canal in a male fetus at 34 weeks.

(Fig. 53.7). Undescended testes may be physiological until 32 weeks but the testes should be intrascrotal near term.

In girls, although the vulvar structure can be identified at 15 weeks and the vulva is clearly seen at 22 weeks, a detailed analysis of a vulvar anomaly is usually not feasible until 24 weeks (Fig. 53.6). In the third trimester, the external genitalia are large and can be easily explored. The identification of the uterus is not always possible, even late in gestation.

The fetal sacrum is an indirect but useful marker of the harmonious development of the fetal pelvis. It curves progressively during the second trimester (Fig. 53.8, 53.9). The anal sphincter can also be identified (Fig. 53.10).

Urinary tract anomalies

Prenatal diagnosis of fetal urinary tract anomalies is relatively easy based on the identification of transonic images corresponding to the dilated urinary tract. However, it is not always possible to ascertain the exact mechanism of the uropathy in utero, because an obstructive process often cannot be imaged directly, and because urinary tract dilatations resulting from a vesicoureteral reflux do not differ from dilatations above a true urinary outflow obstruction. Nevertheless, the accuracy of the pathophysiological diagnosis is not crucial before birth, since a satisfactory repair can be achieved by postnatal surgery in most cases, resulting in a good paediatric outcome provided that renal function is not altered and that there is no associated malformation. Therefore prenatal management of fetal uropathies mainly consists of ruling out associated anomalies or renal failure, thereby providing an adequate prognostic evaluation to the parents. This process is fundamental in order to organize prenatally a rational perinatal management plan in collaboration with paediatric surgeons and neonatologists.

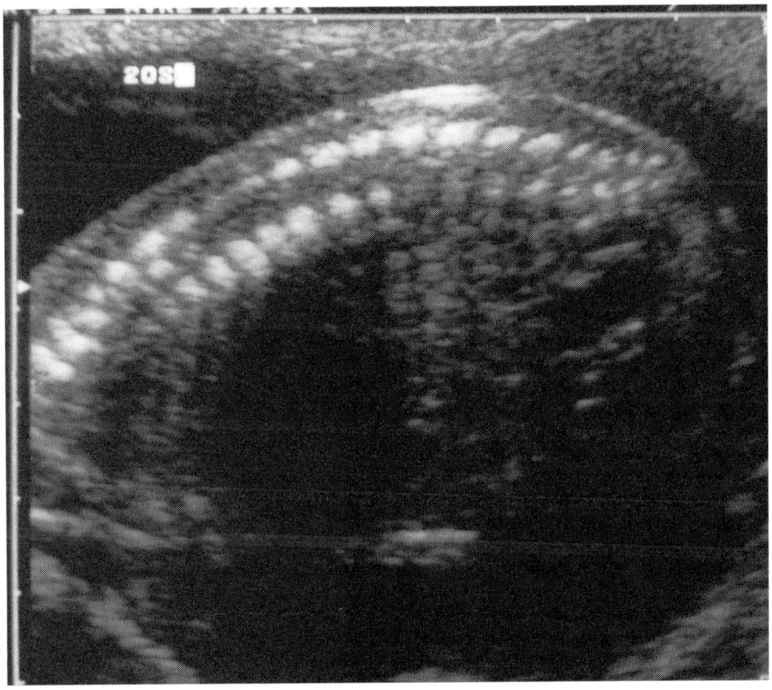

Fig. 53.8 Normal sacrum at 20 weeks. Note that the fifth and sixth sacral vertebrae are difficult to see.

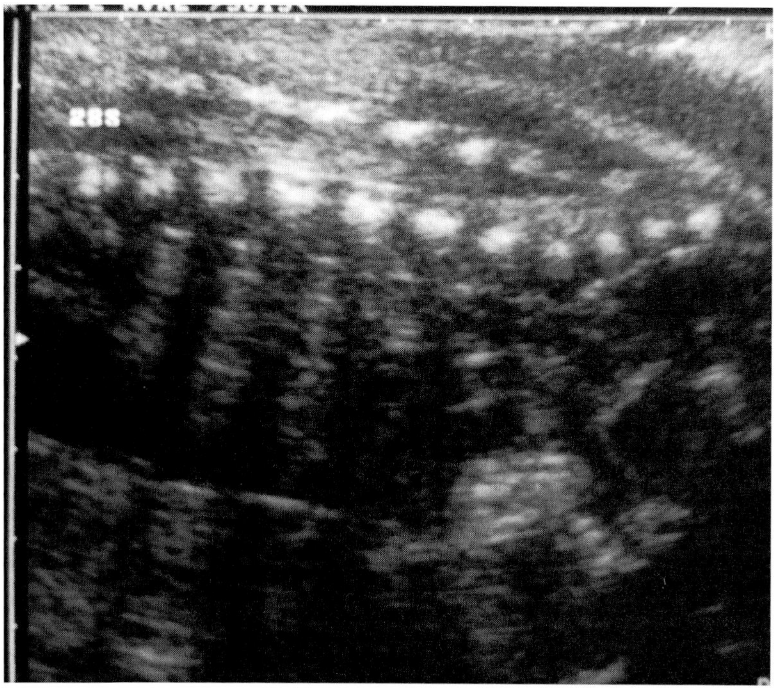

Fig. 53.9 Normal sacrum at 28 weeks; all vertebrae are seen.

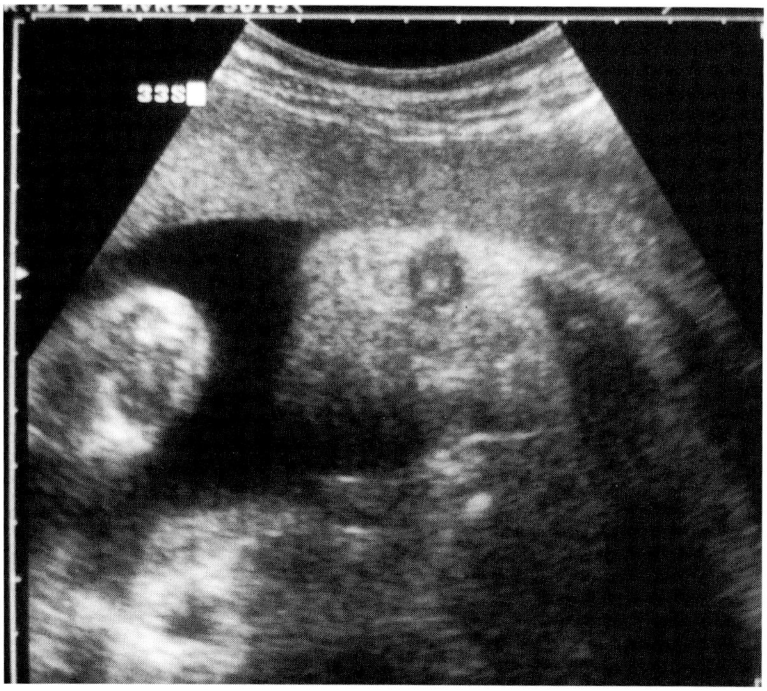

Fig. 53.10 Anal sphincter at 32 weeks.

NOSOLOGICAL CLASSIFICATION AND PATHOLOGY

Fetal urinary tract dilatations may result either from overdistension above an obstructive lesion or from increased urinary output occurring as a consequence of reflux.

NEPHROLOGICAL CONSEQUENCES OF FETAL UROPATHIES

In cases with no associated anomaly, the prognosis depends on renal function, since renal dysplasia may be associated with obstructive uropathies. It is not definitely established whether dysplasia results from an early increase in the renal urinary pressure or whether it results from an abnormal embryological process simultaneous to the obstruction but not occurring as a true consequence of it. If the latter hypothesis was eventually true, the attempts at intrauterine therapy based on uroamniotic shunting of the overdistended urinary cavities would be meaningless. However, a number of experimental data have suggested that at least in the fetal lamb, renal lesions similar to those encountered in the human can be reproduced by ligating the fetal urinary tract during the first half of gestation and can be prevented by fetal urinary diversion[16–21].

Nevertheless, it is clear that the question of renal function is only raised in bilateral forms, which are less numerous that the unilateral cases. In severe bilateral obstructions, a localized lesion such as posterior urethral valves or urethral atresia may be extremely deleterious. In the most severe forms, the uropathy is associated with terminal renal failure early in the second trimester. Fetal anuria results in severe oligohydramnios, fetal urine being the main source of amniotic fluid production in the second and third trimester of pregnancy. Due to the absence of amniotic fluid the fetus is compressed in the uterus. This prevents the expansion of its thorax and results in severe pulmonary hypoplasia, which is lethal postnatally. Fetal demise may also occur in utero due to cord compression. In addition, the absence of amniotic fluid causes a combination of anomalies usually referred to as 'Potter's sequence'. The absence of fetal movements due to severe oligohydramnios results in a variety of limb deformations and specific dysmorphic features. There are prominent epicanthic folds that form characteristic semicircles arising on the forehead, a flattened nose, low set ears, bowing of the legs with inward rotation of the feet, and large spade-shaped hands[22].

In some cases, fetal anuria may occur in the third trimester. Pulmonary hypoplasia is then unusual, but neonatal demise often results from terminal neonatal renal failure. This bad outcome can be predicted when ultrasound shows dysplastic kidneys, and should be confirmed by fetal urinalysis. However, when the kidneys appear non-dysplastic and urinalysis is reassuring, renal function may be good despite third-trimester oligohydramnios.

In more moderate cases, the amniotic fluid volume remains normal or only suboptimal during pregnancy. Prenatal sonography may reveal moderately abnormal features in the structure of the renal parenchyma such as a mild hyperechogenicity. When sonography is inconclusive analysis of fetal urine is required to diagnose abnormal renal function. Neonatally, high serum creatinine values may be found, but are expected to decrease after the obstruction is relieved. However, in the neonatal period, it is not possible to predict the evolution of renal function throughout childhood and adolescence. This underscores the need for long-term postnatal follow-up of these patients.

Nevertheless, it should be remembered that the great majority of fetuses with urinary tract dilatation will have normal renal function postnatally. This is of course the case for all unilateral lesions, for most bilateral lesions of the upper urinary tract, and for a substantial number of posterior urethral valves. These cases with a good postnatal outcome are characterized prenatally by normal amniotic fluid volume, the persistence of normal structure in the renal parenchyma, and if fetal urine sampling is indicated, by normal urinalysis. It should be emphasized that the size of the pelvic dilatation is not a bad prognostic marker and that huge dilatation may be associated with normal urine output and low urinary pressure resulting from high compliance of the urinary tract walls.

OBSTRUCTIONS TO THE URINARY OUTFLOW

Obstructions at the ureteropelvic junction

Ureteral obstruction at the ureteropelvic junction[23] is the most common lesion of the fetal urinary tract. The obstruction may rarely be associated with compression by an ectopic vessel. It may also be seen in duplication or ectopy.

Megaureter

True megaureter is the result of a dysfunction at the ureterovesical junction. Spontaneous relief of this dysfunction often occurs in the first years of life[24].

Ureterocele

Ureterocele is a cystic dilatation of the distal intravesical ureter. Most ureteroceles arise from an abnormal location of the ureteral meatus in the bladder and are therefore termed ectopic. They are often associated with a double ureter, the ureterocele at the lower ureteric orifice draining the upper pole of the duplex kidney. The lesion is associated with obstruction accounting for the dilatation of the corresponding ureter and/or renal pelvis. A large ureterocele can even obstruct the bladder neck, the disease then resembling an infravesical obstruction.

Obstruction of the bladder outlet

Obstruction of the bladder outlet usually occurs in the urethra and can lead to bladder dilatation with muscle hypertrophy, and hydronephrosis. The kidneys may also be dysplastic, resulting in a varaiable degree of renal failure[25]. The degree of outflow obstruction is thought to determine the gestational age of presentation and the ultimate outcome (see 'Nephrological Consequences of Fetal Uropathies' above).

The most common cause of bladder obstruction are posterior urethral valves. The valves consist of folds of mucosa along the posterior wall of the urethra, most often extending from the verumontanum, resulting in a very narrow urethral lumen. Urethral atresia is less common and results in lethal lesions with fetal anuria in the early second trimester.

REFLUX

Vesicoureteral reflux is a common disorder, usually diagnosed postnatally. Occasionally, it may be diagnosed before birth based on a dilatation of the upper urinary tract. Direct imaging of the reflux is sometimes possible. In the most severe cases, the bladder and ureters appear dilated due to a functional increase of the urinary outflow. The potential benefit of prenatal diagnosis of such cases is to avoid postnatal urinary infection and subsequent kidney damage. Postnatal surgery may be required in the severe forms of reflux.

COMPLEX CLOACAL ANOMALIES

These anomalies result from the failure of the urogenital sinus to divide properly. Therefore fistulae form in vesicovaginal or urethrovaginal locations in females or urethrorectal locations in males. The association with anorectal atresia is frequent.

PRUNE BELLY SEQUENCE

The prune belly sequence was described as the association of deficient abdominal wall musculature, vesical distension with renal dysplasia, absence of prostatic tissue, and cryptorchidism[26]. A patent urachus is common. The uropathy usually consists of urethral obstruction or dysfunction resulting in megacystis and bilateral megaureter. In males, hypoplasia of the prostate is very often observed. This syndrome occurs rarely in females in whom the uropathy and the abdominal wall defect are associated with vaginal atresia, rectovaginal or rectovesical fistula, and bicornuate uterus. As for any uropathy, the prognosis depends on the amount of functional renal tissue.

URACHAL DIVERTICULUM

The urachus connects the bladder to the anterior wall in utero. The intrafunicular part of this canal can remain open in utero[27] and result in a transonic cystic mass located in the cord, next to its fetal insertion. Although the cyst itself may disappear in utero, it may result in a vesicocutaneous fistula that should be managed appropriately in the neonatal period.

SONOGRAPHIC PRENATAL DIAGNOSIS OF FETAL UROPATHIES

Diagramatically, the fetal uropathies may be classified according to the level of the dilatation[28–33]. In upper lesions, only the renal pelves are dilated, while the ureters are also involved in midlevel lesions. Upper and mid uropathies can be categorized as uni- or bilateral, an important feature from a prognostic point of view, since postnatal renal function will always be normal in unilateral cases. Dilatations of the upper urinary tract may correspond either to a ureteropelvic junction obstruction or to a ureteropelvic reflux. Similarly, a midlevel uropathy may be the morphological manifestation of a vesicoureteral reflux as well as a congenital megaureter.

The bladder is involved in low-level lesions, which comprise mainly posterior urethral valves. However, a dilated bladder may also be the hallmark for major vesicoureteral reflux, which increases the urine output through the bladder and therefore its volume. More complex urinary malformations, for example cloacal malformations, may be revealed by a bladder dilatation. This latter aetiology is relatively more common in females.

PELVIC DILATATIONS AND HYDRONEPHROSIS

There is no universally accepted definition and grading of upper urinary tract dilatation in the fetus. Diagramatically, one could define pyelectasis as a pelvic dilatation without calyceal involvement (Fig. 53.11), hydronephrosis being defined by the finding of dilated calyces. Grading systems

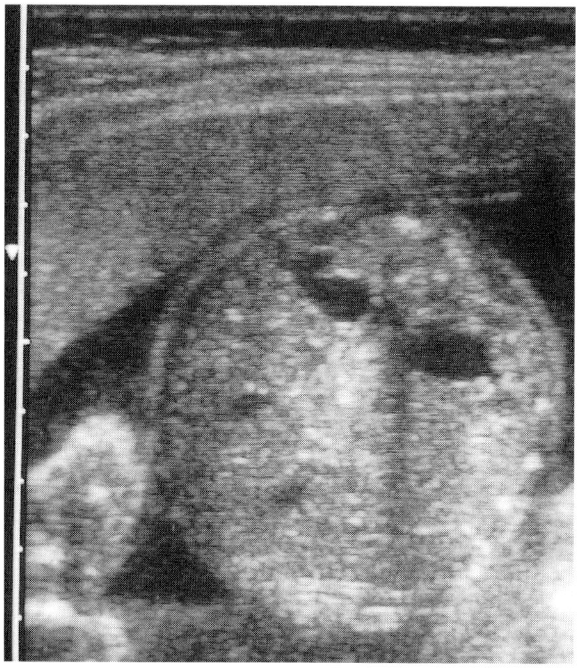

Fig. 53.11 Pyelectasis at 23 weeks; transverse cross-section.

have been proposed[34,35]. For instance[35], grade I corresponds to normal fetuses, grade II to pyelectasis (pelvis < 1.5 cm), and grades III to V to hydronephrosis (pelvis > 1.5 cm).

Pyelectasis

Moderate dilatation of the pelvic cavities is diagnosed by routine sonography in up to 2% of pregnancies (Fig. 53.11). In the literature, pyelectasis is defined by an antero-posterior pelvic diameter exceeding 4 to 6 mm in the second trimester on a cross-sectional view and 8–10 mm in the third[36–42]. We believe that the quantitative definition of fetal pyelectasis should be stringent enough to avoid generating iatrogenic consequences due to an unacceptable rate of false positive diagnosis.

In most cases, isolated fetal pyelectasy is physiological. However, it may correspond to a mild reflux or to a uretero-pelvic junction syndrome. Sonographic prenatal follow up should check that the dilation does not increase throughout gestation[43]. Postnatal evaluation is usually limited to a renal sonography by 1 to 2 weeks of age. In case of unexplained symptoms such as fever occurring postnatally, the prenatal history should be kept in mind in order not to overlook a urinary tract infection[28,44,45]. However, the sensitivity of prenatal ultrasound remains low for the screening of reflux, and most cases are picked up based only on postnatal symptoms.

Hydronephrosis

Diagramatically, fetal hydronephrosis may be defined by an anteroposterior pelvic size of more than 1.5 cm and/or calyceal involvement[35]. In mild hydronephrosis (grade III), the calyces are slightly dilated (Figs 53.12, 53.13). In larger dilatations of the upper urinary tract (grade IV) the calyces become round in shape (Fig. 53.14), but the transonic calyceal images are distributed regularly and are connected with the renal pelvis, in contrast to the irregular pattern of a multicystic kidney in which the cysts are independent from the pelvis. In more severe cases (grade V), the calyceal images are no longer identified from the pelvis, because the calyces become involved in a large single transonic image (Fig. 53.15). The renal parenchyma may be considered as exceedingly thinned when it becomes less than 3 mm thick. However, this latter feature is not necessarily ominous, since large dilations with a thin parenchyma may be associated with a normal renal function.

At the parenchymal level, the presence or absence of a corticomedullary differentiation should be recorded, as well as the echogenicity of the parenchyma and the presence of cysts. Although subjective[46–50] the evaluation of the sonographic structure of the renal parenchyma may be a useful predictor of renal function, but it is less sensitive than urinalysis to predict postnatal survival with altered renal function[7].

HYDROURETER

The ureter is normally not seen. A dilated ureter appears as a convoluted transonic image, located between the kidney and the bladder (Fig. 53.16). Peristaltic activity is suggestive of a megaureter, but a dilated ureter may also be due to a vesicoureteral reflux[51].

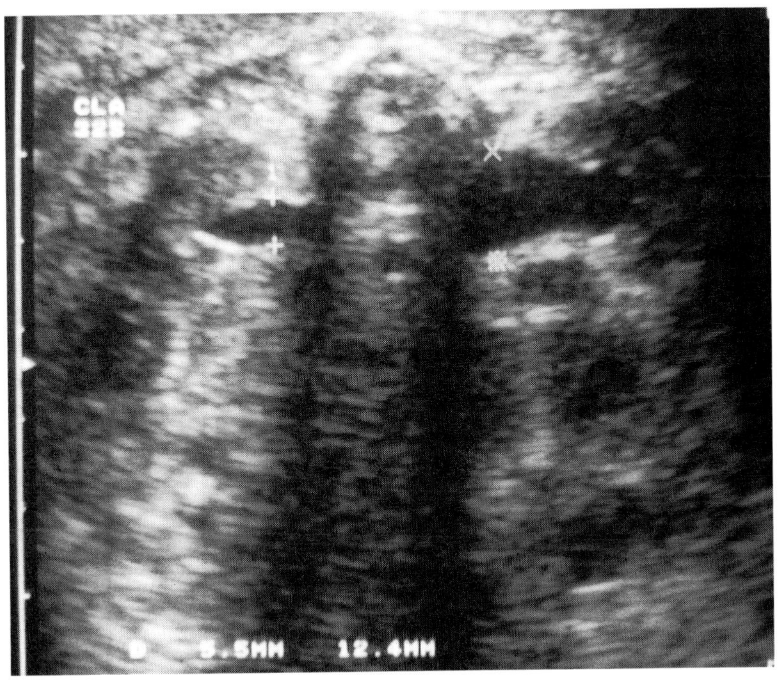

Fig. 53.12 Mild unilateral hydronephrosis in a 32-week fetus with ureteropelvic junction obstruction (grade III); transverse cross-section.

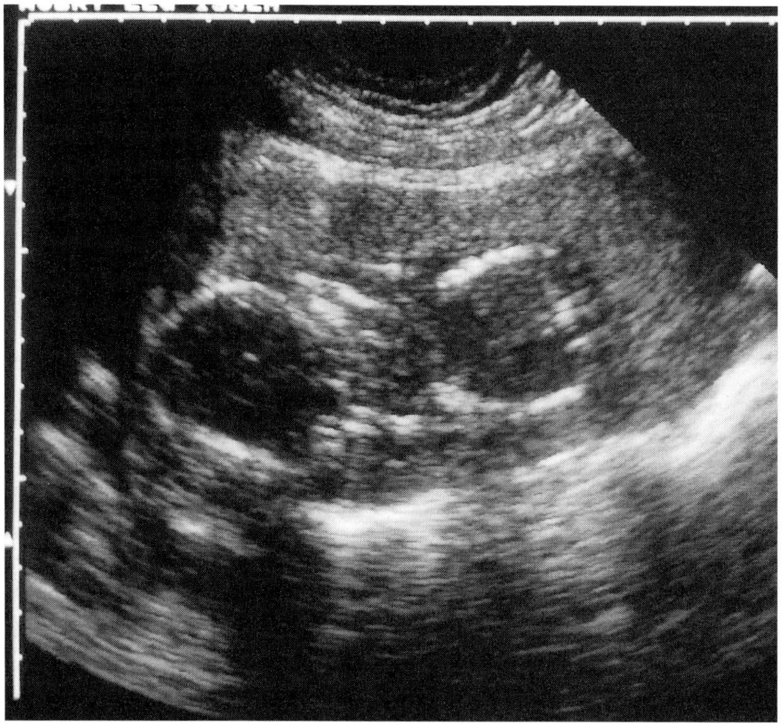

Fig. 53.36 Severe oligohydramnios at 20 weeks.

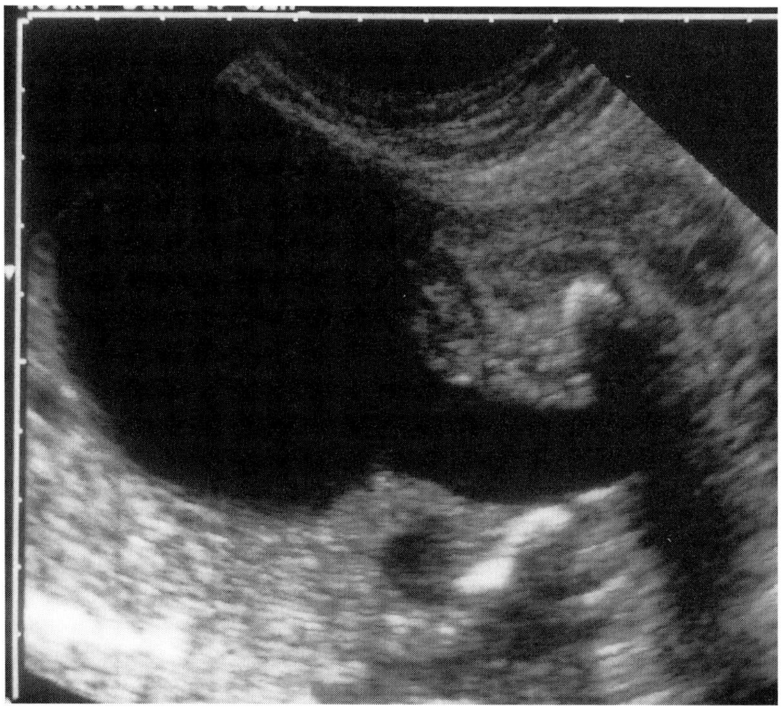

Fig. 53.37 Major bladder dilatation, recessus, and severe oligohydramnios at 24 weeks (posterior urethral valves).

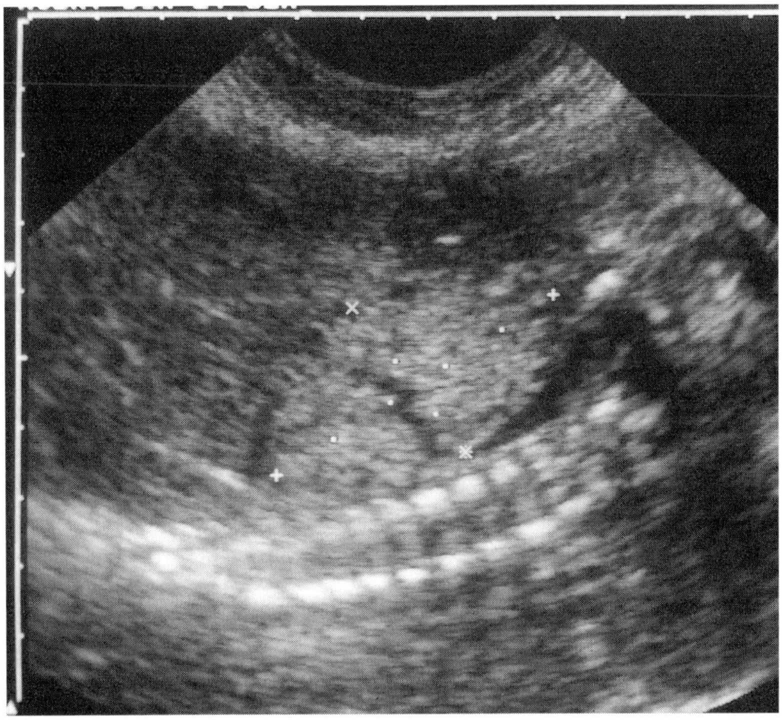

Fig. 53.38 Hyperechogenic renal parenchyma with microcysts and loss of the normal corticomedullary differentiation at 24 weeks (same patient as Fig. 53.37).

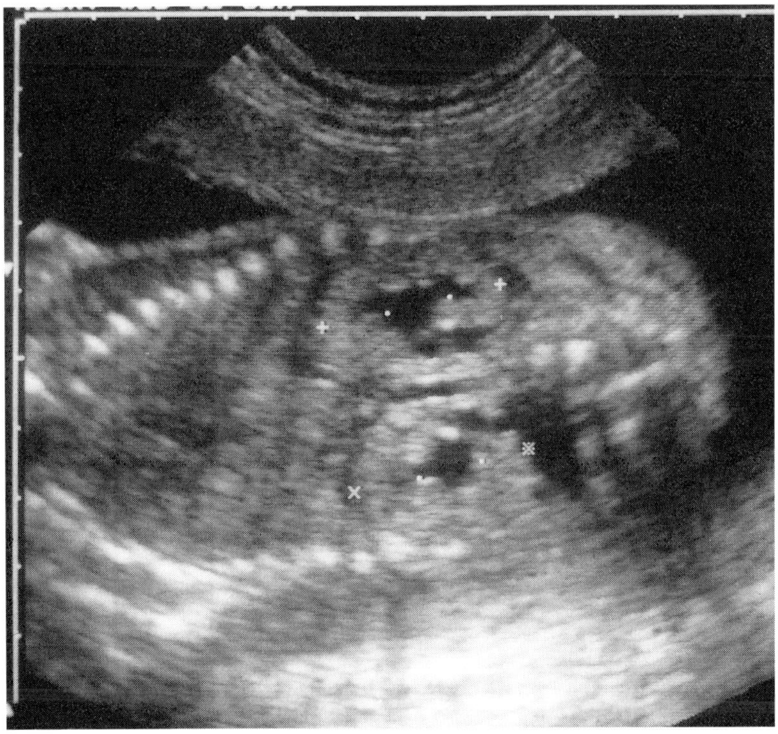

Fig. 53.39 Mild dilatation of the upper urinary tract, but hyperechogenic renal parenchyma at 22 weeks (posterior urethral valves, same patient as Fig. 53.18).

prognosis suggested by sonography. The most clinically relevant question is probably to identify among the children who will survive, i.e. grossly those with normal or slightly decreased amniotic fluid volume, which are at risk for developing postnatal renal failure and which will have normal renal function following surgical repair.

Establishing the prognostic value of any marker is made difficult by the fact that renal failure may occur relatively late, for instance during adolescence, which underscores the need for long-term follow-up of children in whom fetal urine analysis was performed in utero. Until such studies are completed, we must base our prenatal evaluation of renal function on cohorts with a shorter follow-up. Therefore we made the assumption that children with a fetal uropathy and a serum creatinine less than 1 SD above the mean (50 µmol/L) between 1 and 2 years were less likely to develop renal failure later than those with higher creatinine values, and could therefore be considered as having a normal renal function[9]. We were able to demonstrate that prenatal fetal urinary assessment of sodium and beta 2 microglobulin were reasonably good predictors of postnatal outcome, as defined above by serum creatinine at 1–2 years. Diagramatically, fetuses with a normal urinary sodium but a urinary beta 2 microglobulin above the 95th percentile are at increased risk for having a high serum creatinine in infancy. When both compounds are abnormally high, neonatal renal failure is likely. In contrast, a good postnatal outcome is anticipated when both compounds are within normal range (Fig. 53.40). When biochemical data are difficult to interpret, serial sampling could be helpful[82,92].

MANAGEMENT OPTIONS

Once the prognosis has been established, management options should be considered with the parents, including postnatal care and follow-up, termination of pregnancy, and occasionally fetal therapy.

Termination of pregnancy

In the most severe cases, i.e. babies with multiple malformations or terminal renal failure, the prognosis is unequivocally poor and most patients elect to have their pregnancy terminated. However, for a variety of reasons some parents would rather consider a conservative management resulting in perinatal death. In any of these situations, it is important to ensure that postmortem examination can be implemented in order to provide genetic counselling subsequently.

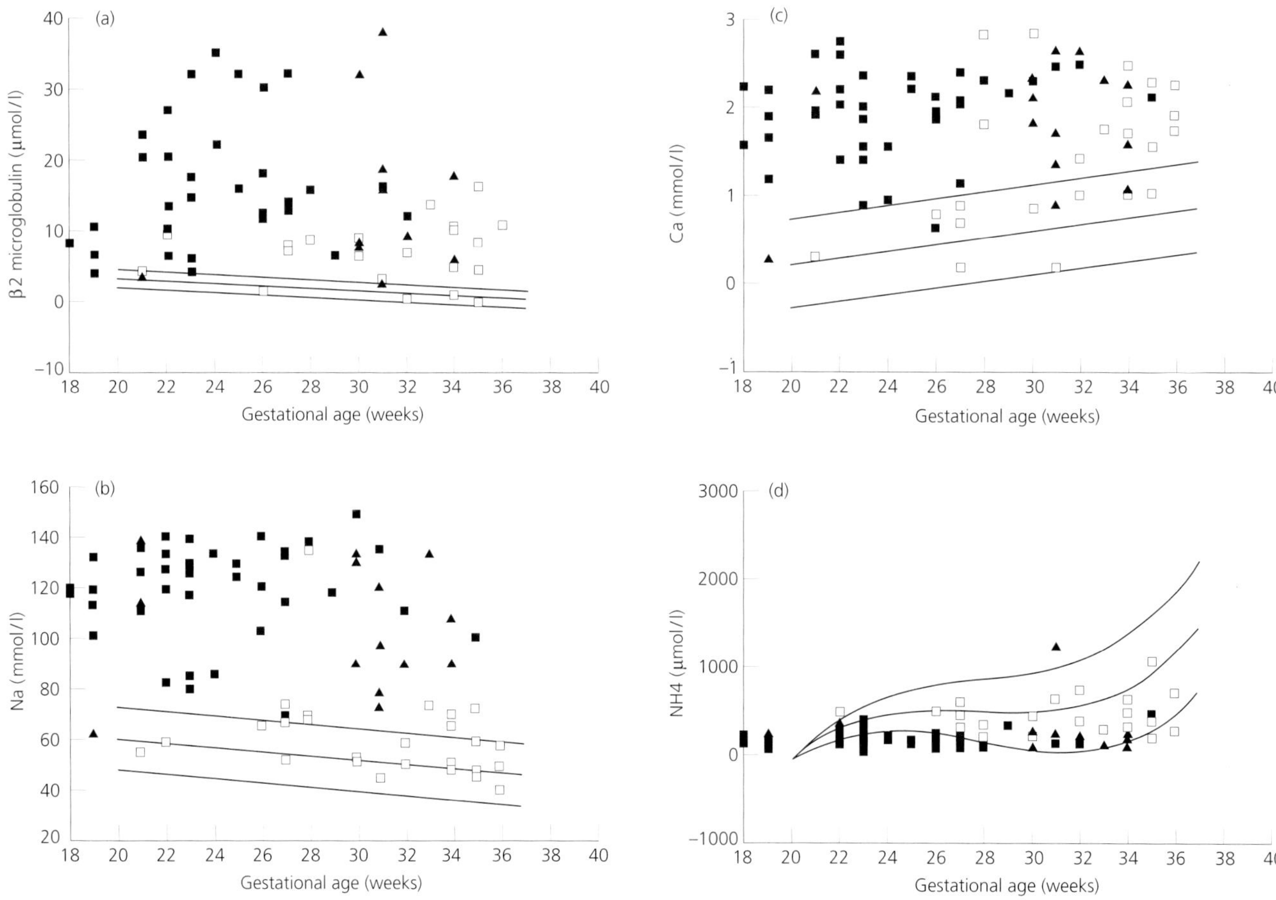

Planning postnatal therapy

In contrast, when the uropathy is isolated and the renal parenchyma is not damaged, the parents should be encouraged to continue the pregnancy. The fact that normal renal function is confirmed by fetal urinalysis may be an important argument for the parents to consider conservative management. During pregnancy, contact with the paediatrician who will be in charge of the baby postnatally is extremely useful to relieve the stress occasioned to the parents by the announcement of a fetal anomaly, even with a good prognosis. In cases in which no specific surgical therapy is likely to be performed, such as pyelectasis, the couple is usually referred to the paediatrician in charge of the maternity hospital in which the mother intends to deliver. In more severe cases, we tend to refer the couple prenatally to the paediatric urologist who will later be in charge of the baby. This allows direct information concerning the timing of postnatal investigations, and also the anticipated surgical procedures. In this respect, the identification of posterior urethral valves is important prenatally, because this anomaly requires emergency endoscopic or surgical therapy. The option of delivery near to a neonatal surgical centre should be offered to the mother, to avoid transferring the neonate elsewhere.

However, in many uropathies, no specific therapy is needed in the neonatal period, allowing the mother to deliver in the maternity hospital of her choice.

Fetal therapy

Fetal therapy for uropathies has been considered because obstruction of the urinary tract, although potentially lenitive by relatively simple postnatal procedures may be associated with severe renal lesions which occur before birth[93].

Although experimental data suggest that renal dysplasia can be induced by experimental urinary tract obstruction in the fetal lamb, and reversed by urinary decompression[17–19, 94–96] there is no conclusive evidence of the effectiveness of fetal therapy in human fetal uropathies[85,97–101].

From a technical point of view, restoring a normal urinary outflow in a fetus with posterior urethral valves could be

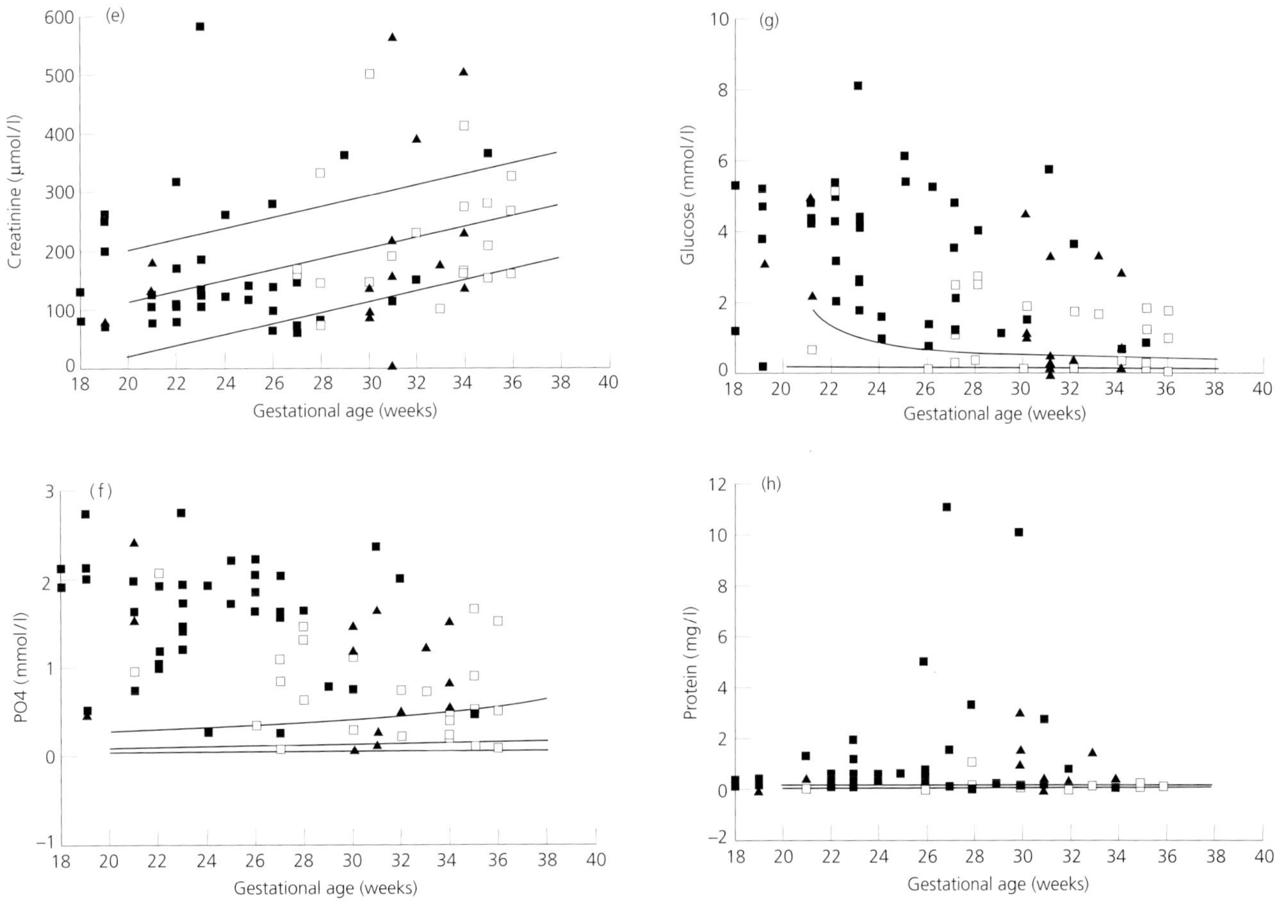

Fig. 53.40 Fetal urinalysis, abnormal cases. Datapoints for 70 cases with poor outcome are superimposed on the 5th, 50th and 95th centile reference regression curves. Full triangles: termination of pregnancy because of absent amniotic fluid and dysplastic kidneys. Full squares: neonatal death caused by renal failure. Open squares: survival with serum creatinine above 50 μmol/L at 1–2 years. (Adapted from Muller et al.[9]).

achieved by different approaches. One could consider the direct destruction of the valves by elecrocoagulation or laser ablation. This has been performed using a transvesical fetoscopic approach, but has many drawbacks[102,103]. First, once the endoscope is introduced into the fetal bladder, the valves are not easy to identify accurately. Second, it is difficult to be certain that surrounding tissue will not be damaged, especially when elecrocoagulation is used in a small fetus. The other approach consists in bypassing the obstruction by a uroamniotic shunt. Theoretically, performing a vesicostomy or a nephrostomy by direct fetal surgery would allow a better control of the quality of the shunt. However, open fetal surgery is extremely invasive and the risk of premature delivery associated with this approach is such that we believe it should not be attempted in the human, at least for uropathies.

The last option consists in percutaneous ultrasound guided uroamniotic shunting. Briefly, one end of a double pigtailed catheter in inserted in a dilated pelvic cavity or into the bladder, the other end of the catheter being left in the amniotic cavity[10]. This approach is clearly less invasive, but sometimes does not achieve urinary drainage successfully mainly due to shunt displacement.

Although vesicocentesis is not a therapeutic approach, early first trimester images of bladder dilatation were reported to have regressed following bladder puncture[104]. These results should be interpreted cautiously since regression of urinary dilatations is also possible spontaneously, for instance in reflux.

Contraindications to fetal therapy

We believe that fetal uroamniotic shunting is not indicated when irreversible renal damage has occurred. Although this approach might avoid neonatal death due to pulmonary hypoplasia by restoring a normal amount of amniotic fluid, it would tend to replace the natural course of a perinatal death by the artificial survival of a baby severely handicapped by neonatal renal insufficiency.

At the opposite end of the spectrum, we believe no invasive therapeutic attempt should be made in these cases in which a spontaneously good prognosis can be demonstrated by sonography, fetal urinalysis or both. Indeed, percutaneous shunting may result in severe complications such as amniotic fluid leakage, premature delivery, or chorioamnionitis, and therefore should not be undertaken without the proof of a compromised outcome in the absence of intervention. Does this mean that shunting should be performed in these borderline cases in which the baby will survive (normal amniotic fluid volume or mild oligohydramnios normal urine sodium), but with an increased risk of renal insufficiency in infancy (borderline parenchyma, moderate elevation of fetal urinary beta 2 microglobulin)?

This question cannot be answered on an objective basis so far. If in utero therapy can be offered to the parents in such cases, it should by no means be imposed on them, since we have no demonstration of the efficacy of this therapeutic approach.

Kidney anomalies

NOSOLOGICAL CLASSIFICATION AND PATHOLOGY

Diagramatically, fetal renal anomalies include anomalies of number, location, size, and structure of the kidney. These malformations are primarily renal and occur in the absence of a urinary tract defect. Some of these are rather common and easy to diagnose, for example renal agenesis or multicystic kidney disease. The diagnosis and prenatal management may be more difficult, however, as in structural anomalies of the kidney presenting prenatally as hyperechogenic enlarged kidneys.

As for uropathies, the prognosis is uniformly good in unilateral lesions, while bilateral anomalies associated with severe oligohydramnios are lethal. In bilateral cases with normal amniotic fluid, the long-term postnatal morbidity is usually impossible to predict. Biochemical markers which have proved predictive of postnatal morbidity in uropathies have not been as helpful in fetal nephropathies.

ANOMALIES OF NUMBER

Renal agenesis

Renal agenesis can be uni- or bilateral. It may result from early degeneration of the ureteric bud, or from failed interaction between the ureteric bud and the blastema (Figs 53.41, 53.42 and Plate 53.1). The corresponding adrenal gland takes a globoid shape and should not be misdiagnosed prenatally for a hypoplastic kidney[105].

Bilateral agenesis is a lethal condition resulting in the oligohydramnios sequence (pulmonary hypoplasia, dysmorphic face, and limb deformities)[106]. However, the amount of amniotic fluid remains normal until the second trimester, when fetal urine becomes the main source of amniotic fluid production[107].

In contrast, fetuses with unilateral renal agenesis will remain asymptomatic during postnatal life, in the absence of associated anomalies.

Minor genital anomalies such as duplicated/hypoplastic uterus, absent fallopian tube, absent epididymis and vas efferens can be found ipsilateral to unilateral renal agenesis. They cannot be diagnosed in utero, but would not alter the prognosis anyway[2].

More complex anomalies can also be associated with renal agenesis such as hypoplastic/atretic bladder and urethra, rectal atresia, lumbosacral vertebra anomalies, tracheo-oesophageal anomalies, congenital heart defects such as tetralogy of Fallot, and single umbilical artery. The combination of these anomalies constitutes syndromes referred to as

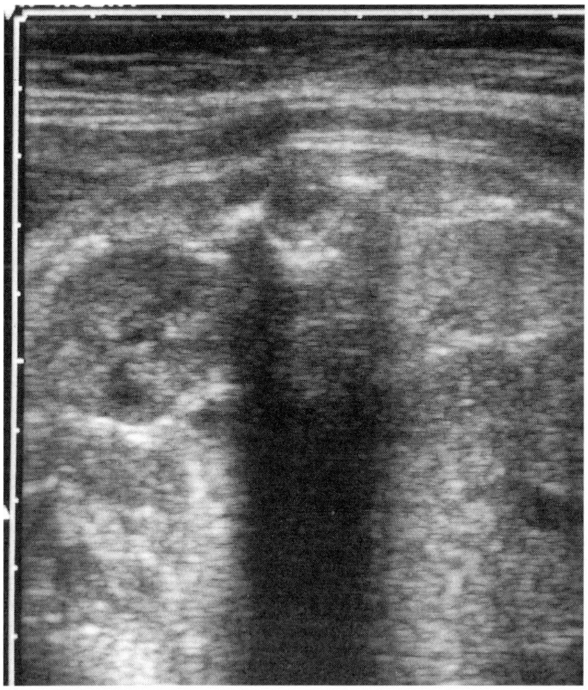

Fig. 53.41 Unilateral renal agenesis. Transverse scan of the fetal abdomen at 35 weeks. Note the ipsilateral enlarged adrenal gland and the normal controlateral kidney.

VATER or VACTERL association. In even more complex anomalies such as caudal regression or syrenomelia, major anomalies of the lower limbs are associated with the defects mentioned above.

Most cases of renal agenesis are sporadic, with a low risk of recurrence among subsequent sibs. However, familial cases have been reported with different types of inheritance[2].

Renal adysplasia is an uncommon condition that should be known by those involved in fetal medicine, in which unilateral renal agenesis is combined with controlateral dysplasia. This underscores the need for careful prenatal evaluation of the development of the controlateral kidney in fetuses with apparently isolated unilateral renal agenesis. The mode of inheritance is autosomal dominant with an incomplete penetrance and a wide variability of expression, ranging from lethal cases with a single dysplastic kidney to unilateral renal agenesis with minor controlateral anomalies such as uretero-pelvic junction obstruction.

Duplex kidney

Duplication of the kidney results from premature division of the ureteric bud before it connects to the nephrogenic mesoderm (Fig. 53.43). This accounts for the association with a double or bifid ureter. The upper ureter usually enters the

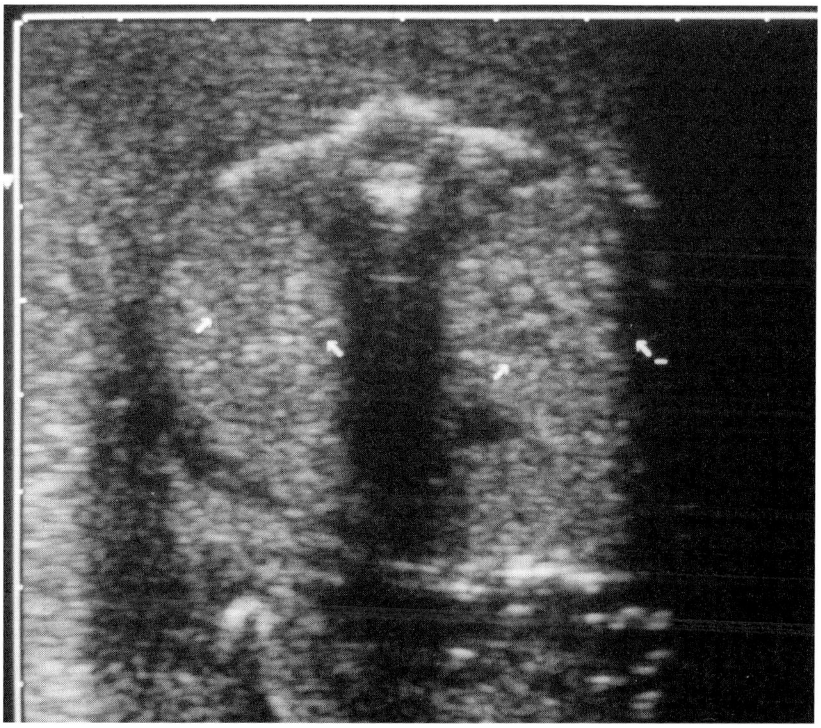

Fig. 53.42 Bilateral renal agenesis at 26 weeks. Severe oligohydramnios. Both adrenal glands differ from kidneys because of the absence of pelvis and of corticomedullary differentiation.

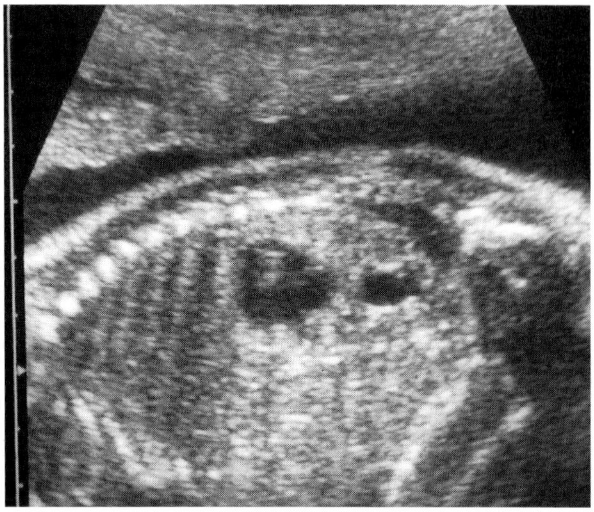

Fig. 53.43 Duplex kidney at 22 weeks.

bladder more caudally, and may also connect ectopically to the urethra, vagina, seminal vesicle, or the rectum.

The upper kidney usually presents with some degree of outflow obstruction and parenchymal dysplasia. Therefore a dilated pelvis or the abnormal structure of the dysplastic part of the kidney can be the hallmark for the prenatal diagnosis of this condition in which a ureterocele may be the marker of the connection of the distal ureter to the bladder[108].

Supernumerary kidney

A third kidney may result from premature branching of the ureteric bud. It has its own ureter and blood supply, and may be complicated by obstruction or dysplasia.

ABNORMALITIES OF POSITION

Renal ectopy

Ectopic kidneys are usually displaced caudally (Fig. 53.44). One or both kidneys may be involved. Their shape can appear abnormal due to malrotation. This condition is asymptomatic, provided the renal parenchyma is well differentiated and free from dysplasia[109]. In crossed renal ectopia, both kidneys are located on the same side and may be fused.

Horseshoe kidney

This anomaly (Fig. 53.45) results from the fusion of the kidneys, usually by their lower poles[110]. Fusion of both upper and lower poles results in ring kidney. When isolated, horseshoe kidneys are usually asymptomatic, but they can be associated with aneuploidy (trisomy 18, Turner syndrome, triploidy).

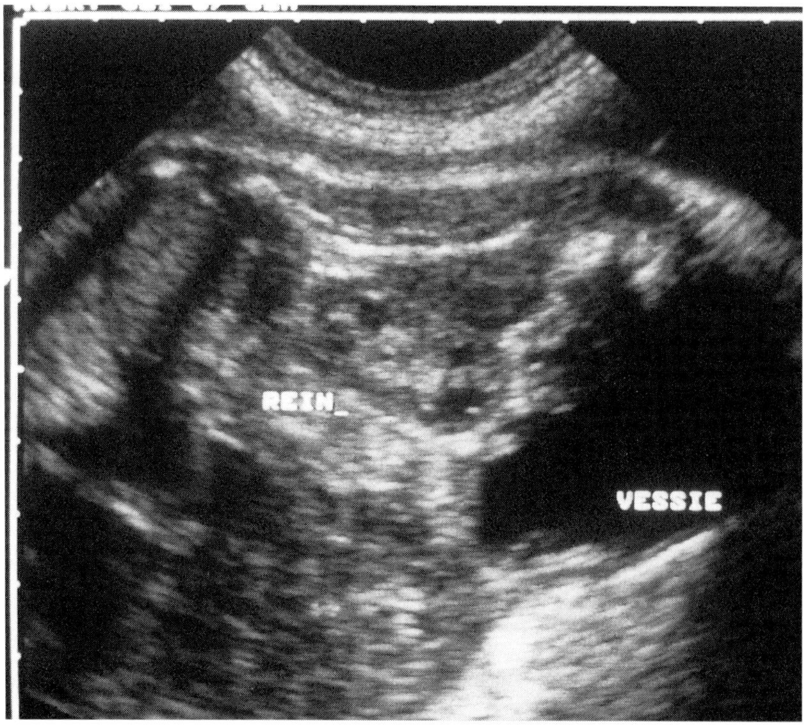

Fig. 53.44 Ectopic kidney at 37 weeks. Renal parenchyma (REIN) is seen next to the fetal bladder (VESSIE).

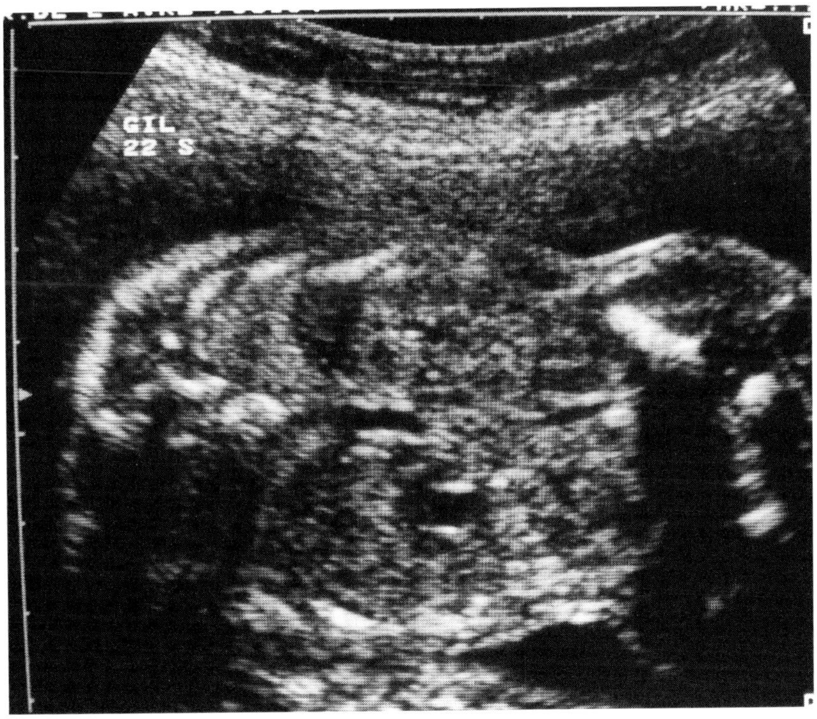

Fig. 53.45 Horseshoe kidney at 22 weeks (trisomy 18). (Coronal section.)

ISOLATED ABNORMALITIES OF SIZE AND/OR STRUCTURE

Although growth charts are available[12,13], the assessment of renal size is usually made by visual examination. However, growth charts may be useful to express the degree of kidney enlargement, for instance in standard deviations above the mean.

Renal hypoplasia

Renal hypoplasia is defined as a kidney mass less than 2 SD below the mean. This condition is usually diagnosed postnatally, except in the most severe forms (Fig. 53.46).

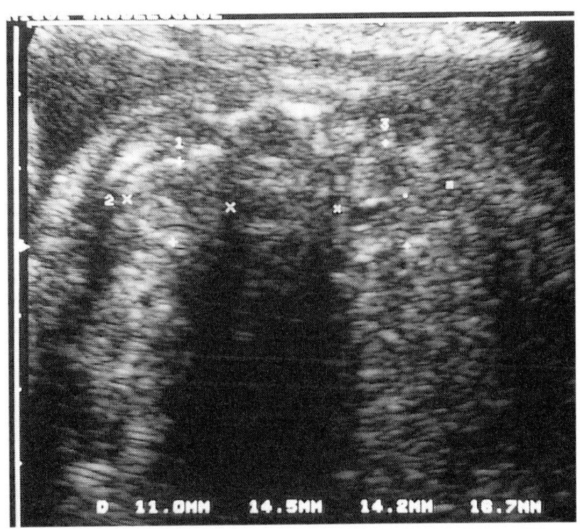

Fig. 53.46 Hypoplastic kidneys at 31 weeks.

Multicystic dysplasia

Idiopathic multicystic dysplasia presents prenatally as kidneys that have lost their normal shape due to cysts of variable diameter (0.5–3 cm or more), which are not connected to each other or to the rest of the urinary tract. Some clusters of tubules, rudimentary glomeruli, primitive ducts, and bars of metaplastic cartilage can be irregularly distributed within the loose mesenchyme. The ureter is usually atretic. While bilateral cases are lethal, unilateral ones carry a good prognosis. Spontaneous involution of the multicystic kidney is usual in postnatal life, and may exceptionally occur in utero. The size of the cysts is usually constant throughout fetal life, but very unusually, extremely large cysts may compress the fetal abdomen or cause dystocia and therefore require intrauterine needling.

These macrocystic lesions (Fig. 53.47) are easy to differentiate from polycystic kidney diseases which present prenatally as enlarged hyperechogenic kidneys. The sonographic pattern of the latter conditions is due to the presence of microscopic cysts in the renal parenchyma[111].

oesophagus from the respiratory tree occurs during the fourth and fifth weeks postconception (pc) and a failure of this process at this point leads to the development of a tracheo-oesophageal fistula. However, a further problem arises from a failure of growth at the cranial end of the of the oesophagus, which is initially a very short tube. This growth is completed by about 7 weeks pc and its velocity matches the rapid elongation of the embryo at this time. The epithelium of the oesophagus proliferates and partially obliterates the lumen, recanalization of which is not complete until the end of the embryonic period.

DEFINITION

Tracheo-oesophageal atresia is a rare condition occurring in about 1 in 5000 births. There are six main types, only two of which are identifiable on ultrasound because they are associated with an absent stomach, there being no communication between the upper gut and trachea[4]. In 80% of cases the oesophagus ends blindly and the stomach is connected to the lower end of the trachea. Figure 54.1 illustrates the common arrangements, with type (b) and type (e) being associated with an absent stomach on ultrasound. Type (a) occurs in about 90% of all cases. Because of the connections between the trachea and the lower end of the oesophagus the abdomen becomes rapidly distended with air, once the baby is delivered.

DIAGNOSIS

Polyhydramnios[5] is the most likely clinical alerting factor but this may not become apparent until the third trimester.

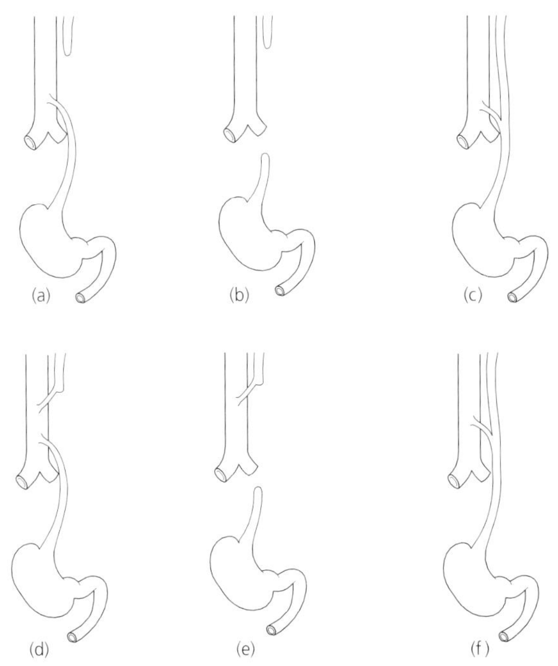

Fig. 54.1 The different types of tracheo-oesophageal fistulae.

Ultrasound will confirm the polyhydramnios and although the fetal stomach may be identified, its presence does not exclude tracheo-oesophageal fistula because of the high chance that the stomach will connect with the trachea. However, the stomach should always be visible at a 20-week screening scan so its absence must prompt a further evaluation at 24 to 26 weeks[6,7].

When tracheo-oesophageal fistula is suspected the presence of associated abnormalities should always be sought and may be found in about 40% to 60% of fetuses[4]. These abnormalities will include cardiovascular defects in about 30%, defects of the anorectal and genitourinary systems each in about 15%. The combination of these abnormalities may amount to the VATER syndrome, which includes vertebral, anorectal, cardiac, oesophageal anomalies, radial aplasia and the presence of a single umbilical artery. Karyotypic abnormalities may also exist and Down syndrome has been reported in tracheo-oesophageal fistula.

The differential diagnosis of the ultrasound appearances is limited. If the absence of a fetal stomach is the only ultrasound feature apart from polyhydramnios, a careful search for the stomach elsewhere, namely in the chest, is important to exclude diaphragmatic hernia. The presence of the stomach on the wrong side is found in situs invertus.

MANAGEMENT

When the condition is suspected, a detailed ultrasound examination should exclude other abnormalities. If appropriate a karyotype should be obtained. In the absence of other abnormalities the prognosis can be favourable with about an 80% survival. The main surgical problem arises from the shortness of the oesophagus so that a staged procedure may be required to achieve anastomosis.

The immediate neonatal management problem stems from the inhalation of milk and this can be prevented by ensuring that a balloon will pass into the stomach before oral feeding is attempted. It is essential that this simple test is performed whenever the possibility of tracheo-oesophageal atresia exists, a suspicion which may arise if there is clinical polyhydramnios.

Genetic counselling should indicate that isolated tracheo-oesophageal fistula is likely to be a sporadic event and that recurrence rates reflect those of the associated conditions. VATER itself is usually regarded as sporadic.

DUODENAL OBSTRUCTION

EMBRYOLOGY

During the development of the foregut, the proliferation of the endothelial lining during the fifth and sixth weeks leads initially to occlusion. Recanalization is usually complete by the end of the embryonic period but a failure in this process will lead to the development of stenosis. Another mechanism for stenosis arises from the presence of an annular pancreas which may compress the duodenum externally and which is found in about 20% of duodenal atresias. Most atresias are found in the second and third part of the duodenum and comprise a web or membrane (Fig. 54.2).

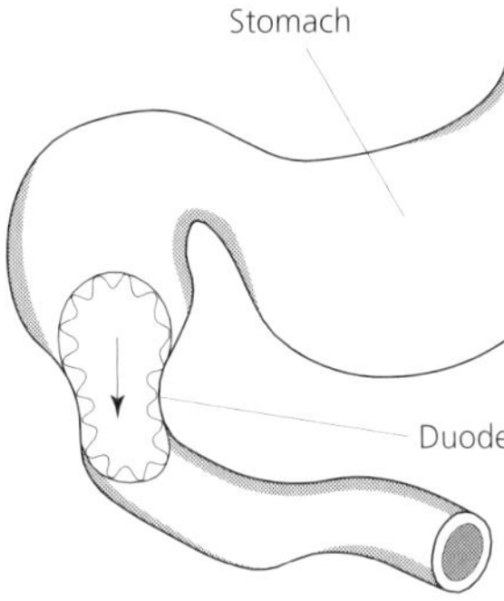

Fig. 54.2 The site of duodenal atresia.

DEFINITION

Duodenal atresia arises in about 1 in 5000 pregnancies and may be associated with abnormalities of the bile duct[8]. The atresia is complete in 40% to 60% of cases, the space between the two parts of the duodenum being filled by pancreas.

DIAGNOSIS

The typical double bubble appearance arises from the enlarged stomach and the duodenal cap which becomes fluid-filled[9,10] (Figure 54.3). Usually the diagnosis is not difficult but interestingly the double bubble is not always apparent at 20 weeks, presumably because the duodenal cap fills later in pregnancy[11]. However, diagnosis in the first trimester has been reported[12]. The pyloric sphincter can usually be identified. Polyhydramnios is a constant finding and is often the initial indication for the scan.

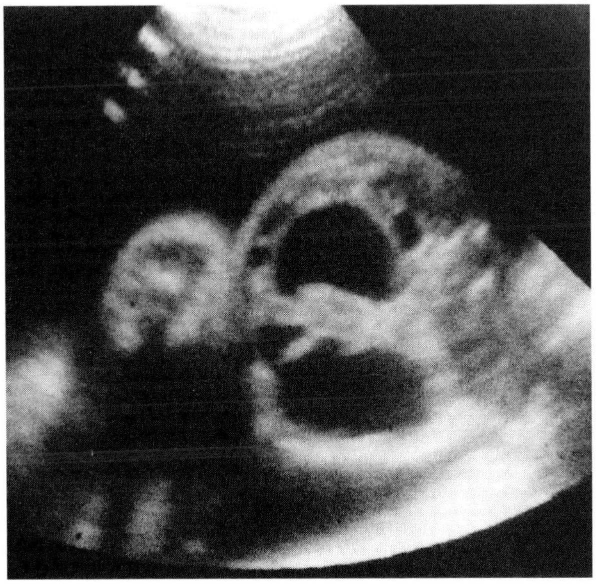

Fig. 54.3 Ultrasound appearance of duodenal atresia – 'double bubble'.

A careful search for other anomalies must be made because duodenal atresia occurs as an isolated abnormality in only about 50% of cases. Cardiac abnormalities may be found in about 10% to 20%, skeletal changes about a third and other intestinal abnormalities in about a quarter. Perhaps the best known association is with trisomy 21, although the literature gives a wide range of incidence, but when the duodenal atresia is isolated the risk of Down syndrome is reported from 15% to 30%[13]. However, the numbers of cases in these studies are very small and caution is required in interpreting these figures.

The diagnosis of duodenal atresia is not usually difficult but other cystic structures may confuse the picture. Thus structures such as a distended gallbladder or a choledochal cyst both lie more anterior than the duodenum but can be mistaken. Gut reduplication cysts or mesenteric cysts may be seen but these are unlikely to cause diagnostic difficulties as they are not usually associated with polyhydramnios. An annular pancreas is one which surrounds the duodenum and may cause obstruction. The clue to its presence is from the presence of a further cyst in the head of the pancreas which is located behind the stomach. This cyst may arise from the abnormal drainage of an accessory pancreatic duct.

MANAGEMENT

In the absence of associated abnormalities the outcome for duodenal atresia is excellent, with about 95% survival. Because the condition has a known association with Down syndrome there is a need to discuss karyotyping, but because the presentation is often late the subsequent management, with a possible prospect of fetocide, can be difficult and distressing for both parents and attendants. Surgical repair of the atresia is performed soon after birth and once the baby is stable[14].

JEJUNAL AND ILEAL ATRESIAS

EMBRYOLOGY

Gut atresias which occur distal to the duodenum are more likely to have a vascular basis rather than a strictly embryological one.

DEFINITION

These are rare conditions which occur with a frequency of about 1 in 10 000 pregnancies. They are probably the consequence of a volvulus, a transparietal constriction or a parietal perforation and the resulting vascular occlusion causes a segment of bowel to become atretic rather than stenotic. Multiple forms may rarely be familial. The apple-peel type[15,16] is seen when the bowel is coiled around a vascular axis and it can be secondary to a volvulus which causes occlusion of the jejunal branches of the superior mesenteric arteries. Other structural fetal abnormalities are rare with jejunal atresia.

About a third of these atresias involve the ilium, and like the jejunum the incidence of other abnormalities is rare, although Down syndrome has been reported in about 1%.

DIAGNOSIS

The classical ultrasonic appearance of jejunal atresia is an intra-abdominal 'triple bubble' (Fig. 54.4). This is a bit of a misnomer since in fact there are more than three 'bubbles', and the phenomenon arises from the effect of the ultrasound 'cut' across the abdomen. The distended loops usually appear large and as with other upper gut problems there is usually polyhydramnios[17].

Ileal atresia may produce similar appearances and although the small bowel distension may produce a typical honeycomb appearance, in fact small and large bowel changes can be difficult if not impossible to distinguish. There is less likely to be polyhydramnios with ileal atresia.

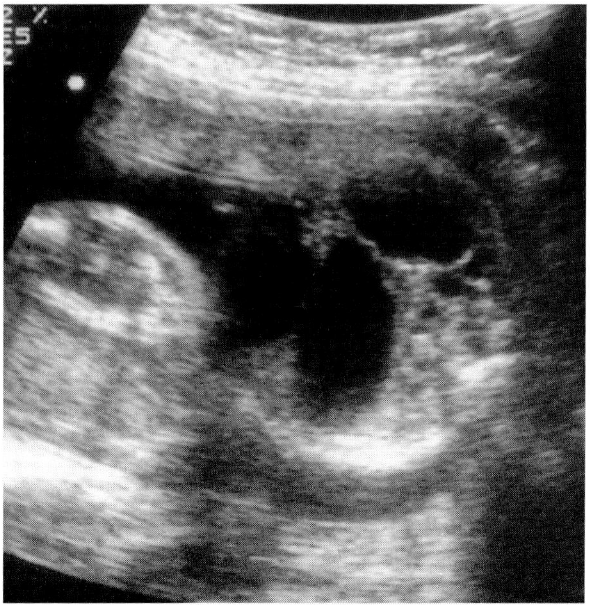

Fig. 54.4 Ultrasound appearance of jejunal atresia – 'triple bubble'.

MANAGEMENT

The prognosis for jejunal and ileal atresias is usually good although dependent on the length of bowel which has to be resected. If very long sections have to be removed, the child may suffer from nutritional deficiencies as he or she gets older. Conversely the rarity of associated problems considerably improves prognosis. Advanced knowledge that the lesions exist also allows a more timely surgical intervention after delivery and before the baby can become unwell from dehydration.

IMPERFORATE ANUS

EMBRYOLOGY

The rectum and anus are developed from the division of the cloaca by the urorectal septum which develops caudally towards the cloacal membrane, fusion occurring by the end of the sixth week. The rectum and anus lie dorsal to the urogenital septum and the urogenital sinus ventrally. The proctodeum develops as a pit, external to the anal membrane which closes the primitive anal canal (Fig. 54.5).

DEFINITION

The commonest abnormality is anal agenesis, which has an incidence of about 1 in 3000 and which is found in about 45% of all cases of imperforate anus. It is more common in males and usually arises as a failure of the urorectal septum to develop normally, this leading to incomplete separation of the cloaca into urogenital and anorectal portions. It is usually associated with a fistula which in females may open in the vulva and in males the urethra. A rare malformation is the 'covered anus', which is due to a failure of the anal membrane to perforate. These conditions are usually isolated but may be found in syndromes such as VATER.

DIAGNOSIS

The ultrasound diagnosis of imperforate anus is unreliable although in some cases distended loops of bowel are observed in the fetal pelvis leading to a fluid-filled, dilated rectum. There is no polyhydramnios unless abnormalities of the upper tract exist as well. Other bowel conditions may cause confusion and both Hirschsprung's disease and colonic atresia may provide similar ultrasound appearances[18–20].

MANAGEMENT

Prenatal diagnosis of imperforate anus is unusual. Firstly, the ultrasound markers are unreliable, and secondly, clinical features do not usually appear – polyhydramnios is not associated with the condition. However, if features compatible with VATER syndrome are apparent, then a careful examination of the fetal pelvis is advisable.

Once the baby is born, clinical examination should be undertaken to confirm the patency of the anus. If obstruction is confirmed, then a defunctioning colostomy procedure or immediate anatomical correction with primary anastomosis is

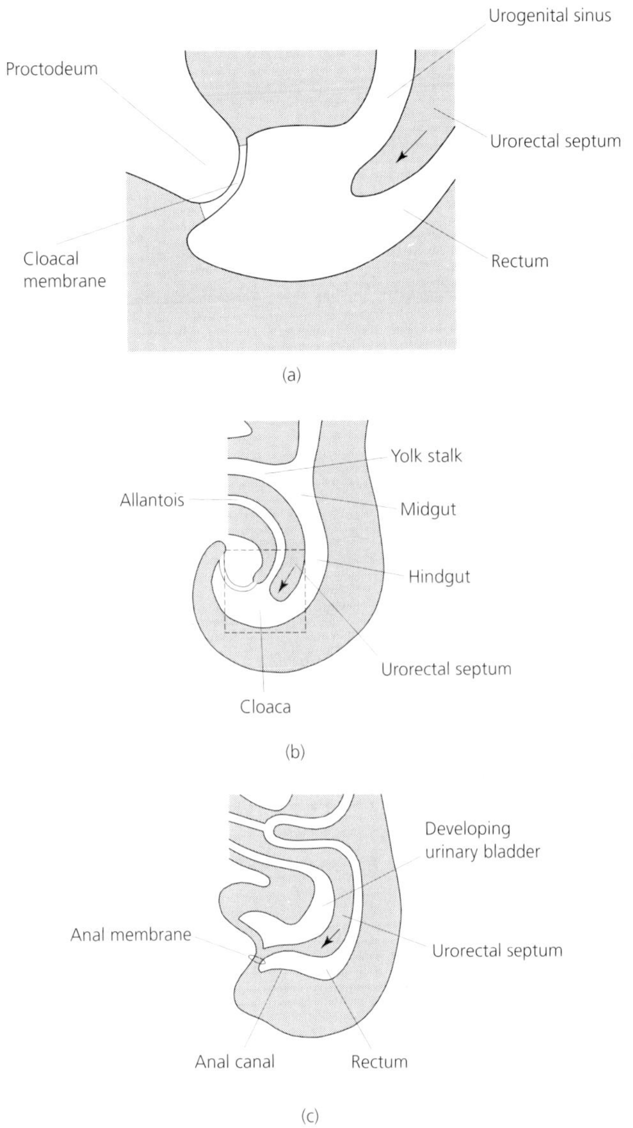

Fig. 54.5 A sequence showing the embryonic development of cloacal structures and showing the progressive downgrowth of the urorectal septum which divides the primitive cloaca.

required. Prognosis is good for low lesions but less certain with high ones, in which the risk of associated problems may be significant.

BLADDER EXTROPHY AND CLOACAL EXTROPHY

EMBRYOLOGY

The embryology has already been described for imperforate anus and it relates to the development of cloacal structures. In bladder extrophy the problem is restricted to the bladder such that there is incomplete retraction of the cloacal membrane and a failure of mesodermal ridges to reinforce the lower abdominal wall. Once the cloacal membrane disintegrates the posterior wall of the primitive bladder becomes exposed and remains so.

The problems seem more profound in cloacal extrophy when disappearance of the cloacal membrane before the urogenital ridge divides the primitive cloaca, leads to exposure of both bladder and rectum.

DEFINITION

Bladder extrophy exists when the anterior wall of the bladder is missing. It has an incidence of about 1 in 30 000 and occurs a little over twice as commonly in boys. It is associated with separation of the pubic bones, low set umbilicus, and abnormalities of the external genitalia.

Cloacal extrophy comprises two hemibladders, each with its own ureter, separated by bowel which often ends blindly at the anus. Exomphalos occurs in about 85% of cases but overall the condition is exceedingly rare, with an incidence of 1 in 300 000.

DIAGNOSIS

Neither of these conditions is readily diagnosed; however, the absence of a fetal bladder on ultrasound is likely to be the most reliable feature[21]. A bladder should always be visible at some time during an examination and a failure to see one should raise suspicion that a serious problem exists. Both bladder and cloacal extrophy may be associated with other abnormalities, the latter particularly so, and it may well be these other features that eventually lead to the diagnosis.

Although ultrasound is the main method of diagnosis, fetoscopy to directly visualize the cloacal area has been attempted.

MANAGEMENT

The affected neonates need immediate treatment to close the defect. Whereas bladder extrophy can be repaired with reasonable success, although several operations may be required, cloacal extrophy is a major surgical challenge. Important peripheral issues may make it necessary to reassign gender in males. Long-term prognosis must be guarded not only from the point of cloacal extrophy itself but also the associated conditions.

INTESTINAL DUPLICATION

DEFINITION

Duplications may be classified into those that are closed and cystic and those that are tubular duplications and which communicate with the intestinal lumen. The former are the most common and probably the ones most likely to be seen in the fetus. They are formed by failure of normal canalization, resulting in two lumina, and lie on the mesenteric side of the intestine.

DIAGNOSIS

Their precise diagnosis in utero is not usually possible although they can look like ovarian cysts so the appearance of such cysts in the male fetus should increase suspicion. Alterations within the duplicated bowel may produce a variety of bizarre changes with calcification of the cyst wall (Fig. 54.6) and visible remnants of the cyst wall[21]. The cyst may become very large.

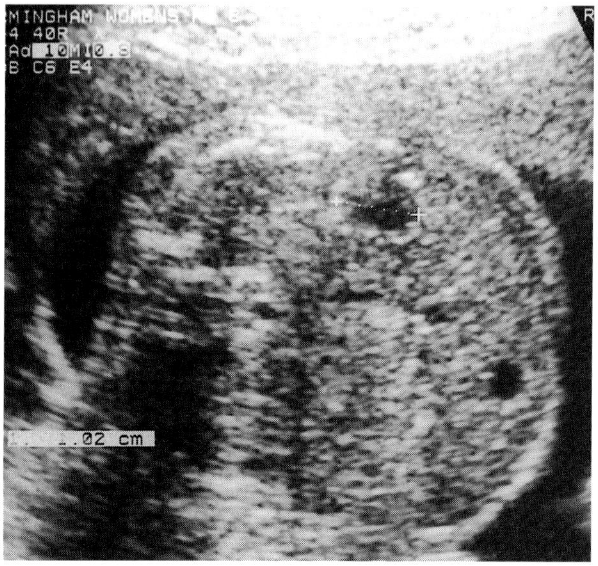

Fig. 54.6 Ultrasound appearances of a bowel duplication cyst in the left fetal hypochondrium.

MANAGEMENT

Simple observation is all that is required in the antenatal period but postnatally careful assessment is advised since these reduplications can be the cause intestinal obstruction.

Functional bowel abnormalities

These are generally very rare conditions which may occasionally be identified during routine ultrasound examinations.

MEGACYSTIS-MICROCOLON-INTESTINAL HYPOPERISTALSIS SYNDROME (MMIHS)

DEFINITION

This abnormality is associated with functional small bowel obstruction, intestinal malrotation, microcolon and an enlarged bladder with a non-obstructed renal tract. The condition is usually fatal in early life and affects predominantly females.

DIAGNOSIS

Ultrasound diagnosis has been described[22]. The striking feature is the grossly distended bladder; dilated bowel is rare. The other odd feature appears to concern amniotic fluid volume, oligohydramnios being noted in early pregnancy but with polyhydramnios in the latter weeks.

MANAGEMENT

Most of these children end in renal failure and the outlook is poor. Prune belly syndrome is a further complication.

CONGENITAL CHLORIDORRHOEA

This is an exceedingly rare condition in which there is impaired chloride transport in the bowel wall leading to gross dilatation of the terminal ilium and colon.

Structural abnormalities of the liver

EMBRYOLOGY

The liver, gallbladder and biliary duct system arise from the foregut as a ventral bud at the fourth week. This hepatic diverticulum extends rapidly in between the layers of the ventral mesentary and divides into a large cranial component which becomes the liver and a smaller caudal one which gives rise to the gallbladder. The cranial portion divides many times to becomes the intrahepatic biliary system and this is surrounded by mesenchyme which differentiates into fibrous and haemopoietic tissue and the Kupffer cells.

The gallbladder arises from the caudal division of the hepatic diverticulum and is attached by the cystic duct to the duodenum. This is initially occluded but later canalizes and its attachment to the duodenum becomes the common bile duct. This lies initially on the ventral aspect of the duodenum, growth and rotation of which eventually places it dorsally. Although variations in liver lobulation are not uncommon, serious congenital malformations of the liver are rare. Abnormalities of the biliary tree, such as extrahepatic biliary atresia, are most serious and may occur in 1 in 20 000 pregnancies arising from a failure of recanalization.

HEPATIC CYST

DEFINITION

The lining of the cyst usually comprises cuboidal or columnar epithelium and presumably arises from canalicular maldevelopment. These cysts seem to be very rare but can potentially be large enough to cause respiratory embarrassment following delivery. The cyst will appear in the right upper abdomen more frequently than the left and it should be possible to see that it is placed within the structure of the liver and separate from other surrounding organs[23]. Hepatic cysts need to be differentiated from other cystic structures, such as those associated with bowel reduplication, although these other cysts are much more likely to be mobile. Choledochal cysts will exist on the right side of the liver usually and pancreatic cysts will lie behind the stomach.

MANAGEMENT

Prior identification alerts the paediatrician to the possibility of respiratory embarrassment. The cysts themselves can be very large but excision is usually possible and the prognosis is good.

Liver tumours are rare and arise mainly from the mesenchymal tissue which form the definitive liver.

HEPATIC HAMARTOMA

These tumours are primarily non-neoplastic malformations containing a variety of tissue types of mesenchymal origin. They are not locally destructive although may produce pressure effects. They are rare but will appear in the liver as cystic spaces which may be septated and very large[24,25].

HEPATIC TERATOMA

Teratomata are rare fetal tumours, the commonest examples being sacrococcygeal tumours. Extragonadal sites, such as the liver, are particularly rare, and in these areas the tumour may arise from both somatic cells or ectopic germ cells. The tumour comprises tissue from all three germ layers and may be cystic or solid. Histologically, teratomata can theoretically be differentiated from fetus in fetu by a lack of a notochord, but this has been disputed, and fetus in fetu may be part of the teratomata spectrum.

HEPATIC HAEMANGIOMA

Small haemangiomata are sometimes found incidentally at the time of necropsy and probably are of little significance. In the fetus very large hepatic haemangiomata can be rarely seen[26,27]. These are benign tumours which will usually resolve following delivery. However, their size and their large vascular interconnections may provoke heart failure in the fetus with the development of hydrops. Under these circumstances a fatal outcome becomes a possibility. Although these tumours will usually be detected incidentally they may sometimes present with polyhydramnios as a secondary feature of hydrops. The appearance of the liver will suggest the diagnosis, and invasive investigations such as biopsy do not seem justifiable.

Structural abnormalities of the biliary tree

GALLSTONES

Gallstones are extremely rare in the fetus and indeed the neonate, although an incidence of about 1.5% is reported in paediatric populations. They may be associated with abnormalities of the biliary tree, haemolytic disease due to sickle cell haemoglobinopathy, thalassaemia or spherocytosis. The presence of echodense material within the gallbladder (sludge) can be clearly identified within the gallbladder on the right side of the liver. Apart from the associated causative factors their presence does not probably have any significance[28,29].

GALLBLADDER ABNORMALITIES

Abnormalities of the gallbladder are rare[30]. Agenesis and bilobing may occur in development, and a left-sided gallbladder has been described. The gallbladder should be visible by 15 to 16 weeks, and its absence may occur in the presence of other anomalies. External biliary atresia may present with an absent gall bladder, and this has a poor prognosis. The simple congenital absence of the gallbladder usually carries a good prognosis.

CHOLEDOCHAL CYST

DEFINITION

Choledochal cysts arise probably as a weakness in the wall of the common bile duct although other parts of the biliary tree, both intra- and extrahepatic, may be involved[31]. It is rare in the Western world, most cases being described from Japan. The cyst usually appears in the right half of the liver and the fetal gall bladder may be separately identified[32–34] (Fig. 54.7). The cyst must be distinguished from duodenal atresia and other cystic structures in the liver, mesentery and omentum. Duodenal atresia will usually be associated with polyhydramnios whilst intra-abdominal cysts will usually appear freely mobile within the abdominal cavity.

MANAGEMENT

There is little that needs to be done antenatally apart from confirmation of the diagnosis. Once the baby is born, further evaluation should establish the exact site of the cyst[35]. Usually it is possible to excise the cyst, but failing this it may be drained into a Roux jejunal loop. Long-term outcome is usually good, but ascending cholangitis, portal hypertension and malignancy in the cyst wall have been described.

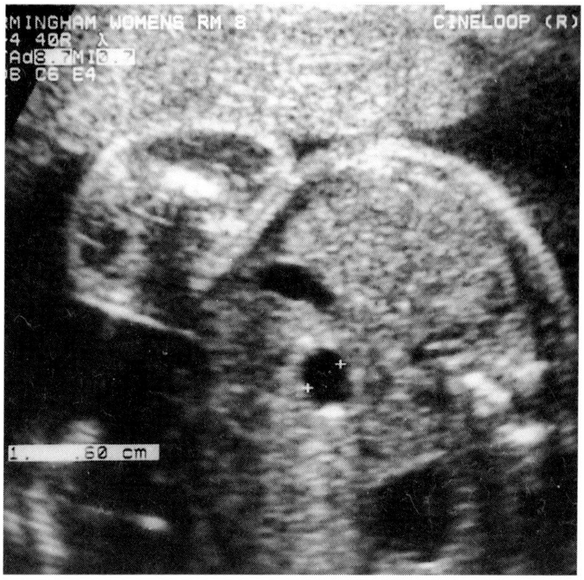

Fig. 54.7 Ultrasound appearances of a choledochal cyst shown between the two + marks.

Intestinal accidents

CONGENITAL VOLVULUS

EMBRYOLOGY

Volvulus arises as a result of malrotation of the gut, and several types exist. One, the so-called left-sided colon, occurs as the result of total non-rotation of the gut, which leaves the gut prone to volvulus. A mixed rotation is one in which the caecum lies just inferior to the pylorus; volvulus in this circumstance leads to duodenal obstruction. In midgut volvulus the intestine is attached to the posterior abdominal wall at only two points and the small intestines hang by a narrow mesentery containing the superior mesenteric arteries, an arrangement which is particularly likely to tort.

DEFINITION

Volvulus may result in the necrosis of a large amount of bowel. The prognosis is poor, with about an 80% mortality. The occurrence of fetal distress in the presence of the condition is recognized and may arise either as a feature of central shock or perhaps shock arising from loss of fluid; intra-abdominal haemorrhage is described.

DIAGNOSIS

The appearance of a complex intra-abdominal mass is typical[36–38]. The bowel will become very distended and sonolucent as the bowel fills with fluid. Particulate matter may be observed within the bowel and peristalsis may cease. Ascites or haemoperitoneum may develop[39]. During the acute phase fetal movements may cease, but if the baby survives, recovery is marked by the return of fetal activity; the affected bowel, however, remains dilated.

MANAGEMENT

The prospects for a successful outcome are poor. If the event occurs before 37 weeks the immediate delivery of the baby is probably not indicated, but presentation after this time may allow the baby to be rescued, although the prognosis is still grave.

INTESTINAL PERFORATION

DEFINITION

Perforation usually occurs as the result of bowel obstruction which may arise as the result of a vascular accident to the bowel such as volvulus, intussusception, or secondary to severe growth retardation. Obstructive problems may also arise from meconium ileus as seen in cystic fibrosis or later in pregnancy Hirschsprung's disease although *intrauterine* perforation in the latter condition is not reported.

DIAGNOSIS

The early diagnosis (15–17 weeks) of intestinal obstruction has been reported although changes may be noted which are normal and only transient[40,41]. Evidence of possible meconium ileus may be seen from the presence of echogenic fetal bowel[3] (Fig. 54.8). The ascites develop (Fig. 54.9) as a result of the peritoneal irritation arising from leaked meconium. There are probably two phases, the first being acute, in which generalized ascites forms, and the second, adhesive when the ascites begins to be walled-off, leading to the development of pseudoascites[42–44]. Under these circumstances the gut often appears bound to the posterior abdominal wall rather than to be freely floating. Calcified deposits may appear on the peritoneal surfaces (Fig. 54.10)[45]. Further obstructive changes may appear but spontaneous resolution is also observed.

The meconium peritonitis which arises from bowel perforation is probably secondary to meconium ileus. The commonest association is with cystic fibrosis (25–40%), an autosomal recessive condition due to a gene deletion on chromosome 7. Why this condition should be associated with spontaneous perforation is unclear but it probably relates to transient obstruction[46]. The meconium which leaks from the bowel acts as an irritant, which produces peritonitis and ascites. Pseudoascites may develop because the ascites becomes walled-off by the inflammatory process. After time the pseudoascites may disperse, in worst cases leaving a scaphoid abdominal wall. Intra-abdominal calcification may remain. Meconium peritonitis is a serious condition with a

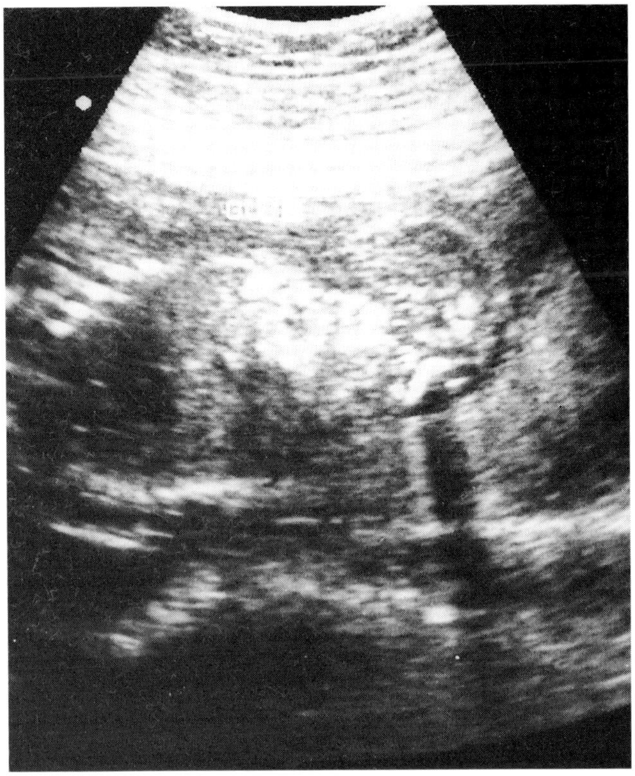

Fig. 54.8 Ultrasound appearances of 'bright gut' seen in some cases of cystic fibrosis.

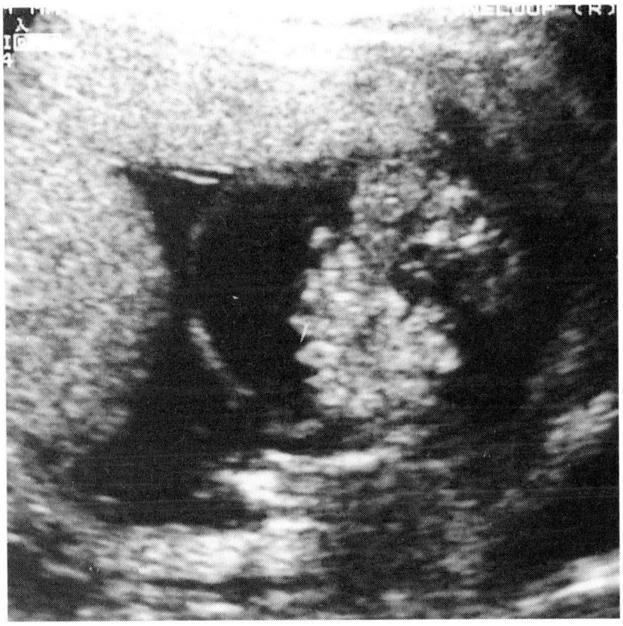

Fig. 54.9 Ultrasound appearances of ascites due to probable bowel perforation.

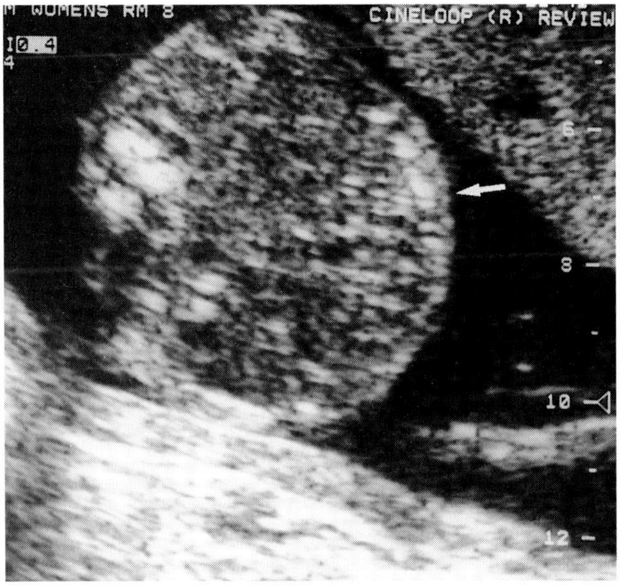

Fig. 54.10 Ultrasound appearance of intra-abdominal calcification.

mortality of about 60% in neonates who undergo surgery. In utero survival rates are hard to establish.

MANAGEMENT

Other causes of ascites need to be excluded and it may be indicated to perform an assessment of fetal karyotype, look for evidence of infection and possibly screen the parents as carriers of cystic fibrosis. There is no particular indication for precipitate delivery and indeed the prevention of prematurity should be the aim. Polyhydramnios is a common complication of meconium perforation and can be reduced often by the use of indomethicin (15 mg orally tds) for 5 days.

Care should be taken at the time of delivery because the continuing presence of ascites may splint the baby's diaphragm and limit respiration to the extent that urgent paracentesis may be required. Following delivery the baby will need careful evaluation and if bowel obstruction persists, laparotomy.

Midline herniations

EXOMPHALOS

DEFINITION

Normally the gut returns to the abdominal cavity by the 10th week pc, undergoing rotation at this time. Exomphalos has an incidence of about 1 in 5000 and results from defective embryological development. The severest conditions are associated with failure of the closure of the lateral fold by about 4 weeks pc. This results in a very large defect in the abdominal wall which may include bladder and cloacal extrophy. In both large and small exomphalos the mass is covered by a layer of peritoneum and amnion. Because the mechanism is faulty by which the rectus muscles approach one another to close the circular defect left once the intestines have returned to the abdomen, babies who have had their exomphalos repaired remain with a totally deficient anterior abdominal wall.

DIAGNOSIS

Exomphalos should not usually be missed by an adequate screening scan[47] (Fig. 54.11). However, minor defects which may amount to a small herniation of the sac into the base of the umbilical cord may be overlooked. This is important, since the small defects may be more likely associated with karyotypic anomalies. A major lesion is one which exceeds 5 cm in diameter at term. The maternal serum alpha-fetoprotein levels may be elevated in about two-thirds of those cases with an exomphalos. Once an exomphalos has been diagnosed a detailed ultrasound examination of the rest of the baby is essential.

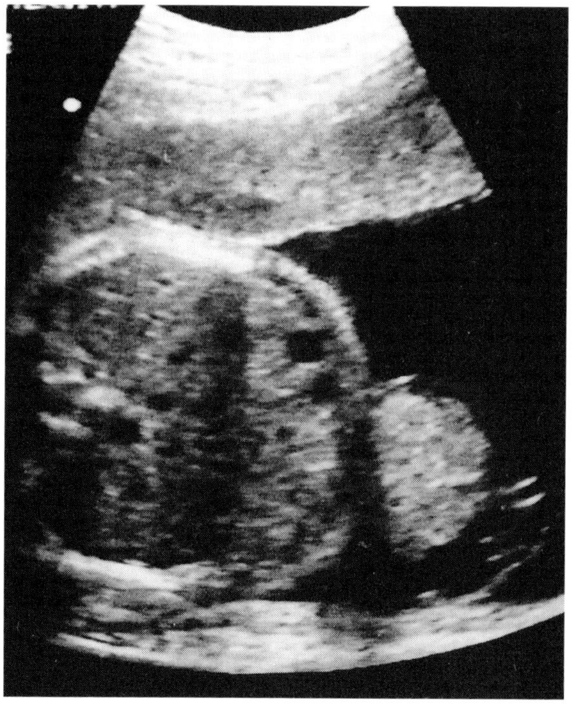

Fig. 54.11 Ultrasound appearance of exomphalos at 20 weeks.

MANAGEMENT

Once identified, the presence of an exomphalos should elicit an intense search for other abnormalities. The parents should be counselled that termination of pregnancy is an option for them but that once it can be established as far as possible that the lesion is isolated the prognosis might be as good as 90%, although not all studies support this figure[48]. It is important to exclude karyotypic and cardiac abnormalities, which are found in about 50% of cases of exomphalos[49,50]. Conditions such as Beckwith–Wiedemann syndrome, which is associated with macrosomia, macroglossia and enlarged, potentially malignant kidneys should be considered. The exclusion of cloacal abnormalities is also important, especially in the absence of a fetal bladder and because ultrasound views of this area may be difficult fetoscopy may have a limited role.

Delivery should be in a unit with appropriate neonatology support. Vaginal delivery is not generally indicated although concerns about major exomphalos and the need to time delivery may indicate a caesarean section.

GASTROSCHISIS

DEFINITION

Gastroschisis may arise from an embryological aberration of the right vitilline vessel. The gut is usually short and malrotated so the aetiology is more complex than merely an abdominal defect. The incidence of the condition appears to be increasing and it is more common among women aged less than 20 years[51]. Smoking and drug abuse are other possible factors. Importantly, other anomalies are rare and may only be found in about 5% of cases. Karyotypic abnormalities do not appear to be increased and occur at the background frequency for the mother's age. The pregnancy must be carefully monitored and evidence of bowel dilatation assessed. Intrauterine death is described, although the underlying aetiology of this is uncertain. Babies with gastroschisis tend to be small for dates, about 30% weighing below the tenth centile.

DIAGNOSIS

Gastroschisis is not usually missed so long as the anterior abdominal wall is carefully scrutinized[52] (Fig. 54.12). The important differential is with exomphalos but in the case of gastroschisis the bowel lies free in the amniotic cavity. The bowel can be some way from the fetus, often around the feet, so the whole amniotic cavity must be scanned. If serum screening is used virtually 100% of gastroschisis will be detected from elevated maternal serum alpha-fetoprotein.

MANAGEMENT

Planned early delivery is not indicated in this condition but careful monitoring of the fetal status is required. Reduced amounts of amniotic fluid seem to be a common feature although the underlying cause of these changes is unclear. Should delivery be indicated then an attempt at vaginal

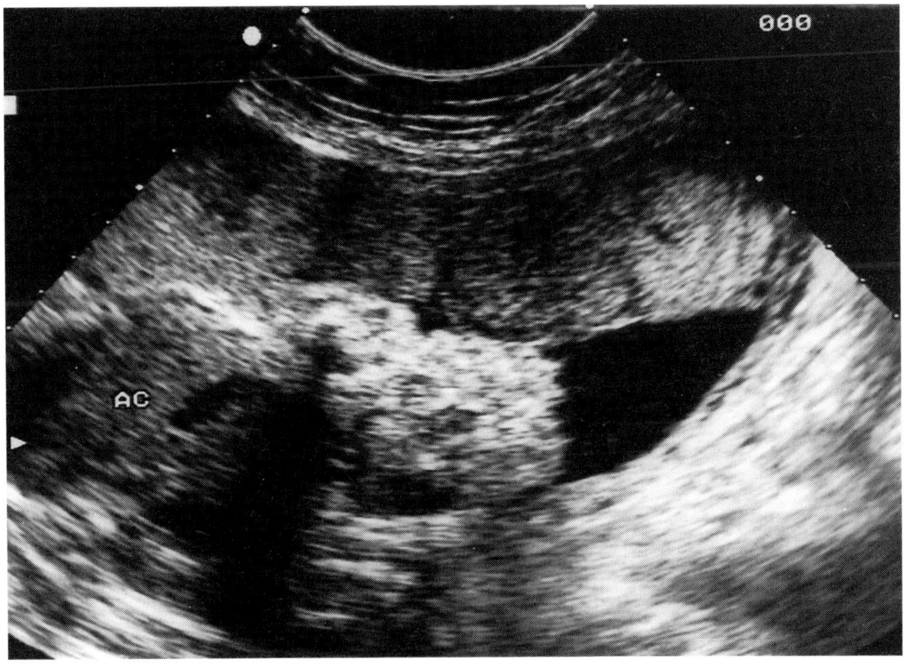

Fig. 54.12 Ultrasound appearances of gastroschisis at 20 weeks.

delivery should be made, there being no substantial evidence to suggest an advantage to caesarean section.

PENTALOGY OF CANTRELL

DEFINITION

The five features of this syndrome are defects of the pericardium, sternum, diaphragm and abdominal wall, together with displacement of the heart. The abnormality probably arises from an embryological defect which occurs between 14 and 18 days pc when there is a failure of ventromedial migration of paired mesodermal structures. Many variants of the syndrome have been described and other parts of the fetus such as the face and cranium can be affected.

DIAGNOSIS

The bizarre collection of abnormalities should indicate the diagnosis[53–55]. The most striking abnormality is the displacement of the fetal heart outside the thorax. The anterior wall defect may be typical of either gastroschisis or exomphalos and may have features of both.

MANAGEMENT

This is an extremely severe abnormality which is likely to be fatal, although survivors are reported, probably in the lesser affected cases. It is likely that most couples may elect to terminate the pregnancy.

REFERENCES

1. Parulekar SG. Sonography of normal fetal bowel. *J Ultrasound Med* **10**:211–220, 1991.
2. Nyberg DA, Mack LA, Patton RM, Cyr DR. Fetal bowel: Normal sonographic findings. *J Ultrasound Med* **6**:3–6, 1987.
3. Chitty LS, Griffen DR. The gastrointestinal tract. In *Ultrasound in Obstetrics and Gynaecology* (eds K. Dewbury, H. Meire & D. Cosgrove) pp. 352–354 London: Churchill Livingstone, 1993.
4. Harvard AC, MacDonald LM. Oesophageal atresia and other disorders with a similar antenatal presentation. *Br J Radiol* **64**:557–558, 1991.
5. Pretorius DH, Drose JA, Dennis MA, Manchester DK, Manco-Johnson ML. Tracheoesophageal fistula in utero. Twenty two cases. *J Ultrasound Med* **6**:509–513, 1987.
6. Estroff JA, Parad RB, Share JC, Benacerraf BR. Second trimester prenatal findings in duodenal and esophageal atresia without tracheoesophageal fistula. *J Ultrasound Med* **13**:375–379, 1994.
7. Akhtar J, Guiney EJ. Congenital duodenal obstruction. *Br J Surg* **79**:133–135, 1992.
8. Athale AS, Vaishnav TV, Jhala PJ, Vohra P. Prenatal diagnosis of duodenal atresia by ultrasound. *Indian J Pediatr* **58**:145–147, 1991.
9. Collier D. Antenatal diagnosis of duodenal atresia by ultrasound; a case report. *Radiography* **48**:102–103, 1982.
10. Nelson LH, Clark CE, Fishburne JI, Urban RB, Penry MF. Value of serial sonography in the in utero detection of duodenal atresia. *Obstet Gynecol* **59**:657–660, 1982.
11. Petrikovsky BM. First trimester diagnosis of duodenal atresia. *Am J Obstet Gynecol* **171**:569–570, 1994.
12. Snijders RMJ, Nicolaides KH. Fetal abnormalities. In *Ultrasound Markers for Fetal Chromosome Defects* (eds R.M.J. Snijders, K.H. Nicolaides et al.), p. 33–35. London: Parthenon Publishing Group, 1996.

13. Grosfeld JL, Rescorla FJ. Duodenal atresia and stenosis; reassessment of treatment and outcome based on antenatal diagnosis, pathological variance and longterm followup. *Wld J Surg* **17**:301–309, 1993.
14. Fletman D, McQuown D, Kanchana Poon V, Gyepes MI. 'Apple peel' atresia of the small bowel: prenatal diagnosis of the obstruction by ultrasound. *Pediar Radiol* **9**:118–119, 1980.
15. Lai PC, Jehng CH, Chiang LM. et al. Jejunal atresia with 'apple peel' deformity; report of one case. *Acta Paediatr Sin* **32**:47–53, 1991.
16. Filkins K, Russo J, Flowers WK. Third trimester ultrasound diagnosis of intestinal atresia following clinical evidence of polyhydramnios. *Prenat Diagn* **5**:215–220, 1985.
17. Shalev E, Weiner E, Zuckerman H. Prenatal ultrasound diagnosis of intestinal calcifications with imperforate anus. *Acta Obstet Gynecol* **62**:95–96, 1983.
18. Hallak M, Reiter AA, Smith LG, Dildy GA, Finegold MJ. Oligohydramnios and megacolon in the fetus with vesicorectal fistula and anal-urethral atresia; a case report. *Am J Obstet Gynecol* **167**:79–81, 1992.
19. Miller SF, Angtuaco TL, Quirk JG, Hairston K. Anorectal atresia presenting as an abdominopelvic mass *J Ultrasound Med* **9**:669–672, 1990.
20. Romero R, Pilu G, Jeanty P, Ghidini A, Hobbins J. Bladder extrophy and cloacal extrophy. In *Prenatal Diagnosis of Congenital Anomalies* (ed. R. Romero), pp. 228–232. New York: Appleton and Large, 1988.
21. Chitty LS, Griffen DR. The gastrointestinal tract. In *Ultrasound in Obstetrics and Gynaecology*. (eds K. Dewbury, H. Meire & D. Cosgrove), p. 359. London: Churchill Livingstone, 1993.
22. Stamm E, King G, Thickman D. Megacystis-microcolon-intestinal hypoperistalsis syndrome: prenatal identification in siblings and review of the literature. *J Ultrasound Med* **10**:599–602, 1991.
23. Chung WM. Antenatal detection of hepatic cyst. *J Clin Ultrasound* **14**:217–219, 1986.
24. Foucar E, Williamson RA, Yiu-Chiu V, Varner MW & Kay BR. Mesenchymal hamartoma of the liver identified by fetal sonography. *Am J Radiol* **140**:970–972, 1983.
25. Hirata GI, Matsunaga ML, Medearis AL, Dixon P, Platt LD. Ultrasonographic diagnosis of a fetal abdominal mass; a case of a mesenchymal liver hamartoma and a review of the literature. *Prenat Diagn* **10**:507–512, 1990.
26. Nakamoto SK, Dreilinger A, Dattel B, Mattrey RF, Key TC. The sonographic appearance of hepatic haemangioma in utero. *J Ultrasound Med* **2**:239–241, 1983.
27. Sepulveda WH, Donetch G, Giuliano A. Prenatal diagnosis of fetal hepatic haemangioma. *Eur J Obstet Gynecol Reprod Biol* **48**:73–76, 1993.
28. Abbitt PL, McIlhenny J. Prenatal detection of gallstones. *J Clin Ultrasound* **18**:202–204, 1990.
29. Heijne L, Ednay D. The development of fetal gallstones demonstrated by ultrasound. *Radiography* **51**:155–156, 1985.
30. Bronshtein M, Weiner Z, Abramovici H, Filmar S, Erlik Y, Blumfeld Z. Prenatal diagnosis of gallbladder anomalies; report of 17 cases. *Prenat Diag* **13**:851–861, 1993.
31. Tsang TM, Tam PK, Chamberlain P. Obliteration of the distal bile duct in the development of congenital choledochal cyst. *J Pediatric Surg* **29**:1582–1583, 1994.
32. Ellia F, Dugue Mrechaud MD, Levrd G, Bonneau D, Magnin G. Choledochal cysts. A rare parental diagnosis. *J Gynecol Obstet Biol Reprod* **24**:400–404 (in French), 1995.
33. Gallivan EK, Crombleholme TM, D'Alton ME. Early prenatal diagnosis of choledochal cyst. *Prenat Diagn* **16**:934–937, 1996.
34. Bancroft JD, Bucuvalas JC, Ryckman FC, Dudgeon DL, Saunders RC, Schwarz KB. Antenatal diagnosis of choledochal cyst. *J Ped Gastero Nutr* **18**:142–145, 1994.
35. Baunin C, Mechinaud-Puget C, Fajadet P, Vaysse P, Guitard J, Moscovici J, Visentin M, Viogt JJ. Management of a biliary cyst disclosed prenatally. 2 cases. *Chir Pediatr* (French) **31**:160–163, 1990.
36. Cloutier MG, Fried AM, Selke AC. Antenatal observation of midgut volvulus by ultrasound. *J Clin Ultrasound* **11**:286–288, 1983.
37. Mercado MG, Bulas DI, Chandra R. Prenatal diagnosis and management of congenital volvulus. *Pediatr Radiol* **23**:601–602, 1993.
38. Samuel N, Dicker D, Feldberg D, Goldman JA. Ultrasound diagnosis and management of fetal intestinal obstruction and volvulus in utero. *J Perinat Med* **12**:333–337, 1984.
39. Witter FR, Molteni RA. Intrauterine intestinal volvulus with hemoperitoneum presenting as fetal distress at 34 weeks gestation. *Am J Obstet Gynecol* **155**:1080–1081, 1986.
40. Bronshtein M, Zimmer EZ. Early sonographic detection of fetal obstruction and possible diagnostic pitfalls. *Prenat Diagn* **16**:203–206, 1996.
41. Slotnick RN, Abuhamad AZ. Prognostic implications of fetal echogenic bowel. *Lancet* **347**:85–87, 1996.
42. Shalev J, Frankel Y, Avigad I, Mashiach S. Spontaneous intestinal perforation in utero; ultrasonic diagnostic criteria. *Am J Obstet Gynecol* **144**:855–857, 1982.
43. Denholm TA, Crow HC, Edwards WH, Simmons GM, Marin-Padilla M, Bartrum RJ. Prenatal sonographic appearance of meconium ileus in twins. *Am J Roentgenol* **143**:371–372, 1984.
44. McGahan JP, Hanson F. Meconium peritonitis with accompanying pseudocyst; prenatal sonographic diagnosis. *Radiology* **148**:125–126, 1983.
45. Dunne M, Haney P, Sun CC. Sonographic features of bowel perforation and calcific meconium peritonitis in utero. *Pediatr Radiol* **13**:231–233, 1983.
46. Shalev J, Navon R, Urbach D, Mashiach S, Goldman B. Intestinal obstruction and cystic fibrosis; antenatal ultrasound appearance. *J Med Genet* **20**:229–230, 1983.
47. Lindfors KK, McGahan JP, Walter JP. Fetal exomphalos and gastroschisis; pitfalls in sonographic diagnosis. *Am J Roentgenol* **147**:797–800, 1986.
48. Morrow R, Whittle MJ, McNay MB, Raine PA, Gibson AA, Crossley J. Prenatal diagnosis and management of anterior abdominal wall defects in the west of Scotland. *Prenat Diagn* **13**:111–115, 1993.
49. Gilbert WM, Nicolaides KP. Fetal omphalocoele: associated malformations and chromosomal defects. *Obstet Gynecol* **70**:633–635, 1987.
50. Snijders RJM, Sebire NJ, Souka A, Santiago C, Nicolaides KH. Fetal exomphalos and chromosomal defects; relationship to maternal age and gestation. *Ultrasound Obstet Gynecol* **6**:250–255, 1995.
51. Tan KH, Kilby MD, Whittle MJ, Beattie BR, Booth IW, Botting BJ. Congenital anterior abdominal wall defects in England and Wales, 1987–1993; retrospective analysis of OPCS data. *Br Med J* **313**:903–906, 1996.
52. Langer JC, Khanna J, Caco C, Dykes EH, Nicolaides KH. Prenatal diagnosis of gastroschisis; development of objective sonographic criteria for predicting outcome. *Obstet Gynecol* **81**:53–56, 1993.
53. Abu-Yousef MM, Wray AB, Williamson RA, Bonsib SM. Antenatal diagnosis of variant of pentalogy of Cantrell. *J Ultrasound Med* **6**:535–538, 1987.
54. Ghidini A, Sirtori M, Romero R, Hobbins JC. Prenatal diagnosis of pentalogy of Cantrell. *J Ultrasound Med* **7**:567–572, 1988.
55. Zimmer EZ, Bronshtein M. Fetal midline disruption syndromes *Prenat Diagn* **16**:65–69, 1996.

Skeletal anomalies

55

G. Pilu, R. Romero and P. Jeanty

Congenital abnormalities of the skeleton include a heterogeneous group of disorders. For a number of reasons, the prenatal diagnosis of these malformations is a particularly challenging task. This chapter will review the birth prevalence and classification of skeletal anomalies and provide an approach to the antenatal sonographic diagnosis, with emphasis upon skeletal dysplasias and limb amputations.

Skeletal dysplasias

BIRTH PREVALENCE AND CONTRIBUTION TO PERINATAL MORTALITY

The birth prevalence of skeletal dysplasias recognizable in the neonatal period has been estimated to be 2.4/10 000 births[1]. In a large series, 23% of affected infants were stillbirths, and 32% died during the first week of life. The overall frequency of skeletal dysplasias among perinatal deaths was 9.1/1000. The birth prevalence of the different skeletal dysplasias and their relative frequency among perinatal deaths in this study are shown in Table 55.1. The four most common skeletal dysplasias found were thanatophoric dysplasia, achondroplasia, osteogenesis imperfecta and achondrogenesis. Thanatophoric dysplasia and achondrogenesis accounted for 62% of all lethal skeletal dysplasias. The most common non-lethal skeletal dysplasia was achondroplasia[1].

In another large series, reporting the prevalence and classification of lethal neonatal skeletal dysplasias in West Scotland, the prevalence was 1.1/10 000 births, and the most frequently diagnosed conditions were thanatophoric dysplasia (1/42 000), osteogenesis imperfecta (1/56 000), rhizomelic chondrodysplasia punctata (1/84 000), campomelic syndrome (1/112 000) and achondrogenesis (1/112 000)[2].

CLASSIFICATION OF SKELETAL DYSPLASIAS

The existing nomenclature for skeletal dysplasias is complicated. There is a lack of uniformity about definition criteria. For example, some disorders are referred to by eponyms (e.g., Ellis–van Creveld syndrome, Larsen dysplasia), by Greek terms describing a salient feature of the disease (diastrophic (twisted), metatropic (changeable) or by a term related to the presumed pathogenesis of the disease (e.g., osteogenesis imperfecta, achondrogenesis). The fundamental problem with any classification of skeletal dysplasias is that the pathogenesis of these diseases is largely unknown. Therefore, the current system relies on purely descriptive findings of either clinical or radiological nature.

In an attempt to develop a uniform terminology, a group of experts met in Paris in 1977 and proposed an International Nomenclature for Skeletal Dysplasias that has been recently revised (Table 55.1)[3]. The system subdivides the diseases into three different groups: osteochondrodysplasias, or abnormalities of cartilage and/or bone growth and development, disorganized development of cartilaginous and fibrous components of the skeleton and idiopathic osteolyses.

A comprehensive description of these diseases is beyond the scope of this chapter. For a complete discussion, the reader is referred to Goldberg's textbook *The Dysmorphic Child*[4]. This chapter will focus primarily on the osteochondrodysplasias that are recognizable at birth. Although more than 200 skeletal dysplasias have been described, and more will probably be identified as distinct entities, the number that can be recognized with the use of sonography in the antepartum period is considerably smaller. Most of these disorders result in short stature, and the term dwarfism has been used to refer to this clinical condition. However, this term carries a negative connotation and for this reason the term dysplasia is used instead.

TABLE 55.1
International nomenclature of constitutional bone disease

Abnormality	Transmission
Osteochondrodysplasias, abnormalities of cartilage and/or bone growth and development	
Defects of the tubular (and flat) bones and/or axial skeleton	
1. Achondroplasia group:	
Thanatophoric dysplasia	AD
Thanatophoric dysplasia – straight femur/cloverleaf skull type	AD
Achondroplasia	AD
Hypochondroplasia	AD
2. Achondrogenesis:	
Type IA	AR
Type B	AR
3. Spondylodysplastic group (Perinatally lethal):	
San Diego type	Sp
Torrance type	Sp
Luton type	Sp
4. Metatropic dysplasia group:	
Fibrochondrogenesis	AR
Schneckenbecken dysplasia	AR
Metatropic dysplasia	AD
5. Short rib dysplasia group (with or without polydactyly):	
SR(P) Type I Saldino–Noonan	AR
SR(P) Type II Majewski	AR
SR(P) Type III Verma–Naumoff	AR
SR(P) Type IV Bermeer–Langer	AR
Asphyxiating thoracic dysplasia	AR
Ellis–van Creveld dysplasia	AR
6. Atelosteogenesis/diastrophic dysplasia group:	
Boomerang dysplasia	Sp
Atelosteogenesis type 1	Sp
Atelosteogenesis type 2 (de La Chapelle)	AR
Omodysplasia I (Maroteaux)	AR
Omodysplasia II (Borochowitz)	AR
Oto-palato-digital syndrome type 2	XLR
Diastrophic dysplasia	AR
Pseudodiastrophic dysplasia	AR
7. Kniest–Stickler dysplasia group:	
Dyssegmental dysplasia – Silverman–Handmaker type	AR
Dyssegmental dysplasia – Rolland–Desbuquois type	AR
Kniest dysplasia	AD
Oto-spondylo-megaepiphyseal dysplasia	AR
Stickler dysplasia (heterogeneous, some not linked to Cole coL2A)	AD
8. Spondyloepiphyseal dysplasia congenita group:	
Langer–Saldino dysplasia (Achondrogenesis type II)	AD
Hypochondrogenesis	AD
Spondyloepiphyseal dysplasia congenita	AD
9. Other spondylo epi-(meta)-physeal dysplasias:	
X-linked spondyloepiphyseal dysplasia tarda	XLD
Other late-onset spondylo epi-(meta)-physeal dysplasias	
Progressive pesudorheumatoid dysplasia	AR
Dyggye–Melchior–Clausen dysplasia	AR
Wolcott–Rallyson dysplasia	AR
Immunoosseous dysplasia	AR
Pseudoachondroplasia	AD
Opismodysplasia	AR
10. Dysostosis multiplex group:	
Mucopolysaccharidosis I-H	AR
Mucopolysaccharidosis I-S	AR
Mucopolysaccharidosis II	AR
Mucopolysaccharidosis III-A	AR
Mucopolysaccharidosis III-B	AR
Mucopolysaccharidosis III-C	AR
Mucopolysaccharidosis III-D	AR
Mucopolysaccharidosis IV-A	AR
Mucopolysaccharidosis IV-B	AR
Mucopolysaccharidosis VI	AR
Mucopolysaccharidosis VII	AR
Fucosidosis	AR
α-Mannosidosis	AR
β-Mannosidosis	AR
Aspartylglucosaminuria	AR
gMI Gangliosidosis, several forms	AR
Sialidosis, several forms	AR
Sialic storage disease	AR
Galactosialidosis	AR
Mucosulfatidosis	AR
Mucolipodisis II	AR
Mucolipodisis III	AR
Mucolipodisis IV	AR
11. Spondylometaphyseal dysplasias:	
Spondylometaphyseal dysplasia – Kozlowski type	AD
Spondylometaphyseal dysplasia – corner fracture type (Sutcliffe)	AD
Spondyloenchondrodysplasia	AR
12. Epiphyseal dysplasias:	
Multiple epiphyseal dysplasias – Fairbanks–Ribbing	AD
13. Chondrodysplasia punctata (Stippled epiphyses) group:	
Rhizomelic type	AR
Conradi–Hunemann type	XLD
X-linked recessive type	XLR
MT-type	Sp
Others include CHILD syndrome; Zellweger syndrome; Warfarin embryopathy; chromosomal abnormalties; fetal alcohol syndrome	
14. Metaphyseal dysplasias:	
Jansen type	AD
Schmid type	AD
Spahr type	AR
McKusick type (CHH)	AR
Metaphyseal anadysplasia	XLR?
Shwachmann type	AR
Adenosine deaminase deficiency	AR
15. Brachyrachia (Short spine dysplasia):	
Brachyolmia, several types	
16. Mesomelic dysplasias:	
Dyschondrosteosis	AD
Langer type	AR
Nievergelt type	AD
Robinow type	AD

TABLE 55.1 *continued*

Abnormality	Transmission
17. Acro/acro-mesomelic dysplasias:	
Acromiric dysplasia	Sp
Geleophysic dysplasia	AR
Acrodysostosis	AD
Tricho-rhino-phalangeal dysplasia type 1	AD
Tricho-rhino-phalangeal dysplasia type 2	AD
Saldino–Mainzer dysplasia	AR
Pseudohypoparathyroidism, several types	AD
	AR?
	XLD?
Cranioectodermal dysplasia	AR
Acromesomelic dysplasia	AR
Grebe dysplasia	AR
18. Dysplasias with significant (but not exclusive) membranous bone involvement:	
Cleidocranial dysplasia	AD
Osteodysplasty, Melnick–Needle	AD
19. Bent bone dysplasia group:	
Camptomelic dysplasia	AR
Kyphomelic dysplasia	AR
Stuve–Wiedemann dysplasia	AR
20. Multiple dislocations syndrome:	
Larsen syndrome	AD
Desbuquois syndrome	AR
Spondylo-epi-metaphyseal dysplasia with joint laxity	AR
21. Osteodysplastic primordial dwarfism group:	
Type 1	AR
Type 2	AR
22. Dysplasias with decreased bone density:	
Osteogenesis imperfecta (several types)	AD
	AD
	AR
Osteopetrosis with pseudoglioma	AR
Idiopathic juvenile osteopetrosis	Sp
Bruck syndrome	AR
Homocystinuria	AR
Singleton–Meren syndrome	Sp
Geroderma osteodysplastica	AR
Menkes syndrome	XLR
23. Dysplasias with defective demineralization:	
Hypophosphatasia	AD
Hypophosphatemic rickets	XLR
Pseudodeficiency rickets, several types	AR
Neonatal hyperparathyroidism	AR
24. Dysplasias with increased bone density:	
Osteopetrosis	
(a) precocious type	AR
(b) delayed type	AD
(c) intermediate type	AR
(d) with renal tubular acidosis	AR
Dysosteosclerosis	AR
Pyknodysostosis	AR
Osteosclerosis – Stanescu type	AD
Axial osteosclerosis including	
(a) osteomesopynesosis	AD
(b) with bamboo hair (Netherton syndrome)	AR
(c) Tricho-thirodystrophy	AR
Osteopoikilosis	AD
Melorheostosis	Sp
Osteopathia striata	AD
Osteopathia striata with cranial sclerosis	AD
Diaphyseal dysplasia – Camurati–Engelmann	AD
Craniodiphyseal dysplasia	AD
	AR
Lenz–Majewski dysplasia	Sp
Craniometadiaphyseal dysplasia	Sp
Endosteal hyperostoses	
(a) van Buchem disease	AR
(b) Sclerosteosis	AR
(c) Worth disease	AD
(d) with cerebellar hypoplasia	AR
Pachydermoperiostosis	AD
Fronto-metaphyseal dysplasia	XLR
Craniometaphyseal dysplasia	
(a) severe type	AR
(b) mild type	AD
Pyle (disease) dysplasia	AR
Osteoectasia with hyperphosphatasia	
Oculo-dento-osseous dysplasia	
(a) severe type	AR
(b) mild type	AD
Familial infantile cortical hyerostosis – Caffey	AD
Disorganized development of cartilaginous and fibrous compenents of the skeleton	
Dysplasia epiphyseal hemimelica	Sp
Multiple cartilaginous exostoses	AD
Enchondromatosis (Ollier)	Sp
Enchondromatosis with hemangiomata (Maffucci)	Sp
Metachondromatosis	AD
Osteoglophonic dysplasia	Sp
Fibrous dysplasia (Jaffe–Lichtenstein)	Sp
Cherubism	AD
Myofibromatosis (generalized fibromatosis)	AR
Idiopathic osteolyses	
1. Predominantly phalangeal:	
Hereditary acrosteolysis, several forms	
Hajdu–Chenev type	AD
2. Predominantly carpal-tarsal:	
Carpal-tarsal osteolysis with nephropathy	AD
Francois syndrome (dernochondro-corneal dystrophy)	AR
3. Multicentric:	
Winchester syndrome	AR
Torg type	AR
Mandibulo-acral dysplasia	AR
4. Other:	
Familial expansile osteolysis	AD

AD = autosomal dominant; AR = autosomal recessive; XLD = X-linked dominant; XLR = X-linked recessive; Sp = sporadic

Source: The International Working Group on Constitutional Diseases of Bone (1992) International classification of osteochondrodysplasias. *Eur. J. Pediatr.* **151**, 407–415

CLINICAL PRESENTATION

The challenge of the antenatal diagnosis of skeletal dysplasias will generally present itself in one of two ways: (1) a patient who has delivered an infant with a skeletal dysplasia and desires antenatal assessment of a subsequent pregnancy or (2) the incidental finding of a skeletal anomaly during a routine sonographic examination, most frequently a shortened, bowed or anomalous extremity. The task is easier when a particular phenotype is looked for in a patient at risk. The inability to obtain reliable information about skeletal mineralization and the involvement of other systems (e.g., skin) with sonography is a limiting factor in the establishment of an accurate diagnosis after the identification of an incidental finding. Another limitation is the paucity of information about the in utero natural history of these disorders.

Despite these difficulties and limitations, there are good medical reasons for attempting an accurate prenatal diagnosis of skeletal dysplasias. A number of these disorders are uniformly lethal, and a confident antenatal diagnosis would present the patient with options for the termination of the pregnancy. Other skeletal dysplasias are associated with mental retardation[5], and this information is important in prenatal counselling. There is a group of disorders associated with thrombocytopenia. Vaginal delivery may expose these infants to the risk of intracranial haemorrhage.

APPROACH TO THE DIAGNOSIS OF SKELETAL DYSPLASIAS

Frequently, the sonographic findings clearly indicate the presence of a skeletal dysplasia; however, the differentiation among the various entities is much more difficult, particularly in cases that have no familial history. Diagnostic difficulties derive from the complexity of the findings and the large number of conditions that must be considered in the differential diagnosis. During the postnatal period, triangulation is commonly used and yields good results[6]. Triangulation is obtained by identifying the major findings in a given case and comparing lists of defects that share the same findings. The radiographic findings that are used after birth, however, differ from those that can be derived sonographically in a fetus. The criteria that are potentially helpful for antenatal diagnosis are listed in Table 55.3 and will be discussed in the following.

TABLE 55.2
Reference values for sonographic measurements of fetal skeleton (in millimetres; SD = standard deviation)

Gestational age	Ulna		Radius		Tibia		Fibula		Femur		Chest circumference	
(weeks)	Mean	SD	Mean	SD	Mean	SD	Mean	SD	Mean	SD	Mean	SD
12	7	3	7	2.4	7	3	6	3	8	3	57	12
13	10	3	10	2.4	10	3	9	3	11	3	66	12
14	13	3	13	2.4	12	3	12	3	14	3	74	12
15	16	3	15	2.4	15	3	15	3	17	3	83	12
16	18	3	18	2.4	17	3	18	3	20	3	91	12
17	21	3	20	2.4	20	3	21	3	23	3	100	12
18	24	3	22	2.4	22	3	23	3	25	3	109	12
19	26	3	24	2.4	25	3	26	3	28	3	118	12
20	29	3	27	2.4	27	3	28	3	31	3	126	12
21	31	3	29	2.4	30	3	31	3	34	3	135	12
22	33	3	31	2.4	32	3	33	3	36	3	143	12
23	36	3	32	2.4	35	3	35	3	39	3	152	12
24	38	3	34	2.4	37	3	37	3	42	3	160	12
25	40	3	36	2.4	40	3	40	3	44	3	168	12
26	42	3	37	2.4	42	3	42	3	47	3	176	12
27	44	3	39	2.4	44	3	44	3	49	3	184	12
28	46	3	40	2.4	46	3	45	3	52	3	192	12
29	48	3	42	2.4	48	3	47	3	54	3	199	12
30	49	3	43	2.4	50	3	49	3	56	3	206	12
31	51	3	44	2.4	52	3	51	3	59	3	212	12
32	53	3	45	2.4	54	3	52	3	61	3	219	12
33	54	3	46	2.4	55	3	54	3	63	3	225	12
34	56	3	47	2.4	57	3	55	3	65	3	230	12
35	57	3	48	2.4	58	3	57	3	67	3	235	12
36	58	3	48	2.4	60	3	58	3	68	3	240	12
37	60	3	49	2.4	61	3	59	3	70	3	244	12
38	61	3	49	2.4	63	3	61	3	71	3	248	12
39	62	3	50	2.4	64	3	62	3	73	3	251	12
40	63	3	50	2.4	66	3	63	3	74	3	254	12

EVALUATION OF LONG BONES

Measurement of the fetal femur is recommended in any standard sonographic examination performed after the midtrimester. The sonographic documentation of a short femur length is the harbinger of skeletal dysplasias in the vast majority of cases, and should prompt a careful investigation of the entire fetal anatomy.

The first step in such cases is to measure all long bones. Long bone biometry has been used extensively in the prediction of gestational age. Nomograms available for this purpose use the long bone as the independent variable and the estimated fetal age as the dependent variable. However, the type of nomogram required to assess the normality of bone dimensions uses the gestational age as the independent variable and the long bone as the dependent variable. For the proper use of these nomograms, the clinician must accurately know the gestational age of the fetus. Therefore, patients at risk for skeletal dysplasias should be advised to seek prenatal care at an early gestational age to assess all clinical estimators of gestational age. Table 55.2 presents nomograms for the assessment of limb biometry for the upper and lower extremities. For those patients presenting with uncertain gestational age, comparisons between limb dimensions and the head perimeter can be used (Table 55.3). Other authors have employed the biparietal diameter for this purpose. The head perimeter has the advantage of being shape independent. A limitation of this approach is that it assumes that the cranium is not involved in the dysplastic process, and this may not be case in some skeletal dysplasias.

The nomograms in Tables 55.2 and 55.3 provide the mean and standard deviations of long bones and chest. While describing restriction of fetal limbs, we suggest to transform the measurements in number of standard deviations (SDs) from the expected mean for a given gestational age. A measurement that falls within 2 SDs from the mean can be considered normal. A value that falls below −4 SDs is almost constantly indicative of a skeletal abnormality, if severe growth retardation can be ruled out. Measurements between −2 and −4 SDs are alarming. They do not necessarily indicate a skeletal disorder, but require a careful evaluation.

Shortening of the extremities can involve the entire limb (micromelia), the proximal segment (rhizomelia), the intermediate segment (mesomelia) or the distal segment (acromelia). The diagnosis of rhizomelia or mesomelia requires the comparison of the dimensions of the bones of the legs and forearm with those of the thigh and arm. Table 55.3 presents skeletal dysplasias characterized by rhizomelia, mesomelia, acromelia and micromelia.

Recently, a multicentric study has addressed the problem of femur growth in fetuses with skeletal dysplasias[7]. The results of this study, with regard to four of the most common anomalies encountered in prenatal studies, are shown in Fig. 55.1. It has been found that most achondroplastic fetuses have measurements that fall into the interval between −2 and −4 SDs in the midtrimester. On the other hand, growth restriction is much more severe in thanatophoric dysplasia and achondrogenesis. Fetuses presenting these anomalies had values falling significantly below −4 SDs at the onset of the second trimester.

A detailed examination of each bone is necessary to exclude the absence or hypoplasia of individual bones (fibula, tibia, scapula, radius), which are frequently absent in certain conditions.

An attempt should be made to characterize the degree of mineralization. This can be assessed by examining the acoustic

TABLE 55.3

Gestational-age-independent nomograms to evaluate the size of the fetal femur from the head circumference (HC) and the size of the chest (CC, chest circumference) from the abdominal circumference (AC) (values in mm, SD = standard deviation)

HC	Femur	SD	AC	CC	SD
150	27	3	150	123	10
155	29	3	155	126	10
160	30	3	160	130	10
165	31	3	165	134	10
170	33	3	170	137	10
175	34	3	175	141	10
180	35	3	180	144	10
185	36	3	185	148	10
190	38	3	190	151	10
195	39	3	195	155	10
200	40	3	200	158	10
205	41	3	205	162	10
210	43	3	210	165	10
215	44	3	215	169	10
220	45	3	220	173	10
225	46	3	225	176	10
230	48	3	230	180	10
235	49	3	235	183	10
240	50	3	240	187	10
245	51	3	245	190	10
250	53	3	250	194	10
255	54	3	255	197	10
260	55	3	260	201	10
265	56	3	265	204	10
270	58	3	270	208	10
275	59	3	275	211	10
280	60	3	280	215	10
285	61	3	285	219	10
290	63	3	290	222	10
295	64	3	295	226	10
300	65	3	300	229	10
305	66	3	305	233	10
310	68	3	310	236	10
315	69	3	315	240	10
320	70	3	320	243	10
325	71	3	325	247	10
330	73	3	330	250	10
335	74	3	335	254	10
340	75	3	340	258	10
345	76	3	345	261	10
350	78	3	350	265	10
355	79	3	355	268	10

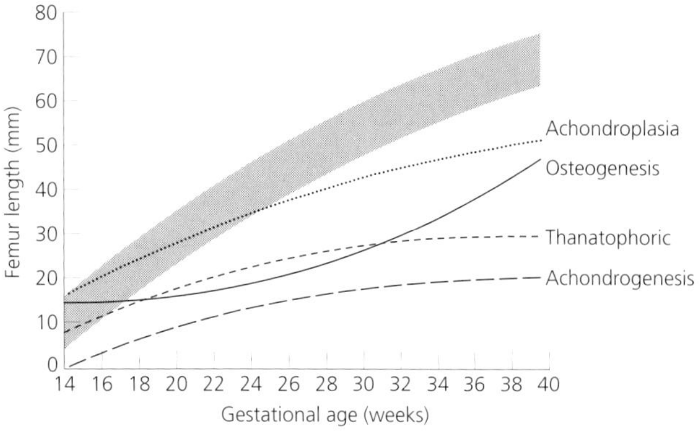

Fig. 55.1 Length of fetal femur in different types of skeletal dysplasias. The curves represent the mean values obtained by polynomial regression analysis of a large group of affected fetuses derived from a multicentric study. The shaded area represents the interval between –2 and –4 SDs derived from the analysis of a group of normal fetuses. In achondrogenesis and thanatophoric dysplasia the length of the femur is expected to deviate significantly from the expected values after 14–16 weeks. With achondroplasia, deviation usually occurs only in the midtrimester. The curve of fetuses with osteogenesis imperfecta reflect probably the heterogeneous presentation of this disease. (Modified from: Goncalvez, L & Jeanty, P. (1994) Fetal biometry of skeletal dysplasias: a multicentric study. *J Ultrasound Med* **13**:977–985.)

shadow behind the bone and the echogenicity of the bone itself. It should be stressed that there are limitations in the sonographic evaluation of mineralization of long bones and that other structures, such as the skull, are perhaps better suited for this assessment. The degree of long bone curvature should be examined. At present, there is no objective means of assessing this sign, and experience is the only means by which the operator can discern the boundary between normality and abnormality. Camptomelia (excessive bowing) is characteristic of certain disorders (e.g., camptomelic dysplasia). Finally, the possibility of fractures should also be considered, as they can be detected in some conditions (e.g., osteogenesis imperfecta). The fractures may be extremely subtle or may lead to angulation and separation of the segments of the affected bone.

EVALUATION OF THORACIC DIMENSIONS

Several skeletal dysplasias are associated with a hypoplastic thorax. Such a finding is extremely important because chest restriction leads to pulmonary hypoplasia, a frequent cause of death in these conditions. The appropriateness of thoracic dimensions can be assessed by measuring the thoracic circumference at the level of the four-chamber view of the heart. The thoracic circumference can be measured or calculated either using the formula:

thoracic circumference = (anteroposterior diameter + transverse diameter) $\times$ 1.57

or using an ellipsoid generated on-screen. Table 55.2 illustrates nomograms used to evaluate the thoracic dimensions that were developed in our laboratory. In many cases, chest restriction in the context of skeletal dysplasia is associated with redundant soft tissue. The nomogram in Table 55.2 was constructed therefore upon measurements obtained by placing the calipers on the rib cage, and excluding the thoracic soft tissues. When gestational age is uncertain, age-independent ratios can be utilized. The thoracic to abdominal circumference ratio (Table 55.3) and the thoracic to head circumference ratio (normal value: 0.56–1.04)[8] permit evaluation of the transverse thoracic dimensions. Another approach is to use the ratio between the cardiac circumference and the thoracic circumference.

Evaluation of thoracic dimensions is a critical part of the diagnostic work-up because the cause of death in most lethal skeletal dysplasias is pulmonary hypoplasia associated with alteration of thoracic dimensions. We have found that a thoracic circumference of less than 2 SDs from the mean in a fetus with abnormal measurements of the long bones is strongly indicative of a skeletal dysplasia with thoracic restriction. The interested reader is referred to a recent review on the use of sonography to predict pulmonary hypoplasia[9].

EVALUATION OF HANDS AND FEET

Several skeletal dysplasias feature alterations of the hands and feet. Polydactyly refers to the presence of more than five digits. It is classified as postaxial if the extra digits are on the ulnar or fibular side and preaxial if they are located on the radial or tibial side. Syndactyly refers to soft tissue or bony fusion of adjacent digits. Clinodactyly consists of deviation of a finger(s). When a skeletal dysplasia is suspected, fetal hands and feet should be examined to exclude polydactyly and syndactyly and also extreme postural deformities such as those seen in diastrophic dysplasia. Table 55.4 displays disorders associated with hand and feet deformities. Disproportion between hands and feet and the other parts of the extremity may also be a sign of a skeletal dysplasia. The femur length/foot length ratio is nearly constant from the 14th to 40th week. The mean is 0.99 (SD = 0.06). A ratio below 0.87 should be considered abnormal[10]. Although fetuses with skeletal dysplasias have been reported to have abnormally low ratios, more experience is required to test the diagnostic value of this method. It is expected that a small proportion of normal fetuses may have an abnormal ratio. As in the case of other limb biometric parameters, large deviations from the lower limit of normal are likely to be significant.

EVALUATION OF FETAL SPINE

Several skeletal dysplasias are associated with abnormalities of the spine. The most common spinal abnormality seen in skeletal dysplasias is platyspondyly, which consists of flattening of the vertebrae. A longitudinal sonogram of the spine has been proposed to evaluate the ratio between the vertebral interspace and the vertebral body height (Fig. 55.2). By using

TABLE 55.4
Antenatal sonographic findings useful for triangulation of skeletal dysplasias

Skeletal dysplasias associated with different types of shortening of long bones

Rhizomelia
- Thanatophoric dysplasia
- Atelosteogenesis
- Chondrodysplasia punctata (rhizomelic type)
- Diastrophic dysplasia
- Congenital short femur
- Achondroplasia

Mesomelia
- Mesomelic dysplasia (Langer, Reinhardt and Robinow type)
- COVESDEM association
- Acromelia
- Ellis–van Creveld syndrome (chondroectodermal dysplasia)

Micromelia
- Achondrogenesis
- Atelosteogenesis
- Short rib polydactyly syndrome (type I and type III)
- Diastrophic dysplasia
- Fibrochondrogenesis
- Osteogenesis imperfecta (type II)
- Kniest dysplasia
- Dyssegmental dysplasia
- Roberts syndrome

Skeletal dysplasias associated with altered thoracic dimensions

Long narrow thorax
- Asphyxiating thoracic dysplasia (Jeune)
- Chondroectodermal dysplasia (Ellis–van Creveld)
- Metatropic dysplasia
- Fibrochondrogenesis
- Atelosteogenesis
- Camptomelic dysplasia
- Jarcho–Levin syndrome
- Achondrogenesis
- Hypophosphatasia
- Dyssegmental dysplasia
- Cleidocranial dysplasia

Short thorax
- Osteogenesis imperfecta (type II)
- Kniest dysplasia (metatropic dysplasia type II)
- Pena–Shokeir syndrome

Hypoplastic thorax
- Short rib polydactyly syndrome (type I, type II)
- Thanatophoric dysplasia
- Cerebro-costo-mandibular syndrome
- Cleidocranial dysostosis syndrome
- Homozygous achondroplasia
- Melnick–Needles syndrome (osteodysplasty)
- Fibrochondrogenesis
- Otopalatodigital syndrome type II

Skeletal dysplasias associated with hand and foot abnormalities

Postaxial polydactyly
- Chondroectodermal dysplasia
- Short rib polydactyly syndrome (type I, type III)
- Asphyxiating thoracic dysplasia
- Otopalatodigital syndrome
- Mesomelic dysplasia Werner type (associated with absence of thumbs)

Preaxial polydactyly
- Chondroectodermal dysplasia
- Short rib polydactyly syndrome type II
- Carpenter syndrome

Syndactyly
- Poland syndrome
- Acrocephalopolysyndactylies (Carpenter syndrome, Apert syndrome)
- Otopalatodigital syndrome type II
- Mesomelic dysplasia Werner type
- TAR syndrome
- Jarcho–Levin syndrome
- Robert syndrome

Brachydactyly
- Mesomelic dysplasia Robinow type
- Otopalatodigital syndrome

Hitchhiker thumb
- Diastrophic dysplasia

Clubfoot deformity
- Diastrophic dysplasia
- Osteogenesis imperfecta
- Kniest dysplasia
- Spondyloepiphyseal dysplasia congenita

Skeletal dysplasias associated with skull and face deformities

Large head
- Achondroplasia
- Achondrogenesis
- Thanatophoric dysplasia
- Osteogenesis imperfecta
- Cleidocranial dysplasia
- Hypophosphatasia
- Camptomelic dysplasia
- Short rib polydactyly syndrome type III
- Robinow mesomelic dysplasia
- Otopalatodigital syndrome

Cloverleaf skull
- Thanatophoric dysplasia (type II)
- Camptomelic dysplasia

Other craniostenosis
- Apert syndrome
- Carpenter syndrome
- Hypophosphatasia

Congenital cataracts
- Chondrodysplasia punctata

Cleft palate
- Asphyxiating thoracic dysplasia
- Kniest dysplasia
- Diastrophic dysplasia
- Spondyloepiphyseal syndrome
- Camptomelic dysplasia
- Jarcho–Levin syndrome
- Chondroectodermal dysplasia
- Short rib polydactyly syndrome type II
- Metatropic dysplasia
- Dyssegmental dysplasia
- Otopalatodigital syndrome type II
- Roberts syndrome

Hypertelorism
- Otopalatodigital syndrome
- Arthrogryposis multiplex congenita
- Larsen syndrome
- Roberts syndrome
- Cleidocranial dysplasia
- Achondroplasia
- Camptomelic dysplasia
- Coffin syndrome
- Klippel–Feil syndrome
- Apert syndrome
- Sprengel's deformity
- Mesomelic dysplasia
- Holt–Oram syndrome

Micrognathia
- Camptomelic dysplasia
- Diastrophic dysplasia
- Otopalatodigital syndrome
- Achondrogenesis
- Mesomelic dysplasia
- Arthrogryposis multiplex congenita
- Nager acrofacial dysostosis
- Oromandibular limb hypogenesis
- Atelosteogenesis

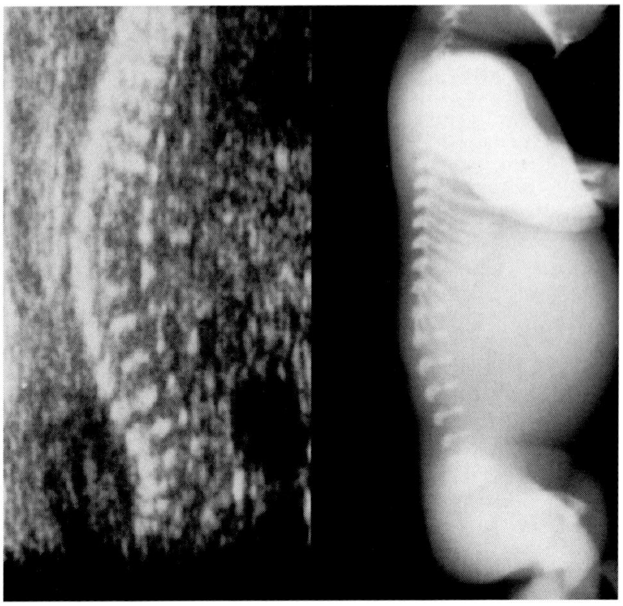

Fig. 55.2 Severe platyspondyly in a fetus with thanatophoric dysplasia. Thinning of the vertebral bodies is evident both in the antanatal sonogram as well as in the postnatal radiographic examination.

this approach, the severe platyspondyly of thanatophoric dysplasia and the milder platysondyly of achondroplasia were detected by about 20 menstrual weeks[11]. Kyphosis and scoliosis can also be identified in utero. Prenatal diagnosis of congenital hemivertebra has also been reported[12].

EVALUATION OF FETAL CRANIUM

Several skeletal dysplasias are associated with defects of membranous ossification and, therefore, affect skull bones. Orbits should be measured to exclude hypertelorism[13].

Other findings which should be searched for are micrognathia[14], short upper lip, abnormally shaped ear[15], frontal bossing and cloverleaf skull deformity. Table 55.4 presents abnormalities of the skull and face in the different skeletal dysplasias.

EXAMINATION OF FETAL MOVEMENTS

Absent fetal movements are pathognomonic of arthrogryposis multiplex congenita. Maternal perception of fetal movements is usually decreased in fetuses with skeletal dysplasias, such as achondrogenesis and thanatophoric dysplasia[16].

DIAGNOSTIC TESTS COMPLEMENTARY TO SONOGRAPHY

Chromosomal studies should be included in all cases, as there is a specific group of constitutional bone disorders associated with cytogenetic abnormalities. Biochemical studies are helpful in rare instances (e.g., hypophosphatasia). DNA restrictions and enzymatic activity assays should be considered in those cases in which the phenotype suggests a metabolic disorder such as a mucopolysaccharidosis. Although a full discussion about such disorders is beyond the scope of this text, they are well known causes of constitutional bone diseases. At present, DNA analysis is becoming available for the specific recognition of an increasing number of osteochondrodysplasias, and will certainly play a major role in the near future[17–19].

PROGNOSTIC ASSESSMENT

It is frequently impossible to identify the precise nature of a skeletal anomaly serendipitously encountered in a fetus, although some findings will allow the outcome to be predicted with reasonable precision. In general, severe thoracic restriction, gross demineralization (fracture of long bones, caput membranaceum) and associated cerebral and/or visceral anomalies are associated with a very poor prognosis.

POSTNATAL DIAGNOSTIC WORK-UP

Despite all efforts to establish an accurate prenatal diagnosis, a careful study of the newborn will be required in all instances. The evaluation should include a detailed physical examination performed by a geneticist or an individual with experience in the field of skeletal dysplasias and radiograms of the skeleton. The latter should include: anterior, posterior, lateral and Towne views of the skull and anteroposterior views of the spine and extremities, with separate films of hands and feet. Examination of the skeletal radiographs will permit precise diagnoses in the overwhelming majority of cases, since the classification of skeletal dysplasias is largely based upon radiographic findings. In lethal skeletal dysplasias, histological examination of the chondro-osseous tissue should be included, as this information may help reach a specific diagnosis.

OSTEOCHONDRODYSPLASIAS

A growing number of skeletal dysplasias have been recognized in utero. A complete account of each disorder is beyond the scope of this chapter, and we refer the reader to texts on the subject for further details[20]. A few of the most common disorders relevant to prenatal diagnosis are discussed here.

THANATOPHORIC DYSPLASIA, FIBROCHONDROGENESIS, ATELOSTEOGENESIS

Thanatophoric dysplasia is the most common lethal skeletal dysplasia in fetuses and neonates. It is characterized by extreme rhizomelia, a normal trunk length with a narrow thorax and a large head with a prominent forehead. It occurs in 0.24–0.69/10 000 births[1]. Thanatophoric dysplasia is associated with abnormal enchondral ossification and approximately 14% of cases show a cloverleaf skull deformity resulting from early synostosis of skull bones. A distinction between thanatophoric dysplasia type I, type II and less common variants ('San Diego', 'Torrance' and 'Luton') has recently been made. Type I is characterized by short curved (telephone receiver) femora and is rarely combined with cloverleaf skull. Type II has straight femora, wider bones and is nearly always associated with a cloverleaf skull deformity (Fig. 55.3)[21]. The differential diagnosis between the two depends upon the radiographic findings and histology. There is no agreement regarding the pattern of inheritance of this condition. The first type seems to have an undetermined pattern of inheritance, and most cases are sporadic. The second type seems to be inherited with an autosomal recessive pattern. As most cases are thought to be sporadic mutations, a risk of recurrence in the range of 1% is presently suggested.

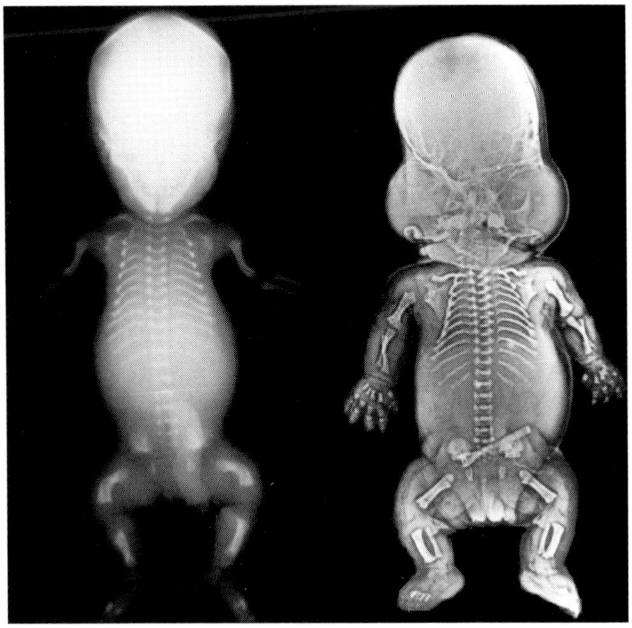

Fig. 55.3 Radiographic appearance of thanatophoric dysplasia type I (left) and type II (right).

The prenatal sonographic findings depend upon the specific variety. In type I, a bowed femur below −4 SDs from the mean will be found after the midtrimester, in association with obvious thoracic hypoplasia (Fig. 55.4) and severe platyspondyly (Fig. 55.2)[22,23]. The association of cloverleaf skull and micromelia is specific for thanatophoric dysplasia type II (Fig. 55.5)[24–26]. The other skeletal dysplasia associated with cloverleaf skull is camptomelic syndrome. However, micromelia is not a feature of this condition. Cloverleaf skull may result from: (1) premature closure of the coronal and lambdoid sutures; (2) defective development of the cranial base with secondary synostosis and (3) a primary developmental disorder of the brain with secondary deformation of the skull. The forehead is prominent, and a saddle nose and hypertelorism may be present. Hydrocephaly and polyhydramnios are frequently present. Thanatophoric dysplasia is a uniformly lethal disorder. Prenatal diagnosis has been documented in several occasions.

Fibrochondrogenesis and atelosteogenesis have a clinical presentation similar to that of thanatophoric dysplasia. A differential diagnosis between these disorders in utero is extremely difficult. Fibrochondrogenesis is a lethal chondrodysplasia inherited with an autosomal recessive pattern and characterized by rhizomelia with significant metaphyseal

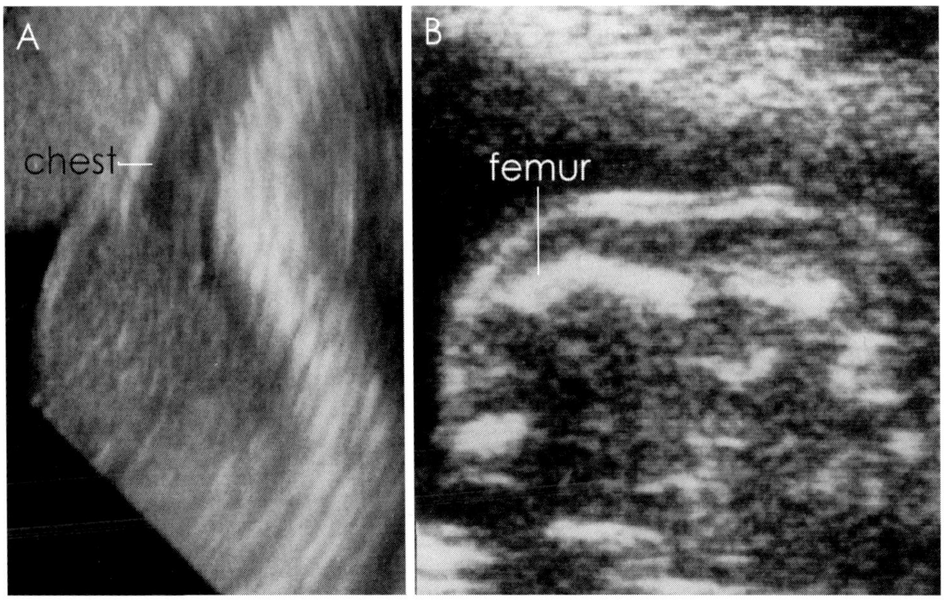

Fig. 55.4 Typical sonographic findings in thanatophoric dysplasia type I: (A) sagittal view of the trunk reveals striking hypoplasia of the chest; (B) the femur is short (−5 SDs from the mean) and bowed.

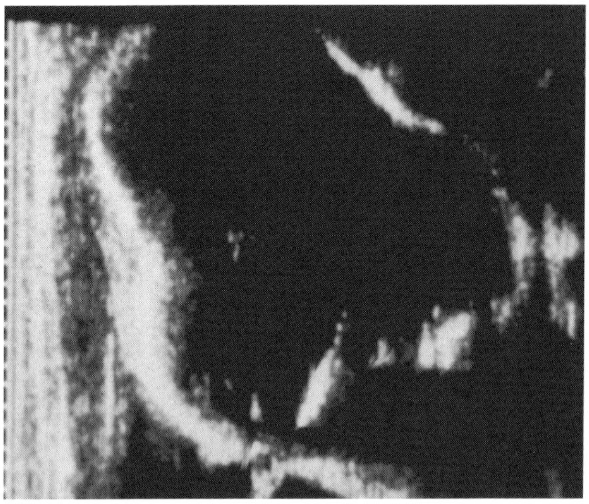

Fig. 55.5 Cloverleaf skull in a fetus with thanatophoric dysplasia type II.

flaring and clefting of the vertebral bodies. Metaphyseal flaring is not a feature of thanatophoric dysplasia[27]. Atelosteogenesis is also a lethal chondrodysplasia characterized by severe micromelia (with hypoplasia of the distal segments of the humerus and femur), bowing of long bones and dislocation at the the level of the elbow and knee. Clubfoot deformities may also be present[28]. Fibrochondrogenesis and atelosteogenesis are extremely rare, and only a few cases of each have been reported.

ACHONDROGENESIS

Achondrogenesis, or anosteogenesis, is a lethal chondrodystrophy, characterized by extreme micromelia, short trunk and macrocrania (Fig. 55.6). The birth prevalence is 0.09–0.23/10 000 births[1]. The traditional classification of achondrogenesis subdivides this disorder into two types. The more severe form, type I (Parenti–Fraccaro), is characterized by partial or complete lack of ossification of the calvarium and spine, very short long bones and multiple rib fractures. Type II (Langer–Saldino) is characterized by a variable degree of calcification of the calvarium and spine and by absence of fractures of the ribs. Hypochondrogenesis had been considered a separate disorder from achondrogenesis. However, recent evidence suggests that hypochondrogenesis and achondrogenesis type II are phenotypic variants of the same disorder[29]. Recently, Whitley and Gorlin have proposed a new classification for achondrogenesis dividing the disease into four types[30]. Prenatal diagnosis should be suspected on the basis of micromelia, lack of vertebral ossification and a large head with various degrees of ossification of calvarium (Fig. 55.7)[31–33]. Polyhydramnios and hydrops have been associated with achondrogenesis. However, sonographic examinations of affected fetuses do not demonstrate fluid accumulation in body cavities. The hydropic appearance of these fetuses and neonates is probably attributable to redundancy of soft-tissue mass over a limited skeletal frame. Achondrogenesis type I is inherited with an autosomal recessive pattern, while most cases of achondrogenesis type II and hypochondrogenesis have been sporadic (new autosomal dominant mutations)[34].

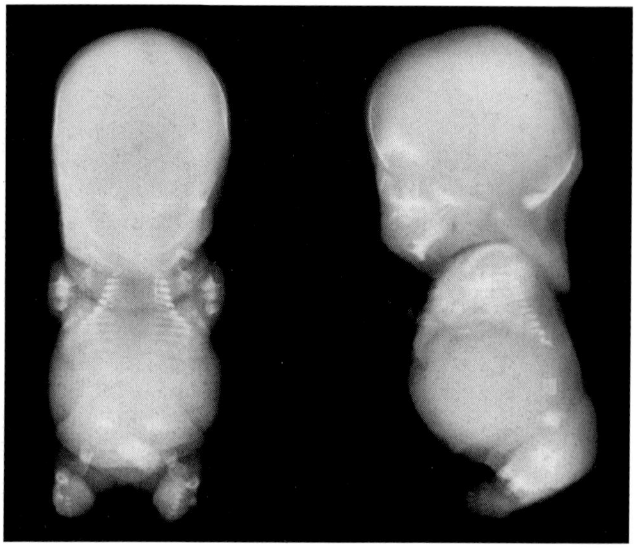

Fig. 55.6 Achondrogenesis. Trunk and limbs are extremely short. The chest is severely hypoplastic; the skull and spine are demineralized.

ACHONDROPLASIA

The most common non-lethal skeletal dysplasia is heterozygous achondroplasia. It is is characterized by rhizomelic dwarfism, limb bowing, lordotic spine and enlarged head. It is inherited with an autosomal dominant pattern, and its prevalence is 1/66 000[1]. Advanced paternal age is a risk factor for achondroplasia. This disease is the result of anomalous growth of cartilage, followed by abnormal endochondral ossification, which is responsible for the shortness of long bones. The bones of the hands and feet are short (brachydactyly). The head is large; a flattened nasal bridge, frontal bossing and a broad mandible are frequent features. In the homozygous state, which is a lethal condition, short limbs are associated with thoracic hypoplasia.

Prenatal diagnosis of heterozygous achondroplasia has been accomplished with sonography upon several occasions. However, most of the cases reported thus far were identified in the third trimester. The problems in the antenatal recognition of heterozygous achondroplasia have been discussed in detail by Kurtz and colleagues[35] and further substantiated by Goncalves and Jeanty[7]. In the midtrimester, the length of the femus usually falls between –2 and –3 SDs from the mean. This finding does represent a diagnostic challenge. Although achondroplasia is immediately suspected, in general ultrasound does not allow a firm diagnosis until late in gestation.

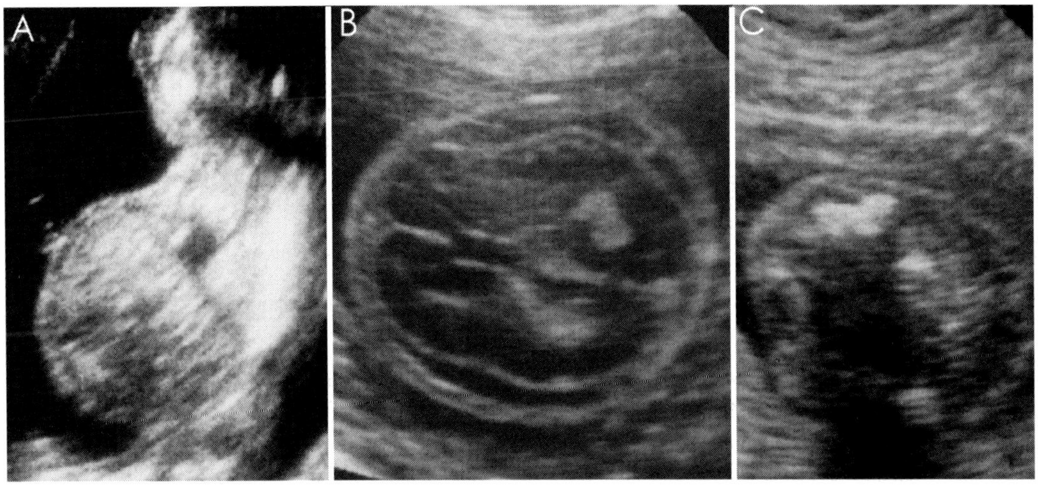

Fig. 55.7 Achondrogenesis. (A) Sagittal view demonstrates a very short trunk; the ribs are mineralized, while the spine is not. (B) Demineralization of the skull is attested by the unusual shape of the calvarium (that was soft and easily compressible by minimal pressures), as well as by the absence of acoustic shadowing and by the enhanced resolution of cerebral anatomy. (C) an extremely shortened femur is demonstrated (12 mm at 24 weeks).

The disproportion between the long bones and the size of the head and foot increases the index of suspicion, but it remains impossible to provide specific risk figures to counsel the couple with. It has been suggested that sonographic demonstration of frontal bossing, depressed nasal bridge and 'trident' hand may be helpful in these cases[36]. It is, however, uncertain whether these findings can be demonstrated in early gestation.

Recently, the achondroplasia gene has been mapped and sequenced[37]. Differently from most other genes, the FGFR3 mutation causally related to achondroplasia is very specific. DNA analysis has been used for the early antenatal diagnosis of homozygous achondroplasia[18]. In one case with dubious sonographic findings at 22 weeks' gestation the diagnosis of heterozygous achondroplasia was firmly established following DNA analysis of fetal blood obtained by funipuncture (Fig. 55.8)[19].

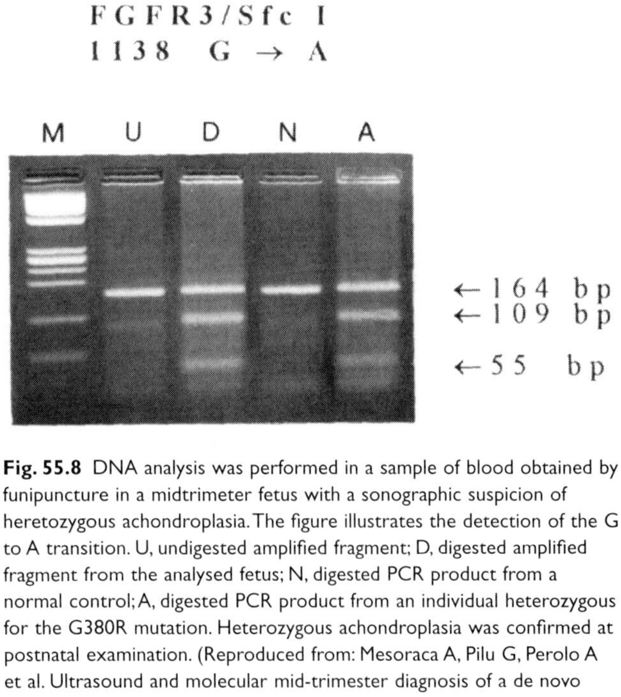

Fig. 55.8 DNA analysis was performed in a sample of blood obtained by funipuncture in a midtrimeter fetus with a sonographic suspicion of heretozygous achondroplasia. The figure illustrates the detection of the G to A transition. U, undigested amplified fragment; D, digested amplified fragment from the analysed fetus; N, digested PCR product from a normal control; A, digested PCR product from an individual heterozygous for the G380R mutation. Heterozygous achondroplasia was confirmed at postnatal examination. (Reproduced from: Mesoraca A, Pilu G, Perolo A et al. Ultrasound and molecular mid-trimester diagnosis of a de novo achondroplasia. *Prenat Diagn*, **16**:764–768, 1996.)

OSTEOGENESIS IMPERFECTA AND HYPOPHOSPHATASIA

These disorders are discussed together because they are characterized by significant skeletal demineralization. Osteogenesis imperfecta (OI) is a heterogeneous group of collagen disorders with a prevalence of 0.18/10 000 births[1]. The traditional classification proposed by Sillence et al.[38] has been recently challenged[39]. At present, OI is regarded as a spectrum of disorders. At one end of the spectrum, there is a neonatal form, frequently lethal, characterized by the presence of multiple fractures at birth, that may be associated with shortness and deformation of long bones and chest and a soft skull (Fig. 55.9). At the other end of the spectrum, there is a tarda form that is manifest with the late appearance of occasional fractures, often in association with blue sclerae. It has been proposed that there two non-lethal forms: one with autosomal dominant transmission with blue sclerae, and one with sporadic occurrence, characterized by severe progressive short stature and pale blue or white sclerae. Autosomal recessive forms are probably very rare, but it has been suggested to assume this mode of inheritance in the severe cases, with perinatal death or severe disability in infancy. Antenatal diagnosis of severe forms of OI has been reported several times. The cases that have been described span in severity from lethal forms, characterized by short limbs, multiple fractures of long bones and ribs and caput membranaceum (Fig. 55.10)[40–43] to less severe forms with either a few fractures or

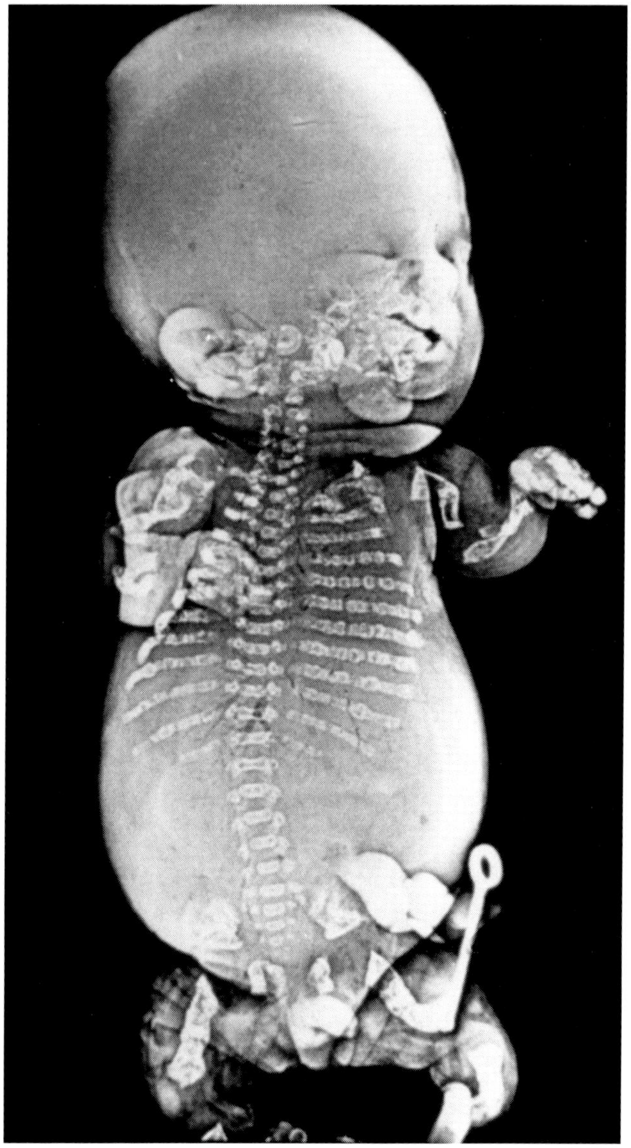

Fig. 55.9 Lethal variety of osteogenesis imperfecta. Note multiple fractures of ribs and long bones, and short limbs.

deformation of long bones[44–48]. Several cases have been described in which the only antenatal sonographic finding was bowing of long bones, mimicking camptomelic dysplasia (Fig. 55.11)[49].

Hypophosphatasia is inherited with an autosomal recessive pattern and is characterized by demineralization of bones and low alkaline phosphatase in serum and other tissues. There are four clinical forms of the disease. Neonatal form (also known as congenital or lethal) is associated with early neonatal death or intrauterine fetal demise may occur. Prenatal diagnosis of this condition has been reported with both ultrasound[50] and by assaying alkaline phosphatase in tissue obtained by chorionic villous sampling[51]. The congenital variety is uniformly lethal.

SKELETAL DYSPLASIAS CHARACTERIZED BY A HYPOPLASTIC THORAX

The dysplastic process involves the ribs and other bones of the rib cages in many skeletal dysplasias. A reduction in thoracic dimensions leads to restriction of lung growth and, consequently, pulmonary hypoplasia. Lung hypoplasia is the main cause of death in lethal skeletal dysplasias. There is a specific group of dysplasias in which thoracic hypoplasia is a cardinal feature. These include asphyxiating thoracic dysplasia, Ellis–van Creveld syndrome and short rib polydactyly syndrome.

Asphyxiating thoracic dysplasia

This skeletal dysplasia, also known as Jeune syndrome, is rare. Its prevalence is 0.14/10 000 births, and it is inherited in an autosomal recessive pattern[1]. It is characterized by a narrow and 'bell-shaped' thorax, with short, horizontal ribs. Long bones are normal or mildly shortened. Polydactyly and cleft lip and/or palate can occur in association[52–55]. The disease is not uniformly lethal, and long-term survivors have been reported[56,57]. We have been able to diagnose this condition prior to viability in five pregnancies at risk. The most striking finding was a small thorax (Fig. 55.12). The femora were below −2 SDs from the mean in only two cases.

Chondroectodermal dysplasia (Ellis–van Creveld syndrome)

Chondroectodermal dysplasia (also referred to as Ellis–van Creveld syndrome) is an autosomal recessive condition characterized by acromelic and mesomelic shortness of limbs, postaxial polydactyly, small chest, ectodermal dysplasia and, in many cases, congenital heart defects (Fig. 55.13). In the late 1970s, chondroectodermal dysplasia was diagnosed antenatally with a combination of ultrasound and fetoscopy, to visualize polydactyly[58]. Current ultrasound technology allows, however, the certain visualization of polydactyly after 15–16 weeks' gestation with standard abdominal sonography, and probably even before by the use of transvaginal probes.

In the midtrimester, the typical findings include shortness of long bones, predominant in the forearms and legs, a small thorax, and polydactyly (Fig. 55.14). Congenital heart defects (most frequently a single atrium or a large atrial defect) are encountered in 60% of cases. In the absence of a positive familial history, distinguishing this condition from other types of skeletal dysplasia with thoracic restriction and polydactyly may be difficult.

Short limb polydactyly syndromes

Short limb polydactyly syndromes are a group of lethal disorders characterized by short limb dysplasia, constricted thorax and postaxial polydactyly. Associated anomalies are

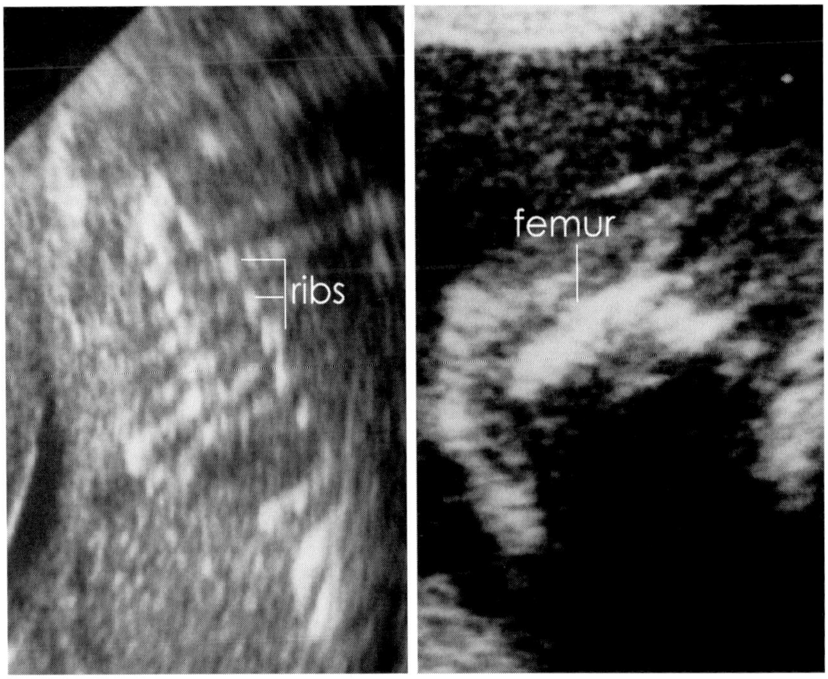

Fig. 55.10 Sonograms from a midtrimester fetus with a very severe form of osteogenesis imperfecta. Obvious fractures of the ribs and femur are present.

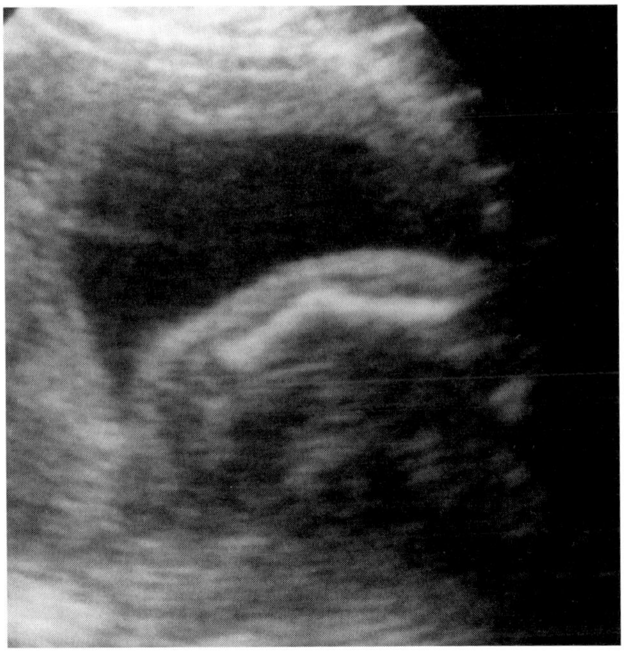

Fig. 55.11 In a third-trimester fetus, bowing of long bones was noted. The image demonstrates the femur. Osteogenesis imperfecta was diagnosed after birth.

frequently found, including congenital heart disease, polycystic kidneys, intestinal atresia. Four different types have been recognized. Type I (Saldino–Noonan) has narrow metaphyses; type II (Majewski) has cleft lip/cleft palate and disproportionally shortened tibiae; type III (Naumoff) has wide metaphyses with spurs; type IV (Beemer–Langer) is characterized by median cleft lip, small chest with extremely short ribs, protuberant abdomen with umbilical hernia and ambiguous genitalia in some 46,XY individuals. The first three types have been identified with prenatal ultrasound[59–61].

CAMPTOMELIC DYSPLASIA

This disease is characterized by bowing of the long bones of the lower extremities, hypoplastic scapulae and several associated anomalies, such as hydrocephalus, cleft palate, micrognathia, hydronephrosis, and congenital heart defects. Camptomelic syndrome has a prevalence of 0.05/10 000 births[1]. The most important feature is bowing of the femur and tibia, while other tubular bones are normal in length. The chest is narrow and can be 'bell-shaped'; the vertebrae are hypoplastic. Differential diagnoses include OI, thanatophoric dysplasia, and hypophosphatasia. Antenatal diagnosis of this dysplasia has been reported in patients at risk[62–64]. The condition is frequently lethal, but some survivors have been reported[65].

DIASTROPHIC DYSPLASIA

Diastrophic dysplasia is characterized by micromelia, clubfoot, hand deformities, multiple joint flexion contractures and scoliosis. This disorder is inherited as an autosomal recessive trait. Due to phenotypic variability, the diagnosis may be difficult at birth, and milder cases are diagnosed later[66]. The clinical features include rhizomelic type micromelia, contractures, hand deformities with abducted position of the thumbs

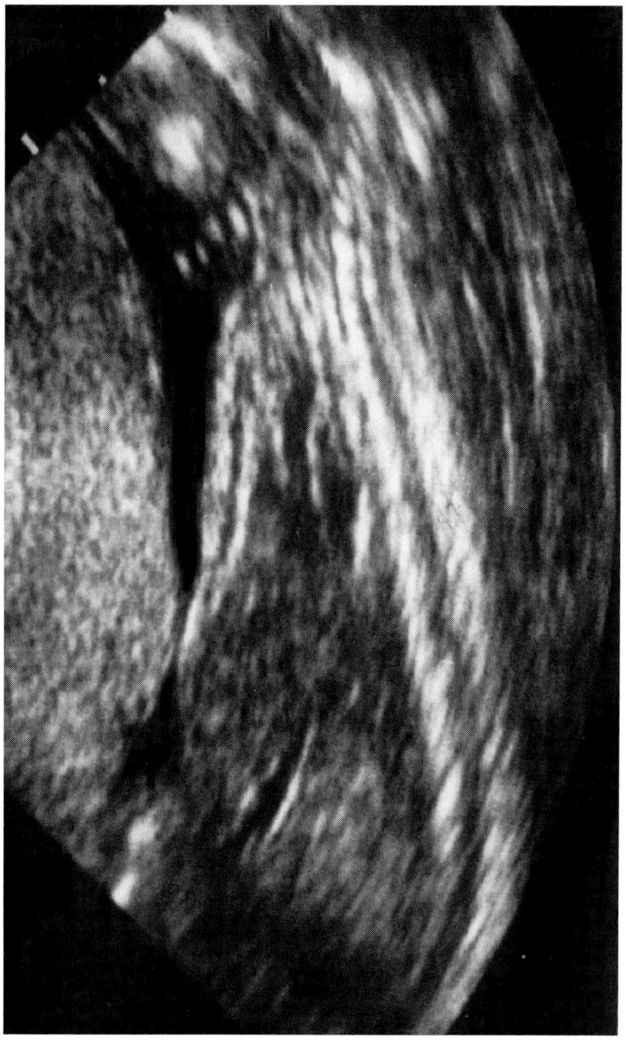

Fig. 55.12 Asphyxiating thoracic dysplasia. A sagittal view of the trunk demonstrates a long and narrow thorax.

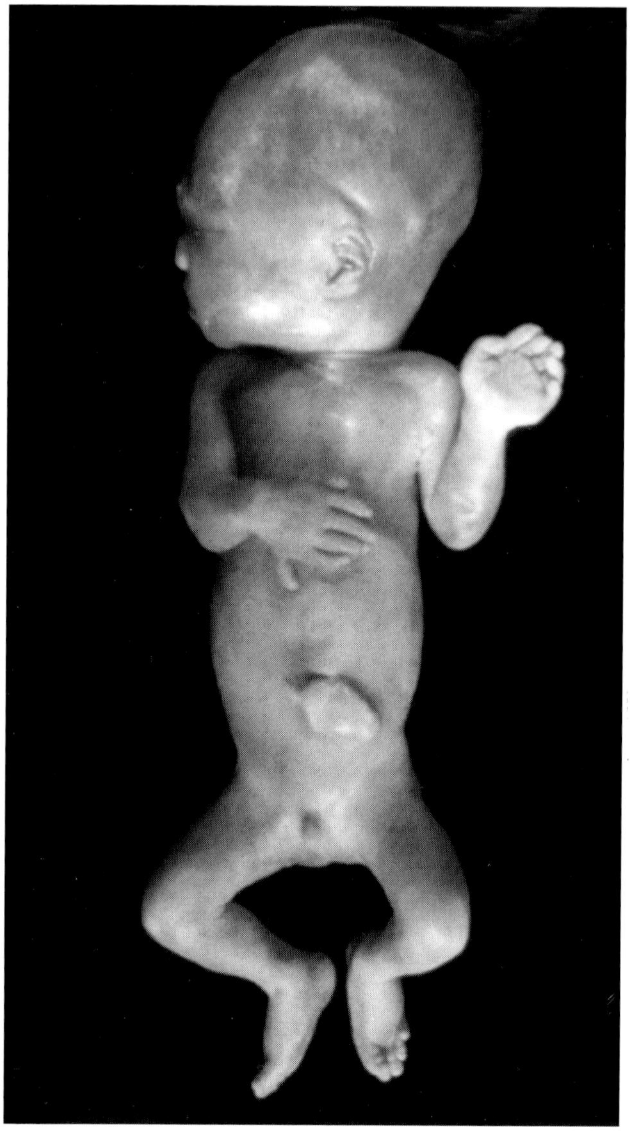

Fig. 55.13 Ellis–van Creveld syndrome. Note the narrow chest, mesomelic shortening of the limbs and postaxial polydactyly.

('hitchhiker thumb') (Fig. 55.15) and severe talipes equinovarus. The head is normal, but micrognathia and cleft palate may be associated. This dysplasia is a generalized disorder of cartilage, with destructive process of cartilage matrix and following formation of fibrous scar tissue and ossification. The latter process is responsible for the contractures. The prenatal diagnosis of diastrophic dysplasia has been found in patients at risk[67–69] based on severe shortening and bowing of all long bones. This disorder has a wide spectrum, and some cases may not be diagnosable in utero. This disease is not lethal, and intellect is not affected.

Limb deficiency or congenital amputations

On occasion, the only identifiable anomaly is the absence of an extremity or a segment of an extremity. These anomalies are referred to as 'limb deficiencies' or 'congenital amputations' (Table 55.5). They constitute a group of disorders different from osteochondrodysplasias. The overall incidence of congenital limb reduction deformities is approximately 0.49/10 000 births[70]. It has been estimated that 51% of these limb reduction defects are simple transverse reduction deficiencies of one forearm or hand without associated anomalies. The remainder consists of multiple reduction deficiencies, with an approximate 23% incidence of additional anomalies of the internal organs of craniofacial structures[70].

Limb deficiencies can present alone or as part of a specific syndrome. An isolated limb deficiency of the upper extremity (e.g., distal segment of an arm) (Fig. 55.16) is generally an isolated anomaly. In contrast, congenital amputation of the leg

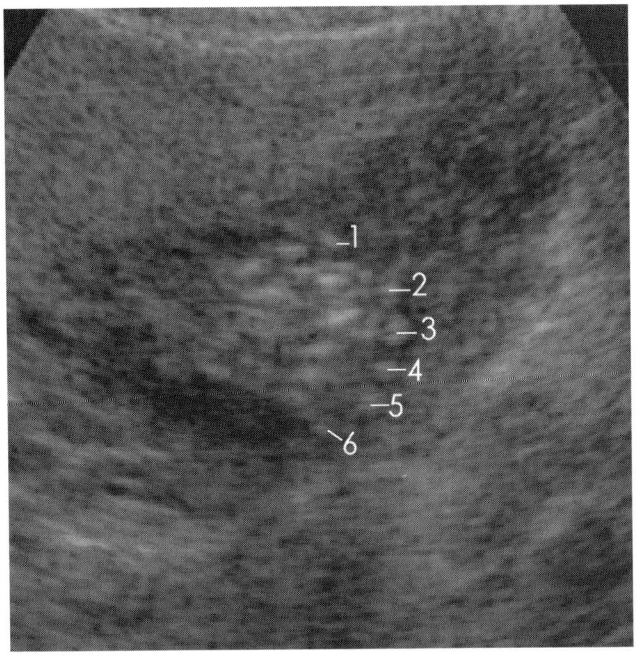

Fig. 55.14 Postaxial polydactyly in an 18-week fetus.

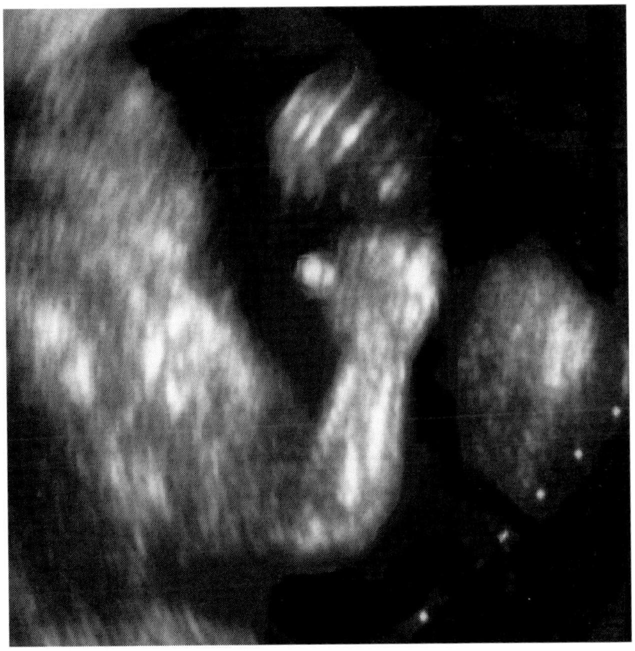

Fig. 55.15 Hitchhiker thumb in a fetus with diastrophic dysplasia.

generally occurs within the context of a syndrome, as do bilateral amputations or reduction of all limbs[4].

Isolated amputation of an extremity can be due to amniotic band syndrome, exposure to a teratogen or a vascular accident. In most cases, the anomaly is sporadic, and the risk of recurrence is negligible. However, recurrence of upper limb deficiencies has been reported[71].

TABLE 55.5
Congenital amputation

Absent limb(s) only
Single absent limb
Multiple absent limbs
Absent limbs with rings
Congenital ring constriction syndrome
Absent limb and face anomaly
Aglossia–adactylia syndrome
Moebius syndrome
Absent limbs with other anomalies
Ichthyosiform skin (CHILD syndrome)
Fibula agenesis–complex brachydactyly (Du Pan syndrome)
Splenogonadal fusion
Skull and scalp defects (*Adams–Oliver* syndrome)
Phocomelia
Thalidomide syndrome
Thrombocytopenia with absent radii (TAR) syndrome
Robert pseudothalidomide–SC syndome
Grebe syndrome
Proxymal femoral focal deficiency
Femoral hypoplasia–unusual facies syndrome
Femur–fibula–ulna complex
Femur–tibia–radius complex
Split hand/split foot (SH/SF) syndrome
SH/SF only
SH/SF and absent long bones
Ectrodactyly, ectodermal dysplasia, cleft lip and palate (EEC syndrome)
Others
Split foot and triphalangeal thumb, autosomal dominant
Split foot, or split hand and central polydactyly
Sh/SF and congenital nystagmus (Karsch–Neugebauer syndrome)
Sh/SF and renal malformations (acrorenal syndrome)
Split foot and mandibulofacial dysostosis (Fontaine syndrome), autosomal dominant

Source: adapted from Goldberg, M.D. (1987) *The Dysmorphic Child: an Orthopedic Perspective.* New York: Raven Press

The syndromes associated with limb deficiencies include aglossia–adactylia syndrome and *Moebius syndrome*. The aglossia–adactylia syndrome (also known as Hanhart syndrome and/or glossopalatine ankylosis) consists of transverse amputations of the limbs and malformations of the mouth (including micrognathia; vestigial tongue; or ankylosis of the tongue to the hard palate, the floor of the mouth or the lips (glossopalatine ankylosis)). The spectrum of anomalies of the extremities is quite variable, ranging from absent digits to severe deficiencies of all four extremities. Intelligence is generally normal. The syndrome is sporadic[72].

The Moebius syndrome consists of a number of facial anomalies attributed to paralysis of the sixth and seventh cranial nerves. Impairment of jaw mobility leads to micrognathia. Ptosis is also a common feature. The Moebius syndrome is generally sporadic[73]. Rare cases of a familial form have been reported[74].

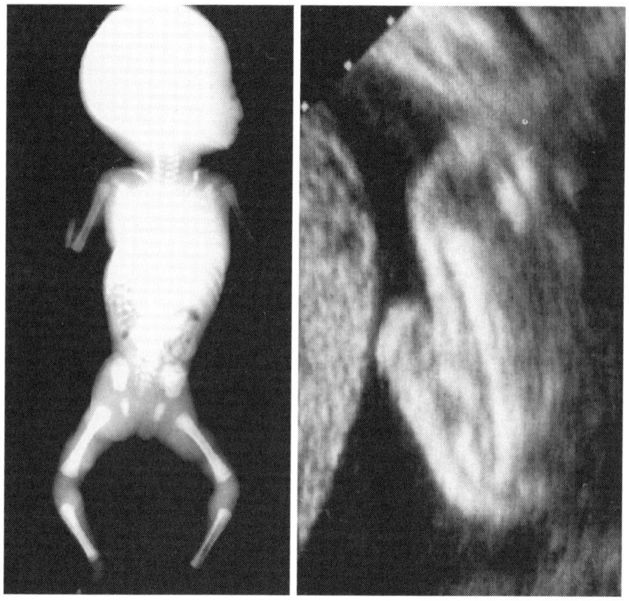

Fig. 55.16 Bilateral amputation of upper limbs. The postnatal appearance is compared with an antenatal sonogram.

The associated limb reduction anomalies are generally present in the upper extremities and range from transverse deficiencies to absent digits.

Limb reduction defects associated with other anomalies are the following: congenital hemidysplasia with ichthyosiform erythroderma and limb defects (CHILD syndrome), a defect characterized by strict demarcation of the skin lesions to one side of the midline. The presence of unilateral defects of long bones is an important feature of the syndrome. Limb deficiencies may vary from hypoplasia of phalanges or metacarpals to complete absence of an extremity. The calvarium, scapulae or ribs may also be involved. Zellweger syndrome and warfarin embryopathy may present with similar findings. Visceral anomalies include: congenital heart disease, unilateral hydronephrosis, hydroureter, unilateral absence of the kidney, fallopian tube, ovaries, adrenal gland and thyroid. The CHILD syndrome predominantly affects females (ratio 19:1)[75].

Fibula aplasia-complex brachydactyly (Du Pan syndrome) is an extremely rare condition characterized by bilateral agenesis of the fibula with abnormalities of the metacarpals and proximal phalanges. Limb reduction defects can involve the lower extremities[76].

The splenogonadal fusion syndrome is characterized by limb reduction defects and splenogonadal fusion. A review of 14 reported cases indicates that there is some overlap between this syndrome and the aglossia–adactylia (Hanhart) syndrome. Most reported cases have occurred in males. Typically, there is a mass in the scrotum, and an ectopic spleen is identified during surgery[77].

The *Adams–Oliver* syndrome is an autosomal dominant disorder characterized by the association of limb reduction defects and scalp defects (aplasia cutis and deficiency of bony calvarium)[78].

In phocomelia, the extremities resemble those of a seal. Typically, the hands and feet are present, but the intervening arms and legs are absent. Hands and feet may be normal or abnormal. Three syndromes must be considered in the differential diagnosis of phocomelia: Roberts syndrome, some varieties of the thrombocytopenia with absent radius (TAR) syndrome and Grebe syndrome. Phocomelia can also be caused by exposure to thalidomide, but this is only of historical interest[79].

Roberts syndrome is an autosomal recessive disorder characterized by the association of tetraphocomelia and facial clefting defects or hypoplastic nasal alae. Hypertelorism may also be present. The upper extremities are generally more severely affected than the lower extremities. The spine is not involved. Polyhydramnios has been noted, and other anomalies associated with the syndrome include horseshoe kidney, hydrocephaly, cephalocele and spina bifida[80].

Grebe syndrome is a condition described among the inbred Indian tribes from Brazil. It is an autosomal recessive disorder characterized by marked hypomelia of upper and lower limbs increasing in severity from proximal to distal segments. In contrast to Roberts syndrome, the lower limbs are more affected than the upper extremities[81].

TAR syndrome is discussed in detail in the section on radial clubhand deformities.

Proximal femoral focal deficiency or congenital short femur consists of a wide variety of congenital developmental anomalies of the femur. The disorder has been classified into five groups: type I, simple hypoplasia of the femur; type II, short femur with angulated shaft; type III, short femur with coxa vara (the most common); type IV, absent or defective proximal femur; and type V, absent or rudimentary femur[82]. One or both femurs can be affected (Fig. 55.17). The right femur is more frequently involved. Anomalies of the upper limbs can also be present and do not exclude the diagnosis[83]. The proximal femoral focal deficiency syndrome may be associated with umbilical or inguinal hernias. If both femurs are affected, it is important to examine the face carefully. The disorder may be femoral hypoplasia and unusual face syndrome[84]. Femoral hypoplasia–unusual facies syndrome consists of bilateral femoral hypoplasia and facial defects, including short nose with broad tip, long philtrum, micrognathia and cleft palate. Long bone abnormalities can extend to other segments of the lower extremity (absent fibula) and also to the upper extremity. The syndrome is sporadic and has been associated with maternal diabetes mellitus. A familial form has been described[85].

If the defect is unilateral, it may correspond to the femur–fibula–ulna or femur–tibia–radius complex. These two syndromes have different implications for genetic counselling; the former is non-familial, while the second has a strong genetic component[86].

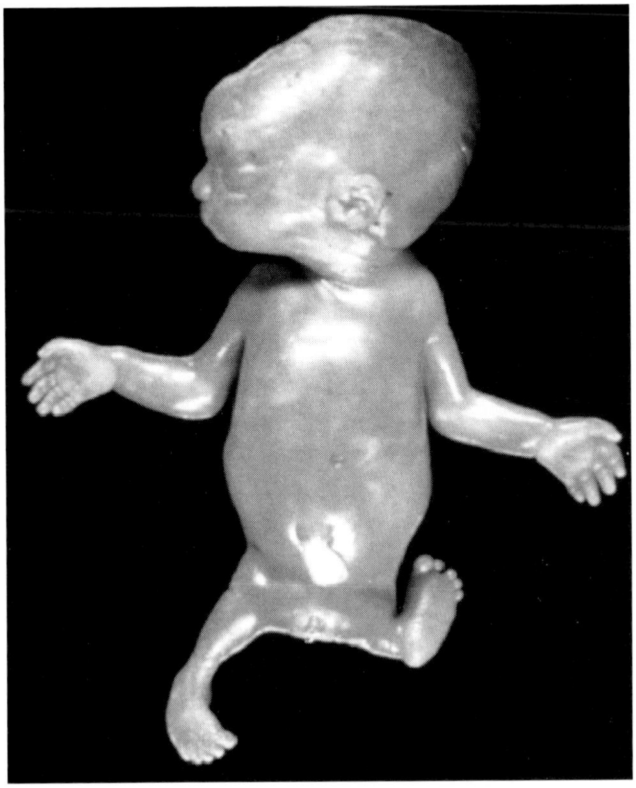

Fig. 55.17 Proxymal femoral deficiency.

The term 'split hand and foot syndrome' is used to refer to a group of disorders characterized by splitting of the hand and foot into two parts. Other terms include lobster-claw deformity, ectrodactyly and aborted fingers. The conditions are classified into typical and atypical varieties[87]. The typical form consists of absence of both the finger and the metacarpal bone, resulting in a deep V-shaped central defect that clearly divides the hand into an ulnar and a radial part. It occurs in 1:90 000 live births and has a familial tendency (usually inherited with an autosomal dominant pattern). The atypical variety is characterized by a much wider cleft formed by a defect of the metacarpals and the middle fingers. As a consequence, the cleft is U-shaped and wide, with only thumb and small finger remaining. It occurs in 1:150 000 live births[88].

A complex system for the classification of these disorders, based upon the distribution of remaining fingers, has been proposed[89]. However, this system is not helpful in differential diagnosis and syndrome classification.

Split hand/foot deformities can occur as isolated anomalies or as part of a more complex syndrome. The syndromic types are the ones more frequently encountered[4].

Several syndromes are associated with split hand/foot deformities. The split hand/foot and absent long bones syndromes include two conditions in which there is split hand and aplasia of the tibia or split foot with aplasia of the ulna. However, skeletal anomalies are not limited to these bones; the clavicle, femur and fibula can also be affected. The pattern of inheritance of these disorders has not been clearly determined. Autosomal dominant, recessive and X-linked recessive patterns have been proposed[90,91]. Ectrodactyly–ectodermal dysplasia–cleft lip/palate syndrome (EEC syndrome) generally involves the four extremities with more severe deformities of the hands. The spectrum of ectodermal defects is wide, including dry skin, sparse hair and dental defects[92]. Defects of the tear duct lead to absence of lacrimal secretions, chronic kerato–conjunctivitis and severe loss of visual acuity. The cleft lip is generally bilateral. Obstructive uropathy can also occur[93]. The pattern of inheritance is autosomal dominant. Intelligence is generally normal[94].

There is a different group of syndromes that involves associations of the split hand/foot deformity with other anomalies. This entity includes split foot and triphalangeal thumb, split foot and hand and central polydactyly, Karsch–Neugebauer syndrome (split hand/foot with congenital nystagmus), acro-renal syndrome and mandibulofacial dysostosis (Fontaine syndrome)[95–98].

Clubhands

Clubhand deformities are classified into two main categories: radial and ulnar. Radial clubhand includes a wide spectrum of disorders that encompass absent thumb, thumb hypoplasia, thin first metacarpal and absent radius (Fig. 55.18). Ulnar clubhand is much less frequent than radial clubhand and ranges from mild deviations of the hand of the ulnar side of the forearm to complete absence of the ulna. While radial clubhand is frequently syndromatic, ulnar clubhand is usually an isolated anomaly[4].

Whenever a clubhand is identified, it is important to conduct a thorough examination of the fetus and newborn to delineate associated anomalies that may suggest a syndrome. Fetal blood sampling procedures and fetal echocardiography are recommended. A complete blood cell count, including platelets, is important to establish the diagnosis of Fanconi's pancytopenia, TAR syndrome and Aase syndrome. A fetal karyotype is indicated because several chromosomal abnormalities (e.g., trisomy 18, 21 and other structural aberrations) have been reported in association with clubhand deformities. Congenital heart disease is an important feature of the Holt–Oram syndrome and the Lewis upper limb–cardiovascular syndrome, and is also present in some cases of TAR syndrome.

The isolated radial clubhand can be present with other anomalies. This constellation may not represent a recognizable or previously described syndrome. Isolated radial clubhand is generally a sporadic disorder[99].

The three syndromes associated with haematologic abnormalities are Fanconi's pancytopenia, TAR syndrome and Aase syndrome. Fanconi's anaemia (pancytopenia) is an autosomal

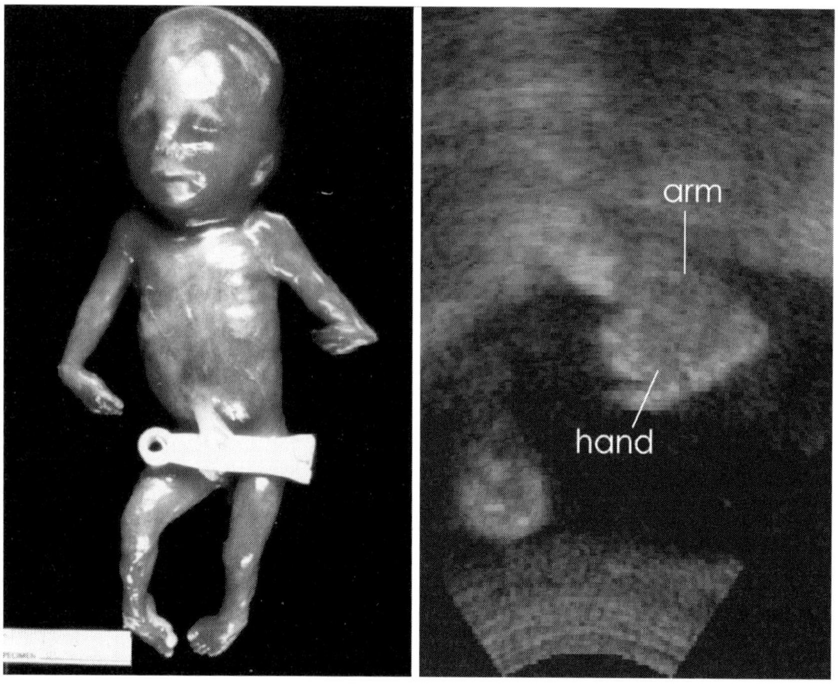

Fig. 55.18 Clubhand in a fetus with trisomy 18.

recessive disease characterized by the association of bone marrow failure (anaemia, leukopenia and thrombocytopenia) and skeletal anomalies, including a radial clubhand with absent thumbs, radial hypoplasia and a high frequency of chromosomal breakage (demonstrated in amniotic fluid cells or fetal lymphocytes after incubation with diepoxybutane)[100]. It can be associated with congenital dislocation of the hip; scoliosis; and cardiac, pulmonary and gastrointestinal anomalies. Intrauterine growth retardation is common. Prenatal diagnosis has been reported many times[101].

TAR syndrome is an autosomal recessive disorder characterized by thrombocytopenia (platelet count of less than 100 000/mm^3) and bilateral absence of the radius. The thumb and metacarpals are always present. The ulna and humerus may be absent, and clubfoot deformities may also be present. Congenital heart disease is present in 33% of the cases (tetralogy of Fallot and and septal defects). Prenatal diagnosis of this condition has been described [102–104]. In couples at genetic risk, ultrasound demonstration of a limb defect is sufficient for a specific diagnosis. In an index case, a combination of ultrasound and cordocentesis, demonstrating a low platelet count has been described.[104] Delivery by caesarean section is recommended, as these fetuses are at risk of intracranial haemorrhage[105].

Aase syndrome is an autosomal recessive condition characterized by congenital hypoplastic anaemia and a radial clubhand with a triphalangeal thumb and a hypoplastic distal radius. Cardiac defects (ventricular septal defects) may be present[106,107]. Other disorders associated with triphalangeal thumbs are Holt–Oram syndrome and Nager syndrome.

Holt–Oram syndrome is an autosomal dominant disorder characterized by congenital heart disease (mainly atrial septal defects, secundum type and ventricular septal defects) and aplasia or hypoplasia of the radius. Limb defects are often asymmetric. There is no correlation between the severity of the limb defects and the cardiac anomaly. Other anomalies include hypertelorism and vertebral defects[108]. This condition has been prenatally diagnosed[109,110]. The upper limb–cardiovascular syndrome described by Lewis et al. is probably not separate from Holt–Oram syndrome[111].

Craniofacial abnormalities and radial clubhand deformities form a different group of syndromes. These syndromes are sporadic and have common features that make a prenatal differential diagnosis difficult. The most common craniofacial anomaly is cleft lip and palate. Uuspaa's study of 3225 cases with orofacial cleft showed a 2.8% association with upper extremity deformities[112].

Radial clubhand is also associated with congenital scoliosis. The three syndromes that should be considered part of the differential diagnosis include: VATER association, some cases of the Goldenhaar syndrome and the Klippel–Feil syndrome[113,114]. The VATER association includes vertebral segmentation (70%), anal atresia (80%), tracheo-oesophageal fistula (70%), oesophageal atresia and radial and renal defects (65% and 53%, respectively). Other anomalies include a single umbilical artery (35%) and congenital heart disease, occurring in nearly 50% of the patients. The VATER association occurs sporadically. The Goldenhaar syndrome, a disorder characterized by alterations in the morphogenesis of the first and second brachial arches (microtia and hypoplasia of the malar, maxillary, and/or mandibular region) can also be associated with radial clubhand[115].

Radial clubhand has been reported in association with several chromosomal anomalies, including trisomies 18 and 21, deletion of the long arm of 13 and ring formation of chromosome 4.

Ulnar clubhand occurs as an isolated, non-syndromic anomaly in most cases. It can also be associated with a variety of syndromes, for example, Poland complex[116–118].

Polydactyly

Polydactyly is the presence of an additional digit. The extra digit may range from a fleshy nubbin to a complete digit with controlled flexion and extension. Polydactyly can be classified as postaxial (the most common form), preaxial, and central. Postaxial polydactyly occurs on the ulnar side of the hand (Figs 55.13, 55.14) and fibular side of the foot. Preaxial polydactyly is present on the radial side of the hand and the tibial side of the foot.

The majority are isolated conditions with an autosomal dominant mode of inheritance. Some of them are part of a syndrome, usually an autosomal recessive one. Preaxial polydactyly, especially triphalangeal thumb, is most likely to be part of multisystem syndrome. Central polydactyly consists of an extra digit that is usually hidden between the long and the ring finger. It is often bilateral and is inherited with an autosomal mode of inheritance. It can be associated with other hand and foot malformations[119–121].

Arthrogryposis

The term arthrogryposis multiplex congenita (AMC) refers to multiple joint contractures present at birth. Normal fetal movement is important for the development of the joints; limitation of the fetal joint motion leads to the development of contractures and AMC[122].

AMC is not a specific disorder but rather a syndrome. Neurologic, muscular, connective tissue, skeletal abnormalities or intrauterine crowding can lead to impaired fetal motion and AMC[123]. In a series of 74 children, Banker found that the most common cause of AMC was a neurogenic disorder followed by myopathic disorders[124]. The condition is present in 0.03% live births[125].

The deformities are usually symmetric. In most cases of AMC, all four limbs are involved, followed by deformities of the lower extremities only, or bimelic involvement. The severity of the deformities increases distally in the involved limb, with the hands and feet typically being the most deformed.

There are many congenital anomalies associated with AMC. The most frequent are micrognathia, cleft palate, Klippel–Feil syndrome, meningomyelocele and congenital heart disease. Ten percent of patients with AMC have associated anomalies of the central nervous system[122].

The prenatal diagnosis of AMC with ultrasound has been reported[126–131]. The cardinal findings are absent fetal movement on real-time examination and severe flexion deformities. Polyhydramnios, chest restriction and micrognathia are frequently found in association (Figs 55.19, 55.20).

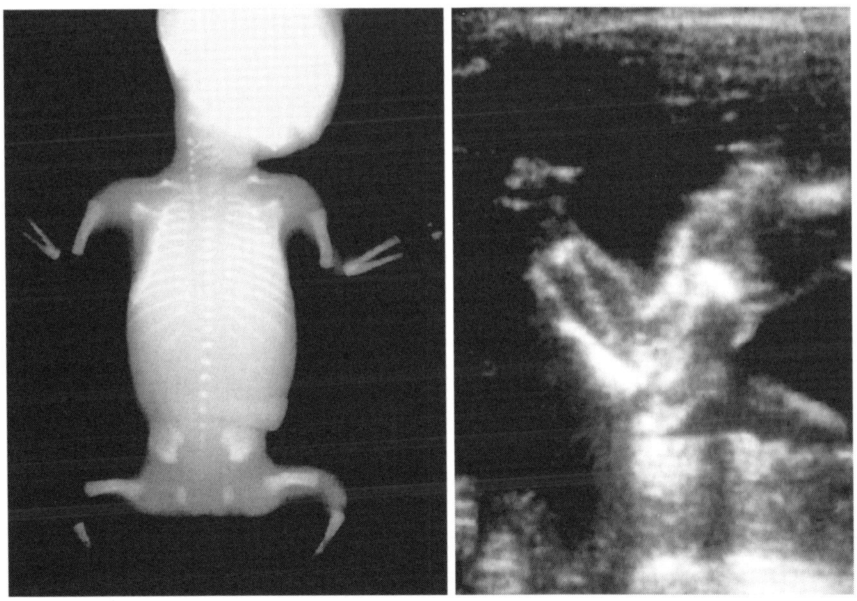

Fig. 55.19 Arthrogryposis multiplex congenita. In a midtrimester fetus, polyhydramnios was associated with absence of fetal movements. The long bones were shortened, particularly in the proximal segments. The limbs were constantly flexed.

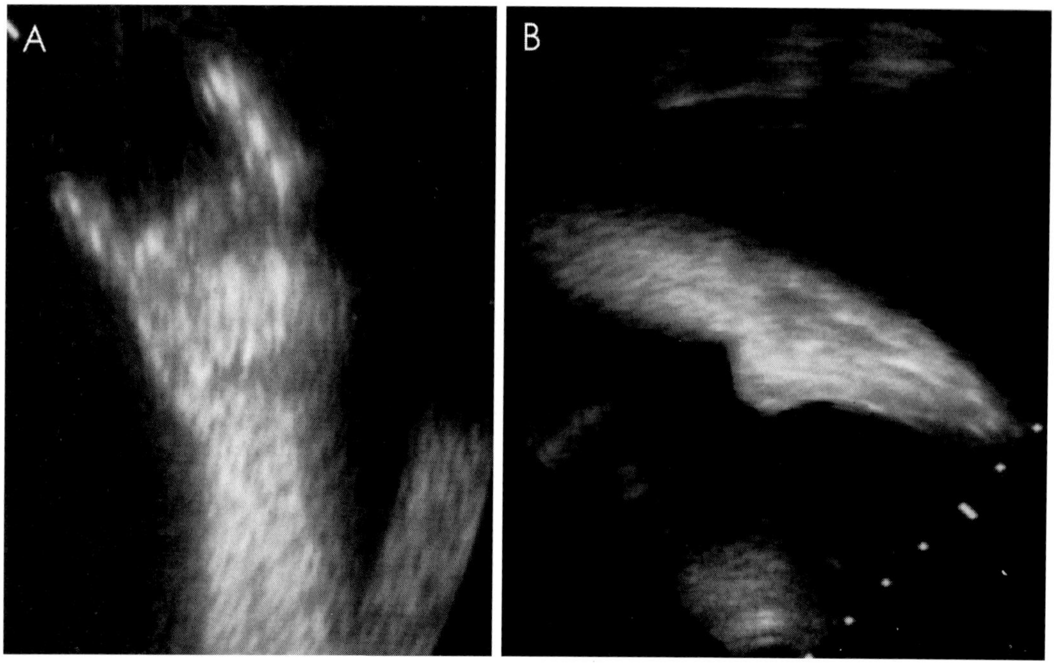

Fig. 55.20 Arthrogryposis multiplex congenita. The diagnosis was inferred by a combination of polyhydramnios, absence of the fetal movements, and by the constantly abnormal posture of the fingers (A) and feet (B).

REFERENCES

1. Camera G, Mastroiacovo P. Birth prevalence of skeletal dysplasias in the Italian multicentric monitoring system for birth defects. In *Skeletal Dysplasias* (eds C.J. Papadatos & C.S. Bartsocas), pp. 441–449. New York: Alan R. Liss, 1982.
2. Connor JM, Connor RA, Sweet EM et al. Lethal neonatal chondrodysplasias in the West of Scotland 1970–1983 with a description of a thanatophoric, dysplasialike, autosomal recessive disorder, Glasgow variant. *Am J Med Genet* **22**:243–253, 1985.
3. International Working Group on Constitutional Diseases of Bone. International classification of osteochondrodysplasias. *Eur J Pediatr* **151**:407–415, 1992.
4. Goldberg MJ. *The Dysmorphic Child: an Orthopedic Perspective*. New York: Raven Press, 1987.
5. Coffin GS, Siris E, Wegienka LC. Mental retardation with osteocartilaginous anomalies. *Am J Dis Child* **112**:205–211, 1966.
6. Poznanski AK. Congenital and developmental anomalies. In *Textbook of Diagnostic Imaging*, 2nd edn (eds C.E. Putnam & C.E. Ravin), pp. 1315–1351. Philadelphia: W.B. Saunders, 1994.
7. Goncalvez L, Jeanty P. Fetal biometry of skeletal dysplasias: a multicentric study. *J Ultrasound Med* **13**:977–985, 1994.
8. Chitkara U, Rosenberg J, Chervenak FA et al. Prenatal sonographic assessment of the fetal thorax: normal values. *Am J Obstet Gynecol* **156**:1069–1074, 1987.
9. Lauria M, Gonik B, Romero R. Pulmonary hypoplasia: pathogenesis, diagnosis and antenatal prediction. *Obstet Gynecol* **86**:466–475, 1995.
10. Campbell J, Henderson A, Campbell S. The fetal femur/foot length ratio: a new parameter to assess dysplastic limb reduction. *Obstet Gynecol* **72**:181–189, 1989.
11. Rouse GA, Filly RA, Toomey F, Grube GL. Short limb skeletal dysplasias: evaluation of the fetal spine with sonography and radiography. *Radiology* **174**:177–180, 1990.
12. Benacerraf BR, Greene MF, Barss VA. Prenatal sonographic diagnosis of congenital hemivertebra. *J Ultrasound Med* **5**:257–259, 1986.
13. Galli G. *Craniosynostosis*. Boca Raton, FL: CRC Press, 1984.
14. Pilu G, Romero R, Reece EA, Jeanty P, Hobbins JC. The prenatal diagnosis of Robin anomalad. *Am J Obstet Gynecol* **154**:630–631, 1986.
15. Pilu G, Reece EA, Romero R, Bovicelli L, Hobbins JC. Prenatal diagnosis of craniofacial malformations with ultrasonography. *Am J Obstet Gynecol* **155**:45–50, 1986.
16. Escobar LF, Bixler D, Weaver DD, Padilla LM, Golichowski A. Bone dysplasias. The prenatal diagnosis challenge. *Am J Med Genet* **36**:488–494, 1990.
17. Francomano CA. The genetic basis of dwarfism. *N Engl J Med* **332**:58–59, 1995.
18. Bellus GA, Escallon CS, Ortiz de Luna R et al. First trimester prenatal diagnosis in couple at risk for homozygous achondroplasia. *Lancet* **344**:1511–1512, 1994.
19. Mesoraca A, Pilu G, Perolo A et al. Ultrasound and molecular midtrimester diagnosis of a de novo achondroplasia. *Prenat Diagn* **16**:764–768, 1996.
20. Romero R, Pilu G, Jeanty P, Ghidini A, Hobbins JC. *Prenatal Diagnosis of Congenital Anomalies*. Norwalk, CT: Appleton & Lange, 1988.
21. Langer LO, Yang SS, Hall JG et al. N. Thanatophoric dysplasia and cloverleaf skull. *Am J Med Genet Suppl* **3**:167–179, 1987.
22. Fink IJ, Filly RA, Callen PW, Golbus MS. Sonographic diagnosis of thanatophoric dwarfism in utero. *J Ultrasound Med* **1**:337–339, 1982.
23. Beetham FGT, Reeves JS. Early ultrasound diagnosis of thanatophoric dwarfism. *J Clin Ultrasound* **12**:43, 1984.
24. Mahony BS, Filly RA, Callen PW, Golbus MS. Thanatophoric dwarfism with the cloverleaf skull: A specific antenatal sonographic diagnosis. *J Ultrasound Med* **4**:151–154, 1985.
25. Elejald BR, de Elejalde MM. Thanatophoric dyplasia: fetal manifestations and prenatal diagnosis. *Am J Med Genet* **22**:669–683, 1985.
26. Weiner CP, Williamson RA, Bonsib SM. Sonographic diagnosis of cloverleaf skull and thanatophoric dysplasia in the second trimester. *J Clin Ultrasound* **14**:463–465, 1986.
27. Whitley CB, Langer LO, Ophoven J et al. Fibrochondrogenesis: lethal, autosomal recessive chondrodysplasia with distinctive cartilage histopathology. *Am J Med Genet* **19**:265, 1984.
28. Chevernak FA, Isaacson G, Rosenberg JC et al. Antenatal diagnosis of frontal cephalocele in a fetus with atelosteogenesis. *J Ultrasound Med* **5**:111, 1986.

29. Borochowitz Z, Ornoy A, Lachman R, Rimoin DL. Achondrogenesis II – hypochondrogenesis: variability versus heterogeneity. *Am J Med Genet* **24**:273–288, 1986.
30. Whitley CB, Gorlin RJ. Achondrogenesis: new nosology with evidence of genetic heterogeneity. *Radiology* **148**:693–697, 1983.
31. Mahony BS, Filly RA, Cooperberg PL. Antenatal sonographic diagnosis of achondrogenesis. *J Ultrasound Med* **3**:333–335, 1984.
32. Benacerraf B, Osathanondh R, Bieber FR. Achondrogenesis type I: ultrasound diagnosis in utero. *J Clin Ultrasound* **12**:357–360, 1984.
33. Glenn LW, Teng SSK. In utero sonographic diagnosis of achondrogenesis. *J Clin Ultrasound* **13**:195, 1985.
34. van der Harten HJ, Brons JTJ, Dijkstra PF. Achondrogenesis, hypochondrogenesis, the spectrum of chondrogenesis imperfecta: a radiologic, ultrasonographic and histopathologic study of 23 cases. *Pediatr Pathol* **8**:571–597, 1988.
35. Kurtz AB, Filly RA, Wapner RJ et al. In utero analysis of heterozygous achondroplasia: variable time of onsets detected by femur length measurements. *J Ultrasound Med* **5**:137–140, 1986.
36. Cordone M, Lituania M, Bocchino G, Passamonti U, Tomà P, Camera G. Ultrasonographic features in a case of heterozygous achondroplasia at 25 weeks' gestation. *Prenat Diagn* **13**:395–401, 1993.
37. Rousseau F, Bonaventure J, Legeai-Mallet L et al. Mutations in the gene encoding fibroblast growth factor receptor-3 in achondroplasia. *Nature* **371**:252–254, 1994.
38. Sillence DO, Senn A, Danks DM. Genetic heterogeneity in osteogenesis imperfecta. *J Med Genet* **16**:101–116, 1979.
39. Wynne-Davies R, Gormley J. Clinical and genetic patterns in osteogenesis imperfecta. *Clin Orthoped Rel Res* **159**:26–35, 1981.
40. Mertz E, Goldhofer W. Sonographic diagnosis of lethal osteogenesis imperfecta in the second trimester: case report and review. *J Clin Ultrasound* **14**:380–382, 1986.
41. Brons JTJ, van der Harten JJ, Wladimiroff JW et al. The prenatal ultrasonographic diagnosis of osteogenesis imperfecta. *Am J Obstet Gynecol* **159**:176–181, 1988.
42. Elejalde BR, Elejalde MM. Prenatal diagnosis of perinatally lethal osteogenesis imperfecta. *Am J Med Genet* **14**:353–359, 1983.
43. Ghosh A, Woo JSK, Wan CW, Wong VCW. Simple ultrasonic diagnosis of osteogenesis imperfecta type II in early second trimester. *Prenat Diagn* **4**:235–240, 1984.
44. Hobbins JC, Bracken MB, Mahoney MJ. Diagnosis of fetal skeletal dysplasias with ultrasound. *Am J Obstet Gynecol* **142**:306–312, 1982.
45. Chervenak FA, Romero R, Berkowitz RL, Mahoney MJ, Hobbins JC. Antenatal sonographic findings of osteogenesis imperfecta. *Am J Obstet Gynecol* **143**:228–230, 1982.
46. Aylsworth AS, Seeds JW, Bonner-Guilford W. Prenatal diagnosis of a severe deforming type of osteogenesis imperfecta. *Am J Med Genet* **19**:707–711, 1984.
47. Robinson LP, Worthen NJ, Lachman RS, Adomian GE, Rimoin DL. Prenatal diagnosis of osteogenesis imperfecta type III. *Prenat Diagn* **7**:7–15, 1987.
48. van der Harten JJ, Brons JTJ, Dijkstra PF. Perinatal lethal osteogenesis imperfecta: radiologic and pathologic evaluation of seven prenatally diagnosed cases. *Pediatr Pathol* **8**:233–252, 1988.
49. Sanders RC, Greyson-Fleg RT, Hogge WA, Blakemore KJ, McGowan KD, Isbister S. Osteogenesis imperfecta and campomelic dysplasia: difficulties in prenatal diagnosis. *J Ultrasound Med* **13**:691–700, 1994.
50. Kousseff BG, Mulivor RA. Prenatal diagnosis of second-trimester skeletal dysplasias: a prospective analysis in a high-risk population. *J Ultrasound Med* **2**:99–107, 1983.
51. Wladimiroff JW, Niermeijer MF, Van der Harken JJ et al. Early prenatal diagnosis of congenital hypophosphatasia: case report. *Prenat Diagn* **5**:47–52, 1985.
52. Elejalde BR, Elejalde MM, Pansch D. Prenatal diagnosis of Jeune syndrome. *Am J Med Genet* **21**:433–435, 1985.
53. Lipson M, Waskey J, Rice J et al. Prenatal diagnosis of asphyxiating thoracic dysplasia. *Am J Med Genet* **18**:273–277, 1984.
54. Schinzel A, Savoldelli G, Briner J, Schuliger G. Prenatal sonographic diagnosis of Jeune syndrome. *Radiology* **154**:777–778, 1985.
55. Skiptunas SM, Weiner S. Early prenatal diagnosis of asphyxiating thoracic dysplasia (Jeune's syndrome): value of fetal thoracic measurement. *J Ultrasound Med* **6**:41–43, 1987.
56. Kozlowski K, Masel J. Asphyxiating thoracic dystrophy without respiratory distress. Report of 2 cases of the latent form. *Pediatr Radiol* **5**:30–35, 1976.
57. Friedman JM, Kaplan HG, Hall JG. The Jeune syndrome (asphyxiating thoracic dystrophy) in an adult. *Am J Med* **59**:857–863, 1975.
58. Mahoney MJ, Hobbins JC. Prenatal diagnosis of chondroectodermal dysplasia (Ellis–Van Creveld syndrome) with fetoscopy and ultrasound. *N Engl J Med* **297**:258–259, 1977.
59. Gembruch U, Hansmann M, Fodish HJ. Early prenatal diagnosis of short rib polydactyly syndrome I (Majewski) by ultrasound in a case at risk. *Prenat Diagn* **5**:357–360, 1985.
60. Wladimiroff JW, Niermeijer MF, Laar J, Jahoda M, Stewart PA. Prenatal diagnosis of skeletal dysplasia by real-time ultrasound. *Obstet Gynecol* **63**:360–366, 1984.
61. Meizner I, Bar Ziv J. Prenatal ultrasonic diagnosis of short rib polydactyly syndrome (SRPS) type III: A case report and a proposed approach to the diagnosis of SRPS and related conditions. *J Clin Ultrasound* **13**:284–288, 1985.
62. Balcar I, Bieber FR. Sonographic and radiologic findings in camptomelic dysplasia. *AJR* **141**:481, 1983.
63. Fryns JP, van der Berghe K, van Assche A et al. Prenatal diagnosis of camptomelic dwarfism. *Clin Genet* **19**:199, 1981.
64. Winter R, Rosenkranz W, Hofmann H et al. Prenatal diagnosis of camptomelic dysplasia by ultrasonography. *Prenat Diagn* **5**:1, 1985.
65. Beluffi G, Fraccaro M. Genetical and clinical aspects of campomelic dysplasia. *Prog Clin Biol Res* **104**:53–57, 1982.
66. Horton WA, Rimoin DL, Lachman RS et al. The phenotypic variability of diastrophic dysplasia. *J Pediatr* **93**:609–613, 1978.
67. Mantagos S, Weiss RR, Mahoney M, Hobbins JC. Prenatal diagnosis of diastrophic dwarfism. *Am J Obstet Gynecol* **139**:111–113, 1981.
68. Gembruch U, Niesen M, Kehrberg H, Hansmann M. Diastrophic dysplasia: a specific prenatal diagnosis by ultrasound. *Prenat Diagn* **8**:539–545, 1988.
69. Gollop TR, Eigier A. Brief clinical report: prenatal ultrasound diagnosis of diastrophic dysplasia at 16 weeks. *Am J Med Genet* **27**:321–324, 1987.
70. Marid BOD, Creizel A, Lenz W. Incidence at birth of different types of limb reduction abnormalities in Hungary, 1975–1977. *Hum Genet* **65**:27–32, 1983.
71. Pilarski RT, Pauli RM, Engber WD. Hand-reduction malformations: genetic and syndrome analysis. *J Pediatr* **5**:274–277, 1985.
72. Tunobileck E, Yalcin C, Atasu M. Aglossia-adactylia syndrome (special emphasis on the inheritance pattern). *Clin Genet* **11**:421–425, 1977.
73. Baraitser M. Genetics of Mobius syndrome. *J Med Genet* **14**:415–419, 1977.
74. Sugarman GI, Stark HH. Mobius syndrome with Poland's anomaly. *J Med Genet* **10**:192–196, 1973.
75. Happle R, Koch H, Lenz W. The CHILD syndrome: congential hemidysplasia with ichthyosiform erthyroderma and limb defects. *Eur J Pediatr* **134**:27–31, 1980.
76. Martin Du Pan CH: Absence congenitale du perone sans deformation du tibia. *Rev D'Orthoped* **3**:227–232.
77. Pauli RM, Greenlaw A. Limb deficiency and splenogonadal fusion. *Am J Med Genet* **13**:81–85, 1982.
78. Bonafede RP, Beighton P. Autosomal dominant inheritance of scalp defects with extrodactyly. *Am J Med Genet* **3**:35–41, 1979.
79. Claus GH, Newman CGH. The thalidomide syndrome: risks of exposure and spectrum of malformations. *Teratology* **13**:555–573, 1986.
80. Waldenmaier C, Aldenhoff P, Klemm T. The Roberts' syndrome. *Hum Genet* **40**:345–351, 1978.
81. Romeo G, Zonana J, Lachman RS et al. Grebe chondrodysplasia and similar forms of severe short-limbed dwarfism. *Birth Defects* **13**:109–115, 1977.
82. Hamanishi C. Congenital short femur. *J Bone Joint Surg* **62**:307–311, 1980.
83. Graham M. Congenital short femur: prenatal sonographic diagnosis. *J Ultrasound Med* **4**:361–365, 1985.
84. Daentl DL, Smith DW, Scott C. Femoral hypoplasia–unusual facies syndrome. *J Pediatr* **86**:107–111, 1975.
85. Gupta DKS, Gupta SK. Familial bilateral femoral focal deficiency. *J Bone Joint Surg* **66-A**:1470–1472, 1984.

86. Tentamy S, McKusick V. Birth defects. National Foundation – *March of Dimes; Vol. XIV, Number 3, March of Dimes*. New York: Alan R. Liss, 1978.
87. Miura T, Suzuki M. Clinical differences between typical and atypical cleft hand. *J Hand Surg* **9**:311, 1984.
88. Barsky AJ. Cleft hand: classification, incidence, and treatment. *J Bone Joint Surg* **46**:1707–1714, 1964.
89. Tada K, Yonenobu K, Swanson AB. Congenital central ray deficiency in the hand – a survey of 59 cases and subclassification. *J Hand Surg* **6**:434–440, 1981.
90. Van den Berghe H, Dequeker J, Fryns JP, David G. Familial occurrence of severe ulnar aplasia and lobster claw feet: a new syndrome. *Hum Genet* **42**:109–113, 1978.
91. Verma IC, Joseph R, Bhargava S, Mehta S. Split-hand and split-foot deformity inherited as an autosomal recessive trait. *Clin Genet* **9**:8–11, 1976.
92. Rudiger RA, Haase W, Passarge E. Association of ectrodactyly, ectodermal dysplasia, and cleft lip-palate. *Am J Dis Child* **120**:160–162, 1970.
93. Leiter E, Lipson J. Genitourinary tract anomalies in lobster claw syndrome. *J Urol* **115**:339–341, 1976.
94. Penchaszadeh VB, De Negrotti TC. Ectrodactyly-ectodermal dysplasia-clefting (EEC) syndrome: dominant inheritance and variable expression. *J Med Genet* **13**:281–284, 1976.
95. Halal F, Homsy M, Perreault G. Acro-renal-ocular syndrome: autosomal dominant thumb hypoplasia, renal ectopia, and eye defect. *Am J Med Genet* **17**:753–762, 1984.
96. Chan KM, Lamb DW. Triphalangeal thumb and five-fingered hand. *Hand* **15**:329–334, 1983.
97. Wood VE. Congenital thumb deformities. *Clin Orthop* **195**:7–25, 1985.
98. Bujdoso G, Lenz W. Monodactylous splithand-splitfoot. *Eur J Pediatr* **133**:207–210, 1980.
99. Carroll RE, Louis DS. Anomalies associated with radial dysplasia. *J Pediatr* **84**:409–411, 1974.
100. Glanz A, Fraser FC. Spectrum of anomalies in Fanconi anaemia. *J Med Genet* **19**:412–416, 1982.
101. Auerbach AD, Sagi M, Adler B. Fanconi anemia: prenatal diagnosis in 30 fetuses at risk. *Pediatrics* **76**:794–800, 1985.
102. Filkins K, Russo J, Bilinki I, Diamond N, Searle B. Prenatal diagnosis of thrombocytopenia absent radius syndrome using ultrasound and fetoscopy. *Prenat Diagn* **4**:139–142, 1984.
103. Luthy DA, Hall JG, Graham CB. Prenatal diagnosis of thrombocytopenia with absent radii. *Clin Genet* **15**:495–499, 1979.
104. Donnenfeld AE, Wiseman B, Lavi E, Weiner S. Prenatal diagnosis of thrombocytopenia absent radius syndrome by ultrasound and cordocentesis. *Prenat Diagn* **10**:29–35, 1990.
105. de Vries LS, Connell J, Bydder GM et al. Recurrent intracranial haemorrhages in utero in an infant with alloimmune thrombocytopenia case report. *Br J Obstet Gynaecol* **95**:299–302, 1988.
106. Higginbottom MC, Jones KL, Kung FH. The Aase syndrome in a female infant. *J Med Genet* **15**:484–486, 1978.
107. Jones B, Thompson H. Triphalangeal thumbs associated with hypoplastic anemia. *Pediatrics* **52**:609–612, 1973.
108. Zhang KZ, Sun QB, Tsung OC. Holt–Oram syndrome in China: a collective review of 18 cases. *Am Heart J* **111**:573–577, 1986.
109. Muller LM. The antenatal ultrasonographic detection of the Holt–Oram syndrome. *S Afr Med J* **68**:313–315, 1985.
110. Brons JTJ, van Geijn HP, Wladimiroff JW et al. Prenatal ultrasonographic diagnosis of the Holt–Oram Syndrome. *Prenat Diagn* **8**:175–181, 1988.
111. Lewis KB, Bruce RA, Baum D. The upper limb–cardiovascular syndrome. *JAMA* **193**:1080–1086, 1965.
112. Uuspaa V. Upper extremity deformities associated with the orofacial clefts. *Scand J Plast Reconstr Surg* **12**:157–162, 1978.
113. Chemke J, Nisani R, Fischel RE. Absent ulna in the Klippel–Feil syndrome: an unusual associated malformation. *Clin Genet* **17**:167–170, 1980.
114. Tentamy SA, Miller JD. Extending the scope of the VATER association: definition of a VATER syndrome. *J Pediatr* **85**:345, 1974.
115. Setzer ES, Reiz-Castaneda N, Severn C, Ryden S, Frias JL. Etiologic heterogeneity in the oculoauriculo vertebral syndrome. *J Pediatr* **98**:88–90, 1981.
116. Swanson AB, Tada K, Yonenubo K. Ulnar ray deficiency: its various manifestations. *J Hand Surg* **9A**:658–664, 1984.
117. Gausewitz SH, Meals RA, Setocuchi Y. Severe limb deficiency in Poland's syndrome. *Clin Orthop* **185**:9–13, 1984.
118. David TJ. Preaxial polydactyly and the Poland complex. (Letter to the editor.) *Am J Med Genet* **13**:333–334, 1982.
119. Lowry RB. Variability in the Smith–Lemli–Opitz syndrome: overlap with the Meckel syndrome. *Am J Med Genet* **14**:429–433, 1983.
120. Goodman RM, Sternberg M, Shem-Tob Y. Acrocephalopolysyndactyly type IV: a new genetic syndrome in 3 sibs. *Clin Genet* **15**:209–214, 1979.
121. Khaldi F, Bennaceur B, Hammou A. An autosomal recessive disorder with retardation of growth, mental deficiency, ptosis, pectus excavatum and camptodactyly. *Pediatr Radiol* **18**:432–435, 1988.
122. Hageman G, Willemse J. Arthrogryposis multiplexa congenita: review with comments. *Neuroped* **14**:6–10, 1983.
123. Swinyard CA, Bleck EE. The etiology of arthrogryposis (multiple congenital contracture). *Clin Orthop* **194**:15–20, 1985.
124. Banker BQ. Neuropathologic aspects of arthrogryposis multiplex congenita. *Clin Orthop* **194**:30–34, 1985.
125. Thompson GH, Bilenker RM. Comprehensive management of arthrogryposis multiplex congenita. *Clin Orthop* **194**:6–14, 1985.
126. Miskin M, Rothberg R, Rudd N, Benzie R, Shine J. Arthrogryposis multiplex congenita – prenatal assessment with diagnostic ultrasound and fetoscopy. *J Pediatr* **95**:463–465, 1979.
127. Socol ML, Sabbagha RE, Elias S et al. Prenatal diagnosis of congenital muscular dystrophy producing arthrogryposis. *N Engl J Med* **313**:1230–1235, 1985.
128. Goldberg JD, Chervenak FA, Lipman RA, Berkowitz RL. Antenatal sonographic diagnosis of arthrogryposis multiplex congenita. *Prenat Diagn* **6**:45–49, 1986.
129. Kirkinen P, Herva R, Leisti J. Early prenatal diagnosis of a lethal syndrome of multiple congenital contractures. *Prenat Diagn* **7**:189–196, 1987.
130. Gorczyca DP, McGahan JP, Kindfors KK, Ellis WG, Grix A. Arthrogryposis multiplex congenita: prenatal ultrasonographic diagnosis. *J Clin Ultrasound* **17**:40–44, 1989.
131. Hall JG. Genetic aspects of arthrogryposis. *Clin Orthop* **194**:44–47, 1985.

Fetal hydrops and tumours

56

U. Nicolini

Fetal hydrops

INTRODUCTION

Fetal hydrops is the end stage of a variety of conditions leading to the accumulation of fluid in fetal tissues and/or body cavities. In its most severe form, the fetus has subcutaneous oedema, ascites, hydrothorax and pericardial effusion (Fig. 56.1). The umbilical cord and placenta may also be oedematous, with placental thickening, and polyhydramnios is often associated. Most studies of fetal hydrops, however, include cases in which the fluid accumulation is not present in all compartments. It is generally assumed, in fact, that the aetiology is the same and that these cases represent an earlier stage of the same pathological condition. Although this is true for some, other pathologies lead to accumulation of fluid in only some compartments (i.e. isolated ascites, or isolated hydrothorax etc.), without clear progression to generalized hydrops. There is also considerable overlapping in the literature between hydrops, nuchal cystic hygroma, and accumulations of lymph fluid in body cavities caused by obstruction of major lymphatic vessels.

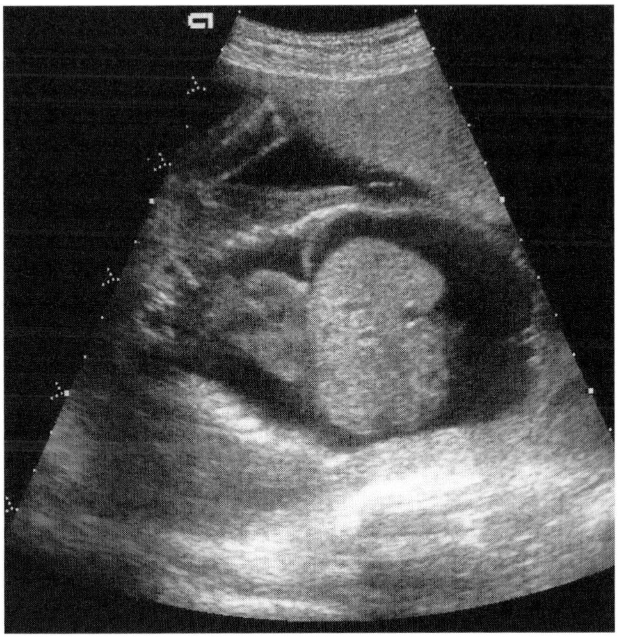

Fig. 56.1 Longitudinal section of the fetal chest and abdomen showing bilateral hydrothorax and ascites.

Fetal hydrops is defined as 'immune' or 'non-immune', based on whether there is evidence of fetomaternal blood group incompatibility (fetomaternal alloimmunisation). This chapter is not going to deal with immune hydrops, which is covered in the section on red cell alloimmunization. However, it must be stressed that an indirect Coombs test to rule out fetomaternal alloimmunization always needs to be included within the initial investigations to be carried out when fetal hydrops is diagnosed.

During the last three decades, following the introduction of anti-D prophylaxis, the proportion of non-immune/immune type of fetal hydrops has steadily increased. The incidence of non-immune hydrops varies according to population selection. In studies carried out in tertiary referral centres, the incidence of non-immune hydrops can be as high as 0.5%[1]. Neonatal series reported incidences ranging from 1:1475[2]–1:3538[3]. These figures are likely to be underestimations due to the high rate of intrauterine demise. In the past, ultrasonic series reported diagnoses of fetal hydrops mainly in the second and third trimester, but more recent studies have described cases at 11–17 weeks' gestation[4]. The widespread use of early ultrasound screening will reveal an incidence of fetal hydrops which is probably higher than that previously estimated. Regional variations are also expected, reflecting the varying frequencies of genetic disorders in different populations. For example, in Southeast Asia the commonest cause of fetal hydrops is homozygous α-thalassaemia, which is rare in other ethnic groups, but probably remains the most frequent aetiology worldwide.

A large number of maternal, placental and fetal disorders may cause fetal hydrops. Table 56.1 (modified from Machin[5]) displays the causes of 1585 reported cases of fetal hydrops[1,2,4,6–12] subdivided into broad categories. The aetiology remained undetermined in 20% of them. Taking into consideration that these series were mainly reported from tertiary referral centres, the proportion of cases which remain without a cause is likely to be higher overall. This has obvious consequences as far as counselling for future pregnancies is concerned, and the lack of a diagnosis may mean missing the opportunity for prenatal treatment in some instances. For example, we recently received a patient referred with a diagnosis of 'unexplained' fetal hydrops at 20 weeks' gestation who had had an intrauterine death in the previous pregnancy. The postmortem at the time had revealed a hydropic fetus and routine investigations had ruled out fetomaternal alloimmunization and chromosomal abnormalities. The patient had been counselled about the unlikelihood of a recurrence of the condition but fetal blood sampling allowed diagnosis of congenital dyserythropoietic anaemia which was treated by serial intravascular transfusions and resulted in the delivery of a live child[13]. Since most cases of fetal hydrops are diagnosed in peripheral hospitals and intrauterine death often ensues, a protocol which allows extensive and rapid investigations needs to be defined, requiring collaboration between the referral and the referring centres.

TABLE 56.1
Causes of fetal hydrops in 1585 reported cases

Cause	No.	%
Cardiovascular	370	23.3
Chromosomal	209	13.2
Thoracic	152	9.6
Anaemia	114	7.2
Hygroma	97	6.1
Twinning	93	5.9
Fetal infections	67	4.2
Urinary tract malformations	44	2.8
Peritonitis	41	2.6
Fetal hypomobility	23	1.5
Liver disorders	13	0.8
Genetic metabolic diseases	10	0.6
Miscellaneous	34	2.1
Unknown	318	20.1

PRENATAL DIAGNOSIS OF FETAL HYDROPS

Irrespective of the aetiology, ultrasonic definition of fetal hydrops requires a skin oedema >5 mm, measured at the level of the skull[14], associated with different serous effusions, and/or polyhydramnios, and/or increased placental thickness[9,14–16]. Skin oedema can obviously be seen also in the abdomen, chest and limbs, but it is easiest to identify in the skull, since the scalp is usually closely approximate to the bone. In order to monitor changes with time, it is best to always measure the scalp oedema in the same area, i.e. the occiput. The presence of serous effusions is usually easy to diagnose, but some care must be taken in order to avoid common errors. Occasionally, the abdominal or dorsal musculature may produce a hypoechogenic rim around the bowel which may be mistaken as ascites. True ascites is evident around the whole of the abdominal circumference and remains clearly identifiable from all incident angles (Fig. 56.2). Similar pitfalls may occur with the diagnosis of pericardial effusion. The hypoechogenic myocardium mimics the presence of fluid around the heart. A pericardial effusion is present if the pericardium is distended and does not move with cardiac activity.

The presence of hydrothorax is easy to diagnose, and it should be noted whether it is bilateral or unilateral. At times, following intrauterine pleuroamniotic shunting for unilateral hydrothorax, pleural effusion may develop on the opposite side. In these instances, one has to postulate that the contralateral hydrothorax prevented the collection of pleural fluid due to higher pressure and an unbalanced lymphatic obstruction. In male fetuses, an obvious fluid collection in the scrotum often precedes massive ascites. Placental oedema is diagnosed when placental thickness is >6 cm in depth from chorionic plate to base[9], and the definition of polyhydramnios is best based on the measurement of the amniotic fluid index[17].

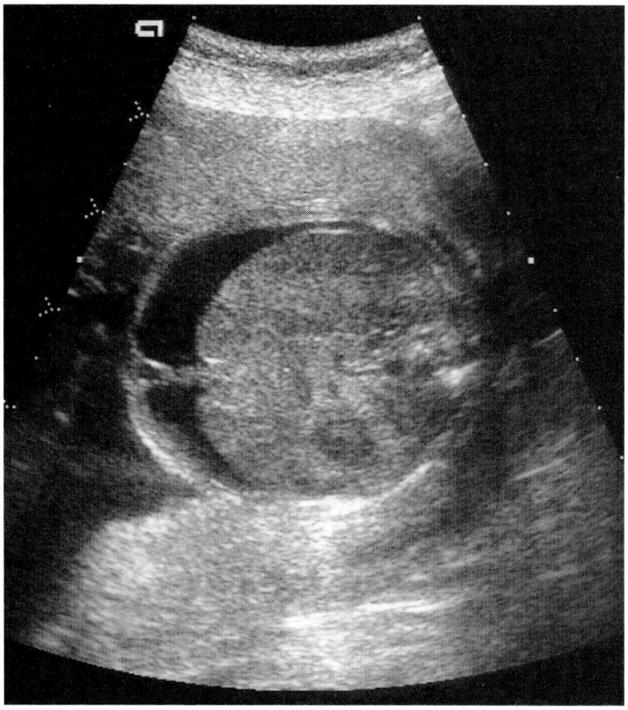

Fig. 56.2 Fetal ascites.

All possible combinations of the various findings which define fetal hydrops may occur. Saltzman et al.[9] have demonstrated, although in a small number of cases (No = 26), that there are typical combinations in hydropic fetuses with or without anaemia: pleural effusion or marked skin oedema are significantly more common in non-anaemic fetuses, whereas the absence of hydrothorax and a moderate subcutaneous oedema, as well as a thickened placenta, occur more frequently with anaemia-associated hydrops. In practice, a fetus with ascites and significant pleural effusion (unilateral or bilateral) is unlikely to have anaemia as the cause of hydrops.

In pregnancies at risk of α-thalassaemia-1 (although frank hydrops develops at 12–14 weeks' gestation in only 7%, and at 17–18 weeks in 33%[18]) a cutoff level of >0.5 for a cardiothoracic ratio allows diagnosis of 75% of the affected fetuses at 13–14 weeks and of all homozygous fetuses at 17–18[19]. Since fetuses affected by α-thalassaemia-1 develop anaemia early in gestation, these data show that the initial changes leading to the full picture of fetal hydrops are cardiomegaly and, to a lesser extent, placentomegaly[20].

MECHANISMS OF FETAL HYDROPS

The pathway to the development of hydrops in the fetus is not different from that which occurs postnatally. Hydrops is a disorder of the body's water, the pathogenesis of which may be attributed to three main mechanisms:

- Altered lymphatic flow
- Increased intravascular hydrostatic pressure
- Decreased intravascular osmotic pressure

Disorders which lead to any of these mechanisms result in the accumulation of fluid in the interstitial fluid. This is a large space in continuous dynamic balance with the intravascular compartment. Under normal conditions, there is a net flow of fluid at the capillary level from the intravascular compartment into the interstitial space, which is directly proportional to the intravascular hydrostatic pressure and the osmotic pressure in the interstitial fluid, and inversely related to the interstitial hydrostatic pressure and the plasma colloid osmotic pressure. This excess of fluid in the interstitial space is transported back into the vascular circulation by an adequate lymphatic flow[21]. It must be noted that, in the fetus, the intravascular space is in balance, via the placenta, with the maternal vascular compartment, which provides virtually unlimited fluid supply. This peculiarity leads to a situation which is similar to that of an adult with, for example, cardiac failure, who is continually infused intravascular crystalloids. Early in pregnancy, before the skin becomes keratinized, the amniotic fluid can be considered an extention of the interstitial fluid, which may explain the relative rarity of generalized hydrops prior to 16–18 weeks' gestation. Further fetal peculiarities are the low colloid osmotic pressure compared to the adult, an extracellular fluid which is larger than the intracellular one[22] and hypotonic urine[23]. This latter physiological characteristic of the fetus corroborates the finding that polyhydramnios due to polyuria often precedes the development of hydrops.

Fetal anaemia, hypoproteinaemia, cardiac failure and obstruction to the lymphatic flow are the intermediate changes which are found in most cases of fetal hydrops. Anaemia may cause hydrops through the combination of various mechanisms. Heteroptopic erythropoiesis in the liver is associated with hypoproteinaemia and a consequent decrease in colloid osmotic pressure; tissue hypoxia and its arterial vasoactive response may lead to myocardial insufficiency and cardiac failure; endothelial damage due to hypoxia increases capillary permeability to water and colloids[24]. If less protein is synthetized in the liver or more is lost by the kidney, and hypoproteinaemia develops, there is a redistribution of proteins between the intravascular and interstitial compartments, which maintains the transcapillary colloid osmotic gradient. Subsequently, however, especially if there is an endothelial leakage, the interstitial volume rises following even small increases in the hydrostatic pressure[25]. Some congenital cardiac malformations and/or dysrrhythmias and thoracic space-occupying lesions may cause haemodynamic compromise with obstruction of the venous return to the right atrium, distension of the venous circulation, and decreased peripheral tissue perfusion. The combination of these changes leads to increased hydrostatic pressure, hepatomegaly with impaired liver function, and hypoxaemia. Lymphatic vascular dysplasia reduces the return of the excess interstitial fluid into the intravascular space, thus producing accumulation of fluid in a specific area of the body, if the obstruction is limited to a peripheral lymphatic area, or systemically, when the thoracic duct is obstructed.

It must be underlined, however, that in some instances, no clear mechanism can be identified, even after extensive investigations. In addition, the cause of hydrops in some congenital infections and inherited metabolic disorders often remains obscure.

CONDITIONS ASSOCIATED WITH FETAL HYDROPS

Cardiovascular disorders are the most frequent cause of fetal hydrops (Table 56.1). Of these, cardiac malformations account for approximately 40%, tachyarrhythmias for 25%, high output cardiac failure for 15%, and bradyarrhythmias for 7%[5]. Table 56.2 lists the conditions which fall into the category of cardiovascular abnormalities. With cardiac malformations, the presumed mechanism leading to hydrops is raised systemic venous pressure, due either to the obstruction of the right heart output or to the transmission of systemic arterial pressure to the right heart. With aortic valve or arch obstruction, for example, the left ventricular and atrial pressures increase, with consequent reduced shunting at the level of the foramen ovale. This in turn leads to raised right atrial pressure and systemic venous congestion. Fetal cardiac malformations

TABLE 56.2
Cardiovascular abnormalities which may lead to fetal hydrops

Cardiac malformations/lesions
Left ventricular hypoplasia[a]
Atrioventricular canal[a]
Right ventricular hypoplasia[a]
Primary closure of foramen ovale
Single ventricle
Transposition of great vessels
Ventricular septal defect
Atrial septal defect
Tetralogy of Fallot
Ebstein anomaly
Premature closure of ductus arteriosus
Subaortic stenosis
Tricuspid/pulmonary/mitral/aortic valve stenosis/atresia
Endocardial fibroelastosis
Cardiomyopathy
Myocarditis
Myocardial infarction
Rhabdomyoma
Pericardial/intrapericardial/intracardial teratoma
Atrial haemangioma
Conduction system hamartoma
Tachyarrhythmias
Atrial flutter[a]
Supraventricular tachycardia[a]
Wolff–Parkinson–White syndrome[a]
High cardiac output failure
Sacrococcygeal teratoma[a]
Large placental chorioangioma[a]
Bradyarrhythmias
Complete heart block[a]
Non-conducted premature atrial contractions
Others
Arterial calcification
Aneurysm of the vein of Galen
Atresia of the umbilical vein
Peripheral artery thrombosis

[a]Most common conditions

account for 10–20% of all congenital defects and their incidence can be as high as 1.2% in an unselected population[26]. Although ultrasonographic screening yields disappointingly low sensitivity if only the four chamber view is obtained[27], fetal echocardiography including visualization of the left and right ventricular outflow tracts, and of the main pulmonary artery and its branches allows detection of 86% of major cardiac abnormalities in a low risk population[28]. With fetal hydrops, a thorough echocardiographic investigation will eventually identify cardiovascular abnormalities in approximately one of four to five cases. Colour Doppler investigation, demonstrating atrioventricular valve regurgitation, and venous Doppler blood flow studies, showing a pulsatile velocity pattern[29], may also confirm that congestive heart failure is the main cause of hydrops.

A thickened endocardium with decreased contractility would suggest endocardial fibroelastosis. Cardiac rhabdomyomas are easy to visualize (Fig. 56.3), but 50% of them are associated with tuberous sclerosis. Since 50–80% of the cases of tuberous sclerosis are due to a new mutation, family history and investigation of the parents will remain inconclusive, leaving prognosis undetermined until after birth.

Abnormalities of cardiac rhythm (supraventricular tachycardia, atrial flutter and heart block) are best studied by M-mode or Doppler echocardiography, which may also reveal the reduction of stroke volume as seen during runs of fetal tachycardia/flutter. The pathogenesis of hydrops is thought to be related to inability of the lymphatics to return interstitial fluid into the vascular compartment because of the increased venous pressure[30]. The finding of a sinus rhythm at the time of ultrasound diagnosis of fetal hydrops, in the absence of other abnormalities, should prompt repeated observations in order to rule out intermittent episodes of tachycardia as the primary cause. Prolonged fetal bradycardia may be related to non-conducted premature atrial contractions or complete heart block, which occurs in association with cardiac structural malformations or as an isolated dysrrythmia. Since the association between isolated heart block and maternal connective tissue disorders, even in the absence of clinical symptoms, has long been established[31], the presence of maternal anti-Ro or anti-La (anti-SSA, anti-SSB) antibodies should be investigated. In these cases, histology shows fibrous replacement of the conducting tissue, whereas left atrial isomerism with displacement or absence of the sinus node can be demonstrated in most fetuses/neonates with heart block associated with structural malformations[32].

Sacrococcygeal teratomas and large placental chorioangiomas may lead to fetal hydrops by acting as a peripheral arteriovenous shunt causing increased fetal cardiac output, cardiac hypertrophy and congestive heart failure. Anaemia and disseminated coagulopathy have also been reported in fetuses with both teratomas and chorioangiomas[33–35]. It is uncertain whether these haematological changes precede or follow cardiac failure, but anaemia might arise from chronic microangiopathy and be an independent cause of hydrops. Colour and energy (power) Doppler are invaluable tools to identify other rare causes of cardiovascular disorders associated with fetal hydrops. For example, large cerebral arteriovenous malformations and aneurysm of the great vein of Galen may lead to systolic and diastolic right to left shunting through the ductus arteriosus causing continuous retrograde flow in the transverse aortic arch and congestive heart failure[36]. Agenesis of the umbilical vein with the oxygenated blood from the placenta flowing into one of the two umbilical arteries (Fig. 56.4) may cause ascites and hydrops, probably by increasing inferior vena cava pressure.

Chromosomal abnormalities are the second commonest cause of fetal hydrops. Turner and Down syndrome together account for approximately 75% in all[2,5], but other anomalies (trisomy 18, 13, 15, 16, triploidy, tetraploidy, 46,XX/XY

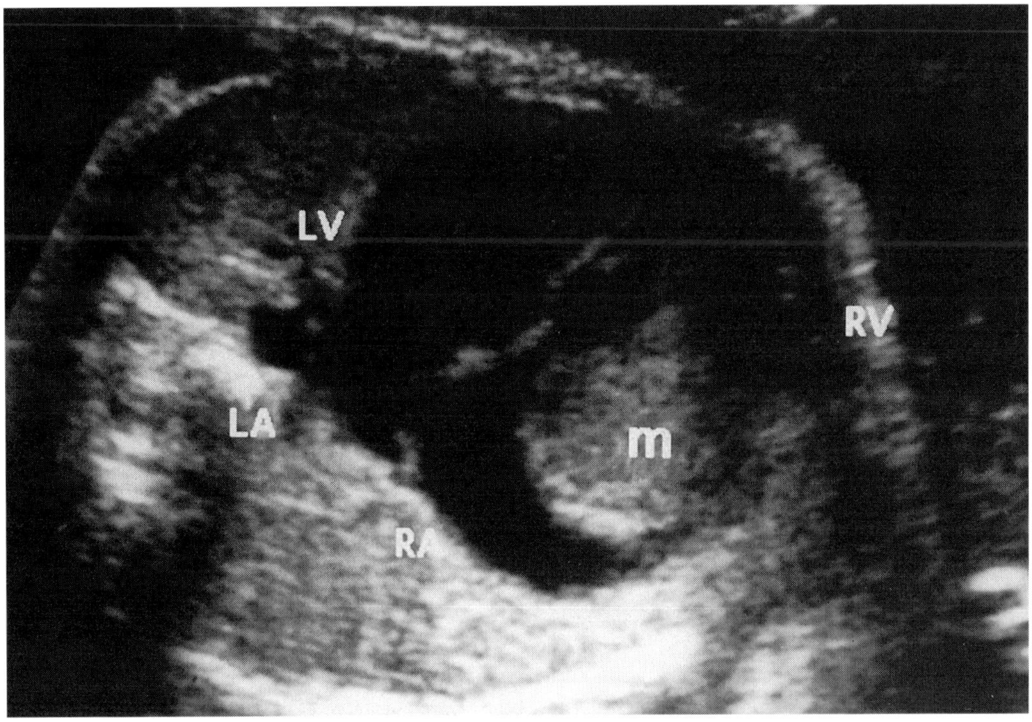

Fig. 56.3 Transverse section of fetal chest and heart showing the right atrium (RA) occupied by a large protruding mass (m).

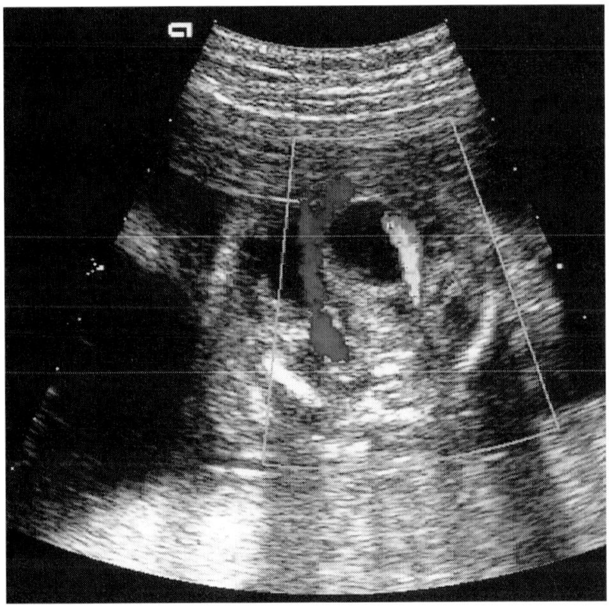

Fig. 56.4 Agenesis of the umbilical vein with venous blood flowing from the placenta into the right umbilical artery.

mosaicism, partial duplication of chromosomes 11, 15, 17, 18, partial deletion of the short arm of chromosomes 13 and 18, rearrangement of the long arm of chromosome 22) have been reported as well[37]. Recent evidence from chromosomally abnormal fetuses diagnosed at 10–14 weeks' gestation suggests that the narrowing of the aortic isthmus may be a common denominator causing increased nuchal translucency and eventually full hydrops[38]. Since most fetuses with Turner syndrome have tubular coarctation and aortic valve stenosis, which may lead to cardiac failure, it is not unexpected that hydrops is commonest with this chromosomal abnormality. Vice versa, hydrops is rare with trisomy 13, while, with other abnormalities, some lymphatic dysfunction may be the main responsible mechanism. This might explain why spontaneous resolution of serous effusions may occur in some fetuses with trisomy 21 and even in some with Turner syndrome[39]. In view of the high incidence of chromosomal abnormalities, rapid karyotyping is indicated as the primary investigation of fetuses with cardiac malformations, congenital pleural effusion[40], cystic hygroma, and hydrops without obvious reasons at the initial ultrasound examination.

Fetal hydrothorax and thoracic anomalies may be isolated ultrasonic findings or be associated with generalized hydrops. Fetal pleural effusion (s) may occur secondary to intrathoracic abnormalities such as diaphragmatic hernia[41], pulmonary sequestration[42] (Fig. 56.5), thyroid teratoma[43], congenital goitre[44], and cystic adenomatoid malformation of the lung[45]. All these conditions may increase intrathoracic pressure and impair fetal venous return. In addition, the compression of the mediastinum may obstruct fetal swallowing, which leads to polyhydramnios. Once the presence of intrathoracic space-occupying masses has been excluded, and rapid karyotyping has ruled out chromosomal abnormalities, primary fetal hydrothorax, with or without associated generalized hydrops, can be assumed to be the result of accumulation of lymphatic

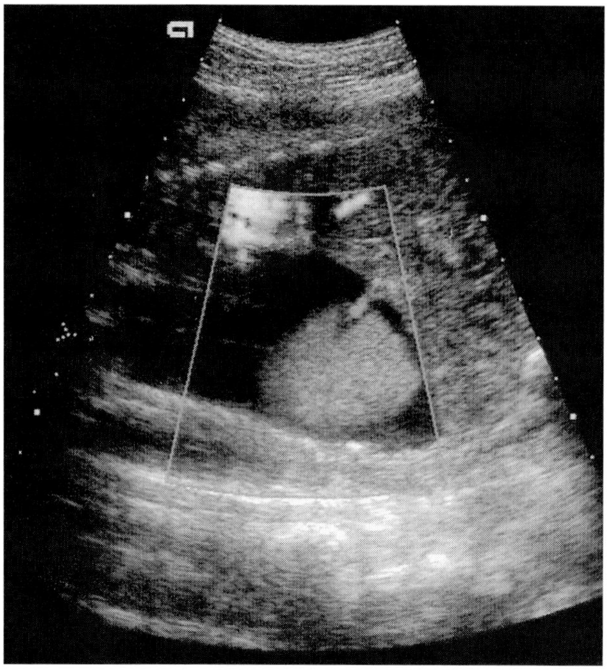

Fig. 56.5 Pulmonary sequestration and hydrothorax.

fluid in the pleural cavity (Fig. 56.6). Alternatively, pleural effusion may be secondary to generalized fluid retention from another cause. In the neonate, the most common cause of pleural effusion is chylothorax, which is characterized by a typical milky appearance of the pleural fluid. In the fetus,

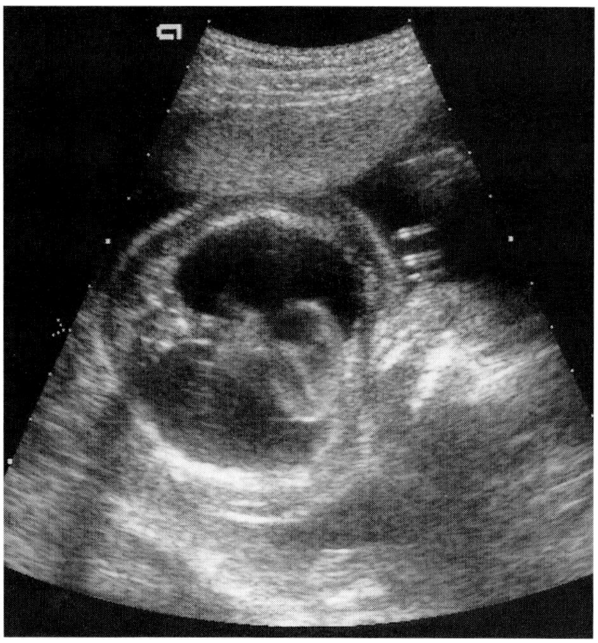

Fig. 56.6 Bilateral hydrothorax: the lungs and mediastinum are compressed.

however, the fluid collected at thoracentesis is non-specifically gold-yellow. Although lymphocyte counts above 80% have been proposed as an index of primary fetal hydrothorax[46], similar percentages are expected in most pleural fluids, irrespective of the aetiology, due to physiological fetal lymphocytosis. Prolonged compression by pleural effusion(s) may cause lung hypoplasia, which, together with prematurity caused by uterine overdistension due to polyhydramnios, and low-output cardiac failure, are the underlying causes of the poor prognosis in fetuses with early onset of primary hydrothorax[47]. Congenital pulmonary lymphangiectasia, which is generally fatal in the neonatal period and may have a familial occurrence[48], is indistinguishable prenatally from those more benign forms of primary pleural effusions which may be caused by thoracic duct pathology[49]. Such anatomical defects in the lymphatic circulation, however, are difficult to demonstrate, even at postmortem examination. On the other hand, in most neonates pleural effusion resolves spontaneously, probably because of the lung distension which occurs with the first breaths.

Fetal anaemia is the mechanism leading to immune hydrops, but the absence of atypical antibodies in the maternal serum does not rule out that other causes of fetal anaemia are involved. Actually, the opposite is true: the presence of antibodies cannot exclude other reasons for the development of anaemia in the fetus. We recently had a patient with mild anti-D immunization, in whom serial ultrasound scans had not detected signs of anaemia during the course of the whole pregnancy. The finding of an abnormal heart rate pattern during spontaneous labour at 37 weeks' gestation prompted an ultrasound examination which revealed a grossly hydropic fetus and oligohydramnios. A Kleihauer–Betke test on maternal blood collected prior to delivery allowed diagnosis of massive fetomaternal haemorrhage as the cause of fetal anaemia, which otherwise would have been attributed erroneously to haemolysis because of maternal antibodies. Fetomaternal haemorrhage is found occasionally to be the primary cause of fetal hydrops[50,51], but a maternal sample has to be taken before fetal blood sampling is performed, because the invasive procedure itself may provoke bleeding from the fetus into the maternal circulation[52], thus making impossible to ascertain whether anaemia is due to other causes. Fetuses with homozygous α-thalassaemia, but not those with β-thalassaemia, are invariably anaemic and hydropic at birth. Contrary to fetomaternal alloimmunization, anaemia due to homozygous α-thalassaemia is often associated with oligohydramnios[53], which suggests reduced renal perfusion due to decreased blood volume and/or placental failure, possibly related to the high oxygen affinity of Hb-Bart which leads to generalized hypoxic tissue damage. Glucose-6-phosphate dehydrogenase (G6PD)[54,55], glucose phosphatase isomerase deficiency[56], and congenital dyserythropoietic anaemia[13] are genetic disorders which have been reported to cause fetal anaemia and hydrops only in a handful of cases. Similarly rare conditions leading to anaemic hydrops are fetal leukaemia[57] and Gaucher's disease[58], which may cause infiltration of the bone marrow and suppression of erythropoiesis. Intrauterine bleeding, such as in cases of intracranial haemorrhage[59], causes transitional anaemia which may be severe enough to cause hydrops[60]. However, the most frequent cause of non-immune anaemic hydrops is probably congenital parvovirus B19 infection. Parvovirus B19 specifically affects the erythroid series, but a transient decrease in neutrophil and platelet counts may also occur[61]. The virus binds to the P antigen, or globoside, which is present on the surface of erythrocytes, erythroblasts, megakaryocytes, endothelial cells, placenta, fetal liver and heart cells[62]. The rate of transplacental passage of parvovirus B19 has been estimated to be 33% in one study involving 190 women with serologically confirmed infection in pregnancy[63]. However, the true risks of fetal infection and perinatal loss cannot be assessed precisely, given the high frequency with which maternal infection occurs asymptomatically. In the two prospective studies which recruited mainly symptomatic women, the percentage of live healthy neonates ranged from 84–95%[63,64]. This contrasts with seven hydropic fetuses and one fetal death out of 22 maternal infections ascertained during 1993 in the Avon area in UK[65]. Fetal hydrops has been diagnosed at as early as 12 weeks' gestation following maternal infection with parvovirus B19[66], but spontaneous resolution may occur[67]. Diagnosis of fetal parvovirus infection relies on the combination of fetal anaemia, maternal exposure to the infection, maternal B19 seroconversion of IgG and IgM antibodies detected by radioimmunoassay and enzyme-linked immunoabsorbent assay, identification of parvovirus-specific DNA in fetal tissues, and of nuclear inclusions in the fetal red blood cell precursors. Active erythropoiesis, as shown by high reticulocyte and nucleated red cell counts on fetal blood, may be taken as evidence of recovery from the viral damage to the bone marrow, despite the persistence of hydrops[67]. If maternal infection in pregnancy is documented, serial ultrasound scans are indicated to detect the eventual development of fetal hydrops, and assessment of the fetal P phenotype might be considered in selected cases. The absence of P antigen should rule out any possibility of future risks to the fetus/neonate, independent of transplacental passage of the virus.

Cystic hygroma results from abnormal development of the lymphatic system. This may consist of reduced or absent development of peripheral lymphatics or of delayed or absent connections between the lympatic and venous circulations. Cystic hygroma of neck is the most obvious manifestation of lymphatic dysplasia and represents the most extreme form of nuchal oedema. The rate of chromosomal abnormalities found in these cases is higher (up to 70%) than for any other structural abnormality, but even if the karyotype is normal, nuchal cystic hygroma may be the epiphenomenon of a variety of genetic syndromes (see below). Data from the literature are confusing, since many series do not distinguish between nuchal oedema and nuchal cavitation, which appears on ultrasound as a cystic space with multiple septa (Fig. 56.7). Increased nuchal translucency may be considered as a minimum degree of lymphatic dysplasia. Screening for increased nuchal translucency at 10–14 weeks' gestation allows diagnosis of 70–80% of all fetuses with chromosomal abnormalities[68]. Whether chromosomally normal or abnormal, many cases of cystic hygroma resolve spontaneously, leaving some fetuses with residual mechanical deformities such as neck skin webbing, hypoplastic heart and aortic arches, and pulmonary hypoplasia. Careful ultrasonic monitoring of the whole fetal anatomy needs to be carried out also in cases of transitionally increased nuchal translucency, in which associated structural abnormalities may be diagnosed only after birth[69].

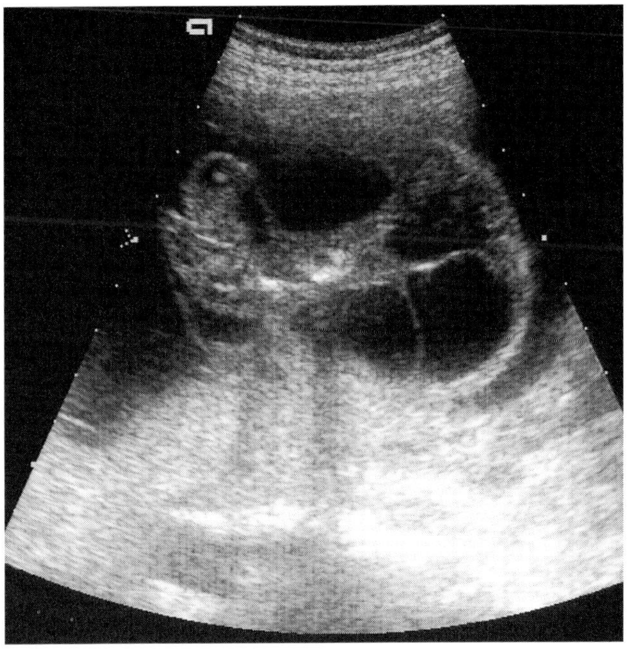

Fig. 56.7 Nuchal cystic hygroma with multiple septa.

In *monochorionic twin pregnancies* complicated by twin-to-twin transfusion syndrome (TTTS), non-immune hydrops may develop both in the recipient and in the donor fetus. Although vascular anastomoses are present in virtually all monochorionic placentas[70], TTTS, no matter which criteria are adopted for its definition, complicates only a minority of monochorionic twin pregnancies. The combination of polyhydramnios in one sac and severe oligohydramnios in the other (the 'stuck twin' sign) is probably the most typical feature of both acute and chronic TTTS[71], the pathophysiology of both phenomena being an abnormality of fetal urine production. Chronic fluid overload in the recipient twin causes enhanced release of atrial natriuretic peptide, which in turn leads to increased fetal diuresis[72,73]. In contrast, in the smaller fetus, urine output is markedly decreased[73]. Consequently, the bladder of the larger twin is often persistently enlarged, and that of the donor twin is consistently small on serial ultrasound scans. All available tests aimed at diagnosing TTTS rely on indirect evidence of the two dichotomies: decreased/increased blood volume and anaemia/polyglobulia. Although in one study the assessment of fetal blood viscosity was found to correlate with survival[74], most reported twins investigated by blood sampling had similar values of haemoglobin/haematocrit, and a variable distribution of hypoxaemia/acidaemia between donor and recipient twins[75–77]. The mechanism leading to hydrops in the recipient twin is the sequence hypervolaemia – cardiac hypertrophy (Fig. 56.8) – cardiac failure. In the donor twin, on the other hand, the reason for the development of hydrops is not necessarily the most obvious, i.e. anaemia, which is rarely found at fetal blood sampling. Inversion of the roles between the twin fetuses may in fact occur, with the donor, hypovolaemic twin becoming suddenly hypervolaemic because of reversed flow through the placental anastomoses. A similar phenomenon (acute exsanguination into the dying cotwin) is now considered the mechanism responsible for the development of ascites/hydrops and eventually neurological abnormalities and death in the survivor of a monozygotic twin pair in which one intrauterine death occurs[78].

The acardiac twin malformation, first described by Benedetti in 1553[79], has since been reported under different names, which either refer to the anatomical abnormality (holoacardius, hemiacardius, acardiac monster), or to what is reputed to be its pathophysiological basis (twin reversed arterial perfusion sequence, TRAP). This rare anomaly probably develops during the early stages of embryogenesis, as a result of extensive artery to artery and vein to vein anastomoses within a monochorionic placenta[80]. Secondary atrophy of the heart and other tissues occurs in the perfused twin, whereas the 'pumping' normal cotwin may be susceptible to cardiac failure. Perinatal mortality in the normal twin is as high as 55%, primarily related to prematurity[81]. Survivors may experience congestive heart failure, with right ventricular hypertrophy and relative pulmonary stenosis, poor liver function and hypoalbuminaemia, which are often corollaries of fetal hydrops.

Fetal infections by streptococci, coxsackie virus, leptospirosis, cytomegalovirus, rubella virus, varicella virus, respiratory syncytial virus, parvovirus B19, hepatitis virus, herpes simplex, *toxoplasma gondii*, *treponema pallidum* and *trypanosoma cruzi* (Chagas disease) have all been described as possible causes of hydrops. The reason for hydrops being a common denominator to such a heterogeneous group of infections is unclear. However, infected fetuses, whatever the infectious agent (with the exception of parvovirus B19, which causes fetal anaemia – see above), tend to present similar biochemical, haematological and immunological alterations[82–85]. In particular, liver derangement, as testified by elevated γGT, AST and ALT levels, seems to be constant with severe intrauterine infections, possibly because the liver is the first organ to be reached by the microorganism during the haematogenous dissemination after crossing the placenta[25]. The typical ultrasonic findings which suggest intrauterine infection are, in fact, gross ascites, out of proportion with other serous effusions, and hepatomegaly.

Urinary tract abnormalities may be associated with ascites, but rarely with generalized hydrops. Lower urinary tract obstruction is the most frequent malformation of the uropoietic system where ascites may be present. Bladder overdistension, due to posterior urethral valves or urethral atresia, may lead to spillage into the peritoneal cavity with the formation of urinary ascites (Fig. 56.9)[86]. The ultrasonic diagnosis relies on the association of ascites, oligohydramnios (due to the

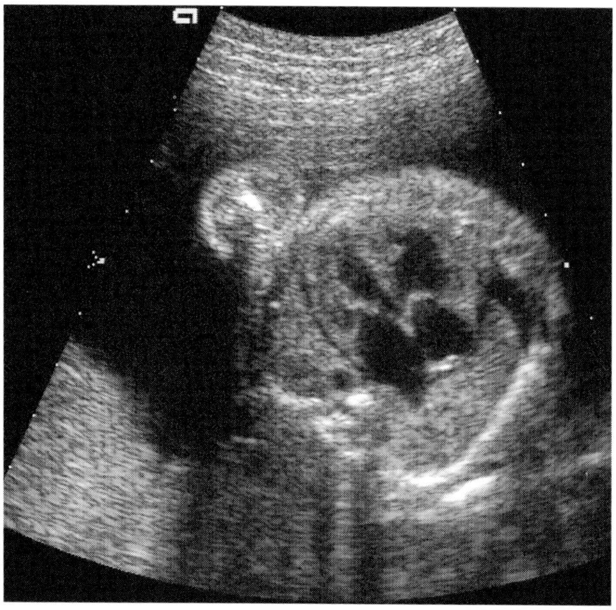

Fig. 56.8 Cardiac hypertrophy in the recipient fetus of a twin-to-twin transfusion syndrome.

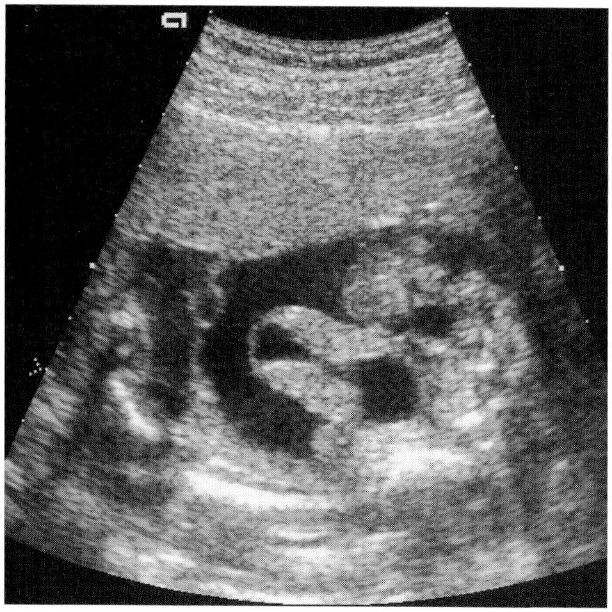

Fig. 56.9 Ascites due to spillage of urine from a grossly hypertrophic bladder in a case of lower urinary tract obstruction.

obstruction of fetal micturition), a thick bladder wall, dilated ureters, and hydronephrosis and/or hyperechogenic kidneys. Urinary ascites may also occur with spontaneous or iatrogenic (following fetal urine sampling) rupture of a dilated renal pelvis. In this case, however, the ensuing accumulation of urine is more often limited to the retroperitoneal space.

Hydrops has been reported in association with Wilms tumour and with congenital nephroblastomatosis, a rare condition in which the enlarged kidney contains areas of embryonic renal blastoma, which appear as focal calcifications on ultrasound[87]. Ascites may also occur with fetal renal vein thrombosis. This diagnosis may be suggested by the finding of unilateral gross enlargement of the kidney and is facilitated by using colour Doppler.

It must be noted that increased fetal diuresis may be the cause of polyhydramnios in some cases of hydrops. In these fetuses, the renal pelvises, and, at times, the bladder, appear moderately dilated. This ultrasonic finding should not mislead one to suspect a urinary tract abnormality, but rather raise the suspicion that fetal hypervolaemia, leading to compensatory polyuria, may be the primary reason for cardiac failure and hydrops.

Meconium peritonitis may be indistinguishable from other serous effusions limited to the abdominal cavity. If a dilated portion of the bowel has been recorded prior to the ultrasonic finding of ascites, the most likely diagnosis is that intestinal perforation has occurred. Lumps of meconium in the peritoneum appear as echogenic plaques, which should lead to suspect meconium peritonitis, even in the absence of dilated portions of intestine. The possibility that cystic fibrosis is the primary condition should be considered.

Genetic conditions which may be associated with fetal hydrops are listed in Table 56.3 (from Jones[37] and POSSUM[37a]). However large, the number of genetic conditions susceptible to cause fetal hydrops is likely to be incomplete and to increase in the future. While for some disorders it is possible to hypothesize which mechanism is responsible for the insurgence of hydrops, for others it is not. For example, compression of the inferior vena cava by a large hydrometrocolpos, which also leads to urinary tract obstruction, may be postulated in the McKusick–Kaufman syndrome. The cardiac malformations and frequent bradycardia of the polysplenia syndrome may cause cardiac failure. In glucose phosphate isomerase deficiency and sialic acid storage disorder, fetal anaemia is the most likely explanation for generalized hydrops, etc. In the absence of a family history or of structural malformations which may lead to diagnosis, and without anatomical/functional/haematological clues to the cause of hydrops, most cases of genetic disorders are likely to remain undiagnosed and to enter the large group of 'unexplained hydrops'. The routine use of blood sampling as a means of investigating hydropic fetuses allows to storage fetal blood for later investigations, if intrauterine demise occurs[88]. Numerous skeletal dysplasias may be associated with fetal hydrops. This underlines the need for systematic radiological

TABLE 56.3
Genetic conditions which may be associated with fetal hydrops

Condition	Inheritance
Generalized syndromes	
Arthrogryposis multiplex congenita	Sp
Cornelia de Lange syndrome	AD
Fanconi syndrome type III	AR
Hypophosphatasia	AR
Kasabach–Merritt syndrome	AD
Klippel–Trenaunay–Weber syndrome	Sp
Lethal congenital contracture syndrome, Finnish type	AD
Lethal multiple pterygium syndrome	AR
Maroteaux–Lamy syndrome	AR
Kaufman–McKusick syndrome	AR
Myotonic dystrophy (neonatal Steinert disease)	AD
Neu–Laxova syndrome	AR
Noonan syndrome	DX-L
Optiz–Frias syndrome	AD, DX-L
Oro-facial-digital syndrome type II (Mohr syndrome)	AR
Pena–Shokeir syndrome	AR
Polysplenia syndrome (Ivemark syndrome)	AR
Simpson–Golabi–Behmel syndrome	RX-L
Tuberous sclerosis	AD
Metabolic disorders	
Carnitine deficiency	AR
Galactosialidosis (Goldberg syndrome)	AR
GM1 gangliosidosis (Morquio disease)	AR
Gaucher disease	AR
Glucose phosphate isomerase (GPI)	AD
Hurler syndrome	AR
Mucolipidosis type I and II	AR
Mucopolysaccharidosis type IVA (Morquio syndrome) and VII	AR
Niemann–Pick disease type A and C	AR
Pyruvate kinase deficiency of erythrocyte	AR
Sialic acid storage disorder (sialuria)	AR
Skeletal dysplasias	
Achondrogenesis type I and IA	AR
Achondrogenesis, Langer–Saldino	AR
Achondroplasia	AR
Asphyxiating thoracic dystrophy	AR
Beemer syndrome	AR
Boomerang dysplasia	AD
Chondrodysplasia, Blomstrand type	AR
Chondrodysplasia punctata, Conradi–Hunermann type	DX-L
Dappled metaphyseal dysplasia	AD, AR?
Fryns syndrome	AR
Greenberg dysplasia	AR
Koide's osteochondrodystrophy	AR
Lethal Kniest-like dysplasia	AR
Lethal osteopetrosis	AR
Majewski type of short rib–polydactyly syndrome	AR
Osteogenesis imperfecta type II	AD
Pyknoachondrogenesis	AR
Saldino–Noonan type of short rib–polydactyly syndrome	AR
Thanatophoric dwarfism	AD, AR
Verma-Naumoff type of short rib–polydactyly syndrome	AR

AR = autosomal recessive; AD = autosomal dominant; DX-L = dominant X-linked; RX-L = recessive X-linked; Sp = sporadic

investigation of aborted fetuses and of those which died in utero. The risk of recurrence in future pregnancies may be under- or overestimated if this information is missing. Several genetic conditions associated with hydrops have the common denominator of fetal akinesia or hypomobility. The ultrasonographer examining a fetus with hydrops should, therefore, pay attention to whether there are normal movements of flexion of the limbs, and the pathologist should look for signs of joint contractures.

As with genetic conditions, the list of *other causes* of fetal hydrops is likely to grow with time. Under the label of 'miscellaneous' are included conditions which may or may not have a causal relationship with fetal hydrops. One example is represented by haemorrhagic endovasculitis of the placenta[89]. This is a histopathological finding, the incidence of which varies from 0.7%[90]–2.1%[89]. It is a vasodestructive process of unknown cause, characterized by occlusion of chorionic vessels by myointimal proliferation with mural non-exudative necrosis and intraluminal thrombi. Haemorrhagic endovasculitis of the placenta has been described in association with cases of fetal hydrops without other apparent causes, but also in other instances in which there was a clear reason for the development of hydrops.

Torsion of an ovarian cyst may cause rupture into the peritoneum, which will appear filled with ascites. Angiomyxoma of the umbilical cord, aneurysm of the umbilical artery, cord vein thrombosis, and anomalies of the umbilical cord, such as torsion and true knots, are other conditions described in association with hydrops. Similarly, the administration of drugs to the mother, such as indomethacin, which may cause closure of the ductus arteriosus, or maternal conditions, such as hyperthyroidism, with transplacental passage of organ-specific antibodies leading to sustained fetal tachycardia, are all situations characterized by negative cardiovascular effects, the end result of which may be fetal hydrops.

MATERNAL COMPLICATIONS

In its most severe forms, fetal hydrops may be associated with the maternal 'mirror' syndrome. This is a type of preeclampsia, which is characterized by having an extremely rapid onset and rapid deterioration. In one series, pregnancy-induced hypertension occurred in 46% of 26 pregnant women with fetal hydrops[91]. In our experience, this serious complication occurs only if the placenta is grossly oedematous, while it is rare if the fluid accumulation is limited to the fetal body. Other peculiarities are that, contrary to that which occurs with the 'normal' preeclampsia, the maternal blood volume is not decreased, and, if an effective treatment is instituted and hydrops is ameliorated[92], the maternal signs and symptoms may disappear without the need to deliver the patient. As with hydatidiform mole, hyperplacentosis and increased chorionic gonadotropin production may be associated with the development of ovarian thecalutein cysts and transitional hyperthyroidism in the mother[93]. A higher than expected rate of postpartum haemorrhage and amniotic fluid embolism has also been reported[2].

MANAGEMENT

Perinatal mortality in pregnancies complicated by non-immune fetal hydrops remains frustratingly high. Holzgreve reported an overall mortality of 81% in 128 cases of non-immune hydrops[12]. In another series, there were only two survivors out of 25 fetuses diagnosed during a 20-year period (1967–1987)[2]. More recently, McCoy et al.[94] reviewed their experience with 82 fetuses: perinatal mortality was 87%, but as high as 95% if only cases diagnosed prior to 24 weeks' gestation were considered. In a series of 45 fetuses with non-immune hydrops, whose gestational age at diagnosis ranged from 11–17 weeks, Iskaros et al.[4] reported 43 (96%) terminations of pregnancy, intrauterine or neonatal deaths. One case study, however, described a prospective protocol to select cases which might benefit from prenatal treatment: having excluded chromosomal and structural abnormalities, five of six fetuses survived without sequelae[95]. This underlines the fact that the goal of a thorough investigation of pregnancies complicated by non-immune hydrops is the identification of those fetuses for which some antenatal therapy is indicated. Equally important, however, is to define whether there is a risk of recurrence in future pregnancies, or whether the primary cause of fetal hydrops is a sporadic event. Table 56.4 summarizes the essential investigations which may help to reach a diagnosis in pregnancies complicated by fetal hydrops. If intrauterine demise occurs, X-ray of the fetus and meticulous pathological examination of fetus and placenta will undoubtedly achieve a more precise anatomical evaluation than that which can be obtained by prenatal ultrasound. However, the obstetrician has the task of acquiring data which, otherwise, would be missed once the pregnancy is concluded. It is certainly possible to obtain fetal karyotype on the placenta or fetal tissues after termination, but if the interval from intrauterine death and delivery is prolonged, this crucial information may be lost. Whether the hydropic fetus was anaemic or not can be inferred from the histological finding of heterotopic erythropoiesis, but this is common to severe hypoxaemia. Even maternal data cannot always be retrieved a posteriori: a positive Kleihauer–Betke test will fade with time and, vice versa, evidence of fetomaternal haemorrhage after delivery is not conclusive of that being the cause of hydrops, since the delivery itself might have provoked bleeding from the fetus into the maternal circulation. In the absence of a significant family/personal history, the diagnosis of any one of the many genetic syndromes and congenital metabolic disorders which are associated with fetal hydrops is unlikely to be reached antenatally. If intrauterine or early neonatal death ensues, the availability of stored fetal tissues may become invaluable to diagnose or rule out some conditions which subsequent data would reveal as the possible causes of hydrops.

TABLE 56.4
A flow chart for the investigation of pregnancies complicated by fetal hydrops

Diagnostic tests	Questions
1. Detailed ultrasound scan echocardiography Doppler (colour energy) studies	Is the serous collection isolated (ascites, pleural effusion etc.) or is it generalized hydrops? Is the placenta increased in thickness? Is there polyhydramnios? Does the combination of findings suggest fetal anaemia (ascites ± subcutaneous oedema without pleural effusion)? Are there signs of fetal hypervolaemia (dilated renal pelvises/bladder) Are there signs of cardiac failure (tricuspid regurgitation, pulsatile umbilical venous flow etc.)? Are there fetal structural malformations (including cardiac defects)? Is the heart rate normal (consider repeating the scan)? Are there placental, cord, and fetal vascular abormalities? Is the fetus hypoxaemic (absent end diastolic velocities in the umbilical artery)?
2. Tests on maternal blood	Has the mother atypical antibodies (indirect Coombs test)? Is the mother a carrier of haematological disorders (complete blood count ± Hb electrophoresis and, in case, G6PD and piruvate kinase carrier status)? Has there been feto-maternal haemorrhage (Kleihauer–Betke test)? Is there a risk of fetal infection (VDRL and TORCH titres, if not already done)? Is there hyperplacentosis or placental failure (serum β-HCG and AFP)? Do the family or personal history suggest any specific risk (specific tests as indicated)?
3. Invasive fetal testing	Is the fetus anaemic/thrombocytopenic or recovering from anaemia (full blood count, platelet, erythroblast and reticulocyte counts)? Is the fetus chromosomally normal (karyotype on fetal blood/villi or amniotic fluid)? Is the fetus hypoxaemic/acidaemic (acid–base balance) Are there signs of liver damage (γGT, AST, ALT, bilirubin)? Is the fetus infected (specific tests as suggested by the maternal immunological status, parvovirus tests if the fetus is anaemic, aspecific tests such as total IgM and lymphocyte subpopulations)? Is the fetus hypoproteinaemic (total proteins)? Is the fetus affected by a specific condition suggested by the family/maternal history (specific tests as indicated)?

Store maternal blood, fetal blood, amniotic fluid, and possibly extract fetal DNA for subsequent investigations, if the indication arises

In view of the many severe chromosomal, structural and infectious causes of hydrops, it is not surprising that termination of pregnancy is the most frequent outcome of the investigative process[2,4,12,94,95]. Spontaneous resolution of hydrops may occur, but this is not necessarily reassuring as far as the absence of severe abnormalities is concerned[39]. However, the possibility that hydrops is transitory must always be considered, especially when evaluating the effect of any antenatal intervention. Success has been claimed in some cases of 'idiopathic' hydrops by empirically infusing albumin to the fetus[96] or by administering digoxin to the mother[97]. These results have to be viewed with some scepticism. Fetal hydrops is a symptom and not a defined clinical entity. Therefore, any attempts of treatment need to be aimed at correcting the mechanism which has caused hydrops, rather than at the resolving hydrops per se. Bearing this in mind, there are a few conditions that are amenable to antenatal therapy:

- *Fetal anaemia* can be treated by intravascular/intraperitoneal transfusion[13,50,51,98]
- *Fetal tachycardia*[99,100] and bradycardia[101,102] may be corrected by administering specific drugs to the mother or directly to the fetus[8,103]
- *Primary hydrothorax* can be resolved by pleuroamniotic shunting[47,104,105],
- *Hypervolaemia and cardiac hypertrophy* in the recipient twin may resolve if the fluid imbalance in TTTS is treated effectively with serial decompressive amniocenteses or laser ablation of vascular communications[106–108],
- *Fetal and placental tumours*, with congestive heart failure may improve following removal of the tumour (see below). The latter two are conditions in which the aetiology is identified, and direct treatment is instituted.
- *Congenital hyperthyroidism* is another example of direct treatment of the primary cause[109].

Although transplacental transfer of drugs is thought to be impaired if the placenta is hydropic, cardioversion to sinus rhythm by variable combinations of digoxin, verapamil, flecainide, propranolol, amiodarone, and quinidine in fetuses with atrial flutter/supraventricular tachycardia may achieve resolution of hydrops in up to 80% of cases[99]. Less effective are the strategies used to increase heart rate in fetuses with congenital heart block. The administration of fluorinated steroids, dexamethasone and beta-mimetics to the mother have been reported as being able to correct hydrops in only a handful of fetuses[101,102,110]. Intramuscular injections of digoxin and furosemide directly to the fetus have been shown to be effective in a few grossly hydropic fetuses with supraventricular tachycardia[111] or atrioventricular block[112], in which therapeutic concentrations of the drugs could not be achieved via the mother, due to poor transplacental passage.

Intrauterine transfusion is a proven effective treatment for severe fetal anaemia. Contrary to immune hydrops, in which continuous transplacental passage of antierythrocyte antibodies require serial transfusions up until delivery, fetomaternal haemorrhage and parvovirus infection, the commonest causes which lead to non-immune anaemia and hydrops, are acute events. Intrauterine transfusion might depress the natural compensatory erythropoiesis and increase further the fetal/neonatal risk. Congenital red cell aplasia, resulting in one death at 9 months of age and in two transfusion dependencies, has indeed been reported in three infants who underwent repeated transfusions following diagnosis of intrauterine parvovirus infection[113]. The management of the fetus with non-immune anaemia is therefore not defined. In the case of hydrops, the benefit of intrauterine transfusion needs to be balanced against the risks of the procedure and the possibility of further suppressing the bone marrow. Active erythropoiesis, as shown by a high reticulocyte and nucleated red cell counts on fetal blood, may be taken as evidence of recovery, despite the persistence of hydrops[67].

Weber and Philipson[47] reviewed the English literature and found 124 reported cases of fetal hydrothorax. In their meta-analysis they proved that antenatal therapy is significantly associated with a better outcome. The number of treated fetuses was too small to allow comparison between thoracentesis and pleuroamniotic shunting, but the latter approach allows continuous drainage of pleural fluid. Conversely, reaccumulation of fluid usually occurs within a maximum of 10 days, and often within a few hours, following thoracentesis, which, therefore, needs to be repeated until delivery. Insertion of a double pigtail shunt (Rocket, London, UK) (Fig. 56.10) may allow prolongation of pregnancy up to 20 weeks and resolution of hydrops and polyhydramnios, usually within 10–15 days[43,104]. On the other hand, if lung expansion does not occur following thoracentesis or shunting, and the pleural effusion persists, this suggests that prolonged compression, at an early and crucial stage of development, has caused lung hypoplasia[104]. There is a clear benefit of antenatal therapy if the fetus is hydropic and before 32 weeks of gestation[47]. Therafter, potential complications of intrauterine shunting, such as premature rupture of membranes, infection, and amniotic fluid leakage into the maternal peritoneal cavity[114], need to be balanced against the possibility of delivering the patient after performing percutaneous drainage of fetal hydrothorax to facilitate neonatal resuscitation.

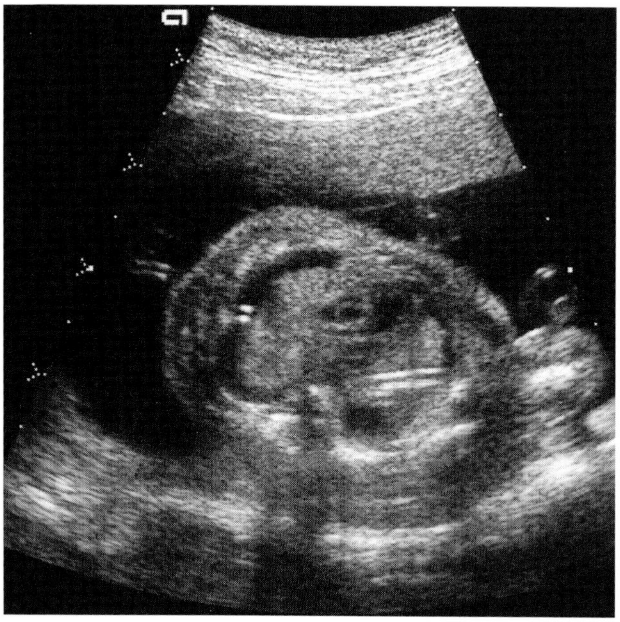

Fig. 56.10 Fetus with primary hydrothorax which underwent bilateral shunting.

Fetal tumours

Congenital tumours can be defined as 'a mass of tissue that has grown in locations or to amounts that diverge from the normal pattern of development and that do not duplicate, partially or completely, any normal structure of the body'[115]. Diagnosis of malignancy in the fetus and neonate poses peculiar microscopic difficulties since, due to the rapid growth of the embryo, normal organs and tissues are characterized by enhanced mitotic activity and include immature structures which may be similar to those found within malignant tumours. Therefore, fetal tumours are more often classified as malignant or not, based on the postnatal clinical course rather than on strict histological criteria. Of 427 congenital and neonatal tumours reported by five surveys, and reviewed by Isaacs[115], neuroblastoma (32%), teratoma (18%), leukaemia (14%) and sarcoma (13%) were the commonest types, followed by brain (9%), renal (5%) and liver (4%) tumours; retinoblastoma accounted for 5% and other rarer forms for 9% of the total.

Regarding the aetiology, congenital tumours are probably related to the same poorly understood causes which lead to cancer in general. However, there is a well-recognized association between some congenital malformations and syndromes and the development of tumours[116]. Examples of this are Wilms tumour and the Beckwith–Wiedemann, Perlman and Drash syndromes; leukaemia and Poland and Bloom syndromes etc. Some chromosomal abnormalities are also known to cause increased risk of specific tumours: with trisomy 18 and the 11p13 deletion there is a high incidence of Wilms tumour, with trisomy 21 of leukaemia, and with the 13q14 deletion of retinoblastoma and osteosarcoma. Links between hydantoin and neuroblastoma[117], and viral infections and malignant tumours[118] have also been proposed. Fetal metastases occur only rarely. Although placental metastases have been reported in women with a variety of malignant tumours, melanoma is probably the only instance of transplacental passage to the fetus.

An extensive review of all the tumours which can develop in the fetus is beyond the remit of this chapter. Most relevant tumours which pertain to a specific system are dealt with in the corresponding section. Neuroblastoma, teratoma, ovarian cyst and placental chorioangioma are discussed here as they represent relatively common tumours which pose specific diagnostic challenges and/or raise controversies on perinatal management.

NEUROBLASTOMA

Neuroblastoma is the commonest congenital malignant tumour with a clinical incidence of one in 10 000–30 000[119,120]. It derives from undifferentiated neural tissue of the adrenal medulla or sympathetic ganglia in the abdomen, thorax, pelvis or head and neck. Neuroblastic nodules, however, can be found within the adrenal gland in almost all second-trimester fetuses[121]. Diagnosis of neuroblastoma has been achieved in a number of fetuses, the ultrasonographic findings being quite variable[122]. In 90% of cases, the tumour involves the adrenal gland, ranging in size from millimetres to a few centimetres, and it typically appears on ultrasound as a combination of cystic and solid areas. The vast majority are tumours in situ or at stage I or II. However, three fetuses with advanced stages of the disease had liver metastases and developed hydrops, and in two cases, diagnosed and treated as stage I, hepatic and liver metastases developed later[123,124]. Purely cystic masses have been described, but these are associated with a favourable prognosis. In fact, clinical cystic neuroblastomas are rare and probably represent neuroblastomas in situ of no clinical significance[125]. The typical finding which would suggest fetal neuroblastoma is a suprarenal mass associated with hepatomegaly. Since metastases in the placenta can occur, careful assessment of placental structure is indicated. On the other hand, the finding of a liver mass should prompt investigation of the renal and suprarenal areas where most primary neuroblastomas arise. More rarely, fetal tumours which would later be diagnosed as neuroblastoma, might be found in the chest, neck or paravertebral regions. Fetomaternal transplacental passage of catecholamines leading to maternal symptoms such as sweating, hot flushes, palpitations and hypertension has also been reported[126].

TERATOMA

Teratoma is a germ cell tumour which is thought to derive from isolation of one or more blastomeres, fertilization of a polar body or parthogenetic development of an egg. Fetus in fetu is the most extreme form of this type of tumour; it is an embryonic duplication, which presents as an abdominal, scrotal or intracranial mass with an axial skeleton. Prenatal diagnosis of fetus in fetu has been made[127].

Teratomas are composed of tissues which originate from each of the three layers of the embryonic disc, with the ectodermal component, especially brain tissue, being the most represented. Mesodermal-derived tissues, such as fat, cartilage, bone and muscle are also present in most congenital teratomas. Although teratomas may be located in the brain, pineal gland, the retroperitoneal and mediastinal space, heart and pleura, pharynx, thyroid, spine, base of the skull and subcutaneous tissue, by far the commonest sites are the sacrococcygeal and presacral regions and the neck.

Sacrococcygeal teratoma has an incidence of one in 35 000–40 000 live births[128] and is found four times more frequently in female than in male fetuses, in whom, however, malignant changes occur more commonly[129]. Type I tumours, which are predominantly external with only a minimal presacral component, are the most common (46%); type II tumours, with a significant intrapelvic extension, account for 36% of the total; the remainder consists of type III and IV teratomas, which have the largest portion, or the whole of the tumour, within the pelvis and up to the abdominal cavity[130]. Sacrococcygeal teratoma can grow rapidly to reach very large dimensions and appear on ultrasound as solid, mixed solid/cystic, or entirely cystic masses which are extremely vascularized, as shown by colour Doppler. Only a minority of teratomas are malignant, although the presence of histologically immature tissue is common[129]. Malignant changes, which are more likely with intrapelvic tumours[130], are a bad prognostic sign, since these neoplastic elements are both radioresistant and respond poorly to chemotherapy. On the other hand, metastatic teratomas have never been reported. Overall, the most important variables which correlate with perinatal outcome are gestational age at diagnosis and size. Non-immune hydrops, secondary to high output cardiac failure, is, in fact, more common when teratomas develop early in gestation and reach large dimensions[125,131]. Predominantly cystic tumours have a better prognosis, probably due to a lower incidence of intratumoral haemorrhage and vascular steal[132]. The literature provides conflicting evidence on whether long-term complications are associated with the intrapelvic extension of the tumour[133,134]. Faecal and urinary incontinence, and weakness of the lower limbs, secondary to sciatic nerve palsy, are functional sequelae which can be found in up to 40% of infants[133] and 12% of adults[134] who were operated on for a benign sacrococcygeal teratoma. In neonates with sacrococcygeal teratoma diagnosed at birth, however, the chances of survival are extremely good, following prompt excision of the tumour and the coccyx. The primary cause of death is malignant invasion. In contrast, the mortality rate in prenatally diagnosed cases is exceedingly high, with very few of the fetuses with hydrops and placentomegaly surviving the perinatal period[135]. Prematurity consequent to uterine distention due to polyhydramnios and the large size of the tumour, cardiac failure and haemorrhage at delivery from the exsanguinating tumour are the main causes of fetal/neonatal loss. Elective classical caesarean section may prevent rupture and avulsion of the tumour and serial decompressive amniocenteses may prolong gestation by reducing the amniotic fluid volume. No conventional treatment, however, is available to prevent the high output cardiac failure related to the large volume of blood which supplies the vast majority of sacrococcygeal teratomas. Fetal surgery after hysterotomy has been attempted in a few cases[136,137], but only temporary improvement of the fetal condition has been achieved. Robertson et al.[138] have proposed devascularization of sacrococcygeal teratoma by ligating the middle sacral and internal iliac arteries in a premature neonate. This procedure allowed rapid correction of the hyperdynamic state, while awaiting for complete resection of the tumour. In the future, this less invasive approach might be attempted in utero.

Teratoma of the neck occurs less commonly than in the sacrococcygeal and presacral areas, but 150 cases had already been reported in 1994[122]. Although some malignant tumours have been reported[139], the vast majority are benign. The typical ultrasonic appearance is that of a unilateral, asymmetric, multiloculated, well-demarcated mass extending cranially up to the mandible and mastoid, and caudally to the clavicle and sternum. The fetal head is often laterally flexed and hyperextended. Oesophageal compression impairs fetal swallowing, leading to polyhydramnios. Due to the increased incidence of malpresentation, caesarean section is often required. Airway obstruction causing prolonged neonal hypoxia may occur in up to 39% of cases[140]. Since immediate intubation may be difficult, tracheostomy or in utero intubation[141] should be considered.

OVARIAN CYST

Small non-neoplastic cysts of the fetal ovary are not uncommon, especially during the third trimester. Histologically, they are benign cysts of germinal or graafian epithelium. The underlying mechanisms are not fully understood, but the influence of fetal gonadotropins, maternal oestrogens and placental chorionic gonadotropin has been suggested[142]. Cysts larger than 1 cm are uncommon, but this possibility should be considered whenever an abdominal fluid filled mass, not related to the urinary tract, is seen in a female fetus. As in neonates, the most common complication of ovarian cysts is torsion, which may be seen in up to 40% of cases[143]. Brandt et al.[142] reported that in more than 90% of neonates who were thought to have torsion, there was evidence of torsion (the ultrasonic appearance was that of a complex rather than simple unilocular cyst), either at prenatal or at the first postnatal ultrasound examination. In order to prevent ovarian tissue necrosis, antenatal decompression has been proposed, but the criteria to perform such a procedure have not been established. As many as 50% of fetal ovarian cysts may in fact resolve spontaneously. Crombleholme et al. have recently suggested that in utero aspiration should be considered in cases of female fetuses with simple anechoic cysts larger than 4 cm, or increasing in size >1 cm/week[144]. No prospective randomized study has been carried out so far, but, in view of the relative safety of transbdominal needle aspiration of an abdominal cyst in the third trimester, these criteria seem to be a reasonable option for the time being.

PLACENTAL CHORIOANGIOMA

Placental chorioangioma is a benign vascular tumour arising from chorionic tissue. Small chorioangiomas are found in 0.01–1.3% of examined placentas and are clinically irrelevant. In contrast, large masses (more than 4–5 cm in diameter) occur in one in 3000–9000 births[145] and may lead to polyhydramnios, maternal and fetal coagulopathy, preeclampsia, preterm labour, intrauterine growth retardation, fetomaternal transfusion and fetal hydrops[135]. Prenatal diagnosis of placental chorioangioma relies on the typical ultrasound appearance (Fig. 56.11). Colour flow and pulsed Doppler may demonstrate that vascular channels in the tumour are continuous with the fetal circulation, ruling out other possible diagnoses such as a degenerating fibroid, placental teratoma and patient hydatidiform mole. Abnormalities of amniotic fluid volume are common. Polyhydramnios, which is reported in approximately 30% of large chorioangiomas, is thought to develop due to the combination of increased transudation of fluid through the vascular surface of the tumour and obstructed venous return. However, since oligohydramnios can also occur, the mechanism of fluid imbalance remains elusive. It is possible that differences in histology and vessel structure of the tumour play a role in the aetiology of fluid exchanges. Alternatively, reduced amniotic fluid volume might be related to relative placental failure and fetal growth restriction, both the consequence of a large fraction of fetal blood perfusing a

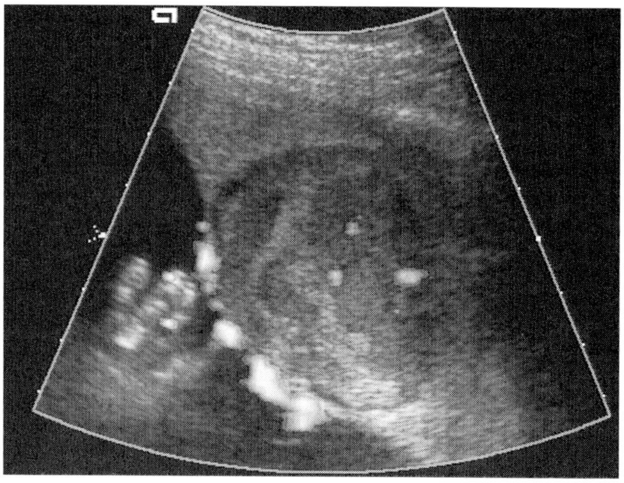

Fig. 56.11 Placental chorioangioma.

placental area unavailable for maternal–fetal exchanges. Chorioangiomas may act as a peripheral arteriovenous shunt leading to increased fetal cardiac output, cardiac hypertrophy, congestive heart failure and fetal hydrops. Severe anaemia has been previously reported in association with chorioangioma in neonates, as well as in a fetus at prenatal blood sampling[146]. It is unclear, however, whether the haematological modifications precede or follow cardiac failure. Anaemia might in fact arise from chronic microangiopathy, and be an independent cause of hydrops. Prenatal evaluation of fetal haematological status might therefore be indicated in cases of large chorioangiomas associated with ultrasound findings suggestive of impending hydrops. Intrauterine transfusion has been performed in one such case with improvement in fetal condition[146]. More recently, alcoholization of the major vessels within a large chorioangioma has achieved resolution of polyhydramnios (U. Nicolini, unpublished observation).

Since the negative effects to the fetus caused by large fetal tumours are related to increased total blood volume and consequent high output cardiac failure, attempts of antenatal therapy should try to reduce tumour vascularization. Alcoholization, thermocoagulation or endoscopic ligation of the vessels supplying the tumour are new procedures which may be entertained in selected cases.

REFERENCES

1. Santolaya J, Alley D, Jaffe R, Warsof SL. Antenatal classification of hydrops fetails. *Obstet Gynecol* **79**:256–259, 1992.
2. Poeschmann RP, Verheijen RHM, Van Dongen PWJ. Differential diagnosis and causes of nonimmunological hydrops fetalis: a review. *Obstet Gynecol Surv* **46**:223–231, 1991.
3. MacAfee CAJ, Fortune DW, Beischer NA. Non-immunological hydrops fetalis. *J Obstet Gynaecol Br Commonw* **77**:226–237, 1970.
4. Iskaros J, Jauniaux E, Rodeck CH. Outcome of nonimmune hydrops fetalis diagnosed during the first half of pregnancy. *Obstet Gynecol* **90**:321–325, 1997.
5. Machin GA. Hydrops, cystic hygroma, hydrothorax, pericardial effusions and fetal ascites. In *Potter's Pathology of the Fetus and Infant* (ed. E Gilbert-Barness), pp. 163–181. St Louis: Mosby–Year Book, 1997.
6. Machin GA. Hydrops revisited: literature review of 1414 cases published in the 1980s. *Am J Med Genet* **34**:366–390, 1989.
7. Boyd PA, Keeling JW. Fetal hydrops. *J Med Genet* **29**:91–97, 1992.
8. Hansmann M, Gembruch U, Bald R. New therapeutic aspects of nonimmune hydrops based on 402 prenatally diagnosed cases. *Fetal Ther* **4**:29–37, 1989.
9. Saltzman DH, Frigoletto FD, Harlow BL, Barss VA, Benacerraf BR. Sonographic evaluation of hydrops fetalis. *Obstet Gynecol* **74**:106–111, 1989.
10. Ruiz Villaespesa A, Suarez Mier MP, Lopez Ferrer P, Alvarez Baleriola I, Rodriguez Gonzalez JI. Nonimmunologic hydrops fetalis: an ethiopathogenetic approach through the postmortem study of 59 patients. *Am J Med Genet* **35**:274–279, 1990.
11. Shimokawa H, Hara K, Maeda H, Miyamoto S, Koyanagi T, Nakano H. Intrauterine treatment of idiopathic hydrops fetails. *J Perinat Med* **16**:133–138, 1988.
12. Holzgreve W. The fetus with nonimmune hydrops. In *The unborn patient: Prenatal Diagnosis and Treatment*, 2nd edn. (eds MR Harrison, MS Golbus & RA Filly), pp. 228–245. Philadelphia: WB Saunders, 1991.
13. Cantu'-Rajnoldi A, Zanella A, Conter U et al. A severe transfusion-dependent congenital dyserythropoietic anaemia presenting as hydrops fetalis. *Br J Haematol* **96**:530–533, 1997.
14. Fleischer AC, Killam AP, Boehm FH et al. Hydrops fetalis: sonographic evaluation and clinical implications. *Radiology* **141**:163–168, 1981.
15. Mahoney BS, Filly RA, Callen PW, Chinn DH, Golbus MS. Severe nonimmune hydrops fetalis; sonographic evaluation. *Radiology* **151**:757–761, 1984.
16. Watson J, Campbell S. Antenatal evaluation and management in nonimmune hydrops fetalis. *Obstet Gynecol* **67**:589–593, 1986.
17. Moore TR, Cayle JE. The amniotic fluid index in normal human pregnancy. *Am J Obstet Gynecol* **162**:1168–1173, 1990.
18. Lam YH, Ghosh A, Tang MHY, Lee CP, Sin SY. Second-trimester hydrops fetalis in pregnancies affected by homozygous α-thalassaemia-1. *Prenat Diagn* **17**:267–269, 1997.
19. Lam YH, Ghosh A, Tang MHY, Lee CP, Sin SY. Early ultrasound prediction of pregnancies affected by homozygous α-thalassaemia-1. *Prenat Diagn* **17**:327–332, 1997.
20. Ghosh A, Tang MHY, Lam YH, Fung E, Chan V. Ultrasound measurement of placental thickness to detect pregnancies affected by homozygous α-thalassaemia-1. *Lancet* **344**:988–989, 1994.
21. Fadnes HO, Oian P. Transcapillary fluid balance and plasma volume regulation: a review. *Obstet Gynecol Surv* **44**:769–773, 1989.
22. Hutchinson AA. Pathophysiology of hydrops fetalis. In *Fetal and Neonatal Cardiology* (ed. W.A. Long). Philadelphia: WB Saunders, 1990.
23. Nicolini U, Fisk NM, Beacham J, Rodeck CH. Fetal urine biochemistry: An index of renal maturation and dysfunction. *Br J Obstet Gynaecol* **99**:46–50, 1992.
24. Rodeck CH, Santolaya J, Nicolini U. The fetus with immune hydrops. In The *Unborn Patient: Prenatal Diagnosis and Treatment* 2nd edn. (eds M.R. Harrison, M.S. Golbus & R.A. Filly), pp. 215–227. Philadelphia: WB Saunders, 1991.
25. Santolaya-Forgas J, Warsof SL. Hydrops and associated anomalies. In *Prenatal Diagnosis and Screening* (eds D.J.H. Brock, C.H. Rodeck & M.A. Ferguson-Smith), pp. 329–347. Edinburgh: Churchill Livingstone, 1992.
26. Tegnander E, Eik-Nes SH, Johansen OJ et al. Prenatal detection of heart defects at the routine fetal examination at 18 weeks in a non-selected population. *Ultrasound Obstet Gynecol* **5**:372–380, 1995.
27. Todros T, Faggiano F, Chiappa E et al. Accuracy of routine ultrasonography in screening heart disease prenatally. *Prenat Diagn* **17**:901–906, 1997.
28. Achiron R, Glaser J, Gelernter I, Hegesh J, Yagel S. Extended fetal echocardiographic examination for detecting cardiac malformations in low risk pregnancies. *Br Med J* **304**:671–674, 1992.
29. Gudmundsson S, Huhta JC, Wood DC, Tulzer G, Cohen AW, Weiner S. Venous Doppler ultrasonography in the fetus with nonimmune hydrops. *Am J Obstet Gynecol* **164**:33–37, 1991.
30. Gest AL, Hansen TN, Moise AA, Hartley CJ. Atrial tachycardia causes hydrops in fetal lambs. *Am J Physiol* **258**:159–163, 1990.
31. Scott JS, Maddison PJ, Taylor PV, Esscher E, Scott O, Skinner RP. Connective tissue disease, antibodies to ribonucleoprotein, and congenital heart block. *N Engl J Med* **312**:98–100, 1985.
32. Machado MVL, Tynan MJ, Curry PVL, Allan LD. Fetal complete heart block. *Br Heart J* **60**:512–515, 1988.
33. Langer JC, Harrison MR, Schmidt KG et al. Fetal hydrops and death from sacrococcygeal teratoma: rationale for fetal surgery. *Am J Obstet Gynecol* **160**:1145–1150, 1989.
34. Bauer CR, Fojaco RM, Bancalari E, Fernandez-Rocha L. Microangiopathic hemolytic anemia in a neonate associated with a large placental chorioangioma. *Pediatrics* **62**:574–577, 1978.
35. Zoppini C, Acaia B, Lucci G, Pugni L, Tassis B, Nicolini U. Varying clinical course of large placental chorioangiomas. *Fetal Diagn Ther* **12**:61–64, 1997.
36. Johnson W, Berry JM, Einzig S, Bass JL. Doppler findings in nonimmune hydrops fetalis and cerebral arteriovenous malformation. *Am Heart J* **115**:1138–1140, 1988.
37. Jones DC. Nonimmune fetal hydrops: diagnosis and obstetrical management. *Sem Perinatol* **19**:447–461, 1995.

37a. P.O.S.S.U.M. Picture of standard and undiagnosed malformations. Melbourne: Murdoch Institute for Research into Birth Defects, Royal Children's Hospital, 1997.
38. Hyett J, Moscoso G, Nicolaides KH. Abnormalities of the heart and great arteries in first trimester chromosomally abnormal fetuses. *Am J Med Genet* **69**:207–216, 1997.
39. Mostello DJ, Bofinger MK, Siddiqi TA. Spontaneous resolution of fetal cystic hygroma and hydrops in Turner syndrome. *Obstet Gynecol* **73**:862–865, 1989.
40. Vaughan JI, Fisk NM, Rodeck CH. Fetal pleural effusions. In *Invasive Fetal Testing and Treatment* (ed. C.R. Harman), pp. 218–239. Boston: Blackwell Scientific Publications, 1995.
41. Whittle MJ, Gilmore DH, McNay MB, Turner TL, Raine PAM. Diaphragmatic hernia presenting in utero as a unilateral hydrothorax. *Prenat Diagn* **9**:115–118, 1989.
42. Evans MG. Hydrops fetalis and pulmonary sequestration. *J Pediatr Surg* **31**:761–764, 1996.
43. Nicolaides KH, Azar GB. Thoraco-amniotic shunting. *Fetal Diagn Ther* **5**:153–164, 1990.
44. Sinniah D, Sivanesan S. Sporadic congenital goiter and pleural effusion. *Am J Dis Child* **122**:245–246, 1971.
45. Adzick NS. The fetus with a cystic adenomatoid malformation. In *The Unborn Patient: Prenatal Diagnosis and Treatment* 2nd edn. (eds M.R. Harrison, M.S. Golbus & R.A. Filly), pp. 320–327. Philadelphia: WB Saunders, 1991.
46. Longaker MT, Laberge JM, Dansereau J et al. Primary fetal hydrothorax: natural history and management. *J Pediatr Surg* **24**:573–576, 1989.
47. Weber AM, Philipson EH. Fetal pleural effusion: a review and meta-analysis for prognostic indicators. *Obstet Gynecol* **79**:281–286, 1992.
48. Scott-Emuakpor AB, Warren ST, Kapur S, Quiachon EB, Higgins JV. Familiar occurrence of congenital pulmonary lymphangiectasias. Genetic implications. *Am J Dis Child* **135**:532–534, 1981.
49. Gates GF, Dore EK, Kanchanapoom V. Thoracic duct leakage in neonatal chylothorax visualized by ^{198}Au lymphangiography. *Radiology* **105**:619–620, 1972.
50. Tannirandorn Y, Nicolini U, Nicolaidis P, Nasrat H, Letsky E, Rodeck CH. Intrauterine death due to fetomaternal haemorrhage despite successful treatment of fetal anemia. *J Perinat Med* **18**:233–235, 1990.
51. Montgomery LD, Belfort MA, Adam K. Massive fetomaternal hemorrhage treated with serial combined intravascular and intraperitoneal fetal transfusions. *Am J Obstet Gynecol* **173**:234–235, 1995.
52. Nicolini U, Kochenour NK, Greco P et al. Consequences of feto-maternal haemorrhage following intrauterine transfusion. *Br Med J* **297**:1379–1381, 1988.
53. Hsieh FJ, Chang FM, Ko TM, Chen HY. Percutaneous ultrasound-guided fetal blood sampling in the management of nonimmune hydrops fetalis. *Am J Obstet Gynecol* **157**:44–49, 1987.
54. Perkins RP. Hydrops fetalis and stillbirth in a male glucose-6-phosphate dehydrogenase-deficient fetus possibly due to maternal ingestion of sulfisoxazole. *Am J Obstet Gynecol* **111**:379–381, 1971.
55. Mentzer WC, Collier E. Hydrops fetalis associated with erythrocyte G-6PD deficiency and maternal ingestion of fava beans and ascorbic acid. *J Pediatr* **86**:565–567, 1975.
56. Ravindranath Y, Paglia DE, Warrier I, Valentine W, Nakatani M, Brockway RA. Glucose phosphate isomerase deficiency as a cause of hydrops fetalis. *N Engl J Med* **316**:258–261, 1987.
57. Watson J, Campbell S. Antenatal evaluation and management in nonimmune hydrops fetalis. *Obstet Gynecol* **64**:589–593, 1986.
58. Ginsburg SJ, Groll M. Hydrops fetalis due to infantile Gaucher's disease. *J Pediatr* **82**:1046–1048, 1973.
59. Vergani P, Strobelt N, Locatelli A et al. Clinical significance of fetal intracranial hemorrhage. *Am J Obstet Gynecol* **175**:536–543, 1996.
60. Bose C. Hydrops fetalis and in utero intracranial hemorrhage. *J Pediatr* **93**:1023–1024, 1978.
61. Potter CG, Potter AC, Hatton CSR et al. Variation of erythroid and myeloid precursors in the marrow and peripheral blood of volunteer subjects infected with human parvovirus B19. *J Clin Invest* **79**:1486–1492, 1987.
62. Brown KE, Anderson SM, Young NS. Erythrocyte P antigen: cellular receptor for B19 parvovirus. *Science* **262**:114–117, 1993.
63. Public Health Laboratory Service Working Party on Fifth Disease. Prospective study of human parvovirus (B19) infection in pregnancy. *Br Med J* **300**:1166–1170, 1990.
64. Rodis JF, Quinn DL, Gary GW et al. Management and outcomes of pregnancies complicated by human B19 parvovirus infection: a prospective study. *Am J Obstet Gynecol* **163**:1168–71, 1990.
65. Smoleniec JS, Pillai M, Caul EO, Usher J. Subclinical transplacental parvovirus B19 infection: an increased fetal risk? *Lancet* **343**:1100–1101, 1994.
66. Petrikovsky BM, Baker D, Schneider E. Fetal hydrops secondary to human parvovirus infection in early pregnancy. *Prenat Diagn* **16**:342–344, 1996.
67. Morey AL, Nicolini U, Welch CR, Economides D, Chamberlain PF, Cohen BJ. Parvovirus B19 infection and transient fetal hydrops. *Lancet* **337**:496, 1991.
68. Pandya PP, Snijders RJM, Johnson SP, Brizot M, Nicolaides KH. Screening for fetal trisomies by maternal age and fetal nuchal translucency thickness at 10 to 14 weeks of gestation. *Br J Obstet Gynaecol* **102**:957–962, 1995.
69. Moselhi M, Thilaganathan B. Nuchal translucency: a marker for the antenatal diagnosis of aortic coarctation. *Br J Obstet Gynaecol* **103**:1044–1045, 1996.
70. Robertson EG, Neer KJ. Placental injection studies in twin gestation. *Am J Obstet Gynecol* **147**:170–173, 1983.
71. Chescheir NC, Seeds JW. Polyhydramnios and oligohydramnios in twin gestations. *Obstet Gynecol* **71**:882–884, 1988.
72. Wieacker P, Wilhelm C, Prompeler H, Petersen KG, Schillinger H, Breckwoldt M. Pathophysiology of polyhydramnios in twin transfusion syndrome. *Fetal Diagn Ther* **7**:87–92, 1992.
73. Rosen DJD, Rabinowitz R, Beyth Y, Fejgin MD, Nicolaides KH. Fetal urine production in normal twins and in twins with acute polyhydramnios. *Fetal Diagn Ther* **5**:57–60, 1990.
74. Ludomirsky A, Weiner S, Capraro F, Bhutani V. Twin to twin transfusion syndrome: role of Doppler flow and fetal hyperviscosity in predicting outcome. *Am J Obstet Gynecol* **164** (SPO abstr 5):243, 1991.
75. Fisk NM, Borrell A, Hubinont C, Letsky EA, Nicolini U, Rodeck CH. Feto-fetal transfusion syndrome: do the neonatal criteria apply in utero? *Arch Dis Child* **65**:657–661, 1990.
76. Saunders NJ, Snijders RJM, Nicolaides KH. Twin-twin transfusion syndrome during the 2nd trimester is associated with small intertwin hemoglobin differences. *Fetal Diagn Ther* **6**:34–36, 1991.
77. Nicolini U. Invasive testing and opportunity for therapy in multiple gestation. In *Invasive Fetal Testing and Treatment* (ed. C.R. Harman), pp. 315–338. Boston: Blackwell Scientific Publications, 1995.
78. Nicolini U, Pisoni MP, Cela E, Roberts A. Fetal blood sampling immediately prior to and within 24 hours of death in monochorionic twin pregnancies complicated by single intrauterine death. *Am J Obstet Gynecol* **179**:800–803, 1998.
79. Benedetti A. *De Singulis Corpori Humani Morbis a Capite ad Pedem.* Venezia, 1553.
80. Nicolaidis P, Nasrat H, Tannirandorn Y. Fetal acardia: aetiology, pathology and management. *J Obstet Gynaecol* **10**:518–525, 1990.
81. Moore TR, Gale S, Benirschke K. Perinatal outcome of forty-nine pregnancies complicated by acardiac twinning. *Am J Obstet Gynecol* **163**:907–912, 1990.
82. Nicolini U, Kustermann A, Tassis B et al. Prenatal diagnosis of congenital human cytomegalovirus infection. *Prenat Diagn* **14**:903–906, 1994.
83. Hohlfeld P, Vial Y, Maillard-Brignon C, Vaudaux B, Fawer CL. Cytomegalovirus fetal infection: prenatal diagnosis. *Obstet Gynecol* **78**:615–618, 1991.
84. Daffos F, Forestier F, Capella-Pavlosky M et al. Prenatal management of 746 pregnancies at risk for congenital toxoplasmosis. *N Engl J Med* **318**:271–275, 1988.
85. Nicolini U, De Julio C, Roberts A et al. Maternal and fetal lymphocyte subpopulations in pregnancies at risk of congenital infections. (submitted for publication).
86. Cheng HH, Nicolaides KH. Renal and urinary tract abnormalities. In *Prenatal Diagnosis and Screening* (eds D.J.H. Brock, C.H. Rodeck & M.A. Ferguson-Smith), pp. 257–270. Edinburgh: Churchill Livingstone, 1992.
87. Ambrosino MM, Hernanz-Schulman M, Horri SC, Raghavendra BN,

Genieser NB. Prenatal diagnosis of nephroblastomatosis in two siblings. *J Ultrasound Med* **9**:49–51, 1990.
88. Lalatta F, Salmona S, Fogliani R, Rizzuti T, Nicolini U. Prenatal diagnosis of genetic syndromes may be facilitated by serendipitous findings at fetal blood sampling. *Prenat Diagn* **18**:941–946, 1998.
89. Novak PM, Sander CM, Yang SS, von Oeyen PT. Report of fourteen cases of nonimmune hydrops fetalis in association with hemorrhagic endovasculitis of the placenta. *Am J Obstet Gynecol* **165**:945–950, 1991.
90. Shen-Schwarz S, MacPherson TA, Mueller-Heubach E. The clinical significance of hemorrhagic endovasculitis of the placenta. *Am J Obstet Gynecol* **159**:48–51, 1988.
91. Graves GR, Baskett TR. Nonimmune hydrops fetalis: antenatal diagnosis and management. *Am J Obstet Gynecol* **148**:563–565, 1983.
92. Duthie SJ, Walkinshaw SA. Parvovirus associated fetal hydrops: reversal of pregnancy induced proteinuric hypertension by in utero fetal transfusion. *Br J Obstet Gynaecol* **102**:1011–1013, 1995.
93. Lao TT, Chin RKH, Chan A. Transient hyperthyroidism in a pregnancy with hydrops fetalis. Case report. *Br J Obstet Gynaecol* **95**:624–625, 1988.
94. McCoy MC, Katz VL, Gould N, Kuller JA. Non-immune hydrops after 20 weeks' gestation: review of 10 years' experience with suggestions for management. *Obstet Gynecol* **85**:578–582, 1995.
95. Ayida GA, Soothill PW, Rodeck CH. Survival in non-immune hydrops fetalis without malformation or chromosomal abnormalities after invasive treatment. *Fetal Diagn Ther* **10**:101–105, 1995.
96. Shimokawa H, Hara K, Maeda H, Mijamoto S, Koyanagi T, Nakano H. Intrauterine treatment of idiopathic hydrops fetalis. *J Perinat Med* **16**:133–138, 1988.
97. Chavkin Y, Kupfersztain C, Ergaz Z, Guedj P, Finkel AR, Stark M. Successful outcome of idiopathic nonimmune hydrops fetalis treated by maternal digoxin. *Gynecol Obstet Invest* **42**:137–139, 1996.
98. Fairley CK, Smoleniec J, Caul OE, Miller E. Observational study of effect of intrauterine transfusions on outcome of fetal hydrops after parvovirus B19 infection. *Lancet* **346**:1335–1337, 1995.
99. Van Engelen AD, Weijtens O, Brenner JL, Kleinman CS, Copel JA, Stoutenbeek P, Meijeboom EJ. Management, outcome and follow up of fetal tachycardia. *J Am Coll Cardiol* **24**:1371–1375, 1994.
100. Naumburg E, Riesenfeld T, Axelsson O. Fetal tachycardia: intrauterine and postnatal course. *Fetal Diagn Ther* **12**:205–209, 1997.
101. Buyon JP, Waltuck J, Kleinman C, Copel J. In utero identification and therapy of congenital heart block. *Lupus* **4**:116–121, 1995.
102. Groves AM, Allan LD, Rosenthal E. Therapeutic trial of sympathomimetics in three cases of complete heart block in the fetus. *Circulation* **92**:3394–3396, 1995.
103. Anandakumar C, Biswas A, Chew SS, Chua D, Wong YC, Ratnam SS. Direct fetal therapy for hydrops secondary to congenital atrioventricular heart block. *Obstet Gynecol* **87**:835–837, 1996.
104. Rodeck CH, Fisk NM, Fraser DI, Nicolini U. Long-term in utero drainage of fetal hydrothorax. *N Engl J Med* **319**:1135–1138, 1988.
105. Chan V, Greenough A, Nicolaides KN. Antenatal and postnatal treatment of pleural effusion and extra-lobar pulmonary sequestration. *J Perinat Med* **24**:335–338, 1996.
106. Trespidi L, Boschetto C, Caravelli E, Villa L, Kustermann A, Nicolini U. Serial amniocenteses in the management of twin-twin transfusion syndrome: when is it valuable? *Fetal Diagn Ther* **12**:15–20, 1997.
107. Ville Y, Hyett K, Hecher K, Nicolaides KH. Preliminary experience with endoscopic surgery for severe TTTS. *N Engl J Med* **332**:224–227, 1995.
108. Fesslova V, Villa L, Nava S, Mosca F, Nicolini U. Fetal and neonatal echocardiographic findings in twin-twin transfusion syndrome. *Am J Obstet Gynecol* **179**:1056–1062, 1998.
109. Treadwell MC, Sherer DM, Sacks AJ, Ghezzi F, Romero R. Successful treatment of recurrent non-immune hydrops secondary to fetal hyperthyroidism. *Obstet Gynecol* **87**:838–840, 1996.
110. Copel JA, Buyon JP, Kleinman CS. Successful in utero therapy of fetal heart block. *Am J Obstet Gynecol* **173**:1384–1390, 1995.
111. Hallak M, Neerhof MG, Perry R, Nazir M, Huhta JC. Fetal supraventricular tachycardia and hydrops fetalis: combined intensive, direct, and transplacental therapy. *Obstet Gynecol* **78**:523–525, 1991.
112. Anandakumar C, Biswas A, Chew SSL, Chia D, Wong YC, Ratnam SS. Direct fetal therapy for hydrops secondary to congenital atrioventricular heart block. *Obstet Gynecol* **87**:835–837, 1996.
113. Brown KE, Green SW, Antunez de Mayolo J et al. Congenital anemia after transplacental B19 parvovirus infection. *Lancet* **343**:895–896, 1994.
114. Ronderos-Dumit D, Nicolini U, Vaughan J, Fisk NM, Chamberlain PF, Rodeck CH. Uterine-peritoneal amniotic fluid leakage: an unusual complication of intrauterine shunting. *Obstet Gynecol* **78**:913–915, 1991.
115. Isaacs H. Tumors. In *Potter's Pathology of the Fetus and Infant* (ed. E. Gilbert-Barness), pp. 1242–1339. St. Louis: Mosby–Year Book, 1997.
116. Isaacs H. *Tumors of the Newborn and Infant*. St. Louis: Mosby–Year Book, 1991
117. Pendergrass TW. Fetal hydantoin syndrome and neuroblastoma. *Lancet* **2**:150, 1976.
118. Fine PEM, Adelstein AM, Snowman J, Clarkson JA, Evans SM. Long term effects of exposure to viral infections in utero. *Br Med J* **290**:509–511, 1985.
119. Bader JL, Miller RW. U.S. cancer incidence and mortality in the first year of life. *Am J Dis Child* **133**:157–159, 1979.
120. Isaacs H. Congenital and neonatal malignant tumors: a 28 year experience at Children's Hospital in Los Angeles. *Am J Pediatr Hematol Oncol* **9**:121–129, 1987.
121. Turkel SB, Habashi HH. The natural history of neuroblastic cells in the fetal adrenal gland. *Am J Pathol* **76**:225–244, 1974.
122. Garmel SH, Crombleholme TM, Semple JP, Bhan I. Prenatal diagnosis and management of fetal tumors. *Sem Perinatol* **18**:350–365, 1994.
123. Fenart D, Deville A, Donzeau M, Bruneton JN. Neuroblastome retroperitoneal diagnostique in utero. *J Radiol* **64**:359–361, 1983.
124. Ferraro EM, Fakhry J, Aruni JA, Bracero LA. Prenatal adrenal neuroblastoma. *J Ultrasound Med* **7**:275–278, 1988.
125. Crombleholme TC, Murray TA, Harris BH. Diagnosis and management of fetal neuroblastoma. *Curr Opin Obstet Gynecol* **6**:199–202, 1994.
126. Newton ER, Louis F, D'Alton MF, Feingold M. Fetal neuroblastoma and catecholamine-induced hypertension. *Obstet Gynecol* **65**:49–52, 1985.
127. Nicolini U, dell'Agnola CA, Ferrazzi E, Motta G. Ultrasonic prenatal diagnosis of fetus in fetu. *J Clin Ultrasound* **11**:321–322, 1983.
128. Schiffer MA, Greenberg E. Sacrococcygeal teratoma in labor and the newborn. *Am J Obstet Gynecol* **72**:1054–1062, 1956.
129. Carney JA, Thompson DP, Johnson CL, Lynn HB. Teratomas in children: clinical and pathologic aspects. *J Pediatr Surg* **7**:271–282, 1972.
130. Altman RP, Randolph JG, Lilly JR. Sacroccocygeal teratoma: American Academy of Pediatrics surgical section survey. *J Pediatr Surg* **9**:389–398, 1974.
131. Holzgreve W, Willital GH. Fetal tumors. In *Ultrasound in Obstetrics and Gynecology* (eds F.A. Chervenak, G.C. Isaacson & S. Campbell), pp. 1009–1025. St Louis: Mosby–Year Book, 1993.
132. Hogge WA, Thiagarajah S, Barber VG, Rodgers BM, Newman BM. Cystic sacro-coccygeal teratoma: ultrasound diagnosis and perinatal management. *J Ultrasound Med* **6**:707–710, 1987.
133. Malone PS, Spitz L, Kiely EM, Brereton RJ, Duffy PG, Ransley PG. The functional sequelae of sacrococcygeal teratoma. *J Pediatr Surg* **25**:679–680, 1990.
134. Rintala R, Lahdenne P, Lindahl H, Siimes M, Heikinheimo M. Anorectal function in adults operated for a benign sacrococcygeal teratoma. *J Pediatr Surg* **28**:1165–1167, 1993.
135. Bond SJ, Harrison MR, Schmidt KG et al. Death due to high-output cardiac failure in fetal sacrococcygeal teratoma. *J Pediatr Surg* **25**:1287–1291, 1990.
136. Langer JC, Harrison MR, Schmidt KG et al. Fetal hydrops and death from sacrococcygeal teeratoma: rationale for fetal surgery. *Am J Obstet Gynecol* **160**:1145–1150, 1989.
137. Flake AW. Fetal sacrococcygeal teratoma. *Semin Pediatr Surg* **2**:113–120, 1993.
138. Robertson FM, Crombleholme TM, Frantz ID, Shephard BA, Bianchi DW, D'Alton ME. Devascularization and staged resection of giant sacrococcygeal teratoma in the premature infant. *J Pediatr Surg* **30**:309–311, 1995.
139. Baumann FR, Nerlich A. Metastasizing cervical teratoma of the fetus. *Pediatr Pathol* **13**:21–27, 1993.
140. Azizkhan RG, Haase GM, Applebaum H et al. Diagnosis, management and outcome of cervicofacial teratomas in neonates: a children's cancer group study. *J Pediatr Surg* **30**:312–316, 1995.

141. Graf J, Mychaliska G, Albanese C, Jennings R, Harrison M. The Ex Utero Intrapartum Treatment (EXIT) procedure. Presented at the 16th Annual Meeting of IFMSS. Girdwood, Alaska, 1–5 June, 1997.
142. Brandt ML, Luks FI, Filiatrault D, Garel L, Desjardins JG, Youssef S, Surgical indications in antenatally diagnosed ovarian cysts. *J Pediatr Surg* **26**:276–281, 1991.
143. Meizner I, Levy A, Katz M, Maresh AJ, Glezerman M. Fetal ovarian cysts: prenatal ultrasonographic detection and postnatal evaluation and treatment. *Am J Obstet Gynecol* **164**:874–878, 1991.
144. Crombleholme TM, Craigo SD, Garmel S, D'Alton ME. Fetal ovarian cyst decompression to prevent torsion. *J Pediatr Surg* **32**:1447–1449, 1997.
145. Lopez HBB, Kristoffersen SE. Chorioangioma of the placenta. *J Obstet Invest* **28**:108–110, 1989.
146. Hirata GI, Masaki DI, O'Toole M, Medearis AL, Platt LD. Color flow mapping and doppler velocimetry in the diagnosis and management of a placental chorioangioma associated with nonimmune fetal hydrops. *Obstet Gynecol* **81**: 850–852, 1993.

57 Operative fetoscopy

R.A. Quintero and C. Carreño

Introduction

The diagnosis of surgically correctable birth defects and certain high-risk conditions represents a dilemma to parents and physicians. A fundamental decision must be made as to whether prenatal intervention is either necessary or possible. This decision in turn must balance the risks/benefits to the mother and/or fetus of performing or withholding therapy.

Conditions and criteria used to consider fetal surgery are:

- Accurate diagnosis
- Absence of other major anomalies
- Normal karyotype
- Knowledge of the natural history of the disease
- Previability
- Feasibility of the proposed treatment
- Fetal benefits outweigh maternal and fetal risks

The risk/benefit to the fetus will depend on the likelihood that the particular condition will either disappear, remain stable, or worsen during the course of the pregnancy, i.e., on the knowledge of the natural history of the disease in utero. Pleural effusions and certain cases of cystic adenomatoid malformation of the lung may have a transient course[1] and call for prudent expectant management until resolution. Certain conditions may persist, yet lack of in utero treatment may not compromise the outcome. This is the case of most fetuses with gastroschisis or ovarian cysts, and definitive treatment may be deferred until after birth[2,3]. On the other hand, prenatal intervention should be seriously considered for those conditions where fetal death or damage may occur unless treatment is undertaken before birth, as with many cases of obstructive uropathy[4], diaphragmatic hernia[5], or acardiac twins[6]. Once the medical necessity for intervening has been established, the risks to the mother and/or fetus of the proposed procedure will depend on the nature of the proposed intervention.

Unfortunately, and despite the many advances in prenatal ultrasound and prenatal diagnosis, the fetus remains a relatively inaccessible patient. The limitations are obviously posed by the intrauterine–intraamniotic location of the fetus, and by our relative lack of understanding of the factors responsible for the onset of normal and pathological labour and for the intact preservation of the fetal membranes. Despite these limitations, the fetus has increasingly become the subject of different therapeutic approaches. The transplacental route has been used for the delivery of antiarrhythmic agents for the management of complex fetal arrhythmias[7,8], and hyperimmune immunoglobulin for alloimmune thrombocytopenia[9]. Minimally invasive procedures involve the intravascular placement of thin needles under ultrasound guidance, such as for the treatment of fetal anaemia[10]. These procedures constitute one of the most successful forms of fetal therapy. The placement of pleuroamniotic[11] and vesicoamniotic[12–14] shunts for the treatment of pleural effusions and obstructive uropathy respectively, constitute the second major forms of minimally invasive fetal therapies. Major fetal anomalies, such as diaphragmatic hernia, sacrococcygeal teratoma, and cystic adenomatoid malformation of the lung can only be treated via a more direct access to the fetus as they involve more complicated surgical tasks. The need to perform more complicated surgical procedures led to the development of open fetal surgery.

All forms of fetal therapy have their advantages and limitations. In general, the less invasive the procedure, the less likely that it will elicit an untoward response from the uterus[15]. In this sense, for the past 4 years we have explored the possibility of using minimally invasive endoscopic methods to treat the human fetus. This approach intends to address the limitations of other forms of fetal therapy, while offering unique therapeutic options. In this chapter we will examine the advantages, disadvantages, and applications of endoscopy for the management of human fetal disease.

The fetus as a surgical patient: open fetal surgery

Attempts to perform open fetal surgery date back to the 1960s[16,17]. Since then, several groups have conducted extensive research to establish the scope and limitations of this approach[18]. In open fetal surgery, the mother undergoes laparotomy and hysterotomy. The fetus is extracted partially, undergoes surgery, and is subsequently returned into the amniotic cavity. The uterus and membranes are then closed. The fetus is ultimately delivered by caesarean section a few weeks later. The conditions in which open fetal surgery has been performed are:

- Repair of diaphragmatic hernia
- Tracheal ligation for diaphragmatic hernia
- Cystostomy or ureterostomy for osbtructive uropathy
- Ligation of sacrococcygeal teratoma
- Selective fetectomy for acardiac twin or twin transfusion syndrome

Although most of the experience has been gained in the management of fetuses with congenital diaphragmatic hernia[19], other conditions such as obstructive uropathy[20] and sacrococcygeal teratoma[21] have also been addressed using this approach.

A number of concepts have been drawn from the vast experience of these groups:

- Prenatal intervention is justified in certain conditions and under certain circumstances to prevent further organ damage or death, as elegantly shown in animal models of fetal obstructive uropathy[22]
- Surgical healing within the amniotic cavity seems to differ from that which occurs in the extrauterine environment, such that scar formation is either absent or significantly reduced[23]
- The placenta and the intrauterine environment provide stable and ideal postoperative conditions for the fetus in terms of temperature and nutrient supplies, but probably have a limited ability to respond to acute haemodynamic or hydrostatic changes
- The incidence of uterine contractions, preterm labour and rupture of membranes is directly related to the degree of trauma to the uterus and membranes[15]
- Most fetal and maternal complications are directly related to preterm labour, which has been difficult or impossible to control

The complications associated with open fetal surgery,

- Preterm labour
- Premature rupture of membranes
- Abruptio placenta
- Amniotic bands
- Fetal intracranial haemorrhage
- Maternal pulmonary oedema
- Need to deliver by caesarean section

are mostly related to the 'unforgiving nature' of the pregnant uterus to the injury inflicted by the scalpel, and they have limited the scope in which this approach can be applied. These limitations, and the significantly invasive nature of this type of surgery, are also responsible for the lack of widespread acceptance of this approach for the management of complex congenital anomalies.

Endoscopic fetal surgery: operative fetoscopy

Historically, fetal endoscopy preceded ultrasound and several other diagnostic and therapeutic modalities in fetal medicine. Originally described in 1954 in an isolated report[24], fetoscopy reached its height in the late 1970s and mid 1980s as a technique to visualize the fetus, and to aid in obtaining tissue samples or fetal blood (Fig. 57.1). Despite its initial promise, fetoscopy was only performed in selected centres throughout the world. The invasive nature of the procedure, the limited field and depth of view, particularly if intraamniotic bleeding occurred, limited its use. The development and widespread use of diagnostic ultrasound and of ultrasound-guided invasive procedures quickly displaced fetoscopy as a diagnostic and therapeutic tool.

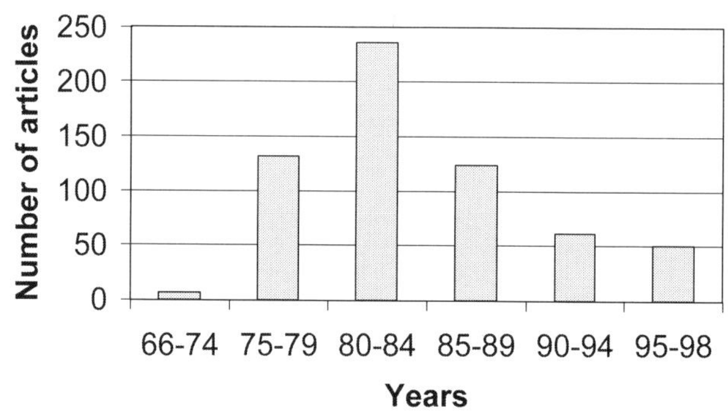

Fig. 57.1 Distribution of publications in fetoscopy in the last 20 years.

Beginning in 1980, an endoscopic revolution began to take place in medicine as a result of the advances made in visualization technology and surgical instruments. The use of bipolar electrocoagulation, the addition of video, and the development of endoscopic surgical instruments changed the outlook of virtually every surgical speciality. These advances have been particularly prominent in general surgery, with the laparoscopic performance of relatively complex operations such as cholecystectomies[25]. Such progress has been more slowly incorporated into gynaecological surgery, but has steadily gained acceptance and support.

Given that most complications associated with open fetal surgery are related to the degree of trauma to the uterus and membranes, it is only logical to assume that an endoscopic approach to surgically correctable fetal disorders, with its attending lesser degree of trauma to the uterus and fetal membranes, should be associated with better outcomes. The same basic principles that guide endoscopic surgery in other fields, i.e., minimal invasiveness and lesser morbidity, take on a different meaning from the savings in cost or length of hospital stay when extrapolated into endoscopic fetal surgery. Indeed, less morbidity in operative fetoscopy is synonymous with a greater likelihood that the pregnancy will not be lost as a consequence of the intervention. Therefore, the efforts in fetal surgery should concentrate on developing endoscopic or minimally invasive techniques to correct birth defects currently managed by open fetal surgery, and to address others that may have seemed impossible to address until now.

Developing endoscopic surgical techniques to operate inside the pregnant uterus practically entails developing a whole new surgical field. The unique working environment – the amniotic fluid, the access methods, the operating instruments – all constitute areas that need research and development. The following sections address the progress made in these areas by ourselves and other groups, and some clinical applications of these concepts.

Animal experimentation

A number of animal experiments have been performed using endoscopic techniques, some specific to the treatment of a particular condition, others addressing the endoscopic techniques themselves. We have performed endoscopic procedures in the non-pregnant rabbit under a fluid level (hydrolaparoscopy) using custom-designed 2 mm instruments[26]. The use of such small instruments within a limited space has allowed us to extrapolate our experience more readily into clinical human work. In this model, dissection, electrocoagulation, and extracorporeal knots were performed with excellent results. Estes et al. have used endoscopy and custom-designed 5 mm instruments to repair an experimentally created cleft lip in the fetal lamb. Healing of the lip incision was virtually unnoticeable at birth[27]. De Lia used a YAG-laser to photocoagulate placental surface vessels in a pregnant non-human-primate model[28]. This experience has been extrapolated to humans for the management of pregnancies affected by twin–twin transfusion syndrome[29–32], and acardiac twins (Ville, and Quintero, International Fetal Medicine Society, Antwerp, Belgium, unpublished results).

Luks et al. have created an endoscopic model of urinary tract obstruction in the lamb by ligating the urachus and the fetal urethra of male fetuses. The urinary tract obstruction was subsequently treated endoscopically with a cystostomy[33]. This group has also performed fetal laryngoscopy and bronchoscopy to occlude the trachea[34]. This accomplishment is quite promising for the management of fetuses with diaphragmatic hernia, as will be discussed below.

Concepts

A number of concepts and conclusions have been derived from the animal work. However, a direct application of many of these concepts into human clinical applications may not be feasible. For example, most animal surgery has been performed with 5 mm instruments[27,34,35]. The use of these relatively wide instruments in the human uterus is likely to be associated with greater maternal and fetal morbidity. Secondly, most animal work has been performed through a laparotomy, without the use of ultrasound, which, as will be seen, is essential for clinical work. Therefore, additional concepts need to be incorporated to make human endoscopic fetal surgery possible.

ACCESS

Entry into the amniotic cavity can be performed percutaneously, or through a small laparotomy. The percutaneous approach is less traumatic, can be performed as an outpatient procedure, and can be used provided that the size of the instruments is small (usually less than 3 mm). In the technique described by us, 2 mm instruments are used, which require a minimal skin incision[36]. If a minilaparotomy is done to access the uterus, a 2–3 cm incision is made in the maternal abdomen[31], and the trocar is introduced through the myometrium into the amniotic cavity. A purse string is tied around the entry site to avoid amniotic fluid leakage.

There are no trocars specifically designed to enter the amniotic cavity. Currently available trocars for adult or pediatric laparoscopy are at least 5 mm in inner diameter (6–7 mm outer diameter). In addition, most rigid endoscopes are equipped with thick protecting sheaths that keep them from bending. In order to facilitate human work, we have developed special 2–3 mm trocars in varying lengths. A checkflow valve at the hub of the trocar prevents amniotic fluid leakage. In addition, a plastic side arm with a valve allows the infusion of fluid or removal of amniotic fluid as desired.

THE WORKING ENVIRONMENT: FLUID OR GAS

Laparoscopy uses gas as a distension medium. Fetoscopic work within a gaseous medium, as opposed to liquid, would have several advantages. Firstly, the techniques used in laparoscopy would be more easily translated into operative fetoscopy. Secondly, visualization under gas is superior to that under fluid, particularly if the amniotic fluid cavity is turbid or if intraamniotic bleeding has occurred. Unfortunately, fetal acidosis has been reported in fetal lambs when endoscopic work was performed under a CO_2/fluid medium[27,35]. An additional limitation of using gas in the amniotic cavity is that it would not allow the concomitant use of ultrasound. Therefore, a fluid environment appears to be necessary, and unique techniques need to be developed to operate within this medium.

VISUALIZATION

The exchange of amniotic fluid for lactated Ringer's is a necessity for several reasons. We and others have found that light transmission through human amniotic fluid is significantly less than through air or physiological solution[37,38]. In addition to the baseline limitations, visualization through amniotic fluid may be further hindered by previous blood-staining from preoperative cordocentesis, from intraamniotic bleeding during surgery, or from excessive vernix.

The infusion of fluid into the amniotic cavity has been used clinically with protocols designed to decrease the incidence of abnormal fetal heart rate patterns in labour[39], for the prevention of meconium aspiration syndrome[40] and in the management of certain fetuses with oligohydramnios[41]. Extrapolating from this experience, we have developed a technique to exchange the amniotic fluid during endoscopic fetal surgery. In our current technique, a suction/irrigation pump with manual pressure calibration is attached to the sideports of the trocars. This system can rapidly clear the amniotic fluid in cases of intraamniotic bleeding, without altering the total amniotic fluid volume. Different ports are preferred for irrigation and suction, although the exchange can also be performed in an alternative fashion through a single port.

IMAGE DISPLAY

Given the restrictions in the instrument size, the panoramic view provided by larger endoscopes (e.g., 10 mm) cannot be enjoyed in operative fetoscopy. Instead, one is limited to the small field of view provided by relatively small endoscopes (1.9 mm). To offset this limitation, we use ultrasound to guide the insertion of the instruments into the amniotic cavity, and for orientation during surgery. To coordinate both images, we use a videomixer, a device that displays simultaneously or selectively the endoscopic and the sonographic image on a single monitor (Plate 57.1). By definition, the videomixer reduces by half the number of monitors needed in the room. As with videolaparoscopy, we place a monitor on each side of the patient's bed so that all members of the surgical team can monitor the procedure adequately.

ENDOSCOPES

Naturally, the endoscopes are a key element in performing endoscopic fetal surgery. A number of endoscopes are currently available in different specialities, but no endoscope is specifically designed for fetoscopic surgery at the present time. Table 57.1 shows a classification of available endoscopes according to their characteristics. We have concluded in fact that different endoscopes are necessary for different procedures[36]. The smallest endoscope is chosen whenever possible. For diagnostic procedures we prefer to use either a 0.7 mm flexible endoscope (Intramed Laboratories, San Diego, CA), or a 1.9 mm rigid scope (Richard Wolf Inc., Vernon Hills, IL), but we have used endoscopes as large as 2.5 mm, and 5 mm. Wider fibreoptic endoscopes may not be necessarily associated with a better image, as they often retain the same optical resolution but increase the scope diameter with irrigation or working channels.

TABLE 57.1
Functional characteristics of currently available endoscopes that can be used in operative fetoscopy

Constitution	Consistency	Function	Manoeuvrability
Fibreoptic	Flexible	Diagnostic	Passive
Solid rod lens	Rigid	Operating	Steerable
Multilens	—	—	—

The length of the endoscope is also important. It must be longer than the trocars, so that it can reach the amniotic cavity, and preferably be able to span the length of the whole amniotic cavity. This is particularly important if the fetus changes position during the operation. Figure 57.2 shows

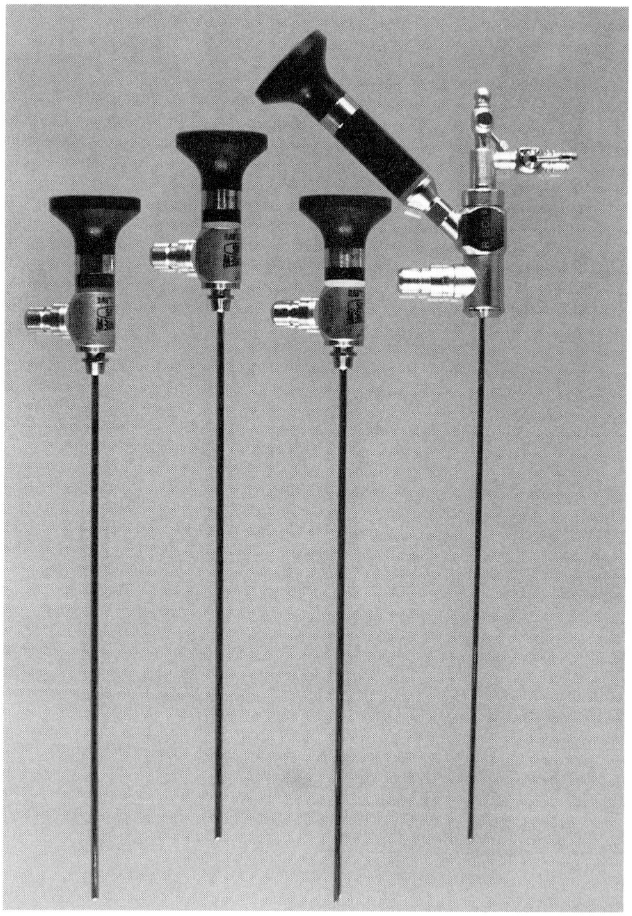

Fig. 57.2 Selection of endoscopes currently in use. Modifications of working ports, construction materials, and other technical aspects are often necessary to improve performance.

some of the endoscopes we currently use, including some specifically designed by us.

SURGICAL INSTRUMENTS

As with the endoscopes, there is currently no given set of instruments specifically designed for operative fetoscopy. Therefore, a significant amount of research time is devoted to either identifying available products that may be adapted to operative fetoscopy, or actually designing them (Table 57.2). Unfortunately, only a small selection of instruments at or below the 3 mm range is currently available. If the instruments are 1 mm or less in diameter, they can be introduced through the working channel of some endoscopes (operating endoscopes), obviating the need for a second port. If 5 mm instruments could be safely used for intrauterine surgery, a wider variety of instruments are available.

TABLE 57.2
Instruments designed and adapted for operative fetoscopy

Designed	Adapted
Trocars	Forceps
Blunt probe	Scissors
Knot pushers	Electrodes
Knot cutters	Wire guides
Bipolar electrocautery scapel	Laser fibres
Bipolar forceps	
Monopolar electrodes	

PRESSURE/VOLUME REGULATION

The amniotic fluid pressure rises linearly by 1 mmHg per litre of physiological fluid infused[42]. In our procedures, we maintain a baseline level of amniotic fluid, unless it is abnormally high or low to begin with. In our initial cases we monitored the intraamniotic pressure several times during surgery. As we did not notice significant variations (1–2 mmHg), we have not continued this practice. However, as many of our cases were performed under general anaesthesia, this may have blunted any possible pressure changes. In our current technique, an even exchange of amniotic fluid is performed to diminish the likelihood of significant pressure changes.

SAFETY

The potential for maternal or fetal injury exists, particularly when wide trocars (e.g., 3.5 mm) are used. As stated, some investigators perform a minilaparotomy when using these relatively large endoscopes to avoid injuring uterine vessels, as well as to place a purse string stitch around the endoscope to prevent fluid leakage.

Data regarding the pregnancy loss rate associated with fetoscopy is limited to the few series that have been performed in ongoing pregnancies. Hobbins and Mahoney reported two losses among 65 patients (3%) in continuing pregnancies[43]. They used an endoscope of 1.7 mm in diameter inserted transabdominally through a 2.2 × 2.7 mm cannula in patients at risk for haemoglobinopathies and other genetic disorders. Rodeck, using a similar endoscope, had a 3.7% pregnancy loss rate among 108 patients who underwent transabdominal fetoscopy for fetal blood sampling, skin biopsy, or evaluation for suspected anomalies[44]. An additional 37 patients underwent pregnancy termination based on the results of the examination. Therefore, a 3.0–3.7% figure likely approximates a corrected pregnancy loss rate associated with transabdominal fetoscopy.

Approximately 5–7% of patients in the above mentioned series experienced amniotic fluid leakage, though the majority had a successful outcome[43,44]. The corresponding figure of 1% to 1.3% associated with second trimester amniocentesis[45], probably reflects the use of a smaller bore instrument in this latter technique.

The potential teratogenic effect of light or heat on the developing concepts has been mentioned since the inception of fetoscopy. However, there is a scarcity of literature evaluating this issue. Hyperthermia is a known human teratogen, primarily affecting the central nervous system, with the most significant manifestations (neural tube defects) occurring if exposure takes place during the 21th–28th day postconception period. A threshold of approximately 1.5–2.5°C is required before effects are seen. A considerable amount of heat can be generated at the light cord/endoscope interface. We have not been able to show any significant temperature elevation at the tip of the endoscope in a water bath, using a 2.7 mm endoscope for over 30 min[38]. In addition, embryoscopy or fetoscopy are performed after the period of neural tube closure. Therefore, it is unlikely that the use of endoscopes inside the amniotic cavity would be associated with heat teratogenicity.

The potential harmful effect of light on the developing visual pathway has also been a concern for over 20 years. The human optic vesicle is visible from the sixth to ninth week of menstrual age. The eyelids are fused beyond 9–10 weeks. Experiments using red laser light focused on the optic vesicles of chick embryos at stages 10–20 have resulted in several anomalies, including microphthalmia, and anophthalmia[46]. Other experiments, using white light, have shown alterations in the pineal gland of chick embryos[47]. In our own experiments, we have used a 2.7 mm endoscope and a 300 W xenon light source for 5 min directed at the optic vesicle of chick embryos at stage E10, equivalent to 10–12 weeks of gestation in the human. In this setting, we have been unable to show any histological alterations in the retina, nor any alteration in the pattern of neurotransmitter transport from the retina to the optic colliculi[48]. Chick embryos exposed to the above conditions, when allowed to hatch, were able to feed normally when the unexposed eye was covered. Based on these results, white light as provided by an endoscope probably lacks any teratogenic potential on the developing visual organs. Vandenberghe et al. have performed light exposure experiments in the fetal lamb, showing no obvious damage to the fetal retina[37]. Despite these negative results, we suggest that fetal endoscopy should probably be performed beyond the time of the fusion of the eyelids, i.e., at approximately 9–10 weeks' gestation (menstrual age), as the actual threshold at which endoscopic white light may cause visual damage has not been established.

Clinical applications

In the following sections, we will discuss the specific entities in which operative fetoscopy has been used, as well as those in which this approach could be potentially applied.

TWIN-TO-TWIN TRANSFUSION SYNDROME

Twin-to-twin transfusion syndrome appears to result from a net unbalanced flow of blood between two fetuses sharing a common placenta. In the classic model, an artery from one twin supplies a placental cotyledon, which in turn is drained by a vein to the cotwin[49]. Therefore, blood is shunted from one twin, the donor; and transfused to the cotwin, the recipient, through placental vascular anastomoses. Monochorionic placentas usually exhibit various degrees of shared fetal circulation[50]. Injection studies of twin placentas[51] have shown that these anastomoses are almost universally present in monochorionic placentas but are rare in dichorionic placentas. In the case of monochorionic placentas these anastomoses commonly take the form of arterioarterial anastomoses, but sometimes venous anastomoses can also be found[52]. The anastomoses can be superficial, deep, or both superficial and deep, but eventually all vessels come to the surface of the placenta. The most common superficial types are artery-to-artery (28%) in conjunction with artery-to-vein anastomoses (28%), followed by arteriovenous anastomoses (11%). An average of 3.1 anastomoses per placenta are present in each twin pair.

In twin-to-twin transfusion syndrome the anastomoses generally take the form of artery-to-vein communications[52]. These shunts may be single or multiple and result in a net transfer of blood from one twin to the other. Both acute and chronic forms of the twin-to-twin transfusion syndrome have been described[53,54]. The acute form results in a hypovolaemic, anaemic donor twin and a hypervolaemic, plethoric recipient twin of similar birthweight, due to a rapid transfer of blood through superficial artery-to-artery or vein-to-vein anastomoses during labour and delivery. The chronic form has been attributed to a gradual antepartum transfusion mostly through deep artery-to-vein connections.

Vascular anastomoses are probably formed when angiogenesis of the placenta is taking place, but may become functional during any stage of the pregnancy, during labour and delivery, or not at all. An anastomosis may cease to function after the death of one fetus, when the shared circulation stops. Likewise, these anastomoses may insidiously function producing the chronic form of the syndrome and/or abruptly become permeable, leading to acute and frequently fatal transfusion.

Despite the high frequency of occurrence of vascular anastomoses in monochorionic placentation, twin-to-twin transfusion syndrome occurs only in 5.5–17.5%[51,53,55–57] of monochorionic gestations. It is important to point out that this variation may be related to the criteria used to make the diagnosis of the syndrome in the neonatal period. Standard diagnostic criteria for chronic twin-to-twin transfusion syndrome are an intertwin haemoglobin difference >5 g/dL[58] and a birthweight difference >20%[53]. However, in a study done by Danskin and Neilson[59] on 178 twin pairs, only four pairs had a haemoglobin difference >5 g/dL and a weight difference >20%, and none of these pregnancies showed evidence of polyhydramnios or oligohydramnios. Therefore, the standard criteria used in clinical obstetrics do not permit a definitive diagnosis of twin-to-twin transfusion.

Sonographic criteria for the syndrome have also been proposed. Wittman et al. suggested that the diagnosis be based on a discrepancy greater than 10 mm of either the biparietal diameter or the transverse diameter of the trunk between the twins, and on the hydramnios surrounding the larger twin[60]. Brennan et al. suggested that the presence of same sex, disparity in size or in the number of vessels in the umbilical cords, single placenta with different echogenicity of the cotyledons supplying the two cords, and evidence of hydrops in either twin or congestive heart failure in the recipient be added to the criteria[56]. In the extreme presentation, there is polyhydramnios in the sac of one twin, and severe oligohydramnios in the sac of the other, such that this latter fetus appears pressed against the uterine wall (stuck twin syndrome).

Doppler studies have been equivocal in the prenatal diagnosis of twin-to-twin transfusion syndrome. Farmakides et al.[57] found that the umbilical artery systolic/diastolic (UA S/D) ratio was low in the recipient and high in the donor in two twin pairs. An intertwin difference greater than 0.4 in the UA S/D ratio was associated with a growth discordance of at least 350 g. Pretorius et al.[61] found abnormal blood flow in the umbilical artery and vein and tricuspid insufficiency in eight twin transfusion cases. Giles et al.[62] reported differences of less than 1 (mean 0.4 ± 0.2) in the UA S/D ratio of 11 pairs of twins with twin-to-twin transfusion syndrome, indicating that the UA S/D ratios were concordant even in the presence of discordant fetal size. Ishimatsu et al.[63] reported that umbilical artery blood flow velocity is not useful to diagnose twin transfusion syndrome or to differentiate donor and recipient fetus, but that cardiomegaly may be an early sign of haemodynamic change in the recipient fetus. Yamada et al.[64] showed a positive correlation between the difference in pulsatility index and in estimated fetal weight in cases of twin-to-twin transfusion syndrome, but not in discordant or concordant twins.

Cordocentesis to assess fetal anaemia and zygosity has also been used in twin transfusion syndrome. An intertwin Hb concentration difference greater than 0.5 g/dL was found by Fisk et al. in only one of three twin pairs sampled[65]. Saunders et al. found only a mean difference of 1.7 g/dL in four twin pairs[66]. Tanaka et al.[67] have suggested infusion of pancuronium bromide into one cord to produce paralysis of the other fetus ('pancuronium test') to demonstrate transplacental communications. However, as some form of communication is virtually universally present, this finding does not establish the diagnosis by itself.

Expectant or medical management of twin-to-twin transfusion syndrome has been associated with virtually 100% perinatal mortality[68]. Treatment with digoxin or with indomethacin has been attempted, with little success[69,70]. Given these poor results, invasive treatment options have been proposed. These include serial amniocentesis[71,72], coagulation of surface placental vessels[29–31], selective feticide[73], or selective fetectomy[74]. Serial amniocentesis in the sac of the recipient twin (polyhydramnios) occasionally results in expansion of the sac of the stuck twin, presumably through improved circulation and increased urine production of this fetus. An overall 50–60% survival rate has been reported with serial amniocentesis[75]. Despite initial enthusiasm, the support for this approach has dwindled, because it does not correct the underlying problem, requires multiple procedures, and is unlikely to be successful in cases far from viability. Additional problems include infection, rupture of membranes, disruption of the dividing membrane, and placental abruptio due to quick removal of large amounts of amniotic fluid. In addition, death of one of the twins may result in death of the other fetus, or porencephalic cysts and other major neurological complications in the other twin[76–79]. Originally, these complications were thought to result from the release of thromboplastic substances from the dead twin into the surviving twin. More recently, however, acute anaemia has been documented in the surviving twin, suggesting that perhaps hypotension from acute bleeding into the dead twin may be responsible for the observed complications[80,81].

If the underlying pathophysiological mechanisms are indeed an uneven sharing of blood between the fetuses, it would only seem logical that interruption of the vascular communications between the fetuses through the placenta would correct the problem. De Lia first advocated the use of neodymium:YAG laser under endoscopic control to photocoagulate surface-communicating vessels between the two placental areas[28]. To access the amniotic cavity, he performed a minilaparotomy and placed a purse string suture around the trocar to prevent amniotic fluid leakage. Patients with an anterior placenta were excluded. In his last report[82] 22 patients had been treated, and results were available on 19. Overall 56% (20 of 38) of fetuses survived. Recently, Ville et al., using a percutaneous approach, reported at least one survivor in 70% of cases (21 of 30) with YAG laser photocoagulation, versus 44% (11 of 25) of those treated with amniodrainage, a difference that was statistically significant[32]. We have had experience with photocoagulation in 14 patients with twin-to-twin transfusion syndrome, most of which had an anterior placenta. To target vessels in anterior placentas, we use flexible steerable endoscopes. As with other operative fetoscopic procedures, we use a percutaneous approach and combined sonographic–endoscopic guidance with a videomixer. Forty-three percent of our cases were also complicated by hydrops of the recipient twin. Despite this very high risk group, our survival rates are 50% for at least one fetus surviving. Table 57.3 compares the outcome of fetuses with twin-to-twin transfusion syndrome treated expectantly, with amniodrainage, or with laser photocoagulation.

TABLE 57.3
Treatment of twin–twin transfusion

Treatment	n	Both alive	One alive	None alive
Conservative[a]	106	0	5 (4.7%)	101
Amniocentesis[b]	103	39 (37.8%)	22 (21.4%)	42 (40.7%)
Laser[c]	52	17 (32.6%)	22 (42.3%)	13 (25%)

Comparison between serial amniocentesis and laser treatment shows a trend towards better outcome (survival of at least one fetus) for the latter modality (chi squared = 3.0995, df = 1, p = 0.07, 95% confidence limits: 0.92–4.64)

[a]Data from reference 66
[b]Data from references 66 and 71, and Pinette, M.G. Pan, Y., Pinette, S.G. et al. (1993) Treatment of twin–twin transfusion syndrome. *Obstet. Gynecol.* **82**, 841; Mahony, B.S., Petty, C.N., Nyberg, D.A. et al. (1990) The 'stuck twin' phenomenon: ultrasonographic findings, pregnancy outcome, and management with serial amniocentesis. *Am. J. Obstet. Gynecol.* **163**, 1513
[c]Data from references 30, 32 and 82

Selective feticide has also been proposed in selected cases of twin-to-twin transfusion syndrome when one of the fetuses is deemed non-viable. Because of the presence of placental vascular communications, injection of potassium chloride into the cord of this twin may result in the death of both twins[83]. Cardiac tamponade has been successful in one report[84], but this technique may carry risks similar to those of potassium chloride injection. An extravascular approach to interrupt the circulation of one of the fetuses avoids the complications of intravascular potassium chloride or coil injections. The technique of umbilical-cord ligation developed by us may be used in these cases. The procedure may be performed with combined sonographic–endoscopic guidance[85] or with the use of ultrasound alone[86,87]. We have treated three cases with this technique. In every case, the recipient twin was severely hydropic, with evidence of marked heart failure and poor heart contractility, and amniodrainage had been performed unsuccessfully several times at the referring institutions. The donor twin tolerated the procedure well. Umbilical cord ligation is probably the best alternative method for selective feticide in this context, allowing one fetus to survive. In addition, it eliminates the likelihood of postmortem feto-fetal haemorrhage and its attendant morbidity. However, this technique should only be considered if there is reasonable evidence that one of the fetuses will spontaneously die.

ACARDIAC TWINS

Twin reverse arterial perfusion sequence (TRAP sequence) affects 1% of monozygotic twins or 1:35 000 births[88] or 1:30 triplets. The proposed pathophysiology for this condition is that in the presence of artery-to-artery and vein-to-vein anastomoses in a monozygotic placenta, a haemodynamically advantaged twin (pump twin) perfuses the other twin (perfused twin) via retrograde flow[89]. Inadequate perfusion of the recipient twin is responsible for the development of a characteristic and invariably lethal set of anomalies including acardia and acephalus. The diagnosis of acardiac twin is made by pulsed and colour Doppler by demonstrating arterial blood flow perfusing the acardiac twin in a retrograde fashion. Typically, the pump twin is structurally normal, but it is at risk for developing in utero cardiac failure, and without treatment dies in 50–75% of cases, particularly if the acardiac/pump twin size ratio is greater than 50%[6]. Subtle signs of haemodynamic decompensation in the pump twin include enlarged right atrium, increased reverse flow in the inferior vena cava, reverse flow in the ductus venosus, or pulsatile flow in the umbilical vein, all of which may occur prior to the appearance of ascites and oedema.

The therapeutic goal of interrupting the vascular communication between the two twins, although simple in concept[90], has been difficult to accomplish. Prior to our description of the technique of umbilical-cord ligation, selective delivery of the acardiac twin – or sectio parva – was the preferred method of treatment[91–93]. Sectio parva requires a laparotomy and hysterotomy and the patient must subsequently be delivered by caesarean section. Abruptio placenta, preterm labour, preterm birth and prolonged maternal hospitalization are other complications of this technique. Ultrasound-directed percutaneous thrombosis of the umbilical cord of the acardiac twin with thrombogenic coils or fibrin superglue has also been proposed[94–97]. Unfortunately, although technically easier, this method has been associated with death of both twins and recanalization of the umbilical arterial flow after the procedure[95,97].

We proposed a percutaneous extravascular approach to ligate the cord of the acardiac twin[85]. The ports are introduced into the amniotic cavity under ultrasound guidance. Ultrasound is essential to identifying the correct cord, as well as to identify placental-free areas through which the trocars can be introduced. An endoscope is delivered intraamniotically to monitor the surgical procedure. As the acardiac twin usually lacks any amniotic fluid, access to the umbilical cord may be hindered by the amniotic membrane of this twin. Therefore, an amnioinfusion or amniorrhexis of this sac needs to be performed in order to reach the umbilical cord. Through the other port, a 3–0 Vicryl suture is passed with a small grasper beneath the umbilical cord (Plate 57.2). The suture is grasped on the opposite side of the cord and retrieved outside the maternal abdomen. An extracorporeal knot is tied and delivered intraamniotically with a knot-pusher to occlude the cord[98]. The procedure is repeated for safety, and the suture is cut with small scissors inside the amniotic cavity.

Endoscopic umbilical-cord ligation is the first surgical procedure to be performed in a human pregnancy using more than one port. It exemplifies many of the concepts needed to perform operative fetoscopy, including the combined use of ultrasound, videomixer, amnioinfusion, suture material, and specialized instruments.

AMNIOTIC BAND SYNDROME

The differential diagnosis of the sonographic identification of echoreflective membranes within the amniotic cavity includes amniotic band syndrome (ABS), amniotic sheets or shelves, amniochorion separation, and subchorionic haematomas[99]. Useful differential diagnostic criteria have been proposed to distinguish between all of these conditions[100–102]. The sonographic diagnosis of ABS is suggested by the presence of eccentric encephaloceles, cleft lip/palate, abdominal or thoracic wall defects, or amputation of extremities, in addition to restriction of fetal movements or evidence of membrane attachment to the fetus.

The aetiology of ABS is not well understood. Streeter[103] suggested that the amniotic bands are secondary to an in utero vascular insult, which is also responsible for the associated fetal anomalies. This theory is supported by the finding of concomitant anomalies of internal organs in the fetus, which cannot be explained by amniotic constrictions[104–106]. On the other hand, Torpin argued that rupture of the amnion early in pregnancy could be associated with limb amputations and other characteristic birth defects; this theory was based on placental pathological analyses[107]. A third theory suggests that the disorder may be of genetic origin, as occurs with a strain of mice in whom the presence of a Disorganization gene has been proposed[108]. A familial occurrence of ABS has also been reported[109].

Some fetuses with ABS may show signs of venous stasis and oedema of an extremity without evidence of amputation. It is thought that in such cases endoscopic release of the amniotic bands could be of benefit. We have had the opportunity to examine two fetuses thought to have ABS[36]. Endoscopic visualization of the membranes revealed no signs of entrapment or impending fetal danger in one case, but significant limitation of movement of the mouth in a second case. Hydrodissection of the membranes in the latter case demonstrated webbing of membranes into the fetal mouth. In addition, a tight membrane could be identified arising from the umbilical cord. The first fetus was born without anomalies. The second fetus showed a constriction ring in one of the extremities. In both cases, the addition of fetoscopy aided in establishing the correct diagnosis.

It is conceivable that selected fetuses affected by ABS may warrant endoscopic release of the bands. Further experience in this area is needed to evaluate the indications and limitations of operative fetoscopy in these cases.

LOWER OBSTRUCTIVE UROPATHY

Fetal lower urinary tract obstruction is a sporadic condition that affects 1:5000–8000 males[110]. Untreated, the obstruction may lead to hydronephrosis, renal dysplasia, and perinatal death[4,111]. Prenatally diagnosed cases of posterior urethral valves have a 30–50% mortality. Death is attributable to pulmonary hypoplasia and/or renal dysplasia.

The sonographic diagnosis of fetal lower urinary tract obstruction is suggested by the presence of a dilated and thickened bladder, hydroureters, hydronephrosis, and oligohydramnios[112]. These findings, in the presence of a male fetus, are highly suggestive of posterior urethral valves. However, other aetiologies, such as urethral stricture or atresia, urethral agenesis, ureteral reflux, persistent cloaca, and megalourethra, can present with a very similar sonographic image[112,113]. Thus, precise diagnosis can only be made after birth.

The management of patients with sonographic findings of lower urinary tract obstruction (LUTO) is outlined in Fig. 57.3. A careful ultrasound examination is performed to rule out associated major congenital anomalies[112]. Sonographic evidence of renal cystic dysplasia and the volume of amniotic fluid are also noted, as they have prognostic value (Table 57.4)[114]. Serial vesicocenteses are performed to assess the functional status of the fetal kidneys[115,116]. A single vesicocentesis may not adequately reflect the renal reserve, such that two consecutive samples may be on different sides of the normal cutoff level[117]. Table 57.5 shows the fetal urinary cutoff values used to predict a normal or abnormal neonatal outcome.

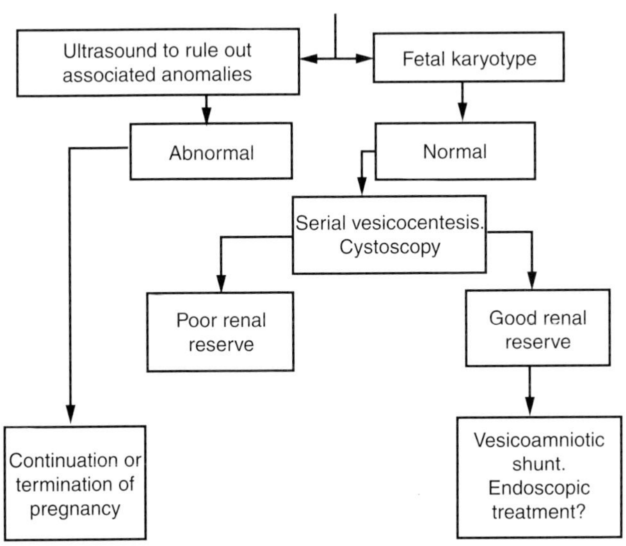

Fig. 57.3 Algorithm used for the management of fetuses with sonographic evidence of lower obstructive uropathy. The value of fetal cystoscopy in the diagnosis and possible treatment of these fetuses is presently being evaluated.

TABLE 57.4
Prognostic sonographic findings in fetuses with obstructive uropathy

	Sensitivity	Specificity	Positive pred. V.	Negative pred. V
Renal cysts	44	100	100	44
Hyperechogenic renal parenchyma	73	80	89	57
Hydronephrosis	41	73	78	35
Oligohydramnios	35	96	86	69

Modified from reference 114 and Muller, F., Dommergues, M., Mandelbrot, L. et al. (1993) Fetal urinary biochemistry predicts postnatal renal function in children with bilateral obstructive uropathies. *Obstet. Gynecol.* **82**:813

TABLE 57.5
Ability of biochemical threshold values to predict absence of renal dysplasia

	Sensitivity	Specificity	Positive pred. V	Negative pred V.
Na^+ < 100 mg/dL	56	64	56	88
Ca^{++} < 8 mg/dL	100	27	43	100
Osmolality < 200 mOsm/L	83	82	71	90
β-2-μglobulin < 4 mg/L	17	36	100	44
Total protein < 20 mg/dL	67	91	80	83

Data from reference 117

Ultrasound-guided vesicoamniotic shunts have been suggested for the treatment of fetuses with LUTO since 1982[12–14]. The deviation of fetal urine into the amniotic cavity serves a dual purpose: it prevents the renal damage that may result from the urinary obstruction, and it allows normal pulmonary development. The rationale for this therapy is based on animal studies in which ligation of the ureters[118] or of the urethra and urachus[119] of fetal lambs in midgestation produced renal dysplasia, and pulmonary hypoplasia. Decompression of the obstruction resulted in resolution of the urinary obstruction and improved pulmonary status at birth[120]. Experience with percutaneous vesicoamniotic shunting in humans, collected at the International Fetal Surgery Registry, shows a 5% procedure-related loss, and a 48% survival rate (40 of 83 treated fetuses). Of the treated fetuses, 74% with posterior urethral valves survived, in contrast to a 45% fetal loss rate reported in untreated fetuses with posterior urethral valves[4]. Survivors with total urethral obstruction, as with urethral atresia or agenesis, are extremely rare[121].

Treatment of fetuses with LUTO with urinary diversion procedures has significant limitations. First, they are palliative measures that defer the final treatment of the obstruction until the birth of the child. Second, vesicoamniotic shunts may become obstructed or displaced in up to 25% of cases[122], requiring additional interventions to replace the shunt, with their attendant complications. Fetal vesicostomy or ureterostomy via open fetal surgery have been proposed[123] to overcome the problems associated with the percutaneous shunts, but they have not gained support.

We have introduced the concept of performing percutaneous fetal cystoscopy to evaluate fetuses affected with LUTO[124,125]. This procedure uses the same techniques and skills as fetal vesicocentesis. A thin endoscope is passed through the lumen of the needle or trocar to observe the fetal bladder at the time of the vesicocentesis. The elements in the trigone can be identified, and the diagnosis of urethral obstruction can be confirmed or ruled out. The endoscope is then removed, and the bladder is drained. Fetal cystoscopy may also be used therapeutically. Indeed, we have performed ablation of posterior urethral valves in a fetus at 24 weeks of gestation[124]. To accomplish this, we inserted an operating endoscope towards the posterior urethra, and advanced an electrode through the operating channel of the endoscope. The valves were electrocauterized under direct endoscopic visualization, and urethral patency was confirmed by instilling physiological solution into the amniotic cavity transurethrally. We have subsequently used YAG laser energy to ablate the valves on eight additional cases, with documentation of urethral patency (Plate 57.3). Unfortunately, there are no survivors at the present time, but one patient is undelivered and doing well.

We hypothesize that percutaneous fetal cystoscopy may allow a more precise prenatal diagnosis and prognosis in fetuses with lower urinary tract obstruction. Since this procedure can be performed at the time of diagnostic vesicocentesis, it should not pose additional risks to the standard assessment of fetal renal function. In addition, those fetuses truly identified as having posterior valves may fare better if the obstruction can be eliminated in utero, avoiding the complications of vesicoamniotic shunts or the morbidity of open fetal surgery.

CHORIOANGIOMA

Chorioangiomas are the most common placental tumour, occurring approximately in 1% of microscopically examined placentas. The incidence of chorioangioma is higher than realized, because many small lesions are overlooked on routine examinations of the placenta[126]. Chorioangiomas large enough for recognition at delivery occur approximately once in 13 000 deliveries[127], while careful sectioning of fixed placentas at 0.5 cm intervals followed by microscopic examinations of all macroscopic lesions detected chorioangiomas in five out of 500 unselected placentas. Chorioangiomas arise from angioblastic tissue. Histologically, they are not considered to be a true neoplasm, but rather a hamartoma.

Most tumours are located on the fetal surface of the placenta[128]. A few have been noted at the base of the umbilical cord entirely separated from the placenta, some emerging from the cord[129,130]. The vascular supply to the tumour is established by vessels that come from the umbilical cord vessels[131] or other vessels arising from the placenta. Occasionally a vascular pedicle approaching the tumour has been identified[127,132–134]. However, the blood supply of these tumours has not been well studied. Chorioangiomas differ in no essential respects from haemangiomas in other bodily sites[135].

Most tumours are asymptomatic[136] especially if small (<4 cm in diameter). Larger tumours may be clinically significant, and occur in approximately 1:3500 to 1:9000 births[137,138]. The most frequent clinical presentation is the onset of acute polyhydramnios, characterized by a rapid increase of amniotic fluid and marked uterine distension[139]. Common maternal complaints are abdominal pain, nausea, vomiting and dyspnoea in a previously normal pregnancy.

Large chorioangiomas have been associated with several fetal complications including polyhydramnios (18–35%), oligohydramnios[140], non-immune fetal hydrops[141], cardiomegaly with/or heart failure, growth retardation, dystocia[142], premature labour (10%), fetal thrombocytopenia[143], fetal malformations, microangiopathic haemolytic anaemia[144], and intrauterine fetal death (16%)[145]. Maternal complications include thrombocytopenia, coagulopathy[138], toxaemia[146], abruptio placentae, fetomaternal transfusion, haemolysis and haemoglobinuria[147].

Several potential pathophysiological mechanisms have been proposed to explain the maternal and fetal complications associated with large chorioangiomas. These include excessive transfer of fluid into the amniotic cavity from an increased tumoral vascular area, venous obstruction or functional insufficiency within the placenta, and fetal heart failure. Fetal heart failure may result from poorly oxygenated blood returning to the fetus following circulation through the non-functioning placental tissue. In addition, hypoalbuminaemia and anaemia may also be implicated. Antepartum haemorrhage has been reported in 15–20%[147] of these patients, possibly due to retroplacental bleeding or rupture of the vascular pedicle of the tumour[148]. Intrauterine fetal death may result from congestive heart failure, anaemia, or placental bleed. Neonatal mortality associated with large tumours has been estimated to range between 30% and 40%[144].

Chorioangiomas can be diagnosed with ultrasound as uniform and non-uniform echogenic, multicystic masses, or as complex masses. Colour Doppler[149] can be used to confirm the vascular nature of the mass. The flow pattern varies with the location of the tumour, and the size and number of vascular communications within the tumour. Hirata et al.[150]

demonstrated pulsatile blood flow in a placental chorioangioma using colour flow imaging and Doppler velocimetry. In addition, pulsed Doppler can help to differentiate in utero between maternal and fetal vascular placental abnormalities. Alphafetoprotein has also been used in the early detection of these tumours[151,152].

Management of patients with chorioangiomas should be individualized. Since maternal and fetal complications may lead to premature termination of the pregnancy or to premature birth, serial ultrasound examinations including fetal echocardiography are suggested to determine the optimal time of delivery. Premature labour, acute onset of polyhydramnios may require hospitalization, and the use of tocolytic agents.

Most patients diagnosed with chorioangiomas have been managed expectantly. A review of the literature shows an overall mortality rate of approximately 30%, half of which are due to intrauterine fetal demises. These figures are undoubtedly biased, as bad outcomes are less likely to be reported. Of the available reports, the most frequent cause of death was prematurity, followed by evidence of fetal heart failure or hydrops. However, since 1986, only two of 17 fetuses (11%) with chorioangioma have died. Specific risk factors associated with a higher risk of fetal or neonatal death have not been identified, particularly since many diagnoses have been made retrospectively, and standard parameters of evaluation have not been established. Nonetheless, it is fair to say that fetuses with overt signs of failure diagnosed prior to viability constitute the highest risk group, and in whom in utero intervention is more clearly indicated.

To date, cordocentesis has been used to manage three patients with chorioangiomas. Two fetuses were transfused and delivered within 24 h for fetal distress[153]. A third case was managed with serial intrauterine transfusions[150]. In this latter case, a 8.5 cm chorioangioma was diagnosed at 28 weeks. The patient complained of uterine contractions. Ultrasound showed a fetus with scalp oedema, and a small pericardial effusion. Colour Doppler studies confirmed the vascular nature of the tumour. Serial cordocenteses and intravascular fetal transfusions were performed, raising the initial haematocrit from 17% to 53%. The scalp oedema disappeared. The patient delivered prematurely 25 days later at approximately 32 weeks, and the fetus survived. De Lia in 1993[154] suggested an alternative treatment for these angiomatous tumours with fetoscopic laser photocoagulation of vessels nurturing the tumour. We recently had a patient with a large chorioangioma (9 cm) and a hydropic fetus at 24 weeks of gestation. Colour Doppler disclosed a large artery and vein located subchorionically. Haemodynamic evaluation of the fetus revealed signs of overt heart failure with pulsatile venous blood flow, enlarged right atrium, and tricuspid regurgitation. Cordocentesis revealed moderate fetal anaemia and hypoalbuminaemia. The vessels feeding the tumour appeared too large to be photocoagulated with neodynium:YAG laser. Endoscopically, the artery was dissected from the surface of the placenta, and a suture was placed around this vessel. Remaining vessels were obliterated with bipolar electrocautery. Unfortunately, the fetus did not tolerate the surgery and died 3 days later. Despite the untoward outcome, this case illustrates the possibility of interrupting the blood supply to the chorioangioma, and eliminating the shunt through this mass. We speculate that perhaps a combination of intravascular fetal transfusions and endoscopic coagulation or ligation of the feeding vessels may be warranted for severe cases detected prior to fetal viability.

Limitations of operative fetoscopy

The limitations that we have identified in performing operative fetoscopy are:

- Placental location
- Access
- Visualization
- Instruments
- Fetal position
- Premature rupture of membranes

The need for better instrumentation cannot be overemphasized. As Kurt Semm, a leader in gynaecological laparoscopy, has said, laparoscopic surgery should not be performed with any lesser availability of instruments than open surgery. As no specific instruments are available for operative fetoscopy, this statement is more so relevant, and should stress the need to continue to develop the necessary tools for this type of surgery.

Fetal position may be particularly limiting, and techniques to correct it are not available. Occasionally, external manoeuvres may change the position of the fetus in the uterus, but these are neither effective nor reliable. We have attempted to correct the fetal position from within the amniotic cavity with limited success. Further efforts to address this issue are being pursued.

The location of the placenta may also hinder the performance of operative fetoscopy. In open fetal surgery, if the placenta is anterior, the uterus is entered posteriorly. Although this technique is significantly more involved, it could be considered for operative fetoscopy in selected cases as well. Although we have been able to avoid entering the placenta in most cases, we have had one instance in which no space free of placenta could be found, and in which bleeding from transplacental insertion of the trocars, though not resulting in fetal morbidity, forced us to abandon the procedure.

Some conditions may never become amenable to an endoscopic approach. Such may be the case of cystic adenomatoid malformation of the lung, pulmonary sequestrations, large fetal tumours, or other complex fetal anomalies. These cases should probably continue to be managed by teams with significant expertise in open fetal surgery.

Future of operative fetoscopy

A great deal of interest in the management of fetuses with diaphragmatic hernia has been generated recently. Wilson and others have shown that tracheal ligation in fetal lambs with iatrogenic diaphragmatic hernias reverses the pathophysiologic effects of pulmonary hypoplasia[155–157]. The net accumulation of fluid in the tracheobronchial tree resulted in expanded lungs. Histological, molecular, and functional analysis of these lungs demonstrated cell proliferation and lack of arrest of pulmonary development. Using this experience, Harrison et al. have recently reported three cases of fetuses with diaphragmatic hernias, who underwent tracheal obstruction through open fetal surgery (International Fetal Medicine Society Meeting, Antwerp, Belgium, 1994, unpublished results). One fetus survived, requiring minimal ventilatory support at birth, and intubation for a few weeks after birth due to tracheal instability. The other two fetuses died from postoperative complications. These animal and clinical experiences are extremely encouraging, and may completely change our approach to fetuses with diaphragmatic hernias. If an endoscopic procedure could be devised to obstruct the fetal trachea, it is likely that better results with lesser morbidity would be achieved.

Other conditions for which endoscopic fetal surgery could be potentially used are:

- Urinary tract obstruction
- Diaphragmatic hernia
- Sacrococcygeal teratoma and other fetal tumours
- Laryngeal atresia
- Acqueductal stenosis
- Spina bifida
- GI obstruction

While much research is still needed to understand how these disorders could be addressed endoscopically in utero, it is clear that the list of conditions potentially amenable to in utero surgery is expanding as a result of the lesser morbidity associated with this technique. Further development of operative fetoscopy should make the fetus become a true endoscopic surgical patient.

REFERENCES

1. Kerr-Wilson R, Duncan A, Hume R et al. Prenatal pleural effusion associated with congenital pulmonary lymphangiectasia. *Prenat. Diagn.* **5**:73, 1985.
2. Carpenter M, Curci M, Dibbins A et al. Perinatal management of ventral wall defects. *Obstet. Gynecol.* **64**:646, 1984.
3. Muraji T, Twugawa C, Nishijima E et al. Gastroschisis: a 17-year experience. *J. Pediatr. Surg.* **24**:343, 1989.
4. Nakayama D, Harrison M & deLorimier A. Prognosis of posterior urethral valves present at birth. *J. Pediatr. Surg.* **21**:43, 1986.
5. Harrison M, Adzick N, Estes J et al. A prospective study of the outcome for fetuses with diaphragmatic hernia. *JAMA* **2**(271 (5)):382, 1994.
6. Moore T, Gale S & Benirschke K. Perinatal outcome of forty-nine pregnancies complicated by acardiac twinning. *Am. J. Obstet. Gynecol.* **163**:907, 1990.
7. Kerenyi T, Miller J, Steinfeld L et al. Transplacental cardioversion of intrauterine supraventricular tachycardia with digitalis. *Lancet* **2**:393, 1980.
8. Dumesic D, Silverman N, Tobias S et al. Transplacental cardioversion of fetal supraventricular tachycardia with procainamide. *N. Engl. J. Med.* **307**:1128, 1982.
9. Bussel J, Berkowitz R, McFarland J et al. Antenatal treatment of neonatal alloimmune thrombocytopenia. *N. Engl. J. Med.* **319**:1373, 1988.
10. Grannum P, Copel J, Plaxe S et al. In utero exchange transfusion by direct intravascular injection in severe erythroblastosis fetalis. *N. Engl. J. Med.* **314**:1431, 1986.
11. Rodeck C, Fisk N, Fraser D et al. Long-term in utero drainage of fetal hydrothorax. *N. Engl. J. Med.* **319**:1135, 1988.
12. Golbus M, Harrison M, Filly R et al. In utero treatment of urinary tract obstruction. *Am. J. Obstet. Gynecol.* **142**:383, 1982.
13. Berkowitz R, Glickmann M, Smith G et al. Fetal urinary tract obstruction: what is the role of surgical intervention in utero? *Am. J. Obstet. Gynecol.* **144**:367, 1982.
14. Rodeck C & Nicolaides K. Ultrasound guided invasive procedures in obstetrics. *Clin. Obstet. Gynecol.* **10**:515, 1983.
15. Nakayama D, Harrison M, Seron-Ferre M et al. Fetal surgery in the primate II. Uterine electromyographic response to operative procedures and pharmacologic agents. *J. Pediatr. Surg.* **19**:333, 1984.
16. Adamson K, Fetal surgery. *N. Engl. J. Med.* **275**:204, 1966.
17. Asensio S. Surgical treatment of erythroblastosis fetalis. In *Diagnosis and Treatment of Fetal Disorders* (ed. K. Adamson), p. 264. New York: Springer-Verlag, 1969.
18. Harrison M, Golbus M, Filly R et al. Fetal treatment. *N. Engl. J. Med.* **307**:1651, 1982.
19. Harrison M, Adzick N, Flake A et al. Correction of congenital diaphragmatic hernia in utero: VI. Hard-earned lessons. *J. Pediatr. Surg.* **28**:1411, 1993.
20. Harrison M, Golbus M, Filly R et al. Fetal hydronephrosis: selection and surgical repair. *J. Pediatr. Surg.* **22**:556, 1987.
21. Langer J, Harrison M, Schmidt K et al. Fetal hydrops and demise from sacrococcygeal teratoma: rationale for fetal surgery. *Am. J. Obstet. Gynecol.* **160**:1145, 1989.
22. Harrison M. *The Unborn Patient* (eds M. Harrison, M.S. Golbus & R.A. Filly), p. 159. Philadelphia, PA: W.B. Saunders Company, 1991.
23. Krummel T & Longaker M. Fetal wound healing. In *The Unborn Patient* (eds M.R. Harrison, M.S. Golbus & R.A. Filly), p. 526. Philadelphia, PA: W.B. Saunders Company, 1991.
24. Westin B, Hysteroscopy in Early Pregnancy. *Lancet* **2**:872, 1954.
25. Club, TSS. A prospective analysis of 1518 laparoscopic cholecystectomies. *N. Engl. J. Med.* **324**:1073, 1991.
26. Quintero R, Puder K, Bardicef M et al. Hydrolaparoscopy in the rabbit: a fine model for the development of operative fetoscopy. *Am. J. Obstet. Gynecol.* **171**:1139, 1994.
27. Estes J, Szabo Z & Harrison M. Techniques for in utero endoscopic surgery. *Surg. Endosc.* **6**:215, 1992.
28. De Lia J, Cukierski M, Lundergan D et al. Neodymium: yttrium–aluminum–garnet laser occlusion of rhesus placental vasculature via fetoscopy. *Am. J. Obstet. Gynecol.* **160**:485, 1989.
29. Ville Y, Hyett J, Hecher K et al. Management of severe twin–twin transfusion: amniodrainage compared to endoscopic surgery. *Ultrasound Obstet. Gyecol.* **4**(suppl 1):130, 1994.
30. Quintero R, Goncalves L, Guevara F et al. Color-Doppler guided coagulation of abnormal communicating vessels in twin–twin transfusion. *Ultrasound Obstet. Gynecol.* **4**(suppl. 1):93 (abstract), 1994.
31. De Lia J, Cruikshank D & Keye W. Fetoscopic neodymium: YAG laser occlusion of placental vessels in severe twin–twin transfusion syndrome. *Obstet. Gynecol.* **75**:1046, 1990.

32. Ville Y, Hyett J, Hecher K et al. Preliminary experience with endoscopic laser surgery for severe twin–twin transfusion syndrome. *N. Engl. J. Med.* **332**:224–227, 1995.
33. Luks F, Deprest J, Vandenberghe K et al. A model for fetal surgery through intrauterine endoscopy. *J. Pediatr. Surg.* **29**:1007, 1994.
34. Luks F, Deprest J, Vandenberghe K et al. Fetoscopy-guided fetal endoscopy in a sheep model. *J. Am. Coll. Surg.* **178**:609, 1994.
35. Luks F, Deprest J, Marcus M et al. Carbon dioxide pneumoamnios causes acidosis in fetal lamb. *Fetal Diagn. Ther.* **9**:105, 1994.
36. Quintero R, Reich H, Puder K et al. Operative fetoscopy: a new frontier in fetal medicine. *Am. J. Obstet. Gynecol.* **179**(1, part 2):297 (abstract), 1994.
37. Vandenberghe K. Fetal endoscopic surgery, lessons from animal experiment. *Ultrasound Obstet. Gynecol.* **4**(suppl 1):129, 1994.
38. Quintero R, Puder K & Cotton D. Embryoscopy and fetoscopy. *Obstet. Gynecol. Clin. N. Am.* **20**:563, 1993.
39. Miyazaki F & Nevarez F. Saline amnioinfusion for relief of repetitive variable decelerations: a prospective randomized study. *Am. J. Obstet. Gynecol.* **153**:301, 1985.
40. Wenstrom K & Parsons M. The prevention of meconium in labor using amnioinfusion. *Obstet. Gynecol.* **73**:647, 1989.
41. Quetel T, Mejides A, Salman F et al. Amnioinfusion: an aid in the ultrasonographic evaluation of severe oligohydramnios in pregnancy. *Am. J. Obstet. Gynecol.* **167**:333, 1992.
42. Fisk N, Giussani D, Parkes M et al. Amnioinfusion increases amniotic pressure in pregnant sheep but does not alter fetal acid-base status. *Am. J. Obstet. Gynecol.* **165**:1459, 1991.
43. Hobbins J & Mahoney M. Clinical experience with fetoscopy and fetal blood sampling. In *Intrauterine Fetal Visualization, a Multidisciplinary Approach* (eds M.M. Kaback & Valenti), pp. 164–170. Amsterdam: Excerpta Medica, 1976.
44. Rodeck C. Fetoscopy guided by real-time ultrasound for pure fetal blood samples, fetal skin samples, and examination of the fetus in utero. *Br. J. Obstet. Gynaecol.* **87**:449, 1980.
45. Group TNNRfAS. Midtrimester amniocentesis for prenatal diagnosis. Safety and accuracy. *J. Am. Med. Ass.* **236**:1471, 1976.
46. Sanchez del Campo F, Puchades A, Panchon A et al. Action of laser light on the ocular development of chick embryos. *Anatomisch Anzeig* **169**:253, 1989.
47. Aige-Gil V & Murilli-Ferrol N. Effects of white light on the pineal gland of the chick embryo. *Histol. Histopathol.* **7**:1, 1992.
48. Quintero R, Crossland W & Cotton D. Effect of endoscopic white light on the developing visual pathway: a histologic, histochemical, and behavioral study. *Am. J. Obstet. Gynecol.* **171**:1142, 1994.
49. Schatz F. Eine besondere Art von einseitiger Polyhydramnie mit anderseitiger Oligohydramnie bei eineügen Zwillingen. *Arch. Gynaekol.* **19**:329, 1882.
50. Benirschke K. Multiple gestation: incidence, etiology and inheritance. In *Maternal–Fetal Medicine* (eds R.K. Creasy & P. Resnik), p. 511. Philadelphia, PA: W.B. Saunders, 1984.
51. Roberston E & Neer K. Placental injection studies in twin gestation. *Am. J. Obstet. Gynecol.* **147**:170, 1983.
52. Benirschke K & Driscoll S. *The Pathology of the Human Placenta*. New York: Springer-Verlag, 1967.
53. Tan K, Tan R & Tan A. The twin transfusion syndrome. *Clin. Pediatr.* **18**:111, 1979.
54. Klebe J & Ingomar C. The fetoplacental circultation during parturition illustrated by the interfetal transfusion syndrome. *Pediatrics* **49**:112, 1972.
55. Benirschke K. Twin placenta in perimortality. *NY State J. Med.* **61**:1499, 1961.
56. Brennan J, Diwan R, Rosen M et al. Fetofetal transfusion syndrome: prenatal ultrasonographic diagnosis. I. *Radiology* **143**:535, 1982.
57. Farmakides G, Schulman H, Saldana L et al. Surveillance of twin pregnancy with umbilical arterial velocimetry. *Am. J. Obstet. Gynecol.* **153**:789, 1985.
58. Rausen A, Seki M & Strauss L. Twin transfusion syndrome. *J. Pediatr.* **66**:613, 1965.
59. Danskin F & Neilson J. Twin-to-twin transfusion syndrome: what are appropriate diagnostic criteria? *Am. J. Obstet. Gynecol.* **161**:365–369, 1989.
60. Wittman B, Baldwin V & Nichol B. Antenatal diagnosis of twin transfusion syndrome by ultrasound. *Obstet. Gynecol.* **58**:123, 1981.
61. Pretorius D, Manchester D, Barkin S et al. Doppler ultrasound of twin transfusion syndrome at 18 weeks of gestation. *J. Clin. Ultrasound* **11**:442, 1983.
62. Giles W, Trudinger B, Cook C et al. Doppler umbilical artery studies in the twin–twin transfusion syndrome. *Obstet. Gynecol.* **76**:1097, 1990.
63. Ishimatsu J, Yoshimura O, Manabe A et al. Ultrasonography and Doppler studies in twin-to-twin transfusion syndrome. Asia-Oceania *J. Obstet. Gynecol.* **18**:325, 1992.
64. Yamada A, Kasugai M, Ohno Y et al. Antenatal diagnosis of twin–twin transfusion syndrome by Doppler ultrasound. *Obstet. Gynecol.* **78**:1058, 1991.
65. Fisk N, Borrell A, Hubinont C et al. Fetofetal transfusion syndrome: do the neonatal criteria apply in utero? *Arch. Dis. Child.* **65**:657, 1990.
66. Saunders N, Snijders R & Nicolaides K. Twin–twin transfusion syndrome during the 2nd trimester is associated with small intertwin hemoglobin differences. *Fetal Diagn. Ther.* **6**:34, 1991.
67. Tanaka M, Natori M, Ishimoto H et al. Intravascular Pancuronium bromide infusion for prenatal diagnosis of twin–twin transfusion syndrome. *Fetal Ther.* **7**:36, 1992.
68. Weir P, Ratten G & Beischner N. Acute polyhydramnios: A complication of monozygous twin pregnancy. *Br. J. Obstet. Gynaecol.* **86**:849, 1979.
69. De Lia J, Emery M, Sheafor S et al. Twin transfusion syndrome: successful in utero treatment with digoxin. *Int. J. Gynecol. Obstet.* **23**:197, 1985.
70. Jones J, Sbarra A, Dilillo L et al. Indomethacin in severe twin-to-twin transfusion syndrome. *Am. J. Perinatol.* **10**:24, 1993.
71. Montan S, Jorgensen C & Sjoberg N. Amniocentesis in treatment of acute polyhydramnios in twin pregnancies. *Acta. Obstet. Gynecol. Scand.* **64**:537, 1985.
72. Elliot J, Urig M & Clewell W. Aggressive therapeutic amniocentesis for treatment of twin–twin transfusion syndrome. *Obstet. Gynecol.* **77**:537, 1991.
73. Chitkara U, Berkowitz R, Wilkins I et al. Selective second-trimester termination of the anomalous fetus in twin pregnancies. *Obstet. Gynecol.* **73**:690–694, 1989.
74. Urig M, Simpson G, Elliot J et al. Twin–twin transfusion syndrome. The surgical removal of one twin as a treatment option. *Fetal Ther.* **3**:185–188, 1988.
75. Urig M, Clevell W & Elliot J. Twin–twin transfusion syndrome. *Am. J. Obstet. Gynecol.* **163**:1522, 1990.
76. Bejar R, Vigliocco G, Gramajo H et al. Antenatal origin of neurologic damage in newborn infants. Part II. Multiple gestations. *Am. J. Obstet. Gynecol.* **162**:1230, 1990.
77. Melnick M. Brain damage in survivor after in utero death in monozygous co-twin. *Lancet* **2**:128, 1977.
78. Schinzel A, Smith D & Miller J. Monozygotic twinning and structural defects. *J. Pediatr.* **95**:921, 1979.
79. Yoshioka H, Kadomoto Y, Mino M et al. Multicystic encephalomalacia in liveborn twin with a still-born macerated co-twin. *J. Pediatr.* **95**:798, 1979.
80. Dudley D & D'Alton M. Single fetal death in twin gestation. *Semin. Perinatol.* **10**:65, 1986.
81. Okamura K, Murotsuki J, Tanigawars S et al. Funipuncture for evaluation of hematologic and coagulation indices in the surviving twin following co-twin's death. *Obstet. Gynecol.* **83**:975, 1994.
82. De Lia J, Kuhlman R, Harstad T et al. Twin–twin transfusion syndrome treated by fetoscopic neodymium:YAG laser occusion of chorioangioagus. *Am. J. Obstet. Gynecol.* **168**(1, p 2):308, 1993.
83. Evans M, Goldberg J, Dommergues M et al. Efficacy of second-trimester selective termination for fetal abnormalities: international collaborative experience among the world's largest centers. *Am. J. Obstet. Gynecol.* **171**:90, 1994.
84. Wittman B, Farquharson D, Thomas W et al. The role of feticide in the management of severe twin transfusion syndrome. *Am. J. Obstet. Gynecol.* **155**:1023, 1986.
85. Quintero R, Reich H, Puder K et al. Brief Report: Umbilical-cord ligation of an acardiac twin by fetoscopy at 19 weeks of gestation. *N. Engl. J. Med.* **330**:469, 1994.
86. Lemery D. Ligation of the cord under ultrasound guidance: is endoscopy necessary? *Ultrasound Obstet. Gynecol.* **4**(suppl. 1):130, 1994.

87. Quintero R, Goncalves L, Berry S et al. Endoscopic and ultrasound-guided umbilical cord ligation in abnormal monochorionic twin gestations. *Ultrasound Obstet. Gynecol.* **4**(suppl. 1):93 (abstract), 1994.
88. James W. A note on the epidemiology of acardiac monsters. *Teratology* **16**:211, 1977.
89. Van Allen M, Smith D & Shepard T. Twin reversed arterial perfusion (TRAP) sequence: A study of 14 twin pregnancies with acardius. *Semin. Perinatol.* **7**:285, 1983.
90. Platt L, DeVore G, Bieniarz A et al. Antenatal diagnosis of acephalus acardia: A proposed management scheme. *Am. J. Obstet. Gynecol.* **146**:857, 1983.
91. Fries M, Goldberg J & Golbus M. Treatment of acardiac-acephalus twin gestations by hysterotomy and selective delivery. *Obstet. Gynecol.* **79**:601, 1992.
92. Ginsberg N, Applebaum M, Rabin S et al. Term birth after midtrimester hysterotomy and selective delivery of an acardiac twin. *Am. J. Obstet. Gynecol.* **167**:33, 1992.
93. Robie G, Payne G & Morgan M. Selective delivery of an acardiac, acephalic twin. *N. Engl. J. Med.* **320**:512, 1989.
94. Hamada H, Okane M, Koresawa M et al. Fetal therapy in utero by blockage of the umbilical blood flow of acardiac monster in twin pregnancy. *Nippon Sanka Fujinka Gakkai Zasshi* **41**:1803, 1989.
95. Roberts R, Shah D, Jeanty P et al. Twin, acardiac, ultrasound-guided embolization. *Fetus* **1**(7615):5–10, 1991.
96. Porreco R, Barton S & Haverkamp A. Occlusion of umbilical artery in acardiac, acephalic twin. *Lancet* **337**:326, 1991.
97. Grab D, Schneider V, Keckstein J et al. Twin, acardiac, outcome. *Fetus* **2**(7615):11–13, 1992.
98. Clarke H. Laparoscopy: new instruments for suturing and ligation. *Fertil. Steril.* **23**:274, 1972.
99. Abuhamad A, Romero R & Schaffer W. The value of Doppler flow analysis in the prenatal diagnosis of amniotic sheets. *J. Ultrasound Med.* **11**:623, 1992.
100. Mahony B, Filly R, Callen P et al. The amniotic band syndrome: antenatal sonographic diagnosis and potential pitfalls. *Am. J. Obstet. Gynecol.* **152**:63, 1985.
101. Finberg H. Uterine synechiae in pregnancy: expanded criteria for recognition and clinical significance in 28 cases. *J. Ultrasound Med.* **10**:547, 1991.
102. Randel S, Filly R, Callen P et al. Amniotic sheets 1. *Radiology* **166**:633, 1988.
103. Streeter G. Focal deficiencies in fetal tissues and their relation to intrauterine amputation. *Cont. Embryol. Carneg. Inst.* **22**:1, 1930.
104. Higginbottom M, Jones K, Hall B et al. The amniotic band disruption complex: timing of amniotic rupture and variable spectra of consequent defects. *J. Pediatr.* **95**:544, 1979.
105. Donnai D & Winter R. Disorganization: a model for 'early amnion rupture'? *Med. Genet.* **26**:421, 1989.
106. Hunter A & Carpenter B. Implications of malformations not due to amniotic bands in amniotic band sequence. *Am. J. Med. Genet.* **24**:691, 1986.
107. Torpin R. Amniochorionic mesoblastic fibrous strings and amniotic bands. *Am. J. Obstet. Gynecol.* **91**:65, 1965.
108. Hummel K. Developmental anomalies in mice resulting from action of the gene, disorganization, a semi-dominant lethal. *Pediatrics* **23**:212, 1959.
109. Lubinsky M, Sujansky E, Sanger W et al. Familial amniotic bands. *Am. J. Med. Genet.* **14**:81, 1983.
110. Reuss A, Wladimiroff J & Niermeyer M. Antenatal diagnosis of renal tract anomalies by ultrasound. *Pediatr. Nephrol.* **1**:546, 1987.
111. Harrison M, Filly R, Parer J et al. Management of the fetus with a urinary tract malformation. *JAMA* **246**:635, 1981.
112. Grannum P. The genitourinary tract. In *Diagnostic Ultrasound of Fetal Anomalies* (eds D.A. Nyberg, B.S. Mahony & D.H. Pretorius), p. 453. St. Louis: CV Mosby, 1990.
113. Noia G, Masini L, Caruso A et al. Prenatal diagnosis of congenital uropathies. *Fetal Ther.* **4**:40, 1989.
114. Mahony B, Filly R, Callen P et al. Fetal renal dysplasia: sonographic evaluation. *Radiology* **152**:143, 1984.
115. Evans M, Sacks A, Johnson M et al. Sequential invasive assessment of fetal renal function and the intrauterine treatment of fetal obstructive uropathies. *Obstet. Gynecol.* **77**:545, 1991.
116. Nicolini U, Tannirandorn Y, Vaughan J et al. Further predictors of renal dysplasia in fetal obstructive uropathy: bladder pressure and biochemistry of 'fresh' urine. *Prenat. Diagn.* **11**:159, 1991.
117. Johnson M, Bukowski T, Reitelman C et al. In utero surgical treatment of fetal obstructive uropathy: a new comprehensive approach to identify appropriate candidates for vesicoamniotic shunt therapy. *Am. J. Obstet. Gynecol.* **170**:1770–1776, 1994.
118. Beck A. The effect of intrauterine urinary obstruction upon the development of the fetal kidney. *J. Urol.* **105**:784, 1971.
119. Harrison M, Nakyama D, Noall R et al. Correction of congenital hydronephrosis in utero. II. Decompression reverses the effects of obstruction of the fetal lung and urinary tract. *J. Pediatr. Surg.* **17**:965, 1982.
120. Nakayama D, Glick P & Villa R. Experimental pulmonary hypoplasia due to oligohydramnios and its reversal by relieving thoracic compression. *J. Pediatr. Surg.* **18**:347, 1983.
121. Steinhardt G, Hogan W, Wod E et al. Long-term survival in an infant with urethral atresia. *J. Urol.* **143**:336, 1990.
122. Elder J, Duckett J & Snyder H. Intervention for fetal obstructive uropathy: Has it been effective? *Lancet* **ii**:1007–1010, 1987.
123. Cromblehome T, Harrison M, Langer J et al. Early experience with open fetal surgery for congenital hydronephrosis. *J. Pediatr. Surg.* **23**:1114, 1988.
124. Quintero R, Hume R, Smith C et al. Percutaneous fetal cystoscopy and endoscopic fulguration of posterior urethral valves. *Am. J. Obstet. Gynecol.* **172**:206–209, 1995.
125. Quintero R, Johnson M, Romero R et al. In-utero percutaneous cystoscopy in the management of fetal lower obstructive uropathy. *Lancet* **346**:537–540, 1995.
126. Siddall R. Chorioangiofibroma (Chorioangioma). *Am. J. Obstet. Gynecol.* **8**:554, 1924.
127. Fox H. Haemangiomata of the placenta. *J. Clin. Pathol.* **19**:133, 1966.
128. Cash J & Powell D. Placental chorioangioma. Presentation of a case with electronmicroscopic and immunochemical studies. *Am. J. Surg. Pathol.* **4**:87, 1980.
129. Barry F, McCoy C, Callahan W et al. Hemangioma of the umbilical cord. *Am. J. Obstet. Gynecol.* **62**:675, 1951.
130. Baylis M, Jones R & Hughes M. Angiomyxoma of the umbilical cord detected by ultrasound. *J. Obstet. Gynecol.* **4**:243, 1984.
131. Davies D. A benign tumour of the placenta. *J. Obstet. Gynaecol. Br. Emp.* **55**:44, 1948.
132. Fisher J. Chorioangioma of the placenta. *Am. J. Obstet. Gynecol.* **40**:439, 1940.
133. Eldar-Geva T, Hochner-Celnikier D, Ariel I et al. Fetal high output cardiac failure and acute hydramnios caused by large placental chorioangioma. Case report. *Br. J. Obstet. Gynaecol.* **95**:1200, 1988.
134. Burrows S, Gaines J & Hughes F. Giant chorioangioma. *Am. J. Obstet. Gynecol.* **15**:579, 1973.
135. Reiner L & Fries E. Chorangioma associated with arteriovenous aneurysm. A study on hamartoma. *Am. J. Obstet. Gynecol.* **93**:58, 1965.
136. Grundy H, Byer L, Walton S et al. Antepartum ultrasonographic evaluation and management of placental chorioangioma. A case report. *J. Reprod. Med.* **31**:520, 1986.
137. Marchetti A. A consideration of certain types of benign tumors of the placenta. *Surg. Gynecol. Obstet.* **68**:733, 1939.
138. Limaye N & Tchabo J. Asymptomatic thrombocytopenia associated with chorioangioma of placenta. *Am. J. Obstet. Gynecol.* **161**:76, 1989.
139. Panaccione J, Esposito W & Haller J. Acute polyhydramnios associated with chorioangioma. A case report. *J. Reprod. Med.* **36**:210, 1991.
140. Resnick L. Chorioangioma with a report of a case associated with oligohydramnios. *S. Afr. M. J.* **27**:57, 1953.
141. Tonkin I, Setzer S & Ermocilla R. Placental chorioangioma: A rare cause of congestive heart failure and hydrops fetalis in the newborn. *Am. J. Roentgenol.* **134**:181, 1980.
142. Emge L. Dystocia caused by a hemangioma of the placenta. *Am. J. Obstet. Gynecol.* **14**:35, 1927.
143. Fox H. Pathology of the placenta. In *Major Problems in Pathology* (ed. J.L. Bennington), p. 343. Philadelphia, PA: W.B. Saunders, 1978.
144. Bauer C, Fojaco R, Bancalari E et al. Microangiopathic hemolytic anemia and thrombocytopenia in a neonate associated with a larger placental chorioangioma. *Pediatrics* **62**:574, 1978.
145. Asadourian L & Taylor H. Clinical significance of placental hemangiomas. *Obstet. Gynecol.* **31**:551, 1968.

146. Heggtveit H, De Carvalho R & Nuyens A. Chorioangioma and toxemia of pregnancy. *Am. J. Obstet. Gynecol.* **91**:291, 1965.
147. Stiller A & Skafish P. Placental chorioangioma: a rare cause of fetomaternal transfusion with maternal hemolysis and fetal distress. *Obstet. Gynecol.* **67**:296, 1986.
148. Asokan S, Chadalavada K, Gardi R et al. Prenatal diagnosis of placental tumor by ultrasound. *J. Clin. Ultrasound* **6**:180, 1978.
149. Chou M, Ho E, Hwang S et al. Prenatal diagnosis of placental chorioangioma: contribution of color Doppler ultrasound. *Ultrasound Obstet. Gynecol.* **4**:332, 1994.
150. Hirata G, Masaki D, O'Toole M et al. Color flow mapping and Doppler velocimetery in the diagnosis and management of a placental chorioangioma associated with nonimmune fetal hydrops. *Obstet. Gynecol.* **81**:850, 1993.
151. Mann L, Alroomi L, McNay M et al. Placental haemangioma. Case Report. *Br. J. Obstet. Gynaecol.* **90**:983, 1983.
152. Salafia C, Silberman L, Herrera N et al. Placental pathology at term associated with elevated midtrimester maternal serum alpha-fetoprotein concentration. *Am. J. Obstet. Gynecol.* **158**:1064, 1988.
153. Hubinont C, Bernard P, Khalik N et al. Fetal liver hemangioma and chorioangioma: two unusual cases of severe fetal anemia detected by ultrasonography and its perinatal management. *Ultrasound Obstet. Gynecol.* **4**:330, 1994.
154. De Lia J, Kuhlmann R, Cruikshank D et al. Current topic: placental surgery: a new frontier. *Placenta.* **14**:477, 1993.
155. Wilson J, DiFiore J & Peters C. Experimental fetal tracheal ligation prevents the pulmonary hypoplasia associated with fetal nephrectomy: possible application for congenital diaphragmatic hernia. *J. Pediatr. Surg.* **28**:1433, 1993.
156. Di Fiore J, Fauza D, Slavin R et al. Experimental fetal tracheal ligation reverses the structural and physiological effects of pulmonary hypoplasia in congenital diaphragmatic hernia. *J. Pediatr. Surg.* **29**:248, 1994.
157. Hedrick M, Estes J, Sullivan K et al. Plug the lung until it grows (PLUG): a new method to treat congenital diaphragmatic hernia in utero. *J. Pediatr. Surg.* **29**:612, 1994.

SECTION

8

Diagnosis and management of other fetal conditions

The management of intrauterine growth restriction

58

M.J. Whittle

Introduction

Intrauterine growth restriction (IUGR) remains an important problem in perinatal medicine today. The exact incidence of the condition is uncertain, but it may occur in about 3–5% of pregnancies, although this depends on the population examined. Confusion arises from the frequent error of using the term 'IUGR' synonymously with 'small for dates' which is a statistical description of a population rather than a pathological condition. Traditionally, 'small for dates' has been used as an important end-point in perinatal medicine in the evaluation of predictive tests of fetal well-being and this has led to enormous difficulties in understanding the efficacy of these investigations. It is clear, of course, that some, possibly even the majority, of small-for-dates babies are indeed growth restricted but by no means all, and future progress in this area demands a clear appreciation of the difference between these two terms.

The implications of IUGR may be serious. It is likely that about a quarter of the babies who weigh less than 2.5 kg at birth and contribute to perinatal mortality figures, are growth restricted[1]. The Registrar General's OPCS data are difficult to interpret in this regard but if birthweight is taken alone, then 60% of all deaths occur in babies weighing less than 2.5 kg[2]. In addition, it is possible that babies who suffer with severe IUGR may be overrepresented in those children who develop long-term handicap[3,4]. However, this has been disputed and outcome may be more a function of maturity at the time of delivery[5,6]. Finally, the work of Barker would suggest that the influence of being born small may extend into adulthood in the form of the development of hypertension, diabetes and possibly stroke[7].

Control of fetal growth

The control of fetal growth is undoubtably a complex problem which has occupied the thoughts of many researchers over the years. Whilst it may be possible to control confounding factors with some success in animal experiments, the situation in humans is almost infinitely variable. For example, maternal height and socio-economic group are factors which may relate to the size of the baby[8]. Thus, small women from certain ethnic groups are more likely to have small babies but not necessarily ones with IUGR. However, it seems likely that the impact of other factors which affect fetal size such as smoking and, for example, hypertension is likely to be greatest amongst those women who have constitutional factors which influence fetal size. The challenge in maternal–fetal medicine is to develop techniques which will successfully separate out these different components.

At a biological level fetal growth depends upon only two components: genomic potential and substrate supply. The genomic potential is derived from both of the parents, although it can be modified by a number of factors. Indeed, the best evidence that the mother's size may influence the size of her fetus comes from the classic Shire horse experiments in which female ponies were sired by Shire horses, the resulting foals being more appropriate for the size of the mare than for the stallion[9]. Other genetic influences are seen from fetal size based on sex. Many studies indicate that the male fetus is heavier at birth than his sister. Why this should be is unclear, although presumably the growth potential is to some extent influenced by the Y chromosome. Aneuploidy has also been associated with the birth of small babies and in these cases the chromosome disorder itself effectively reduces the genetic fetal growth potential. The genetic control is undoubtably mediated through a complex series of mechanisms which include the switching on and off of growth factors such as insulin-like growth factors. Both intracellular and extracellular matrix factors are involved in a complex interchange of signals to produce both growth and differentiation[10] (see Chapter 12).

An adequate substrate supply is essential regardless of the genetic mechanisms controlling growth. This supply depends on both the placenta and uterine and placental vascular integrity. The placenta is currently the subject of a great deal of research in this area, the results of which may suggest that it has the ability to modify and control the growth of the fetus. This makes good teleological sense since it confers on the placenta the role of matching the rate of fetal growth to the available substrate supply. Evidence that this may be the case is accumulating, and substances such as hepatocyte growth factor (HGF) and placental growth factor, which are produced by the placenta, may be important[11,12]. Thus mice which are bred without the ability to express HGF (genetic knock-out experiments) show severe growth restriction and, usually, death. Similar studies involving the HGF receptor 'c-met' have been shown to produce the same effect[13]. Identical results are seen for angiotensin which implies that the placenta does indeed secrete substances which might influence the growth of both the placenta and the fetus and that there is the potential for a mechanism which matches fetal growth rate with substrate supply. Placental mass experiments[14] clearly show that the size of the 'placenta' dictates the size of the fetus. In carunclectomied sheep those fetuses with adequate placentae grew satisfactorily whilst those with depleted placentae did not. This demonstrated that the intrauterine environment itself may not be a significant factor in all cases of IUGR. Why a particular placenta should be small is uncertain but may relate to some of the factors described above.

One further interesting observation relates to the effect of confined placental mosaicism[15] often involving chromosome 16 or 22 in which the placenta is small and probably dysfunctional – the fetus is usually severely growth restricted. Uniparental disomy in which a chromosome pair is derived from the same parent is also associated with IUGR[16,17]. Disappointingly, this mechanism does not seem to be a significant cause of IUGR although work in this area continues.

The adequacy of the blood supply to the fetus may be determined as early as the time of implantation which, of course, begins soon after the fertilised ovum enters the uterine cavity and which is discussed by other authors in this book. The local changes required to enable this to occur successfully are currently largely a mystery, but are undoubtedly crucial to our understanding of IUGR. The process occurs probably in several stages, but as far as the vascular changes are concerned, the initial trophoblastic invasion of the maternal spiral arteries is probably complete by about 16 weeks[18]. A secondary invasion is complete by about 22–24 weeks[19]. A failure of these processes increases the chances that IUGR, and/or conditions such as pre-eclampsia, may complicate the pregnancy probably as a result of inadequate blood supply to the placental bed. The reduced blood supply then leads to further problems within the placental vasculature which ultimately reflect themselves in inadequate growth of both the placenta and the fetus.

Some of the best evidence for the effects of failure of vascular supply on the mother's side comes from sheep experiments undertaken back in the early 1980s in which pregnant ewes underwent embolisation of their uterine arteries[20]. Interestingly, although the blood flow in the uterine artery appeared unaltered, quite gross changes were noted in the fetal circulation. The implication of this experimental finding was that changes in the supply of blood through the spiral arteries to the placental bed which were insufficient to interfere with overall uterine blood flow, produced local areas of hypoxia in the placenta leading to a modification of blood flow in the placental vascular circulation. The best analogy for this phenomenon is the lung in which perfusion is withdrawn from areas of reduced ventilation such as seen in pneumonia.

These observations led to the concept that the placental vasculature was under humoral control and recently a number of vasoactive agents have been identified[21]. Probably the best known of these is nitric oxide which is a locally secreted vasoactive substance derived from the vascular endothelium and which has vasodilatory effects. However, there is a large number of other substances all of which may be involved in controlling this vasculature such as angiotensin, bradykinin and vascular endothelial growth factor (VEGF) and placental growth factor (PlGF). There may be others and it is becoming increasingly apparent that these substances do not work in isolation, but are orchestrated to act in a way which controls the placental vasculature. In a physiological sense, it is quite difficult to understand why there are so many different substances, both agonists and antagonists, and it may be that this complex humoral system has been devised with multiple 'backup' mechanisms to prevent vasoconstriction of this vital circulation which lacks neurogenic control. It is possible that such complexity may represent primitive vascular control such as was required before the evolution of neurogenic control mechanisms.

The most recent area of interest in terms of fetal growth comes from the work of Barker and the concept of growth programming. Whether programming is a physiological event which occurs in all pregnancies or is yet another example of an adaptation to unfavourable circumstances which may arise from failed or inadequate implantation remains to be seen. Undoubtably programming has many guises. For example, by as early as 18 weeks, maternal haemoglobin levels may be influencing eventual placental size[22]. It can also be demonstrated that alterations in maternal nutrition may also influence fetal size[23,24]. If this is indeed the case, the potential for therapy to correct or modify IUGR in later pregnancy is markedly diminished. It would seem that most of the effort to ensure adequate fetal growth must be applied to the first half, or even the first quarter, of pregnancy. Our understanding of programming is currently poor, but human evidence for its possible existence comes from such studies that existed from the Dutch famine in the Second World War in which the mothers who were starved and from supplementation studies[23].

Aetiology of IUGR

The management of IUGR depends not only on our ability to identify the affected pregnancy but also a clear idea about the possible underlying cause.

GENETIC

Fetal abnormality may be associated with IUGR or small for dates (SFD). Some old data suggest that about a third of SFD babies weighing less than 1500 g may be congenitally abnormal[25]. Aneuploidy may be a cause and two trisomies likely to be associated with small-for-dates babies are trisomy 18 (Edward syndrome) and 13 (Patau syndrome). Down syndrome itself is not characteristically associated with delivery of a small baby.

In general, babies that are dysmorphic, not necessarily due to a genetic problem, also tend to be small. Thus when a small fetus is found with apparently normal amounts of amniotic fluid the possibility that the baby has aneuploidy or is dysmorphic should always be considered.

INFECTION

The growth potential of a fetus may be severely impaired as a result of infection, particularly when this is due to a virus. The classic example is rubella and, although this is now uncommon in the UK due to widespread and virtually complete immunisation, it remains a problem worldwide. Rubella is an important embryopathic virus and when infection occurs in the first trimester the fetus is at considerable risk of developing profound abnormalities such as blindness, cardiac malformations and deafness. The virus appears to have the potential to interfere with the genomic drive to growth which leads, almost universally, to a growth-restricted baby.

Other viral infections may also be responsible for growth restriction, although the time at which they infect the baby is probably crucial. Both cytomegalovirus (CMV) and, more recently described, varicella (chickenpox) have been shown to be associated with growth restriction when they infect the fetus in the early weeks of pregnancy. In general, the role of viral infections and their effect on pregnancy has not been well studied and it is an area of some considerable research currently.

Infections with other agents such as bacteria and protozoa do not appear to affect fetal growth and this is probably because they are unlikely to cross the placenta to infect the fetus in early pregnancy because of their size. It is also possible that certain infections with bacteria are likely to provoke miscarriage.

Infections with agents, such as *Treponema pallidum*, are uncommon in the UK but, on a worldwide basis, are a significant cause of growth problems. Because of its size the spirochaete does not cross the placenta until late in the second trimester but it does infect the placenta, perhaps adversely affecting placental function.

It is important to understand the potential effect of infection on fetal growth so that the appropriate investigations can be undertaken in the presence of a growth-restricted fetus.

MATERNAL DISEASE

It is well recognised that certain maternal diseases such as hypertension, renal disease, autoimmune disorders and microvascular disease associated with long-standing insulin-dependent diabetes place the fetus at risk of IUGR. These conditions influence fetal growth because they lead primarily to reduced blood supply, via the uterine arteries, which arises from inadequate changes in the maternal spiral arteries at the time of placentation and in the subsequent weeks. This lack of change results in unaltered spiral arteries which then remain as resistance vessels restricting the flow of blood to the placental bed. The presence of these unaltered vessels in association with maternal hypertension and IUGR has been recognised for many years[19]. However, one important distinction is that the phenomenon is not necessarily all or none and the extent to which it does occur relates to the influence it has on blood supply to the placental bed. Not only do the blood vessels remain unaltered, but they also undergo secondary changes which have been described as acute atherosis, a process which narrows them still further. These changes conspire to restrict blood supply and, therefore, substrate delivery to the placental bed and the situation will be exacerbated by the presence of pre-existing vascular disease.

When the pathology in the spiral arteries is critical, the mother is at particular risk of developing pregnancy-induced hypertension or more likely pre-eclampsia. The mechanism by which this occurs is unclear, but probably relates to local placental ischaemia. Whilst it was always said that characteristic changes in the placenta were not seen in pre-eclampsia, it is now apparent that typical features can be observed. Not only does the placenta tend to be grossly small, but in addition the number of vessels in the tertiary villi appear to be depleted[26,27]. Whether this occurs because of defective angiogenesis, or because the vessels are steadily destroyed over time, remains unclear. The author's preference is for the latter since in the sheep experiments described by Clapp[20] the vascular insult on the maternal side was capable of influencing the feto-placental flow even though the placental vessels were presumably originally intact. It would seem likely that local hypoxia may lead to closure of vessels within the placenta, a process which if prolonged causes these tiny vessels to be absorbed; histological examination of the tertiary villi reveals that they are depleted of vessels[26,27].

The vascular consequence of these changes would be a rise in the placental vascular resistance, something which may be determined from examination of the umbilical artery Doppler waveforms. The correlation between abnormal waveforms, in which the diastolic velocities are reduced, and depleted placental vasculature, has been shown by several different groups and has recently been reviewed[28]. The concept that the changes noted occur through hypoxia has been challenged and the possibility that they arise from increased oxygen locally and its free radicals, has been raised. It seems reasonable to propose that the vascular changes in the placenta are progressive since it has also been shown that umbilical artery waveform changes deteriorate steadily as the fetal condition worsens.

The fundamental problem therefore which arises from the maternal conditions discussed above is vascular, affecting the maternal spiral arteries. This leads to a secondary problem in the feto-placental vasculature both of which conspire to deprive substrate supply to the fetus and so restrict growth.

Maternal illness can indirectly produce growth problems in the fetus, not so much from the illness, but from the drugs required to control it. Probably the best example is anticonvulsant therapy, the hydantoins, such as phenytoin, being the most clearly recognised to produce IUGR as part of the hydantoin syndrome. Other anticonvulsants have also been implicated in IUGR but the mechanism is uncertain. Presumably the anticonvulsants affect cellular mechanisms, rather than substrate supply, since the condition is most frequently associated with symmetrical growth retardation.

TOXINS

Both smoking and excessive alcohol are well recognised as being associated with growth restriction. Smoking may have its effect both from the vasoconstrictive effect of nicotine in the maternal circulation and because of the displacement of oxygen from haemoglobin by carbon monoxide.

The effects of alcohol are much less certain, although it is possible that excessive alcohol taken in early pregnancy may act as a cellular poison so reducing the fetal potential to growth. Perversely, small amounts of alcohol may act as a vascular dilator and it is possible may well encourage growth, although this too would be debatable. The Royal College of Obstetricians and Gynaecologists have recently recommended that no more than 15 units a week should be consumed during pregnancy[29].

Drug abuse in the form of cocaine and crack are potent vasoconstrictors which may have sufficient influence on the uterine vasculature to be a potential cause of severe IUGR[30].

The identification of at-risk groups

SCORING SYSTEMS

A number of different scoring systems have been devised to identify groups of women who may be particularly at risk of an IUGR baby. Whilst these scoring systems may have some value, they have not proved to be particularly sensitive or specific, although they may provide some guide[31]. More powerful prediction comes from the identification of one of the aetiological components discussed above, the presence of which would be sufficient to place a woman in a high-risk category[32]. Thus if she herself has hypertension, has had a previously small baby, is undernourished or smokes heavily, then her risk of having an IUGR baby is high although difficult to quantify.

Unfortunately, in spite of this approach, IUGR still remains often unanticipated and generally only between a third and a half of cases of IUGR are identified antenatally. Thus ironically the apparently normal pregnancy with a baby that has 'silently' failed to reach its growth potential may be at greater risk than the woman who develops hypertension at 32 weeks with an identified IUGR fetus requiring immediate delivery. It is possible that OPCS data from 1986 to 1995 reflect this phenomenon in that whilst unexplained antenatal death has tended to rise, when the cause is known loss has fallen (Fig. 58.1). This implies that outcome is likely to be better when a condition has been identified or anticipated.

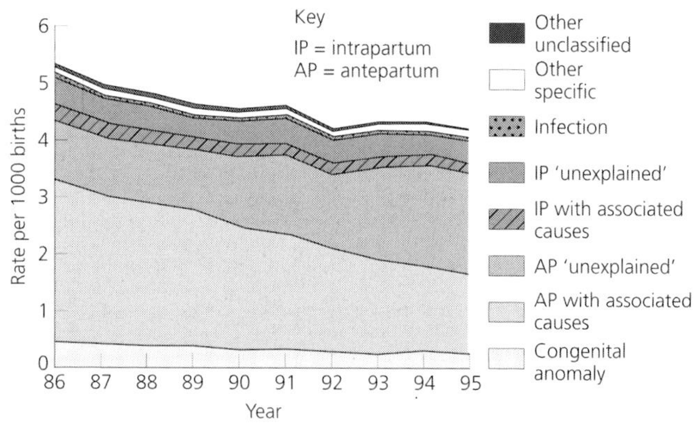

Fig. 58.1 Trends in different categories of stillbirths in England and Wales 1986 to 1995 (CESDI 1997).

SCREENING PROCEDURES

A number of techniques have been devised to screen for fetal growth problems. It would be true to say that enormous doubt exists as to the efficacy of all these methods, but some are still in common use and all need to be discussed.

SERIAL WEIGHT MEASUREMENTS

Traditionally maternal weight has been measured at each antenatal visit. Normal maternal weight gain in pregnancy has a wide range but on average is between 10 and 12 kg and some place considerable importance on both excessive weight gain and weight loss. It is also recognised that mothers who have a booking weight of below 45 kg, or above 100 kg, can be regarded as having a risk factor in their pregnancy. Low-weight mothers will, of course, tend to have smaller babies and some feel that serial ultrasound biometry in this group is worthwhile. The Cochrane database contains no randomised studies to establish whether serial maternal weight measurement in pregnancy confers advantage.

FUNDAL HEIGHT

The laying on of hands has been the obstetrician's stock in trade for generations. Most often, and until recently, the aim of this simple procedure was to establish gestational age and uterine size in most of the older textbooks was described (Fig. 58.2) in terms of the gestational age of the pregnancy. Fundal height was deemed compatible with gestational age unless gross discrepancies existed but, in general, this approach has proved to be a fairly pointless exercise.

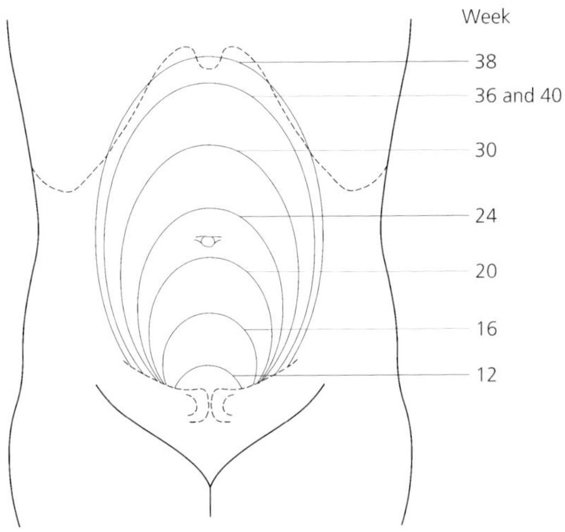

Fig. 58.2 Uterine height at advancing gestation.

In the 1970s, the idea that the fundal height should be assessed with a tape measure began to find favour and indeed many obstetric systems now use fundal height measurements as the first sign of impending fetal growth problems (Fig. 58.3). The literature is uncertain as to whether this is a worthwhile procedure or not and a randomised study did not find the procedure to be effective[33].

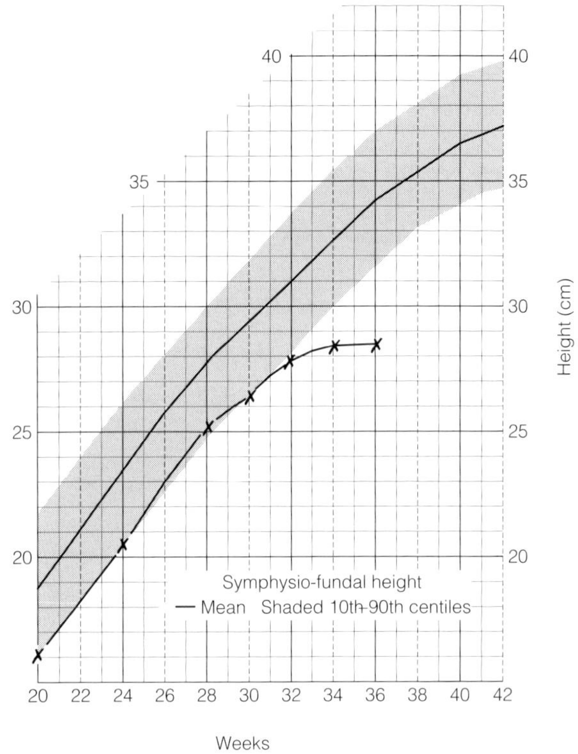

Fig. 58.3 A symphysiofundal height (cm) chart illustrating possible IUGR.

ULTRASOUND SCREENING

Whereas the measurement of weight and fundal height are both subjective, ultrasound biometry provides the opportunity of objectivity. One of the first studies was by Neilson *et al.*[34] who used a static scanner to measure both the fetal crown–rump length and the trunk area; crown–rump length measurement in late pregnancy is not now a measurement which would be easy to undertake on a real-time scanner. The scan was performed at two screening windows, one between 26 and 30 weeks and the other between 34 and 36 weeks and was highly sensitive and specific. In spite of this, the randomised control trial failed to show any advantage to the procedure in terms of perinatal mortality, but the study was small[35].

In the UK, about 5% of departments undertake an ultrasound scan in the third trimester, primarily to estimate fetal size. However, since no obvious advantage accrues from this procedure, it cannot, based on current evidence, be recommended[36].

The inability of ultrasound used in this way to improve outcome of IUGR is disappointing and to some extent surprising. It probably reflects the fact that size alone is not the important arbiter and that there are other factors, including the dynamics of growth and evidence of impending fetal demise, which are more important.

The most effective method of identifying the small-for-dates fetus, and certainly superior to Doppler velocimetry studies of the umbilical artery, is by measuring the change in the estimated fetal weight over a period of two weeks[37]. To some extent, this observation is self-evident because a failure to reach the growth velocity over a period of two weeks would be tantamount to diagnosing IUGR. The main problem is one of practicality, since obstetricians are often faced with the need to make a decision on whether or not a particular fetus has IUGR over a period of a few days, not weeks. However, when the fetal situation is not dire, a longer period of observation can be effective. Indeed charts such as those devised by Gardosi *et al.* may prove effective as a screening test for growth potential and the technique should be subjected to a randomised controlled trials (RCT).

DOPPLER

Doppler was one of the great hopes for the effective screening for growth problems. Since it appears reasonable to assume that an abnormal umbilical artery Doppler indicates some disturbance in the placental vasculature, it would follow that umbilical artery Doppler waveforms should provide a useful predictive screening test for those babies likely to develop IUGR.

There are now a number of RCTs involving the umbilical artery which suggest that, at least, in the low-risk groups umbilical artery Doppler information does not confer an advantage. Conversely, meta-analysis for high-risk groups suggests a marginal advantage for the use of umbilical artery Doppler (odds ratio 0.71{0.5–1.01})[38]. The number of patients now in the meta-analysis of RCTs is in the region of 8000. However, for studies to have sufficient power to show whether there is an advantage to the use of a technique with the potential to improve perinatal outcome will require around 30 000 cases[39]. In spite of the slightly tenuous advantage noted with the use of umbilical artery Doppler, which is still the most extensively evaluated test in perinatal medicine, it is in widespread use.

The situation is different for the uterine artery Doppler for which studies are much fewer. However, most suggest that abnormal Doppler waveforms in the uterine artery may indicate that the pregnancy could be at added risk of developing hypertension and/or IUGR because they reflect the failure of the normal physiological changes in the spiral arteries described above. These Doppler studies are undertaken usually on two occasions, once at 20 weeks and, if abnormal, again at around 24–26 weeks[40]. The uterine artery studies are rather more difficult to perform, in contrast to those involving the umbilical artery, and examinations take longer and have, therefore, greater resource implications. If the uterine artery Doppler is abnormal at the 20-week scan, then a second scan preferably using colourflow equipment at 24 weeks is required and this, for many units, would be both expensive and inconvenient. There does need to be a large randomised study looking at the use of uterine artery Doppler not only in terms of its efficacy, but also in terms of practicality. In addition, it is not clear what advantage would accrue from the knowledge that the pregnancy is at risk apart from providing the opportunity of extra surveillance. However, a recent publication does suggest that the identification of an abnormal uterine artery Doppler by 24 weeks does allow the use of low dose aspirin as an intervention to reduce the incidence of PET and/or IUGR but the study is small and needs to be repeated using larger numbers[41].

BIOCHEMICAL MONITORING

Few units, if any now, in the world undertake biochemical monitoring using unconjugated oestriol or human placental lactogen. These two analytes formed the mainstay of fetal assessment in the 1960s and 1970s and were replaced by biophysical methods because it was thought that they had little place in modern obstetric practice. Whilst this may be the case, it should perhaps be recognised that the studies themselves were flawed because the end-point used was merely that of small for dates, without separate recognition of IUGR. One of the first randomised controlled studies undertaken in obstetric practice was in fact for human placental lactogen and the study clearly showed that when the result was revealed to the obstetrician, outcome of pregnancy was improved[42]. It is true to say that these observations were made in hypertensive pregnancies, but the results were more clear-cut than those of many of the other techniques used today.

PLACENTAL GRADING

Placental grading was first described by Grannum *et al.*[43] and indicated that senescent changes occurred in the placenta which could be of some value in assessing the pregnancy. Although this technique is rarely used nowadays in a practical sense, a small randomised controlled study did suggest that when it was revealed that senescence was present at 32 weeks appropriate intervention could reduce the incidence of meconium, for example, during labour[44]. This was a small study which should be repeated because the technique itself is relatively easy to undertake and could provide a useful screen for potential perinatal problems.

Those procedures that are described above have been used in the management and screening of a general population. The majority of these techniques appear to have limited value when used in an unselected or low-risk population, but when used in an at-risk population, perhaps in which hypertension exists, they are more effective. This certainly applies to Doppler studies of the umbilical artery and probably also for various fetal biometric measurements. The problem is always one of identifying the at-risk group and the conclusion from the data above is that no single effective screening test for growth restriction exists. In practice, of course, obstetricians tend to use a variety of different strategies to establish whether risk exists, but it is sobering to realise that in spite of immense effort a reliable method to identify the majority of IUGR pregnancies is still not available.

Management of IUGR

Probably the majority of IUGR pregnancies are recognised because of complications in the mother, usually hypertension. This alerts either obstetrician or midwife that the fetus may be at risk of growth restriction and is the initiating factor which leads to a series of appropriate investigations. The management of these cases is relatively straightforward since the aetiology is obvious, but significant difficulties may arise in other cases in which the small-for-dates problem is identified without maternal risk factors when detailed investigations may be required to establish the underlying aetiology.

Aetiology is best established through a stepwise investigation process.

HISTORY

The history should include the outcome of previous pregnancies, past medical history and maternal health in the current pregnancy. The particular clues to be established here include a history of a previous small-for-dates baby. Evidence of a poor obstetric history such as repeated miscarriage in the first trimester or, more significantly, a second trimester loss should raise the suspicion that an immunological disorder, such as the antiphospholipid syndrome, exists.

The current obstetric history is also important and here the possibility of maternal infection should be sought. This is not usually a reliable area in which to question the patient, but occasionally there is evidence that the mother has suffered a significant, but perhaps non-specific illness during the current pregnancy which would be typical of something like cytomegalovirus.

Of course, all mothers should undergo a complete physical examination with special reference to their cardiovascular system and evidence of renal and immunological disease.

FETAL BIOMETRY

The importance of the measurement of the fetus has already been alluded to. As far as the evaluation of IUGR is concerned, the main measurements are those of the head and abdominal circumference and the long bones. Using a variety of different formulae and various parameters it is possible to calculate an estimate of the fetal weight, remembering that result is only accurate to between ±10 and 15%. It is important that it is realised that this is only an estimate of weight and not growth, the latter requiring sequential measurements usually spaced about 10–14 days apart[37]. Using these measurement parameters, however, allows the size of the fetus to be placed against the usual growth charts which are available widely in many books and indeed in many obstetric notes; an example is shown (Fig. 58.4).

In general, combinations of, rather than single, measurements are often more helpful in biological problems and the traditional evaluation is that of the head–trunk (H:T) ratio. This gives information about the pattern of growth and whether or not growth is symmetrical or asymmetrical. There has been criticism of these terms, but in a practical sense they do have some value. Asymmetrical IUGR, for example, is usually found when the baby is suffering from intrauterine 'starvation' usually as a result of deficient substrate supply as seen in maternal hypertension. Under these circumstances the fetal head continues to grow but the abdominal circumference increases more slowly in size, remains static or even shrinks. The reason for this is that the major contributor to the abdominal circumference is the fetal liver, the size of which reflects, amongst other things, the state of its glycogen stores. These stores either fail to accumulate or become depleted as a feature of the starvation process.

Symmetrically small babies have previously been considered to be merely constitutionally small, but this is incorrect and in fact some of the most severely growth restricted babies

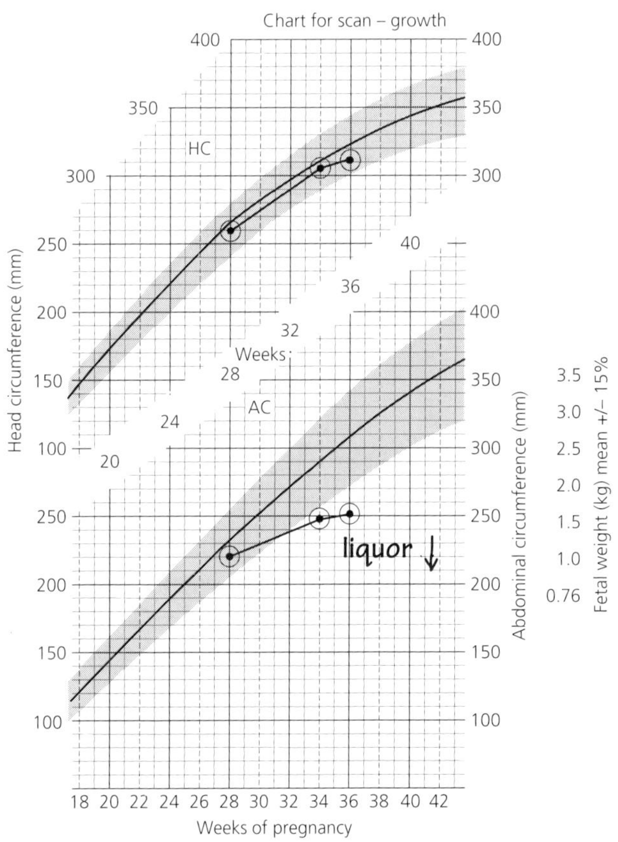

Fig. 58.4 A typical chart to plot ultrasound measurements. It shows a fall-off of abdominal growth compatible with asymmetrical IUGR.

show a symmetrical pattern of growth of their head–trunk ratios (Fig. 58.5). Thus the fact that the baby is symmetrically small does not exclude the possibility of severe IUGR and should not be regarded as an indication that all is well.

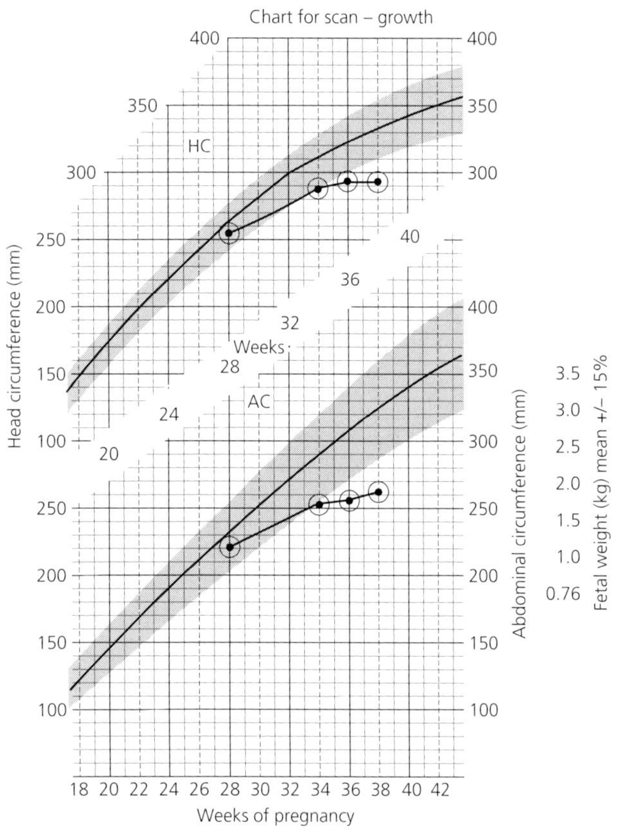

Fig. 58.5 Ultrasound growth chart showing a symmetrically small fetus.

ASSESSMENT OF FETAL WELL-BEING

There is a need to determine the chronicity of the problem which affects the fetus. The first examination provides a baseline against which to judge the rate of deterioration of the fetal condition. Probably the best indication of the duration of the growth-restricting problem is the amniotic fluid volume. After about 20 weeks, amniotic fluid is largely the product of the fetal urine output and reductions in amniotic fluid volume probably represents a fall in fetal renal blood flow as a result of chronic hypoxia[45]. In fact, there is considerable debate about the exact mechanism by which amniotic fluid decreases but it is possible that the fetal responses to chronic hypoxia include the redistribution of blood flow away from non-vital areas such as the kidney, gut and peripheral tissue. However, animal work has suggested that in prolonged hypoxaemia, fetal renal output is maintained but that amniotic fluid falls, suggesting that an alternative mechanism for oligohydramnios exists[46].

Nevertheless, the amniotic fluid volume has proved a useful guide in fetal evaluation. The problem with amniotic fluid volume estimations is that they are difficult to do and generally not very reproducible. Several methods have been adopted, namely the measurement of deepest pool, the amniotic fluid index and indeed just an overall impression of the adequacy of the amniotic fluid. It is helpful when repeated observations are being made over a short period of several days that measurements of the amniotic fluid index are made. Sequential data of a numeric nature are likely to be more helpful than single observations. A more recent evaluation involves correlated centiles, but this does require measurements to be made about two weeks apart, which in the usually semi-acute circumstance in which these evaluations are being undertaken, may not be valuable[47]. When there is particular concern daily evaluation of the amniotic fluid is worthwhile and certainly amniotic fluid volumes can fall very rapidly in cases that are becoming seriously compromised. Changes of this sort should be taken seriously and careful consideration should be given to deliver.

Other ultrasound evidence of developing chronic hypoxia may be found from changes in certain fetal organs, for example the fetal gut, which may become bright presumably as a result of oligaemia, although there is no strong evidence for this[48]. This observation is consistent with concepts about the fetal responses to hypoxia discussed above and evidence does exist that these changes in the gut can be correlated with an increased incidence of necrotising enterocolitis in the delivered baby.

Although changes in amniotic fluid volume provide some clues about the duration of the hypoxic insult, acute markers are to be found in other components of what has been described as the biophysical profile. First described by Manning *et al.*[49] as a method of dealing with post-dates pregnancies, it has become incorporated into methods of evaluating IUGR, although, in fact, it may not prove particularly effective under these circumstances. Its components, which include the assessment of amniotic fluid volume, comprise both chronic and acute markers which in spite of the method's shortcomings can prove valuable as an overall assessment.

The acute changes may be identified from reductions in gross body movements and fetal breathing movements. In fact, it is possible that a loss of fetal breathing movements is the first indication of hypoxia[50]; however, this feature has a very high false-positive rate and so is of little clinical value. Nevertheless, a steady decline in fetal activity in general, together with loss of fetal breathing, is likely to be very significant. Loss of fetal tone is the final stage and although data do not exist specifically for IUGR, about 70% of fetuses in general will be acidotic by this stage[51].

Little work has been done on the use of biophysical profile in the specific circumstance of IUGR. One small randomised study suggested that biophysical profile was more effective than cardiotocography, but this was not necessarily in growth-restricted pregnancies[52]. However, it is usually reckoned that as much information as possible should be gleaned from the ultrasound examination and it seems reasonable at least to evaluate amniotic fluid volume and probably fetal breathing.

Cardiotocography, which is also a component of the biophysical profile, is another evaluation which has been used for many years. In fact, the randomised studies which are available for it do not suggest it confers advantage, and indeed one interpretation could be that the test is positively dangerous[53]. The studies, however, are small and, again, do not really address the specific issue of IUGR.

The use of computerised cardiotocography, again, has not been evaluated in a randomised trial, but is widely available. In this technique, which was first described by Dawes *et al.*, not only the presence of reactivity, but also the background variation of the trace are taken into account. It is said to be a more sensitive guide to the presence of hypoxia, but has not been looked at specifically in growth-restricted babies, neither has it been subjected to trial. However, it does seem to provide a more objective and consistent method of evaluation[54].

DOPPLER EVALUATION OF THE FETUS

The use of Doppler to evaluate the small-for-dates fetus has never been specifically studied but the evidence that exists concerning umbilical artery Doppler in high-risk pregnancies may suggest an advantage to its use[38]. What is uncertain is how it should be used and the literature is unclear. Serial measures of the waveform velocity perhaps weekly or twice weekly seem appropriate, the development of absent or particularly, reversed, diastolic velocities being an indication either for closer monitoring or, often, delivery. The presence of abnormal Doppler may be associated with about a 70% chance that the fetus is acidotic[55]. It is usually considered that reduced velocity waveforms are the result of increased downstream resistance in the placental vasculature rather than hypoxia per se[56]. Whatever the aetiology, the loss of diastolic velocities is generally considered to be a serious development.

More recently, there has been interest in the pulsations in the ductus venosus as providing a significant indication of impending fetal demise[57]. However, whether these signs enhance the use of Doppler as a diagnostic tool remains to be seen.

The use of Doppler to examine other circulations is even less clear. The fetal cerebral circulation has been extensively studied but the use of middle cerebral artery Doppler has not been subjected to trial. In this circulation, the hypoxic fetus shows a loss of downstream impedance such that the diastolic velocities increase. However, it has been shown that as hypoxia deepens impedance increases so that a U-shaped curve is seen as oxygen levels fall. This fact makes interpretation difficult although relating the middle cerebral artery and umbilical artery resistances does help to indicate the increasingly hypoxic fetus[58].

The uterine arteries may give a clue that uteroplacental vascular failure is likely to be the cause of the growth failure. This knowledge aids the decision concerning both investigations and management but does not help in determining the timing or necessity for delivery.

FETAL NORMALITY

As discussed above, it is clear that the IUGR, or severely small-for-dates baby is at risk of congenital abnormality. A detailed structural review of the fetus is essential in these circumstances. This can be difficult given the possible associated oligohydramnios, and if doubt exists, the mother should be referred for review. The use of amnioinfusion may need to be considered especially if good views of the fetal kidneys are not possible.

The presence of structural abnormalities increases the risk of aneuploidy to the extent that there is a clear indication for karyotyping and this can be done either by cordocentesis[59] or by chorionic villus biopsy. Both procedures carry an enhanced risk of perhaps 5–10% of fetal loss in the presence of IUGR but the advantage of blood sampling is that in addition, it will be possible to screen for fetal infection and, if indicated, obtain fetal blood gases. It is felt that it is not justified to undertake the procedure merely to obtain the fetal acid–base status[60].

The investigations described should enable the obstetrician not only to decide the underlying aetiology but also provide an impression of the current fetal status. The investigations available allow the small fetus to be categorised into the following groups;

- Uteroplacental failure
  - High H:T ratio
  - Reduced amniotic fluid volume
  - Abnormal umbilical artery Doppler
  - Notched uterine artery Doppler
  - Structurally normal fetus
- Infection
  - Probably normal or decreased H:T ratio
  - Normal amniotic fluid volume
  - Possible fetal markers, i.e. hydrops, cerebral changes
  - Umbilical/uterine Doppler normal
- Fetal abnormality
  - Normal or markedly increased H:T ratio
  - Normal amniotic fluid volume
  - Possible structural abnormalities
  - Umbilical artery Doppler may be abnormal
  - Uterine artery Doppler normal

These are generalisations but the plan helps to identify the specific groups. When there are mixed results, it is important that all investigations are completed before delivery is contemplated.

MANAGEMENT PLANNING

IUGR can present the obstetrician with several major problems most of which relate to the difficulty of trading increased maturity with risk of intrauterine demise. The extent of these problems is reflected by the need for the current Growth Restriction Intervention Trial (GRIT)[61]. This trial is attempting to address these difficult issues which are particularly severe before 28 weeks. Recent data may suggest a more aggressive approach is beneficial but the study was relatively small[62].

In essence gestational age can be divided into five bands each provoking a different response.

BEFORE 26 WEEKS

The outcome in this group of babies is usually extremely poor. The combination of severe growth restriction and prematurity means that survival is about 30% and long-term handicap around 30–50%[63,64]. It seems likely that the best incubator at this gestation is the uterus and it seems unlikely that the baby would do better if delivered. Of course, if the mother has an additional problem such as hypertension, the baby may need to be delivered for her sake. However, in the absence of such pressure, delay is probably correct. It may be worth administering steroids to the mother in any case.

26 TO 28 WEEKS

This is an area of great uncertainty and possibly the one in which the results of the GRIT study will provide most enlightenment. So long as the fetus is not clearly moribund delivery, following the use of maternal steroids, would seem usually appropriate. The results are reasonable both in terms of mortality (85% survival) and morbidity (about 15%) and the additional risk to the mother of delivery by caesarean section seems justifiable. However, it remains true that whether prolonged intrauterine life confers advantage is still unclear.

28 TO 32 WEEKS

At this gestational age, the indications to deliver the IUGR fetus are fairly clear although steroids should always be given for 48 hours if at possible. The closer to 32 weeks, the easier becomes the decision to deliver but hasty delivery should be avoided unless the indications to do so are clear, since neonatal respiratory problems can still prove a significant problem at these gestational ages.

32 TO 36 WEEKS

When severe problems of IUGR are found at this stage, delivery should be recommended. Steroids should be given if possible but delivery should not be delayed for this if the baby is clearly in difficulties.

37 WEEKS AND OVER

IUGR at this stage should be the indication for delivery as soon as is practically possible. There is no justification to wait and the route of delivery will be by caesarean section unless the cervix is favourable.

Outcome

SHORT TERM

IUGR babies have a number of significant problems. They have difficulties in temperature control because of their small body mass to surface area, lack of glycogen stores and usually absent brown fat which reduces their non-shivering thermogenesis. The adaptation to prolonged intrauterine hypoxia makes them prone to necrotising enterocolitis. Respiratory problems relate more to the gestational age at delivery than IUGR and although there have always been suggestions that IUGR enhances lung maturity the evidence is not secure.

The care of these babies can, therefore, be complex and requires sophisticated neonatal support. Such babies should, therefore, be delivered at tertiary centres especially if prematurity is an additional factor.

MEDIUM TERM

The subsequent development of these children depends both on the extent and aetiology of the IUGR and the gestational age at delivery. Outcome data with respect to survival and long-term handicap show the significance of gestational age at the time of delivery[64]. However, it has been suggested that being born small for dates may interfere more with intellectual development[65] than being born early which had an additional effect on motor function. Those children who were severely IUGR at birth, typically symmetrically small, did not illustrate the catch-up growth seen when IUGR has arisen from a relatively short spell of uteroplacental insufficiency[66].

LONG TERM

The work of Barker and his group indicates the possibility that those babies born small for dates are prone to develop hypertension and non-insulin dependent diabetes as adults and the subject has been extensively reviewed[67]. Whether this arises from programming or as a response to intrauterine hypoxia is not clear. Certainly the babies that are 'rescued' nowadays from hostile intrauterine environments would almost certainly not have survived in the era in which those cases under study in Barker's work were born. It was the effect of low birthweight rather than IUGR which formed the basis of his studies and although these babies may be part of a continuum, this remains uncertain. Nevertheless, the fact that intrauterine environment may influence adult development is a critical and important observation which does offer some opportunity for useful intervention.

Conclusions

IUGR remains a major obstetric and neonatal challenge. The investigations which are now available allow aetiology to be more precisely established but the appropriate timing of delivery is often difficult to judge. Evidence is emerging that some forms of IUGR may be preordained early in pregnancy such that their recognition may provide the opportunity for effective intervention. However, in most the diagnosis is late in the process and likely to remain so in the foreseeable future. At the moment, therefore, we must concentrate on establishing an accurate diagnosis and carefully planning delivery, with neonatologists, to optimise outcome.

REFERENCES

1. Whitfield CR, Smith NC, Cockburn F, Gibson AAM. Perinatally related wastage – a proposed classification of primary obstetric factors. *Br J Obstet Gynaecol* **93**:694–703, 1986.
2. *OPCS Mortality statistics. Perinatal and infant: social and biological factors. Reviews of the Registrar General on deaths in England and Wales, 1990.* Series DH3. London: HMSO. 1990.
3. Harvey D, Prince J, Bunton J, Parkinson C, Campbell S. Ability of children who were small for gestational age babies. *Paediatrics* **69**:296–300, 1982.
4. Chiswick M. IUGR. *BMJ* **291**:845–848, 1985.
5. Powls A, Botting N, Cooke RWI, Marlow N. Motor impairment in children 12 to 13 years old with a birthweight of less than 1250 g. *Arch Dis Childh* **72**:62–66, 1995.
6. Murphy DJ, Sellars S, MacKenzie IZ, Yudkin PL, Johnson AM. Case–control study of antenatal and intrapartum risk factors for cerebral palsy in very preterm singleton babies. *Lancet* **346**:1449–1453, 1995.
7. Barker DJP, Bull AR, Osmond C, Simmonds SJ. Fetal and placental size and risk of hypertension in adult life. *BMJ* **301**:259–262, 1990.
8. Gardosi J, Mongelli M, Wilcox M, Chang A. An adjustable fetal weight standard. *Ultrasound Obstet Gynecol* **6**:168–174, 1995.
9. Walton A, Hammond J. The maternal effects on growth and conformation in Shire horse–Shetland pony crosses. *Proc R Soc* **174**:647–651, 1954.
10. Hill DJ, Han VKM. Control of cellular multiplication and differentiation. In *Fetal Growth* (eds F. Sharp & R.D.G. Milner), pp. 83–98. London: RCOG, 1989.
11. Kilby MD, Afford S, Li XF, Strain AJ, Ahmed A, Whittle MJ. Localisation of HGF and its receptor (c-met) protein and mRNA in human term placenta. *Growth Factors* **13**:1–7, 1996.
12. Khaliq A, Li XF, Shams M *et al.* Localisation of placenta growth factor (PlGF) in human term placenta. *Growth Factors* **13**:243–250, 1996.
13. Uehara Y, Minowa O, Mori C, Shiota K, Kuno J, Noda T, Kitamura N. Placental defect and embryonic lethality in mice lacking HGF/Scatter factor. *Nature* **373**:702–705, 1995.
14. Robinson JS, Kingston JE, Jones CT, Thorburn GD. Studies on experimental growth retardation in sheep. The effect of removal of endometrial caruncles on fetal size and metabolism. *J Dev Physiol* **1**:379–398, 1979.
15. Kalousek DK, Barrett I. Genomic imprinting related to prenatal diagnosis. *Pren Diag* **14**:1191–1201, 1994.
16. Robinson WP, Barrett IJ, Bernard L *et al.* Meiotic origin of trisomy in confined placental mosaicism is correlated with the presence of fetal uniparental disomy, high levels of trisomy in trophoblast and increased risk of fetal IUGR. *Am J Hum Genet* **60**:917–927, 1997.
17. Moore GE, Ali Z, Khan RU, Blunt S, Bennett PR, Vaughan JI. The incidence of uniparental disomy associated with IUGR in a cohort of 35 severely affected babies. *Am J Obstet Gynecol* **176**:294–299, 1997.
18. Khong TY, De Wolf F, Robertson WB, Brosens I. Inadequate maternal vascular response to placentation in pregnancies complicated by pre-eclampsia and small for gestational age infant. *Br J Obstet Gynaecol* **93**:1049–1059, 1986.
19. Khong TY. The Robertson–Brosens–Dixon hypothesis: evidence for the role of haemochorial placentation in pregnancy success. *Br J Obstet Gynaecol* **98**:1195–1199, 1991.
20. Clapp JF, Szeto HH, Larrow R, Hewitt J, Mann LI. Umbilical blood flow response to embolization of the uterine circulation. *Am J Obstet Gynecol* **138**:60–67, 1980.
21. Myatt L. Control of vascular resistance in the human placenta. *Placenta* **13**:329–341, 1992.
22. Howe DT, Wheeler T, Osmond C. The influence of maternal haemoglobin and ferritin on mid-pregnancy placental volume. *Br J Obstet Gynaecol* **102**:213–219, 1995.
23. Rush D. Effects of changes in maternal energy and protein intake during pregnancy with special reference to fetal growth. In *Fetal Growth* (eds F. Sharp & R.B. Fraser), pp. 203–229. London: RCOG. 1989.
24. Godfrey K, Robinson S, Barker DJP, Osmond C, Cox V. Maternal nutrition in early and late pregnancy in relation to placental and fetal growth. *BMJ* **312**:410–414, 1996.
25. Drillien CM. Prenatal and perinatal factors in etiology and outcome of low birthweight. *Clin Perinatol* **1**:197–211, 1974.
26. Macara L, Kingdom JCP, Kohnen G, Bowman AW, Greer IA, Kaufmann P. Elaboration of stem villous vessels in growth restricted pregnancies with abnormal umbilical artery Doppler waveforms. *Br J Obstet Gynaecol* **102**:807–812, 1995.
27. Krebs C, Macara LM, Leiser R, Bowman AW, Greer IA, Kingdom JCP. IUGR with absent end-diastolic flow velocity in the umbilical artery in association with maldevelopment of the placental terminal villous tree. *Am J Obstet Gynecol* **175**:1534–1542, 1996.
28. Kingdom JCP, Burrell SJ, Kaufman P. Pathology and clinical implication of abnormal umbilical artery Doppler waveforms. *Ultrasound Obstet Gynecol* **9**:271–286, 1997.
29. RCOG *Alcohol consumption in pregnancy. Guideline 9.* 1996.
30. MacGregor SN, Keith LG, Chasnoff IJ *et al.* Cocaine use during pregnancy: adverse perinatal outcome. *Am J Obstet Gynecol* **157**:686–690, 1987.
31. Hobel CJ. Risk assessment in perinatal medicine. In *High Risk Obstetrics* (ed. E.L. Makowski), Vol. 21 pp. 287–295, MD: Harper and Row, 1978.
32. James DK. Organization of prenatal care and identification of risk. In *High Risk Pregnancy* (eds D.K. James, P.J. Steer, C.P. Weiner & B. Gronik), pp. 21–33. London: WB Saunders 1994.
33. Linhard A, Nielsen PV, Mouritsen LA, Zachariassen A, Sorensen HU, Roseno H. The implications of introducing the symphysial–fundal height measurement. A prospective RCT. *Br J Obstet Gynaecol* **97**:675–680, 1990.
34. Neilson JP, Whitfield CR, Aitchison TC. Screening for the small for dates fetus: a two stage ultrasound examination schedule. *BMJ* **228**:1203–1206, 1980.
35. Neilson JP, Munjanja SP, Whitfield CR. Screening for the small for dates fetus; a controlled trial. *BMJ* **289**:1179–1182, 1984.
36. Neilson JP, Grant A. Ultrasound in pregnancy. In *Effective Care in Pregnancy and Childbirth* (eds I. Chalmers, M. Enkin & M.J.N.C. Keirse), p. 426. Oxford: Oxford University Press, 1989.
37. Chang TC, Robson SC, Spencer JA, Gallivan S. Prediction of perinatal morbidity at term in small fetuses; comparison of fetal growth and Doppler ultrasound. *Br J Obstet Gynaecol* **101**:422–427, 1994.
38. Neilson JP. Alfisevic Z. Doppler ultrasound in high risk pregancies. In *Pregnancy and Childbirth Modules of the Cochrane Database of Systematic Reviews* (eds J.P. Neilson, C.A. Crowther, E.D. Hodnett, G.J. Haffmeyr

& M.J.N.C. Keirse). The Cochrane Collaboration Issue 3. Oxford: Update Software, 1997.
39. De Bono M, Fawdry RDS, Lilford RJ. Size of trials for evaluation of antenatal tests of fetal wellbeing in high risk pregnancy. *J Perinat Med* **18**:77–87, 1990.
40. Bower S, Bewley S, Campbell S. Improved prediction of pre-eclampsia by two stage screening of uterine arteries using the early diastolic notch and colour Doppler imaging. *Obstet Gynecol* **82**:78–83, 1993.
41. Bower S, Harrington KF, Schuchter K, McGinn C, Campbell S. Prediction of pre-eclampsia by abnormal uterine Doppler ultrasound and modification by aspirin. *Obstet Gynecol* **103**:625–629, 1996.
42. Spellacy WN, Buhi WC, Birk SA. The effectiveness of HPL measurements as an adjunct in decreasing perinatal deaths. *Am J Obstet Gynecol* **121**:835–843, 1975.
43. Grannum PAT, Berkowitz RL, Hobbins JC. The ultrasound changes in the maturing placenta and their relation to fetal pulmonic maturity. *Am J Obstet Gynecol* **133**:915–922, 1979.
44. Proud J, Grant A. Third trimester placental grading by ultrasound as a test of fetal wellbeing. *BMJ* **294**:1641–1644, 1987.
45. Vyas S, Nicolaides KH, Campbell S. Renal artery flow velocity waveforms in normal and hypoxaemic fetuses. *Am J Obstet Gynecol* **161**:168–172, 1989.
46. Cock ML, McCrabb GJ, Wlodek ME, Harding R. Effects of prolonged hypoxemia on fetal renal function and amniotic fluid volume in sheep. *Am J Obstet Gynecol* **176**:320–326, 1997.
47. Owen P, Ogston S. Conditional centiles for the serial analysis of amniotic fluid index. *J Obstet Gynecol* **17** (Supplement) **1**:511, 1997.
48. Ewer AK, McHugo JM, Chapman S, Newell SJ. Fetal echogenic gut: a marker of intrauterine gut ischaemia. *Arch Dis Childh* **69**:510–513, 1993.
49. Manning FA, Platt LD, Sipos L. Antepartum fetal evaluation. Development of a fetal biophysical profile. *Am J Obstet Gynecol* **136**:787–795, 1980.
50. Vintzileos AM, Campbell WA, Ingordia CJ, Noachinson DJ. The fetal biophysical profile and its predictive value. *Obstet Gynecol* **62**:271–278, 1983.
51. Vintzileos AM, Gaffney SE, Salinger LM, Kontopoulis VG, Campbell WA, Noachinson DJ. The relationships among the fetal biophysical profile umbilical cord pH and Apgar scores. *Am J Obstet Gynecol* **157**:627–631, 1987.
52. Manning EA, Lange IR, Morrison I, Harman CR. Fetal biophysical score and the non-stress test: a comparative trial. *Obstet Gynecol* **64**:325–331, 1984.
53. Mohide P, Kierse MJNC. Biophysical assessment of fetal well-being. In *Effective Care in Pregnancy and Childbirth* (eds I. Chalmers, M. Enkin & M.J.N.C. Kierse), pp. 485–488. Oxford: Oxford University Press, 1989.
54. Dawes GS, Moulden M, Redman CWG. Improvements in computerised fetal heart rate analysis antepartum. *J Perinatal Med* **24**:25–36, 1996.
55. Tyrell S, Obaid AH, Lilford RJ. Umbilical artery Doppler velocimetry as a predictor of fetal hypoxia and acidosis at birth. *Obstet Gynecol* **74**:332–336, 1989.
56. Morrow RJ, Adamson SL, Bull SB, Ritchie JWK. Acute hypoxemia does not affect the umbilical artery flow velocity waveform in fetal sheep. *Obstet Gynaecol* **75**:590–593, 1990.
57. Kiserud T, Eik-Nes, SH, Blaas HG, Hellevik LR, Simensen B. Ductus venosus blood velocity and the umbilical circulation in the seriously growth retarded fetus. *Ultrasound Obstet Gynecol* **4**:109–114, 1994.
58. Arias F. Accuracy of the middle cerebral to umbilical artery resistance index ratio in the prediction of neonatal outcome in patients at high risk for fetal and neonatal complications. *Am J Obstet Gynecol* **171**:1541–1545, 1994.
59. Morrison JJ, Rodeck CH. Fetal blood sampling: does it have a place? *Curr Obstet Gynaecol* **7**:93–97, 1997.
60. Nicolini U, Rodeck CH, Fisk NM. Limited role of fetal blood sampling in prediction of outcome in IUGR. *Lancet* **336**:768–772, 1990.
61. The GRIT Study Group. When do obstetricians recommend delivery for a high risk preterm growth retarded fetus? *Eur J Obstet Gynecol* **67**:121–126, 1996.
62. Schapp AHP, Wolf H, Bruinse HW *et al.* Influence of obstetric management on outcome of extremely preterm growth retarded infants. *Arch Dis Childh* **77**:95–99, 1977.
63. Murphy DJ, Hope PL, Johnson A *et al.* Neonatal risk factors for cerebral palsy in very preterm babies: a case–control study. *Lancet* **314**:404–408, 1997.
64. Fanaroff AA, Wright LL, Stevenson DK *et al.* Very low birthweight outcomes of the National Institute of Child Health and Human Development Neonatal Research Network. May 1991 through December 1992. *Am J Obstet Gynecol* **173**:1423–1431, 1995.
65. Hutton JL, Pharoah POD, Cooke RWI, Stevenson RC. Differential effects of preterm birth and small for gestational age on cognitive and motor development. *Arch Dis Childh* **76**:75–81, 1997.
66. Leger J, Levy-Marchal C, Bloch J *et al.* Reduced final heights and indication for insulin resistance in 20 year olds born small for gestational age: regional cohort study. *BMJ* **15**:341–347, 1997.
67. Barker DJP (ed.) *Fetal and Infant Origins of Adult Disease*. London: BMJ. 1992.

Red cell alloimmunisation

59

C.H. Rodeck and A. Deans

Introduction

Over the last 25 years, the incidence of severe haemolytic disease of the fetus and newborn (HDFN) caused by red cell alloimmunisation has dramatically fallen due to the widespread use of prophylactic anti-D immunoglobulin. In 1971, when anti-D immunoglobulin became generally available in the UK to be given to all unsensitised rhesus Rh(D)-negative women after termination of pregnancy or delivery of a rhesus-positive baby, the stillbirth and neonatal death rate attributable to Rh(D) alloimmunisation was around 120 per 100 000 births[1]. By 1992, this figure had fallen to 1.3 per 100 000 births[2]. Despite such successes, around 600–700 new Rh(D) immunisations occur each year in the UK[3]. The main reasons for failure of immunoprophylaxis include the administration of an insufficient dose of anti-D and failure to give anti-D after potentially sensitising events. Immunisation occurring in the last few weeks of uncomplicated pregnancy is now the single commonest identifiable cause suggesting that antenatal prophylaxis of all Rh(D)-negative women might reduce the maternal immunisation rate still further[4]. In North America, where such policy is routinely employed, there has been a more dramatic decline in the number of sensitised Rh(D)-negative women[5]. While Rh(D) alloimmunisation remains the most prevalent, there are also a small number of women who develop antibodies to other Rhesus antigens or to atypical antigens, such as Kell (K), Duffy (Fy^a) and Kidd (Jk^a, Jk^b). Fetal and newborn deaths attributable to haemolytic disease due to these antibodies have remained stable at around six cases per year in the UK[2].

The reduction in perinatal deaths due to HDFN has also occurred as a result of the great advances made in neonatal care and in the management of the affected fetus over the last few years. The introduction of high-resolution real-time ultrasound and the development of *in utero* fetal blood transfusion, in combination with increasing knowledge of the pathophysiology of the disease process, has meant that even in severely alloimmunised women, the prognosis can be optimistic. However, fetal haemolytic disease continues to be a significant cause of perinatal morbidity.

History

In 1941, Levine *et al.* demonstrated that maternal Rh antibodies were responsible for causing erythroblastosis fetalis, a condition characterised by hydrops fetalis, icterus gravis and severe anaemia of the newborn[6]. Such ominous features had been recognised for centuries but had only been attributed to a single disease process, together with hepatosplenomegaly and erythroblastosis (increased nucleated red blood cell count), when described in the medical literature in 1932[7]. Soon after this, exchange transfusion was shown to improve the prognosis for affected neonates[8]. It was also discovered that early delivery improved perinatal survival and work by Bevis showed that the severity of the fetal haemolytic disease could be predicted by serial amniocentesis[9]. A major therapeutic breakthrough though came in 1963 when Liley successfully performed the first intraperitoneal blood transfusions in severely affected fetuses *in utero* using adult red blood cells[10]. At about the same time, several attempts were made at intravascular transfusion but this required hysterotomy and the fetal and maternal risks were deemed too high. Twenty years later, Rodeck *et al.* reported a percutaneous technique for intravascular fetal blood transfusion using fetoscopy[11]. Refinements of these techniques remain the basis for successful treatment of the severely affected fetus today. Fortunately, most Rh(D)-negative women will never require such intervention due to the work of Clarke's group which led to the development of anti-D immunoglobulin in 1961[12].

Mechanism of red cell alloimmunisation

PATHOPHYSIOLOGY

Red cell membranes contain numerous surface antigens including those of the ABO and Rhesus groups. Maternal IgG red cell antibodies can be raised against most of the blood group specificities following exposure to an adequate quantity of foreign red blood cell antigen, either as a result of transplacental haemorrhage from the fetus to the mother or after heterologous blood transfusion. It has been demonstrated using Kleihauer testing that around 75% of women have fetal red cells in their circulation at some time during pregnancy and delivery although the number of fetal red cells varies considerably depending on gestation[13]. Anti-A,B antibodies in group O women are the commonest antibodies found in the UK but are very rarely seen to cause significant problems for the fetus or require intrauterine transfusion. For practical purposes anti-Rh(D), anti-c, anti-E and anti-Kell should be considered as the antibodies likely to have the potential to cause moderate to severe HDFN[14]. Other antibodies such as anti-Fy^a (Duffy) and Kidd (Jk^a, Jk^b) rarely cause significant problems.

Initial exposure to foreign red blood cell antigen leads to a weak primary immune response in the mother whereby predominantly IgM is produced after a latent period of some weeks. Since IgM cannot cross the placenta, the fetus is unaffected although the presence of these antibodies can be detected in maternal blood for up to a year after the primary event thus indicating maternal sensitisation. On subsequent exposure of the mother to similar antigenic red cells (usually in a subsequent pregnancy) her previously primed memory B cells act swiftly to produce IgG antibody. Considerably less antigenic stimulus is required for this secondary response compared to the first exposure and results in much higher antibody titres being produced. Maternal IgG antibodies are actively transported across the placenta via receptors to the Ig Fc portion located on the synctiotrophoblast. IgG immunoglobulin directed against a red cell antigen will bind to fetal red cells that express that antigen, so causing their sequestration. Red cell destruction appears to be mediated by subclasses IgG1 and IgG3 only[17]. IgG-sensitised red cells bind, via the Fc part of the antibody molecule, to Fcγ receptors (FcγR) on mononuclear phagocytes in the fetal reticuloendothelial system so triggering erythrocyte destruction by phagocytosis and/or cytolysis[15]. Three distinct classes of Fcγ receptor have been identified[16]. Recent work shows that in the fetus high affinity FcγR1 plays a major role in the IgG anti-D-mediated attachment to, and phagocytosis by, circulating monocytes and splenic mononuclear phagocytes[17]. The latter cells also have high expression of FcγR111 which is primarily involved in target ingestion. Monoclonal antibody to FcγR1 will almost completely inhibit the effector function of fetal or newborn monocytes and markedly reduce that of fetal splenic mononuclear phagocytes *in vitro*. It is possible that this could be the basis for a new therapeutic intervention for HDFN.

FcγR-mediated phagocytosis by monocytes and macrophages appears to be well developed by the early second trimester, i.e. some time before the onset of even the most severe Rh(D) haemolytic disease at 17–18 weeks[17]. Although placental transfer of maternal IgG has been shown to occur as early as 6–10 weeks' gestation, it is not until later in the second trimester that significant amounts are found in the fetal circulation[18,19]. Before this gestation, there is insufficient maternal anti-D transfer to cause severe fetal red cell haemolysis. By the end of pregnancy, a significantly higher concentration of IgG1 has accumulated in the fetus compared to that found in maternal blood whilst levels of the other IgG subclasses are similar in both mother and fetus[20]. Sensitised mothers carrying an Rh(D)-positive anaemic fetus demonstrate higher maternal levels of IgG1 compared to control pregnancies. In addition, there appears to be a preferential accumulation of IgG1 in those fetuses affected by the haemolytic process along with significantly lower levels of fetal IgG3 than are found in fetuses not at risk of HDFN. When measuring antibody levels in maternal serum for the purpose of predicting the severity of fetal haemolytic disease, the results are not normally corrected to allow for this discrepancy in IgG1 and IgG3 levels between mother and fetus. Furthermore, recent work suggests that the quantitative composition of IgG1 and IgG3 in the maternal serum, as determined by flow cytometry or enzyme-linked immunosorbent assay (ELISA), is important in determining the severity of haemolysis in the fetus[21,22]. Although the IgG3 subclass has a higher potential for inducing phagocytosis and monocyte adherence *in vitro*, IgG1 has a greater influence on the severity of HDFN *in vivo* than IgG3. Some laboratory anti-D assays currently in use display higher functional activities with IgG1 + IgG3 Rh(D) antibodies than with purely IgG1 antibodies and may fail to predict severe HDFN where serum antibodies comprise mainly of IgG1 antibodies[23].

Without a programme of anti-D prophylaxis, approximately 1% of Rh(D)-negative women will have detectable anti-D in their serum by the end of their first pregnancy with an Rh(D)-positive baby. A further 7–9% of these women will have detectable antibodies six months following delivery of that pregnancy and roughly the same number again will develop antibodies during a second pregnancy carrying an Rh(D)-positive fetus; thus around 17% Rh(D)-negative women are immunised by a single Rh(D)-positive pregnancy[24]. ABO incompatibility between the mother and fetus offers a protective effect against alloimmunisation because fetal cells entering the maternal circulation are quickly destroyed by maternal ABO antibodies before the Rh(D) antigen can be recognised by the maternal immune system. This reduces the chances of maternal sensitisation by around 20%[25]. The risk of Rh(D) alloimmunisation during pregnancy increases with advancing gestation because of the increasing incidence of fetomaternal transplacental haemorrhage (TPH) and the likelihood that larger amounts of incompatible red cells will enter the maternal circulation. Using the Kleihauer acid elution technique, it has been shown that during the first-trimester TPH is rare (3% of pregnancies) and involves only 0.03 ml of fetal blood whereas in the third trimester the frequency is as high as 45% of pregnancies with amounts as great as 25 ml recorded[13]. It is important to note that, whereas miscarriage in the first trimester carries a risk of sensitisation of less than 1%, surgical termination is associated with a much higher risk in the order of 20–25%. Bleeding in pregnancy, abdominal trauma, fetal blood sampling (FBS) amniocentesis, external cephalic version and chorionic villus sampling (CVS) should be regarded as potentially high-risk situations. Amniocentesis is associated with a 2% risk of maternal sensitisation even when performed under ultrasound guidance[26]. CVS carries a higher risk than amniocentesis, possibly as high as 50%, although the amount of fetomaternal haemorrhage that is associated with the procedure is dependent on the operator and technique used[27,28].

Being Rh(D) negative does not mean that the formation of maternal anti-Rh(D) antibodies and subsequent Rh(D) HDFN is inevitable in the event of prophylaxis being unavailable. Some Rh(D)-negative women are poor responders to the Rh(D) antigen while others may produce anti-Rh(D) that has a low potency or poor efficacy at mediating Fc receptor interaction with phagocytic cells. In addition, there is the protective effect of ABO incompatibility and the fact that some women will have partners who are heterozygous for Rh(D) so may deliver Rh(D)-negative babies. When maternal sensitisation with anti-RH(D) does occur it is estimated that around 50% of affected infants will have mild or no anaemia, 25–30% of fetuses will have a moderate anaemia which will require treatment in the neonatal period while the remaining 20–25% will develop hydrops, likely to lead to intrauterine death or neonatal death, unless antenatal fetal therapy is undertaken[29].

HYDROPS FETALIS

Ascites, pericardial and pleural effusions, subcutaneous oedema and placentomegaly are the classical sonographic features of hydrops although the precise mechanism behind their development remains speculative. The affected fetus becomes progressively anaemic due to red cell haemolysis and compensates with cardiovascular adjustments and by increasing erythropoiesis. Initially, to maintain tissue oxygenation, cardiac output, rather than heart rate, is increased as a consequence of the fall in peripheral resistance secondary to vasodilatation and decreased blood viscosity[30]. Evidence to support this comes from Doppler blood flow–velocity measurements of the umbilical artery and fetal descending aorta which correlate inversely with the degree of fetal anaemia[31,32]. A similar relationship is found between mean blood flow velocities in the middle cerebral artery and fetal haemoglobin (as measured at FBS) which appears to hold true irrespective of the pulsatility index value (PI) or whether there is fetal hypoxaemia suggesting that the hyperdynamic circulation is primarily as a consequence of decreased blood velocity[33].

In response to mild or moderate degrees of anaemia (fetal haemoglobin deficit of 2–7 g/dl for gestational age), intramedullary haematopoiesis is stimulated through increased erythropoietin production; analysis of fetal blood at this stage reveals an increased fetal reticulocyte count, in the absence of erythroblastosis[34]. Excessive and prolonged haemolysis results in marked erythroid hyperplasia of the bone marrow. As severe anaemia develops (haemoglobin deficit > 7 g/dl) large areas of extramedullary haematopoiesis are recruited in the liver which is characterised by an erythroblastosis or increased nucleated red blood cell count in fetal blood[35]. Pronounced leukocytosis may be present as a result of increased activity of the reticuloendothelial system. Fetal thrombocytopenia can occur although levels less than 80 × 10^9 are rare. Occasionally, in a severely hydropic fetus, widespread haemopoietic failure is indicated by a leukopenia and absence of a reticulocytosis or erythroblastosis[36].

Fetal haemoglobin concentration rises with gestational age and hydrops tends to occur at higher haemoglobin levels at later gestations compared to early on in pregnancy (Fig. 59.1)[37]. It is therefore more appropriate to relate severity of fetal disease to the haemoglobin deficit for gestational age rather than to the actual fetal haemoglobin or haematocrit value. The presence of hydrops indicates a fetal haemoglobin deficit ≥ 7 g/dl which, in the second trimester, means a haematocrit of under 15% or haemoglobin of 4 g/dl or less[34,38]. However, even at these levels, the fetus may not become hydropic. There are several possible explanations for the genesis of hydrops at this degree of anaemia including cardiac failure, increased capillary permeability caused by

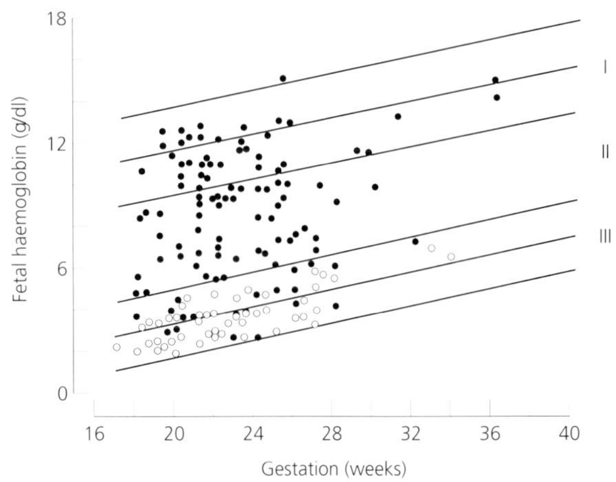

Fig. 59.1 Fetal haemoglobin concentration in Rh-alloimmunised pregnancies with (○) and without (●) fetal hydrops plotted on the normal range: mean and 95% data intervals. (Reproduced from Nicolaides *et al.* with permission from *Lancet* Ltd[37].)

chronic tissue hypoxia and decreased colloid oncotic pressure due to hypoproteinaemia secondary to liver dysfunction.

It has been suggested that hydrops is secondary to hypoproteinaemia caused by disruption of protein synthesis as the liver parenchyma becomes extensively infiltrated by erthyropoietic tissue. This now seems doubtful because, although hypoproteinaemia and hypoalbuminaemia are found in hydropic fetuses (total protein concentration < 3 g/dl, albumin < 2 g/dl) together with liver enlargement and significantly elevated liver transaminases, when compared to controls such findings are not unique to the hydropic state and can also be present in severely anaemic but non-hydropic fetuses[39–41]. Nicolini *et al.* have reported that in both hydropic and non-hydropic fetuses aspartate transaminase levels correlate with the erythroblast count indicating liver dysfunction to be a direct result of the fetal anaemia rather than a consequence of hydrops[41]. Correction of anaemia by transfusion causes fetal transaminases to revert to normal. After the first intrauterine transfusion rises in fetal γ-glutamyl transpeptidase can be demonstrated to directly correlate with the amount of blood transfused[41]. This appears to be more marked in hydropic fetuses and may indicate portal hypertension following the transfusion of a large blood volume. An alternative hypothesis is that the enlarged erythropoietic tissue causes a mechanical compression of the portal and umbilical veins altering substrate uptake and rate of synthesis[42]. Portal or umbilical hypertension with intrahepatic venous stasis secondary to such compression seems unlikely, though, in view of the hyperdynamic circulation demonstrated by Doppler ultrasound.

The fetus is able to tolerate mild-to-moderate anaemia by increasing blood flow to the tissues. However, with progressive anaemia, oxygen delivery to the tissues falls and, at a critical level, there is redistribution of blood flow to vital organs such as the brain and heart. Severe anaemia causes tissue hypoxia and fetal haemoglobin levels correlate significantly with umbilical artery blood acid–base values[43]. Since haemoglobin is the principal buffer in fetal blood, at a critical level, a metabolic acidaemia and hyperlactic acidaemia occurs. Soothill *et al.* have demonstrated when the fetal haemoglobin drops below 8 g/dl umbilical artery lactate concentrations increase although umbilical vein hyperlactataemia is not evident until haemoglobin levels of 4 g/dl or under are reached[35]. At this point, placental capacity for lactate clearance appears to be saturated so leading to fetal metabolic acidosis. In this environment, it seems reasonable to postulate that myocardial dysfunction occurs and leads to congestive cardiac failure and fluid retention in a manner similar to myocardial ischaemia in the adult.

Hypervolaemia related to a high-output cardiac failure has also been put forward as a reason for extravasation of fluids into the tissues. Very high levels of atrial natriuretic factor are found in association with immune hydrops implying an expanded intravascular volume[44]. Increased amniotic fluid volume is a recognised finding preceding the onset of hydrops which raises the possibility that the normoxaemic severely anaemic fetus is able to compensate by increasing urine production. However, estimations of fetoplacental blood volume before the first intrauterine blood transfusion in both hydropic and non-hydropic fetuses have failed to show any significant difference between the two groups[45]. A more credible theory is that hypoxia and its arterial vasoactive response leads to myocardial insufficiency and relative cardiac failure. Weiner *et al.* have reported elevated umbilical venous pressure (assumed to be an approximation of fetal central venous pressure) in two fetuses with immune hydrops immediately prior to first intrauterine transfusion while, in the same study, all anaemic non-hydropic fetuses had pressure values within the normal range[46]. These elevated levels rapidly corrected within 24 hours of intrauterine transfusion, although the hydrops took longer to resolve. This would support the suggestion that correction of hypoxia by infusion of blood increases the oxygen carrying capacity of the blood so improving myocardial function. Further evidence comes from pulsed Doppler measurement of ductus venosus blood flow before fetal transfusion which indicates that cardiac preload is increased in severely anaemic fetuses, possibly reflecting imminent congestive cardiac failure[47]. Hypoxia may affect not only the cardiac efficiency but also capillary endothelial cells, increasing their permeability to water and colloids.

GENETICS

The Rh blood group antigens are carried by a series of at least three very similar but distinct transmembrane proteins scattered across the red cell surface[48]. Two Rhesus antigens have immunologically distinguishable isoforms Cc and Ee but there is no evidence of an isoform d for the major antigen D. The Rhesus gene locus is located on chromosome 1p34–p36[49]. It consists of two closely linked, highly homologous (96% identical) genes, each 10 exons in length[50]. One gene is designated RhCcEe encoding both the Cc and Ee proteins by alternate splicing of a primary transcript, and a second gene, RhD, encodes the major antigen RhD (Fig. 59.2). An individual may be homozygous or heterozygous for Cc,Dd and Ee inheriting one set from each parent with d indicating an absence of the RhD gene. Being serologically Rh(D) negative means the absence of the major D antigen on the red cell surface either as a result of homozygous absence of Rh(D) gene or, as has been recently described, partial deletion of exons 7 to 9 or a stop codon exon 5 of the Rh D gene[51]. There are as many as 40 other Rh antigens but the RhD epitope is the most immunogenic of the Rh system, followed by Rhc which is more than 20-fold less potent. The use of 'Rhesus negative' or 'Rhesus positive' is best abandoned in favour of the more accurate and precise terms of Rh(D) negative and Rh(D) positive. A few individuals have an abnormality of the D antigen and are termed D^u positive. In some cases, part of the D antigen is missing and these women could form anti-D if exposed to a normal D antigen[52]. There

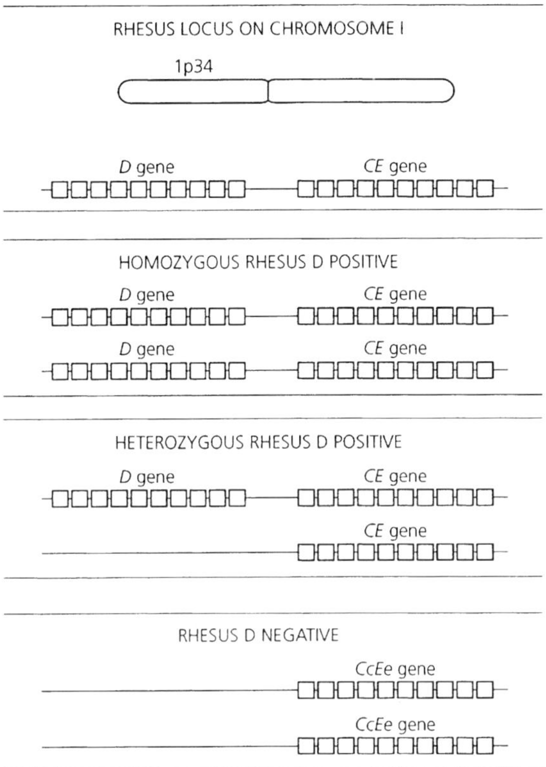

Fig. 59.2 RhD gene locus on chromosome 1. (Reproduced from Van den Veyver *et al.* with permission from the C.V. Mosby Company.)

is increasing evidence that they should receive anti-D immunoglobulin in appropriate circumstances[4].

Around 15% of the white Caucasian population are Rh(D) negative, apart from the Basque population where the incidence is as high as 30% giving rise to the hypothesis that the mutation originated there. In the Afro-Caribbean black population, the incidence is around 7–8% and drops to less than 1% in Chinese and Japanese peoples; 56% of Rh(D)-positive whites are heterozygous for the Rh(D) antigen and thus have a 50% chance of an Rh(D)-positive offspring from a partnership with an Rh(D)-negative woman.

The fetal genotype in respect to Rh(D) status can now be rapidly determined using a polymerase chain reaction (PCR) method on small amounts of fetal DNA in amniotic fluid and chorionic villous cells[53]. Initially, Bennett *et al.* developed two pairs of DNA primers, one pair to amplify a region common to the RhCcEe and RhD genes (exon 7), thus acting as an internal control, and one pair to amplify an area specific to exon 10 of the RhD gene. Analysis of 135 amniocenteses using these primers indicated a 1.5% false-negative rate for PCR Rh(D) genotyping of amniotic fluid as two of the 36 fetuses classified as Rh(D)-negative were subsequently found to be Rh(D)-positive after birth[54]. Contamination of amniotic fluid with maternal cells is a possibility where a fetus is incorrectly typed as Rh(D) negative. Contamination of the sample by Rh(D)-positive DNA at any point from collection onwards can also lead to errors, making it vital to handle the any such samples carefully. However, differences between serological and DNA primer Rh(D) typing also arise because of variations in the structure of the Rh(D) gene. There are examples of individuals who are serologically Rh(D) negative but because they have retained exon 10 of an internally deleted Rh(D) gene are typed as Rh(D) positive by PCR whilst other individuals are serologically Rh(D) positive but because they have a partial deletion of the Rh(D) gene or substitution of Cc,Ee sequences into Rh(D) gene exons they are typed as Rh(D)-negative by PCR[51]. Because of the far reaching implications of incorrect prenatal Rh(D) testing most groups now use two independent primer sets, designed from different parts of the RhCcEe and D genes, for instance using one set of primers specific for exons 4 and 5 and another specific for exon 10 of the RhD gene[55].

The DNA amplification technique has several advantages over serological fetal RhD typing which was carried out on erythrocytes obtained by fetal blood sampling (FBS) or chorionic villus sampling (CVS)[56]. It can be performed on amniotic fluid thus potentially reducing the fetal loss rate associated with FBS and CVS. Amniocentesis carries a lower risk of fetomaternal haemorrhage so there is less likelihood of the test causing an increase in maternal antibody levels and thus worsening fetal anaemia[57]. Rh(D) typing of the fetus can be performed at the first amniocentesis for ΔOD_{450} measurement (see below) and values in the mild-to-unaffected range interpreted in the light of fetal Rh(D) status. The potential of CVS to worsen alloimmunisation by inducing antibodies secondary to TPH means that CVS testing is, for the most part, best reserved for women with a history of very severe alloimmunisation who are planning to possibly terminate an Rh(D)-positive fetus. Women who have a history of alloimmunisation and a partner who is heterozygous for Rh(D), should be offered amniocentesis at 15–16 weeks. If the fetus is found to be Rh(D) negative, further investigations and invasive procedures are avoided whereas for the Rh(D)-positive fetus, there can be more rational planning of therapeutic intervention[58]. By this means RhD typing can also be carried out before the earliest onset of fetal hydrops.

The isolation of fetal cells from the cervix using techniques such as mucus aspiration, endocervical lavage and cytobrush has meant that it may be possible to routinely determine fetal RhD type by less-invasive methods in the future[59]. Adinolfi *et al.* have shown that fetal RhD sequences can be detected in this manner but with insufficient reliability at present to be used in clinical practice[60]. Alternatively, the discovery that fetal red cells are present in the maternal circulation at around 7 weeks of gestation raises the possibility of fetal Rh(D) typing by isolating fetal cells from maternal blood[61]. Preliminary work has demonstrated low success rates but this may reflect the rapid clearance of RhD cells from the circulation of sensitised Rh(D)-positive women[62]. There is a small subgroup of sensitised Rh(D)-negative women, with heterozygous Rh(D) positive partners, who have suffered repeated pregnancy losses or serial transfusions in previous pregnancies due to RhD alloimmunisation. It is theoretically possible to offer *in vitro* fertilisation with pre-implantation determination of embryonic Rh(D) type so that only Rh(D)-negative embryos are transferred.

A PCR-based approach to prenatal determination of RhCc and RhEe type has also become possible recently[63,64]. In the case of women with Rh(c) alloimmunisation, there is an 80% chance of her partner being positive for Rh(c) with a 60% likelihood that he is heterozygous. It is still not possible at the time of writing to use DNA techniques to determine the homozygous or heterozygous state for Rh(D) gene. Serology is required to determine Cc and Ee status and then, because these antigens are closely linked to the D locus, population studies enable further evaluation as to an Rh(D)-positive individual's likely zygosity.

Monitoring a pregnancy at risk

Routine antenatal management for all women should include first-trimester determination of their ABO blood group and Rhesus status together with a red cell antibody screen. For those women who are Rh(D) positive, it is reasonable to repeat the antibody screen at the beginning of the third trimester to detect red cell antibodies other than anti-Rh(D) that may have developed during the course of the pregnancy. In the UK, it is standard practice to repeat the antibody screen at 28 and 34 weeks' gestation for Rh(D)-negative women who have no relevant previous history and no evidence of sensitisation at booking. Nearly a third of women who subsequently have evidence of Rh alloimmunisation in a pregnancy do not demonstrate antibodies on initial testing of their blood[65]. Repeated testing is therefore important although antibodies detected early on are more likely to cause severe fetal disease. Paternal blood group testing, and the reduction of maternal surveillance should the partner prove to be Rh(D) negative, is useful as long as there are no doubts regarding paternity.

Once a woman is known to be alloimmunised, several factors can be used to predict the course of the disease. The management of red cell alloimmunisation is similar regardless of the inciting antigen, with the exception of Kell which will be discussed later, but for the sake of clarity we will refer to Rh(D) immunisation here.

PREVIOUS OBSTETRIC HISTORY

In the first sensitised pregnancy, the risk of fetal disease is very low with significant fetal anaemia and hydrops being unlikely to occur. With subsequent pregnancies, the severity of the fetal disease remains the same or, much more commonly, becomes progressively worse with onset of fetal anaemia at an earlier gestational age. In general, for patients with a previous affected pregnancy, it is aimed to perform the first intervention at approximately 10 weeks before the earliest previous fetal or neonatal death, fetal transfusion or birth of a severely affected baby as this is likely to be the time when the fetus has become anaemic but not hydropic. Fetal death or hydrops due to alloimmunisation before 18 weeks is exceptionally rare. If hydrops has occurred in one pregnancy, then it is likely to occur in subsequent pregnancies carrying an Rh-incompatible fetus if treatment is not undertaken.

ANTIBODY LEVELS

Serial measurement of maternal serum red cell antibody levels has traditionally been an important part of monitoring because of the well-established association between maternal antibody concentration and outcome of pregnancy. Routine antibody testing is by the indirect Coombs method. This technique involves incubating the patient's serum with red blood cells carrying the antigen against which the patient's antibodies are thought to be directed. Antihuman antiglobulin is then added, which causes agglutination of the red cells if they have absorbed the patient's antibodies. The antibody titre is expressed as a reciprocal of the highest dilution of serum that causes agglutination. Many laboratories now use an automated system that quantifies the concentration of anti-Rh(D). Although this is less subjective and related to an international standard, the most reproducible results are best obtained by testing all samples from one individual in the same laboratory.

Unfortunately, antibody levels do not always correlate well with the severity of fetal disease, probably reflecting the fact that the quality of the antibodies, i.e. the IgG subclass, and number of IgG bound molecules is important. The trend, e.g. a sudden rise in antibodies, is more significant than the absolute value, especially in more severely affected pregnancies where antibody titres do not distinguish between hydropic and non-hydropic fetuses. However, for those women in their first affected pregnancy, or with only a previous mildly affected pregnancy, maternal haemolytic antibody levels are reasonably reliable and should be measured at 2–4-weekly intervals. MacKenzie *et al.* have reported from a series of more than 1200 Rh(D) sensitised pregnancies[66]. They demonstrate that, where antibody levels are persistently below 4 IU/ml this indicates insignificant or, at the most, mild fetal haemolysis and that it is safe to allow the fetus to deliver spontaneously at term. Management of such cases is associated with a less than 5% risk of requiring an exchange transfusion for hyperbilirubinaemia. Moreover, the authors found that it was very rare for the cord haemoglobin level to be less than 10 g/dl at birth if the maternal antibody levels had been under 10 IU/ml during the week prior to delivery (only 2 babies out of 800 cases where antibodies demonstrated this pattern) although neonatal exchange transfusion was required for treatment of neonatal hyperbilirubinaemia in more than half of this group. It was recommended that invasive testing or delivery (if the pregnancy had reached 36 weeks' gestation) should only be undertaken at antibody levels greater than 10 IU/ml More recently, Nicolaides and Rodeck, in a cross-sectional study of 237 pregnancies with Rhesus alloimmunisation between 17 and 38 weeks, found that as long as the maternal anti-D concentration was < 15 IU/ml the fetus was, at the most, mildly anaemic (Hb deficit < 3 g/dl) on cordocentesis[67]. On this basis, it seems reasonable therefore to reserve invasive testing for those pregnancies where the antibody levels are above 15 IU/ml. Similarly, a sudden rise in antibody levels is often indicative of increasing severity of disease and may require intervention. Laboratories using titres will have a 'critical titre' at which there is a significant risk of fetal hydrops, typically between 1:8 and 1:32 dilutions.

A recent retrospective analysis of 120 mothers with anti-c antibodies, of whom 100 gave birth to a c-positive infant, showed that when the level of anti-c was below 7.5 IU/ml then the fetus was unlikely to be seriously affected[68]. However, above this level, prediction of fetal disease was difficult, maternal anti-c levels over 9.5 IU/ml being associated with exchange transfusion in 14 babies but with no treatment or phototherapy in 15 babies. Anti-Kell antibody levels should not be relied upon to determine the degree of fetal illness as fetal hydrops has been reported at indirect Coombs titres as low as 1:4[69].

The problem is that, although it is possible to decide upon a 'cut-off' level below which severe fetal disease does not occur, quantification of maternal antibody levels does not accurately predict fetal anaemia once this level has been exceeded. A number of workers have investigated the use of *in vitro* assays, such as the monocyte monolayer assay (MMA), antibody-dependent cell-mediated cytotoxicity assay (ADCC) and monocyte chemiluminescence (CL) test, which measure the ability of the anti-D antibodies to mediate red cell destruction through haemolysis and activation of effector cells. Some have demonstrated that these tests are superior to routine quantification of antibodies by indirect Coombs when it comes to predicting the severity of HDFN and the need for neonatal exchange transfusion but similar claims in respect to predicting fetal anaemia and determining when to perform invasive testing are not proven.[21,70,71]

ULTRASOUND ASSESSMENT

Ultrasound assessment of the at-risk fetus is important for detecting fetal hydrops. Weekly ultrasonography is appropriate in high-risk cases. The sonographic features of hydrops fetalis have been well described and include ascites, pericardial and pleural effusions, subcutaneous and scalp oedema, polyhydramnios and placentomegaly. There is no standard definition of hydrops and classification in terms of mild, moderate and severe is subjective. A fetus with hydrops will be severely anaemic with a haemoglobin deficit of 7 g/dl or more. Even so, the presence or absence of hydrops is still not totally reliable as only two-thirds of fetuses with a haemoglobin this low will demonstrate fetal ascites. The earliest indicators of hydrops include the first signs of fetal ascites, such as the 'bowel halo' sign of free fluid within the peritoneal cavity or the ability to visualise both sides of the fetal bowel, and the presence of fluid within the pericardial space[72].

It is important to be able to identify those fetuses whose condition is deteriorating but who have not yet developed hydrops. The earliest sonographic feature of haemolytic disease has been said to be enlargement of the heart, in particular the right atrium, as the fetal circulation adjusts to decreasing haemoglobin value[73]. An increase in amniotic fluid is often seen before the development of hydrops although an explanation for the pathophysiology of this finding is still lacking. Sonographic measurement of parameters such as extrahepatic and intrahepatic umbilical vein diameter, placental thickness, abdominal circumference, intraperitoneal volume and the ratio between the head and abdominal circumference have been investigated as to their usefulness in diagnosing anaemia but have now been shown to be unreliable in predicting fetal haematocrit in the absence of hydrops[74]. On the other hand, measurement of fetal liver length (as measured in a parasagittal plane) and fetal spleen perimeter (measured by tracing round the spleen in the same cross-sectional plane as the fetal stomach) appear to show some potential in evaluating fetal anaemia, enlargement of these dimensions reflecting the increased extramedullary erythropoietic mass[75–77]. Reference ranges for these two parameters have been established which we currently use in our unit[78].

DOPPLER STUDIES

The use of fetal Doppler ultrasound in the evaluation of severe alloimmunisation is appealing in view of the correlation between fetal haemoglobin and the increased maximum systolic flow velocities found in various parts of the fetal circulation as a consequence of elevated cardiac output and decreased blood viscosity. There is considerable literature describing various arterial and venous Doppler velocity measurements from fetal vessels such as the umbilical vein, descending thoracic aorta, middle cerebral artery, common carotid artery in relationship to the degree of fetal anaemia[31–33,79–82]. Intracardiac Doppler evaluation and demonstration of increased outflow tract velocities provide evidence of increased cardiac work with worsening anaemia[83,84]. In practice, the accurate prediction of fetal anaemia using such non-invasive assessment has not been demonstrated. The reasons for this are complex. These studies have been generally cross-sectional performed at the time of invasive testing. We are still unclear about the precise nature of the haemodynamic changes as anaemia progresses, for instance, what happens to peripheral resistance with impending hydrops. Our current practice is to measure the maximum umbilical vein velocity (V_{max}) as a means of non-invasive assessment of the fetal haematocrit in the non-hydropic fetus. The nomogram is shown in Fig. 59.3.

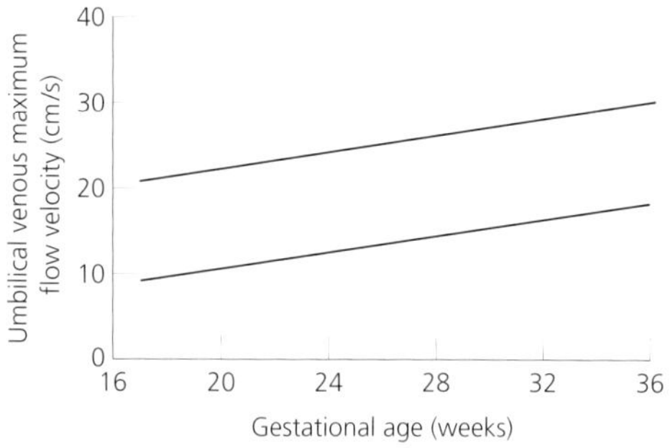

Fig. 59.3 Nomogram for umbilical vein maximal flow velocity (after Oepkes 1993)[78].

OTHER NON-INVASIVE TECHNIQUES FOR ASSESSMENT

Fetal movement counting is of some value and a reported change in the frequency of fetal movements should prompt further investigation. A reduction in fetal movements in association with the ultrasound findings of hydrops indicates a severely distressed fetus, although fetal movements have been said to be present until almost the time of death[85,86]. Sporadic or absent breathing movements may also be an ominous sign. Cardiotocographic (CTG) assessment of the fetus is not particularly helpful. A decrease in fetal heart rate (FHR) reactivity and baseline variability may be the first CTG indicators of anaemia but these FHR changes, along with CTG abnormalities such as a sinusoidal patterns or late decelerations, tend only occur once the fetus is severely compromised and hypoxic[87]. CTG patterns do not appear to allow for accurate prediction of mild-to-moderate fetal anaemia[88]. Measurement of fetal cardiac conduction times may be more helpful in the light of work correlating prolonged QRS complexes with anaemia at birth[89].

Invasive testing of the fetus

There are two methods of assessing the degree of fetal anaemia: indirectly by spectrophotometric assessment of the amount of bilirubin in the amniotic fluid around the fetus; or directly by haematological studies on a fetal blood sample (FBS). When to proceed to invasive testing should be a decision based on previous obstetric history, the duration of the pregnancy, maternal antibody levels and the results of non-invasive tests. The aim of management is to allow the pregnancy to continue to a safe gestational age, ideally 37 completed weeks or more, when a fetus who is not severely anaemic or hydropic can be delivered. This requires particular expertise and referral to a specialist fetal medicine centre is advisable once invasive testing is being contemplated. In many units there has been a decline in the number of amniocenteses performed in favour of non-invasive assessment and fetal blood sampling.

AMNIOCENTESIS

The end product of fetal red cell destruction is bilirubin. Fetal bilirubin has been shown to be raised in fetuses affected with haemolytic anaemia[90]. Most bilirubin is removed from the fetus via the placenta but small amounts enter the amniotic fluid in fetal urine and pulmonary fluid during the second and third trimester and increases in the bilirubin level in amniotic fluid correlate with the degree of fetal red cell destruction[9]. The amniotic bilirubin concentration can be quantified spectrophotometically by assessing the change in optical density at the wavelength 450 nm[91]. This is expressed as the ΔOD_{450} value (see Fig. 59.4). Contamination of the amniotic fluid with blood or meconium can lead to erroneous results as these substances can also produce peaks at these wavelengths. It is also important to transport specimens in light-proof containers and to send them immediately to the laboratory for analysis to avoid degradation of the bilirubin. Each amniocentesis has the potential to worsen maternal sensitisation. To reduce the risk of fetomaternal haemorrhage ultrasound guidance during the procedure is essential to avoid passage of the needle through the placenta.

In 1961, Liley devised a system for managing pregnancies complicated by rhesus alloimmunisation based on his observation that amniotic fluid ΔOD_{450} values between 27 and 35 weeks' gestation correlated with newborn outcome[91]. Essentially the same graph, the Liley chart, is in use today with ΔOD_{450} values plotted against gestational age and divided into three zones: a lower zone indicating mildly affected or unaffected fetuses, a mid-zone indicating mildly to moderately

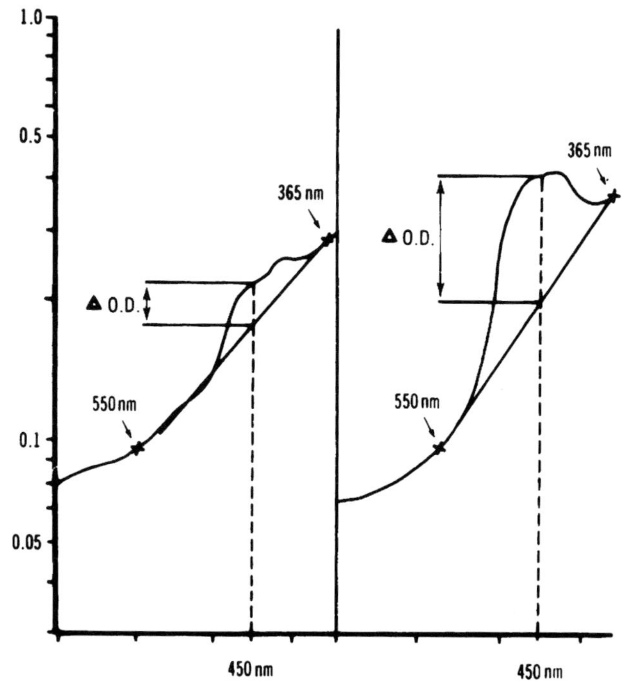

Fig. 59.4 Measurement of ΔOD_{450} at 450 nm, using a baseline drawn between the OD reading at 365 nm and 550 nm. The size of the peak at 450 nm is proportional to the amount of bilirubin present.

affected fetuses and an upper zone indicating those who are severely affected and require treatment or delivery (see Fig. 59.5). Very high ΔOD_{450} values confidently anticipate hydrops and, from 27 weeks onwards, accuracy of levels in zone 1 at predicting severe haemolysis have been reported as high as 96% and are an indication for intervention by FBS, transfusion or delivery[92]. However, several groups have demonstrated that ΔOD_{450} measurements can be inaccurate particularly in zone 2 where there can be considerable overlap with mildly and severely affected fetuses[93–95]. This is to be expected because ΔOD_{450} values merely indicate the amount of haemolysis that is occurring and the likely outcome in the untreated fetus rather than the fetal haematopoietic response and resulting haematocrit. Serial amniocenteses are usually recommended to gauge the trend of ΔOD_{450} measurements in the third trimester when initial results lie in zone 3 or zone 2. Higher levels will require FBS or delivery.

Confidence in the reliability of serial amniocentesis in the third trimester does not extend to its use in the second trimester. Liley's original work only examined pregnancies beyond 27 weeks. Nicolaides *et al.* have shown that the backward extrapolation of the Liley lines is of little value in accurately separating severely affected from mildly affected fetuses prior to this gestation[96]. The wide scatter and fluctuation of ΔOD_{450} values leads to a 68% false-negative rate for severely affected fetuses between 18 and 25 weeks. A number of

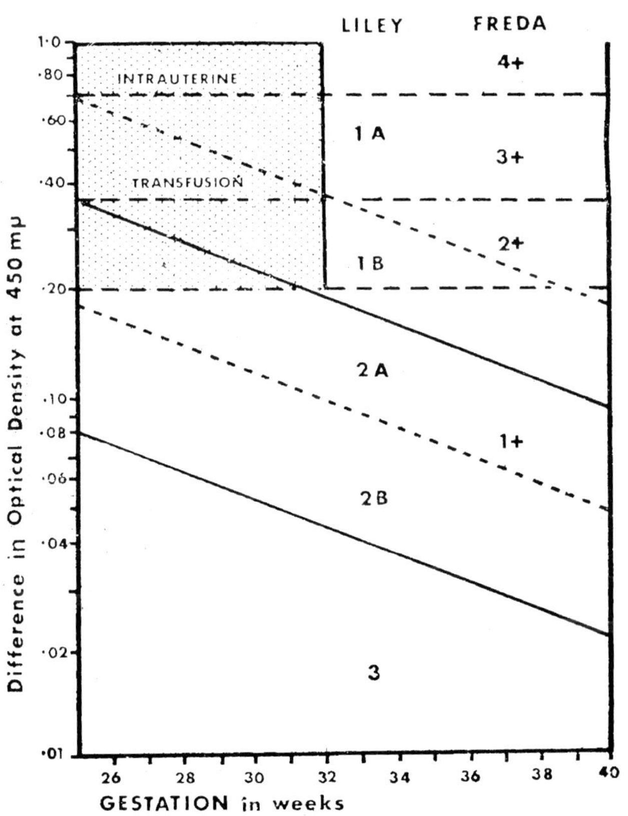

Fig. 59.5 Liley's chart showing ΔOD_{450} values in amniotic fluid against gestational age (Freda's classification is also included).

modified charts have been proposed using data from pregnancies sampled during the mid trimester and these suggest a curvilinear pattern to amniotic bilirubin levels during this time[97–99]. Extensive prospective use of this data in the management of affected fetuses is still awaited and at present an FBS rather than amniocentesis is the invasive test of choice if a fetus is likely to be at risk of severe disease in the early or mid second trimester.

FETAL BLOOD SAMPLING

The obvious advantage of obtaining fetal blood is to measure fetal haemoglobin and haematocrit. The first experimental attempts at FBS were during hysterotomy and were reported in 1973[100]. Five years later, Rodeck and Campbell demonstrated that pure fetal blood could be reliably obtained from umbilical cord vessels at the placental or fetal insertion using fetoscopy[101]. Nowadays, FBS has become a routine procedure under ultrasound guidance following its introduction by Daffos *et al.* in 1983 and in skilled hands is usually performed from around 18 weeks[102]. Depending on fetal position, the umbilical vein is needled either at the placental insertion or in the intrahepatic portion. By having a Coulter counter close at hand, the fetal haematocrit can be obtained within one minute and treatment, by intravascular transfusion, can be given through the same needle. FBS also allows for measurement of other haematological and biochemical parameters[37,90,103]. Knowledge of the fetal reticuloctye count and direct Coombs test can be helpful in predicting the course of the fetal anaemia. The fetal ABO group and Rhesus status can be determined in the event of the fetus proving not to be anaemic. Some fetal medicine centres advocate the use of FBS in cases previously managed by serial amniocentesis but this policy is not without risk to the fetus. In the largest reported series (606 cases), the fetal loss rate following FBS by skilled operators was 1.9%, although severely affected fetuses or those at early gestations are at greater risk[104,105]. Complications of FBS include exsanguination, intra-amniotic bleeding, fetal bradycardia, cord tamponade and failure to obtain a sample[104,105]. There is also the potential to worsen the degree of alloimmunisation as fetomaternal haemorrhage occurs in 70% of cases where the placenta is transgressed[106].

Management

WHEN TO PERFORM THE FIRST INVASIVE TEST

Broadly speaking, red cell alloimmunised women can be grouped into four categories which determine the type of management that they require. For the sake of clarity, Rh(D) will be used but can refer to the other red cell antigens.

1. *Women with a partner who is heterozygous for Rh(D)*
   They should be offered an amniocentesis for fetal genotyping in the early second trimester. If the fetus is Rh(D)-negative then no further action need be taken.

2. *Women with a previously mild history with a homozygous partner*
   In the presence of stable antibody levels, absence of sonographic signs and normal Doppler umbilical vein V_{max} measurements, expectant management can be pursued. However, once antibody levels exceed a threshold level, e.g. 15 IU/ml or a titre of 1 in 128, or if there has been a rapid rise in levels, then unless the fetus is at a suitable gestation for delivery (36 weeks or more) invasive testing is indicated with a view to proceeding to treatment as necessary. Whether invasive testing is by amniocentesis or cordocentesis depends partly on the specialist unit managing the woman and on the gestation of the pregnancy. Before 27 weeks' gestation, a fetal blood sample is the more reliable means of accurately assessing fetal anaemia. After 27 weeks, some centres favour amniocentesis to identify those fetuses who are likely to be severely anaemic, before proceeding to FBS and possible fetal blood transfusion. Others favour serial FBS as a more precise way of assessing the fetal condition despite the potential risk of worsening the alloimmunisation[106].

SERIAL FBS

If the haematocrit is less than 2 SD below the mean-for-gestational age intrauterine blood transfusion is indicated where delivery of the fetus is not a valid option. If the anaemia is only mild, e.g. the haematocrit is > 30%, then the direct Coombs titre and reticuloctye count give further useful information. A high reticuloctye count or strongly positive Coombs test in the presence of a normal haematocrit value would suggest the fetus is at risk of anaemia and we would advise repeating the FBS in 1–2 weeks. If all three parameters are normal, then repeating in 5–6 weeks may be more appropriate. These judgements are made in the light of the results of non-invasive testing.

3. *Severe previous history/homozygous partner*
   If the woman has had a severely affected fetus in a previous pregnancy, an FBS should be planned for approximately 10 weeks before the time of the earliest previous fetal or neonatal death, fetal transfusion or birth of a severely affected fetus but not before 20 weeks unless signs of hydrops are present. Ultrasound monitoring of the fetus should begin around 16 weeks to monitor for the development of hydrops. At the first FBS, the fetus is either transfused immediately and has regular transfusions until delivery or, depending on the haematological results, serial FBS is planned.
4. *Exceptional cases – death of an affected fetus before 20 weeks' gestation*
   In these women fetal blood transfusion will be necessary before 20 weeks' gestation. The risks of intravascular transfusion are high before this time (14% procedure related loss) and early intraperitoneal transfusion is preferable[107].

INTRAUTERINE BLOOD TRANSFUSION

Intrauterine transfusion is indicated when an FBS shows the fetal haematocrit is low or the fetus is hydropic. Either intravascular or intraperitoneal transfusion, or a combination of the two methods, can be performed depending on circumstances and operator preference as will be discussed below.

BACKGROUND

Fetal intravascular exchange transfusions were first attempted in the 1960s by open cannulation of fetal vessels, such as the femoral artery[108], saphenous vein[109] or chorionic plate vasculature[110], but these techniques required hysterotomy and fetal loss rates were high. A more successful and safer technique pioneered at this time was percutaneous intraperitoneal transfusion, first described by Liley in 1963 and to remain the only practical method for intrauterine transfusion for the next 20 years[10]. Without the benefit of ultrasound, Liley relied on fluoroscopic screening to correctly position the transfusion needle and catheter in the fetal peritoneal cavity. Urografin was injected into the amniotic cavity and the fetal bowel was visualised using X-rays as the fetus swallowed the contrast medium. Introduction of ultrasound-assisted intraperitoneal transfusion increased survival rates by avoiding the risk of fetal death from traumatic complications, such as damage to intra-abdominal and intrathoracic viscera, which accounted for up to 50% of the total mortality rate[111].

By the early 1980s, intrauterine intraperitoneal blood transfusion was firmly established as a treatment for fetuses identified by amniotic fluid ΔOD_{450} estimation as being severely affected but who were too immature for delivery (i.e. under 32–34 weeks). The outlook for fetuses with hydrops under 26 weeks of gestation, however, remained extremely poor so most centres did not perform transfusions before this gestation[112]. The presence of ascites appeared to prevent adequate absorption of erythrocytes[113]. In order to overcome these problems, Rodeck *et al.* in 1981 described a technique for intravascular transfusion by needling the umbilical artery under direct fetoscopic vision[11]. Following this type of treatment, the same group reported a survival rate of 84% in 19 fetuses, both hydropic and non-hydropic, who received their first transfusion on or before 25 weeks' gestation, some as early as 19 weeks[114]. Ultrasound-guided techniques for direct intravascular transfusion into the intrahepatic portion of the umbilical vein[115,116], the umbilical cord at the placental insertion[117] and the heart[118] were reported soon afterwards and became established practice, being less invasive and easier to use compared to fetoscopic methods. Several groups have published their experiences showing that repeated intravascular transfusions from as early as 18 weeks' gestation to up to 36 weeks' gestation are associated with survival rates ranging from 76 to 96%[117,119–122]. Delivery can be delayed until near term (in practice 36–37 weeks) so reducing the need for caesarean section and prolonged, expensive neonatal care.

PATHOPHYSIOLOGY

The anaemic fetus has a reduced capacity for tissue oxygenation. Compensatory mechanisms such as redistribution of blood flow to vital organs and fall in oxygen delivery to other fetal tissues allow the fetus to maintain normal blood gas and acid–base indices until the haemoglobin falls under 30% of normal (4–6 g/dl depending on gestational age), at which point tissue hypoxia is present[43]. Severe fetal anaemia is treated by infusing adult haemoglobin to increase the oxygen capacity of the blood. After the third or fourth transfusion, fetal erythrocytes will have been completely replaced by adult red blood cells in the fetal circulation.

Infusion of packed cells into anaemic non-hypoxic fetuses (haemoglobin > 4 g/dl) produces only a slight fall in pH and change in base excess, despite the fact that donor blood is relatively acidic (mean pH 6.76) with a high P_{CO_2} content, because of the buffering effect of the feto-maternal circulation[123]. Once the fetal circulation contains predominantly adult haemoglobin, fetal umbilical artery blood is more acidotic with a higher base deficit compared to when only fetal haemoglobin is present[124]. In the fetal umbilical venous circulation, P_{O_2} is around 5 mmHg higher with predominantly adult haemoglobin[124]. This suggests that oxygen delivery to the tissues is better with fetal haemoglobin, most likely to be due to the differences in the oxygen dissociation curves of fetal and adult haemoglobin. The relative acidosis found in association with adult haemoglobin would shift the oxygen dissociation curve to the right and promote oxygen release. The high umbilical venous P_{O_2} found in association with adult haemoglobin indicates greater oxygen transfer across the placenta. In situations where the fetus has pre-existing acidosis, transfusion could worsen the acidosis and be responsible for the higher rate of adverse outcome seen in such cases. In addition, at low P_{O_2} levels adult haemoglobin has a smaller reserve and releases less oxygen than fetal haemoglobin in response to the same fall in P_{O_2} which would be worse in the presence of fetal hypoxia.

INTRAVASCULAR VS. INTRAPERITONEAL TRANSFUSION

Intravascular transfusion (IVT)

Advantages

Intravascular transfusion offers a number of advantages over the intraperitoneal route, including:

- determination of the fetal blood group; the fetus may be Rhesus negative so rendering further investigation unnecessary
- direct assessment of the haematocrit and haemoglobin
- measurement of the pre- and post-transfusion haematocrit
- allows the appropriate amount of blood to be transfused
- blood is transfused into the fetal circulation, avoiding the lymphatic transport from the peritoneal cavity
- more effective correction of anaemia when fetus is hydropic
- reversal of hydrops *in utero*
- avoids trauma to fetal intraperitoneal organs
- allows for timing of subsequent transfusions and optimum time for delivery by calculation of the fall in haematocrit per day
- treatment can be continued until well into the third trimester so avoiding the complications of premature delivery and exchange transfusions at birth.

Technique

Initially a 20 gauge spinal needle is passed under ultrasound guidance to obtain a fetal blood sample in the normal manner. A Teflon-coated needle may be superior[125]. Ideally three trained personnel are required: an experienced operator who performs the needling of the fetal vasculature and monitors the transfusion throughout by visualisation on the ultrasound screen, an assistant who administers the blood and a third person who acts as a 'runner' performing the blood tests and calculations.

Premedication. In general, fetal transfusions are performed as an outpatient procedure and are associated with only minimal maternal discomfort. Although maternal anxiety can usually be allayed by appropriate counselling, very occasionally it may be necessary to administer a premedication. This will also sedate the fetus.

Site for transfusion. Most operators favour the umbilical cord at its placental insertion. The umbilical vein is used for a number of reasons. It is wider in diameter than the artery and is more easily targeted. It is less likely to go into spasm during the procedure and cause a fetal bradycardia. Its use allows the operator to watch the flow of transfused blood sonographically confirming the correct placement of the needle and so avoids the potentially fatal complication of cord tamponade should the needle slip and blood be injected into the Wharton's jelly. If fetal lie and placental position prevents safe access to this site then an alternative approach is to needle the intrahepatic vein. Unlike some, we would not advocate use of a free portion of umbilical cord because of the potential for needle slippage. Cardiac puncture is rarely used because of the potential hazards such as cardiac tamponade, haemopericardium and arrhythmia including asystole[118].

Fetal paralysis. If the fetus moves during an IVT procedure, this can cause needle displacement, haemorrhage or fetal trauma. If the fetus is very active and the placenta is posterior temporary paralysis may be advisable. Various neuromuscular blocking agents have been used including intramuscular or intravenous pancuronium bromide and curare[126,127].

Volume and rate of transfusion. On obtaining access to the fetal circulation, a 1-ml sample of fetal blood is promptly obtained in order to determine the fetal haematocrit. Our unit has a Coulter counter adjacent to the procedure room so that the result is obtained within a few seconds, during which time the tip of the needle remains in the fetal vessel. Mean fetal haemoglobin varies with gestation (Fig. 59.1). If the fetal haematocrit is less than 2 SD below the mean for gestation, in practice below 30%, then an *in utero* transfusion is undertaken. The needle is first connected to a three-way stop-cock via extension tubing so that the blood transfusion can be administered with minimal chance of movement of the needle during the procedure (Fig. 59.6). If transfusion is not necessary because the haematocrit is normal, then the needle can be withdrawn and conservative management by non-invasive monitoring be pursued.

The volume of blood transfused is determined by three factors: the pretransfusion fetal haematocrit, the estimated fetoplacental blood volume and the haematocrit of the donor blood. Nomograms have been constructed to provide an estimation of the volume of donor blood required to raise the fetal haematocrit to 40% (Fig. 59.7)[117]. Alternatively a simple calculation can be performed:

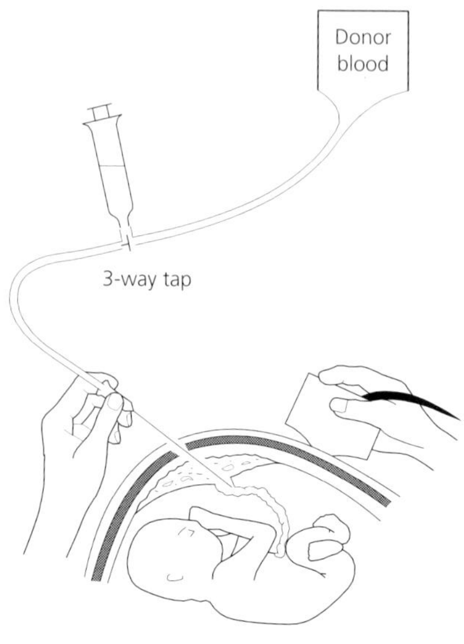

Fig. 59.6 Fetal blood transfusion into the umbilical vein at the placental cord insertion.

We aim to raise the fetal haematocrit to supraphysiological levels, i.e. to 35–40% in the early mid trimester and to 45–50% later on in pregnancy. Sometimes, a sample of fetal blood is aspirated mid-way during the transfusion to check the fetal haematocrit and to confirm the amount of blood to be further transfused. At the end, a final sample of fetal blood is taken to estimate the post-transfusion fetal haematocrit and

$$\text{Volume to be transfused} = \frac{\text{Donor haematocrit} - \text{Desired haematocrit}}{\text{Desired haematocrit} - \text{Fetal haematocrit}} \times \text{Fetal blood volume}$$

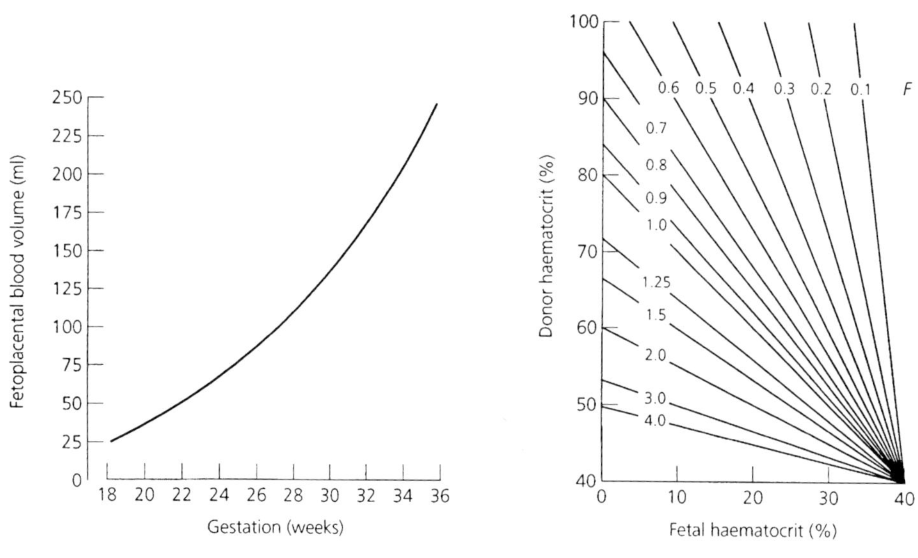

Fig. 59.7 Nomogram for intravascular transfusion. To calculate the volume of donor blood necessary to achieve a fetal haematocrit of 40%, the estimated fetoplacental blood volume (left, e.g. 100 ml at 27 weeks) is multiplied by *F* (right, e.g. 0.8 for a pretransfusion haematocrit of 10% and a donor haematocrit of 80%). (Reproduced from Nicolaides *et al.* with permission from S. Karger AG.)

for a Kleihauer–Betke test to determine the proportion of adult red blood cells now present in the fetal circulation.

The blood is transfused at a rate of 5 to 10 ml per minute. During the procedure the flow of blood is continuously visualised on the ultrasound screen to confirm that the needle remains correctly placed and the fetal heart periodically checked for arrhythmias, in particular fetal bradycardia. In our unit we use a free-hand technique rather than a needle guide so allowing independent movement of the ultrasound transducer.

Donor blood. The blood used should be adult group O RhD-negative blood which has been collected within 24 hours and cross-matched with the maternal blood. It should have been screened for hepatitis B and C, cytomegalovirus and HIV as well as irradiated to remove the white blood cells to avoid 'graft-versus-host'-like complications in the fetus. The blood is packed to a haematocrit of 75–85% to minimise the volume of blood that needs to be transfused.

'Top-up' vs. exchange transfusion. Concerns have been voiced that by directly transfusing blood into the fetus without removing any blood, the so-called 'top-up' transfusion, there might be a danger of volume overload and cardiac embarrassment. Some groups have reported a technique of exchange transfusion whereby small amounts of blood are aspirated from the fetus at regular intervals during its blood transfusion with the intention of preventing hypervolaemia especially in the hydropic fetus whose myocardium may be already overstressed[119,128]. Others suggest that the umbilical venous pressure should be routinely monitored and if the change in pressure exceeds 10 mmHg then blood should be removed and replaced with an equal volume of saline as such changes in pressure are associated with fetal demise[129]. In practice, although umbilical venous pressure can be demonstrated to rise significantly during transfusion (mean increase 4.6 mmHg), the fetus appears to tolerate 'top-up' transfusions of 100–150% of its fetoplacental blood volume[46,117,130]. Pressure increments in the umbilical vein of up to 12 mmHg have been recorded after transfusion without complication[131]. 'Top-up' transfusions have the advantage of being quicker than exchange transfusions, which reduces the risk of needle displacement, bacterial contamination and umbilical vein thrombosis. Fetal blood viscosity is probably a more important consideration than volume infused, particularly at earlier gestations. Post-transfusion fetal blood viscosity tends to be above the 95th centile for gestational age following IVT[132]. Radunovic *et al.* reported on 19 severely anaemic, hydropic fetuses receiving their first intravascular transfusion in the mid trimester where seven fetuses (36.8%) died 24–72 hours after transfusion despite no evidence of fetal distress associated with the procedure[133]. There were no significant differences in gestational age, in the total blood volume infused or volume transfused as a percentage of total fetoplacental blood volume between survivors and those who died. The only significant difference was in the relative increase in haematocrit. It was 5.5-fold in those who died compared to 3.5-fold in the survivors. Such acute increases in haematocrit represent substantial increases in fetal blood viscosity and confirm our opinion that it is this that leads to fetal demise rather than volume overload.

Timing of subsequent transfusions

The second transfusion should be performed not later than 2 weeks after the first transfusion. In cases of severe anaemia or where a small first transfusion has been given then the second transfusion will need to be performed after one week. The mean fall in haematocrit is around 1% per day but there can be a wide variation (SD 0.44)[134]. This rate of fall is particularly unpredictable during the interval between the first and second transfusions when the percentage of fetal erythrocytes left in the fetal circulation and suppression of erythropoiesis in the fetus after the initial transfusion are variable. The general tendency is for a less marked fall between the second and third transfusion with the exception of a few fetuses who show active erythropoiesis after the first transfusion. In these latter cases, the Kleihauer test indicates that there is an increase in the percentage of fetal erythrocytes at the start of the second transfusion compared to at the end of the first transfusion, thus alerting one to the likelihood that the fall in haematocrit will be higher in the subsequent than previous interval due to more cells being haemolysed. After the second and third transfusions, the rate of fall in haematocrit per day is usually very constant for an individual fetus. The fetal circulation now contains adult red blood cells almost exclusively (as shown by the Kleihauer test), fetal erythropoiesis is suppressed (fetal reticuloctye count < 1%) and fall in haematocrit is due to fetal growth and plasma expansion, not due to haemolysis. One can plot the pre- and post-transfusion haematocrit values on a graph. By calculating the rate of fall during transfusions one can predict when the next IVT should be scheduled in order to prevent the development of hydrops. This means maintaining the fetal haematocrit above the critical level of one-third of the normal mean for the gestational age (haematocrit 20–25%) and usually leads to an IVT every 3 weeks. Maintaining the longest possible interval between transfusions reduces the overall number needed and reduces risk of procedure-related loss (Fig. 59.8).

Complications. The fetal loss rate per IVT ranges from 0.6 to 4%[134,135]. The risks are greatest before 20 weeks, procedure-related losses being as high as 14% in this group[107]. The most common complication is that of a transient fetal bradycardia which occurs in around 8% of procedures although this rarely requires delivery of the fetus[122]. Other potentially fatal complications include cord accidents, such as cord tamponade resulting from a cord haematoma, endothelial dissection of the fetal vessel, umbilical artery spasm, haemorrhage from the

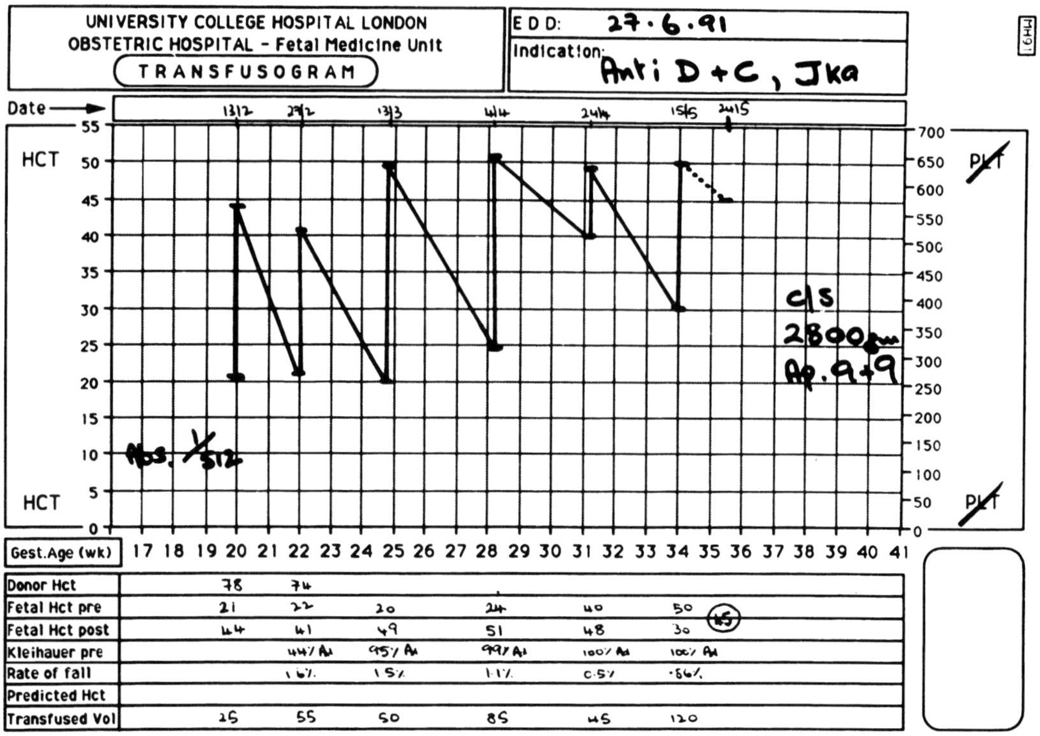

Fig. 59.8 An example of a patient who had a successful programme of IVTs.

puncture site, thromboembolism and overload of the fetal circulation[117,121,122,136]. Chorioamnionitis, preterm rupture of the membranes and preterm labour can occur but are infrequent. The intravascular route has the potential to cause feto-maternal haemorrhage, particularly if the placenta is traversed, thus worsening the degree of maternal sensitisation.

Fetal surveillance. Following administration of an IVT we recommend monitoring the fetal heart rate by cardiotocography for 1 hour. It should be pointed out that, if the fetus has been given pancuronium bromide during the procedure, the fetal heart rate variability is often poor because there are no fetal movements[137]. The mother should be given a fetal-movement chart and attend for weekly monitoring by ultrasonography and umbilical artery Doppler waveform assessment until the next transfusion.

Consequences of transfusion. After *in utero* transfusion, the fetal circulation will contain adult red blood cells and, after a number of transfusions (usually three transfusions) the Kleihauer–Betke test will show that there are virtually no fetal erythrocytes present. Fetal erythropoiesis will have been suppressed. At birth, the fetal blood group will be group O RhD negative. It can take several weeks for complete resumption of erythropoiesis and parents should be warned that 'top-up' blood transfusions may be necessary, anaemia developing as the baby grows, and that this should not be regarded as a failure. Regular monthly haemoglobin estimations until 6 months of age are advisable. In the future, exogenous erythropoietin may prove to be effective in preventing late anaemia[138]. Babies born after intrauterine transfusion do not appear to have an increased risk of compromise at birth. Normal growth and normal neurological and development patterns have been reported[139,140].

Rh-alloimmunised fetuses have been shown to have high serum ferritin levels – often above the normal reference range[141]. Serial *in utero* transfusions are associated with further increase in these levels to concentrations that would be considered to represent iron overload in children. One case of liver disease consistent with iron overload has been reported in an infant after *in utero* transfusion therapy[142]. It is recommended that serum ferritin levels are monitored in the neonatal and infant period and iron supplementation withheld until levels are within the normal range.

Intraperitoneal transfusion (IPT)

As described earlier, Liley successfully pioneered this method of transfusion over 30 years ago but since the development of intravascular techniques many have advocated intravascular transfusion as the treatment of choice[114,122,135]. Intraperitoneal transfusion relies on placing the donor red cells into the peritoneal cavity so that they become absorbed into the fetal circulation via the subdiaphragmatic lymphatics and thoracic duct. However, the presence of ascites reduces the efficacy of this process. For this reason in the hydropic fetus intravascular transfusion is considerably more successful at reversing hydrops and ensuring survival in the neonatal period. In a case–control study by Harman *et al.*, 18/21 (86%) of hydropic fetuses survived after IVT compared to 10/21 (48%) who had IPT[135]. The situation, however, is less clearcut when considering non-hydropic fetuses as survival rates for both IVT and IPT are in the region of 80–100% when ultrasound is routinely employed.

Advantages

- Method of choice if treatment becomes necessary at very early gestations, under 18 weeks when direct access to the fetal vasculature is difficult and hazardous.
- Enables transfusion when fetal lie and position of the placental cord insertion technically precludes access to the fetal circulation.
- When combined with IVT, allows an increased blood volume to be given (so lengthening time between transfusions) without overloading the fetal circulation.

Disadvantages

- Not suitable for the hydropic fetus.
- Cannot obtain pre- and post-transfusion haemoglobin so have to estimate blood volume to be transfused based on gestational age.
- Danger of trauma to fetal abdominal organs although this has been greatly reduced by the use of ultrasound.
- Inadvertent transfusion into fetal bowel, liver or abdominal wall can occur.
- Increased intraperitoneal pressure can compromise venous return to the heart resulting in fetal bradycardia.

Technique

The mother is prepared in a similar manner for IVT. A 20 or 18 gauge spinal needle is inserted into the fetal abdomen under ultrasound guidance. Ideally, the needle should enter the fetal abdominal cavity through the anterior abdominal wall, below the umbilical vein but above the fetal bladder, thus avoiding trauma to the fetal liver which may well be enlarged. To verify that the needle is correctly positioned, the operator should either aspirate ascitic fluid if the fetus is hydropic or, in the absence of ascites, can infuse a bolus of saline solution into the peritoneal cavity while observing the tip of the needle sonographically. Pancuronium bromide can be given intraperitoneally if there is a concern that the fetus may move and dislodge the needle. The needle can then be connected via a three-way tap to the infusion tubing and donor blood administered at a rate of about 10 ml/min, as described for IVT. Throughout the infusion, the tip of the needle is monitored sonographically to observe the flow of blood entering the peritoneal cavity and the fetal heart rate observed in case is persistent bradycardia indicates the transfusion should be discontinued.

The amount of donor blood to be given is calculated using the following empirical formula:

$$(\text{gestation in weeks} - 20) \times 10 \text{ ml}$$

It should be noted that this means that the quantity of blood being infused is related to the gestational age of the fetus rather than the degree of anaemia. If a large amount of ascitic fluid is present, this should be removed.

Combined IVT and IVP transfusions

In view of the procedure-related risks for both IVT and IPT techniques, it would clearly be beneficial to maintain the longest possible interval between transfusions. One way to achieve this is to combine both techniques as this permits a high-volume transfusion to be given without overloading the fetal circulation. Animal studies and our own personal observation indicate that intraperitoneal blood is absorbed over a few days[143]. Data from Nicolini *et al.* reporting on 31 fetuses who had a total of 99 intrauterine transfusions, of which 59 were combined intravascular and intraperitoneal procedures, showed a significantly longer interval between transfusions when blood was given both intravascularly and into the peritoneal cavity compared to when only intravascular transfusion was given[134]. Although the increase in time interval between the combined IVT–IPT and single IVT technique was only 3 days, the initial haematocrit at subsequent transfusions was a mean of 3.9 g/dl higher with the combined procedure. There is no overall difference in the percentage fall in haematocrit indicating that, effectively, all the intraperitoneal blood is absorbed.

The technique used is the same for IVT. Enough donor blood is given intravascularly to raise the fetal haematocrit to 40%, as confirmed by a post-transfusion haematocrit. The same spinal needle is then used to perform an IPT, particularly easy if the intrahepatic portion of the umbilical vein has been used[144], with the amount of donor blood transfused intraperitoneally being the same as that amount that would be required intravascularly to raise the haematocrit to 60%.

Outcome of treatment

At University College Hospital, London, between 1992 and 1994, 46 fetuses underwent 169 intrauterine transfusion of whom 8 (17%) were hydropic at the first transfusion. The fetal loss rate per transfusion was 2.4% and the overall survival rate was 87% (92% for non-hydropic fetuses and 88% for hydropic fetuses). Ten fetuses had their first transfusion at 20 weeks or earlier and in this group the survival rate was 80%. There were no losses in those fetuses who had their first transfusion after 29 weeks' gestation. The last transfusion should be performed so when delivery occurs, ideally 37–38 weeks, the fetal haematocrit is not less than 20–25%.

OTHER TREATMENTS OF RED CELL ALLOIMMUNISATION

A variety of alternative treatments for alloimmunisation have been proposed with varying success. Plasmapheresis has been reported as reducing maternal anti-D levels but there is little evidence that severe fetal disease can be prevented by doing this[145,146]. The technique is costly and time-consuming, involving the removal of large volumes of plasma several times a week, and is not without complications. The use of high-dose intravenous immunoglobulin (IVIG) has been described in two series where pregnancies were complicated by severe Rh alloimmunization[147,148]. Although there is some evidence for its efficacy before 28 weeks' gestation, it does not appear to alleviate the need for IVT. Promethazine, in large doses, has been cited as decreasing red cell phagocytosis and decreasing antibody production but the evidence for the effectiveness of such treatment remains unproven[149].

OTHER ANTIGEN SENSITISATION

There are numerous minor antigens found in addition to the D antigen on the surface of red blood cells. Antibodies raised to these antigens have become relatively more common in pregnancy as Rh(D) sensitisation has become less frequent due to the use of anti-D immunoglobulin. In the majority of cases sensitisation to these minor antigens can be traced back to a blood transfusion which the mother has received; blood banks do not routinely test for compatibility other than for the ABO and Rh(D). Those antigens which can cause severe haemolytic disease of the newborn include anti-c, anti-E and anti-Kell. Anti-Fy^a (Duffy) rarely causes more than mild HDFN but recent data indicate that pregnancies where anti-Fy^a titres are found in excess of 64 are at significant risk of severe anaemia[150]. Fetal genotyping may be appropriate where the father is known to be heterozygous and antibody titres are high or rising. Multiple antibodies may be present and can also occur in combination with anti-Rh(D). In a 12-year study in Sweden investigating the prevalence of red cell antibodies, 0.57% of mothers tested in routine antenatal screening had red cell antibodies with 0.24% being clinically significant[151]. Multiple antibodies occurred in 8.2%.

Management of minor antigen sensitivity is, in essence, the same as that undertaken for Rh(D) disease. Regular measurement of maternal antibody titres should be performed throughout the pregnancy and significant rises in antibody titres should lead to further assessment similar to that described for anti-Rh(D) alloimmunisation. Unfortunately, maternal antibody titres may not be reliable indicators for predicting the severity of the haemolytic disease in the newborn nor is it possible to easily establish a critical titre for antenatal intervention. Van Dijk *et al.*, reporting on a retrospective study of 418 pregnancies complicated by red cell alloantibodies, showed that at titres of 1 in 16 for anti-c, anti-E and anti-Kell only 4% of newborn required transfusion compared to 20% with anti-D[152]. In the future, assays to measure cytotoxic lysis or phagocytosis may be more helpful. With anti-C levels below 7.5 IU/ml, the fetus is unlikely to be seriously affected; above this, intervention may be necessary[153]. DNA-based RhEe genotyping is possible on amniotic and CVS samples[154].

ANTI-KELL

Around 10% of the population are Kell positive. The vast majority of Kell-negative women who develop Kell antibodies do so as a consequence of receiving a transfusion of Kell-positive blood. Anti-Kell antibodies can cause severe fetal anaemia and hydrops *in utero*. The frequency of affected neonates is 1 in 10 000[155].

Maternal antibody titres are unreliable at predicting whether the fetus is Kell positive (large rises in antibody titres have been reported in the presence of a Kell-negative fetus) or at indicating the severity of fetal disease[156,157]. A recent study of 11 fetuses who were anaemic due to maternal anti-Kell alloimmunisation showed them to have a significantly lower reticulocyte count and reduced erythroblastosis when compared to anaemic fetuses (matched for haematocrit, gestational age, hydrops and perinatal outcome) where the mother was alloimmunised to anti-D[158]. These findings suggest that erythroid suppression, rather than haemolysis, is the predominant mechanism in producing fetal anaemia secondary to maternal Kell alloimmunisation. The authors found that amniotic fluid bilirubin concentrations correlated poorly with fetal haematocrit which is consistent with reduced haemolysis. Amniocentesis is therefore not helpful in predicting fetal anaemia.

Our approach to mothers with anti-Kell sensitisation is firstly to determine the paternal antigen status with regards to Kell. If he is Kell negative, then the fetus should be as well. No further investigation is needed although serial ultrasound monitoring for hydrops may still be advisable as paternity cannot always be guaranteed. If he is Kell positive, only 3% of such people are homozygous positive so the fetus may still be Kell negative despite the fact that maternal anti-Kell titres are elevated. In these cases, early FBS for Kell grouping and assessment of fetal anaemia, followed by frequent non-invasive ultrasound assessment and further FBS as necessary is usually indicated. DNA-based Kell genotyping is now also possible.

The future

Advances in the management of fetal disease caused by red cell alloimmunisation has meant that sensitised women, who in the past would have suffered multiple fetal and neonatal losses, can now be optimistic about achieving a successful pregnancy outcome and completing their families. Some couples choose to go through two or even three pregnancies that require serial *in utero* blood transfusion, although it should not be forgotten that each pregnancy does involve considerable commitment by both parents and medical staff as well as not being completely risk-free for both mother and fetus.

There are further inroads to be made into the antenatal prevention of red cell sensitisation: namely, the adoption of the routine administration of anti-D immunoglobulin to Rh-negative mothers during the antenatal period and routine assessment of donor–recipient compatibility for atypical red blood cell antigens that could cause alloimmunisation when blood transfusion is planned for women of child-bearing age.

There are new therapeutic interventions on the horizon. One possibility is the development of monoclonal antibody therapy directed against the FcγR1 receptor that is so important in mediating the attachment of IgG anti-D to, and phagocytosis by, fetal monocytes during the Rh(D) haemolytic process. Another possibility would be the use of fetal stem cell transfusions from an antigen negative donor, although this has not yet been proved to be successful[159].

REFERENCES

1. Clarke CA & Whitfield AGW. Deaths from rhesus haemolytic disease in England and Wales in 1977: accuracy of records and assessment of anti-D prophylaxis. *BMJ* **i**:1665–1669, 1979.
2. Clarke C & Hussey RM. Decline in deaths from Rhesus haemolytic disease of the newborn. *J. R. Col. Physicians Lond.* **28**:310–311, 1994.
3. Tovey LAD. Haemolytic disease of the newborn and its prevention. *BMJ* **300**:313–316, 1990.
4. Hughes RG, Craig JIO, Murphy WG & Greer IA. Causes and clinical consequences of Rhesus(D) haemolytic disease of the newborn: a study of a Scottish population, 1985–1990. *Br. J. Obstet. Gynaecol.* **101**:297–300, 1994.
5. Walker RH, Batton DG & Morrison M. The current rarity of RhD haemolytic disease of the newborn in a community hospital. *Am. J. Clin. Pathol.* **100**:340–341, 1993.
6. Levine P, Katrin EM & Burnham L. Isoimmunization in pregnancy: Its possible bearing on the etiology of erythroblastosis foetalis. *JAMA* **116**:825–830, 1941.
7. Diamond LK, Blackfan KD & Baty JM. Erythroblastosis fetalis and its association with universal edema of the fetus, icterus gravis neonatorum and anemia of the newborn. *J. Pediatr.* **1**:269–274, 1932.
8. Wallerstein H. Treatment of severe erythroblastosis by simultaneous removal and replacement of the blood of the new born infant. *Science* **103**:583–584, 1946.
9. Bevis DCA. The antenatal prediction of haemolytic disease of the newborn. *Lancet* **ii**:395–398, 1952.
10. Liley AW. Intrauterine transfusion of the foetus in haemolytic disease. *B.M.J.* **2**:1107–1109, 1963.
11. Rodeck CH, Holman CA, Karnicki J, Kemp JR, Whitmore DN & Austin MA. Direct intravascular fetal blood transfusion by fetoscopy in severe rhesus isoimmunization. *Lancet* **i**:625–627, 1981.
12. Finn R, Clarke CA, Donohoe WTA *et al.* Experimental studies on the prevention of Rh haemolytic disease. *Br. Med. J.* **i**:486–490, 1961.
13. Bowman JM, Pollock JM & Penston LE. Fetomaternal transplacental haemorrhage during pregnancy and after delivery *Vox Sang.* **51**:117–125, 1986.
14. Walker RH & Hartrick MB. Non-ABO clinically significant erythrocyte allo-antibodies in Caucasian obstetric patients. *Transfusion* **31**:52S, 1991.
15. Weiner E. The ability of IgG subclasses to cause elimination of targets *in vivo* and to mediate their destruction by phagocytosis/cytolysis *in vitro*. In *The Human IgG Subclasses* (ed. F. Shakib), pp. 135–160. Oxford: Pergamon Press, 1990.
16. Schreiber AD, Rossman MD & Levinson AI. The immunobiology of human Fc receptors on hemopoietic cells and tissue macrophages. *Clin. Immunol. Immunopathol.* **62**:566–572, 1992.
17. Wiener E, Mawas F, Dellow RA, Singh I, Rodeck CH. A major role of class I Fcγ receptors in immunoglobulin G anti-D mediated red blood cell destruction by fetal mononuclear phagocytes. *Obstet. Gynecol.* **86**:157–162, 1995.
18. Chown B. On a search for rhesus antibodies in very young fetuses. *Arch. Dis. Childh.* **30**:237, 1955.
19. Gitlin D. Development and metabolism in the immune globulins. In *Immunological Incompetence* (eds B.M. Kaga & E.R. Stiehm) Chicago: Year Book, 1971.
20. Lubenko A, Contreras M, Rodeck CH, Nicolini U, Savage J & Chana H. The transplacental IgG subclass concentrations in pregnancies at risk of haemolytic disease of the newborn. *Vox Sang.* **67**:291–298, 1994.
21. Garner SF, Gorick BD, Lai WY, Brown D, Taverner J, Hughes-Jones, Contreras M & Lubenko A. Prediction of the severity of haemolytic disease of the newborn. Quantitative IgG anti-D subclass determinations explain correlation with functional assay results. *Vox Sang.* **69**:169–176, 1995.
22. Thomas NC, Shirey RS, Blakemore K & Kickler TS. A Quantitative assay for subclassing IgG alloantibodies implicated in hemolytic disease of the newborn. *Vox Sang.* **69**:120–125, 1995.
23. Report from nine collaborating laboratories. Results of tests with different cellular bioassays in relation to severity of RhD haemolytic disease. *Vox. Sang.* **60**:225–229, 1991.
24. Mollison PL, Engelfriet CP & Contreras M. *Blood Transfusion in Clinical Medicine*, 9th edn. Oxford: Blackwell Scientific Publications, 1993.
25. Contreras M & de Silva M. The prevention and management of haemolytic disease of the newborn. *J. Roy. Soc. Med.* **87**:256–258, 1994.
26. Bowman JM & Pollack JM. Transplacental fetal hemorrhage after amniocentesis. *Obstet. Gynecol.* **66**:749–755, 1985.
27. Blakemore KJ, Baumgarten A, Schoenfeld-Dimaio M, Hobbins JC, Mason EA & Mahoney MJ. Rise in maternal serum α-fetoprotein concentration after chorionic villus sampling and the possibility of isoimmunization. *Am. J. Obstet. Gynecol.* **155**:988–993, 1986.
28. Rodeck CH, Sheldrake A, Beattie B & Whittle MJ. Maternal serum alpha-fetoprotein after placental damage in chorionic villous sampling *Lancet* **341**:500, 1993.
29. Nicolaides KH & Rodeck CH. Rhesus disease: the model for fetal therapy. *Br. J. Hosp. Med.* **34**:141–148, 1985.
30. Huikeshoven FJ, Hope ID, Power GG, Gilbert RD & Longo LD. A comparison of sheep and human fetal oxygen delivery systems with the use of mathematical model. *Am. J. Obstet. Gynecol.* **151**:449–455, 1988.
31. Kirkinen P, Jouppila P & Eik-Nes S. Umbilical vein blood flow in rhesus-isoimmunization *Br. J. Obstet. Gynaecol.* **90**:640–644, 1983.
32. Rightmire DA, Nicolaides KH, Rodeck CH & Campbell S. Midtrimester fetal blood velocities in Rh isoimmunisation: Relationship to gestational age and to fetal haematocrit. *Obstet. Gynecol.* **68**:233–236, 1986.
33. Vyas S, Nicolaides KH & Campbell S. Doppler examination of the middle cerebral artery in anaemic fetuses *Am. J. Obstet. Gynecol.* **162**:1066–1068, 1990.
34. Nicolaides KH, Thilaganathan B, Rodeck CH & Mibashan RS. Erythroblastosis and reticulocytosis in anemic fetuses. *Am. J. Obstet. Gynecol.* **159**:1063–1065, 1988.
35. Soothill PW, Nicolaides KH, Rodeck CH, Clewell WH & Lindridge J. Relationship of fetal hemoglobin and oxygen content to lactate

concentration in Rh isoimmunized pregnancies. *Obstet. Gynecol.* **69**:268–270, 1987.

36. Rodeck CH, Santolaya J & Nicolini U. The fetus with immune hydrops. In *The Unborn Patient – Prenatal Diagnosis and Treatment* (eds M.R. Harrison, M.S. Golbus & R.A. Filley), USA: WB Saunders, 1991.
37. Nicolaides KH, Soothill PW, Clewell WH, Rodeck CH, Miboshan RS & Campbell S. Fetal haemoglobin measurement in the assessment of red cell isoimmunisation. *Lancet* **i**:1073–1075, 1988.
38. Nicolaides KH, Rodeck CH, Millar DS & Mibashan RS. Fetal haematology in rhesus isoimmunization. *Br. Med. J.* **290**:661–663, 1985.
39. Nicolaides KH, Warenski JC & Rodeck CH. The relationship of fetal plasma protein concentration and hemoglobin level in the development of hydrops in rhesus isoimmunization. *Am. J. Obstet. Gynecol.* **152**:341–344, 1985.
40. Roberts A, Mitchell J, Pattison NS. Fetal liver length in normal and isoimmunized pregnancies. *Am. J. Obstet. Gynecol.* **161**:42–46, 1989.
41. Nicolini U, Nicolaidis P, Tannirandorin Y, Fisk NM, Nasrat H & Rodeck CH. Fetal liver dysfunction in Rh alloimmunization. *Br. J. Obstet. Gynaecol.* **98**:287–293, 1991.
42. Bowman JM. The management of Rh isoimmunization. *Obstet. Gynecol.* **53**:1, 1978.
43. Soothill PW, Nicolaides KH & Rodeck CH. Effect of anaemia on fetal acid–base status. *Br. J. Obstet. Gynaecol.* **84**:880–883, 1987.
44. Robillard JE & Weiner CP. Atrial natriuretic factor in the human fetus – effect of volume expansion. *J. Pediatr.* **113**:552–555, 1988.
45. Nicolaides KH, Clewell WH, Rodeck CH. Measurement of fetoplacental blood volume in erythroblastosis fetalis. *Am. J. Obstet. Gynecol.* **157**:60, 1987.
46. Weiner CP, Pelzer GD, Heilskoy J, Wenstrom KD & Williamson RA. The effect of intravascular transfusion on umbilical venous pressure in anemic fetuses with and without hydrops *Am. J. Obstet. Gynecol.* **161**:1498–1501, 1989.
47. Oepkes D, Vandenbussche FP, Van Bel F & Kanhai HH. Fetal ductus venosus blood flow velocities before and after transfusion in red-cell alloimmunized pregnancies. *Obstet. Gynecol.* **82**:237–241, 1993.
48. Blanchard D, Bloy C, Hermand P, Cartron JP, Saboan AM, Smith BC & Agre P. Two-dimensional idopeptide mapping demonstrated that erythrocyte RhD, c, and E polypeptides are structually homologous but nonidentical. *Blood* **72**:1424–1427, 1988.
49. Cherif-Zahar B, Mattei MG, Le Van Kim C, Bailly P, Cartron JP & Colin Y. Localization of the human Rh blood group gene structure to chromosome region 1p34–1p36 by *in situ* hybridization. *Hum. Genet.* **86**:398–400, 1991.
50. Colin Y, Cherif-Zahar B, Le Van Kim C, Raynal V, Van Huffel V & Cartron JP. Genetic basis of the RhD-positive and RhD-negative blood group polymorphism as determined by Southern analysis. *Blood* **78**:2747–2752, 1991.
51. Carritt B, Steers FJ & Avent ND. Prenatal determination of fetal RhD type. *N. Engl. J. Med.* **344**:205–206, 1994.
52. Lacey PA, Caskey CR, Werner DJ & Moulds JJ. Fatal haemolytic disease of the newborn due to anti-D in an Rh-positive Du variant mother. *Transfusion* **23**:91–94, 1983.
53. Bennett PR, Le Van Kim C, Colin Y, Warwick RM, Cherif-Zahar B, Fisk NM & Cartron J-P. Prenatal determination of fetal RhD type by DNA amplification. *N. Engl. J. Med.* **329**:607–610, 1993.
54. Lighten A, Overton T, Sepulveda W, Warwick RM, Fisk NM & Bennett PR. Accuracy of prenatal determination of RhD type status by polymerase chain reaction using amniotic cell in RhD-negative women. *Am. J. Obstet. Gynecol.* **173**:1182–1185, 1995.
55. Rossiter JP, Blakemore KJ, Kickler TS, Kasch LM, Khouzami AN, Pressman EK, Sciscione AC & Kazazian HH. The use of polymerase chain reaction to determine fetal RhD status. *Am. J. Obstet. Gynecol.* **171**:1047–1051, 1994.
56. Spence WC, Maddalena A, Demers DB & Bick DP. Molecular analysis of the RhD genotype in fetuses at risk for RhD hemolytic disease *Obstet. Gynecol.* **85**:296–298, 1995.
57. Bowell PJ, Selinger M, Ferguson J, Giles J & MacKenzie IZ. Antenatal fetal blood sampling for the management of alloimmunized pregnancies: effect on maternal anti-D potency levels. *Br. J. Obstet. Gynaecol.* **95**:759–764, 1988.
58. Fisk NM, Bennett P, Warwick RM, Letsky EA, Welch R, Vaughan JI & Moore G. Clinical utility of fetal RhD typing in alloimmunized pregnancies by means of polymerase chain reaction on amniocytes or chorionic villi. *Am. J. Obstet. Gynecol.* **171**:50–54, 1994.
59. Rodeck C, Tutschek B, Sherlock J & Kingdom J. Methods for the transcervical collection of fetal cells during the first trimester of pregnancy. *Prenatal. Diag.* **15**:933–942, 1995.
60. Adinolfi M, Sherlock J, Kemp T, Carritt B, Soothill P, Kingdom J & Rodeck C. Prenatal detection of fetal RhD DNA sequences in transcervical samples. *Lancet* **345**:318, 1995.
61. Thomas MR, Tutschek B, Frost A, Rodeck CH, Yazdani N, Craft I & Williamson R. The time of appearance and disappearance of fetal DNA from the maternal circulation. *Prenatal. Diag.* **15**:641–646, 1995.
62. Lo YMD, Bowel PJ, Sellinger M *et al.* Prenatal determination of fetal RhD status by analysis of peripheral blood of Rhesus negative mothers. *Lancet* **341**:1147, 1993.
63. Le Van Kim C, Mouro I, Brossard Y, Chavinie J, Cartron JP & Colin Y. PCR-based determination of Rhc and RhE status of fetuses at risk of Rhc and RhE haemolytic disease. *Br. J. Haematol.* **88**:193–194, 1994.
64. Spence WC, Potter P, Maddalena A, Demers DB, Bick DP. DNA-based prenatal determination of the RhEe genotype. *Obstet. Gynecol.* **86**:670–672, 1995.
65. Bowell PJ, Allen DL & Entwistle CC. Blood group antibody screening tests during pregnancy *Br. J. Obstet. Gynaecol.* **93**:1038–1043, 1986.
66. MacKenzie IZ, Selinger M & Bowell PJ. Management of red cell isoimmunization in the 1990s. In *Progress in Obstetrics and Gynaecology* Vol. 9 (ed. J. Studd) Edinburgh: Churchill Livingstone, 1991.
67. Nicolaides KH & Rodeck CH. Maternal serum anti-D antibody concentration and assessment of rhesus isoimmunisation. *BMJ* **304**:1155–1156, 1992.
68. Kozlowski CL, Lee D, Shwe KH & Love EM. Quantification of anti-c in haemolytic disease of the newborn. *Transfus. Med.* **5**:37–42, 1995.
69. Bowman JM, Pollock JM, Manning FA, Harman CR & Menticoglou S. Maternal Kell blood group alloimmunization. *Obstet. Gynecol.* **79**:239–244, 1992.
70. Noble AL, Poole GD, Anderson N, Lucas GF & Hadley AG. Predicting the severity of haemolytic disease of the newborn: an assessment of the clinical usefulness of the chemiluminescence test. *Br. J. Haematol.* **90**:718–720, 1995.
71. Moise KJ, Perkins JT, Sosler SD *et al.* The predictive value of maternal serum testing for detection of fetal anemia in red blood cell alloimmunization. *Am. J. Obstet. Gynecol.* **172**:1003–1009, 1995.
72. Benacerraf BR & Frigoletto FD. Sonographic sign for the detection of early fetal ascites in the management of severe isoimmune disease without intrauterine transfusion *Am. J. Obstet. Gynecol.* **152**:1039–1041, 1985.
73. Queenan JT. Current management of the Rh-sensitised patient. *Clin. Obstet. Gynecol.* **25**:293–301, 1982.
74. Nicolaides KH, Fontanarosa M, Gabbe SG & Rodeck CH. Failure of ultrasonographic parameters to predict the severity of fetal anaemia in rhesus isoimmunization. *Am. J. Obstet. Gynecol.* **158**:920–926, 1988.
75. Vintzileos AM, Campbell WA, Storlazzi E, Mirochnick MH, Escoto DT & Nochimson DJ. Fetal liver ultrasound measurements in isoimmunized pregnancies. *Obstet. Gynecol.* **68**:162–167, 1986.
76. Roberts AB, Mitchell JM & Pattison NS. Fetal liver length in normal and isoimmunized pregnancies. *Am. J. Obstet. Gynecol.* **161**:42–46, 1989.
77. Oepkes D, Meerman RH, Vandenbussche FPHA, van Kamp IL, Kok FG & Kanhai HHH. Ultrasonographic fetal spleen measurements in red blood cell alloimmunized pregnancies. *Am. J. Obstet. Gynecol.* **169**:121–128, 1993.
78. Oepkes D, Ultrasonography and Doppler in the Management of Red Cell Alloimmunized Pregnancies. MD thesis University of Leiden, 1993.
79. Nicolaides KH, Bilardo CM & Campbell S. Prediction of fetal anaemia by measurement of the mean blood velocities in the fetal aorta. *Am. J. Obstet. Gynecol.* **162**:209–212, 1990.
80. Oepkes D, Brand R, Vandenbussche FP, Meerman RH & Kanhai HHH. The use of ultrasonography and Doppler in the prediction of fetal haemolytic anaemia: a multivariant analysis. *Br. J. Obstet. Gynaecol.* **101**:680–684, 1994.
81. Hecher K, Snijders R, Campbell S, Nicolaides KH. Fetal venous, arterial and intracardiac blood flows in red cell isoimmunization. *Obstet. Gynecol.* **85**:122–128, 1995.

82. Steiner H, Schaffer H, Spitzer D, Batka M, Graf AH & Staudach A. The relationship between peak velocity in the fetal descending aorta and hematocrit in rhesus isoimmunisation. *Obstet. Gynecol.* **85**:659–662, 1995.
83. Copel JA, Grannum PA & Green JJ. Fetal cardiac output in the isoimmunized pregnancy: a pulsed Doppler–echocardiographic study of patients undergoing intravascular transfusion. *Am. J. Obstet. Gynecol.* **161**:361–365, 1989.
84. Oepkes D, Vandenbussche FP, Van Bel F & Kanhai HHH. Fetal ductus venosus blood flow velocities before and after transfusion in red cell alloimmunized pregnancies. *Obstet. Gynecol.* **82**:237–241, 1993.
85. Gordon H. The diagnosis of hydrops fetalis. *Clin. Obstet. Gynecol.* **14**:548, 1971.
86. Sadovsky E, Laufer N & Beyth Y. The role of fetal movements: Assessment in cases of severe Rh immunized patients. *Acta Obstet. Gynecol. Scand.* **58**:313–316, 1979.
87. Visser G. Antepartum sinusoidal and decelerative heart rate patterns in Rh disease. *Am. J. Obstet. Gynecol.* **143**:538, 1982.
88. Nicolaides KH, Sadovsky G & Cetin E. Fetal heart rate patterns on red blood cell isoimmunized pregnancies. *Am. J. Obstet. Gynecol.* **161**:351–356, 1989.
89. Brambati B & Pardi G. The intraventricular conduction time of the fetal heart in pregnancies complicated by rhesus haemolytic disease. *Br. J. Obstet. Gynaecol.* **88**:1233–1240, 1981.
90. Weiner CP. Human fetal bilirubin and fetal hemolytic disease. *Am. J. Obstet. Gynecol.* **116**:1449–1454, 1992.
91. Liley AW, Liquor amnii analysis in the management of the pregnancy complicated by rhesus sensitization. *Am. J. Obstet. Gynecol.* **82**:1359–1370, 1961.
92. Bowman JM & Pollock JM. Amniotic fluid spectrophotometry and early delivery in the management of erythroblastosis fetalis. *Pediatrics* **35**:815–820, 1965.
93. Pridmore BR, Robertson EG & Walker W. Liquor bilirubin levels and false prediction of severity in rhesus haemolytic disease. *Br. Med. J.* **iii**:136–139, 1972.
94. Fairweather DVI, Whyley GA & Millar MD. Six years experience of the prediction of severity in rhesus haemolytic disease. *Br. J. Obstet. Gynaecol.* **83**:698–706, 1976.
95. MacKenzie IZ, Bowell PJ, Castle BM, Selinger M & Ferguson JF. Serial fetal blood sampling for the management of pregnancies complicated by severe rhesus(D) isoimmunization. *Br. J. Obstet. Gynaecol.* **95**:753–758, 1988.
96. Nicolaides KH, Rodeck CH, Mibashan RS & Kemp JR. Have Liley charts outlived their usefulness? *Am. J. Obstet. Gynecol.* **155**:90–94, 1986.
97. Queenan JT, Tomai TP, Ural SH & King JC. Deviation in the amniotic fluid optical density at a wave length of 450 nm in Rh-immunized pregnancies from 14–40 weeks gestation: a proposal for clinical management. *Am. J. Obstet. Gynecol.* **168**:1370–1376, 1993.
98. Whitfield CR. A three-year assessment of an action-line method of timing intervention in Rhesus isoimmunization. *Am. J. Obstet. Gynecol.* **108**:1239–1244, 1970.
99. Ananth U, Warsof SL, Coulehan JM, Wolf Ph & Queenan JT. Mid trimester amniotic fluid delta optical density at 450 nm in normal pregnancies. *Am. J. Obstet. Gynecol.* **155**:664–666, 1986.
100. Valenti C. Antenatal detection of haemoglobinopathies. A preliminary report. *Am. J. Obstet. Gynecol.* **115**:851–853, 1973.
101. Rodeck CH & Campbell S. Sampling pure fetal blood by fetoscopy in second trimester of pregnancy *Br. J. Med.* **ii**:728–730, 1978.
102. Daffos F, Capella-Pavlovsky M & Forestier F. A new procedure for fetal blood sampling *in utero*. *Prenat. Diagn.* **3**:271–274, 1983.
103. Nicolaides KH, Thilaganathan B & Mibashan RS. Cordocentesis in the investigation of fetal erythropoiesis *Am. J. Obstet. Gynecol.* **161**:1197–2000, 1989.
104. Daffos F, Capella-Pavlovsky M & Forestier F. Fetal blood sampling during pregnancy with the use of a needle guided by ultrasound a study of 606 consecutive cases. *Am. J. Obstet. Gynecol.* **153**:655–660, 1985.
105. Weiner CP. Cordocentesis for diagnostic indications: two years' experience. *Obstet. Gynecol.* **70**:664–667, 1987.
106. Nicolini U, Kochenour NK, Greco P, Letsky EA, Johnson RD, Contreras M & Rodeck CH. Consequences of fetomaternal haemorrhage after intrauterine transfusion. *Br. Med. J.* **297**:1379–1381, 1988.
107. Vaughan JI & Rodeck CH. Interventional procedures. In *Ultrasound in Obstetrics and Gynaecology* (eds K. Dewbury, H. Meire & D. Cosgrove). Edinburgh: Churchill Livingstone. 1993.
108. Freda VJ & Adamsons K. Exchange transfusion *in utero*. *Am. J. Obstet. Gynecol.* **89**:817–821, 1964.
109. Asensio SH, Figueroa-Longo JG & Pelegrina IA. Intrauterine exchange transfusion. *Am. J. Obstet. Gynecol.* **95**:1129–1133, 1966.
110. Seelen J, Van Kessel H, Eskes T *et al.* A new method of exchange transfusion *in utero*. Cannulation of vessels on the fetal side of the human placenta. *Am. J. Obstet. Gynecol.* **95**:872–876, 1966.
111. Harman CR, Manning FA, Bowman JM & Lange IR. Severe Rh-disease – poor outcome is not inevitable. *Am. J. Obstet. Gynecol.* **145**:823–829, 1983.
112. Frigoletto FD, Umansky I, Birnholtz J, Acker D, Easterday CL, Harris GBG & Griscom NT. Intrauterine transfusion in 365 fetuses during 15 years. *Am. J. Obstet. Gynecol.* **139**:781–790, 1981.
113. Lewis M, Bowman JM, Pollock J & Lowen B. Absorption of red cells from the peritoneal cavity of an hydropic twin. *Transfusion* **13**:37–40, 1973.
114. Rodeck CH, Nicolaides KH, Warsof SL, Fysh WJ, Gamsu HR & Kemp JR. The management of severe rhesus isoimmunization by fetoscopic intravascular transfusions. *Am. J. Obstet. Gynecol.* **150**:769–774, 1984.
115. Bang J, Bock JE & Trolle D. Ultrasound-guided fetal intravascular transfusion for severe rhesus haemolytic disease *Br. Med. J.* **284**:373–374, 1982.
116. de Crespigny LC, Robinson HP, Quinn M, Doyle L, Ross A & Cauchi M. Ultrasound-guided fetal blood transfusion for severe rhesus isoimmunization. *Obstet. Gynecol.* **66**:529–532, 1985.
117. Nicolaides KH, Soothill PW, Rodeck CH & Clewell W. Rh disease: Intravascular fetal blood transfusion by cordocentesis. *Fetal Therapy* **1**:185–192, 1986.
118. Westgren M, Selbing A & Stangenberg M. Fetal intracardiac transfusions in patients with severe rhesus isoimmunization. *Br. Med. J.* **298**:885–886, 1988.
119. Berkowitz RL, Chitkara U, Wilkins IA, Lynch L, Plosker H & Bernstein HH. Intravascular monitoring and management of erythroblastosis fetails. *Am. J. Obstet. Gynecol.* **158**:783–795, 1988.
120. Sampson AJ, Permezel M, Doyle LW, de Crespigny L, Ngu A & Robinson H. Ultrasound-guided fetal intravascular transfusions for severe eythroblastosis, 1984–1993. *Aust. NZ J. Obstet. Gynecol.* **34**(2):125–130, 1994.
121. Poissonnier HM, Brossard Y, Demedeiros N *et al.* Two hundred intrauterine exchange transfusions in severe blood incompatibilites. *Am. J. Obstet. Gynecol.* **161**:709–713, 1989.
122. Weiner CP, Williamson RA, Wenstrom KD, Sipes SL, Widness JA, Grant SS & Estle L. Management of fetal hemolytic disease by cordocentesis. II. Outcome of treatment. *Am. J. Obstet. Gynecol.* **165**:1302–1307, 1991.
123. Nicolini U, Santolaya J, Fisk NM, Hubinont C, Kochenour NK, Greco P & Rodeck CH. Changes in fetal acid–base status during intravascular transfusion. *Arch. Dis. Childh* **63**:710–714, 1988.
124. Soothill PW, Nicolaides KH, Rodeck CH & Bellingham AJ. The effect of replacing fetal with adult haemoglobin on blood gas and acid/base parameters in human fetuses *Am. J. Obstet. Gynecol.* **158**:66–69, 1988.
125. Welch CR, Talbert DG, Warwick RM, Letsky EA & Rodeck CH. Needle modifications for invasive fetal procedures. *Obstet. Gynecol.* **85**:113–117, 1995.
126. Moise KJ, Deter RL, Kirshon B, Karolina A, Patton DE & Carpenter RJ. Intravenous pancuronium bromide for fetal neuromuscular blockade during intravascular transfusion for red-cell alloimmunization. *Obstet. Gynecol.* **74**:905–908, 1989.
127. de Crespigny LC, Robinson HP, Ross AW & Quinn M. Curarisation of fetus for intrauterine procedures *Lancet* **i**:1164, 1985.
128. Ronkin S, Chayen B & Wapner RJ *et al.* Intravascular exchange and bolus transfusion in the severely isoimmunized fetus. *Am. J. Obstet. Gynecol.* **160**:407–411, 1989.
129. Hallak M, Moise KJ, Hesketh DE, Cano LE & Carpenter RJ. Intravascular transfusion of fetuses with rhesus incompatibility: prediction of fetal outcome by changes in umbilical venous pressure. *Obstet. Gynecol.* **80**:286–290, 1992.
130. Nicolini U & Rodeck CH. A proposed scheme for planning

intrauterine transfusion in patients with severe Rh-immunization. *J. Obstet. Gynecol.* **9**:162–163, 1988.
131. Nicolini U, Talbert DG, Fisk NM & Rodeck CH. Pathophysiology of pressure changes during intrauterine transfusion. *Am. J. Obstet. Gynecol.* **160**:1139–1145, 1989.
132. Welch R, Rampling MW, Anwar A, Talbert DG & Rodeck CH. Changes in hemorheology with fetal intravascular transfusion. *Am. J. Obstet. Gynecol.* **170**:726–732, 1994.
133. Radunovic N, Lockwood CJ, Alvarez M, Plecas D, Chitkara U & Berkowitz RL. The severely anaemic and hydropic isoimmune fetus: changes in fetal haematocrit associated with intrauterine death. *Obstet. Gynecol.* **79**:390–393, 1992.
134. Nicolini U, Kochenour NK, Greco P, Letsky E & Rodeck CH. When to perform the next intra-uterine transfusion in patients with Rh allo-immunization: Combined intravascular and intraperitoneal transfusion allows longer intervals. *Fetal. Ther.* **4**:14–20, 1989.
135. Harman CR, Bowman JM, Manning FA & Menticoglou SM. Intrauterine transfusion – intraperitoneal versus intravascular approach: a case control comparison. *Am. J. Obstet. Gynecol.* **162**:1053–1059, 1990.
136. Hajek Z, Prokop M, Campr V, Kulovany E & Cech E. Thromboembolization of axillary artery after intrauterine blood transfusion – case report. *J. Maternal–Fetal Investig.* **6**:231–232, 1996.
137. Spencer JAD, Ryan G, Ronderos-Dumit D, Nicolini U & Rodeck CH. The effect of neuromuscular blockade on human fetal heart rate and its variation. *Br. J. Obstet. Gynaecol.* **101**:121–124, 1994.
138. Scaradavou A, Inglis S, Peterson P, Dunne J, Chervenak F & Bussel J. Suppression of erythropoiesis by intrauterine transfusions in hemolytic disease of the newborn: use of erythropoietin to treat the late anaemia. *J. Pediatrics* **123**:279–284, 1993.
139. Roberts A, Grannum P, Belanger K, Pattison N & Hobbins J. Fetal growth and birthweight in isoimmunized pregnancies after intravenous intrauterine transfusion. *Fetal. Diagn. Ther.* **8**:407–411, 1993.
140. Doyle LW, Kelley EA, Rickards AJ, Ford GW & Callanan C. Sensorineural outcome at 2 years for survivors of erythroblastosis treated with fetal intravascular transfusions. *Obstet. Gynecol.* **81**:931–935, 1993.
141. Nasrat HA, Nicolini U, Nicolaidis P, Letsky EA, Gau G & Rodeck CH. The effect of intrauterine intravascular blood transfusion on iron metabolism in fetuses with Rh alloimmunization *Obstet. Gynecol.* **77**:558–562, 1991.
142. Lasker MR, Eddleman K & Toor AH. Neonatal hepatitis and excessive hepatic iron deposition following intrauterine blood transfusion. *Am. J. Perinatol.* **12**:14–17, 1995.
143. Harman CR, Biehl DR & Pollock JM. Intrauterine transfusion: Kinetics of absorption of donor cells in fetal lambs. *Am. J. Obstet. Gynecol.* **145**:830–836, 1983.
144. Nicolini U, Nicolaidis P, Fisk NM, Tannirandorn Y & Rodeck CH. Fetal blood sampling from the intrahepatic vein: analysis of safety and clinical experience with 214 procedures. *Obstet. Gynecol.* **76**:47–53, 1990.
145. Graham-Pole J, Barr W & Willoughby ML. Continuous-flow plasmapheresis in management of severe rhesus disease. *Br. J. Med.* **i**:1185–1188, 1977.
146. Erkkola R, Ekblad U, Piiroinen O, Kero P, Rajamaki A, Karanko M & Katka K. Plasma exchange and intrauterine transfusion in the management of severe rhesus isoimmunization. *Int. J. Feto-Maternal Med.* **2**:11–14, 1989.
147. Chitkara U, Bussel J, Alvarez M, Lynch L, Meisel RL & Berkowitz RL. High dose gamma globulin: does it have a role in the treatment of severe erythroblastosis fetalis? *Obstet. Gynecol.* **76**:703–708, 1990.
148. Margulies M, Voto LS, Mathet E & Margulies M. High dose intravenous IgG for the treatment of severe Rhesus alloimmunization. *Vox Sang.* **61**:181–189, 1991.
149. Charles AG & Blumenthal LS. Promethazine hydrochloride therapy in severely Rh-sensitised pregnancies. *Obstet. Gynecol.* **60**:627–630, 1982.
150. Goodrick MJ, Hadley AG & Poole G. Haemolytic disease of the fetus and newborn due to anti-Fy^a and the potential clincal value of Duffy genotyping in pregnancies at risk. *Transfus. Med.* **7**:301–304, 1997.
151. Fillbey D, Hanson U & Wesstrom G. The prevalence of red cell antibodies in pregnancy correlated to the outcome of the newborn: a 12 year study in central Sweden. *Acta Obstet. Gynaecol. Scand.* **74**:686–692, 1995.
152. van Dijk BA, Dororen MC & Overbeeke MA. Red cell antibodies in pregnancy: there is no 'critical' titre. *Transfus. Med.* **5**:199–202, 1995.
153. Kozlowski CL, Lee D, Shwe KH & Love EM. Quantification of anti-c in haemolytic disease of the newborn. *Transfus. Med.* **5**:37–42, 1995.
154. Spence WC, Potter P, Maddalena A, Demers DB & Bick DP. DNA-based perinatal determination of the RhEe genotype. *Obstet. Gynecol.* **86**:670–672, 1995.
155. Tovey LAD. Haemolytic disease of the new born – the changing scene. *Br. J. Obstet. Gynaecol.* **93**:960–966, 1986.
156. Copel JA, Scioscia A, Grannum PA *et al.* Percutaneous umbilical blood sampling in the management of Kell immunisation. *Obstet. Gynecol.* **67**:288–290, 1986.
157. Leggat HM, Gibson JM, Barron SL & Reid MM. Anti-Kell in pregnancy. *Br. J. Obstet. Gynaecol.* **98**:162–165, 1991.
158. Vaughan JL, Warwick R, Letsky E, Nicolini U, Rodeck CH & Fisk NM. Erythropoietic suppression in fetal anaemia because of Kell alloimmunisation. *Am. J. Obstet. Gynecol.* **171**:247–252, 1995.
159. Linch DC, Rodeck CH, Nicolaides KH, Jones HM & Brent L. Attempted bone marrow transplantation in a 17 week fetus. *Lancet* **i**:1402–1405, 1986.

Diagnosis and management of fetal platelet disorders

60

L. Porcelijn and H.H.H. Kanhai

Introduction

Fetal thrombocytopenia is both a rare and potentially devastating condition. In contrast to thrombocytopenia in newborns, the exact frequency of the condition in fetuses is unknown. The overall incidence of thrombocytopenia (< 150 × 10^9/l) in newborns is approximately 0.9%[1]. In 0.3% of the newborns, thrombocytopenia with an immunological origin is encountered[1].

Most patients at risk for a fetal platelet disorder are identified when a baby is born with a low platelet count. In order to institute proper management in the next pregnancy, it is important to identify the cause of the thrombocytopenia. Fetal platelet disorders may be caused by several conditions including severe growth retardation, congenital malformations (e.g. thrombocytopenia–absent radius (TAR) syndrome, trisomy 21), infections (e.g. parvo- or cytomegalovirus), red cell alloimmunization, maternal autoimmune thrombocytopenia and alloimmune thrombocytopenia (Table 60.1). Thrombocytopenia in the mother due to cocaine abuse, pre-eclampsia and systemic lupus erythematosus are poorly correlated to fetal platelet counts. Haemorrhagic disorders of pregnancy such as Von Willebrand's disease and haemophilia may lead to other abnormalities in coagulation in the fetus (see Chapter 42).

Alloimmune thrombocytopenia (AITP), also known as neonatal alloimmune thrombocytopenia (NAITP) and autoimmune thrombocytopenia, also called idiopathic or isoimmune thrombocytopenic purpura (ITP), are immune-mediated thrombocytopenias.

In the last 15 years, the knowledge about several aspects of immune-mediated thrombocytopenia has grown substantially. The value of the different tests for each disorder has become clear and thus resolving most of the serological problems. The molecular genetics and the exact position on the glycoproteins of most of the important antigens is known (Fig. 60.1). In this chapter, ITP and AITP, being the most frequent causes of fetal platelet disorders, will be discussed. Since severely affected fetuses are predominantly born to mothers

TABLE 60.1
Non-immunological causes for thrombocytopenia in the fetus/newborn.

- Prematurity
- Dysmaturity
- Asphyxia
- Pre-eclampsia
- Congenital malformations (e.g. TAR syndrome, trisomy 21)
- Hepatomegaly/splenomegaly
- Congenital infection
- Hypoglycaemia
- Red cell alloimmunization

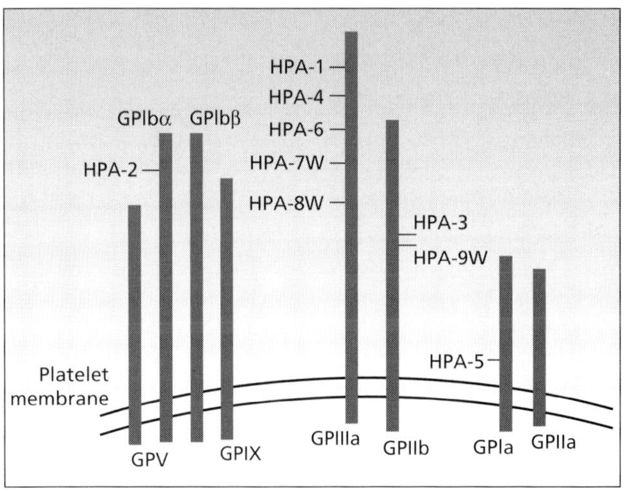

Fig. 60.1 HPA-glycoprotein association.

with alloimmune platelet antibodies[2], this condition will be described in more detail.

Autoimmune or idiopathic thrombocytopenia (ITP)

ITP in the mother is defined as thrombocytopenic purpura without responsible exogenous factors or causal disorders. Two different forms of ITP can be distinguished: the acute and the chronic form. Acute ITP is mainly a disorder of children, mostly preceded by a viral infection, with a higher incidence in the autumn and winter. The platelet-specific autoantibodies in this disorder are more often of the IgM class. The thrombocytopenia in the acute form resolves within weeks or months. Chronic ITP is mostly seen in adults, without any seasonal preference.

ITP is an autoimmune process, which means that the patient (the mother) produces antibodies against antigens located on her platelets. The disease can occur in isolation or associated with other organ-specific or generalised autoimmune disorders. Platelet-associated autoantibodies can cause increased platelet destruction but also abnormal platelet function. In the large majority of the chronic ITP patients the autoantibodies are of the IgG class[3]. Most antibodies are bound to platelets, whereas in a minority of patients free circulating antibodies are also detectable.

NATURAL HISTORY

ITP is more a problem of the mothers than of the fetuses. The clinical symptoms in ITP mothers can vary from none or slight to severe haemorrhagic diathesis. Haemorrhage due to thrombocytopenia is unlikely if the platelet count is $> 50 \times 10^9/l$[4]. Along with thrombocytopenia, an elevated mean platelet volume as a sign of increased platelet production can be present. Normal or elevated megakaryocyte numbers are found in the bone marrow. The plasma thrombopoietin levels in ITP patients are normal or only slightly elevated. In the acute ITP form, signs of infection may still be present.

ITP in pregnancy may cause neonatal thrombocytopenia. The antibodies, mostly of the IgG class, can pass the placenta and bind to the fetal platelets. The reported incidence of severe neonatal thrombocytopenia ($< 50 \times 10^9/l$) in ITP mothers varies between 10 and 30%[4,5]. The nadir of the platelet count in the affected newborn mostly occurs within 7 days after birth[6]. Unfortunately, there are no reliable predictive parameters for the severity of the neonatal thrombocytopenia caused by the maternal platelet autoantibodies. No correlation exists between the platelet count in the mother and in her child. However, both the early and nadir neonatal platelet counts of the second newborns correlate well with those of the siblings[6]. In addition, in the neonate, the clinical symptoms can vary from slight to severe haemorrhagic diathesis. The reported incidence of intracranial haemorrhage in the perinatal period is low and varies between 0 and 1.2%[7–9]. In a review of 288 cases and in recently reported large series of patients[6,10] no infant with major morbidity and no spontaneous fetal *in utero* haemorrhage, in the absence of labour, has been described.

DIAGNOSIS

The diagnosis of ITP in the mother is mainly made clinically. The suggested diagnostic evaluation of ITP, based principally on medical history, physical examination and investigation of the peripheral blood is based on the exclusion of other causes of thrombocytopenia[11]. Recently, it has become possible to distinguish platelet production disorders from platelet destruction disorders, by measuring the plasma thrombopoietin (TPO) level in the thrombocytopenic patient. TPO levels in ITP patients are normal or only slightly elevated, contrasting with the elevated levels in patients with platelet production disorders[12–15].

The laboratory diagnosis of ITP can be difficult. The platelet immunofluorescence test (PIFT; see Fig. 60.2), frequently used to detect platelet-specific autoantibodies, has both a low sensitivity and specificity[3,16,17]. It is possible to determine the glycoprotein-specificity of autoantibodies in the monoclonal antibody immobilisation of platelet antigens (MAIPA, see Fig. 60.3) test[18]. In different studies a varying sensitivity is observed for the detection of autoantibodies in the MAIPA[19–22]. In a recent study, including 100 serologically and clinically well-defined ITP patients, we detected glycoprotein specific autoantibodies in only 25% of patients[17]. These specific autoantibodies are almost always directed against the glycoproteins V, IIb/IIIa and/or Ib/IX (unpublished data).

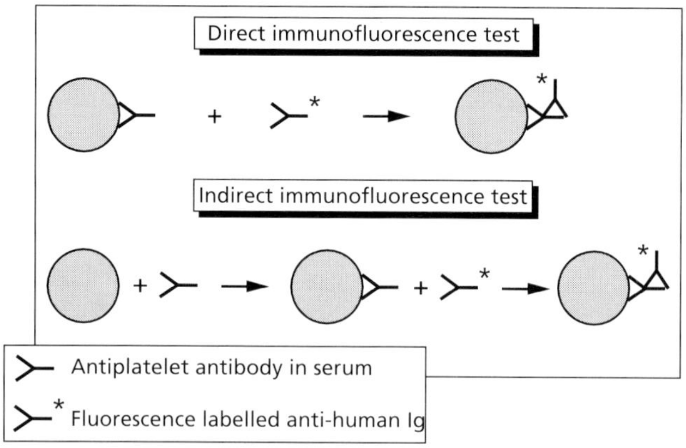

Fig. 60.2 Direct and indirect immunofluorescence tests.

TREATMENT

For pregnant patients with severe thrombocytopenia, corticosteroids are the first-choice therapy. In the rare cases resistant to corticosteroid therapy, intravenous immunoglobulins,

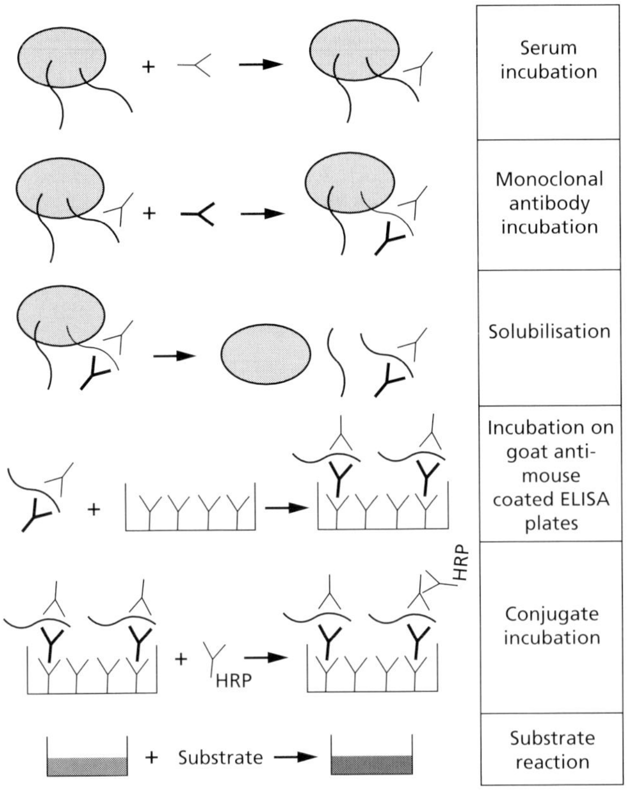

Fig. 60.3 MAIPA.

plasmapheresis or, very rarely, splenectomy are used. Platelet transfusions should only be considered in ITP mothers with very low platelet counts and risk for intracerebral haemorrhage. Maternal therapy with, for example, corticosteroids or immunoglobulins has not proven to benefit the infant.

Initially, the management of delivery in ITP patients was based on the fear of intracranial haemorrhage (ICH) in the thrombocytopenic neonate, secondary to vaginal birth trauma. Therefore caesarean delivery was preferred in fetuses with a platelet count of $< 50 \times 10^9$/l. For this purpose, fetal scalp blood sampling and, in recent years, cordocentesis was applied. Fetal scalp or breech blood sampling during delivery is cumbrous and appeared to yield falsely low counts in a substantial proportion of cases[23]. Predelivery cordocentesis, on the other hand, produces a reliable fetal platelet count but has a risk of fetal loss and severe morbidity. Moreover, platelet counts may decrease in the time interval between cordocentesis and delivery[10].

The previously mentioned arguments, in combination with the low incidence of perinatal bleeding and the fact that the route of delivery (vaginal or caesarean section) does not affect the incidence of ICH[24], lead to the following recommendations for management in pregnancy and during delivery. Cordocentesis is not indicated as a routine procedure in ITP patients. It can be considered in nulliparous women with an increased risk for perinatal intracranial haemorrhage and in multigravidas with a previous infant who suffered intracranial haemorrhage in the perinatal period. Caesarean section in ITP patients should only be performed for obstetric indications.

Alloimmune thrombocytopenia (AITP)

Alloimmune thrombocytopenia in the fetus or newborn is the result of a disease process, in which the mother produces an antibody-mediated response against a platelet-specific antigen present on the fetal but not on her own platelets. Advances in immunology, molecular biology, fetal ultrasound and fetal therapy, in the last decades, have resulted in substantial progress in the diagnosis and management of AITP.

PLATELET ALLOANTIGENS

Platelet alloantigens are located on glycoprotein structures on the platelet membrane (Fig. 60.1). These membrane glycoproteins play an important role in platelet adhesion and aggregation by serving as receptors for specific ligands (Table 60.2).

TABLE 60.2
Platelet membrane adhesive glycoproteins

Family/subfamily	Member	CD	Ligands
Integrins			
VLA	GPIa/IIa (VLA-2, α_2, β_1)	CD49b/29	Col
	GPIc/IIa (VLA-5, α_5 β_1)	CD49e/29	Fn
	GPIc′ IIa (VLA-6, α_6 β_1)	CD49f/29	Lm
Cytoadhesion	GPIIb/IIIa (αIIbβ_3)	CD41/61	Fb, Fn, vWF, Vn
	VNR ($\alpha^v\beta_3$)	CD51/61	Fb, Fn, vWF, Vn, Tsp
Leucine-rich glycoproteins	GPIbα	CD42b	vWF
	GPIbβ	CD42a	
	GPIX	CD42c	
	GPV	CD42d	

CD = cluster designation; Col = collagen; Lm = laminin; Fb = fibrinogen; Fn = fibronectin; GP = glycoprotein; Tsp = thrombospondin; VLA = very late antigen; Vn = vitronectin; VNR = vitronectin receptor; vWF = von Willebrand factor.

A distinction between platelet-specific antigens and antigens that are shared with other blood cells can thus be made. Antigens shared with other blood cells are the human leucocyte antigens (HLA)-A, -B and -C and the red cell antigens, ABH, Lewis, I, i and P antigens[25–30]. The presence of human leucocyte antigens (HLA class I) on platelets is partly due to adsorption of HLA antigens from plasma. Although some of the red cell antigens and most of the HLA class antigens can invoke an alloantibody response, their role in AITP is controversial. HLA antibodies are not believed to enter the fetal circulation because they are adsorbed onto placental tissues[31–34]. The specific human platelet antigens (HPA) defined so far are all known to be able to cause AITP and are shown in Table 60.3. Also shown are the glycoproteins (GP) upon which the antigens are located, the position of the polymorphism and the amino acid change. For example, as first described in 1989 by Newman *et al.*[35], a polymorphism at base 196 of platelet GPIIIa DNA, and a nucleotide substitution (C ↔ T) resulted in an amino acid change leucine ↔ proline on amino acid position 33, which in turn is responsible for the HPA-1a or HPA-1b phenotype.

Although it was originally thought that these specific antigens could only be found on platelets and platelet precursors, recent findings have shown that the GPIIIa structures, with the alloantigen systems HPA-1 and HPA-4, are also expressed by endothelial cells, vascular smooth muscle cells and foreskin fibroblasts and that the GPIa/IIa structures with HPA-5 are also expressed on endothelial cells and activated T-lymphocytes[36–40].

The proportion of individuals belonging to a particular platelet antigen type varies according to the race involved. Some of these differences in frequencies of HPA alloantigens in different populations are shown in Table 60.4[41–44]. Remarkable differences in antigen frequencies for the different populations may be found. Firstly, Caucasians, compared to other populations, have a relatively low (97.9%) frequency of the HPA-1a antigen. In Caucasians AITP is mostly caused by alloimmunization against HPA-1a[45–50a]. (Table 60.5)

A second important difference is the relatively high number of Orientals that are positive for the HPA-4b antigen and low number that are negative for HPA-1a. Because of this, AITP in the Oriental populations is less often caused by alloimmunization against HPA-1a and more often by alloimmunization against HPA-4b. HPA-4b is not found in Caucasians.

TABLE 60.3
Human platelet alloantigens

System	Alternative names	Glycoprotein	Nucleotide change	Amino acid change	Molecular name
HPA-1a	Zw^a, Pl^{A1}	GPIIIa	T^{196}	Leu^{33}	GPIIIa–Leu-33
HPA-1b	Zw^b, Pl^{A2}		C^{196}	Pro^{33}	GPIIIa–Pro-33
HPA-2a	Ko^b	GPIbα	T^{524}	Thr^{145}	GPIbα–Thr-145
HPA-2b	Ko^a, Sib^a		C^{524}	Met^{145}	GPIbα–Met-145
HPA-3a	Bak^a, Lek^a	GPIIb	T^{2622}	Ile^{843}	GPIIb–Ile-843
HPA-3b	Bak^b		G^{2622}	Ser^{843}	GPIIb–Ser-843
HPA-4a	Yuk^b, Pen^a	GPIIIa	A^{526}	Arg^{143}	GPIIIa–Arg-143
HPA-4b	Yuk^a, Pen^b		G^{526}	Gln^{143}	GPIIIa–Gln-143
HPA-5a	Br^b, Zav^b	GPIa	G^{1648}	Glu^{505}	GPIa–Glu-505
HPA-5b	Br^a, Zav^a, Hc^a		A^{1648}	Lys^{505}	GPIa–Lys-505
HPA-6W	Ca^a, Tu^a	GPIIIa	C^{1564}	Gln^{489}	GPIIIa–Gln-489
			G^{1564}	Arg^{489}	(GPIIIa–Arg-489)
HPA-7W	Mo^a	GPIIIa	G^{1317}	Ala^{407}	GPIIIa–Ala-407
			C^{1317}	Pro^{407}	(GPIIIa–Pro-407)
HPA-8W	Sr^a	GPIIIa	C^{2004}	Cys^{636}	GPIIIa–Cys-636
			T^{2004}	Arg^{636}	(GPIIIa–Arg-636)
HPA-9W	Max^a	GPIIb	A^{2603}	Met^{837}	GPIIb–Met-837
			G^{2603}	Val^{837}	(GPIIb–Val-1837)
HPA-10W?	La^a	GPIIIa	A^{281}	Gln^{62}	GPIIIa–Gln-62
			G^{281}	Arg^{62}	(GPIIIa–Arg-62)
Private antigens					
–	Gro^a	GPIIIa	A^{1996}	His^{633}	GPIIIa–His-633
–			G^{1996}	Arg^{633}	(GPIIIa–Arg-633)
–	Va^a	GPIIIa	–	–	–
–	Iy^a	GPIb	G^{141}	Gly^{15}	GPIb–Gly-15
–			A^{141}	Glu^{15}	(GPIb–Glu-15)
–	Pe^a	GPIb	–	–	–
–	Sit^a	GPIb	$C^{2531}A/G^{2532}$	Thr^{799}	GPIb–Thr-799
–			T^{2531} G^{2532}	Met^{799}	(GPIb–Met-799)
–	Oe^a	GPIIIa	–	–	–
–	Pl^T	GPV	–	–	–
–	Vis	GPIV	–	–	–
–	Gov^a	Cdw109	–	–	–
	Gov^b	–	–	–	

TABLE 60.4
Human platelet alloantigen frequencies

Antigens	Percentage frequency						
	Caucasians	Japanese	Koreans	Blacks	Indians	Indonesians	Chinese
HPA-1a	97.9	>99.9	>99.9	99.9	99.9	>99.4	>99.9
HPA-1b	28.6	3.7	11.5	16.0	n.t.	n.t.	n.t.
HPA-2a	>99.9	n.t.	99.0	97.0	n.t.	n.t.	n.t.
HPA-2b	13.2	25.4	25.0	33.0	n.t.	n.t.	n.t.
HPA-3a	80.9	78.9	91.0	85.0	89.3	72.9	78.6
HPA-3b	69.8	70.7	57.0	60.0	n.t.	80.7	71.9
HPA-4a	>99.9	99.9	>99.9	100.0	99.9	>99.4	>99.9
HPA-4b	0.0	1.7	1.6	0.0	0.9	0.6	0.17
HPA-5a	99.0	n.t.	96.0	96.0	n.t.	>99.4	99.3
HPA-5b	19.7	n.t.	6.0	38.0	4.9	9.3	17.7

TABLE 60.5
Antibodies involved in AITP. Literature review

Authors	Number of patients	Antibodies detected
Von dem Borne *et al.* (1981)[45]	35	83% anti HPA-1a
Reznikoff-Etievant *et al.* (1988)[46]	30	90% anti HPA-1a
Mueller-Eckhardt *et al.* (1989)[47]	36	78% anti HPA-1a 19% anti HPA-5b
Kuijpers *et al.* (1993)[49]	45	80% anti HPA-1a 5% anti HPA-1b 5% anti HPA-3a 6% anti HPA-5b
Porcelijn *et al.* (1995)[50]	72	75% anti HPA-1a 3% anti HPA-1b 4% anti HPA-3a 15% anti HPA-5b 3% anti Priv.Ag
Bussel *et al.* (1996)[48]	55	95% anti HPA-1a

NOMENCLATURE

Several different names for platelet alloantigen systems have been proposed in the past. The first platelet antigen system which was discovered in 1959 by Van Loghem *et al.*[51], was named Zw after the two first letters of the patient's family name. Zw^a was discovered first, later the allelic antigen Zw^b was discovered. In 1964 Shulman *et al.*[52] described PL^{A1}, which appeared to be identical to Zw^a. They proposed to change the symbol Zw into PL, a more uniform platelet antigen symbol. Thus the two alleles were named PL^{A1} and PL^{A2}, a nomenclature still often used by Americans. The International Platelet Antigen Working Party suggested another nomenclature[53]. In Table 60.3, this nomenclature of the human platelet alloantigens (HPA) is depicted together with the alternative nomenclature. The present nomenclature is based on the chronological numbering of alloantibodies in the order of their discovery. The letters 'a' or 'b' are assigned to the high-frequency and low-frequency allele respectively. A 'W' is used to mark an HPA system of which only one allele has been identified so far. Also nine family or 'private' antigens are shown in Table 60.3. These antigens have been identified on platelets of members of only one family so far and therefore have not received an HPA number.

The molecular unravelling of the platelet antigens involved in AITP has raised the question whether the HPA nomenclature is still useful. Consequently nomenclatures based on the antigen location on the glycoprotein structures and the polymorphisms responsible for these antigen structures have been proposed[54]. One supplementary nomenclature which implements both the glycoprotein and the amino acid change is also shown in Table 60.3 as 'molecular name'.

PLATELET ALLOANTIBODIES

The immune response to alloantigens is mediated by HLA class II molecules. Antigen-presenting cells (APC) such as dendritic cells, macrophages and B-lymphocytes, process the antigens into small peptides, which are presented by the HLA class II antigens on their surface. CD4-positive T-helper lymphocytes can recognize the peptide–HLA complex, leading to the activation of the T-cell. Activated T-cells then interact with B-lymphocytes, initiating antibody production[55–59].

The development of anti-HPA-1a antibodies is associated with certain HLA antigens. The strongest association is with HLA DR52a (DRB3*0101 in the most recent nomenclature). At least 80% of mothers who developed anti-HPA-1a antibodies were HLA DR52a positive[60–66]. HLA-B8 and HLA-DR3 are also positively correlated with the development of anti-HPA-1a antibodies[32,62,65,67–70]. Of interest is that in (rare) cases of HPA-1b alloimmunization, no particular HLA type seems to be involved. Thus, HLA restriction seems to play a role in enhancement of the immune response.

Since 1953, when Harrington *et al.*[71] suggested an alloimmune aetiology for AITP and 1959 when Van Loghem *et al.*[51] described the first case together with the Zw system, at least 14 different platelet specific alloantigens and alloantibodies have been discovered. Most of these alloantibodies were discovered during laboratory tests performed for neonatal thrombocytopenia. These antibodies are of the IgG class and capable of crossing the placenta. In Caucasians, anti-HPA-1a is responsible for the majority (75–95%) of cases of AITP[45–50] (Table 60.5). This is a striking finding if we consider that only about 2% of the pregnant (Caucasian) women are negative for HPA-1a (Table 60.4). Only about 5–25% of AITP is caused by other anti-HPA antibodies, most frequently anti HPA-5b, anti HPA-3a and anti HPA-1b (Table 60.5).

As discussed earlier, in the Japanese population, the incidence of AITP caused by anti HPA-1a is very rare, whereas anti-HPA 4 is involved in a substantial number of cases[72,73].

INCIDENCE OF AITP

The reported incidence of AITP in the literature varies widely[23,32,52,62,65,74–78]. In the reported pregnancies (*n* = 51 302) the mean incidence was 1 : 1425. The wide variation in the literature is most likely caused by both different definitions of AITP and serological methods used by the authors.

Results of the largest prospective antibody screening programme, including ± 16 000 pregnant women, were recently published by Williamson *et al.*[78,79]. They found anti-HPA-1a antibodies in 44 of 385 HPA-1a negative women (± 1 : 350) which resulted in 8 neonates with a platelet count < 50 × 10^9/l and 10 neonates with a mild (50–110 × 10^9) thrombocytopenia. In this study, no screening for the presence of other anti-HPA antibodies was performed.

The reported incidence of ICH in AITP has a wider range of variation than the reported incidence of AITP (overall). AITP is reported to have a 2–20% chance of ICH in the fetus[47,49,80–84].

NATURAL HISTORY AND PATHOPHYSIOLOGY

There is surprisingly little information about both the pathophysiology and natural history of AITP. AITP is considered as the platelet equivalent of haemolytic disease of the newborn. However, in contrast to red cell alloimmunization, AITP is induced in the first pregnancy in over 50% of cases[47]. Since no screening for anti-HPA antibodies is performed in pregnancy, an affected first child in a family is usually totally unexpected. After crossing the placenta, the specific platelet antibodies (IgG) may cause platelet destruction in the fetus. However, there is a lack of correlation between the maternal antibody levels and the seriousness of the AITP[85,90]. Results of a recent study suggest that maternal IgG3 anti-HPA-1a has predictive value for severe thrombocytopenia of the neonate[86]. As discussed earlier, HPA-1a is considered the most immunogenic antigen (Table 60.5).

The severely thrombocytopenic fetus is at risk of ICH. This risk is at its highest during or soon after delivery but spontaneous ICH may occur *in utero*. Most cases of intrauterine ICH have been reported between 30 and 35 weeks of gestation, but ICH has rarely been observed before 20 weeks[87,88].

The recurrence rate of AITP in subsequent, incompatible pregnancies is high and varies from 75 to 90%[47,81,82,84,89,90]. Bussel *et al.* found that in 50% of their cases with affected siblings the initial platelet count at cordocentesis, performed between 20 and 28 weeks, was ≤ 20 × 10^9/l[91]. There are a few observations of worsening AITP with successive pregnancies, resulting in a progressively earlier occurrence of ICH[88,92,93].

However, in the large majority of cases, those with a prior thrombocytopenic sibling without ICH, both the prevalence and the time of occurrence of ICH are not precisely known. This implies that in cases where the previous infant was thrombocytopenic but without signs of haemorrhage, an assessment of the risk of ICH *in utero* in a subsequent pregnancy is difficult to make.

DIAGNOSIS

AITP should be considered in cases of thrombocytopenia (platelet count < 100 × 10^9/l) of the newborn. Other potential causes of neonatal thrombocytopenia should be excluded (Table 60.1).

Techniques for the detection of antibodies are based on different principles. Initially, the methods depended on a secondary result of the platelet–antibody interaction such as agglutination and the activation of complement. Because of the low sensitivity and specificity of these techniques for detecting platelet antibodies, they are no longer in use.

Current methods are based on the detection of antibody binding to platelets. The platelet immunofluorescence test (PIFT) described by Von dem Borne *et al.* in 1978 is based on the use of fluorescence-labelled antiglobulin reagents to detect the binding of antibodies[16]. Although this technique is relatively insensitive (i.e a positive reaction is defined as being > 1000 molecules of IgG bound to a platelet, whereas > 450 molecules of IgG bound can already cause platelet destruction), it has been proven to be very valuable. In the PIFT, it is possible to test for both platelet-bound antibodies and free antibodies in the plasma (direct and indirect PIFT, Fig. 60.2).

The monoclonal antibody-specific immobilization of platelet antigens assay (MAIPA) described by Kiefel *et al.* in 1987 is based on a sandwich ELISA technique (Fig. 60.3) and has become possible by the development of glycoprotein-specific monoclonal antibodies[18]. This assay is sensitive in the detection of specific alloantibodies. However, this assay is also sometimes not sensitive enough. In our laboratory, no anti-HPA-1a antibodies were detectable in the MAIPA in 4 of 45 (9%) HPA-1a-negative women with HPA-1a-positive children who were suspected of having AITP.

It is essential to differentiate antibodies associated with autoimmune (idiopathic) thrombocytopenia (ITP) from antibodies causing alloimmune thrombocytopenia (AITP). In addition, it is necessary to differentiate between anti-HPA and anti-HLA antibodies. For this purpose, chloroquine-treated platelets are used. With chloroquine treatment, the β_2-microglobulin part of the HLA antigens is removed, causing the 44-kDa band (carrying all HLA-class I antigens) to unfold and so preventing the binding of anti-HLA antibodies.

In our laboratory, the following procedures are performed when AITP is expected to be the cause of neonatal thrombocytopenia.

- Screening for anti-HPA antibodies in the maternal serum with typed donor platelets in the PIFT and in the MAIPA.
- Cross-matching of untreated and cloroquine-treated paternal platelets with maternal serum.
- HPA phenotyping of mother and father.
- Testing for autoantibodies on maternal platelets, in the maternal serum and in an eluate made of maternal platelets.
- Testing for autoantibodies on the paternal platelets (this can cause false-positive reactions in the cross-matches).

If anti-HPA antibodies are detected, the antibodies are specified with a large panel of typed donor platelets in the MAIPA.

For the management of pregnancies, it is important to know if the father is homozygous or heterozygous for the offending antigen. In case of heterozygosity of the father, it might be useful to perform genotyping of the fetus via analysis of amniocytes or chorionic villi by the polymerase chain reaction (PCR). Genotyping for all important HPAs has become possible. Several molecular genetic methods are used to genotype the different HPA systems. Most familiar are the allele-specific primer amplification and the allele-specific restriction enzyme analysis[44,94–99]. Finally, pre-implantation diagnosis using single cells of blastomeres has become technically possible[100].

Unfortunately, monitoring anti-HPA antibodies does not accurately predict the severity of fetal thrombocytopenia[85,90]. Fetal blood sampling is currently the only available tool to monitor the severity of the disease. However, it can bear a high risk for procedure-related complications in those cases with a low fetal platelet count. In particular, puncture in a posteriorly located umbilical cord insertion or in a free loop can be hazardous. During the course of a multicentre study, a series of losses occurred at the time of fetal blood sampling in fetuses with a low platelet count[48,101].

Special safety precautions can lower the risk of haemorrhage in these patients considerably. At the Leiden University Medical Centre (LUMC), the protocol for cordocentesis includes the following:

1. Cordocenteses in AITP pregnancies are performed by the most experienced members of the fetal medicine unit.
2. Using a cell counter in the operating room, platelet count and histogram are obtained within 2 minutes.
3. Before each cordocentesis, maternal platelets are collected, washed and resuspended in AB plasma, irradiated (20 Gy) and infused at cordocentesis, if necessary, to achieve a platelet count of > 100×10^9/l before withdrawal of the needle.

With the use of this protocol bleeding complications were not observed in our series of patients[102]. Fetomaternal haemorrhage, tested by α-fetoprotein and Kleihauer tests, occurred less frequently than in cordocentesis for other indications without fetal thrombocytopenia[102,103].

TREATMENT

In contrast to the management of the neonate, there is divergence of opinion about the antenatal management of AITP. The management of AITP in the neonate is straightforward and includes intravenous immunoglobulin (ivIG) administration and (if necessary) transfusion of washed maternal or donor platelets. The antenatal management protocols in AITP are based on the prevention of ICH. In order to diagnose fetal thrombocytopenia as early as possible, various centres have designed protocols for routine invasive assessment beginning as early as 20 weeks[104,105]. In addition, ultrasound is performed on regular (e.g. biweekly) intervals.

Patients with fetal thrombocytopenia are being treated with weekly transfusion of platelets or corticosteroids or with high-dose maternal ivIG with or without corticosteroids. Combinations of these options are also in use. Bussel *et al.*[81] reported in 1988 that weekly maternal ivIG (1.0 g/kg maternal weight) was effective at elevating the fetal platelet count. Others, however, reported at the same time failure of this treatment[90,102,106,107]. There is one report in the literature of a multicentre prospective randomized trial, comparing ivIG with or without dexamethasone in fetuses with AITP[48]. Fifty-four mothers with thrombocytopenic fetuses, identified by cordocentesis, were randomized to intravenous immunoglobulins 1 g/kg/week with or without 1.5 mg/day of dexamethasone. Non-responders after 4–6 weeks received continued ivIG plus prednisone at 60 mg/day ('salvage treatment'). Fetal thrombocytopenia was documented by means of cordocentesis. During the course of the study, an increased risk of fetal exsanguination was noted when cordocentesis was performed on severely thrombocytopenic fetuses[102]. These fetuses were not included in the study. The overall results of the trial showed a mean platelet increase from the first to the second fetal blood sampling of 36 000/μl and from the first fetal blood sampling to birth of 69 000/μl. A total of 62–85% of fetuses responded. Dexamethasone did not enhance the effect of ivIG. There were no intracranial haemorrhages even though 10 of the infants had a previous sibling who had an intracranial haemorrhage of which 3 were known to have occurred *in utero*. 'Salvage treatment' increased the platelet count in 5 of 10 non-responders to ivIG. The authors concluded that ivIG treatment is appropriate for a thrombocytopenic fetus due to AITP. Although the results of this study are encouraging, some points of criticism on the study design can be made. One of the response criteria was defined as 'a platelet decrease no more than 10×10^9/l from that obtained at first fetal blood sampling and a fetal platelet count $\geq 40 \times 10^9$/l'. Since little is known about the natural course of the disease, it is conceivable that in some cases a marginal decrease (or even increase) of platelets can occur without any treatment. Also, the results of the study might be influenced by the fact that the participating centres were free to perform cordocenteses on, for example (bi-)weekly basis and transfuse platelets in case of fetal thrombocytopenia.

In the antenatal management of AITP, it is important to realise that the majority of at-risk patients are those having a sibling with a history of severe thrombocytopenia but without internal bleeding. The risk of ICH haemorrhage in this category of patients is difficult to estimate but appears to be low. Therefore, it seems unnecessary to perform cordocenteses in these patients. Non-invasive strategies, including ivIG or corticosteroids, might be appropriate. In the (exceptional) case of a sib with ICH and a father homozygous for the offending antigen, however, the recurrence risk is considered to be high. At the LUMC, in recent years the antenatal management of patients with a thrombocytopenic sib (without ICH), has moved towards a less invasive approach. In the first series[103] the management included 39 cordocenteses. In a comparable group of patients, thereafter, a reduction of 50% in cordocenteses and the prophylactic use of ivIG resulted in a favourable outcome (unpublished data). Our current management protocol is depicted in Fig. 60.4.

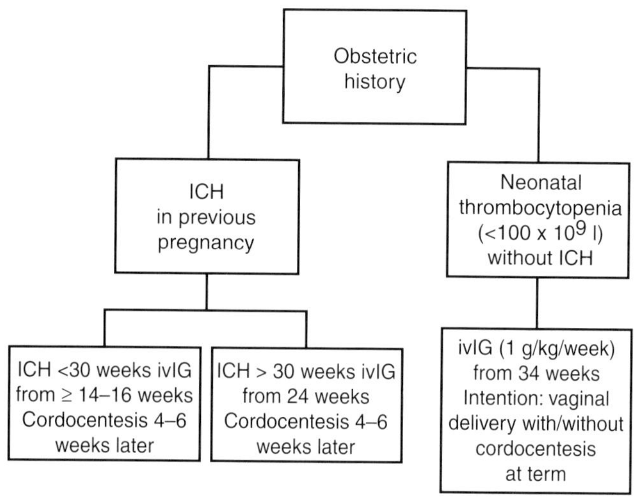

Fig. 60.4 Care for patients at risk for AITP. Protocol Leiden University Medical Centre.

Conclusion

In ITP patients, the low risk for perinatal ICH does not justify routine invasive fetal testing. Platelet counts of second newborns correlate well with those of their siblings. At present, caesarean section is recommended only for an obstetric reason.

Although advances in immunology, molecular biology and fetal medicine has facilitated the diagnosis and treatment of AITP, little is known about the natural history of the disease. It is generally accepted that pregnant women who have previously given birth to an infant with ICH have a high recurrent risk. Both invasive and non-invasive strategies are used in order to prevent ICH in these fetuses. There is controversy about the risk of ICH in those fetuses who have a thrombocytopenic sibling without ICH. A non-invasive strategy including treatment with immunoglobulin should be considered in these cases. Consideration should also be given to starting ivIG treatment 2–4 weeks before the first planned cordocentesis in high-risk cases. The safety precautions used in severely thrombocytopenic fetuses and described in this chapter prevent bleeding complications of cordocentesis. Because of both its rarity and seriousness, the treatment of this disorder should be undertaken in a centre experienced in invasive fetal procedures and with expert laboratory and blood-bank back-up.

Thus far, a final conclusion on the optimal prenatal management of AITP cannot yet be drawn since there are still too many questions about the pathophysiology and management which remain unanswered. Results from laboratory, epidemiological and clinical research on the course of the disease are necessary to optimize the management.

REFERENCES

1. Dreyfus M, Kaplan C, Verdy E, Schlegel N, Durand-Zaleski I & Tchernia G. Immune Thrombocytopenia Working Group. Frequency of immune thrombocytopenia in newborns: a prospective study. *Blood* **89** (12), 4402–4406, 1997.
2. Burrows RF & Kelton JG. Fetal thrombocytopenia and its relation to maternal thrombocytopenia. *N. Engl. J. Med.* **329** (20), 1463–1466, 1993.
3. von dem Borne AEGK, Helmerhorst EM, Leeuwen EF, Pegels HG, Riesz E & Engelfriet CP. Autoimmune thrombocytopenia: Detection of platelet autoantibodies with the Suspension Immunofluorescence Test. *Br. J. Haematol.* **45**, 319–327, 1980.
4. Samuels P, Bussel JB, Braitman LE, Tomaski A, Druzin M, Mennuti M & Cines D. Estimation of the risk of thrombocytopenia in the offspring of pregnant women with presumed immune thrombocytopenia purpura. *N. Engl. J. Med.* **323** (4), 229–235, 1990.
5. Burrows RF & Kelton JG. Pregnancy in patients with idiopathic thrombocytopenic purpura: Assessing the risks for the infant at delivery. *Obst. Gynec. Surv.* **48** (12), 781–788, 1993.
6. Christiaens GCML, Nieuwenhuis K & Bussel JB. Comparison of platelet counts in first and second newborns of mothers with immune thrombocytopenic purpura. *Obstet. Gynecol.* **90**, 546–552, 1998.
7. Burrows RF & Kelton JG. Fetal thrombocytopenia and its relation to maternal thrombocytopenia. *N. Engl. J. Med.* **329**, 1463–1466, 1993.

8. Bussel J, Kaplan C & McFarland J. Recommendations for the evaluation and treatment of neonatal autoimmune and alloimmune thrombocytopenia. *Thromb. Haemost.* **65**, 631–634, 1991.
9. Bussel JB, McFarland JG & Berkowitz RL. Antenatal management of fetal alloimmune and autoimmune thrombocytopenia. *Transfus. Med. Rev.* **4**, 149–162, 1990.
10. Berry SM, Leonardi MR, Wolfe HM, Dombrowski M, Lanouette J & Cotton D. Maternal thrombocytopenia; predicting neonatal thrombocytopenia with cordocentesis. *J. Reprod. Med.* **42**, 276–280, 1997.
11. George JN, Woolf SH, Raskob GE *et al.* Idiopathic thrombocytopenic purpura: A practice guideline developed by explicit methods for the American Society of Hematology. *Blood* **88**, 3–40, 1996.
12. Emmons RV, Reid DM, Cohen RL *et al.* Human thrombopoietin levels are high when thrombocytopenia is due to megakaryocyte deficiency and low when due to increased platelet destruction. *Blood* **87**, 4068–4071, 1996.
13. Kosugi S, Kurata Y, Tomiyama Y *et al.* Circulating thrombopoietin level in chronic immune thrombocytopenic purpura. *Br. J. Haematol.* **93**, 704–706, 1996.
14. Porcelijn L, Folman CC, Bossers B *et al.* The diagnostic value of thrombopoietin level measurements in thrombocytopenia. *Thromb. Haemost.* **79**, 1101–1105, 1998.
15. Tahara T, Usuki K, Sato H *et al.* A sensitive sandwich ELISA for measuring thrombopoietin in human serum: serum thrombopoietin levels in healthy volunteers and in patients with haemopoietic disorders. *Br. J. Haematol.* **93**, 783–788, 1996.
16. von dem Borne AEGK, Verheugt FWA, Oosterhof F, von Riesz E, Brutel de la Riviere A & Engelfriet CP. A simple immunofluorescence test for the detection of platelet antibodies. *Br. J. Haematol.* **39**, 195–207, 1978.
17. Porcelijn L, Huiskes E, & von dem Borne AEGK. Glycoprotein V plays an important role in ITP. Unpublished data, 1998.
18. Kiefel V, Santoso S & Weisheit M. Monoclonal antibody-specific immobilization of platelet antigens (MAIPA): A new tool for the identification of platelet reactive antibodies. *Blood* **70**, 1722–1726, 1987.
19. Brighton TA, Evans S, Castaldi PA, Chesterman CN & Chong BH. Prospective evaluation of the clinical usefulness of an antigen-specific assay (MAIPA) in idiopathic thrombocytopenic purpura and other immune thrombocytopenias. *Blood* **88**, 194–201, 1996.
20. Kiefel V, Santoso S, Kaufmann E & Mueller-Eckhardt C. Autoantibodies against platelet glycoprotein Ib/IX: A frequent finding in autoimmune thrombocytopenic purpura. *Br. J. Haematol.* **79**, 256, 1991.
21. Joutsi L & Kekomaki R. Comparison of the direct platelet immunofluorescence test (direct PIFT) with a modified direct monoclonal antibody-specific immobilization of platelet antigens (direct MAIPA) in detection of platelet-associated IgG. *Br. J. Haematol.* **96**, 204–209, 1997.
22. de Moerloose P, Boehlen F, Extermann P & Hohlfeld P. Neonatal thrombocytopenia: incidence and characterization of maternal antiplatelet antibodies by MAIPA assay. *Br. J. Haematol.* **100**, 735–740, 1998.
23. Christiaens GCML & Helmerhorst FM. Validity of intrapartum diagnosis of fetal thrombocytopenia. *Am. J. Obstet. Gynecol.* **157**, 864–865, 1987.
24. Kagan R & Laros RK Jr. Immune thrombocytopenia. *Clin. Obstet. Gynecol.* **26**, 537–540, 1983.
25. Lalezari P & Murphy GB. Cold reacting leukocyte agglutinins and their significance. In *Histocomp Testing* (eds E.S. Curtoni, P. L. Mattiuz & R.M. Tosi), p. 421. Copenhagen: Munksgaard, 1967.
26. Shumak KH, Rachkewich RA, Crookston MC & Crookston JH. Antigens of the Ii system on lymphocytes. *Nature (New Biol.)* **231**, 148, 1971.
27. Dunstan RA & Simpson MB. Heterogeneous distribution of antigens on human platelets demonstrated by fluorescence flow cytometry. *Br. J. Haematol.* **61**, 603–609, 1985.
28. Dunstan RA, Simpson MB, Knowles RW & Rosse WF. The origin of ABH antigens on human platelets. *Blood* **65**, 615–619, 1985.
29. Kools A, Collins J & Aster RH. Studies of the ABO antigens of human platelets. (Abstract.) *Transfusion* **21**, 615–616, 1981.
30. Kelton JG, Hamid C, Aker S & Blajchman MA. The amount of blood group A substance on platelets is proportional to the amount in the plasma. *Blood* **59**, 980–985, 1982.
31. Taaning E & Skibsted L. The frequency of platelet alloanti-bodies in pregnant women and the occurrence and management of neonatal alloimmune thrombocytopenia purpura. *Obst. Gynecol. Surv.* **45**, 521–525, 1990.
32. Sternbach MS, Malette M & Nadon F. Severe alloimmune neonatal thrombocytopenia due to specific HLA antibodies. *Curr. Stud. Hematol. Blood Transfus.* **59**, 97–103, 1986.
33. Skacel PO & Contreras M. Neonatal thrombocytopenia. *Blood Rev.* **3**, 174–179, 1989.
34. Sharon R & Amar A. Maternal anti-HLA antibodies and neonatal thrombocytopenia. *Lancet* **i**, 1313, 1981.
35. Newman PJ, Derbes RS & Aster RH. The human platelet alloantigens, Pl^{A1} and Pl^{A2}, are associated with a $leucine^{33}/proline^{33}$ amino acid polymorphism in membrane glycoprotein IIIa, and are distinguishable by DNA typing. *J. Clin. Invest.* **83**, 1778–1781, 1989.
36. Ginsberg MH, Loftus JC & Plow EF. Cytoadhesins, integrins and platelets. *Thromb. Haemost.* **59**, 1–6, 1988.
37. Giltay JC, Brinkman HJM & Modderman PW. Human vascular endothelial cells express a membrane protein complex immunochemically indistinguishable from the platelet VLA-2 (glycoprotein Ia–IIa) complex. *Blood* **73**, 1235–1241, 1989.
38. McEver RP, Beckstead JM & Moore KL. GMP-140, a platelet alpha-granule membrane protein, is also synthesized by vascular endothelial cells and is localized in Weibel-Palade bodies. *J. Clin. Invest.* **84**, 92–99, 1989.
39. Sugiyama T, Pidard D, Wautier MP & Wautier JL. Comparative immunochemical analysis of membrane proteins from human platelets and endothelial cells. *Nouv. Rev. Fr. Hematol.* **32**, 199–205, 1990.
40. Zhong CH & Jacques PC. Are megakaryocytes and endothelial cells sisters? *J. Lab. Clin. Med.* **121**, 821–825, 1993.
41. Williamson LM, Lubenko A, Hadfield R *et al.* Large-scale genotyping of platelet donors for the platelet-specific alloantigens HPA-1, 2 and 3. *Br. J. Haematol.* **84**, 7, 1993.
42. Kim HO, Jin Y, Kickler TS, Blakemore K, Kwon CH & Bray PF. Gene frequencies of the five major human platelet antigens in African American, white, and Korean populations. *Transfusion* **35**, 863–867, 1995.
43. Urwijitaroon Y, Barusrux S, Romphruk A & Puapairoj C. Frequency of human platelet antigens among blood donors in northeastern Thailand. *Transfusion* **35**, 868–870, 1995.
44. Simsek S, Faber NM, Bleeker PM *et al.* Determination of human platelet antigen frequencies in the Dutch population by immunophenotyping and DNA (allele-specific restriction enzyme) analysis. *Blood* **81**, 835–840, 1993.
45. von dem Borne AEGK, van Leeuwen EF, von Riesz LE, van Boxtes CJ & Engelfriet CP. Neonatal alloimmune thrombocytopenia: detection and characterization of the responsible antibodies by the platelet immunofluorescence test. *Blood* **57**, 649–656, 1981.
46. Reznikoff-Etievant MF. Management of alloimmune neonatal and antenatal thrombocytopenia. *Vox Sang.* **55**, 193–201, 1988.
47. Mueller-Eckhardt C, Kiefel V, Grubert A *et al.* 348 cases of suspected neonatal alloimmune thrombocytopenia. *Lancet* **i**, 363–366, 1989.
48. Bussel JB, Berkowitz RL, Lynch L *et al.* Antenatal management of alloimmune thrombocytopenia with intravenous gamma-globulin: A randomized trial of the addition of low-dose steroid to intravenous gamma-globulin. *Am. J. Obstet. Gynecol.* **174**, 1414–1423, 1996.
49. Kuijpers RWAM. Neonatal Alloimmune Thrombocytopenia: Relation between Serological Parameters and Clinical Picture. Thesis: Maastricht University, 1993.
50. Porcelijn I, Huiskes E & von dem Borne AEGK. Antibodies involved in NAIT. Unpublished data, 1997.
51. van Loghem JJ, Dorfmeijer H, van der Hart M & Schreuder F. Serological and genetical studies on a platelet antigen (Zw). *Vox Sang.* **4**, 161–169, 1959.
52. Shulman NR, Nader VJ, Hiller MC & Collier EM. Platelet and leucocyte isoantigens and their antibodies. Serologic and clinical studies. *Progr. Haematol.* **4**, 222, 1964.
53. von dem Borne AEGK & Decary F. ICSH/ISBT Working Party on Platelet Serology. Nomenclature of platelet-specific antigens. *Vox Sang.* **58**, 176, 1990.

54. Newman PJ. Nomenclature of human platelet alloantigens: a problem with the HPA system? *Blood* **83**, 1447, 1994.
55. Lanzavecchia A. Clonal sketches of the immune response. EMBO J. **7**, 2945–2951, 1988.
56. Rudensky AY, Preston-Hurlburt P, Hong SC, Barlow A & Janeway CA. Sequence analysis of peptide bound to MHC class II molecules. *Nature* **353**, 622–627, 1991.
57. Marrack P & Kappler J. The T cell receptor. *Science* **238**, 1073–1079, 1987.
58. Trowsdale J, Ragoussis J & Campbell RD. Map of the human MHC. *Immunol. Today* **12**, 443–446, 1991.
59. Tsuji K. *Proceedings of the Eleventh International Histocompatibility Workshop and Conference held in Tokyo, Japan*, pp. 1167–1168. Oxford: Oxford University Press, 1992.
60. de Waal LP, van Dalen CM, Engelfriet CP & von dem Borne AEGK. Alloimmunization against the platelet-specific Zw (a) antigen, resulting in neonatal alloimmune thrombocytopenia or posttransfusion purpura, is associated with the supertypic DRw52 antigen including DR3 and DRw6. *Human Immunol.* **17**, 45–53, 1986.
61. Valentin N, Vergracht A, Bignon JD *et al.* HLA-DRw52a is involved in alloimmunization against PL-A1 antigen. *Human Immunol.* **27**, 73–79, 1990.
62. Reznikoff-Etievant MF, Kaplan C, Muller JY, Daffos F & Forestier F. Allo-immune thrombocytopenias, definition of a group at risk; a prospective study. *Curr. Stud. Hematol. Blood Transf.* **55**, 119–124, 1988.
63. L'Abbé D, Tremblay L, Goldman M, Décary F & Chartrand P. Alloimmunization to platelet antigen HPA-1a (Zwa) association with HLA-DRw52a is not 100%. *Transf. Med.* **2**, 251, 1992.
64. Taaning E. HLA antigens and maternal antibodies in alloimmune neonatal thrombocytopenia. *Tissue Antigens* **21**, 351–359, 1983.
65. Mueller-Eckhardt C, Mueller-Eckhardt G, Willen Ohff H *et al.* Immunogenicity of an immune response to human platelet antigen Zw (a) is strongly associated with HLA-B8 and DR3. *Tissue Antigens* **26**, 71–76, 1985.
66. Mueller-Eckhardt G & Mueller-Eckhardt C. Alloimmunization against the platelet specific Zw (a) antigen associated with HLA-DRw52 and/or DRw6? *Human Immun.* **18**, 181–182, 1987.
67. Reznikoff-Etievant MF, Dangu C & Lobet R. HLA-B8 antigens and anti-PL (A1) alloimmunisation. *Tissue Antigens* **18**, 66–68, 1981.
68. L'Abbé D, Tremblay L, Filion M *et al.* Alloimmunization to platelet antigen HPA-1a (PL-A1) is strongly associated with both HLA-DRB3* 0101 and HLA-DQB1*0201. *Human Immunol.* **34**, 107–114, 1992.
69. Reznikoff-Etievant MF, Muller JY, Julien F & Patereau C. An immune response gene linked to HLA in man. *Tissue Antigens* **22**, 312–313, 1983.
70. Reznikoff-Etievant MF, Muller JY, Kaplan C *et al.* L'immunisation contre l'antigène plaquettaire zw (a) (PL (A1)): groupe à risque, prévention des complications a propos de 132 cas. *Path. Biol.* **341**, 783–787, 1986.
71. Harrington WJ, Sprague CC, Minnich V, Moore CV, Aulvin RC & Dubach R. Immunologic mechanisms in idiopathic and neonatal thrombocytopenic purpura. *Ann. Intern. Med.* **38**, 433–469, 1953.
72. Shibata Y, Miyaji T, Ickikawa Y & Matsuda I. A new platelet antigen system, Yuk (a)/Yuk (b). *Vox Sang.* **51**, 334–336, 1986.
73. Shibata Y, Matsuda I, Miyaji T & Ickikawa Y. Yuk (a), a new platelet antigen involved in two cases of neonatal alloimmune thrombocytopenia. *Vox Sang.* **50**, 177–180, 1986.
74. Blanchette VS, Peters MA & Pegg-Feige K. Alloimmune thrombocytopenia review from a neonatal intensive care unit. *Curr. Stud. Hematol. Blood Transf.* **52**, 87–96, 1986.
75. Blanchette VS, Chen L, Salomon de Friedberg Z, Hogan VA, Trudel E & Décary F. Alloimmunization to the Pl-A1 platelet antigen: results of a prospective study. *Br. J. Haematol.* **74**, 209–215, 1990.
76. Panzer S, Auerbach L, Cechnova E *et al.* Maternal alloimmunization against fetal platelet antigens: a prospective study. *Br. J. Haematol.* **90**, 655–660, 1995.
77. Doughty HA, Murphy ME, Metcalfe P & Waters AH. Antenatal screening for fetal alloimmune thrombocytopenia: the results of a pilot study. *Br. J. Haematol.* **90**, 321–325, 1995.
78. Williamson IM, Hackett GA, Rennie JM *et al.* The natural history of fetomaternal alloimmunization to the platelet-specific antigen HPA-1a (PL^{A1}, Zw^{a}) as determined by antenatal screening. *Blood* **92**, 2280–2287, 1995.
79. Williamson LM, Hadfield R, Maciver C & Ouwehand WH. An antenatal screening programme to detect pregnancies at risk of neonatal alloimmune thrombocytopenia due to anti-HPA-1a. *Vox Sang.* **67**, 3, 1994.
80. Herman JH, Jumbelic MI, Ancona RJ & Kickler TS. *In utero* cerebral hemorrhage in alloimmune thrombocytopenia. *Am. J. Pediatr. Hematol. Oncol.* **8**, 312–317, 1986.
81. Bussel JB, Richard MD, Berkowitz L, McFarland JG, Lynch L & Chitkara U. Antenatal treatment of neonatal alloimmune thrombocytopenia. *N. Engl. J. Med.* **319**, 1374–1378, 1988.
82. Muller JY, Reznikoff-Etievant MF, Patereau C, Dangu C & Chesnel N. Thrombopénies néo-natales allo-immunes étude clinique et biologique de 84 cas. *La Presse Médicale* **14**, 83–86, 1985.
83. Bussel JB. Neonatal alloimmune thrombocytopenia (NAITP): a prospective case accumulation study. *Pediatr. Res.* **23**, 337A, 1988.
84. Kaplan C, Morel-Kopp MC, Kroll H *et al.* HPA-5b (Bra) neonatal alloimmune throbocytopenia: clinical and immunological analysis of 39 cases. *Br. J. Haematol.* **78**, 425–429, 1991.
85. Proulx C, Filion MM, Goldman M, Bradley A, Devine D, Decary F & Chartrand P. Analysis of immunoglobulin class IgG subclass and titre of HPA-1a antibodies in alloimmunized mothers giving birth to babies with or without neonatal alloimmune thrombocytopenia. *Br. J. Hematol.* **87**, 813–817, 1994.
86. Mawas F, Wiener E, Williamson LM & Rodeck CH. Immunoglobulin G subclasses of anti-human platelet antigen 1a in maternal sera: relation to the severity of neonatal alloimmune thrombocytopenia. *Eur. J. Hematol.* **59**, 287–292, 1997.
87. Giovangrandi Y, Daffos F, Kaplan C, Forestier F, MacAleese J & Moirot M. Very early intracranial haemorrhage in alloimmune fetal thrombocytopenia. *Lancet* **ii**, 310, 1990.
88. Murphy MF, Metcalfe P, Waters AH, Ord J, Hambley H & Nicolaides K. Antenatal management of severe feto-maternal alloimmune thrombocytopenia: HLA incompatibility may affect responses to fetal platelet transfusions. *Blood* **81**, 2174–2179, 1993.
89. Martemagno R, Soothill PW, Scarelli M, O'Brien P & Rodeck CH. Detection of alloimmune thrombocytopenia a cause of isolated hydrocephalus by fetal blood sampling. *Lancet* **343**, 1300–1301, 1994.
90. Kaplan C, Daffos F, Forestier F *et al.* Management of alloimmune thrombocytopenia: antenatal diagnosis and *in utero* transfusion of maternal platelets. *Blood* **72**, 340–343, 1988.
91. Bussel JB, Zabusky MR, Berkowitz RL & McFarland JG Fetal alloimmune thrombocytopenia. *N. Engl. J. Med.* **337**, 22–24, 1997.
92. de Vries LS, Connell J, Bydder GM *et al.* Recurrent intracranial haemorrhages *in utero* in an infant with alloimmune thrombocytopenia. Case report. *Br. J. Obstet. Gynaecol.* **95**, 299–302, 1988.
93. Khouzami AN, Kickler TS, Callan NA, Shumway JB, Perlman EJ & Blakemore KJ. Devastating sequelae of alloimmune thrombocytopenia: an entity that deserves more attention. *J. Maternal–Fetal Med.* **5**, 137–141, 1996.
94. Kuijpers RWAM, Faber NM, Kanhai HHH & von dem Borne AEGK Typing of platelet alloantigens when platelets are not available. *Lancet* **336**, 1319, 1990.
95. Simsek S & von dem Borne AEGK. Molecular genetic aspects of human platelet antigen system. *Infusionsther. Transfusionsmed.* **21**, (suppl. 3), 29, 1994.
96. Simsek S, Christiaens GC, Kanhai HH *et al.* Human platelet antigen-1 (Zw) typing of fetuses by analysis of polymerase chain reaction-amplified genomic DNA from amniocytes. *Transfus. Med.* **4**, 15–19, 1994.
97. Simsek S & von dem Borne AE. Molecular genetics of human platelet antigens. *Infusionsther. Transfusionsmed.* **21**, (Suppl. 3), 29–33, 1994.
98. Simsek S, Bleeker PM, Heeremans J & von dem Borne AE. Human platelet antigen-5 (Br) genotyping by ASPA: allele-specific primer amplification (PCR-SSP) [published erratum appears in *Br. J. Haematol.* **88** (4), 898]. *Br. J. Haematol.* **88**, 659–661, 1994.
99. Simsek S, Gallardo D, Ribera A & von dem Borne AE. The human platelet alloantigens, HPA-5 (a+, b−) and HPA-5 (a−, b+), are associated with a Glu505/Lys505 polymorphism of glycoprotein Ia (the alpha 2 subunit of VLA-2). *Br. J. Haematol.* **86**, 671–674, 1994.

100. van den Veyver IB, Chong SS & Kristjansson K. Molecular analysis of human platelet antigen on single cells can be applied to preimplantation genetic diagnosis for prevention of alloimmune thrombocytopenia. *Am. J. Obstet. Gynecol.* **170**, 807–812, 1994.
101. Paidas MJ, Berkowitz RL, Lynch L *et al.* Alloimmune thrombocytopenia: fetal and neonatal losses related to cordocentesis. *Am. J. Obstet. Gynecol.* **172**, 475–479, 1995.
102. Kanhai HHH, Porcelijn L, van Zoeren D *et al.* Antenatal care in pregnancies at risk of alloimmune thrombocytopenia: report of 19 cases in 16 families. *Eur. J. Obstet. Gynecol. Reprod. Biol.* **68**, 67–73, 1996.
103. van Selm M, Kanhai HHH & van Loon AJ. Detection of fetomaternal haemorrhage associated with cordocentesis using serum alpha fetoprotein and the Kleihauer technique. *Prenat. Diagn.* **15**, 313–316, 1995.
104. Lynch L, Bussel JB, McFarland JG, Chitkara U & Berkowitz RL. Antenatal treatment of alloimmune thrombocytopenia. *Obstet. Gynecol.* **80**, 67–71, 1992.
105. Kelsey HC & Rodeck CH. Prenatal management of fetal alloimmune thrombocytopenia. International Forum. *Vox Sang.* **65**, 183–184, 1993.
106. Nicolini U, Tannirandorn Y, Gonzalez P *et al.* Continuing controversy in alloimmune thrombocytopenia: fetal hyperimmunoglobulinemia fails to prevent thrombocytopenia. *Am. J. Obstet. Gynecol.* **163**, 1144–1146, 1990.
107. Mir N, Samson D, House MJ & Kovar IZ. Failure of antenatal high-dose immunoglobulin to improve fetal platelet count in neonatal allo-immune thrombocytopenia. *Vox Sang.* **55**, 188–189, 1988.

Fetal cardiac arrhythmias

61

D.C. Wood and J.C. Huhta

Introduction

The estimation of fetal well-being by auscultation of the fetal heart rate has long been a standard of clinical obstetrical practice. Indeed, the term 'fetal distress' refers to abnormalities of fetal heart rate[1]. Whereas accelerations in fetal heart rate near term greater than 15 bpm for longer than 15 seconds are associated with fetal well-being, a baseline tachycardia may be associated with progression toward hydrops fetalis[2]. The introduction of external electronic fetal monitoring by continuous-wave Doppler instruments has contributed to the awareness of the possibilities of various heart rate and rhythm disturbances. Electrocardiographic recordings of the fetal heart would be ideal to differentiate the various patterns of arrhythmias, but to date, transabdominal recordings are unable to reliably show fetal atrial P-wave morphology and the use of scalp electrode electrocardiography is only available at the time of delivery. However, the widespread use of ultrasound during pregnancy combined with the recognition of an abnormality of rate or rhythm has led to the development of echocardiographic techniques to further enhance and delineate the nature of the disturbance[3]. This chapter will discuss and demonstrate the methods of studying fetal rate and rhythm patterns and disorders, maternal–fetal associations of fetal arrhythmias and possible treatment regimens for tachycardias and bradyarrhythmias.

CONDUCTION

The early muscle layers of the atrium and the ventricle are continuous. Peristaltic movement of blood through the primitive heart tube has been recognized on about day 21 of embryonic development[4]. Whereas the atrial portion of the tube acts as the first pacemaker, the sinoatrial node, originally located in the right wall of the sinus venosus, becomes incorporated into the wall of the right atrium near the entrance of the superior vena cava and begins the activation of the cardiac cycle[5]. Cells from the left wall of the sinus venosus are found near the base of the interatrial septum anterior and adjacent to the ostium of the coronary sinus. Together with cells from the atrioventicular canal region, they combine to form the atrioventricular node and the bundle of His[6].

By week 16 of gestation, the conduction system of the fetal heart is functionally mature[7]. The conduction system extends from the sinus node to the atrial and ventricular myocardium. The sinus node is a fusiform structure which is supported by a collagen framework. The primary cells are P cells, considered to be the true pacemaker cells. The central cluster is supported by the sinus node artery, the largest on the atrial surface, and is surrounded by other P cells and smaller transitional cells. The borders of the sinus node are completely surrounded by the transitional cells and are considered to be the site of sinoatrial entrance and exit block[8]. Although there is some evidence from studies of electrophysiologic conduction times that normal conduction may travel via internodal tracts including along the interatrial septum through the limbus of the fossa ovalis and into the crista terminalis, Gillette *et al.* suggest that conduction spreads radially and syncytially from the sinus node to the atrioventricular node (AV) by the fastest route[9].

The AV node lies between the right atrium and right ventricle at the central fibrous body between the ostium of the coronary sinus and the annulus of the tricuspid and mitral valves. This compact node is mostly transitional cells interwoven with collagen to form a longitudinal bundle of fibres which penetrate the central fibrous body to form the bundle of His. The bundle bifurcates to the left and right fascicles. The left fascicles run along the inflow and outflow portions on the surface of the left ventricle. The right bundle runs subendocardially to the septal band and then into the moderator band to the right ventricular free wall. Initially, the fascicles, made up of Purkinje cells, are surrounded by connective-tissue sheaths and therefore do not come into contact with the ventricular muscle. The fascicles terminate in Purkinje fibres which branch out to the ventricular endocardium.

Transmission of a current through the conduction system occurs by means of change in the electrical potential of adjacent cell membranes. When a resting cell membrane is stimulated, the sodium permeability increases dramatically causing a rapid depolarization or change from negative to positive inside the cell. This is followed by different phases of repolarization during which the cell cannot be restimulated, known as the refractory period. The pacemaker cells in the sinus node possess automaticity which allows these cells to depolarize spontaneously. The pacemaker cells are also found to a lesser extent in the AV node and in other atrial and ventricular tissue. The rate of slow diastolic depolarization decreases from the sinus node down to the Purkinje fibres, such that the sinus node returns to normal resting potential the fastest, with subsequent resetting of the pacemaker cells at longer time intervals down to the ventricle cells, which return to normal resting potential the slowest. The current from the depolarization of the sinus node passes through the other conduction tissue, driving all of the subordinate pacemaker cells to threshold before they could fire themselves automatically. When the pacemaker cells are driven faster than their automatic rate, there is a mechanism of overdrive suppression of the repolarization which results in a prolonged diastolic period, as when a premature beat is followed by a compensatory pause. Abnormal automaticity of the depolarization and/or blocked conduction though the sinus node to the Purkinje fibre system leads to cardiac arrhythmias[10].

Between week 4 and 5, the heart rate climbs from a mean of 90 bpm to 124 bpm and continues to increase until a maximum average of 180 bpm in weeks 8 to 10. The average fetal heart rate declines to approximately 140 bpm between weeks 18 and 24 and continues to drop until term to a rate of 130 bpm. This was shown in a number of studies compared by Dubose[11]. Normal variations in heart rate may typically be ±15 bpm during a complete ultrasound examination or during a non-stress test.

CARDIAC RHYTHMS

We may presume that the normal sequential timing of contractions seen as atrial and venticular wall motions and Doppler flow patterns seen as inflow and outflow blood velocities across the atrioventicular and semi-lunar valves recorded during fetal echocardiography represent the electrical activity of normal sinus rhythm (see M-mode and Doppler rhythm images). The average heart rate of the typical fetus between weeks 18 and 22 of gestation is 140 bpm. Sinus rhythm occurs when the sinus node begins the cardiac cycle which is conducted normally through the AV node and His–Purkinje system and then repeated. The automaticity of the sinus node is more rapid than the other potential pacemaker sites along the conduction system, resulting in the sinus rhythm as the fastest normal atrioventricular sequential rhythm. When the sinus node is suppressed such as by a vagal stimulus, an impulse will originate from the next fastest location of pacemaker cells, which may be in the atria, the AV node or the Purkinje fibres. These escape beats, when occurring together, produce a rhythm that would be slower than the intrinsic sinus rate in a hierarchy defined by the origin of the rhythm: atrial rhythm at 100 to 120 bpm; AV nodal or junctional rhythm at 70 to 100 bpm; and ventricular rhythm at a rate of 45 to 70 bpm. Junctional and ventricular rhythms occur typically when there is a lack of normal conduction from the sinus node or there is a block between the atrial impulse and the nodal or ventricular impulse, such that the atrial rate will be faster than and dissociated from the ventricular rate. A premature beat is defined as a depolarization of the atrium, AV node or ventricle that occurs earlier than the automatic rate of the sinus node or site of origin of the intrinsic rhythm. Therefore, a premature beat comes earlier than the expected beat to beat interval, while an escape beat comes later or at the normal rate for the site of origin.

Sinus node disorders include sinus tachycardia, sinus bradycardia, sinus arrhythmia and sino-atrial block. A fetal sinus tachycardia is seen at a rate over 180 bpm, usually with a 5 to 15 bpm variability. Causes include heart failure, increased cardiac output, hypovolaemia, early fetal hypoxia, maternal anxiety, maternal fever and exposure to certain medications such as atropine and scopolamine[12]. Sinus bradycardia is common in the fetus and may be caused by head or cord compression, maternal hypotension and exposure to medications including propranolol, reserpine and paracervical block anaesthesia. Sino-atrial block may occur with severe cord or head compression or hyperkalaemia, resulting in slower escape rhythms.

Supraventicular tachycardias (SVT) can be classified as automatic from an ectopic focus or re-entrant with or without an accessory bypass tract. Re-entrant mechanisms are more likely to have sudden paroxysmal onset following a premature depolarization and be transient in duration. Ectopic tachycardias occur due to enhanced or altered automaticity and may occur continuously[13]. They may occur with excess catecholamines or changes in electrolytes. In re-entry tachycardia with 1 : 1 AV conduction, there are two distinct pathways with different conduction periods and refractory periods in use during each cardiac cycle. Simply stated, conduction down the antegrade pathway may trigger conduction in the retrograde pathway and back into the atrium, causing early firing of the atrium before the normal automatic rate. This persists in a circus rhythm. We have recently observed this phenomena in two cases of maternal Graves' disease with fetal rates from 175 to 200 bpm. Currently, the nature of SVT in the fetus remains undefined by non-invasive ultrasound techniques. However, approximately 15% of fetal SVT will manifest as Wolff–Parkinson–White pathway at some time postnatally[14].

Bradycardias detected by auscultation may occur with several possible mechanisms. They may represent transient sinus bradycardia associated with cord compression or vagal stimulus or various degrees of atrioventricular block, such as with a bigeminal atrial rhythm where every other sinus beat is blocked before ventricular stimulation, second-degree heart block where the ventricular rate is half or less than atrial rate and complete heart block where there is dissociation between atrial and ventricular conduction. In addition, atrial and ventricular bigeminal rhythms may occur where the ventricular response appears slowed only because the second conducted beat occurs prior to complete filling of the ventricle. The volume and force of contraction of these early beats are lessened and thus may not be detected by auscultation (see Doppler rhythm images). These apparent bradycardias are usually transient arrhythmias often associated with variable response premature beats.

CIRCULATORY EFFECTS OF FETAL ARRHYTHMIAS

Detection of a fetal arrhythmia is an indication for fetal echocardiography. After the discovery of a fetal arrhythmia on routine obstetrical examination, those patients referred for fetal echocardiography receive a complete segmental analysis of the fetal heart and viscera by two-dimensional ultrasound to rule out major structural defects of congenital heart disease and/or signs of fetal heart failure. Arrhythmias associated with structural defects are rare with the exception of complete heart block associated with left atrial isomerism or corrected transposition of the great arteries[15–17].

Premature atrial contractions (PACs), reflecting the mechanical action of atrial extrasystoles, typically cause a change in the timing of and an increase in the reversal wave seen in the immediate peripheral venous Doppler flow patterns such as the inferior vena cava and hepatic veins. An atrial premature beat will cause a low-velocity abnormally timed reversal wave in the venous flow patterns while a ventricular premature beat may be seen indirectly as relatively higher pattern of the normally timed atrial reversal wave as it reflects atrial contraction against the closed atrioventricular valves. Conducted atrial premature beats and ventricular extrasystoles produce a diminished forward-flow pattern in the arterial circulation. These early conducted beats are generally followed by a compensatory pause before the return of normal atrioventricular rhythm[18]. The postextrasystolic potentiation or increased volume and ejection force of the forward wave flow pattern in the delayed beat following the atrial or ventricular ectopic beat suggests that the Frank–Starling mechanism of increased ventricular filling causes a stretching of the myocardial tissue, resulting in an augmented stroke volume[19].

Supraventricular tachycardias dramatically alter the peripheral venous and cardiac valve flow patterns. Whereas extrasystoles may affect the continuously forward flow in the ductus venosus as seen by an augmented atrial waveform, there is significant reversal of flow back toward the umbilical vein during even short bursts of SVT. With persistent SVT, this reversal can be seen to continue as pulsatile umbilical venous flow in fetuses with persistent SVT and may lead to hydrops fetalis and fetal demise due to decreased cardiac output[20,21].

Complete atrioventricular dissociation or complete heart block (CHB) may occur with complex congenital heart disease and with maternal collagen disease including antibodies against the Ro SSA and La SSB antigen systems (Sjögren's syndrome)[22]. Machado *et al.* reported on 37 fetuses with CHB, 11 of whom were found to have non-immune hydrops[23]. In our laboratory, we have seen fetuses with isolated CHB associated with signs of fetal heart failure including pericardial effusion, cardiomegaly, biventricular hypertrophy and semilunar valve insufficiency. Several fetuses have manifested endocardial or valvular echogenicity possibly due to the inflammatory changes of Sjögren's syndrome.

Methods of evaluation

Most abnormalities of fetal cardiac rhythm are referred because of fetal heart rate disturbances detected on routine obstetrical auscultation. Each fetus receives a complete cardiac ultrasound evaluation consisting of two-dimensional imaging augmented by M-mode recordings and Doppler insonation of cardiac and peripheral vascular flow patterns[24]. Colour Doppler is used extensively to both identify and align the particular vessel or intracardiac area so that the cursor is in the most parallel direction to the flow, so as to achieve the highest velocity deflection pattern. Pulsed and colour Doppler are used with a power of less than 100 mW/cm^3. Continuous-wave Doppler is used when the velocity of the flow being measured exceeds the limit of the pulsed Doppler scale.

A thorough segmental approach to the fetal heart is begun with two-dimensional imaging of the fetus for fetal lie. The image-density settings are adjusted to include a low persistence with a relatively high contrast and low grey scale. We primarily use a 5- or 7-MHz sector scanner for our studies. The fetal heart is isolated by utilizing a high-resolution zoom mode over the thorax. A transverse section of the heart is then obtained and a slow sweep is made through the abdomen to the head of the fetus to establish cardiac position. During the sweep, the fetal heart is observed for approximately one minute while the relative positions and proportions of the four valves and chambers are identified with close scrutiny paid to the direction of the outflow tracts and great arteries as they arise from the heart. A sagittal section of the thorax is then obtained to identify the relative size and location of the inferior vena cava and superior vena cava as they enter into the right atrium and the position and sizes of the aortic and ductal fetal arches. Specific measurements during two-dimensional imaging include the diameters of the valves and the atria, inferior vena cava (IVC) at the right atrial junction and the ratio of the circumferences of the heart and thorax from the transverse view while imaging the four cardiac chambers. Pulmonary venous ostia and the size, shape and position of the flap of septum primum tissue at the fossa ovalis are typically identified during observation of the four-chamber view. All of this is recorded on video tape for later review as the fetus is likely to suddenly move out of the imaging plane during the examination.

Our protocol includes two-dimensionally directed M-mode recordings of wall thickness made of the ventricular myocardium at the level of the left ventricular papillary muscles such that the interventricular septum is easily seen between the two opposing ventricular free walls (Fig. 61.1). This image is obtained either from a short axis or long axis view of the ventricles. Timing-interval measurements are made by determining the distance against time of recurring contractile or movement elements in consecutive cardiac cycles. When an irregular rhythm is detected, the M-mode cursor is placed through the atrial wall for comparison of atrioventricular movement with either a ventricular free wall or the opening of a semilunar valve (Figs 61.2 and 61.3). It is most useful to record through the right atrial wall near the superior vena cava (SVC) so as to obtain the maximal atrial wall motion. When obtainable, this has remained the method of choice for relating identifiable cardiac wall movements to various arrhythmias. M-mode analysis is relatively easy to perform at any age after 9 weeks' gestation using modern ultrasound systems[25–27]. Colour Doppler imaging may be placed over the fetal heart in order to obtain persistent directional colour movements on the M-mode strip, which may be useful in differentiating very fast atrial rhythms with variable ventricular response, such as in atrial flutter with 2 : 1 block.

In observing the normal sinus rhythm atrioventricular M-mode recording, there will be a single atrial wall movement at the activation of the atrium closely followed by a single ventricular wall movement or semilunar valve cusp opening after the activation of the ventricle. An ectopic atrial contraction will occur as an earlier than normal atrial wall motion which will be followed by the ventricular motion when conducted to the ventricle. There will be no ventricular wall motion response if the ectopic beat is blocked. Premature ventricular beats in the fetus will occur without prior atrial wall motion and will typically not have an atrial wall motion following closely after the ventricular ectopic beat. In both cases of single ectopic beats, there will be a postextrasystolic compensatory pause in wall motion, followed by the expected wall motion interval of the normal atrioventricular sequential rhythm. M-mode wall motion interval measurements through both atria are particularly useful in evaluating the very high rates of atrial flutter and fibrillation (Fig. 61.2).

Two-dimensionally directed pulsed Doppler insonation of the inflow and outflow tracts of the left ventricle and of adjacent venous and arterial structures have been used successfully in determining the nature of arrhythmias, especially when obtaining appropriate M-mode recordings is limited or difficult secondary to fetal lie or maternal habitus[28]. With the fetus in a spine up or spine down position in a transverse view of the thorax (Fig. 61.4), the four chambers of the fetal heart

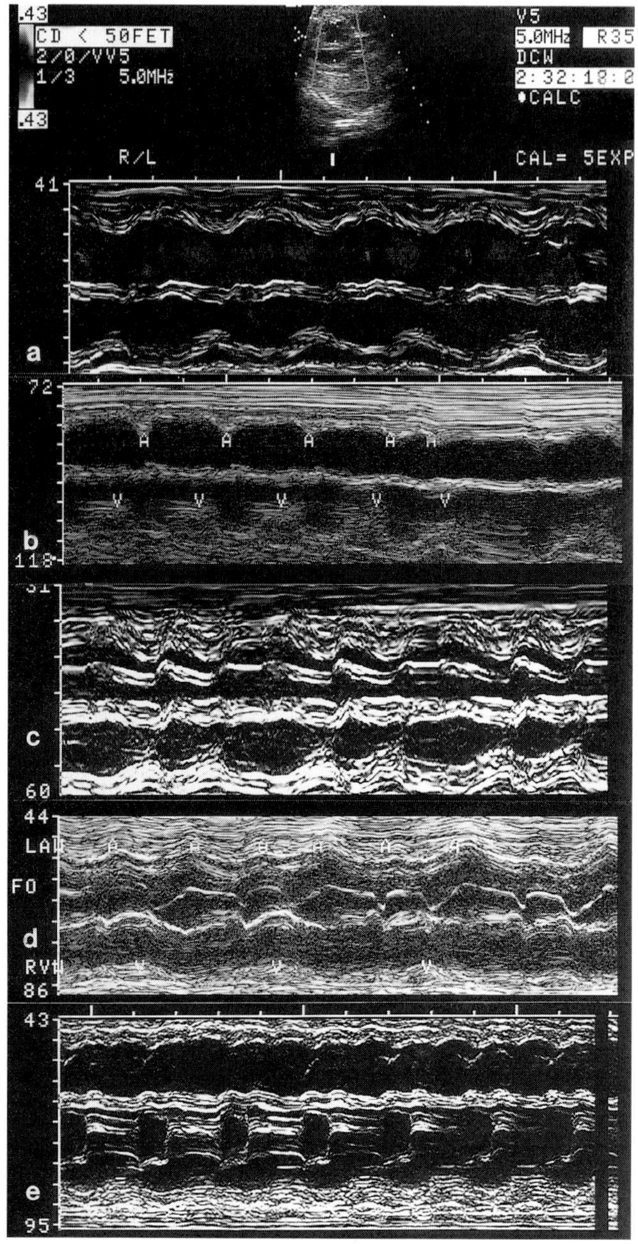

Fig. 61.1 The two-dimensionally directed M-mode strip-chart recording is used for timing of cardiac wall movements and detecting abnormal atrioventricular sequences. The taller timing markers are 1 second intervals while the shorter markers are 0.2 seconds. (a) RV, septum and LV walls showing normal rate of 140 bpm. (b) RA, septum and LV walls showing a conducted PAC with a postextrasystolic pause. (c) RV, TV, septum and LV showing conducted atrial bigeminy. (d) LA, fossa ovalis, septum and RV walls showing 2 : 1 AV block or blocked atrial bigeminy with a ventricular rate of 86 bpm. (e) RA, ventricular septum, MV and LV showing 2 : 1 AV block with an atrial rate of 300 and ventricular rate of 150 bpm. (Abbreviations: A = atrium; V = ventricle; IVC = inferior vena cava; RA = right atrium; RAW = right atrial wall; RV = right ventricle; IVS = interventricular septum; LA = left atrium; LAW = left atrial wall; LV = left ventricle; TV = tricuspid valve; MV = mitral valve; AoV = aortic valve, FO = fossa ovalis, the flap of septum primum; SVT = supraventricular tachycardia; AF/F = atrial flutter or fibrillation; L/R = left ventricle over right ventricle; CHB = complete heart block. See text.)

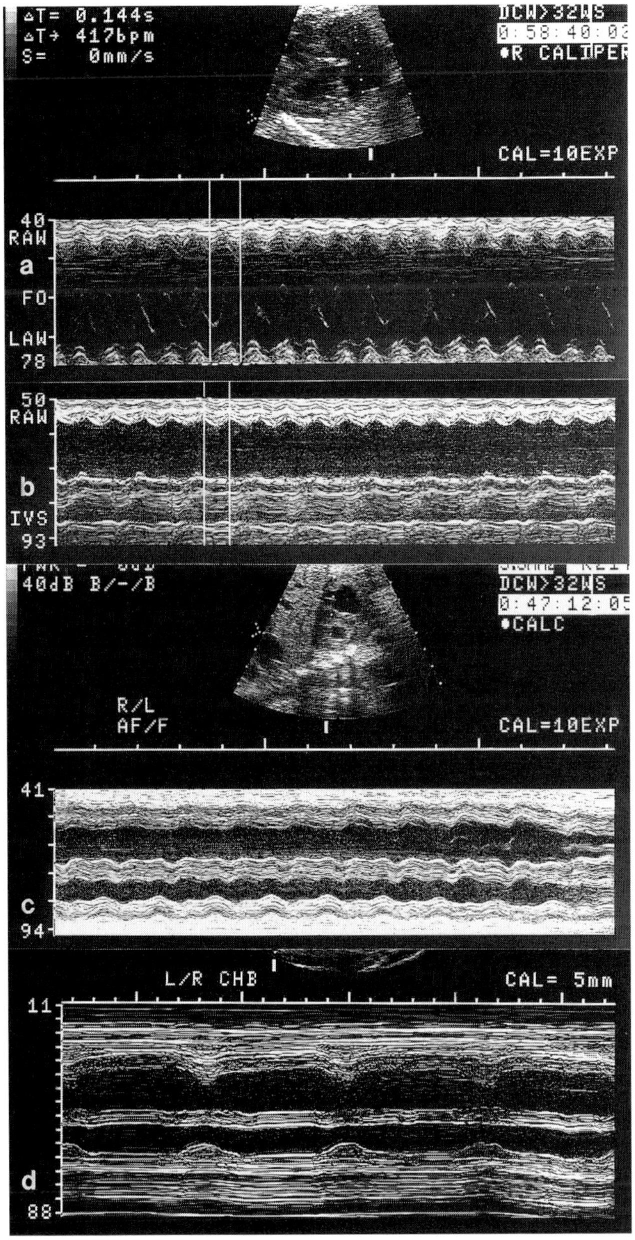

Fig. 61.2 The two-dimensionally directed M-mode recording is used for timing of cardiac wall movements in four separate fetuses. (a) RA and LA walls showing an atrial rate of 417 bpm. (b) RA and ventricular septum showing 2 : 1 AV conduction. (c) RV, septum and LV showing 2 : 1 AV conduction and flutter waves. (d) LV, septum and RV walls in CHB with the ventricular rate of 46 bpm. (See Abbreviations, Fig. 61.1.)

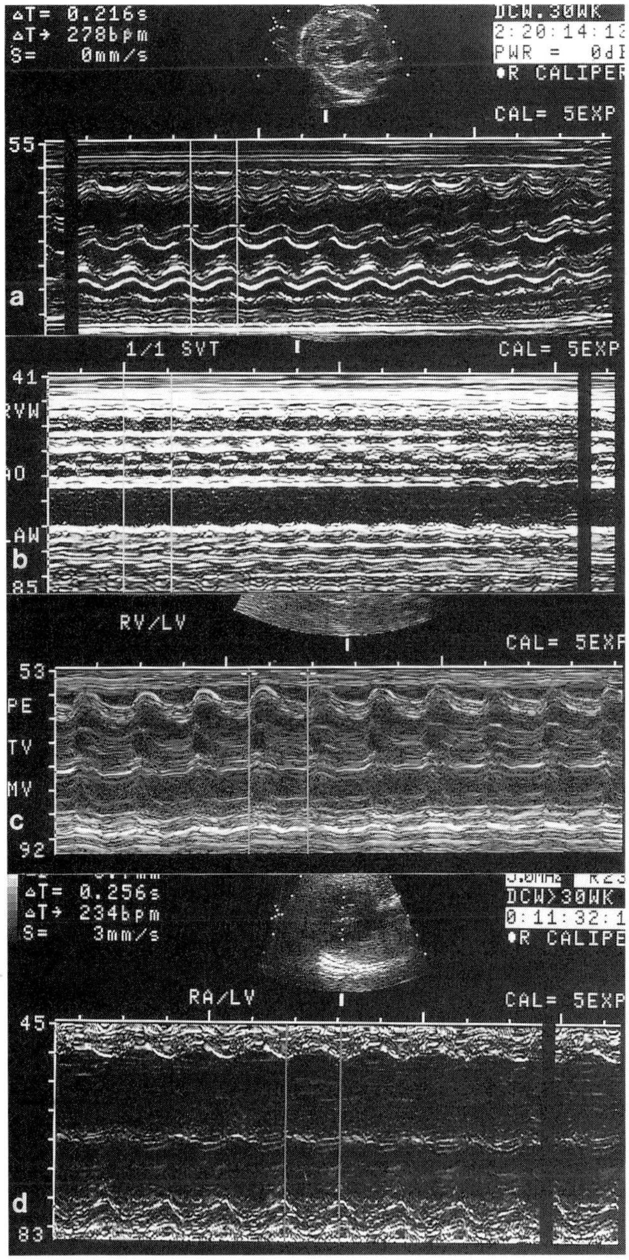

Fig. 61.3 These two-dimensionally directed M-mode recordings are used for timing of cardiac wall movements in four different fetuses with SVT. (a) RV and LV walls showing SVT at a rate of 278 bpm. (b) RA, aortic valve and LA showing 1 : 1 conduction SVT at 270 bpm. (c) M-mode through the tricuspid and mitral valves at a rate of 205 bpm. Note the pericardial effusion (PE). (d) RA, septum and LV walls in SVT at 234 bpm. (See Abbreviations, Fig. 61.1.)

can be imaged, such that a minimal cephalic angulation of the scanner will open up the left ventricular outflow tract (LVOT). Recordings are usually made at 100 mm/s. Placing a large sample volume of the pulsed Doppler cursor between the mitral valve and the interventricular septum permits the insonation of the inflow and outflow of the left ventricular blood volume (Fig. 61.5). The first peak (E wave) of the 'M' shape of the inflow pattern represents passive diastolic filling while the second peak (A wave) follows atrial contraction. This is followed by flow in the opposite direction of the outflow pattern, which represents systolic ventricular ejection. An estimate of the electrocardiographic PR interval can be made by timing the beginning of the upstroke of the A wave to the beginning of the upstroke of the ventricular ejection wave. Premature atrial contractions (PACs) can be seen as an early A wave and the determination of whether the

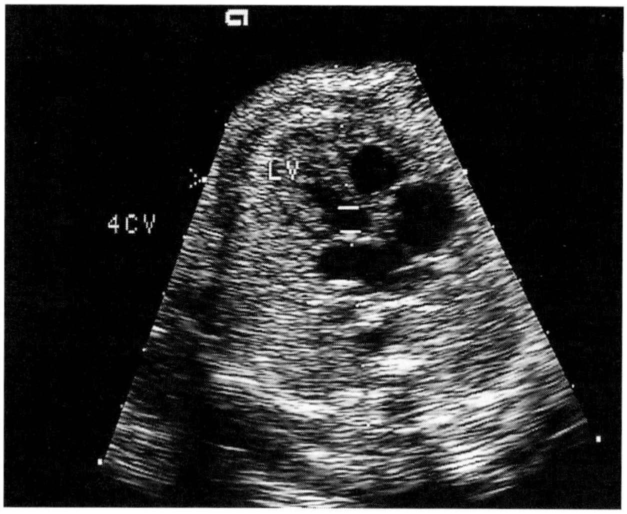

Fig. 61.4 Transverse thoracic two-dimensional ultrasound image showing the placement of the pulsed Doppler cursor in the left ventricular outflow tract between the mitral valve and ventricular septum just below the area of the aortic valve.

premature contraction was blocked or conducted can be easily made. Similarly, early ventricular beats can be seen as occurring prior to a normal A-wave interval. In cases of atrial bigeminal rhythm, early conducted beats may occur to early to allow adequate ventricular filling. During auscultation, either blocked or early atrial bigeminy will be heard as a slower rhythm. This can be seen on the tracings obtained from the umbilical artery (Fig. 61.6).

If the fetus is in a spine to the side position, the left ventricular flow patterns will be perpendicular to the Doppler beam and will give less than optimal flow patterns for arrhythmia interpretation. We and others have found that insonating the pulmonary artery and vein will give a similar back-and-forth pattern to the LVOT and is easily obtained with low-frequency colour Doppler imaging by placing the cursor just posterior and lateral to the atrial wall. We have also found the combined flow patterns in adjacent structures such as the ascending aorta and superior vena cava or descending aorta and inferior vena cava useful in differentiating arrhythmias when the fetus is in a position where these vessels are parallel to the Doppler beam (Fig. 61.7). Our protocol requires multiple M-mode and Doppler tracings to support the diagnosis and the nature or variety of rhythm disturbances.

In those cases of occasional or frequent (more than 10/min) PACs, especially when increased fetal breathing activity is present, it may be difficult to obtain sharp M-mode or Doppler tracings. Insonating the lower segment of the IVC or within one of the hepatic veins will give excellent images of early and typically larger atrial deflections (Fig. 61.8).

The size and shape of the tissue of the septum primum at the fossa ovalis is closely observed as redundancy or aneurysm

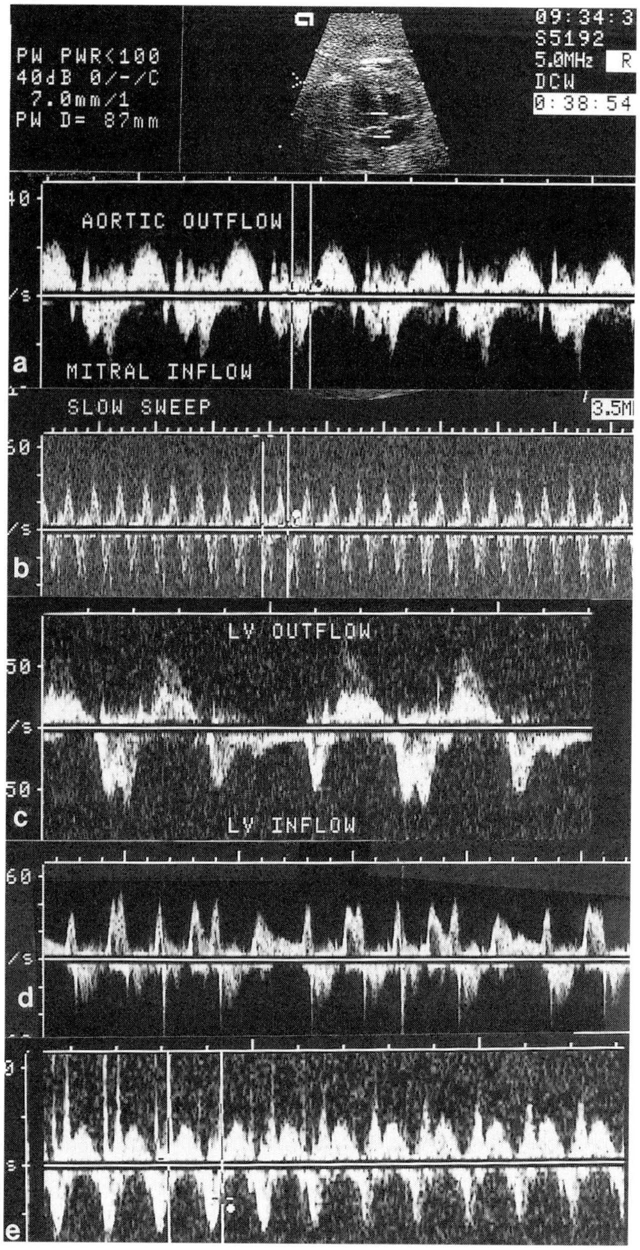

Fig. 61.5 Left ventricular outflow Doppler patterns used to show atrioventricular time intervals and sequencing. The orientation for blood flow toward the fetal left ventricular apex in (a), (b) and (c) is below the baseline and above the baseline in (d) and (e). (a) Normal inflow and outflow patterns used to show normal atrioventricular sequence. (b) The use of a slow sweep rate in an attempt to capture occasional arrhythmias. (c) Pulsed Doppler sampling of the LV inflow and outflow in a fetus with atrial trigeminy showing every third atrial beat is a blocked PAC. (d) Similar inflow–outflow pattern showing variable blocked and conducted PACs. (e) Similar inflow–outflow pattern showing SVT with 1 : 1 conduction at a rate 272 bpm. (See Abbreviations, Fig. 61.1.)

of this structure has been implicated in causing PACs (Fig. 61.9)[29,30]. It is also necessary to look carefully for other free-floating structures that may be seen within the heart, as reported by Clements *et al.* who described a polyp-like structure related to the Chiari's network of tissue near the inferior

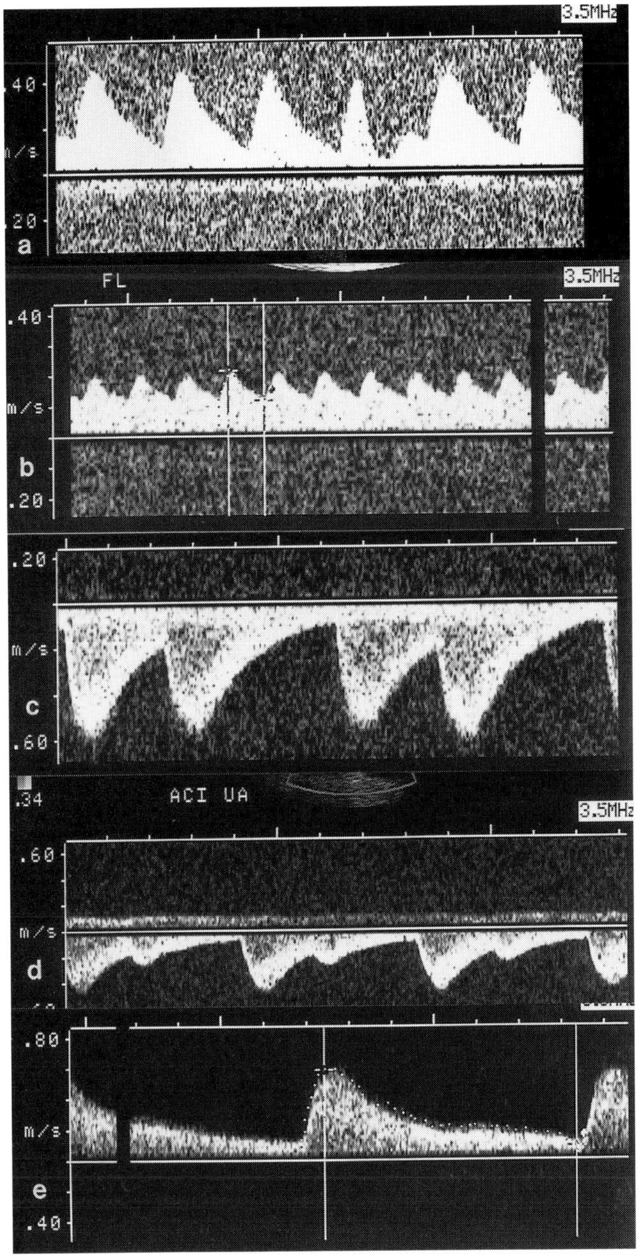

Fig. 61.6 Doppler flow patterns obtained from the umbilical artery (UA) from near the abdominal insertion (ACI) or in a free loop (FL) of the cord. The orientation for blood flow toward the placenta in (a), (b) and (e) is above the baseline and below the baseline in (c) and (d). (a) Normal rhythm showing the effect of a hiccup on the flow pattern. (b) Supraventricular tachycardia at a rate of 310 bpm in a hydropic fetus at 28 weeks' gestation. (c) Blocked atrial trigeminy in an otherwise well 32-week fetus. (d) Conducted atrial bigeminy resulting in a perceived bradycardia at 75 bpm. (e) Complete heart block at 45 bpm in a fetus with SSA antibodies at 25 weeks' gestation.

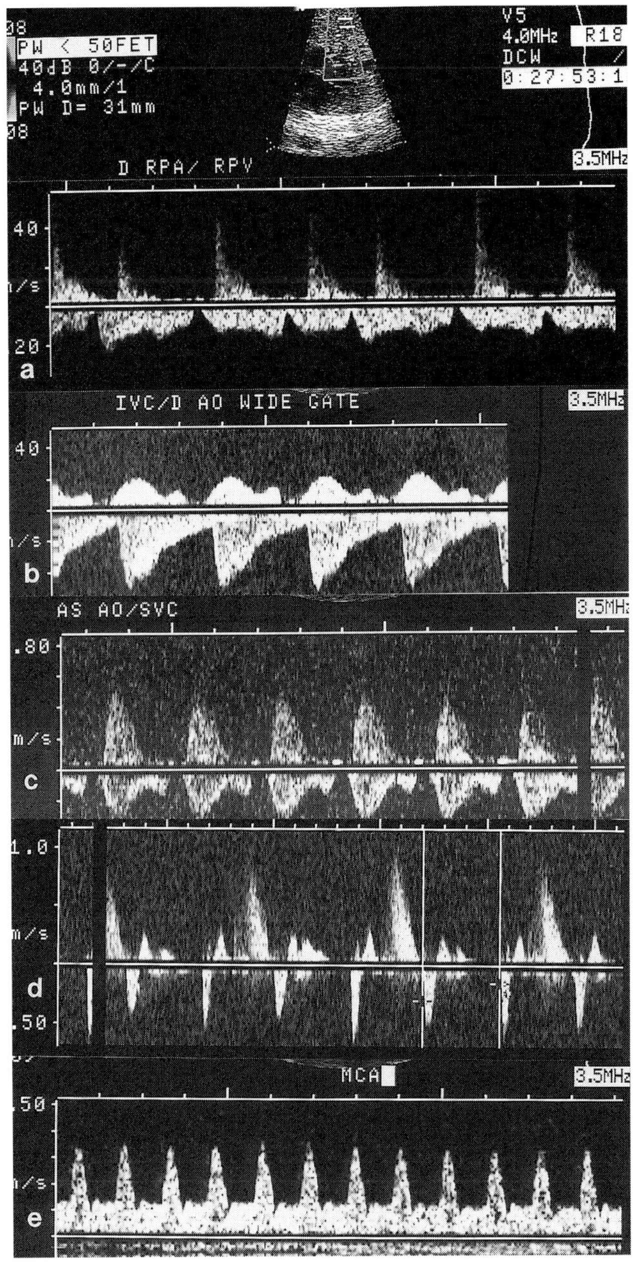

Fig. 61.7 Pulsed Doppler recordings in vascular spaces using a wide sample gate placement to obtain atrioventricular timing interval relationships. The orientation for blood flow toward the fetal heart in (a), (c) and (e) is below the baseline and above the baseline in (b) and (d). (a) Distal right pulmonary artery and vein showing conducted atrial trigeminy. The deep notches in the venous pattern represents the atrial contractions. (b) Inferior vena cava and descending aorta showing normal conduction. (c) Superior vena cava and ascending aorta showing normal conduction. (d) Tricuspid valve regurgitation and inflow in complete heart block. (e) Middle cerebral artery showing a ventricular rate of 300 bpm in supraventricular tachycardia with increased diastolic flow.

vena cava and which caused both atrial and ventricular premature contractions[31].

Doppler-waveform patterns of the ductus venosus may be particularly useful in evaluating the effects of arrhythmia on the fetal circulation. By following the abdominal vein to where it curves and becomes the portal vein, the right angle take off of the ductus venosus may be found aiming towards the IVC/right atrium junction. This structure is typically the highest velocity fetal venous structure and may easily be insonated with the use of colour Doppler imaging. Normal

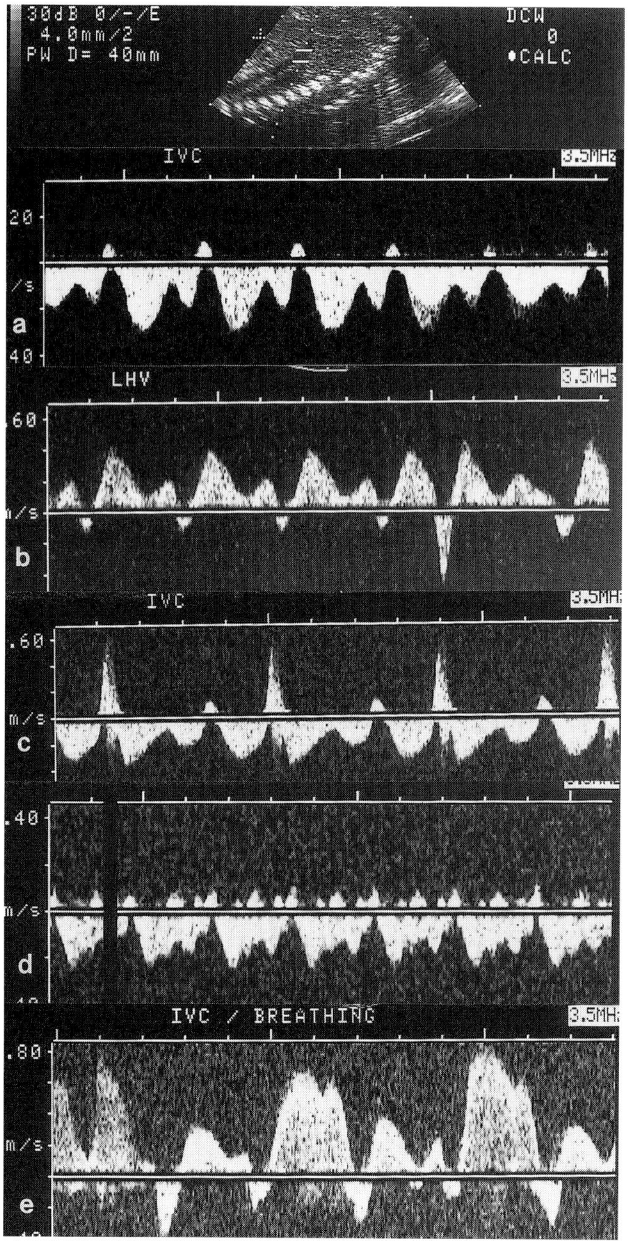

Fig. 61.8 Typical venous flow patterns seen by pulsed Doppler insonation. The orientation for blood flow toward the fetal heart in (a), (c) and (d) is below the baseline. (a) Normal inferior vena cava pattern of normal sinus rhythm showing the atrial wave above the baseline at a rate of 142 bpm. (b) Left hepatic vein showing an early atrial beat (PAC). (c) Inferior vena cava showing atrial bigeminy. (d) Atrial fibrillation waves above the baseline with relatively normal forward flow below the baseline in the proximal inferior vena cava. (e) The effects of fetal breathing movements on the normal Doppler flow patterns in the inferior vena cava showing increased velocities above the line during inspiration and normal rhythm.

flow is continuous forward towards the atrium but will show reversal of direction with atrial contractions if a PAC occurs when the tricuspid valve is closed or when the atrial pressure exceeds the umbilical venous pressure for part of the cardiac cycle (Fig. 61.10). Doppler flow patterns may also be useful to

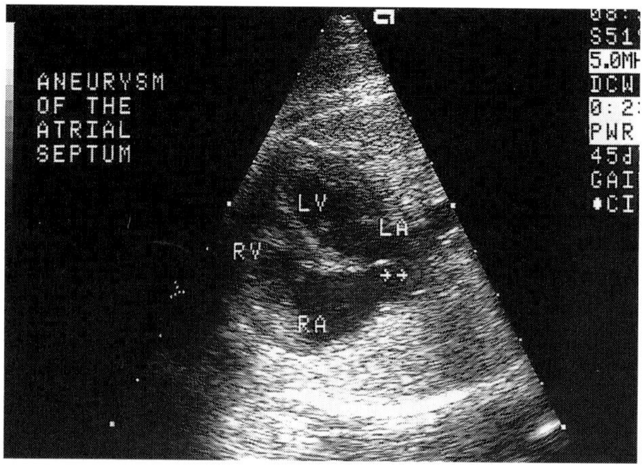

Fig. 61.9 Two-dimensional image of a sac-like redundancy (arrows) of the tissue of the septum primum as it approaches the left atrial wall in an otherwise normal fetus whose post-natal course was normal. Aneurysms of the atrial septum have been associated with premature atrial contractions.

indicate signs of heart failure such as with umbilical venous pulsations associated with hydrops with or without SVT (Fig. 61.11).

The fetal heart rate may be slowed following inadvertent compression of the umbilical cord between the uterine wall and fetus, which was also reported by Mendoza *et al.*[32]. Relaxing pressure on the transducer will allow the fetal rate to return to normal. While caution is required to prevent cord compression during routine cardiac studies, vagally-mediated bradycardias may be of diagnostic use in the fetus presenting with SVT. We have successfully applied this manoeuvre to achieve at least momentary conversion to normal rhythm in older fetuses with paroxysmal SVT in fashion similar to that reported by Fernandez *et al.* and Martin *et al.*[33,34].

Prior to definitive diagnosis and possible treatment, we categorize our ultrasound findings of fetal arrhythmias based on somewhat overlapping heart rate criteria:

- Normal AV rhythm — 110 to 180 bpm
- Bradycardia — 70 to 120 bpm (age dependent)
- Bigeminal and trigeminal rhythms:
  - Effective (ventricular) pulse rate — 70 to 100 bpm
- Isolated extrasystoles
  - Rare — <1/minute
  - Occasional — 2–9/minute
  - Frequent — >10/minute
- Tachycardia — >180 bpm
  - AV tachycardia — 170 to 220 bpm
  - SVT — >200 bpm
- Ventricular tachycardia — Dissociated AV conduction >180 bpm (V>A)

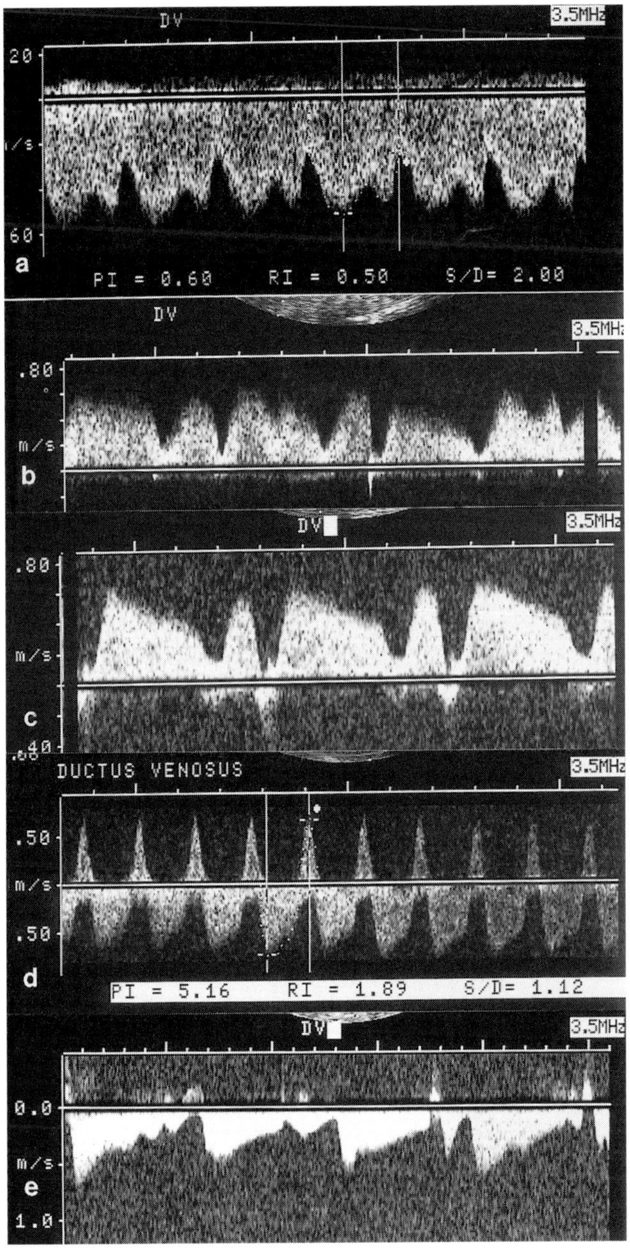

Fig. 61.10 The ductus venosus Doppler waveform pattern is useful in estimating the right atrial pressure relative to the umbilical venous pressure during different parts of the cardiac cycle. The orientation for blood flow toward the fetal heart in (a), (d) and (e) is below the baseline and above the baseline in (b) and (c). (a) Normal forward flow from the umbilical vein to the ductus venosus is continuous. Note that the pulsatility index is below 1.0. (b) Atrial reversal waves are seen with premature atrial contractions suggesting momentary right atrial pressure elevation above the umbilical venous pressure. (c) Atrial bigeminy effects on ductus venosus forward flow. (d) Supraventricular tachycardia at 300 bpm shows significant reversal of blood and is associated with hydrops in this fetus of 29 weeks' gestation. Note that the pulsatility index (PI) exceeds 1.0. (e) Atrial reversal occurs in the ductus venosus in complete heart block when the atrium contracts against the closed tricuspid valve. Reversal can also occur when severe heart failure is present.

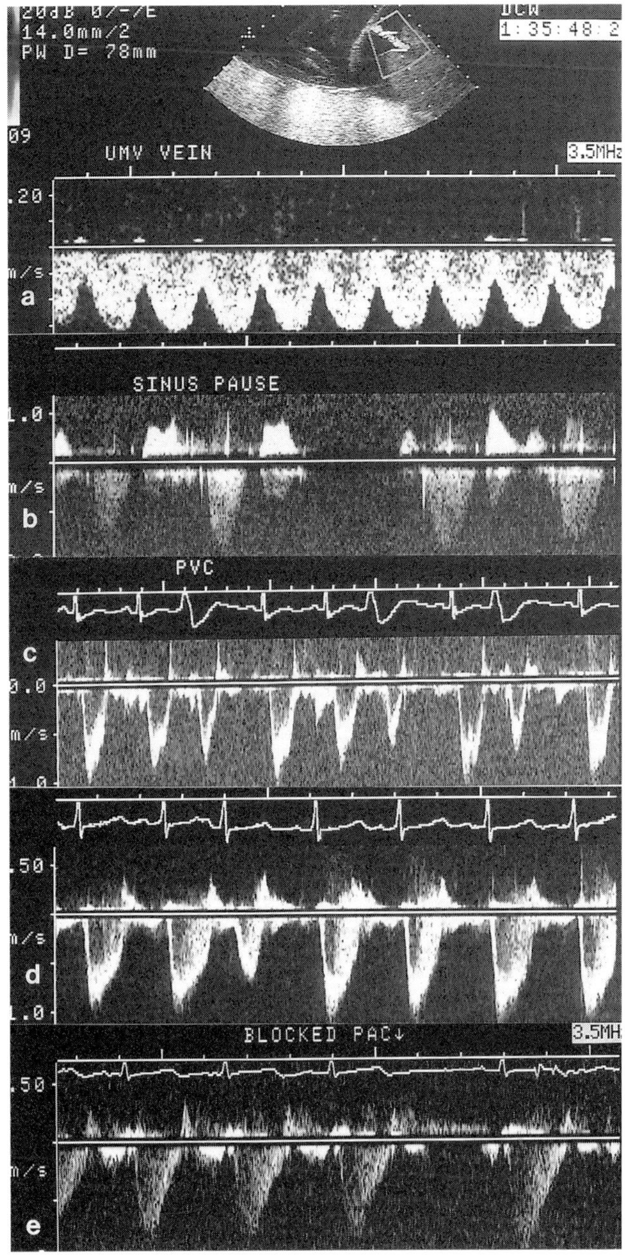

Fig. 61.11 Doppler flow patterns can be used to indicate the physiological effects of arrhythmias on the circulation. (a) Pulsatility in the abdominal umbilical vein with supraventricular tachycardia and congestive heart failure. Note the two-dimensional image showing significant ascites and polyhydramnios. (b) Doppler patterns from the left ventricular outflow tract image showing increased volume and ventricular ejection time following a sinus pause. Images (b) through (e) show the effects of the Frank–Starling mechanism of postextrasystolic potentiation on ejection time, volume and velocity. (c) Doppler flow in the main pulmonary artery in a newborn with ventricular premature beats. (d) Doppler flow in the main pulmonary artery in a newborn with a conducted premature atrial contraction. (e) Doppler flow in the main pulmonary artery in a newborn with a blocked atrial contraction.

- Self-limiting SVT — >3 consecutive PACs, breaking to normal rhythm
- Persistent SVT — Presenting with heart rate >210 bpm
- Atrial flutter — Atrial rate >400 bpm with 2:1 AV block
- Atrial fibrillation — Atrial rate above 400 bpm with variable ventricular rate

Management of fetal arrhythmias

Approximately 90% of studies in which fetal arrhythmias are detected involve isolated extrasystoles or bigeminal rhythm. These are considered benign with the recommendation of weekly auscultation to detect tachycardia and monthly routine ultrasound evaluation for development of hydrops. SVT occurs in 1–3% of fetuses with isolated atrial ectopic beats. It is suggested that the woman avoids caffeine and other stimulants during pregnancy. A newborn electrocardiogram may be ordered prior to discharge from the hospital. Sinus tachycardia without signs of tricuspid insufficiency or hydrops is followed in a similar fashion with the addition of investigation for maternal hyperthyroidism. Fetuses with bradycardia and bigeminal rhythms perceived as bradycardia similarly are recommended to have frequent evaluation of the fetal heart rate and, if the bradycardia persists, monthly ultrasound studies to evaluate for signs of fetal heart failure and cardiomegaly.

Supraventricular tachycardias are closely followed to determine whether they are persistent or paroxysmal and for signs of heart failure. In a recent two-year period we examined the risk factors and indications for transplacental therapy for sustained SVT. In a group of 34 fetuses with heart rate above 200 bpm (20–41 weeks' gestation, mean age of 31 weeks), we found 21 with SVT at rates of 200–325 bpm, 11 with atrial flutter with ventricular rates of 210–300 bpm and 2 with sinus tachycardia with rates of 200–205 bpm. All had history of a persistent tachycardia at the first fetal echocardiogram. Each received in-hospital fetal monitoring prior to therapy except 4 who presented with hydrops and in whom therapy was immediately initiated. Treatment was based on our criteria of fetal heart failure which includes cardiomegaly, tricuspid valve regurgitation, abnormal venous pulsations in the ductus venosus and umbilical vein and hydrops fetalis[35,36] When indicated, initial treatment was digoxin with procainamide added after two days if SVT persisted with adequate maternal digoxin levels. Three of these fetuses received direct *in utero* digoxin by transabdominal intramuscular injections to supplement transplacental attempts when achieving therapeutic levels of that drug was difficult in the mother[37]. In the group with SVT, two mothers were found to have Graves' disease and were treated with propylthiouracil in addition to transplacental therapy. One mother with hyperthyroidism suffered nausea after the addition of procainamide. The treatment was continued with oral digoxin and oral procainamide where indicated. All of the fetuses survived and did well after delivery. In one group, 8 received no treatment (mean age at presentation was 34.5 weeks' gestation); *in utero* conversion to normal rhythm was achieved in 18 of 26, and 8 of 26 were successfully converted after birth.

In a separate group of 2/11 fetuses with atrial flutter refractory to digoxin and procainamide, either flecainide or propranolol was administered to the mother under close in-hospital surveillance. All fetuses converted *in utero* to normal rhythm and were maintained on oral maternal digoxin until delivery. One mother developed mild diplopia and one mother suffered nausea, vomiting and blurred vision after administration of flecainide. A decrease in ventricular function was attributed to flecainide use in one fetus and was therefore discontinued. We no longer use flecainide. If SVT or flutter is refractory to digoxin and procainamide, we will proceed quickly to amiodarone administered orally to the mother.

In a multicentre retrospective study of management outcome of fetal tachycardias in Baltimore, New Haven and Utrecht, Netherlands, covering the years 1985 to 1992, 50 patients with fetal tachycardia were followed, 34 of which were treated by transplacental antiarrhythmia therapy[38]. The treated group was divided into 15 hydropic and 19 non-hydropic fetuses. As in our experience, those with hydrops usually required the addition of drugs beyond the original digoxin, or in 4 of their patients, flecainide. The median number of days for acceptable control of the arrhythmia was 3 days in the non-hydropic group (84% conversion) and 12.5 days in the group with hydrops (80% conversion). Three fetuses were not able to be controlled during gestation. Of the 48 fetuses surviving into infancy, 22 showed a relapse of tachycardia with 3 requiring continued therapy at three years of age. The most difficult to control patients in the series had permanent junctional reciprocating tachycardia or Wolff–Parkinson–White syndrome.

Complete heart block is also closely followed for signs of cardiomegaly and the development of hydrops. We reviewed seven fetuses diagnosed in a two-year period diagnosed by fetal echocardiography. Five had complex congenital heart disease (CHD) associated with left atrial isomerism and in 2 the mother had SS-A/SS-B antibodies. Hydrops was present in 6, all of whom showed umbilical venous pulsations. All were treated with beta-agonist therapy (6 terbutaline and 1 fenoterol) and were followed weekly. The 2 with SS-A/SS-B also received steroid therapy (4 mg dexamethasone, daily). The fetal heart rate improved immediately in 6/7 from 56 bpm to 87 bpm (mean 30 bpm) and hydrops improved in 4 fetuses. In a subsequent fetus with SS-A/SS-B, a trial without terbutaline returned the fetal heart rate to baseline. The heart rate improved by 10% after restarting the terbutaline. One fetus with congenital heart disease died *in utero* and 2 died at surgery. All 3 with SSA/SSB received pacemaker implantation shortly after birth and are doing well[39].

Aggressive management of the fetus with complete heart block can lead to successful outcome, although those with complex CHD carry a guarded prognosis. Copel reported on 5 cases of SS-A/SS-B with structurally normal hearts who underwent treatment with dexamethasone[40]. Hydrops in 3 of the fetuses resolved after treatment. They commented on the difficulty of predicting which fetuses would need to have neonatal pacemaker therapy, although Karpawich and the Texas Children's Hospital group recommended that any child, regardless of age, with a persistent ventricular rate less than 50 bpm be considered for pacemaker therapy[41]. *In utero* pacemaker therapy has been attempted without survival[42,43].

It must be emphasized that each new case of tachy- or bradyarrhythmia demands individual attention and deserves appropriate interaction between the referring obstetrician, the perinatologist and the perinatal cardiologist. The timing of delivery should be a team effort which includes the neonatologist and, when immediate pacemaker insertion is indicated, the surgical team. Appropriate counselling of the parents is critical. They should be actively involved in the decision process as well as any decisions regarding medical therapy. The timing of follow-up visits and maternal blood sampling for therapeutic levels of antiarrhythmic drugs should be part of the initial protocol for management. We have not found it necessary to use the umbilical venous route for either blood sampling or for the administration of antiarrhythmic medications.

Conclusion

As many as 15% of patients referred to our laboratories for fetal echocardiography have abnormalities of fetal heart rate and rhythm. The nature of the arrhythmia as well as structural defects can be delineated from segmental analysis of the fetal heart and vasculature and from careful timing of either fetal cardiac wall-movement events or from Doppler blood velocity patterns. The majority of arrhythmias are isolated atrial premature contractions which were originally detected at routine obstetrical ausculation and will have a benign course. Both brady- and tachyarrhythmias may be associated with fetal heart failure and hydrops and should be aggressively managed.

REFERENCES

1. Gilstrap III LC, Hauth JC, Toussaint S. Second stage fetal heart rate abnormalities and neonatal acidosis. *Obstet. Gynecol.* **62**(2):209–213, 1984.
2. Patrick J, Carmichael L, Chess L, Probert C, Staples C. The distribution of accelerations of the human fetal heart rate at 38 to 40 weeks' gestation. *Am. J. Obstet. Gynecol.* **151**:283–287, 1985.
3. Cameron A, Nicholson S, Nimrod C, Harder J, Davies D, Fritzler M. Evaluation of fetal cardiac dysrhythmias with two-dimensional, M-mode and pulsed Doppler ultrasonography. *Am. J. Obstet. Gynecol.* **158**:286–290, 1988.
4. Sissman N. Developmental landmarks in cardiogenic morphogeneses: Comparative chronology. *Am. J. Cardiol.* **25**:141–148, 1970.
5. Moore K. The circulatory system. In *The Developing Human: Clinically Oriented Embryology* (ed. K. Moore) 3rd edn. pp. 318–319. Philadelphia: WB Saunders, 1982.
6. Anderson R, Taylor I. Development of the atrioventicular specialized tissue in the human heart. *Br. Heart J.* **34**:1205, 1972.
7. Shenker L. Fetal Cardiac Arrhythmias. *Obstet. Gynecol. Surv.* **34**:561–572, 1979.
8. Garson A. Arrhythmias. In *The Electrocardiogram in Infants and Children: A Systematic Approach* p. 237. Philadelphia: Lea & Febiger, 1983.
9. Gillette P, El-Said G, Silvarajan N. Electrophysiologic abnormalities after Mustard's operation for transposition of the great arteries. *Br. Heart J.* **36**:186–191, 1974.
10. Cranefield P, Wit A, Hoffman B. Genesis of cardiac arrhythmias. *Circulation* **47**:190–197, 1973.
11. Dubose T. Heart rate. In *Fetal Sonography*, pp. 263–274. Philadelphia: W.B. Saunders, 1996.
12. Shenker L. Fetal Cardiac Arrhythmias. *Obstet. Gynecol. Surv.* **34**:561–572, 1979.
13. Garson A. Arrhythmias. In *The Electrocardiogram in Infants and Children: A Systematic Approach*, p. 237. Philadelphia: Lea & Febiger, 1983.
14. Bergmans M, Jonker G, Kock H. Fetal supraventricular tachycardia: review of the literature. *Obstet. Gynecol. Sury.* **55**:61–68, 1985.
15. Stewart P, Tonge H, Wladimiroff J. Arrhythmia and structural abnormalities of the fetal heart. *Br. Heart J.* **50**:550–554, 1983.
16. Kleinman C, Donnerstein R, Jaffe C, *et al.* Fetal echocardiography. A tool for the evaluation of cardiac arrhythmias and monitoring of *in utero* therapy: analysis of 71 patients. *Am. J. Cardiol.* **52**(2):237–243, 1983.
17. Allen L, Anderson R, Sullivan I, Campbell S, Holt D, Tynan M. Evaluation of fetal arrhythmias by echocardiography. *Br. Heart J.* **50**:240–244, 1983.
18. Maulik D, Nanda N, Saini V. Fetal Doppler echocardiography: Methods and characterization of normal and abnormal hemodynamics. *Am. J. Cardiol.* **53**:572–578, 1984.
19. Lingman G, Marsal K. Circulatory effects of fetal cardiac arrhythmias. *Pediatr. Cardiol.* **7**:67–74, 1996.
20. Tulzer G, Gudmundsson S, Wood D, Cohen A, Weiner S, Huhta J. Doppler in non-immune hydrops fetalis. *Ultrasound. Obstet. Gynecol.* **4**:279–283, 1994.
21. Reed KR, Appleton C, Anderson CF, Shenker L, Sahn DJ. Doppler studies of normal vena cava flows in human fetuses. *Circulation* **81**:498–505, 1990.
22. Vielle JC, Sunderland C, Bennet M. Complete heart block in a fetus associated with maternal Sjögren's syndrome. *Am. J. Obstet. Gynecol.* **151**:660–661, 1985.
23. Machado MV, Tynan M, Curry PV, Allen L. Fetal complete heart block. *Br. Heart J.* **60**:512–515, 1988.
24. Steinfeld L, Rappaport HL, Rossbach HC, Martinez E. Diagnosis of fetal arrhythmias using echocardiographic and Doppler techniques. *J. Am. Coll. Cardiol.* **9**:1425–1433, 1986.
25. DeVore G, Siassi B & Platt L. Fetal echocardiography III: The diagnosis of arrhythmias using real-time-directed M-mode ultrasound. *Am. J. Obstet. Gynecol.* **146**:792–799, 1983.
26. Crowley D, Dick M, Rayburn W, Rosenthal A. Two-dimensional and M-mode echocardiographic evaluation of fetal arrhythmia. *Clin. Cardiol.* **8**:1–10, 1985.
27. Silverman N, Enderline M, Stanger P, Teitel D, Heyman M, Golbus M. Recognition of fetal arrhythmias by echocardiography. *J. Clin. Ultrasound* **13**:255–263, 1985.
28. Huhta J, Strasburger J, Carpenter R, Reiter A, Abinader E. Pulsed fetal echocardiography. *J. Clin. Ultrasound* **13**:247–254, 1985.
29. Rice M, McDonald R, Keller D. Fetal atrial septal aneurysm: a cause of atrial arrhythmias. *J. Am. Coll. Cardiol.* **12**:1292–1297, 1988.
30. Stewart P, Wladimiroff J. Fetal atrial arrhythmia associated with redundancy/aneurysm of the foramen ovale. *J. Clin. Ultrasound* **16**:643–650, 1988.
31. Clements J, Sobotka-Plojhar M, Exalto N, van Geijn H. A connective tissue membrane in the right atrium (Chiari's network) as a cause of fetal cardiac arrhythmia. *Am. J. Obstet. Gynecol.* **142**:709–712, 1982.

32. Mendoza G, Almeida O, Steinfeld L. Intermittent fetal bradycardia induced by midpregnancy fetal ultrasonography study. *Am. J. Obstet. Gynecol.* **160**:1038–1040, 1989.
33. Martin Jr C, Nijhius J, Weijer A. Correction of fetal supraventricular tachycardia by compression of the cord: Report of a case. *Am. J. Obstet. Gynecol.* **150**:324–326, 1984.
34. Fernandez C, De Rosa G, Guevara E *et al.* Reversion by vagal reflex of a paroxysmal atrial tachycardia detected by echocardiography. *Am. J. Obstet. Gynecol.* **159**:860–861, 1988.
35. Gudmundsson S, Huhta J, Wood D, Tulzer G, Cohen A, Weiner S. Venous Doppler ultrasonography in the fetus with nonimmune hydrops. *Am. J. Obstet. Gynecol.* **164**:33–37, 1991.
36. Tulzer G, Gudmundsson S, Rotondo K, Wood DC, Cohen A, Huhta J. Doppler in the evaluation and prognosis of fetuses with tricuspid regurgitation. *J. Matern. Fetal Invest.* **1**:15–18, 1991.
37. Hallek M, Neerhof M, Perry R, Nazir M, Huhta JC. Fetal supraventricular tachycardia and hydrops fetalis: confined intensive and direct transplacental therapy. *Obstet. Gynecol.* **78**:523–525, 1991.
38. van Engelen AD, Weijtens O, Brenner J *et al.* Management outcome and follow-up of fetal tachycardia. *J. Am. Coll. Cardiol.* **24**:1371–1375, 1994.
39. Hare J, Huhta J, Weil-Chalker S, Stauffer N, Cuneo B, Respondek M. Beta agonist therapy of fetal complete heart block. *Am. J. Obstet. Gynecol.* **172**:426, 1995.
40. Copel J, Buyon J, Kleinman C. Successful *in utero* therapy of fetal heart block. *Am. J. Obstet. Gynecol.* **173**:1384–1390, 1995.
41. Karpawich P, Gillette P, Garson A *et al.* Congenital complete atrioventricular block: clinical and electrophysiologic predictors of need for pacemaker insertion. *Am. J. Cardiol.* **48**:1098–1102, 1981.
42. Carpenter Jr R, Strassburger J, Garson A *et al.* Fetal ventricular pacing for hydrops secondary to complete atrioventricular block. *J. Am. Coll. Cardiol.* **8**:1434–1436, 1986.
43. Walkinshaw S, Welsh C, McCormack J, Walsh K. *In utero* pacing for congenital complete heart block. *Fetal Diagn. Ther.* **9**:183–185, 1994.

Fetal endocrine disorders

62

P. Lewis, Y. Yaron and M.I. Evans

Introduction

Before the advent of modern prenatal diagnostic techniques, the discovery of congenital endocrine disorders could not be made until delivery of an affected newborn. Permanent and irreversible adverse consequences were common. With developments and improvements in ultrasonography, invasive fetal diagnostic techniques and molecular biology, early fetal diagnosis and treatment of such endocrinopathies have become possible. This chapter reviews the diagnosis and treatment of the common fetal endocrine disorders chiefly of the adrenal and thryoid, and possible employment of these principles for the diagnosis and treatment of similar disorders.

Adrenal gland

The adrenal gland comprises two distinct endocrine tissues, the cortex and the medulla, each having a different embryonic origin. The adrenal cortex originates from the coelomic mesoderm, in close association with the primordial genital ridge, and is ultimately responsible for biosynthesis and secretion of steroid hormones. The adrenal medulla arises from the primitive ganglia of the coeliac plexus of the autonomic nervous system, which is derived from the neural crest. It is responsible for the biosynthesis and secretion of catecholamines[1].

The most common and the best described adrenal abnormality affecting the fetus is congenital adrenal hyperplasia (CAH). This consists of a group of autosomal recessive disorders characterized by a deficiency in one or more of the five enzymes required for cortisol biosynthesis. The most common abnormality (responsible for greater than 90% of CAH[2] is caused by a deficiency of the enzyme 21-hydroxylase (21-OH), also known as p450c21. Other, less common, causes for CAH include enzyme deficiencies in 11β-hydroxylase, 17α-hydroxylase, and p450scc deficiency, 3β-OH-dehydrogenase.

Diminished 21-OH activity results in accumulation of 17-hydroxyprogesterone (17-OHP) due to a decrease in its conversion to 11-deoxycorticosterone (Fig. 62.1). The excess 17-OHP is then converted via androstenedione to androgens, the levels of which increase by as much as several hundred-fold. In the presence of androgen excess, the undifferentiated female external genitalia undergo masculinization, the degree of which can vary from clitoral hypertrophy to complete formation of a phallus and scrotum. Conversely, genital formation in male fetuses is normal although signs of androgen excess may develop in childhood, resulting in precocious masculinization, and accelerated growth and development (Fig. 62.2)

21-OH deficiency is a relatively common disorder, occurring in 1 in 5000 to 1 in 15 000 births in most populations. However, some ethnic groups, such as the Yupic Eskimos, manifest an incidence of about 1 in 500. There are two major forms of 21-OH deficiency: 'classical' and 'non-classical'. The classical form involves an almost complete block of enzyme activity and is clinically present at birth. It occurs at a frequency of 1 in 14 000 births. The non-classical form involves only partial blockade of the enzymatic activity and is usually clinically apparent later in life. This form has a gene frequency of 1 in 100 in the general white population, and an increased incidence in certain ethnic groups (Table 62.1)[3,4].

21-OH deficiency is inherited as an autosomal recessive trait in close linkage to the HLA major histocompatability complex on the short arm of chromosome 6. The simple virilizing form is associated with HLA-B5. The non-classic disease is associated with HLA-B14,DR1, and a salt-wasting form of the disease is associated with the haplotypes HLA-A3, Bw47, DR7 and HLA-Bw60[2,5–7]. Before the advent of molecular techniques, prenatal diagnosis relied upon such

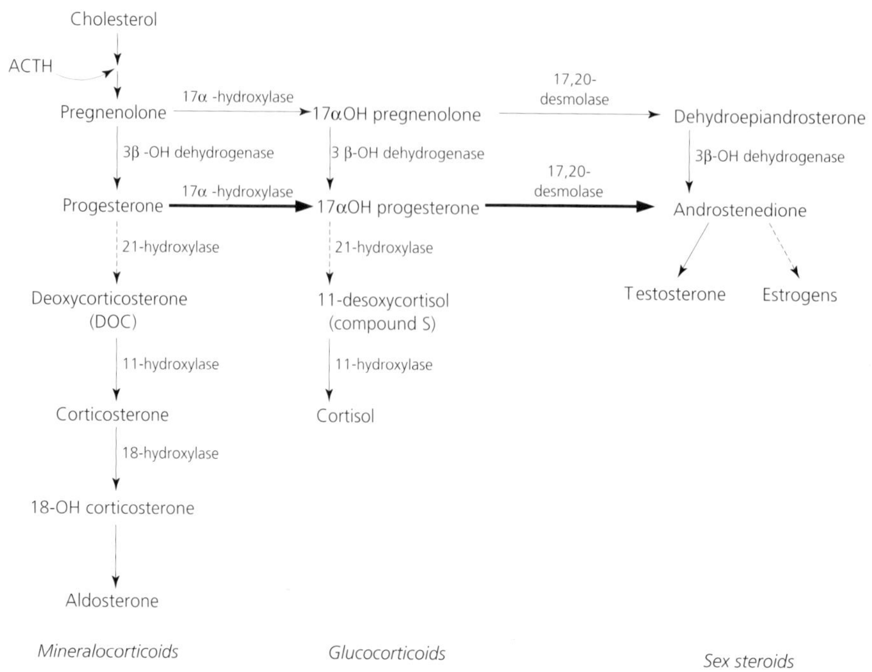

Fig. 62.1 Androgen production in 21-hydroxylase deficiency.

TABLE 62.1
The incidence and the heterozygous carrier rate of non-classical congenital adrenal hyperplasia (CAH). (Modified from Speroff et *al.*[34])

Ethnicity	Non-classical disease	Heterozygous carrier
Eastern European Jews	1 in 30	1 in 3
Hispanics	1 in 40	1 in 4
Yugoslavs	1 in 50	1 in 5
Italians	1 in 333	1 in 9
Others	1 in 1000	1 in 14

linkage studies. The gene for 21-OH (*CYP21B*) has been mapped and was found to have a pseudogene counterpart (*CYP21A*)[8]. These are located immediately adjacent to a respective gene encoding a component of serum complement (C4A and C4B). The orientation of this gene group is *C4A-CYP21A-C4B-CYP21B*, and it is located specifically within the HLA-DR region on the short arm of chromosome 6. This conformation is most likely a result of gene duplication and divergence.

DIAGNOSIS

As with most autosomal recessive disorders, most couples are known to be 'at risk' only after having an affected child. Historically, in the late 1970s and early 1980s, diagnosis of CAH had been made by the finding of elevated levels of 17-OHP in amniotic fluid. With the development of chorionic villus sampling (CVS) in the 1980s, linkage-based diagnosis in the first trimester became available. Diagnosis entailed a two-step process. First, the fetal sex was determined. If the fetus was a female, then linkage analysis would be performed. Since discovery and mapping of the allelic variants in the 1980s direct DNA analysis has become the routine approach. Nevertheless, in some families the mutations are not known, requiring sequencing of the whole gene or linkage studies. Still in other instances, linkage studies are not informative and biochemical analysis is still necessary. In addition, the sonographic detection of an abnormally enlarged phallus should alert the physician to investigate for CAH[9].

TREATMENT

In an attempt to prevent the birth of virilized females, Evans *et al.* first administered dexamethasone at a dose of 0.25 mg q.i.d. to a mother known to be at risk for CAH, beginning at 10 weeks of gestation[10]. Serial maternal oestriol and cortisol levels indicated that adrenal gland suppression had been achieved. The fetus, ultimately found to be affected, was born at 39 weeks' gestation with normal external genitalia. Forrest and David then employed a similar protocol beginning at 9 weeks' gestation to treat several fetuses known to be at risk for CAH[11]. Subsequently, those female fetuses confirmed to be clinically affected with the severe form of CAH were spared masculinization of the external genitalia.

Since the differentiation of the external genitalia begins at

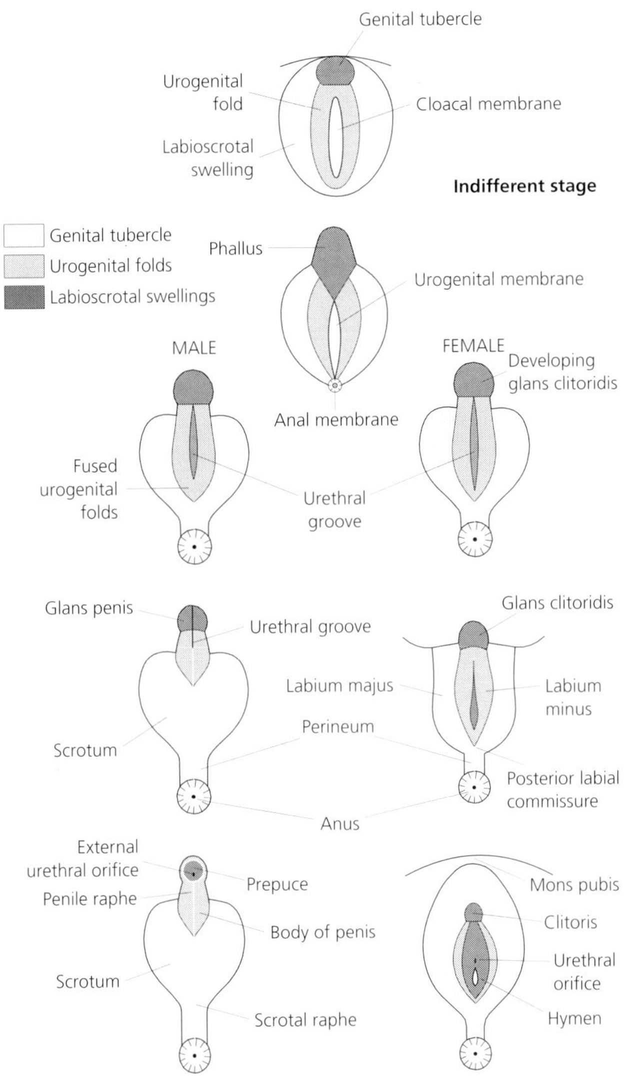

Fig. 62.2 Diagrammatic illustration of the embryonic development of the external genitalia in males and females.

about 7 weeks of gestation, diagnosis by amniocentesis or even CVS comes too late to prevent masculinization. Thus, for patients at risk of having an affected fetus, pharmacological therapy has to be initiated prior to sex assignment. This implies that therapy needs to be administered to all patients at risk despite the fact that the chance of an affected female fetus for carrier parents is only 1 in 8 (i.e. 1 in 4 affected × 1 in 2 females). It is currently recommended to start the therapy at 7 weeks' gestation as a few cases of masculinization have been reported when treatment was initiated only at 9 weeks' gestation. Direct DNA diagnosis or linkage studies may then be performed by CVS in the first trimester. Thus, for 7/8th of patients, therapy can be discontinued as soon as the diagnosis of CAH is ruled out. If the fetus is an affected female, then therapy is continued throughout gestation. Stress-dose corticosteroids should be given to the patient during labour and then tapered gradually post-partum. If, however, the fetus is a male, or is unaffected, then therapy is discontinued at the time of diagnosis.

Although this therapy is widely accepted it is still considered experimental. A recently published commentary written in *JAMA* advocates Institutional Review-Board approval be obtained on all patients offered this treatment. As long term follow-up has not been documented on individuals who received *in utero* steroid treatment for CAH, a registry has been proposed by the Lawson Wilkins Pediatric Endocrine Society for studies in North America[12]. This should help to assess the long-term outcome of fetuses exposed to high-dose steroids.

Thyroid

INTRODUCTION

The thyroid gland is the first endocrine gland to develop in the fetus. During the week 4 of gestation, it appears as a median endodermal thickening in the floor of the early pharynx. With further development, it is displaced caudally and reaches its final anatomic location in front of the hyoid bone and the laryngeal cartilages by week 7 of gestation. At 12 weeks' gestation, colloid-filled follicles appear, and iodide accumulation can be detected within the gland. Fetal triiodothyronine (T_3) and thyroxine (T_4) are synthesized by week 15 of gestation. Fetal thyroid-stimulating hormone (TSH) can first be detected at about 11 weeks' gestation; its level gradually increases to reach a maximum at about 30–35 weeks' gestation, after which it decreases until birth. Thyroxine-releasing hormone (TRH) can be detected in the fetal hypothalamus by 12 weeks' gestation[13].

HYPOTHYROIDISM

Fetal hypothyroidism may have severe fetal and neonatal consequences. Fetal oesophageal obstruction, secondary to a goitre, can lead to polyhydramnios and may result in preterm delivery. Furthermore, a fetal goitre can cause extension of the fetal neck leading to dystocia. Without treatment, postnatal growth delay and severe mental retardation can ensue. Even with immediate diagnosis and treatment at birth, long-term follow-up of children with congenital hypothyroidism has shown them to have lower scores on perceptual-motor, visuospatial and language tests[14].

Fetal hypothyroidism may be have numerous aetiologies (Table 62.2). Maternal hyperthyroidism is often associated with fetal hypothyroidism. This may be secondary to the suppression of the fetal thyroid by maternally administered propylthiouracil (PTU). Conversely, fetal hypothyroidism may also result from transplacental passage of maternal blocking antibodies. These antibodies, known as TB1Ab or (TBII), block TSH binding. Occasionally, fetal hypothyroidism is the result of inadvertent use of ^{131}I in the pregnant

TABLE 62.2
Aetiology of thyroid dysfunction. (After Thorpe-Beeston and Nicolaides[16]).

Duration	Hypothyroidism	Hyperthyroidism
Permanent		
	Thyroid dysgenesis	Maternal autoimmune disease
	athyreosis	Graves' disease
	hypoplastic disease	Hashimoto's disease
	ectopic	
	Biochemical	
	Immunological	
	Iatrogenic	
Transient		
	Iatrogenic	
	iodine administration	
	antithyroid drugs	
	Iodide deficiency	
	Idiopathic	

women, maternal ingestion of amiodarone or lithium, or excessive maternal iodine intake, sometimes in the form of vaginal douching.

Fetal hypothyroidism caused by an intrinsic fetal abnormality is uncommon, occuring in 1 in 4000–5000 births[15]. The most common form of such permanent hypothyroidism in infants is thyroid dysgenesis. This may include hypoplastic and ectopic thyroid, or the total absence of thyroid tissue (athyreosis) which is associated with undetectable levels of thyroglobulin. Congenital hypothyroidism is only rarely associated with errors of thyroid hormone synthesis, TSH insensitivity or absence of the pituitary gland.

DIAGNOSIS

Inquiry regarding a history of maternal hypothyroidism is considered as routine. In patients with this history, routine maternal thyroid hormone levels as well as blocking immunoglobulin levels should be measured. In addition, all women with a history of any thyroid disease (both hypothyroidism and hyperthyroidism) are advised to have monthly fetal ultrasound to screen for goitre, polyhydramnios or fetal tachycardia[16].

Fetal goitrous hypothyroidism is initially identified by ultrasound. Most commonly, the indication for the ultrasonographic scan is a fundal height greater than expected by gestational age. In such cases the increased uterine size is caused by polyhydramnios, resulting from oesophageal obstruction and impaired swallowing, and this may be a cause of preterm labour. The hyperextension of the neck caused by the goitre may lead to dystocia. Sometimes, a fetal goitre is discovered incidentally on a routine scan. Finally, some cases are diagnosed on serial scans in fetuses with either known elevated maternal thyroid immunoglobulins, or maternal treatment with antithyroid medications.

FETAL THERAPY

Before the advent of cordocentesis, amniotic fluid levels of TSH and fetal T_4 were used as potential indicators of fetal thyroid function. However, these proved inconsistent[17]. Currently, with cordocentesis, fetal thyroid status can be directly and accurately evaluated[18,19], and fetal response to therapy reliably measured, using available nomograms (Figs 62.3–62.5)[20]. Fetal hypothyroidism is diagnosed by measuring fetal serum levels of free T_4, total T_4, free T_3 and TSH. *In utero* treatment was initially suggested by Van Herle *et al.* using intramuscular (i.m.) injection of levothyroxine sodium[21]. Subsequent studies, however, have indicated that intraamniotic administration of thyroxine is superior. The doses commonly used for treatment range from 200–500 μg given intraamniotically every week[22]. More recently, it has been recommended that the dosage be adjusted for the fetal weight using 10 μg/kg, similar to the recommended dose for neonates[23]. With this regimen, fetal goitres have been shown to regress, and fetal and newborn TSH levels have normalized.

HYPERTHYROIDISM

Neonatal hyperthyroidism is rare with an incidence of 1 in 4000 to 1 in 40 000[24]. In these cases, fetal thyrotoxic goitre is usually secondary to maternal autoimmune disease, principally Graves' disease or Hashimoto's thyroiditis. It is estimated that 1.5–12% of infants of mothers with a known history of Graves' disease are affected with neonatal thyrotoxicosis. This may even occur despite the fact that the mother is currently euthyroid[25]. As with hypothyroidism, inherent to the underlying mechanism is the transplacental passage of maternal IgG antibodies. In this case the antibodies, known as TSAb (or TSI), are predominantly directed against the TSH receptor.

Fetal hyperthyroidism can be a cause of fetal morbidity and mortality because of goitre (see above). Fetal hyperthyroidism may also cause growth retardation, tachycardia, hydrops associated with cardiac failure and craniosynostosis[24–26].

Premature delivery occurs in up to 90% of cases with fetal hyperthyroidism and the perinatal death rate is 12–50%[25]. Consequently, it is paramount that the clinician be aware of any maternal history of thyroid disease. As with fetal hypothyroidism associated with maternal thyroid disease, such patients require evaluation of maternal thyroid function tests and immunoglobulin status (specifically TBIAb and TSAb). A fetal ultrasound is recommended every 4 weeks to screen for development of goitre, hydrops and tachycardia.

DIAGNOSIS

Usually, the investigation of fetal hyperthyroidism begins only after the discovery of fetal goitre. Often, the goitre is diagnosed on ultrasound in patients referred due to elevated thyroid-stimulating antibodies. In some cases, fetal goitres are realized serendipitously on routine ultrasonography. Others may be discovered in patients referred for scan because fundal height measures greater than expected by gestational age. Once a fetal goitre is identified, biochemical evaluation is

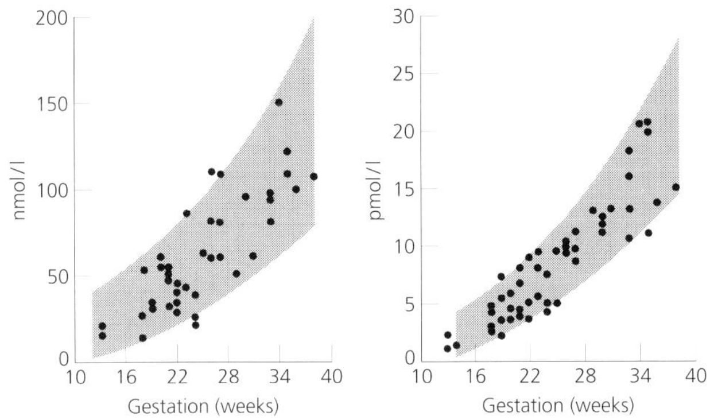

Fig. 62.3 Fetal T_4 (left) and fetal free T_4 (right).

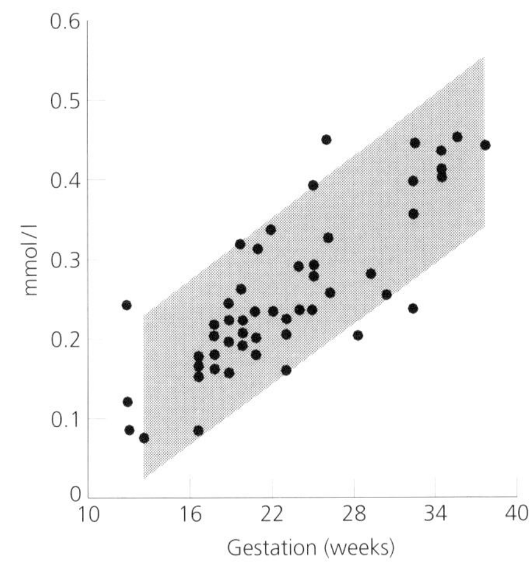

Fig. 62.4 Fetal thyroid binding goitre.

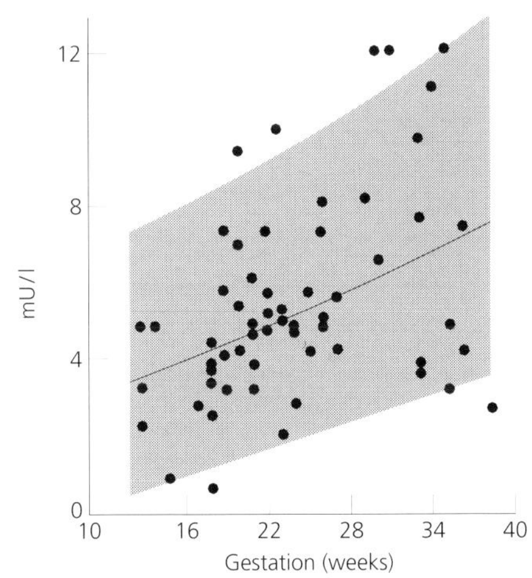

Fig. 62.5 Fetal TSH.

indicated and treatment planned according to the results (Figs 62.3–62.5).

Fetal therapy

Once the diagnosis of fetal hyperthyroidsm is confirmed, fetal treatment should be initiated. Authors have attempted treating fetal hyperthyroidism with maternally administered antithyroid drugs. Porreco and Bloch have reported maternal treatment of fetal thyrotoxicosis with propylthiouracil which led to a good outcome[27]. The initial dose used was 100 mg orally three times a day, which was later decreased to 50 mg orally three times a day. Wenstrom *et al.* described a favourable outcome using maternal methimazole to treat fetal hyperthyroidism in a patient who could not tolerate propylthiouracil[28]. Hatjis also treated fetal goitrous hyperthyroidism with a maternal dose of 300 mg propylthiouracil. This patient, however, required supplemental synthroid to remain euthyroid. There was good fetal outcome in this case as well[29].

Possibilities for the future

In 1990, the Human Genome Project was initiated with the goal of mapping all 50 000 to 100 000 genes that comprise the human genome by the year 2005. It is currently estimated that this goal will be reached even before the scheduled date. Undoubtedly, more genes responsible for fetal endocrine *disorders* will be discovered, thus offering early fetal diagnosis. Moreover, recent advances in gene therapy and fetal stem cell transfer[30,31] are very promising and may provide therapeutic options and even definitive cures. As an example, four forms of inherited growth hormone deficiency (IGHD) have been described[32]: IGHD Types IA and IB are inherited as autosomal recessive disorders; IGHD type II is inherited as an autosomal dominant and is caused by splice site, dominant negative mutations; finally, IGHD type III is an X-linked disorder, often associated with hypogammaglobulinaemia. Several kindred with multiple affected siblings have been described. With the mapping of the growth hormone gene to chromosome 17q22–q24, and the description of characteristic deletions, it is now conceivable to apply DNA testing on CVS culture. Moreover, Archer *et al.*[33] were able to transfer replication-defective retroviruses encoding the human growth hormone gene into the mammary gland of goats for the purpose of producing growth in the goat milk. Theoretically, similar approaches may be used *in vivo* to treat such growth hormone-deficient fetuses diagnosed *in utero*.

With the identification of more gene loci responsible for endocrinopathies, prenatal diagnoses of more genetic disorders, using early CVS will be made possible. Finally, the development of pre-implantation diagnosis of the morular-stage embryo offers potential diagnoses prior to implantation and possible correction by gene transfer.

REFERENCES

1. Moore KL. *Before We are Born: Basic Embryology and Birth Defects*, 3rd edn, pp. 185–187. Philadelphia: W.B. Saunders, 1989.
2. New MI, White PC & Pang S *et al.* The adrenal hyperplasias. In *The Metabolic Basis of Inherited Disease* (eds C.R. Scriver, A.L. Beaudet, W.S. Sly & D.Valle) 6th edn., pp. 1881–1917. New York: McGraw Hill, 1994.
3. New MI. 21-Hydroxylase deficiency congenital adrenal hyperplasia. *J. Steroid Biochem. Molec. Biol.* **48**(1), 12–22, 1994.
4. Speiser PW, Dupont B, Rubinstein P, Piazza A, Kastelan A & New MI. High frequency of nonclassical steroid 21-hydroxylase deficiency. *Am. J. Hum. Genet.* **37**, 650–657, 1985.
5. Dupont B, Oberfield SE, Smithwick EM *et al.* Close genetic linkage between HLA and congenital adrenal hyperplasia (21-hydroxylase deficiency). *Lancet* **ii**, 1309–1311, 1977.
6. Levine LS, Zachman M, New ML *et al.* Genetic mapping of the 21-hydroxylase deficiency gene within the HLA linkage group. *N. Engl. J. Med.* **299**, 911–915, 1978.
7. Klouda PT, Harris R & Price DA. Linkage and association between HLA and 21-hydroxylase deficiency. *J. Med. Genet.* **17**, 337–341, 1980.
8. White PC, Grossberger D, Onufer BJ *et al.* Two genes encoding steroid 21-hydroxylase are located near the fourth complement component in man. *Proc. Natl. Acad. Sci. USA* **82**, 1089–1093, 1985.
9. Mandell J, Bromley B, Peters CA & Benacerraf BR. Prenatal sonographic detection of genital malformations. *J. Urol.* **153**(6), 1994–1996, 1995.
10. Evans MI, Chrousos GP, Mann DL, Larsen JW Jr, Green I, McCluskey J *et al.* Pharmacologic suppression of the fetal adrenal gland *in utero:* attempted prevention of abnormal external genital masculinization in suspected congenital adrenal hyperplasia. *JAMA* **253**, 1015, 1985.
11. Forrest M & David M. Prenatal treatment of congenital adrenal hyperplasia due to 21-hydroxylase deficiency. *7th International Congress of Endocrinology, Quebec, Canada.* Abstract y11, 1984.
12. Seckl JR & Miller WL. How safe is long-term prenatal prenatal glucocorticoid treatment? *JAMA* **13**, 1077–1079, 1997.
13. McDougall IR. Hyperthyroidism and maternal–fetal thyroid hormone metabolism. In *Endocrine Disorders in Pregnancy* (eds S. Brody & K. Ueland), pp. 151–163. Norwalk, CT: Appleton & Lange, 1989.
14. Rovet J, Ehrlich R & Sorbara D. Intellectual outcome in children with fetal hypothyroidism. *J. Pediatr.* **110**, 700–704, 1987.
15. Trainer TD & Howard PL. Thyroid function tests in thyroid and nonthyroid disease. *CRC Crit. Rev. Clin. Lab. Sci.* **19**, 135–171, 1983.
16. Thorpe-Beeston JG & Nicolaides KH. *Maternal and Fetal Thyroid Function in Pregnancy*, p. 61. New York: Parthenon, 1996.
17. Sack J, Fisher DA, Hobel CJ & Lam R. Thyroxine in human amniotic fluid. *J. Pediatrics* **87**, 364–368, 1975.
18. Thorpe-Beeston JG, Nicolaides KH & McGregor AM. Fetal thyroid function. *Thyroid* **2**, 207–217, 1992.
19. Ballabio M, Nicolini U, Jowett T, Ruiz de Elvira MC, Ekins RP & Rodeck CH. Maturation of thyroid function in normal human fetuses. *Clin. Endocrinol.* **31**, 565–571, 1989.
20. Thorpe-Beeston JG, Nicolaides KH, Felton CV, Butler J & McGregor AM. Maturation of the secretion of thyroid hormone and thyroid stimulating hormone in the fetus. *N. Engl. J. Med.* **324**, 532–536, 1991.
21. Van Herle AJ, Young RT, Fisher DA, Uller RP & Brinkman CR. III. Intra-uterine treatment of a hypothyroid fetus. *J. Clin. Endocrinol. Metab.* **40**, 474–477, 1973.
22. Abuhamad AZ, Fisher DA, Warsof SL, Slotnik RN, Pyle PG, Wu SY & Evans AT. Antenatal diagnosis and treatment of fetal goitrous hypothyroidism: case report and review of the literature. *Ultrasound Obstet. Gynec.* **6**(5), 368–371, 1995.
23. Hadi HA & Strickland RT. *In utero* treatment of fetal goitrous hypothyroidism caused by maternal Graves' disease. *Am. J. Perinatol.* **12** (6), 455–458, 1995.
24. Fisher DA. Neonatal thyroid disease of women with autoimmune thyroid disease. *Thyroid Today* **9**, 1–7, 1986.
25. Bruinse HW, Vermeulen-Meiners C & Wit JM. Fetal treatment for thyrotoxicosis in non-thyrotoxic pregnant women. *Fetal Therapy* **3**, 152–157, 1988.
26. Ramsey I. Attempted prevention of neonatal thyrotoxicosis. *Br. Med. J.* **2**, 1110, 1976.
27. Porreco RP & Bloch CA. Fetal blood sampling in the management of intrauterine thyrotoxicosis. *Obstet. Gynecol.* **76**, 509–512, 1990.
28. Wenstrom KD, Weiner CP, Williamson RA & Grant SS. Prenatal diagnosis of fetal hyperthyroidism using funipuncture. *Obstet. Gynecol.* **76** (3 Pt. 2), 513–517, 1990.
29. Hatjis CG. Diagnosis and successful treatment of fetal goitrous hyperthyroidism caused by maternal Graves' disease. *Obstet. Gynecol.* **81** (5 Pt. 2), 837–839, 1993.
30. Flake AW, Puck JM, Almieda-Porada G *et al.* Successful *in utero* correction of X-linked recessive severe combined immuno-deficiency (X-SCID): Fetal intraperitoneal transplantation of CD34 enriched paternal bone marrow cells (EPPBMC). *N. Engl. J. Med.* **335** (24), 1806–1810, 1996.
31. Yaron Y, Kramer R, Johnson MP & Evans MI. Gene therapy: Is the future here yet? *Obstet. Gynecol. Clin. North Am.* **24**, 179–199, 1997.
32. Phillips JA III & Cogan JD. Genetic basis of endocrine disease. 6: Molecular basis of familial human growth hormone deficiency. *J. Clin. Endocrin. Metab.* **78**, 11–16, 1994.
33. Archer JS, Kennan WS, Gould MN & Bremel RD. Human growth hormone (hGH) secretion in milk of goats after direct transfer of the *hGH* gene into the mammary gland by using replication-defective retrovirus vectors. *Proc. Natl. Acad. Sci.* **91**, 6840–6844, 1994.
34. Speroff L, Glass RH & Kase NG. *Clinical Gynecologic Endocrinology and Infertility*, p. 391. Baltimore: Williams & Wilkins, 1989.

Early pregnancy loss

63

E. Jauniaux, P. Kaminopetros and H. El-Rafaey

Introduction

Spontaneous abortion is the commonest complication of pregnancy. The diagnosis of a specific anomaly in cases of early spontaneous abortion has important epidemiological value and may help to elucidate unclear mechanisms implicated in some early pregnancy failure. Recent years have seen an expansion in the availability of prenatal diagnosis. In particular, during the last decade, great advances have been made in ultrasound imaging enabling the investigation of the pregnancy from 3 weeks after conception. At the end of the first trimester, major fetal abnormalities that use to be diagnosed around mid-gestation can now be detected accurately.

As the availability of new and improved prenatal diagnosis techniques increases, so does the relevance of the emotional impact on the couple of an early pregnancy failure. In this chapter, we will present the different techniques available for the investigation of the aetiopathology of early pregnancy failure. We include sections on the clinical aspects of pregnancy miscarriage, the pathological examination of the specimen and on the diagnostic tools. The chapter also contains a section discussing the role of an organized unit to support pregnant women with early pregnancy complication.

Clinico-pathology

An early pregnancy loss (EPL) is defined as a miscarriage or spontaneous abortion occurring within the first 12 weeks of gestation. There are four different clinical forms of EPL.

A THREATENED ABORTION

This is defined as painless vaginal bleeding occurring any time between implantation and 24 weeks of pregnancy according to the WHO nomenclature[1]. Probably a quarter of all pregnancies are complicated by threatened abortion, although many patients may be unaware of their pregnancy at the time they present with vaginal bleeding. It is certainly one of the most common indications (together with suspected ectopic pregnancy) for emergency referral of a young woman to a casualty department. The bleeding may resolve spontaneously in a few days, never to recur. It may also continue, or stop and start over several days or weeks. It is only when abdominal cramps supervene that the process may move in the direction of inevitability, in particular if the cervix opens. It usually happens between 6 and 9 weeks of gestation when the definitive placenta forms.

The diagnosis is usually based on clinical examination. The role of ultrasound and endocrinology in predicting this type of early pregnancy complication remains controversial. Nevertheless, the evaluation of the size of the gestational sac or the embryo and demonstration of embryonic heart action are important to the management of this common pregnancy complication. Within this context, ultrasound plays probably its most important role in reassuring the patient that the embryo/fetus is alive and developing normally.

AN INEVITABLE ABORTION

This can be complete or incomplete depending on whether or not all fetal and placental tissues have been expelled from the uterus. The typical features of incomplete abortion are heavy (sometimes intermittent) bleeding with passage of clots and tissue together with lower abdominal cramps. If these symptoms improve spontaneously, a complete abortion is more likely.

Ultrasound examination is important in determining the absence or persistence of conception products inside the uterine cavity, thus guiding the management of this complication (Fig. 63.1).

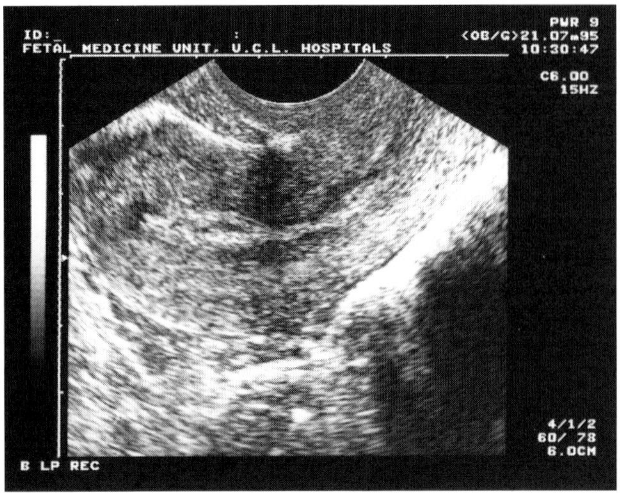

Fig. 63.1 Ultrasound scan showing a thickened endometrial line after a complete abortion at 8 weeks' gestation.

A MISSED ABORTION

This is a gestational sac containing a dead embryo/fetus before 20 weeks of gestation without clinical symptoms of expulsion[1]. The diagnosis is usually made by failure to identify fetal heart action on ultrasound. Within this context, the mother often complains of chronic but slight vaginal bleeding.

With the introduction of transvaginal ultrasound, the diagnosis of missed abortion can now be made from as early as 6 weeks of gestation. When the gestational sac is more than 25 mm in diameter and no embryonic/fetal part can be seen, the terms 'blighted ovum' or 'anembryonic pregnancy' have often been used by pathologists and more commonly by ultrasonographers, suggesting that the sac may have develop without an embryo (Fig. 63.2). Recent data have demonstrated that the explanation for this feature is the early death and resorption of the embryo with persistence of the placental tissue rather than a pregnancy originally without an embryo. Thus, most pregnancies traditionally classified as anembryonic gestation result from early embryonic demise, the embryo having developed for at least up to 14 days after ovulation corresponding to the stage of embryonic life when the secondary yolk sac starts to form[2].

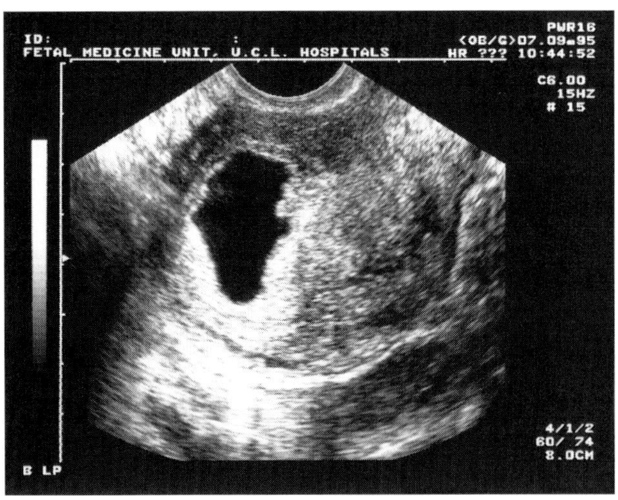

Fig. 63.2 Transvaginal ultrasound scan showing an anembryonic sac at 10 weeks of gestation. The outline of the gestational sac is irregular and no fetal pole or yolk sac was identified.

A RECURRENT ABORTION

This is defined as three or more consecutive spontaneous abortions. The aetiologies of recurrent pregnancy failure are diverse, not well understood and will be discussed later. They may present clinically as any of the previously described forms of EPL.

Incidence of pregnancy loss in humans

It has been estimated that about 60% of all fertilised ova are lost before the end of the first trimester is reached[3]. Most of them are lost during the first month after the last menstrual period and are often ignored as conceptions, particularly if they occur around the time of an expected menstrual period.

DURING THE FIRST MONTH OF GESTATION

A recent prospective study of 200 presumably fertile couples desiring to achieve pregnancy over 12 menstrual cycles has shown that 82% conceived and that the maximal fertility rate was 30% per cycle in the first two cycles[4]. Pregnancy wastage during the first three cycles accounted for 31% of the pregnancies detected. About 40% of these losses were seen only by urine human chorionic gonadotropin (hCG) testing.

AFTER THE FIRST MONTH

The rate of pregnancy loss is known to decrease with gestational age (Table 63.1). The precise incidence of EPL at different periods of gestation has been more clearly defined with the routine use of transvaginal ultrasound. In a prospective study of 232 women with positive urinary pregnancy tests and no antecedent history of vaginal bleeding, pregnancy loss was virtually complete by the end of the embryonic period (70 days after the onset of the last menstrual period)[5]. Once a gestational sac has been documented on scan subsequent loss of viability in the embryonic period is still of 11.5%. If an embryo has developed up to 5 mm, subsequent loss of viability still occurs in 7.2%. Loss rates drop rapidly after that to 3.3% for embryos of 6–10 mm and to 0.5% for embryos over 10 mm. No pregnancies were lost between 8.5 and 14 menstrual weeks. The fetal loss rate after 14 weeks was 2%. The ultrasound screening of a large group of women with pregnancies between 10 and 13 weeks' gestation has con-

TABLE 63.1
Incidence of early pregnancy failure

Variable*	Percentage
Total loss of conceptions	50–70%
Total clinical miscarriages	25–30%
Before 6 weeks' gestation	18%
Between 6 and 9 weeks' gestation	4%
After 9 weeks' gestation	3%
EPF in primigravidas	6–10%
Risk of EPF after three miscarriages	25–30%
Risk of EPF of 40-year-old women	30–40%
Ectopic pregnancies per live births	1–2%

*EPF = early pregnancy failure.

firmed that the prevalence of EPL at the end of first trimester is around 2–3%[6].

Pathophysiology of EPL

Although EPL is a common disorder, very little is known about its pathological basis and mechanism of occurrence and this for some causes only. Theoretically, a variety of fetal and maternal conditions may lead to a miscarriage. However, epidemiological studies are fraught with pitfalls and often reflect the widespread medical belief that there is little to gain from the investigation of an isolated first trimester abortion. It is only after three similar pregnancy losses or when the abortion occurs after 12 weeks that a detailed investigation including cytogenetics of the conceptus and maternal biology may be started. Thus it is still impossible to judge whether the investigation of all miscarriages would be cost-effective or beneficial either from a psychological or medical perspective.

The only well-established epidemiological fact about spontaneous abortion is that about half of them are associated with a chromosomal defect of the conceptus and that the frequency of abnormal chromosomal complement increases when the embryonic demise occurs earlier in gestation[7,8]. The other causes of EPL include endocrine diseases, anatomical abnormalities of the female genital tract, infections, immune factors, chemical agents, hereditary disorders, trauma, maternal diseases and psychological factors. None of these aetiologies can quantitatively be shown to cause more than a small percentage of pregnancy losses in general. Aetiologies such as exposure to certain toxins should be rare in the general population although this may become an important issue in the context of ecological disasters. Some other causes may be relatively more frequently found in recurrent aborters, such as psychological factors, luteal phase deficiency and traumas.

The two most common factors are that the risk of pregnancy loss increases with maternal age (i.e. a 40-year-old woman carrying twice the risk of a 20-year-old woman) and past obstetric history. The pregnancy loss rate among primigravidae is 6% whereas for three or more losses the risk increases to 25–30%). These risks apply for all women with recognised losses between 5 and 12 weeks[9].

AETIOLOGY

CHROMOSOMAL ABNORMALITIES

These represent at least 50% of clinically recognized EPL[10]. Chorionic villus sampling at the time of ultrasound diagnosis of fetal demise, increasing the success rate of karyotyping, indicates an even higher frequency of chromosomal abnormalities with values ranging between 75 and 90%[11]. Autosomal trisomies are the most common with an incidence of 30–35% followed by triploidies and monosomies X[10,12]. All possible autosomal trisomies have been described in cytogenetically abnormal abortions except trisomy 1 which has only been reported in an eight-cell embryo[13]. Triploidy and tetraploidy are frequent but are extremely lethal chromosomal abnormalities and are therefore rarely found in late miscarriages. Triploid conceptions may result from fertilization of a haploid ovum by either a single sperm that undergoes reduplication, or two sperm (diandry) or are due to a double maternal contribution when the ovum fails to undergo the first or second meiotic division before fertilization (digyny). A supernumerary paternal haploid set is thus imparted to the ovum, giving a total of 69 chromosomes with three possible sex chromosomes permutations of XXX, XXY and XYY[12]. Unlike other common chromosomal abnormalities, triploidy of paternal origin may affect the mother with persisting trophoblastic disease.

The frequency of most trisomies is influenced by maternal age at any gestation suggesting that autosomal trisomies are predictably more likely to arise cytologically in maternal meiosis (90%) than in paternal meiosis[9,14]. This is true for trisomy 21 and for all the acrocentric chromosomes. In particular, trisomy 16 is exclusively attributable to errors in maternal meiosis I whereas trisomy 18 usually arises at maternal meiosis II[15–17].

Chromosomal complements of successive miscarriages in a given family are more likely to be either recurrently normal or recurrently abnormal. If the complement of the first miscarriage is abnormal, the chromosomal complement of the subsequent one will be abnormal in up to 80% of the cases and the recurrent abnormality is usually a trisomy[18]. This can be supported by the observation that the risk of liveborn trisomy 21 following an aneuploid abortus is about 1–2% compared to 1 in 800 in the general population[19].

Structural chromosomal rearrangements such as translocation or inversions are present in only 1.5% of abortuses in the general population but are a significant cause of repetitive spontaneous abortions. Translocation are observed in about 5% of couples experiencing repeated losses[20,21]. Individuals with balanced translocations are phenotypically normal, but miscarriages or abnormal liveborns may show chromosomal duplications or deficiencies as a result of normal meiotic segregation. About 60% of the translocations detected are reciprocal; 40% are Robertsonian. Females are about twice as likely as males to show a balanced translocation.

MATERNAL AGE AND INFERTILITY

These are indirect factors of EPL. The incidence of EPL after confirmation of early fetal heart activity by transvaginal ultrasound scan is substantially greater in infertile patients than previously reported, when considered as a function of maternal age. In infertile women of less than 35 years old[22], the rate of spontaneous abortion is 2.1% which is similar to the background rate of EPL after 8 weeks in the general population[7]. This rate increases rapidly to 16.1% for patients > 36 years old and 20% for patients > 40 years old. Overall, there is a fivefold increase in EPL in women of 40 years or more compared to women 31–35 years which is independent from the infertility diagnosis, mode of insemination and ovulation induction protocol[22].

IATROGENIC CAUSES

These mainly involve the different invasive procedures used to obtained a fetal karyotype. The diagnostic procedure before 14 weeks of gestation would be either chorionic villus sampling or an early amniocentesis. Either can cause a miscarriage, the excess risk is about 1–2% compared to late amniocentesis (at about 16 weeks) which has been evaluated to be 1%[23]. As the availability and demand for first-trimester prenatal diagnosis is increasing rapidly, especially among women of advanced maternal age, the impact of invasive techniques is also increasing. The procedure-related accident is obviously related to the type of equipment used and operator experience and in particular to the number of attempts needed to obtain a sufficient villus sample. This particular factor is rarely considered in epidemiological studies or in economic evaluation of the benefits and costs of prenatal diagnosis.

MEDICAL AND ENDOCRINE DISORDERS

These may influence the implantation of the blastocyst resulting in early miscarriage. Luteal phase deficiency (LPD), for example, has been used to describe the endometrium manifesting an inadequate progesterone effect. Recent observations have suggested a relationship between fetal loss and either oligomenorrhoea or polycystic ovary disease (PCO)[24], either of which could reflect ovarian–endometrial dysynchrony. It has also been suggested that women with hypersecretion luteinizing hormone (LH) may experience a higher rate of pregnancy loss[25,26]. Unfortunately, suppression of high LH levels with gonadotrophin-releasing hormone analogues combined with human menopausal gonadotrophin stimulation is ineffective in improving the pregnancy outcome in these women[25]. By contrast, hypothyroidism, diabetes and lupus anticoagulant and antiphospholipid antibodies are associated with decreased conception rates and increased fetal losses and should be treated before the patient is considering a pregnancy or from conception.

PELVIC ANATOMICAL ABNORMALITIES

These are rare causes of EPL. Leiomyomas, uterine septa or endometrial adhesions can interfere with implantation or with early embryonic development but their impact in the incidence of EPL is often overestimated by the medical establishment. Uterine anomalies such as fibroids are so common (10–25% of the women) that observed adverse outcomes are probably only coincidental. Relatively few women with congenital or acquired uterine anatomical anomalies develop symptoms requiring medical or surgical therapy. Women with these anomalies may more often manifest infertility related to hypomenorrhoea or amenorrhoea than recurrent abortions. Mullerian tract fusion and cervical abnormalities are well accepted causes of second trimester losses, but the association of these abnormalities with EPL is uncertain.

INFECTIONS

Infections are accepted causes of late fetal wastage, and have been blamed for early fetal loss as well. Among the many infection reported to have been associated with spontaneous abortion are *Salmonella typhi*, malaria, cytomegalovirus, *Brucella*, *Toxoplasma*, *Mycoplasma hominis*, *Chlamydia trachomatis* and *Ureaplasma urealyticum*. Transplacental infection doubtless occurs with each of these, and sporadic losses could be caused theoretically by any. However, prospective epidemiological surveys suggest that the attributable risk of infection in first-trimester spontaneous abortion is small[27]. A role for a specific organism could still exist in selective women with repetitive abortions. Of the organisms implicated in repetitive abortion, *Ureaplasma* and *Chlamydia* seem most likely because they exist in an asymptomatic state and their virulence is not always severe enough to cause infertility due to fallopian tube occlusion[28]. Data are less compelling for other organisms.

CHEMICAL AGENTS

Chemicals have been claimed to be associated with fetal losses, but consensus seems to be settling around a selected few[29]. These include anaesthetic gases, arsenic, aniline dyes, benzene, solvents, ethylene oxide, formaldehyde, pesticides and certain divalent cations (lead, mercury, cadmium). Among workers at greatest risk are those in rubber industries, battery factories and chemical production plants and personnel handling chemotherapeutic agents. External irradiation and internal radionucleotides in high doses are proven abortifacients but rare events. Pelvic X-ray exposure of up to 10 rads are common but places a woman's fetus at little to no increased risk as actual doses to the conceptus are usually far less. Finally, some authors[30] have found an increased abortion rates in smokers, independent of maternal age and independent of alcohol consumption.

THE ROLE OF MORPHOLOGICAL ANALYSIS

DIAGNOSING THE CAUSE OF AN EPL

Consideration of the pathology of EPL has often led to the conclusion that morpholological studies have relatively little to offer to our understanding of the aetiology or pathogenesis of EPL. This is not surprising as histopathological analysis of 'abortus specimens' is often delegated to the most junior pathologist of the team. However, the histopathological investigation of a first-trimester conceptus is particularly difficult not only because of the limited amount of material available but also because the specimens are often fragmented or macerated. Around one-half of early spontaneous abortion specimens contain no embryonic or fetal part and about 12% consist of maternal decidua only[31]. Thus, more often, small amounts of placental tissue are the only material available for routine pathological examination which must be in part responsible for a certain lack of enthusiasm in examining these specimens.

STUDYING THE AETIOPATHOLOGY OF EPL

Normal placentation requires a progressive transformation of the spiral arteries and infiltration of the placental bed by trophoblastic cells. These physiological changes normally extend down into the inner third of the myometrium and in normal pregnancies all the spiral arteries are transformed in uteroplacental arteries before 20 weeks of gestation. In most cases of early pregnancy failure as in pregnancy-induced hypertension there is inadequate placentation and in particular, a defective transformation of the spiral arteries[32,33]. Reduced trophoblastic penetration into the decidua and into the spiral arteries together with a thinner and discontinuous trophoblastic shell has also been shown in spontaneous abortions, whereas in normal first-trimester pregnancies the physiological changes are always present. These findings suggest that one of the functions of trophoblastic plugging of spiral arteries is to restrict maternal blood flow into the intervillous space in normal early pregnancy. The premature entry of a lot of maternal blood into the intervillous space at this stage of pregnancy disrupts the placental shell and is probably the mechanical cause of abortion[34].

The extent of the placentation deficit in first-trimester complicated pregnancies seems not to be linked to a specific aetiology. However, the defective transformation of the spiral arteries and the poor trophoblastic infiltration of the placental bed are more pronounced in pregnancies complicated by partial and complete hydatidiform moles[35]. This could explain the early onset of pregnancy-induced hypertension in these cases. In non-molar pregnancies complicated by hypertension, there is probably a relationship between the severity of the disease and the degree of inadequate placentation. If one extrapolates this concept to the first trimester of pregnancy, recurrent miscarriage in pregnancy disorders known to be associated with a defect of placentation such as in lupus or thrombophilia could represent the earliest form of this phenomenon.

SCREENING FOR GESTATIONAL TROPHOBLASTIC DISORDERS (GTD)

The diagnosis of partial mole is initially based on the ultrasound appearance of the placenta *in utero* or gross examination of the placenta at delivery during the second or third trimester of pregnancy. If there is no further microscopic examination showing some form of trophoblastic hyperplasia, the patient will not be entered in the follow-up registry. In most European countries, spontaneous abortions are not routinely investigated for partial mole and/or diandric (paternally inherited) triploidy and it is mainly second- or third-trimester partial moles which have been registered for follow-up. As diandric triploidies are much more common in the first trimester, a large group of women at risk of persistent GTD theoretically escape detection and if treatment is required, it would only be started at a later stage of the disease. In this context, those women who develop a persistent GTD may experience several subsequent episodes of uterine bleeding before the diagnosis eventually is made. Diandric triploidy is less often associated with molar changes in the first trimester of pregnancy than in the second or third trimester[12]. The majority of diandric triploid miscarriages, therefore, escape detection on the base of ultrasound or macroscopic examination. The use of standardized criteria for detection by microscopic examination is both accurate and reproducible and should play a pivotal role in screening women at risk of persistent GTD.

Clinical assessment of EPL

Before ultrasound became widely available, the obstetrician–gynaecologist had to rely essentially on clinical symptoms in the assessment of an EPL. Endocrinological tests were evaluated repeatedly over the last three decades but so far only serum hCG brings direct information into the management of EPL and the differential diagnosis of causes of bleeding in early pregnancy. Transvaginal ultrasound examination has become the 'gold standard' in the clinical management of early pregnancy complications. There have been concerns about the potential side-effect of ultrasound on the developing embryo/fetus but data in general are limited and often inconclusive. The very different results observed in these studies can be explained by the fact that different protocols, equipment, selection criteria and follow-up methods have been used. So far there has been no investigation showing any effect of ultrasound in the first trimester of pregnancy.

THE ROLE OF ENDOCRINOLOGY

Maternal serum levels of many proteins and hormones of fetal and placental origin have been tested to predict the outcome of women with vaginal bleeding in early pregnancy. The fact that, before the appearance of any clinical symptoms, some forms of early pregnancy failure may be associated with abnormal serum levels of specific placental protein, is still the matter of debate. In general, the concentration of placental products is reduced in threatened miscarriage in which the outcome is fetal loss, but normal in cases in which pregnancy proceeds[36]. As a clinical predictive tool, measurement of these compounds is unnecessary if fetal life can be demonstrated by ultrasound[37]. In particular, if the fetal heart beat is not evident ultrasonically after 7 weeks of gestation, then abnormally low levels of any fetoplacental products will not provide additional information. However, a small proportion of fetuses with a heart beat will subsequently spontaneously abort and a single serum free β-hCG measurement taken in early pregnancy has a 88% sensitivity and 83% positive predictive value in the diagnosis of early pregnancy failure and long-term prognosis of viability[38]. In this small group of patients, the levels of pregnancy associated plasma protein A (PAPP-A) and pregnancy specific β1-glycoprotein (SP-1) are reduced before fetal death[36]. Low progesterone levels and low β-hCG levels at 4–7 weeks' gestation have been shown to have 59% and 68% sensitivity in the prediction of EPL[39]. This suggests that there may be a relationship between trophoblast dysfunction and some forms of miscarriage. Furthermore, the pattern of the reduction in the circulating levels of the placental proteins in later miscarriages suggests the function of specific cell types may be impaired in these cases[40].

Other factors have been tested at an experimental level. An early pregnancy factor has been studied in sera of women with unexplained spontaneous abortion. It was found that low levels of this factor are associated poor prognosis[41]. Inhibin, relaxin and progesterone have also been studied in the luteal phase of cycles stimulated by gonadotropins and it has been found that pregnancies resulting in a miscarriage have low inhibin and progesterone levels[42]. Finally, in women with recurrent pregnancy loss serum LH concentrations are raised inappropriately in 81% of the cases. High LH levels may have adverse effects on the developing oocyte or endometrium either directly or indirectly by causing an elevation in testosterone and oestrogen levels[43]. High pre-pregnancy LH levels in spontaneous and induced cycles and high oestrogen levels in cycles induced by gonadotropins are also associated with EPL[44].

ULTRASOUND CRITERIA USED TO DIAGNOSE EPL

About one-third of normal embryos with a crown–rump length of less than 5 mm have no demonstrable cardiac activity[45,46]. Thus, the diagnosis of missed abortion should not be made in embryos smaller than this (Fig. 63.3). The sonographic features of a missed abortion include the presence of a gestational sac, which sometimes appears collapsed, and a dead fetus (Fig. 63.4) whereas the sonographic diagnosis of anembryonic pregnancy is based on the absence of embryonic echoes within a gestational sac large enough for such structures to be visible (Fig. 63.2). Provided that both operator and equipment are technically adequate, a mean gestational sac diameter greater than 1.5 cm (using transvaginal probe) or 1.7 cm (using transabdominal probe) are necessary before diagnosing this anomaly[47]. Careful clinical analysis is also required to distinguish an empty

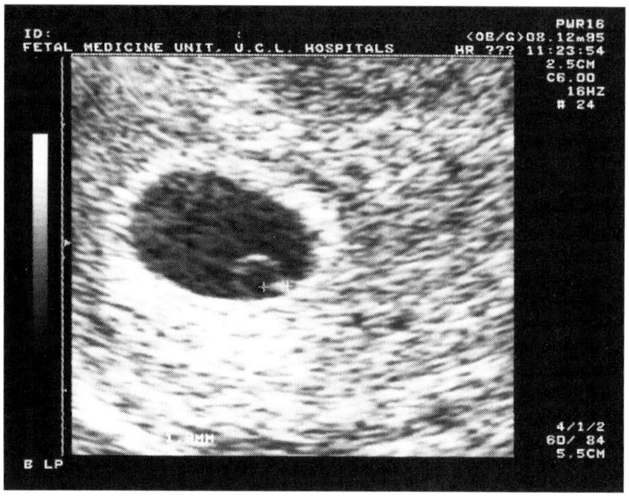

Fig. 63.3 Transvaginal ultrasound scan of a pregnancy sac at 5 weeks' gestation showing a 1.9-mm embryo under a secondary yolk sac. No cardiac activity could be detected at this stage.

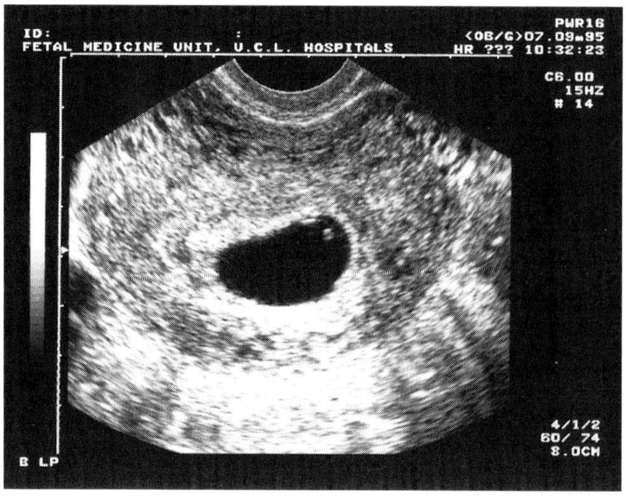

Fig. 63.4 Ultrasound scan of a missed abortion at 7 weeks' gestation. The gestational sac contains a small embryonic remnant in the upper right corner.

gestational sac from the pseudosac of an ectopic pregnancy as the sonographic features may not be accurate enough. The sonographic appearance of incomplete abortion is of thick irregular echoes in the midline of the uterine cavity. However, this is often not diagnostic of retained products as blood clots may look remarkably similar on scan. Conversely, the finding of a well-defined regular endometrial line can effectively exclude this diagnosis. The reliability of ultrasonography in the detection of complete abortion is high, enabling correct identification in 98% of patients with an empty uterus (complete abortion) and 69% of patients with retained products[48].

With the widespread use of transvaginal ultrasound equipment, an increasing number of instances in which fetal death was erroneously diagnosed by ultrasound examination was reported within the context of medical litigation. As a consequence, the Board of the Faculty of Clinical Radiology of the Royal College of Radiologists and the Council of the Royal College of Obstetricians and Gynaecologists issued guidelines on the use of ultrasound diagnostic criteria in early pregnancy[45]. The following important points were highlighted:

1. An ultrasound scan should be transvaginal if any doubt exists.
2. If the gestational sac has a mean diameter greater than 20 mm, with no evidence of an embryo or yolk sac, this is highly suggestive of missed abortion.
3. If the embryo has a crown–rump length greater than 6 mm, with no evidence of heart pulsations, this is highly suggestive of a missed abortion.
4. When the mean gestation sac is less than 20 mm in diameter or the crown–rump length is less than 6 mm, a repeat examination should be performed at least one week later, both to assess growth of the gestation sac and the embryo, and to establish whether heart activity exists.
5. If the gestation sac is smaller than expected for gestational age the possibility of incorrect dates should always be considered, especially in the absence of clinical feature suggestive of threatened abortion. Under these circumstances, a repeat scan should be arranged after a period of at least 7 days and be performed by an experienced operator.

ULTRASOUND CRITERIA USED TO PREDICT AN EPL

Strong relationships exist between the occurrence of a spontaneous abortion and the following ultrasound criteria: fetal bradycardia, discrepancy between the diameter of the gestational sac and the crown–rump length, and discrepancy between menstrual and sonographic age of more than one week. The risk of EPL is 6% when none of the above risk factors were present and is as high as 84% when all were present[49].

GESTATIONAL SAC SIZE

This has often been studied as possible marker of impending EPL but its significance has not been extensively documented. A small gestational or chorionic sac in the first trimester is a predictor of poor pregnancy outcome, even in the presence of embryonic cardiac activity[50,51]. A small sac, with measurements below the 50th centile, is present in all anembryonic pregnancies and in 62% of all missed abortions[52]. It has also been reported that in twin pregnancies with a difference of more than 3 mm between the diameters of the two sacs there is a 54% risk of subsequent loss of one of the twins. A decrease in the ratio between the mean amniotic sac diameter to crown–rump length indicates a poor outcome with a high sensitivity and specificity and a low false-positive rate in predicting EPL[52].

INTRAUTERINE HAEMATOMAS

These can be subchorionic (between the membranes and the uterine wall) and retroplacental (between the placenta and the myometrium), or both. The incidence of haematomas in the general population of early pregnancies varies greatly between studies ranging from 4 to 48%[53]. Their aetiology remains unclear. Even large haematomas in the first trimester are not considered to pose a serious threat to the pregnancy[54]. Much emphasis has been put on the volume of an intrauterine haematoma and/or on the presence of vaginal bleeding but not on the location of the haemorrhage. It is likely, that if the bleeding occurs at the level of the definitive placenta (under the cord insertion), it may result in placental separation and subsequent abortion. By contrast, a subchorionic haematoma only detaching the membrane opposite to the cord insertion can probably reach a significant volume before it affects normal pregnancy development (Fig. 63.5).

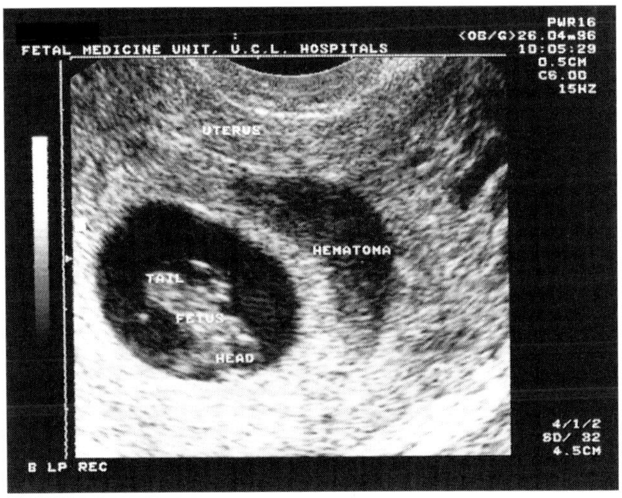

Fig. 63.5 Transvaginal ultrasound examination of an 8-week pregnancy presenting as a threatened abortion, demonstrating a large mixed subchorionic and retroplacental haematoma.

SECONDARY YOLK SAC

This is known to play a major role in embryonic nutrition, biosynthesis and haemopoiesis. Because of its close interrelationship with the embryo, impairment of the function of the secondary yolk sac must affect embryonic development. However, the predictive value of secondary yolk sac measurements in determining the long-term outcome of an early pregnancy is limited. Indeed, most pregnancies that subsequently abort (between 8 and 12 weeks) have normal secondary yolk sac measurements at their initial scan before 8 weeks of gestation. Furthermore, changes in secondary yolk sac shape and echogenicity (Fig 63.6) can be found in uncomplicated pregnancy, whereas most complicated pregnancies, even those with an abnormal karyotype, are associated with yolk sac measurements within normal limits. Finally, it is usually the yolk sac that is found to persist inside the gestational sac after the embryo has disappeared. Therefore, variations of the yolk sac size and sonographic appearance in most abnormal pregnancies are probably the consequence of poor embryonic development or embryonic death (Fig. 63.7), rather than being the primary cause of early pregnancy failure. Nevertheless, in the ultrasound evaluation of threatened abortion, a smaller or larger than expected secondary yolk sac may provide additional information about the immediate pregnancy outcome. However, recent evidence suggests that even the absence of a yolk sac in the first trimester is not an accurate predictor of poor pregnancy outcome[54]. Calcification of the yolk sac has been associated with intrauterine demise in the first trimester but can also be found in normal pregnancies, in particular after 9 weeks' gestation. In monochorionic twins the absence of one yolk sac is associated with monoamnionicity[55].

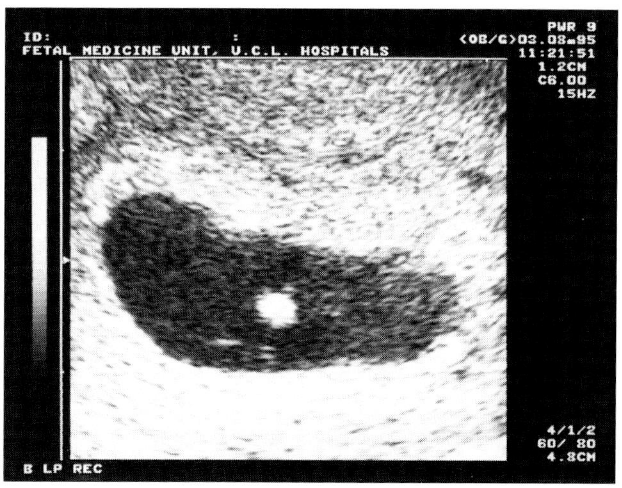

Fig. 63.6 Transabdominal ultrasound scan demonstrating a calcified yolk sac in a normal pregnancy at 10 weeks of gestation.

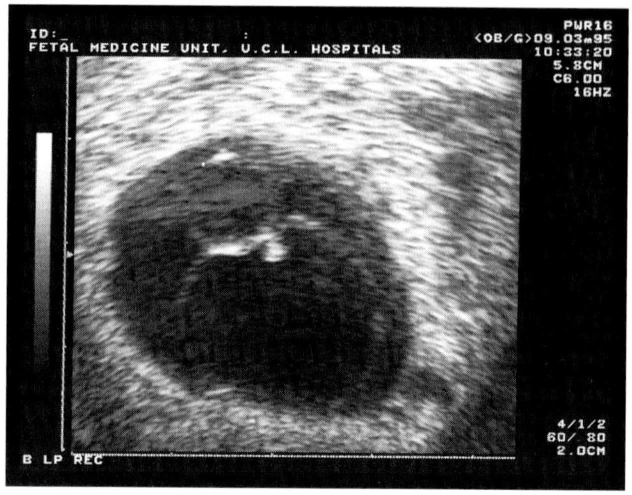

Fig. 63.7 Missed abortion at 8 weeks' gestation. Note the 'double' sac appearance due to the enlargement of the secondary yolk sac on top of the embryo and amniotic cavity.

EMBRYONIC GROWTH DELAY

This is classically described in association with poor outcome in women with threatened abortion[56] and in pregnancies complicated by diabetes[57]. The absence of fetal cardiac activity at 6 weeks and 5 days together with a smaller than expected embryonic size are highly sensitive and specific parameters in the diagnosis of an EPL[54].

ABNORMALITIES OF FETAL AND PLACENTAL CIRCULATION DEVELOPMENT

These are increasingly investigated in the context of EPL. Theoretically, cardiac activity should always be evident when the embryo is over 2 mm. However, in around 5–10% of embryos of between 2 and 4 mm, it cannot be demonstrated, although the corresponding pregnancies will have a normal outcome. It is, therefore, recommended in these cases to perform a follow-up scan within 3–5 days. Absence of embryonic heart pulsations by 32 days after conception using transvaginal ultrasound or serum hCG greater than 21 000 mIU/ml predicts reliably spontaneous abortion[58–62]. From 6–9 weeks of gestation, there is a rapid increase in the mean heart rate from 125 to 175 beats per minute (bpm). Thereafter the heart rate gradually decreases to around 160 bpm at 14 weeks. The rise in the heart rate parallels the increase in crown–rump length (CRL) and is probably required to meet the demands of the growing conceptus at this stage of pregnancy. An abnormal developmental pattern of embryonic heart rate and/or bradycardia has been found in pregnancies that subsequently aborted. A single observation of an abnormally slow heart rate does not necessarily indicate subsequent embryonic death, but a continuous decline of embryonic heart activity is inevitably associated with EPL. Determination of the heart rate correlated with CRL is useful in predicting spontaneous abortion before any invasive procedure is performed during the first trimester. Embryonic tachycardia has also been reported to have a high sensitivity in predicting EPL[59–62].

It has been demonstrated that there is no apparent difference in the resistance to blood flow in the uterine arteries, as assessed by Doppler ultrasound, between complicated and normal early pregnancies[34]. Thus, unlike the fetal heart rate, the investigation of the placental circulations is of limited use for patient at risk of EPL. However, a recent study has indicated that the presence of an intervillous circulation before the end of the first trimester gestation may be an indicator of subsequent pregnancy complications such as pre-eclampsia[63].

FIRST-TRIMESTER MARKERS OF ANEUPLOIDY

There is an increasing interest in the predictive value of early ultrasound markers of aneuploidy in pregnancies reaching the end of first trimester. This may be of particular interest as aneuploidies are strongly associated with a high incidence of late pregnancy loss.

GESTATIONAL SAC AND YOLK SAC SIZE

These have been rarely investigated within this context. Triploidy and trisomy 16 seem to be more often associated with a smaller chorionic sac before 9 weeks of gestation than other aneuploidies[51,64]. A larger yolk sac than normal has been reported in association with triploidy[65].

EMBRYONIC GROWTH DELAYS

These have been reported in association with triploidy, and aneuploidy and in particular trisomy 18[66,67]. The comparison of CRL measurements with gestational age calculated from the last menstrual period indicates that a CRL smaller than dates is associated with a higher risk of chromosomal anomalies than expected for maternal age. The larger the discrepancy, the higher the possibility that the aneuploidy affecting the fetus is of the severe (trisomy 18 or 13) or lethal type (triploidy)[66]. By contrast, in early pregnancy, the growth of fetuses affected by trisomy 21 or sex chromosome abnormalities does not differ from that of euploid fetuses[67].

EARLY FETAL ANATOMICAL DEFECTS

These can be markers of a chromosomal abnormality. Recent investigations have suggested that some second trimester ultrasound markers of aneuploidy could be accurately detected from the end of the first trimester. Within this context, the following markers may be evaluated routinely at 12–14 weeks of gestation:

- *For trisomy 21:* Nuchal fold thickening, generalized hydrops, atrioventricular septal defects, duodenal atresia and hydronephrosis.
- *For trisomy 18:* Choroid plexus cyst, enlarged cisterna magna, meningomyelocele, nuchal fold thickening, generalised oedema, tetralogy of Fallot, diaphragmatic hernia, omphalocoele, hydronephrosis and syndactyly.
- *For trisomy 13:* Holoprosencephaly, cleft lip, atrioventricular septal defects, polycystic kidneys, omphalocoele, post-axial polydactyly and syndactyly.
- *For triploidy:* Partial molar transformation of the placenta, holoprosencephaly, atrioventricular septal defects, syndactyly.
- *For monosomy X:* Large nuchal lymphoedema, generalised oedema and cardiac defects.

To date, existing data on the ultrasound diagnosis and epidemiological significance of most of these fetal abnormalities in early pregnancy are derived from case reports or small retrospective series. The following markers have been evaluated prospectively in large populations of women with pregnancies between 10 and 14 weeks gestation:

- *Nuchal fold thickening:* If >3 mm (Fig. 63.8) may enable the early detection of up to 70% of fetuses with chromosomal abnormalities[68,69]. The lethality rate in the first 2 weeks after a nuchal translucency measurement ranges from 5.3% for those with translucency of 1–3 mm to 23.5% for translucency more than 7 mm[70]. Septated nuchal cystic hygromata can be reliably differentiated from increased nuchal translucency and are associated with an increased incidence of chromosomal abnormalities including monosomy X.
- *Omphalocoele:* This is associated with chromosomal defects in 39.4% of the cases at 12 weeks' gestation decreasing to 27.5% at 20 weeks and 14.4% in live births. This decrease is due to fetal wastage of aneuploid fetuses with other major abnormalities[70].

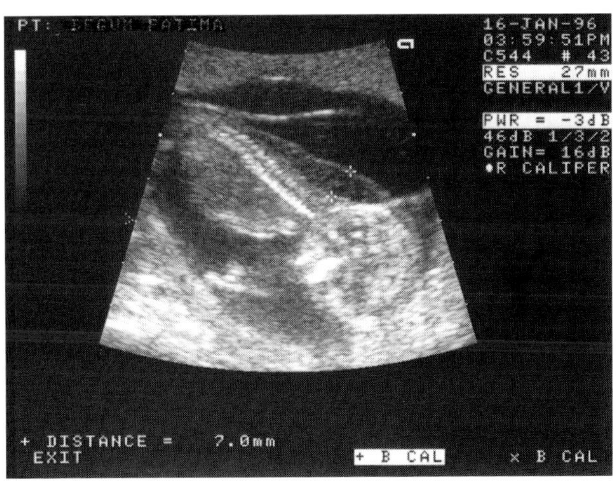

Fig. 63.8 Increased nuchal translucency thickness and generalised skin oedema in an 11-week fetus with trisomy 21.

CHANGES IN FETAL HEART RATE AND UMBILICAL ARTERY FLOW VELOCITY WAVEFORM CHARACTERISTICS

These are currently being investigated for the early screening of aneuploidies. Sporadic cases of fetus with Down syndrome presenting with an abnormally low heart rate in the first trimester of pregnancy have been reported. However, Van Lith *et al.*[71] in a study of 10 chromosomally abnormal fetuses between 6 and 16 weeks, including 5 fetuses with trisomy 21, found no difference in the fetal heart rate compared to normal fetuses. In a recent study, a stable and significant increase in the mean fetal heart rate in trisomy 21 pregnancies was reported[72]. No significant difference was found for the other variables between the aneuploidy and the control group. In chromosomally normal fetuses with an increased nuchal thickness, the development of fetal heart rate and compliance of the umbilicoplacental circulation were within the normal ranges. Some fetuses with trisomy 18 or triploidy may present with an increased resistance to blood flow in the umbilical artery which is probably due to an abnormal development of the villous vasculature in these cases.

The management of early pregnancy loss

THERAPEUTIC APPROACH

Spontaneous miscarriage is the most common complication of pregnancy and probably accounts for 50 000 admissions in the UK each year. Generally, the management is a well-established routine that has changed little compared to other areas of gynaecological practice. Miscarriage currently accounts for about three-quarters of emergency gynaecological admissions[73] and the following options are available to the patient.

SURGICAL MANAGEMENT

Surgery, in particular the dilatation and curettage (D&C) of the uterus for the evacuation of retained products of conception (ERPC), is seen as simple procedure that is usually performed by junior doctor. Although complications are uncommon, they do still happen. Mechanical dilatation of the cervical canal with tapered metal dilators of increasing diameters may be associated with a variety of possible injuries such as cervical tears, uterine perforation and the creation of false passage. Some of these complications are prevented by cervical preparation and the use of ultrasound guidance. Prostaglandin analogue pessaries have been used for that purpose but so far not uniformly. They should be used when a difficult cervical dilatation is anticipated. Misoprostol, a prostaglandin E_1 analogue which was originally marketed by Searle Pharmaceuticals for the management of peptic ulcer disease, has recently been introduced to the field of cervical preparation before surgery. This drug has been shown to be a potent cervical priming agent when used vaginally, prior to surgical induction of abortion. A dose of 600 μg of misoprostol administered vaginally two hours before surgery has been shown to be as effective as gemeprost (16,16-dimethyl-*trans*-Δ^2-PGE_1) in achieving presurgical dilatation of the cervix. The cost of the former is less than £1 per patient while the latter may cost up to £20. Misoprostol is also thermostable and therefore more applicable in developing countries.

MEDICAL MANAGEMENT

This has been made possible with the introduction of prostaglandins into gynaecological practice. Prostaglandin analogues were first studied within that context[74–79] but overall the results were disappointing because, when administered vaginally (1 mg 3 hourly up to 5 mg), complete evacuation of the uterus was achieved in only 55% of the cases and because of the long interval required to achieve evacuation of the uterus. The introduction of mifepristone in gynaecology in 1988 opened a new chapter in this area. Mifepristone (RU486) is a progesterone competitive antagonist that was licensed for induction of abortion. The combination of mifepristone and prostaglandin analogues has been shown to be effective in abortion induction up to 63 days' amenorrhoea. The success rate of 600 mg mifepristone followed by 1 mg gemeprost 48 hours later is up to 95%. When misoprostol is used instead of gemeprost, a similar efficacy is obtained. Developments in medical induction of abortion were quickly applied in the field of miscarriage[77–79]. The combination of oral 600 mg of mifepristone followed by oral 600 μg misoprostol 36–48 hours later has been reported to be successful in 95% of the cases of anembryonic pregnancies[79].

The oral route of administration of misoprostol makes this prostaglandin analogue particularly attractive. Unlike pregnancy termination, vaginal bleeding is common in cases of EPL and this may interfere with the absorption of the prostaglandins by the vaginal route. Further work in the field of induction of abortion has shown that higher oral dosages (800 μg) are well tolerated. However, the vaginal administration of misoprostol seems more potent than oral administration in medical induction of abortion. Whether the vaginal route will also be suitable for cases of miscarriage despite vaginal bleeding remains to be investigated. Anembryonic pregnancies or blighted ova seem to respond well to a regimen of mifepristone and misoprostol. Incomplete abortion, on the other hand, seems to respond successfully to misoprostol only. 'Incomplete abortion' is a term that is widely used by clinicians without clear specification whether it is a clinical or ultrasonic diagnosis. Misoprostol 400 μg was effective in the management of cases where the ultrasound scan showed thickened endometrial shadows with no pregnancy sac in the presence of vaginal bleeding. In a study involving 60 patients, 58 did not require surgical curettage. The differentiation between anembryonic pregnancy and incomplete abortion can therefore lead to different therapeutic strategies in the management of EPL.

EXPECTANT MANAGEMENT

This is another option and most cases of early EPL could be managed conservatively. Historically, D&C was used in a completely different context than that of today. The operation was developed at a time when backstreet abortion was widely practised due to the legal restrictions on the procedure. It was difficult for clinicians to differentiate between those women presenting to hospitals with incomplete abortion due to miscarriage and those presenting with complications of a backstreet abortion. Faced with this situation, D&C developed as a routine operation for all cases of incomplete abortion.

A recent trial of expectant versus surgical management of patients with incomplete abortion showed that in selected cases this is both feasible and safe. All patients included in the study had a pregnancy of less than 13 weeks' gestation and the ultrasound scan demonstrated that the retained tissue or blood clots were less than 1.5–2.5 mm in thickness[80]. Although the size of the population studied was small (103 women), the trial showed that the rate of infection, of anaemia, severity and duration of pain and length of convalescence was not different between the two groups. The duration of bleeding was 1.3 days longer in the group with conservative management. Transvaginal ultrasonography can help in refining the management by identifying reliably women with minimal residual tissue in the uterine cavity which can safely be treated expectantly[81].

THE ROLE OF THE EARLY PREGNANCY UNIT

Early pregnancy units (EPU) are dedicated units for the assessment, diagnosis, treatment, psychological support and counselling of patients with early pregnancy complications. It has been shown that an EPU offers improved quality of care and produces considerable savings in financial and staff resources[82,83]. Furthermore, patients feel that their condition is a priority to the staff. Their condition is usually diagnosed in less than 2 hours and treatment completed in less than a day. Patients are also spared the anxiety of unnecessary admission to the hospital, which can cause domestic problems, especially if they have other children.

The on-call work for junior medical staff during the night can be decreased and close supervision by senior staff can be achieved during the day time. Counselling is also provided more effectively. The principal disadvantages are that admission to hospital is delayed for a few hours, although immediate admission is possible when clinically necessary, and that a doctor and nurse must devote up to the first 3 hours of the working day to dealing with the assessment of these cases.

A dedicated EPU makes easier the attempts of the staff to reduce the anxieties of women who may be prone to miscarriage by screening them early and offering same-day results. Furthermore, an EPU can help in reducing dissatisfaction with healthcare services concerned with EPL problems and resulting from inadequate information, misunderstanding, insensitivity, lack of control over decisions and treatment and discontinuity of care.

Health workers can develop high standards of communication skills, which can improve interactions between women and healthcare workers and prevent unnecessary distress. Counselling about the diagnostic evaluation processes, treatments required, prognosis and risks for future pregnancies should always be offered. Counselling should be patient-focused with the helper's and patient's roles clearly defined within a particular timeframe. The aims of counselling are communication, to enable women to be well informed, to offer support and encouragement. The ideal helping relationship is a partnership in which there is genuine empathy, mutual participation and respect. Even in the initial contact, consideration should be given to ensure privacy and adequate time, which should be free of interruptions and distractions. By ensuring appropriate settings and trained staff, a dedicated EPU can help in ensuring good standards of practice. Genetic counselling should be offered to all couples with a balanced translocation or a chromosomal variant. Although not treatable, the prognosis for future pregnancies is directly dependent on the type of abnormality and on which of the parents carries it.

REFERENCES

1. FIGO News. List of gynaecologic and obstetric terms and definitions. *Int. J. Gynaecol. Obstet.* **14**, 570–576, 1976.
2. Jauniaux E, Gulbis B, Jurkovic D, Gavriil, P & Campbell S. The origin of alpha-fetoprotein in first-trimester anembryonic pregnancies. *Am. J. Obstet. Gynecol.* **173**, 1749–1753, 1995.
3. Edmonds DK, Lindsay KS, Miller JF, Williamson E & Wood P. Early embryonic mortality in woman. *Fertil. Steril.* **38**, 447–453, 1982.
4. Zinaman MJ, Clegg ED, Brown CC, O'Connor J & Selevan SG. Estimates of human fertility and pregnancy loss. *Fertil. Steril.* **65**, 503–509, 1996.
5. Goldstein SR. Embryonic death in early pregnancy: A new look at the first trimester. *Obstet. Gynecol.* **84**, 294–297, 1994.
6. Pandya P, Snijders RJM, Psara N, Hibert L & Nicolaides KH. The prevalence of non-viable pregnancy at 10–13 weeks of gestation. *Ultrasound Obstet. Gynaecol.* **7**, 170–173, 1996.
7. Edwards RG. Causes of early embryonic loss in human pregnancy. *Hum. Reprod.* **1**, 185–198, 1986.
8. Barnea E. Epidemiology, etiology of early pregnancy disorders. In *The First Twelve Weeks of Gestation* (eds E. Barnea, J. Hustin & E. Jauniaux), pp. 263–279. Heidelberg: Springer-Verlag, 1992.
9. Simpson JL, Gray RH, Queenan JT *et al.* Risk of recurrent spontaneous abortion for pregnancies discovered in the fifth week of gestation [Letter]. *Lancet* **344**, 964, 1994.
10. Simpson JL & Bombard AT. Chromosomal abnormalities in spontaneous abortion: Frequency, pathology and genetic counselling. In

Spontaneous Abortion (eds K. Edmonds & M.J. Bennett), pp. 51–76. London: Blackwell, 1987.
11. Sorokin Y, Johnson MP, Uhlman WR, Zador IE, Drugan A, Koppitch FC, Moody J & Evans MI. Postmortem chorionic villus sampling: correlation of cytogenetic and ultrasound findings. *Am. J. Med. Genet.* **39**, 314–316, 1991.
12. Jauniaux E, Brown R, Snijders JM, Noble P & Nicolaides KH. Early prenatal diagnosis of triploidy. *Am. J. Obstet. Gynecol.* **176**, 550–554, 1997.
13. Watt JL, Templeton AA, Messinis I, Bell L, Cunningham P & Duncan RO. Trisomy I in an eight cell human pre-embryo. *J. Med. Genet.* **24**, 60–64, 1987.
14. Zaragoza MV, Jacobs PA & James RS. Nondisjunction of human acrocentric chromosomes: studies of 432 trisomic fetuses and liveborns. *Hum. Genet.* **19**, 411–417, 1994.
15. Warburton D, Kline J, Stein Z, Hutzler M, Chin A & Hassold T. Does the karyotype of a spontaneous abortion predict the karyotype of a subsequent abortion? Evidence from 273 women with two karyotyped spontaneous abortions. *Am. J. Hum. Genet.* **41**, 465–483, 1987.
16. Fisher JM, Harvey JF, Morton NE & Jacobs PA. Trisomy 18: studies of the parent and cell division of origin and the effect of aberrant recombination on nondisjunction. *Am. J. Hum. Genet.* **56**, 669–675, 1995.
17. Delhanty JDA & Handyside AH. The origin of genetic defects in the human and their detection in the preimplantation embryo. *Hum. Reprod. Update* **1**, 201–215, 1995.
18. Warburton D, Kline R, Stein Z, Hutzler M, Chin A & Hassold T. Does the karyotype of a spontaneous abortion predict the karyotype of a subsequent abortion? *Am. J. Hum. Genet.* **41**, 465–483, 1987.
19. Alberman ED. The abortus as a predictor of future trisomy 21. In *Trisomy 21 Down Syndrome* (eds F.F. De la Cruz & P.S. Gerald), pp. 69–78. Baltimore MD: University Park Press, 1981.
20. De Braekeleer M & Dao TN. Cytogenetic studies in couples experiencing repeated pregnancy losses. *Hum. Reprod.* **5**, 519–528, 1990.
21. Stephenson MD. Frequency of factors associated with habitual abortion in 197 couples. *Fertil. Steril.* **66**, 24–29, 1996.
22. Smith KE & Buyalos RP. The profound impact of patient age on pregnancy outcome after early detection of fetal cardiac activity. *Fertil. Steril.* **65**, 35–40, 1996.
23. Jauniaux E. A comparison of chorionic villus sampling and amniocentesis for prenatal diagnosis in early pregnancy. *In Screening for Down syndrome in the first trimester* (eds J.G. Grudzinskas & R.H.T. Ward), pp. 259–269. London: RCOG Press, 1997.
24. Li TC. Recurrent miscarriage: principles of management. *Hum. Reprod.* **13**, 478–482, 1998.
25. Sagle M, Bishop K, Ridley N, Alexander IM, Michel M, Bonney RC, Beard RW & Franks S. Recurrent early miscarriage and polycystic ovaries. *Br. Med. J.* **297**, 1027–1028, 1988.
26. Regan L, Owen EJ & Jacobs HS. Hypersecretion of lutenising hormone, infertility, and miscarriage. *Lancet* **336**, 1141–1143, 1990.
27. Simpson JL, Mills JL, Kim H, Holmes L, Lee J, Metzger B & Knopp R. Infectious processes; an infrequent cause of first trimester spontaneous abortions. *Human Reprod.* **3**, 668–672, 1996.
28. Witkin SS & Ledger WJ. Antibodies to *Chlamydia trachomatis* in sera of women with recurrent spontaneous abortions. *Am. J. Obstet. Gynecol.* **167**, 135–139, 1992.
29. Savitz DA, Sonnenfeld NL & Olshan AF. Review of epidemiologic studies of paternal occupational exposure and spontaneous abortion. *Am. J. Ind. Med.* **25**, 361–383, 1994.
30. Kline J, Shrout P, Stein ZA, Susser M & Warburton D. Drinking during pregnancy and spontaneous abortion. *Lancet* **2**, 176 180, 1980.
31. Kalousek DK. Anatomic and chromosome anomalies in specimens of early spontaneous abortion: & seven-years experience. *Birth Defects* **23**, 153–168, 1987.
32. Khong TY, Liddell HS & Robertson WB. Defective haemochorial placentation as a cause of miscarriage. A preliminary study. *Br. J. Obstet. Gynaecol.* **94**, 649–655, 1987.
33. Hustin J, Jauniaux E & Schaaps JP. Histological study of the materno-embryonic interface in spontaneous abortion. *Placenta* **11**, 477–486, 1990.
34. Jauniaux E, Zaidi J, Jurkovic D, Campbell S & Hustin J. Comparison of colour Doppler feature and pathological findings in complicated early pregnancy. *Human Reprod.* **9**, 2432–2437, 1994.
35. Jauniaux E, Kadri R & Hustin J. Partial mole and triploidy: screening in patients with first trimester spontaneous abortion. *Obstet. Gynecol.* **88**, 616–619, 1996.
36. Salem HT, Ghaneimah SA, Shaaban MM & Chard T. Prognostic value of biochemical tests in the assessment of fetal outcome in threatened abortion. *Br. J. Obst. Gynaecol.* **81**, 382–385, 1984.
37. Stabile I, Campbell S & Gruzinskas G. Ultrasound and circulating placental protein measurements in complications of early pregnancy. *Br. J. Obstet. Gynaecol.* **96**, 1182–1191, 1989.
38. Al-Sebai MAH, Diver M & Hipkin LJ. The role of a single free β-human chorionic gonadotropin measurement in the diagnosis of early pregnancy failure and the prognosis of fetal viability. *Hum. Reprod.* **11**, 881–888, 1996.
39. Lower AM & Yovich JL. The value of serum levels of oestradiol, progesterone and beta-human chorionic gonadotrophin in the prediction of early pregnancy loss. *Hum. Reprod.* **7**, 711–717, 1992.
40. Johnson MR, Riddle AF, Sharma V, Collins WP, Nicolaides KH & Grudzinskas JG. Placental and ovarian hormones in anembryonic pregnancy. *Hum. Reprod.* **8**, 112–115, 1993.
41. Shu-Xin H & Zhen-Qun ZA. Study of early pregnancy factor activity in the sera of patients with unexplained spontaneous abortion. *Am. J. Reprod. Immunol.* **29**, 77–81, 1993.
42. Norman DJ, Barry JM & Fischer S. The beneficial effect of pretransplant third-party blood transfusions on allograft rejection in HLA identical sibling kidney transplants. *Transplant* **41**, 125–126, 1986.
43. Watson H, Kiddy DS, Hamilton Fairley D, Scanlon MJ, Barnard C, Collins WP, Bonney RC & Franks S. Hypersecretion of luteinizing hormone and ovarian steroids in women with recurrent early miscarriage. *Hum. Reprod.* **8**, 829–833, 1993.
44. Lam SY, Baker HW, Evans JH & Pepperell RJ. Factors affecting fetal loss in induction of ovulation with gonadotropins: increased abortion rates related to hormonal profiles in conceptual cycles. *Am. J. Obstet. Gynecol.* **160**, 621–628, 1989.
45. RCR/RCOG. *Guidance on ultrasound procedures in early pregnancy*. pp. 1–8. Royal College of Radiologists/Royal College of Obstetricians and Gynaecologists, 1995.
46. Pennell RG, Needleman L, Pajak T, Baltarowich O, Vilaro M, Goldberg BB & Kurz AB. Prospective comparison of vaginal and abdominal sonography in normal early pregnancy. *J. Ultrasound. Med.* **10**, 63–67, 1991.
47. deCrespigny L. Early diagnosis of pregnancy failure with transvaginal ultrasound. *Am. J. Obst. Gynecol.* **159**, 408–409, 1988.
48. Rulin MC, Bornstein SG & Campbell JD. The reliability of ultrasonography in the management of spontaneous abortion, clinically thought to be complete: a prospective study. *Am. J. Obstet. Gynecol.* **168**, 12–15, 1993.
49. Falco P, Milano V, Pilu G, David C, Grisolia G, Rizzo N & Bovicelli L. Sonography of pregnancies with first trimester bleeding and a viable embryo: a study of prognostic indicators by logistic regression analysis. *Ultrasound Obstet. Gynaecol.* **7**, 165–169, 1996.
50. Bromley B, Harlow BL, Laboda LA & Benacerraf BR. Small sac size in the first trimester: a predictor of poor fetal outcome. *Radiology* **178**, 375–377, 1991.
51. Dickey RP, Gasser R, Olar TT, Taylor SN, Curole DN, Rye PH & Matulich EM. Relationship of initial chorionic sac diameter to abortion and abortus karyotype based on new growth curves for 16th to 49th post-ovulation day. *Human Reprod.* **9**, 559–565, 1994.
52. Tadmor OP, Achiron R, Rabinowiz R, Aboulafia Y, Mashiach S & Diamant YZ. Predicting first-trimester spontaneous abortion. Ratio of mean sac diameter to crown–rump length compared to embryonic heart rate. *J. Reprod. Med.* **39**, 459–462, 1994.
53. Pearlstone M & Baxi L. Subchorionic haematoma: A review. *Obstet. Gynecol. Sur.* **48**, 65–68, 1993.
54. Jauniaux E, Gavriil P & Nicolaides KH. Ultrasonographic assessment of early pregnancy complications. In *Ultrasound and Early Pregnancy* (eds D. Jurkovic & E. Jauniaux), pp. 53–65. Carforth: Parthenon, 1996.
55. Bromley B & Benacerraf B. Using the number of yolk sacs to determine amnionicity in early first trimester monochorionic twins. *J. Ultrasound. Med.* **14**, 415–419, 1995.
56. Mantoni M & Pedersen JF. Fetal growth delay in threatened abortion: an ultrasound study. *Br. J. Obstet. Gynecol.* **89**, 525–527, 1982.
57. Pedersen JF, Molsted-Pedersen L & Mortesen HB. Fetal growth delay

and haemoglobin A1c in early diabetic pregnancy. *Obstet. Gynecol.* **64**, 351–354, 1984.
58. Howe RS, Isaacson KJ, Albert JL & Coutifaris CB. Embryonic heart rate in human pregnancy. *J. Ultrasound Med.* **10**, 367–371, 1991.
59. Achiron R, Tadmor O & Mashiach S. Heart rate as a predictor of first-trimester spontaneous abortion after ultrasound-proven viability. *Obstet. Gynecol.* **78**, 330–334, 1991.
60. May DA & Sturtevan NV. Embryonal heart rate as a predictor of pregnancy outcome: a prospective analysis. *J. Ultrasound Med.* **10**, 591–593, 1991.
61. Merchiers EH, Dhont M, De Sutter PA, Beghin CJ & Vanderkerckhove DA. Predictive value of early embryonic cardiac activity for pregnancy outcome. *Am. J. Obstet. Gynecol.* **165**, 11–14, 1991.
62. Wisser J & Dirschedl P. Embryonic heart rate in dated human embryos. *Early Human Dev.* **37**, 107–115, 1994.
63. Jaffe R, Dorgan A & Abramowicz JS. Color Doppler imaging of the uteroplacental circulation in the first trimester: value in predicting pregnancy failure or complication *Am. J. Roentgenol* **164**, 1255–1258, 1995.
64. Dickey RP, Olar TT, Taylor SN, Curole DN, Rye PH, Matulich EM & Dickey MH. Incidence and significance of unequal gestational sac diameter or embryo crown–rump length in twin pregnancy. *Hum. Reprod.* **7**, 1170–1172, 1992.
65. Zalel Y, Shalev E, Yanay N, Schiff E & Weiner EA. Large yolk sac: a possible clue to early diagnosis of partial hydatidiform mole. *J. Clin. Ultrasound.* **22**, 519–521, 1994.
66. Drugan A, Johnson MP, Isada NB, Holzgreve W, Zador IE, Dombrowski M, Sokol RJ, Hallak M & Evans MI. The smaller than expected first-trimester fetus is at increased risk for chromosome anomalies. *Am. J. Obstet. Gynecol.* **178**, 1525–1528, 1992.
67. Kuhn P, Brizot ML, Pandya PP, Snijders RJ & Nicolaides KH. Crown–rump length in chromosomally abnormal fetuses at 10 to 13 weeks' gestation. *Am. J. Obstet. Gynecol.* **172**, 32–35, 1995.
68. Nicolaides KH, Brizot ML & Snijders RMJ. Fetal nuchal translucency: Ultrasound screening for fetal trisomy in the first trimester of pregnancy. *Br. J. Obstet. Gynaecol.* **101**, 782–786, 1994.
69. Taipale P, Hilesmaa V, Salonen R & Ylostalo P. Increased nuchal translucency as a marker for fetal chromosomal defects. *N. Engl. J. Med.* **337**, 1654–1658, 1997.
70. Snijders RJM, Johnson S, Sebire NJ, Noble P & Nicolaides KH. First trimester ultrasound screening for chromosomal defects. *Ultrasound Obstet. Gynaecol.* **7**, 216–226, 1996.
71. van Lith JMM, Visser GHA, Matingh A & Beekhuis JR. Fetal heart rate in early pregnancy and chromosomal disorders. *Br. J. Obstet. Gynaecol.* **99**, 741–744, 1992.
72. Jauniaux E, Gavriil P, Khun P, Kurdi W, Hyett J & Nicolaides KH. Fetal heart rate and umbilicoplacental Doppler flow velocity waveforms in early pregnancies with a chromosomal abnormality and/or increased nuchal translucency thickness. *Hum. Reprod.* **11**, 435–439, 1996.
73. Macrow P & Elstein M. Managing miscarriage medically. *Br. Med. J.* **306**, 876, 1993.
74. Henshaw RC, Cooper K, El-Rafaey H, Smith NC & Templeton AA. Medical management of miscarriage: non-surgical uterine evacuation of incomplete and inevitable abortion. *Br. Med. J.* **306**, 894–895, 1993.
75. Chung TKH, Cheung LP, Lau WC, Haines CJ & Chang AMZ. Spontaneous abortion: a medical approach to management. *Aust. NZ. J. Obstet. Gynaecol.* **4**, 432–436, 1994.
76. Lelaidier C, Baton-Saint-Mleux C, Fernandez H, Bourget P & Frydman R. Mifepristone (RU486) induces embryo expulsion in the first trimester non-developing pregnancies: a prospective randomised trial. *Human Reprod.* **8**, 492–495, 1993.
77. El-Rafaey H, Hinshaw K, Henshaw R, Smith N & Templeton A. Medical management of missed abortion and anembryonic pregnancy *Br. Med. J.* **305**, 1399, 1992.
78. Henshaw RC, Naji A, Russell IT & Templeton AA. Comparison of medical abortion with surgical vacuum aspiration: women's preferences and acceptability of treatment. *Br. Med. J.* **307**, 714–717, 1993.
79. El-Rafaey H, Rajasekar D, Abdalla M, Calder L & Templeton A. Early induction of abortion with mifepristone (RU486) and misoprostol: a randomised comparison between the oral and vaginal administration of misoprostol. *N. Eng. J. Med.* **332**, 983–987, 1995.
80. Nielsen S & Hahlin M. Expectant management of first trimester spontaneous abortion. *Lancet* **345**, 84–86, 1995.
81. Haines CJ, Chung T & Leung DY. Transvaginal sonography and the conservative management of spontaneous abortion. *Gynecol. Obstet. Invest.* **37**, 14–17, 1994.
82. Hunter M. Providing information and support. In *Counselling in Obstetrics and Gynaecology* (ed. M. Hunter), pp. 87–104. London: British Psychological Society, 1994.
83. Birigg MA & Read MD. Management of women referred to early pregnancy assessment unit: care and cost effectiveness. *Br. J. Med.* **302**, 577–579, 1992.

Fetal infection

64

J. Yankowitz and C.P. Weiner

Introduction

Several parasites and a growing number of viruses are now known to cause clinically significant fetal infection resulting in miscarriage, intrauterine death or long-term sequelae secondary to structural and neurodevelopmental abnormalities. This chapter focuses on syphilis, toxoplasmosis, cytomegalovirus, varicella, rubella, human immunodeficiency virus and other recently defined viral agents. Limited background is provided for each virus, as the main thrust of the chapter is to focus on recent data. Several chapters or entire texts are available for the reader desiring additional information[1–5].

The possibility of a viral aetiology should be considered for most ultrasound abnormalities. These include, but are not limited to, fetal growth restriction, amniotic fluid volume disorders, intracranial or intrahepatic calcifications, hydrocephalus, microcephaly, isolated ascites, pericardial or pleural effusions, and non-immune hydrops[5,6]. There are benefits and pitfalls of the various tools used to determine the presence of a viral infection. These tools include maternal and fetal serology, various culture techniques and determination of other fetal haematological parameters including complete blood count, blood gases and liver function tests[6]. Each gold standard is good for a decade or so until knowledge outpaces it. There are also several techniques available to obtain fetal samples for testing including amniocentesis, chorionic villus sampling and fetal blood sampling[7,8].

Syphilis

Congenital defects secondary to syphilis were first recognized at least five hundred years ago[9,10]. The triad for late congenital syphilis of notched incisor teeth, interstitial keratitis and VIIIth cranial nerve deafness was first described by Sir Jonathan Hutchinson in 1858[9,10]. Congenital syphilis itself was first described over 40 years ago[11]. The rate is increasing despite adequate treatment per recommendations of the U.S. Centers for Disease Control and because of failure to adhere to treatment guidelines[10,12]. Socioeconomic factors contributing to the increase include lack of timely prenatal care and drug abuse[13,14]. The rise in congenital syphilis mirrors the rising rates of primary and secondary syphilis[15].

ORGANISM

Syphilis is caused by the spirochaete *Treponema pallidum*. Too narrow to be visible under light microscopy, the spirochaete is best seen using dark-field. The cell wall contains muramic acid and *N*-acetylglucosamine as do bacteria, rendering the organism sensitive to penicillin and other antibiotics[1]. Outer membrane non-protein constituents include diphosphatidylglycerol (cardiolipin) which is the antigen that stimulates production of the Venereal Disease Research Laboratory (VDRL) antibody. The cardiolipin does not appear to be synthesized by the organism; rather, it is incorporated from damaged host tissues[9].

CLINICAL MANIFESTATIONS

The primary lesion appears 10–90 days after exposure. It is a painless, ulcerated chancre with a raised border and indurated base which persists for 2–8 weeks. Painless inguinal adenopathy may also be present. The secondary or parasitic stage of syphilis consists of condyloma latum and a generalized maculopapular rash involving the palms and soles. This stage resolves spontaneously in 2–6 weeks when the patient enters the asymptomatic, latent stage of syphilis. Periodic exacerbations may occur during the early latent stage (less than 4 years). While infectivity by sexual transmission ceases during the late latent stage, transplacental transmission still occurs. Without treatment, one-third of patients develop tertiary syphilis characterized by gummas or vasculites involving the cardiovascular, central nervous or musculoskeletal systems as well as other organs.

Transplacental passage of the spirochaetes occurs throughout gestation, but fetal clinical manifestations require immunocompetency which occurs around 16 weeks. Transmission is more likely during the primary or secondary phase of disease when the parasite load is high.

DIAGNOSIS

Since 1983, the incidence of syphilis in the adult female has increased[13,15]. The prevalence in the United States in 1990 was approximately 15 per 100 000[16]. Screening remains cost-effective as long as the prevalence is greater than 5 cases per 100 000 population[17]. All pregnant women should be screened at the first prenatal visit; rescreening of high-risk populations is recommended at 28–34 weeks[18]. A cost-benefit analysis performed in 1983 revealed a favourable benefit–cost ratio of 3.8 for first trimester screening and 1.7 for the combined screening when the cost of testing and treatment is compared to the cost of prematurity and care of affected children[19].

Screening (Fig. 64.1) begins with a non-treponemal test such as the rapid plasma reagin (RPR) test or the VDRL (Venereal Disease Research Laboratory). These tests detect antibodies against the mammalian membrane lipid cardiolipin. A positive test is followed by a treponema-specific test such as the *T. pallidum* immobilization (TPI) test, the fluorescent treponemal antibody absorption (FTA–ABS) test, or the microhaemagglutination test for *T. pallidum* (MHA–TP). All are positive within 4 weeks of the chancre's appearance. However, they may be negative at the time the chancre first appears when only the dark-field examination is diagnostic.

TREATMENT

Treatment recommendations for syphilis have changed little since the advent of long-acting penicillin G preparations in the early 1950s (Fig. 64.1). The U.S. Centers for Disease Control (CDC) recommends that patients with early syphilis (including primary, secondary or latent syphilis of less than 1 year's duration) receive benzathine penicillin G, 2.4 million units intramuscularly. Treatment failure rates range from 5 to 14%[9,20]. Pregnant patients should be retested monthly after treatment. A fourfold decline in titre indicates successful treatment. Patients with later disease stages or HIV should receive benzathine penicillin G 7.2 million units total (2.4 million units i.m. weekly for three consecutive weeks). Patients with neurosyphilis require intravenous penicillin for 10–14 days. Treatment of penicillin-allergic women during pregnancy should not be withheld. Penicillin-allergic patients should undergo desensitization and treatment. Therapeutic success depends on the interaction between the host immune system and the antibiotic[20,21].

A drug-dependent lifestyle, use of cocaine and lack of or late prenatal care, or failure to complete treatment and obtain follow-up are important risk factors for congenital disease[22,23].

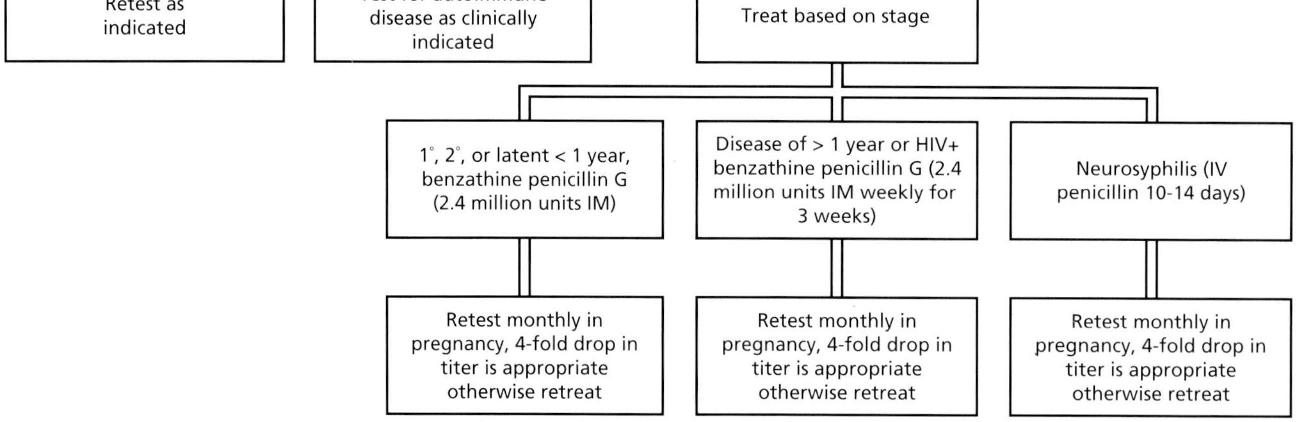

Fig. 64.1 Flow chart outlining screening, diagnosis and treatment for syphilis during pregnancy.

McFarlin *et al.*[12] noted that there was no difference in the rate of congenital infection among women with disease of less than 1-year duration if the treatment was one dose or three doses of benzathine penicillin (26.7% versus 30%). They interpreted this finding to mean there was a very high rate of reinfection. However, differentiating between a treatment failure and reinfection is difficult because diagnosis is based on serologic testing. Whether treatment failure or reinfection accounts for 'relapse' in other populations such as those with HIV is unclear[24]. Inappropriate drug therapy or dose also contributes to congenital disease.

CONGENITAL DISEASE

Congenital syphilis can lead to preterm delivery and may be associated with growth restriction, hydrops or placentomegaly. The affected neonate may fail to thrive, and have rhinitis (snuffles), jaundice, hepatosplenomegaly, haematological manifestations, mucocutaneous manifestations, bony lesions, central nervous system manifestations and ocular manifestations. Most neonates have hepatosplenomegaly and the one-third with jaundice have syphilitic hepatitis. Mucocutaneous manifestations such as rhinitis occur in 15–60% of infants. Cerebrospinal fluid abnormalities indicative of CNS involvement are found in 60% of infants with congenital syphilis. Later findings include the effects of ongoing inflammation causing interstitial keratitis, deafness and mulberry molars.

Toxoplasmosis

Congenital toxoplasmosis affects 1 per 500 to 1 per 10 000 births depending on geographic location and personal hygiene habits[25–29]. Infection of a healthy parturient is generally benign with non-specific findings. The HIV-infected woman may have severe multisystem disease[25–28]. Screening is standard in central Europe but not in the United States[30–32]. Routine screening with a favourable cost–benefit ratio depends on how common the infection is, how many susceptible women there are, and how easily the serology can be interpreted[33]. A recent study in the United States showed that to detect one case of toxoplasmosis, 12–18 normal pregnancies would be lost secondary to the invasive procedures performed for diagnosis in women who have seroconverted during pregnancy[34]. Concern over toxoplasmosis was the major stimulus for the development of cordocentesis[35].

ORGANISM

Toxoplasma gondii is an intracellular parasite with three life stages. The oocysts are formed in the intestines of the cat family. Excreted in the faeces, they remain viable in moist soil for long periods. The tachyzoite is present in the acute stage of infection and the tissue cyst is formed within the host cell[7,25–28]. Transmission usually occurs by the ingestion of infected meat or from contaminated soil (or cat litter) that contains infective oocysts. The undercooked meat is usually from sheep or swine since cattle have low rates of positivity for *T. gondii*[25–28].

Thirty-nine percent of pregnant women in the United States have serological evidence of past infection[29]. The prevalence of seropositivity varies markedly by geographical location with only 3.3% of women in Denver versus 30% of women in Los Angeles. Worldwide rates also vary greatly from 2% in India to over 70% in France. These prevalence rates reflect different rates of exposure to cats, variations in food preparation as well as hygienic and eating habits. A recent prospective study revealed a congenital infection rate of about 1 per 12 000 births in Massachusetts and New Hampshire; most infants had clinically inapparent infection[36,37].

CLINICAL MANIFESTATIONS

Acute toxoplasmosis is usually asymptomatic. When present, symptoms include lymphadenopathy and fatigue. Occasionally fever, headache, sore throat and myalgias are present. Maternal parasitaemia results in seeding of the placenta and subsequent fetal infection. The later in gestation maternal infection occurs, the shorter the latency period between placental seeding and fetal infection. The time between placental infection and spread to the fetus depends on inoculum size, the virulence of the specific strain and the developmental stage of the placenta. The rate of congenital infection of untreated pregnancies increases from 10–15% in the first trimester and 25% in the second trimester, to over 60% in the third trimester[38,39]. However, the severity of the congenital infection is greatest with early infection[40]. By the third trimester, almost all infected newborns are asymptomatic. Maternal treatment decreases the rate of fetal infection.

Women infected prior to pregnancy are at virtually no risk of an offspring with congenital toxoplasmosis unless they are immunosuppressed. Immunosuppressed patients at risk for chronic infection include those with HIV, Hodgkin's disease or systemic lupus erythematosus on corticosteroid therapy[40].

DIAGNOSIS

The diagnosis of primary infection during pregnancy is made by maternal *Toxoplasma*-specific serology. The Sabin–Feldman dye test is the current gold standard for evaluating IgG. The dye test is based on observation that organisms mixed with normal serum stain deeply blue with methylene blue while organisms exposed to antibody-containing serum appear thin, distorted and do not stain. The result is reported as a titre or in international units based on the dilution of millilitres of serum. The Sabin–Feldman dye test measures IgG by evaluation of lysis of the organism in the presence of IgG and complement. Several types of tests for IgM are available. They have different sensitivities and specificities and are extensively reviewed in other texts[2]. Reproducibility is a problem and the tests are best performed in reference laboratories.

Generally, high titres and a positive dye test indicate acute infection. With lower values, it may be necessary to evaluate serial IgM and IgG titres 3 weeks apart. IgM becomes positive 1–2 weeks after infection. Serial rising titres 3 weeks apart confirm acute infection even if the IgM is positive since IgM persists for months or years. IgG appears early after infection and peaks at about 2 months. While titres decline, they remain measurable for years.

Persistence of IgM and IgG makes the diagnosis of acute versus past infection problematic. The evaluation of specific IgG-isotypes or acute-phase IgG can help[41]. Recently, it was shown that IgA antibodies appear at the end of the first month of infection and usually disappear between 3 to 7 months[42]. IgE antibodies appear at the same time as the IgA and typically disappear by 8 months[43]. Thus, complete evaluation of a patient with a question of a primary toxoplasmosis infection during pregnancy may involve measurement of IgM, IgG, IgA and IgE antibodies in two samples at least 3 weeks apart (Fig. 64.2).

Fetal diagnosis should be offered to any woman who has acquired toxoplasmosis during pregnancy. The presence of *Toxoplasma*-specific IgM or non-specific indicators of fetal infections such as leukocyte count, eosinophil count, platelet count, total IgM, specific IgM, lactic dehydrogenase or γ-glutamyltransferase can by sought in fetal blood[32,44]. But this approach is problematic in that all tests have significant risk or false-negative and false-positive results[45]. Serial ultrasound examinations may show sequelae of infection such as ventricular dilation, cerebral or hepatic calcifications, ascites,

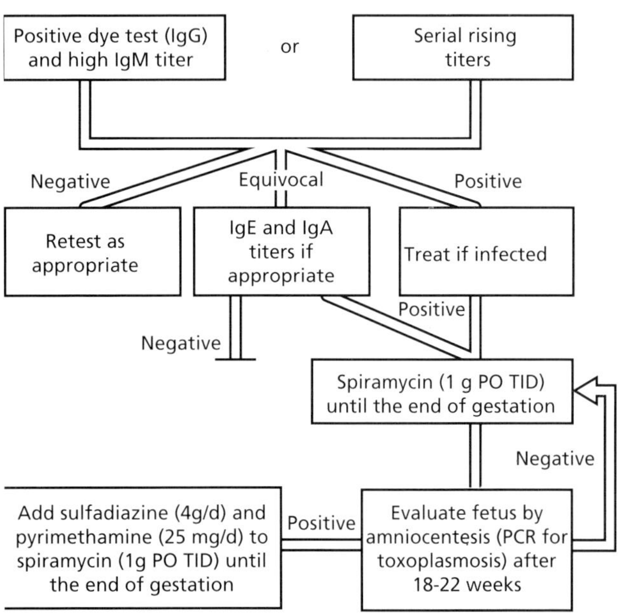

Fig. 64.2 Flow chart outlining screening, diagnosis and treatment for toxoplasmosis during pregnancy.

hydrops or other abnormalities. Polymerase chain reaction (PCR) testing for *Toxoplasma gondii* has been available for several years[32,46,47]. PCR analysis of the amniotic fluid appears highly accurate in identifying fetal infection[48]. Hohlfeld *et al.* applied PCR to amniotic fluid samples and compared it to the standard evaluation by inoculation of mice with amniotic fluid and fetal blood, tissue culture of amniotic fluid, or the identification of specific IgM in fetal blood. PCR was more sensitive and equally specific as conventional methods. There was only a single false-negative and no false-positive results[38]. Most centres in France now rely on PCR for prenatal diagnosis.

TREATMENT

Spiramycin (1 g every eight hours) is initiated when acute infection is identified (Fig. 64.2). The antenatal treatment of women who acquire toxoplasmosis during pregnancy reduces the incidence of fetal infection and the likelihood of sequelae if fetal infection takes place[32,49]. Spiramycin is only available in the United States on request from the Food and Drug Administration. Its release requires confirmation of the diagnosis by a reference laboratory. It is readily available outside the United States. Spiramycin is continued until delivery whether the fetus is infected or not since the placenta remains infected for the duration of pregnancy. Sulfadiazine (4 g/day) and pyrimethamine (25 mg/day) are added if fetal infection is confirmed[32]. This treatment regimen appears to reduce the risk of severe congenital infection.

Overly pessimistic counselling by medical staff of patients with both seroconversion before 26 weeks and evidence of fetal infection, has led many patients to choose abortion[32]. Most pregnancies will result in little long-term problems after delivery if the women received appropriate treatment[32]. Therefore termination may be an extreme response that is not warranted by outcome[50].

Prevention would be the most effective type of 'treatment' and primary prevention of disease has been advocated in the pregnant woman. Pregnant women should be educated to avoid contact with materials potentially contaminated by cat faeces and to wear gloves if contact is necessary. Pregnant women should wear gloves while gardening, cook meat thoroughly, wash fruits and vegetables before eating, avoid contact with mucous membranes while preparing uncooked meat or unwashed fruits and vegetables, and wash kitchen surfaces thoroughly after contact with these materials.

Secondary prevention of congenitally affected neonates born to women with primary infection during pregnancy requires serological screening. Parturients in high-risk areas are tested early in pregnancy, and seronegative women are retested thereafter at varying intervals[30,31]. Screening can reduce the rate of congenital toxoplasmosis from 50–70 per 10 000 births to 1 per 10 000 births[31]. The cost-effectiveness of such a screening programme depends on the frequency and cost of serological tests, cost of subspeciality referrals, costs of prenatal diagnosis and the costs of affected children. While cost-effective in France or Austria, such a programme may not be in the UK where the seropositivity rate is lower[51]. An evaluation of the cost–benefit ratio of a prevention programme in Norway is also underway[52]. Primary prevention could reduce the rate of seroconversion during pregnancy by over 60%, and secondary prevention could provide further reduction in congenital toxoplasmosis[35,53]. Screening is not cost effective in the United States.

CONGENITAL DISEASE

Findings of congenital infection include hydrops fetalis, extensive necrosis of brain parenchyma due to vascular involvement and periventricular nodules with calcium deposition, hydrocephalus, chorioretinitis, inner-ear inflammation, pneumonia, myocarditis, hepatosplenomegaly, renal lesions and others. Most children with congenital toxoplasmosis appear normal at birth. Central nervous system or eye findings may not appear for years[39,54]. Up to 85% of asymptomatic neonates have chorioretinitis by age 20 years.

The rate of congenital infection in the United States has been studied. Guerina *et al.* screened 635 000 neonates in Massachusetts and New Hampshire from 1986 to 1992[36]. Congenital infection was suggested in 100 neonates and confirmed on follow-up in only 50. Thus the rate of congenital infection in this area approximates 1 per 10 000 neonates. This is a tenth of the incidence in France (1–2 children per 1000 births).

In one study of 89 fetuses with proven toxoplasmosis, 32 had abnormal ultrasound findings. The findings included ventricular dilatation often of rapid onset, intracranial densities, increased placental thickness or hyperdensity, intrahepatic densities, ascites and pericardial and pleural effusion[55].

Cytomegalovirus

ORGANISM

Cytomegalovirus (CMV) is a double-stranded DNA virus of the herpesvirus family which includes varicella-zoster, herpes simplex and Epstein–Barr virus. The virus may be excreted weeks, months or years after a primary infection. A latency period eventually occurs but reactivation and reinfection are possible[56]. The prevalence of seropositivity varies by age and many demographic factors. One study of over 21 000 women attending a prenatal clinic in London revealed marked variation in the rate by race (White, 46%; Asian, 88%; and Black, 77%), parity (increasing seropositivity with increasing parity) and socioeconomic status[57,58]. Among mostly middle-income women in Alabama, 54% were seropositive with Whites having a lower rate than Blacks[59]. The incidence of seroconversion in women of childbearing age approximates 2% in high socioeconomic groups and up to 6% in lower socioeconomic groups.

Primary infection occurs in 2.2% of women during pregnancy[60]. Serological or culture evidence of *in utero* CMV infection is present in 0.2–2.2% of all liveborns[59]. Thus, congenital CMV infection is a major health problem and is thought to be the most common congenital infection in the United States[56,61,62].

CLINICAL MANIFESTATIONS

Maternal infection is generally asymptomatic. Occasionally it manifests as a mononucleosis-like syndrome with leukocytosis, lymphocytosis, abnormal liver function tests, spiking fever and malaise, myalgias and chills. Congenital disease is also often asymptomatic at birth. Severe disease may cause hepatosplenomegaly, jaundice, thrombocytopenia purpura, microcephaly, deafness, chorioretinitis, cerebral calcifications and later, mental retardation. Intrauterine growth restriction is described. CMV is the most common cause of congenital sensorineural hearing loss which may not be detected because most neonates are otherwise aymptomatic[63].

DIAGNOSIS

Fifty percent of reproductive age women have antibody to CMV, thus paired specimens are often necessary if seroconversion from negative to positive has not been documented. A significant rise in titre is consistent with a primary infection. IgM-specific antibody is usually present for 4–8 months following a primary infection but can increase periodically or persist at low titre for years.

In utero infection may be diagnosed by either the detection of an elevated fetal anti-CMV IgM obtained by cordocentesis[64] or by the culture of amniotic fluid. A prospective evaluation of 1771 pregnant Belgian women by serial serology and culture of urine, saliva, and cervical secretions at each prenatal visit revealed a seronegative rate of 49%. Seroconversion occurred in 20 susceptible women (2.3%). Seven of the 20 agreed to a fetal evaluation by cordocentesis and amniocentesis. Five of the 7 had positive amniotic fluid cultures for CMV; 3 of these 5 had fetal IgM for CMV. Pathological confirmation of CMV in fetal tissues was confirmed after termination, supporting the authors' contention that amniotic fluid culture is superior to fetal IgM in diagnosing fetal infection[65]. Others have reported lack of fetal CMV seropositivity for IgM. Thus, amniotic fluid culture or PCR analysis of amniotic fluid is superior to CMV-specific IgM[66,67]. There have been reports of false-negative amniotic fluid cultures as ascertained by neonatal shedding, but the relationship of these apparent negative results to the timing of infection and to long-term sequelae are unclear. Culture failure may be related to performance of amniocentesis too close to the time of initial maternal infection, or too early in gestation[68–70]. PCR or nested PCR evaluation of amniotic fluid may aid in detection of infected fetuses, but all techniques have false-negative results making counselling a difficult endeavour[71,72].

Some, but not all, infected fetuses have sonographic abnormalities, anaemia, thrombocytopenia and elevated liver function tests[73,74]. The natural history of the disease has been followed antenatally by serial ultrasound and cordocentesis in at least one case[75]. Hyperechoic bowel can precede development of ventriculomegaly, intrauterine growth retardation (IUGR), hydrops and fetal death in infected fetuses[76].

TREATMENT

No effective therapy is yet available. Work on a CMV vaccine has been in progress for 20 years and has not yet produced a good option[77]. Ganciclovir has been administered into the umbilical vein of a fetus at about 27 weeks. Dosage was 10 mg/day for 5 days, 15 mg/day for 3 days and 20 mg/day for 4 days. Several episodes of bradycardia were noted after administration. While the viral load in amniotic fluid decreased dramatically over the time of treatment and the liver function tests improved, a demise was noted at 32 weeks[78]. Whether direct administration of antiviral agents to the fetus to treat CMV will be an acceptable treatment awaits more work.

CONGENITAL DISEASE

Congenital CMV infection can be the result of both primary and recurrent infection. Serial ultrasound and fetal blood sampling have shown the natural history of fetal CMV infection in at least one case[75]. Among infected neonates, 90–95% are asymptomatic at birth, but almost 30% develop sensorineural hearing loss, mental retardation, chorioretinitis and other subtle late complications in the first years of life[59]. Saliva may be a better means of detecting congenital CMV infection than urine screening for viral antigen[79].

The rate of congenital infection depends on whether the maternal infection is primary or secondary. Among low socioeconomic groups, secondary infection is more likely to cause congenital infection than among higher socioeconomic patients for reasons not understood[80]. The risk of sequelae is about three times higher with primary infection during pregnancy than with recurrent infection[81]. The severity of sequelae is greater following primary infection as opposed to secondary infection. While deafness is typically the most severe sequelae following secondary infection, mental retardation and other central nervous system effects are part of the congenital picture following primary maternal infection (Fig. 64.3).

Varicella

The original description of the congenital varicella syndrome was made by Laforet and Lynch in 1947[82] where the woman contracted varicella during week 8 of pregnancy. The neonate delivered at term with well-defined reddish pigmented areas, 3–5 mm in diameter on a leg. The right leg was thin with bony hypoplasia. Hydrocephalus was present and there was optic nerve atrophy.

ORGANISM

The varicella-zoster virus is a member of the herpesvirus family. Transmission of the disease is probably by respiratory

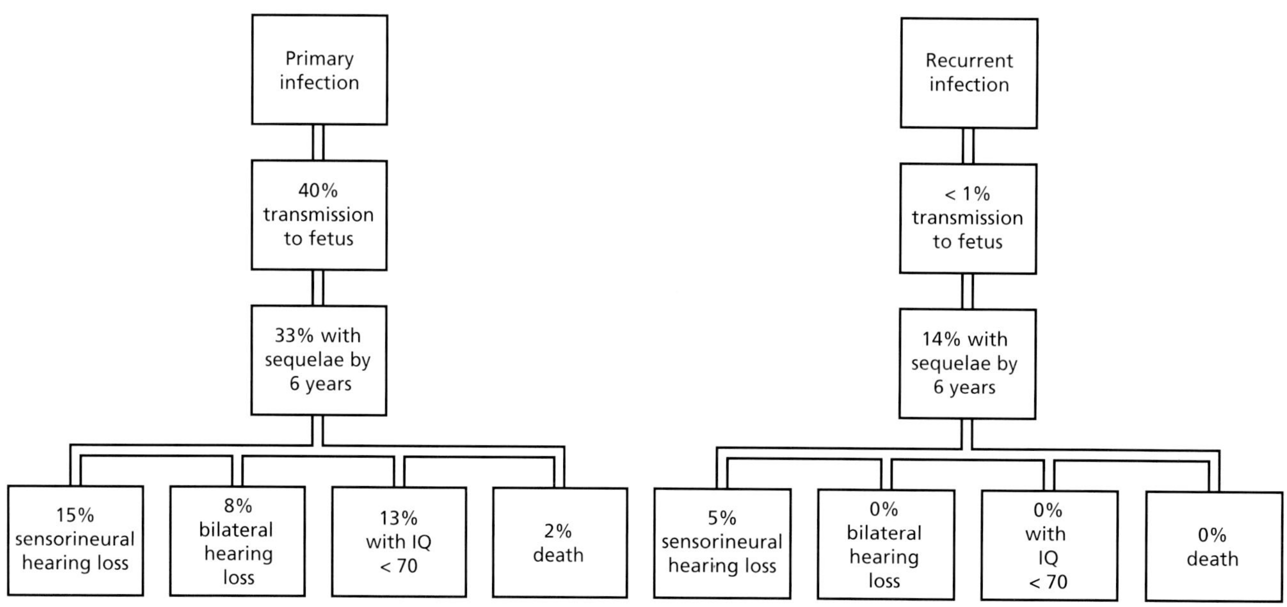

Fig. 64.3 Chart outlining risk of congenital disease secondary to cytomegalovirus. Some children may have more than one complication as listed at the bottom of the chart. All complications are not listed.

droplets carrying virus from mucosal vesicles or close personal contact[83].

CLINICAL MANIFESTATIONS

Acute varicella infection, or chickenpox, is a contagious disease characterized by an exanthem consisting of vesicles which evolve to pustules, crusts and scabs occurring 10–21 days after exposure. Patients are contagious 1–2 days before the onset of the rash and for up 10 days after it first appears until the lesions dry and crust over. The attack rate is high, over 90% of susceptible household contacts becoming infected. This generally mild childhood disease is much more severe in adults. Only 1.8% of cases are reported in adults, yet 25% of deaths occur after the second decade[83]. Zoster, or shingles, is caused by reactivation of virus that has lain dormant in dorsal root ganglia. It usually affects segmental dermatomes upon reactivation; 70–80% of young adults report a history of varicella. Over 90% of adults are seropositive for varicella[84]. However, over 20% of individuals giving a history of varicella do not have serological evidence of a past infection[84]. Among adults with no history of varicella, only about 25% are actually susceptible. Among pregnant women with a negative or indeterminate history of varicella, 80% have serology indicative of previous infection[85]. It has been estimated that there are about 7000–9000 cases of varicella during pregnancy in the United States annually[83,86]. One study of over 250 000 members of the Harvard Community Health Program showed a higher incidence of varicella in persons over 14 years of age and with more complications than previously reported[87].

DIAGNOSIS

Serological tests are available to measure both IgM and IgG anti-varicella antibodies. While culture of the virus from vesicular fluid or Tzanck smear preparations are the classical means of diagnosis, DNA diagnostic methods are emerging as a powerful tool[88]. The presence of anti-varicella IgM or a fourfold increase in varicella antibody titre is proof of a recent infection.

Documentation of congenital varicella is problematic. Total and specific IgM can be detected in fetal blood by 19 weeks though it may not persist until birth[6]. Virus can also be cultivated from amniotic fluid and identified by DNA probes. Unfortunately, serology may be negative in fetuses destined to have severe infection and positive serology[89] or PCR results[90] show only that virus was or is present and do not predict severity of disease. All sonographic abnormalities manifest within 20 weeks of maternal infection. The authors of one study suggest that if an early ultrasound is normal, a follow-up be performed at least 5 weeks after maternal infection to detect later sequelae[91].

Pathological evaluation of tissue specimens can be facilitated by DNA hybridization[92] or the PCR which can detect varicella genomic material in tissue[93].

TREATMENT

Seronegative women exposed to infected patients can be given varicella-zoster immune globulin (VZIG) to reduce the likelihood of severe symptomatology. Rouse and colleagues have shown that immune testing is more cost effective than universal administration of VZIG to women who are presumed seronegative by history[94]. Acyclovir is the drug of choice for treatment of varicella infection. Its use during pregnancy is usually reserved for cases complicated by, or at high risk of, pneumonia. Neither VZIG nor acyclovir demonstrably reduce the risk of congenital malformations.

The development of a live varicella virus vaccine (Varivax, Merck)[95,96] administered as a childhood immunization should reduce the pool of susceptible reproductive age women. The vaccine, developed from the Oka strain, was first produced in the 1970s and has been used in over 2 million children in Japan and Korea conferring immunity for at least 8 years[77,97]. Vaccination appears cost-effective for young children and there is a 'catch-up' programme for 12-year olds if the coverage rate for younger ages is low[98]. One evaluation showed a very favourable benefit – cost ratio of 6.9 using vaccination at 15 months of age[99]. No consensus concerning the risk–benefit ratio in reproductive age women is available.

CONGENITAL DISEASE

Congenital varicella is associated with a syndrome of skin scarring, limb hypoplasia and eye and brain damage. Atrophy of an extremity, specifically a leg, is the most distinguishing feature. Specific central nervous system findings includes cerebral atrophy, hydranencephaly, cerebellar aplasia and optic atrophy. Lambert *et al.* recently described 3 cases with bulbar palsy, mild hemiparesis, cicatricial skin lesions, development delay, chorioretinitis, optic atrophy or hypoplasia, congenital cataract and Horner's syndrome[100]. The period of highest risk is stated to only extend through the first half of pregnancy. Although small, early studies had placed the risk of congenital varicella syndrome at 9% (1 of 11 infants)[101], two more recent, large studies report that the risk of the syndrome approximates 2% with maternal infection at less than 20 weeks[102–104]. Maternal reactivation (i.e. zoster) poses little risk of causing embryopathy in the absence of disseminated viraemia[101,102]. With later infections, manifestations are less common but occur[104,105].

RUBELLA

The description of congenital cataracts and heart disease following maternal rubella infection is a classic demonstration of a virus acting as a teratogen[106].

ORGANISM

Rubella, also called German measles, three-day measles and third disease, is an exanthematous disease caused by a single-stranded RNA virus of the Togaviridae family.

CLINICAL MANIFESTATIONS

Rubella is acquired via respiratory droplet exposure and manifests after a 2–3-week incubation period. German measles is only modestly contagious, leaving many children uninfected after epidemic outbreaks. Patients becoming ill develop a rash which spreads from the face to the trunk and extremities, lasting about 3 days. Fever, arthralgias and postauricular and suboccipital lymphadenopathy are characteristic. Rubella infection, both in adults and children, is usually a mild illness; rare but severe complications include encephalitis, bleeding diathesis and arthritis. Besides the fact that the maculopapular rash resembles that caused by other viruses, overt clinical symptoms occur in only 50–75% of rubella-infected patients, thus invalidating clinical history as a useful method of documenting prior illness.

DIAGNOSIS

Acute infection is diagnosed by isolation of virus from the blood or throat. Prior infection produces lifelong immunity and is diagnosed by the presence of IgG antibodies. Women with confirmed infection are counselled based on risks and types of congenital abnormalities. Reverse transcription PCR has similar sensitivity and specificity to virus isolation in pharyngeal swab specimens and products of conception[107]. This technique can also detect the presence of viral RNA even when the fetal rubella virus-specific IgM obtained by fetal blood sampling is negative[108]. Prenatal diagnosis of fetal rubella infection can be made by fetal blood sampling and measurement of rubella specific IgM or chorionic villus sampling and dot-blot analysis.[109,110]. The specificity and sensitivity of amniotic fluid culture, assessment of fetal blood for specific IgM or use of the PCR are low enough that counselling based on gestational age related risk of congenital infection provides equally good information about the risk of severe disease.

TREATMENT

None currently available.

CONGENITAL DISEASE

The major defects associated with congenital rubella infection include congenital heart disease, cataracts, deafness and mental retardation. Defects involving virtually every organ have been reported. A fifty-year follow-up of 50 patients born in 1939–43[111] showed that of the 40 alive, all had hearing impairment. Severe hearing impairment was present in 36 of the 40. Twenty-three had eye defects related to the rubella.

Risk of fetal infection and resultant congenital anomalies in the first trimester may be over 80%[112,113] and is at least 25% in the second trimester. The risk of severe congenital abnormalities due to fetal infection probably declines through the second trimester. The rate of neonatal seropositivity increases again with third trimester maternal infection, probably due to increased fetal immunocompetence[114].

A recent report describes a potential association between *in utero* rubeola infection and later development of Crohn's disease[115]. This potential relationship does not warrant attempts at antenatal diagnosis of fetal infection.

Human immunodeficiency virus

ORGANISM

Human immunodeficiency virus (HIV) type I is the most common HIV virus. These are DNA retroviruses that cause fetal disease by affecting the immune and central nervous systems. Selective depletion of CD4$^+$ helper T-lymphocytes is the pathognomonic finding. Risk factors for acquiring the disease include multiple sex partners and parenteral drug abuse.

CLINICAL MANIFESTATIONS

Clinical manifestations are complex and varied depending on the stage of the disease. The patient may be completely asymptomatic early in the course. Women with advanced disease are at great risk of multiple opportunistic infections. Acquired immunodeficiency disease (AIDS) was one of the five leading causes of death among women 15–44 years in 1991[116].

DIAGNOSIS

Infection is usually diagnosed by an enzyme-linked immunosorbent assay (ELISA). The ELISA detects HIV-specific antibodies in the serum. An ELISA to detect p24 core antigen is also sometimes used. After two sequentially positive ELISA screening tests, a Western blot must be performed to confirm the patients infection[117].

TREATMENT AND CONGENITAL DISEASE

No clear fetal syndrome associated with maternal HIV infection has been reported. Treatment is based on maternal health and a desire to decrease transmission to the fetus[118]. Lowering maternal antigen level and maternal/neonatal treatment with zidovudine reduces transmission[119] by two-thirds (26% to 8%)[120]. These results were confirmed across a range of CD4 counts[121]. All HIV-positive pregnant women should be offered treatment with zidovudine[122,123] since HIV is lethal and zidovudine poses no teratogenic risk to the developing fetus[124–126]. The treatment regime consists of zidovudine 100 mg orally five times per day antepartum, 2 mg/kg body weight intravenously over 1 hour followed by 1 mg/kg/hour intravenously intrapartum until delivery, and the neonate receives 2 mg/kg orally every 6 hours for 6 weeks starting at

8–12 hours of life[120]. These studies provide a strong argument for routine maternal screening at the time of the first prenatal visit. There is concern that there may be long-term effects on the *in utero* exposed fetus that must be followed through infancy and childhood as a significant number of drug exposed fetuses would never become infected[127].

Several other obstetrical interventions may reduce vertical transmission of HIV such as caesarean section (compared to vaginal delivery)[128–132], maternal nutritional status, particularly vitamin A deficiency, which may increase vertical transmission of HIV-1[133] and length of ruptured membranes with increasing perinatal infection beyond 4 hours[134]. While interesting, the latter two possibilities have not been thoroughly evaluated enough to change current practice.

Recently, viral load has been shown to be important in terms of disease progression in the general population and predictive of perinatal transmission risk in the obstetric population. Higher maternal viral load is associated with greater perinatal transmission of HIV 1[135–139] and a higher load in the neonate is associated with more rapid disease progression[140].

Parvovirus B19

ORGANISM

A member of the family Parvoviridae, parvovirus B19 is a single-stranded DNA virus discovered in 1975[141]. It infects only humans and is transmitted via aerosolized droplets. B19 preferentially replicates in actively dividing cells such as erythroid progenitors; 30–50% of reproductive age women have serological evidence of past infection[5,141–143]. Several reviews concerning human disease caused by parvovirus are available[144,145].

CLINICAL MANIFESTATIONS

The incubation period before symptoms or rash is 4–20 days[141]. Childhood infection is characterized by erythema infectiosum (fifth disease or slapped-cheek disease). Most adult infection is asymptomatic. The rash, though usually facial, can also appear on the trunk and extremities. The rash results from immune complex deposition and the patient is no longer infectious when it appears. Viraemia occurs 6–8 days after exposure and persists for 4–7 days. The rash develops 16 days after exposure or 8 days after the viraemia. A drop in haematocrit can be detected 2–3 weeks after exposure in the adult or about a week following the viraemia. The associated reticulocytopenia lasts for 7–10 days[146,147]. Arthritis is also a common manifestation, affecting as many as 80% of adults but only 10% of children[148]. In some individuals with chronic haemolytic anaemias (e.g. sickle cell and hereditary spherocytosis) parvovirus infection produces a transient aplastic crisis[149]. Other clinical manifestations of B19 infection include chronic anaemia, encephalitis, meningitis and vasculitis[150,151].

In one study of 134 women infected during pregnancy, 66 were between 10 and 18 weeks. There were 11 fetal deaths (17%) in this group of 66 but no deaths in the 13 women infected between 19 and 27 weeks[142]. During a large outbreak in Connecticut, 39 pregnant women were found to have serological evidence of recent infection with no evidence of hydrops, but only 11 women were in the higher risk period between 13 and 18 weeks[152]. The rate of acute infection during pregnancy was 3.7% in one large study, with only a 1.7% rate of fetal loss (1 per 60 maternal infections)[143].

DIAGNOSIS

B19-specific IgM is a marker of recent primary infection appearing 14 days after inoculation or 3 days after the start of symptoms. It remains present for 3–4 months[147]. B19-specific IgG appears in week 3 and is present life-long[147]. The absence of maternal IgM and IgG indicates no previous infection and a susceptible individual. The presence of only B19 IgG indicates previous infection at least 4 months ago. The presence of only B19 IgM indicates very recent (<7 days) infection and the presence of both IgM and IgG indicates recent infection (7 days to 4 months).

PCR or DNA dot-blot can now detect the presence of parvovirus in maternal serum, fetal blood or amniotic fluid[153–156].

TREATMENT AND CONGENITAL DISEASE

There is a 33% transplacental transmission rate following maternal infection based on serology. Hydrops may result from aplastic anaemia, myocarditis or chronic fetal hepatitis. Many cases of fetal hydrops have been reported following maternal infection[156–158]. Stillbirth with maternal B19 infection has occurred 1–12 weeks following infection. However, hydrops is unlikely to occur later if fetal anaemia and hydrops have not developed by 8 weeks following infection. For this reason, we perform weekly ultrasound evaluations for 4–8 weeks after maternal exposure or infection. A careful history must be obtained because adults can have two symptomatic periods following exposure: fever, malaise and other flu-like symptoms occur during the viraemia, and the rash which occurs 17–18 days after exposure[147]. If maternal rash is used as the starting point, surveillance should be instituted 2–3 weeks earlier than for the viraemia. If hydrops with significant anaemia develops, intrauterine transfusion can be performed and appears to benefit the fetus[159]. The fetus with anaemia and reticulocytosis as ascertained by fetal blood sampling may already be recovering and not need transfusion as hydrops has been observed to resolve spontaneously[155,160,161]. Though some advocate observation of the hydropic fetus, this entails significant risk since no sonographic finding other than the hydrops predicts demise. Overall, it appears that the risk of fetal death following maternal infection is under 10%[162]. Parvovirus B19 may account for 10–18% of cases of non-immune hydrops[163–165] depending on patient mix and how one determines whether B19 was truly the causative agent. At least 2 cases of malformations associated with parvovirus B19 infection have been described, but these reports do not clearly implicate the parvovirus as the causative agent[166].

Enterovirus, adenovirus and others

The potential role of enterovirus (specifically the echovirus and coxsackievirus) in causing fetal infection and congenital disease was first extensively evaluated by Evans and Brown in 1963[167]. Based on serological assessment for coxsackievirus and echovirus in stored blood samples from over 800 pregnancies complicated by congenital abnormalities and 23 000 controls, they showed a relationship between congenital heart disease, urogenital abnormalities and digestive system anomalies in the neonate and increase in titre in the mother[168,169]. Burch *et al.* showed that a high percentage of infants with histological evidence of interstitial myocarditis had infection with coxsackievirus B[170]. Echovirus 11 has been implicated in a fetal death at 29 weeks[171]. The patient's 18-month-old son had a confirmed echovirus 11 infection 3 weeks before the demise and the virus was present in multiple fetal tissues at autopsy. A study in Sweden observed that mothers of children who developed diabetes are more likely to have had enteroviral-specific antibodies during their pregnancy than women whose children did not develop diabetes. The authors hypothesized that enteroviral infection during pregnancy predisposes the fetus to later diabetes[172].

Adenovirus was implicated in a case of fetal anasarca with massive ascites, scalp and skin oedema and pericardial and pleural effusions. There appeared to be a cardiomyopathic process based on ultrasound evaluation. Delivery occurred at 34 weeks due to preterm labour. Cardiomyopathy was documented after delivery. Adenoviral genomic material was found using PCR in maternal, fetal and neonatal blood[173]. PCR-detectable adenovirus genomic material is present in 68% of myocardial biopsies or blood samples obtained from children with viral myocarditis[174] and could thus be a potential cause of *in utero* myocardial dysfunction. A recent report indicated an association between adenovirus and fetal hydrops and supraventricular tachycardia[175].

Lymphocytic choriomeningitis virus (LCMV) is a member of the Arenaviridae family and is maintained in nature by vertical infection in mice. Human infection is usually acquired by contact with infected mice, hamsters or their excreta. A 2898-g infant with microphthalmia, anterior chamber abnormalities and retinitis was found to have hydrocephalus. Serum and CSF evaluation were consistent with intrauterine LCMV infection[176]. Seropositivity rates vary by geographic location (5.1% in Alabama, 0% in Texas and 1.54–3.07% in Argentina)[177,178] and may depend on rates of house mice infection[179]. LCMV causes hepatitis in mice[180] and primates[181,182] and whether this will be true in congenital infections awaits further work.

Current work carried out in our facility, in collaboration with others, is evaluating the presence of viral genomic material in samples from both anomalous and control fetuses. Preliminary findings suggest a high association of viral genomic material in pregnancies with an abnormal ultrasound[183]. The field of virology as related to congenital anomalies and fetal loss, is clearly in its infancy despite reports of a relationship for over 30 years[167–170]. We look forward to rapid strides in diagnosis, treatment and reduction of sequelae of intrauterine infection as a result of development of powerful techniques such as PCR and easier access to the fetus. Hopefully, the next steps will lead to efficacious treatments to reduce the risks of intrauterine viral infection.

REFERENCES

1. Isada NB & Grossman JH. Perinatal Infections. In *Obstetrics: Normal and Problem Pregnancies* (eds S.G. Gabbe, J.R. Niebyl & J.L. Simpson), 2nd edn. New York: Churchill Livingstone, 1991.
2. Remington JS & Klein JO. (eds) *Infectious Diseases of the Fetus and Newborn Infant*, 4th edn. Philadelphia: W.B. Saunders, 1995.
3. Gibbs RS & Sweet RL. Maternal and fetal infections: clinical disorders. In *Maternal–Fetal Medicine: Principles and Practice*, 3rd edn (eds R.K. Creasy & R. Resnik), pp. 656–725. Philadelphia: W.B. Saunders, 1994.
4. Minkoff HL. Human immunodeficiency virus. In *Maternal–Fetal Medicine: Principles and Practice*, 3rd edn. (eds R.K. Creasy & R. Resnik). Philadelphia: W.B. Saunders, 1994.
5. Giovangrandi Y, Weiner CP, Smoleniec J & Brettes JP. Fetal infection. In *High Risk Pregnancy* (eds D.K. James, P.J. Steer, C.P. Weiner & B. Gonik), pp. 841–870. London: W.B. Saunders, 1994.
6. Weiner CP, Grose CF & Naides SJ. Diagnosis of fetal infection in the patient with an ultrasonographically detected abnormality but a negative clinical history. *Am. J. Obstet. Gynecol.* **168**, 6–11, 1993.
7. Grose C, Itani O & Weiner CP. Prenatal diagnosis of fetal infection: advances from amniocentesis to cordocentesis – congenital toxoplasmosis, rubella, cytomegalovirus, varicella virus, parvovirus and human immunodeficiency virus. *Pediatr. Infect. Dis. J.* **8**, 459–468, 1989.
8. Valente P & Sever J. *In utero* diagnosis of congenital infections by direct fetal sampling. *Isr. J. Med. Sci.* **30**, 414–420, 1994.
9. Ingall D, Sánchez PJ & Musher DM. Syphilis. In *Infectious Diseases of the Fetus and Newborn Infact*, 4th edn. (eds J.S. Remington & J.O. Klein). Philadelphia: W.B. Saunders, 1995.
10. Berry MC & Dajani AS. Resurgence of congenital syphilis. *Infect. Dis. Clin. North Am.* **6**, 19–29, 1992.
11. Stokes JH, Beerman H & Ingraham NR. The present status of penicillin in the treatment of syphilis in pregnancy and infantile congenital syphilis. *Am. J. Med. Sci.* **219**, 433–442, 1950.
12. McFarlin BL, Bottoms SF, Dock BS & Isada NB. Epidemic syphilis: Maternal factors associated with congenital infection. *Am. J. Obstet. Gynecol.* **170**, 535–540, 1994.
13. Mascola L, Pelosi R, Blout JH, Binkin NJ, Alexander CE & Cates W. Congenital syphilis. Why is it still occurring? *JAMA* **252**, 1719–1722, 1984.

14. Rawstron SA & Bromberg K. Failure of recommended maternal therapy to prevent congenital syphilis. *Sex. Transm. Dis.* **18**, 102–106, 1991.
15. Rolfs RT & Nakashima AK. Epidemiology of primary and secondary syphilis in the United States, 1981 through 1989. *JAMA* **264**, 1432–1437, 1990.
16. Sweet RL & Gibbs RS. *Infectious Diseases of the Female Genital Tract*, 2nd edn, pp. 119–126. Baltimore: Williams & Wilkins, 1990.
17. Center for Disease Control. Policy guidelines for the prevention and control of congenital syphilis. *MMWR* **37** (Suppl. S-1), 1–13, 1988.
18. Dunn RA, Webster LA & Nakashima AK. Surveillance for geographic and secular trends in congenital syphilis – United States, 1983–1991. *MMWR* **42**, 59–71, 1993.
19. Stray-Pedersen B. Economic evaluation of maternal screening to prevent congenital syphilis. *Sex. Transm. Dis.* **10**, 167–172, 1983.
20. Musher DM. How much penicillin cures early syphilis? *Ann. Intern. Med.* **109**, 849–851, 1988.
21. Centers for Disease Control. Sexually transmitted diseases treatment guidelines. *MMWR* **38** (Suppl. 8), September 1, 1989.
22. Webber MP, Lambert G, Bateman DA & Hauser WA. Maternal risk factors for congenital syphilis: a case-control study. *Am. J. Epidemiol.* **137**, 415–422, 1993.
23. Ricci JM, Fojaco RM & O'Sullivan MJ. Congenital syphilis: The University of Miami/Jackson Memorial Medical Center experience, 1986–1988. *Obstet. Gynecol.* **74**, 687–693, 1989.
24. Malone JL, Wallace MR, Hendrick BB *et al.* Syphilis and neurosyphilis in a human immunodeficiency virus type-1 seropositive population: Evidence for frequent serologic relapse after therapy. *Am. J. Med.* **99**, 55–63, 1995.
25. Guerina NG. Congenital infection with *Toxoplasma gondii*. *Pediatr. Ann.* **23**, 138–151, 1994.
26. Holliman RE. Congenital toxoplasmosis: prevention, screening and treatment. *J. Hosp. Infect.* **30** (Suppl.), 179–190, 1995.
27. Hall SM. Congenital toxoplasmosis. *BMJ* **305**, 291–297, 1992.
28. Wong S-Y & Remington JS. Toxoplasmosis in pregnancy. *Clin. Infect. Dis.* **18**, 853–862, 1994.
29. Sever JL, Ellenberg JH, Ley AC, Madden DL, Fuccillo DA, Tzan NR & Edmonds DM. Toxoplasmosis: Maternal and pediatric findings in 23 000 pregnancies. *Pediatrics* **82**, 181–192, 1988
30. Thulliez P. Screening programme for congenital toxoplasmosis in France. *Scand. J. Infect. Dis.* (Suppl. 84), 43–45, 1992.
31. Aspöck H & Pollak A. Prevention of prenatal toxoplasmosis by serological screening of pregnant women in Austria. *Scand. J. Infect. Dis.* (Suppl. 84), 32–38, 1993.
32. Daffos F, Forestier F, Capella-Pavlovsky M, Thulliez P, Aufrant C, Valenti D & Cox WL. Prenatal management of 746 pregnancies at risk for congenital toxoplasmosis. *N. Engl. J. Med.* **318**, 271–275, 1988.
33. Foulon W, Naessens A & Derde MP. Evaluation of the possibilities for preventing congenital toxoplasmosis. *Am. J. Perinat.* **11**, 57–62, 1994.
34. Bader TJ, Macones GA & Asch DA. Prenatal screening for toxoplasmosis. *Obstet. Gynecol.* **90**, 457–464, 1997.
35. Daffos F, Capella-Pavlovsky M & Forestier F. Fetal blood sampling during pregnancy with use of a needle guided by ultrasound: A study of 606 consecutive cases. *Am. J. Obstet. Gynecol.* **153**, 655–660, 1985.
36. Guerina NG, Hsu H-W, Meissner HC *et al.* Neonatal serologic screening and early treatment for congenital *Toxoplasma gondii* infection. *N. Engl. J. Med.* **330**, 1858–1863, 1994.
37. Hsu H-W, Grady GR, Maguire JH, Weiblem BJ & Hoff R. Newborn screening for congenital toxoplasmosis infection: Five years experience in Massachusetts, USA. *Scand. J. Infect. Dis.* (Suppl. 84), 59–64, 1992.
38. Hohlfeld P, Daffos F, Costa J-M, Thulliez P, Forestier F & Vidaud M. Prenatal diagnosis of congenital toxoplasmosis with a polymerase-chain-reaction test on amniotic fluid. *N. Engl. J. Med.* **331**, 695–699, 1994.
39. Koppe JG & Rothova A. Congenital toxoplasmosis. A long-term follow-up of 20 years. *Int. Ophthalmol.* **13**, 387–390, 1989.
40. Lynfield R & Eaton RB. Teratogen update: Congenital toxoplasmosis. *Teratology* **52**, 176–180, 1995.
41. Thulliez P, Daffos F & Forestier F. Diagnosis of *Toxoplasma* infection in the pregnant woman and the unborn child: Current problems. *Scand. J. Infect. Dis.* **84**, 18–22, 1992.
42. Bessières MH, Roques C, Berrebi A, Barre V, Cazaux M & Séguéla JP. IgA antibody response during acquired and congenital toxoplasmosis. *J. Clin. Pathol.* **45**, 605–608, 1992.
43. Wong S-Y, Hajdu M-P, Ramireq R *et al.* Role of specific immunoglobulin E in diagnosis of acute *Toxoplasma* infection and toxoplasmosis. *J. Clin. Microbiol.* **31**, 2952–2959, 1993.
44. Pratlong F, Boulot P, Issert E *et al.* Fetal diagnosis of toxoplasmosis in 190 women infected during pregnancy. *Prenat. Diagn.* **14**, 191–198, 1994.
45. Holliman RE, Johnson JD, Constantine G, Bissenden JG, Nicolaides K & Savva D. Difficulties in the diagnosis of congenital toxoplasmosis by cordocentesis: Case report. *Br. J. Obstet. Gynaecol.* **98**, 832–834, 1991.
46. Burg JL, Grover CM, Pouletty P *et al.* Direct and sensitive detection of a pathogenic protozoan, *Toxoplasma gondii* by polymerase chain reaction. *J. Clin. Microbiol.* **27**, 1787, 1989.
47. van de Ven E, Melchers W, Galama J *et al.* Identification of *Toxoplasma gondii* infections by *B1* gene amplification. *J. Clin. Microbiol.* **29**, 2120, 1991.
48. Casenave J, Forestier F, Bessieres MH, Broussin B & Begueret J. Contribution of a new PCR assay to the prenatal diagnosis of congenital toxoplasmosis. *Prenat. Diagn.* **12**, 119–127, 1992.
49. Stray-Pedersen B. Treatment of toxoplasmosis in the pregnant mother and newborn child. *Scand. J. Infect. Dis.* (Suppl. 84), 23–31, 1992.
50. Berribi A, Kobuch WE, Bessieres MH *et al.* Termination of pregnancy for maternal toxoplasmosis. *Lancet* **344**, 36–39, 1994.
51. Joynson DH. Epidemiology of toxoplasmosis in the UK. *Scand. J. Infect. Dis.* **84**, 65–69, 1992.
52. Stray-Pedersen B & Jenum P. Economic evaluation of preventive programmes against congenital toxoplasmosis. *Scand. J. Infect. Dis.* (Suppl. 84), 86–96, 1992
53. Foulon W. Congenital toxoplasmosis: Is screening desirable? *Scand. J. Infect. Dis.* (Suppl. 84), 11–17, 1992.
54. Koppe JG, Loewer-Sieger DH & de Roever-Bonnet H. Results of 20 year follow-up of congenital toxoplasmosis. *Lancet* **i**, 254–256, 1986.
55. Hohlfeld P, MacAleese J, Capella-Pavlovski M, Giovangrandi Y, Thulliez P, Forestier F & Daffos F. *Ultrasound. Obstet. Gynecol.* **1**, 241–244., 1991
56. Raynor BD. Cytomegalovirus infection in pregnancy. *Sem. Perinat.* **17**, 394–402, 1993.
57. Tookey PA, Ades AE & Peckham CS. Cytomegalovirus prevalence in pregnant women: the influence of parity. *Arch. Dis. Childh.* **67**, 779–783, 1992.
58. Peckham CS, Coleman JC, Hurley R, Chin KS, Henderson K & Preece PM. Cytomegalovirus infection in pregnancy: Preliminary findings from a prospective study. *Lancet* **i**, 1352–1355, 1983.
59. Stagno S, Pass RF, Cloud G *et al.* Primary cytomegalovirus infection in pregnancy. *JAMA* **256**, 1904–1908, 1986.
60. Yow MD, Williamson DW, Leeds LJ *et al.* Epidemiologic characteristics of cytomegalovirus infection in mothers and their infants. *Am. J. Obstet. Gynecol.* **158**, 1189–1195, 1988.
61. Stagno S & Whitley RJ. Herpesvirus infections of pregnancy. Part I: Cytomegalovirus and Epstein–Barr virus infections. *N. Engl. J. Med.* **313**, 1270–1274, 1985.
62. Demmler GJ. Infectious Diseases Society of America and Centers for Disease Control summary of a workshop on surveillance for congenital cytomegalovirus disease. *Rev. Infect. Dis.* **13**, 315–329, 1991.
63. Hicks T, Fowler K, Richardson M, Dahle A, Adams L & Pass R. Congenital cytomegalovirus infection and neonatal auditory screening. *J. Pediatr.* **123**, 779–782, 1993.
64. Lange I, Rodeck CV, Morgan-Capner P, Simmons A & Kangro HO. Prenatal neurological diagnosis of intra-uterine cytomegalovirus infection. *BMJ* **284**, 1673–1674, 1982.
65. Lamy ME, Mulongo KN, Gadisseux J-F, Lyon G, Gaudy V & Lierde MV. Prenatal diagnosis of fetal cytomegalovirus infection. *Am. J. Obstet. Gynecol.* **166**, 91–94, 1992.
66. Hogge WA, Buffone GJ & Hogge JS. Prenatal diagnosis of cytomegalovirus (CMV) infection: A preliminary report. *Prenat. Diagn.* **13**, 131–136, 1993.
67. Xu W, Sundqvist V-A, Brytting M & Linde A. Diagnosis of cytomegalovirus infections using polymerase chain reaction, virus isolation and serology. *Scand. J. Infect. Dis.* **25**, 311–316, 1993.
68. Catanzarite V & Dankner WM. Prenatal diagnosis of congenital cytomegalovirus infection: False-negative amniocentesis at 20 weeks' gestation. *Prenat. Diagn.* **13**, 1021–1205, 1993.

69. Nicolini U, Kustermann A, Tassis B *et al.* Prenatal diagnosis of congenital human cytomegalovirus infection. *Prenat. Diagn.* **14**, 903–906, 1994.
70. Conner C, Liesnard C, Brancart F & Rodesch F. Accuracy of amniotic fluid testing before 21 weeks' gestation in prenatal diagnosis of congenital cytomegalovirus infection. *Prenat. Diagn.* **14**, 1055–1059, 1994.
71. Revello MG, Baldanti F, Furione M, Sarasini A, Percivalle E, Zavattoni M & Gerna G. Polymerase chain reaction for prenatal diagnosis of congenital human cytomegalovirus infection. *J. Med. Virol.* **47**, 462–466, 1995.
72. Ruellan-Eugene G, Barjot P, Campet M *et al.* Evaluation of virological procedures to detect fetal human cytomegalovirus infection: Avidity of IgG antibodies, virus detection in amniotic fluid and maternal serum. *J. Med. Virol.* **50**, 9–15, 1996.
73. Hohlfeld P, Vial Y, Mallard-Brignon C, Vaudaux, B & Fawer C-L. Cytomegalovirus fetal infection: Prenatal diagnosis. *Obstet. Gynecol.* **78**, 615–618, 1991.
74. Lynch L, Daffos F, Emanuel D *et al.* Prenatal diagnosis of fetal cytomegalovirus infection. *Am. J. Obstet. Gynecol.* **165**, 714–718, 1991.
75. Watt-Morse ML, Laifer SA & Hill LM. The natural history of fetal cytomegalovirus infection as assessed by serial ultrasound and fetal blood sampling: A case report. *Prenat. Diagn.* **15**, 567–570, 1995.
76. Peters MT, Lowe TW, Carpenter A & Kole S. Prenatal diagnosis of congenital cytomegalovirus infection with abnormal triple-screen results and hyperechoic fetal bowel. *Am. J. Obstet. Gynecol.* **173**, 953–954, 1995.
77. Plotkin SA. Vaccines for varicella-zoster virus and cytomegalovirus: Recent progress. *Science* **265**, 1383–1385, 1994.
78. Revello MG, Rercivalle E, Baldanti F, Gerna G, Kustermann A, Nava S & Nicolini U. Prenatal treatment of congenital human cytomegalovirus infection by fetal intravascular administration of ganciclovir. *Clin. Diagn. Virol.* **1**, 61–67, 1993.
79. Balcarek KB, Warren W, Smith RJ, Lyon MD & Pass RF. Neonatal screening for congenital cytomegalovirus infection by detection of virus in saliva. *J. Infect. Dis.* **167**, 1433–1436, 1993.
80. Stagno S, Pass RF, Dworsky ME, Henderson RE, Moore EG, Walton PD & Alford CA. Congenital cytomegalovirus infection: the relative importance of primary and recurrent maternal infection. *N. Engl. J. Med.* **306**, 945–949, 1982.
81. Fowler KB, Stagno S, Pass RF, Britt WJ, Boll TJ & Alford CA. The outcome of congenital cytomegalovirus infection in relation to maternal antibody status. *N. Engl. J. Med.* **326**, 663–667, 1992.
82. Laforet EG & Lynch CL. Multiple congenital defects following maternal varicella. *N. Engl. J. Med.* **236**, 534–537, 1947.
83. Chapman S & Duff P. Varicella in pregnancy. *Semin. Perinat.* **17**, 403–409, 1993.
84. Struewing JP, Hyams KC, Tueller JE & Gray GC. The risk of measles, mumps, and varicella among young adults: A serosurvey of US Navy and Marine Corps recruits. *Am. J. Publ. Health* **83**, 1717–1720, 1993.
85. McGregor JA, Mark S, Crawford GP & Levin MJ. Varicella zoster antibody testing in the care of pregnant women exposed to varicella. *Am. J. Obstet. Gynecol.* **157**, 281–284, 1987.
86. Brunell PA. Varicella in pregnancy, the fetus, and the newborn. Problems in management. *J. Infect. Dis.* **166** (Suppl. 1), S42–47, 1992.
87. Choo PW, Donahue JG, Manson JE & Platt R. The epidemiology of varicella and its complications. *J. Infect. Dis.* **172**, 706–712, 1995.
88. Nahass GT, Goldstein BA, Zhu WY, Serfling U, Penneys NS & Leonardi CL. Comparison of Tzanck smear, viral culture, and DNA diagnostic methods in detection of herpes simplex and varicella-zoster infection. *JAMA* **268**, 2541–2544, 1992.
89. Lécuru F, Taurelle R, Bernard J-P, Parrat S, Lafay-Pillet M-C & Rozenberg F. Varicella zoster virus infection during pregnancy: the limits of prental diagnosis. *Eur. J. Obstet. Gynecol.* **56**, 67–68, 1994.
90. Isada NB, Paar DP, Johnson MP, Evans MI, Holzgreve W, Qureshi F & Straus SE. *In utero* diagnosis of congenital varicella zoster virus infection by chorionic villus sampling and polymerase chain reaction. *Am. J. Obstet. Gynecol.* **165**, 1727–1730, 1991.
91. Pretorius DH, Hayward I, Jones KL & Stamm E. Sonographic evaluation of pregnancies with maternal varicella infection. *J. Ultrasound Med.* **11**, 459–463, 1992.
92. Scharf A, Scherr O, Enders G & Helftenbein E. Virus detection in the fetal tissue of a premature delivery with congenital varicella syndrome. *J. Perinat. Med.* **18**, 317–322, 1990.
93. Puchhammer-Stöckl E, Kunz C, Wagner G & Enders G. Detection of varicella zoster virus (VZV) DNA in fetal tissue by polymerase chain reaction. *J. Perinat. Med.* **22**, 65–69, 1994.
94. Rouse DJ, Gardner M, Allen SJ & Goldenberg RL. Management of the presumed susceptible varicella (chickenpox)-exposed gravida: a cost-effectiveness/cost–benefit analysis. *Obstet. Gynecol.* **87**, 932–936, 1996.
95. Anonymous Licensure of varicella virus vaccine, live. *JAMA* **273**, 1253, 1995.
96. Committee on Infectious Diseases Recommendations for the use of live attenuated varicella virus. *Pediatrics* **95**, 791–796, 1995.
97. Krause PR & Klinman DM. Efficacy, immunogenicity, safety, and use of live attenuated chickenpox vaccine. *J. Pediatr.* **127**, 518–525, 1995.
98. Lieu TA, Cochi SL, Black SB, Halloran E, Shinefield HR, Holmes SJ *et al.* Cost-effectiveness of a routine varicella vaccination program for US children. *JAMA* **271**, 375–381, 1994.
99. Preblud SR. Varicella. Complications and costs. *Pediatrics* **78**, 728–735, 1986.
100. Lambert SR, Taylor D, Kriss A, Holzel H & Heard S. Ocular manifestations of the congenital varicella syndrome. *Arch. Ophthalmol.* **107**, 52–56, 1989.
101. Paryani SG & Arvin AM. Intrauterine infection with varicella-zoster virus after maternal varicella. *N. Engl. J. Med.* **314**, 1542–1546, 1986.
102. Enders G, Miller E, Cradock-Watson J, Bolley I & Ridehalgh M. Consequences of varicella and herpes zoster in pregnancy: prospective study of 1739 cases. *Lancet* **343**, 1547–1550, 1994.
103. Pastuszak AL, Levy M, Schick B *et al.* Outcome after maternal varicella infection in the first 20 weeks of pregnancy. *N. Engl. J. Med.* **330**, 901–905, 1994.
104. Jones KL, Johnson KA & Chambers CD. Offspring of women infected with varicella during pregnancy: A prospective study. *Teratology* **49**, 29–32, 1994.
105. Michie CA, Acolet D, Charlton R *et al.* Varicella-zoster contracted in the second trimester of pregnancy. *Pediatr. Infect. Dis. J.* **11**, 1050–1053, 1992.
106. Gregg N. Congenital cataract following German measles in the mother. *Trans. Ophthalmol. Soc. Aust.* **3**, 35, 1941.
107. Bosma TJ, Corbett KM, O'Shea S, Banatvala JE & Best JM. PCR for detection of rubella virus RNA in clinical samples. *J. Clin. Microbiol.* **33**, 1075–1079, 1995.
108. Tanemura M, Suzumori K, Yagami Y & Katow S. Diagnosis of fetal rubella infection with reverse transcription and nested polymerase chain reaction: A study of 34 cases diagnosed in fetuses. *Am. J. Obstet. Gynecol.* **174**, 578–582, 1996.
109. Terry GM, Ho-Terry L, Warren R, Rodeck CH, Cohen A & Rees K. First trimester prenatal diagnosis of congenital rubella: a laboratory investigation. *BMJ* **292**, 930–933, 1986.
110. Daffos F, Forestier F, Grangeot-Keros L, Capella-Parlovsky M, Lebon P, Chartier M & Pillot J. Prenatal diagnosis of congenital rubella. *Lancet* **ii**, 1–3, 1984.
111. McIntosh EDG & Menser MA. A fifty-year follow-up of congenital rubella. *Lancet* **340**, 414–415, 1992.
112. Centers for Disease Control Congenital rubella syndrome among the Amish – Pennsylvania 1991–1992. *JAMA* **268**, 859–860, 1992.
113. Mellinger AK, Cragan JD, Atkinson WL, Williams WW, Kleger B, Kimber RG & Tavris D. High incidence of congenital rubella syndrome after a rubella outbreak. *Pediatr. Infect. Dis. J.* **14**, 573–578, 1995.
114. Miller E, Cradock-Watson JE & Pollock TM. Consequences of confirmed maternal rubella at successive stages of pregnancy. *Lancet* **ii**, 781–785, 1982.
115. Ekbom A, Daszak P, Kraaz W & Wakefield AJ. Crohn's disease after *in utero* measles virus exposure. *Lancet* **348**, 515–517, 1996.
116. Lindsay MK. Human immunodeficiency virus and the obstetrician. *Clin. Obstet. Gynecol.* **36**, 821–831, 1993.
117. Centers for Disease Control Update: serologic testing for antibody to human immunodeficiency virus. *MMWR* **36**, 833–840, 1988.
118. Peckham C & Gibb D. Mother-to-child transmission of the human immunodeficiency virus. *N. Engl. J. Med.* **333**, 298–302, 1995.
119. Boyer PJ, Dillon M, Navaie M, Deveikis A, Keller M, O'Rouke S & Bryson YJ. Factors predictive of maternal-fetal transmission of HIV-1. *JAMA* **271**, 1925–1930, 1994.

120. Connor EM, Sperling RS, Gelber R *et al.* Reduction of maternal–infant transmission of human immunodeficiency virus type 1 with zidovudine treatment. *N. Engl. J. Med.* **331**, 1173–1180, 1994.
121. Matheson PB, Abrams EJ, Thomas PA *et al.* Efficacy of antenatal zidovudine in reducing perinatal transmission of human immunodeficiency virus type 1. *J. Infect. Dis.* **172**, 353–358, 1995.
122. Centers for Disease Control Recommendations of the U.S. Public Health Service Task Force on the use of zidovudine to reduce perinatal transmission of human immunodeficiency virus. *MMWR* **43**, 1–20, 1994.
123. Anonymous Zidovudine for the prevention of HIV transmission from mother to infant. *JAMA* **271**, 1567–1568, 1994.
124. Anonymous Birth outcomes following zidovudine therapy in pregnant women. *JAMA* **272**, 17, 1995.
125. Kumar RM, Hughes PF & Khurranna A. Zidovudine use in pregnancy: A report on 104 cases and the occurrence of birth defects. *J. Acquir. Imm. Def. Syndr.* **7**, 1034–1039, 1994.
126. Centers for Disease Control Birth outcomes following zidovudine therapy in pregnant women. *MMWR* **43**, 409–416, 1994.
127. Anonymous Zidovudine for mother, fetus, and child: home or poison? *Lancet* **344**, 207–209, 1994.
128. Tovo P-A. Caesarean section and perinatal HIV transmission: what next? *Lancet* **342**, 630, 1993.
129. European Collaborative Group Caesarean section and risk of vertical transmission of HIV-1 infection. *Lancet* **343**, 1464–1467, 1994.
130. Minkoff H & Mofenson LM. The role of obstetric interventions in the prevention of pediatric human immunodeficiency virus infection. *Am. J. Obstet. Gynecol.* **171**, 1167–1175, 1994.
131. Kuhn L, Bobat R, Coutsoudis A, Moodley D, Coovadia HM, Tsai W-Y & Stein ZA. Cesarean deliveries and maternal–infant HIV transmission: Results from a prospective study in South Africa. *J. Acq. Immune Defic. Syndr. Hum. Reprod.* **11**, 478–483, 1996.
132. Tovo P-A, de Martino M, Gabiano C *et al.* Mode of delivery and gestational age influence perinatal HIV-1 transmission. *J. Acq. Immune Defic. Syndr. Hum. Reprod.* **11**, 88–94, 1996.
133. Semba RD, Miotti PG, Chiphangwi JD, Saah AJ, Canner JK, Dallabetta GA & Hoover DR. Maternal vitamin A deficiency and mother-to-child transmission of HIV-1. *Lancet* **343**, 1593–1597, 1994.
134. Landesman SH, Kalish LA, Burns DN *et al.* Obstetrical factors and the transmission of human immunodeficiency virus type 1 from mother to child. *N. Engl. J. Med.* **334**, 1617–1623, 1996.
135. Dickover RE, Garratty EM *et al.* Identification of levels of maternal HIV-1 RNA associated with risk of perinatal transmission. *JAMA* **275**, 599–605, 1996.
136. Sperling RS, Shapiro DE & Coombs RW *et al.* Maternal viral load, zidovudine treatment, and the risk of transmission of human immunodeficiency virus type 1 from mother to infant. *N. Engl. J. Med.* **335**, 1621–1629, 1996.
137. Coll O, Hernandez M, Boucher CA *et al.* Vertical HIV-1 transmission correlates with a high maternal viral load at delivery. *J. Acq. Immune Defic. Syndr. Hum. Reprod.* **14**, 26–30, 1997.
138. Mayaux MJ, Dussaix E, Isopet J *et al.* Maternal virus load during pregnancy and mother-to-child transmission of human immunodeficiency virus type 1: The French perinatal cohort studies. *J. Infect. Dis.* **175**, 172–175, 1997.
139. Pitt J, Brambilla D, Reichelderfer P *et al.* Maternal immunologic and virologic risk factors for infant human immunodeficiency virus type 1 infection. Findings from the Women and Infants Transmission Study. *J. Inf. Dis.* **175**, 567–575, 1997.
140. Shearer WT, Quinn TC, LaRussa P *et al.* Viral load and disease progression in infants infected with human immunodeficiency virus type 1. *N. Engl. J. Med.* **336**, 1337–1342, 1997.
141. Anderson LJ. Role of parvovirus B19 in human disease. *Pediatr. Inf. Dis. J.* **6**, 711–718, 1987.
142. Shmoys S & Kaplan C. Parvovirus and pregnancy. *Clin. Obstet. Gynecol.* **33**, 268–275, 1990.
143. Gratacós E, Torres P-J, Vidal J *et al.* The incidence of human parvovirus B19 infection during pregnancy and its impact on perinatal outcome. *J. Infect. Dis.* **171**, 1360–1363, 1995.
144. Thurn J. Human parvovirus B19: Historical and clinical review. *Rev. Infect. Dis.* **10**, 1005–1011, 1988.
145. Boley TJ & Popek E. Parvovirus infection in pregnancy. *Sem. Perinat.* **17**, 410–419, 1993.
146. Rodis JF, Hovick TJ, Quinn DL, Rosengren SS & Tattersall P. Human parvovirus infection in pregnancy. *Obstet. Gynecol.* **72**, 733–738, 1988.
147. Anderson MJ. Parvoviruses as agents of human disease. *Prog. Med. Virol.* **34**, 55–69, 1987.
148. Pattison JR. Human parvovirus B19. *BMJ* **308**, 918–919, 1994.
149. Rao KRP, Patel AR, Anderson MJ, Hodgson J, Jones SE & Pattison JR. Infection with parvovirus-like virus and aplastic crisis in chronic hemolytic anemia. *Ann. Intern. Med.* **98**, 930–932, 1983.
150. Török TJ. Parvovirus B19 and human disease. *Adv. Int. Med.* **37**, 431–455, 1992.
151. Cohen B. Parvovirus B19: an expanding spectrum of disease. *BMJ* **311**, 1549–1552, 1995.
152. Rodis JF, Quinn DL, Gary W *et al.* Management and outcomes of pregnancies complicated by human B19 parvovirus infection: A prospective study. *Am. J. Obstet. Gynecol.* **163**, 1168–1171, 1990.
153. Kovacs BW, Carlson DE, Shahbahrami B & Platt LD. Prenatal diagnosis of human parvovirus B19 in nonimmune hydrops fetails by polymerase chain reaction. *Am. J. Obstet. Gynecol.* **167**, 461–466, 1992.
154. Schwarz TF, Jäger G, Holzgreve W & Roggendorf M. Diagnosis of human parvovirus B19 infections by polymerase chain reaction. *Scand. J. Infect. Dis.* **24**, 691–696, 1992.
155. Török TJ, Wang Q-Y, Gary GW, Yang C-F, Finch TM & Anderson LJ. Prenatal diagnosis of intrauterine infection with parvovirus B19 by the polymerase chain reaction technique. *Clin. Infect. Dis.* **14**, 149–155, 1992.
156. Nikkari S & Ekblad U. A rapid and safe method to detect fetal parvovirus B19 infection in amniotic fluid by polymerase chain reaction: Report of a case. *Am. J. Perinatol.* **12**, 447–449, 1995.
157. Maeda H, Shimokawa K, Satoh S, Nakano H & Nunoue T. Nonimmunologic hydrops fetalis resulting from intrauterine human parvovirus B-19 infection: Report of two cases. *Obstet. Gynecol.* **72**, 482–485, 1988.
158. Samra J, Obhrai MS & Constantine G. Parvovirus infection in pregnancy. *Obstet. Gynecol.* **73**, 832–834, 1989.
159. Fairley CK, Smoleniec JS, Caul OE & Miller E. Observational study of effect of intrauterine transfusions on outcome of fetal hydrops after parvovirus B19 infection. *Lancet* **346**, 1335–1337, 1995.
160. Sheikh AU, Ernest JM & O'Shea M. Long-term outcome in fetal hydrops from parvovirus B19 infection. *Am. J. Obstet. Gynecol.* **167**, 337–341, 1992.
161. Pryde PG, Nugent CE, Pridjian G, Barr M & Faix RG. Spontaneous resolution of nonimmune hydrops fetalis secondary to human parvovirus B19 infection. *Obstet. Gynecol.* **79**, 859–861, 1992.
162. Centers for Disease Control Risks associated with human parvovirus B19 infection. *MMWR* **38**, 81–97, 1989.
163. Yaegashi N, Okamura K, Yajima A, Murai C & Sugamura K. The frequency of human parvovirus B19 infection in non-immune hydrops fetalis. *J. Perinat. Med.* **22**, 159–163, 1994.
164. Yaegashi N, Okamura K, Tsunoda A, Nakamura M, Sugamura K & Yajima A. A study by means of a new assay of the relationship between an outbreak of *erythema infectiosum* and non-immune *hydrops fetalis* caused by human parvovirus B19. *J: Infect.* **31**, 195–200, 1995.
165. Jordan JA. Identification of human parvovirus B19 infection in idiopathic nonimmune hydrops fetalis. *Am. J. Obstet. Gynecol.* **174**, 37–42, 1996.
166. Tiessen RG, van Elsacker-Niele AMW, Vermeij-Keers C, Oepkes D, van Roosmalen J & Gorsira MCB. A fetus with a parvovirus B19 infection and congenital anomalies. *Prenat. Diagn.* **14**, 173–176, 1994.
167. Evans TN & Brown GC. Congenital anomalies and virus infections. *Am. J. Obstet. Gynecol.* **87**, 749–761, 1963.
168. Brown GC & Evans TN. Serologic evidence of coxsackievirus etiology of congenital heart disease. *JAMA* **199**, 183–187, 1967.
169. Brown GC & Karunas RS. Relationship of congenital anomalies and maternal infection with selected enteroviruses. *Am. J. Epidemiol.* **95**, 207–217, 1972.
170. Burch GE, Sun S-C, Chu K-C, Sohal RS & Colcolough HL. Interstitial and coxsackievirus B myocarditis in infants and children. *JAMA* **203**, 1–8, 1968.
171. Johansson ME, Holmström S, Abebe A, Jacobsson B, Ekman G, Samuelson A & Wirgart BZ. Intrauterine fetal death due to echovirus 11. *Scand. J. Infect. Dis.* **24**, 381–385, 1992.

172. Dahlquist GG, Ivarsson S, Lindberg B & Forsgren M. Maternal enteroviral infection during pregnancy as a risk factor for childhood IDDM. *Diabetes* **44**, 408–413, 1995.
173. Towbin JA, Griffin LD, Martin A *et al.* Intrauterine adenoviral myocarditis presenting as nonimmune hydrops fetalis: diagnosis by polymerase chain reaction. *Pediatr. Infect. Dis. J.* **13**, 144–150, 1994.
174. Martin AB, Webber S, Fricker FJ *et al.* Acute myocarditis: Rapid diagnosis by PCR in children. *Circulation* **90**, 330–339, 1994.
175. Ranucci-Weiss D, Uerpairojkit B, Bowles N, Towbin JA & Chan L. Intrauterine adenovirual infection associated with fetal non-immune hydrops. *Prenat. Diagn.* **18**, 182–185, 1998.
176. Larsen PD, Chartrand SA, Tomashek KM, Hauser LG & Ksiazek TG. Hydrocephalus complicating lymphocytic choriomeningitis virus infection. *Pediatr. Infect. Dis. J.* **12**, 528–531, 1993.
177. Stephensen CB, Blount SR, Lanford RE, Holmes KV, Montali RJ, Fleenor ME & Shaw JFE. Prevalence of serum antibodies against lymphocytic choriomeningitis virus in selected populations from two U.S. cities. *J. Med. Virol.* **38**, 27–31, 1992.
178. Ambrosio AM, Feuillade MR, Gamboa GS & Maiztegui JI. Prevalence of lymphocytic choriomeningitis virus infection in a human population of Argentina. *Am. J. Trop. Med. Hyg.* **50**, 381–386, 1994.
179. Childs JE, Glass GE, Korch GW, Ksiazek TG & Leduc JW. Lymphocytic choriomeningitis virus infection and house mouse (*Mus Musculus*) distribution in urban Baltimore. *Am. J. Trop. Med. Hyg.* **47**, 27–34, 1992.
180. Löhler J, Gossmann J, Kratzberg T & Lehmann-Grube F. Murine hepatitis caused by lymphocytic choriomeningitis virus-I. The hepatic lesions. *Lab. Invest.* **70**, 263–278, 1994.
181. Montali RJ, Connolly BM, Armstrong DL, Scanga CA & Holmes KV. Pathology and immunohistochemistry of Callitrichid hepatitis, an emerging disease of captive New World primates caused by lymphocytic choriomeningitis virus. *Am. J. Pathol.* **148**, 1441–1449, 1995.
182. Stephensen CB, Park JY & Blount SR.cDNA sequence analysis confirms that the etiologic agent of Callitrichid hepatitis is lymphocytic choriomeningitis virus. *J. Virol.* **69**, 1349–1352 , 1995.
183. Van den Veyver IB, Ni J, Bowles N *et al.* Detection of intrauterine viral infection using the polymerase chain reaction (PCR). *Molec. Genet. Metab.* **63**, 85–89, 1998.

Twins and polyhydramnios

65

M. Denbow and N. Fisk

Introduction

The incidence of twin pregnancies is geographically dependent and ranges from as low as 4.3 per thousand births in Japan to as high as 54 per thousand in Nigeria[1]. In the UK the current rate is 12.5 per thousand births[2], an increase of 25% compared to the early 1980s. The incidence is highest in older women (19.1 per thousand in women aged 35–39 in 1992) among whom the greatest increase (25%) occurred as a result of assisted reproductive techniques (ART). Three-quarters of twin pregnancies are dizygotic (DZ). The incidence of monozygotic (MZ) twinning is 3–5 per thousand pregnancies, a rate which is largely independent of geography and maternal age. Evidence is emerging, however, that MZ twinning rates, long believed to be fairly constant throughout the world, are now increasing. Some have related the rise in MZ twinning rates to the increased use of the combined oral contraceptive pill, although this may simply represent a temporal rather than causal relationship. Similarly, there is some evidence that the rate of monozygous twinning is increased by ART. Indeed, one group found that the incidence of monochorionic twins following all forms of ART was eight times the population rate[3]. These findings further confirm previous work that post-implantation embryo cleavage does occur[4]. The mechanism for this phenomenon remains unclear, although it has long been known in fish that alterations in local environment, such as oxygen supply and temperature, can increase the MZ twinning rate[5]. In mammals, both a delay in implantation[6], and exposure of the blastocyst to a culture environment[7], can precipitate monozygotic embryonic cleavage.

This small increase in frequency of multiple pregnancy will have a disproportionate effect on perinatal mortality and morbidity. Twins have an eightfold increased risk of cerebral palsy and there is a 47-fold increase in triplets[8]. Perinatal mortality and morbidity are highest in same sex pregnancies, suggesting increased risk in the perinatal period in the presence of monozygosity[2]. There is increasing evidence that much of this risk is attributable to the two-thirds of MZ twins that are monochorionic (MC).

The temporal sequence of the splitting of the early cell mass in MZ conceptions determines chorionicity. Splitting on post-fertilization days 1 to 3 results in dichorionic, diamniotic (DCDA) placentation, whereas when the twinning process occurs at a later gestational age the fetuses will be firstly monochorionic, diamniotic (MCDA) (days 3 to 8), and then monochorionic monoamniotic (MCMA) (days 8 to 10); thereafter twinning becomes much less likely because of the enlarging embryonic/placental masses. Conjoined twins may develop during a narrow window of time soon after the primitive stalk is formed, with incomplete division of the embryonic cell mass[9]. Older theories of the possible fusion of the embryos at a point after the twinning process[10] have not been substantiated.

Perinatal morbidity and mortality in monochorionic (MC) twins is three- to fivefold higher than in dichorionic (DC) twins[11–13]. Much of the increase in risk is due to the presence of vascular anastomoses which are implicated in feto-fetal transfusion syndrome (FFTS) and the co-twin sequelae after intrauterine death of one twin.

Polyhydramnios

CONTROL OF AMNIOTIC FLUID VOLUME

Amniotic fluid volume regulation remains poorly understood. In the first trimester, amniotic fluid is considered initially a maternal dialysate, and then a fetal transudate, since its composition resembles that of maternal and then fetal serum[14]. After 15 weeks with progressive impermeability of fetal skin, amniotic fluid becomes increasingly hypotonic with greater concentrations of urea and creatinine, implicating fetal urine as the major contributor[15]. In addition, there is a net outflow of lung liquid although fetal swallowing accounts for much of this volume[16].

The major routes of amniotic fluid clearance include fetal swallowing and transmembranous flow. Human fetuses with lesions preventing swallowing often develop polyhydramnios[17], a phenomenon confirmed in animal experiments following oesophageal occlusion[18]. Bulk flow of fluid across permeable membranes between maternal, fetal and amniotic compartments occurs in response to osmotic[19] and hydrostatic gradients[20]. Consistent with this is the correlation between maternal plasma and amniotic fluid volume in human pregnancies with both normal and abnormal quantities of amniotic fluid[21].

It is not known whether the intramembranous pathway (from the amniotic cavity via vascularised membranes into the fetal circulation) documented in sheep plays a role in amniotic fluid volume control in the human fetus. The fetus is known to be able to alter its urine production by releasing vasoactive peptides such as vasopressin and atrial natriuretic peptide (ANP) in response to changes in maternal and fetal intravascular volume[22]. This suggests that alterations in amniotic fluid volume in response to changes in maternal fluid balance occur via their effect on fetal fluid balance[23]. Amniotic fluid arises from secondary partitioning of water within the fetoplacental extracellular space and reflects fetal fluid balance. Polyhydramnios develops as a result of the loss of control of the normal pathways involved in amniotic fluid balance.

CAUSES OF POLYHYDRAMNIOS

Polyhydramnios has been associated in singletons with a number of either fetal or maternal conditions. Disorders of the gastrointestinal, musculoskeletal and central nervous systems are the main fetal anomalies implicated with polyhydramnios[24,25], where impairment of fetal swallowing seems the predominant mechanism. Recent improvements in the management of diabetic pregnancies has resulted in the sharp decrease of polyhydramnios in affected pregnancies, with a recent review of 10 000 births showing an incidence of polyhydramnios of only 0.6%[26]. The most common cause was fetal malformation accounting for over a quarter of cases. There were also significantly higher frequencies of diabetic, aneuploid, virally-infected and multiple pregnancies in the polyhydramnios group. Maternal drug administration may also affect fetal urinary output, most notably with maternal lithium therapy. Lithium, which is widely used to treat bipolar affective disorders, can induce a nephrogenic diabetes insipidus-type polyuria both in the mother and also in the fetus, leading to polyhydramnios[27].

The most common cause of polyhydramnios in multiple gestations is FFTS which is characterised by the poly-/oligohydramnios sequence in monochorionic twins. Rarer causes include the twin reversed arterial perfusion sequence (TRAP) or thoracopagus conjoined twins where fetal swallowing in one or both twins may be impaired. Finally, a multiple pregnancy may be discordant for any of the fetal causes for polyhydramnios.

EFFECTS OF POLYHYDRAMNIOS

Polyhydramnios is associated with preterm labour; a rate corrected for congenital anomalies of 22% has been reported[28]. In many cases, premature rupture of membranes (PROM) precedes the onset of preterm labour[29]. Because amniotic pressure is raised in polyhydramnios[30], these complications have all been attributed to uterine overdistension. However, others have proposed that the aetiology of the polyhydramnios itself, rather than the excess of fluid/increased amniotic pressure, is a greater determinant of outcome[31]. In addition, severe polyhydramnios may produce maternal abdominal discomfort, respiratory embarrassment, renal failure and uterine irritability[29,32].

The increased incidence of congenital malformations, preterm labour and asphyxial complications such as abruption, cord prolapse and placental insufficiency result in perinatal mortality rates as high as 13–29%[25,26,28]. Three main variables influence perinatal survival in polyhydramnios: the presence of congenital anomalies, gestational age at delivery and severity of polyhydramnios. In a series of 537 singletons with polyhydramnios, perinatal mortality was 61% in the presence of fetal or placental malformations, 10% with maternal diabetes and only 2.4% in their absence[33]. In severe FFTS, the untreated perinatal mortality rate exceeds 80% when detected before 28 weeks[34,35]. Acute polyhydramnios complicating FFTS accounts for 17% of overall perinatal mortality in twins[36].

In addition to the specific complications of preterm delivery and congenital malformations, there also is an excess of unexplained stillbirths seen in fetuses with normal anatomy. It has been suggested that raised amniotic pressure in polyhydramnios impairs uteroplacental perfusion[37] based on observations of changes in fetal condition during iatrogenic polyhydramnios from intrapartum amnioinfusion. Indeed, in a study of fetuses with polyhydramnios investigated by blood sampling, fetal pH and P_{O_2} were inversely correlated with amniotic pressure[38].

DIAGNOSIS OF POLYHYDRAMNIOS

Liquor volume is assessed ultrasonographically. The measurement of a single deepest vertical pool (DVP) has now largely been replaced by the semiquantitative amniotic fluid index (AFI). The AFI is the sum of the DVP in each of four quadrants of the uterus. When measuring the AFI, care should be taken to ensure that the transducer is held in a vertical plane and that undue pressure is not used[39]. Polyhydramnios is defined as an AFI >25 cm[40], and so the severity of polyhydramnios can be quantified, both as a baseline and for prognosis. Several studies have confirmed that this method is fairly reproducible and is a reasonable indicator of actual amniotic fluid volume[41–46]. Nevertheless, the AFI overestimates the incidence of oligohydramnios and underestimates that of polyhydramnios[42].

A detailed ultrasound is performed for structural malformations with particular emphasis on the upper gastrointestinal tract and its associated structures. Neurological function is assessed by observing fetal movements and in twin pregnancies, chorionicity is determined if not previously done.

Polyhydramnios is associated with aneuploidy in 5% of cases[47], rising to 13% in the presence of a congenital malformation[48], and therefore we recommend karyotyping. In MC twins, and in the absence of any other pathology, the likely cause for polyhydramnios will be FFTS, particularly if there is oligohydramnios around the co-twin. Rarely, it may be secondary to TRAP, which is readily recognised by the presence of the grossly abnormal acardiac recipient twin.

TREATMENT OF POLYHYDRAMNIOS

The goal in treating polyhydramnios is the safe and effective reduction in amniotic fluid volume, and hence pressure, in an attempt to relieve maternal discomfort and to prolong further the pregnancy. In all cases, the cause for the polyhydramnios should be sought and if possible corrected; however, if this is not successful both surgical and medical therapies are available.

AMNIOREDUCTION

Amnioreduction was first described over 50 years ago[49], and seems successful in reducing maternal symptoms and prolonging gestation in both singleton and twin pregnancies. Most workers were initially conservative in the selection of the amniotic volume to be removed in view of concerns regarding precipitation of abruption or preterm labour[50,51]. Indeed, raised amniotic pressure in severe polyhydramnios is restored to normal by removal of relatively small volumes[52]. However, with rapid re-accumulation of fluid, it seems likely that amniotic pressure soon rises again. Accordingly, one group[35] considered restitution of normal amniotic fluid volume the more important goal and drained much larger volumes, up to 5000 ml in 29 procedures. Their promising results using 'aggressive therapeutic amniocentesis' with reversal of hydrops in the recipient and of oligohydramnios in the donor support their claim[53].

In a large series of 200 amnioreductions, the complication rate was 1.5%[54], with only one case of abruption which followed removal of 10 litres of amniotic fluid. It may be prudent therefore to limit the volume removed to 5–6 litres and perhaps less before 20 weeks' gestation. Patients having contractions at the time of amnioreduction are known to have a greater risk of preterm delivery following the procedure[55]. Ideally, amnioreduction should be performed before the onset of contractions or cervical dilatation.

To avoid supine hypotension, the patient is wedged in the left lateral position and care taken to make the patient as comfortable as the procedure may take up to one hour. A sterile technique, together with prophylactic intravenous antibiotics, is employed. A large amniotic pocket is located by ultrasound slightly lateral and midway down the uterus. The needle entry site is chosen both to avoid the placenta and allow maximal flexibility of the needle to minimise maternal discomfort and contractions as the relationship between the overlying skin, uterus and amniotic cavity changes greatly during drainage. Local anaesthetic is instilled and the skin pierced with a scalpel blade. An 18-gauge needle is inserted into the pool under ultrasound guidance, and following the removal of the trochar, intra-amniotic pressure is measured. A 50-ml syringe is then attached to the three-way tap and fluid is aspirated continuously until the AFI is decreased into the normal range (DVP <8 cm). We have recently shown a linear relationship between the ΔAFI and volume of fluid removed, so that the volume required to be drained may be estimated before the amnioreduction to obviate the need for multiple intraprocedural amniotic fluid estimations[46] (Fig. 65.1). The fluid is removed as rapidly as possible to avoid a lengthy procedure and thus discomfort to the mother. At the end of the procedure, the intra-amniotic pressure is remeasured. Thereafter the patient is monitored two or three times per week by ultrasound; repeat amnioreductions as with the first are then indicated in the presence of maternal symptoms or an AFI >40 cm (or DVP >12 cm).

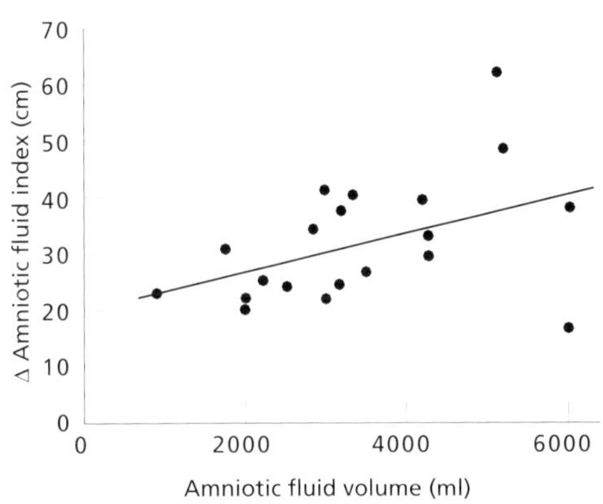

Fig. 65.1 Linear relationships between ΔAFI and volume removed at amnioreduction in twin pregnancies complicated by severe polyhydramnios ($y = 0.0034x + 20.14$). (Data adapted from Denbow, M., Sepulveda, W., Ridout, D., Fisk, N. (1997) Relationship of the change in amniotic fluid index with the volume of fluid removed at amnioreduction. *Obstet. Gynecol.* **90**, 529–532).

PROSTAGLANDIN SYNTHASE INHIBITOR DRUGS

The evidence of decreased urinary flow rates in neonates given indomethacin[56] led to the demonstration of reduced hourly fetal urine production[57] and subsequent amniotic fluid volume[57–60]. Indomethacin appears effective in treating symptomatic polyhydramnios when the underlying aetiology is associated with increased urine output. The response is limited when polyhydramnios is secondary to poor fetal swallowing such as neuromuscular disorders or gastrointestinal obstruction[61].

Two mechanisms by which indomethacin reduces urine output have been proposed[62]. Urine production may be altered by blood flow being directed away from the inner and more mature nephrons. Although Doppler studies of the renal artery are unchanged by treatment[63], in fetal sheep exposed to indomethacin renal blood flow overall is unchanged, but flow to the inner cortex is reduced[64]. Another mechanism is reduced inhibition of arginine-vasopressin by prostaglandin E in the renal collecting duct[65]. Concomitant administration of an arginine-vasopressin V_2-receptor antagonist with indomethacin in sheep blocks the oliguric and free-water clearance effect of indomethacin alone[66].

The side-effects of indomethacin have raised concern. Maternal side-effects after oral or rectal administration have mainly been limited to the gastrointestinal tract, although cases of renal insufficiency, cholestatic jaundice and pulmonary oedema have been reported[67]. The predominant concern, however, is with the fetal side-effects, in particular oligohydramnios[68], premature closure of the ductus arteriosus[69] and cerebral vasoconstriction[70]. Monitoring ductal patency by Doppler has been recommended, particularly when treatment lasts longer than 72 hours, as neonatal pulmonary hypertension and persistent fetal circulation are presumed to occur in fetuses with prolonged ductal constriction *in utero*[69]. Neonatal complications from premature closure of the ductus *in utero* appear very rare, and indeed overall only 26% of exposed fetuses develop abnormal ductal waveforms[71]. However, 50% of fetuses will demonstrate ductal constriction and/or tricuspid regurgitation by 32 weeks' gestation[72] and therefore therapy is not recommended beyond this gestation. Fetal echocardiography in patients on long-term indomethacin is recommended 24 hours after starting treatment and weekly thereafter[72]. The dose should be reduced if ductal constriction and/or tricuspid regurgitation occur, and if necessary stopped in order to achieve reversal[73]. Others have reported rarer fetal complications including neonatal renal failure[74,75], neonatal patent ductus arteriosus, necrotising enterocolitis[76] and fetal pleural effusions[77]. The relatively long period of time for a normal amniotic fluid volume to be attained with the sole use of indomethacin has led to one group advocating an initial amnioreduction prior to maternal indomethacin administration[61]. Indomethacin may also be useful in moderate polyhydramnios to avoid the need for amnioreduction. Indomethacin is not recommended in FFTS because of concern about further jeopardising renal function in the already oliguric donor[74].

Other prostaglandin synthase inhibitors, similar in structure to indomethacin, have recently been introduced. Sulindac has been shown successfully to reduce amniotic fluid volume in three sets of monoamniotic twins in the second trimester to reduce gross fetal movements and avoid further cord entanglement. Amniotic fluid volume was reduced from normal to relative oligohydramnios and there was no evidence of ductal constriction during therapy[78]. Sulindac therefore appears to have a role in treating polyhydramnios, and although in comparison to indomethacin it may have a less pronounced effect on fetal urine production, the constrictive effects on the ductus arteriosus seem less likely.

Polyhydramnios in dichorionic twins

Discordancy for polyhydramnios in a dichorionic multiple pregnancy is most commonly secondary to structural abnormality in one of the fetuses. Rarely, both fetal sacs may have excessive amniotic fluid, as in the example of twins concordant for any of the above abnormalities, or in the presence of maternal causes such as poorly controlled diabetes.

DIAGNOSIS

The diagnosis of polyhydramnios is made on the usual parameter of an AFI >28 cm. In twins, this is commonly measured as a total for the whole pregnancy, with subjective or objective (in the form of each sac's maximal DVP) quantification for each sac. Individual AFI measurements are less usually made for the four quadrants of each twin's sac. Detailed anomaly scanning of both fetuses is then indicated in an attempt to elucidate the cause for polyhydramnios. As in singletons, particular attention is paid to the exclusion of abnormal fetal tone/movement (arthrogryposis), neck attitude (goitre), absent stomach (oesophageal atresia) and absent cranial development (anencephaly). Other markers for aneuploidy should be excluded, but even in their absence, invasive karyotypic assessment is offered.

TREATMENT

The choice of treatment for dichorionic twins discordant for polyhydramnios can be difficult, and is often governed by the legal gestational limit for termination of pregnancy. In 1994, the collaborative experience of second trimester selective termination from nine worldwide centres was published[79], reviewing the outcome of over 180 procedures, the majority of which employed intracardiac potassium chloride administration. Complete abortion occurred in 12.6%, with an increased loss rate if the procedure was performed after 16 weeks' gestation. Forty-two percent of the remaining fetuses delivered preterm, but only 16% were before 32 weeks' gestation. These results were similar to the one-third rate of preterm labour, and over 80% survival rate reported by another group in an earlier review of 22 cases[80]. The loss rate following selective fetocide in one of two MC twins in these series was over 85% (7 of 8 fetuses). These studies therefore showed that selective termination as then performed was contraindicated in MC twins. However, the development of occlusive termination techniques, to prevent the acute transfusion of the surviving twin into its dead co-twin, has allowed the cautious use of selective fetocide in MC twins (see below).

Twins discordant for anencephaly represent a dilemma for the clinician, where the choice is whether to intervene or pursue conservative management. On the one hand, selective termination places the unaffected twin at risk of miscarriage, while on the other hand, conservative management may allow severe polyhydramnios to develop with the attendant risk of preterm labour and amniorrhexis. In a review of 14 cases of dichorionic twins discordant for anencephaly, Lipitz and colleagues argue the case for conservative management[81]. They found polyhydramnios occurred in fewer than half the cases (43%), and that only 21% of the pregnancies were delivered before 35 weeks' gestation. Overall, the outcome was good for the unaffected twin, with just one infant death secondary to unrelated causes. In countries where termination of pregnancy is permitted for severe fetal abnormality, a third option of management may be pursued. It is our practice to follow expectant management, but if severe polyhydramnios develops, a selective termination can then be performed at the time of the first amnioreduction to negate the need for repeated amnioreductions, therefore reducing the overall risk to the unaffected twin. Indeed, in a review of 36 cases where selective fetocide was performed after 24 weeks' gestation, there was only one co-twin pregnancy loss, with over 80% of the remaining pregnancies extending beyond 34 weeks[82].

Placental vascular anastomoses in dichorionic twins have been reported but are exceedingly rare[83]. Some have argued that their presence should be excluded prior to fetocide to preclude the chance of acute transfusion from the healthy twin into its terminated co-twin. Potential intertwin transfusion in the direction from the unaffected to affected twin can only be identified by injection at fetal blood sampling of a marker substance, such as adult blood[84] with confirmation of its passage into the affected twin at a further fetal blood sampling. More recent alternatives such as pancuronium[85] or an ultrasound microbubble contrast agent[86] (Plate 65.1) injection into the unaffected twin, require sampling of only one twin. The procedure, however, carries a further chance of loss in addition to those associated with selective termination[79], which in our view outweighs the remote chance of anastomotic intertwin blood flow, and therefore is not recommended.

Polyhydramnios in monochorionic twins

The overwhelming majority of cases of polyhydramnios in monochorionic twins will be secondary to FFTS. Rarer causes include TRAP, and thoracopagus conjoined twins where fetal swallowing may be impaired.

FETO-FETAL TRANSFUSION SYNDROME

FFTS complicates 4–35% of MCDA twin pregnancies[87,88] and accounts for 15–17% of overall perinatal mortality in twins[36,89]. It has classically been attributed to transfusion of blood via placental vascular anastomoses between the two fetuses' circulations, causing anaemia and growth restriction in the twin denoted the 'donor', and polycythaemia with circulatory overload in the 'recipient'[90,91].

Presentation in the mid-trimester has until recently been associated with an 80–100% perinatal wastage rate, mainly from preterm delivery secondary to polyhydramnios[34,89]. Recent treatments such as serial amnioreduction[92], amniotic septostomy[93], laser ablation of placental vessels[94] and selective fetocide[95] have resulted in an approximate halving of these rates; nevertheless neurological, cardiac and renal sequelae are common in survivors.

DIAGNOSIS OF FFTS

Initially, a diagnosis of FFTS was based on neonatal criteria, comprising a difference in cord blood haemoglobin concentrations >5 g/dl, and a difference in birthweights ≥20%[90,91,96]. However, with the widespread availability of diagnostic ultrasonography, these criteria have now been abandoned. Furthermore, it is now clear that severe FFTS, without intervention, leads to amniorrhexis and preterm labour/miscarriage with a perinatal mortality rate approaching 100%. This implies that many of the cases of 'FFTS' diagnosed by the neonatal criteria may in fact either be describing mild disease, unassociated with severe polyhydramnios, or cases within the normal spectrum for MC twins. This is supported by several findings.

Firstly, these criteria are frequently satisfied by discordant growth restriction in twins. Impaired fetal growth is a known cause of polycythaemia, and indeed more than half the cases of haemoglobin (7 of 13) and weight discordance (14 of 26) in one series occurred in DC pregnancies[97]. Even in known MC placentae, one-third of cases with both haemoglobin and birthweight discordance had polycythaemia in the smaller twin[98]. Secondly, Raussen found that 15% of MC twins without FFTS had a haemoglobin difference >5 g/dl, in contrast to 46 DC twin pairs, which all had a difference <3.3 g/dl[90]. Thirdly, fetal blood sampling studies have shown that the previously-considered requisite haemoglobin difference is rarely present *in utero*[99,100]. These studies were done predominantly in the mid-trimester, whereas the neonatal studies were done in the third trimester, when they may also have been influenced by labour. Fetal blood sampling data from Queen Charlotte's and Chelsea Hospital and Milan show that a haemoglobin difference between donor and recipient ≥5 g/dl is present in only approximately 20% of cases of FFTS *in utero*[101]. The situation also appears relatively dynamic as we have anecdotally observed relatively acute changes in haemoglobin difference within periods as short as 1–14 days. Other authors conclude that significant, albeit lesser, haemoglobin differences do in fact exist *in utero* with one group advocating a haemoglobin discordancy of >2.4 g/dl as diagnostic of the condition[102].

In contrast, most cases of FFTS do have estimated fetal weight discordance *in utero*[99,103]. Weight estimates are, however, subject to the usual 10–15% measurement error, and accordingly are difficult to use diagnostically. Differences <15% are unusual. There is some evidence that the prognosis worsens with increasing change in abdominal circumference measurements[104], cumulatively reflecting the severity of overload/early hydrops in the recipient and growth restriction in the donor.

The syndrome presents in the second trimester with discordant amniotic fluid volume. The donor twin becomes oliguric, with consequent oligohydramnios, hence appearing enshrouded within its membrane and finally stuck to the uterine wall. In addition, neither the urinary bladder nor the stomach are usually visible, once anhydramnios is present. The growth velocity of the donor may follow the asymmetrical pattern seen with fetuses affected by intrauterine growth restriction. Furthermore, it may also exhibit abnormal umbilical and middle cerebral artery velocities, with absent/reversed flow in the former, and redistribution in the latter[105].

The overloaded recipient develops polyuria and severe polyhydramnios. The bladder becomes chronically distended, and only voids incompletely. Venous Doppler studies in the recipient fetus deteriorate in accordance with the disease process. There may be evidence of pulsatile venous flow, progressing to reverse end-diastolic flow within the ductus venosus[106]. The development of tricuspid regurgitation indicates worsening of the right-sided cardiac failure.

We recommend fetal echocardiography, both to document cardiac dysfunction and to look for congenital heart disease, for which these fetuses are at increased risk by virtue of being monozygotic. Aneuploidy is rare in FFTS, but if it is suspected in MC twins with fetal anomalies, genetic risk counselling should be based on the 'double-or-nothing' risk for MZ twins, i.e. either both or neither twins will be affected.

Surveillance of fetal well-being can be difficult, but is of great importance should there be any concern that either twin might die *in utero*. Perceived fetal movements may be decreased, because the donor's movements are restricted, and the polyhydramnios may sometimes mask the usually active recipient fetus. Therefore, regular ultrasonographic and Doppler assessment are important in the management of these pregnancies.

The diagnosis of mid-trimester FFTS should be restricted to MC pregnancies with complete discordance of amniotic fluid volume. This is because there are no other known pathologies in MC twins that result in severe oligohydramnios in one and severe polyhydramnios in the other sac. This statement, however, does not preclude some other pathology such as discordant congenital abnormality or infection initiating feto-fetal transfusion[107].

VASCULAR BASIS OF FFTS

Many authors have erroneously considered the presence of anastomoses, or indeed the demonstration of intertwin transfusion, as diagnostic of FFTS. However, it is now evident that anastomoses and intertwin transfusion are simply diagnostic of MC placentation.

The anatomy of MC placentae, and in particular the presence of intertwin vascular anastomoses, was first described over a century ago[108]. Subsequent work has confirmed that these anastomoses are usually multiple, and of different types, either superficial or deep (Fig. 65.2). The superficial anastomoses lie on the surface of the chorionic plate, and are direct vascular connections between the two fetal circulations; they may be either artery-to-artery (A-A) or vein-to-vein (V-V). The so-called 'deep anastomoses' in fact describe a shared cotyledon, which derives its arterial supply from one twin and drains its venous flow to the other (A-V).

It seems likely, therefore, that intertwin transfusion is a normal event in most MC pregnancies, but can lead to specific disease states should significant imbalance in flow occur. Anastomoses were previously believed never to occur in DC placentae, although they have been identified with extreme rarity[83].

Intertwin transfusion has been shown *in vivo*, by the injection of marker substances, either adult erythrocytes or pancuronium, into one twin with the subsequent identification of the presence of the marker in the co-twin[84,85,99]. These studies, however, are based on small numbers, predominantly of MC pregnancies with FFTS, and the degree of intertwin

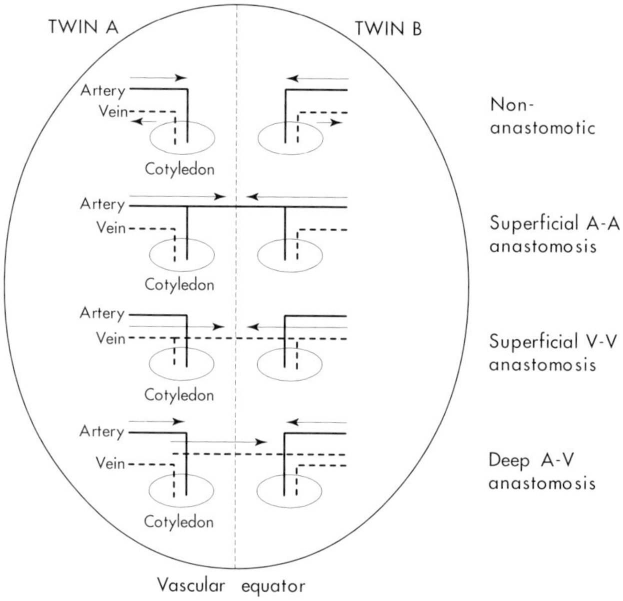

Fig. 65.2 The vascular configuration of anastomoses within monochorionic placentae. From top to bottom: non-anastomotic; superficial A-A anastomosis; superficial V-V anastomosis; deep A-V anastomosis.

transfusion in MC pregnancies uncomplicated by FFTS remains unknown. Superficial anastomoses can be visualised by power Doppler, and the bidirectional flow velocity waveforms have recently been shown by computer analysis to reflect the summation of arterial waveforms of different heart rates from opposing directions[109]. These are indicative of intertwin transfusion, and we have recently shown that they are present in the majority of MC pregnancies[110].

Theoretically, only A-V channels should produce unidirectional flow from one twin to the other. However, superficial A-A or V-V anastomoses could also produce unidirectional flow, when a disturbance in the respective twins' circulatory pressures results in a shift of the zero-flow area along the A-A anastomosis away from the vascular equator, enabling the one twin to recruit cotyledons from the other, thus producing a functional A-V anastomosis. In this way, the superficial vessels have been implicated in the sequelae of co-twin intrauterine death[111], as the initially healthy twin transfuses blood into the dead twin's circulation[112,113]. This results in a 25% incidence of necrotic neurological and renal lesions in co-twin survivors[111], and a similar risk of intrauterine death in the initially healthy co-twin, which we have recently estimated as 20–25%, based on 49 affected MC pregnancies (Fusi *et al.*, unpublished observations).

More than 90 years ago, Schatz proposed that the circulatory imbalance in FFTS was the result of deep A-V anastomoses[114]. However, attempts at correlating MC vascular anatomy with neonatal outcome proved inconclusive for several reasons, including the small numbers inherent in these studies, the use of the now discredited neonatal diagnostic criteria and in the absence of ultrasound, the inability to exclude FFTS in any control population[88,114–116].

These deficiencies were addressed in a prospective placental perfusion study[103], in which both control and FFTS pregnancies were monitored with serial ultrasound, and the diagnostic criterion for FFTS was markedly discordant amniotic fluid volume. Postnatal placental vascular anatomy was characterised in controlled experiments, with dye-contrast perfusion delineating the anastomoses. Anastomoses in MC pregnancies with mid-trimester FFTS were significantly fewer in number (median one versus six respectively), and more likely to be solitary and of deep A-V type, than those without FFTS. In general, FFTS placentae were characterised by a paucity of superficial anastomoses. Control non-FFTS placentae had multiple anastomoses of all three types, and the majority with multiple A-V anastomoses had these running in both directions. This study, recently confirmed by another group[117], supports the concept that although intertwin transfusion occurs in almost all MC twin pregnancies, it is likely to be bidirectional and therefore balanced in pregnancies that do not develop FFTS. The *in utero* identification of A-A anastomoses in 71% of 28 unaffected MC twin pregnancies, but in one of 12 cases of FFTS[110], further supports the hypothesis that superficial anastomoses compensate for the haemodynamic imbalance set up by the deep ones[108,118], and thus protect against the development of FFTS. The absence of A-A anastomoses on rigorous Doppler study should allow prospectively for prediction of pregnancies at risk of FFTS.

PATHOPHYSIOLOGY OF FFTS

Excessive amniotic fluid volume in the one sac is attributed to ANP-mediated polyuria in the recipient. Rosen *et al.* reported that hourly fetal urine production rates in three FFTS recipients exceeded the 95th centile for gestation in singletons, whereas that in control twins did not[119]. Indeed, in clinical practice the recipient's bladder is seen to be chronically full, and to empty frequently and incompletely. ANP has been shown to be elevated in cord blood of most recipient but not donor fetuses, albeit in small series[120,121]. The extent to which this results from raised right atrial pressure versus hypoxia is not known[122]. ANP has been shown to rise with the volume load of intravascular transfusion in some but not all human fetuses[123,124], while in sheep, acute hypoxia appears the more potent stimulus to ANP release[125].

Understanding of the pathophysiology of FFTS has been limited both by the relative inaccessibility of the human fetus, and by the lack of a suitable animal model with MC placentation. Accordingly, our group developed a computer model of MC twins linking known fetal and placental physiological variables in a dynamic model of haemotological, hydro-osmotic and metabolic relationships. The clinical features of FFTS could be reproduced by intertwin transfusion along placental vascular anastomoses between twins with otherwise identical physiology[126]. In particular, various experimental combinations of interplacental A-V anastomoses were introduced, to determine which combination led to the most florid sequelae. The direction and symmetry of A-V anastomoses determined the net hydrostatic and osmotic gradients and thus FFTS severity, with the more extreme findings occurring with increasing numbers of unidirectional anastomoses in the same direction only. These findings support the theory that FFTS is caused by net imbalance in flow between the fetuses, which is set up by the unidirectional A-V anastomoses.

The recipient fetus may develop hydrops, the mechanism of which has been assumed to be volume overload. Doppler studies have shown that severe cases are often associated with venous waveform patterns consistent with raised central venous pressure[106,127]. Typically recipient fetuses with cardiac dysfunction develop cardiomegaly, tricuspid regurgitation, ventricular hypertrophy and right ventricular outflow tract obstruction (RVOT)[128]. The RVOT obstruction could simply be attributed to the cardiac sequelae of transfusional volume overload, although recent work suggests in contrast that raised afterload may be present. Firstly, umbilical venous pressure is not raised in all hydropic recipients[129]. Next, plasma levels of endothelin-1, a potent endothelially-derived vasoconstrictor are two- to threefold higher in recipient fetuses compared to donor and control fetuses[130]. This would be consistent with observations of relative hypertension in recipient twins in the neonatal period[131]. Furthermore, using colour Doppler, we have anecdotally observed reversed flow in the pulmonary duct of a recipient fetus with right ventricular dysfunction. In recipient twins, therefore, the increased afterload with elevated pressure in the systemic circulation leads to high pressure in the ductus arteriosus and obstructed outflow to the right ventricle, resulting in the development of congestive heart failure and right ventricular hypertrophy, which could secondarily mediate RVOT.

THERAPEUTIC OPTIONS FOR FFTS

A variety of treatments including transplacental drug therapy, selective fetocide, amnioreduction, laser ablation of the intertwin placental anastomoses, and intrauterine venesection and exchange transfusion, have been attempted, with varying degrees of success. There continues to be little consensus on the optimal treatment, and current therapies remain far from ideal.

Drug Treatment

Maternal administration of digoxin in a single case of FFTS with recipient cardiac failure appeared effective in improving recipient cardiac failure[132], although this has not been confirmed. Prostaglandin synthase inhibitors like indomethacin and sulindac, which act on the fetal kidney to reduce fetal urine output, are contraindicated in FFTS, because of their concomitant but harmful effects on renal function in the already oliguric donor, which may manifest as renal failure in the neonatal period[74].

Amniotic Septostomy

Amniotic septostomy, in which an artificial aperture is created within the septum, has also been suggested as a possible treatment[93]. This is based on the anecdotal improvement in condition when the septum was first inadvertently ruptured at amnioreduction, and on the observation that FFTS is extremely rare in monoamniotic twins. The mechanism by which this treatment might work is unclear, but by allowing oral rehydration, the donor fetus may be able to correct its hypovolaemia. It, however, seems unlikely that if the chain of intertwin transfusion is not broken then the recipient fetus will continue to be overloaded with all the known sequelae. The only series, of nine pregnancies, treated by septostomy has reported a perinatal survival of 83%[133]. Although cord entanglement from post-septostomy functionally-monoamniotic twins has been a concern, no evidence of cord entanglement was found in this series following single-needle puncture of the septum. Further work is now indicated to assess the role of this promising technique in the treatment of FFTS.

Serial Amnioreduction

Serial amnioreduction remains the current treatment of choice, with an overall perinatal survival rate in the region of 60–65% in the available albeit uncontrolled series (Table 65.1)[139]. Although amnioreduction aims primarily to control polyhydramnios to allow prolongation of gestation, there is some evidence in FFTS that it may ameliorate fetal condition and the disease process. However, the small number of cases seen in any one centre renders it unlikely that the efficacy of this procedure can ever be evaluated adequately without a randomised multicentre trial.

Several groups have reported maintenance of normal amniotic volume, and/or resolution of hydrops, after amnioreduction[53,135,140]. Rosen *et al.* reported less divergence in hourly fetal urine production rates following serial amnioreduction[119]. Two conclusions are possible. Firstly, this apparent amelioration could simply be a gestational age effect, as recur-

TABLE 65.1
Data from the published trials of amnioreduction for the treatment of FFTS from proven monochorionic twin pregnancies, together with our own unpublished experience at Queen Charlotte's Hospital (QCH)

Authors	Number of pregnancies	Gestational age at diagnosis (weeks)	Volume	Survival
Urig *et al.* (1990)[35]	5	21–25	1000–5000 ml	6/10 (60%)
Mahony *et al.* (1990)[135]	8	16–28	300–5500 ml	11/16 (69%)
Elliott *et al.* (1991)[53]	17	16–28	225–5000 ml	27/34 (79%)
Saunders *et al.* (1992)[104]	19	17–25	500–6700 ml	14/38 (37%)
Pinette *et al.* (1993)[135]	9	20–26	300–8500 ml	15/18 (83%)
Weiner & Ludomirski (1994)[136]	11	21–27	1000–2000 ml	11/22 (50%)
QCH (1995)	23	17–30	925–6000 ml	31/46 (67%)
Mari *et al.* (1996)[137]	26	14–32	N.S.*	33/52 (63%)
Trespidi *et al.* (1997)[138]	23	18–26	1000–6000 ml	26/46 (57%)
Total	141	14–32	225–8500 ml	174/282 (62%)

N.S. = not stated.

rence of severe polyhydramnios necessitating drainage is rare after 30 weeks, as indeed is initial presentation with discordant amniotic fluid volume. Alternatively, it could be a true treatment effect although any mechanism must remain speculative.

We have anecdotally observed one case of FFTS sampled before and after amnioreduction, in which drainage was associated with a marked improvement in fetal P_{O_2} and pH[30]. Together with anecdotal observation of changes in fetal condition during iatrogenic intrapartum polyhydramnios[37], this led us to speculate that amnioreduction may improve uteroplacental perfusion. Recently it has been shown that amnioreduction in patients with FFTS was associated with a 74% median increase in uterine blood flow[141]. In addition, fetal middle-cerebral artery pulsatility indices fall acutely with amnioreduction in both recipient and donor fetuses[142].

Serial aggressive amniocenteses has become the mainstay of management of this condition. However, concerns that the perinatal mortality still remains relatively high, and that no attempt was being made to affect the disease process itself, led to the development of experimental procedures intent on cure.

Selective Fetocide

Selective fetocide has been suggested to have a role in the management of FFTS by a number of groups. In its favour, the procedure may be performed once the *in utero* death (IUD) of one of the twins appears imminent, or once all other treatment options have failed. Indeed, this usually allows the parents to feel that the procedure is absolutely necessary to allow even a single twin to be saved. However, to the procedure's detriment, this delay may allow some degree of insult to happen to the surviving fetus, before its co-twin is terminated.

In order to be a safe and effective procedure, the possibility of acute transfusion of the remaining twin into the terminated twin must be avoided. Placental injection studies suggest that FFTS is characterised by a lack of the superficial anastomoses[103], implicated in acute transfusion which follows single IUD in MC twins[13]. It follows therefore that when one dies *in utero*, fetuses from pregnancies complicated by FFTS should be at relatively low risk of acute transfusion, and its clinical sequelae of neurological and renal lesions, and co-twin death. Nevertheless, it seems likely that a degree of acute transfusion may occur along unidirectional anastomoses, albeit only in the one direction, and of a lesser volume, as unlike with superficial anastomoses transfusion along deep anastomoses must pass through the cotyledonary capillary network.

In FFTS, either the donor or the recipient fetus may become preterminal. The donor may be severely growth restricted with grossly abnormal arterial Doppler studies, and may show acidaemia at fetal blood sampling. Alternatively, the recipient may be hydropic, with poor ventricular function, and abnormal venous Doppler waveforms, and similarly be found to be compromised at blood sampling. A common placental finding in FFTS is of one deep A-V anastomosis passing from the donor to the recipient; it follows, therefore, with this pattern that if the donor is terminated, there should be no route by which the recipient fetus should exsanguinate into its co-twin.

Selective fetocide ideally should involve an occlusive technique, to prevent any residual possibility of the surviving twin exsanguinating into the terminated twin's circulation. In MC twins discordant for fetal abnormality, several methods have been tried with varying degrees of success, including vascular occlusion with histoacryl gel injection[143] or thrombogenic coils[144], or the initiation of cardiac asystole by saline-induced cardiac tamponade[95]. In these situations the optimal technique would simultaneously occlude both umbilical artery and vein – the artery to prevent flow from the remaining twin via an A-A anastomosis passing retrogradely up the umbilical arteries and the vein to prevent similar retrograde venous flow. A review of the reports of selective fetocide in the management of FFTS, together with our unpublished experience, indicates a successful outcome in the remaining twin in over 85% of cases (Table 65.2).

It would seem prudent to perform serial ultrasonography on the surviving twin's brain to exclude evidence of cortical

TABLE 65.2
Outcome following selective fetocide for FFTS from published trials and our unpublished experience at Queen Charlotte's Hospital (QCH)

Authors	Number of cases	Terminated fetus	Indication	Co-twin survival
Wittmann (1986)[95]	1	Donor	Severe IUGR	1/1
Weiner (1987)[145]	1	Donor	Severe IUGR	1/1
Dommergues (1995)[143]	3	Recipient	Hydrops	2/3
	1	Donor	Ascites/Cytomegaly	1/1
QCH (1996)	1	Donor	Severe IUGR	1/1
	1	Recipient	Hydrops	1/1
Total	8			7/8

damage. Nevertheless, there remains a role for selective fetocide in the management of FFTS, particularly when first-line treatments have failed.

Laser ablation

The technique of laser coagulation of placental vessels was first developed in animals in 1985[146] and later applied to human pregnancies with FFTS[94,147]. All surface chorionic vessels crossing the intertwin septum are photocoagulated by a neodymium:yttrium–aluminium–garnet (Nd:YAG) laser. Theoretically laser should be an ideal treatment if FFTS is due to the presence of anastomoses, and these can be selectively ablated. The results, however, are disappointing. Perinatal survival was only 53% in each of the two large series of laser plus amnioreduction[147,148], which is empirically lower than that with serial amnioreduction alone. The overall experience with laser is that both babies survive in one-third of cases, one baby survives in a further one-third, while both babies die in the remaining one-third. Alternatively, the technique could be viewed as an incompletely effective form of selective fetocide, with the donor fetus dying in approximately 50% of procedures, but at the cost that both fetuses may die as a result of the treatment in one-third of cases. It is, by definition, an occlusive technique which remains a prerequisite for effective selective fetocide, as indicated by the full-width chorionic plate necrosis seen after the delivery of the placenta. However, the significant chance of both fetuses dying as a result of the procedure often precludes its uptake by the parents.

High procedural loss rates can be explained by an understanding of the placental anatomy. Both groups advocating this procedure describe ablating 6–10 communicating vessels crossing the intertwin septum[94,149], which is in contrast with placental injection studies that suggest that FFTS is characterised by a paucity of superficial anastomoses (usually one or none)[103,117]. As the site of the intertwin septum bears little relation to the vascular equator[103] it appears that many normal chorionic plate vessels are instead being ablated[150]. This would explain the full-thickness placental necrosis seen after laser[94] and the high rate of intrauterine death within 24 hours of the procedure.

Notwithstanding this, development of a technique whereby the implicated deep anastomosis, or the superficial chorionic plate vessels either supplying or draining them, is identified and selectively ablated, remains the long-term goal in the treatment of this condition.

LONG-TERM SEQUELAE OF FFTS

There are scant data available at present on longer term sequelae of FFTS. Cerebral white-matter lesions are increased in MC twin pregnancies overall, both with or without FFTS, and this has been attributed to haemodynamic imbalance due to the shared circulation[13]. In addition to white-matter changes, lenticulostriate vasculopathy, an abnormal ultrasonographic appearance of the basal ganglia vasculature, has also been reported in FFTS[151]. Lenticulostriate vasculopathy is a non-specific finding also seen in viral infections, trisomy and congenital heart disease, but may be considered as a marker for antenatal insult; the long-term significance of this appearance, however, is uncertain. Our group have recently shown an incidence of 35% of antenatally-acquired neurological lesions in surviving twins from pregnancies complicated by severe FFTS, although with the exception of one case, these lesions were relatively subtle, and thus of uncertain longterm significance[152]. Both donors and recipients seem to be at risk. It may be that the raised haematocrit, and hence the potential for intravascular sludging, may cause local ischaemia, with subsequent cortical damage in the recipient fetuses. The mechanism in the donor fetus may be secondary to anaemia and/or hypoxaemia both of which may occur *in utero*[102]. In addition, cardiac sequelae, especially RVOT (see above), are common among surviving recipient fetuses.

One group has suggested that laser ablation, with effective isolation of the two fetal circulations, may protect against this, as they reported a higher incidence of cerebral palsy in their historical amnioreduction group, compared to their laser-treated group. Further work is, however, indicated as this comparison with small numbers took no account of prematurity, a known risk factor for cerebral palsy, nor was a specific endpoint for the diagnosis of cerebral palsy established. Notwithstanding this, cerebral lesions are certainly known to be common in 'unaffected' MC twins[13] mediated through superficial anastomoses which are known to be almost universal in the absence of FFTS. Furthermore the probability that some degree of subthreshold ischaemic injury occurs in the face of a procedure with a 50% fetal loss rate seems likely, and the frequency of hydrocephalus in survivors further supports this.

TWIN REVERSED ARTERIAL PERFUSION SEQUENCE

TRAP, otherwise termed 'acardiac twinning', is an extreme form of FFTS, occurring in approximately 1% of MC pregnancies.

DIAGNOSIS AND PATHOPHYSIOLOGY

The condition is characterised by the presence of an acardiac 'perfused' twin, and its co-twin denoted as the 'pump' twin. The perfused twin receives the majority of its blood supply through an arterio-arterial anastomosis from the other twin. The blood enters via the arterial side of its circulation, and, by definition, is deoxygenated. The combination of this retrograde flow of deoxygenated blood has a devastating effect upon the development of the perfused twin, with absent or rudimentary development of structures, particularly in the upper body. The pump twin may also develop the cardiovascular sequelae seen in FFTS recipient fetuses, namely congestive heart failure[153]. Sixty-five per cent of these pregnancies are complicated by polyhydramnios and preterm labour, with an overall perinatal mortality for the pump twin of 50%[154]. The ratio between the estimated fetal weights influences prognosis, with a worse outcome associated with a proportionately larger perfused twin.

TREATMENT

Management is now focused on occlusive fetocidal techniques that interrupt the intertwin communication, as separation of the twins' cardiovascular systems will cure the disease, although the perfused twin will never be viable. This may be achieved in a number of ways. Hysterotomy with selective delivery of the perfused twin has been reported, but the inherent complications of preterm labour and both long- and short-term maternal morbidity render a safer and less-invasive option preferable. Fetoscopic cord occlusion has been reported, either with a ligation technique, or with a YAG laser (see Chapter 57). However, both these methods involve a relatively large bore trochar to be inserted into the uterus and hence the risks of preterm labour and amniorrhexis (ca. 30% as discussed in Chapter 57) persist at a significant level. The use of the lesser invasive ultrasound-guided techniques therefore has gained favour. Various approaches have been employed: injection of absolute ethanol to achieve total occlusion of the vessel has been reported[155,156]; others have used thrombogenic coils[144], cord diathermy[157] and ligation techniques[158–160] with mixed results.

The management of this condition is challenging, and the timing of a fetocidal technique has remained a matter for debate. There are essentially two options available to the physician: either to follow expectant management, with intervention only if the pump twin becomes haemodynamically unstable; or if amniotic fluid volume control is lost. Alternatively, a prophylactic fetocidal procedure may be performed when the diagnosis of TRAP is first made. There are few data to support either approach; however, the latter seems favourable for two reasons. Firstly, the risk of co-twin abortion following selective fetocide is lower if the procedure is performed before 16 weeks[79]. Secondly, an early procedure may preempt any *in utero* event that might result in serious long-term sequelae, most notably the occurrence of neurological damage secondary to an episode of acute intertwin transfusion.

Drug treatment with digoxin has been reported, with resolution of subcutaneous oedema in one case[161]. Prostaglandin synthase inhibitors may be used in the management of polyhydramnios here as, unlike in FFTS, the acardiac twin's renal function is of no clinical concern[162].

Conclusion

Polyhydramnios arises following the loss of one of its several complex control mechanisms. The identification of a twin pregnancy discordant for polyhydramnios is a relatively common finding, with the majority in MC twins secondary to FFTS. In cases of discordant fetal abnormality in DC twins, the management choice between selective termination and conservative expectancy will depend on the lethality of the anomaly, parental wishes and local practice relating to termination.

Optimal management for FFTS remains controversial, although amnioreduction with selective fetocide for treatment failure would seem the preferred strategy at present. Notwithstanding recent encouraging experience with amniotic septostomy, and the poor results with laser to date, the long-term curative goal remains selective identification and ablation of shared cotyledons without damage to surrounding cotyledons. In the future, early prediction and diagnosis of the condition may allow less-/non-invasive and potentially pre-emptive treatments to be attempted.

Acknowledgement

Dr Denbow was supported by the Richard and Jack Wiseman Trust and Action Research.

REFERENCES

1. MacGillvray I. Epidemiology of twin pregnancy. *Semin. Perin.* **10**, 4–8, 1986.
2. O.P.C.S. Birth Statistics *Review of the Register General on births and patterns of family building in England and Wales, 1992*. London: HMSO, 1992.
3. Wenstrom KD, Syrop CH, Hammitt DG & Van-Voorhis BJ. Increased risk of monochorionic twinning associated with assisted reproduction. *Fertil. Steril.* **60**, 510–514, 1993.
4. Yovich JL, Stanger JD, Grauaug A *et al.* Monozygotic twins from *in vitro* fertilization. *Fertil. Steril.* **41**, 833–837, 1984.
5. Stockard C. Developmental rate and structural expression: An experimental study of twins, 'double monsters' and single deformities, and the interaction among embryonic organs during their origin and development. *Am. J. Anat.* **27**, 115–262, 1921.
6. Vorherr H & Vorherr UF. Suckling-induced delay of implantation and increased fecundity in rats. *Gynecol. Obstet. Invest.* **17**, 106–110, 1984.
7. Hsu YC & Gonda MA. Monozygotic twin formation in mouse embryos *in vitro*. *Science* **209**, 605–606, 1980.
8. Petterson B, Nelson KB, Watson L & Stanley F. Twins, triplets, and cerebral palsy in births in Western Australia in the 1980s. *BMJ* **307**, 1239–1243, 1993.
9. Benirschke K & Kim CK. Multiple pregnancy. II. *N. Engl. J. Med.* **288**, 1329–1336, 1973.
10. Aird I. Conjoined twins – further observations. *BMJ* **1**, 1313–1315, 1959.
11. Benirschke K & Kim CK. Multiple pregnancy. I. *N. Engl. J. Med.* **288**, 1276–1284, 1973.

12. Neilson JP, Danskin F & Hastie SJ. Monozygotic twin pregnancy: diagnostic and Doppler ultrasound studies. *Br. J. Obstet. Gynaecol.* **96**, 1413–1418, 1989.
13. Bejar R, Vigliocco G, Gramajo H *et al.* Antenatal origin of neurologic damage in newborn infants. *Am. J. Obstet. Gynecol.* **162**, 1230–1236, 1990.
14. Lind T, Kendall A & Hytten FE. The role of the fetus in the formation of amniotic fluid. *J. Obstet. Gynaecol. Br. Commonw.* **79**, 289–298, 1972.
15. Lind T, Billewicz WZ & Cheyne GA. Composition of amniotic fluid and maternal blood through pregnancy. *J. Obstet. Gynaecol. Br. Commonw.* **78**, 505–512, 1971.
16. Harding R, Bocking AD, Sigger JN & Wickham PJ. Composition and volume of fluid swallowed by fetal sheep. *Q. J. Exp. Physiol.* **69**, 487–495, 1984.
17. Moya F, Apgar V, James L & Berrien C. Hydramnios and congenital anomalies. *JAMA* **173**, 1552–1556, 1960.
18. Fujino Y, Agnew CL, Schreyer P, Ervin MG, Sherman DJ & Ross MG. Amniotic fluid volume response to esophageal occlusion in fetal sheep. *Am. J. Obstet. Gynecol.* **165**, 1620–1626, 1991.
19. Gilbert WM & Brace RA. Increase in fetal hydration during long-term intraamniotic isotonic saline infusion. *Am. J. Obstet. Gynecol.* **159**, 1413–1417, 1988.
20. Ross MG, Ervin MG, Leake RD, Oakes G, Hobel C & Fisher DA. Bulk flow of amniotic fluid water in response to maternal osmotic challenge. *Am. J. Obstet. Gynecol.* **147**, 697–701, 1983.
21. Goodlin RC, Anderson JC & Gallagher TF. Relationship between amniotic fluid volume and maternal plasma volume expansion. *Am. J. Obstet. Gynecol.* **146**, 505–511, 1983.
22. Lumbers ER & Stevens AD. Changes in fetal renal function in response to infusions of a hyperosmotic solution of mannitol to the ewe. *J. Physiol. (Lond.)* **343**, 439–446, 1983.
23. Stevens AD & Lumbers ER. The effect of maternal fluid intake on the volume and composition of fetal urine. *J. Dev. Physiol.* **7**, 161–166, 1985.
24. Ben-Chetrit A, Hochner-Celnikier D, Ron M & Yagel S. Hydramnios in the third trimester of pregnancy: a change in the distribution of accompanying fetal anomalies as a result of early ultrasonographic prenatal diagnosis. *Am. J. Obstet. Gynecol.* **162**, 1344–1345, 1990.
25. Queenan JT & Gadow EC. Polyhydramnios: chronic versus acute. *Am. J. Obstet. Gynecol.* **108**, 349–355, 1970.
26. Yaman C, Arzt W, Tulzer G & Tews G. The polyhydramnios symptom: analysis of 56 cases. *Geburtshilfe Frauenheilkd.* **56**, 287–290, 1996.
27. Ang MS, Thorp JA & Parisi VM. Maternal lithium therapy and polyhydramnios. *Obstet Gynecol* **76**, 517–519, 1990.
28. Hill LM, Breckle R, Thomas ML & Fries JK. Polyhydramnios: ultrasonically detected prevalence and neonatal outcome. *Obstet. Gynecol.* **69**, 21–25, 1987.
29. Cardwell MS. Polyhydramnios: a review. *Obstet. Gynecol. Surv.* **42**, 612–617, 1987.
30. Fisk NM Tannirandorn Y, Nicolini U, Talbert DG & Rodeck CH. Amniotic pressure in disorders of amniotic fluid volume. *Obstet. Gynecol.* **76**, 210–214, 1990.
31. Many A, Hill LM, Lazebnik N & Martin JG. The association between polyhydramnios and preterm delivery. *Obstet. Gynecol.* **86**, 389–391, 1995.
32. Vintzileos AM, Turner GW, Campbell WA, Weinbaum PJ, Ward SM & Nochimson DJ. Polyhydramnios and obstructive renal failure: a case report and review of the literature. *Am. J. Obstet. Gynecol.* **152**, 883–885, 1985.
33. Desmedt EJ, Henry OA & Beischer NA. Polyhydramnios and associated maternal and fetal complications in singleton pregnancies. *Br. J. Obstet. Gynaecol.* **97**, 1115–1122, 1990.
34. Gonsoulin W, Moise K, Jr, Kirshon B, Cotton DB, Wheeler JM & Carpenter R Jr. Outcome of twin–twin transfusion diagnosed before 28 weeks of gestation. *Obstet. Gynecol.* **75**, 214–216, 1990.
35. Urig MA, Clewell WH & Elliott JP. Twin–twin transfusion syndrome. *Am. J. Obstet. Gynecol.* **163**, 1522–1526, 1990.
36. Steinberg LH, Hurley VA, Desmedt E & Beischer NA. Acute polyhydramnios in twin pregnancies. *Aust. NZ J. Obstet. Gynaecol.* **30**, 196–200, 1990.
37. Tabor BL & Maier JA. Polyhydramnios and elevated intrauterine pressure during amnioinfusion. *Am. J. Obstet. Gynecol.* **156**, 130–131, 1987.
38. Fisk NM, Vaughan J & Talbert D. Impaired fetal blood gas status in polyhydramnios and its relation to raised amniotic pressure. *Fetal. Diagn. Ther.* **9**, 7–13, 1994.
39. Flack NJ, Dore C, Southwell D, Kourtis P, Sepulveda W & Fisk NM. The influence of operator transducer pressure on ultrasonographic measurements of amniotic fluid volume. *Am. J. Obstet. Gynecol.* **171**, 218–222, 1994.
40. Moore TR. Superiority of the four-quadrant sum over the single-deepest-pocket technique in ultrasonographic identification of abnormal amniotic fluid volumes. *Am. J. Obstet. Gynecol.* **163**, 762–767, 1990.
41. Moore TR & Cayle JE. The amniotic fluid index in normal human pregnancy. *Am. J. Obstet. Gynecol.* **162**, 1168–1173, 1990.
42. Dildy GR, Lira N, Moise K Jr, Riddle GD & Deter RL. Amniotic fluid volume assessment: comparison of ultrasonographic estimates versus direct measurements with a dye-dilution technique in human pregnancy. *Am. J. Obstet. Gynecol.* **167**, 986–994, 1992.
43. Croom CS, Banias BB, Ramos-Santos E, Devoe LD, Bezhadian A & Hiett AK. Do semiquantitative amniotic fluid indexes reflect actual volume? *Am. J. Obstet. Gynecol.* **167**, 995–999, 1992.
44. Magann EF, Nolan TE, Hess LW, Martin RW, Whitworth NS & Morrison JC. Measurement of amniotic fluid volume: accuracy of ultrasonography techniques. *Am. J. Obstet. Gynecol.* **167**, 1533–1537, 1992.
45. Sepulveda W, Flack NJ & Fisk NM. Direct volume measurement at midtrimester amnioinfusion in relation to ultrasonographic indexes of amniotic fluid volume. *Am. J. Obstet. Gynecol.* **170**, 1160–1163, 1994.
46. Denbow M, Sepulveda W, Ridout D & Fisk N. The relationship of the change in amniotic fluid index with the volume of fluid removed at amnioreduction. *Obstet. Gynecol.* **90**, 529–532, 1997.
47. Landy HJ, Isada NB & Larsen J Jr. Genetic implications of idiopathic hydramnios. *Am. J. Obstet. Gynecol.* **157**, 114–117, 1987.
48. Stoll CG Alembik Y & Dott B. Study of 156 cases of polyhydramnios and congenital malformations in a series of 118 265 consecutive births. *Am. J. Obstet. Gynecol.* **165**, 586–590, 1991.
49. Rivett L. Hydramnios. *J. Obstet. Gynaecol. British Emp.* **40**, 522–525, 1933.
50. Feingold M, Cetrulo CL, Newton ER, Weiss J, Shakr C & Shmoys S. Serial amniocenteses in the treatment of twin to twin transfusion complicated with acute polyhydramnios. *Acta. Genet. Med. Gemellol. Roma.* **35**, 107–113, 1986.
51. Cabrera-Ramirez L & Harris RE. Controlled removal of amniotic fluid in hydramnios. *South. Med. J.* **69**, 239–240, 1976.
52. Fisk N, Tannirandorn Y, Nicolini U, Talbert D & Rodeck C. Amniotic pressure in disorders of amniotic fluid volume. *Obstet. Gynecol.* **76**, 210–214, 1990.
53. Elliott JP, Urig MA & Clewell WH. Aggressive therapeutic amniocentesis for treatment of twin–twin transfusion syndrome. *Obstet. Gynecol.* **77**, 537–540, 1991.
54. Elliott JP, Sawyer AT, Radin TG & Strong RE. Large-volume therapeutic amniocentesis in the treatment of hydramnios. *Obstet. Gynecol.* **84**, 1025–1027, 1994.
55. Caldeyro-Barcia R, Pose S & Alvarez H. Uterine contractility in polyhydramnios and the effects of withdrawal of the excess of amniotic fluid. *Am. J. Obstet. Gynecol.* **73**, 1238–1254, 1957.
56. Cifuentes RF, Olley PM, Balfe JW, Radde I.C & Soldin SJ. Indomethacin and renal function in premature infants with persistent patent ductus arteriosus. *J. Pediatr.* **95**, 583–587, 1979.
57. Kirshon B, Moise K Jr, Wasserstrum N, Ou CN & Huhta JC. Influence of short-term indomethacin therapy on fetal urine output. *Obstet. Gynecol.* **72**, 51–53, 1988.
58. Cabrol D, Landesman R, Muller J, Uzan M, Sureau C & Saxena BB. Treatment of polyhydramnios with prostaglandin synthetase inhibitor (indomethacin). *Am. J. Obstet. Gynecol.* **157**, 422–426 , 1987.
59. Mamopoulos M, Assimakopoulos E, Reece EA, Andreou A, Zheng XZ & Mantalenakis S. Maternal indomethacin therapy in the treatment of polyhydramnios. *Am. J. Obstet. Gynecol.* **162**, 1225–1229, 1990.
60. Lange I.R, Harman CR, Ash KM, Manning FA & Menticoglou S. Twin with hydramnios: treating premature labor at source. *Am. J. Obstet. Gynecol.* **160**, 552–557, 1989.
61. Kirshon B, Mari G, Moise K, Jr. Indomethacin therapy in the treatment of symptomatic polyhydramnios. *Obstet. Gynecol.* **75**, 202–205, 1990.

62. Millard RW, Baig H & Vatner SF. Prostaglandin control of the renal circulation in response to hypoxemia in the fetal lamb *in utero*. *Circ. Res.* **45**, 172–179, 1979.
63. Mari G, Moise K, Deter R, Kirshon B & Carpenter R. Doppler assessment of the renal blood flow velocity waveform during indomethacin therapy for preterm labour and polyhydramnios. *Obstet. Gynecol.* **75**, 199–201, 1990.
64. Stevenson KM & Lumbers ER. Effects of indomethacin on fetal renal function renal and umbilicoplacental blood flow and lung liquid production. *J. Dev. Physiol.* **17**, 257–264, 1992.
65. Seyberth HW, Rascher W, Hackenthal R & Wille L. Effect of prolonged indomethacin therapy on renal function and selected vasoactive hormones in very-low-birth-weight infants with symptomatic patent ductus arteriosus. *J. Pediatr.* **103**, 979–984, 1983.
66. Walker MP, Moore TR & Brace RA. Indomethacin and arginine vasopressin interaction in the fetal kidney: a mechanism of oliguria. *Am. J. Obstet. Gynecol.* **171**, 1234–1241, 1994.
67. Kramer WB, Van den Veyver IB & Kirshon B. Treatment of polyhydramnios with indomethacin. *Clin. Perinatol.* **21**, 615–630, 1994.
68. Hendricks SK, Smith JR, Moore DE & Brown ZA. Oligohydramnios associated with prostaglandin synthetase inhibitors in preterm labour. *Br. J. Obstet. Gynaecol.* **97**, 312–316, 1990.
69. Moise K Jr, Huhta JC, Sharif DS *et al.* Indomethacin in the treatment of premature labor. Effects on the fetal ductus arteriosus. *N. Engl. J. Med.* **319**, 327–331, 1988.
70. Cowan F. Indomethacin, patent ductus arteriosus, and cerebral blood flow. *J. Pediatr.* **109**, 341–344, 1986.
71. Respondek M, Weil SR & Huhta JC. Fetal echocardiography during indomethacin treatment. *Ultrasound Obstet. Gynecol.* **5**, 86–89, 1995.
72. Moise K Jr. Effect of advancing gestational age on the frequency of fetal ductal constriction in association with maternal indomethacin use. *Am. J. Obstet. Gynecol.* **168**, 1350–1353, 1993.
73. Kirshon B, Mari G, Moise K, Jr & Wasserstrum N. Effect of indomethacin on the fetal ductus arteriosus during treatment of symptomatic polyhydramnios. *J. Reprod. Med.* **35**, 529–532, 1990.
74. Buderus S, Thomas B, Fahnenstich H & Kowalewski S. Renal failure in two preterm infants: toxic effect of prenatal maternal indomethacin treatment? *Br. J. Obstet. Gynaecol.* **100**, 97–98, 1993.
75. van der Heijden BJ, Carlus C, Narcy F, Bavoux F, Delezoide AL & Gubler MC. Persistent anuria, neonatal death, and renal microcystic lesions after prenatal exposure to indomethacin. *Am. J. Obstet. Gynecol.* **171**, 617–623, 1994.
76. Norton ME, Merrill J, Cooper BA, Kuller JA & Clyman RI. Neonatal complications after the administration of indomethacin for preterm labor. *N. Engl. J. Med.* **329**, 1602–1607, 1993.
77. Murray H, Stone P, Strand L & Flower J. Fetal pleural effusion following maternal indomethacin therapy. *Br. J. Obstet. Gynaecol.* **100**, 277–282, 1993.
78. Peek M, McCarthy A, Kyle P, McCarthy A, Sepulveda W & Fisk N. Medical amnioreduction with sulindac to reduce cord complications in monoamniotic twins. *Am. J. Obstet. Gynecol.* **176**, 334–336, 1997.
79. Evans M, Goldberg J, Dommergues M *et al.* Efficacy of second-trimester selective termination for fetal abnormalities: international collaborative experience among the world's largest centers. *Am. J. Obstet. Gynecol.* **171**, 90–94, 1994.
80. Golbus MS, Cunningham N, Goldberg JD, Anderson R, Filly R & Callen P. Selective termination of multiple gestations. *Am. J. Med. Genet.* **31**, 339–348, 1988.
81. Lipitz S, Meizner I, Yagel S, Shapiro I, Achiron R & Schiff E. Expectant management of twin pregnancies discordant for anencephaly. *Obstet. Gynecol.* **86**, 969–972, 1995.
82. Lipitz S, Shalev E, Meizner I, *et al.* Late selective termination of fetal abnormalities in twin pregnancies: a multicentre report. *Br. J. Obstet. Gynaecol.* **103**, 1212–1216, 1996.
83. King AD, Soothill PW, Montemagno R, Young MP, Sams V & Rodeck CH. Twin-to-twin blood transfusion in a dichorionic pregnancy without the oligohydramnios–polyhydramnios sequence. *Br. J. Obstet. Gynaecol.* **102**, 334–335, 1995.
84. Bruner JP & Rosemond RL. Twin-to-twin transfusion syndrome: a subset of the twin oligohydramnios–polyhydramnios sequence. *Am. J. Obstet. Gynecol.* **169**, 925–930, 1993.
85. Tanaka M, Natori M, Ishimoto H, Kohno H, Kobayashi T & Nozawa S. Intravascular pancuronium bromide infusion for prenatal diagnosis of twin–twin transfusion syndrome. *Fetal Diagn. Ther.* **7**, 36–40, 1992.
86. Denbow M, Blomly M, Cosgrove D & Fisk N. Ultrasound microbubble contrast angiography in monochorionic twin fetuses. *Lancet* **349**, 773, 1997.
87. Patten RM, Mack LA, Harvey D, Cyr DR & Pretorius DH. Disparity of amniotic fluid volume and fetal size: problem of the stuck twin – US studies. *Radiology* **172**, 153–157, 1989.
88. Robertson EG & Neer KJ. Placental injection studies in twin gestation. *Am. J. Obstet. Gynecol.* **147**, 170–174, 1983.
89. Weir PE, Ratten GJ & Beischer NA. Acute polyhydramnios – a complication of monozygous twin pregnancy. *Br. J. Obstet. Gynaecol.* **86**, 849–853, 1979.
90. Rausen AR, Seki M & Strauss L. Twin transfusion syndrome. *J. Pediatr.* **66**, 613–627, 1965.
91. Tan KL, Tan R, Tan SH & Tan AM. The twin transfusion syndrome. Clinical observations on 35 affected pairs. *Clin. Pediatr. (Phil.)* **18**, 111–114, 1979.
92. Reisner DP, Mahony BS, Petty CN *et al.* Stuck twin syndrome: outcome in thirty-seven consecutive cases. *Am. J. Obstet. Gynecol.* **169**, 991–995, 1993.
93. Hubinont C, Bernard P, Mwebesa W, Magritte J & Donnez J. Nd:YAG laser and needle disruption of the interfetal septum: a possible therapy in severe twin-to-twin transfusion syndrome. *J. Gynecol. Surg.* **12**, 183–189, 1996.
94. De Lia JE, Cruikshank DP & Keye WR Jr. Fetoscopic neodymium: YAG laser occlusion of placental vessels in severe twin–twin transfusion syndrome. *Obstet. Gynecol.* **75**, 1046–1053, 1990.
95. Wittmann BK, Farquharson DF, Thomas WD, Baldwin VJ & Wadsworth LD. The role of feticide in the management of severe twin transfusion syndrome. *Am. J. Obstet. Gynecol.* **155**, 1023–1026, 1986.
96. Abraham JM. Intrauterine feto-fetal transfusion syndrome. *Clin. Pediatr.* **6**, 405–410, 1967.
97. Danskin FH & Neilson JP. Twin-to-twin transfusion syndrome: what are appropriate diagnostic criteria? *Am. J. Obstet. Gynecol.* **161**, 365–369, 1989.
98. Wenstrom KD, Tessen JA, Zlatnik FJ & Sipes SL. Frequency, distribution, and theoretical mechanisms of hematologic and weight discordance in monochorionic twins. *Obstet. Gynecol.* **80**, 257–261, 1992.
99. Fisk NM, Borrell A, Hubinont C, Tannirandorn Y, Nicolini U & Rodeck CH. Fetofetal transfusion syndrome: do the neonatal criteria apply *in utero*? *Arch. Dis. Childh.* **65**, 657–661, 1990.
100. Saunders NJ, Snijders RJ & Nicolaides KH. Twin–twin transfusion syndrome during the 2nd trimester is associated with small intertwin hemoglobin differences. *Fetal Diagn. Ther.* **6**, 34–36 , 1991.
101. Denbow M Fogliani R, Kyle P, Letsky E, Nicolini U & Fisk N. Haematological indices at fetal blood sampling in monochorionic pregnancies complicated by feto-fetal transfusion syndrome. *Prenat. Diagn.* **18**, 941–946, 1998.
102. Berry SM, Puder KS, Bottoms SF, Uckele JE, Romero R & Cotton DB. Comparison of intrauterine hematologic and biochemical values between twin pairs with and without stuck twin syndrome. *Am. J. Obstet. Gynecol.* **172**, 1403–1410, 1995.
103. Bajoria R, Wigglesworth J & Fisk NM. Angioarchitecture of monochorionic placentas in relation to the twin–twin transfusion syndrome. *Am. J. Obstet. Gynecol.* **172**, 856–863, 1995.
104. Saunders NJ, Snijders RJ & Nicolaides KH. Therapeutic amniocentesis in twin–twin transfusion syndrome appearing in the second trimester of pregnancy. *Am. J. Obstet. Gynecol.* **166**, 820–824, 1992.
105. Hecher K Ville Y & Nicolaides KH. Fetal arterial Doppler studies in twin–twin transfusion syndrome. *J. Ultrasound Med.* **14**, 101–108, 1995.
106. Hecher K, Ville Y, Snijders R & Nicolaides K. Doppler studies of the fetal circulation in twin–twin transfusion syndrome. *Ultrasound Obstet. Gynecol.* **5**, 318–324, 1995.
107. Weiner CP & Naides SJ. Fetal survival after human parvovirus B19 infection: spectrum of intrauterine response in a twin gestation. *Am. J. Perinatol.* **9**, 66–68, 1992.
108. Schatz F. Zur Frage über die Quelle des Fruchtwassers und über Embryones papyracei. *Arch. Gynäkol.* **19**, 329, 1882.

109. Hecher K, Jauniaux E, Campbell S, Deane C & Nicolaides K. Artery-to-artery anastomosis in monochorionic twins. *Am. J. Obstet. Gynecol.* **171**, 570–572, 1994.
110. Denbow M, Cox P, Talbert D & Fisk N. Colour Doppler energy insonation of placental anastomoses in monochorionic twins: absent arterio-arterial anastomoses in association with twin-to-twin transfusion syndrome. *Br. J. Obstet. Gynaecol.* **105**, 760–765, 1998.
111. Fusi L & Gordon H. Twin pregnancy complicated by single intrauterine death. Problems and outcome with conservative management. *Br. J. Obstet. Gynaecol.* **97**, 511–516, 1990.
112. Fusi L, McParland P, Fisk N, Nicolini U & Wigglesworth J. Acute twin–twin transfusion: a possible mechanism for brain-damaged survivors after intrauterine death of a monochorionic twin. *Obstet. Gynecol.* **78**, 517–520, 1991.
113. Okamura K, Murotsuki J, Tanigawara S, Uehara S & Yajima A. Funipuncture for evaluation of hematologic and coagulation indices in the surviving twin following co-twin's death. *Obstet. Gynecol.* **83**, 975–978, 1994.
114. Schatz F. *Klinische Beiträge zur Physiologie des Fetus*. Berlin: Hirschwald, 1900.
115. Strong S & Corney G. *The Placenta in Twin Pregnancy*. Oxford: Pergamon Press, 1966.
116. Aherne W, Strong SJ & Corney G. The structure of the placenta in the twin transfusion syndrome. *Biol. Neonat.* **12**, 121–135, 1968.
117. Machin G, Still K & Lalani T. Correlations of placental vascular anatomy and clinical outcomes in 69 monochorionic twin pregnancies. *Am. J. Med. Genet.* **61**, 229–236, 1996.
118. Benirschke K. Accurate recording of twin placentation: a plea to the obstetrician. *Obstet. Gynecol.* **18**, 334–347, 1961.
119. Rosen DJ, Rabinowitz R, Beyth Y, Fejgin MD & Nicolaides KH. Fetal urine production in normal twins and in twins with acute polyhydramnios. *Fetal Diagn. Ther.* **5**, 57–60, 1990.
120. Nageotte MP, Hurwitz SR, Kaupke CJ, Vaziri ND & Pandian MR. Atriopeptin in the twin transfusion syndrome. *Obstet. Gynecol.* **73**, 867–870, 1989.
121. Wieacker P, Wilhelm C, Prompeler H, Petersen KG, Schillinger H & Breckwoldt M. Pathophysiology of polyhydramnios in twin transfusion syndrome. *Fetal Diagn. Ther.* **7**, 87–92, 1992.
122. Moya FR, Grannum PA, Riddick L, Robert JA & Pinheriro J. Atrial natriuretic factor in hydrops fetalis caused by Rh isoimmunisation. *Arch. Dis. Childh.* **65**, 683–686, 1990.
123. Fisk NM, Tannirandorn Y, Nicolini U, Hubinont C, Rodeck CH & Meliagros L. Atrial natriuretic peptide in fetal disease. *Br. J. Obstet. Gynaecol.* **97**, 545–546, 1990.
124. Panos MZ, Nicolaides KH, Anderson JV, Economides DL, Rees L & Williams R. Plasma atrial natriuretic peptide in human fetus: response to intravascular blood transfusion. *Am. J. Obstet. Gynecol.* **161**, 357–361, 1989.
125. Cheung CY & Brace RA. Fetal hypoxia elevates plasma atrial natriuretic factor concentration. *Am. J. Obstet. Gynecol.* **159**, 1263–1268, 1988.
126. Talbert D, Bajoria R, Sepulveda W, Bower S & Fisk N. Hydrostatic and osmotic pressure gradients produce manifestations of fetofetal transfusion syndrome in a computerised model of monochorial twin pregnancy. *Am. J. Obstet. Gynecol.* **174**, 598–608, 1996.
127. Rizzo G, Arduini D & Romanini C. Cardiac and extracardiac flows in discordant twins. *Am. J. Obstet. Gynecol.* **170**, 1321–1327, 1994.
128. Zosmer N, Bajoria R, Weiner E, Rigby M, Vaughan J & Fisk NM. Clinical and echographic features of *in utero* cardiac dysfunction in the recipient twin in twin–twin transfusion syndrome. *Br. Heart. J.* **72**, 74–79, 1994.
129. Weiner CP. Umbilical pressure measurement in the evaluation of nonimmune hydrops fetalis. *Am. J. Obstet. Gynecol.* **168**, 817–823, 1993.
130. Bajoria R, Sullivan M & Fisk N. Plasma endothelin concentrations and echocardiographic features in feto-fetal transfusion syndrome. *Israel J. Obstet. Gynecol.* **5**, 25, 1994.
131. Tolosa J, Zoppini C, Ludomirsky A, Bhutani V, Weil S & Huhta J. Fetal hypertension and cardiac hypertrophy in the discordant twin syndrome. SPO abstracts. *Am. J. Obstet. Gynecol.* **168**, 292, 1993.
132. De Lia J, Emery MG, Sheafor SA & Jennison TA. Twin transfusion syndrome: successful *in utero* treatment with digoxin. *Int. J. Gynaecol. Obstet.* **23**, 197–201, 1985.
133. Berry D, Montgomery L, Johnson A, Saade G & Moise K. Amniotic septostomy for the treatment of the stuck twin sequence. SPO abstracts. *Am. J. Obstet. Gynecol.* **176**, S19, 1997.
134. Mahony BS, Petty CN, Nyberg DA, Luthy DA, Hickok DE & Hirsch JH. The 'stuck twin' phenomenon: ultrasonographic findings, pregnancy outcome, and management with serial amniocenteses. *Am. J. Obstet. Gynecol.* **163**, 1513–1522, 1990.
135. Pinette MG, Pan Y, Pinette SG & Stubblefield PG. Treatment of twin–twin transfusion syndrome. *Obstet. Gynecol.* **82**, 841–846, 1993.
136. Weiner CP & Ludomirski A. Diagnosis, pathophysiology, and treatment of chronic twin-to-twin transfusion syndrome. *Fetal Diagn. Ther.* **9**, 283–290, 1994.
137. Mari G, Abuhamad A, Verpairojkit B, Jones D, Gomez K, Bahado-Singh K, Soper R & Copel JA. Treatment of twin-to-twin transfusion syndrome. Is the therapeutic amniocentesis still a good management option? SPO abstracts. *Am. J. Obstet. Gynecol.* **174**, 487, 1996.
138. Trespidi L, Boschetto C, Caravelli E, Villa L, Kustermann A & Nicolini U. Serial amniocentesis in the management of twin–twin transfusion syndrome: when is it valuable? *Fetal Diagn. Ther.* **12**, 15–20, 1997.
139. Fisk NM & Denbow ML. Fetal surgery in twin–twin transfusion syndrome: amnioreduction as optimal treatment. In *Proceedings of the 4th European Society for Gynaecological Endoscopy, Brussels, Belgium, December 1995*. pp. 9–18. Bologna: Monduzzi Editore, 1996.
140. Wax JR, Blakemore KJ, Blohm P & Callan NA. Stuck twin with cotwin nonimmune hydrops: successful treatment by amniocentesis. *Fetal Diagn. Ther.* **6**, 126–131, 1991.
141. Bower S, Flack N, Sepulveda W, Talbert D & Fisk N. Uterine artery blood flow response to correction of amniotic fluid volume. *Am. J. Obstet. Gynecol.* **173**, 502–507, 1995.
142. Mari G, Wasserstrum N & Kirshon B. Reduction in the middle cerebral artery pulsatility index after decompression of polyhydramnios in twin gestation. *Am. J. Perinatol.* **9**, 381–384, 1992.
143. Dommergues M, Mandelbrot L, Delezoide AL *et al.* Twin-to-twin transfusion syndrome: selective feticide by embolization of the hydropic fetus. *Fetal Diagn. Ther.* **10**, 26–31, 1995.
144. Bebbington MW, Wilson RD, Machan L & Wittmann BK. Selective feticide in twin transfusion syndrome using ultrasound-guided insertion of thrombogenic coils. *Fetal. Diagn. Ther.* **10**, 32–36, 1995.
145. Weiner CP. Diagnosis and treatment of twin to twin transfusion in the mid-second trimester of pregnancy. *Fetal Ther.* **2**, 71–74, 1987.
146. De Lia JE, Rogers JG & Dixon JA. Treatment of placental vasculature with a neodymium–yttrium–aluminum–garnet laser via fetoscopy. *Am. J. Obstet. Gynecol.* **151**, 1126–1127, 1985.
147. Ville Y, Hyett J, Hecher K & Nicolaides K. Preliminary experience with endoscopic laser surgery for severe twin–twin transfusion syndrome. *N. Engl. J. Med.* **332**, 224–227, 1995.
148. De Lia JE, Kuhlmann RS, Harstad TW & Cruikshank DP. Fetoscopic laser ablation of placental vessels in severe previable twin–twin transfusion syndrome. *Am. J. Obstet. Gynecol.* **172**, 1202–1208, 1995.
149. Ville Y, Hecher K, Ogg D, Warren R & Nicolaides K. Successful outcome after Nd:YAG laser separation of chorioangiopagus-twins under sonoendoscopic control. *Ultrasound Obstet. Gynecol.* **2**, 429–431, 1992.
150. Fisk NM, Bajoria R & Wigglesworth J. Twin–twin transfusion syndrome. *N. Engl. J. Med.* **333**, 388–389, 1995.
151. de Vries L, Beek F & Stoutenbeek P. Lenticulostriate vasculopathy in twin-to-twin transfusion syndrome: sonographic and CT findings. *Pediatr. Radiol.* **25**, 41–42, 1995.
152. Denbow ML, Battin MR, Cowan F, Azzopardi D, Edwards AD & Fisk NM. Neonatal cranial ultrasound findings of twins from pregnancies complicated by severe feto-fetal transfusion syndrome. *Am. J. Obstet. Gynecol.* **478**, 479–483, 1998.
153. Moore TR, Gale S & Benirschke K. Perinatal outcome of forty-nine pregnancies complicated by acardiac twinning. *Am. J. Obstet. Gynecol.* **163**, 907–912, 1990.
154. Van-Allen MI, Smith DW & Shepard TH. Twin reversed arterial perfusion (TRAP) sequence: a study of 14 twin pregnancies with acardius. *Semin Perinatol.* **7**, 285–293, 1983.
155. Sepulveda W, Bower S, Hassan J & Fisk N. Ablation of acardiac twin by alcohol injection into the intra-abdominal umbilical artery. *Obstet. Gynaecol.* **86**, 680–681, 1995.

156. Holzgreve W, Tercanli S, Krings W & Schuierer G. A simpler technique for umbilical-cord blockade of an acardiac twin. *N. Engl. J. Med.* **331**, 56–57, 1994.
157. Rodeck CH, Deans A & Jauniaux E. Thermocoagulation for the early treatment of pregnancy with an acardiac twin. *N. Engl. J. Med.* **339**, 1293–1295, 1998.
158. Foley MR, Clewell WH, Finberg HJ & Mills MD. Use of the Foley Cordostat grasping device for selective ligation of the umbilical cord of an acardiac twin: a case report. *Am. J. Obstet. Gynecol.* **172**, 212–214, 1995.
159. Quintero RA, Reich H, Puder KS *et al.* Brief report: umbilical-cord ligation of an acardiac twin by fetoscopy at 19 weeks of gestation. *N. Engl. J. Med.* **330**, 469–471, 1994.
160. Lemery DJ, Vanlieferinghen P, Gasq M, Finkeltin F, Beaufrere AM & Beytout M. Fetal umbilical cord ligation under ultrasonographic guidance. *Ultrasound Obstet. Gynecol.* **4**, 399–401, 1994.
161. Donnenfeld AE, van de Woestijne J, Craparo F, Smith CS, Ludomirsky A & Weiner S. The normal fetus of an acardiac twin pregnancy: perinatal management based on echocardiographic and sonographic evaluation. *Prenat Diagn.* **11**, 235–244, 1991.
162. Ash K, Harman CR & Gritter H. TRAP sequence – successful outcome with indomethacin treatment. *Obstet. Gynecol.* **76**, 960–962, 1990.

Pregnancy reduction and selective termination in multifetal pregnancies

66

M. Dommergues, M.C. Aubry, D. Mahieu-Caputo, M.I. Evans and Y. Dumez

Introduction

Multifetal pregnancy reduction (MFPR) and selective termination both involve termination of pregnancy in a multiple gestation. However, these techniques are based on radically different concepts. Selective termination results from prenatal diagnosis in a multiple pregnancy, usually twins, in which only one of the fetuses is affected. The aim of selective termination is to allow for selective birth of the unaffected baby by avoiding termination of the pregnancy as a whole. In contrast in MFPR, none of the fetuses is abnormal, but the outcome of the pregnancy is considered potentially compromised by obstetrical complications associated with multiple gestations of high rank. Therefore, a multifetal pregnancy of high order may be reduced to twins or to a singleton pregnancy to avoid these complications, and mainly the deleterious consequences of prematurity.

Multifetal pregnancy reduction

Multiple pregnancies of high order almost always result from infertility therapies, including ovulation induction by parenteral gonadotropins[1,2] with or without assisted reproductive technologies such as GIFT, IVF and also less powerful agents such as clomifene citrate[3,4]. Perinatal mortality and morbidity are positively correlated to the number of fetuses[5], mainly due to a high rate of premature deliveries. The aim of MFPR is to improve perinatal outcome of multiple pregnancies of high order by reducing the risk of premature delivery. MFPR can be achieved by several techniques including transcervical aspiration and intrathoracic potassium chloride (KCl) injection either transabdominally or transvaginally.

Large series of MFPR are now available, allowing for a quantitative evaluation of the risk and benefits of the procedure. However, MFPR remains a major moral stress in patients who under go infertility treatment. After prenatal diagnosis of a multiple pregnancy of high order, it is probably more helpful to listen carefully to the emotional response of couples than to rush into offering management options such as MFPR. Indeed, the proposition of performing MFPR may be perceived as inappropriate and even extremely shocking by infertility patients who would not even think of undergoing any kind of termination of pregnancy. The decision process leading to MFPR is complex and should always include thorough information regarding the possibility of a conservative alternative. This is particularly true for triplet pregnancies, in which the benefits expected from MFPR are arguable, while mortality associated with premature delivery tends to decrease due both to the use of prenatal corticosteroids and to improvements in neonatal care.

PRE-OPERATIVE COUNSELLING

The need for careful counselling prior to MFPR should not be underestimated. It is important to provide information both on the natural history of multiple pregnancies and on the expected obstetrical and perinatal results of MFPR, including the risk of premature delivery associated with multiple pregnancies of high order. Obstetrical benefits of MFPR should be weighed against potential drawbacks of the procedure including fetal loss and maternal stress. The motivation of the couples should also be evaluated and medical history should be taken into account. For example, the subjective experience of a triplet pregnancy is likely to be extremely different in a young fertile multipara following a cavalier ovulation induction as opposed to a couple with a long history of infertility.

TECHNIQUES

All MFPR techniques are ultrasound guided and can be performed under local anaesthesia on an outpatient basis. However, this technique is feasible in multichorial gestations only.

The choice of a particular technique cannot be based on objective criteria only. While we and others have had better results with transabdominal MFPR than with transcervical aspiration[3,6], this has not been universally confirmed[7]. Whatever technique is used, the experience of the operator is an important factor of safety and we believe MFPR should be performed by experienced physicians.

Although there is no definitive consensus regarding the optimal gestational age for MFPR, our opinion is that it is optimally done at 10–11 weeks. At this gestational age, the odds for spontaneous death *in utero* of one of the embryos are small, and some gross birth defects can be identified or suspected, which may contribute to the choice of which embryos should be terminated.

ULTRASOUND GUIDANCE

The aim of pre-operative sonography is to assess the number of live embryos and their growth, to map their respective locations and to check for interovular membranes (monochorial versus multichorial type). The embryos not to be terminated should be precisely identified to avoid any trauma of their ovular cavities throughout the procedure. Careful mapping of the embryos to be reduced is also crucial since survival after a failed attempt can potentially result in survival with sequels. Therefore, any attempt should be thoroughly completed. If there are no fetal abnormalities, the choice of the embryos to be terminated is mainly based on topographical criteria, and the easiest to reach should be chosen. If a set of monochorial embryos is recognised within a multiple pregnancy, both monochorial fetuses should be terminated.

TRANSCERVICAL ASPIRATION

This technique was first published by Martene-Duplan *et al.*[8] in the early 1980s and we used it routinely until 1987[9].

The patient is placed in the lithotomy position and ultrasound control is obtained using an abdominal probe. The uterine cervix is exposed by a single valve speculum, cleansed and grasped using a Pozzi tenaculum. Progressive cervical dilatation is achieved using Hegar dilators. A Karman cannula, connected to a 20-ml syringe, is then inserted transcervically and brought in contact with the embryo located nearest to the internal cervical os. The embryo is aspirated by a brisk vacuum operated manually. The corresponding placenta is not aspirated. The operation can be repeated if more than one embryo is to be terminated[3,7–9].

This technical approach has many disadvantages. Cervical dilatation is often required. Significant peroperative bleeding may occasionally occur. The procedure is easier with smaller embryos, i.e. at 9 weeks or earlier, a gestational age at which screening for fetal anomaly is not possible. In our hands, the miscarriage rate of the whole pregnancy using this method was twice that of the transabdominal route[3]. However, some authors have reported good results following transcervical MFPR[7].

TRANSABDOMINAL NEEDLING

Under sonographic guidance by an abdominal probe, a 20-gauge needle is inserted through the mother's abdomen into the thorax of the embryo. In the earliest attempts, fetal demise was achieved by mechanical trauma or the injection of air or saline. However, mechanical trauma and saline injections were not always effective and air injection altered sonographic images. Therefore, nowadays, transabdominal MFPR is achieved by KCl injection[6,10–12], at a concentration of 1.3–2 mEq/ml. Fundal embryos are usually easier to needle than lower-lying ones. After the needle has been inserted into the embryo's heart or thorax 1–2 ml of KCl are injected. Occasionally, the fluid injected into the embryo can be seen as a transonic image in the fetal mediastinum and pleura. When the needle is correctly inserted, fetal heart stops within a few seconds following the injection. The success of the procedure should be checked by ultrasound a few hours later or the following day, to avoid the risk of misdiagnosing a failed attempt.

TRANSVAGINAL NEEDLING

This approach is similar to the latter technique, but the needle is inserted through a transvaginal needle guide attached to a vaginal ultrasound probe and advanced through the vaginal and uterine wall into the gestational sac.

Although transvaginal needling can be done at earlier gestational ages, it is usually performed at 9½–10 weeks. Originally a 17–19-gauge needle was inserted manually through the vagina and the myometrium into the embryo, and KCl was then injected into the fetal thorax. More recently, a thinner 21-gauge needle has been used, and insertion by an automated spring-loaded device has been described[13].

Earlier in gestation, at 7–8 weeks, MFPR can be achieved by mechanical trauma using the same transvaginal route. The tip of a 25-cm-long needle with an external diameter of 1.6 mm connected by a catheter to a 20-ml syringe is placed in contact with the embryo. A brisk suction is applied, resulting in cessation of fetal heart activity[14]. This technique has the potential disadvantage of being performed at a gestational age at which sonographic evaluation of the structure of the embryo is not yet possible. However, performing MFPR earlier may be more psychologically acceptable by some patients. In addition, preliminary reports suggested that the fetal loss rate was lower in early transvaginal procedures[15].

POSTOPERATIVE FOLLOW UP

Spotting is usually noticed following transcervical aspiration, but not after transvaginal or transabdominal MFPR. The usefulness of prophylactic antibiotics, tocolytic agents or cervical suture has not been demonstrated. The major goal of subsequent obstetrical follow-up is to achieve prevention of prematurity. Since the risks of premature delivery are decreased but not completely eliminated by MFPR, this concern should be clearly explained to the patients. Psychological support is also useful. In addition, centres performing MFPR should obtain extensive perinatal follow-up of all their cases in order to provide continuous self-evaluation.

OBSTETRICAL AND PERINATAL RESULTS

FETAL LOSS AND MATERNAL MORBIDITY

Following MFPR, spontaneous death *in utero* of one of the surviving embryos is infrequent. In contrast, miscarriage of the whole pregnancy before 24 weeks occurs in a significant number of cases (9–15%)[11], and these miscarriages often take place 4–8 weeks' post-procedure. However, this relatively high pregnancy loss rate must be compared with the incidence of miscarriages in multiple pregnancies of high order. For example, in our institution, pregnancy loss before 24 weeks occurs in up to 10% of triplet pregnancies without MFPR.

The risk of miscarriage following MFPR has been shown to increase not only with the initial number of embryos, but also with the number of fetuses reduced[11]. It should also be stressed that there is a learning curve and that the miscarriage rate decreases with the experience of the operator[16].

While maternal complications are not infrequent in multiple pregnancies of high order, no significant maternal morbidity is associated with MFPR, apart from miscarriages. The use of local anaesthesia is recommended to avoid the potential side-effects of general anaesthesia, which is not used by the majority of centres.

PREMATURITY

Since prematurity is the major factor of paediatric morbidity in multiple pregnancies, gestational age at birth should be the prominent criteria to evaluate the efficacy of MFPR. MFPR has not been found to be associated with an increase in the incidence of intrauterine growth retardation or malformations in surviving fetuses. In the absence of MFPR, prematurity, as well as neonatal mortality and morbidity associated with multiple pregnancies, are correlated to the number of fetuses[5]. Nearly all quadruplets are delivered before 37 weeks, and 30–40% of them are born before 32 weeks[17]. In our institution, 78% of potentially viable triplets deliver before 37 weeks, and 21% before 32 weeks. Similar results have been found by others[1].

The obstetrical follow-up of over 1000 MFPR performed since 1981[11,16,18] has shown that among potentially viable deliveries (≥24 weeks), mean gestational age at birth was 36 menstrual weeks. However, nearly half of the patients delivered after 37 completed weeks and more than 85% delivered later than 33 weeks.

The major factor correlated with gestational age at birth is the number of embryos left following MFPR[3,11]. Following MFPR to a number of three embryos, 89% of the patients delivered before 37 weeks and 33% before 32 weeks. With a final number of two embryos, 52% of the MFPR patients delivered before 37 weeks and 13% before 32 weeks. In contrast, with a final number of one embryo, 30% of the MFPR patients delivered before 37 weeks and 10% before 32 weeks.

These data and the results presented above suggest that MFPR clearly provides a major decrease in the risk of premature delivery in quadruplets or more (Fig. 66.1). Benefits can also be expected from MFPR in triplets but this is more debatable than in pregnancies of higher order (Fig. 66.2).

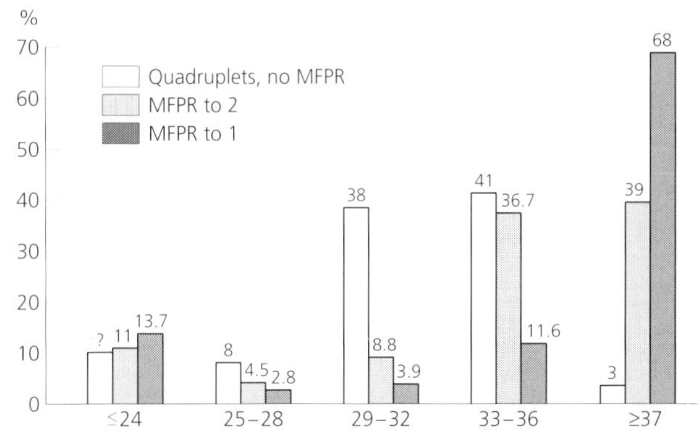

Fig. 66.1 The distribution of gestational ages (weeks) at delivery is given after MFPR to either one or two embryos, as calculated from a sample of 1789 procedures collected in a multicentre study[18]. This is compared to a survey conducted among of 65 mothers affiliated to the Association Nationale d'Entraide aux Parents de Naissances Multiples (French Association of Families with Multiple Deliveries) who did not undergo MFPR and who delivered quadruplets between 1972 and 1988[17]. Although deliveries ≤ 24 weeks were not taken into account in this series, the figure was built with an estimated miscarriage rate of 10%, based on our experience in triplets.

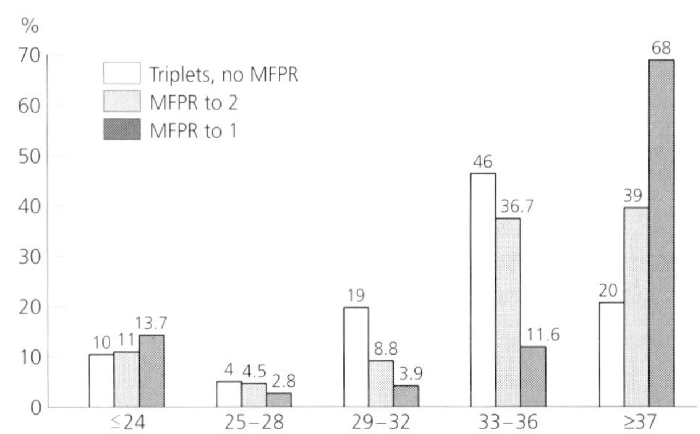

Fig. 66.2 The distribution of gestational ages at delivery is given after MFPR to either one or two embryos, as calculated from a sample of 1789 procedures collected in a multicentre study[18], and is compared to that of a continuous series of 80 triplet pregnancies followed in the Maternité Port Royal between 1981 and 1992 and who did not undergo MFPR.

Therefore, we feel that MFPR should be offered to patients with quadruplet pregnancies. In the case of triplets, parental autonomy should be given a high priority in the decision process after thorough counselling on the potential risks and benefits of MFPR. We do not perform MFPR in twins except in very exceptional circumstances.

The final number of embryos to be left following MFPR has also been debated. While leaving a single embryo is the most effective way of preventing prematurity, this approach is associated with a higher risk of miscarriage. Moreover, most couples with a long history of infertility wish to keep twins despite an increased risk of premature delivery.

CONCLUSION

MFPR has a tremendous emotional impact on couples who are distressed following the diagnosis of a high order multiple pregnancy. In most cases, the pregnancy is much wanted by the parents who often have undergone stressful and expensive infertility therapies, sometimes over many years. However, the birth of triplets or quadruplets may be perceived negatively by these parents. Many couples originally consider MFPR mainly for 'social' or personal reasons and do not realise that maternal and paediatric outcomes may be significantly compromised in multiple pregnancies of high order. The burden of guilt experienced by these parents may be at least partly relieved when they get accurate information. On the other hand, physicians should be careful not to urge patients to undergo MFPR when this option is not in accordance with their ethical beliefs or their emotional feelings. This is particularly true when the diagnosis of a triplet pregnancy after induction of ovulation is perceived as a positive event by the mother and as a side effect of infertility therapy by the physician.

In conclusion, despite the relatively good results of MFPR, it must be stressed that this technique reduces, but does not completely eliminate, the increased risk of prematurity associated with multiple pregnancies of high order. Therefore, our major goal remains prevention of iatrogenic multiple pregnancies. During IVF, this can be easily achieved by limiting the number of embryos transferred. However, despite careful monitoring, induction of ovulation can result in the recruitment of multiple follicles. In such cases, follicle aspiration is a potential alternative. It is clear that to obviate the need for MFPR, infertility specialists must continue to be vigilant in the use of fertility drugs.

Selective termination of pregnancy

When prenatal diagnosis techniques such as routine sonography, fetal karyotyping, or screening for genetic disorders in at-risk families are applied to multiple pregnancies, one of the fetuses can be affected by a severe disorder while the other is normal. In dizygous twins, the probability that both fetuses are affected is far smaller than the odds of discordance for a given disorder (Tables 66.1 and 66.2). In such a situation, the parents may wish to have the affected fetus selectively terminated and allow the unaffected twin to survive to term[19]. Selective termination may also be indicated when obstetrical complications, such as polyhydramnios, occur as a consequence of a severe malformation of one fetus which may jeopardise the pregnancy as a whole. In monochorionic pregnancies selective termination is potentially harmful to the surviving twin because of the presence of placental vascular anastomoses. In contrast, it is now established that selective feticide can be a reasonably safe procedure in dichorionic pregnancies, i.e. without placental vascular shunts, at least in trained hands. However, a good perinatal outcome of the normal twin should remain the major goal in the management of a pregnancy with an abnormal twin, underscoring the need to weigh the expected benefits of selective termination against its potential side-effects.

TABLE 66.1
Genetic risk in dizygotic twins: autosomal recessive disorder

Affected fetuses	Risk calculation	Calculated risk
Both	p^2	6.25%
None	q^2	56.25%
One out of two	$2pq$	37.50%

p: probability that a fetus is affected by a genetic disorder.
q: probability that a fetus is not affected by a genetic disorder.
For mendelian recessive disorder: $p = 0.25, q = 0.75$.
In a dizygotic pregnancy, the risks can be easily calculated, based on the concept that for each fetus, the probability of being affected is independent from the status of the other twin. This can be expressed as:

$$(p + q) \times (p + q) = p^2 + q^2 + 2pq = 1$$

in which p^2 is the probability for both fetuses to be affected, q^2 for both to be unaffected, 2-pq for one fetus affected and the other unaffected. However, because zygocity is not known *a priori* in a bichorial pregnancy, the above risks should be weighed to take into account the chances of a bichorial pregnancy to be dizygotic eventually.

TABLE 66.2
Genetic risk in dizygotic twins: aneuploidy and maternal age

Maternal age	Risk for a singleton (per 100)	Risk for both twins affected (per 100 000)	Risk for 1 twin affected (per 100)
35 years	0.4	1.6	0.8
36 years	0.5	2.5	1
38 years	1.0	10	2
42 years	2.6	67.6	5

The risk calculation is detailed in Table 66.1. Note that the probability of having both twins affected is extremely low, while the probability of one affected fetus in a set of twins is grossly twice that of a singleton.

TECHNIQUE

Psychological support based on adequate preoperative counselling should be considered as an important part of the whole process of selective termination. From a technical point of view, two issues are absolute prerequisites before considering selective termination

- the absence of placental vascular shunts must be documented; and
- the affected twin must be identified accurately.

PRE-OPERATIVE COUNSELLING

As for any termination of pregnancy, the prognosis of the disorder affecting one of the fetuses must have been thoroughly explained to the parents. This may require the advice of a paediatric subspecialist or a geneticist and a specialist in a fetal medicine centre. In France, before each medical termination of pregnancy, the law requires that the patient should be reviewed by two experts[20]. One of these medical experts should belong to a centre of fetal medicine accredited by the national Ministry of Health, while the other is a medical doctor appointed by the law court[21]. The goal of this procedure is to check that adequate information was provided to the parents, and that 'there is a high probability that the fetus is affected by a severe disorder which is not accessible to therapy at the time of prenatal diagnosis'. In addition, the procedure and the expected obstetrical outcome should be explained to the couple. We believe that adequate pre-operative counselling is the basis of effective psychological support of the parents who are put in the stressful situation of twins discordant for a severe anomaly.

PLACENTAL VASCULAR SHUNTS

In practice, placental vascular shunts can be considered as absent when there is unarguable evidence that the placenta is dichorionic.[22] This can be established when either two separate chorions or a thick dividing membrane are documented by first-trimester ultrasound (Fig. 66.3). Later in gestation, the identification of a three- to four-layer dividing membrane could bring an additional evidence for a dichorial pregnancy (Fig. 66.4). However, this latter approach has been evaluated on a limited number of patients only so far[23]. In the absence of conclusive sonographic evidence, it may be impossible to demonstrate the absence of vascular shunts[24,25], unless the fetuses are found to be dizygotic and thereby dichorionic. Zygosity can sometimes be easily demonstrated in cases discordant for fetal sex, fetal karyotype, blood group, or for a

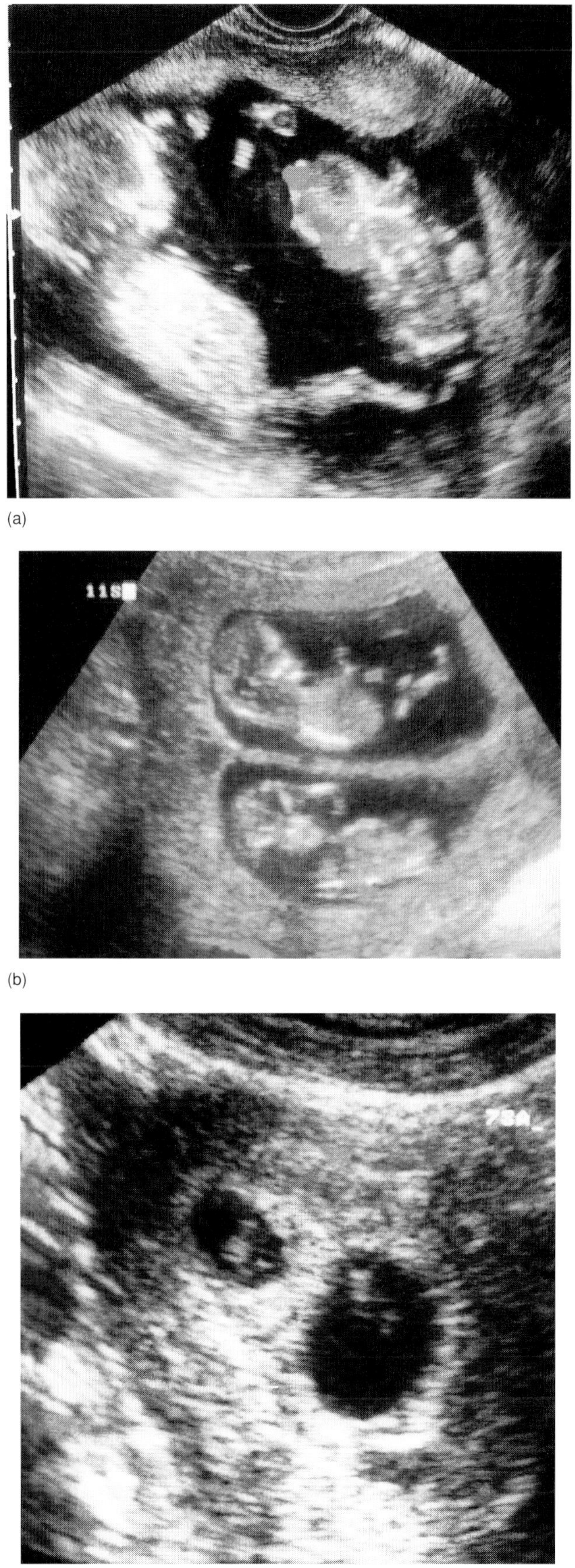

Fig. 66.3 First-trimester prenatal diagnosis of chorionicity.
(a) Monochorial pregnancy at 14 weeks. (b) Thick dividing membrane in a bichorial pregnancy at 11 weeks. (c) Separate chorions in a bichorial pregnancy at 7 weeks.

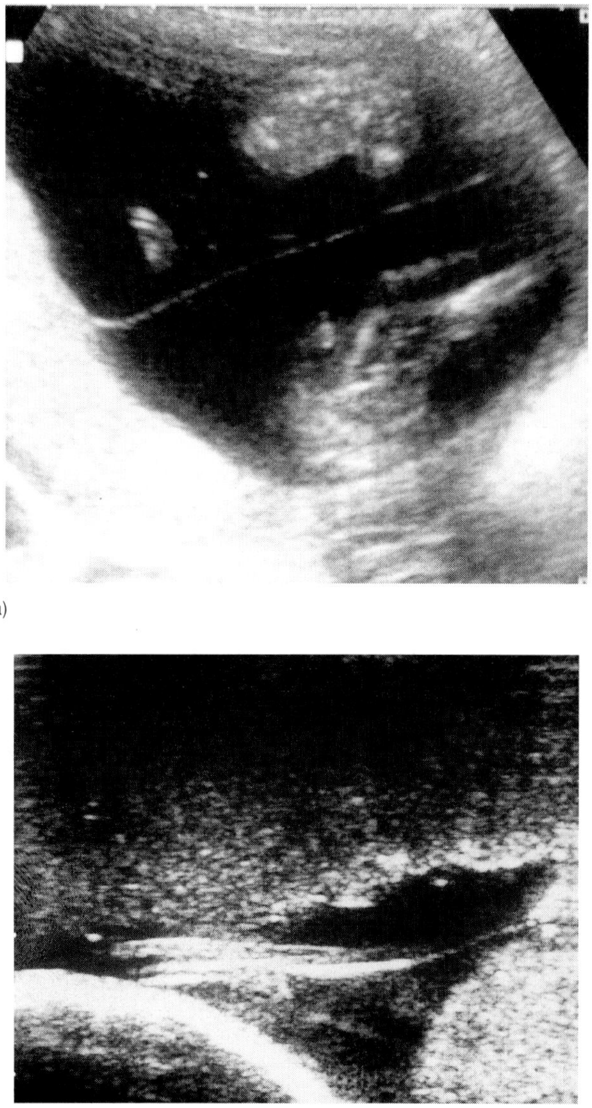

(a)

(b)

Fig. 66.4 Second- and third-trimester prenatal diagnosis of chorionicity. (a) Single layer dividing membrane in a monochorial pregnancy at 16 weeks. (b) Three- to four-layer membranes in a bichorial pregnancy at 31 weeks.

given inborn error of metabolism. In difficult cases, for instance in twins of the same sex who are discordant for a sonographic anomaly with normal karyotypes, a genetic fingerprint approach can be useful to demonstrate dizygosity based on fetal DNA obtained by amniocentesis or fetal blood sampling.[26–28]

IDENTIFICATION OF THE ABNORMAL TWIN

The unequivocal identification of the affected twin is crucial. This may seem trivial when the affected twin can be recognised by ultrasound, for instance in case of a fetal structural defect or when the gender of the fetus affected by a karyotypic or genetic anomaly is different from that of the normal co-twin. In other cases, it may be difficult to identify the affected fetus. Therefore, the location of each fetus must be carefully mapped at the time of amniocentesis or chorionic villus sampling. Placental location, cord insertions and position of the dividing membranes should be recorded precisely. The samples should also be labelled unequivocally before being processed to the laboratory. Despite all these precautions, the topography of the pregnancy may have changed when biological results become available. If there is any doubt regarding the location of the affected fetus, this must be checked using a rapid technique, for instance karyotyping on fetal blood or chorionic villi.

INTRAUTERINE FETOCIDE

The procedure is conducted under continuous ultrasound guidance and should be performed only by specialists trained in interventional fetal medicine. After the maternal abdomen has been cleaned and draped, the affected twin is identified by sonography, the probe being wrapped in a sterile bag. Fetal cardiac arrest is obtained by the injection of KCl into the fetal heart using a 20-gauge needle inserted through the maternal abdomen under local anaesthesia although a variety of other techniques have been used in the past[1,29,30]. Prior to this, fetal sedation should be obtained by injection of diazepam or pethidine into the fetal circulation.

Following the procedure, bed rest is not needed unless otherwise indicated. However, the mother should be informed that selective termination does not reduce the risk of premature delivery associated with twin pregnancies and that precautions aiming at preventing premature labour should not be discontinued.

Within a few weeks following selective termination, the amniotic fluid volume of the terminated twin progressively decreases, while the growth of the other twin remains normal at follow-up sonograms. Maternal coagulation tests have been performed, but no significant abnormality was reported in large series of selective terminations[31]. The delivery process is usually uneventful. When selective termination was performed in the first or early second trimester, delivery is similar to that of a singleton pregnancy, and the remnant of the terminated fetus is usually found attached to the placenta of the normal twin.

PERINATAL RESULTS

There has been much concern about the risk of premature labour, rupture of membranes, or amnionitis potentially associated with selective fetocide. Early reports[32] as well as more recent collaborative studies[31] showed that selective termination was associated with an overall risk of pregnancy loss of 13%, and a risk of premature delivery of 35% of potentially viable pregnancies. These figures should be interpreted with caution. Twin pregnancy *per se* carries a substantial risk of

TABLE 66.3
Gestational age at birth in twins: selective termination vs. natural history

Gestational age at birth or pregnancy loss	Selective termination performed at ≤ 16 weeks (*n* = 37)	Selective termination performed at > 16 weeks* (*n* = 146)	Natural history** (*n* = 119)
≤ 20 weeks	2 (5.4%)	5 (3.4%)	2 (1.7%)
21–24 weeks		16 (11%)	2 (1.7%)
25–28 weeks		7 (4.8%)	4 (3.4%)
29–32 weeks	2 (5.4%)	17 (11.6%)	15 (12.6%)
33–36 weeks	11 (29.7%)	30 (20.5%)	37 (31%)
≥ 37 weeks	22 (59.5%)	71 (48.6%)	59 (49.6%)

*After Evans *et al.*,[31] who collected a multicentre survey of 183 cases of selective terminations for severe fetal anomalies in 169 twins, 11 triplets and 3 quadruplets.
**Twin gestations without selective termination followed in one of the centres which contributed to the above survey (Maternité Port Royal, Paris 1989–1991).

premature delivery, that might be increased by the presence of an abnormal fetus[33]. This suggests that some of the complications observed after selective fetocide are not due to the procedure itself (Table 66.3).

However, the risk of miscarriage seems lower when selective termination is performed before 16 weeks than when the procedure is performed later in gestation (Table 66.3). This underscores the potential interest of early first trimester prenatal diagnosis in multiple gestations. Overall, if the risk of premature delivery after selective termination is higher than that of normal singletons, it compares favourably with twin gestations without selective termination[34].

INDICATIONS

Because selective termination remains an invasive procedure, its potential risks should be weighed against the expected benefits. When a twin is affected by a disorder which is lethal in the early neonatal period, the indication for performing a selective termination is debatable. The option of preparing the couple for a natural neonatal demise may be preferable to performing a second-trimester selective termination, since this procedure is likely to increase the risk of pregnancy loss. This situation may be encountered, for instance when anencephaly is diagnosed by 20–22 weeks. Nevertheless, clinical and sonographic follow-up should pick up complications such as polyhydramnios of the abnormal twin, which may jeopardise the pregnancy as a whole and therefore make selective termination desirable for the sake of the normal co-twin. However, when a lethal anomaly is detected during the early first trimester, the good obstetrical outcome of early selective terminations favours performing this procedure.

When one twin is affected by a non-lethal anomaly associated with severe postnatal morbidity, some parents may elect to perform a selective termination to avoid the birth of a severely handicapped child. In such cases, we believe that parental autonomy should be respected provided adequate information has been given to the family concerning both the postnatal prognosis of the affected fetus and the obstetrical outcome of selective termination.

SELECTIVE TERMINATION IN MONOCHORIAL TWINS

A monochorial placenta is a contraindication to selective fetocide, because the lethal injection to one fetus may reach the co-twin through placental vascular shunts and because of the possibility of haemodynamic instability (see below). Therefore, some authors have considered alternative approaches. Creating a tamponade in the affected twin[35] is not a satisfactory approach since the acute events occurring during fetal death might cause major haemodynamic variation in the normal twin's circulation and in turn account for cerebral ischaemic lesions[36–38]. Although theoretically safer, other techniques such as embolisation[39], endoscopic cord ligation[40], or open fetal surgery[41] seem very invasive and the cases reported are too few to allow for appropriate evaluation. Percutaneous coagulation of the umbilical cord is currently being evaluated.

From a practical point of view, situations in which selective fetocide is considered are rare in monochorial pregnancies, but raise such technical difficulties that the early first-trimester determination of placentation appears to be a high priority in the management of twin pregnancies.

CONCLUSION: IMPLICATIONS FOR PRENATAL DIAGNOSIS IN TWINS

When a major fetal anomaly is diagnosed in one twin, selective termination may be indicated to avoid the birth of a severely handicapped child. This may also be required when obstetrical complications such as polyhydramnios occur as a consequence of a lethal malformation in one twin and jeopardise the pregnancy as a whole. However, selected fetocide should not be undertaken unless the following criteria are met:

- absence of placental vascular shunts;
- adequate identification of the affected twin; and
- thorough pre-operative counselling of the couple.

In addition, because the obstetrical outcome is improved when selective termination is performed in the first trimester, we believe that prenatal diagnosis should be implemented as early as possible in twins. This underscores the importance of performing a first sonographic evaluation at 12–13 menstrual weeks, in order to identify multiple gestations, to determine chorionicity, and to screen for fetal structural anomalies. In families at high risk for a mendelian disorder, chorionic villus sampling is probably the best approach to prenatal diagnosis in twins. However, in dichorial pregnancies, one must be certain that each trophoblast is sampled separately, and this can be based only on the quality of ultrasound guidance. As for aneuploidy screening in relatively lower risk situations such as elevated maternal age, early amniocentesis might be the method of choice, since cytogenetic results may be difficult to interpret after chorionic villus sampling due to mosaicism.

REFERENCES

1. Holcberg G, Biale Y, Lewenthal H & Insler V. Outcome of pregnancy in 31 triplet gestations. *Obstet. Gynecol.* **59**:472–479, 1982.
2. Schenker JG, Yarkoni S & Granat M. Multiple pregnancies following induction of ovulation. *Fertil. Steril.* **35**:105–123, 1981.
3. Dommergues M, Nisand I, Mandelbrot L, Isfer E, Radunovic N & Dumez Y. Embryo reduction in the management of multifetal pregnancies following infertility therapy: obstetrical risks and perinatal benefits are related to the operative strategy. *Fertil. Steril.* **55**:801–811, 1991.
4. Evans MI, Fletcher JC & Zador IE. Selective first trimester termination in octuplet and quadruplet pregnancies: clinical and ethical issues. *Obstet. Gynecol.* **71**:289–296, 1988.
5. Botting BH, McDonald Davies I & McFarlane AJ. Recent trends in the incidence of multiple births and associated mortality. *Arch. Dis. Childh.* **62**:941–950, 1987.
6. Berkowitz R, Lynch L & Chitkara U. Selective reduction of multifetal pregnancies in the first trimester. *N. Engl. J. Med.* **318**:1043–1047, 1988.
7. Salat-Baroux J, Aknin J, Antoine JM & Alamowitch R. The management of multiple pregnancies after induction for superovulation. *Human Reprod.* **3**:399–401, 1988.
8. Martene-Duplan J, Aknin AJ & Alamowitch R. Aspiration embryonnaire partielle au cours de grossesses multiples. *Contraception, Fertilité, Sexualité* **11**:745–748, 1983.
9. Dumez Y & Oury JF. Method for first trimester selective abortion in multiple pregnancy. *Contr. Gynaecol. Obst.* **15**:50–53, 1986.
10. Bessis R, Milanese C & Frydman R. Partial termination of pregnancy. 2nd Congress on the Fetus as a Patient, Jerusalem, May 1985.
11. Evans MI, Dommergues M, Wapner RJ *et al.* Efficacy of transabdominal multifetal pregnancy reduction – collaborative experience among the world's largest centers. *Obstet. Gynecol.* **82**:61–66, 1993.
12. Jeny R & Leroy B. Réduction sélective en cas de grossesses multiples. *Ann. Radiol.* **26**:446, 1983.
13. Timor-Tritsch IE, Peisner DB, Monteagudo A, Lerner JP & Sharma S. Multifetal pregnancy reduction by transvaginal puncture – evaluation of the technique used in 134 cases. *Am. J. Obstet. Gynecol.* **168**:799–804, 1993.
14. Itskovitz J, Boldes R, Thaler I, Bronstein M, Erlik Y & Brandes J. Transvaginal ultrasonography guided aspiration of gestational sacs for selective abortion in multiple pregnancy. *Am. J. Obstet. Gynecol.* **160**:215–217, 1989.
15. Itskovitz-Eldor J, Drugan A, Levron J, Thaler I, Brandes JM. Transvaginal embryo aspiration – a safe method for selective reduction in multiple pregnancies. *Fertil. Steril.* **58**:351–355, 1992.
16. Evans M, Dommergues M, Timor-Tritch I *et al.* Transabdominal versus transcervical/vaginal multifetal pregnancy reduction: international collaborative study of more than 1000 cases. *Am. J. Obstet. Gynecol.* **170**:902–909, 1994.
17. Pons JC, Le Moal S, Dephot N & Papernik E. La grossesse quadruple en France. In *Les Grossesses Multiples.* (ed. E. Papernik), pp. 319–328. Paris Doin, 1991.
18. Evans M, Dommergues M, Wapner R *et al.* International collaborative experience of 1789 patients having multifetal pregnancy reduction: a plateauing of risks and outcome. *J. Soc. Gynecol. Invest.* **3**:23–26, 1996.
19. Aberg A, Mitelman F, Cantz M, Gehler J. Cardiac puncture of fetus with Hurler's disease avoiding abortion of the affected co-twin. *Lancet* **2**:990–991, 1978.
20. *Journal Officiel de la République Française, 17 January 1975* Law 75.17.
21. *Journal Officiel de la République Française, 29 July 1994* Law 94.647.
22. Benirschke K & Driscoll SG. *The Pathology of the Human Placenta.* Berlin: Springer Verlag. 1967.
23. Vayssiere CF, Heim N, Camus EP, Hillion YE & Nisand IF. Determination of chorionicity in twin gestations by high frequency abdominal ultrasonography: counting the layer of the dividing membrane. *Am. J. Obstet. Gynecol.* **175**:1529–1533, 1996.
24. Townsend R & Filly RA. Sonography of nonconjoined monoamniotic twin pregnancies. *J. Ultrasound Med.* **7**:665–670, 1988.
25. Mahony BS, Filly RA & Callen PW. Amnionicity and chorionicity in twin pregnancies: prediction using ultrasound. *Radiology* **155**:205–209, 1985.
26. Hill AVS & Jeffreys AJ. Use of minisatellite DNA probes for determination of twin zygocity at birth. *Lancet* **ii**:1394, 1985.
27. Azuma C, Kamiura S, Nobunaga T, Negoro T, Séaji F & Tanizawa O. Zygosity determination of multiple pregnancy by deoxyribonucleic acid fingerprints. *Am. J. Obstet. Gynecol.* **160**:734–736, 1989.
28. Kovacs B, Shahbahrami MS, Platt LD & Commings DE. Molecular genetic prenatal determination of twin zygocity. *Obstet. Gynecol.* **72**:954–956, 1988.
29. Kereny TD & Chitkara U. Selective birth in twin pregnancy with discordance for Down syndrome. *N. Engl. J. Med.* **304**:1525–1527, 1981.
30. Rodeck CH, Mibashan RS, Abramowicz J & Campbell S. Selective feticide of the affected twin by fetoscopic air embolism. *Prenat. Diagn.* **2**:189–194, 1982.
31. Evans MI, Goldberg DG, Dommergues MD *et al.* Efficacy of second-trimester selective termination for fetal abnormalities: international collaborative experience among the world's largest centers. *Am. J. Obstet. Gynecol.* **171**:90–94, 1994.
32. Chitkara U, Berkowitz RL, Wilkins IA, Lynch L, Mehalek KE & Alvarez M. Selective second trimester termination of the anomalous fetus in twin pregnancies. *Obstet. Gynecol.* **73**:690–694, 1989.
33. Malone FD, Craigo SD, Chelmow D & Dalton ME. Outcome of twin gestations complicated by a single anomalous fetus. *Obstet. Gynecol.* **88**:1–5, 1996.
34. Lynch L, Berkowitz RL, Stone J, Alvarez M & Lapinski R. Preterm delivery after selective termination in twin pregnancies *Obstet. Gynecol.* **87**:366–368, 1996.
35. Wittmann BK, Farquharson DF, Thomas WDS, Baldwin VJ & Wadsworth, LD. The role of feticide in the management of severe twin transfusion syndrome. *Am. J. Obstet. Gynecol.* **155**:1023–1026, 1986.
36. Larroche JC. Fetal encephalopathies of circulatory origin. *Biol. Neonate.* **50**:61–74, 1986.
37. Blickstein I. The twin–twin transfusion syndrome. *Obstet. Gynecol.* **76**:714–722, 1990.
38. Fusi L, McFarland P, Fisk N, Nicolini U & Wigglesworth J. Acute twin–twin transfusion. A possible mechanism for brain damaged survivors after intrauterine death of a monochorionic twin. *Obstet. Gynecol.* **78**:517–520, 1991.
39. Dommergues M, Aubry MC, Delezoide AL *et al.* Fetal embolization for twin to twin transfusion syndrome. *Fetal Diagn. Ther.* **10**:26–31, 1995.
40. Crombleholme TM, Robertson F, Marx G, Varnell R & Dalton ME. Fetoscopic cord ligation to prevent neurological injury in monozygous twins. *Lancet.* **348**:191, 1996.
41. Robie GF, Payne GG & Morgan MA. Selective delivery of an acardiac acephalic twin. *N. Engl. J. Med.* **320**:512–513, 1989.

In utero haematopoietic stem cell transplantation

67

A.W. Flake

The engraftment and clonal proliferation of a relatively small number of normal haematopoietic stem cells (HSC) can sustain normal haematopoiesis for a lifetime. This observation provides the compelling rationale for bone-marrow transplantation (BMT) and is now supported by thousands of long-term survivors of BMT who would otherwise have succumbed to lethal haematological disease. However, the current success of BMT can only be viewed as the tip of a massive therapeutic iceberg. Realization of the full potential of BMT continues to be limited by a critical shortage of immunologically compatible donor cells, the inability to specifically control the recipient or donor immune response, and the requirement for recipient myeloablation to achieve engraftment[1–3]. The price of human leukocyte antigen (HLA) mismatch remains high: the greater the mismatch, the higher the incidence of graft failure, graft-versus-host disease (GvHD) and delayed immunological reconstitution. Current methods of myeloablation result in increased morbidity and mortality[4]. In combination, these problems remain prohibitive for the majority of patients who might benefit from BMT. A theoretically attractive alternative, which can potentially address many of the limitations of BMT, is *in utero* transplantation of HSC. This approach is potentially applicable to any congenital haematopoietic disease which can be diagnosed prenatally and can be cured or improved by engraftment of normal HSCs.

Ontogeny of haematopoiesis

Understanding the biology of *in utero* stem-cell transplantation requires familiarity with normal haematopoietic and immunologic ontogeny. Fetal haematopoiesis is characterized by an orderly series of migrational events proceeding from the yolk sac, to the fetal liver and finally to the bone marrow[5] (Fig. 67.1). This process is presumably controlled by sequential expression and/or downregulation of homing receptors

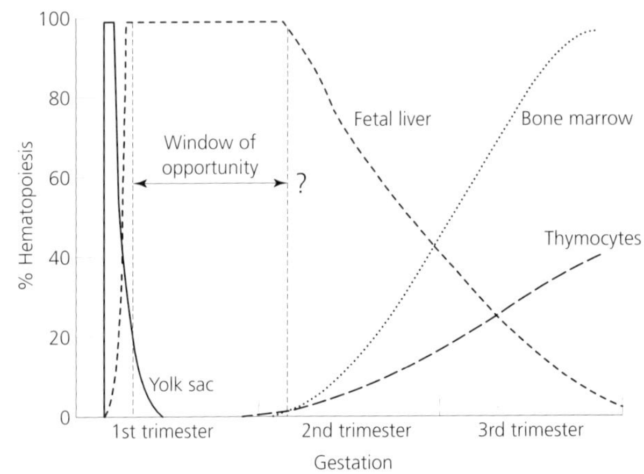

Fig. 67.1 Schematic of normal haematopoietic ontogeny depicting the 'window of opportunity' for *in utero* transplantation. The late limit for tolerance induction is relatively unknown, particularly for the immunodeficiency conditions.

and their corresponding ligands on the surface of microenvironmental cells and HSCs. Thus, the migration of fetal haematopoiesis is probably best viewed as a sequential development of organ specific microenvironmental 'niches' of increasing HSC affinity.

In humans the bone marrow begins as a cartilaginous matrix[6]. Calcification and breakdown of the matrix accompany the arrival of osteoclasts at around 10 weeks' gestation. The marrow cavity becomes populated by macrophages and other stromal elements prior to the migration of haematopoietic elements and contains only stromal elements at 12 weeks' gestation. The first haematopoietic elements begin to appear around 15 weeks' gestation and the migration of HSC from the fetal liver to the bone marrow is not largely complete until around 34 weeks' gestation[7–10]. Thus, there is a prolonged period during gestation when the bone marrow is forming new 'niches' and is receptive to the engraftment of circulating HSC.

Normal immunologic ontogeny includes a period of immunological 'immaturity' characterized by the ability to induce antigen-specific tolerance. Evidence is now overwhelming that the fetal thymic microenvironment plays a primary role in determination of self-recognition and repertoire of response to foreign antigen[11]. Pre-T-cells undergo a series of maturational steps in the fetal thymus that are controlled by thymic stromal cells. Expression of the clonally expressed, heterodimeric T-cell receptor (TCR) occurs early by somatic rearrangement of the genes for the α- and β-chain subunits that bind antigen. The cell surface accessory molecules, CD8 and CD4, are then expressed to create a TCR^{lo} double positive and as yet immature cell[12,13]. This cell is positively selected by interaction with thymic stromal epithelial cells for recognition of major histocompatibility complex (MHC) class I or class II antigen to create $CD8^+$ or $CD4^+$ cells, respectively[13]. These cells are now capable of immunologic reaction and undergo a process of negative selection (deletion) by interaction with thymic self antigen presenting dendritic cells[14,15]. The end result is deletion of T-cell clones with high affinity for self antigen in association with self-MHC, and preservation of a T-cell repertoire against foreign antigen. The timing of these events is of critical importance for clinical application of *in utero* HSC transplantation. The first haematopoietic cells begin to appear in the human fetal thymus at 8–9 weeks' gestation. The first appearance of significant numbers of single positive-reactive T-lymphocytes in the fetal thymus occurs around 13–14 weeks' gestation and these cells appear in the circulation (post-thymic) at 15–16 weeks gestation[16,17].

Rationale for *in utero* transplantation

The rationale for *in utero* transplantation is to take advantage of the 'window of opportunity' created by normal ontogeny. There is a period, prior to population of the bone marrow, and prior to thymic processing of self antigen when the fetus should theoretically be receptive to engraftment of foreign HSC, without rejection, and without the need for myeloablation. In the human fetus, the ideal window would appear to be prior to 14 weeks' gestation, before release of mature T-lymphocytes into the circulation and while the bone marrow is just beginning to develop sites for haemopoiesis. It may certainly extend beyond that in immunodeficiency states, particularly when T-cell development is abnormal. During this time, presentation of foreign antigen by thymic dendritic cells should theoretically result in clonal deletion of reactive T-cells during the negative selection phase of thymic processing. Recent advances in prenatal diagnosis have made possible the diagnosis of a large number of congenital diseases during the first trimester[18]. Technical advances in fetal intervention make transplantation feasible by 10–12 weeks' gestation. The ontological 'window of opportunity' (Fig. 67.1) falls well within these diagnostic and technical constraints making application of this approach a realistic possibility.

Because of the unique fetal environment, prenatal HSC transplantation could theoretically avoid many of the current limitations of postnatal BMT (Table 67.1). There would be no requirement for HLA matching, resulting in expansion of the donor pool. Transplanted cells would not be rejected and space would be available in the bone marrow, eliminating the need for toxic immunosuppressive and myeloablative drugs. The mother's womb is the ultimate sterile isolation chamber, eliminating the high risk and costly 2–4 months of isolation required, after postnatal BMT, prior to immunological reconstitution. Finally, prenatal transplantation would preempt the clinical manifestations of the disease, avoiding the recurrent infections, multiple transfusions, growth retardation and other complications which cause immeasurable suffering for the patient and often compromises postnatal treatment.

TABLE 67.1
***In utero* HSC transplants**

Advantage	Effect
Immunological tolerance	No HLA-restriction/immunosuppression
Bone-marrow space available	No myeloablation
Sterile 'isolation'	No post-transplant isolation
Proliferative environment	Potential competitive advantage – normal cells
Preempts clinical disease	Avoids complicating morbidity/suffering

Experimental support for *in utero* HSC transplantation

The most convincing experimental support for the efficacy of prenatal HSC transplantation comes from an experiment of nature. The observation that dizygotic cattle twins which share cross-placental circulation are permanent haematopoietic chimeras[19] and exhibit specific transplantation tolerance for skin or organ transplants from their siblings[20,21], is directly relevant, and led to Billingham, Brent and Medawar's classic studies on 'acquired' immunological tolerance[22]. These experiments in rodents demonstrated that preimmune exposure to foreign antigen results in specific transplantation tolerance under defined circumstances. Over the past decade, we have performed a large number of experiments in the fetal lamb model which support the feasibility and define the biology of in utero HSC transplantation.

THE ALLOGENEIC SHEEP MODEL

The sheep is particularly tolerant of prenatal manipulations and because of its large size and long gestation (term = 145 days), transplantation is technically feasible at a relatively early stage of gestation development. Intraperitoneal transplantation of HSC can be performed as early as 45 days' gestation which is well within the preimmune phase of immunological ontogeny. In the allogeneic sheep model, preimmune transplantation of fetal liver derived haematopoietic cells results in long-term, multilineage haematopoietic chimerism[23]. Donor hemoglobin levels as high as 30% have been achieved after a single prenatal injection and engraftment and donor cell expression has remained relatively stable for over five years after transplantation, without immunosuppression and without the occurrence of GvHD[24]. Timing of transplantation is critical to successful engraftment. To define the gestational limitations of tolerance in the sheep model we performed transplantation of fetal donor cells into recipients of varying gestational age (Table 67.2). We found that the incidence of chimerism decreases significantly with advancing gestational age and that few, if any, fetuses older than 90 days' gestation exhibited donor cell engraftment. This supports the concept of a 'window of opportunity' limited by immunological development, for successful application of *in utero* HSC transplantation.

TABLE 67.2
Relationship of recipient gestational age to engraftment

Age (days)		No. transplanted	No. alive at term	No. chimeric at birth
Recipient	Donor			
48–68	50–53	16	9	7
75–80	50–53	16	11	5
90–110	50–53	11	8	2
120	50–53	4	4	0

THE HUMAN–SHEEP XENOGENEIC MODEL

The fetal tolerance phenomenon also applies to xenogeneic transplantation[25-27]. We developed the human–sheep model to better define the biology of *in utero* HSC transplantation and as an animal model for the study of human haematopoiesis. Because of the availability of reagents for human cell markers, and the availability of techniques for human HSC enrichment, the human–sheep model allows insight into questions which cannot be answered in the allogeneic sheep model. In this model, transplantation of preimmune fetal lambs (48–54 days' gestation) by intraperitoneal injection of human fetal liver (12–15-week gestation) derived haematopoietic cells ($2 \times 10^9 - 1 \times 10^{10}$ cells/kg estimated fetal body weight) results in stable, multilineage, human cell engraftment in a subset of the transplanted animals[28]. The human–sheep chimerism created in the original experiments has now persisted for over four years (Fig. 67.2). The primary differences between allogeneic and xenogeneic models are the requirement for transplantation of a higher dose of xenogeneic cells to achieve

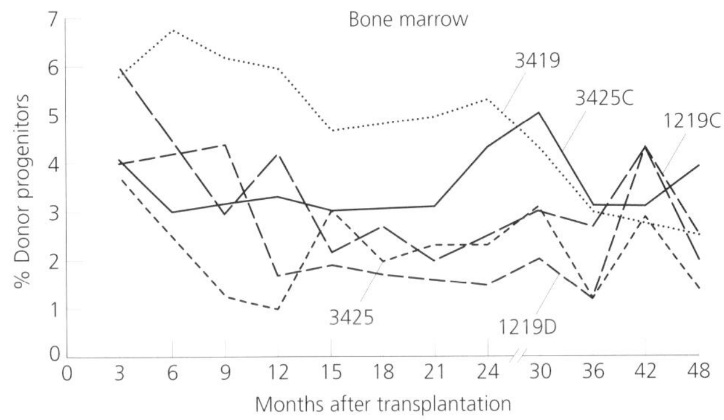

Fig. 67.2 Percent human progenitors in bone marrow of human–sheep chimeras at intervals after birth. Human cells have remained detectable for over four years after transplantation.

engraftment, and subsequently, relatively low levels of peripheral donor cell expression in the xenogeneic model.

HAEMATOPOIETIC STEM-CELL ENGRAFTMENT

Although, long-term, multilineage, donor-cell expression suggests engraftment of true pluripotent HSC, it is not absolute proof. Unequivocal proof of HSC engraftment requires the presence of long-term multilineage engraftment as well as the ability to achieve multilineage repopulation after retransplantation into a second-generation recipient. Since *in utero* transplantation would be performed at an early age, and donor cells must persist for a human lifetime, it was particularly important to prove HSC engraftment in our model. To examine this question we harvested bone marrow from three long-term human–sheep chimeras at 3.2–3.6 years after transplantation[29]. At the time of harvest, all three donors exhibited multilineage, human-cell expression in the bone marrow. Human cells were isolated by positive selection for the human CD45 antigen by panning, pooled and reinjected into six preimmune fetal lambs (4.8×10^6 cells/fetus). At birth, two of the six recipients had detectable human-cell engraftment. Subsequent analysis has confirmed human-cell multilineage expression in the bone marrow and peripheral blood which has persisted for over a year after birth (Table 67.3). The presence of multilineage, long-term engraftment in second-generation chimeras is conclusive evidence for the

TABLE 67.3
Distribution of human cells after retransplantation

		CD45⁺ cells (%)			
Animal #	Tissue	3 weeks	24 weeks	46 weeks	68 weeks
G 27	Blood	0.8	3.2	<0.5	1.7
	Marrow	2.9	8.8	4.6	6.3
G 28	Blood	<0.5	1.6	1.1	0.8
	Marrow	3.7	5.7	6.2	7.9

engraftment of 'immortal' HSCs confirming the potential of *in utero* HSC transplantation for lifelong reconstitution of fetuses with haematopoietic disease.

SOURCE OF DONOR CELLS

The source of donor cells may be critical to the success of engraftment. The most obvious advantage of the use of fetal cells is the absence of mature T-cells in fetal liver-derived populations prior to 14 weeks' gestation[30]. This alleviates any concern about GvHD and avoids the necessity of T-cell depletion which detrimentally influences engraftment. Other advantages of fetal cells are now being appreciated. As alluded to above, there may be ontological differences in the expression of homing receptors/ligands on the surface of HSC. In addition, there is increasing evidence of ontological differences in proliferative and differentiative capacity of fetal versus adult HSC. In a murine model of transplacental injection of fetal- or adult-derived allogeneic cells into W/W^v genetically anaemic mice, Fleischman and Mintz found that adult derived cells had a more limited capacity for self-renewal than fetal liver-derived cells[31]. In *in vitro* studies an increased replating potential of umbilical cord blood derived $CD34^+$ cells compared to those derived from adult bone marrow has been observed[32]. In another study, Lansdorp *et al.*[33] reported striking differences between primitive haematopoietic cells purified from adult bone marrow, umbilical cord blood and fetal liver in cytokine-supplemented, serum-free cultures. In such cultures, both the fraction of responding cells and their ability to produce $CD34^+$ progenitor cells decreased markedly with the age of the cell donor. These results document extensive, ontogeny-related functional differences between primitive haematopoietic cells. In addition to functional differences, there may be ontological differences in developmental potential between adult and fetal HSC. Ikuta *et al.*[34] have shown that only fetal-derived HSC are capable of differentiation into $V\gamma3^+$ T-cells in seeded fetal thymic cultures, whereas adult marrow-derived HSC have lost that capacity. B-lymphocyte differentiation pathways also appear to differ depending upon the ontological age of the B-cell progenitors. Most isolated pro-B cells from fetal liver give rise to $CD5^+$ B-cells, whereas few adult pro-B cells ultimately express CD5 when examined either *in vitro* or in severe combined immunodeficiency disease (SCID) mice[35]. This would suggest that the source of cells for fetal transplantation might not only influence homing and engraftment of donor cells but also the ultimate lineages of donor cell expression.

Although there may be important homing, proliferative and developmental advantages to the use of fetal cells, there are practical and ethical advantages to the use of cord blood or postnatal HSC sources. There are legitimate ethical concerns regarding the use of fetal tissue for transplantation which need to be addressed[36–38]. In addition, fetal tissue obtained by the usual methods has a high degree of microbial contamination[39]. The transplantation of transmissible viral, fungal or bacterial disease could have disastrous consequences for the recipient fetus or mother. Finally, although the fetal liver is a rich source of HSC, small size limits total cell yield, and at the current time, the specific donor cells are not renewable. In contrast, the use of adult-derived cells would allow a renewable, relatively infection free, ethically acceptable source of donor cells. One appealing strategy would be tolerance induction by the *in utero* transplantation of highly purified adult bone-marrow HSC, from a living related donor, followed by a single or multiple postnatal 'booster' injections.

Experimental data for preimmune transplantation of cells of peri- or postnatal derivation is limited but encouraging. Early studies using unprocessed adult marrow in the allogeneic sheep model resulted in engraftment but the occurrence of uniformly lethal GvHD[40]. Efforts to T-cell deplete adult marrow resulted in failure of engraftment. Partial reconstitution of T-cell depleted donor cells with peripherally derived mature T-cells restored engraftment and GvHD in a T-cell dose-dependent fashion[41]. Transplantation of various populations of highly enriched human adult bone-marrow-derived cells ($CD34^+HLADR^-$, $CD34^+lin^-CD38^-$) has resulted in long-term multilineage engraftment at somewhat lower levels than fetal cell transplants, without GvHD[42–44]. Comparison of level of engraftment in these separate experiments is relatively uninformative because they were not standardized for progenitor or HSC content. To compare the relative efficacy of cells derived from various sources we recently transplanted cell inoculums standardized for progenitor content derived from various pre- and postnatal sources in the allogeneic and xenogeneic sheep models[45,46]. Although donor-cell engraftment was similar in all groups, survival to term was reduced in all groups relative to the fetal liver group. In addition, with the exception of the fetal liver group, all surviving chimeric animals developed lethal GvHD. Comparable studies using enriched populations of adult cells have not been performed.

These studies suggest that, at the present time, the risk of transmissible infectious disease inherent in the use of fetal tissue outweigh its theoretical advantages (Table 67.4). In addition, the potential for increasing engraftment with postnatal

TABLE 67.4
Donor cell source

	Pros	Cons
Fetal liver	Proliferation/homing? No GvHD	Safety Ethics? Non-renewable
Adult bone marrow	Safe Renewable	GvHD Proliferation/homing?
Enriched bone marrow	Safe Renewable No GvHD	Proliferation/homing?

transplants using cells from the same donor compensates for the theoretical disadvantages of adult tissue. Using modern methods of bone-marrow enrichment, populations of adult cells markedly enriched for HSC content, with very few residual T-cells, can be obtained. Until fetal tissue or cord blood can be meaningfully expanded in culture and preserved for future use, enriched adult bone marrow is probably the safest, most practical, and most efficacious source of donor cells for prenatal transplantation.

HOMING AND ENGRAFTMENT AFTER PRENATAL TRANSPLANTATION

In tracking studies in the allogeneic and xenogeneic sheep models homing and engraftment of fetal liver derived cells *in vivo* was dependent upon the gestational stage of the recipient[47]. Before the development of the bone marrow, transplanted HSC (liver- or marrow-derived) homed exclusively to the liver/spleen. With the development of marrow, around day 60 of gestation (term = 145 days), homing also occurred to the nascent marrow, and by day 80 transplanted cells homed exclusively to the marrow. These findings support the concept of microenvironmental determination of homing with bone marrow having greater affinity for circulating HSC than fetal liver.

Engraftment of HSC is dependent upon homing to a receptive haematopoietic environment. The concept of bone-marrow 'niches' composed of nests of nurturing stromal elements and extracellular matrix appears to apply to ontogeny. A clear temporal progression is observed in the developing fetal bone marrow from stroma alone to stroma and haematopoietic elements. If this model is correct, the engraftment of donor HSC would be determined by the availability of open niches and the relative affinity of homing interactions of donor-versus-host-derived HSC. If homing affinity of donor and host HSC were equal, engraftment would be directly competitive. Timing of transplantation, dose of donor HSC, or differences in homing affinity of donor HSC, might therefore dramatically influence engraftment. A relevant model has recently been described by Stewart *et al.*[48]. In normal, non-myeloablated mice, transplantation of normal syngeneic cells in repetitive doses results in incremental increases in long-term engraftment. Multiple injections of the same total cell dose results in higher levels of engraftment than a single injection. An explanation of these results is that a percentage of bone-marrow niches are open, even in normal postnatal bone marrow, at any particular time, and that they obey saturation kinetics with respect to engraftment of transplanted cells. In the allogeneic sheep model, transplantation of increasing numbers of donor cells results in a modest increase in engraftment, but this plateaus in a manner consistent with saturation of open niches (Fig. 67.3). If this is true, one potential method of improving engraftment is to deliver donor cells in divided doses over time rather than as a single large bolus.

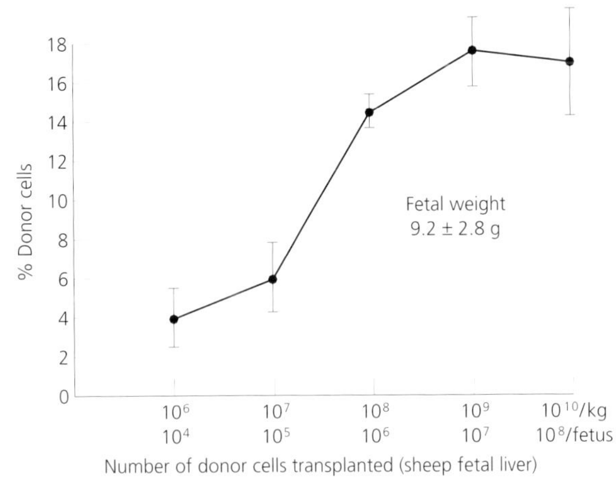

Fig. 67.3 Levels of engraftment plateau with transplantation of increasing numbers of donor cells consistent with saturation of available sites for engraftment.

Diseases amenable to prenatal treatment

A partial list of prospective diseases treatable by prenatal HSC transplantation is given in Table 67.5. Generally speaking, any disease which can be diagnosed early in gestation, which is improved by BMT, and for which postnatal treatment is not entirely satisfactory, is a target disease. However, some diseases are far more likely to benefit from prenatal transplantation than others. The list can be divided into three general categories: haemoglobinopathies, immunodeficiency disorders and inborn errors of metabolism. It is important to emphasize that each of the diseases has unique considerations for treatment, and in fact each individual disease may respond differently. Of particular relevance to the prenatal approach where experimental levels of engraftment have been relatively low, is the observation that in many of the target diseases, engrafted normal cells would be predicted to have a significant survival advantage over diseased cells. This would have the clinical effect of amplification of the level of engraftment in the peripheral circulation. In addition, even with minimal levels of engraftment, specific tolerance for donor antigen should be induced, allowing additional cells from the same donor to be given to the tolerant recipient after birth.

HAEMOGLOBINOPATHIES

The sickle-cell anaemia and thalassaemia syndromes make up the largest patient groups potentially treatable by prenatal stem-cell transplantation. Both groups can be diagnosed within the first trimester. Both have been cured by postnatal BMT, but BMT is not routinely recommended because of its prohibitive mortality, and the relative success of modern medical management. In both diseases the success of BMT is indirectly related to the morbidity of the disease, i.e. the younger the patient, the fewer transfusions received, and the less organ

TABLE 67.5
Congenital diseases potentially amenable to *in utero* stem-cell transplantation (incomplete list)

Haemoglobinopathies
- β-Thalassaemia major
- α-Thalassaemia major
- Sickle-cell anaemia

Immunodeficiency diseases
- Severe combined immunodeficiency syndrome (SCID)
- Bare lymphocyte syndrome
- Chronic granulomatous disease
- Wiskott–Aldrich syndrome
- Chediak–Higashi syndrome
- Infantile agranulocytosis (Kostman's syndrome)
- Lazy leukocyte syndrome (neutrophil actin deficiency)
- Neutrophil membrane GP-180 deficiency
- Agammaglobulinaemia
- X-linked lymphoproliferative syndrome
- X-linked hyper-IgM syndrome

Inborn errors of metabolism
- *Mucopolysaccharidoses*
  - Hurler's disease (MPS-I) (α-iduronidase deficiency)
  - Hurler–Scheie syndrome
  - Hunter disease (MPS-II) (iduronate sulfatase deficiency)
  - Sanfillipo B (MPS-IIIB) (α-glycosaminidase deficiency)
  - Morquio (MPS-IV) (hexosamine-6-sulfatase deficiency)
  - Maroteaux–Lamy syndrome (MPS-VI) (arylsulfatase B deficiency)
  - Sly syndrome (MPS-VII) (β-glucuronidase deficiency)
- *Mucolipidoses*
  - Fabry disease (α-galactosidase A deficiency)
  - Gaucher disease (glucocerebrosidase deficiency)
  - Krabbe disease (galactosylceramidase deficiency)
  - Metachromatic leukodystrophy (arylsulfatase A deficiency)
  - Niemann–Pick disease (sphingomyelinase deficiency)
  - Adrenal leukodystrophy
  - I-cell mucolipidosis II

Other haematopoietic disease
- Osteopetrosis
- Diamond–Blackfan syndrome
- Fanconi anaemia

compromise from iron overload, the better the results[49–51]. With both diseases, the primary questions relevant to prenatal transplantation are 'What levels of normal peripheral cell expression are necessary to alleviate clinical disease' and 'Can adequate levels of donor cell engraftment be achieved by *in utero* HSC transplantation?' At present, only indirect evidence exists to answer these questions.

In sickle-cell disease, the pathophysiology is directly related to the concentration of HbS within red cells which results in marked rheological abnormality including hyperviscosity, cellular adherence and sickling, with an end result of vaso-occlusion and tissue ischaemia. In examining the *in vitro* relationships between haematocrit and viscosity using mixtures of sickle and normal red blood cells (RBCs) Schmalzer *et al.*[52] observed that the primary determinant of viscosity is the sickle haematocrit (fraction of RBCs that contain HbS). Adverse effects of haematocrit on viscosity were seen at a sickle haematocrit level in the low 20s. Oxygen delivery, as gauged by the maximal point on the haematocrit versus viscosity curve, was markedly improved by exchanging normal for sickle RBCs (even when the total haematocrit was held constant). The clinical correlate of this *in vitro* information is chronic exchange transfusion therapy which is indicated after cerebrovascular accidents in sickle-cell disease. Maintenance of the percent HbS below 30% reduces the risk of recurrent stroke from 60–90% to less than 10%[53]. The maximal HbS that effectively prevents stroke is unknown but a transfusion regimen maintaining a HbS of 50% was found to be effective in preventing recurrent stroke in a small study group of sickle-cell disease patients[54].

The clinical manifestations of thalassaemia are secondary to hypoxia related to severe anaemia and ineffective erythropoiesis. It is now standard therapy to chronically transfuse patients with thalassaemia major from an early age which suppresses endogenous erythropoiesis and maintains oxygen delivery. When instituted at an early age, this effectively prevents the bone-marrow expansion and secondary bony changes as well as the haemodynamic and cardiac manifestations of the disease. The necessary normal haemoglobin level required is controversial but good results have been achieved with maintenance of a hemoglobin of 9 g/dl[50,55,56].

Although these levels of normal haemoglobin are higher than we have achieved experimentally (30% donor haemoglobin-maximal), there would be a significant survival advantage of normal cells in both diseases. In sickle-cell disease, erythrocytes have a circulating half-life of 10–20 days (normal = 120 days) prior to destruction. In thalassaemia, most (80%) cells never leave the bone marrow and also have shortened survival in the periphery. Therefore, engraftment of even a few normal stem cells could result in significantly amplified levels of peripheral donor-cell expression.

IMMUNODEFICIENCY DISEASES

These represent an extremely heterogeneous group of diseases which differ in their likelihood of cure by achievement of haematopoietic chimerism. Once again, the most likely to benefit from even low levels of donor-cell engraftment are those diseases in which a survival benefit exists for normal cells. The best example of this situation is severe combined immunodeficiency syndrome (SCID). A number of different molecular causes of SCID have been identified with approximately two-thirds of cases being of X-linked recessive inheritance (X-SCID)[57]. The genetic basis of X-SCID has been recently defined[58] as a mutation of the gene encoding the common γ-chain (γ_c) which is a common component of several members of the cytokine receptor superfamily including those for IL-2, IL-4, IL-7, IL-9, IL-15 and possibly IL-13[59–61]. Children affected with X-SCID therefore have simultaneous inactivation of multiple cytokine systems resulting in a block in thymic T-cell development and diminished T-cell response. B-cells, although present in normal or even increased numbers, are dysfunctional, either secondary to the lack of helper T-cell function, or due to an intrinsic defect in B-cell maturation. Another form of SCID is secondary to adenosine deaminase (ADA) deficiency[62]. Clinical experience with HLA-matched sibling bone marrow or fetal liver/thymus transplantation generally has been successful without myeloablative therapy which suggests that the lymphoid progeny of relatively few engrafted normal HSC have a selective growth advantage *in vivo* over genetically defective cells[63,64]. The competitive advantage of non-affected cells in X-SCID is best supported by the finding of skewed X-inactivation in female carriers[65,66]. Only T-cells containing the normal X-chromosome are present in the circulation. Evidence that ADA production confers a survival advantage derives from the early experience with gene therapy for ADA deficiency SCID[67]. *ADA* gene-corrected autologous T-cells have persisted for prolonged periods despite discontinuation of the T-cell infusions. Transfer of *ADA* gene-corrected cells versus uncorrected cells from the same SCID patient into an immunodeficient BNX mouse results in survival of the corrected cells and death of the uncorrected cells confirming a survival advantage for ADA-producing cells even when there is normal ADA production in the surrounding environment[68]. Unfortunately, other diseases such as chronic granulomatous disease would not be expected to provide a competitive advantage for donor cells. Nevertheless, in all these conditions, even a partial reconstitution of the defective cell or component would at least partially ameliorate the clinical manifestations of the disease and should result in donor-specific tolerance. If higher levels of engraftment are needed, further HSC transplants from the same donor could be performed after birth without fear of rejection.

INBORN ERRORS OF METABOLISM

This is an even a more heterogeneous group of diseases which are caused by a deficiency of a specific lysosomal hydrolase and which results in the accumulation of substrates such as mucopolysaccharide, glycogen or sphingolipid. Depending upon the specific enzyme abnormality and the compound(s) which accumulate, specific patterns of tissue damage and organ failure occur[69]. These include central nervous system deterioration, growth failure, dysostosis multiplex and joint disability, hepatosplenomegaly, myocardial or cardiac disease, upper-airway obstruction, pulmonary infiltration, corneal clouding and hearing loss. The potential efficacy of prenatal HSC transplantation for the treatment of these diseases must be considered on an individual disease basis. The purpose of BMT in these diseases is to provide HSC-derived mononuclear cells which can repopulate various organs in the body including the liver (Kupffer cells), skin (Langerhan's cells), lung (alveolar macrophages), spleen (macrophages), lymph nodes, tonsils and the brain (microglia). Those which have been corrected by postnatal BMT such as Gaucher's disease or Maroteaux–Lamy syndrome (minimal CNS involvement) are certainly reasonable candidates for prenatal treatment[70]. In many cases postnatal BMT has corrected the peripheral manifestations of the disease and has arrested the neurological deterioration, but not reversed preexisting neurological injury, i.e. metachromatic leukodystrophy and Hurler's disease[71]. In these cases, the neurological injury may begin before birth. Postnatal maturation of the blood–brain barrier restricts access to the CNS of transplanted cells or the deficient enzyme. These considerations suggest that prenatal treatment may be a necessity to cure the disease. The primary question is whether donor HSC-derived microglial elements would populate the CNS providing the necessary metabolic correction within the blood–brain barrier. In the author's opinion, these represent the least likely group of diseases of benefit from *in utero* HSC transplantation.

Clinical experience

In spite of the absence of practical limitations, reported clinical experience has been limited. There have been 21 *in utero* haematopoietic stem-cell transplants reported or discussed in the literature including the initial report by Linch in 1986[72–84]. As shown in Table 67.6 they have been performed for a variety of indications, at various gestational ages, using different donor-cell sources and preparations. In most cases, no engraftment was achieved. In many instances, the timing, dose or source of donor cells has been suboptimal providing an explanation for failure. There have been no successful cases reported with the exception of immunodeficiency disease. Touraine[73–75] has reported two cases: one patient with 'bare lymphocyte syndrome' and the other patient a female with presumed autosomal SCID. In both cases, fetal liver- and thymus-derived donor cells were used and analysis is complicated by multiple transplants from different donors including postnatal transplants in the SCID patient. There has been minimal engraftment data published on these patients, particularly beyond one year of age, but they are reported to be healthy. Two cases of successfully treated X-linked SCID have recently been reported. One of these is very preliminary (3.5 months of age) and contains very little data on immunologic function[84]. The other, as described below, has documented evidence of donor progenitor cells in the bone marrow, with complete T-lymphocyte reconstitution, and remains healthy at 22 months of age[83]. In both cases, CD34-enriched paternal bone-marrow cells were transplanted into the peritoneal cavity.

This limited experience, and our experience discussed below, offers hope for the future clinical application of prenatal HSC transplantation. The experimental challenge in the future will be to unravel the biology of HSC transplantation so that maximal advantage may be taken of the unique fetal environment. In the absence of animal models mimicking

TABLE 67.6
Clinical experience with *in utero* HSC transplantation

Gestational age (weeks)	Donor-cell source*	Disease treated*	No. cases	Postnatal outcome*	Reference
17	Maternal TCD BM	Rh disease	1	Survived with no engraftment	72
28	Fetal liver and	Bare lymphocyte	1	Clinically normal, 26% donor	
26	fetal thymus	syndrome		HLA expression at 1 year	
		SCID	1	Alive, engrafted by PCR for Y	
12	Fetal liver	β-thalassaemia major	1	Alive, not engrafted	73–75
19	Fetal liver	β-thalassaemia major	1	Intrauterine death	
34, 23, 25	Paternal TCD BM	MCLD	2	No evidence of engraftment,	
	Sibling TCD BM	β-thalassemia	1	clinical status consistent with primary disease	76
19		SCID	1	Terminated at 26 weeks, no engraftment	
26	Maternal TCD BM	Chediak–Higashi	1	No engraftment at birth	77
18		α-thalassaemia	1	Terminated at 24 weeks, + donor cells in extramedullary haematopoiesis	
12	Maternal TCD BM	Rh disease	1	No detectable engraftment + tolerance	78
14	Fetal liver	β-thalassemia major	1	Septic abortion	79
14	Fetal liver	Hurler's Disease	1	Low-level engraftment, death at age 1 year from complications of the disease	80
15	Paternal CD34 enriched	CGD	1	Alive, no detectable engraftment	80
15	Cryopreserved	α-thalassaemia	1		
13	fetal liver	Sickle-cell disease	1	No detectable engraftment	81
18		β-thalassaemia major	1		
13	Paternal CD34 enriched	MCLD	1	Intrauterine death at 20 weeks, extensive donor cell infiltration	82
16	Paternal CD34 enriched	X-linked SCID	1	Alive at 18 months. Normal immune function, split chimerism	83
20	Paternal CD34 enriched	X-linked SCID	1	Alive at 3.5 months, split chimerism	84

*TCD = T-cell depleted; BM = bone marrow; MCLD = metachromatic leukodystrophy; SCID = severe combined immunodeficiency disease; CGD = chronic granulomatous disease; HLA = human leukocyte antigen; PCR = polymerase chain reaction.

human disease, the efficacy of prenatal HSC transplantation for some conditions can only be answered by ethically performed clinical studies.

SUCCESSFUL TREATMENT OF X-LINKED SCID

We have recently reported the first unequivocally successful treatment of a genetic disease by prenatal cellular therapy.

CASE REPORT

T.D., now a 22-month-old boy, is the second son of a 28-year-old female known to carry an X-SCID mutation. The first son was initially healthy but died at 7 months of age, with a clinical diagnosis of SCID. X-inactivation analysis of the mother's lymphocytes demonstrated skewed X-inactivation confirming the X-SCID genotype. Genetic analysis of trophoblast material from chorionic villus sampling performed at 12 weeks' gestation of the second pregnancy confirmed that the male fetus was affected. After extensive, non-directive counselling and consultation with a variety of specialists, the family elected to undergo the *in utero* transplant procedure. The father underwent bone-marrow harvest and the bone-marrow cells were enriched for $CD34^+$ cells resulting in a cell population containing >98% $CD34^+$ cells and <0.5% $CD3^+$ cells. The fetus received three transplants at 16, 17.5 and 18.5 weeks' gestation of 14.8×10^6, 2×10^6 and 1.8×10^6 enriched cells, respectively, by ultrasound guided-intraperitoneal injection. Estimated fetal weight at the time of the injections based on fetal biometry, was 130, 225 and 290 g giving a dose per injection of 1.14×10^8, 8.9×10^6 and 6.2×10^6 $CD34^+$ cells/kg estimated fetal weight.

The postnatal clinical course of the patient has been uneventful. He was discharged home at 2 weeks of age on prophylactic Bactrim and has remained at home since discharge. An incarcerated inguinal hernia was repaired at 2 months of age. He has had normal growth and development with no hospitalizations and no significant infections since birth.

Donor-cell engraftment and function

Analysis of the patient's cord blood after birth by a variety of methodologies including polymerase chain reaction (PCR) analysis for donor Class II HLA antigen, IL2RG sequence analysis of cord blood and cord blood-derived lineages for mutant sequence, and Class I HLA analysis by flow cytometry (Fig. 67.4), were all consistent with high levels of donor-cell engraftment in a pattern of 'split

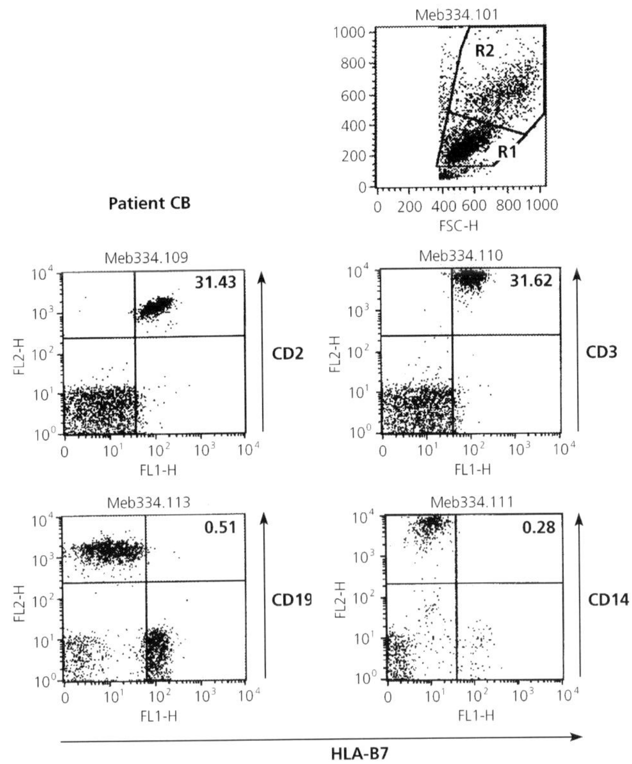

Fig. 67.4 HLA-B7 and phenotypic analysis of cord blood by dual colour flow cytometry. Embedded numbers on scans represent percent gated events which were lineage R2 gated). Essentially all of the CD2 and CD3+ cells (T-cells) are HLA-B7+ (donor in origin) whereas CD19+ (B-cells) and CD14+ (monocytes) cells are all HLA-B7− (recipient origin). TCL = T-cell line, CB = cord blood.)

chimerism'. Essentially, 100% of T-lymphocytes were donor in origin and all of the patients monocytes and B-cells were host in origin. Sequential analysis over time confirmed persistence of this pattern of engraftment and progressive improvement of the patient's lymphocyte counts and subsets into the normal range. He has normal mitogen response relative to age-matched controls, and T-cell lines derived from cord blood have comparable IL-2 and anti-CD3 response to paternal T-cell lines. Mixed-lymphocyte reactions of the patient's cells with paternal, maternal and fourth-party antigens clearly show donor-specific tolerance at a polyclonal level (Table 67.7). The patient's humoral response has shown progressive improvement with low normal IgG levels and evidence of specific response to vaccinations at the time of writing. Finally, we have documented the presence of a donor-derived haematopoietic stem-cell candidate population (CD34+ CD38−) in the patient's bone marrow suggesting engraftment of true HSC.

Summary

From a clinical perspective, prenatal transplantation has tremendous potential to broaden the current indications for reconstitution therapy and to offer a safe, efficacious and cost-effective alternative to conventional postnatal BMT for a large number of congenital haematopoietic diseases. Experimental work and limited clinical experience offer hope for the future. The primary experimental challenges will be to unravel the biology of *in utero* HSC transplantation so that the approach will be safe and broadly applicable. This will require strategies to improve engraftment, safely and effectively utilize alternative sources of cells and develop techniques for procurement, *ex vivo* expansion and tissue banking of safe donor cells. The clinical challenges in the future will be to identify recipients most likely to benefit from the approach, and to further define clinical and ethical guidelines for its application.

TABLE 67.7
Mixed-lymphocyte reaction to maternal, paternal (donor) and fourth-party allogeneic cells

	Medium	S.D.	Patient	S.D.	Father	S.D.	Mother	S.D.
Medium	77	19	2,028	815	529	119	642	333
Patient PBL	90	42	1,382	243	23,346	3,872	39,321	10,683
Father's PBL	77	38	2,193	320	1,101	172	25,344	4,504
Mother's PBL	69	12	7,048	1,541	11,261	4,983	321	158
23 PBL	114	15	24,294	1,572	64,525	8,187	75,396	9,913
58 PBL	109	6	15,111	1,103	23,555	9,255	53,619	4,537
86 PBL	86	24	22,844	4,025	36,142	8,638	73,721	13,628

Fresh cells all donors; PBMC, 1×10^5 cells/well; pulsed at day 5–6. Data expressed as counts per minute. PBL = peripheral blood lymphocytes.

REFERENCES

1. Hansen JA, Anasetti C, Petersdorf E, Clift RA, Martin PJ. Marrow transplants from unrelated donors. *Transplant. Proc.* **26**(3):1710–1720, 1994.
2. Hiemenz JW, Greene JN. Special considerations for the patient undergoing allogeneic or autologous bone marrow transplantation. *Hem. Oncol. Clin. North Am.* **7**(5):961–1002, 1993.
3. Rowe JM, Ciobanu N, Ascensao J *et al.* Recommended guidelines for the management of autologous and allogeneic bone marrow transplantation. A report from the Eastern Cooperative Oncology Group (ECOG). *Ann. Intern. Med.* **120**(2):143–158, 1994.
4. Locatelli F, Giorgiani G, Pession A, Bozzola M. Late effects in children after bone marrow transplantation: a review. *Haematologica* **78**(5):319–328, 1993.

5. Metcalf D, Moore MAS. Embryonic aspects of haemopoiesis. In *Haemopoietic Cells Frontiers in Biology*, Vol. 24 (eds A. Neuberger & E.L. Tatum). Amsterdam: North-Holland.
6. Tavassoli M. Embryonic and fetal hemopoiesis: an overview. *Blood Cells* **17**(2):269–281, 1991.
7. Djaldetti M, Ovadia J, Bessler H, Fishman P, Halbrecht I. Ultrastructural study of the erythropoietic events in human embryonic livers. *Biol. Neonate.* **28**:367–374, 1975.
8. Bessler H, Djaldetti M. Ultrastructural studies on bone marrow development in embryonic mice. *Biol. Neonate.* **61**(4):243–252, 1992.
9. Sminia T, Dijkstra CD. The origin of osteoclasts: an immunohistochemical study on macrophages and osteoclasts in embryonic rat bone. *Calcif. Tissue Int.* **39**:263–266, 1986.
10. Hunn IM, Bodger MP, Hoffbrand AV. Development of pluripotent hematopoietic progenitor cells in the human fetus. *Blood* **62**:118–123, 1983.
11. Blackman M, Kappler J, Marrack P. The role of the T-cell receptor in positive and negative selection of developing T-cells. *Science* **248**:1335–1342, 1990.
12. Kraft DL, Weissman IL, Waller EK. Differentiation of CD3-4-8-human fetal thymocytes *in vivo*: characterization of a CD3-4+8-intermediate. *J. Exp. Med.* **178**:265–267, 1993.
13. Guidos CJ, Danska JS, Fathman CG, Weissman IL. TCR-mediated negative selection of autoreactive T lymphocyte precursors occurs after commitment to the CD4 or CD8 lineages. *J. Exp. Med.* **172**:835–845, 1990.
14. Kappler JW, Roehm N, Marrack P. T-cell tolerance by clonal elimination in the thymus. *Cell* **49**:273–280, 1987.
15. Sha WC, Nelson CA, Newberry RD *et al.* Positive and negative selection of an antigen receptor on T-cells in transgenic mice. *Nature* **336**:73–76, 1988.
16. Haynes BF, Martin ME, Kay HH, Kurtzberg J. Early events in human T-cell ontogeny. Phenotypic characterization and immunohistologic localization of T-cell precursors in early human fetal tissues. *J. Exp. Med.* **168**:1061–1080, 1988.
17. Lobach DF, Hensley LL, Ho W, Haynes BF. Human T-cell antigen expression during early stages of fetal thymic maturation. *J Immunol* **135**:1752–1759, 1985.
18. Fetal diagnosis: Finding defects before birth. In *The Unborn Patient. Prenatal Diagnosis and Treatment*, 2nd edn. (eds M.R. Harrison, M.S. Golbus & R.A. Filly) pp. 39–154. Philadelphia: W.B. Saunders, 1990.
19. Owen RD. Immunogenetic consequences of vascular anastomoses between bovine cattle twins. *Science* **102**:400–401, 1945.
20. Simonsen M. The acquired immunity concept in kidney homotransplantation. *Ann. NY Acad Sci.* **59**:448–452, 1955.
21. Cragle R, Stone W. Preliminary results of kidney grafts between cattle chimeric twins. *Transplantation* **5**:328–335, 1967.
22. Billingham R, Brent L, Medawar PB. Actively acquired tolerance of foreign cells. *Nature* **172**:603–607, 1953.
23. Flake AW, Harrison MR, Adzick NS, Zanjani ED. Transplantation of fetal hematopoietic stem cells *in utero*: the creation of hematopoietic chimeras. *Science* **233**(4765):776–778, 1986.
24. Flake AW, Zanjani ED. *In utero* transplantation of hematopoietic cells. *Crit. Rev. Oncol. Hemat.* **15**:35–48, 1993.
25. Hedrick MH, Rice HE, Sachs DH, Zanjani ED, Flake AW. Creation of pig–sheep xenogeneic hematopoietic chimerism by the *in utero* transplantation of hematopoietic stem cells. *Transplant. Sci* **3**:23–26, 1993.
26. Pallavicini MG, Flake AW, Madden D *et al.* Hemopoietic chimerism in rodents transplanted *in utero* with fetal human hemopoietic cells. *Transplant. Proc.* **24**(2):542–543, 1992.
27. Rice HE, Hedrick MH, Flake AW. *In utero* transplantation of rat hematopoietic stem cells induces xenogeneic chimerism in mice. *Transplant. Proc.* **26**(1):126–128, 1994.
28. Zanjani ED, Pallavicini MG, Ascensao JL *et al.* Engraftment and long-term expression of human fetal hemopoietic stem cells in sheep following transplantation *in utero*. *J. Clin. Invest.* **89**(4):1178–1188, 1992.
29. Zanjani ED, Flake AW, Rice H, Hedrick M, Tavassoli M. Long-term repopulating ability of xenogeneic transplanted human fetal liver hematopoietic stem cells in sheep. *J. Clin. Invest.* **93**(3):1051–1055, 1994.
30. Royo C, Touraine JL, de Bouteiller O. Ontogeny of T lymphocyte differentiation in the human fetus: acquisition of phenotype and functions. *Thymus* **10**(1–2):57–73, 1987.
31. Fleischman RA, Mintz B. Development of adult bone marrow stem cells in H-2 compatible and noncompatible mouse fetuses. *J. Exp. Med.* **159**:159–169, 1984.
32. Lu L, Xiao M, Shen RN, Grigsby S, Broxmeyer HE. Enrichment, characterization, and responsiveness of single primitive CD34^{+++} human umbilical cord blood hematopoietic progenitors with high proliferative and replating potential. *Blood* **81**:41, 1993.
33. Lansdorp P, Dragowska W, Mayani H. Ontogeny-related changes in proliferative potential of human hematopoietic cells. *J. Exp. Med.* **178**:787–791, 1993.
34. Ikuta K, Kina T, MacNeil L *et al.* Developmental switch in thymic lymphocyte maturation potential occurs at the level of hematopoietic stem cells. *Cell* **62**:863–874, 1990.
35. Hardy RR, Hayakawa K. A developmental switch in B lymphopoiesis. *Proc. Natl. Acad. Sci. USA* **88**(24):11550–11554, 1991.
36. Cohen CB, Jonsen AR. The future of the fetal tissue bank. *Science* **262**:1663–1665, 1993.
37. Fine A. Human fetal tissue research: Practice, prospects, and policy. *Cell Transplant* **3**:113–145, 1994.
38. Garry DJ, Caplan AL, Vawter DE, Kearney W. The use of fetal tissue in research on Parkinson's disease. *N. Engl. J. Med.* **327**:1591–1595, 1992.
39. Rice HE, Hedrick MH, Flake AW, Donegan E, Harrison MR. Bacterial and fungal contamination of human fetal liver collected transvaginally for hematopoietic stem cell transplantation. *Fetal Diagn. Ther.* **8**(2):74–78, 1993.
40. Zanjani ED, Lim G, McGlave PB *et al.* Adult haematopoietic cells transplanted to sheep fetuses continue to produce adult globins. *Nature* **295**:244–246, 1982.
41. Crombleholme TM, Harrison MR, Zanjani ED. *In utero* transplantation of hematopoietic stem cells in sheep: the role of T cells in engraftment and graft-versus-host disease. *J. Pediatr. Surg.* **25**(8):885–892, 1990.
42. Srour EF, Zanjani ED, Cornetta K *et al.* Persistence of human multilineage, self-renewing lymphohematopoietic stem cells in chimeric sheep. *Blood* **82**(11):3333–3342, 1993.
43. Srour EF, Zanjani ED, Brandt JE *et al.* Sustained human hematopoiesis in sheep transplanted *in utero* during early gestation with fractionated adult human bone marrow cells. *Blood* **79**(6):1404–1412, 1992.
44. Civin CJ, Lee MJ, Hedrick M, Rice H, Zanjani ED. Purified CD34^{+} lineage-/38^{-} cells contain hematopoietic stem cells. *Blood* **82**(Suppl 1), 180a (abstract 707), 1993.
45. Flake AW, Porada CD, Tavassoli M, Zanjani ED. Comparison of potential for *in utero* engraftment and graft vs. host disease (GvHD) of hematopoietic stem cells (HSC) from fetal, neonatal, and adult sources. *Blood* **82**(Suppl 1):299a (abstract 1182), 1993.
46. Zanjani ED, Flake AW, Rice HE, Hedrick MH, Tavassoli M. An *in vivo* comparison of potential human donor hematopoietic stem cell sources for bone marrow transplantation using the human/sheep xenograft model. *Blood* **82**(Suppl. 1):655a (abstract 2605). 1993.
47. Zanjani ED, Ascensao JL, Tavassoli M. Homing of liver-derived hemopoietic stem cells to fetal bone marrow. *Trans. Assoc. Am. Physic.* **105**:7–14, 1992.
48. Stewart FM, Crittenden RB, Lowry PA, Pearson-White S, Quesenberry PJ. Long-term engraftment of normal and post-5-fluorouracil murine marrow into normal nonmyeloablated mice. *Blood* **81**:2566–2571, 1993.
49. Lane PA. Sickle hemoglobinopathies [published erratum appears in *Curr Opin. Pediatr.* **5**(2):244, 1993.] *Curr. Opin. Pediatr.* **5**(1):74–79, 1993.
50. Piomelli S, Loew T. Management of thalassemia major (Cooley anemia). *Hem./Onc. Clin. North Am.* **5**:557–569, 1991.
51. Steingart R. Management of patients with sickle cell disease. *Med. Clin. North Am.* **76**:669–682, 1992.
52. Schmalzer E, Lee J, Brown A *et al.* Viscosity of mixtures of sickle and normal red cells at varying hematocrit levels: implications for transfusion. *Transfusion* **27**:228–235, 1987.
53. Russell M, Goldberg H, Hodson A *et al.* Effect of transfusion therapy on arteriographic abnormalities and on recurrence of stroke in sickle cell disease. *Blood* **63**:162–169, 1984.
54. Cohen A, Martin M, Silber J *et al.* A modified transfusion program for prevention of stroke in sickle cell disease. *Blood* **79**:1657–1665, 1992.
55. Propper R, Button L, Nathan D. New approaches to the transfusion management of thalassemia. *Blood* **55**:55–60, 1980.

56. Ohene-Frempong K, Rappaport E, Schwartz E. Thalassemia syndromes, recent advances. *Hem./Onc. Clin. North Am.* **1**:503–519, 1987.
57. Puck JM. Prenatal diagnosis and genetic analysis of X-linked immunodeficiency disorders. *Pediatr. Res.* **33**(Suppl), S29–33; discussion S33–34, 1993.
58. Noguchi M, Yi H, Rosenblatt HM *et al.* Interleukin-2 receptor gamma chain mutation results in X-linked severe combined immunodeficiency in humans. *Cell* **73**(1):147–157, 1993.
59. Leonard WJ, Noguchi M, Russell SM, McBride OW. The molecular basis of X-linked severe combined immunodeficiency: the role of the interleukin-2 receptor gamma chain as a common gamma chain, gamma c. *Immunol. Rev.* **138**:61–86, 1994.
60. Matthews DJ, Clark PA, Herbert J *et al.* Function of the interleukin-2 (IL-2) receptor gamma-chain in biologic responses of X-linked severe combined immunodeficient B cells to IL-2, IL-4, IL-13, and IL-15. *Blood* **85**(1):38–42, 1995.
61. Giri JG, Anderson DM, Kumaki S, Park LS, Grabstein KH, Cosman D. IL-15, a novel T cell growth factor that shares activities and receptor components with IL-2. *J. Leukocyte. Biol.* **57**(5):763–766, 1995.
62. Markert ML. Molecular basis of adenosine deaminase deficiency. *Immunodeficiency Review* **5**(2):141–157, 1994.
63. O'Reilly R, Keever C, Small T *et al.* The use of HLA-non-identical T-cell depleted marrow transplants for the correction of severe combined immunodeficiency disease. *Immunodef. Rev.* **1**:273–309, 1989.
64. Buckley RH, Schiff SE, Schiff RI *et al.* Haploidentical bone marrow stem cell transplantation in human severe combined immunodeficiency. *Sem. Hemat.* **30**(Suppl. 4):92–101, 1993.
65. Puck JM, Stewart CC, Nussbaum RL. Maximum-likelihood analysis of human T-cell X chromosome inactivation patterns: normal women versus carriers of X-linked severe combined immunodeficiency. *Am. J. Hum. Genet* **50**(4):742–748, 1992.
66. Hendriks RW, Kraakman ME, Schuurman RK. X chromosome inactivation patterns in haematopoietic cells of female carriers of X-linked severe combined immunodeficiency determined by methylation analysis at the hypervariable DXS255 locus. *Clin. Genet.* **42**(3):114–121, 1992.
67. Blaese RM. Development of gene therapy for immunodeficiency: adenosine deaminase deficiency. *Pediatr. Res.* **33**(Suppl.):S49–53, 1993.
68. Ferrari G, Rossini S, Giavazzi R *et al.* An *in vivo* model of somatic cell gene therapy for human severe combined immunodeficiency. *Science* **251**:1363–1366, 1991.
69. Moses S. Pathophysiology and dietary treatment of the glycogen storage diseases. *J. Pediatr. Gastr. Nutrit.* **11**:155–174, 1990.
70. Hobbs J. Displacement bone marrow transplantation for some inborn errors. *J. Inher. Metab. Dis.* **13**:572–596, 1990.
71. Krivit W, Shapiro E, Kennedy W *et al.* Treatment of late infantile matachromatic leukodystrophy by bone marrow transplantation. *N. Engl. J. Med.* **322**:28–32, 1990.
72. Linch D, Rodeck C, Nicolaides K *et al.* Attempted bone marrow transplantation in a 17 week fetus. *Lancet* **i**:1382, 1986.
73. Touraine JL, Raudrant D, Royo C *et al.* *In utero* transplantation of stem cells in bare lymphocyte syndrome. *Lancet* **i**(8651):1382, 1989.
74. Touraine JL. Stem cell transplantation in primary immunodeficiency, with special reference to the first prenatal, *in utero*, transplants. *Allergol. Immunopathol. (Madrid)* **19**(2):49–51, 1991.
75. Touraine JL, Raudrant D, Rebaud A *et al.* *In utero* transplantation of stem cells in humans: immunological aspects and clinical follow-up of patients. *Bone Marrow Transplant.* **1**:121–126, 1992.
76. Slavin S, Naparstek E, Ziegler M *et al.* Clinical application of intrauterine bone marrow transplantation for treatment of genetic disease – feasibility studies. *Bone Marrow Transplant.* **1**:189–190, 1992.
77. Diukman R, Golbus MS. *In utero* stem cell therapy. *J. Reprod. Med.* **37**(6):515–520, 1992.
78. Thilaganthan B, Nicolaides K. Intrauterine bone-marrow transplantation at 12 weeks' gestation. *Lancet* **342**:243, 1993.
79. Cowan M, Golbus M. *In utero* hematopoietic stem cell transplants for inherited disease. *Am. J. Pediatr. Hem. Onc.* **16**:35–42, 1994.
80. Flake AW & Zanjani ED. Unpublished data, 1995.
81. Westgren M, Ringden O, Sturla E-N *et al.* Lack of evidence of permanent engraftment after *in utero* fetal stem cell transplantation in congenital hemoglobinopathies. *Transplantation* **61**:1176–1179, 1996.
82. Barmbach BJ, Moser HW, Blakemore K *et al.* Engraftment following *in utero* bone marrow transplantation for globoid cell leukodystrophy. *Bone Marrow Transplantation* **19**:399–402, 1997.
83. Flake A, Roncarolo M-G, Puck J *et al.* Treatment of X-linked severe combined immunodeficiency by *in utero* transplantation of paternal bone marrow. *N. Engl. J. Med.* **335**:1806–1810, 1996.
84. Wengler G, Lanfranchi A, Frusca T *et al.* *In utero* transplantation of parental CD34 haematopoietic progenitor cells in a patient with X-linked severe combined immunodeficiency (SCIDX1). *Lancet* **348**:1484–1487, 1996.

Fetal gene therapy

68

L.S. Lashford and L.J. Fairbairn

The prospect of fetal gene therapy raises some important ethical, biological and technical questions. Not all of these are unique to the prenatal period but are also issues in mature subjects and include the need to obtain efficient gene transfer as well as adequate and durable gene expression in target tissues. Many of these technical questions are being addressed in children and adults before extrapolating the technology into the fetus. However, there are some unique biological features both in terms of cell biology and the evolution of disease processes that will only be determined by studies undertaken in the prenatal period. This chapter initially concentrates on the general principles that underpin attempts at genetic therapy before focusing on some of the unique features of fetal treatment.

Gene transfer

VECTOR DESIGN

There are a variety of potential approaches to transferring genetic material into cells. Historically, and largely for experimental purposes, gene transfer has been achieved in the laboratory by physical measures which temporarily perturb the cell membrane including electroporation, lipofection and calcium phosphate precipitation. As a general principle, these methods are only suitable for *ex vivo* use as they cause significant collateral cytotoxicity and produce low levels of gene transfer[1]. Moreover, because the genetic material is rarely integrated into the genome, gene expression and protein production persists for a relatively short period of time. This situation is unsatisfactory for many inherited diseases where it is important that efficient and durable gene expression is achieved. Consequently, the key to fetal gene therapy is the identification of delivery systems which have the capacity to transfer genetic material into cells at high frequency and which subsequently results in stable gene expression.

RETROVIRAL VECTORS

The first generation of vectors for clinical use has exploited the capacity of viruses to enter, transfer and replicate their own genome in human cells. To produce safer delivery systems, the viruses have been modified so that their initial infectivity is maintained but their normal ability to replicate in target cells is lost. The most widely studied vectors are retroviruses (RNA viruses) which have the capacity to infect a broad range of human cell types, transcribe their RNA genome into a DNA copy (provirus) and integrate into the host chromosome in an essentially random manner[2]. Vectors for clinical use have been largely derived from murine type C oncoviruses, most notably the murine Moloney leukaemia virus (MuMoLV). To create sufficient capacity for gene transfer and provide a replication-incompetent virus, the genes coding for viral structural and envelope proteins as well as the viral enzyme reverse transcriptase are removed. This leaves a 'cassette' with specialised terminal regions containing viral promoter and enhancer sequences (long terminal repeats, LTRs) as well as a packaging signal (psi) which controls assembly of viral structural proteins into a virion. In order to function, this minimal vector contains a small number of additional RNA sequences between the viral LTRs including a primer binding site to which cellular tRNA binds and acts as a primer for reverse transcriptase-driven DNA synthesis. The human cDNA of interest is cloned into the cassette at an engineered multicloning site, and infectious particles produced through transfection of the vector into a packaging cell line which expresses viral proteins from non-packageable sequences. Those viral proteins then package the viral cassette producing an infective, but replication-incompetent pseudovirus. Viral particles containing the 'therapeutic' gene bud into the extracellular medium producing a viral supernatant for subsequent gene transfer.

The resultant viral vector has a number of practical limitations. The first of these is a finite capacity for carrying

DNA. In practice, it is possible to insert approximately 7–10 kb of DNA into many retroviruses and although this is satisfactory for a number of therapeutic purposes some genes require co-transfer of sizeable regulatory sequences to enable efficient transcription. The most notable example of this, and relevant to the treatment of beta-thalassaemia, is the beta-globin gene which needs a locus control region (LCR) to provide adequate and position-independent gene expression[3].

Secondly, although retroviruses are able to infect a wide range of primary cells, the fact that they only integrate during mitosis makes it unlikely that satisfactory levels of gene expression will be achieved in tissues with a low growth fraction. This problem is compounded in relatively undifferentiated cells such as embryonic stem cells and haemopoietic progenitors by rapid downregulation of gene expression. A number of mechanisms contribute to this phenomenon, including repressive influences of the site of integration, suppressive sequences within the therapeutic cDNA[4], repression from the viral primer binding sites and direct silencing effects of marker genes[6] which are frequently incorporated into the genetic construct to improve selection of cells expressing the transfected gene. The general result of these effects is methylation of the viral LTR with consequent loss of the viral promoter and enhancer activities. A number of strategies are being developed to try to overcome such problems, including the selection of retroviruses with enhanced ability to express in embryonic stem cells and identification of additional regulatory sequences which remain active both in pluripotent stem cells and their committed progeny[7–9]. For example, Ostertag and colleagues have selected retroviruses such as the spleen focus forming virus and the myeloproliferative sarcoma virus, which are particularly potent at driving transcription in primitive cells, and have combined their enhancer regions with a leader sequence from the murine embryonic stem cell virus to create composite vectors with improved performance in primitive haematopoietic progenitors and embryonic stem cells. These hybrid vectors certainly appear to improve the level of expression of specific genes in lymphoid and myeloid cells, although as yet there is no definitive data on the effect of these modifications on the durability of protein production.

Other important factors which will influence the performance of retroviral vectors include the immune response of the host. Most murine retroviruses are highly sensitive to the effects of human complement and are rapidly inactivated *in vivo*[10]. This is not simply an effect of serum activity but is also seen when vectors are introduced into amniotic fluid[11]. The inactivation of retroviruses by human complement is not a universal phenomenon, with other species-specific viruses such as the feline leukaemia virus (FeLV) appearing relatively resistant[12]. The resistance is attributable to the composition of the viral protein envelope and this knowledge has been exploited to engineer packaging cell lines which produce a composite vector with a MuMoLV core but contain additional envelope proteins from the feline endogenous virus RD114[13]. In addition to conferring resistance to human complement, this strategy demonstrates the potential for engineering vectors with a degree of cellular specificity. The idea has been developed to include the incorporation of single-chain antibodies[14] and peptide growth factors in the viral envelope[15], producing 'targeted' but so far, low-titre vectors.

Whilst these novel approaches are likely to improve the efficacy and specificity of retroviral mediated gene transfer, there are important concerns regarding their safety. One worrying issue is the potential for recombination between the vector and packaging line sequences, producing a replication competent wild-type virus. Replication competent virus has the potential to spread within the genome, produce a large number of random integration events and subsequently inactivate or enhance activity of adjacent genes with both mutagenic and potentially teratogenic effects. One aspect of this issue has been highlighted by the experimental work of Donohue *et al.* who exposed primate bone marrow to high levels of replication-competent retrovirus and reintroduced the bone marrow into immunosuppressed monkeys[16]. Although it is noteworthy that the monkeys were highly immunosuppressed by the effects of total body irradiation, three out of eight animals rapidly developed a T-cell lymphoma. The occurrence of such events can be minimised by engineering packaging cell lines so that the 3′ LTR as well as the viral packaging sequence is deleted or by splitting the viral genes into separate constructs[17,18]. Both strategies significantly reduce the chance of a recombination event producing a replication-incompetent virus and although there remains a finite risk, this is felt to be quite small.

ADENOVIRAL VECTORS

To overcome some of these difficulties, vector design has taken a number of parallel directions: the generation of non-integrating or site-specific integrating viral vectors and the development of artificial self-assembling delivery systems. The best example of the first approach is vectors based on adenoviral subtypes. Unlike retroviruses, these are DNA viruses which express their genetic material as an episome. They are able to infect a broad range of cell types including postmitotic cells and have been used for transferring genetic material into neurons and respiratory epithelium[19,20]. Unfortunately, the episome is lost at the time of cell division, making them unsuitable for permanent reconstitution of dividing cells. However, although permanent reconstitution cannot be achieved, it is possible to obtain expression for many weeks under appropriate conditions. A major contributory factor to loss of expression is a marked inflammatory response to the vector. The clinical relevance of this effect was demonstrated in the first human studies where four patients with cystic fibrosis received 2–4 ml of a solution containing an adenoviral vector carrying the cDNA for the cystic fibrosis transmembrane conductance regulator (CFTR)[21]. Whilst three out of four patients did not experience any serious adverse events, a single patient suffered a pneumonitic illness which was accompanied by a rise in serum interleukin-6. The study was stopped and further investigations undertaken into the possible modes of lung damage.

These more extensive studies have demonstrated that a number of the viral proteins are highly immunogenic and induce antigen-dependent cell-mediated immunity[22,23]. Unfortunately, the resulting chronic inflammation is not only toxic but adds to the rapid elimination of virus from the host and consequent loss of transgene expression.

These effects may also be relevant to fetal gene transfer as similar problems have been encountered in preclinical experiments in fetal lambs[24,25]. Using a vector in which the E1a, E1b and E3 regions had been deleted, Vincent and colleagues examined the effect of transferring the beta-galactosidase gene into the trachea during the latter third of gestation. The lungs of treated animals were examined for histological evidence of gene expression and lung fluid sampled for evidence of an inflammatory reaction. Transient staining for beta-galactosidase was found throughout the pulmonary epithelium with maximal intensity noted 3–12 days after administration of the virus and which had disappeared by 14 days. Loss of expression was accompanied by a significant inflammatory reaction comprising diffuse interstitial thickening and an intraluminal neutrophilia. Although there have been some additional studies suggesting that severe inflammation is not a universal corollary of adenoviral gene transfer in the fetus, there is also important evidence indicating that that it should be possible to reduce the risks of an inflammatory reaction by removing alternative portions of the viral genome such as the E2a or E4 regions[26,27]. This work is very much in the developmental stage whilst the optimal combination of deleted sequences is found and a balance is struck between reducing viral immunogenicity, identifying appropriate promoters to drive gene expression and optimising viral production.

LIPOSOMES

An alternative approach is to exploit the sort of liposomal technology that has been developed for systemic carriage and delivery of toxic drugs. In principle, liposomes or cationic lipid complexes might be less toxic and have the potential for delivering quite large genetic constructs. Both approaches essentially trap plasmid DNA in a lamellar lipid structure which enters cells through endocytic pathways. Unfortunately, the liposomes are often trapped and degraded in the acidic environment of the endosomal compartment thus reducing the translocation of DNA to the nucleus[28]. There are a number of strategies which are potentially helpful in overcoming these problems. For example, concurrent administration of the lysomotropic drug chloroquine reduces the endosomal pH, inhibits the activity of degradative enzymes and can improve gene expression[29]. Unfortunately, such drugs are often quite toxic, even in the postnatal period, such that investigators have looked at modifying the vector to increase the chance of endosomal escape. A widely applied method is to incorporate elements of viruses into the lipid structure, which have the capacity to destabilize the endosome. This might include complexing the HA2 peptide of the influenza virus to polylysinated DNA[30], or the construction of fusogenic liposomes through direct coupling of a virus such as Sendai virus[31] or adenovirus[32] to the liposomal formulation. These methods increase the release of genetic material into the cytosol and improve initial gene expression.

At present, there are some early clinical studies investigating the safety and efficacy of these physical methods of gene delivery. Most notable of these are the attempts to express the *CFTR* gene in the respiratory epithelium of patients with cystic fibrosis where it has been shown that it is possible to obtain transient expression of the *CFTR* gene in the nasal epithelium of affected individuals[33]. Despite the transient nature of transgene expression, it has been possible to demonstrate a quantifiable biological effect with detectable changes in ion flux across cell membranes. As it is quite feasible to repeatedly administer a non-immunogenic liposome to the respiratory tract, this approach may prove to be of worthwhile benefit in patients with cystic fibrosis. In the fetus, where it may be important to obtain more durable protein expression, further modifications to synthetic systems are needed which might include the addition of nuclear localisation signals to increase the probability of nuclear targeting and integration in host DNA. For example, addition of a nuclear binding protein such as a histone has significantly increased the expression of a reporter gene in cell lines[34]. This technology is in its infancy but developments such as these are likely to significantly advance the field, producing safer vectors which are capable of delivering adequate and durable gene expression.

In summary, there is a major research effort being undertaken in the field of vector design to enable satisfactory transfer of genetic material to target tissues. At present, all of the available vectors for clinical use have either safety or efficacy issues which make them broadly unsuitable for fetal use. Considerably more developmental work will need to be undertaken in the postnatal period before testing in the prenatal period. However, a wide range of strategies have been identified which suggests that this approach may become technically feasible.

Tissue targets

Whilst vector design is crucial in mediating gene transfer, there are a number of cellular characteristics which will also determine gene expression. As was alluded to in the discussion on modifying retroviral vectors, differential factors operate to regulate transcription during cellular development. The importance of this is illustrated by the improved expression levels achieved from the hybrid retroviral vector FMEV which is attributable to the gain of a binding site for a ubiquitous cellular transcription factor Spl, and altered affinity for another family of transcription factors.

In addition, it must be borne in mind that there is little prospect of gaining any fine control over gene expression with the current generation of vectors. Consequently, the targeted cell needs to be tolerant of dysregulated protein production. This is not generally seen as a problem given the generally low levels of gene transfer achieved *in vivo* and the capacity for many tissues to recover from a toxic insult. However, it should be noted that at least experimentally it has been shown that dysregulated protein production can lead to secondary pathology[35]. For example, overexpression of the lysosomal enzyme α-L-iduronidase in fibroblasts of patients affected by this enzyme deficiency (mucopolysaccharidosis type 1 or Hurler's syndrome), can result in secondary lowering of other lysosomal enzyme levels producing an alternative pathology. In this case, the problem is attributed to saturation of the lysosomal transport system by α-L-iduronidase at the expense of other enzymes.

Problems such as these need to be worked through on an individual basis and the theoretical consequences for the fetus considered within its developmental context. However, a major issue that crosses all pathologies is the identification and targeting of cells with the capacity to transfer the genetic correction to subsequent generations, and to maintain the effect in a population of long-lived progenitors, the so-called 'stem cell pool'.

TARGETING STEM CELLS

HAEMATOPOIETIC PROGENITORS – THE PARADIGM

The best characterised of these target populations for gene transfer is the haemopoietic stem cell (HSC) which can be defined functionally by its ability to regenerate all haematopoietic lineages in lethally irradiated recipients, and to a lesser extent both phenotypically (contained within the $CD34^+$, $CD38^-$, HLA-DR-progenitor fraction) and by *in vitro* characteristics such as the identification of the long-term culture initiating cells (LTC-IC) and high proliferative potential colony-forming cells. The clinical rationale for attempting gene transfer into these primitive subpopulations comes from the number of single-gene disorders which arise as primary haematological defects, such as the haemoglobinopathies and the primary immunodeficiencies, as well as a number of metabolic disorders which can be ameliorated by allogeneic bone-marrow transplantation (e.g. the lysosomal disorders).

In the human fetus, primitive erythroblasts appear at 3–4 weeks' gestation and are derived from yolk-sac progenitors. HSCs migrate from the yolk sac to establish haemopoiesis in the fetal liver at about 5–7 weeks' gestation. This remains the main site of haematopoietic activity until the third trimester although HSCs begin to seed the preformed bone-marrow stroma at around week 16 of gestation. Transfer of HSCs to bone marrow is completed at approximately 34 weeks of gestation. Several studies have looked at the size of the circulating progenitor compartment in the fetus and it is evident that there are high levels of circulating progenitors in all blood samples taken at different times in gestation and that these high levels are sustained until birth[36,37]. These progenitors have a high proliferative capacity and have at least a limited capacity to self-renew as identified by the ability to repeatedly form colonies following sequential replating. Such features indicate that fetal blood could be an important biological target for gene transfer.

The evidence that these primitive cells can be transduced has largely been established in the postnatal period, using either bone marrow, peripheral blood progenitors or umbilical cord blood as a source of HSCs. The methods for obtaining efficient transduction have been established using either animal models where it is possible to test transduction through the ability of transduced cells to engraft in lethally irradiated recipients, or in *in vitro* models of human haemopoiesis such as the modified Dexter culture system. This *in vitro* model has been adapted for measuring gene transfer and expression in progenitor populations obtained both from peripheral blood and from the umbilical cord. The general concensus of a range of experiments is that it is possible to obtain successful retroviral mediated gene transfer into approaching 70% of progenitors under defined culture conditions[38,39]. Moreover, despite concerns regarding repression of retrovirally-driven transcription, protein production has been detected throughout the lifetime of the long-term cultures[39] and in the case of animal studies, transduced bone marrow has successfully reconstituted irradiated mice and with protein production continuing up to six months following transplantion[40].

A small number of studies have investigated the feasibility of targeting fetal HSCs. Proof of principle was established by Kantoff *et al.* who withdrew fetal blood from 93–105-day fetal sheep, transferred the neomycin resistance gene using a retroviral vector N2, and reinfused the transduced cells[41]. Unfortunately, there was a high procedural mortality as well as a large number of early postnatal deaths. Despite a very low initial efficiency of gene transfer, a number of the animals dying in the postnatal period showed evidence of transgene persistence, which was also evident in a single sheep reaching two years of age. Given the high numbers of circulating progenitors in fetal blood, it should be expected that a much higher efficiency of gene transfer might be achieved. In a comparative study, Ekhterae investigated the ease of transducing fetal- and adult-derived HSCs with a neomycin reporter gene using the same standard MuMoLV vector, N2, and confirmed the expectation that there would be a numerical advantage in transducing fetal HSCs with at least a 100% increase in the successful expression of transgene in the colony-forming population[42].

A number of programmes are underway to assess the efficacy of HSC transduction in an appropriate clinical setting. These include retroviral transduction of peripheral blood progenitors as treatment for Gaucher's disease and chronic granulomatous disease, bone marrow in Hurler's syndrome (Mucopolysaccharidosis type I) as well as studies investigating the benefit of transducing long-lived, terminally-differentiated cells such as T-lymphocytes (adenosine deaminase deficiency [ADA] and Hunter's syndrome). The results of these studies are eagerly awaited so that informed decisions can be made about moving studies into the fetus. However, it is already pertinent to examine the rationale for taking fetal gene transfer forward.

RATIONALE FOR FETAL HSC TRANSDUCTION

The most compelling argument for prenatal gene therapy through manipulation of HSCs centres on the necessity of preventing irreversible organ damage in the fetus. There are a few situations where this criterion can be clearly applied. In Hurler's syndrome, where allogeneic bone-marrow transplant (BMT) in the postnatal period has a role to play in ameliorating the disease process, there is already established skeletal damage at birth. However, this complication remains a problem even after early BMT (during infancy), so that it is not clear whether the continuing problems are due to an absolute or relative failure of the haematological graft to deliver corrective levels of enzyme. Consequently, one cannot be sure that a fetal transplant would prevent the emergence of bony pathology and in this situation more fundamental work on the pathogenesis of the disease is needed.

For many metabolic disorders including Hurler's syndrome, the site of damage is more often the central nervous system (CNS). In this disease, allogeneic HSC transplant has been shown to prevent or reduce the CNS effects of enzyme deficiency provided it is undertaken before there is clinical evidence of developmental impairment. The mechanism for CNS enzyme transfer is largely through the bone-marrow derived microglial population which presumably have either the capacity to secrete enzyme into the interstitial space or to transfer enzyme through direct cellular interaction. These mechanisms have been well characterised for other cellular populations[43] and the role of the microglial population has been shown experimentally in animal studies of gene transfer for Gaucher's disease (glucocerebrosidase deficiency). Once again, using the N2 vector, Krall and colleague transplanted transduced bone marrow into lethally irradiated mice and showed that with the passage of time there was an increase of microglia containing enzyme within the CNS of treated animals. This reached 20% of cells by six months with the majority of the enzyme located in perivascular tissue[44].

Several factors need to be considered when weighing up the value of fetal HSC transplantion in attaining corrective levels of enzyme in conditions which have pre-established CNS impairment at birth. On the positive side, the majority of animal studies show that the earlier transplantion is undertaken the greater the influence on subsequent disease pathology. However, all of the successful preclinical studies have used myeloablative conditioning regimes to correct tissue abnormalities, with a clear relationship between increasing radiation dose and better levels of functional enzyme[45,46]. It is not known whether the beneficial role of the conditioning is through facilitating engraftment or through tissue injury which in turn stimulates trafficking of the bone marrow-derived microglia. It must also be borne in mind that, although immature microglia can be detected in the fetal CNS from relatively early in gestation, fully differentiated forms are detectable only after establishing haematopoiesis from the bone marrow, i.e. at around 34 weeks' gestation[47]. Such factors emphasise the relative uncertainty around the biological rationale for early HSC transplantion in many metabolic disorders which affect the CNS, and further preclinical work is necessary to dissect out its potential value, both in conditions where there is some evidence of a postnatal benefit from HSC transplantion and perhaps in some where there is not.

Given the level of uncertainty around many of these issues, the earliest clinical studies of prenatal gene therapy will clearly build on evidence from fetal allogeneic transplantion in life-threatening, primary haematological conditions.

A further important rationale resides in the opportunity to take advantage of the immunological tolerance of the early fetus. It has been recently shown in animal models of various lysosomal storage disorders that animals with a null phenotype, and which are administered exogenous recombinant protein, produce an immune response to the protein[48,49]. Consequently, one concern surrounding postnatal gene therapy is the emergence of an immune response to the transgene product in the most severely affected patients, who have undetectable protein levels. There is the potential to overcome this problem by introducing the transgene at a time when the fetus is establishing tolerance to self antigens. In essence, this means targeting HSCs before week 18 of gestation. It might be argued that the same result would be achieved by an allogeneic transplant undertaken at the same time point, either from fetus to fetus or adult donor to fetus. Despite some encouraging animal work demonstrating the receptiveness of the early fetus to allogeneic transplants both within and across species barriers, human studies are still in a relatively early stage with major problems related to fetal loss during the procedure and lack of adequate levels of donor engraftment[50,51]. The first successful fetal transplant was in the condition 'bare lymphocyte syndrome' where lymphocytes do not express MHC antigens. This initial success may have been fortuitous, as most subsequent successful transplants seem to have been achieved when the recipient has had a primary immunodeficiency. Consequently, despite the theoretical and experimental rationale for transplantation during a 'window' of tolerance, fetuses without a primary immunodeficiency frequently fail to engraft. However, this observation is based on a small number of transplanted fetuses and work will undoubtedly continue in this area until it becomes clear over the coming decade whether allogeneic transplantion or genetic manipulation and subsequent reinfusion of autologous HSCs are technically possible and which technique will be of most clinical benefit. The risk–benefit analysis may be influenced by the decision as to whether genetic modification of HSCs takes place *in vivo* or *in vitro*, since *in vivo* transduction might also induce tolerance to elements in the viral vector, potentially leaving the recipient vulnerable to a later wild type infectious viral challenge.

ALTERNATIVE SOMATIC TISSUE TARGETS

There is an increasing body of evidence from postnatal studies indicating that, despite the limitations of current vector systems, useful levels of transgene expression will eventually be obtained and assessed in some clinical situations. This would include expression of CFTR in the respiratory epithelium of patients with cystic fibrosis, the use of muscle to express a range of secreted proteins such as clotting factors, and in hepatocytes where clinical trials investigating expression of the low-density lipoprotein receptor are already underway. Some of these tissues, which are lead targets for postnatal gene therapy, also have complementary programmes in the fetus. As has been alluded to, prenatal studies are underway to assess transfer of the *CFTR* gene into the fetal respiratory epithelium and, although there is no evidence of prenatal lung damage in this condition, earlier targeting perhaps with integrating vectors may lead to a more durable correction of the disorder. Initial studies using a retroviral vector to carry a reporter gene into the trachea of fetal lambs have been disappointing[52]. Although it was possible to demonstrate gene transfer, this was not evident in the more distal airways and was associated with considerable toxicity including epithelial desquamation, inflammatory infiltrates and fetal loss.

Other investigators have concentrated on gene transfer through amniotic fluid, relying on fetal swallowing and respiratory mechanisms to disperse the vector through the gastrointestinal tract and lung[53]. So far, the results have been quite variable between infected fetuses, producing a rather patchy distribution of transgene expression and with a tendency for most of the expression to be confined to the upper airways and the proximal gastrointestinal tract, namely oesophagus, stomach and duodenum.

Not suprisingly, given its pivotal role in fetal health, the placenta is also under scrutiny as target for genetic manipulation[54]. To date, investigators have looked at the ability of adenovirus to mediate gene transfer in the placenta and have shown that it is possible to transduce the human cytotrophoblast *in vitro* although it became quite difficult to achieve this when the cells underwent terminal differentiation into multinucleate syncytiotrophoblasts. The block on gene expression appeared to be at the level of infection rather than gene transcription and is in keeping with the clinical observation that adenoviral infection of the fetus is a rare event.

The uncertainty surrounding microglia as suitable vehicles for gene transfer in the CNS has already been discussed, and although there are still relatively few fetal studies examining the potential for CNS gene transfer, preclinical studies in postnatal animals are moving ahead. The strategies revolve around many of the issues that have already been highlighted and in particular involve the development of adenoviruses which have the capacity to infect neurons but also demonstrate immunogenicity within the CNS[55]. Herpes simplex virus is also under consideration, but so far clinical development is constrained by concerns over safety, particularly viral reactivation, as well as the identification of efficient promoters which can maintain gene expression in a vector which is otherwise transcriptionally inactive in its latent state[56,57]. A particularly interesting development and offering an approach more closely allied to HSC transplant has been the exploration of neural progenitors for gene transfer and expression.

A key advance has been the demonstration that human fetal tissue is capable of engrafting and forming neural connections. Fetal tissue has been successfully engrafted into patients with Parkinson's disease and has shown evidence of clinical effect. Such experiments indicate the potential for grafting cells in the CNS, but these do not achieve the diffuse repopulation achieved with microglia and are presumably only of value for treatment of site-specific lesions. In animal studies, investigators have immortalised cells from the external granular layer of the cerebellum by transducing with cellular oncogenes such as *myc*. Following injection into the ventricular system, these lines have been shown to engraft throughout the CNS and can differentiate into both neurons and glia[58]. In an animal model of the metabolic disorder mucopolysaccharidosis type VII (Sly syndrome), intracranial grafts have been formed without conditioning, enzyme activity has been detected and animals did not develop the usual behaviour associated with neurodegeneration[59]. Similar experiments have been undertaken for one form of Tay–Sachs disease and, following the general trend of other animal work, highest levels of enzyme activity were achieved when transplantation was undertaken in fetal tissue[60].

Of course, the value of this approach in human subjects, either as an allogeneic graft or as a vehicle for gene transfer, must remain highly speculative, not least because of safety concerns regarding the potential for secondary tumour induction from immortalised cell lines. The alternative approach of expanding primary neural progenitors is probably technically feasible but, so far, such cells have failed to engraft.

Summary

There are a significant number of biological and clinical issues which need to be addressed before taking forward genetic manipulation of somatic cells into the fetus. These issues vary, but key problems include the interaction of the vector with the host to produce safe and effective gene expression, which should also take account of the factors influencing gene expression at different developmental stages. In determining the value of taking such a strategy forward, gene therapy must be weighed against alternative therapeutic options which include the timing of the therapeutic intervention and other possible transplantation strategies.

REFERENCES

1. Neil GA & Zimmerman U. Electro injection. *Methods Enzymol.* **221**, 339–361, 1993.
2. Coffin JM. Retroviral DNA integration. *Dev. Biol. Stand.* **76**, 141–151, 1992.
3. Grosveld F, Dillon N & Higgs D. The regulation of human globin gene expression. *Baillière's Clin. Haematol.* **6**(1), 31–55 , 1993.
4. Koeberl D, Halbert C, Krumm A & Miller A. Sequences within the coding regions of clotting factor VIII and CFTR block transcriptional elongation. *Hum. Gene. Ther.* **6**, 469–479, 1995.
5. Grez M, Akgun E, Hilberg F & Ostertag W. Embryonic stem cell virus, a recombinant murine retrovirus with expression in embryonic stem cells. *Proc. Natl. Acad. Sci. USA* **87**(23), 9202–9206, 1990.
6. Artelt P, Grannemann R, Stocking C *et al.* The prokaryotic neomycin resistance encoding gene acts as a transcriptional silencer in eukaryotic cells. *Gene* **99**(2), 249–254, 1991.
7. Beck Engeser G, Stocking C, Just U *et al.* Retroviral vectors related to the myeloproliferative sarcoma virus allow efficient expression in haematopoietic stem and precursor cell lines, but retroviral infection is reduced in more primitive cells. *Hum. Gene. Ther.* **2**(1), 61–70, 1991.
8. Baum C, Hegewisch-Becker S, Eckert HG, Stocking C & Ostertag W. Novel retroviral vectors for efficient expression of multidrug resistance (*mdr-1*) gene in early haematopoietic cells. *J. Virol.* **69**(12), 7541–7547, 1995.
9. Baum C, Eckert HG, Stockshlader M *et al.* Improved retroviral vectors for haematopoietic stem cell protection and *in vivo* selection. *J. Hematother* **5**(4), 323–329, 1996.
10. Welsh RJ, Cooper NR, Jensen FC & Oldstone MB. Human serum lyses RNA tumour viruses. *Nature* **257**, 612–614, 1975.
11. Douar AM, Themis M, Sandig V, Friedmann T & Coutelle C. Effect of amniotic fluid on cationic lipid mediated transfection and retroviral infection. *Gene. Ther.* **3**, 789–796, 1996.
12. Takeuchi Y, Cosset F, Lachman P *et al.* Type C retrovirus inactivation by human complement is determined by both the viral genome and producer cell. *J. Virol.* **68**, 8001–8007, 1994.
13. Cosset FL, Takeuchi Y, Battini JL, Weiss RA & Collins MK. High-titer packaging cells producing recombinant retroviruses resistant to human serum. *J. Virol.* **69**(12), 7430–7436, 1995.
14. Russell SJ, Hawkins RE & Winter G. Retroviral vectors displaying functional antibody fragments. *Nucleic Acids Res.* **21**(5), 1081–1085, 1993.
15. Cosset FL, Morling F, Takeuchi Y *et al.* Retroviral retargeting by envelopes expressing an N-terminal binding domain. *J. Virol.* **69**, 7430–7436, 1995.
16. Donohue RE, Kessler SW, Bodine D *et al.* Helper virus induced T cell lymphoma in non-human primates for retroviral mediated gene transfer. *J. Exp. Med.* **176**, 1125–1138, 1992.
17. Markowitz D, Goff S & Bank A. A safe packaging line for gene transfer; separating viral genes on two different plasmids. *J. Virol.* **62**(4), 1120–1124, 1988.
18. Danos O & Mulligan RC. Safe and efficient generation of recombinant retroviruses with amphotropic and ecotropic host ranges. *Proc. Natl. Acad. Sci. USA* **85**, 6460–6464, 1988.
19. Le-Gal-La-Salle G, Robert JJ, Berrard S *et al.* An adenovirus vector for gene transfer into neurons and glia in the brain. *Science* **259**(5097), 988–990, 1993.
20. Rosenfeld MA, Chu CS, Seth P *et al.* Gene transfer to freshly isolated human respiratory epithelial cells *in vitro* using a replication-deficient adenovirus containing the human cystic fibrosis transmembrane conductance regulator cDNA *Hum. Gene. Ther.* **5**(3), 331–342, 1994.
21. Crystal RG, McElvaney NG, Rosenfeld MA *et al.* Administration of an adenovirus containing the human CFTR DNA to the respiratory tract of individuals with cystic fibrosis. *Nature Genet.* **8**, 42–51, 1994.
22. Yang Y, Su Q & Wilson JM. Role of viral antigens in distinctive immune responses to adenovirus vector transduced cells in mouse lungs. *J. Virol.* **70**, 7209–7219, 1996.
23. De Matteo RP, Chu G, Ahn M *et al.* Immunologic barriers to hepatic adenoviral gene therapy for transplantation. *Transplantation* **63**(2), 315–319, 1997.
24. McCray PB, Armstrong K, Zabner J *et al.* Adenoviral-mediated gene transfer to fetal pulmonary epithelia *in vitro* and *in vivo*. *J. Clin. Invest.* **95**(6), 2620–2632, 1995.
25. Vincent MC, Trapnell BC, Baughman RP *et al.* Adenovirus mediated gene transfer to the respiratory tract of fetal sheet *in utero*. *Hum. Gene. Ther.* **6**(8), 1019–1028, 1995.
26. Gorziglia MI, Kadan MJ, Yei S *et al.* Elimination of both E1 and E2 from adenovirus vectors further improves prospects for *in vivo* human gene therapy. *J. Virol.* **70**(6), 4173–4178, 1996.
27. Armentano D, Zabner J, Sacks C *et al.* Effect of the E4 region on the persistence of transgene expression from adenovirus vectors. *J. Virol.* **71**(3), 2408–2416, 1997.
28. Zabner J, Fasbender AJ, Moninger T, Poellinger KA & Welsh MJ. Cellular and molecular barriers to gene transfer by a cationic lipid. *J. Biol. Chem.* **270**(32), 18997–19007, 1995.
29. Cotten M, Langle-Rouault F, Kirlappos H *et al.* Transferrin-polycation mediated introduction of DNA into human leukemic cells: stimulation by agents that affect the survival of transfected DNA or modulate transferrin receptor levels. *Proc. Natl. Acad. Sci. USA* **87**(11), 4033–4037, 1990.
30. Wagner E, Plank C, Zatloukal K, Cotten M & Birnstiel ML. Influenza virus hemagglutinin HA2 N-terminal fusogenic peptides augment gene transfer by transferrin–polylysine–DNA complexes: toward a synthetic virus-like gene-transfer vehicle. *Proc. Natl. Acad. Sci. USA* **89**(17), 7934–7938 , 1992.
31. de Fiebre CM, Bryant SO, Notabartolo D, Wu P & Meyer EM. Fusogenic properties of Sendai virosome envelopes in rat brain preparations. *Neurochem. Res.* **18**(10), 1089–1094, 1993.
32. Cotten M, Wagner E, Zatloukal K *et al.* High efficiency receptor mediated delivery of small and large (48 kilobase gene constructs) using the endosome disruption activity of defective or chemically inactivated adenovirus particles. *Proc. Natl. Acad. Sci. USA* **89**(13), 6094–6098, 1992.
33. Caplen NJ, Alton EW, Middleton PG *et al.* Liposome mediated CFTR gene transfer to the nasal epithelium of patients with cystic fibrosis. *Nature Med.* **1**(1), 39–46, 1995.
34. Chen J, Stickles RJ & Daichendt KA. Galactosylated histone mediated gene transfer and expression. *Hum. Gene. Ther.* **5**(4), 429–435, 1994.
35. Anson DS, Bielicki J & Hopwood JJ. Correction of mucopolysaccharidosis type 1 fibroblasts by retroviral mediated transfer of the human alpha-L-iduronidase gene. *Hum. Gene Ther.* **3**(4), 371–379, 1992.
36. Migliaccio G, Baiocchi M, Hamel N, Eddleman K & Migliaccio AR. Circulating progenitor cells in human ontogenesis: response to growth factors and replating potential. *J. Hematother.* **5**(2), 161–170, 1996.
37. Eddleman KA, Chervenak FA, George-Siegel P, Migliaccio G & Migliaccio AR. Circulating hematopoietic stem cell populations in human fetuses: implications for fetal gene therapy and alterations with *in utero* red cell transfusion. *Fetal Diagn. Ther.* **11**(4), 231–240, 1996.
38. Xu LC, Luepfel Stahl S & Blanco M. Growth factors and stromal support generate very efficient retroviral transduction of peripheral blood CD34$^+$ cells from Gaucher patients. *Blood* **86**(1), 141–146, 1995.

39. Fairbairn LJ, Lashford LS, Spooncer E *et al.* Long term *in vitro* correction of alpha- L-iduronidase deficiency (Hurler syndrome) in human bone marrow. *Proc. Natl. Acad. Sci. USA* **93**(5), 2025–2030, 1996.
40. Ohashi T, Boggs S & Robbins P. Efficient transfer and sustained high expression of the human glucocerebrosidase gene in mice and their functional macrophages following transplantation of bone marrow transduced by a retroviral vector. *Proc. Natl. Acad. Sci. USA* **89**(23), 11332–11336, 1992.
41. Kantoff PW, Flake AW, Eglitis MA *et al. In utero* gene transfer and expression. A sheep transplantation model. *Blood* **73**, 365–369, 1990.
42. Ekhterae D, Crumbleholme T, Karson E *et al.* Retroviral vector mediated transfer of the bacterial neomycin resistance gene into fetal and adult sheep and human hematopoietic progenitors *in vitro*. *Blood* **75**(2), 365–369, 1990.
43. Olsen I, Muir H, Smith R, Fensom A & Watt DJ. Direct enzyme transfer from lymphocytes is specific. *Nature* **306**, 75–77, 1983.
44. Krall WJ, Challita PM, Perlmutter LS, Skelton DC & Kohn DB. Cells expressing human glucocerebrosidase from a retroviral vector repopulate macrophages and central nervous system microglia after murine bone marrow transplantation. *Blood* **83**(9), 2737–2748, 1994.
45. Birkenmeier EH, Barker JE, Vogler CA *et al.* Increased life span and correction of metabolic defects in murine mucopolysaccharidosis Type VII after syngeneic bone marrow transplantation *Blood* **78**, 3081–3092, 1991.
46. Sands MS, Barker JE, Vogler C *et al.* Treatment of murine mucopolysaccharidosis Type VII by syngeneic bone marrow transplantation in neonates. *Lab. Invest.* **68**, 676–686, 1993.
47. Esiri MM, al-Izzi MS & Reading MC. Macrophages, microglial cells and HLA-DR antigens in fetal and infant brain. *J. Clin. Pathol.* **44**(2), 102–106, 1991.
48. Shull RM, Kakkis ED, McEntee MF *et al.* Enzyme replacement in a canine model of Hurler syndrome. *Proc. Natl. Acad. Sci. USA* **91**, 12937–12941, 1994.
49. King BM, Crawley AC, Byers S *et al.* Immune response to enzyme replacement therapy in MPS VI cats. *Proceedings 4th International Symposium on Mucopolysaccharide and Related Diseases*, Wollongong NSW, Australia, 1996.
50. Touraine JL. Treatment of human fetuses and induction of immunological tolerance in humans by *in utero* transplantation of stem cells into fetal recipients. *Acta Haematol.* **96**(3), 115–119, 1996.
51. Westgren M, Ringden O, Eik-Nes S *et al.* Lack of evidence of permanent engraftment after *in utero* fetal stem cell transplantation in congenital hemoglobinopathies. *Transplantation* **61**(8), 1176–1179, 1996.
52. Pitt BR, Schwarz MA, Pilewski JM *et al.* Retrovirus mediated gene transfer in lungs of living fetal sheep. *Gene Ther.* **2**, 344–350, 1995.
53. Holzinger A, Trapnell BC, Weaver TE, Whitsett JA & Iwamoto HS. Intraamniotic administration of an adenoviral vector for gene transfer to fetal sheep and mouse tissues. *Pediatr. Res.* **38**(6), 844–850, 1995.
54. MacCalman CD, Furth EE, Omigbodun A *et al.* Transduction of human trophoblast cells by recombinant adenoviruses is differentiation dependent. *Biol. Reprod.* **54**(3), 682–691, 1996.
55. Byrnes AP, MacLaren RE & Charlton H. Immunological instability of persistent adenovirus vectors in the brain: peripheral exposure to vector leads to renewed inflammation, reduced gene expression and demyelination. *J. Neurosci.* **16**, 3045–3055, 1996.
56. Wood MJA, Byrnes AP, Pfaff DW, Rabkin SD & Charlton HM. Inflammatory effects of gene transfer into the CNS with defective HSV-1 vectors. *Gene Ther.* **1**, 283–291, 1994.
57. Latchman DS. Molecular biology of herpes simplex virus latency. *J. Exp. Pathol.* **71**, 133–141, 1990.
58. Snyder EY, Deitcher DL, Walsh C *et al.* Multipotent neural cell lines can engraft and participate in development of mouse cerebellum. *Cell* **68**, 33–50, 1992.
59. Snyder EY, Taylor RM & Wolfe JM. Neural progenitor cell engraftment corrects lysosomal storage throughout the MPS VII mouse brain. *Nature* **374**, 367–370, 1995.
60. Lacorazza HD, Flax JD, Snyder EY & Jendoubi M. Expression of human beta hexosaminidase alpha subunit gene (the gene defect of Tay–Sachs disease) in mouse brains upon engraftment of transduced progenitor cells. *Nature Med.* **2**, 424–429, 1996.

SECTION 9

Methods of fetal monitoring

Antenatal cardiotocography

69

Z. Alfirevic and G.J. Hofmeyr

Introduction

Auscultation of fetal heart sounds has been used for clinical purposes for more than 150 years[1,2]. However, the era of modern antenatal cardiotocography began with the work of Hammacher, who developed the first phonocardiograph and described fetal heart rate characteristics associated with antepartum fetal compromise[3]. During the last two decades Doppler cardiotocography has been the most commonly used method for recording antenatal fetal heart rate patterns. Early equipment was based on the principle of 'peak detection' of Doppler frequency shift. This technique had a relatively low signal-to-noise ratio, high signal loss and many artefacts. Initial disappointment with the clinical performance of antenatal cardiotocography[4] has been often attributed to these technical 'teething' problems[5]. A new generation of instruments introduced during the 1980s was equipped with autocorrelation, a method of processing Doppler signals to derive the best estimate of pulse signals, and range gates that improves the signal-to-noise ratio and record quality. The relative simplicity of this non-invasive method of fetal assessment was virtually impossible to resist, and antenatal cardiotocography has become a standard method for assessment of fetal well-being. It is most commonly performed as an initial screening test in complicated pregnancies (non-stress test). Several refinements have been introduced into clinical practice (computerized cardiotocography, oxytocin challenge test, vibroacoustic stimulation, biophysical testing), mainly as second-line tests following equivocal non-stress cardiotocography.

THE PHYSIOLOGICAL BASIS OF FETAL HEART RATE PATTERNS

Short-term ('beat-to-beat') heart rate variability is thought to be mainly a reflection of fluctuating parasympathetic (vagal) tone[6], which is constantly being altered in response to fluctuating inputs such as baroreceptor tone. It is eliminated by parasympathetic blockade. It is increased during fetal breathing activity[7–9], during quiet sleep in the lamb (high-voltage slow-wave electrocortical activity)[9] and during active sleep in the human. In the fetal lamb, variability is also increased by induced hypoxaemia[7,9] or catecholamine infusion[9,10]. The possibility that high catecholamine levels might account for persistent variability despite acidaemia in human fetuses has not been confirmed[11]. In the human fetus, short-term variability is usually reduced in the compromised fetus, and is virtually always absent prior to fetal death in utero[12,13].

Long-term fetal heart rate variability (heart rate fluctuations occurring three to six times per minute) is thought to reflect fluctuating sympathetic and parasympathetic tone. It is also commonly reduced in response to fetal compromise.

Variable fetal heart rate decelerations (abrupt slowing of the heart rate with rapid recovery, not always related to uterine contractions and varying in shape) are usually an appropriate, protective fetal response to umbilical cord compression. As 45% of the fetal cardiac output flows through the umbilical vessels, obstruction of these vessels might cause considerable increase in blood pressure. Blood pressure fluctuations are particularly dangerous in the fetus (and preterm neonate) because of the propensity to rupture of the germinal matrix vasculature lining the cerebral ventricles. This is prevented by abrupt slowing of the heart rate as a vagal response to baroreceptor stimulation[14]. Usually the umbilical vein is compressed more than the arteries, causing a brief compensatory tachycardia in response to reduced venous return to the heart. The resistance to flow is quickly transmitted back via the placental vessels to the umbilical arteries, resulting in variable deceleration as described above. When the compression is relieved, there may be a drop in blood pressure causing a brief compensatory tachycardia ('overshoot'). This pattern is referred to as 'shouldering'.

Early decelerations (concomitant with a uterine contraction and recovering within 30 s of the end of the contraction) are probably also vagal in origin, resulting from cord compression or pressure on the fetal head during a contraction.

Late decelerations take more than 30 s to recover after the end of a uterine contraction. This lag phase implies biochemical rather than neurological mechanisms alone. The most common mechanism is probably a protective mechanism whereby oxygen is conserved during episodes of reduced oxygen supply, analogous to the diving reflex of aquatic mammals. The fetal lamb responds to induced hypoxia, detected by carotid chemoreceptors, by stopping breathing and body movements, and a redistribution of blood flow in favour of the essential organs, the heart, brain, adrenals and placenta, with vasoconstriction in all other tissues[15]. The overall effect is increased peripheral resistance, increased arterial pressure and a compensatory bradycardia. In the human a similar mechanism probably accounts for most cases of late decelerations (maternal blood flow to the placenta is arrested when the intrauterine pressure exceeds 35 mmHg), or other causes of hypoxia such as aortocaval compression in the supine position. The recovery lag phase represents the time taken for reoxygenation of the placenta and transfer of oxygen to the fetus. In many cases this pattern represents an appropriate response of non-acidaemic fetuses, and baseline heart rate and variability are normal. Late decelerations alone should not be considered evidence of fetal asphyxia[16]. However, late decelerations may also occur in acidaemic fetuses, when variability may also be reduced, with or without baseline tachycardia.

A different pattern of deceleration appears to occur in severely compromised fetuses, usually associated with absence of fetal movements and reduced short-term variability, ascribed to loss of autonomic control of the fetal heart rate[13]. This is similar to the very flat heart rate pattern seen in adults with autonomic blockade, the so-called intrinsic heart rate[17]. Interference with energy synthesis in the myocardium may cause slowing of the intrinsic heart rate[18]. In the fetal lamb, progressive myocardial glycogen depletion is associated with a fall in the intrinsic heart rate[19]. This mechanism may explain the prolonged shallow decelerations observed after Braxton–Hicks uterine contractions in the terminal fetal heart rate pattern, as well as the terminal bradycardia prior to fetal death in utero[13] (Figs 69.1, 69.2). It has also been postulated to account for the true sinusoidal fetal heart rate pattern[20], when in the presence of cardiac failure and severe tissue hypoxia, myocardial energy availability may 'teeter' about a critical threshold[21].

Fetal heart rate accelerations (15 beats/min increase lasting 15 s) are thought to be due to sympathetic discharge. Most are associated with fetal movements, though not all movements are noticed by the mother. Accelerations are considered a sign of fetal well-being (Fig. 69.3).

NON-STRESS TEST

This term should be reserved for the antenatal cardiotocography which is performed according to an established clinical protocol[22], which should include standards for test interpretation. Unfortunately, there is no consensus about the minimum duration of monitoring and criteria for normality. Most clinicians use an arbitrary 30 min time span in which normal heart rate variability must be accompanied by at least two accelerations.

With appropriate equipment the non-stress test can be performed at home. Signals are transmitted by telecommunication to the nearest hospital for assessment. A small study[23] which compared the quality of recordings generated at home

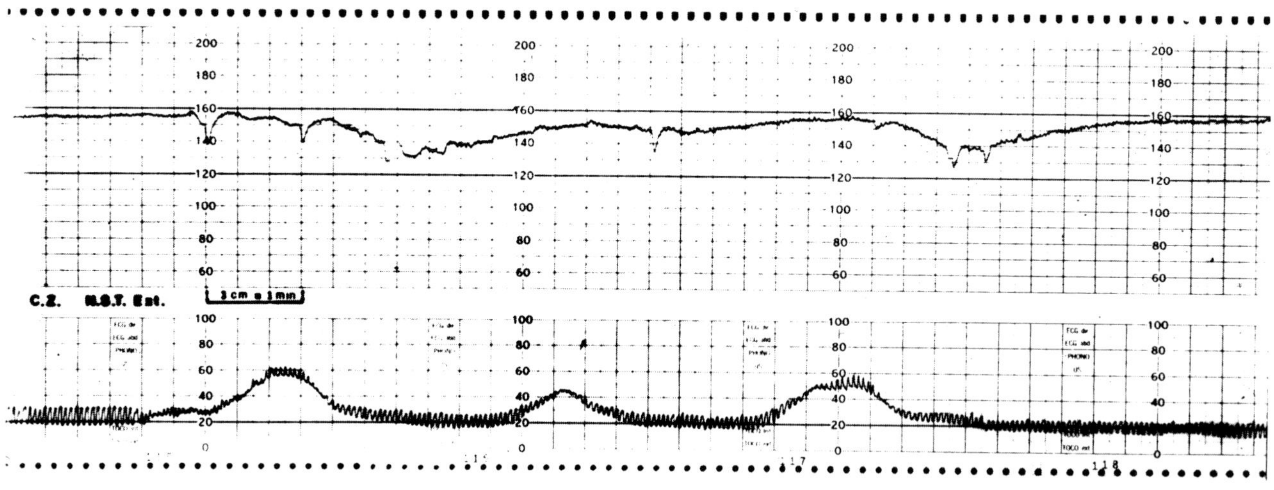

Fig. 69.1 A prelabour terminal fetal heart rate pattern showing normal baseline heart rate, greatly reduced short-term and long-term variability and prolonged shallow late decelerations following spontaneous (Braxton–Hicks) contractions. Fetal movements were absent. This pattern probably represents loss of autonomic control of the heart rate due to central nervous system depression and heart rate slowing due to direct myocardial depression following contractions.

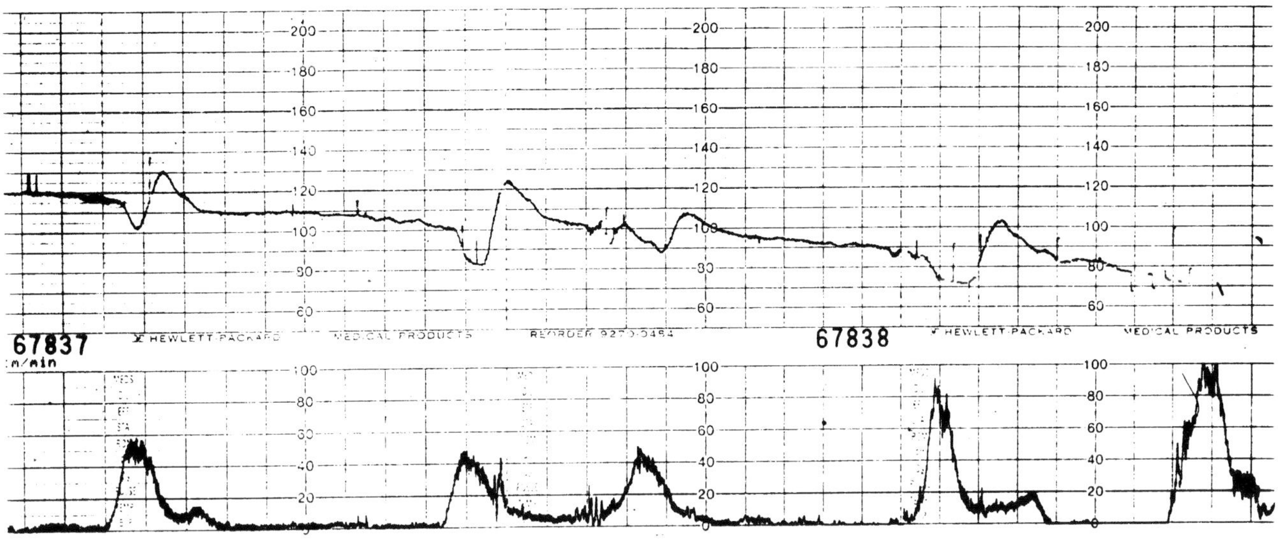

Fig. 69.2 A fetal heart rate pattern immediately prior to intrauterine death. Autonomic control of the heart rate has probably been lost due to central nervous system depression. Progressive bradycardia is probably due to direct myocardial depression as hypoxia and acidosis become more profound.

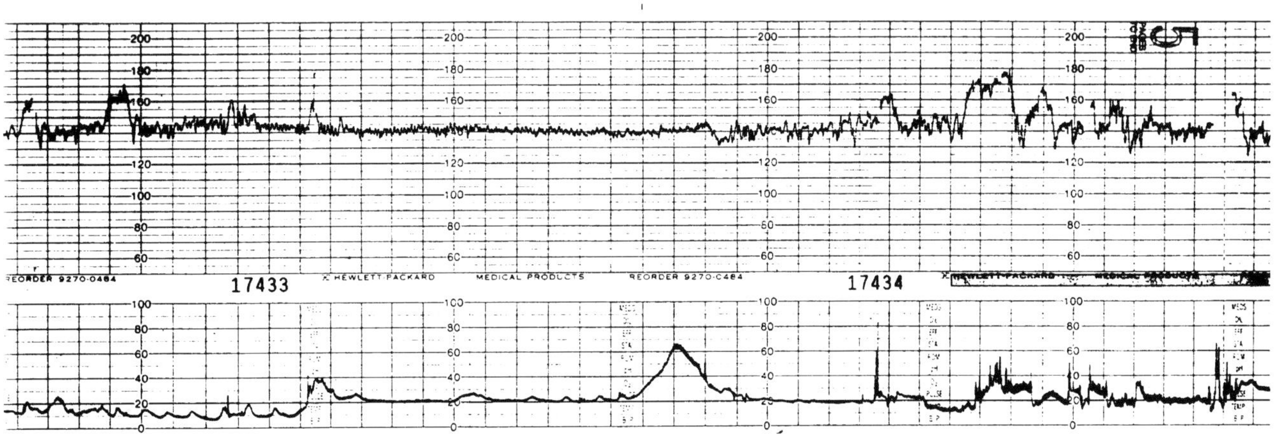

Fig. 69.3 Fetal sleep cycles are illustrated in this tracing showing a 15 min episode of non-reactivity with reduced variability preceded and followed by a reactive pattern with accelerations (active sleep).

and in hospital within 1 h showed that home monitoring is feasible. However, the question whether such monitoring is reassuring or anxiety generating and whether it leads to unnecessary interventions remains unanswered.

STRESS TEST

The contraction stress test historically preceded the 'non-stress test' (unstressed antepartum cardiotocography). The first 'stress' used was maternal exercise, based on the observation of fetal bradycardia following exercise in hypertensive pregnancies[24]. The observation in animals that maternal blood flow to the intervillous space was interrupted during uterine contractions[25] led to the development of the contraction stress test[26,27].

The basis of the test is to assess the fetal heart rate response to uterine contractions as is done during labour. At least three contractions per 10 min lasting at least 45 s are induced using syntocinon infusion or nipple stimulation[28]. The occurrence of 'late' fetal heart rate decelerations is assumed to indicate reduced placental reserve. Two possible mechanisms have been proposed[29]: an autonomic reflex to mild hypoxia, in which PO_2 values below 17 mmHg stimulate carotid chemoreceptors leading to alpha-sympathetic stimulation, vasoconstriction in non-essential organs, increased peripheral resistance, baroreceptor stimulation and compensatory vagal bradycardia, and direct myocardial depression in the presence of metabolic acidosis[30]. The test has largely been replaced by the 'non-stress test', but may be useful in women with persistent non-reactive (inconclusive) non-stress tests. It has been argued that the contraction stress compares favourably to the non-stress test because it gives earlier warning of fetal compromise[31].

It is essential to ensure that fetal movements or baseline heart rate variability are present before commencing uterine stimulation, and to have a tocolytic available in case of excessive fetal response. We have observed a case of fetal death following the second induced uterine contraction in a women with an unrecognized 'terminal' fetal heart rate pattern.

FETAL AROUSAL

In an attempt to improve its diagnostic performance, antenatal cardiotocography has been combined with physical or auditory stimulation of the fetus. The most commonly used stimuli are manual shaking and vibroacoustic stimulation.

Because of the expense of electronic fetal heart rate monitors, attempts have been made to use maternal perception of fetal movements evoked by auditory or physical stimulation[32–34]. Vibroacoustic stimulators, even using an electric toothbrush or razor, are relatively expensive. A sound pressure very similar to that generated by the commercial vibroacoustic stimulators has been generated by placing the base of an empty soft drink can against the woman's abdomen, steadying the top rim with the thumb and third finger, depressing the ring opener with the second finger and allowing it to snap back to give a vibratory sound[35]. The effectiveness of these low-cost methods of fetal assessment for preliminary screening in well-resourced environments, or definitive testing in underresourced environments, is yet to be established.

COMPUTERIZED CARDIOTOCOGRAPHY

Many obstetricians simply do not believe that the cardiotocogram (CTG) can be accurately interpreted by a computer. CTG analysis is often perceived as an 'art' for which years of clinical experience and a full understanding of the underlying clinical picture are mandatory. However, numerous studies have confirmed poor agreement between experts in assessing various components of antenatal CTGs[36–38], with some improvement if a formal scoring system was introduced[36–39]. An even more powerful argument in favour of objective, computerized analysis is the unquestionable need for antenatal CTG to detect recognizable patterns linked to fetal conditions like acidosis, anaemia or cerebral damage. If such patterns exist, software should be able to identify them.

The most advanced commercially available expert system for CTG analysis has been developed in Oxford by Dawes *et al.*[40,41]. The analysis includes several criteria which cannot be assessed by a naked eye (Table 69.1).

The main emphasis in the analysis is placed on fetal heart rate variation. The average pulse interval (in milliseconds) is recorded for each epoch lasting one-sixteen of a minute (3.75 s). The minute range is the difference between the smallest and largest epochs over 1 min, excluding recognized decelerations. Accelerations thus contribute to the minute range. The mean minute range is the average of the minute ranges over the period recorded. Accelerations and decelerations, the main focus of visual analysis, are given much less weight, because their presence or absence has been shown to be an unreliable guide to fetal outcome[42,43].

One of the main advantages of the described system is that the results are presented numerically and the gestational age dependent limits for normality are calculated from the large database. Strict management protocols can be put in place based on the published observational data (Table 69.2).

Finally, such protocols can be tested in randomized trials. Computerized cardiotocography will only fulfil its potential if a management package triggered by the described analysis

TABLE 69.1
Definitions used in the computerized CTG analysis developed by Dawes *et al.*[41,44]

Feature	Definition	Normal criteria
High variation	A section of the trace where the 1 min 'peak-to-peak' variation is above predefined threshold for 5 out of 6 consecutive minutes. Identified high variation episodes must have an average peak to peak variation that is greater than the 1st centile for gestation (10.7 beats/min at 24 weeks; 11 beats/min at 38 weeks)	At least one episode
Decelerations	The deceleration area is calculated and expressed as the number of 'lost beats'. Any deceleration of more than 20 'lost beats' is considered significant and counted	No decelerations of more than 20 'lost beats'
Basal heart rate	Average fetal heart rate calculated from all episodes of low variation or from the baseline fitted algorithm. Not the same as a baseline	116–160 beats/min
Short-term variation	Each minute is divided into 16 epochs (3.75 s). The mean heart rate for each epoch is expressed as a pulse interval in milliseconds. The differences between pulse intervals are used to compute the short-term variation	3 msec or greater

TABLE 69.2
The management protocol based on computerized cardiotocography (Sonicaid System 8002) suitable for evaluation in prospective randomized trials[44]

High variation	Large decelerations	Short-term variation (ms) ≥5.0	4–4.9	3–3.9	2.6–2.9	<2.5	Action
Normal	No	Yes					Normal. Follow-up depends on clinical presentation
Normal	Yes	Yes					Minor deviation. Repeat within 24 h. Consider induction after 38 weeks
Normal	Yes		Yes				Minor deviation. Repeat within 24 h. Consider induction after 38 weeks
Normal	Yes			Yes			Minor deviation. Repeat within 24 h. Consider induction after 38 weeks
Unreactive	No	Yes					Suboptimal. Repeat within next 24 h. Consider induction after 40 weeks
Unreactive	No		Yes				Suboptimal. Repeat within next 24 h. Consider induction after 40 weeks
Unreactive	No			Yes			Moderate deviation. Repeat within 6 h. If persists after 36 weeks then deliver. Before 36 weeks repeat every 12 h
Unreactive	Yes/No				Yes		Severe deviation. Deliver after 34 weeks. If delivery deferred before 34 weeks repeat every 6 h
Unreactive	Yes	Yes					Minor deviation. Repeat within 24 h. Consider induction after 38 weeks
Unreactive	Yes		Yes				Moderate deviation. Repeat within 6 h. If persists after 36 weeks deliver. Before 36 weeks repeat every 12 h
Unreactive	Yes			Yes			Severe deviation. Deliver after 34 weeks. If delivery deferred before 34 weeks repeat every 6 h
Unreactive	Yes/No					Yes	Terminal. Deliver after 28 weeks. If delivery deferred repeat every 4 h

is capable of improving perinatal outcomes that matter to parents and health care purchasers. Several large perinatal trials have been successfully completed recently, demonstrating that it should be possible to recruit the tens of thousands of women needed to reliably assess the effectiveness of computerized cardiotocography in reducing serious perinatal morbidity.

Evaluation of effectiveness

Antenatal cardiotocography is firmly entrenched in routine obstetric clinical practice. Furthermore, its ability to predict and prevent adverse perinatal outcomes is a yardstick against other tests of fetal well-being are measured. Over the years only a few dissenting voices advocated caution[4,45] and suggested that the test should be properly evaluated in a research setting before its widespread clinical use. The aim of this review is to establish to what extent a widespread belief that antenatal cardiotocography can predict and prevent serious adverse perinatal outcomes is based on sound scientific evidence. Perinatal mortality will be the main outcome of interest throughout this review. We assume that an anticipated reduction in unexplained stillbirths and early neonatal deaths is the main motivation for using modern monitoring equipment in pregnancy. Only if this goal is achievable can the ever increasing intensity of fetal monitoring be justified.

ABILITY TO PREDICT ADVERSE FETAL OUTCOME

Ideally, antepartum cardiotocography should have been evaluated by compiling the receiver operator curve (ROC) curve for important endpoints in studies in which the test results are concealed from the clinicians[46]. A plea to study endpoints such as perinatal death and suboptimal neurodevelopmental outcome rather than doubtful surrogate measures including fetal distress, hypoxaemia and low Apgar scores is understandable. However, the need to conceal the test results during evaluation of antenatal cardiotocography has been largely ignored by researches in the field[45]. Lack of blinding has been accepted almost as the norm in the evaluation of tests of fetal well-being. This should not come as a surprise.

Most clinicians find it impossible to ignore what is accepted as an 'abnormal' CTG result, to satisfy methodological purity. Unfortunately, this also means that the performance of cardiotocography may be falsely inflated, given that an abnormal CTG may lead to preterm delivery and death of a baby that would have survived if untested. A knee-jerk reaction to react to an 'unusual' fetal heart rate tracing may not be as ethical as it seems. Let us examine this so called 'treatment paradox' in more detail.

Mrs N.O., a 28-year-old primigravida, was found to have a fetus with mild unexplained oligohydramnios at 20 weeks. The subsequent fetal growth curve assessed by serial ultrasound, persistent mild oligohydramnios and raised Doppler indices in the umbilical artery were compatible with impaired intrauterine growth. However, there was a pocket of amniotic fluid >2 cm, end diastolic velocities in the umbilical arteries were present and fetal movements were satisfactory. At 29 weeks, the estimated fetal weight was 810 g, corticosteroids for lung maturation were given and outpatient antenatal cardiotocography was commenced on alternate days. At 29 + 5 weeks a non-stress test showed reduced variability with unprovoked decelerations (Fig. 69.4). The non-stress test result was a 'trigger' for an immediate elective delivery. A male infant was born by caesarean section weighing 844 g with cord pH = 7.302, cord lactates = 2.52 mmol/L and Apgar 9 at 5 min. His subsequent progress through neonatal intensive care was largely uneventful.

The non-stress test performance is falsely improved by the decision to deliver

The non-stress test has accurately predicted low birthweight, preterm delivery, caesarean section for 'fetal distress' and admission to special care baby unit (SCBU) which are common surrogate measures for adverse perinatal outcome. However, it is possible that the diagnosis of 'fetal distress', preterm delivery by caesarean section and admission to SCBU are all direct consequences of antenatal CTG. It is possible that, if CTG was not performed and the decision was based on Doppler ultrasound, maternal perception of fetal movements and possibly biophysical profile, these outcomes would have been avoided.

In the absence of randomized controls it is not possible to know whether antenatal CTG and the intervention that followed benefited or harmed the infant. Not surprisingly, clinicians were praised by the parents for 'accurate' interpretation of a complex test and timely delivery of their baby. Even in cases where the outcome is death, the decision to perform a test that resulted in preterm delivery is hardly ever questioned.

The non-stress test performance may also be falsely worsened

Let us say that a 'true' abnormal non-stress test led to an effective intervention (caesarean section) and a good outcome. This CTG would appear as a false positive for abnormal pH, low Apgar score and all 'hard' perinatal adverse outcomes.

The ability of the non-stress test to predict subsequent presence or absence of adverse perinatal outcomes has been summarized in an excellent review by Mohide and Keirse[45]. However, clinically useful interpretation of these results is

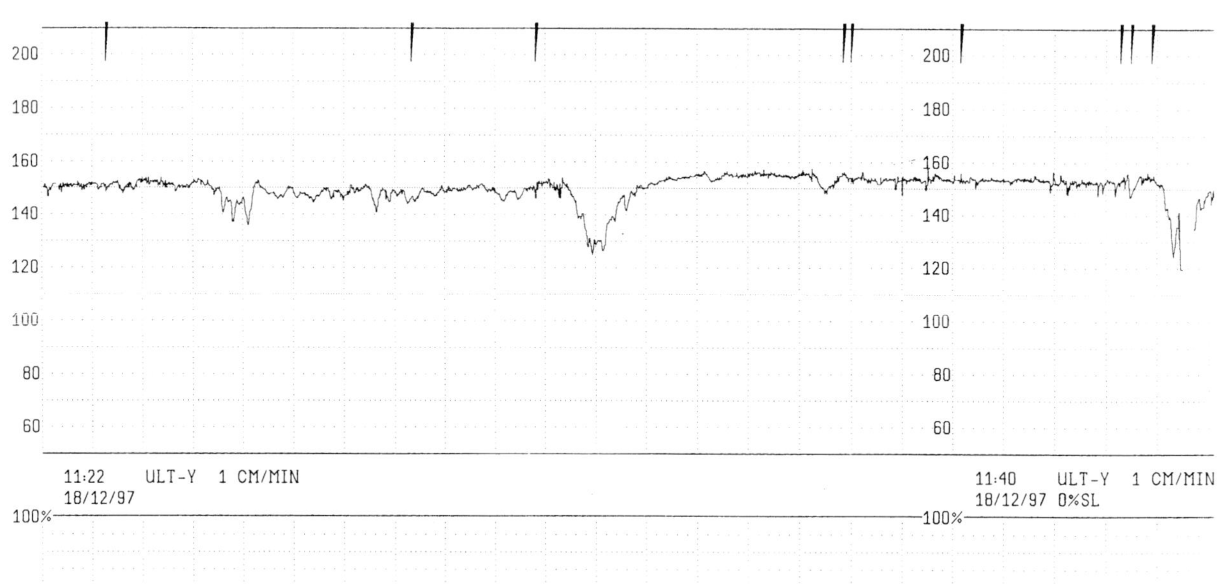

Fig. 69.4 Non-reactive CTG at 29 weeks' gestation in a fetus with intrauterine growth restriction. By conventional criteria this a pathological tracing because of reduced short-term variability, unprovoked decelerations and lack of accelerations. According to computerized analysis (Oxford Sonicaid 8002) calculated area of deceleration(s) was less than 20 'lost beats' and therefore not significant. Short-term variability was 3.0 ms which gives an estimated likelihood of metabolic acidaemia or intrauterine death of 29%[44].

TABLE 69.3
Diagnostic test properties for antepartum cardiotocography[45]

Outcome	Sensitivity (%)	Specificity (%)	Likelihood ratio Positive	Likelihood ratio Negative
Perinatal death	0–100	70–100	0–7.6	0–100
Fetal distress	6–100	78–98	2–30.3	0–100
Low Apgar score	12–59	78–97	2.1–4.5	50–90
Low pH	20–100	72–94	1.6–3.6	0–90
Neonatal morbidity	13–74	87–95	2.6–5.6	30–90
Combined adverse outcomes	7–83	82–97	2.1–40	20–100

very difficult. Statistical methods (meta-analysis) for pooling the sensitivity, specificity and likelihood ratios are now being developed, but even these pooled values are unlikely to be very helpful. The considerable heterogeneity of the test performance (Table 69.3) and lack of blinding to the test results makes any attempt to perform formal meta-analysis unwise.

One point about the diagnostic performance of antenatal cardiotocography highlighted by Mohide and Keirse[45] deserves to be emphasized. It is often suggested that the main value of the non-stress test lies in its high negative predictive value. In other words, the reported high specificity may be seen as proof that a normal CTG provides important reassurance about fetal well-being and minimizes the risk of serious perinatal morbidity. Unfortunately, this is incorrect. It should be noted that most of the published literature on antenatal fetal monitoring studied populations with a relatively low background incidence of death or poor neurodevelopmental outcome (<5%). Under those circumstances an uneducated guess about the state of fetal well-being would have specificity of 94.7% even if all fetuses with subsequent poor outcome were missed (sensitivity = 0%) (Table 69.4).

TABLE 69.4
Performance of a hypothetical diagnostic test of fetal well-being ('wild guess') in pregnancies with an overall prevalence of serious perinatal morbidity and mortality of 5%

Wild guess	Perinatal outcome Abnormal	Normal	Total
Abnormal outcome	0	50	50
Normal outcome	50	900	950
Total	50	950	1000

Sensitivity = 0/50 (0%)
Specificity = 900/950 (94.7%)
Positive predictive value = 0
Negative predicative value = 94.7%

Ability to prevent adverse fetal outcome

A diagnostic test has to be linked to an effective intervention in order to improve perinatal outcome. Evaluation of clinical effectiveness and safety of such a 'package' is more complex than evaluation of its components. Increasingly, clinicians are prepared to change their practice only if the evidence comes from randomized controlled trials, because only interpretation based on the 'intention to treat' is free of bias. However, randomized trials of diagnostic tests do have a problem with generalizibility, particularly if there is no evidence of beneficial effect. Proponents of a certain diagnostic test will often dismiss a negative result, arguing that the diagnostic test was inadequately interpreted or the intervention triggered by test (or lack of it) was inappropriate. Furthermore, constant refinements in the interpretation of the diagnostic tests may make fairly robust evidence obsolete very soon. Randomized controlled trials of antepartum cardiotocography are a good example of these problems.

Four randomized trials[47–50] have evaluated the impact of antenatal cardiotocography on the management of high-risk pregnancies (Table 69.5). It is difficult to make any firm conclusion based on data from only 1579 randomized women. Despite some methodological shortcomings, particularly in the methods of randomization, these four trials still represent the best available evidence on the effectiveness of antenatal cardiotocography in the prevention of adverse perinatal outcomes. They suggest that the availability of antenatal cardiotocography does not make an impact on caesarean section rate, admissions to the neonatal intensive care units (NICU) and the incidence of abnormal neonatal neurological signs (Table 69.6).

The observed increase in perinatal mortality in the CTG groups has been largely ignored by practising obstetricians in the belief that this was a chance finding. Seven out of 10 perinatal deaths amongst 795 pregnancies where CTG findings were revealed appear to be potentially preventable. However, there is no definitive evidence that the false reassurance by a normal CTG was a contributing factor to these deaths. Nevertheless, the fact that higher perinatal mortality in the CTG group was observed in all four trials is a matter of concern. Given the current evidence one has to conclude that the indiscriminate use of antenatal CTGs in pregnant women with an anticipated perinatal mortality of around 1% is best avoided.

The performance of the antenatal cardiotocography is likely to be enhanced in severe antepartum haemorrhage,

TABLE 69.5
Details of published randomized controlled trials of antepartum cardiotocography

Study	Women	Risk	Weeks	Action	Additional fetal monitoring	PM
Brown[47]	353	Age (32%); Hypertension (19%); Low *HPL* (18%); History of stillbirth or IUGR (12%); IUGR (10%); bleeding (8%)	32–36	Weekly CTG scored and then concealed or revealed	Cardiff 'Count of Ten'; Urinary oestrogens; placental lactogen; fetal growth	0.6%
Flynn[48]	300	*PET* (26%); Post-term (33%); IUGR (16%); bad history (4%)	Any	Weekly CTG either revealed or concealed	Urinary oestriol, HPL, ultrasound	0.7%
Lumley[49]	530	Hypertension/PET; diabetes (2%); IUGR (13%); bleeding; medical problems; abnormal serum oestriol and HPL	26–41	Weekly CTG or no CTG	Serum oestriol, HPL, Pregnancy specific glycoprotein, ultrasound, Fetal movements count	2%
Kidd[50]	396	Hypertension (38%); bleeding (13%); preterm labour (12%); IUGR (11%); medical disorders (8%)	Any	Daily CTG either revealed or concealed	Not specified	0.7%

PM = perinatal mortality; HPL = human placental lactogen; IUGR = intrauterine growth restriction; PET = pre-eclamptic toxaemia

TABLE 69.6
The impact of serial antenatal cardiotocography on important perinatal outcomes from four randomized controlled studies in high-risk pregnancies[46–49]

	CTG	Control	Pooled odds ratio	95% CI
Perinatal death	14/795	4/784	3.01	1.19–7.62
Caesarean section	182/795	169/784	1.07	0.84–1.36
Abnormal neurological signs[a]	27/588	27/584	0.98	0.57–1.71
Admission to NICU[a]	121/588	115/584	1.05	0.79–1.41

[a]Data for Kidd *et al.*[50] not available

suspected placental abruption and severe intrauterine growth restriction and other complications where the risk for the fetus is high. In these cases antenatal cardiotocography is indicated primarily to exclude imminent fetal death. If a fetus is alive the need for and the choice of further antenatal testing remains controversial. The choice lies between no further tests, the non-stress test, some form of stress test, umbilical artery Doppler measurements, ultrasound scan, formal biophysical profile or a combination of these tests. In the absence of published randomized comparisons of these approaches and lack of evidence that any form of follow-up will improve fetal outcome, local policies will vary. The choice is determined by the availability of equipment, type of antenatal care, resources and, most importantly, view of the local opinion leaders.

Implications for research

It appears that the opportunity to properly evaluate the test performance of antenatal cardiotocography has passed. The method has been accepted as the 'Gold Standard' for assessment of fetal well-being and the 'window of opportunity' to undertake large studies where clinicians are blinded to the CTG results has disappeared. Alternative research strategies are needed to provide evidence-based antenatal fetal monitoring. New modifications of currently used tests should be evaluated by comparing their receiver-operator curves for perinatal deaths and long-term neurodevelopmental outcomes. It is critically important that clinicians are blinded to the test results under evaluation. As far as antenatal cardiotocography is concerned several comparisons should be tested in randomized controlled trials:

- Visual versus computerized analysis followed by the same intervention package
- High-frequency monitoring (12–48 h) versus low-frequency monitoring (weekly or less)
- Different monitoring policies in women with decreased fetal movements, impaired fetal growth including oligohydramnios, diabetes and preterm prelabour rupture of membranes

In the absence of these studies, clinical practice will continue to be guided by the personal views of opinion leaders in the field.

Evidence-based guidelines on the use of antenatal cardiotocography

- Indiscriminate use of antenatal cardiotocography where the background risk of serious adverse perinatal outcomes is low (≤1%) should be avoided. (recommendation based on the evidence from randomized trials)
- Normal cardiotocography does not provide adequate reassurance about fetal well-being. If the clinical indication for antenatal testing persists, use of alternative fetal monitoring methods is recommended despite repeatedly normal CTGs (recommendation based on non-randomized evidence)
- A formal method of CTG assessment, either by visual scoring or computer assisted analysis, is preferred to 'eyeballing' (recommendation based on non-randomized evidence)
- Every unit should be encouraged to develop CTG-triggered management protocols which are indication and gestation dependent (recommendation based on non-randomized evidence)

REFERENCES

1. Patel NB & Owen P. Fetal assessment in the third trimester: biophysical methods. In *Turnbull's Obstetrics.* (ed. G. Chamberlain), pp. 231–251. London: Churchill Livingstone, 1996.
2. Wulf KH. History of fetal heart rate monitoring. In *Fetal Heart Rate Monitoring* (ed. W. Kunzel), pp. 3–15. Berlin: Springer-Verlag, 1985.
3. Hammacher K. Neue Methode zur selektiven Registrierung der fetalen Herzschlagfrequenz. *Geburtsch. Frauenheilk.* **22**, 1542–1543, 1962.
4. Neilson JP. Cardiotocography for antepartum fetal assessment. In *The Cochrane Pregnancy and Childbirth Database.* The Cochrane Collaboration, Issue 2. Oxford: Update Software. (Available from BMJ Publishing Group, London.), 1995
5. Mandruzzato GP, Dawes GS & Meir YJ. Computerized evaluation of cardiotocography and its clinical role. In *Fetus as a Patient* (eds A. Kurjak & F.A. Chervenak), pp. 195–206. London: The Parthenon Publishing Group, 1994.
6. Parer JT, Laros RK, Keilbron DC & Krueger JR. The roles of parasympathetic and beta-adrenergic activity in beat-to-beat fetal heart rate variability. *Physiological Science* Vol 8, *Cardiovascular Physiology* (eds A.G.B. Kovac, E. Namos, G. Rubanyi), pp. 327–335. New York: Pergamon Press, 1981.
7. Dalton KJ, Dawes GS & Patrick JE. Diurnal, respiratory and other rhythms of fetal heart rate in lambs. *Am. J. Obstet. Gynecol.* **127**, 414–424, 1977.
8. Compogrande M, Alemanno MG, Viora E & Bussolini S. *J. Perinat. Med.* **10**, 203–208, 1982.
9. Hofmeyr GJ, Bamford OS, Dawes GS & Parkes MJ. High-frequency heart rate variability in the fetal lamb. In *The Physiological Development of the Fetus and Newborn* (eds C.T. Jones & P.W. Nathaneilsz), pp. 493–444. London: Academic Press, 1985.
10. Jones CT & Robinson RO. Plasma catecholamines in fetal and adult sheep. *J. Physiol.* **248**, 15–33, 1975.
11. Hofmeyr GJ, Esser J, Nikodem VC, Lowson M Kramer T & Gulmezoglu AM. Do fetal catecholamine levels affect heart rate variability and meconium passage during labour? *S. Afr. Med. J.* **83**, 739–742, 1993.
12. Parer JT. *Handbook of Fetal Heart Rate Monitoring.* Philadelphia: Saunders, 1983.
13. Cetrulo CL & Schifrin BS. Fetal heart rate patterns preceding death in utero. *Obstet. Gynecol.* **48**, 521–527, 1976.
14. Itskovitz J, La Gamma EF & Rudolph AM. Baroreflex control of the circulation in chronically instrumented fetal lambs. *Circ. Res.* **52**, 589–596, 1983.
15. Jensen A, Bamford OS, Dawes GS, Hofmeyr GJ & Parkes MJ. Changes in organ blood flow between high and low voltage electrocortical activity and during isocapnic hypoxia in intact and brain stem transected fetal lambs. In *The Physiological Development of the Fetus and Newborn* (eds C.T. Jones & P.W. Nathanielsz), pp. 605–610. London: Academic Press, 1985.
16. Krebs HB, Petres RE, Dunn LJ & Segreti A. Intrapartum fetal heart rate monitoring. IV Observations on elective and nonelective fetal heart rate monitoring. *Am. J. Obstet. Gynecol.* **138**, 213, 1980.
17. Jose AD & Taylor RR. Autonomic blockade by propranolol and atropine to study intrinsic myocardial function in man. *J. Clin. Invest.* **48**, 2019–2031, 1969.
18. Jose AD & Stitt F. The effects of hypoxia and metabolic inhibitors on the intrinsic heart rate and myocardial contractility in dogs. *Circ. Res.* **25**, 53–66, 1969.
19. Hokegard KH, Eriksson BO, Kjellmer I, Magno R & Rosen KG. Myocardial metabolism in relation to electro-cardiographic changes and cardiac function during graded hypoxia in the fetal lamb. *Acta. Physiol. Scand.* **113**, 1–7, 1981.
20. Hofmeyr GJ & Sonnendecker EWW. Pseudosinusoidal fetal heart rate patterns, *Br. J. Obstet. Gynaecol.* **90**, 1193–1194, 1983.
21. Hofmeyr GJ & Sonnendecker EWW. Heart rate changes after acute fetal haemorrhage: A basis for the pathophysiology of the sinusoidal pattern. *S. Afr. J.* **64**, 23–25, 1983.
22. Devoe LD. The nonstress test. *Obstet. Gyn. Clin. N. Am.* **17**, 111–128, 1990.
23. Reece EA, Hagay Z, Garofalo J & Hobbins JC. A controlled trial of self-nonstress test versus assisted nonstress test in the evaluation of fetal well-being. *Am. J. Obstet. Gynecol.* **166**, 489–492, 1992.
24. Hon EH & Wohlgemuth R. The electronic evaluation of fetal heart rate. IV The effect of maternal exercise. *Am. J. Obstet. Gynecol.* **81**, 361–371, 1961.
25. Hendricks CH. Amniotic fluid pressure recordings. *Clin. Obstet. Gynecol.* **9**, 535, 1966.
26. Spurrett B. Stressed cardiotocography in late pregnancy. *J. Obstet. Gynaecol. Br. Commonw.* **78**, 894, 1971.
27. Ray M, Freeman RK, Pine S & Hesselgesser R. Clinical experience with oxytocin challenge test. *Am. J. Obstet. Gynecol.* **114**, 1–9, 1972.
28. Lenke RR & Nemes JM. Use of nipple stimulation to obtain contraction stress test. *Obstet. Gynecol.* **63**, 345–348, 1984.
29. Myers RE, Mueller-Huebach E & Adamsons K. Predictability of the state of fetal oxygenation from a quantitative analysis of the components of late deceleration. *Am. J. Obstet. Gynecol.* **115**, 1083–1094, 1973.
30. Martin DB, de Haan J, van der Wildt B *et al.* Mechanism of late deceleration in the fetal heart rate. *Eur. J. Obstet. Reprod. Biol.* **9**, 361, 1979.
31. Freeman RK, Anderson G & Dorchester W. A prospective multi-institutional study of antepartum fetal heart rate monitoring. II. Contraction stress test versus nonstress test for primary surveillance. *Am. J. Obstet. Gynecol.* **143**, 778–781, 1982.
32. Luz NP. Auditory evoked responses of the human fetus: simplified methodology. *J. Perinat. Med.* **19**, 177–183, 1991.
33. Nyman M, Arulkumaran S, Jakobsson J & Westgren M. Vibro-acoustic stimulation in high-risk pregnancies: maternal perception of fetal movements, fetal heart rate and fetal oucome. *J. Perinat Med.* **20**, 267–274, 1992.
34. Strong TH, Jordan TL & Marden DW. The fetal recoil test. *Am. J. Obstet. Gynecol.* **167**, 1382–1383, 1992.
35. Hofmeyr GJ, Lawrie T & DeJager M. Primary care fetal assessment – low-cost fetal arousal testing. *S. Afr. Med. J.* **87**, 171–172, 1997.
36. Trimbos JB & Keirse MJNC. Observer variability in assessment of antepartum cardiotocograms. *Br. J. Obstet. Gynaecol.* **85**, 900–906, 1978.

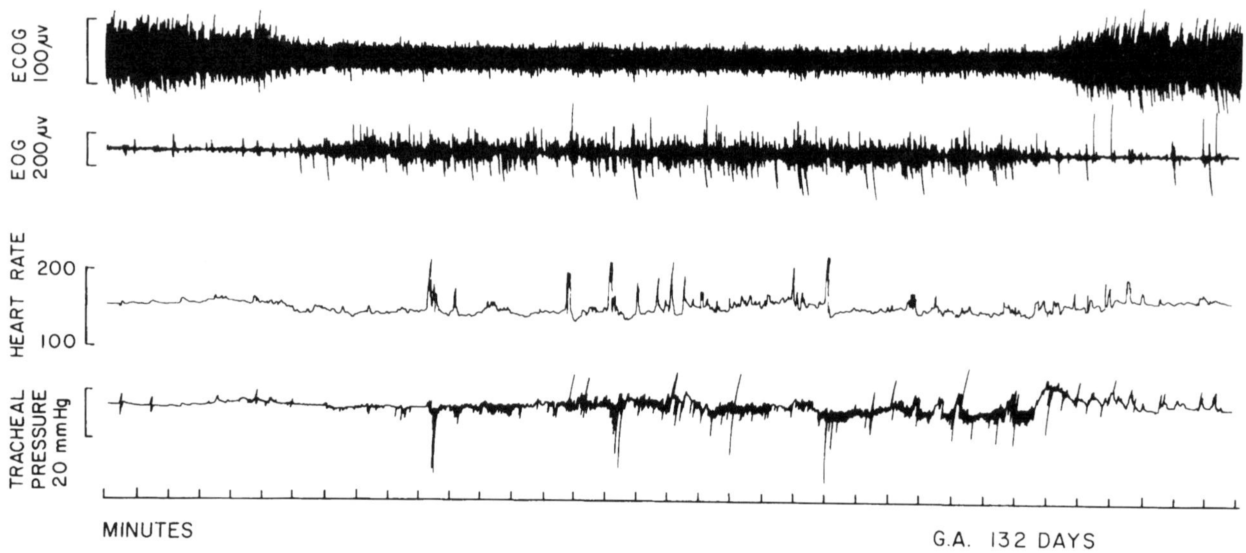

Fig. 70.1 Chart recording demonstrating that electroocular activity (EOG) and fetal breathing movements normally occur during times of low-voltage electrocortical activity (ECoG).

BODY MOVEMENTS

There has been limited study of fetal body movements using fetal animal preparations; again most information has been obtained from the ovine fetus. Dawes et al.[1] provided one of the first descriptions in sheep near term delivered into a warm saline bath with intact umbilical cords. Three different types of movement activity were observed. In the first, the lamb appeared awake, moved its limbs, raised its head, and opened its eyes. The second type involved only slow gentle extension of the limbs and seemed to correspond to non-REM sleep. The third type appeared to correspond to REM sleep, since it entailed movements of the eyes and intermittent twitching of ears, lips and limbs. Fetal movement activity has subsequently been characterized by use of electromyography (EMG) leads and/or transit time ultrasonography on different skeletal muscles including forelimb, neck (postural muscle activity) and trunk[9–11]. Simple fetal movements such as extension of the head and flexion or extension of the limbs have been identified, as have complex movements characterized by two to three repetitive elements involving combined movements of neck, limb and trunk.

A close association between skeletal muscle activity, as measured by EMG from nuchal and limb muscle groups, and fetal heart rate (FHR) accelerations is reported for the ovine fetus near term[12,13]. When skeletal muscle activity is abolished by neuromuscular blockade, the number of FHR accelerations is decreased by approximately a third, although there is no change in the frequency distribution of amplitude or duration of FHR accelerations[12]. These results suggest that, in the ovine fetus, the majority of FHR accelerations occur in association with movement as a consequence of central neuronal output affecting both the cardioaccelerator neuronal processes and the skeletal muscle motor neurons simultaneously, rather than the movement causing the FHR acceleration.

Ovine fetal movement activity is also affected by the behavioural state, although the relationship is much less clear than that reported for breathing movements. Simple fetal movements, although episodic in nature, are seen during both high-voltage and low-voltage electrocortical activity characteristic of non-REM and REM sleep, respectively[9,10]. Complex movements likewise usually occur in clusters and are particularly prevalent during the transition between electrocortical states, although this can also occur both in high-voltage and to a lesser extent, during low-voltage electrocortical activity. Near term the ovine fetus also demonstrates short periods of wakefulness characterized by low-voltage electrocortical activity and nuchal muscle tone and a marked increase in gross movement activity. As with breathing movements, a circadian rhythm in body movements has also been observed characterized by an increase in gross movement activity overnight which becomes more pronounced near term with the establishment of the awake state[9].

OTHER MOVEMENTS

Fetal swallowing movements have been recorded in the ovine fetus during the last third of gestation using oesophageal flow probes and EMG[14–16]. These studies reveal a consistent pattern of fetal swallowing in which the majority of fluid is ingested during 'bouts' of intense activity with a number of propagated swallows over 2–3 min duration and occurring at varying intervals from approximately 30 min[16] to 2.3 h[15] dependent in part on the muscle groups recorded and the criteria used to define a 'bout'. Fetal EMG confirmed that episodes of intense repetitive laryngeal adduction were associated with oesophageal fluid flow and EMG activity. Of note, while EMG-propagated swallow activity and swallowing bout characteristics are quite consistent among fetuses, net oesophageal fluid intake is considerably more variable[16].

Fetal bladder contractions have also been studied in the ovine fetus during the latter part of gestation using implanted catheters[17,18]. Increases in bladder pressure exceeding intraperitoneal pressure by at least 5 mmHg for at least 30 s duration, are associated with voiding via the urethra and/or urachus to the amniotic and allantoic fluid sacs, respectively[17]. Fetal bladder contractions and thus voiding episodes as measured, were found to occur with a frequency of two to four per hour[17,18]. There was no diurnal variation in this number as monitored throughout the day.

In the ovine fetus, episodes of repeated swallowing and bladder contractions are also influenced by behavioural state. Near term, both of these fetal activities mainly occur during the low-voltage electrocortical activity state in association with eye movements, breathing movements, and increased nuchal muscle activity, suggesting a state of heightened activity resembling wakefulness[15,18]. However, while associated with the low-voltage electrocortical state, these activities occur with significantly different frequencies and are temporally unrelated[18], suggesting that neural control mechanisms are likewise probably unrelated.

DEVELOPMENTAL CHANGES

BREATHING MOVEMENTS

Developmental changes in fetal breathing activity are noted for the ovine species and are clearly dependent on the means by which this activity is measured. Whereas the incidence of fetal breathing movements as measured from tracheal pressure changes is lower in the younger gestational aged fetus (occurring approximately 20% of the time at 90 days of gestation; term 147 days), diaphragmatic EMG activity is almost continuous with increasing apnoeic modulation as gestation advances[19,20]. However, the diaphragmatic EMG activity of the fetus of younger gestational age is primarily tonic in nature with a prolonged burst duration. With advancing gestation, phasic diaphragmatic activity becomes more pronounced in keeping with the increased incidence of fetal breathing movements as measured by tracheal pressure change in animals near term.

A developmental change in the pattern of breathing is also noted for the ovine fetus and appears to be related to the development of episodic variations in electrocortical activity characteristic of sleep states[21]. Before 105 days of gestation and with electrocortical activity still undifferentiated, breathing movements are non-episodic and occur over short durations at frequent intervals. Thereafter, breathing movements become distinctly episodic and are associated with REM as the electrocorticogram begins to differentiate into high- and low-voltage patterns. A change in the pattern of breathing over the last third of gestation has also been reported for the fetal baboon whereby the amplitude and inspiratory time of fetal breaths increases, while the rate and variability in rate of fetal breathing decreases[8].

BODY MOVEMENTS

A developmental change in the pattern of nuchal muscle activity is evident for the ovine fetus and appears to be related to behavioural state development[21]. Prior to 105 days of gestation and with electrocortical activity still undifferentiated, nuchal muscle activity is almost continuous and without obvious pattern or relationship to the other biophysical variables. Thereafter, nuchal muscle activity becomes episodic and, with the distinct differentiation of electrocortical activity after 120 days' gestation, becomes clearly related to the high-voltage state. Gross body movement activity is also increased in the last few days prior to birth and probably relates to the appearance at this time of fetal wakefulness[9,11].

OTHER MOVEMENTS

In the sheep fetus, swallowing movements have been elicited as early as 0.5 of gestation[22], but there is little information on the volume and pattern of swallowing until the last third of pregnancy. Over this period of gestation, swallowing 'bouts' would appear to become more regular and at closer intervals, consistent with the development of behavioural state activity and its affect[14–16]. Conversely, the number of bladder contractions per hour in the ovine fetus appears to be unaffected by gestational age and developmental changes in behavioural state, at least as studied from 120 days of gestation until term[18].

PARTURITION

BREATHING MOVEMENTS

The incidence of breathing movements in the sheep fetus decreases 2 or 3 days before the onset of labour and remains significantly reduced until delivery, despite fetal blood gas and glucose concentrations within the normal range[23,24]. The mechanism for this decrease in fetal breathing activity may relate to increasing concentrations of prostaglandin E_2, which is thought to play an important role in the onset of labour in sheep[25] and is known to diminish fetal breathing activity[26]. Such a mechanism is further supported by the findings of Patrick et al.[24], during the last 12 h before the onset of ACTH-induced labour in sheep, of a significant negative relationship between fetal arterial prostaglandin E_2 concentrations and the incidence of fetal breathing movements which fell to approximately 15% of the time during early labour.

BODY MOVEMENTS

In the ovine fetus, forelimb movements, although decreased by approximately 50%, continue to be evident throughout labour and linked to behavioural state activity[10]. As labour becomes well established, movements are often associated with uterine contractions.

OTHER MOVEMENTS

While there has been limited study on the changes in other movements in relation to labour and delivery, a decrease in the number of bladder contractions has been noted in the ovine fetus over the last 5 days before the onset of spontaneous labour at term[18].

HYPOXIA AND ASPHYXIA

BREATHING MOVEMENTS

Neuromuscular blockade in the ovine fetus results in an approximate 20% decrease in O_2 consumption, presumably due in part to a decrease in breathing activity and other movements[27]. Conversely, fetal O_2 consumption is increased to a similar extent during periods of fetal breathing movements when compared to apnoeic periods[28]. As such, a decrease in fetal movements when oxygenation becomes compromised may serve as a protective mechanism whereby energy expenditure and thus O_2 requirements are also decreased.

In the near-term ovine fetus, moderate hypoxaemia of short-term duration (reduction of arterial pO_2 from approximately 24 to 14 mmHg for 1–2 h) results in a decrease in fetal breathing movements to less than 10% of the time[2,29]. Similar responses to fetal hypoxaemia are observed in chronic rhesus monkey preparations[7,30]. However, if this degree of hypoxaemia is maintained in the absence of onsetting metabolic acidaemia, movement activity returns toward normal after several hours, indicating an adaptive process[31,32]. With sustained hypoxaemia of a moderate to severe degree and leading to metabolic acidosis, fetal breathing movements are again markedly decreased and more so than for other biophysical activities[33] (Fig. 70.2). As such, fetal breathing movements would appear to be a more sensitive biophysical indicator for worsening hypoxaemia. However, with the removal of the asphyxial insult there is a rapid normalization of biophysical activity including that of breathing movements for those animals surviving[33], although some of these animals will subsequently demonstrate neuropathological change[34]. With prolonged and graded reductions in fetal oxygenation over several days, a marked decrease in fetal movement activity is only seen as the degree of hypoxaemia approaches the level at which acidaemia becomes apparent[35] (Fig. 70.3). Fetal breathing assessment should thus be seen as a marker for moderate to severe hypoxaemic changes, with heightened surveillance required for the extremely 'high risk' pregnancy as the time course for alteration prior to fetal demise may be relatively short. It should also be noted that a maturational process is apparent for the biophysical response of the ovine fetus to hypoxic insults, with the preterm fetus showing less reduction in breathing activity at 0.7 to 0.8 of gestation[21,29] and no

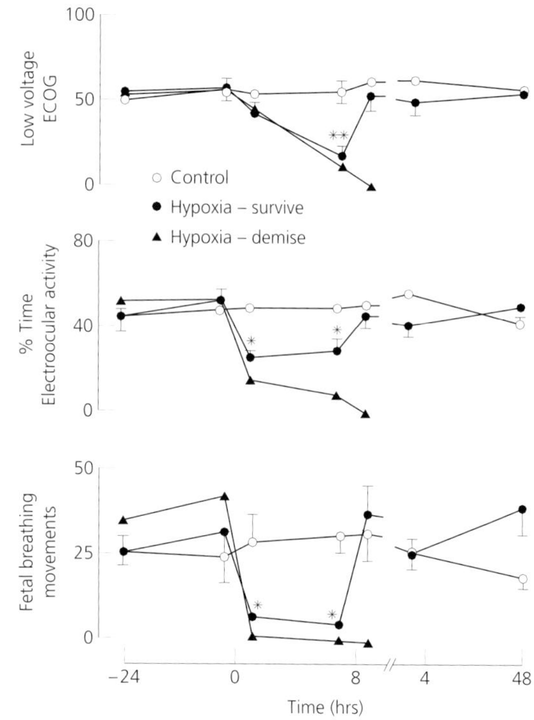

Fig. 70.2 Percentage time with low-voltage electrocortical activity (ECoG), electroocular activity, and fetal breathing movements plotted for 2 h time intervals before, during, and after experimental period (0 to approximately 8 h). Values are mean ± SE. Asterisk, $p < 0.05$; two asterisks, $p < 0.01$ versus control group values. Statistical analysis was not performed for hypoxia, death group. (From: Matsuda, Y., Patrick, J., Carmichael, L., Fisher, L & Richardson, B. (1994) Recovery of the ovine fetus from sustained hypoxia: effects on endocrine, cardiovascular and biophysical activity. *Am. J. Obstet. Gynecol.* **170**, 1433–1441.)

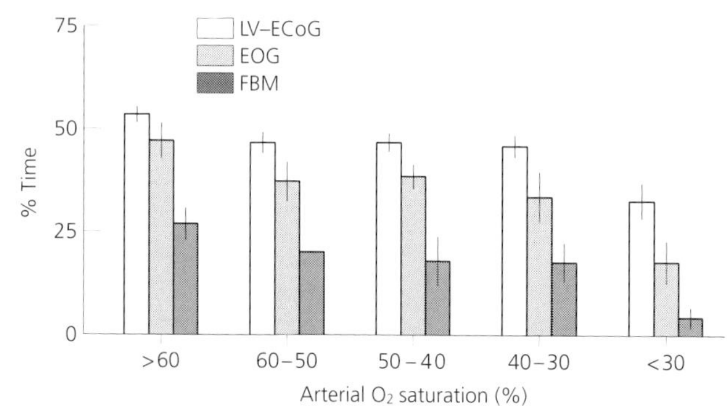

Fig. 70.3 Percentage of time with low-voltage electrocortical activity (LV-ECoG), electroocular activity (EOG) and fetal breathing movements (FBM) during graded reductions in fetal arterial oxygen saturation over 5 days of study. (From: Richardson, B. (1991) Metabolism of the fetal brain: biological and pathological development. In *The Fetal and Neonatal Brain Stem*, pp. 87–105. Cambridge, UK: Cambridge University Press.

reduction in breathing activity at 0.6 of gestation[20]. This may then impact on survival as well as the success of antenatal assessment protocols.

BODY MOVEMENTS

In the unanaesthetized sheep fetus, moderate hypoxaemia of short-term duration (reduction of arterial pO_2 from approximately 22 mmHg to 14 mmHg for 1–2 h), induced by either reducing maternal inspired oxygen[10] or by reducing uterine blood flow[29] results in a decrease in fetal forelimb and nuchal muscle activity to less than 30% of control values. It should be noted that this degree of hypoxaemia is sufficient to result in metabolic acidaemia. With mild hypoxaemia (reduction of arterial pO_2 to approximately 16 mmHg), nuchal muscle activity is decreased by only 10–15% from control values[36]. Although of probable biological significance and representing a protective adaptive mechanism, this small fall in fetal movement activity would be of little clinical use as an indicator of mild fetal hypoxaemia. Fetal body movements should also be seen as a marker for moderate to severe hypoxaemic change and, when markedly decreased, probably reflects a degree of hypoxaemia close to that required for the onset of metabolic acidaemia.

OTHER MOVEMENTS

In the near-term ovine fetus, moderate hypoxaemia of short-term duration results in an immediate decrease in the percentage time swallowing (from approximately 10% of the time to 1% of the time) and the volume swallowed (from approximately 20 ml/30 min to 5 ml/30 min)[37]. However, after 3–4 h with this degree of hypoxaemia, fetal swallowing movements gradually increase, but only to one-half control levels when studied through 24 h[38]. Fetal bladder contractions and/or voiding are likewise significantly decreased with moderate hypoxaemia of short-term duration[39,40], but return to normal levels by 6 h of hypoxia[38].

INTRAUTERINE GROWTH RESTRICTION

BREATHING MOVEMENTS

Growth is known to account for a consequential fraction of the total substrate consumption of fetal sheep near term[41]. With both prolonged reduction in fetal O_2 delivery over several days[42] and induced intrauterine growth restriction (IUGR)[43], total O_2 consumption by the fetus is reduced approximately 20%. This decrease in oxidative metabolism represents the energy 'savings' from decreased tissue growth but also will reflect, in part, changes in movement activity and associated energy requirements. The ovine fetus thus demonstrates a rapid adaptation to a limitation in substrate delivery with a decrease in growth rate and movement activity and thereby substrate needs, resulting in remarkable metabolic normality with a variable degree of hypoxaemia and usually little evidence of metabolic acidosis or anaerobic metabolism[43,44]. Of note, if decreased fetal growth is sufficient, the fall off in O_2 consumption may balance that for O_2 delivery such that fetal oxygen levels are in fact normalized[45]. As such, movement activity in some IUGR fetuses may be little affected.

Worthington et al.[44] have studied the effects of reduction of placental size in sheep with resultant asymmetrical IUGR and chronic hypoxaemia without acidaemia. The incidence of fetal breathing movements was marginally decreased, occurring approximately 20% of the time. This finding was statistically significant, but involved 24 h periods of observation which would limit the effects of other influencing factors including the diurnal and periodic nature of breathing activity.

OTHER FACTORS AFFECTING BIOPHYSICAL ACTIVITY

Numerous other factors alter movement activity in chronic fetal animal preparations. These factors are outlined in Table 70.1.

HUMAN STUDIES

PHYSIOLOGY AND BIOLOGICAL PATTERNS

BREATHING MOVEMENTS

In the mid-1970s it became possible to quantify fetal breathing and body movements by means of linear-array real-time imaging techniques with most investigators documenting visual interpretations of movements by means of an event marker from echoes displayed on a video screen[65]. Human fetal breathing movements are most readily visualized on longitudinal scanning, thus permitting visualization of both anterior fetal chest and abdominal wall echoes. During each fetal breathing movement, the anterior chest wall echoes move inward 0.5 to 5 mm and the anterior abdominal wall echoes move outward in the opposite direction about 3 to 8 mm. These paradoxical movements of the chest and abdominal wall echoes permit identification of each breath. As in the ovine fetus, the amplitude of chest and abdominal wall movements during episodes of fetal breathing is variable. Likewise, the fetal diaphragm appears to be the primary muscular force generating these movements, as echoes that represent this structure descend into the fetal abdomen during and return after each fetal breath. The incidence of human fetal breathing movements has been shown to correlate with induced changes in maternal end-tidal pCO_2, increasing with maternal breathing of 2% and 4% carbon dioxide and decreasing with maternal hyperventilation[66]. This would again suggest the existence of functional fetal chemoreceptors as previously noted for the ovine fetus.

TABLE 70.1
Factors affecting movement activity in fetal sheep

Factor	Effects
Breathing movements	
Vibroacoustic stimulation	Increased FBM with change to low-voltage ECoG state[46]
Glucose concentration:	
Hypoglycaemia	Decreased FBM[47]
Glucose infusion	Increased FBM in fetuses with low blood glucose; no effect in normoglycaemic fetuses[48]
Temperature:	
Increased core temperature	Increased FBM for 2–3 h[49]
Barbiturates:	
Phenobarbitone	Decreased FBM in mature fetuses[50]
Caffeine	Increased FBM for 10–15 min[51,52]
Catecholamines	Increased FBM[47]
Cocaine	Increased FBM during labour[53]
Diazepam	Decreased FBM[51]
Doxapram	Increased FBM[52,54]
Ethanol	Variable effect on FBM depending on acute or chronic exposure[55,56]
General anaesthesia	Total suppression of FBM[57]
Narcotics:	
Methadone, morphine	Initial decrease followed by an increase in FBM with acute exposure[58–60]
Prostaglandin E_2	Arrest of FBM[26]
Prostaglandin inhibitors	
Indomethacin/meclofenamate	Increased FBM for 12–19 h[61,62]
Theophylline	Increased FBM[63]
Body movements	
Vibroacoustic stimulation	Increased nuchal muscle activity with change to low-voltage ECoG state suggesting wakefulness[46]
Cocaine	Increased nuchal muscle activity during labour[53]
Doxapram	Increased nuchal muscle activity suggesting arousal[52]
Methadone	Increased nuchal and quadriceps muscle activity suggesting arousal[58]
Other movements	
Plasma hyperosmolality	Increased swallowing movements[64]

FBM = fetal breathing movements
ECoG = electrocortical activity

Breathing movements made by healthy human fetuses are episodic and separated by periods of apnoea. Measurements of breath-to-breath intervals over the last 10 weeks of pregnancy reveals that only 3% of these intervals are 6 s or longer[67]. Therefore, in the absence of gross fetal body movements, it is reasonable to define fetal apnoea as a period of 6 s or longer in humans. Human fetal breathing movements are seen to occur approximately 30% of the observed time over the last 10 weeks of pregnancy[65,68]. Near term there is a clustering of fetal breathing and gross body movements into episodes lasting 20–60 min and recurring every 60–90 min, suggesting a relationship to behavioural state activity as previously noted for the animal studies (Fig. 70.4)[65,68]. This behavioural state relationship has been quantified by Junge and Walter[69], with breathing movements reported to be present approximately 30% of the time during fetal 'active' periods (analogous to the REM state) as determined by coincident recording of heart rate and body movements. Although breathing movements are decreased, they are still present approximately 14% of the time during fetal 'quiet' periods (analogous to the non-REM state). The character of fetal breathing is also affected by sleep states, as Nijhuis *et al.*[70] report fetal breathing rhythm to be more regular during 'quiet' periods than during 'active' periods.

As a result of the episodic nature of human fetal breathing movements, the percentage of time spent breathing can be substantially altered by the length of recording time. It is thus necessary to record for a long enough period to be certain that the recording interval does not entirely consist of a normal period of fetal apnoea. Twenty-four-hour observation studies of healthy patients over the last 10 weeks of pregnancy have demonstrated that approximately 25% of 5 min intervals, 15% of 15 min intervals, and 8% of 30 min intervals contained no fetal breathing movements[65–68] (Fig. 70.5). It was also evident from such study that episodes of fetal apnoea of up to 2 h can occasionally occur in healthy human fetuses when recordings are made without attention to time of day or the relationship to maternal meals.

Throughout the last 10 weeks of pregnancy the percentage of time a fetus spends breathing is increased significantly during the second and third hours following maternal meals, with the increase appearing to follow the normal postprandial increase in maternal blood glucose concentration[65,68] (Fig. 70.6). A prolonged and significant increase in fetal breathing movements is also observed overnight while mothers are alseep[65,68,71] (Fig. 70.6). This may represent a circadian rhythm in fetal breathing activity, as previously described for the ovine fetus.

BODY MOVEMENTS

Human fetal body movements have been systematically studied over the last half of pregnancy by Patrick and colleagues using linear-array real-time imaging techniques, as previously described for the study of human fetal breathing movements. These studies of fetal activity in healthy pregnancies have relied upon longitudinal scanning of the fetus, thus permitting the simultaneous measurement of fetal breathing activity. Although providing for the accurate measurement of fetal rolling and stretching movements, isolated movements of the fetal limbs are not as well visualized.

Human fetal gross body movements occur approximately 10% of the time over the last 10 weeks of pregnancy with an average of 31 movements per hour over a 24 h period[72]. As previously noted, near term there is a clustering of fetal breathing and gross body movements, suggesting a relationship to behavioural state activity (Fig. 70.4)[65,68,73]. Studies by Nijhuis *et al.*[73] have now identified an inextricable linkage

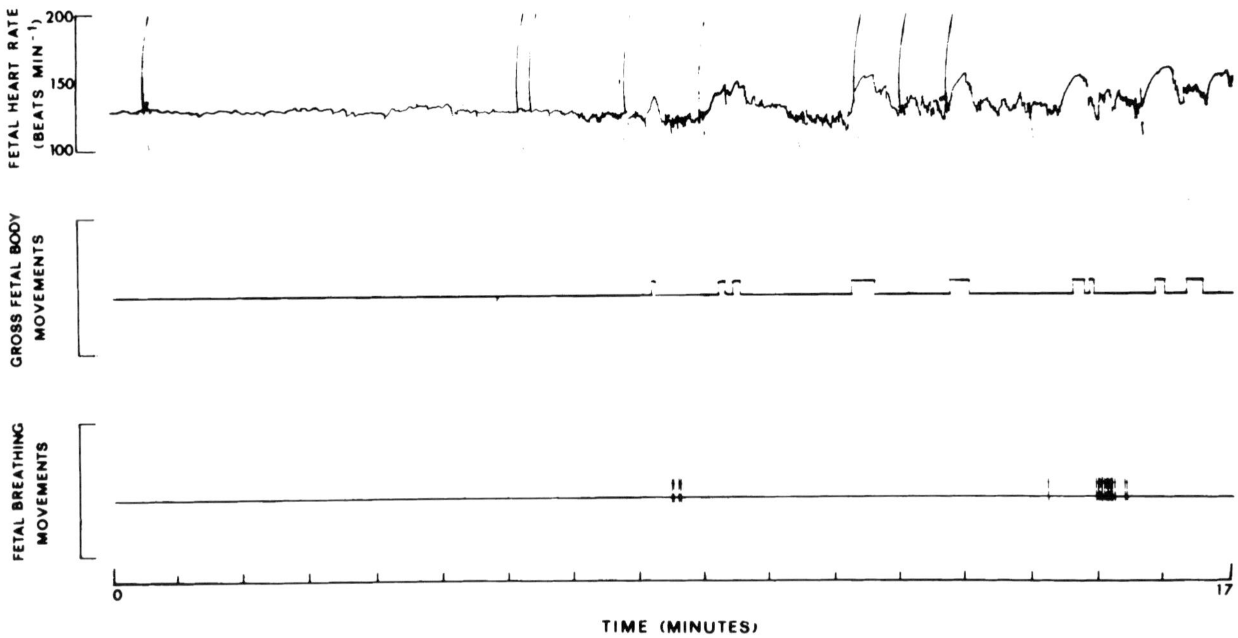

Fig. 70.4 Chart recording of fetal heart rate, gross fetal body movements, and fetal breathing movements over a 17 min observation period. For the first 8 min there were no gross fetal body movements and the fetal heart rate demonstrated no significant accelerations or decelerations. From 8 to 17 min a normal episode of gross fetal body movements accompanied by accelerations in the fetal heart rate occurred. (From: Richardson B, Campbell K, Carmichael L & Patrick J. (1981) Effects of external physical stimulation on fetuses near term. *Am. J. Obstet. Gynecol.* **139**, 344–352.)

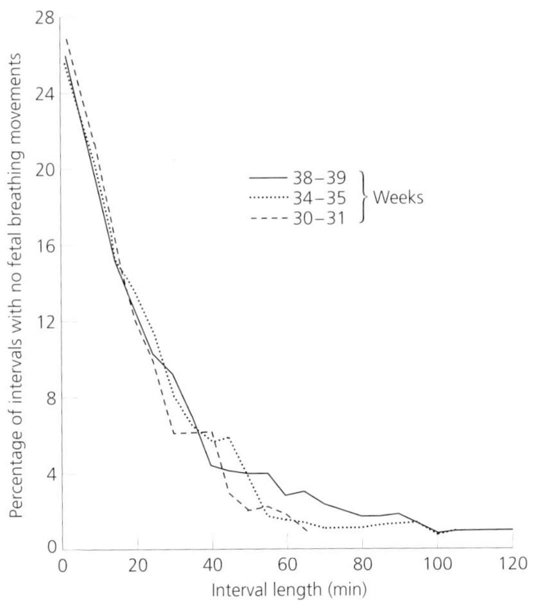

Fig. 70.5 Composite plot of the percentage of intervals with no fetal breathing movements in nine fetuses at 30 to 31 weeks, 11 at 34 to 35 weeks, and 11 at 38 to 39 weeks, demonstrating a similar distribution at these different gestational ages. The longest apnoeic interval was 65 min at 30–31 weeks, 105 min at 34–35 weeks, and 120 min at 38–39 weeks. (From: Patrick J, Campbell K, Carmichael L, Natale R & Richardson B. (1980) A definition of human fetal apnea and the distribution of fetal apneic intervals during the last 10 weeks of pregnancy. *Am. J. Obstet. Gynecol.* **136**, 471–477.)

of gross body movement activity to other behavioural parameters, thus firmly establishing the existance of fetal behavioural states. Fetal body movements are frequent during state 2F (active periods analogous to the REM state), whereas they are much reduced or absent during state 1F (quiet periods analogous to the non-REM state). This gives rise to an 'activity-quiescent' cycle with a duration of approximately 60 min by term, although with considerable variability. An additional 'active' fetal period has been described, termed state 4F, which is characterized by frequent and vigorous gross body movements and, by inference from human neonatal studies, appears to represent periods of fetal wakefulness. These are usually seen no more than 10% of the time and are of relatively short duration (5–10 min).

As a result of the episodic nature of human fetal gross body movements, it is again important to record for a long enough period to be certain that the recording interval does not entirely consist of a normal period of fetal quiescence. From our 24 h observation studies on healthy pregnant patients through the last 10 weeks of pregnancy, we have determined that approximately 25% of 5 min intervals, 10% of 15 min intervals, and 5% of 30 min intervals contain no gross body movement activity (Fig. 70.7)[72]. It was also evident that episodes of fetal quiescence of up to 75 min can occasionally occur in healthy human fetuses when recordings are made without attention to time of day.

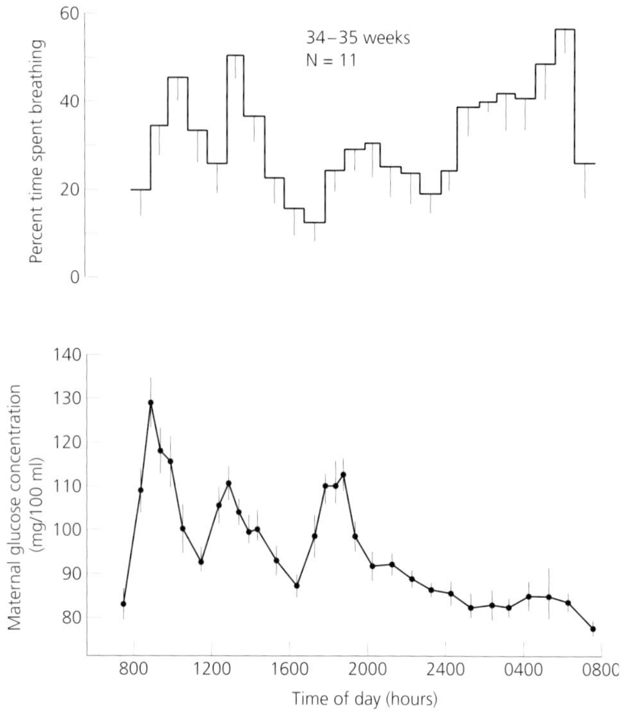

Fig. 70.6 Percentage of time spent breathing by 11 fetuses at 34–35 weeks each hour of the day. Mothers were given meals at 0800, 1200, and 1700 h. Fetuses made breathing movements a greater percentage of the time during the second and third hours following breakfast, lunch, and dinner. There was a prolonged significant increase in the percentage of time spent breathing between 0100 and 0700 h. Peak glucose concentrations occurred at 0900, 1300, and 1800. (From: Patrick J, Natale R & Richardson B. (1978) Patterns of human fetal breathing activity at 34 to 35 weeks gestational age. *Am. J. Obstet. Gynecol.* **132**:507–513.)

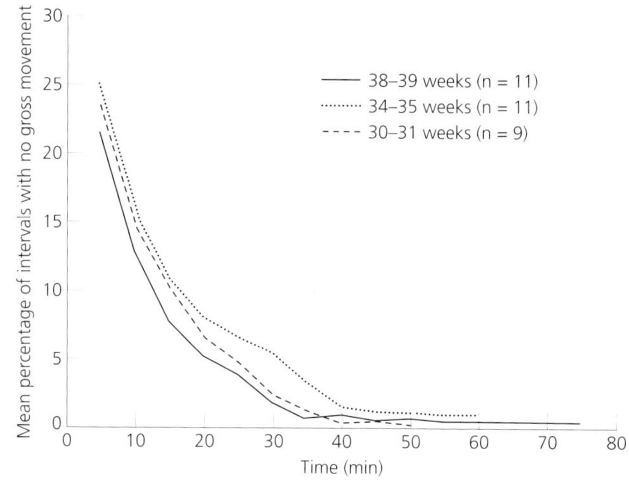

Fig. 70.7 Composite plot of the percentage of intervals with no gross fetal body movements in nine fetuses at 30–31 weeks, 11 at 34–35 weeks, and 11 at 38–39 weeks, demonstrating a similar distribution at these different gestational ages. The longest period of fetal quiescence was 70 min at 30–31 weeks, 75 min at 34–35 weeks, and 50 min at 38–39 weeks. (From: Patrick J, Campbell K, Carmichael L, Natale R & Richardson B. (1982) Patterns of gross fetal body movements over 24-hour observation intervals during the last 10 weeks of pregnancy. *Am. J. Obstet. Gynecol.* **142**, 363–371.)

Near term there is an increase in the incidence and number of gross fetal body movements in the late evening and this increase may correspond to increased periods of wakefulness (Fig. 70.8)[72]. In contrast to fetal breathing movements, gross body movements are not influenced by maternal plasma glucose concentrations or maternal meals during the day (Fig. 70.8).

RELATIONSHIP OF BODY MOVEMENTS TO FHR ACCELERATIONS

The relationship of fetal body movements to heart rate accelerations is an important one and provides the basis for non-stress heart rate testing. Timor-Tritsch et al.[74], using strain gauges placed on the maternal abdomen wall, reported that 99.8% of all fetal movements of greater than 3 s duration are associated with fetal heart rate accelerations (>10 bpm). Patrick and co-workers[75], using real-time ultrasound and abdominal electrocardiographic (EKG) methods, reported that near term 92% of all evident gross body movements were associated with fetal heart rate accelerations (≥10 bpm and lasting ≥10 s), whereas 95% of all accelerations occurred in association with body movements. Thus quantitative observations of fetal movements would appear to be interchangeable with fetal heart rate accelerations over the last few weeks of pregnancy. However, it remains to be determined whether the compromised fetus with a non-reactive non-stress test has a loss of fetal heart rate acceleration with body movement or rather becomes inactive and stops moving.

OTHER MOVEMENTS

Swallowing movements in the human fetus have been characterized with the use of colour-flow Doppler signals superimposed on grey-scale imaging of the upper gastrointestinal and respiratory tracts[76]. An inital stage of sucking movements with the introduction of amniotic fluid into the oral cavity is then followed by low-frequency tongue movements, upward laryngeal and epiglottic movements, and narrowing of the lumen of the pharynx, directing the fluid bolus downward into the oesophagus.

Real-time ultrasound scanning has made it possible to visualize the changes in size of the human fetal bladder, and Rabinowitz et al.[77] have reported that over the last half of gestation there is a cyclic filling and emptying, with the cycle length variable, but usually less than 60 min. While filling of the fetal bladder takes place at a relatively uniform rate, emptying occurs quickly and over a period of a few seconds. As in the ovine fetus, a linkage to behavioural state activity when established is again apparent as bladder emptying

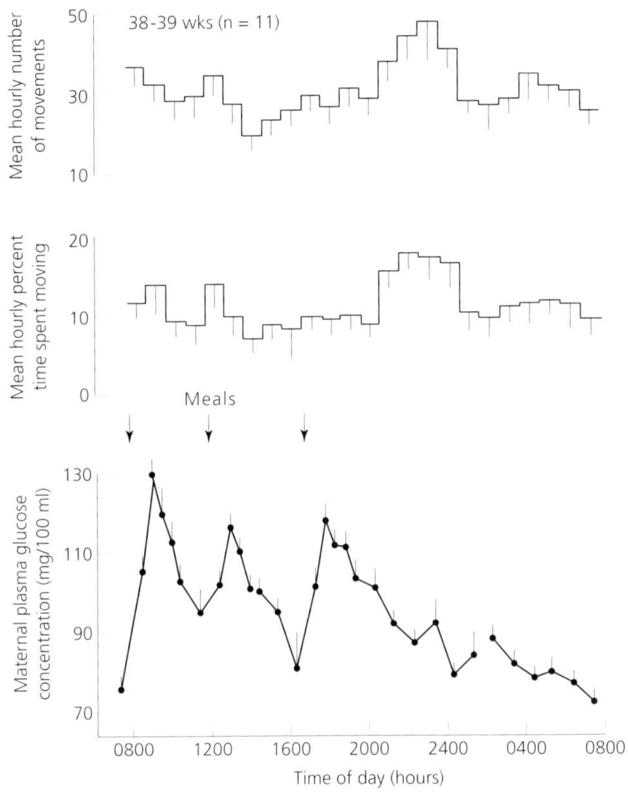

Fig. 70.8 Maternal glucose concentrations, the average number of movements, and the percentage of time spent moving by fetuses plotted each hour of the day (± SEM) in 11 fetuses at 38–39 weeks gestational age. There was a peak in activity between 2100 and 0100 h. (From: Patrick J, Campbell K, Carmichael L, Natale R & Richardson B. (1982) *Am. J. Obstet. Gynecol.* **142**, 363–371.)

usually occurs after a change from an episode of low to high heart rate variation[78], indicating a change from state 1F to 2F.

DEVELOPMENTAL CHANGES

BREATHING MOVEMENTS

Rhythmic breathing movements can be observed from 10 weeks of gestation onward, with a trend toward an increase in incidence thereafter, although they are still only evident 6% of the recording time by 19 weeks of gestation[79,80]. Continuous 24 h recordings of fetal breathing activity at 24 to 28 weeks' gestation have been reported by Natale et al.[71], with the mean incidence found to be 14%. Fetal breathing activity was now distinctly episodic and clustered with other behavioural variables, but the longest period of apnoea was only 14 min, which is significantly less than that seen during the last 10 weeks of pregnancy. This would suggest that different normal values need to be used in the evaluation of fetal health at earlier gestations. Although the overall percentage of time the fetus spends breathing remains little changed between 30 and 40 weeks of gestation, differences in patterns of breathing activity and in distributions of breath-to-breath intervals are evident[67]. The mean rate of fetal breathing movements at 30 to 31 weeks is 58 and falls to 41 breaths per minute at 38 to 39 weeks. The distribution of breath-to-breath intervals is much broader at 30 to 31 weeks than at 38 to 39 weeks when breath-to-breath intervals are more regular. These changes in respiratory rate and variability over this period suggest a maturation in the control of fetal breathing movements, which probably reflects the emergence of behavioural state influences.

BODY MOVEMENTS

Longitudinal study of fetal movement activity over the first half of pregnancy reveals that movements even of the young fetus appear to be specific and with recognizable patterning[79,80]. The majority of these movements, however, seem to occur at no regular interval with fetal quiescence usually no longer than 5–10 min. Continuous 24 h recordings of gross fetal body movements at 24 to 28 weeks of gestation have been reported by Nasello-Paterson et al.[81] who found the mean incidence to be approximately 13%, which is similar to the incidence reported over the last 10 weeks of pregnancy[72]. However, the total number of movements per hour shows a maturational decrease, suggesting that fetuses between 24 and 28 weeks' gestation move significantly more often but with a shorter duration of movement than do fetuses between 30 and 39 weeks' gestation. Although fetal movement activity is now becoming episodic and clustered with other behavioural variables, the longest period of quiescence was only 24 min, which is significantly less than observed during the last 10 weeks of pregnancy, again suggesting that different norms need to be used in the evaluation of fetal health at earlier gestations. This group also noted a maturational change in the relationship of body movements to heart rate accelerations whereby the proportion of larger amplitudes of fetal heart rate accelerations (i.e. ≥15 bpm) increase with gestational age and the proportion of total heart rate accelerations associated with fetal body movements shifted from low-amplitude types of acceleration (i.e. <15 bpm) to accelerations of higher amplitude (i.e. ≥15 bpm) as fetuses reached 32 weeks' gestation (Fig. 70.9)[82]. These maturational changes have obvious implications for non-stress test scoring. As periods of coincidence of behavioural parameters give rise to clearly defined behavioural states, a maturational change in the duration of the so called 'activity-quiescence' cycle is seen with a progressive increase from approximately 20 min at 28 weeks of gestation to approximately 60 min by term, which is in fact similar in length to the sleep state cycling of the newborn infant[73,83].

OTHER MOVEMENTS

The human fetus demonstrates swallowing movements as early as 11 weeks' gestation, with a gradual increase in incidence as measured through the first half of pregnancy[79,80].

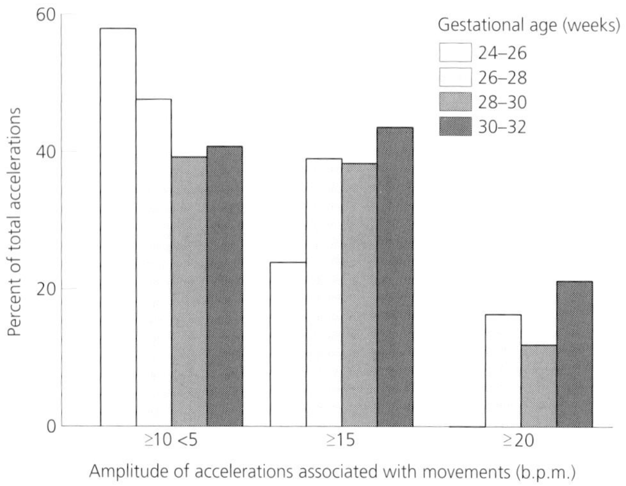

Fig. 70.9 Frequency distribution of the amplitudes of fetal heart rate accelerations associated with fetal body movements. Significantly larger proportions of fetal heart rate accelerations ≥15 bpm and ≥20 bpm are associated with fetal body movements at 30 to 32 weeks' gestation than at 24–26 weeks' gestation ($p < 0.05$). (From: Natale R, Nasello-Paterson C & Turliuk R. (1985) Longitudinal measurements of fetal breathing, body movements, heart rate, and heart rate accelerations and decelerations at 24–32 weeks of gestation. *Am. J. Obstet. Gynecol.* **151**, 256–263.)

More complex sucking movements can be identified at 18–20 weeks[84]. Bladder emptying has been reported from 20 weeks' gestation[77,85] and becomes correlated with the active phase of the fetal heart rate cycle from 28 weeks' gestation onward, and with REM and fetal breathing movements from 34 weeks' gestation onward[86].

PARTURITION

BREATHING MOVEMENTS

A number of reports indicate that patterns of human fetal breathing movements are changed in relation to labour at term. In healthy patients with either spontaneous or induced labour and subsequently shown to have normal outcomes, fetal breathing movements are decreased to less than 10% of the time on average during the latent phase of labour and are further decreased during the active phase of labour[87–89]. In 24 h studies of fetal activity at term, a decrease in fetal breathing movements is also noted in those patients subsequently entering spontaneous labour within 3 days, when compared to those patients delivering more than 7 days following study[90]. These data would additionally indicate that a significant decrease in breathing activity normally occurs in the days immediately preceding the onset of labour at term.

ASSESSMENT OF PRETERM LABOUR

Since fetal breathing activity is known to decrease during labour, its incidence has been proposed as a means of predicting fetuses at risk of preterm delivery in women who present in hospital with signs of premature labour. Several studies have now shown that fetal apnoea of 20–60 min duration is a reliable indicator of true premature labour with subsequent premature delivery within 48–72 h in almost all of these patients[91–94]. However, these patients also have a lower success rate with tocolytic therapy[91,94], suggesting that they were in more advanced premature labour. This suggestion is further supported by our study results for electively induced labour at term, when prolonged fetal apnoea was only evident during active labour[87]. In those same clinical studies of prematurely labouring patients, the presence of fetal breathing movements did not appear to be as reliable in predicting false premature labour, with a number of patients still delivering within the subsequent 48–72 h. Given the wide range in the incidence of fetal breathing movements when monitored over short time intervals and the finding that fetal apnoea is only consistently seen in advanced labour, the observation of a decrease in this activity is unlikely to be clinically useful in the management of women with preterm labour.

BODY MOVEMENTS

Gross fetal body movements, although somewhat reduced, continue to be evident throughout labour with a periodicity suggestive of 'activity-quiescence' cycling[87]. Unlike fetal breathing movements, the incidence of gross body movements remains unchanged during the last 3 days prior to spontaneous labour at term[90].

PREMATURE RUPTURE OF THE MEMBRANES AND CHORIOAMNIONITIS

Rupture of the membranes per se, whether prematurely or at term, would not appear to affect either fetal breathing movements or body movements as measured from an incidence standpoint and/or component parts of biophysical profile scoring[87,95]. With associated increases in uterine contractility and those endocrine events leading to the onset of labour, there is a decrease in fetal breathing movements and to a lesser extent in body movements[91,94], as previously discussed in relation to parturition. A number of clinical studies on patients with preterm rupture of the membranes have also noted a decrease in fetal breathing movements and/or body movements or in biophysical profile scores (especially absent fetal breathing and non-reactive non-stress testing) in those patients with subsequent positive amniotic fluid testing for infection, clinical chorioamnionitis or neonatal sepsis[95–99]. This may relate to the fetal response to bacterial products whereby 'inflammatory' cytokines are released in turn, impacting on fetal behavioural activity. As such, biophysical profile monitoring of fetal activity has been proposed for patients with preterm rupture of membranes as a screen for whether or not amniotic fluid testing for infection is required[96,97] and as an indicator of an onsetting infective process and thus the need for delivery[95–97]. However, studies to date have reported varying sensitivities in the prediction of intrauterine infection[95–101] which probably relates to the severity of the infective process, the degree of any fetal 'inflammatory' response, and the proximity of activity testing to the time of delivery. Additionally, some of these patients will show a decrease in fetal breathing and movement activity in relation to impending labour and without subsequent evidence of infection, contributing to a lowered specificity for such testing as also reported in a number of these studies[91,94,98–101]. The monitoring of fetal activity is thus unlikely to be clinically useful in the management of women with preterm rupture of the membranes.

INTRAUTERINE GROWTH RESTRICTION

BREATHING MOVEMENTS

The human fetus also undergoes intrauterine growth restriction (IUGR) in response to limitations in substrate availability including that of oxygen. Cordocentesis data indicate variable degrees of hypoxaemia[102–104], although in many instances blood gas values are within the normal range, suggesting a degree of normalization with the fall-off in growth. In patients with IUGR, the incidence of fetal breathing movements is reported to be variably decreased and appears dependent on the severity of IUGR (<10th percentile versus <3rd percentile) and the conditions and duration of study[105–110]. Although of probable biological importance with an associated decrease in energy expenditure, there is considerable overlap with population norms, which would limit the usefulness of this parameter – at least as used clinically – as a marker of intrauterine growth restricition. Maternal hyperoxia (inspired oxygen concentration of 50%) has been shown to increase the incidence of breathing movements in the IUGR fetus with no such increases noted for the well-grown fetus[106,108–110]. Although implicating fetal hypoxaemia as the basis for the reduced incidence of breathing movements in the IUGR fetus, the induced increase in such activity is to a level similar to that of the well-grown fetus and, given the inherent periodicity of fetal breathing activity, is again unlikely to serve as a useful clinical marker.

BODY MOVEMENTS

The incidence and number of gross body movements is also variably decreased in patients with IUGR[108,109,111,112]. Although of probable biological significance with a decrease in energy expenditure and thus oxygen requirements anticipated, considerable overlap with population norms is again evident, as previously discussed for fetal breathing movements. It is controversial whether maternal hyperoxia increases the incidence of these movements to a level similar to that of the well grown fetus[108,109]. Given the inherent periodicity of fetal movement activity, this again is unlikely to serve as a useful clinical marker.

ASSESSMENT OF FETAL HEALTH

BREATHING ACTIVITY AND BODY MOVEMENTS

The present use of fetal breathing and body movements in the assessment of fetal health is largely confined to their component parts in biophysical profile scoring (Table 70.2) and has been extensively reported on by both Manning[113–116] and Vintzileos[117–120] and their colleagues. As used in the biophysical profile, fetal movement activity has been scored in an 'all or none' manner and related to a number of outcomes, including subsequent intrauterine demise, fetal distress in labour requiring operative intervention, abnormal 5 min Apgar score, abnormal umbilical cord gases and/or

TABLE 70.2
Criteria for scoring biophysical parameters according to Manning *et al.*[113]

Variable	Score 2	Score 0
Fetal breathing movements	The presence of at least 30 s of sustained fetal breathing movements in 30 min of observation	Fewer than 30 s of fetal breathing movements in 30 min
Fetal movements	Three or more gross body movements in 30 min of observation. Simultaneous limb and trunk movements are counted as a single movement	Two or fewer gross body movements in 30 min observation
Fetal tone	At least one episode of motion of a limb from a position of flexion to extension and rapid return to flexion	Fetus in a position of semi- or full limb extension with no return to flexion with movement. Absence of fetal movement is counted as absent tone
Fetal reactivity	The presence of two or more fetal heart rate accelerations of at least 15 bpm, lasting at least 15 s, and associated with fetal movement in 40 min	No acceleration or fewer than two accelerations in the fetal heart rate in 40 min of observation
Qualitative amniotic fluid volume	A pocket of amniotic fluid that measures at least 1 cm in two perpendicular planes	Largest pocket of amniotic fluid measures < 1 cm in two perpendicular planes
Maximum score	10	—
Minimum score	—	0

pH, and IUGR. While these endpoints differ somewhat, the physiological basis for the use of fetal activity in the biophysical assessment of fetal health is the same; that is, with a compromise in oxygenation leading to hypoxaemia with or without associated acidosis, fetal movement activity will decrease as an adaptive response whereby energy expenditure is also decreased.

As presently scored within the biophysical profile, fetal breathing movements are more likely to be falsely abnormal or positive at 26–33 weeks' gestation when compared to 34–41 weeks[121]. This is in keeping with the lower incidence of breathing activity in younger fetuses[71], and emphasizes the need to establish population norms reflecting the biological patterns and known factors affecting this activity. Likewise, non-stress testing is more likely to be falsely non-reactive prior to 32 weeks' gestation[122], again reflecting well described maturational changes whereby the amplitude in fetal heart rate acceleration in association with body movements is normally less prior to this gestational age[82].

The negative predictive value for a normal perinatal outcome is high and similar among the three dynamic biophysical variables – fetal breathing movements, gross body movements, and non-stress heart rate testing – and in the order of 95% with little improvement when test results are combined[113,123,124]. However, the positive predictive value for an abnormal perinatal outcome is improved and the false positive rate decreased when test results are combined. For the dynamic fetal variables, the monitoring of body movements would appear to improve the positive predictive value of the biophysical profile more than the monitoring of breathing movements or non-stress testing[117,125], although a report by Manning et al.[115] would suggest the same for non-stress testing. However, as noted by Devoe et al.[126], such comparisons are without statistical relationship to physiological incidence data, as the unweighted and somewhat arbitrary scoring system currently used does not provide for the quantification of the dynamic fetal variables and their normal population standards. In the 24 h observation studies of Patrick et al.[67,72] on healthy patients through the last 10 weeks of pregnancy, the percentage of 30 min intervals with no fetal breathing movements was close to 8% on average, while that for no gross fetal body movements was only 4% on average (Figs 70.5 and 70.7). Moreover, sequential rather than concurrent monitoring of these fetal activities, as used in biophysical profile scoring, does not respect the interdependence of these variables with behavioural state organization. Given the cyclic nature of fetal behavioural activity, 70 min of observational testing with biophysical profile scoring should be more predictive of a poor fetal outcome than either 30 min of ultrasound scanning or 40 min of non-stress testing alone. It has yet to be determined whether prolongation of the monitoring interval for any of the dynamic variables, as previously suggested for non-stress testing[127] would be equally successful in improving the positive predictive value for poor perinatal outcome. Despite such concerns, a more recent study by Devoe et al.[128] in high-risk pregnant patients with concurrent biophysical testing and using established population norms, again found the monitoring of body movements to have a better positive predictive value for adverse perinatal outcome than the other dynamic variables.

Fetal movement activity in the high-risk obstetrical patient has also been related to umbilical cord gases and/or pH as obtained at the time of subsequent delivery by elective caesarean section[119,120,129] or by cordocentesis[116,130]. From these studies it would appear that decreased fetal heart rate reactivity and absence of breathing movements are earlier manifestations of fetal hypoxaemia with onsetting acidaemia (Fig. 70.10). With more severe hypoxaemia, hypercapnia, and acidaemia, fetal body movements and tone also become abnormal. This would imply a hierarchy within the fetal brain for the control of these activities in response to onsetting hypoxaemia and/or acidaemia. Although this may be true, as suggested by studies in the ovine fetus[35], the clinical evidence to date shows considerable overlap of blood gas and pH values among test groupings and is again largely based on arbitrary standards without relation to normal values for a given population. In a longitudinal study of IUGR fetuses, Ribbert et al.[131] observed that fetal heart rate reactivity was reduced with the onset of hypoxaemia and was followed by a gradual decrease in fetal body movement. The percentage time fetal breathing was within the normal range with chronic hypoxaemia and normal pH, but fell to zero with the onset of acidaemia. Thus, as fetal oxygenation becomes compromised, body movements may be decreased prior to that in breathing

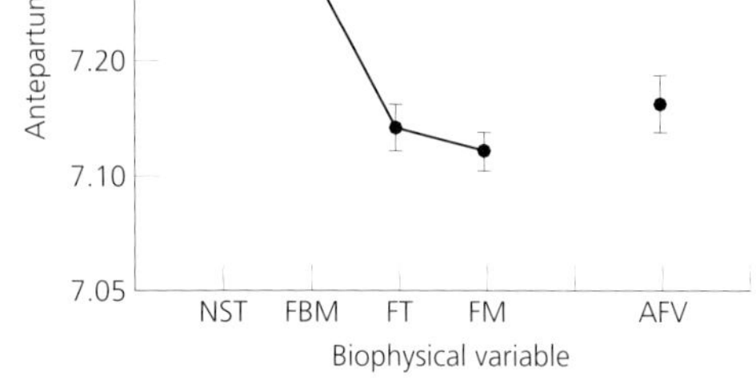

Fig. 70.10 Relationship between individual biophysical parameters and mean (±2 SD) umbilical venous fetal pH: Open circles correspond to normal and closed circles to abnormal biophysical parameters. NST = non-stress test; FBM = fetal breathing movement; FT = fetal tone; FM = fetal movements; AFV = amniotic fluid volume. (From: Manning FA, Snijders R, Harman CR, Nicolaides K, Menticoglou S & Morrison I. (1993) Fetal biophysical profile score. VI. Correlation with antepartum umbilical venous fetal pH. *Am. J. Obstet. Gynecol.* **169**, 755–763.)

movements, but continue to be evident for longer as the decrease in body movements is gradual while that for breathing movements is more abrupt. Nonetheless, as clinically used in biophysical profile scoring, the increased sensitivity of non-reactive non-stress testing and absent fetal breathing movements for predicting adverse perinatal outcome[117], is in keeping with their earlier occurrence as fetal oxygenation worsens.

While the negative predictive value for a normal perinatal outcome is high with biophysical profile scoring, there continues to be a small number of patients with adverse perinatal outcome that is not predicted on the basis of dynamic fetal monitoring[114]. This serves to emphasize that the monitoring of fetal movement activity allows only for the assessment of fetal health, at the time of testing, from which a probability of continued health may be formulated. An improvement in negative predictive value might occur with more frequent testing, but the time course over which these variables become abnormal with a compromise in fetal oxygenation may well vary with different pregnancy complications and their severity. Anecdotal clinical reports indicate that in some instances, deterioration in scoring profiles can occur over as short a time interval as 2–3 days[114,124]. The marked decrease in fetal movement activity required for an abnormal biophysical profile score with the 'all or none' criteria, would appear to be a marker for moderate to severe hypoxaemic change with onsetting acidaemia as determined by related changes in umbilical cord gases and pH[116,119,120,129,130]. This is similar to that discussed for the ovine fetus with prolonged and graded reductions in oxygenation[35], and again suggests the need for heightened surveillance in the extremely high-risk pregnancy, perhaps with daily monitoring as metabolic deterioration may occur rapidly as acidaemia worsens.

Although biophysical profile scoring in the assessment of fetal health has mainly been used antepartum, there has been some study on its use intrapartum[132,133]. While fetal breathing and body movements may be observed throughout labour and meet the criteria for normal biophysical profile scoring[133], their decreased incidence normally observed will contribute to an increased false positive testing[87–89]. Furthermore, in the study of Sassoon et al.[132], metabolic acidaemia at the time of delivery was not well predicted with intermittent biophysical profile testing, which may relate to the rapid deterioration which can occur in the high-risk fetus during labour, thus requiring continuous monitoring. Given the logistical difficulties of such monitoring and the increased false positive and negative rates as noted, biophysical profile scoring in the assessment of fetal health is unlikely to be clinically useful in the management of patients intrapartum.

Fetal body movements and associated heart rate accelerations have also been used in the assessment of fetal health with the so called 'modified biophysical profile' whereby non-stress testing as an acute measure of fetal well-being is combined with amniotic fluid assessment as a measure of longer-term well-being. Such testing is logistically easier than complete biophysical profile assessment and should provide for an effective 'first test' in the high-risk pregnant patient, given the increased sensitivity of non-stress testing for predicting adverse perinatal outcome[117] and the high negative predictive value for all dynamic testing, whether used individually or combined[113,123,124]. Studies to date which have used this testing and with complete biophysical profile assessment when the non-stress test is non-reactive, have reported outcome results comparable to that of the biophysical profile[134,135].

Maternally perceived fetal movement activity has additionally been used as a means of fetal surveillance. Recording of movement by the mother is simple, inexpensive, readily available, and does not require technical skill or sophisticated equipment. However, maternal perception of fetal activity can be misleading, as some movements go undetected and others are wrongly recorded, instead representing Braxton–Hicks contractions or maternal aortic pulsation and respiration. This contributes to the large intrapatient and interpatient variation in the monitoring of fetal movements and the difficulty in establishing population norms.

Connors et al.[136] have studied maternal perception of fetal activity from 24 weeks' gestation until term. Although large interpatient variation in movement counts per hour was evident, only 2% (28–40 weeks) to 4% (24–27 weeks) of 1 h observation periods were without perceived movement. When the observation period was extended to two consecutive hours, only five observations in one patient contained no movement. These findings correlate closely with the objective ultrasonography data reported by Patrick[72] and suggest that 2 h is a sufficient period of time to allow for the normal periodicity of fetal movement activity. While the ideal number of movements to be counted has not been defined, perception of 10 distinct movements in a period of up to 2 h is considered reassuring[137]. In the absence of a reassuring count, a biophysical means of fetal assessment with either non-stress testing or ultrasound scanning for fetal movements, should be used.

FETAL MOVEMENTS VERSUS OTHER MEANS OF FETAL SURVEILLANCE

The different means of fetal surveillance which test for a compromise in oxygenation basically involve testing for causative factors – placental insufficiency with altered umbilical flow velocity waveform patterns as measured with Doppler ultrasound; testing for level of oxygenation directly – umbilical cord blood gases and pH as measured with cordocentesis; and testing for reactive/adaptive responses – a decrease in growth as measured with ultrasound, and decreases in fetal movement activity as measured with biophysical profile scoring and non-stress testing. Whether or not these tests become abnormal will depend in part on the causative role of placental insufficiency versus other factors; the degree of fetal hypoxaemia and onsetting acidaemia; and, the time available for reactive/adaptive responses. Maternal isoimmunization leading to fetal hydrops will compromise fetal oxygenation but without an increase in the umbilical resistance indices. Studies in the ovine fetus[41,43–45] and with supporting evidence from the human[102–104], indicate that IUGR is an adaptive response whereby energy expenditure is decreased and if balanced against the compromise in oxygenation, may lead to a normalization of blood gas values. Impairments in fetal oxygenation which operate acutely over minutes or hours, or subacutely over days, will affect movement activity but will not affect growth, at least as measured clinically with serial ultrasound assessment. It is against this complex interaction between causative factors for fetal hypoxia and reactive/adaptive responses that the different means of fetal surveillance are compared, with additional consideration for the normative range of test values, the biological factors also affecting these values, and the outcomes to be determined.

A number of clinical studies in high-risk pregnant patients have evaluated the changes in fetal movement activity (incidence data, biophysical profile scoring, or non-stress testing) versus umbilical Doppler velocimetry in relation to umbilical cord gases and/or pH, or other outcome determinants[138–142]. In general, these studies indicate that with a chronic compromise in oxygenation that is of placental origin, umbilical Doppler velocimetry is usually the first surveillance test to be abnormal with an increase in the resistance indices[138,140,142]. With continued placental insufficiency, fetal growth becomes demonstrably retarded and is associated with a decrease in fetal movement activity and heart rate variation, but which are still within the population norms[138,140]. With advanced placental insufficiency and a marked decrease in oxygenation, fetal movement activity also becomes abnormal, initially as manifest with non-reactive non-stress testing and absent fetal breathing movements and finally, with absent fetal body movements[138–140,142]. In these studies, umbilical Doppler velocimetry and ultrasound measurements of growth variably relate to given degrees of hypoxaemia and/or acidaemia dependent in part on the extent to which oxygenation is normalized by the fall off in growth as previously discussed for the ovine fetus[43–45]. Fetal movement activity, on the other hand, would appear to be a more direct marker for the level of oxygenation, with abnormalities in testing seen with moderate to severe hypoxic change and onsetting acidaemia as also seen in the ovine fetus[35]. However, it should again be noted that there are large interfetal differences reflecting the complex interaction of the factors discussed.

OTHER FACTORS AFFECTING BIOPHYSICAL ACTIVITY

Numerous other factors alter movement activity in the human fetus. These factors are outlined in Table 70.3.

TABLE 70.3
Factors affecting movement activity in the human fetus

Factor	Effects
Breathing movements	
Vibroacoustic stimulation	Decreased and more irregular FBM after 36 weeks' gestation suggesting wakefulness[143]
Glucose concentration:	
Glucose infusions	Increased FBM in patients who have fasted[144]
Cigarette smoking	Increased frequency of FBM although incidence unchanged[145,146]
Caffeine	Increased FBM with chronic exposure; no effect with acute exposure[147]
Ethanol	Dramatic decrease in FBM[148,149]
Methadone	Decreased FBM with chronic exposure[150]
Tocolytics	Dramatic increase in FBM[151]
Other drugs	Small-series reports have appeared on the effects of amylobarbital, diazepam, meperidine, methyldopa, salbutamol, and terbutaline (for a review see Lewis and Boylan[152])
Body movements	
Vibroacoustic stimulation	Increased gross body movements after 33 weeks' gestation suggesting wakefulness[143,153]

FBM = fetal breathing movements

FETAL GROWTH AND DEVELOPMENT

The abundance of *in utero* movement activity in the healthy fetus and the poor outcome associated with its restriction in animal experimentation and in the human fetus support an important role for movement activity in fetal growth and development.

BREATHING MOVEMENTS

Evidence from animal experimentation and from observations of human fetuses has indicated that fetal breathing movements are important for the normal development of the fetal lungs. Studies in fetal rabbits[154] and sheep[155] have shown that, following section of the upper cervical spinal cord and elimination of phasic respiratory movements of the diaphragm, the DNA content of the lungs was reduced. Circumstantial evidence from anomalous development of human fetuses also supports the conclusion that loss of fetal breathing movements plays a role in abnormal lung growth with pulmonary hypoplasia, although loss of thoracic volume may be just as important if not more so[156]. Although the mechanisms whereby fetal breathing movements effect lung growth are not well understood, phasic distortion of the lungs leading to pulmonary cell division and the maintenance of lung liquid volume and/or distension appear to be important[157].

Since fetal breathing movements are important for lung growth, they have been studied in patients with oligohydramnios in relation to the subsequent development of pulmonary hypoplasia[158–161]. While fetal breathing movements appear to be variably decreased or absent in those fetuses who are subsequently shown to have pulmonary hypoplasia[160,161], this may depend upon the gestational age studied. Fetuses with preterm rupture of the membranes and oligohydramnios, as studied during the latter half of pregnancy, are certainly capable of making breathing movements[87,95]. Moreover, fetuses with renal agenesis and oligohydramnios and subsequently shown to have pulmonary hypoplasia, but studied after 28 weeks of gestation, are also seen to make breathing movements[158]. As such, fetal breathing movements may be seen as decreased or absent in the younger fetus with oligohydramnios as a result of developing pulmonary hypoplasia and increased 'lung stiffness'. With advancing gestation and an increase in the stimuli for respiratory movements and chest wall excursion, breathing movement activity may now be evident despite underlying pulmonary hypoplasia. However, it is also possible that oligohydramnios of a marked degree mechanically restricts chest wall movement in the younger fetus, in turn contributing to the development of pulmonary hypoplasia.

BODY MOVEMENTS

The neural activity of fetal motility and its motor effects may contribute to the development of muscles, joints, and even the fine structure of the central nervous system itself[162]. However, there has been little study, either experimentally or of a clinical nature, in this area to date.

OTHER MOVEMENTS

Fetal swallowing and gastrointestinal absorption may be important for normal gastrointestinal development and maturation[163,164] and possibly for fetal somatic growth[165]. Although of interest from a developmental standpoint, these findings have had little clinical applicability to date.

BEHAVIOURAL STATE ACTIVITY

The use of chronic catheterization techniques in fetal animals, primarily sheep, and the use of high-resolution ultrasound equipment for the study of the human fetus, have firmly established the existence of activity or behavioural states near term that have similarities to postnatal sleep states[11,73,166]. Moreover, a developmental process is evident whereby once behavioural state activity is clearly distinguished, the REM state predominates[11,73], indicating that the immature being has a high requirement for this activity state and that the REM state itself might play an additional role in fetal/neonatal growth and development.

Cerebral metabolism has been studied in the ovine fetus in relation to behavioural state development; a significant increase has been measured during the low-voltage ECoG state or REM state when compared to the high-voltage ECoG state or non-REM state[167,168] (Fig. 70.11). Blood flow velocity waveform studies in the human fetus using Doppler ultrasound suggest a similar relationship[169] given the close correlation between cerebral blood flow and cerebral metabolism. The increased metabolic rate of the brain during the REM state may reflect increased neuronal activity or synthetic processes and supports an important role for the increased incidence of this state during the accelerated growth and development of the brain during the perinatal period. It is thus possible that alterations in behavioural state activity and associated changes in cerebral metabolism during this critical period may provide a mechanism whereby pathological factors give rise to abnormal brain growth and development.

As behavioural state activity characterizes the healthy fetus, disturbances in the ontogeny or organization of these states may also be a potential indicator for central nervous system dysfunction. The appearance of well-defined behavioural states is delayed in the intrauterine growth restricted fetus and the 4F or active (awake) state is less evident than in the healthy fetus[107,170]. Assessment of behavioural states may also indicate delayed development of brain function in the fetuses of diabetic pregnancies[171,172]. Abnormal state organization has additionally been documented in fetuses exposed to alcohol[173] and cocaine[174] throughout pregnancy.

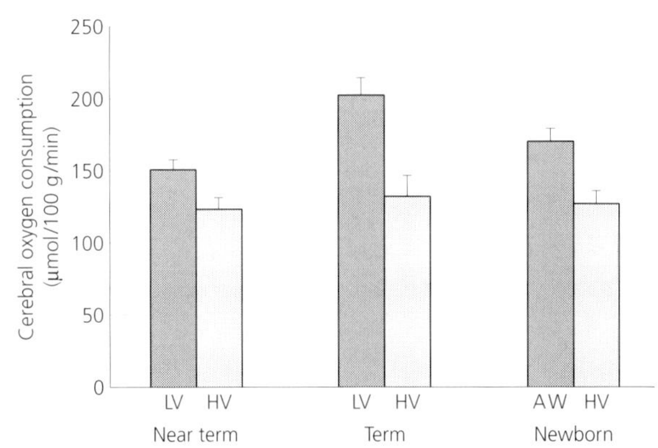

Fig. 70.11 Measurements of cerebral oxygen consumption in the ovine fetus near term (~130 days' gestation), at term (~140 days' gestation), and at 24 h after birth. Cerebral oxidative metabolism shows no significant change with age. A coupling to behavioural state is evident as oxygen consumption significantly increases during both the perinatal low-voltage (LV) ECoG state and the awake (AW) state at 24 h. HV = high voltage electrocortical state. (From: Richardson B. (1994) Ontogeny of behavioural states in the fetus. In *Textbook of Fetal Physiology*, pp. 322–328. Oxford, UK: Oxford Medical Publications.)

REFERENCES

1. Dawes GS, Fox HE, Leduc BM, Liggins GC & Richards RT. Respiratory movements and rapid eye movement sleep in the foetal lamb. *J. Physiol.* **220**:119–143, 1972.
2. Boddy K, Dawes GS, Fisher R, Pinter S & Robinson JS. Foetal respiratory movements, electrocortical and cardiovascular responses to hypoxaemia and hypercapnia in sheep. *J. Physiol.* **243**:599–618, 1974.
3. Hohimer AR & Bissonnette JM. Effect of metabolic acidosis on fetal breathing movements *in utero*. *Respir. Physiol.* **43**:99–106, 1981
4. Hohimer AR, Bissonnette JM & Machida CM. Central chemical regulation of fetal breathing movements in fetal lambs. *Respir. Physiol.* **52**:99–111, 1983.
5. Murai DT, Lee CCH, Wallen LD & Kitterman JA. Denervation of peripheral chemoreceptors decreases breathing movements in fetal sheep. *J. Appl. Physiol.* **59**:575–579, 1985.
6. Boddy K, Dawes GS & Robinson JS. A 24-hour rhythm in the foetus. In *Foetal and Neonatal Physiology (Proceedings of the Sir Joseph Barcroft Centenary Symposium)*, pp. 63–66. Cambridge, UK: Cambridge University Press. 1973.
7. Martin CB, Murata Y, Petrie RH & Parer JT. Respiratory movements in fetal rhesus monkeys. *Am. J. Obstet. Gynecol.* **119**:939–948, 1974.
8. Stark RI. Daniel SS, Kim YI, Leung K, Rey HR & Tropper PJ. Patterns of development in fetal breathing activity in the latter third of gestation of the baboon. *Early Hum. Dev.* **32**:31–47, 1993.
9. Ruckebusch Y, Gaujoux M & Eghbali B. Sleep cycles and kinesis in the foetal lamb. *Electroenceph. Clin. Neurophysiol.* **42**:226–237, 1977.
10. Natale R, Clewlow F & Dawes GS. Measurement of forelimb movements in the lamb in utero. *Am. J. Obstet. Gynecol.* **140**:545–551, 1981.
11. Szeto HH & Hinman DJ. Prenatal development of sleep-wake patterns in sheep. *Sleep* **8**:347–355, 1985.
12. Bocking AD, Harding R & Wickham PJD. Relationship between accelerations and decelerations in heart rate and skeletal muscle activity in fetal sheep. *J. Develop. Physiol.* **7**:47–54, 1985.
13. Clewlow F & Dawes GS. The association between cardiac accelerations and movements in fetal sheep. *J. Dev. Physiol.* **7**:281–287, 1985.
14. Bradley RM & Mistretta M. Swallowing in fetal sheep. *Science* **179**:1016–1017, 1983.
15. Harding R, Sigger JN, Poore ER & Johnson P. Ingestion in fetal sheep and its relation to sleep states and breathing movements. *Q. J. Exp. Physiol.* **69**:477–486, 1984.
16. Sherman DJ, Ross MG, Day L & Ervin MG. Fetal swallowing: correlation of electromyography and esophageal fluid flow. *Am. J. Physiol.* **258** (Regulatory Integrative Comp. Physiol. 27): R1386–R1394, 1990.
17. Wlodek ME, Challis JRG & Patrick J. Urethral and urachal urine output to the amniotic and allantoic sacs in fetal sheep. *J. Dev. Physiol.* **10**:309–310, 1988.
18. Wlodek ME, Thorburn GD & Harding R. Bladder contractions and micturition in fetal sheep: their relation to behavioural states. *Am. J. Physiol.* **357** (Regulatory Integrative Comp. Physiol. 26): R1526–R1532, 1989.
19. Ioffe S, Jansen AH & Chernick V. Maturation of spontaneous fetal diaphragmatic activity and fetal response to hypercapnia and hypoxemia. *J. Appl. Physiol.* **62**:609–622, 1987.
20. Matsuda Y, Patrick J, Carmichael L, Challis J & Richardson B. Effects of sustained hypoxemia on the sheep fetus at midgestation: endocrine, cardiovascular, and biophysical responses. *Am. J. Obstet. Gynecol.* **167**:531–540, 1992.
21. Clewlow F, Dawes GS, Johnston BM & Walker DW. Changes in breathing, electrocortical and muscle activity in unanaesthetized fetal lambs with age. *J. Physiol.* **341**:463–476, 1983.
22. Duncan DL & Phillipson AT. The development of motor responses in the stomach of the foetal sheep. *J. Exp. Biol.* **28**:32–40, 1951.
23. Berger PJ, Walker AM & Horne R, et al. Phasic respiratory activity in the fetal lamb during late gestation and labour. *Respir. Physiol.* **65**:55–68, 1986.
24. Patrick J, Challis JRG, Cross J, Olson DM, Lye SJ & Turliuk R. The relationship between fetal breathing movements and prostaglandin E_2 during ACTH-induced labour in sheep. *J. Dev. Physiol.* **9**:287–294, 1987.
25. Thorburn GD & Challis JRG. Endocrine control of parturition. *Physiol. Rev.* **59**:863–918, 1979.
26. Kitterman JA, Liggins GC, Fewell JE & Tooley WH. Inhibition of breathing movements in fetal sheep by prostaglandins. *J. Appl. Physiol.* **54** (Environ. Exercise Physiol. 54):687–692, 1983.
27. Rurak DW & Gruber NC. The effect of neuromuscular blockade on oxygen consumption and blood gases in the fetal lamb. *Am. J. Obstet. Gynecol.* **145**:258–262, 1983.
28. Rurak DW & Gruber NC. Increased oxygen consumption associated with breathing activity in fetal lambs. *J. Appl. Physiol.* **54**:701–707, 1983.
29. Bocking AD & Harding R. Effects of reduced uterine blood flow on electrocortical activity, breathing, and skeletal muscle activity in fetal sheep. *Am. J. Obstet. Gynecol.* **154**:655–662, 1986.
30. Manning FA, Martin CBV, Murata Y, Miyaka K & Danzler G. Breathing movements before death in the primate fetus (*Macaca mulatta*). *Am. J. Obstet. Gynecol.* **135**:71–76, 1979.
31. Bocking AD, Gagnon R, Milne KM & White SE. Behavioural activity during prolonged hypoxemia in fetal sheep. *J. Appl. Physiol.* **65**:2420–2426, 1988.
32. Koos BJ, Kitanaka T, Matsuda K, Gilbert RD & Longo LD. Fetal breathing adaptation to prolonged hypoxaemia in sheep. *J. Dev. Physiol.* **10**:161–166, 1988.
33. Matsuda Y, Patrick J, Carmichael L, Fraher L & Richardson B. Recovery of the ovine fetus from sustained hypoxia: effect on endocrine, cardiovascular, and biophysical activity. *Am. J. Obstet. Gynecol.* **170**:p1433–1441, 1994.
34. Penning DH, Grafe MR, Hammond R, Matsuda Y, Patrick J & Richardson B. Neuropathology of the near-term and midgestation ovine fetal brain after sustained in utero hypoxemia. *Am. J. Obstet. Gynecol.* **170**:1425–1432, 1994.
35. Richardson BS, Carmichael L, Homan J & Patrick JE. Electrocortical activity, electroocular activity, and breathing movements in fetal sheep with prolonged and graded hypoxemia. *Am. J. Obstet. Gynecol.* **167**:553–558, 1992.
36. Woudstra BR, Aarnoudse JG, de Wolf THM & Zijlstra WG. Nuchal muscle activity at different levels of hypoxemia in fetal sheep. *Am. J. Obstet. Gynecol.* **162**:559–564, 1990.
37. Sherman DJ, Ross MG, Day L, Humme J & Ervin MG. Fetal swallowing: response to graded maternal hypoxemia. *J. Appl. Physiol.* **71**:1856–1861, 1991.
38. Brace RA, Wlodek ME, McCrabb GJ & Harding R. Swallowing and urine flow responses of ovine fetuses to 24 h of hypoxia. *Am. J. Physiol.* **266** (Regulatory Integrative Comp. Physiol. 35):R1345–R1352, 1994.
39. Daniel SS, Yeh MN, Bowe ET, Fukunaga A & James LS. Renal response of the lamb fetus to partial occlusion of the umbilical cord. *J. Pediatr.* **87**:788–794, 1975.
40. Nakamura KT, Ayres NA, Gomez RA & Robillard JE. Renal responses to hypoxemia during renin-angiotensin system inhibition in fetal lambs. *Am. J. Physiol.* **249** (Regulatory Integrative Comp. Physiol. 18):R116–R124, 1985.
41. Battaglia FC & Meschia G. Principal substrates of fetal metabolism. *Physiol. Rev.* **58**:499–527, 1978.
42. Anderson DF, Parks CM & Faber JJ. Fetal O_2 consumption in sheep during controlled long-term reductions in umbilical blood flow. *Am. J. Physiol.* **250** (Heart Circ. Physiol. 19):H1037–H1042, 1986.
43. Clapp JF, Szeto HH, Larrow R, Hewitt J & Mann LI. Fetal metabolic response to experimental placental vascular damage. *Am. J. Obstet. Gynecol.* **140**:446–451, 1981.
44. Worthington D, Piercy WN & Smith BT. Effects of reduction of placental size in sheep. *Obstet. Gynecol.* **58**:215–221, 1981.
45. Mostello D, Chalk C, Khoury J, Mack CE, Siddiqi TA & Clark KE. Chronic anaemia in pregnant ewes: maternal and fetal effects. *Am. J. Physiol.* **261** (Regulatory Integrative Comp. Physiol. 30):R1075–R1083, 1991.
46. Parkes MJ, Moore PJ, Moore DR, Fisk NM & Hanson MA. Behavioural changes in fetal sheep caused by vibroacoustic

stimulation: the effects of cochlear ablation. *Am. J. Obstet. Gynecol.* **164**:1336–1343, 1991.
47. Boddy K & Dawes GS. Fetal breathing. *Br. Med. Bull.* **31**:3–6, 1975.
48. Richardson B, Hohimer AR, Mueggler P & Bissonnette J. Effects of glucose concentration on fetal breathing movements and electrocortical activity in fetal lambs. *Am. J. Obstet. Gynecol.* **142**:678–683, 1982.
49. Walker DW. Effects of increased core temperature on breathing movements and electrocortical activity in fetal sheep. *J. Dev. Physiol.* **10**:513–523, 1988.
50. Boddy K, Dawes GS, Fischer RL, Pinter S & Robinson JS. The effects of pentobarbitone and pethidine on foetal breathing movements in sheep. *Br. J. Pharmacol.* **57**:311–317, 1976.
51. Piercy WN, Day MA, Neims AH & Williams RL. Alteration of ovine fetal respiratory-like activity by diazepam, caffeine, and doxapram. *Am. J. Obstet. Gynecol.* **127**:43–49, 1977.
52. Jansen AH, Ioffe S & Chernick V. Drug-induced changes in fetal breathing activity and sleep state. *Can. J. Physiol. Pharmacol.* **61**:315–324, 1983.
53. Derks JB, Owiny J, Sadowski D, Ding XY, Wentworth R & Nathanielsz PW. Effects of repeated administration of cocaine to the fetal sheep in the last days of pregnancy. *Am. J. Obstet. Gynecol.* **168**:719–723, 1993.
54. Hogg MIJ, Golding RH & Rosen M. The effect of doxapram on fetal breathing in the sheep. *Br. J. Obstet. Gynecol.* **84**:48–50, 1977.
55. Patrick J, Richardson B, Hasen G et al. Effects of maternal ethanol infusion on fetal cardiovascular and brain activity in lambs. *Am. J. Obstet. Gynecol.* **151**:859–867, 1985.
56. Smith GN, Brien JF, Carmichael L, Homan J, Clarke DW & Patrick J. Development of tolerance to ethanol-induced suppression of breathing movements and brain activity in the near-term fetal sheep during short-term maternal administration of alcohol. *J. Dev. Physiol.* **11**:180–197, 1989.
57. Maloney JE, Adamson TM, Brodecky V, Dowling MH & Ritchie BC. Modification of respiratory center output in the unanesthetized fetal sheep 'in utero'. *J. Appl. Physiol.* **39**:552–558, 1975.
58. Szeto HH. Effects of narcotic drugs on fetal behavioural activity: Acute methadone exposure. *Am. J. Obstet. Gynecol.* **146**:211–216, 1983.
59. Bennet L, Johnston BM & Gluckman PD. The central effects of morphine on fetal breathing movements in the fetal sheep. *J. Dev. Physiol.* **8**:297–305, 1986.
60. Hasan SU, Lee DS, Gibson DA et al. Effect of morphine on breathing behaviour in fetal sheep. *J. Appl. Physiol.* **64**:2058–2065, 1988.
61. Kitterman JA, Siggins GC, Clements JA & Tooley WH. Stimulation of breathing movements in fetal sheep by inhibitors of prostaglandin synthesis. *J. Dev. Physiol.* **1**:453–466, 1979.
62. Patrick J, Challis JRG & Cross J. Effects of maternal indomethacin administration on fetal breathing movements in sheep. *J. Dev. Physiol.* **9**:295–300, 1987.
63. Bissonnette JM, Hohimer AR, Chao CR, Knopp SJ & Notoroberto NF. Theophylline stimulates fetal breathing movements during hypoxia. *Pediatr. Res.* **28**:83–86, 1990.
64. Ross MG, Sherman DJ, Ervin MG, Day L & Humme J. Stimuli for fetal swallowing: Systemic factors. *Am. J. Obstet. Gynecol.* **161**:1559–1565, 1989.
65. Patrick J, Natale R & Richardson B. Patterns of human fetal breathing activity at 34 to 35 weeks' gestational age. *Am. J. Obstet. Gynecol.* **132**:507–513, 1978.
66. Connors G, Hunse C, Carmichael L, Natale R & Richardson B. The role of carbon dioxide in the generation of human fetal breathing movements. *Am. J. Obstet. Gynecol.* **158**:322–327, 1988.
67. Patrick J, Campbell K, Carmichael L, Natale R & Richardson B. A definition of human fetal apnea and the distribution of fetal apneic intervals during the last ten weeks of pregnancy. *Am. J. Obstet. Gynecol.* **136**:471–477, 1980.
68. Patrick J, Campbell K, Carmichael L, Natale R & Richardson B. Patterns of human fetal breathing during the last 10 weeks of pregnancy. *Obstet. Gynecol.* **56**:24–30, 1980.
69. Junge HD & Walter H. Behavioural states and breathing activity in the fetus near term. *J. Perinat. Med.* **8**:150–157, 1980.
70. Nijhuis JG, Martin CB, Gommers S, Bouws P, Bots RSGH & Jongsma HW. The rhythmicity of fetal breathing varies with behavioural state in the human fetus. *Early. Hum. Dev.* **9**:1–7, 1983.
71. Natale R, Nasello-Paterson C & Connors G. Patterns of fetal breathing activity in the human fetus at 24 to 28 weeks' gestation. *Am. J. Obstet. Gynecol.* **158**:317–321, 1988.
72. Patrick J, Campbell K, Carmichael L, Natale R & Richardson B. Patterns of gross fetal body movements over 24-hour observation intervals during the last 10 weeks of pregnancy. *Am. J. Obstet. Gynecol.* **142**:363–371, 1982.
73. Nijhuis JG, Prechtl HFR, Martin CB & Bots RSGM. Are there behavioural states in the human fetus? *Early. Hum. Dev.* **6**:177–195, 1982.
74. Timor-Tritsch IE, Dierker LJ, Zador I, Hertz RH & Rosen MG. Fetal movements associated with fetal heart rate accelerations and decelerations. *Am. J. Obstet. Gynecol.* **131**:276–280, 1978.
75. Patrick J, Carmichael L, Chess L & Staples C. Accelerations of the human fetal heart rate at 38 to 40 weeks gestational age. *Am. J. Obstet. Gynecol.* **148**:35–41, 1984.
76. Petrikovsky BM, Kaplan GP & Pestrak H. The application of color Doppler technology to the study of fetal swallowing. *Obstet. Gynecol.* **86**:605–608, 1995.
77. Rabinowitz R, Peters MT, Sanjay V, Campbell S & Nicolaides KH. Measurement of fetal urine production in normal pregnancy by real-time ultrasonograph. *Am. J. Obstet. Gynecol.* **161**:1264–1266, 1989.
78. Visser GHA, Goodman JDS, Levine DH & Dawes GS. Micturition and the heart period cycle in the human fetus. *Br. J. Obstet. Gynaecol.* **88**:803–805, 1981.
79. de Vries JIP, Visser GHA & Prechtl HFR. The emergence of fetal behaviour. I. Qualitative aspects. *Early Hum. Dev.* **7**:301–322, 1982.
80. de Vries JIP, Visser GHA & Prechtl HFR. The emergence of fetal behaviour. II. Qualitative aspects. *Early Hum. Dev.* **12**:99–120, 1985.
81. Nasello-Paterson C, Natale R & Connors G. Ultrasonic evaluation of fetal body movements over twenty-four hours in the human fetus at twenty-four to twenty-eight weeks' gestation. *Am. J. Obstet. Gynecol.* **158**:312–316, 1988.
82. Natale R, Nasello-Paterson C & Turliuk R. Longitudinal measurements of fetal breathing, body movements, heart rate, and heart rate accelerations and decelerations at 24–32 weeks of gestation. *Am. J. Obstet. Gynecol.* **151**:256–263, 1985.
83. Drogtrop AP, Ubels R & Nijhuis JG. The association between fetal body movements, eye movements and heart rate patterns in pregnancies between 25 and 30 weeks of gestation. *Early Hum. Dev.* **23**:67–73, 1990.
84. Diamant NE. Development of the esophageal function. *Am. Rev. Respir. Dis.* **131**(suppl):29–32, 1985.
85. Kurjak A, Kirkinen P, Latin V & Ivankovic D. Ultrasonic assessment of fetal kidney functions in normal and complicated pregnancies. *Am. J. Obstet. Gynecol.* **141**:266–270, 1981.
86. Arduini D, Rizzo G, Giorlandino C, Valensise H, Dell'Acqua S & Romanini C. The development of fetal behavioural states: a longitudinal study. *Prenatal. Diagn.* **6**:117–124, 1986.
87. Richardson B, Natale R & Patrick J. Human fetal breathing activity during electively induced labor at term. *Am. J. Obstet. Gynecol.* **133**:247–255, 1979.
88. Wittmann BK, Davison BM, Lyons E & Towell ME. Real-time ultrasound observation of fetal activity in labor. *Br. J. Obstet. Gynaecol.* **86**:278–281, 1979.
89. Boylan P & Lewis PJ. Fetal breathing in labor. *Obstet. Gynecol.* **56**:35–38, 1980.
90. Carmichael L, Campbell K & Patrick J. Fetal breathing, gross fetal body movements, and maternal and fetal heart rates before spontaneous labor at term. *Am. J. Obstet. Gynecol.* **148**:675–679, 1984.
91. Castle BM & Turnbull AC. The significance of preterm breathing. In *Preterm Labour and its Consequences*. pp. 53–57. London: Royal College of Obstetricians and Gynaecologists, 1985.
92. Boylan P, O'Donovan P & Owens OJ. Fetal breathing movements and the diagnosis of labor: A prospective analysis of 100 cases. *Obstet. Gynecol.* **66**:517–520, 1985.
93. Besinger RE, Compton AA & Hayashi RH. The presence or absence of fetal breathing movements as a predictor of outcome in preterm labor. *Am. J. Obstet. Gynecol.* **157**:753–757, 1987.
94. Devoe LD, Youssef AE, Croom CS & Watson J. Can fetal biophysical observations anticipate outcome in preterm labor or preterm rupture of membranes? *Obstet. Gynecol.* **84**:432–438, 1994.

95. Vintzileos AM, Campbell WA, Nochimson DJ, Connolly MR, Fuenfer MM & Hoehn GJ. The fetal biophysical profile in patients with premature rupture of the membranes – an early predictor of fetal infection. *Am. J. Obstet. Gynecol.* **152**:510–516, 1985.
96. Vintzileos AM, Campbell WA, Nochimson DJ, Weinbaum PJ, Mirochnick MH & Escoto DT. Fetal biophysical profile versus amniocentesis in predicting infection in preterm premature rupture of the membranes. *Obstet. Gynecol.* **68**:488–494, 1986.
97. Goldstein I, Romero R, Merrill S *et al.* Fetal body and breathing movements as predictors of intraamniotic infection in preterm premature rupture of membranes. *Am. J. Obstet. Gynecol.* **159**:363–368, 1988.
98. Gauthier DW, Meyer WJ & Bieniarz A. Biophysical profile as a predictor of amniotic fluid culture results. *Obstet. Gynecol.* **80**:102–105, 1992.
99. Carroll SG, Papaioannou S & Nicolaides KH. Assessment of fetal activity and amniotic fluid volume in the prediction of intrauterine infection in preterm prelabour amniorrhexis. *Am. J. Obstet. Gynecol.* **172**:1427–1435, 1995.
100. Miller JM, Kho MS, Brown HL & Gabert HA. Clinical chorioamnionitis is not predicted by an ultrasonic biophysical profile in patients with premature rupture of membranes. *Obstet. Gynecol.* **76**:1051–1054, 1990.
101. Rosemond RI, Glass CA & Wingo CE. Daily fetal movement and breathing assessments in the management of preterm membrane rupture. *J. Matern. Fetal Invest.* **5**:236–239, 1995.
102. Pardi G, Buscaglia M, Ferrazzi E *et al.* Cord sampling for the evaluation of oxygenation and acid-base balance in growth-retarded human fetuses. *Am. J. Obstet. Gynecol.* **157**:1221–1228, 1987.
103. Soothill PW, Nicolaides KH & Campbell S. Prenatal asphyxia hyperlacticaemia, hypoglycaemia, and erythroblastosis in growth retarded fetuses. *Br. Med. J.* **294**:1051–1053, 1987.
104. Cox WL, Daffos F, Forestier F *et al.* Physiology and management of intrauterine growth retardation: a biologic approach with fetal blood sampling. *Am. J. Obstet. Gynecol.* **159**:36–41, 1988.
105. Luther ER, Gray JH, Scott K, Allan A & Stinson D. The effect of maternal glucose infusion on breathing movements in human fetuses with intrauterine growth retardation. *Am. J. Obstet. Gynecol.* **142**:600–605, 1982.
106. Dornan JC & Ritchie JWK. Fetal breathing movements and maternal hyperoxia in the growth-retarded fetus. *Br. J. Obstet. Gynaecol.* **90**:210–213, 1983.
107. van Vliet MAT, Martin CB, Nijhuis JG & Prechtl HFR. The relationship between fetal activity and behavioural states and fetal breathing movements in normal and growth-retarded fetuses. *Am. J. Obstet. Gynecol.* **153**:582–588, 1985.
108. Ruedrich DA, Devoe LD & Searle N. Effects of maternal hyperoxia on the biophysical assessment of fetuses with suspected intrauterine growth retardation. *Am. J. Obstet. Gynecol.* **161**:188–192, 1989.
109. Gagnon R, Hunse C & Vijan S. The effect of maternal hyperoxia on behavioural activity in growth-retarded human fetuses. *Am. J. Obstet. Gynecol.* **163**:1894–1899, 1990.
110. Bekedam DJ, Mulder EJH, Snijders RJM & Visser GHA. The effects of maternal hyperoxia on fetal breathing movements, body movements and heart rate variation in growth retarded fetuses. *Early Hum. Dev.* **27**:223–232, 1991.
111. Bekedam DJ, Visser GHA, de Vries JJ & Prechtl HFR. Motor behaviour in the growth retarded fetus. *Early Hum. Dev.* **12**:155–165, 1985.
112. Gagnon R, Hunse C, Fellows F, Carmichael L & Patrick J. Fetal heart rate and activity patterns in growth-retarded fetuses: changes after vibratory acoustic stimulation. *Am. J. Obstet. Gynecol.* **158**:265–271, 1988.
113. Manning FA, Platt LD & Sipos L. Antepartum fetal evaluation: development of a fetal biophysical profile. *Am. J. Obstet. Gynecol.* **136**:787–795, 1980.
114. Manning FA, Morrison I, Harman CR, Lange IR & Menticoglou S. Fetal assessment based on fetal biophysical profile scoring: experience in 19,221 high-risk pregnancies. II. An analysis of false-negative fetal deaths. *Am. J. Obstet. Gynecol.* **157**:880–804, 1987.
115. Manning FA, Morrison I, Harman CR & Menticoglou SM. The abnormal fetal biophysical profile score. V. Predictive accuracy according to score composition. *Am. J. Obstet. Gynecol.* **162**:918–927, 1990.
116. Manning FA, Snijders R, Harman CR, Nicolaides K, Menticoglou S & Morrison I. Fetal biophysical profile score. VI. Correlation with antepartum umbilical venous fetal pH. (Transactions of the Thirteenth Annual Meeting of the Society of Perinatal Obstetricians.) *Am. J. Obstet. Gynecol.* **169**:755–763, 1993.
117. Vintzileos AM, Campbell WA, Ingardia CJ & Nochimson DJ. The fetal biophysical profile and its predictive value. *Obstet. Gynecol.* **62**:271–278, 1983.
118. Vintzileos AM, Campbell WA, Nochimson DJ & Weinbaum PI. The use and misuse of the fetal biophysical profile. *Am. J. Obstet. Gynecol.* **156**:527–533, 1987.
119. Vintzileos AM, Gaffney SE, Salinger LM, Kontopoulos VG, Campbell WA & Nochimson DJ. The relationship among the fetal biophysical profile, umbilical cord pH, and Apgar scores. *Am. J. Obstet. Gynecol.* **157**:627–631, 1987.
120. Vintzileos AM, Fleming AD, Scorza WE *et al.* Relationship between fetal biophysical activities and umbilical cord blood gas values. *Am. J. Obstet. Gynecol.* **165**:707–713, 1991.
121. Baskett TF. Gestational age and fetal biophysical assessment. *Am. J. Obstet. Gynecol.* **158**:332–334, 1988.
122. Vintzileos AM, Feinstein SJ, Lodeiro JG, Campbell WA, Weinbaum PJ & Nochimson DJ. Fetal biophysical profile and the effect of premature rupture of the membranes. *Obstet. Gynecol.* **67**:818–823, 1986.
123. Schifrin BS, Guntes V, Gergely RC, Eden R, Roll K & Jacobs J. The role of real-time scanning in antenatal fetal surveillance. *Am. J. Obstet. Gynecol.* **140**:525–530, 1981.
124. Baskett TF, Gray JH, Prewett SJ, Young LM & Allen AC. Antepartum fetal assessment using a fetal biophysical profile score. *Am. J. Obstet. Gynecol.* **148**:630–633, 1984.
125. Platt LD, Eglinton GS, Sipos L, Broussard PM & Paul RH. Further experience with the fetal biophysical profile. *Obstet. Gynecol.* **61**:480–485, 1983.
126. Devoe LD, Castillo RA, Searle N & Searle JS. Prognostic components of computerized fetal biophysical testing. *Am. J. Obstet. Gynecol.* **158**:1144–1148, 1988.
127. Brown R, Patrick J. The nonstress test: how long is enough? *Am. J. Obstet. Gynecol.* **141**:646–651, 1981.
128. Devoe LD, Youssef AA, Gardner P, Dear C & Murray C. Refining the biophysical profile with a risk-related evaluation of test performance. *Am. J. Obstet. Gynecol.* **167**:346–352, 1992.
129. Ribbert LS, Nicolaides KH & Visser GHA. Prediction of fetal acidaemia in intrauterine growth retardation: comparison of quantified fetal activity with biophysical profile score. *Br. J. Obstet. Gynaecol.* **100**:653–656, 1993.
130. Ribbert LSM, Snijders RJM, Nicolaides KH & Visser GHA. Relationship of fetal biophysical profile and blood gas values at cordocentesis in severely growth-retarded fetuses. *Am. J. Obstet. Gynecol.* **163**:569–571, 1990.
131. Ribbert LSM, Visser GHA, Mulder EJH et al. Changes with time in fetal heart rate variation, movement incidences and haemodynamics in intrauterine growth-retarded fetuses. A longitudinal approach to the assessment of fetal well-being. *Early Hum. Dev.* **31**:195–208, 1993.
132. Sassoon DA, Castro LC, Davis JL, Bear M & Hobel CJ. The biophysical profile in labor. *Obstet. Gynecol.* **76**:360–365, 1990.
133. Ash KM, Morrison I & Manning FA. Observations of intrapartum fetal activities. *Am. J. Obstet. Gynecol.* **168**:760–764, 1993.
134. Nageotte MP, Towers CV, Asrat T & Freeman RK. Perinatal outcome with the modified biophysical profile. *Am. J. Obstet. Gynecol.* **170**:1672–1676, 1994.
135. Miller DA, Rabello YA & Paul RH. The modified biophysical profile: antepartum testing in the 1990s. *Am. J. Obstet. Gynecol.* **174**:812–817, 1996.
136. Connors G, Natale R & Nasello-Paterson C. Maternally perceived fetal activity from twenty-four weeks' gestation to term in normal and at risk pregnancies. *Am. J. Obstet. Gynecol.* **160**:932–938, 1989.
137. Moore TR & Piacquadio K. A prospective evaluation of fetal movement screening to reduce the incidence of antepartum fetal death. *Am. J. Obstet. Gynecol.* **160**:1075–1080, 1989.
138. Visser GHA, Bekedam DJ & Ribbert LSM. Changes in antepartum

heart rate patterns with progressive deterioration of the fetal condition. *Int. J. Biomed. Comput.* **25**:239–246, 1990.

139. Vintzileos AM, Campbell WA, Rodis JF, McLean DA, Fleming AD & Scorza WE. The relationship between fetal biophysical assessment, umbilical artery velocimetry, and fetal acidosis. *Obstet. Gynecol.* **77**:622–626, 1991.
140. James DK, Parker MJ & Smoleniec JS. Comprehensive fetal assessment with three ultrasonographic characteristics. *Am. J. Obstet. Gynecol.* **166**:1486–1495, 1992.
141. Yoon BH, Romero R, Rob CR, et al. Relationship between the fetal biophysical profile score, umbilical artery Doppler velocimetry, and fetal blood acid-base status determined by cordocentesis. *Am. J. Obstet. Gynecol.* **169**:1586–1594, 1993.
142. Pardi G, Cetin I, Marconi AM et al. Diagnostic value of blood sampling in fetuses with growth retardation. *New. Engl. J. Med.* **328**:692–696, 1993.
143. Gagnon R, Hunse C, Carmichael L, Fellows F & Patrick J. Human fetal responses to vibratory acoustic stimulation from twenty-six weeks to term. *Am. J. Obstet. Gynecol.* **157**:1375–1381, 1987.
144. Natale R, Patrick J & Richardson B. Effects of maternal venous plasma glucose concentrations on fetal breathing movements. *Am. J. Obstet. Gynecol.* **132**:36–41, 1978.
145. Fox HE & Hohler CW. Fetal evaluation by real-time imaging. *Clin. Obstet. Gynecol.* **20**:339–349, 1977.
146. Thaler JS, Goodman JDS & Dawes GS. The effect of maternal smoking on fetal breathing rate and activity patterns. *Am. J. Obstet. Gynecol.* **138**:282–287, 1980.
147. McGowan J, Devoe LD, Searle N & Altman R. The effects of long- and short-term maternal caffeine ingestion on human fetal breathing and body movements in term gestations. *Am. J. Obstet. Gynecol.* **157**:726–729, 1987.
148. Fox HE, Steinbrecher M, Pessel D, Inglis J, Medvid L & Angel E. Maternal ethanol ingestion and the occurrence of human fetal breathing movements. *Am. J. Obstet. Gynecol.* **132**:354–358, 1978.
149. McLeod W, Brien J, Loomis C, Carmichael L, Probert C & Patrick J. Effect of maternal ethanol ingestion on fetal breathing movement, gross body movements, and heart rate at 37 to 40 weeks' gestational age. *Am. J. Obstet. Gynecol.* **145**:251–257, 1983.
150. Richardson BS, O'Grady JP & Olsen GD. Fetal breathing movements and the response to carbon dioxide in patients on methadone maintenance. *Am. J. Obstet. Gynecol.* **140**:400–405, 1984.
151. Hallak M, Moise KJ, Lira N, Dorman KF, O'Brian Smith E & Cotton DB. The effect of tocolytic agents (indomethacin and terbutaline) on fetal breathing and body movements: a prospective, randomized, double-blind, placebo-controlled clinical trial. *Am. J. Obstet. Gynecol.* **167**:1059–1063, 1992.
152. Lewis P & Boylan P. Fetal breathing: a review. *Am. J. Obstet. Gynecol.* **134**:587–599, 1979.
153. Gagnon R, Hunse C, Carmichael L, Fellows F & Patrick J. Effects of vibratory acoustic stimulation on fetal human fetal breathing and gross fetal body movements near term. *Am. J. Obstet. Gynecol.* **155**:1227–1240, 1986.
154. Wigglesworth JS & Desai R. Effects on lung growth of cervical cord section in the rabbit fetus. *Early Human. Dev.*, **3**:51–65, 1979.
155. Harding R, Hooper SB & Han VKM. Abolition of fetal breathing movements by spinal cord transection leads to reductions in fetal lung liquid volume, lung growth and IGF-II gene expression. *Pediatr. Res.* **34**:148–153, 1993.
156. Liggins GC. Growth of the fetal lung. *J. Dev. Physiol.* **6**:237–248, 1984.
157. Harding R. Development of the respiratory system. In *Textbook of Fetal Physiology* (eds G.D. Thorburn & R. Harding), pp. 140–167. Oxford, UK: Oxford University Press, 1994.
158. Fox HE & Moessinger AC. Fetal breathing movements and lung hypoplasia: preliminary human observations. *Am. J. Obstet. Gynecol.* **151**:531–533, 1985.
159. Moessinger AC, Fox HE, Higgins A & Rey HR. Fetal breathing movements are not a reliable predictor of continued lung development in pregnancies complicated by oligohydramnios. *Lancet* **ii**:1297–1300, 1987.
160. Blott M, Greenough A, Nicolaides KH & Campbell S. The ultrasonographic assessment of the fetal thorax and fetal breathing movements in the prediction of pulmonary hypoplasia. *Early Hum. Dev.* **21**:143–151, 1990.
161. Blott M, Greenough A & Nicolaides KH. Fetal breathing movements in pregnancies complicated by premature membrane rupture in the second trimester. *Early Hum. Dev.* **21**:41–48, 1990.
162. Prechtl HFR. Perinatal development of postnatal behaviour. In *Psychobiology and Early Development* (eds H. Rauh & H. Steinhausen), pp. 231–238. North-Holland: Elsevier Science Publishers BV, 1987.
163. Mulvihill SJ, Stone MM, Fonkalsrud EW & Debas HT. Trophic effect of amniotic fluid on fetal gastrointestinal development. *J. Surg. Res.* **40**:291–296, 1986.
164. Trahair JF, Harding R, Bocking AD, Silver M & Robinson PM. The role of ingestion in the development of the small intestine in fetal sheep. *Q. J. Exp. Physiol. Cogn. Med. Sci.* **71**:99–104, 1986.
165. Pierro A, Colarossi GC, Irving IM, Pierce AM & Lister J. Does fetal gut obstruction cause hydramnios and growth retardation? *J. Pediatr. Surg.* **22**:454–467, 1987.
166. Ioffe S, Jansen AH, Russell BJ & Chernick V. Sleep, wakefulness and the monosynaptic reflex in fetal and newborn lambs. *Eur. J. Physiol.* **338**:149–157, 1980.
167. Richardson BS, Patrick JE & Abduljabbar H. Cerebral oxidative metabolism in the fetal lamb. Relationship to electrocortical state. *Am. J. Obstet. Gynecol.* **153**:426–431, 1985.
168. Richardson BS, Carmichael J, Homan J & Gagnon R. Cerebral oxidative metabolism in lambs during perinatal period: relationship to electrocortical state. *Am. J. Physiol.* **257** (Regulatory Integrative Comp Physiol 26):R1251–R1257, 1989.
169. Wladimiroff JW & van Bel F. Fetal and neonatal cerebral blood flow. *Semin. Perinatol.* **11**:335–346, 1987.
170. Arduini D, Rizzo G, Caforio L, Boccolini MR, Romanini C & Mancuso S. Behavioural state transitions in healthy and growth retarded fetuses. *Early Hum. Dev.* **19**:155–165, 1989.
171. Dierker LJ, Pillay S, Sorokin Y & Rosen MG. The change in fetal activity periods in diabetic and nondiabetic pregnancies. *Am. J. Obstet. Gynecol.* **143**:181–185, 1982.
172. Mulder EJH, Visser GHA, Bekedam DJ & Prechtl HFR. Emergence of behavioural states in fetuses of type-1-diabetic women. *Early Hum. Dev.* **15**:231–251, 1987.
173. Mulder EJH, Kamstra A, O'Brien MJ, Visser GHA & Prechtl HFR. Abnormal fetal behavioural state regulation in a case of high maternal alcohol intake during pregnancy. *Early Human Develop.* **14**:321–326, 1986.
174. Hume RF, O'Donnell KJ, Stranger CL, Killam AP & Gingras JL. In utero cocaine exposure: Observations of fetal behavioural state may predict neonatal outcome. **161**:685–690, 1989.

Fetal biometry

71

J.P. Newnham and S.F. Evans

The need for ultrasound biometry

Traditionally, gestational age has been calculated from the date of the onset of the last menstrual period. This determination is based on an assumption that ovulation will occur on the 14th day of the cycle. Thus, the menstrual age is calculated as 2 weeks greater than the conceptional age. Reliance on the calculation of menstrual age may produce misleading information for several reasons. Firstly, cycle length and the date of ovulation vary widely, and may not be consistent for each woman. By measuring urinary luteinizing hormone, Walker and colleagues[1] observed that ovulation can occur at any time from day 8 to 31 after the first day of the last menstrual period. Ovulation occurred after day 18 in one-third of cycles, and many of these late ovulations would not have been suspected from the menstrual histories. Moreover, cycle length was not a predictor of the date of ovulation, dismissing the age-old belief that menstruation will follow ovulation by 14 days if conception does not occur.

Secondly, many women are uncertain about the date of their last menstrual period, and even in those who are certain, early biparietal diameter measurements often do not agree with their dates. In a study of 2507 singleton pregnancies[2], it was shown that 80% of women were certain of their last menstrual period within 1 week, but ultrasound biometry performed before 18 weeks' gestation confirmed these dates within 7 days in only 76%. In those pregnancies with certain dates and in which the menstrual calculation and ultrasound biometry differed by more than 7 days, the menstrual dates underestimated the gestational age in 44% and overestimated the age in 56%. Overall, only 60.5% of women could accurately date their gestational age by their menstrual dates. In those women who were uncertain about their dates, their gestational age calculation was still within seven days in 48%, overestimated in 40% and underestimated in 12%.

These sources of error are in general skewed to overestimating the gestational age. For cases requiring obstetric intervention this bias may lead to iatrogenic and unexpected preterm birth, and in other pregnancies may lead to an incorrect and apparently higher proportion of post-term gestational ages. In a review of 427 581 consecutive singleton births in Sweden between 1976 and 1980, Bergsjo and coworkers[3] observed that for those pregnancies in which the date of the last menstrual period was known, the rate of delivery after 294 days was 10%. In studies in which the gestational age has been ascertained by ultrasound biometry, the rate in a comparable population was held to be 4%. A reduction in the rate of induction of labour for supposed post-term gestational age is one of the principal benefits of obstetric scanning and its effectiveness in this regard has been demonstrated by a randomized controlled trial[4].

When compared with calculation from the date of the last menstrual period, other traditional methods of estimating gestational age may be even more misleading. Fundal height estimation in the second and third trimesters will ascertain age with an error of up to 8 weeks[5] and maternal perception of fetal movements is known to first occur at any time between 14 and 24 weeks' gestation.

Ultrasound estimation of gestational age provides an accurate and effective method of estimating the time since conception and is based primarily on measurement of fetal size. As for any three-dimensional object, fetal size can be determined by mass, volume or surface area[6]. Mass cannot be determined by current scanning technology and surface area measurements may be feasible in the future but are awaiting developments in three-dimensional scanning techniques. Volume can be calculated from measurements of diameters, but is prone to error because shapes within the fetus are not consistently regular. Greater use has come from simple measurements which can be made from standard two-dimensional images.

Imaging principles

RESOLUTION

Resolution is the ability of an ultrasound system to display structural details and has the following components.

- *Axial resolution*: the minimum separation of two objects within the image along the axis of the beam. The principal determinant of axial resolution is the ultrasonic pulse length; a shorter pulse length produces greater axial resolution
- *Lateral resolution*: the minimum separation of two objects within the image at the same range from the transducer. In other words, lateral resolution is the ability to delineate echoes from structures lying side-by-side across the ultrasound beam. The principal determinant of lateral resolution is the effective width of the ultrasound beam at that site, and is related to focusing of the beam and the position of the target within the beam
- *Contrast resolution:* the ability of the ultrasound system to display neighbouring tissues in different shades of grey. Many factors influence contrast resolution, such as power and transducer frequency, but the major determinant is the scan converter which translates echoes into grey shades
- *Temporal resolution*: the ability of the ultrasound system to separate events in time. The principal determinant of temporal resolution is the frame rate of the system. Measurements are typically taken from frozen images, precluding a role for temporal resolution in their precision

In most ultrasound imaging, axial resolution is superior to lateral resolution and it is deficiencies in lateral resolution which most degrade the image. Measurements of biparietal diameter are based on axial resolution and thus are relatively accurate[7]. In comparison, femur length measurements are based on lateral resolution and are less precise.

Resolution, and hence the precision of measurements, is increased by increasing the frequency of the transducer. At higher frequencies, the ultrasound pulse is shorter and the beam width narrower. Our ability to use transducers of high frequency is restricted by the fact that attenuation of ultrasound in tissue increases with increasing frequency. Thus, the transducer to be chosen should be of the highest frequency which will give the necessary penetration.

TECHNIQUE

The single greatest source of error in fetal biometry is the operator. There is no substitute for training and experience, and any person performing obstetric scanning should have appropriate qualifications and receive continuing education.

Scanning technique is important. An optimal image requires high quality equipment; selection of a transducer of appropriate frequency; a measurement system which has been accurately calibrated; correct adjustment of the output and gain controls to produce a well balanced image; avoidance of artefacts; and choice of the largest feasible scale.

Mathematical principles

SOURCES OF ERROR

There are several sources of error in any measurement or in any study which aims to develop a reference range for clinical use. First, is the actual measurement error, which is the inability of an instrument to accurately perform the measurement. This error is minimized by optimal training and equipment. In the field of biometry, this source is relatively minor for most clinical situations. Secondly, there is operator error, which can be minimized by adequate training and technique. Quality assurance programmes can quantify this source of error by measurement of inter- and intraoperator variability. Thirdly, there is within subject error, which is the variability in size of a measurement in any individual at any given time. Within subject error will be relatively small for measurements of bone length and diameter, but may be troublesome for measurements of soft tissue which are dependent on fetal posture. Fourthly, there is between subject error, which is the variability between different individuals. This error is usually the largest source of variation because a myriad of factors affect the size of an individual, most of which are normal confounding variables. Minimizing this error involves the construction of reference ranges which account for as many confounding variables as feasible. Fifthly, there are systematic errors, which may arise from inaccuracies or deficiencies in the study design or manner in which the measurements are performed. Systematic errors are minimized by improving the study design, rather than increasing the sample size. Finally, there is random error, which arises in the development of reference ranges when a sample is used in the hope that it faithfully represents the whole population. Random errors are sometimes referred to as sampling errors or experimental errors and may be viewed as arising from the operation of a large number of uncontrolled factors, conveniently described by 'chance'. This type of error arises particularly when we draw repeated random samples from a universal population, and then calculate a particular statistic, such as an arithmetic mean, from each sample. These sample means will be different and will distribute themselves below and above the 'true' population parameter, with small deviations between the statistic and the parameter occurring relatively frequently, and large deviations occurring relatively infrequently. The word 'true' has quotation marks around it because it refers to the parameter that would be obtained if we could measure the whole universal population. Differences between the means of particular samples and their population means are said to be random errors. The size of the differences indicate reliability or precision, and in general, decrease as sample sizes increase.

VARIABILITY

The variability of the observations in a population of data is referred to as the variance, and the square root of this is known as the standard deviation. The variance is the average of all the squared differences between values of a sample and the expected sample mean, while the measure of dispersion of the sample, or standard deviation, is the square root of the variance. Standard deviations have the same units of measurement as the original measure. When a set of observations has a 'normal' or Gaussian distribution (the standard bell-shaped curve) multiples of the standard deviation mark certain limits on the scatter of the observations. For instance 1.96 (or approximately two) standard deviations above and below the mean, mark the points within which 95% of the observations lie.

If we draw a series of samples, and calculate the means of each sample, then we have a series of means which also has a standard deviation. The standard error of the mean of one sample is an estimate of the standard deviation of the series of means from the whole population, and so two standard errors on either side of the sample mean represents the 95% confidence limit for the 'true' population mean.

REGRESSION

When a set of observations or samples is collected over time, it is usual to plot the observations or 'dependent' variables on the y (or vertical) axis, and the time, or 'independent' variable on the x (or horizontal) axis. The relationship between these variables is described as regression of y on x, and the regression equation representing this relationship shows how much y changes with each unit change of x. In the case of a linear relationship, this is represented by the formula: $y = a + bx$, where b represents the regression coefficient or slope of the line, and a represents the intercept on the y axis (or the value of y when $x = 0$). The variance around a regression line is calculated in the same manner as the variance of a sample. Note that regression is used to estimate a dependence relationship, and the term is prone to being misused.

CONFIDENCE AND PREDICTION INTERVALS

For a given x value, we assume a normal distribution of possible y values around the regression line, with the mean of such a distribution being referred to as the conditional mean and its standard deviation as the conditional standard deviation. Interval estimates for a conditional mean are usually referred to as confidence intervals, i.e. in 95% of instances, any future sample would have a mean which was between these limits. Estimates which involve predicting an individual value of the dependent variable y are referred to as prediction intervals. Such single values cannot be predicted with as much precision as a conditional mean, although the estimated value is the same; this arises because the sampling error in predicting an individual value of y is greater than the sampling error in estimating a conditional mean value of y.

Setting up confidence intervals for conditional means is appropriate whenever we are interested in estimating the average value of y for a given x. On the other hand, prediction intervals for individual forecasts are appropriate when we are interested in predicting an individual y value for a given x. In terms of statistical theory, when we estimate a conditional mean, we estimate the value of a parameter, but when we predict an individual value of y, we predict the value of a random variable. In the former case, we are trying to estimate a point on the regression line, but in the latter case we are predicting an individual value for y.

The usefulness of confidence intervals or prediction intervals depends on the purposes for which they are used. In ultrasound biometry, curves presenting confidence limits for the population are used to estimate appropriate size, whilst curves representing prediction intervals should be used to estimate gestational age, given a parameter measure.

MISUSE OF REGRESSION INFORMATION IN BIOMETRY

Misuse of regression occurs when the technique is inappropriately used:

- To predict y variables for values of the x variable at the limits of, or outside the range of, the original data set
- To infer a straight line relationship through lack of data, when more information would show some curvature
- To use a y on x regression equation to predict x from y (as in dating curves). For example, if data have been collected for crown–rump length values in a sample of normal subjects with known ovulation dates, and a regression curve is plotted as the dependence of crown–rump length on gestational age, then this reference range should only be used to predict crown–rump length values (with 95% confidence limits) given a gestational age collected in the same manner. In order to predict gestational age from the crown–rump length data, it is necessary to construct a regression equation in which gestational age is the dependent or y variable and crown–rump length is the independent or x variable
- To use a confidence interval instead of a prediction interval or vice versa
- To ignore departures from independence and the problems of autocorrelation
- To ignore increasing variance over the range of gestational ages in the graph (heteroscedasticity)

We will illustrate these points using crown–rump length data collected from 324 pregnancies between 7 and 13 weeks' gestation (Fig. 71.1). As is customary, we have plotted the crown–rump length information as the dependent variable on the y axis, with the gestational age on the x axis, and it can be seen that the relationship is approximately linear. Regressing crown–rump length (CRL) on gestational age (GA) (assuming we know the gestational age for these pregnancies) gives a regression equation:

$$\text{CRL} = -60.49 + 9.64(\text{GA})$$

plotted in Fig 71.1 as the central dotted line. However, for dating purposes, we assume the gestational age is unknown, and we regress gestational age on crown–rump length, giving the regression equation

$$\text{GA} = 6.48 + 0.098(\text{CRL})$$

plotted as the central solid line. These two lines are related through the correlation coefficient, so the greater the correlation, the closer the lines will be. Values near the mean of our data for gestational age and crown–rump length will not incur much penalty for regressing the wrong way; however, it is easy to see that values near the extremities do become inaccurate, varying in this case by several days.

Assuming these data were being used to predict unknown gestational age, then we would plot the latter regression curve. Note we do not have to turn the graph around so that the dependent variable is still on the y axis – it is acceptable to plot the graph in the conventional manner with gestational age on the x axis, provided it is clearly stated that the regression was gestational age on crown–rump length. Figure 1 also shows the 95% prediction interval for crown–rump length regressed on gestational age as the outer dotted lines and the 95% prediction interval for predicting an unknown gestational age from the regression of gestational age on crown–rump length as the outer solid lines. The divergence amounts to an incorrect estimate of 1–2 days.

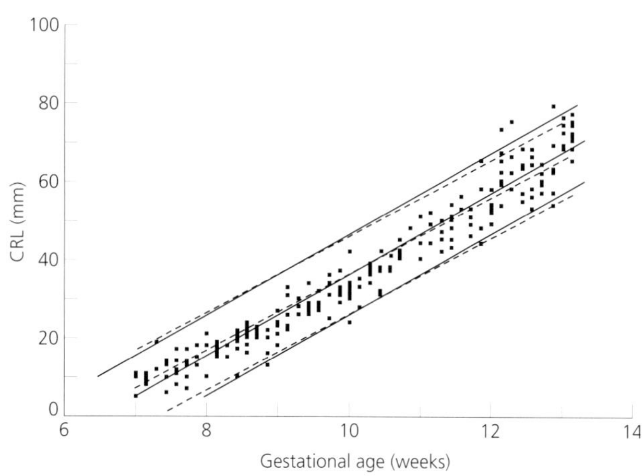

Fig. 71.1 Mean and 95% prediction intervals plotted for regressions of crown–rump length on gestational age (dotted line) together with regression of gestational age on crown–rump length (solid line). The divergence at the extremities of the data reflect the inaccuracy arising from using inappropriate regressions.

It is useful for a variety of reasons to study the residuals in a regression analysis. We can analyse these deviations of actual values from predicted values to determine the magnitude of prediction errors, to check on autocorrelation and heteroscedasticity, and to make diagnoses about how to continue. Particularly in time series, we must ensure that the assumptions of regression analysis are not violated. Residuals are the difference between the observed values and the expected values ($y - y$) for any value of x. The autocorrelation assumption means that a low (or high) value for a particular observation, does not imply that the next y observation will also be low (or high). The validity of this assumption for cross-sectional data is virtually assured because of random sampling; however, care must be taken in the analysis of longitudinal data. Plots of the residuals versus the independent variable should not show a pattern. If the variance of the residuals increases (or decreases) as the values of the independent variable increase, this indicates that the assumption of homoscedasticity has been violated.

CROSS-SECTIONAL VERSUS LONGITUDINAL DATA

Ultrasound biometry curves are in general used for two principal purposes – to estimate gestational age and to assess the appropriateness of size when the age is known. Construction of reference ranges to enable these two different uses of ultrasound biometry require different techniques. The data may be collected in one of two ways: cross-sectional in which each subject is observed at a single time point and longitudinal in which subjects are observed several times over the course of the pregnancy. Cross-sectional data can be used to develop gestational age ranges or size assessment ranges, while only longitudinal data collection should be used for growth assessment curves. Data used in the construction of reference ranges are best collected prospectively and it is beneficial if the same pregnancies are used for all size measurements at the same time. Other confounding variables, such as the racial group of the fetus, also need consideration and specific reference ranges have been developed for some populations.

CROSS-SECTIONAL STUDIES

These are studies in which only one observation for each fetus is included in the regression model, and are the easiest to perform and analyse[8]. Cross–sectional data collection has the advantage of avoiding the autocorrelation issues which complicate longitudinal studies. Altman and Chitty[8] have recommended random allocation of each pregnancy to the gestational age at which measurements will be taken to avoid any potential bias due to 'surviving' populations, and to ensure approximate equality throughout the range of gestational ages. The reference ranges presented by these authors are the only published data which have incorporated this design in their development and are the ranges used in this text.

Regression analysis is then straightforward, and usually involves regression of fetal measurements on known gestational ages. Attention must also be given to the shape of the residual curve. Many authors unfortunately have averaged values and their variation at various intervals during pregnancy, in order to construct an 'average' curve. This methodology is unacceptable because there are too few points in such cases to produce an accurate range. Ranges recommended in this text have used appropriate techniques to model the variance in relation to gestational age.

LONGITUDINAL STUDIES

Longitudinal studies are often thought to provide better estimates of size and growth, since the change of the measurement function with time can be estimated directly, and usually shows more curvature than cross-sectional analysis. Size is measured at only one point in time, but assessment of growth requires serial observations over time[9]. As a consequence of repeatedly measuring the same subjects, special statistical methods are needed to account for both within-subject and between-subject variability and potential autocorrelation between measurements[10]. For example, an observation that the biparietal diameter of a fetus lies below the regression curve at one time point may increase the chance of a low measurement at the next time point, and allowance must be made for this tendency.

Fetal measurements

The first sonographic feature of intrauterine pregnancy is the gestation sac, followed soon after by appearance of the embryo, from which crown–rump length measurements can be made. The precision with which ultrasound biometry may be used to estimate gestational age is inversely proportional to the time which has elapsed since conception. Rate of growth, and consistency of size between individuals, is greatest in the early weeks of pregnancy.

MEASUREMENT OF THE GESTATION SAC

A sac, surrounded by its characteristic decidual echoes, can be imaged from as early as the 25th day after the last menstrual period, corresponding to a gestational age since conception of 11 days. Measurements of the average sac diameter, calculated from the mean of two or three diameters, was popular in the early days of ultrasound imaging[11].

Sac measurements include both the amniotic cavity and the extra-embryonic coelom. The amniotic membrane can almost always be imaged separately until the extra-embryonic coelom is obliterated by fusion of the amnion and chorion, a process which can occur at any time up to 16 weeks' gestation.

The mean sac diameter at 6 weeks menstrual age is 13 mm, increasing to 50 mm at 12 weeks. However, the value of this measurement is diminished by alterations in sac shape induced by bladder distension and uterine contractions, rendering a prediction error of at least ±2 weeks[12]. Greater precision can be obtained by measurement of sac volume using a planimetric technique. With this method, Robinson observed that sac volume increased exponentially from 1 ml at 6 weeks' gestation to 31 ml at 10 weeks, and then to 100 ml at 13 weeks. However, the variance was large, rendering prediction of gestational age to ±9 days[13].

Measurement of sac diameter and volume were soon replaced by the more accurate crown–rump length. If a role remains for any of the measures of sac size, it would be at 5–6 weeks' gestation before the embryo itself may be imaged. However, an estimation of gestational age in this circumstance would remain provisional until a subsequent scan has confirmed the presence of an intrauterine embryo.

CROWN–RUMP LENGTH MEASUREMENTS

The crown–rump length (CRL) is the maximum measurement of the embryo or fetus, not including the limbs (Fig. 71.2). Care must be taken to exclude the yolk sac from the measurement, as it can easily be mistaken for part of the embryo or fetus. The embryo can first be visualized by the 34th day after the last menstrual period, corresponding to a conceptional age of 20 days. Heart motion will be seen either at this time, or within a few days.

The first report of CRL measurements was by Robinson in 1973[14,15]. His study was based on the images obtained by a static scanner with a simple bistable display. Modern real-time scanners provide a much more convenient measurement system by allowing for rapid adjustment of the imaging plane when the embryo or fetus moves. Numerous charts and formulae have been developed for estimating gestational age

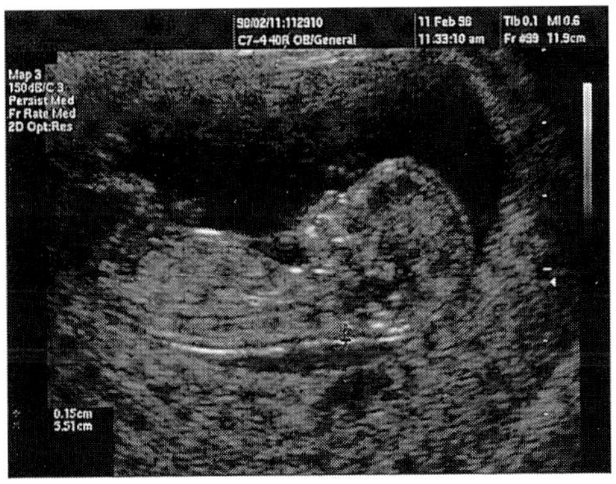

Fig. 71.2 Ultrasound image in the sagittal plane of a fetus at 12 weeks' gestation. Calipers are placed to measure the crown–rump length (55 mm) and the depth of nuchal translucency (1.5 mm).

using measurement of the CRL[15–21] and these methods have remarkable consistency when one considers the changes in technology which have occurred during the time of their development. However, the chart published by Robinson in 1973[14] remains one of the most popular, attesting to the precision of the original work.

CRL measurements should be made with the embryo or fetus imaged in the sagittal rather than the coronal plane. This approach produces a clearer demarcation of the rump, displays any transient flexion of the body which would result in an erroneously small measurement, and also enables an assessment of nuchal translucency, this being one of the markers of aneuploidy. To aid precision in placement of the calipers, the embryo or fetus should occupy at least two-thirds of the image. The measure should be taken with the fetus in its usual posture and not at times of sudden flexion or extension. If an overdistended bladder appears to compress the fetus and influence its flexion, the most appropriate action is to re-examine with less bladder distension.

At the earliest ages at which the CRL can be imaged, the shape is almost circular. Nevertheless, the maximum length should be sought.

CRL is the most suitable method of estimating gestational age between 5 and 12 weeks' gestation. After this age, the measurement is markedly affected by the degree of flexion and its precision is diminished. Head size then becomes a more appropriate measurement.

At the early stage in life when CRL measurements are used, there are only a few factors which will impact on embryonic and fetal growth. Pedersen has reported that the average CRL after 8 weeks' gestation in males in 2 mm greater than in females[22], and there have also been reports of possible differences in diabetic pregnancies[23], congenital anomalies[24], and threatened abortion[25]. However, none of these influencing factors is sufficiently large to warrant consideration when estimating early gestational age, although delayed embryonic and fetal growth may manifest as one of the early signs of aneuploidy.

CRL is the most precise and robust measurement of fetal size for the prediction of gestational age. When Drumm and colleagues[16] applied their equation for estimating gestational age from CRL data to pregnancies in which the age had been calculated from known dates of ovulation, they observed that all gestational age assessments were within 3 days of the predicted value; and that the mean error in the assessment was −0.2 days with a standard deviation of 1.3 days.

The accuracy of CRL measurements is largely due to the rapid growth at this time in development. At 6–7 weeks' gestation, embryonic growth is almost 1 mm per day, and by 11–12 weeks fetal growth is approximately 2 mm each day. Hence, for a measurement at 7 weeks' gestation to be in error by 20% and inaccurately reported as 12 mm rather than 10 mm, the error confronting the clinician is no more than 3 days.

EMBRYONIC/FETAL TRUNK CIRCUMFERENCE

Between 7 and 12 weeks' gestation, measurement of the circumference of the fetal body at a point just caudal to the heart provides an alternative to the CRL method[21]. Both this measure and CRL have curvilinear associations with gestational age and are reported to have similar precision. However, the ease of measuring the CRL has led to its greater popularity. Abdominal circumference and femur length can also be measured from 10 weeks' gestation onwards and at this early age their efficacy has been shown to be comparable, but not superior, to either CRL or biparietal diameter measurement[26].

BIPARIETAL DIAMETER

The biparietal diameter (BPD) is the width of the fetal head, arbitrarily defined to be at the level of the thalami (Figs 71.3 and 71.4). This measurement is made in an axial plane and should display the falx cerebri anteriorly and posteriorly, the cavum septi pellucidi and the thalamic nuclei in the midline, and the Silvian fissure laterally. The cavum septi pellucidi is a space between the anterior hemispheres which is obliterated after birth and which provides an echogenic landmark. At this axial plane, part of the choroid plexus may be seen in the lateral ventricles. In later pregnancy, the maximum width of the fetal head may no longer be at this level; however, convention dictates the thalami to be the level chosen and all charts have been developed as such.

Measurement of the BPD is made from the outer table of the proximal skull to the inner table of the distal skull. This technique is usually referred to as 'outer-to-inner' and overcomes artefacts in axial resolution which confound any measure at the supposed centre of the skull table or at the bone most distal from the transducer. As a consequence of this methodology, the BPD as defined for use in ultrasonic measurements is less than the true maximum diameter of the fetal head which must negotiate the pelvic inlet in vaginal birth. Some authors have described BPD measurements from

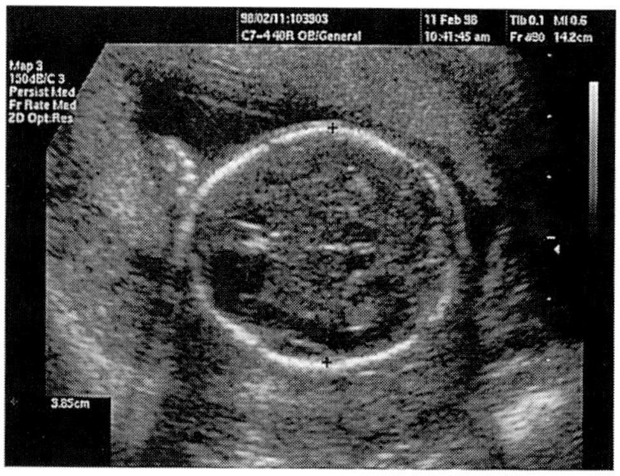

Fig. 71.3 Ultrasound image in an axial plane demonstrating measurement of the biparietal diameter at 18 weeks' gestation.

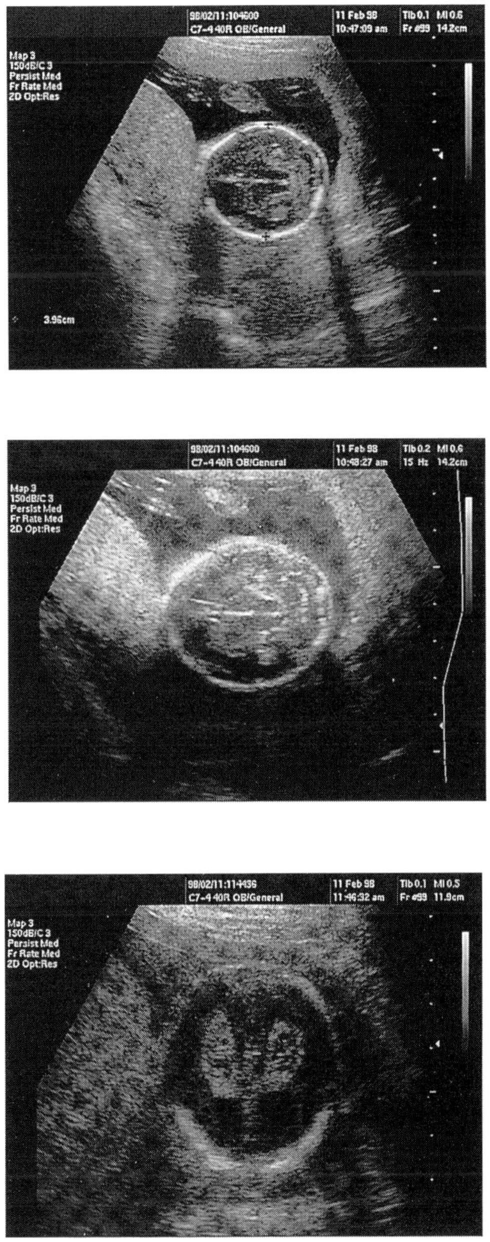

(a) (b) (c)

Fig. 71.4 Ultrasound images demonstrating poor technique in measurement of the biparietal diameter. (a) Errors may involve too small an image of the fetal head which increases error with placement of calipers. (b) Incorrect adjustment of the gain controls shown here as excessive gain in the near field. (c) Fetal head in an occipitoanterior position which precludes adequate imaging of the appropriate landmarks and renders caliper placement inaccurate due to poor lateral resolution at the lateral margins of the skull.

'outer-to-outer' in order that head circumference calculations may be more accurate.

BPD was historically the first measurement used for estimation of gestational age[27]. Early A-mode scanning could delineate the two skull tables and measurements were made from the leading edge of each.

There are now many reference ranges for BPD measurements and the various charts which have been developed are based on a variety of techniques. These include data from cross-sectional studies[28,29]; a combination of single and repeated measures on a cohort of pregnancies[30]; longitudinal study[31]; and randomization to the gestational age at which the measurement will be taken with one data point for each fetus and analysis including separate modelling of variance[32].

For the linear part of the curve, and as a very rough rule of thumb, the BPD in centimetres from 4 cm onwards, if multiplied by four, gives the approximate gestational age in weeks.

Several factors may alter the usual ovoid shape of the fetal skull. Flattening, or elongation of the head is termed dolichocephaly. This finding is a frequent feature of breech presentation, transverse lie, or oligohydramnios. In these conditions the head is subjected to lateral forces not present when the presentation is cephalic. 'Roundness' of the head, known as brachycephaly, is sometimes present in aneuploidy, including Down syndrome, and in fetuses of oriental and southeast Asian parents. There are several methods available to account for these alterations in fetal head shape, as follows.

CEPHALIC INDEX

Firstly, the cephalic index may be calculated. This index is the ratio of the BPD to the occipitofrontal diameter (OFD). The OFD is the longest axis of the head and is measured at the same axial plane as the BPD.

$$\text{Cephalic index} = \frac{\text{BPD}}{\text{OFD}} \times 100$$

There has been controversy over several years as to whether the caliper placement in OFD measurement should be outer-to-outer or middle-to-middle. Since OFD measurements are made on the same image as BPD measurements, and the fetal head is usually in an occipitolateral position with the OFD parallel to the transducer, the outer extremities of the anterior and posterior skull tables are often very imprecise due to poor lateral resolution at the edges of the beam. Middle-to-middle measurement overcomes some of this inaccuracy, and presents the best compromise[31]. The mean cephalic index, using outer-to-inner BPD measurement and middle-to-middle OFD measurement, is 80.6 with a standard deviation of 5.0[31]. Thus, a reference range based on the mean plus or minus two standard deviations is 70.6 to 90.6. BPD measurement should not be used to predict gestational age or fetal weight when the cephalic index is near the extremes of this reference range.

CORRECTED BPD

The second approach to account for alterations in head shape is to adjust the BPD to the value expected if the head shape were in the normal range. This method, proposed by Doubilet and Greenes[33], is best done by accounting for the geometric shape of the normal fetal head using the following formula:

$$OFD = 1.265 \times BPD$$

Thus, the 'corrected BPD' (BPD′) is given by the following formula:

$$BPD' = \left(\frac{BPD \times OFD}{1.265} \right)^{1/2}$$

HEAD CIRCUMFERENCE

The third method which can be used to account for alterations in head shape is measurement or calculation of head circumference (HC)[34,35]. Measurements are taken at the same axial plane as described for BPD and may be made by tracing the perimeter of the skull with electronic calipers. Alternatively, the circumference may be calculated from the width (BPD) and length (OFD) using the traditional formula for an ellipse:

$$HC = \frac{BPD + OFD}{2} \pi$$

This formula may be simplified to:

$$HC = (D1 + D2) \times 1.57$$

D1 and D2 are the two diameters at right angles to each other.

As a general principle, any method which employs direct measurement and has calculated the gestational age regressed on that measurement, must be superior to those techniques in which the values are inferred from an elliptical approximation. Technically, calculation of HC requires the width and length measurements to be made from the outer-to-outer skulls tables, to describe the true outer circumference. However, in practice, modern ultrasound machines often perform this calculation automatically from the BPD and OFD measurements which have been recorded using the techniques described previously.

ACCURACY OF HEAD MEASUREMENTS

The ability to estimate gestational age using measurements of the fetal head, or indeed any measure of fetal size, diminishes with advancing age. For a BPD of 42 mm the 50th percentile is 18 weeks, with an age of 16^6 weeks at the 5th centile and 19^2 weeks at the 95th centile (see Appendix). In late gestation, measurements are typically used to reflect growth rather than age and estimating gestational age becomes inaccurate. Thus, a BPD of 90 mm has an age of 34^5 weeks as the 50th centile with 5th and 95th centiles of 31^5 weeks and 37^6 weeks respectively.

Recommended charts for use of head measurements can be found in the Appendix. For estimation of gestational age, the reference range for BPD calculated by de Crespigny *et al.*[29] is recommended because the methodology involved a large number of pregnancies (719); only a single measurement was included from each, thus avoiding any problems from non-interdependence; the modelling was based on regression analysis of age on the measurement; and the variance was modelled to allow for heteroscedasticity. There are no HC data which have been developed using techniques of such rigour. For determining the appropriateness of size for gestational age by BPD and HC, the reference ranges calculated by Chitty and colleagues[32] are recommended because the methodology also involved a large number of pregnancies (594); only a single measurement was included from each fetus; each pregnancy had been allocated at random to the age at which the measurement was taken; the curves were modelled by regression of the measurement on age; the variance was modelled to allow for heteroscedasticity; and appropriate plots of residuals and actual measurements were presented.

Comparison of the variance in BPD and HC reference ranges indicates that at each gestational age, the standard deviation for HC is a lower percentage of the mean value than for BPD. This observation indicates there is relatively less scatter about the mean regression line for HC than BPD, rendering HC a superior predictor of size than BPD.

ABDOMINAL CIRCUMFERENCE

The abdominal circumference (AC) is measured from an axial section of the fetal trunk at a specified level which is superior to the umbilicus and inferior to the heart[36–39] (Figs 71.5 and 71.6). At this level, the umbilical segment of the left portal vein, and its intersection with the right portal vein to join the ductus venosus, is seen as a 'J' shaped echo lucency. This vascular image should be located one-third of the way posterior from the anterior abdominal (Fig. 71.2). If the vessel is seen adjacent to the skin of the anterior abdominal wall, then the

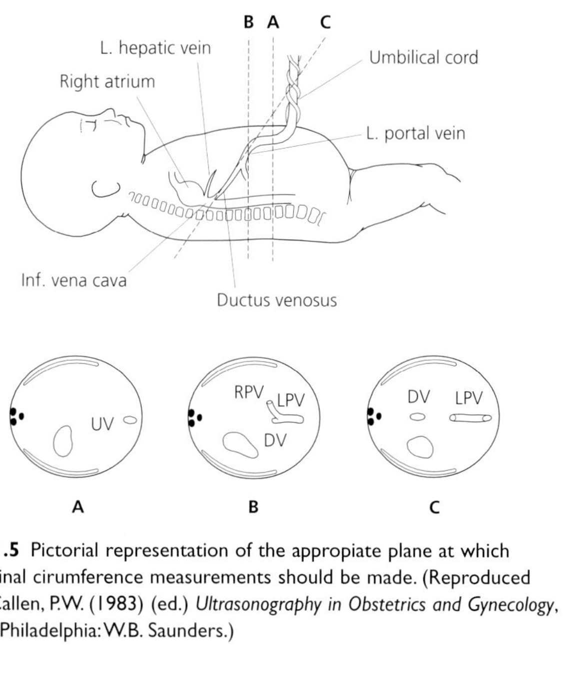

Fig. 71.5 Pictorial representation of the appropiate plane at which abdominal cirumference measurements should be made. (Reproduced from Callen, P.W. (1983) (ed.) *Ultrasonography in Obstetrics and Gynecology*, p. 126. Philadelphia: W.B. Saunders.)

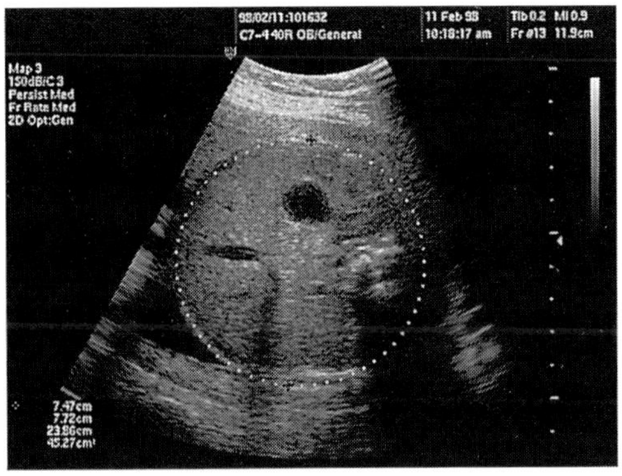

Fig. 71.6 Ultrasound image in an axial plane demonstrating abdominal circumference measurement at 20 weeks' gestation. The intrahepatic umbilical vein, stomach and spine are shown.

plane is too inferior. An oblique cut may present as a vessel running in continuity from the midsection of the trunk to the skin at the umbilicus. The fetal stomach and spine will also be imaged at the correct plane, although imaging the umbilical/portal venous complex is required to be certain the correct axial level has been achieved.

In order to obtain the correct image, it often is best to commence with a plane perpendicular to the longitudinal axis of the fetus and the fetal aorta parallel to the transducer. The centre of the image should then be aligned with the plane midway between the heart and the umbilicus, and an orthogonal plane then achieved by rotating the transducer 90° to this plane. This technique is particularly useful when the fetal lie is displaced from its typical position by alterations in amniotic fluid volume or in multiple pregnancies.

As a method of determining gestational age in early pregnancy, AC has less precision than measurements of the head and has similar efficacy to femur length measurement[26]. However, at later gestational ages, AC is the most powerful biometric descriptor of growth[40–42]. The measurement reflects both liver size and subcutaneous fat, each of which is a sensitive marker of fetal nutrition.

There are several other important sources of error in AC measurements[43]. The shape of the abdomen is not always circular or elliptic. In such instances, the software in many of the modern ultrasound machines will be unable to accurately place an ellipse over the image and the operator should revert to directly tracing the outline by one of the manual methods which are offered. Caution should also be exercised when comparing pre- and postnatal AC measurements. Paediatricians typically measure the AC close to the level of the umbilicus[44], while prenatal measurements are made at a level virtually midway between the umbilicus and the heart. Comparison of these measurements, without appreciation of the different planes at which they are taken, will produce a systematic bias. Further, Deter and colleagues have shown that AC measurement performed in the week before delivery carries a 6% systematic overestimation when compared with postnatal measurement, mainly resulting from the differences between intrauterine and extrauterine posture and breathing[43].

A recommended reference range for AC measurements can be found in the Appendix. For estimating the appropriateness of size for a given gestational age, the data from Chitty and colleagues[39] are recommended because the methodology involved a large number of pregnancies (594); only a single measurement from each fetus was included; each pregnancy had been allocated at random to the gestational age at which the measurement would be made; the curves were modelled by regression of the measurements on the gestational ages; the variance was modelled to allow for heteroscedasticity; and appropriate plots of residuals and actual measurements have been presented.

FEMUR LENGTH

The length of the fetal femur is a readily available measurement which can be used to estimate gestational age or assess growth of the skeletal system[45–50]. Indeed, any long bone can be used[51] but the femur, which is the longest, will provide the greatest precision. The humerus is the best alternative if for any reason the femur cannot be measured with accuracy.

The measurement should be made with the shaft of the femur parallel to the transducer (Fig. 71.7). Care must be taken to ensure the entire diaphysis of the femur is measured. The measurement is made from the midpoint of the ends of the profile and any curvature of the shaft is ignored[48]. Using a tangential section will produce too short a measurement; incorrectly long estimates can result from including non-osseous portions of the femur. The echogenic epiphyses which can be incorrectly included in the measurement are the proximal epiphysial cartilage, which will become the future greater trochanter, and the distal femoral epiphysial

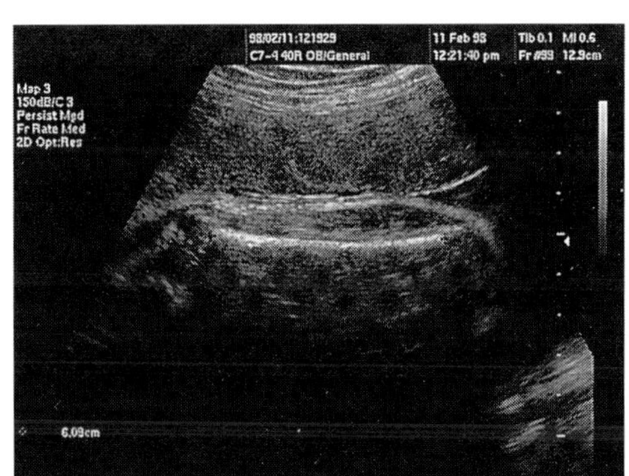

Fig. 71.7 Ultrasound image demonstrating measurement of a fetal femur at 34 weeks' gestation. The measurement includes only the length of the shaft and does not include the femoral head proximally or the distal epiphysis distally. Calipers should be placed on the extremities of the shaft of the long bone at their midpoints.

cartilage, which will become the distal femoral condyles. Images from a dissected postmortem specimen have shown that the echoes which can be seen to continue beyond the distal femoral shaft are not part of the osseous femur, but probably represent a specular reflection from the lateral surface of the distal epiphysis[52] (Fig. 71.8). These echoes, as well as those from the femoral head, are not included in the measurement, leading some authors to describe this measure as the femur diaphysis length (FDL)[52].

Femur length can be measured from 10 weeks' gestation onwards and provides an important adjunct to head and abdominal measurements for gestational age assessment. In addition, measurement of this bone is of prime importance in evaluating fetuses at risk of skeletal dysplasias, for which tabulated data are available.

Recommended reference ranges for femur length are shown in the Appendix. For estimating gestational age the data published by Warda and colleagues[48] are recommended because:

- The methodology involved a reasonable number of pregnancies (254)
- A single measurement from each fetus was included
- The modelling was based on regression of gestational age on the measurements
- The variance was modelled to allow for heteroscedasticity

For estimating the appropriateness of size for a given gestational age, the calculation of Chitty and colleagues[50] is recommended because:

- The methodology involved a large number of pregnancies (649)
- A single measurement from each fetus was included
- Each pregnancy had been allocated at random to the gestational age at which the measurement would be taken
- The modelling was based on regression of the measurement on gestational age

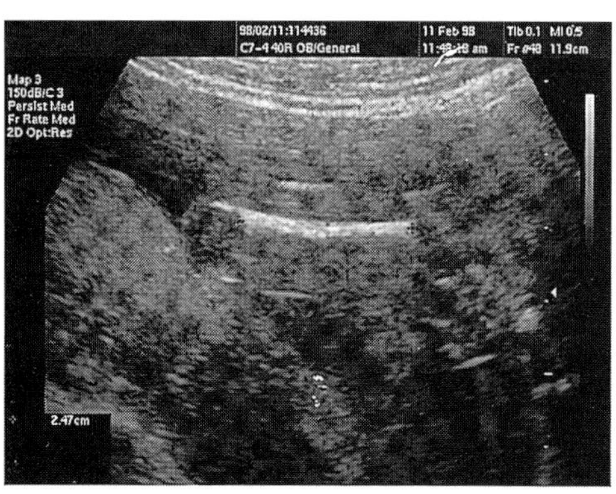

Fig. 71.8 Ultrasound image of a fetal femur showing echoes continuing beyond the distal femoral shaft which are not part of the osseous femur and must not be included in the measurement. The echoes probably represent specular reflection from the lateral surface of the distal epiphysis.

- The variance was modelled to allow for heteroscedasticity
- Appropriate plots of residuals and actual measurements were presented

THIGH CIRCUMFERENCE

Thigh circumference (ThC) has been proposed as a method to describe a mass of fetal soft tissue. Growth restricted fetuses are known to have reductions in subcutaneous and muscle masses, and measurement of ThC provides an opportunity to measure this reduction independent of liver size which so heavily influences AC measurements. The measurement is best made at the junction of the proximal one-third and distal two-thirds of the shaft of the femur, at which point the bone profile changes from polygonal to oval[53]; this plane is at the level of the proximal nutrient foramen of the femur. In contrast, postnatal measurements of ThC are usually made at the midpoint of the thigh, producing a systematic difference between prenatal and postnatal measurements. Measurements of the fetal calf circumference can also be made and the appropriate level is just below the knee[54]. Since thigh and calf circumferences are smaller measures than AC, they should not be considered as alternatives to measurement of the abdomen. Rather, they should be viewed as complementary and may prove to be of some use in improving the accuracy of fetal weight estimation.

A further role for thigh and calf circumferences may come from their use in ratios. Calculations of fetal femur length/thigh circumference and tibial length/calf circumference produce ratios which are relatively constant and independent of gestational age, at least in normal pregnancies[54]. For those cases in which the gestational age is uncertain, such ratios may be of assistance in describing fetal growth, although their efficacy is limited by the small sizes of these measures when compared with the abdominal circumference. Composite measurements of fetal limbs based on bone lengths, transverse and anteroposterior dimensions, and subcutaneous thicknesses, have been used to estimate limb volume[55]. Volumes of the arm and leg are strongly correlated with gestational age, but a role for these calculations in describing fetal growth is limited by the complexity of measurement and the imprecision resulting from small measures.

TRANSVERSE CEREBELLAR DIAMETER

The cerebellum can be measured in an axial plane using the transverse outer-to-outer margins (Fig. 71.9). There is a high degree of correlation between transverse cerebellar diameter and gestational age[56]. Prior to 24 weeks, the transverse cerebellar diameter in millimetres is equivalent to the gestational age in weeks, following which there is a flattening of the growth curve. The relationship between transverse cerebellar diameter and age is best described by a third order polynomial equation.

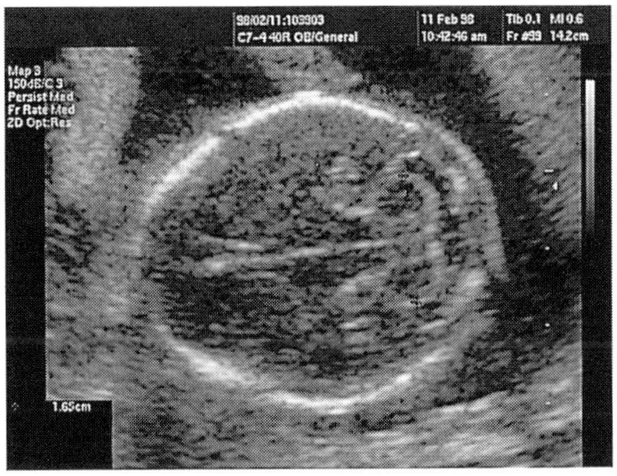

Fig. 71.9 Ultrasound image of a fetal head in the axial plane at 17 weeks' gestation showing measurement of the transverse cerebellar diameter.

Measurement of transverse cerebellar diameter is of use in the evaluation of cases of fetal growth restriction. This diameter is unaffected in asymmetric growth restriction, providing an independent indicator of gestational age against which other measures of fetal size may be compared[57]. The sparing of cerebellar growth probably results from conservation of blood flow to this region at times of fetal undernutrition. Under these conditions, the fetus preferentially shunts blood to the brain at the expense of other organs, and cerebellar perfusion is even conserved at times of asphyxia when flow to the cerebral cortex may be diminished[58].

Calculations made from fetal measurements

The clinical usefulness of fetal biometry can be increased by a variety of calculations which either estimate fetal weight or generate ratios which characterize growth patterns.

ESTIMATED FETAL WEIGHT

Estimation of the weight of a fetus is highly desired by many clinicians who are involved in perinatal decision making. Perinatal morbidity and mortality are increased at the extremes of fetal growth. In the upper weight ranges, weight estimation may influence mode of delivery when the fetus is presenting by the breech or if shoulder dystocia is anticipated. At the lower end of the spectrum, fetal weight estimation may assist in differentiating those fetuses too small to survive after birth from those in which intensive care during birth is appropriate. Within the field of fetal therapy, knowledge of fetal mass is important when calculating drug doses or volumes for red cell or platelet transfusion.

Numerous formulae have been developed which provide an estimation of fetal weight based on fetal biometric measurements. The first of these formulae was reported in 1977 by Warsof and colleagues[59] and was based on measurements of biparietal diameter and abdominal circumference in 85 pregnancies from 17 to 41 weeks' gestation. Their formula to estimate fetal weight was developed using multiple multivariate linear regression analyses and concluded that fetal weight is a logarithmic function of abdominal, and to a lesser extent, head measurements. Biparietal diameter and abdominal circumference in their formula predicted birthweight within 48 h of measurement with a standard deviation of 106 g/kg body weight. Since then, other authors have proposed formulae developed on measurements of the abdomen, head, femur length, and thigh circumference in a variety of combinations. Each of these systems has important sources of error which arise for several reasons.

- The measurements do not involve the entire fetal body. Early work describing fetal volume with static scanning techniques by taking multiple serial planes was cumbersome and impractical. Unfortunately, inclusion of additional measurements such as thigh circumference has made only a small impact on improving accuracy
- The relationship between fetal volume and mass is not linear[60]. Density of the fetus is influenced by the proportion of fat and the relative size of the head and other organs, each of which has a different weight per unit volume. It has been estimated that in normal fetuses, knowledge of the volume with certainty will still lead to errors in weight estimates of 8–21%. This source of error is further compounded by the effects of growth restriction and macrosomia in which differences in body proportions are magnified
- Accurate prediction of weight is limited by the fact that we are attempting to estimate the size of a three-dimensional object by using one-dimensional (biparietal diameter, femur length) or two-dimensional (head circumference, abdominal circumference) measurements. Further improvements in accuracy can be expected to follow advances in imaging capabilities

Abdominal circumference appears to be the single most important component in estimation of fetal weight because it represents such a large proportion of the body[59]. Use of head measurements alone is of little value. Estimation of fetal weight based on calculation of head circumference, abdominal circumference, femur length and thigh circumference produces only a marginal benefit over head circumference, abdominal circumference and femur length. The formula of Hadlock and colleagues has achieved widespread popularity and its calculation was based on log birthweight regressed on measurements of the fetal head, abdomen and femur[61–63] (See the chart of estimation of fetal weight in the Appendix, pp. 1139–1140).

An evaluation of the effectiveness of the available formulae has been performed and indicates systematic errors resulting in underestimation of the weight of large-for-gestational age fetuses, overestimation of the weight of small-for-gestational-age fetuses, and unbiased estimates for fetuses of appropriate size for their age[63]. Formulae dedicated to fetuses in the lower weight ranges have been described but have not produced meaningful improvements in prediction[64,65].

Overall, estimation of fetal weight can be expected to have an error of approximately ± 15%. The clinical implications of this error are important and must not be underestimated. In the lower weight ranges, a prediction of fetal weight of 1000 g will truly represent a weight ranging from 850–1150 g and this degree of precision is probably of clinical value. However, it must be appreciated that for preterm births, survival and morbidity are more closely related to maturity than to birthweight, rendering gestational age assessment a more vital factor than estimation of fetal weight.

At higher weight ranges, a predicted fetal weight of 4000 g will truly represent a weight somewhere between 3400 and 4600 g. This lack of precision must be acknowledged and caution should be exercised when using clinical protocols in which mode of delivery is dictated by estimations of fetal weight.

BODY PROPORTIONALITY

The ratios of various fetal measurements can be used to delineate growth characteristics. In general, circumferences are preferable to diameters as they are less affected by shape and can be related more easily to measurements made after birth. Calculation of the ratio of head circumference to abdominal circumference has been used to evaluate head sparing in fetal undernutrition. When faced with a chronic reduction in nutrient supply, which most frequently results from placental insufficiency, the fetus responds by preferentially shunting blood to the brain at the expense of many other organs including the liver and subcutaneous fat. This response increases the head circumference/abdominal circumference ratio and is manifest as asymmetric growth restriction. By contrast, growth restriction arising from fetal disorders such as viral infection or aneuploidy produces growth delay in a symmetrical manner, with an unaltered head circumference/abdominal circumference ratio. In principle, the head circumference/abdominal circumference ratio should be of great benefit, but is limited by a wide variance in normal fetuses, reducing its clinical usefulness[66].

An alternative ratio is one that attempts to produce an in-utero ponderal index. This index is often used after birth to describe the relative amounts of soft tissue and skeletal length and is given by the formula:

$$\text{Ponderal index} = \frac{\text{Birthweight}}{(\text{Birth length})^3} \times 100$$

To produce an intrauterine equivalent, Vintzileos[67] observed that femur length has a linear relationship with crown–heel length and that these two parameters have the following relationship:

$$\text{Fetal length} = 6.18 + 5.9 \times \text{Femur length}$$

Estimated fetal weight can then be divided by either this estimated fetal length, or the femur length itself, to produce an in utero ponderal index[68,69]. Unfortunately, fetal ponderal index suffers from both the limitations of the indirect estimations of weight and length which are employed, and the fact that cubing the length increases the error. This index, and other measures such as femur length/head circumference ratio, and femur length/abdominal circumference ratio have not been shown to add significantly to direct measures of fetal size when describing the appropriateness of size for a given gestational age[70].

Potentially, these ratios may be of greater use in those cases in which the gestational age is not known. Ratios of head parameters to measures of body size decrease with advancing gestational age, but those ratios which do not involve head measurements tend to remain constant in the latter half of pregnancy. Ratios of potential use include the femur length/abdominal circumference and the femur length/thigh circumference[54]. The ratio of estimated fetal weight/femur length also tends to be independent of age[69]. Ratios may also be of use in evaluating structural abnormalities. The femur length/head circumference ratio is of particular value in evaluating skeletal dysplasias in which long bones will be shortened, and in disorders of head growth such as microcephaly or macrocephaly[71]. A relative reduction in femur length is also of some use in screening for Down syndrome[72].

Optimizing the utility of biometric data

AGE DETERMINATION

COMPOSITE AGE DETERMINATION

Of the various parameters, which should be used to estimate gestational age? In normally formed fetuses, there is no reason to sacrifice information provided by any of the measurements. A composite assessment may be made using BPD, head circumference, abdominal circumference and femur length in a weighted regression equation or by simply taking the average of all four parameters[73]. However, these methods must be adjusted if there is any reason why one or more of the parameters is altered by a pathological condition. For example, head measurements may be altered by hydrocephaly or microcephaly, abdominal circumference decreased by growth restriction or abdominal wall defects, and femur length reduced in skeletal dysplasias. In such cases, the affected measurement should not be included in the regression equation or average.

GROWTH ASSESSMENT

Biometry provides a wealth of information about fetal size, but translation into clinical practice for the purpose of evaluating fetal growth is not necessarily straightforward and involves consideration of several options. The most widespread technique to express the adequacy of size is to plot the value for the measured parameter on a reference range developed for that population, and then to describe the measure either as a percentile, or as a value lying between stated norms, such as 'between the 10th and 90th percentiles'. It is important to note that such charts should not be referred to as 'normal ranges' but rather as 'reference ranges' or 'reference intervals'.

Several techniques have been proposed to enhance the clinical utility of biometric data and to describe growth rather than just size at a given point in time. These systems are based either on predicting future growth by using its preceding measures as the control, by plotting the value on a chart customized by accounting for physiological variables known to influence fetal growth, or by calculating growth velocity based on two or more fetal weight estimations.

GROWTH CURVE TECHNIQUE

This technique is based on an expectation that each fetus will grow along its biologically determined rank as defined by population-derived centile charts. Thus, measurements in early pregnancy are used to predict subsequent growth. To quantify the expected growth, measurements are required at two time points, typically in the second trimester[74]. At each of these times, the measurement is expressed as the percentile for that gestational age, and the predicted growth calculated as the mean of the two percentiles. Thus if the percentile T1 is the first measurement and percentile T2 is the second measurement, then:

$$\text{Predicted percentile} = \frac{\text{T1} + \text{T2}}{2}$$

For example if, for abdominal circumference measurements at 18 and 27 weeks,

T1 = 55th percentile
T2 = 45th percentile

then

$$\text{Predicted percentile} = \frac{55 + 45}{2} = \text{50th percentile}$$

This model is based on an assumption that a fetus growing normally will follow a population profile in a manner similar to that of the mean.

MATHEMATICAL MODEL OF ROSSAVIK

This technique is based on prediction of growth in the third trimester by measurements made at two time points prior to 30 weeks' gestation[75–77]. The model treats each fetus as an individual, and does not compare the fetus with population standards or account for other physiological variables. Each fetus acts as its own control by predicting future growth as a function of the previous measurements.

The equation used in this technique was developed by Rossavik and Deter and is based on several coefficients determined by regression analysis, using data obtained from two scans in the second trimester:

$$P = ct^{(k + st)}$$

where

- P is the measurement being predicted (e.g. biparietal diameter)
- c and s are individual growth constants specific to each fetus and the parameter being tested
- t is the duration of growth between the two second-trimester measurements, calculated in menstrual weeks from the starting point (SP) and the second time point (T2)
- k is a constant specific to the anatomical parameter being predicted

The constants are calculated as:

$$\text{In}(c) = a_0 + a_1 \times \text{In(slope)}$$
$$s = b_0 + b_1\ (c)$$

(adapted from references 74–76). Third-trimester predictions can be made for biparietal diameter, head circumference, abdominal circumference, femur length, estimated fetal weight, head volume or abdominal volume. The method has also been labelled as the growth potential realization index (GRPI)[78] or individualized growth assessment (IGA)[79], to express the individual nature of the fetal growth assessment with each fetus acting as its own control independent of the population. Prediction of third-trimester growth by measurements as early as 17 weeks and as late as 26 weeks' gestation requires the assumption that all fetuses start their growth within a close range of gestational ages; have the same pattern of growth, with the same slope over the same time period; and that growth disturbances would not have already occurred.

CUSTOMIZED ANTENATAL GROWTH CHARTS

Charts have been developed which account for physiological variables known to influence fetal growth[80]. The calculations used in the production of these charts were based on previously recorded cross-sectional birthweight data, with multiple regression analysis used to identify significant covariates. The variables found to significantly influence fetal growth were maternal weight at the first antenatal visit, height, ethnic group and parity. Pathological variables such as smoking, undernutrition and socioeconomic status were not included. Analyses of variance were then used to determine means and variance for each subgroup. Tenth, 50th and 90th percentiles defined the reference ranges and a programme developed such that a customized chart could be printed for any given pregnancy using a standard personal computer. Similarly, allowance for physiological variables has also been included to develop growth trajectories to predict optimal birthweight[81].

Evaluation of these techniques suggests that allowance for physiological variables reduces the frequency of diagnosis of small for gestational age. Conversely, some babies classified as having normal growth by standard population charts will be shown to be small for gestational age when customized charts are used.

FETAL GROWTH VELOCITY

Individual growth velocities have been calculated by regression using standard deviation scores from at least two ultrasound examinations at least 42 days apart and expressed as weight gain per 28 days[82,83]. The error of estimation is too high for this system to be used in individual clinical cases, but is of value when describing groups for research purposes.

The future

This chapter has reviewed the physical and mathematical principles involved in ultrasonic fetal measurement. As technology advances and measurement systems improve, these techniques will evolve. All health care workers in this field need to understand the principles which underpin new measurement systems and the standards which must be achieved before new systems qualify for introduction into their clinical practice[84]. As the consequences of disordered fetal growth are now known to extend into both child and adult life, it can be anticipated that diagnostic testing systems which evaluate the intrauterine environment will increase in importance in the coming years.

REFERENCES

1. Walker EM, Lewis M, Cooper W, Marnie M & Howie PW. Occult biochemical pregnancy: fact or fiction? *Br. J. Obstet. Gynaecol.* **95**, 659–663, 1988.
2. Williams LA, Evans SF & Newnham JP. Factors influencing the relative weights of the fetus and placenta. *Br. Med. J.* **314**, 1864–1868, 1997.
3. Bergsjo P, Denman DW, Hoffman HJ & Meirik O. Duration of human singleton pregnancy. A population-based study. *Acta Obstet. Gynecol. Scand.* **69**, 197–207, 1990.
4. Eik-Nes SH, Okland SH & Aure JC. Ultrasound screening in pregnancy: a randomized controlled trial. *Lancet* **I**, 1347–1348, 1984.
5. Beazley JM & Underhill RA. Fallacy of the fundal height. *Br. Med. J.* **4**, 404–406, 1970.
6. Deter RL, Harrist RB, Hadlock FP & Carpenter RJ. The use of ultrasound in the assessment of normal fetal growth: A review. *J. Clin. Ultrasound* **9**, 481–493, 1981.
7. Pretorius DH, Nelson TR & Manco-Johnson ML. Fetal age estimation: the impact of measurement errors. *Radiology* **152**, 763–766, 1984.
8. Altman DG & Chitty LS. Charts of fetal size: 1. Methodology. *Br. J. Obstet. Gynaecol.* **101**, 29–34, 1994.
9. Mahadevan N, Pearce M & Steer P. The proper measure of intrauterine growth retardation is function, not size. *Br. J. Obstet Gynaecol.* **101**, 1032–1035, 1994.
10. Laird NM, Donnelly C & Ware JH. Longitudinal studies with continuous responses. *Statist. Meth. Med. Res.* **1**, 225–247, 1992.
11. Hellman LM, Kobayashi M, Fillisti L, Lavenhar M & Cromb E. Growth and development of the human fetus prior to the twentieth week of gestation. *Am. J. Obstet. Gynecol.* **103**, 789–800, 1969.
12. Kohorn EI & Kaufman M. Sonar in the first trimester of pregnancy. *Obstet. Gynecol.* **44**, 473–483, 1974.
13. Robinson HP. 'Gestation sac' volumes as determined by sonar in the first trimester of pregnancy. *Br. J. Obstet. Gynaecol.* **82**, 100–107, 1975.
14. Robinson HP. Sonar Measurement of fetal crown–rump length as a means of assessing maturity in first trimester of pregnancy. *Br. Med. J.* **4**, 28–31, 1973.
15. Robinson HP & Fleming JE. A critical evaluation of sonar 'crown–rump length' measurements. *Br. J. Obstet. Gynaecol.* **82**, 702–710, 1975.
16. Drumm JE, Clinch J & MacKenzie G. The ultrasonic measurement of fetal crown–rump length as a method of assessing gestational age. *Br. J. Obstet. Gynaecol.* **83**, 417–421, 1976.
17. Drumm JE. The prediction of delivery date by ultrasonic measurement of fetal crown–rump length. *Br. J. Obstet. Gynaecol.* **84**, 1–5, 1977.
18. Kurjak A, Cecuk S & Breyer B. Prediction of maturity in first trimester of pregnancy by ultrasonic measurement of fetal crown–rump length. *J. Clin. Ultrasound.* **4**, 83–84, 1976.
19. Bovicelli L, Orsini LF, Rizzo N, Calderoni P, Pazzaglia FL & Michelacci L. Estimation of gestational age during the first trimester by real time measurement of fetal crown–rump length and biparietal diameter. *J. Clin. Ultrasound*, **9**, 71–75, 1981.
20. Pedersen J. Fetal crown–rump length measurement by ultrasound in normal pregnancy. *Br. J. Obstet. Gynaecol.* **89**, 926–930, 1982.
21. Reece EA, Scioscia AL, Green J, O'Connor TZ & Hobbins JC. Embryonic trunk circumference: a new biometric parameter for estimation of gestational age. *Am. J. Obstet. Gynecol.* **156**, 713–715, 1987.
22. Pedersen JF. Ultrasound evidence of sexual difference in fetal size in first trimester. *Br. Med. J.* **281**, 1253, 1980.
23. Pedersen JF & Molsted-Pedersen L. Early growth retardation in diabetic pregnancy. *Br. Med. J.* **1**, 18–19, 1979.
24. Pedersen J & Molsted-Pedersen L. Early fetal growth delay detected by ultrasound marks increased risk of congenital malformation in diabetic pregnancy. *Br. Med. J.* **283**, 269–271, 1981.
25. Mantoni M & Pedersen JF. Fetal growth delay in threatened abortion: an ultrasound study. *Br. J. Obstet. Gynaecol.* **89**, 525–527, 1982.
26. Selbing A. Conceptual dating using ultrasonically measured fetal femur length and abdominal diameters in early pregnancy. *Br. J. Obstet. Gynaecol.* **93**, 116–121, 1986.
27. Campbell S & Newman AB. Growth of the fetal biparietal diameter during normal pregnancy. *J. Obstet. Gynaecol. Br. Commonw.* **78**, 513–519, 1971.
28. Hadlock FP, Deter RL, Harrist RB & Park SK. Fetal biparietal diameter: a critical re-evaluation of the relation to menstrual age by means of real-time ultrasound. *J. Ultrasound Med.* **1**, 97–104, 1982.
29. Ch de Crespigny L & Speirs AL. A new look at biparietal diameter. *Aust. NZ. J. Obstet. Gynaecol.* **29**, 26–29, 1989.
30. Shepard M. A standardized plane for biparietal diameter measurement. *J. Ultrasound Med.* **1**, 145–150, 1982.
31. Jeanty P, Cousaert E, Hobbins JC, Tack B, Bracken M & Cantraine F. A longitudinal study of fetal head biometry. *Am. J. Perinatol.* **1**, 118–128, 1984.
32. Chitty LS, Altman DG, Henderson A & Campbell S. Charts of fetal size: 2. Head measurements. *Br. J. Obstet. Gynaecol.* **101**, 35–43, 1994.
33. Doubilet PM & Greenes RA. Improved prediction of gestation age from fetal head measurements. *A.J.R.* **142**, 797–800, 1984.
34. Campbell S & Thoms A. Ultrasound measurement of the fetal head to abdomen circumference ratio in the assessment of growth retardation. *Br. J. Obstet. Gynaecol.* **84**, 165–174, 1977.
35. Hadlock FP, Deter RL, Harrist RB & Park SK. Fetal head circumference: relation to menstrual age. *A.J.R.* **138**, 649–653, 1982.
36. Campbell S & Wilkin D. Ultrasonic measurement of fetal abdomen circumference in the estimation of fetal weight. *Br. J. Obstet. Gynaecol.* **82**, 689–697, 1975.
37. Higginbottom J, Slater J, Porter G & Whitfield CR. Estimation of fetal weight from ultrasonic measurement of trunk circumference. *Br. J. Obstet. Gynaecol.* **82**, 698–701, 1975.

38. Jeanty P & Cousaert E & Cantraine F. Normal growth of the abdominal perimeter. *Am. J. Perinatol.* **1**, 129–135, 1984.
39. Chitty LS, Altman DG, Henderson A & Campbell S. Charts of fetal size: 3. Abdominal measurements. *Br. J. Obstet. Gynaecol.* **101**, 125–131, 1994.
40. Newnham JP, Patterson LL, James IR, Diepeveen DA & Reid SE. An evaluation of the efficacy of Doppler flow velocity waveform analysis as a screening test in pregnancy. *Am. J. Obstet. Gynecol.* **162**, 403–410, 1990.
41. Harding K, Evans S & Newnham J. Screening for the small fetus: a study of the relative efficacies of ultrasound biometry and symphysiofundal height. *Aust. N.Z. J. Obstet. Gynaecol.* **35**, 160–164, 1995.
42. Chang TC, Robson SC, Spencer JAD & Gallivan S. Prediction of perinatal morbidity at term in small fetuses: comparison of fetal growth and Doppler ultrasound. *Br. J. Obstet. Gynaecol.* **101**, 422–427, 1994.
43. Deter RL, Harrist RB, Hadlock FP & Carpenter RJ. Fetal head and abdominal circumferences: 1. Evaluation of measurement errors. *J. Clin. Ultrasound.* **10**, 357–363, 1982.
44. Usher R & McLean F. Intrauterine growth of liveborn Caucasian infants at sea level: standards obtained from measurements in 7 dimensions of infants born between 25 and 44 weeks gestation. *J. Pediatr.* **74**, 901–910, 1969.
45. O'Brien GD, Queenan JT & Campbell S. Assessment of gestational age in the second trimester by real-time ultrasound measurement of the femur length. *Am. J. Obstet. Gynecol.* **139**, 540–545, 1981.
46. Hadlock FP, Harrist RB, Deter RL & Park SK. Fetal femur length as a predictor of menstrual age: Sonographically measured. *A.J.R.* **138**, 875–878, 1982.
47. Jeanty P, Cousaert E, Cantraine F, Hobbins JC, Tack B & Struyven J. A longitudinal study of fetal limb growth. *Am. J. Perinatol.* **1**, 136–144, 1984.
48. Warda AH, Deter RL, Rossavik IK, Carpenter RJ & Hadlock FP. Fetal femur length: a critical re-evaluation of the relationship to menstrual age. *Obstet. Gynaecol.* **66**, 69–75, 1985.
49. Ruvolo KA, Filly RA & Callen PW. Evaluation of fetal femur length for prediction of gestational age in a racially mixed obstetric population. *J. Ultrasound Med.* **6**, 417–419, 1987.
50. Chitty LS, Altman DG, Henderson A & Campbell S. Charts of fetal size: 4. Femur length. *Br. J. Obstet. Gynaecol.* **101**, 132–135, 1994.
51. Jeanty P, Rodesch F, Delbeke D & Dumont JE. Estimation of gestational age from measurements of fetal long bones. *J. Ultrasound Med.* **3**, 75–79, 1984.
52. Goldstein RB, Filly RA & Simpson G. Pitfalls in femur length measurements. *J. Ultrasound Med.* **6**, 203–207, 1987.
53. Warda A, Deter RL, Duncan G, Hadlock FP. Evaluation of fetal thigh circumference measurements: a comparative ultrasound and anatomical study. *J. Clin. Ultrasound* **14**, 99–103, 1986.
54. Vintzileos AM, Neckles S, Campbell WA, Kaplan BM, Andreoli JW & Nochimson DJ. Ultrasound fetal thigh–calf circumferences and gestational age–independent fetal ratios in normal pregnancy. *J. Ultrasound. Med.* **4**, 287–292, 1985.
55. Jeanty P, Romero R & Hobbins JC. Fetal limb volume: a new parameter to assess fetal growth and nutrition. *J. Ultrasound Med.* **4**, 273–282, 1985.
56. Goldstein I, Reece A, Pilu G, Bovicelli L & Hobbins JC. Cerebellar measurements with ultrasonography in the evaluation of fetal growth and development. *Am. J. Obstet. Gynecol.* **156**, 1065–1069, 1987.
57. Reece EA, Goldstein I, Pilu G & Hobbins JC. Fetal cerebellar growth unaffected by intrauterine growth retardation: A new parameter for prenatal diagnosis. *Am. J. Obstet. Gynecol.* **157**, 632–638, 1987.
58. Behrman RE, Lees MH, Peterson EN, de Lannoy CW & Seeds A.E. Distribution of the circulation in the normal and asphyxiated fetal primate. *Am. J. Obstet. Gynecol.* **108**, 956–969, 1970.
59. Warsof SL, Gohari P, Berkowitz RL & Hobbins JC. The estimation of fetal weight by computer-assisted analysis. *Am. J. Obstet. Gynecol.* **128**, 881–892, 1977.
60. Thompson TR & Manning FA. Estimation of volume and weight of the perinate: Relationship to morphometric measurement by ultrasonography. *J. Ultrasound Med.* **2**, 113–116, 1983.
61. Hadlock FP, Harrist RB, Carpenter RJ, Deter RL & Park SK. Sonographic estimation of fetal weight. *Radiology* **150**, 535–540, 1984.
62. Hadlock FP, Harrist RB, Sharman RS, Deter RL & Park SK. Estimation of fetal weight with the use of head, body and femur measurements – a prospective study. *Am. J. Obstet. Gynecol.* **151**, 333–337, 1985.
63. Deter RL & Harrist RB. Assessment of normal fetal growth. In *Ultrasound in Obstetrics and Gynecology* (eds. F.A. Chervenak, G.C. Isaacson & S. Campbell) 1st edn, Vol. 1, pp. 361–385. Boston: Little, Brown and Co., 1993.
64. Weinberger E, Cyr DR, Hirsch JH, Richardson T, Hanson JA & Mack LA. Estimating fetal weights less than 2000 g: an accurate and simple method. *A.J.R.* **142**, 973–977, 1984.
65. Robson SC, Gallivan S, Walkinshaw SA, Vaughan J, Rodeck CH. Ultrasonic estimation of fetal weight: use of targeted formulas in small for gestational age fetuses. *Obstet. Gynecol.* **82**, 359–364, 1993.
66. Colley NV, Tremble JM, Henson GL & Cole TJ. Head circumference/abdominal circumference ratio, ponderal index and fetal malnutrition. Should head circumference/abdominal circumference ratio be abandoned? *Br. J. Obstet. Gynaecol.* **98**, 524–527, 1991.
67. Vintzileos AM, Campbell WA, Neckles S, Pike CL & Nochimson DJ. The ultrasound femur length as a predictor of fetal length. *Obstet. Gynaecol.* **64**, 779–782, 1984.
68. Vintzileos AM, Lodeiro JG, Feinstein SJ, Campbell WA, Weinbaum PJ, Nochimson DJ. Value of fetal ponderal index in predicting growth retardation. *Obstet. Gynecol.* **67**, 584–588, 1986.
69. Yagel S, Zacut D, Igelstein S, Palti Z, Hurwitz A & Rosenn B. In utero ponderal index as a prognostic factor in the evaluation of intrauterine growth retardation. *Am. J. Obstet. Gynecol.* **157**, 415–419, 1987.
70. Benson CB, Doubilet PM, Saltzman DH, Greene MF & Jones TB. Femur length/abdominal circumference ratio: poor predictor of macrosomic fetuses in diabetic mothers. *J. Ultrasound. Med.* **5**, 141–144, 1986.
71. Hadlock FP, Harrist RB, Shah Y & Park SK. The femur length/head circumference relation in obstetric sonography. *J. Ultrasound Med.* **3**, 439–442, 1984.
72. Lockwood C, Benacerraf B, Krinsky A *et al.* A sonographic screening method for Down syndrome. *Am. J. Obstet. Gynecol.* **157**, 803–808, 1987.
73. Hadlock FP, Deter RL, Harrist RB & Park SK. Computer assisted analysis of fetal age in the third trimester using multiple fetal growth parameters. *J. Clin. Ultrasound.* **11**, 313–316, 1983.
74. Shields LE, Huff RW, Jackson GM, Olive DL & Patterson RM. Fetal growth: a comparison of growth curves with mathematical modeling. *J. Ultrasound. Med.* **5**, 271–274, 1993.
75. Rossavik IK & Deter RL. Mathematical modeling of fetal growth: I. Basic principles. *J. Clin. Ultrasound.* **12**, 529–533, 1984.
76. Deter RL, Rossavik IK, Harrist RB & Hadlock FP. Mathematic modeling of fetal growth: development of individual growth curve standards. *Obstet. Gynecol.* **68**, 156–161, 1986.
77. Deter RL & Harrist RB. Growth standards for anatomic measurements and growth rates derived from longitudinal studies of normal fetal growth. *J. Clin. Ultrasound.* **20**, 381–388, 1992.
78. Deter RL, Hill RM & Tennyson LM. Predicting the birth characteristics of normal fetuses 14 weeks before delivery. *J. Clin. Ultrasound* **17**, 89–93, 1989.
79. Simon NV, Deter RL, Kofinas AD, Cavanaugh SH & Shearer DM. Small-for-menstrual-age infants: different subgroups detected using individualized fetal growth assessment. *J. Clin. Ultrasound* **22**, 3–10, 1994.
80. Gardosi J, Chang A, Kalyan B, Sahota D & Symonds EM. Customised antenatal growth charts. *Lancet.* **339**, 283–287, (subsequent correspondence) 878–879, 1992.
81. Mongelli M & Gardosi J. Reduction of false-positive diagnosis of fetal growth restriction by application of customized fetal growth standards. *Obstet. Gynecol.* **88**, 844–848, 1996.
82. Larsen T, Petersen S, Griesen G & Larsen F. Normal fetal growth evaluated by longitudinal ultrasound examinations. *Early Hum. Dev.* **24**, 37–45, 1990.
83. Larsen T, Greisen G & Petersen S. Intrauterine growth correlation to postnatal growth – influence of risk factors and complications of pregnancy. *Early Hum. Dev.* **47**, 157–165, 1997.
84. Newnham JP & Evans SF. Clinical evaluation of ultrasound technology. *Ultrasound. Quart.* **13**, 103–110, 1995).

Doppler ultrasonography

72

B. Trudinger

Introduction

Over recent years there has been intense interest in the application of Doppler ultrasound techniques to the study of maternal and fetal circulations. This non-invasive technique has made it possible to study blood flows to the placenta in human pregnancy. Previously, obstetricians could only speculate on the changes that occurred in health and disease in human pregnancy. The inaccessibility of the fetus has been overcome. Whilst the exact clinical role of the information available from Doppler studies is the subject of debate, randomized control trials have pointed to clinical utility. The indications for performing Doppler studies are becoming clearer.

Doppler studies

Doppler ultrasound techniques have been applied to the study of the fetal and maternal circulation in three ways.

BLOOD FLOW VELOCITY WAVEFORMS

Blood flow velocity waveforms (FVW) are created by displaying the spectral analysis of the Doppler frequency shift in real time on a time base. The envelope of the highest frequencies of the spectral analysis (maximum velocity envelope) represents the highest flow velocity in the sample and its pattern is described by a number of simple indices. The pattern of the FVW will vary with the precise vascular site being studied. In the normal fetus most vessels possess a characteristic pattern so that reproducible waveforms have been described from most large arteries and veins. The waveform pattern is produced by complex interaction of distal impedance, vessel wall elasticity, blood viscosity, upstream pressures and reflected waves.

The circulation is characterized by the haemodynamic parameters pressure, flow and resistance. With each cardiac contraction a time-varying pressure wave spreads down the arterial tree. The pressure gradient between adjacent points along the vascular tree drives the blood flow. Both the pressure gradient or pressure pulse and the flow wave are pulsatile. Both are influenced by the cardiac contraction, the physical properties of the vessel wall and its contained blood and the outflow resistance. Resistance may be thought of as how difficult it is to force blood through the vascular tree. However, the pulsatile character of blood flow means extra energy is required to distend the vascular tree and overcome blood viscosity[1]. For pulsatile flow the term impedance is used as the ratio of pulsatile pressure to pulsatile flow. Pressure and flow waves do not stay synchronous through the cardiac cycle because of the occurrence of reflected waves later in systole[2].

Across the vessel lumen blood flow is not uniform but rather there exists a velocity profile attributed to blood viscosity and shear between adjacent flow lamina. When the velocity profile is flat or uniform then inertial forces are more important than viscous forces. The FVW recorded when the vessel is totally insonnated displays the velocity profile information.

There exists an understandable desire to interpret the FVW in terms of simple haemodynamic parameters. The influence of outflow resistance has been most considered. Waveforms from arteries supplying low impedance vascular beds exhibit relatively high forward velocities throughout the cardiac cycle in systole and diastole. A triphasic waveform shape in which there is a period of reverse flow in diastole is characteristic of high downstream impedance. However, the waveform shape is also influenced by the upstream cardiac contraction, and the effect of this should not be overlooked.

The use of the simple empirical indices of resistance encourages a too simplistic interpretation which ignores the contribution of various factors. The indices do have meaning when the change in one parameter dominates. As an example of this, fetal growth restriction may be due to placental insufficiency with high umbilical placental flow resistance. The high resistance may affect ventricular afterload and the associated hypoxaemia may lead to a redistribution of cardiac output and affect cardiac contractility.

VOLUME FLOW MEASUREMENTS

Volume flow measurements have been described for the umbilical vein and fetal aorta and normal pregnancy values have been defined[3–5]. Volume flow is calculated as the product of mean velocity and vessel area. Whilst this application of pulsed Doppler has provided a great deal of information about fetal cardiac output and other physiological parameters, limits to the accuracy of the measurement and the lack of ready availability of easily operated equipment had prevented its widespread clinical adoption to date. An alternative approach to this was a non-Doppler ultrasound technique to assess volume flow measurement – the Philips® CVI-Q™. This technique uses an autocorrelation function to follow movement of a flowing blood stream characterized by its pattern of reflectors.

COLOUR FLOW MAPPING

This is a technique of visual representation of pulsed Doppler information overlying a B mode ultrasound image. Although much has been written about the role of colour flow mapping (CFM) in obstetric ultrasound it remains principally a tool for rapid localization of vessels which are then studied using spectral Doppler techniques. The successful application of CFM in the diagnosis of vascular malformations, vasa previa and nuchal cords has been described. Another new technique for analysing and displaying topographical Doppler shift information is the 'power Doppler' system or 'ultrasound' angiography. These systems display the power of the Doppler signal rather than the frequency shift at a given point. They are better at producing smooth images of low flow velocities.

Doppler studies of the fetal circulation

THE UMBILICAL PLACENTAL BLOOD FLOW

The umbilical circulation is approximately 40% of the combined ventricular output of the fetus and dominates the fetal cardiovascular system[6,7]. It is a low-resistance vascular bed. It is not innervated and regulation in the placenta is presumed under the control of locally acting mediators. Volume flow can be influenced by changes in heart rate and blood pressure. It is believed that there is little need to precisely regulate flow as the fetus can alter oxygen extraction over a wide range[8]. With control relatively passive the umbilical blood flow is stable and responsive to changes elsewhere in the fetal cardiovascular system. The anatomy of the umbilical circulation also makes it ideal for Doppler study – two arteries which loosely spiral along the umbilical cord surrounded by a sea of amniotic fluid.

NORMAL PREGNANCY

Doppler studies of the umbilical artery FVW with calculation of the indices of resistance reflect the status of the umbilical placental vascular bed. Underpinning these studies is the observation that fetal growth restriction is associated with an increasing resistance[9]. In pregnancy the umbilical artery FVW is characterized by a high diastolic flow relative to the systolic peak velocity. This is a low-resistance flow pattern. With advancing gestation the diastolic flow velocity increases relative to the systolic peak. This change is attributed to decreasing flow resistance with advancing gestation and presumably reflects the growth of the placenta. It would be the expected result from growth of the umbilical placental vascular tree with an increase in the number of vascular channels through the placenta. Three indices have been commonly used to quantitate downstream vascular resistance. These are the systolic/diastolic (*S/D*) ratio, the pulsatility index, and the resistance index (Pourcelot ratio) (Fig. 72.1). These indices are highly correlated, suggesting that they represent a similar haemodynamic finding. All the indices contain the same intrinsic errors[10,11]. A normal range for the systolic/diastolic ratio during pregnancy is shown (Fig. 72.2). During the early part of pregnancy when diastolic flow velocities are low the normal range is wide. Serial studies may be useful at this time as a declining value of the index in normal pregnancy suggests growth and expansion of the placental vascular tree. When diastolic flow velocities are absent the waveform may be quantified by expressing the proportion of the cardiac period during which flow velocity is absent. The umbilical Doppler FVW is influenced by fetal movement and particularly fetal breathing movements. During fetal breathing, blood flow is diverted to the fetal lungs. The fetal heart rate has little influence on the umbilical Doppler indices of resistance over

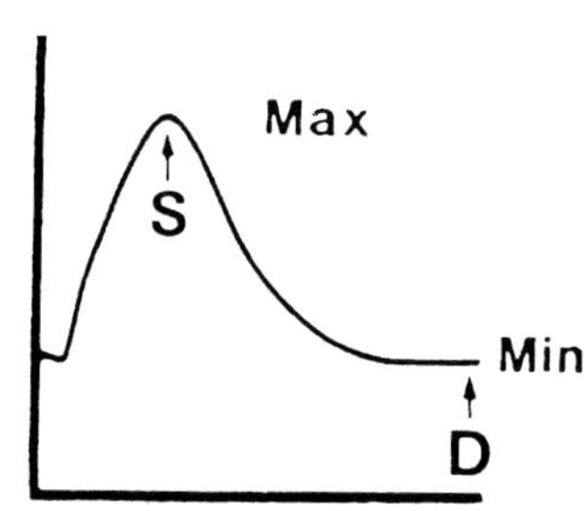

PULSATILITY INDEX $= \dfrac{S - D}{Mean}$

POURCELOT RATIO $= \dfrac{S - D}{S}$

SYSTOLIC/DIASTOLIC RATIO $= S/D$

Fig. 72.1 Three indices of downstream vascular resistance derived from the maximum FVW envelope in common clinical use.

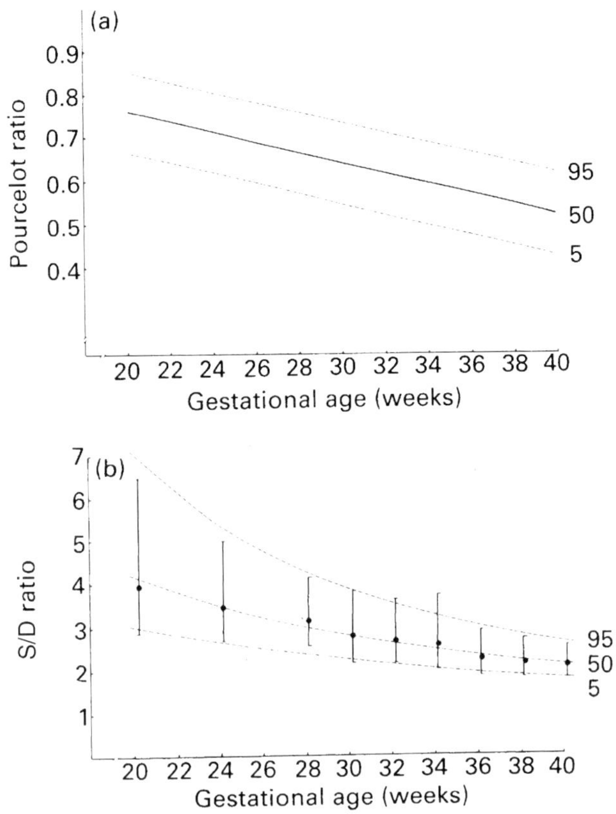

Fig. 72.2 The normal range for the systolic/diastolic ratio and the resistance index (Pourcelot ratio) of the umbilical artery during the second half of the pregnancy[11].

the normal heart range seen in the fetus. It is not necessary to correct for this. Behavioural states do not appear to influence the umbilical Doppler recording. The site of recording along the cord is relevant. The indices of resistance are higher at the fetal end of the umbilical cord and a pattern similar to the fetal aorta may be recorded[12]. Values are lowest at the placental end of the cord. Most advocate that a segment of free-floating loop of cord be used for the Doppler recording. A recording should consist of sequence of five to ten cardiac cycles to confirm a steady state and the absence of variation due to fetal activity and breathing. The sample volume of pulsed Doppler equipment should be large to ensure the whole umbilical artery is insonnated. This ensures that a true maximum FVW is recorded.

THE MEANING OF ABNORMAL UMBILICAL ARTERY FVW PATTERNS

The indices of resistance described in the previous section have been widely applied to studies of the umbilical circulation. These indices should not be equated with volume flow. Rather they relate to downstream resistance. Strictly, the term resistance should only be used for steady flow in rigid pipes. Impedance is the more appropriate term, since blood flow is pulsatile[13]. As stated above, the blood FVW depends not only on the downstream vascular bed, but also the upstream pressure pump, the elasticity or distensibility of vessel walls and the viscous properties of blood. In the umbilical circulation in disease (rather than physiological experiments), the extent, and so the influence, of changes in the downstream vascular bed is so large in comparison to these other considerations that it is the major determinant of changes in the waveform pattern.

Throughout pregnancy the placenta grows with an increase in size and number of villi. The resistance vessels of the placenta are the small arterial and arteriole channels in the tertiary villi[7]. It is across this generation of vessels that the greatest drop in pressure occurs. The decreasing vascular resistance in the umbilical placental circulation seen through pregnancy is attributable to growth and so the increase in the number of these channels. In addition, there is a small increase in the actual number of arterial channels in each of the tertiary stem villi. A study to correlate the umbilical artery FVW pattern with these 'resistance' vessels in the placenta has been carried out[14]. The modal tertiary villus small arterial vessel count was significantly less in a group of patients with abnormal (high resistance index) umbilical artery Doppler FVW patterns in contrast to normal (1–2 to 7–8 arteries/high power field) (Fig. 72.3). This placental lesion of vascular

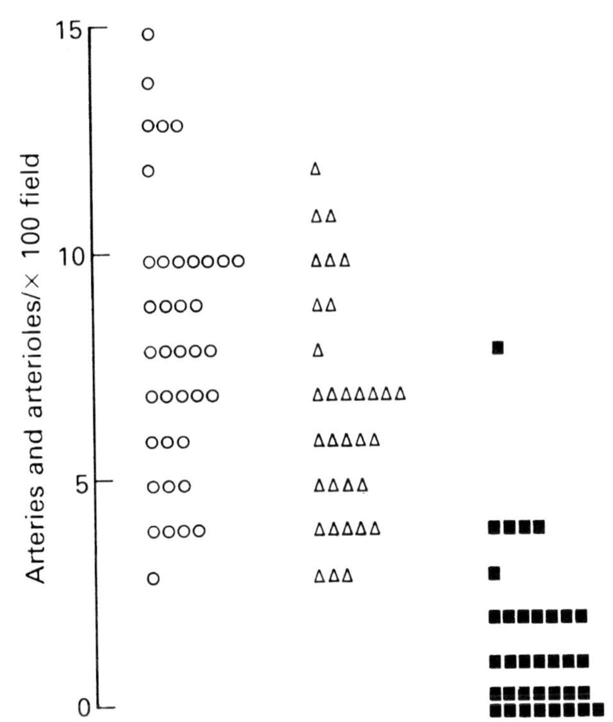

Fig. 72.3 The modal count of 'resistance' vessels (small muscular arteries and arterioles per × 100 microscope field) in the tertiary villi of the fetal placental circulation was significantly less ($p < 0.01$) in pregnancies in which a high-resistance umbilical artery FVW was recorded (■) than in normal pregnancy (○) and at risk pregnancy with normal systolic/diastolic ratio (△)[14].

sclerosis with obliteration of the small muscular arteries of the tertiary villi could be expected to increase flow resistance. It is the Doppler-defined lesion of umbilical placental insufficiency.

There is also support for the concept of a reduction in small arterial channels in the placenta from physical modelling studies. Using a lumped electrical circuit equivalent, Thompson and Stevens[15] developed a computer-based model of the placental vasculature. This has proved to be a very valuable approach and has produced realistic data in a variety of tests. Using this model it can be shown that the pulsatility index of the FVW is related to the size of the downstream vascular bed[16]. This index will increase as the fraction of terminal vessels obliterated is increased, but this is not a linear relationship. Initially there was little change and indeed it was not until the extent of reduction exceeded 50% that the pulsatility index increased beyond the normal range (Fig. 72.4). It is widely believed that umbilical artery Doppler studies provide an early sign of potential fetal compromise. Data from the results of mathematical models of the placenta indicate the extent to which the pathology must be established before clinical detection occurs.

The concept that the various indices of resistance derived from the umbilical Doppler FVW relate to the size (number of vascular channels) of the downstream bed is also supported by experimental studies in fetal lambs[17]. Microsphere embolization of the umbilical cotyledonary circulation produced an increase in these indices.

CLINICAL CORRELATIONS OF ABNORMAL UMBILICAL DOPPLER STUDIES

The use of umbilical Doppler FVW studies in clinical practice can be simply summarized by:

Placental lesion → Fetal effect

As described above, umbilical Doppler studies detect a reduction in the placental vasculature. It is this lesion that is believed to deprive or constrain the fetus. On this basis it can be appreciated that umbilical Doppler studies are not a 'fetal test'. The pregnancies identified as abnormal will include those in which the fetus has been affected and those in which a process is occurring, but the fetus is not yet affected. However, not unexpectedly the most abnormal Doppler results will correlate with the greatest fetal effect (Fig. 72.5).

Many early studies correlated abnormal umbilical artery Doppler results with fetal growth restriction and the birth of an infant small for gestational age[18–22]. However, what matters most to the obstetrician is not the recognition of the small fetus, but rather of the fetus at risk of death in utero, distress in labour, and neonatal morbidity. Umbilical Doppler studies identify this subset of small fetus[23,24]. The author has reviewed the clinical outcome of all studies in high-risk pregnancy in his laboratory (2178 patients) over a five-year period[25]. The significant differences in size at birth and duration of neonatal intensive care remained when

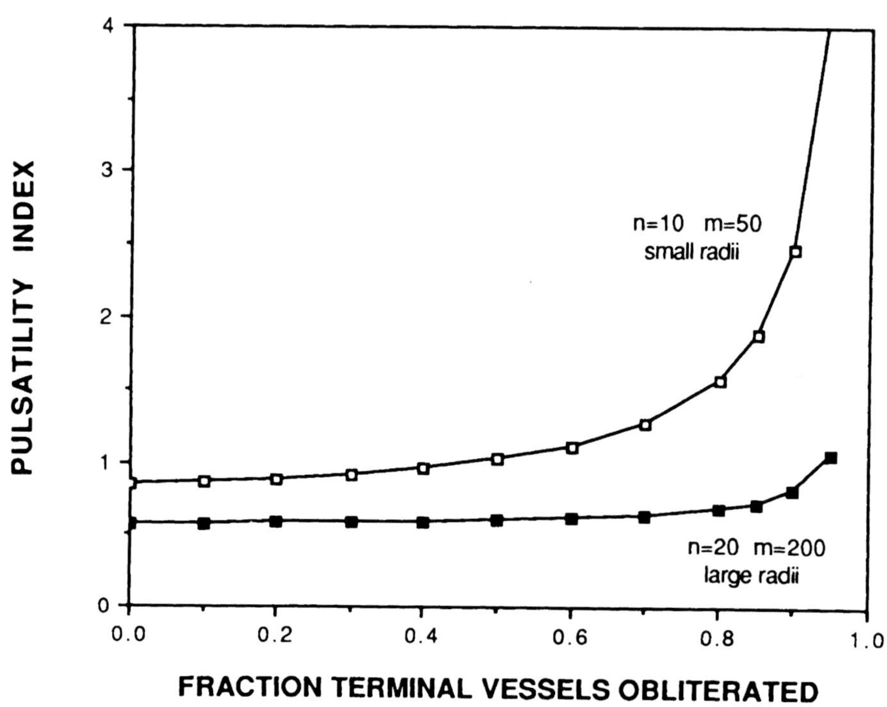

Fig. 72.4 Using a mathematical model of the placenta the calculated change in the pulsatility index of the umbilical artery in response to obliteration of an increasing fraction of the small arterial channels is shown for smaller (□) and a larger (■) umbilical placental vascular bed to demonstrate the theoretical differences in the use of umbilical Doppler at 28 and 40 weeks' pregnancy[16].

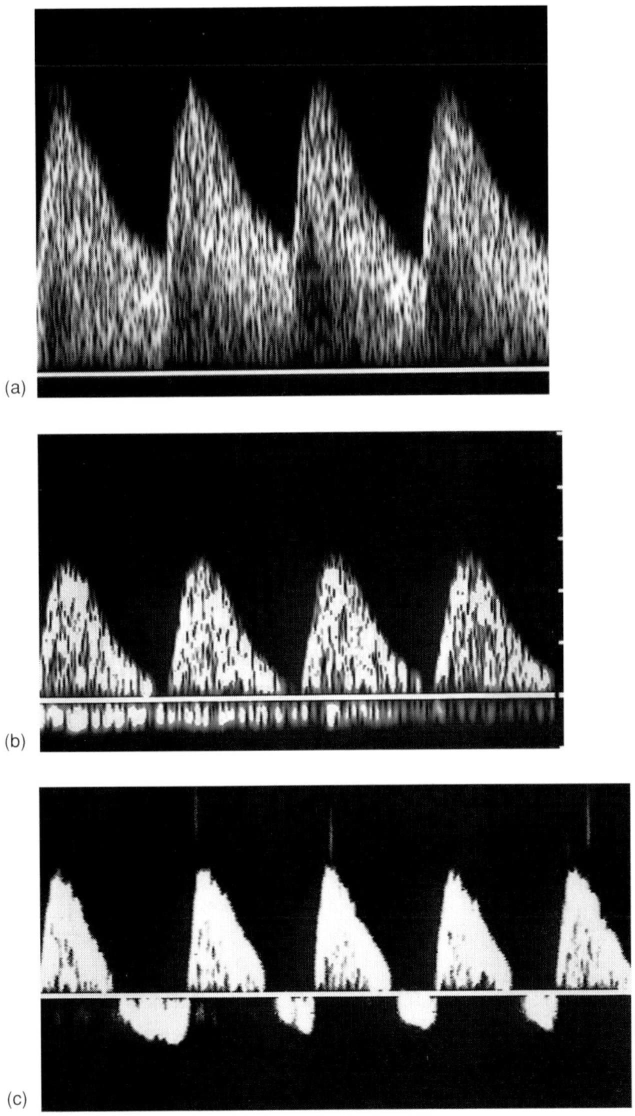

Fig. 72.5 Abnormal high-resistance umbilical artery Doppler FVW recordings showing (a) low diastolic flow velocity, (b) absent end diastolic flow velocity and (c) reversed blood flow in diastole.

analysis of covariance was carried out to eliminate the effects of gestational age.

The author has also analysed the value of using serial studies of the umbilical Doppler FVW to determine a trend[25]. The rationale for this is that an increasing index of resistance suggests vessel obliteration whereas a decrease is indicative of placental growth with vascular expansion. In comparison to the single (abnormal) last study result, the use of an upward trend of serial studies showed stronger correlations for adverse outcome in terms of perinatal mortality or duration of neonatal intensive care nursery stay. In contrast, a downward trend, even if the values were outside the normal range, was associated with an outcome little different from normal.

UMBILICAL DOPPLER STUDIES AND OTHER FETAL ASSESSMENTS

The relationship of change in umbilical Doppler studies to tests of fetal welfare has been reported in a number of studies. In comparison to non-stressed fetal heart rate (FHR) monitoring the umbilical Doppler waveform is a more sensitive indicator of size at birth[26,27]. Although it is important to identify the small fetus it is more important to identify those at risk of morbidity. As stated already, size may not be the most relevant fetal endpoint. Umbilical Doppler study was more sensitive when such measures of 'asphyxia' as operative delivery for fetal distress, low 5 min Apgar score and admission to neonatal intensive care were examined. Non-stressed FHR monitoring and umbilical Doppler had similar predictive values. In current obstetric practice monitoring is widely used to confirm well-being or otherwise in a fetus considered to be at risk. For that reason the published results revealing a higher sensitivity (without additional false positive cases) of umbilical Doppler studies are noteworthy.

Ultrasound biometry is widely used in the third trimester to identify the small for gestational age (SGA) fetus. The abdominal circumference is the most widely measured fetal dimension for this purpose. Not unexpectedly this measurement was shown to be more sensitive than umbilical Doppler in identifying the SGA fetus. However, Doppler studies were shown to identify small fetuses at risk of subsequent perinatal asphyxia and morbidity[28–30]. An investigation designed to screen an unselected population in the third trimester of pregnancy revealed umbilical Doppler ultrasound and ultrasonic measurement of fetal abdominal circumference to be identical in terms of sensitivity, specificity and predictive value when birth weight less than the tenth centile was combined with evidence of fetal hypoxia as endpoint[31].

Fetal blood gas tensions have been measured and the results correlated to umbilical Doppler studies. Such studies are observational and depend upon the existence of a reason for percutaneous umbilical blood sampling. Hypoxaemia is a feature of small fetuses with absent end diastolic flow velocities in the umbilical artery FVW, although not all such fetuses were hypoxaemic[32–34]. Blood gas analysis of cord blood taken at delivery[35] revealed similar findings. Again these data involve a bias in that the fetuses had been selected for elective caesarean section.

UMBILICAL DOPPLER STUDIES IN SPECIFIC PREGNANCY COMPLICATIONS

Information has been collected on umbilical Doppler studies in pregnancies with a particular problem. All published series of high-risk pregnancies include cases with *maternal hypertension*. In these cases it has been demonstrated that an abnormal umbilical Doppler result is associated with the expected increased fetal morbidity and mortality[36]. Interestingly, there was no relationship between the duration of hypertension and the umbilical FVW result. The author has also noted that in many cases the abnormal fetal Doppler result precedes maternal disease. In maternal *diabetes mellitus* fetal size does not correlate well with the Doppler result. Abnormal results predict failure of ultrasonically measured growth or finding a non-reactive, non-stressed FHR tracing[37,38]. In *multiple pregnancy* umbilical Doppler studies are very useful in predicting fetal growth restriction[39–41]. In twin pregnancy growth failure is typically discordant and this is predicted by umbilical Doppler study. In the twin transfusion syndrome, abnormal umbilical Doppler study predicts fetal demise. In this situation umbilical Doppler measurements are more easily performed than ultrasound measurements of size. It is the author's policy to include an umbilical Doppler study at 28 and 34 weeks in the management of all twin pregnancies. In the *antiphospholipid antibody syndrome* placental insufficiency with fetal growth failure and death in utero and severe maternal preeclampsia are common. An abnormal umbilical Doppler study does predict failing fetal growth and deteriorating fetal condition[42].

UMBILICAL DOPPLER – EVIDENCE-BASED MEDICINE

A recently published meta-analysis of randomized trials evaluating the use of umbilical artery Doppler studies in clinical practice[43] has concluded 'there is now compelling evidence that women with high risk pregnancies, including preeclampsia and suspected intrauterine growth retardation, should have access to Doppler ultrasonographic study of umbilical artery waveforms'. Meta-analysis of 12 studies demonstrated that the availability of umbilical Doppler ultrasonography reduced the odds of perinatal death by 38% (95% confidence interval 15% to 55%) This was the primary outcome examined. The result was significant at the 1% level. The reduction in perinatal mortality was observed in all subgroups (still births, neonatal deaths, deaths of normally formed babies). The consistency of results across the trials suggest that the findings are unlikely to be chance. Secondary analyses revealed a significant reduction in the number of antenatal admissions, induction of labour, and caesarean sections for fetal distress in the Doppler groups. Post hoc analyses revealed a statistically significant reduction in elective delivery, intrapartum fetal distress and hypoxic encephalopathy in the Doppler group. In a Committee Opinion the American College of Obstetricians and Gynecologists has endorsed the value of umbilical artery Doppler studies in high-risk pregnancy. It is worth noting that no other test of fetal welfare carries such strong evidence of usefulness.

FETAL ARTERIES STUDIED WITH DOPPLER

Blood flow in the aorta and most of its branches has been studied with Doppler ultrasound. The use of CFM and colour power angiography simplifies vessel identification. The shape of the FVW is influenced by both the upstream pump and the downstream resistance and the simple indices of resistance may not be the best method of waveform analysis and quantification. In the placenta these indices are detecting a gross pathophysiological process of vessel obliteration. Within the fetus the changes in resistance are the result of vasomotor tone redistributing blood flow and unlikely to show the same degree of abnormality as changes in umbilical placental studies. Parameters which reflect volume flow and pressure changes in the fetus may be more valuable in clinical practice.

FETAL AORTA

Several approaches have been taken to the analysis of FVWs recorded from the fetal aorta (Plate 72.1). Indices of resistance used to study umbilical waveforms have been used to examine the aortic FVW[44,45]. Peak and mean flow velocity have also been studied[46,47]. Indices of resistance change little with gestation in the descending thoracic aorta during the second half of pregnancy. Most of the blood flow in the thoracic and abdominal aorta is directed to the placenta. It is not surprising that the low resistance of the umbilical placental circulation dominates the aortic waveform. In fetal growth restriction the indices of resistance are increased. There is no evidence, however, that analysis of the aortic FVW in this way provides different information to that provided by study of the umbilical artery FVW.

Mean flow velocity can be derived from the aortic FVW. This is possible in the aorta since the vessel is straight and clearly imaged and the angle between the ultrasound beam and vessel is measurable. It is not possible in the coiled umbilical circulation. In normal and complicated pregnancy values of the peak mean velocity of the aortic waveform were correlated with fetal hypoxaemia, hypercarbia, hyperlactaemia and acidaemia[32,34]. These last were determined from fetal blood obtained at cordocentesis. Reduction in peak mean velocity correlated with abnormality of these biochemical indices. An explanation for these findings is suggested by experimental work in fetal lambs[48]. Volume blood flow was altered by negative ionotrophic stimulation. Peak and mean aortic flow velocity derived from the Doppler waveform envelope was strongly correlated with volume flow in the descending thoracic aorta. These Doppler parameters therefore reflect aortic flow and ventricular output. It would appear that in the presence of marked fetal hypoxaemia there is a reduction in blood flow in the aorta and this is presumably the result of reduced ventricular output. It is likely that the hypoxaemia affects cardiac contractility. In a comparative analysis of Doppler recordings from various fetal arteries using the statistical technique of principal component analysis it was shown that the reduction of peak mean aortic velocity correlated most strongly with fetal hypoxaemia and fetal hypercarbia[34].

THE CEREBRAL CIRCULATION

The arteries of circle of Willis and the internal carotid artery can be readily imaged using CFM techniques. The FVW can be recorded from these vessels[49–51]. The middle cerebral artery has been most frequently studied. This vessel is usually readily imaged with the ultrasound beam parallel to the direction of the vessel. This maximizes the recording of the FVW (Plate 72.2). Peak and mean velocity are readily determined from this. The cerebral vessels typically show a low resistance pattern. During the third trimester there is a very small decrease in the indices of resistance recorded from these vessels. A normal range for the pulsatility index of the middle cerebral artery lies above a value of 1.1 in the third trimester. FVWs in the cerebral circulation do fluctuate with fetal breathing and fetal activity. They are affected by behavioural state. The normal low resistance pattern of the cerebral circulation has been shown to be accentuated in fetal growth retardation and fetal hypoxaemia[52]. It has been postulated that this results from cerebral vasodilatation as an autoregulatory mechanism to preserve the cerebral oxygenation. In the extremely hypoxic fetus this effect is lost, possibly as the result of cerebral oedema. Before this effect is seen there is much published data suggesting that the more hypoxaemic the fetus the greater is the decrease in the index of resistance. Many cases of fetal hypoxaemia have values in the lower part of the normal range. The use of middle cerebral artery Doppler to make the separation between normal and abnormal values for the fetal oxygen tension therefore is not as complete as was hoped. To enhance the clinical utility of studies of the cerebral FVW a ratio of the cerebral to umbilical resistance index has been used[53]. A ratio of less than one is predictive of neonatal morbidity. It appears that this ratio depends very much on the discrimination by the umbilical artery waveform.

Anaemia is associated with a hyperdynamic circulation and this is seen in the fetus as well as adult. Cerebral blood flow is increased in association with fetal anaemia. The use of peak systolic velocity recorded from the middle cerebral artery in alloimmunization has been promoted[54]. It has been suggested that this may reduce the need for invasive procedures to measure fetal haemoglobin. The correlation between fetal haemoglobin level and increase in peak velocity is hypothesized to be the result of the increase in blood flow in association with anaemia.

OTHER FETAL ARTERIAL CIRCULATIONS

In the fetal external iliac artery there is a small increase in the resistance index reported in fetal growth restriction[55]. In the fetal brachial artery fetal growth restriction and abnormal umbilical Doppler FVW have been associated with an increase in the pulsatility index in the left arm[56].

In the fetal abdomen the renal artery pulsatility index is reported increased in fetal growth restriction and in post-term pregnancy in association wjth oligohydramnios[57]. Small for gestation fetuses have been identified to have a decrease in resistance in the splenic artery[58]. Attempts to correlate the risk of necrotising enterocolitis with superior or inferior mesenteric artery FVW patterns have not been successful.

FETAL VENOUS DOPPLER STUDIES

The great central veins of the fetus, the ductus venosus, the inferior vena cava, the hepatic veins and the umbilical vein have been the subject of recent studies. The FVWs in the central fetal veins are influenced in form by the central venous pressure and this in turn is a reflection of cardiac function. The flow waves have been used as a surrogate for the central venous pressure wave. Preload, afterload and cardiac contractility are important in understanding the form of the central venous flow waveform.

NORMAL PREGNANCY

The form of the FVW of the central fetal veins is best understood by reviewing the shape of central venous pressure waveform. This has recently been recorded from the human fetus using a technique to track vessel wall movement[59]. Four points are identified in the central venous pressure waveform. The *A* crest is associated with atrial contraction. The *X* trough occurs with atrial relaxation in early systole. The *V* crest is the result of rising atrial and venous pressure as the atrioventricular valves are closed in ventricular systole and forward flow is obstructed. The *Y* trough begins as soon as the atrioventricular valves open at the end of the isovolumetric ventricular relaxation.

The same four crests or troughs can be identified on the central venous FVW although flow is inversely related to pressure. Hence a crest of high pressure on the pressure wave is associated with a trough of low flow velocity in the venous flow waveform. High atrial and central venous pressure retards blood flow returning to the heart. The flow patterns of the FVW from the ductus venosus[60] and the inferior vena cava[61] are characteristic of each vessel (Fig. 72.6).

A variety of parameters have been suggested to analyse the venous waveform and provide a numeric index. These indices have been applied to the study of complicated pregnancy[61]. The indices suggested are all derived from the maximum velocity waveform on waveform envelope.

- *Percentage reverse flow.* The time velocity integral for reverse flow expressed as a percentage of the time velocity integral for forward flow
- *Preload index.* The peak velocity of the early systole crest (*X*) minus the least velocity of the atrial contraction (*A*) is the numerator and the denominator is the peak velocity at early systole (*X*)
- *Peak velocity index for vein.* The peak velocity of the early systole crest (*X*) minus the least velocity of atrial contraction (*A*) is the numerator and the denominator is the peak velocity at late systole (*Y*)
- *Pulsatility index for the vein.* The peak velocity of the early systole crest (*X*) minus the least velocity at atrial contraction (*A*) is the numerator and the denominator is the time-averaged mean of the maximum velocity envelope

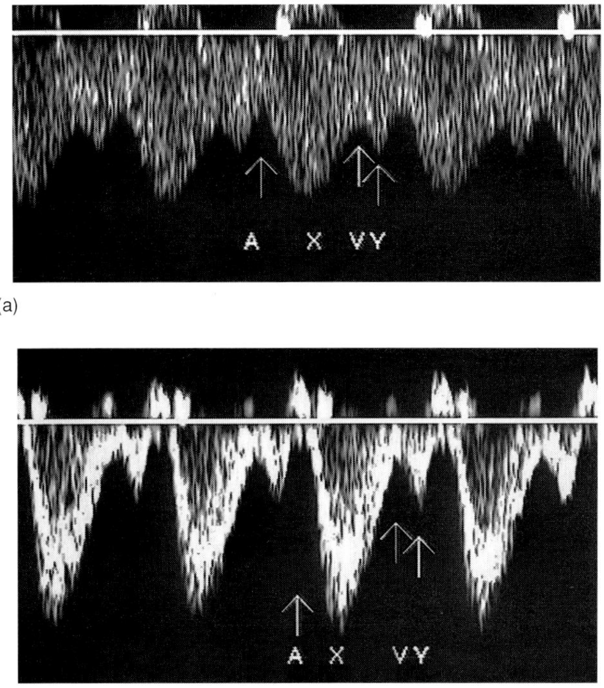

(a)

(b)

Fig. 72.6 FVWs recorded from (a) the ductus venosus and (b) the inferior vena cava with the *A*, *X*, *V* and *Y* waves (see text) shown. The methods in use to quantify the waveform shape are discussed in the text.

In the fetus there are circulation differences in comparison to the extrauterine situation. In the fetus the pulmonary circulation is small and systemic venous return passes to the left heart through the foramen ovale as well as through the right heart. Ventricular outflow from the right heart enters the systemic circulation through the ductus arteriosus. Conceptually there exists a combined ventricular output directed into the systemic circulation so that the afterload for both ventricles is systemic vascular resistance. However, blood from the left ventricle is directed to the head and upper body whereas from the right it is directed to the lower body and placenta. Since 40% of output is directed to the placenta this is a major determinant of right ventricular afterload.

CENTRAL VENOUS FVW IN FETAL COMPROMISE

Doppler studies from the umbilical artery and the intrafetal arterial vessels reflect many of the haemodynamic changes in the growth restricted fetus with placental insufficiency. These in turn influence fetal cardiac function. Umbilical placental resistance is high so that high right ventricle afterload is present. Resistance in the cerebral circulation is low, reducing the left ventricle afterload in the more compromised fetuses. The development of fetal hypoxaemia in association with placental vascular disease ultimately affects cardiac contractility and causes a decrease in cardiac output. The reduction in flow in the fetal aorta in association with fetal hypoxaemia has been commented upon earlier. Studies of the central venous pressure waveform in growth restricted pregnancy demonstrate changes consistent with high right ventricular afterload (giant *A* waves) and at a later stage depressed myocardial function. This appears as a two phase response. The first stage may represent the compensatory response of the right ventricle to the high afterload. The second stage with a low-amplitude pressure waveform is consistent with depressed contractility due to hypoxaemia. The same two-stage response may be inferred from the results of ultrasound measurements of flow around the aortic and pulmonary valves in fetal growth restriction. In severe fetal compromise measurement of volume flow indicates a decrease in output with deterioration of fetal condition[62]. An increase in flow across the pulmonary valve was reported in a less compromised group suggesting a positive myocardial response to the increase in ventricular afterload[63].

In parallel with these changes it does appear that the increase in end diastolic pressure consequent to the increase in right ventricular afterload and later the reduction in cardiac contractility are the major haemodynamic influences which alter the form of the flow velocity waves in the central veins in fetal compromise. Flow velocities during atrial contraction are reduced and may be reversed. The early systolic peak (*X*) is increased. Flow is reduced and may be reversed in late systole (*V* wave) and this is even more pronounced if chamber dilatation and tricuspid regurgitation occurs. In studies of fetal compromise, fetal hypoxia was best predicted from the inferior vena cava FVW by the percentage of reverse flow and the preload index[64,65]. For the ductus venosus waveform the systolic (*X*) to atrial (*A*) contraction peak velocity ratio and the preload index were best. A management plan for high fetal risk pregnancy has been suggested with delivery timed by abnormality in these central venous FVW indices.

Pulsations in the umbilical vein (Fig. 72.6) have been described in association with fetal compromise and fetal growth restriction[66]. They have been associated with the most profound fetal compromise. Two mechanisms have been advanced to explain the occurrence of this phenomenon. In fetal compromise with placental insufficiency there is obliteration and so reduction in small arterial channels in the placenta. This results in a decrease in capacitance in the umbilical placental vascular bed so that compliance (its inverse) is changed. Arterial pulsation in this circumstance can be transmitted through to the venous circulation. This is predicted by placental model studies[16]. The alternative explanation is the retrograde transmission of the giant *A* waves backwards along the venous system.

Doppler studies in the maternal uteroplacental circulation

As Doppler technology was developed there was an early desire to study uterine blood to the placental bed. Both pulsed[67] and continuous wave[68] systems were used for this. Early studies were hampered by problems of vessel identification with uncertainty about the recording site. The introduction of CFM and colour angiography has overcome these difficulties. The main uterine artery and the accurate vessels can be precisely located.

A low-resistance FVW pattern has been recorded from the uterine artery and its placental bed branches throughout the second half of pregnancy. In the first trimester and early second trimester high resistance patterns are seen. Attention has also focused on the presence of an early diastolic notch which has been suggested to be present when downstream resistance is high[68]. The timing of this notch suggests strongly that it is attributable to the presence of a reflected wave.

UTERINE DOPPLER AND PLACENTAL INSUFFICIENCY

Both severe fetal growth restriction and maternal preeclampsia have been associated with uteroplacental waveforms demonstrating high systolic diastolic ratios[69]. The degree of proteinuria, level of maternal uric acid, gestation age at delivery and centile birth weight have all been associated with uterine artery waveform abnormality in hypertensive pregnancy. However, some have disputed this finding in studies of less selected populations[70,71].

The process of trophoblast invasion of the spiral arteries of the decidual and inner third of the myometrium occurs during the first 20 weeks of gestation. The spiral artery is stripped of its musculoelastic coat. It is widely believed that this lowers the resistance to blood flow in the uterine artery branches and so causes higher end diastolic flow velocities. This can be detected early in the second trimester of pregnancy. After 20 weeks of gestation there is little change in the waveform and a high end diastolic velocity relative to peak systolic velocity is seen. The lack of direct evidence linking the trophoblast invasion of the spiral arteries with uterine blood flow or FVWs changes must be appreciated. The standard explanation is presumptive. The early diastolic 'notch' of uteroplacental FVW has been reported in normal pregnancy until approximately 26 weeks' gestation. However, on the same side of the uterus as the placental bed, it has been reported to be rarely found after 20 weeks' gestation. Based on the hypothesis that trophoblast invasion of the spiral arteries causes the change in the FVW pattern of the uterine artery and that trophoblast invasion is less developed in pregnancy hypertension, these studies have been evaluated as a screening test to predict placental insufficiency. The test demonstrated a high sensitivity for prediction of preeclampsia and fetal growth restriction but there was a high false positive rate. Detailed results for evaluation of the use of Doppler ultrasound of the uterine arteries to predict preeclampsia or the delivery of a small for gestational age baby have recently been published[72]. From 1326 pregnancies 214 women were identified at 19–21 weeks. Abnormal Doppler findings were still present in 110 of these women at 24 weeks. Three quarters (77%) of the preeclampsia and one-third of the small for gestational age babies (32%) were selected in this group of 110. The predictive value of 31% and 38% from the 24-week result appears good but would be halved if the denominator for this calculation is the number identified at 19–21 weeks' screening study. Comment has been made that an incidence of 44 in 1326 of proteinuric pregnancy hypertension is high, suggesting a high-risk population of low socioeconomic status. The performance of uterine Doppler in a truly low-risk population remains uncertain. The debate about the clinical value of uterine artery screening is continuing. No adequate randomized controlled trials are available to settle this issue at the present time.

EARLY PREGNANCY UTERINE FLOW STUDIES

The advent of colour Doppler ultrasound leading to precise vessel identification has permitted studies of the early first trimester changes in the uterine artery FVWs. The waveform pattern and the various indices of resistance decrease between 6 and 16 weeks of gestation[73]. In early pregnancy failure (missed abortion, anembryonic pregnancy) there was no difference in these indices of resistance. This finding is interesting as it suggests early pregnancy failure does not result from failure of vascularization[74].

REFERENCES

1. Milnor WR. Pulsatile blood flow. *N. Engl. J. Med.* **187**:27, 1972.
2. Caro CG, Pedley TJ, Schroter CW & Seed WA. *The Mechanics of the Circulation*. London: Oxford University Press, 1978.
3. Gill RW. Pulsed Doppler with B-mode imaging for quantitative blood flow measurement. *Ultrasound Med. Biol.* **5**:223, 1979.
4. Gill RW, Trudinger BJ, Garrett WJ, Kossoff G & Warren PS. Fetal umbilical venous flow measured in utero by pulsed Doppler and B-mode ultrasound. I: Normal pregnancy. *Am. J. Obstet. Gynecol.* **139**:720, 1981.
5. Eik-Nes SH, Brubakk AO & Ulstein MK. Measurement of human fetal blood flow. *Br. Med. J.* **280**:283, 1980.
6. Rudolph AM & Heymann MA. Circulatory changes during growth in the fetal lamb. *Circ. Res.* **26**:289, 1980.
7. Dawes GS. The umbilical circulation. In *Fetal and Neonatal Physiology*, p. 66. Chicago: Year Book Medical Publishers, 1968.
8. Itskovitz J, LaGamma EF & Rudolph AM. The effect of reducing umbilical blood flow on fetal oxygenation. *Am. J. Obstet. Gynecol.* **145**:813, 1983.
9. Trudinger BJ, Giles WB, Cook CM, Bombardieri J & Collins L. Fetal umbilical artery flow velocity waveforms and placental resistance: clinical significance. *Br. J. Obstet. Gynaecol.* **92**:23, 1985.
10. Thompson RS, Trudinger BJ & Cook CM. A comparison of Doppler ultrasound waveform indices in the umbilical artery. I: Indices derived from the maximum velocity waveform. *Ultrasound Med. Biol.* **12**:835, 1986.
11. Thompson RS, Trudinger BJ & Cook CM. Doppler ultrasound waveform indices. AB ratio pulsatility index and Pourcelot ratio. *Br. J. Obstet. Gynaecol.* **95**:581, 1988.

12. Mehalex KE, Rosenberg J, Berkowtiz GS, Chitkara U & Berkowitz RL. Umbilical and uterine artery flow velocity waveforms. Effect of the sampling site on Doppler ratios. *J. Ultrasound Med.* **8**:171, 1989.
13. O'Rourke MF. Vascular impedance in studies of arterial and cardiac function. *Physiol. Rev.* **62**:571, 1982.
14. Giles WB, Trudinger BJ & Baird P. Fetal umbilical artery flow velocity waveforms and placental resistance: Pathological correlation. *Br. J. Obstet. Gynaecol.* **92**:31, 1985.
15. Thompson RS & Stevens RJ. A mathematical mode for interpretation of Doppler velocity waveform indices. *Med. Biol. Eng. Comput.* **27**:269, 1989.
16. Thompson RS & Trudinger BJ. Doppler waveform pulsatility index and resistance, pressure and flow in the umbilical placental circulation: an investigation using a mathematical model. *Ultrasound Med. Biol.* **16**:449, 1990.
17. Trudinger BJ, Stevens D & Connelly A et al. Umbilical artery flow velocity waveforms and placental resistance: the effects of embolization on the umbilical circulation. *Am. J. Obstet. Gynecol.* **157**:1443, 1987.
18. Schulman H, Fleischer A, Stern W, Farmakides G, Jagani N, Blottner P. Umbilical velocity wave ratios in human pregnancy. *Am. J. Obstet. Gynecol.* **148**:986, 1984.
19. Reuwer PJHM, Bruinse HW, Stoutenbeek P, Haspels AA. Doppler assessment of the feto-placental circulation in normal and growth retarded fetuses. *Eur. J. Obstet. Gynaecol. Reprod. Biol.* **18**:199, 1984.
20. Erskine RLA & Ritchie JWK. Umbilical artery blood flow characteristics in normal growth retarded fetuses. *Br. J. Obstet. Gynaecol.* **92**:605, 1985.
21. Gudmundsson S & Marsal K. Umbilical and uteroplacental blood flow velocity waveforms in pregnancies with fetal growth retardation. *Eur. J. Obstet. Gynecol. Reprod. Biol.* **27**:187, 1988.
22. Trudinger BJ, Giles WB & Cook CM. Flow velocity waveforms in the maternal uteroplacental and fetal umbilical placental circulation. *Am. J. Obstet. Gynecol.* **92**:155, 1985.
23. Burke G, Stuart B, Crowley P, Sconaill S & Drumm J. Is intrauterine growth retardation with normal umbilical artery blood flow a benign condition? *Br. Med. J.* **300**:1044–1045, 1990.
24. Reuwer PJHM, Sijmons EA, Rietman GW, Van Tiel MWM & Bruinse HW. Intrauterine growth retardation: prediction of perinatal distress by Doppler ultrasound. *Lancet* **2**:415–418, 1987.
25. Trudinger BJ, Cook CM, Giles WB et al. Fetal umbilical artery velocity waveforms and subsequent neonatal outcome. *Br. J. Obstet. Gynaecol.* **98**:378, 1991.
26. Trudinger BJ, Cook CM, Jones L & Giles WB. A comparison of fetal heart rate monitoring and umbilical artery waveforms in the recognition of fetal compromise. *Br. J. Obstet. Gynaecol.* **93**:171, 1986.
27. Farmakides G, Schulman H & Winter D et al. Prenatal surveillance using non-stress testing and Doppler velocimetry. *Obstet. Gynecol.* **71**:184, 1988.
28. Berkowitz GS, Chitkara U, Rosenberg J et al. Sonographic estimation of fetal weight and Doppler analysis of umbilical artery velocimetry in the prediction of intrauterine growth retardation: a prospective study. *Am. J. Obstet. Gynecol.* **158**:1149, 1988.
29. Chambers SE, Hoskins PR, Haddad NG, Johnstone FD, McDicken WN & Muir BB. A comparison of fetal abdominal circumference measurements and Doppler ultrasound in the prediction of small-for-dates babies and fetal compromise. *Br. J. Obstet. Gynaecol.* **96**:803, 1989.
30. Chang TC, Robson SC, Spencer JAD & Gallivan S. Identification of fetal growth retardation: comparison of Doppler waveform indices and serial ultrasound measurements of abdominal circumference and fetal weight. *Obstet. Gynecol.* **82**:230–236, 1993.
31. Newnham JP, Patterson LC, James IR, Diepeveen DA & Reid SE. An evaluation of the efficacy of Doppler flow velocity waveform analysis as a screening test in pregnancy. *Am. J. Obstet. Gynecol.* **162**:403, 1990.
32. Soothill PW, Nicolaides KH, Bilardo CM & Campbell S. Relation of fetal hypoxia in growth retardation to mean blood velocity in the fetal aorta. *Lancet* **2**:1118, 1986.
33. Nicolaides KH, Bilardo CM, Soothill PW & Campbell S. Absence of end diastolic frequencies in umbilical artery: a sign of fetal hypoxia and acidosis. *Br. Med. J.* **297**:1026, 1988.
34. Bilardo CM, Nicolaides KH, Campbell S. Doppler measurements of fetal and uteroplacental circulations: relationship with umbilical venous blood gases measured at cordocentesis. *Am. J. Obstet. Gynecol.* **162**:115, 1990.
35. Tyrrell S, Obaid AH & Lilford RJ. Umbilical artery Doppler velocimetry as a predictor of fetal hypoxia and acidosis at birth. *Obstet. Gynecol.* **74**:332, 1989.
36. Trudinger BJ & Cook CM. Doppler umbilical and uterine flow waveforms in severe pregnancy hypertension. *Br. J. Obstet. Gynaecol.* **97**:142, 1990.
37. Landon MB, Gabbe SG, Bruner JP & Ludmir J. Doppler umbilical artery velocimetry in pregnancy complicated by insulin-dependent diabetes mellitus. *Obstet. Gynecol.* **73**:961, 1989.
38. Johnstone FD, Steel JH, Haddad NG, Hoskins PR, Green IA & Chambers S. Doppler umbilical artery flow velocity waveforms in diabetic pregnancy. *Obstet. Gynecol.* **99**:135, 1992.
39. Giles WB, Trudinger BJ & Cook CM. Fetal umbilical artery flow velocity time waveforms in twin pregnancies. *Br. J. Obstet. Gynaecol.* **92**:490, 1985.
40. Giles WB, Trudinger BJ, Cook CM & Connelly A. Umbilical artery flow velocity waveforms and twin pregnancy outcome. *Obstet. Gynecol.* **72**:894, 1988.
41. Farmakides G, Schulman H, Saldana LR et al. Surveillance of twin pregnancy with umbilical arterial velocimetry. *Am. J. Obstet. Gynecol.* **153**:789, 1985.
42. Trudinger BJ, Stewart G, Cook CM, Connelly A & Exner T. Monitoring lupus anticoagulant positive pregnancies with umbilical artery flow velocity waveforms. *Obstet. Gynecol.* **72**:215, 1988.
43. Alfirevic Z & Neilson JP. Doppler ultrasonography in high risk pregnancies: systematic review with meta-analysis. *Am. J. Obstet. Gynecol.* **172**:1379–1387, 1995.
44. Jouppila P & Kirkinen P. Increased vascular resistance in the descending aorta of the human fetus in hypoxia. *Br. J. Obstet. Gynaecol.* **91**:853, 1984.
45. Tonge HM, Wladimiroff JW, Noordam MH & van Kooten C. Blood flow velocity waveforms in the descending fetal aorta: comparison between normal and growth retarded pregnancies. *Obset. Gynecol.* **17**:851, 1986.
46. Lingman G & Marsal K. Fetal central blood circulation in the third trimester of normal pregnancy. A longitudinal study. I: Aortic and umbilical blood flow. *Early Hum. Dev.* **13**:137, 1986.
47. Lingman G & Marsal K. Fetal central blood circulation in the third trimester of normal pregnancy. A longitudinal study. II: Aortic blood velocity waveform. *Early Hum. Dev.* **13**:151, 1986.
48. Thompson RS, Trudinger BT, Reed VD & Turner AJ. Aortic Doppler velocity measurements and cardiac function in the fetal lamb. *Ultrasound Med. Biol.* **20**:893–902, 1994.
49. Wladimiroff JW, Tonge HM & Stewart PA. Doppler ultrasound assessment of cerebral blood flow in the human fetus. *Br. J. Obstet. Gynaecol.* **93**:471, 1986.
50. Arbeille Ph, Roncin A, Berson M, Patat F & Pourcelot L. Exploration of the fetal cerebral blood flow by duplex Doppler-linear array system in normal and pathological pregnancies. *Ultrasound Med. Biol.* **13**:329, 1987.
51. Woo JSK, Liang ST, Lo RLS & Chan FY. Middle cerebral artery Doppler flow velocity waveforms. *Obstet. Gynecol.* **70**:613, 1987.
52. Vyas S, Nicolaides KH, Bower S & Campbell S. Middle cerebral artery flow velocity waveform in fetal hypoxaemia. *Br. J. Obstet. Gynaecol.* **97**:797, 1990.
53. Arias F. Accuracy of the middle cerebral to umbilical artery resistance index ratio in the production of neonatal outcome in patients at high risk for fetal and neonatal complications. *Am. J. Obstet. Gynecol.* **171**:1541, 1994.
54. Mari G, Abuhamad AZ, Pirhonen J, Jones DC, Ludomirsky A & Copel JA. Diagnosis of fetal anaemia with Doppler ultrasound in the pregnancy complicated by maternal blood group immunisation. *Ultrasound Obstet. Gynecol.* **5**:400, 1995.
55. Mari G. Arterial blood flow velocity waveforms of the pelvis and lower extremities in normal and growth retarded fetuses. *Am. J. Obstet. Gynecol.* **165**:143–151, 1991.
56. Sepulveda W, Bower S, Nicolaidis P, de Swiet M and Fisk NH. Discordant blood from velocity waveform in left and right brachial arteries in growth retarded fetuses. *Obstet. Gynecol.* **86**:734–738, 1995.
57. Arduini D & Rizzo G. Fetal renal artery velocity waveforms and amniotic fluid volume in growth retarded and post term fetuses. *Obstet. Gynecol.* **77**:370–373, 1991.

58. Abuhamad AZ, Mari G, Bogdan D & Evans AT. Doppler flow velocimetry of the splenic artery in the human fetus: is it a marker of chronic hypoxia? *Am. J. Obstet. Gynecol.* **172**:820–825, 1995.
59. Mori A, Trudinger BJ, Mori R, Reed V & Takeda Y. The fetal central venous pressure waveform in normal pregnancy and in umbilical placental insufficiency. *Am. J. Obstet. Gynecol.* **172**:51–57, 1995.
60. Kiserud T, Eik-Nes S, Blaas H & Hellevik LR. Ultrasonographic velocimetry of the fetal ductus venosus. *Lancet* **338**:1412–1414, 1991.
61. Rizzo G, Capponi A, Talone PE, Arduini D & Romanini C. Doppler indices from inferior vena cava and ductus venosus in predicting pH and oxygen tension in umbilical blood at cordocentesis in growth retarded fetuses. *Ultrasound Obstet. Gynecol.* **7**:401–410, 1996.
62. Rizzo G & Arduini D. Fetal cardiac function in intrauterine growth retardation. *Am. J. Obstet. Gynecol.* **165**:876, 1991.
63. Reed KL, Anderson CF & Shenker L. Changes in intra cardiac Doppler blood flow velocities in fetuses with absent umbilical artery diastolic flow. *Am. J. Obstet. Gynecol.* **157**:774, 1990.
64. Rizzo G, Capponi A, Arduini D, Romanini C. The value of fetal arterial cardiac and venous flow in predicting pH and blood gases in umbilical blood at cordocentesis in growth retarded fetuses. *Br. J. Obstet. Gynaecol.* **102**:963, 1995.
65. Hecher K, Snijders R, Campbell S & Nicolaides S. Fetal venous, intracardiac and arterial blood flow in intrauterine growth retardation. Relationship with blood gases. *Am. J. Obstet. Gynecol.* **173**:10–15, 1995.
66. Indik J, Chen V & Reed KL. Association of umbilical venous with inferior vena cava velocities. *Obstet. Gynecol.* **77**:551, 1991.
67. Cohen-Overbeek T, Pearce JM & Campbell S. The anteantal assessment of utero-placental and feto-placental blood flow using Doppler ultrasound. *Ultrasound Med. Biol.* **11**:329, 1985.
68. Trudinger BJ, Giles WB & Cook CM. Uteroplacental blood flow velocity time waveforms in normal and complicated pregnancy. *Br. J. Obstet. Gynaecol.* **92**:39, 1985.
69. Bower S, Schucther K & Campbell S. Doppler ultrasound screening as part of routine antenatal screening: prediction of preeclampsia and intrauterine growth retardation. *Br. J. Obstet. Gynaecol.* **100**:989–994, 1993.
70. Hanretty KP, Whittle M & Rubin PC. Doppler uteroplacental waveforms in pregnancy induced hypertension: a reappraisal. *Lancet* **1**:850, 1988.
71. Jacobson S-L, Imhof R & Manning N et al. The value of Doppler assessment of the uteroplacental circulation in predicting preeclampsia or intrauterine growth retardation. *Am. J. Obstet. Gynecol.* **162**:110, 1989.
72. Harrington K, Cooper D, Lees C, Hecher K & Campbell S. Doppler ultrasound of the uterine arteries: the importance of bilateral notching in the prediction of preeclampsia, placental abruption or delivery of a small for gestational age baby. *Ultrasound Obstet. Gynecol.* **7**:182–188, 1996.
73. Jauniaux E, Jurkovic D & Campbell S. In vivo investigation of the anatomy and the physiology on early human placental circulations. *Ultrasound Obstet. Gynecol.* **1**:435–445, 1991.
74. Stabile I, Grudzinskas J & Campbell S. Doppler ultrasonographic evaluation of abnormal pregnancies in the first trimester. *J. Clin. Ultrasound* **18**:497–501, 1990.

Day assessment units

73

J.G. Rodriguez, C. Bobrow and P.W. Soothill

Introduction

The term day assessment unit (DAU) describes the organization of antenatal testing into an outpatient unit. Without a DAU the various tests to assess the mother and fetus are often undertaken by different people in different locations. For example, fetal movement monitoring may be by the mother at home, fetal growth, amniotic fluid (AF) volume and biophysical profile (BPP) in the antenatal clinic or ultrasound department and Dopplers in a fetal medicine unit or referral centre. This can make it not only time consuming for the patient but also difficult to obtain all the information at a time when the clinician can counsel the patient and make decisions. Because of this, in the past patients have often been admitted for 'assessment of fetal well-being' simply to help organization.

The tests involved with maternal and fetal assessment can nearly always be done within 90 min and for many clinical indications when the results are normal testing will not need to be repeated. Sometimes serial investigation is required (e.g. every week) but only very rarely is it necessary for testing to be repeated more than once a day. For these reasons, provided the patient is mobile and lives within a reasonable distance from the hospital, assessment of maternal and fetal well-being can nearly always be done on an outpatient basis. This avoids admission to hospital which is expensive and may have serious adverse social consequences for the patient.

In this chapter we discuss the advantages and disadvantages of reorganizing antenatal testing into a DAU and what is required to do so. We then look at some of the indications for referral, the tests used and finally offer some policy suggestions of how to investigate specific problems.

What is a day assessment unit?

A DAU offers a fetal and maternal well-being testing service on an outpatient basis often run by midwives but with the clinical responsibility remaining with the booking consultant. Other terms sometimes used for the same concept include 'antenatal assessment unit' or 'fetal assessment unit'. Referrals come from antenatal clinics, in-patient wards, community midwives, general practitioners or patient self-referrals but whatever the source of the referral, since responsibility remains with the consultant team, any abnormal results must be transmitted to those doctors promptly. The consultant team must counsel the patient about the results and manage any abnormalities. The factors which distinguish a DAU from a fetal medicine unit (FMU) include:

- *Source of referral:* FMUs offer a consultant to consultant referral service for subspecialist advice in complicated pregnancies compared to the wider range of referrals to a DAU
- *Staff in the unit:* whilst DAUs are often operated by midwives with medical staff available to deal with any problems, FMUs tend to have permanent medical staff
- *Range of investigations and treatments offered:* FMUs tend to offer a much wider range of non-invasive and invasive procedures for prenatal diagnosis and also management of diverse fetal conditions often before viability. A DAU is usually for viable pregnancies (e.g. over 24 weeks' gestation) when delivery based on the results may be possible

The improved coordination and organization achieved after setting up a DAU can result in a decrease in the patients' waiting time, the number of admissions to hospital for 'assessment of fetal well-being' and also the length of such admissions when they occur. In one study the opening of a DAU was associated with a decrease of 22% in the antenatal bed occupancy as a result of both a shorter period from admission to delivery and from admission to antenatal discharge still pregnant (Fig. 73.1)[1]. The reason for this decrease in antenatal bed use was that obstetricians were more prepared to discharge antenatal patients from hospital when follow-up was

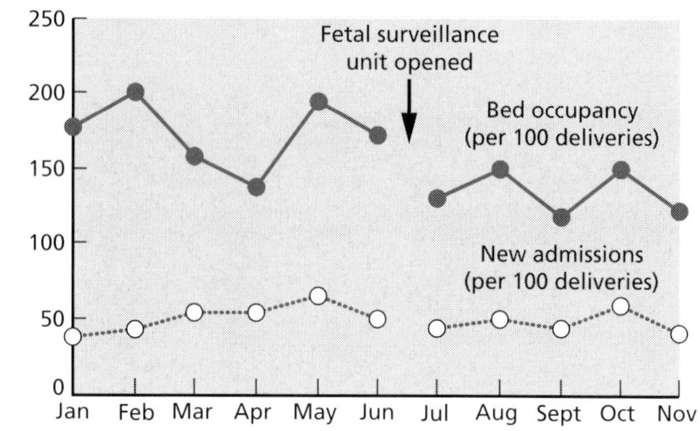

Fig. 73.1 Antenatal admission rate and bed occupancy for 6 months before and 5 months after a day assessment unit was opened[1].

well organized and similarly less likely to admit pregnant women for monitoring when a DAU service was available. Another important advantage of concentrating antenatal testing in one unit is that data can be more easily collected for audit and research. The use of appropriate databases allows collection of information in an organized, planned and prospective way. The concentration of high-risk pregnancies also makes gaining experience and teaching easier so DAUs are a good setting for teaching midwives, medical students and obstetricians.

The potential disadvantages of organizing antenatal testing into a DAU include the risk that the concentration of this work to a few people in each unit could reduce the training, experience and continuing education of generalists. If an obstetrician no longer undertakes the various tests concerned he or she may lose confidence in their use and interpretation. Another important disadvantage is that the patient and professionals can become confused about who is responsible for patient care, especially in DAU in which medical staff work and become known to the patient. As described earlier it is vital that responsibility remains entirely with the patient's obstetric team or alternatively that the DAU is clearly run as a fetal medicine unit. These problems can be avoided by good communication and coordination between the DAU staff, the patient and the patient's obstetric team.

Without great caution the availability of technology can increase investigation, anxiety and even medical intervention. This is especially true in the area of antenatal testing because the sensitivity and specificity of many of the tests used is low with significant false positive rates. Indeed since poor clinical practice can also involve using testing as a way of avoiding clinical decision making or requesting monitoring for inappropriate indications, it is not surprising that there is strong evidence that testing can worsen as well as improve patient care[2].

Resources required

The resources required for a DAU are already available in any hospital that is offering fetal and maternal well-being testing. Setting up a DAU requires a reorganization of existing resources including staff, space, equipment and hospital policies rather than a large new investment. On average for a 4500 deliveries/year maternity unit, one or two full-time midwives with appropriate support staff are required. The unit will occasionally require support from a fetal medicine unit because a DAU usually has no dedicated medical staff, so further equipment or expertise to perform a difficult investigation would need to be available. It is also vital that the unit is supported by the consultant teams and that they or their agreed deputies are available at short notice to review the patients when abnormalities are found.

In many hospitals it has been possible to locate a DAU in rooms previously dedicated to cardiotocography (CTG) or ultrasound or by using part of an existing antenatal ward because of the space saved by reduced antenatal admissions. For the reasons mentioned above it is an advantage if the DAU can be located close to a fetal medicine unit but only if everyone in the hospital understands the fundamentally different roles described in the previous section. An alternative is for the DAU to be close to the obstetric ultrasound scanning department if antenatal testing such as fetal growth measurement are still to be undertaken there.

If CTGs are to be offered there are advantages to obtaining a computerized analysis system such as the Dawes/Redman Sonicaid 8000[3] because these can provide an objective and numerical interpretation of the CTG which allow the unit to agree guidelines for staff and improve record keeping[4]. An imaging ultrasound machine is required for AF volume assessment, BPP and fetal growth measurements. A continuous wave Doppler machine is sufficient for umbilical artery blood velocity studies in singleton pregnancies (>95% of the cases) but for vessels within the fetus, assessment of multiple pregnancies or confirmation of a suspected abnormal continuous wave result a pulsed Doppler machine should be available. In many units pulsed wave Doppler tests are undertaken in the fetal medicine unit, so this expensive equipment could be shared. Adequate data collection and storage is vital and computer hardware and database software are available and important in that they can produce the units' reports and help keep good communication while collecting data for research and audit.

Fetal tests

There are many motives for the enormous effort expended in fetal monitoring, but the main goals should be to decrease perinatal mortality, handicap and unnecessary intervention in pregnancy. The absence at present of in-utero therapy for most fetal diseases means the main interventions available are the best timing of delivery and reassurance. However, while severe fetal growth deficiency, antepartum haemorrhage, preeclampsia, drug taking and infection are risk factors, in a large proportion of pregnancies in which a poor outcome occurs no indication for DAU testing is recognized. Furthermore, in such otherwise uncomplicated pregnancies there is no test which is established to predict injury or sudden intrauterine death.

The main difficulty in evaluating the value of antenatal testing is the absence of good outcome criteria. Mortality is too rare and too late to be useful. Morbidity at birth such as Apgar scores is often used but it is impossible to separate the effects of acute changes in labour or delivery from those present before the onset of labour, which therefore have the potential of being detected in a DAU. Long-term neurodevelopment can be assessed but this is highly multifactorial (including genetic and prenatal and postnatal environmental factors) and the neurodevelopmental tests themselves are subjective with significant inter- and intraobserver variability. For these reasons, events before birth may play a significant but difficult-to-detect part of the total variation in neurodevelopmental scores[5]. Also since these tests are best done when the children are at least 5 years old, by the time the research results are available obstetric and monitoring techniques are likely to have changed anyway.

The tests used in DAUs are described in detail in other parts of this book so in this chapter we will consider the issues relating to the use of each test in a DAU.

NON-STRESS CARDIOTOCOGRAPHY

In the 1980s the antenatal CTG was the main technique of fetal surveillance in many British hospitals[6] but it has been difficult to show any beneficial effect on perinatal outcome despite 13 trials[2]. The CTG has one great advantage in that although it may take 20–40 min to complete, once the trace has been started the DAU midwife can usually leave the patient and continue with other work, only returning every 10 min to see when it can be stopped. The major disadvantage is that while superficially interpretation can seem simple (e.g. reactive or non-reactive defined by the occurrence of two accelerations of at least 15 beats per minute sustained for at least 15 s. within a 20 min period[7]) this is obviously a gross oversimplification. In practice CTG analysis includes baseline variability and rate, and it is vital to assess a CTG in the context of the clinical situation and indication for the test[8]. Therefore it is very hard to provide training or guidelines for midwives working in a DAU as to which CTGs need to be reviewed by the consultant team. Furthermore, the lack of objective patterns of diagnosis and the existence of a paper record which can be disputed at a medicolegal enquiry in the event of bad outcome, make the CTG test dangerous for litigation against the DAU. This can be partially addressed by computer CTG analysers which have the advantage of being objective and closely agreeing with experienced visual assessment[4]. This can allow the unit to develop guidelines for when senior medical staff do not need to be called and so reduce the time pregnant women spend waiting in a DAU. These analysis systems also provide numeric data which can be used in research and reliable record storage for audit.

The second problem about offering CTGs in a DAU is that the predictive value of a positive non-stress antenatal CTG test is below 40% for perinatal mortality and morbidity in most studies[9]. There has rightly been criticism of the application of the CTG in clinical management before it was shown to be beneficial. For example a meta-analysis of the randomized trials assessing the effects of antepartum fetal heart rate testing on fetal outcome and pregnancy management provides:

> no support at all for the use of antepartum CTG as an intermittent supplementary test of fetal well-being in high risk pregnancies[2].

Indeed the analysis showed its use as a prenatal assessment test of fetal well-being was associated with a threefold *increase* of perinatal mortality[2]. Therefore in our view the use of the CTG should be carefully audited and undertaken after informed patient consent. The false positive rate of the contraction stress tests means it is almost never used in the United Kingdom.

AMNIOTIC FLUID VOLUME

Obstetricians who undertake little scanning themselves often do not appreciate how difficult it is to assess the AF volume. There are three techniques; subjective impression (reduced, normal, or increased), measurements of the largest single vertical pocket of fluid, or the AF index which sums the largest vertical fluid pockets in each of the four quadrants of the uterus. All three can be markedly changed by factors including when the fetus alters position, if the fetus empties its bladder, the state of maternal hydration and amniotic fluid leakage. It is therefore not surprising that all these assessments have similar and very low sensitivities in predicting perinatal morbidity[10]. A disadvantage of the subjective method for assessing AF volume compared with quantitative methods is that training is longer and requires greater experience in scanning. Therefore quantitative methods offer some advantages for the training of midwives in AF volume assessment in a DAU.

Polyhydramnios and oligohydramnios are associated with increased perinatal morbidity and mortality because a fetal disease or pregnancy complication is often present[11,12] so these patients should have a fetal medicine assessment first and then the follow up can be done in a DAU. Polyhydramnios is associated with fetal anomalies, preterm labour, diabetes, multiple gestation and twin-to-twin transfusion[11]. Oligohydramnios is associated with uteroplacental insufficiency, premature rupture of membranes, fetal renal disease and post-dates pregnancies. Oligohydramnios associated with placental insufficiency is secondary to fetal oliguria, the degree of reduction in the hourly urine rate correlating with the degree of hypoxaemia[13] and Doppler studies reveal an increase in downstream resistance in the renal artery[14]. In contrast to placental insufficiency, Doppler studies do not support a renovascular mechanism with redistribution of blood flow in post-mature fetuses[15].

BIOPHYSICAL PROFILE

The BPP is a difficult and time-consuming test to undertake in a DAU because the scan of fetal activity may take 30 min and the CTG also required may need another 40 min. Also the patient may have to wait for each of these machines to become available. Other significant problems include that while two of the five factors (body movements, tone) are not independent they are treated as such in the scoring system used and fetal behaviour states can lead to a normal cessation of movements for up to 40 min. In addition the AF volume and CTG assessments have their own problems described in the sections above.

Since fetal death is a rare event the false negative rate for the BPP in predicting mortality is of course low (about 0.7 per 1000). The false positive rate in the same population has been reported to be around 70%, which can be expected to result in unnecessary intervention and its associated maternal and neonatal morbidity and mortality[16]. The relationship between the BPP and outcome (as defined by fetal death, operative intervention for fetal distress, small for gestational age (SGA), 5 min APGAR < 7 and pH < 7.20) appears to be a direct relationship, but since even a borderline BPP is associated with at least 6 fold increase in perinatal mortality[16,17] this test is obviously too late for ideal management.

DOPPLER STUDIES

Doppler of the umbilical artery is a simple, reproducible test which is easily taught to DAU midwives and takes only a few minutes when the operator is skilled. Continuous-wave machines are the simplest and most economic systems, but have the disadvantage that movement anywhere along the path of the sound will be detected. As a result, continuous-wave Doppler can only be used to study vessels which can be reliably identified by their blood velocity waveform patterns, such as the umbilical cord vessels. This is why impedance indices in the umbilical artery are the only Doppler tests used in most DAUs. The pulsatility index is probably the most versatile assessment of this vessel because absent end-diastolic blood flow is a common pathological finding in this circulation and this measurement allows quantification even when the diastolic Doppler shift is zero (see Ch. 72).

Meta-analysis of the published randomized trials shows the use of umbilical artery Doppler ultrasound during high-risk pregnancy is associated with a reduction in perinatal mortality of about 35% when the results are made available to clinicians[18]. In high-risk pregnancies Doppler has good sensitivity and negative predictive values for subsequent fetal distress in appropriately grown and SGA fetuses[19,20]. It has also been shown that umbilical artery Doppler is useful in discriminating between small fetuses at risk of morbidity and those who are healthy but small[21]. Doppler has been evaluated more rigorously and extensively than any other test of fetal health or fetoplacental function. The weight of evidence is now so great that this test should be available in every DAU and in our view further trials of Doppler should probably not include randomization to concealing the results from the clinicians.

Ideally when abnormalities are found in umbilical artery Doppler testing in a DAU with continuous wave equipment, the result should be confirmed with pulsed wave Doppler and probably middle cerebral artery and aorta blood velocity studies before precipitating delivery. Consideration should also be given to causes other than uteroplacental insufficiency such as chromosomal[22] or cardiac abnormality. Furthermore, some fetuses can compensate for a long time and even tolerate labour in chronic hypoxaemia, so for all these reasons cases with abnormal Doppler should be carefully investigated and managed individually.

FETAL GROWTH

An important indication for referral to DAU (about 8% in our series) is when a fetus is thought to be SGA. If the referral is made without first confirming this diagnosis by ultrasound assessment, fetal measurement is obviously the initial test to undertake. Ultrasound abdominal and head circumference measurements are the best way of assessing fetal size and these measurements should be plotted in relation to gestational age. Even in expert hands the estimated fetal weight calculated from ultrasound measurements is only accurate to ±12%, which is clinically useful when the weight is around 1 kg but not when the weight is greater than 3 kg. Fetal growth measurements should be made by experienced sonographers and in many units are better done in the ultrasound department rather than a DAU unless these are combined. Interpretation of the results should include assessment of growth symmetry and growth velocity in addition to the plotted centile position[23,24].

FETAL MOVEMENT COUNTING

Maternal assessment of fetal movements is encouraged in antenatal clinics, especially in those patients who have fetal risk factors, and a 'count-to-ten kick chart' is frequently given to patients as a follow-up after reassessing results in a DAU. The kick-count test is considered abnormal if there are <10 movements between 0800 and 1800 h, at which point the patient is asked to reattend the hospital.

However, fetal movements testing has a number of problems. Biological factors also affect fetal activity, including the developmental stage of fetal behavioural states. Fetal gross body movements occur approximately 10% of the time in the last 10 weeks of pregnancy with an average of 31 movements per hour, but maternal perception of fetal activity can be misleading as some movements go undetected. Similarly Braxton–Hicks contractions, maternal aortic pulsation or respiration can be wrongly recorded. Other important considerations include gestational age, time of day, relationship to maternal food or drug ingestion and obesity. Randomized trials suggest routine fetal movement counting is of no value[25]. However, kick-count charts may be used to reassure patients after obtaining normal results in a woman presenting with decreased fetal movements. More general use of this technique runs the risk of passing the guilt for a bad outcome from the health team to the mother.

BLOOD PRESSURE PROFILE

The measurement of blood pressure is a part of routine antenatal care, and the accuracy of any one recording carries significance for the future management of that patient. However, this is also one of the most difficult clinical measurements and both the British Hypertension Society and the American Heart Association[26,27] have made recommendations as to how it should be done. Blood pressure is recorded while the patient is relaxed in either a sitting or left lateral position. The forearm should be relaxed and supported at the level of the heart and the sphygmomanometer should be placed so that the 90 mmHg mark is at eye level. The correct width of cuff is extremely important and should be equivalent to 40% of the midarm circumference, which for the average adult is 12 cm. The brachial artery should be located to ensure correct placement of the stethoscope bell. The systolic pressure should be estimated before the operator uses the stethoscope by palpation of the brachial artery and inflation of the cuff until the pulsations disappear especially in patients in whom the auscultatory endpoints may be difficult to judge accurately. Ideally, the blood pressure should be measured in both arms and if there is a difference of >10 mmHg in the diastolic or >20 mmHg in the systolic, both should be recorded on each occasion; otherwise the blood pressure can be recorded in either arm.

As a result of the hyperdynamic state of pregnancy, Korotkoff-like sounds may be heard over the brachial artery without any pressure being applied to the cuff. The controversy as to which Korotkoff phase is the best estimate of diastolic blood pressure in pregnancy has led to diverging recommendations and a random use of both measurements. A review[28] of this subject summarized the available evidence regarding Korotkoff phases IV and V in pregnancy concluding that Korotkoff phase V better represents intra-arterial diastolic blood pressure and can be determined in >98% of gravid women. That review also concluded that the measurement of Korotkoff phase IV appears to be accompanied by more observer variability than does phase V and exceeds phase V by a clinically significant amount. For these reason the use of phase IV levels may lead to an inappropriate diagnosis of hypertension in a significant number of women.

When a rise in blood pressure is found it is recommended that at least two auscultatory measurements should be made and if these do not agree further readings should be taken. The reason for this recommendation is the knowledge that sometimes blood pressures recorded by the patients at home are lower than pressures recorded by the physicians in clinics. This 'white coat hypertension' is defined as a persistently elevated clinic pressure with normal blood pressure at other times and occurs in up to 20% of patients with mild hypertension[29]. The difficulty of blood pressure measurements makes it a very sensible test to investigate in a DAU as a 'blood pressure series'. This can be three to five serial measurements done in an expert way over a morning or afternoon.

Fetal management protocols

This section assumes that the DAU is a centralized surveillance unit run by midwives offering the range of tests described above, that the staff do not make obstetric management decisions and that referrals must be after the obstetric team considers the fetus viable, usually after 26 weeks. The most common indications for referral to our DAU are shown in Table 73.1. In this section we make some suggestions about how to use the tests described for the different indications.

TABLE 73.1
Indications for referral in a 6-month period (January–June 1996) to the DAU in St Michael's Hospital, Bristol, which has about 5000 deliveries per year. The figures are for the number of visits to the unit, not the number of new referrals

Indication	Number of visits	%
Post-term pregnancy	320	22
Hypertension	250	17
Decreased fetal movements	187	13
Small for gestational age	115	8
Oligohydramnios/polyhydramnios	97	7
Antepartum haemorrhage	35	2
Maternal diabetes	31	2
Preterm premature rupture of membranes	24	2
Others (obstetric history, anxiety, presentation, etc.)	388	27
Total	1447	100

ALL REFERRALS

Regardless of the indication for referral we use the Fetal Database (Viewpoint, Bildverarbeitung GmbH. Gilching, Germany) at the first visit to record the demographic details, brief obstetric history and review of the obstetric notes (carried by the patients). Basic antenatal maternal variables such as blood pressure, urine testing, measurement of symphysis-fundal height are also noted. The investigations offered include CTG, BPP, AF volume and Doppler studies of the fetoplacental circulation but which tests are done in a particular case depends on the request from the referring team and the indication. All the results are entered into the computer program which produces a clinical spread sheet to be inserted into the notes carried by the patient.

POST-TERM PREGNANCY

By definition, a term pregnancy is 38 to 42 weeks so post-term is when a pregnancy exceeds 294 days or 42 weeks. One of the major problems in delineating the extent of risk beyond term relates to the limited reliability of the last menstrual period as a basis for accurately predicting gestational age and so with routine ultrasound dating the true incidence of post-term gestation is probably lower than previously thought. Nevertheless, virtually all reports suggest a small increase in perinatal morbidity and mortality beyond 42 weeks' gestation. Two key issues remain:

- Is there any antenatal test that can reliably predict complications and so provide reassurance?
- Should all patients who reach 42 weeks' gestational age including those with an unripe cervix be offered induction of labour?

The most common antenatal monitoring approach is to use AF Volume and CTG assessment two to three times a week beginning at 41–42 weeks' gestational age (Fig. 73.2). A possible mechanism of the increased morbidity in this group may be cord compression, so it is reasonable to assess the AF volume[30,31]. Although the CTG is good at detecting decelerations associated with cord compression its use as a single technique to evaluate the post-term gestation is not recommended because the risk of stillbirth within 1 week of a reactive CTG is still high[32]. Most studies reported to date suggest that there is no significant relationship between umbilical artery Doppler blood velocity and outcome in post-term fetuses who are not also SGA and so there seems little point in using this test in these cases.

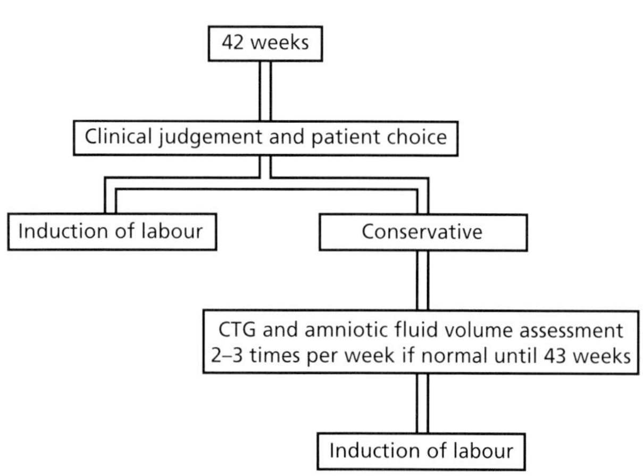

Fig. 73.2 A suggested protocol for DAU monitoring of post-term pregnancies after exclusion of other risk factors.

HYPERTENSION

In women with high blood pressure the main predictor of fetal risk is whether the mother has preeclampsia or chronic hypertension[33] with the former being associated with a much higher fetal risk. This distinction is made by maternal testing as described later under maternal management protocols. Fetal surveillance should include serial ultrasound evaluation of fetal growth, AF volume and umbilical artery Doppler if the fetus is found to be SGA in women with preeclampsia from around 26 weeks. In severe chronic hypertension a similar testing regime may be used from about 34 weeks.

DECREASED FETAL MOVEMENTS

Cessation of maternal perception of fetal movements may be a premortem event. The mother may notice a sharp change in the fetal movements or simply a subconscious sensation of something wrong. What might be normal for one woman – pregnancy–fetus–gestational age combination – may be different for another woman. Provided there is no maternal or fetal condition to explain decreased fetal movements, assessment of the fetus should include an ultrasound scan to confirm normal fetal size, show the fetal movements to the mother and assess the AF volume. A CTG may help, especially if the fetus is found not to be moving on the scan (Fig. 73.3).

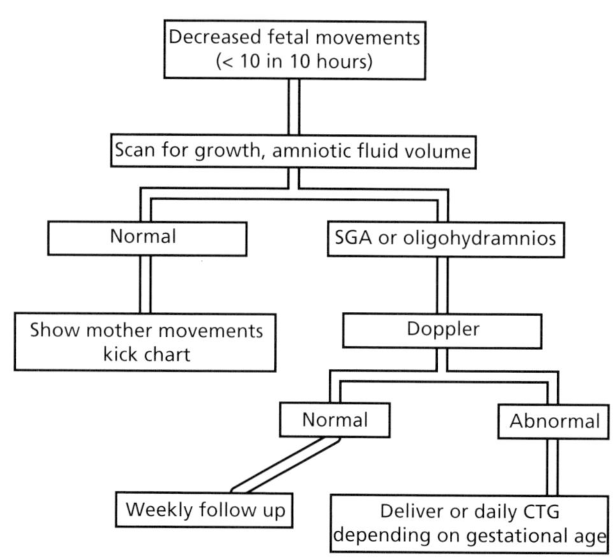

Fig. 73.3 A suggested protocol for the DAU monitoring of pregnancies with decreased fetal movements.

After normal results the mother may wish to monitor the fetal movements with a 'kick chart' although anxiety may be both a cause and complication of some of these cases.

SMALL FOR GESTATIONAL AGE

When ultrasound measurements suggest a fetus is small for gestational age outpatient monitoring in a DAU may be very useful. Since abnormalities in umbilical artery Doppler studies usually occur much earlier than other tests this is the best way of detecting which SGA pregnancies are at highest risk. The frequency with which a normal Doppler needs to be repeated depends on gestational age, background risk factors, presence or absence of maternal vascular disease and the result of the Doppler test itself, but usually this would be once a week. If an abnormal Doppler waveform result is detected with continuous wave equipment it should be confirmed with pulsed Doppler equipment as described in the section on fetal tests. There is no justification to undertake the BPP or CTG in SGA pregnancies if the Doppler and AF volume are normal. We only use the CTG when Doppler testing is abnormal but we are trying to continue the pregnancy as a result of extreme prematurity (Fig. 73.4).

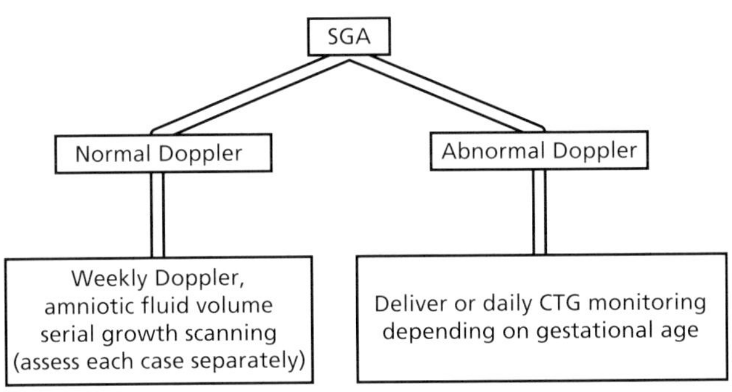

Fig. 73.4 A suggested protocol for the DAU monitoring of pregnancies with small-for-gestational-age fetuses.

OLIGOHYDRAMNIOS/POLYHYDRAMNIOS

Oligohydramnios is associated with premature rupture of membranes, postmaturity, fetal anomalies and hypoxaemia from placental insufficiency and in fewer than 10% of patients with oligohydramnios, an explanation cannot be found. DAU management will depend on the underlying cause and we discuss the fetal testing policies in preterm premature rupture of membranes, intrauterine growth deficiency and postmaturity in other sections of this chapter. Polyhydramnios can be associated with diabetes mellitus, fetal abnormalities such as obstruction of the gastrointestinal tract, neurological impairment of swallowing, twin-to-twin transfusion, high-output cardiac failure and congenital infection. The incidence of idiopathic polyhydramnios is related to the severity, with a cause being identified in 75–91% with a deepest pocket >12 cm versus 17–29% when the deepest pocket is 8–12 cm[34,35]. Maternal testing for diabetes is discussed elsewhere so no DAU protocol is offered. Because of the risk of fetal abnormality in both oligohydramnios and polyhydramnios these patients should be assessed first in a fetal medicine unit.

ANTEPARTUM HAEMORRHAGE

Referral to DAU for antepartum haemorrhage should be after clinical and ultrasound exclusion of placenta praevia and abruption. While this group is at greatly increased risk of perinatal morbidity and mortality this seems to be more related to premature delivery than placental dysfunction. Serial scanning to assess fetal growth and AF volume may be reasonable (Fig. 73.5) but CTG and umbilical artery Doppler are not useful for predicting outcome in patients with unexplained antepartum haemorrhage[36].

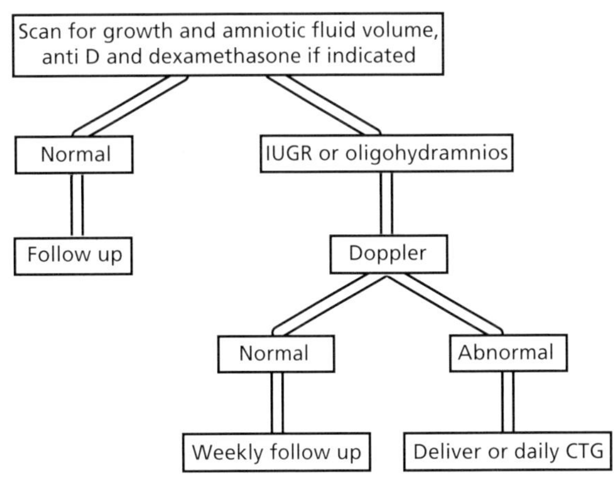

Fig. 73.5 A suggested protocol for DAU monitoring of antepartum haemorrhage.

Maternal management protocols

Most of the issues concerning outpatient antenatal monitoring of the fetal condition also apply to monitoring of the maternal condition. The only exceptions relate to maternal conditions in which a serious complication can occur before the mother could return to hospital, such as in preeclampsia, unstable lie, etc. We now discuss maternal testing in the three commonest maternal indications for referral to DAU; hypertension, diabetes and preterm premature rupture of membranes.

HYPERTENSION

High blood pressure in pregnancy can be classified as preeclampsia or chronic hypertension even if the latter is first revealed by the effects of pregnancy. This is an extremely important distinction because the prognosis and management of these conditions are completely different. Patients with proteinuric hypertension (preeclampsia) should be admitted to hospital, so the DAU would only be involved in the diagnosis of this condition. This is in contrast to chronic and transient hypertension which can be managed on an outpatient basis and are not associated with increased fetal mortality or morbidity. In general preeclampsia occurs after 20 weeks and the diagnosis is based on the association of hypertension (140/90 mmHg) and proteinuria (>300 mg/l in a 24 h urine collection) in the absence of a urinary tract infection. Chronic hypertension is defined as a persistent elevation in blood pressure of 140/90 mmHg or greater which may be called transient if not present before 20 weeks and settles within 6 weeks postpartum[37].

The assessment of a pregnant woman with high blood pressure starts with the medical history including the onset of hypertension, previous medical conditions such as renal disease, migraine, obstetric history, current symptoms (e.g. cerebral or visual disturbances, epigastric pain) and signs such as oedema. Blood tests may include haemoglobin concentration, platelet count, liver function tests (e.g. aspartate amino transferase), renal function tests (e.g. uric acid, urea, creatinine) and urine tests for proteinuria and microbiology are important. If the disease appears severe a coagulation profile (prothrombin time, APTT, fibrinogen) should be assessed. If the diagnosis is preeclampsia the patient should be admitted and managed as an inpatient. Patients with severe chronic hypertension should be managed in a joint medical antenatal clinic with a physician but monitoring periodically in the DAU for assessment of hypertension, blood and urine testing and assessment of fetal well-being may be useful (Fig. 73.6). The frequency of these visits should be determined by the severity, gestational age and other associated clinical conditions.

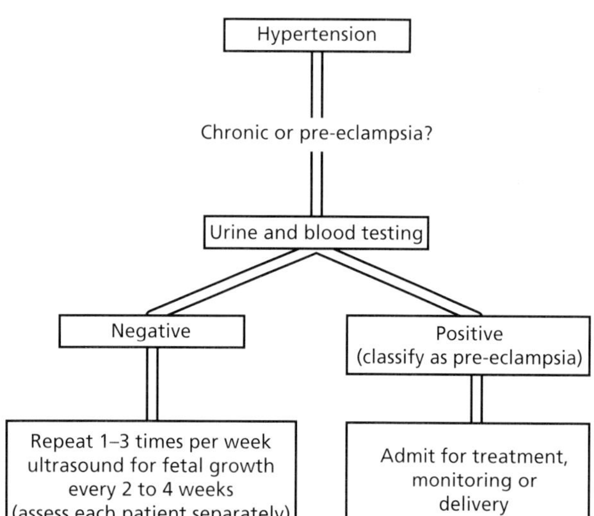

Fig. 73.6 A suggested protocol for DAU monitoring of pregnancies complicated with hypertension.

DIABETES

The management of a mother with diabetes should be shared between a physician and obstetrician. While in some hospitals the DAU may be involved in screening by undertaking glucose tolerance testing or blood glucose monitoring, the main role would be in fetal assessment towards the end of pregnancy.

When a woman has prepregnancy or gestational diabetes, serial scans for measurement of fetal growth and assessment of the AF volume should be performed, but other antenatal testing remains highly controversial. The frequency of assessment depends on how successful the metabolic control has been. Some undertake CTGs twice weekly starting at 32–34 weeks onwards unless fetal growth restriction, maternal hypertension, or oligohydramnios prompt investigation sooner, and daily testing such as fetal movement assessment is used as a adjunct by others. Many centres now use umbilical arterial Doppler velocimetry, especially since diabetic pregnancies are at risk of SGA which may be masked by coexisting fetal macrosomia.

PRETERM PREMATURE RUPTURE OF MEMBRANES

Once the diagnosis of ruptured membranes has been made based on clinical history and speculum examination the patient should be admitted for an initial assessment of AF volume, preterm labour risk and infection. Steroids should be given before 34 weeks to help prevent respiratory distress syndrome in case of preterm delivery. If the patient has not gone into labour after 24–48 h and has no clinical signs of chorioamnionitis, discharge from hospital and management as an outpatient in the DAU should be considered. Continuing admission to hospital may be indicated if there are other complications such as multiple pregnancy, anhydramnios or previous history of preterm delivery.

Management in the DAU may include one or two visits a week for monitoring of signs of chorioamnionitis such as temperature, tachycardia, uterine irritability or abdominal pain and blood tests (white blood cell count, C reactive

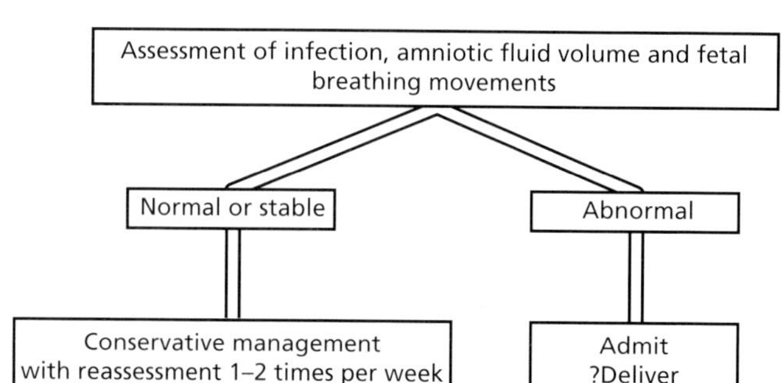

Fig. 73.7 A suggested protocol for the DAU follow-up monitoring of pregnancies with preterm premature rupture of membranes.

protein). Serial speculum vaginal examination is not usually undertaken but swabs for microbiology should be considered in order to treat pathogenic organisms (e.g. Streptococcus B). Fetal assessment is also aimed at the early detection of infection. Scanning for AF volume can be helpful because the risk of infection is lower if the AF volume either is normal or subsequently improves. It may also be worth documenting fetal breathing movements, since these cease quite early in the process of chorioamnionitis-preterm labour[38] (Fig. 73.7).

Conclusion

The experience of hospitals which have opened DAUs indicates that social and financial benefits can be achieved. If obstetricians can be confident of the follow-up arrangements for monitoring they will be more prepared to manage their patients on an outpatient basis. DAUs have also been associated with improvements in organization, efficiency, audit, teaching and research which is especially important since the usefulness and indeed dangers of assessing fetal well-being must be constantly reviewed.

Doppler ultrasound has been more rigorously and extensively evaluated than any other test of fetal health or uteroplacental function and unlike the other tests its use has been shown to reduce perinatal mortality and morbidity. Widely used tests such as CTG and BPP, although they have high positive predictive values, may become abnormal too late in the disease process for corrective intervention and also have such high false positive rates that they can even be dangerous to pregnant women and their unborn babies by causing unnecessary intervention. Organizing antenatal testing into DAU is helping us develop more rational strategies for finding out how this aspect of obstetrics should be undertaken.

REFERENCES

1. Soothill PW, Ajayi R, Campbell S et al. Effect of a fetal surveillance unit on admission of antenatal patients to hospital. *Br. Med. J.* **303**:269–271, 1991.
2. Neilson JP. Cardiotocography for antepartum fetal assessment. In *Pregnancy and Childbirth Module of The Cochrane Database of Systematic Reviews* (eds M.W. Enkin, M.J.N.C. Keirse, M.J. Renfrew & J.P. Neilson) [updated 24 February 1995]. London: BMJ Publishing Group, 1995.
3. Dawes GS, Houghton CRS, Redman CWG & Visser G. Pattern of the normal human fetal heart rate. *Br. J. Obstet. Gynaecol.* **89**:276–844, 1982.
4. Cheng LC, Gibb DMF, Ajayi RA & Soothill PW. A comparison between computerised (mean range) and clinical visual cardiotocographic assessment. *Br. J. Obstet. Gynaecol.* **99**:817–820, 1992.
5. Soothill PW, Ajayi RA, Campbell S, Ross E & Nicolaides KH. Fetal oxygenation at cordocentesis, maternal smoking and childhood neurodevelopment. *Eur. J. Obstet. Gynaecol. Reprod. Biol.* **59**:21–24, 1995.
6. Wheble AM, Gillmer MDG, Spencer JAD & Sykes GS. Changes in fetal monitoring practice in the UK: 1977–1984. *Br. J. Obstet. Gynaecol.* **96**:1140–1147, 1989.
7. ACOG technical bulletin. Antepartum fetal surveillance, p. 1. Washington, DC: American College of Obstetricians and Gynaecologists 1987.
8. Flynn AM, Kelly J, Matthews K, O'Conner M & Viegas O. Predictive value of, and observer variability in, several ways of reporting antepartum cardiotocographs. *Br. J. Obstet. Gynaecol.* **89**:434–440, 1982.
9. Devoe LD, Castillo RA & Sherline DM. The nonstress test as a diagnostic test: a critical reappraisal. *Am. J. Obstet. Gynecol.* **152**:1047, 1985.
10. Ajayi RA & Soothill PW. Ultrasound assessment of amniotic fluid volume: a comparison of the single deepest pool and amniotic fluid index to predict perinatal morbidity. *Ultrasound Obstet. Gynecol.* **1**:401–404, 1991.
11. Barkin SZ, Pretorius DH, Beckett MK, et al. Severe polyhydramnios: incidence of anomalies. *A.J.R.* **148**:155, 1987.
12. Mercer LJ & Brown IG. Fetal outcome with oligohydramnios in the second trimester. *Obstet. Gynecol.* **67**:840–842, 1986.
13. Nicolaides KH, Peters MT, Vyas S, Rabinowitz R, Rosen DJ & Campbell S. Relation of rate of urine production to oxygen tension in small-for-gestational-age fetuses. *Am. J. Obstet. Gynecol.* **162**:387–391, 1990.
14. Vyas S, Nicolaides KH & Campbell S. Renal flow-velocity waveforms in normal and hypoxemic fetuses. *Am. J. Obstet. Gynecol.* **161**:168–172, 1989.
15. Arduini D & Rizzo G. Fetal renal artery velocity waveforms and amniotic fluid volume in growth retarded and post-term fetuses. *Obstetrics and Gynecology* **77**:370–373, 1991.
16. Baskett TF, Allen AC, Gray JH, Young DC & Young LM. Fetal biophysical profile and perinatal death. *Obstet. Gynecol.* **70**:357–360, 1987.
17. Manning FA, Harman CR, Morrison I, Menticoglou SM, Lange IR & Johnson JM. Fetal assessment based on fetal biophysical profile scoring IV. An analysis of perinatal morbidity and mortality. *Am. J. Obstet. Gynecol.* **162**:703–709, 1990.
18. Neilson JP. Doppler ultrasound (all trials). In *Pregnancy and Childbirth Module of the Cochrane Database of Systematic Reviews* [updated 24 February 1995] (eds M.W. Enkin, M.J.N.C. Keirse, M.J. Renfrew & J.P. Neilson.) London: BMJ Publishing Group, 1995.
19. Trudinger BJ, Cook CM, Giles WB, Connelly AJ & Thompson RS. Umbilical artery flow velocity waveforms in high-risk pregnancy: randomised controlled trial. *Lancet* **1**:188–190, 1987.
20. Mason GC, Lilford RJ, Porter J, Nelson E & Tyrell S. Randomised comparison of routine vs highly selective use of Doppler ultrasound in low risk pregnancies. *Br. J. Obstet. Gynaecol.* **100**:130–133, 1993.
21. Soothill PW, Ajayi RA, Campbell S & Nicolaides KH. Prediction of morbidity in small and normally grown fetuses by fetal heart rate variability, biophysical profile score and umbilical artery Doppler studies. *Br. J. Obstet. Gynaecol.* **100**:742–745, 1993.
22. Gabrielli A, Luttichau M, Pittalis C et al. Doppler velocimetry in fetuses with chromosomal abnormalities and intrauterine growth retardation. *Ultrasonica* **5**(1):5–7, 1990.
23. Gardosi J, Chang A, Kalyan B, Sahota D & Symonds EM. Customised antenatal growth charts. *Lancet* **339**:283–287, 1992.
24. Gallivan S, Robson SC, Chang TC, Vaughan J & Spencer JAD. An investigation of fetal growth using serial ultrasound data. *Ultrasound Obstet Gynaecol* **3**:109–114, 1993.
25. Neilson JP. Routine formal fetal movement (FM) counting. In *Pregnancy and Childbirth Module of the Cochrane Database of Systematic Reviews* [updated 24 February 1995] (eds M.W. Enkin, M.J.N.C. Keirse, M.J. Renfrew & J.P. Neilson) London: BMJ Publishing Group, 1995.
26. British Hypertension Society. Blood pressure measurement: techniques recommended by the British Hypertension Society. *J. Hypertens.* **3**:293, 1985.
27. American Heart Association. American Heart Association recommendations for human pressure determination by sphygmomanometers. *Circulation* **62**:1146A–1155A, 1980.
28. Johenning AR & Barron WM. Indirect blood pressure measurement in pregnancy: Korotkoff phase IV versus phase V. *Am. J. Obstet. Gynecol.* **167**:577–580, 1992.

29. Pickering TG. James GD, Boddie C, Harshfield GS, Blank S & Laragh JH. How common is 'white coat' hypertension? *JAMA* **259**:225–228, 1988.
30. Leveno KJ, Quirk JG, Cunningham FG et al. Prolonged pregnancy. I. Observations concerning the causes of fetal distress. *Am. J. Obstet. Gynecol.* **150**:465–473, 1984.
31. Crowley P. Non-quantitative estimation of amniotic fluid volume in suspected prolonged pregnancy. *J. Perinat. Med.* **9**:249–251, 1980.
32. Barss VA, Frigoletto FD & Diamond F. Stillbirth after nonstress testing. *Obstet. Gynecol.* **65**:541–544, 1985.
33. Sibai BM. Chronic hypertension in pregnancy. *Clin. Perinatol.* **18**(4):833–844, 1991.
34. Hill L, Breckle R, Thomas ML & Fries JK. Polyhydramnios: ultrasonically detected prevalence and neonatal outcome. *Obstet. Gynecol.* **69**:21–5, 1987.
35. Barkin SZ, Pretorius DH, Beckett MK, Manchester DK, Nelson TR & Manco-Johnson ML. Severe polyhydramnios: incidence of anomalies. *Am. J. Roentgenol.* **148**:155–159, 1987.
36. Ajayi RA, Soothill PW, Campbell S & Nicolaides KH. Antenatal testing to predict outcome in pregnancies with unexplained antepartum haemorrhage. *Br. J. Obstet. Gynaecol.* **99**:122–125, 1992.
37. Redman CW & Jefferies M. Revised definition of pre-eclampsia. *Lancet* **1**(8589): 809–812, 1988.
38. Turnbull AC. The early diagnosis of impending premature labour. *Eur. J. Obstet. Gynecol. Reprod. Biol.* **33**(1):11–24, 1989.

Admission and stimulation tests in labour

74

S. Arulkumaran and S. Chua

Introduction

The admission test embodies the concept of performing a short period of fetal heart rate (FHR) monitoring or some other test of fetal well-being at the onset of labour to identify fetuses at risk of distress in labour. Any fetus has a potential risk of intrapartum hypoxia which may lead to birth injury, but for most this risk is small. Intrapartum fetal surveillance by continuous electronic heart rate monitoring was introduced with the aim of reducing intrapartum fetal deaths and neonatal mortality and morbidity by identifying all such cases early. There is little evidence to support this in low-risk pregnancies. It may lead to an increase in obstetric intervention in labour producing an increase in caesarean section rates, and deter the emotional satisfaction of childbirth.

Since two-thirds of neonatal death and morbidity is due to congenital malformations and/or prematurity, the number of fetuses that could potentially be salvaged by intrapartum fetal surveillance is small. This was well illustrated by the results of the Dublin randomized study of about 13 000 women. One half had electronic fetal monitoring (EFM), whilst the other had intermittent auscultation. The results in terms of perinatal mortality or morbidity did not show any significant difference[1]. In that study a high-risk group with thick meconium and preterm pregnancies as well as those who had rapid labour were not included. In another large study with adequate numbers to debate this issue (35 000 women), the results of routine or universal monitoring was compared to selective fetal monitoring[2]. Again there was no difference in outcome. The results of these two studies point to the fact that in low-risk labour, intermittent auscultation is as good as EFM. But even after rigorous selection based on known antenatal risk classification systems, fetal morbidity and mortality is present in the so-called low-risk population[3]. The incidence of acidosis at birth is not very different between the low- and high-risk groups[4]. They highlight the need to better identify an 'at risk' group. The 'admission test' (AT) addresses this issue. After selection an optimal standard of intermittent auscultation must be provided. The FHR should be auscultated for 1 min at 15 min intervals, after a contraction in the first stage of labour and after each or every other contraction in the second stage of labour. In centres where such practice is not feasible, continuous or intermittent EFM may be of help.

A good understanding of the features of the FHR tracing in normal and hypoxic situations will help to recognize the fetus at risk with auscultation findings. When doubt arises as to the condition of the fetus, simple stimulation tests can be performed as an alternative to fetal scalp blood sampling.

Admission test

The AT is provided by a small strip of electronic FHR recording for a period of 20 min on admission in labour. It provides more information than auscultation. On auscultation the baseline FHR, accelerations and at times decelerations with or soon after a contraction can be detected. However, the features of reduced baseline variability and shallow decelerations suggestive of a fetus with hypoxia are not discernible to the human ear (Fig. 74.1).

If the AT exhibits a normal baseline rate, baseline variability and two accelerations with no decelerations it is termed reactive and normal. If, during the recording time, one or two contractions are observed these may be evaluated as stressful to the fetus either by reducing the placental perfusion on the maternal side or by compressing the umbilical cord. If no FHR changes are observed with these contractions ('stress') and the trace is reactive and normal, the chance of fetal hypoxia is small in the next few hours of labour[5]. The duration of an AT can be as short as 5 or 10 min if the baseline rate, baseline variability, two accelerations, and two contractions with no FHR changes are observed promptly.

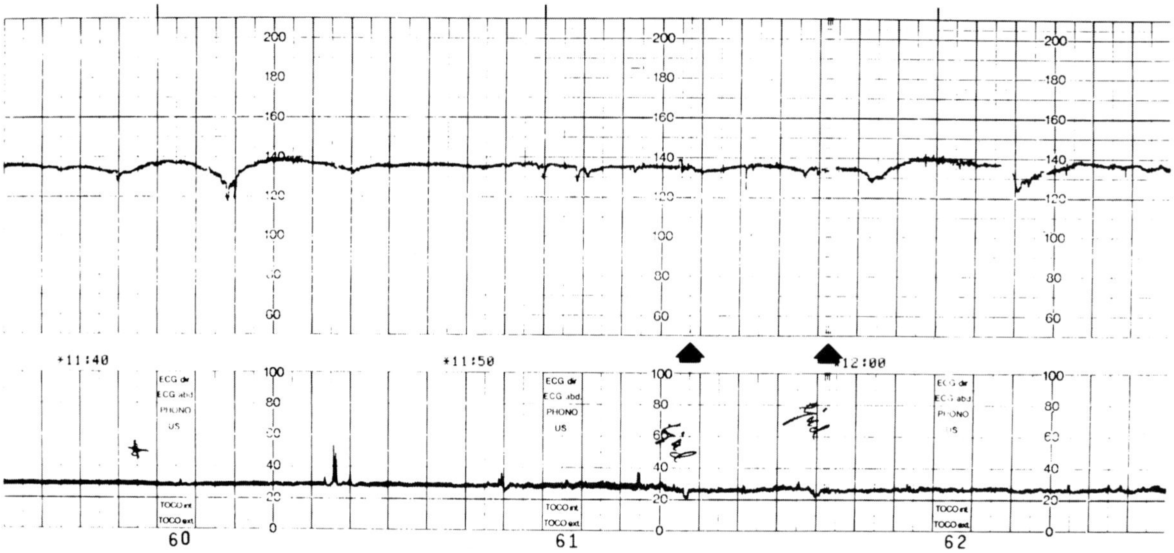

Fig. 74.1 An ominous FHR trace (paper speed 1 cm/min) showing normal baseline rate, reduced baseline variability (<5 bpm), no accelerations and shallow decelerations (<15 beats).

The results of the first study[5] evaluating the AT are given in Table 74.1. For this study a reactive normal trace was defined as one with normal baseline rate, normal baseline variability, two accelerations and no decelerations. A suspicious or equivocal trace was defined as one that had no accelerations in addition to another abnormal feature such as reduced baseline variability, baseline tachy- or bradycardia or some decelerations. A trace was termed ominous when more than one abnormal feature was present in addition to the absence of accelerations. Fetal distress was considered to be present when FHR changes with or without fetal scalp blood sampling led to operative delivery or the fetus was born normally but with an Apgar score <7 at 5 min. Of the 13 who developed fetal distress with a reactive AT, 10 developed fetal distress more than 5 h after admission. Of the three with a reactive AT on admission, who developed fetal distress within 5 h, one had cord prolapse (delivered by CS in good condition) and the other two were preterm and had low Apgar scores when delivered vaginally and needed minimal resuscitation. The above results indicate that a reactive admission test is not predictive of the fetal condition when labour lasts more than 5 h. A negative result (reactive CTG) has limited prognostic value, whilst a positive test (non-reactive CTG/suspicious or abnormal admission test) warrants further action. Statistically, a reactive admission test has a high predictive value of 98.7% and high specificity of 99.4% for fetal well-being. On the other hand, an abnormal admission test has a low predictive value of 40.0% and a low sensitivity of 23.5%. The low sensitivity and predictive values are due to the low prevalence of abnormal tests as well as fetal distress. There was one intrapartum stillbirth (Fig. 74.2) and one neonatal death in the group who had an ominous admission test. The auscultation chart in the case of the fresh stillbirth showed a steady observation of 140 bpm for 2 h at the end of which the fetal heart was not audible. The result of the AT was not disclosed to the clinician. There is debate whether intervention at this stage may result in a neurologically handicapped baby.

TABLE 74.1
Results of AT in relation to the incidence of fetal distress

	Admission test *n* (%)	Fetal distress *n* (%)
Reactive	982 (94.3)	13 (1.4)
Equivocal	49 (4.7)	5 (10.4)
Ominous	10 (1.0)	4 (40.0)

Fetal acoustic stimulation test (FAST) in combination with the admission test (AT)

The equivocal AT can be clarified by using a fetal acoustic stimulation test to provoke accelerations[6]. After a 15–20 min admission test, the fetus can be provoked by a vibroacoustic stimulator (model 5 C electronic larynx or fetal acoustic stimulator by Corometrics) to elicit an FHR acceleration. A fetus which is not hypoxic will exhibit two accelerations (>15 beats for >15 s) or a sustained acceleration lasting >3 min. Four different response patterns can be observed (Fig. 74.3):

Type 1A Prolonged period of acceleration or tachycardia >15 beats above the baseline for >3 min

Type 1B Two accelerations >15 beats for >15 s or one acceleration >1 min

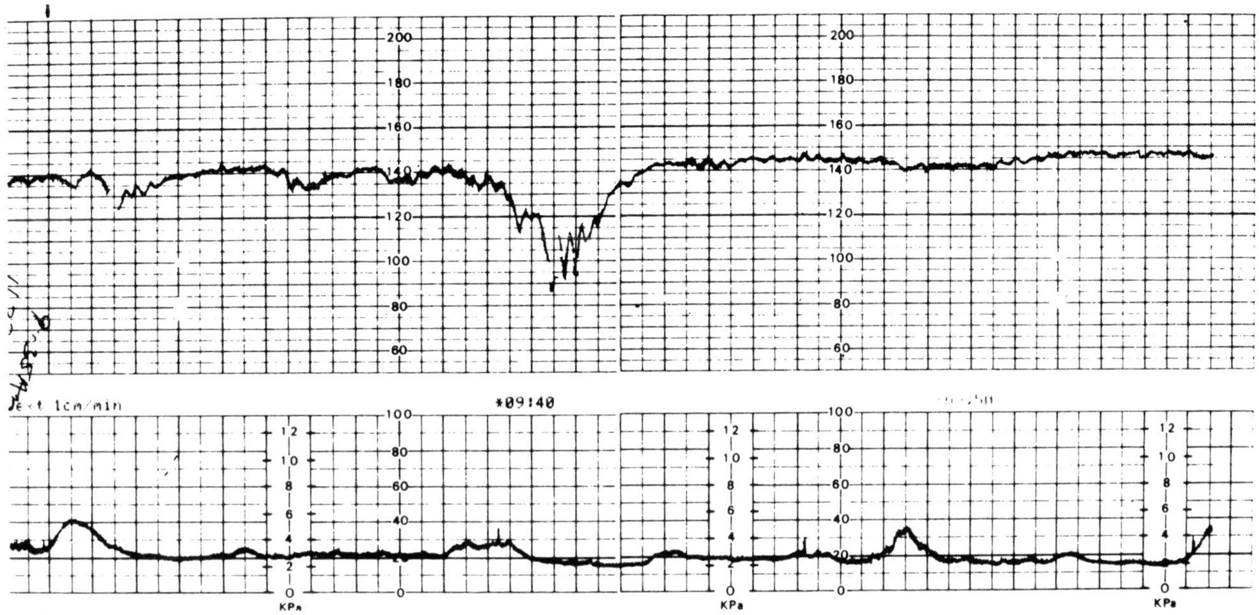

Fig. 74.2 An AT (paper speed 1 cm/min) showing baseline rate of 140 bpm, reduced baseline variability (<5 bpm), no accelerations and subtle decelerations <15 beats suggestive of hypoxia. The findings at intermittent auscultation gave the baseline FHR to be 140 bpm, and was thought to be normal and 2 h later suddenly FH was not heard.

Type 2	A biphasic response with an acceleration followed by a deceleration usually >60 beats from the baseline lasting >60 s
Type 3	No accelerations or accelerations <15 beats from the baseline rate

The results of our study are given in Table 74.2. Type 1A and B reactions were considered to be normal whilst Type 2 and 3 reactions were considered to be abnormal.

Similar to the earlier study fetal distress was defined to be present if an operative delivery was performed for that indication or if the newborn at delivery had low Apgar scores of <5 at 1 min and <7 at 5 min or needed assisted ventilation. When both the AT and FAST were normal the incidence of fetal distress was only 1.7% compared with when both were abnormal when it was 55.6%. FAST appears to give a better predictive value of fetal distress because when it was abnormal even in the presence of a reactive normal AT the incidence of fetal distress was 14.2% compared with 6.1% incidence of fetal distress when the FAST was normal but the AT was suspicious or abnormal. The positive predictive value with a suspicious or an abnormal admission test (58 cases) was 13.8%. The FAST was abnormal in 23 cases of whom seven developed fetal distress giving a positive predictive value of 30.4%. When both tests were abnormal the positive predictive value was 55.6%. The FAST was used to reduce the incidence of equivocal admission tests in 5–6% of the population tested[5]. Forty-six (90.2%) of the 51 cases with equivocal admission test for 15–20 min had type 1 accelerations. In this group only 4.3% developed fetal distress. In the five cases with a type 2 or 3 response to FAST, fetal distress occurred in 40%. Hence a prolonged recording to obtain a reactive pattern is not necessary and FAST can be used to reduce the testing time and to increase the positive predictive value of fetal distress in subsequent labour. Subsequent studies have also shown FAST to be a useful screening test for fetal distress in labour[7–9]. Better discriminatory power with FAST in the antenatal period has been described by Trudinger and Boylan[10].

On the basis of the experience of our unit we recommend, if AT is reactive, intermittent electronic fetal monitoring for 10 to 20 minutes every 3 h and auscultation every 30 minutes for fetal surveillance in labour. If the AT is normal, a gradually developing hypoxia will be reflected by a rising

TABLE 74.2
Frequency of fetal distress in relation to outcome of AT and FAST

	n	Fetal distress *n* (%)
AT, N	708	
FAST, N	694	12 (1.7)
A	14	2 (14.2)
AT, S or A	58	
FAST, N	49	3 (6.1)
A	9	5 (55.6)

N = normal; S = suspicious; A = abnormal

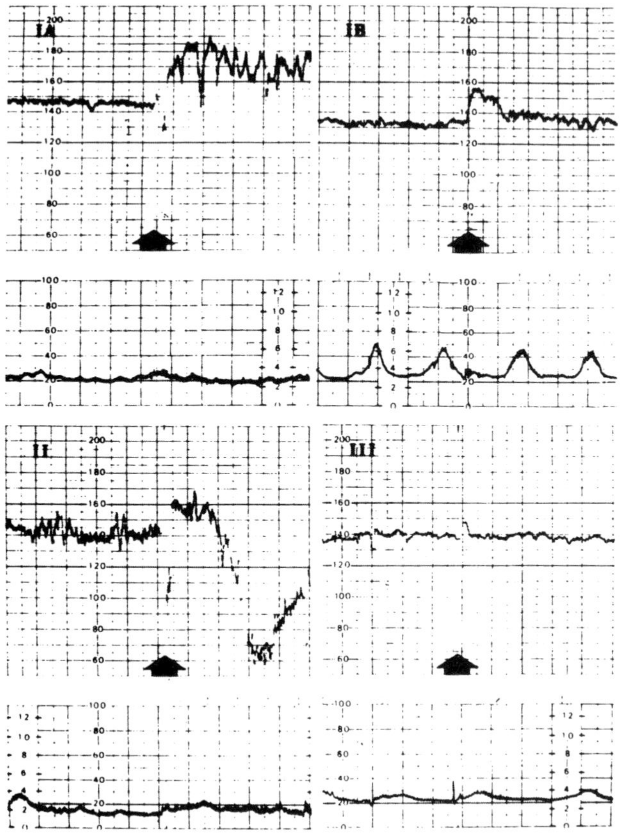

Fig. 74.3 The different types of responses to FAST (paper speed 1 cm/min). Types 1A (acceleration >15 beats for >3 mins) and B (acceleration > 15 beats for > 1 min) are normal; types 2 (deceleration >60 s for > 60 beats following an acceleration) and 3 (response of no acceleration or that <15 beats for <15 s) are abnormal[6].

FHR and should be picked up by auscultation[11]. When there is an increase in baseline FHR on auscultation a small strip of electronic recording should be performed to check for other abnormal features such as absence of accelerations and reduction in the baseline variability which may be associated with hypoxia.

It should be appreciated that if the FHR trace is reactive in a well-grown fetus at term and the amniotic fluid is clear, then fetal compromise is extremely unlikely in the first 3–4 h of labour. It takes time for fetal acidosis to develop. It has been estimated that in such a situation it takes 115 min for 50% of fetuses to become acidotic with repeated late decelerations, 145 min with repeated variable decelerations and 185 min with a flat trace (baseline variability <5 bpm)[12]. The changes in the FHR rate on intermittent auscultation should signify this probability. It is our practice to perform a short strip of electronic FHR recording when suspicion arises on intermittent auscultation. If the trace is abnormal the diagnosis of fetal acidosis can be made by fetal scalp blood sampling (FBS) or likely acidosis excluded by fetal stimulation tests.

Other evaluated admission tests

Studies have been carried out to examine the use of amniotic fluid index and indices of downstream resistance in the umbilical artery blood flow velocity waveform to assess fetal well-being in early labour[13,14]. These tests need expensive equipment and expertise compared with an admission CTG with or without FAST.

ASSESSMENT OF AMNIOTIC FLUID VOLUME

Perinatal mortality and morbidity are increased in the presence of reduced amniotic fluid volume at term[15,16]. A semi-quantitative measurement of amniotic fluid volume in early labour could be used as an adjunct to an admission CTG to triage a fetus to a high or low risk status in early labour[17] provided membranes were intact. In a study[18] involving 120 women in early labour it was found that ultrasound measurement of the vertical depth of two amniotic fluid pockets to be easily and rapidly performed by medical and midwifery staff and that the results were easily reproducible. They found that a vertical depth of two pools of amniotic fluid <3 cm was a useful predictor of significant fetal distress in the first stage of labour. In this study, six women had a vertical depth <3 cm; four of these women had caesarean section in the first stage of labour for fetal distress and in three of the newborns the cord pH was <7.20. None of the women who had amniotic fluid volume >3 cm required caesarean section for fetal distress. In a study of 1092 singleton pregnancies[8], amniotic fluid volume was 'quantified' by measuring the amniotic fluid index (AFI), using the four quadrant technique[19]. AFI < 5 in early labour, even in the presence of a normal admission CTG, was associated with higher operative delivery rates for fetal distress, low Apgar scores, more infants needing assisted ventilation and higher admission rate to neonatal intensive care unit. When the admission CTG was suspicious, an AFI >5 was associated with better obstetric outcome compared with those with AFI < 5. The low AFI < 5 may indicate incipient hypoxia. The stress of cord compression or gradual decline of oxygenation with contractions in labour may be the cause of less optimal outcome.

UMBILICAL ARTERY DOPPLER VELOCIMETRY

Umbilical artery Doppler velocimetry has been used as an AT. It has been shown to be a poor predictor of fetal distress in labour in the low risk population[13,20]. A larger study with 1092 women has shown Doppler velocimetry on admission to be of little value in the presence of a normal admission CTG. However, in cases with suspicious admission CTG, normal Doppler velocimetry was associated with less operative deliveries for fetal distress, better Apgar scores and less need for associated ventilation or admission to the neonatal intensive care unit[8].

TABLE 74.3
Admission FHR findings in 48 neurologically impaired term infants separated on the basis of FHR reactivity[28]

FHR pattern on admission	Up to 120 minutes (*n*)	FHR variability (average) *n* (%)	Decelerations *n* (%)	Tachycardia *n* (%)
Reactive	15	14 (93)	2 (13)	0 (0)
Non-reactive	33	12* (36)	27 (82)	6 (18)

*$P < 0.001$

Relationship of neurologically impaired term infants to results of admission test

There is controversy regarding the value of continuous electronic fetal monitoring, let alone an AT. Other than acute or terminal patterns of prolonged bradycardia or prolonged decelerations of a large magnitude there is little information regarding FHR patterns and neurological handicap at term[21–24] other than some observation of neurological impairment and non-reactivity[25–27] especially in the presence of meconium. In a recent investigation of 48 neurologically impaired singleton term infants the admission FHR findings and the FHR patterns 30 min before delivery were analysed[28]. The findings of this investigation are shown in Tables 74.3 and 74.4.

Based on these Tables, it can be stated that all fetuses with a reactive AT (accelerations) will show the following features prior to becoming hypoxic: all will exhibit decelerations (100%); almost all will have reduced baseline variability (93%), and tachycardia (93%). In one case in which the FHR did not exceed 160 bpm there was an increase in the baseline FHR of 25%. It is clear that if the AT is reactive then it is easy to carry out intermittent auscultation as the gradual rise in the baseline rate and the decelerations can be picked up and action taken. On the other hand, if the FHR tracing on admission is non-reactive the development of further abnormal features with progress of labour is variable and subtle. This is difficult to recognize by intermittent auscultation. Already, hypoxic damage may be present so that the fetus is unable to respond. In those with non-reactive AT on admission 82% had shallow decelerations and the majority with reduced baseline variability (<5 bpm). The baseline heart rate was normal in 82% of cases. The fact that a hypoxic fetus can have a normal baseline heart rate and shallow decelerations of <15 beats in a non-reactive trace when the baseline variability is <5 bpm is not common knowledge to many practitioners (Fig. 74.1).

TABLE 74.4
FHR patterns in the last 30 min before delivery separated on the basis of admission FHR pattern[28]

FHR variability (average) *n* (%)	Decelerations *n* (%)	Tachycardia *n* (%)
1 (7)	15 (100)	14[a] (93)
11* (33)	5 (15)	9** (27)

*$P < 0.05$; ** $P < 0.001$
[a]The baseline FHR in one case did not rise > 160 bpm to be defined as tachycardia but showed an increase in baseline FHR of 25%[28]

Stimulation tests as an alternative to fetal scalp blood sampling

In an unselected population up to 60% of patients can exhibit some FHR changes during labour[29]. This has been the basis for the NIH consensus statement that electronic FHR monitoring is a screening test and not a diagnostic tool to identify fetal acidosis. Historically, fetal scalp blood sampling was practised by Professor Saling in Germany prior to the introduction of electronic FHR monitoring. When the FHR is normal and reactive the chance of fetal acidosis is extremely low[29,30]. Suspicious and abnormal FHR changes are not always associated with acidosis[30–32]. The less experienced the centre is in interpreting the FHR changes the greater is the need to perform FBS. If FHR patterns are properly interpreted, the need to assess pH by FBS for predicting fetal outcome is small[33]. Obstetricians use FBS as an adjunct because the experience of interpreting FHR patterns varies and even with the worst pattern of tachycardia, reduced baseline variability and decelerations only 50–60% of the fetuses are acidotic[30]. It is known that when the FHR pattern exhibits accelerations the chance of fetal acidosis are small, emphasising accelerations as the 'hallmark' of fetal health[30]. Baseline variability is another good indicator of fetal health. When normal baseline variability is observed in the last 20 min prior to delivery, the fetal condition at birth is good regardless of other features of the trace[34]. Fetal acidosis was more common when there was a loss of baseline variability with tachycardia or late decelerations[30,35]. The preservation of normal baseline variability indicates that the autonomic nervous system is not severely affected and the fetus is trying to compensate despite other abnormal features in the trace.

There are two factors contributing to the absence of fetal acidosis in the presence of some cases of FHR abnormality. It takes time for acidosis to develop[12]. The scale of development is related to the status of placental function and the degree of compromise to the perfusion of the placenta, on the maternal or fetal side of the circulation[36].

Despite the usefulness of FBS, expertise and facilities to perform FBS are not available in all centres with electronic fetal monitoring facilities[37,38]. The situation is more of a problem when there is inability to perform FBS because of high head, early cervical dilatation or inexperience of the accoucheur. Therefore any alternatives to FBS should be useful.

A retrospective correlation of the scalp blood pH and to the presence or absence of accelerations at the time of FBS[39] has led to the fetal scalp stimulation test[40,41]. When the scalp is stimulated by a painful stimulus by pinching with an Allice's tissue forceps the presence of an acceleration is unlikely to be associated with a scalp blood pH below 7.20. On the other hand, if there is no acceleration to such a stimulus about 50% have acidotic pH values (<7.20) and a significant proportion had preacidotic values (7.20–7.25) (Table 74.5). This information can be used to identify those who are not at risk of acidosis. It is not as good in predicting those who are acidotic. In centres where facilities do not exist for the performance of FBS, scalp stimulation will be a useful adjunct to reduce the number of unnecessary caesarean sections for 'fetal distress'. In centres where facilities are available, such a test may reduce the number of blood samples required.

The case which showed a positive response and had an acidotic pH was due to respiratory acidosis. This reverses spontaneously once the FHR returns to normal[42]. Although the scalp stimulation test appears to be a suitable alternative to estimation of fetal scalp pH it is not feasible to do frequent vaginal examinations to perform this test because of the risk of introducing infection. There have been several reports showing a fetal response with FHR acceleration to acoustic stimulation in labour in the absence of acidosis[43]. Non-responders had a 50% rate of acidosis. It is difficult to explain why the fetal response of acceleration should be associated with an arbitrary cutoff points to scalp blood pH values. It is known that auditory sensation is one of the first affected by hypoxia and a negative response to acoustic stimulation might warn the possibility of hypoxia. Concern has been raised about safety. To date the studies performed have shown that there is no evidence of catecholamine release with the stimulus[44], no hearing loss[45,46], and no long-term disturbance to the fetal behavioural state studied by FHR variability cycles[47,48]. With these alternative modalities available there is less need for physicians to perform FBS in labour[49]. Care should be exercised, since 50% of fetuses which do not show a reaction to the acoustic or scalp stimulation will not be acidotic (Fig. 74.4). In a centre without facilities for FBS stimulation tests may be a good alternative and may help to reduce unnecessary casesarean sections.

Accelerations are the hallmark of fetal health in the antenatal or intrapartum period. Even in the presence of suspicious or abnormal traces, accelerations induced by external stimuli are indicative of a non-acidotic fetus[40,41,50]. It has been suggested that in the presence of a sinusoidal-like pattern, sound-provoked acceleration would exclude the possibility of a severely anaemic or hypoxic fetus (Fig. 74.4)[51]. In any trace one of the early features that is indicative of hypoxia is the absence of accelerations.

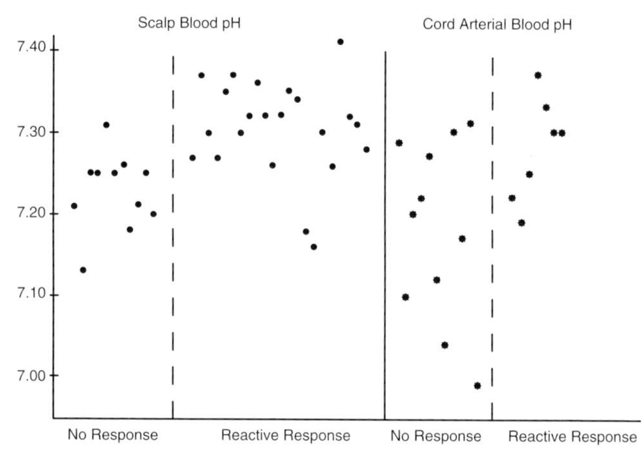

Fig. 74.4 Reactive response to FAST was associated with non-acidotic pH values of >7.20 in scalp blood sample (except two cases of respiratory acidosis) and > 7.15 in umbilical artery blood. In those with no FHR acceleration response to FAST 50% had normal scalp blood or cord arterial pH[50].

TABLE 74.5
Results of scalp stimulation tests in relation to scalp blood pH[40,41]

	Response to scalp stimulation		
Fetal scalp blood pH values	Positive, *n* (%)	Negative, *n* (%)	Total *n* (%)
< 7.20	1[a] (0.4)	40 (44.4)	41 (11.7)
7.20–7.25	33 (12.7)	45 (50.0)	78 (22.3)
> 7.25	226 (86.9)	5 (5.6)	231 (66.0)
Total	260 (100)	90 (100)	350 (100)

[a]Delivered 1½ h later in good condition

Conclusion

Admission test followed by intermittent auscultation is a good method of monitoring low-risk labour. Abnormal FHR changes on auscultation should be confirmed by EFM. The changes observed need to be correlated with the clinical picture in order to rationally take action. In many instances, remedial action like hydration, repositioning of the mother and stopping oxytocin infusion should correct the FHR changes and no further action is necessary. When FHR changes persist despite such action, a positive response of FHR acceleration to a stimulation test will confirm the presence of fetal health. The absence of an acceleratory response is an indication to perform FBS to determine the acid–base balance.

The AT and stimulation tests are techniques to select those who need continuous monitoring and FBS respectively. These techniques will reduce the need for intervention of continuous FHR monitoring, and conduction of FBS in labour and will lead to the more appropriate use of technology in labour. Similar to the debate of the role of EFM in low-risk labour, randomized controlled studies are needed on the role of admission and stimulation tests in labour if they are to be incorporated into routine clinical practice.

REFERENCES

1. MacDonald D, Grant A, Sheridan-Pereira M, Boylan P & Chalmers I. The Dublin randomised control trial of intrapartum fetal heart rate monitoring. *Am. J. Obstet. Gynecol.* **152**:524–539, 1985.
2. Leveno KJ, Cunningham FG & Nelson S. et al. A prospective comparison of selective and universal electronic fetal monitoring in 34,995 pregnancies. *N. Engl. J. Med.* **315**:615–619, 1986.
3. Hobel CJ, Hyvarinen MA, Okada DM & Oh W. Prenatal and intrapartum high-risk screening. I. Prediction of the high risk neonate. *Am. J. Obstet. Gynecol.* **117**:1–9, 1973.
4. Arulkumaran S, Gibb DMF & Ratnam SS. Experience with a selective intrapartum fetal monitoring policy. *Sing. J. Obstet. Gynaecol.* **14**:47–51, 1983.
5. Ingemarsson I, Arulkumaran S, Ingemarsson E, Tambyraja RL & Ratnam SS. Admission test: a screening test for fetal distress in labour. *Obstet. Gynecol.* **69**:800–806, 1986.
6. Ingemarsson I, Arulkumaran S, Paul RH, Ingemarsson E, Tambyraja RL & Ratnam SS. Fetal acoustic stimulation in early labour in patients screened with the admission test. *Am. J. Obstet. Gynecol.* **158**:70–74, 1988.
7. Sarno AP jr, Ahn MO, Phelan JP & Paul RH. Fetal acoustic stimulation in the early intrapartum period as a predictor of subsequent fetal condition. *Am. J. Obstet. Gynecol.* **162**:762–765, 1990.
8. Chua S, Arulkumaran S, Kurup A, Anandakumar C, Norshida S & Ratnam SS. Search for the most predictive tests of fetal well-being in early labour. *J. Perinat. Med.* **76**:606–612, 1993.
9. Tannirandorn Y, Wacharaprechanont T & Phaosavasdi S. Fetal acoustic stimulation for rapid intrapartum assessment of fetal well-being. *J. Med. Assoc. Thai.* **76**:606–612, 1993.
10. Trudinger TJ & Boylan P. Antepartum fetal heart rate monitoring: value of sound stimulation. *Obstet. Gynecol.* **55**:265–268, 1980.
11. Gibb DMF & Arulkumaran S. *Fetal Monitoring in Practice* 2nd edn. Oxford: Butterworth Heinemann, 1997.
12. Fleischer A, Schulman H, Jagani N, Mitchell J & Randolph G. The development of fetal acidosis in the presence of an abnormal fetal heart rate tracing 1. The average for gestational age fetus. *Am. J. Obstet. Gynecol.* **144**:55–60, 1982.
13. Malcus P, Gudmundson S, Marsall K, Kwok HH, Vangadasalam D & Ratnam SS. Umbilical artery Doppler velocimetry as a labour admission test. *Obstet. Gynecol.* **77**:10–16, 1991.
14. Sarno AP jr, Ahn MO, Brar H, Phelan JP & Platt LD. Intrapartum Doppler velocimetry, amniotic fluid volume and fetal heart rate as predictors of subsequent fetal distress. *Am. J. Obstet. Gynecol.* **161**:1508–1511, 1989.
15. Chamberlain PF, Manning FA, Morrison I, Herman CR & Lange I. Ultrasound evaluation of amniotic fluid volume. I. The relationship of marginal and decreased amniotic fluid volumes to perinatal outcome. *Am. J. Obstet. Gynecol.* **150**:245–249, 1984.
16. Crowley P, O'Herlihy C & Boylan P. The value of ultrasound measurement of amniotic fluid volume in the management of prolonged pregnancy. *Br. J. Obstet. Gynaecol.* **91**:444–448, 1984.
17. Chauhan SP, Washburne JF, Magann EF, Perry KG, Martin JN jr & Morrison JC. A randomised study to assess the efficacy of the amniotic fluid index as a fetal admission test. *Obstet. Gynecol.* **86**:9–13, 1995.
18. Teoh TG, Gleeson RP & Darling MR. Measurement of amniotic fluid volume in early labour is a useful admission test. *Br. J. Obstet. Gynaecol.* **99**:859–860, 1992.
19. Phelan JP, Ahn MO, Smith CV, Rutherford SE & Anderson E. Amniotic fluid index measurements during pregnancy. *J. Reprod Med.* **32**:601–605, 1987.
20. Chan FY, Lam C, Lam YH, To WK, Pun TC & Lee CP. Umbilical artery Doppler velocimetry compared with fetal heart rate monitoring as a labour admission test. *Eur. J. Obstet. Gynaecol. Reprod Biol.* **54**:1–6, 1994.
21. Keegan KA jr, Waffarn F & Qulligan EJ. Obstetric characteristics and fetal heart rate patterns of infants who convulse during the newborn period. *Am. J. Obstet. Gynecol.* **153**:732–737, 1985.
22. van der Moer P, Gerretsen G & Visser G. Fixed heart rate pattern after intrauterine accidental decerebration. *Obstet. Gynecol.* **65**:125–127, 1985.
23. Menticoglou SM, Manning FA, Harman CR & Morrison I. Severe fetal brain injury without evident intrapartum trauma *Obstet. Gynecol.* **74**:457–461, 1989.
24. Schields JR & Schifrin BS. Perinatal antecedents of cerebral palsy. *Obstet. Gynecol.* **71**:899–905, 1988.
25. Leveno KJ, William ML, De Palma RT & Whalley PJ. Perinatal outcome in the absence of antepartum fetal heart rate accelerations. *Obstet. Gynecol.* **61**:347–355, 1983.
26. Devoe LD, McKenzie J, Searle NS & Sherline DM. Clinical sequelae of the extended non-stress test. *Am. J. Obstet. Gynecol.* **151**:1074–1078, 1985.
27. Brown R & Patrick J. The non-stress test: how long is long enough? *Am. J. Obstet. Gynecol.* **141**:646–651, 1981.
28. Phelan JP & Ahn MO. Perinatal observations in forty eight neurologically impaired term infants. *Am. J. Obstet. Gynecol.* **171**:424–431, 1994.
29. Ingemarrson E. Routine electronic fetal monitoring during labor. *Acta. Obstet. Gynaecol. Scand. (Suppl)* **99**:1–29, 1981.
30. Beard RW, Filshie GM, Knight CA & Roberts GM. The significance of the changes in the continuous fetal heart rate in the first stage of labour. *J. Obstet. Gynaecol. Br. Cwlth* **78**:865–881, 1971.
31. Zalor RW & Quilligan EJ. The influence of scalp sampling on the Caesarean section rate for fetal distress. *Am. J. Obstet. Gynecol.* **135**:239–246, 1979.
32. Katz M, Mazor M & Insler V. Fetal heart rate patterns and scalp pH as predictors of fetal distress. *Israel. J. Med. Sci.* **17**:260–265, 1981.
33. Parer JT. In defence of FHR monitoring's specificity. *Contemp. Obstet. Gynecol.* **19**:228–234, 1982.
34. Paul RH, Suidan AK, Yeh S-Y, Schifrin BS & Hon EH. Clinical fetal monitoring. VII. The evaluation and significance of intrapartum baseline variability. *Am. J. Obstet. Gynecol.* **123**:206–210, 1975.
35. Schifrin BS & Dame L. Fetal heart rate patterns: prediction of Apgar score. *JAMA* **219**:1322–1325, 1972.
36. Starks GC. Correlation of meconium stained amniotic fluid, early intrapartum fetal pH and Apgar scores as predictors of perinatal outcome. *Obstet. Gynecol.* **56**:604–609, 1980.
37. Gillmer MDG & Combe D. Intrapartum fetal monitoring practice in the United Kingdom. *Br. J. Obstet. Gynaecol.* **86**:753–758, 1979.
38. Wheble AM, Gillmer MDG, Spencer JAD & Sykes GS. Changes in fetal monitoring practice in the UK: 1977–1984. *Br. J. Obstet. Gynaecol.* **96**:1140–1147, 1989.
39. Clarke SL, Gimovsky ML & Miller FC. Fetal heart rate response to scalp blood sampling. *Am. J. Obstet. Gynecol.* **144**:706–708, 1982.
40. Clarke SL, Gimovsky ML & Miller FC. The scalp stimulation test: a clinical alternative to fetal scalp blood sampling. *Am. J. Obstet. Gynecol.* **148**:274–277, 1984.
41. Arulkumaran S, Ingemarsson & Ratnam SS. Fetal heart rate response to scalp stimulation as a test for fetal well being in labour. *Asia. Oceania. J. Obstet. Gynaecol.* **13**:131–135, 1987.

42. Ingemarsson I & Arulkumaran S. Fetal acid base balance in low risk patients in labour. *Am. J. Obstet. Gynecol.* **155**:66–69, 1986.
43. Edersheim TG, Hutson JM, Druzin ML & Kogut EA. Fetal heart rate response to vibratory acoustic stimulation predicts fetal pH in labor. *Am. J. Obstet. Gynecol.* **157**:1557–1560, 1987.
44. Fish NM, Nicolaidis P & Arulkumaran S et al. Vibro-acoustic stimulation is not associated with sudden fetal catecholamine release. *Early Hum. Dev.* **25**:1–17, 1990.
45. Arulkumaran S, Skurr B, Tong H, Kek LP, Yeoh KH & Ratnam SS. No evidence of hearing loss due to fetal acoustic stimulation test. *Obstet. Gynecol.* **78**:282–285, 1991.
46. Arulkumaran S, Talbert D, Hsu TS, Chua S, Anandakumar C & Ratnam SS. The possibility of cochlea cilia damage in the fetus due to in-utero sound levels when vibro-acoustic stimulation is applied to the maternal abdomen. *Br. J. Obstet. Gynaecol.* **99**:43–45, 1992.
47. Spencer JAD, Deans A, Nicolaidis P & Arulkumaran S. Fetal response to vibro-acoustic stimulation during low and high fetal heart rate variability episodes in late pregnancy. *Am. J. Obstet. Gynecol.* **165**:86–90, 1991.
48. Montan S, Arulkumaran S & Ratnam SS. Vibro-acoustic stimulation does not alter the duration of high and low fetal heart rate variability episodes. *J. Perinat. Med.* **20**:331–336, 1992.
49. Clarke SL & Paul RH. Intrapartum fetal surveillance: the role of fetal scalp blood sampling. *Am. J. Obstet. Gynecol.* **153**:717–720, 1985.
50. Ingemarsson I & Arulkumaran S. Reactive FHR response to sound stimulation in fetuses with low scalp blood pH. *Br. J. Obstet. Gynecol.* **96**:562–565, 1989.
51. Arulkumaran S & Tham KF. Sinusoidal-like fetal heart rate pattern: real time ultrasound may help in differential diagnosis. *Acta. Obstet. Gynecol. Scand.* **67**:478, 1988.

Intrapartum fetal monitoring: CTG, ECG and fetal blood sampling

75

K. Greene

It is a truism that 'you are more likely to die on the first day of life than any other – except the last'

Introduction

The purpose of intrapartum monitoring is to ensure the delivery of a fit and healthy infant by the most appropriate means, bearing in mind the safety of the mother. Relative oxygen deficiency is a part of normal labour for the fetus, but at the same time it poses a significant threat to intact survival. Thus, labour is the most hazardous journey of our lifetime. It is to be expected that the healthy fetus has the physiological ability to sustain even stressful labour without handicap. This is not the case for a fetus already partly compromised before labour or for a healthy fetus subject to unusual rigours during labour. It is for these reasons that we need fetal monitoring.

The challenge is to seek to identify the fetus whose physiological defence mechanisms are compromised before permanent damage is sustained using incomplete monitoring systems. It is important to distinguish the effect of acute oxygen lack in a healthy fetus from the same insult in an already compromised fetus (Fig. 75.1). Sepsis, haemorrhage and trauma can contribute to this in labour.

Many of the current problems of intrapartum monitoring stem from a lack of widespread understanding of the physiology, interrelationships and limitations of the different variables, heart rate, acid–base, ECG waveform, Apgar scores and neonatal symptoms, and their relationship to asphyxia and cerebral injury.

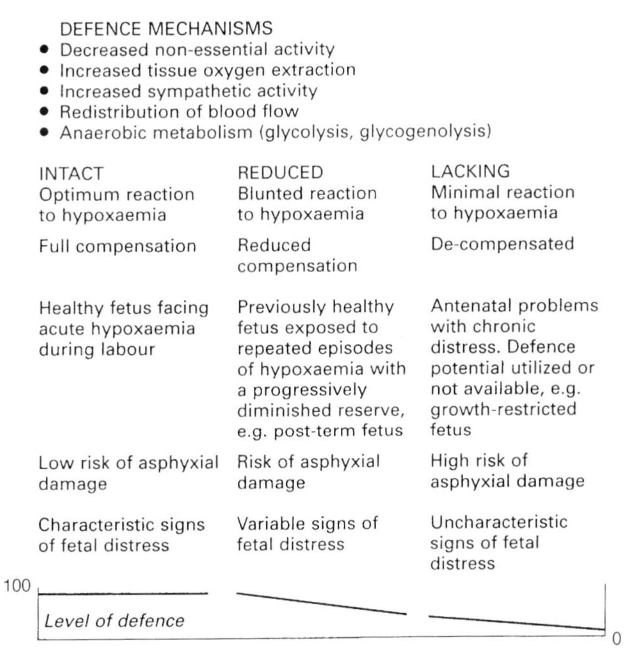

Fig. 75.1 Schematic representation of different responses to intrapartum hypoxaemia dependent on the level of fetal reserve.

Terminology

In the perinatal period *asphyxia* is the combination of oxygen lack and acidosis with impaired organ function. This occurs with a sequence of events over time. First there is *hypoxaemia*, a reduction of oxygen carried in the blood as a result of a decreased pO_2 and decreased oxygen content. This may be compensated for by an increase in blood flow and oxygen extraction to maintain oxygen supply to the tissues. If this oxygen supply is insufficient for the tissue energy requirements, which dictate oxygen consumption, *hypoxia* occurs within the tissues. In the fetus aerobic metabolism is then supplemented by anaerobic metabolism to maintain energy balance. If hypoxia continues, the process of anaerobic metabolism produces lactate and an increase in hydrogen ions so that oxygen lack is accompanied by a metabolic acidosis (Fig. 75.2). There is obviously a critical point in this process when

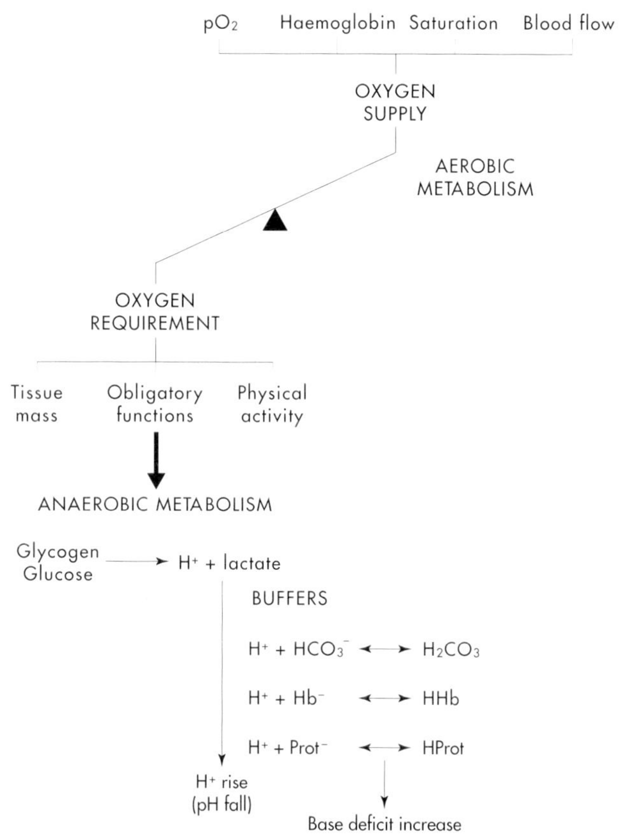

Fig. 75.2 The relationship of aerobic and anaerobic metabolism.

energy balance can no longer be maintained and organ failure occurs with a risk of permanent tissue damage.

How common is the problem?

The reported incidence of intrapartum asphyxia varies because of varying definitions and differences in risk and practice in different parts of the world. The marked decline in intrapartum stillbirth rates in developed countries (now about 0.59/1000[1]) has not been paralleled by a decrease in the incidence of cerebral palsy (2.0–2.5/1000). In fact there has been an increase in cerebral palsy in both preterm and term fetuses[2,3]. The majority of cases are of unknown aetiology and the precipitating event occurs prior to labour[4–6]; but it is possible that current obstetric monitoring and clinical practice has shifted the timing of delivery to favour live handicap rather than perinatal death, as the consequence of both antepartum and intrapartum asphyxia.

It is of great concern that in the UK, 78% of the 873 deaths related to intrapartum events in 1994/95 were considered by the Confidential Enquiry into Stillbirths and Deaths in Infancy to have had suboptimal care[1]. Death and handicap are obviously too late sequelae for clinical practice. We would wish children to be born with good Apgar scores, normal blood gases and to have no abnormal neurological symptoms in the first few days of life. What are the figures? Our unit's incidence of Apgar score less than 3 at 1 min is 20/1000, cord artery acidosis (pH < 7.05) is 21/1000, cord artery metabolic acidosis (pH < 7.05; base deficit > 12 mequiv/L) is 7/1000 and neonatal encephalopathy is about 1.5/1000. It is clear that very large numbers are needed to evaluate monitoring strategies to change these.

Dynamics of labour

It is important to understand the dynamics of human labour to appreciate the impact it can have on the fetal cardiovascular responses, oxygen lack and the process of asphyxia and the difficulties of differentiating these.

The first stage of labour has latent and active phases. The latent phase may last days as the cervix softens and becomes effaced prior to active dilatation. Contractions are usually infrequent and low pressure but may still present a challenge to the compromised fetus. The active phase, recognized by the onset of regular painful contractions and progressive labour, should dilate the cervix at about 1 cm/h to full dilatation at 10 cm. It is associated with uterine contractions of 60–80 mmHg lasting up to 60 s every 3 min. During the second stage intrauterine pressures usually reach 80–100 mmHg and are increased further by maternal effort.

Prior to labour, fetal acid–base status is determined by the maternal acid–base status. During active labour, as the uterus contracts, with intrauterine pressures exceeding 30 mmHg, the arteries supplying the intervillous space of the placenta are constricted so that there is temporarily little flow and therefore temporarily little exchange of oxygen to, or carbon dioxide from the fetus. This can be accommodated by the healthy fetoplacental unit, provided the contractions last no more than 60 s and there is sufficient respite (2 min) between them. If this is not the case there will be a progressive hypoxaemia (which may lead to a metabolic acidosis) and a CO_2 build-up (hypercapnia) to also cause a respiratory acidosis (see later). Too frequent contractions (frequently the result of abuse of oxytocics) also produce low pressure contractions and poor progress, because the strength of a contraction is inversely related to the interval since the last – 'pressure produces progress and frequency produces fetal distress' (Fig. 75.3).

Compression of the cord between uterine wall and fetal body is common during contractions especially with oligohydramnios. This is often associated with a reduction in fetal urine output from decreased renal blood flow with the blood flow redistribution which occurs in growth retardation (see later). In the second stage, as the presenting part moves down through the pelvis, loops of cord which may have become wrapped around the fetal neck or limbs antenatally can tighten, be compressed or produce a functionally short cord with traction on the points of insertion. This affects cardio-

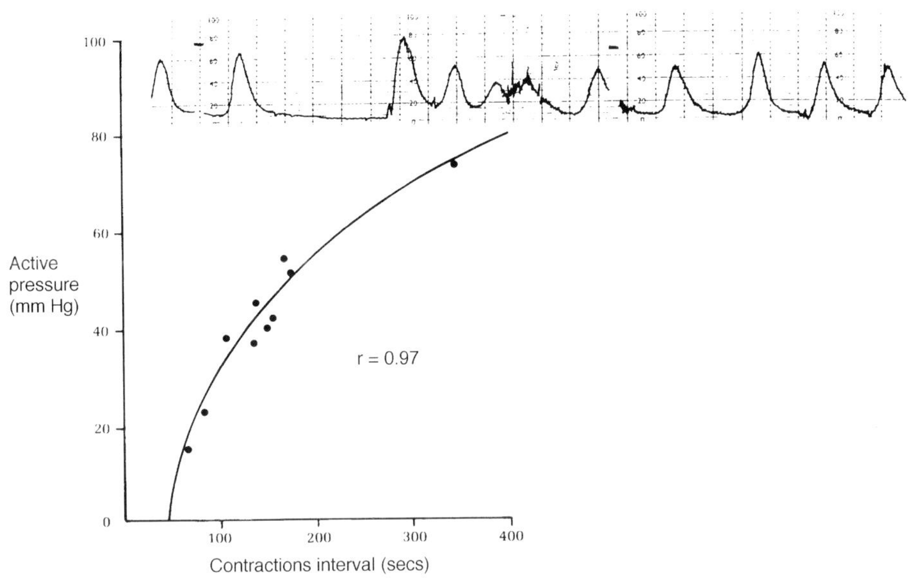

Fig. 75.3 The relationship between contraction frequency and contraction pressure illustrated by calculation from the strip shown above (P.J. Steer, personal communication).

vascular haemodynamics by alterations to preload and afterload and the subsequent changes in cardiac output can impair oxygen delivery to the tissues. The second stage is therefore potentially more hazardous than the first stage.

Other acute events which may occur in labour are placental abruption, maternal hypotension (postural or from fluid loss), and cord prolapse.

Physiological adjustments to hypoxaemia

The fetus is normally able to balance oxygen supply and energy demand to maintain aerobic metabolism despite living at low partial pressures of oxygen. The increased oxygen-carrying capacity of fetal blood is due partly to its higher haemoglobin concentration and partly to the greater affinity of fetal haemoglobin for oxygen. This enables fetal blood to become saturated with oxygen at low partial pressures of oxygen. Tissue oxygen delivery is also determined by blood flow; first to the placenta and then to the individual fetal organs. Fetal cardiac output is four times higher than in the adult per kilogram of body weight, with the majority directed to the placenta[7]. This gives a wide safety margin for adequate oxygen delivery. This oxygen reserve means that fetal oxygen extraction at the tissues can increase by almost 100% when needed[8].

Oxygen requirement is determined by fetal size, fetal activity and essential fetal metabolic processes. Energy demand can be reduced long term by decreased growth. If oxygen supply and requirement are in balance the fetus has adequate oxygen to metabolize glucose aerobically to produce the energy required for organ function.

The healthy fetus is very able to adjust to episodes of hypoxaemia with a synchronized response which involves behavioural, cardiovascular, metabolic and hormonal adjustments[9]. There are some variations in the reflex response related to maturity, but immature fetal tissue is generally more robust. The smaller body mass and therefore lower oxygen requirement relative to placental size also gives a larger oxygen reserve in the premature fetus.

Fetal movements account for a significant proportion of total oxygen consumption[10] and the first response to a reduction in oxygen supply is to decrease energy requirements by a decrease in fetal activity. In the fetus most fetal activity occurs in rapid eye movement (REM) sleep and a reduction in REM state and activity occurs with acute oxygen deficiency[11,12] and prolonged hypoxaemia when the arterial oxygen saturation has fallen to less than 30%[13]. At this level of oxygen saturation the brain still maintains aerobic metabolism[14], so a reduction in REM activity does appear to be a primary response to lower oxidative needs in the brain.

The most important cardiovascular response is the centralization of blood flow to the heart, brain and adrenals with increased oxygen extraction at the placental bed and tissues. Myocardial contractility increases and cardiac output is maintained, or marginally increased. The increase in umbilical blood flow with improved extraction of oxygen from the placental bed ensures aerobic metabolism is maintained until the oxygen content of the arterial blood has fallen by some 70%[14].

If these adjustments fail to maintain adequate oxygen supply to the central organs, aerobic metabolism is supplemented by anaerobic metabolism of glucose and glycogen to maintain cell and organ function. This is most important in the fetal myocardium, where the three-to fivefold increase in coronary blood flow may still be inadequate to compensate for the increase in oxygen consumption caused by the sympatho-adrenergic stimulation of myocardial workload. The importance of anaerobic metabolism to the maintenance of myocardial function and survival of the fetus during asphyxia is long established, and depends on the preasphyxial glycogen content of the myocardium and liver[15,16]. Anaerobic glycolysis produces only 1/15 of the ATP produced aerobically, and it is therefore a short-term emergency measure or a longer-term additional energy source to oxidative metabolism.

The process of anaerobic metabolism produces lactic acid and releases hydrogen ions. The hydrogen ions are buffered primarily by bicarbonate ions, but also by haemoglobin and proteins. As the hydrogen ion concentration increases, these buffers are consumed and a progressive metabolic acidosis develops with a fall in pH and a rise in the base deficit of the extracellular fluid. Glycogen, the long-term store of glucose, is depleted in this process.

Glucose is also the predominant cerebral fuel[17–19]. Alternative cerebral fuels include fatty and amino acids but all require more oxygen than glucose to produce equivalent energy and only glucose can be metabolized in the absence of oxygen.

Hypoxaemic events in labour are often intermittent, so the ability to revert to a normal blood flow distribution and metabolism with normoxia is also important. During prolonged moderate hypoxaemia the acute changes of bradycardia and hypertension at the onset of hypoxaemia are soon followed after about 30 min by fetal adaptation[20]. Haemoglobin, blood volume, erythropoietin, cortisol, catecholamines and heart rate are all increased but by modest amounts, which are are almost indistinguishable from the control state[21,22]. However, the response in these fetuses to further acute episodes of hypoxaemia is likely to be impaired and of smaller magnitude (Fig. 75.1); thus the initial fetal bradycardia in response to acute hypoxaemia is less marked or even abolished in fetuses with modestly elevated catecholamine levels and increased heart rates[22].

These profound alterations of blood flow and metabolism during asphyxia are the result of complex regulatory control by the autonomic nervous system, both neural and humoral. There is an impressive release of catecholamines in the fetus during a normal vaginal delivery[23] and this surge is enhanced many times (to values even greater than in an adult with a phaeochromocytoma) in a fetus that suffers perinatal asphyxia[24]. There is no doubt that this sympathoadrenal response is a fundamental part of the defence mechanism of the fetus and neonate[25].

The case for fetal monitoring

Every woman should have a caring companion with her in labour as evidence finds this decreases the duration of labour with benefits to both mother and fetus[26]. Every woman and her fetus should be monitored during labour. Commonsense suggests that the method of monitoring and clinical response to this should be individualized for the particular woman, particular fetus and particular situation (developed or undeveloped country) and the available resources. Thus in parts of the world it may be better to accept a higher perinatal mortality to avoid caesarean section, and subsequent risk to the mother, whereas in others a high caesarean section rate may be appropriate to avoid any perinatal mortality.

Although there has never been a randomized trial comparing fetal monitoring with no monitoring, there is good observational evidence that intrapartum monitoring prevents perinatal death. Babies are saved by timely intervention for cord prolapse, abruption, disproportion and fetal distress. In deprived communities, with little or no monitoring, fresh intrapartum stillbirths are the major cause of perinatal death[27]. Some would argue this comparison is not justified, since the general standard of nutrition, health and hygiene in these communities is far below that enjoyed in the developed world. Fortunately for cynics, comparable data are available from a natural experiment in Indiana, United States where members of a religious sect, the Faith Assembly, refuse all medical care[28]. They have a maternal mortality rate comparable to Africa but also a perinatal mortality nearly three times that of their Indiana sisters. This is despite the fact that the social status of members is higher than other women in the State and there is some evidence of concealment of perinatal death. It seems reasonable to conclude that some form of intrapartum fetal monitoring does improve fetal outcome.

Fetal monitoring need be no more than evaluating the fetal heart rate (FHR) and the amount and colour of the liquor, together with consideration of the progress of labour. It can be done worldwide. However, it is important to appreciate that recording a variable is one thing, monitoring it requires thought, knowledge and experience coupled with some intuition, and the ability to effect some action.

Fetal heart rate monitoring – what is being measured?

Heart rate may be recorded either intermittently by auscultation with a count of heart beats heard with a Pinard stethoscope or handheld Doppler over an interval traditionally of 1 min. Alternatively, it can be recorded continuously by electronic recording of the interval between heart beats (R–R interval), obtained by ultrasound or ECG clip, and presented as a rate per minute on paper.

It is important to realize what these measurements represent. The physiological event is the interval between cardiac beats which is heart period. This is measured from the same fixed point in the cardiac cycle; most accurately from R wave to R wave of the ECG (R–R interval) but also from valve to valve or cardiac wall movement by ultrasound. The measurement by ultrasound from these less precise loci is obviously less accurate. Heart rate is a derivation; the average number of cardiac beats in a minute either taken as a pulse rate by intermittent auscultation (often counted over 15 s and multiplied by 4) or derived mathematically as the reciprocal of heart period.

Heart rate in beats per minute (bpm) =

$$\frac{1}{\text{Heart period in milliseconds}} \times 60 \text{ (seconds in a minute)} \times 1000 \text{ (milliseconds in a second)}$$

Thus a 500 ms heart period is 120 bpm.

Heart rate variability or variation is the small difference between successive heart periods expressed over time, e.g. beat to beat over two cardiac cycles; 1 min will be over about 120 cycles and so on. This has given rise to the vague terms of short- and long-term variability; both are best avoided. Heart rate variation is most easily measured and compared as the standard deviation (SD) of heart period over a specific, stated, time epoch. Obviously the longer this epoch the greater the SD, particularly if large transient changes (accelerations and decelerations) are not excluded. Heart rate variation is most easily seen as the small perturbations (jitter) in the baseline heart rate on continuous FHR recordings – it can then be expressed as bandwidth, e.g. absent, 5 bpm, 10–25 bpm etc. and this is adequate for clinical interpretation.

There are two important clinical differences between the information obtained from intermittent auscultation and that obtained from continuous FHR records which were appreciated many years ago[29] but are often forgotten. First, the averaging process of a pulse count by intermittent auscultation loses vast amounts of data which may include important transient changes (Fig. 75.4). Second, heart rate variation cannot be assessed by intermittent auscultation. It is now clear that this is as important a physiological variable as heart rate itself.

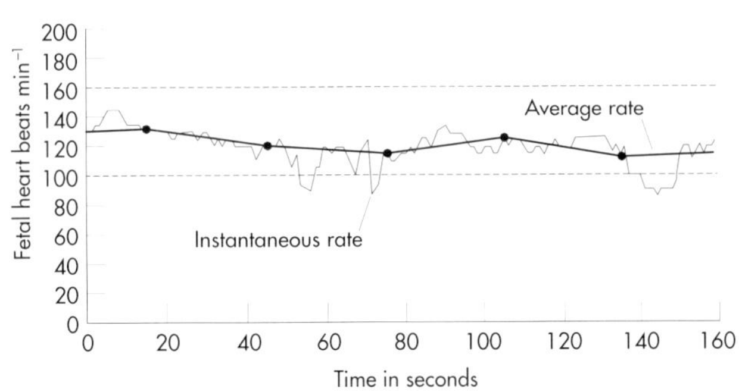

Fig. 75.4 The difference in information obtained by intermittent auscultation compared with continuous heart rate recording.

Fetal heart rate monitoring – the clinical evidence

The question is whether FHR monitoring is best done by intermittent auscultation or continuous electronic fetal monitoring (EFM). EFM was rapidly accepted into clinical practice for fetal monitoring in the developed world soon after its introduction in the late 1960s and without randomized controlled trials (RCTs). Clinical interpretation of changes was largely based on empirical observations of thousands of hours of recordings during human labour[30,31]. In the 1970s there were a large number of observational studies which favourably compared EFM with intermittent auscultation using historical or non-randomized concurrent controls (e.g. Beard *et al.*[31], Paul and Hon[32]). It was impossible to be sure that other factors did not contribute to the improvement noted (e.g. a fall in high parity pregnancy, the impact of termination and improvements in neonatal resuscitation).

The results of the first randomized controlled trial which compared the cardiotocogram (CTG) with intermittent auscultation of the FHR did not appear until 1976 and supported the use of the CTG in high-risk labours[34]. There have now been 12 randomized trials of intrapartum EFM from around the world. Nine of these compare the efficacy of CTG monitoring with intermittent auscultation[34–42]. The other three, which took place in Connecticut, USA[43]; Harare, Zimbabwe[44]; and Lund, Sweden[45], compared the efficacy of alternative approaches with EFM[43–45]. The trials have differed in their entry criteria (variously including 'high risk' or 'low risk' for all or most women), and in whether or not fetal scalp sampling for pH estimation was available as an adjunctive method of assessment of fetal well-being. Meta-analysis[46–48] is much influenced by the very large Dublin trial which specifically excluded meconium and oligohydramnios[40].

The only clear benefit to be demonstrated from the routine use of CTG is a reduction in neonatal seizures. Cumulative analysis suggests there was a protective effect of continuous FHR monitoring on data from the first study but this effect did not become statistically significant until the 1985 Dublin trial and persisted thereafter. Thacker *et al.*'s recent meta-analysis has also found a significant decrease associated with continuous FHR for a 1 min Apgar score of less than 4 (RR 0.82, 95% CI 0.65–0.98) in the seven studies in which this was recorded. This protective effect was only apparent in the non-USA trials and had not been reported previously[48].

The decrease in neonatal seizures and low 1 min Apgar score is at the expense of a significantly increased operative delivery rate both by caesarean section and instrumental vaginal delivery, though this has decreased with time. How much this lowered intervention is the result of increased use of fetal blood sampling, better education or the use of some other modality, such as stimulation testing, is uncertain. Certainly, in the Plymouth trial the use of the ST waveform of the ECG as an additional variable improved the interpretation of the CTG and halved the incidence of operative intervention[49]. Also meta-analysis of the first three trials, in which the option of scalp sampling was not used with EFM, found a fourfold increase in the odds of a caesarean section for fetal distress with no evidence of benefit in fetal outcome[46].

Thus the principal conclusions of the various overviews of RCTs on intrapartum monitoring find that:

- The rate of abdominal and vaginal operative delivery for the mother is increased by continuous CTG monitoring but
- There is reduction in the incidence of neonatal convulsions and some suggestion of fewer Apgar scores less than 4 at 1 min

Whilst a follow-up study of a proportion of children from the Dublin study shows no difference in long-term outcome at 4 years of age[46] and neonatal convulsions are a rare complication, most parents would presumably seek to avoid them. The finding of no detectable difference in long-term outcome does not exclude damage at the time, for the plasticity of the immature brain is well documented. Windle[50] has shown that many monkeys subjected to birth asphyxia lose their clinical neurological deficiencies with time, but remain histologically brain damaged, and the same is probably true of human infants[51].

Ironically there is an increasing argument that the RCTs have been performed too soon because EFM pattern interpretation is unreliable[1] and we are still not certain of appropriate outcome measures[52]. There are now strong recommendations that fetal outcome of labour should be assessed by cord blood gas measurement for pH and base deficit on both artery and vein[53–54] – disappointingly this has not been an outcome measure for evaluation of the efficacy of continuous FHR and intermittent auscultation (IA).

Intermittent auscultation

Whilst the evidence from the randomized trials strongly suggests that IA is as effective a method of monitoring the FHR of healthy fetuses in normal labour as present EFM techniques there has been a loss of confidence in its practice. There are two problems.

First, data from trials unfortunately do not usually reflect routine clinical practice but best practice! At the National Maternity Hospital, Dublin there has subsequently been evidence of a Hawthorne effect with the intrapartum and perinatal mortality rates lower during the trial period than in the 10 years before and since the trial. It seems likely that the quality of intermittent auscultation and EFM was improved during the trial which reduced the chance of detecting a difference between the two monitoring methods.

It has been repeatedly demonstrated that errors in counting the FHR by auscultation can be significant. Observers were more likely to bias baseline counts towards normal when the FHR was fast or slow[55,56] and a significant proportion of decelerations were missed[56–58]. The adoption of written protocols such as that of Sandmire[59] which advocates the setting of a timing device to ensure regular auscultation might improve confidence and ensure more accurate and effective use of IA. In the absence of data to demonstrate optimal time intervals for IA, Sandmire suggested that standard practice should be to evaluate and record the FHR following a contraction at least every 30 min in the active phase of the first stage of labour and at least every 15 min in the second stage of labour. The American College of Obstetricians guidelines are IA every 15 min in the first stage and every 5 min in the second stage of labour[60].

An important practical problem is that most labour wards cannot provide the one-to-one staffing level required to perform auscultation appropriately, however desirable this might be. Even with one-to-one midwifery in a highly motivated group of mothers and midwives there was a two- to sevenfold increase in asphyxia-related perinatal deaths in home delivery cases in South Australia where intrapartum monitoring was by IA[61].

Second, in choosing a monitoring method on the basis of antepartum risk we need to remind ourselves of our inability to identify which pregnancy is high risk or indeed even low risk. There is ample evidence that the concept of deciding intrapartum risk and therefore the method of monitoring on the basis of supposed antenatal risk cannot be supported. Wilson and Schifrin[62], in a summary of five risk assessment papers, found that patients with low antenatal risk contributed 58% of the perinatal mortality and morbidity compared to the 42% contributed by the high-risk group. In a retrospective review of birth asphyxia cases in Oxford 26 of 64 cases (40%) were presumably considered low risk and were not monitored by a CTG[63]. A case controlled study of intrapartum stillbirths in Western Australia failed to identify any antenatal risk factors which predicted these deaths[64]. Current methods of antenatal assessment of risk are poor at identifying the low-risk fetus and the only antepartum factors which are consistently associated with risk of perinatal morbidity and mortality are low birth weight for gestational age, the presence of meconium-stained liquor[65] and antepartum haemorrhage.

It is surely not a difficult concept to accept that risk is individual for any given fetus and, whilst there are maternal factors which can influence this, individual placentation and subsequent growth and development are the more important.

Intrapartum risk for the fetus is best assessed at the onset of labour, or as early as possible thereafter, to determine whether a fetus is healthy with its defence mechanisms intact or whether it is already compromised. This is the rationale for the admission CTG discussed in Ch. 74. If a fetus is normally grown and has a normal reactive strip of CTG in early labour then that fetus will cope with a normal labour without harm[66] and can be monitored by IA.

Another strategy is to regard electronic monitoring as *not* indicated when the fetus is a singleton in cephalic presentation between 37 and 41 weeks, with clear liquor after the spontaneous onset of labour in a pregnancy with no major antenatal complications unless there is an abnormality of the FHR on careful IA. Times of particular risk, for any fetus, are at the end of the first stage and during the second stage for the reasons indicated earlier and it is wise to obtain more careful recordings at these times.

The cardiotocogram

Monitoring may be appropriate by IA in the low-risk fetus but when there is established risk continuous monitoring with the cardiotocogram (CTG) and a fetal blood sampling (FBS) option are indicated[67]. The continuing debate about use of the CTG should not be allowed to cloud the fact that it contains a wealth of important physiological data about the fetus, which *is* useful to clinical practice in the recognition of intrapartum events.

The instruments are recorders of fetal activity; it is the clinicians that are the monitors. It is seldom verbalized that what the obstetrician is really looking for in fetal monitoring is the reassurance to allow labour to continue. What can be said with a good degree of certainty[66,68,69] is that if there is a cyclically reactive heart rate pattern in the range 110–170 (Fig. 75.5) the fetus is not hypoxaemic and does have an ability to respond to the stress of normal labour – it has good sensitivity. This is the basis for advocating a continuous strip of CTG recording early in labour and at regular intervals even in those fetuses being monitored largely by auscultation.

Similarly, when there is a profound and persistent bradycardia or persistent tachycardia with loss of baseline variation and late or large variable decelerations there should be little doubt that the fetus needs delivery by the most expeditious means possible.

It is between these extremes that a variety of other heart rate changes occur (as a result of more frequent contractions, umbilical cord compression, maternal hypotension and pressure on the head as it descends in the pelvis) which are much less readily interpreted as normal or abnormal. It is really no surprise that in widespread clinical practice, if there is no other reassurance of normality, these give rise to much unnecessary intervention (poor specificity).

It is not the intention to discuss FHR patterns in detail here but to draw attention to the important issues. FHR traces should be completely described with consideration of:

- Signal quality – FHR and contraction channel
- Location, duration and frequency of contractions
- Baseline heart rate
- Baseline variation and cyclicity
- Presence or absence of accelerations
- Periodic decelerations; presence, magnitude and timing
- Evolution of patterns

SIGNAL QUALITY – FHR AND CONTRACTION CHANNEL

You cannot monitor with an inadequate CTG signal but in practice this is all too frequent a problem[1]. It is essential to have uterine activity measurement to distinguish the types of deceleration and to recognize abnormal uterine activity. The FHR by ultrasound is more prone to noise and signal dropout than from an ECG clip.

All recorders, particularly when operating from ultrasound, have 'system logic' to prevent triggering by an apparently erroneous signal. In general this improves the quality of the recorded trace but there are times when this cannot be relied upon, e.g. rapid maternal heart rate, fetal heart block or other arrhythmia (see below). The fetal rate should always be checked by auscultation at initial connection. It is also possible to pick up the maternal ECG from a clip to give an apparently bradycardic FHR when the fetus is dead.

The human brain is particularly adapted for pattern recognition and it is important to realize that the pattern of a continuous FHR record looks very different if the vertical (bpm) scale or horizontal (time) scale are different. Unfortunately

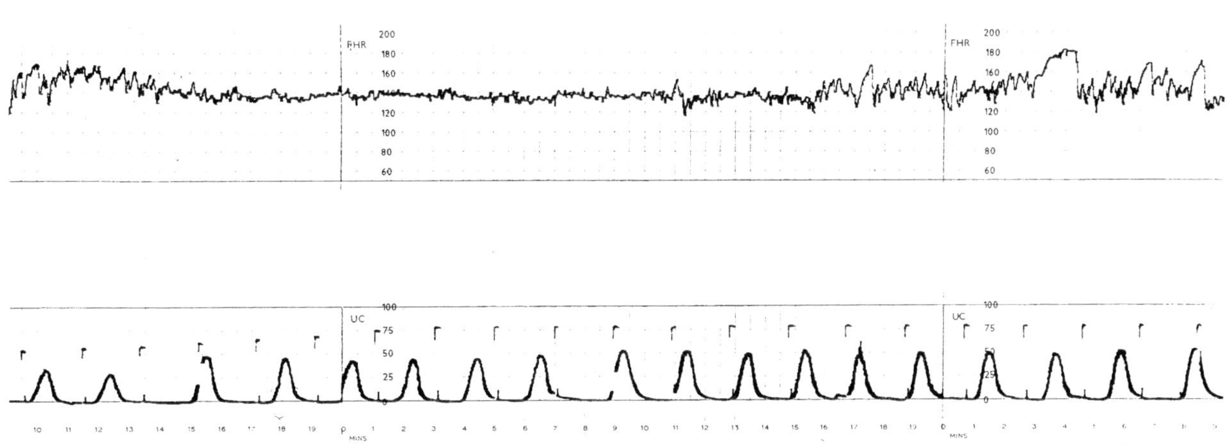

Fig. 75.5 A strip of normal CTG in labour illustrating alternating cycles of reactive and non-reactive heart rate patterns.

the former is not standardized between recorders and there are large differences in the speed of recording in Europe (1 cm/min) and the USA (3 cm/min).

FETAL ARRHYTHMIAS

From time to time a cardiac arrhythmia is detected either by auscultation or more frequently by continuous heart rate monitoring antepartum or during labour. Arrhythmias result from abnormal automaticity, abnormal conduction or a combination of both in some part of the cardiac conduction system. They present with a heart rate of more than 200 bpm, less than 100 bpm or an irregularity of rhythm[70]. An irregularity of rhythm is usually due to atrial or ventricular premature systoles (ectopic foci) which are common, especially in early pregnancy, and are generally benign.

Supraventricular tachyarrhythmias, such as atrial flutter and fibrillation and supraventicular tachycardia, have a 5–10% incidence of congenital heart disease and are prone to fetal and neonatal cardiac failure with ascites and hydrops[71,72].

Persistent bradycardias are usually due to congenital heart block with the rate commonly between 50–70 bpm. Congenital heart block has associations with maternal autoimmune disease[73,74], and there is a 40% incidence of congenital heart disease in the fetus[75]. Again heart failure in not uncommon.

As already noted, these abnormal rates may confuse the logic of heart rate monitors. The definitive diagnosis of an arrhythmia is from the electrocardiogram. Observation of the relative rates and synchrony of atrial and ventricular contraction by ultrasound may determine the nature of the arrhythmia and exclude congenital abnormality and cardiac failure. If the patient labours, serial fetal pH values should be measured to exclude asphyxia as fetuses with supraventricular tachyarrhythmias or heart block may not show the usual heart rate responses to hypoxaemia.

BASELINE

Traditionally, the baseline heart rate has been described as normal between 120–160 bpm. It would not be unusual for it to be 170 or 180 bpm in the preterm and the rate decreases with increasing gestation and maturity of the parasympathetic system so that it may be normal at 110 bpm in the postmature. These rates can therefore be considered normal if all other features of the FHR, and particularly variability/cyclicity, are normal. There is a relationship to the maternal heart rate and there may be a baseline tachycardia with thyrotoxicosis, administration of betamimetics or a baseline bradycardia with the administration of drugs such as betablockers. A tachycardia may also result from a fever with maternal or fetal infection or if the maternal core temperature increases with epidural analgesia which affects the autonomic control of heat loss[76]. Progressive fetal hypoxaemia produces a tachycardia from release of catecholamines whilst an acute event produces a bradycardia from increased vagal tone as a result of stimulation of chemoreceptors sensitive to a fall in pO_2, baroreceptors sensitive to blood pressure change and atrial receptors sensitive to changes in volume of venous return.

Establishing the baseline is the first important step of FHR analysis whether by eye or computer and is done by scanning over a 10 min window excluding transient changes of accelerations or decelerations. On occasions it can be difficult to decide whether there is a normal baseline with accelerations or a baseline tachycardia with decelerations (Fig. 75.6). Getting this wrong results in two diametrically opposite clinical decisions. This can usually be resolved by examining a previous piece of trace, best in a non-reactive cycle, to establish the baseline rate for that particular fetus. If this is at the start of labour then it is useful to remember that there may be previous antenatal CTG records. Clearly the baseline FHR should not be higher antenatally than it is in labour. But if it is be wary, particularly if the variability is reduced and the reactivity absent even if the rate is within the 120–160 level, for this might be a fetus with chronic hypoxaemia and blunted responses.

From time to time obvious sinusoidal patterns (of frequency 1–5 cycles/min) break through the overall FHR pattern. These are usually short-lived and some may be associated with bursts of sucking activity[77]. It has been suggested that one of 5 cycles/min is consistent with thermovasomotor oscillation and may become more obvious in labour if heat loss from the fetus via the placenta is impaired[78]. Persistent sinusoidal patterns occur in a number of different clinical situations associated with fetal anaemia either resulting from an acute bleed[79,80] or rhesus isoimmunization[81] and require immediate action.

BASELINE VARIATION AND CYCLICITY

The most striking feature of long FHR traces in the last third of gestation is of alternating cycles of increased baseline heart rate, increased heart rate variation and accelerations alternating with episodes of decreased heart rate and decreased heart rate variation with few accelerations which when they occur are of low magnitude (Fig. 75.5). These cycles continue throughout normal unsedated labour. Real-time scanning has established that though most fetal movements occur during the episodes of increased variation, movements also occur during the episodes of decreased variation but the modulation of heart rate in association with the fetal movement in these episodes is less marked[82]. Cycles in fetal movement have been observed from 24 weeks' gestation[83] but significant clustering of fetal movement within episodes of high heart rate variation only occurs from 28 weeks onwards[84,85]. Movements are only significantly associated with bursts of acceleration from 34 weeks. From this time too the length of low-variation episodes increases, reaching up to 40 min by term. Thus the relationship of changes in heart rate and variation

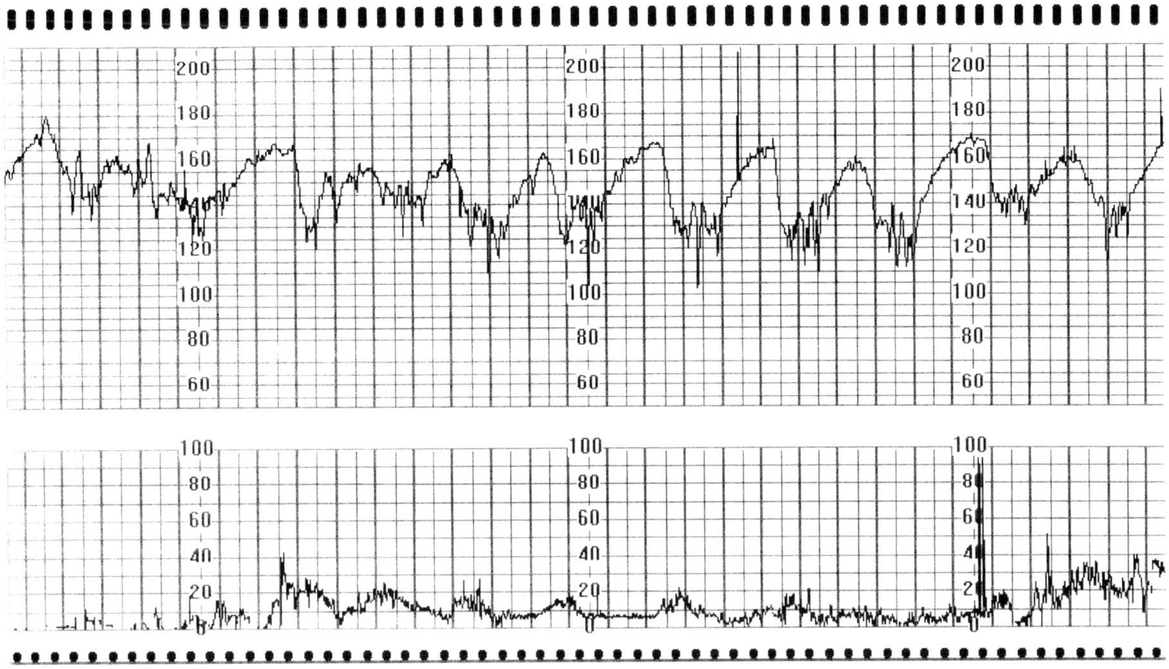

Fig. 75.6 A CTG to illustrate the difficulties and importance of defining baseline – tachycardia with dips or normocardia with accelerations?

with fetal movement seem to reflect a pattern of neurological development and integration. The timing of this is similar to that seen in the ontogeny of sleep states in newborn premature infants[86,87]. Prior to 36 weeks there is no synchronization of cycles of the EEG, rapid eye movements, respiration and tonic activity[88] and it is only after this age that periods of quiet and rapid eye movement (REM) sleep can be consistently identified. Fetal studies with real-time scanners simultaneously observing eye movements, body movements, fetal breathing and swallowing have confirmed that these FHR cycles are related to activity states[89].

Heart rate variation increases with acute hypoxaemia in the fetal lamb[90] and probably also in the human fetus[91] but a more chronic insult reduces the variation to produce a flat trace probably by loss of the episodes of high variation with changes in REM sleep. Such a pattern for more than 60 min duration at term (in the absence of anencephaly or sedation) is suggestive of a compromised fetus, particularly if coupled with decelerations both antepartum and intrapartum[31].

PRESENCE OR ABSENCE OF ACCELERATIONS

Towards the end of gestation the normal FHR trace is dominated by the number and size of accelerations. In fetal sheep the accelerations associated with fetal movement are known to be associated with a blood pressure rise. The fetal movement, whilst contributing to the size of the acceleration, does not initiate it as accelerations persist when the fetus is paralysed with a muscle relaxant[92]. This pattern of increased heart rate, increased blood pressure and limb movement is akin to the fight or flight response of increased sympathetic activity and is a defence reaction. It is the most reassuring sign of ability of the fetus to cope with labour. However, such a reactive CTG cannot exclude prior cerebral damage from an earlier incident in the pregnancy since the origin of these rhythms is likely to be at brain stem level[93]. The absence of accelerations is not associated with an abnormal outcome provided that cycles of increased and decreased heart rate variation remain.

PERIODIC DECELERATIONS: PRESENCE, MAGNITUDE AND TIMING

Decelerations are described as early, late or variable according to their time relationship to the contraction. Early and late decelerations have a symmetrical waveform but very different aetiologies. Early decelerations have the onset and recovery coinciding with the beginning and end of a contraction. They most usually occur when the cervix is 6–7 cm dilated or a high head descends into the pelvis and are more common when the membranes are ruptured. They are vagally mediated and benign. Late decelerations are uniform, usually shallow dips and have their nadir after the nadir of the contraction. They occur either with prolonged contractions, which temporarily reduce oxygenation, or with preexisting hypoxaemia[94] and require attention to improve oxygenation and, if they persist, further evaluation.

Variable decelerations are variable in amplitude, shape and timing to the uterine contraction. Though traditionally thought of as being due to umbilical cord compression[95,96] they also occur with maternal hypotension associated with the supine position and epidural top-ups. The initial onset is vagal, related either to decreased atrial filling with umbilical vein occlusion, or to a rise in fetal blood pressure activating the baroreceptors, to give a reflex bradycardia which is sometimes sufficient to cause a conduction block[97]. If the bradycardia is sustained, there is decreased cardiac output and placental perfusion to cause hypoxaemia. The relationship to asphyxia is therefore also variable, but is related to both their size and duration (dip area). These are the most common and most difficult heart rate patterns to assess.

EVOLUTION OF PATTERNS

The combination and progression of heart rate changes are the most important evidence of problematic hypoxaemia; decelerations in combination with a progressive tachycardia, progressive loss of variability in association with decelerations and tachycardia, progressive widening and deepening of decelerations with lack of recovery to the baseline rate. All these patterns require some action (Table 75.1).

The problems in practice

'For monitoring to be effective, it must be performed correctly, its results must then be interpreted satisfactorily; and this interpretation must provoke an appropriate response'[46]. All these facets have been tested in RCTs to date.

It is the complexity and dynamics of the data provided by the continuous heart rate trace which can be difficult to interpret, particularly by the inexperienced. It requires both knowledge of the physiology and clinical acumen to appreciate important changes over time. These skills are difficult to establish and maintain with rapid staff turnover and they are not available 24 hours a day for all deliveries. The Confidential Enquiry into Stillbirths and Deaths in Infancy[1] found 40% of the deaths in healthy babies that occurred during birth in Britain were linked to suboptimal care by 'human beings' due to insufficient skills, inappropriate attitudes and apparent lack of senior accountability. Failure to react to abnormal cardiotocograms was the commonest reported problem with inadequate monitoring and overdosage with oxytocics as other failings. Nearly two thirds of the intrapartum and early neonatal deaths were attributed to asphyxia. Obstetricians were most commonly criticized for failure to act appropriately, whereas midwives and general practitioners were more likely to have failed to recognize problems. It is usually the most junior member of staff, with the patient, who first has to recognize an abnormality to know that a more experienced further opinion is required. The problem is large, for at least 50% of mothers are monitored by the CTG in the UK.

The difficulties of subjective interpretation and human fallibility have long been recognized and have led to attempts to use CTG computer analysis. Despite their 10–20 years of development, the effectiveness of these systems in labour has yet to be shown. The likely explanation is that conventional computer systems analyse the CTG in isolation from clinical factors. Consideration of the CTG in isolation probably also accounts for much of the reported inter- and intraobserver error[98,99] which is considerably less when the clinical action rather than the interpretation per se is examined[100]. In practice experienced clinicians do not interpret the CTG in isolation but in the context of clinical factors which also affect management. Thus the response to moderate variable decelerations in a primigravida in induced labour at 1 cm dilatation would be different from the same finding in a multigravida in spontaneous labour at 8 cm. More recently research has

TABLE 75.1
A CTG classification protocol with criteria for action, indicating the need for another discriminatory variable (e.g. FBS)

Classification	Baseline	Variability	Decelerations	Action
Normal	110–160 bpm	10–25 bpm	None	Continue recording
Intermediate	100–110 bpm 160–180 bpm	>25 bpm <5 bpm	Early Mild variable[a]	Any two >30 min FBS Repeat 1 h[b]
Abnormal	<100 bpm with accelerations >180 bpm	<5 bpm in the absence of sedation and no accelerations	Severe variable[c] Late	Any one >30 min FBS Any two >15 min FBS Repeat 1 h[b]
Preterminal	Persistent bradycardia, no accelerations exceeding 100 bpm and believe this will persist			Deliver immediately If not FBS

[a]<60 dropped beats, <60 s duration
[b]FBS earlier if CTG deteriorates
[c]>60 dropped beats, >60 s

focused on the possibility of using an expert system approach to support clinical decision making during labour[101–103].

Conventional computing systems manipulate numerical data whilst expert systems manipulate symbolic representations of knowledge. Central to an expert system is a resident rule base representing knowledge derived from clinical experts. The system simulates human reasoning by using this knowledge to assess new incoming data (the CTG, clinical information), to infer relationships and draw conclusions within the 'inference engine'. Since the system is rule-based it can explain and justify how a conclusion was reached allowing a dialogue with the clinician which would allow even an inexperienced one to reach an informed decision rather than blindly accept advice. It therefore has the important capacity not only to monitor but also to teach. Clearly the most difficult aspect of development is rigorous evaluation and validation but this is proceeding apace[100]. There is then the challenge of developing the user interface to ensure meaningful interaction between man and machine in widespread clinical use[103].

Whilst it is possible to derive much information about neurodevelopmental integration and the cardiovascular responses to stress and hypoxia from the CTG, it has always been somewhat naive to think one can judge the condition of the fetus solely on the basis of a sophisticated pulse rate. Even the experienced frequently need more information to determine what the best course of clinical action might be. The addition of another variable does improve the reliability of interpretation when there are uncertain patterns of CTG change. Fetal blood sampling has traditionally been the second variable to judge the level of acidosis but the evoked response is widely used in North America, and the ECG waveform shows considerable promise, whilst pulse oximetry is being widely investigated clinically. The use of other variables can add to interpretational difficulties and emphasize still further the need for decision support tools. However, the CTG will always be the mainstay of intrapartum fetal monitoring.

Fetal blood sampling

ACID–BASE PHYSIOLOGY

As already discussed, the fetus normally derives its metabolic needs by the oxidation of glucose (or glycogen) to water and carbon dioxide in the presence of oxygen with the generation of 38 units of ATP – aerobic metabolism. However, in conditions of hypoxaemia the fetal tissues can still metabolise glucose and glycogen as far as lactic acid in the Kreb cycle with the generation of 2 units of ATP – anaerobic metabolism. This process will occur in some tissues before others as a result of redistribution of oxygen flow from the least dependent tissues to the vital organs of heart, brain and adrenals. Clearly anaerobic metabolism is much more inefficient than aerobic metabolism but it is a very important survival mechanism, particularly to maintain cardiac and brain function. However, in anaerobic metabolism, the accumulation of pyruvic and lactic acid causes an increase in hydrogen ions [H^+] – a metabolic acidosis. Free intracellular hydrogen ions are toxic to cells and are buffered by bicarbonate, haemoglobin and plasma protein. Hydrogen ions can also accumulate (and the availability of bicarbonate to buffer metabolic acidosis decrease) by accumulation of CO_2 – a respiratory acidosis. It is only when the buffers are saturated that there is a marked increase in free [H^+] ions and a fall in pH and acidosis, and this occurs sometime after the onset of hypoxaemia. It is important to realize that pH is a logarithmic function of the [H^+] concentration. Thus a fall in pH from 7.30 to 7.20 is not as significant as a fall from 7.10 to 7.00. In the latter situation there are about twice as many free [H^+] generated. Extracellular levels of pH and pCO_2 can be measured from a blood sample and the buffering capacity (expressed as base deficit, BD, or buffer base, BB) calculated from these. Siggaard-Anderson[104] has shown that a high pCO_2 and the extracellular fluid (ECF) volume can unduly influence these calculations. Since the fetus has a relatively high pCO_2 and an increased ECF compared with the adult and acidosis is usually of both respiratory and metabolic origin (a mixed acidosis) it is increasingly argued[105,106] that buffering capacity in the perinatal period should be calculated in the ECF, not blood, and expressed as BDecf. In cases of a mixed acidosis with pH less than 7.20 the BDblood was about 30% higher than the BDecf[105].

SCALP BLOOD SAMPLING

Fetal blood sampling (FBS) was introduced into clinical practice for pH measurements by Saling in 1962[107]. This was an important step forward in understanding the effect of labour and blood gas homeostasis of the human fetus and in defining the importance of the FHR patterns revealed by continuous FHR measurement techniques. FBS is limited to the skin covering the fetal presenting part. Whilst animal studies have shown a good correlation for pH between scalp blood samples and the carotid artery[108] and between blood from the fetal scalp in the second stage and that of the umbilical vessels[109] there are a number of situations in which scalp pH measurements are inaccurate (e.g. oedema, caput succedaneum) or are misinterpreted.

The technique must be appropriate. Fetal blood can only be obtained with ruptured membranes and the cervix 2–3 cm dilated. Samples should be taken with the mother in the lateral position to avoid supine hypotension, which can produce a profound bradycardia with hypoxaemia and hypercarbia with a mixed acidosis. An amnioscope is passed into the vagina and through the cervix to rest on the presenting part of the fetus with sufficient pressure to exclude amniotic fluid (which would otherwise contaminate the sample) but not sufficient to cause stasis of capillary flow. Fetal skin is cleaned by a swab in a holder and then smeared with silicone gel so that, when the skin is punctured with a 2 mm blade, a droplet of blood forms rather than runs across the surface. An ethyl chloride spray will produce a reactive hyperaemia which aids bleeding. The droplet of blood is allowed to flow into a pre-heparined glass capillary tube, best by capillary action. The sample is then transferred to a blood gas analyser for immediate measurement. Modern blood gas analysers can perform a full analysis on a 40 μl sample to produce a value for pCO_2, pH and the calculated base deficit. The complete acid–base balance should, if possible, be assessed to differentiate between respiratory and metabolic acidosis.

Apart from the inconvenience and practical difficulties of obtaining an accurately measured sample a major problem of FBS is that it is intermittent. The physiology of hypoxaemia and acidosis (see earlier) means that a significant fall in pH can occur a short time after a normal sample has been obtained. Attempts over the last couple of decades to produce a continuous pH measurement have continued to prove unsuccessful.

The acid–base status of the fetus during labour usually mirrors that of the mother but at 0.10 of pH unit less than the maternal venous blood value[110]. Measurement of this difference was used clinically in the past but has fallen from clinical practice. However, it could be usefully reinstituted for there are several situations where consideration of both the maternal and fetal acid–base status is helpful. If a mother is hyperventilating (usually without an epidural and with ineffective pain relief) she will blow off CO_2 and have a respiratory alkalosis with a blood pH value of 7.50 or more. This will raise the fetal pH level and may confound the confirmation of hypoxaemia/acidosis. Similarly if she has a prolonged labour with a ketoacidosis there can be an infusion acidosis to the fetus to lower its pH level without hypoxaemia. In these situations a fetomaternal pH difference of more than 0.20 of a pH unit should be taken as indicative of fetal acidaemia. It is also a good habit to plot serial pH measurements to observe and interpret the trend in conjunction with any FHR abnormalities and the expected duration of labour. Significant hypoxaemia will produce a progressive acidaemia that can be recognized by such repeated measurements and projected to the expected time of delivery from the partogram. Again maternal samples might help *earlier* decision making, for a clear divergence in the graph of fetal from maternal pH (Fig. 75.7) suggests accumulating fetal $[H^+]$ and a significant hypoxaemia.

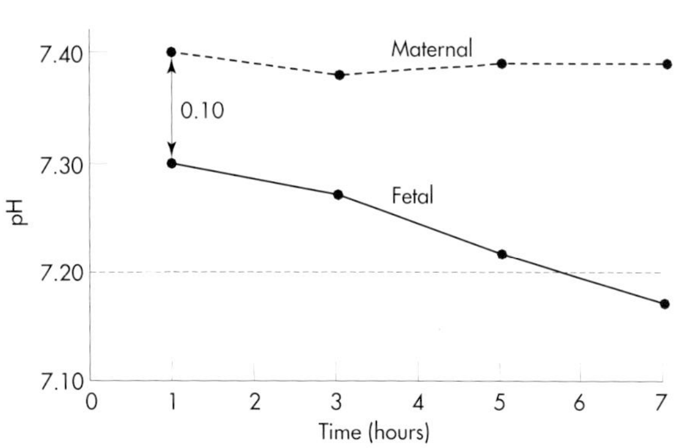

Fig. 75.7 Paired maternal and fetal blood samples plotted to illustrate use of comparison of data to establish a trend, whether there is divergence and its projection over time. This may help overcome some of the limitations of intermittent sampling.

There are also circumstances in which the use of FBS is potentially misleading; a fall in fetal pH is a late event in sepsis which may occur in labour with ascending chorioamnionitis.

LACTATE

There are good physiological reasons to measure lactate as a direct marker of anaerobic metabolism. A simple technique for the measurement in whole blood has recently been developed using just 5 μl of blood on a test strip and providing a lactate result within 1 min by analyses of the strip in a bedside electrochemical device[111].

A recent prospective randomized study compared lactate analysis to pH analysis at fetal scalp blood sampling in 341 cases with ominous FHR patterns[112]. Sufficient blood for lactate analysis was obtained significantly more often than for pH analysis. The failure rate for pH was inversely related to the degree of cervical dilation. The lactate group required fewer scalp incisions to obtain a sample and the result was obtained sooner than for pH (2 min compared with just under 4 min). There appeared to be no difference in the predictive value of either in this small study.

Since reluctance to perform FBS[113,114] is largely related to the difficulties of obtaining and measuring the sample, lactate analysis with this simple disposable test strip may increase the frequency of FBS and even encourage more serial use as a simple monitoring procedure. Further studies in other centres are required.

The effectiveness of FBS in clinical practice is quite another problem. Even with a strict protocol during a research trial[115] 39% of cases had FBS performed unnecessarily and 33% of cases did not have it performed when it was indicated. Murphy *et al.*[63] found similar problems with the selection and timing of FBS in a review of birth asphyxia cases. It is important to appreciate that FBS and the CTG are not independent monitoring methods in that a decision to obtain an FBS is dependent upon the interpretation of the CTG. If the level of CTG interpretation is suboptimal, the value of monitoring by FBS will be limited. Some units[116] advocate high FBS rates and there is evidence that higher rates of sampling are associated with higher mean cord arterial pH at delivery[117]. There is no evidence, however, that this approach will result in a reduction in birth asphyxia and, contrary to the RCT data, some large units with low intervention rates seldom perform FBS, but perhaps rely on fetal stimulation testing [114,118,119]. There is plenty of scope for misinterpretation of FBS results, and an increase in FBS rates without an improvement in knowledge of how to use the information is unlikely to be successful. The real problem, again, is the need for adequate training, knowledge and expertise in the interpretation of CTG changes in the context of the individual patient's labour.

RESPONSE TO FETAL STIMULATION

There is persuasive evidence, which is in keeping with the physiology of behavioural adjustments to hypoxaemia, that it is useful to assess the fetal FHR response to stimulation. Clark and colleagues, in a retrospective study of the FHR response to FBS, found that an acceleration of the heart rate of more than 15 bpm above the baseline rate for more than 15 s only occurred in fetuses with a pH more than 7.20 and in no fetus with a pH less than 7.20[120]. A subsequent prospective study of 100 cases with ominous FHR traces found that this positive response could be used to avoid FBS in 51% of cases. Of the 49 non-responders, 19 had a pH of 7.19 or less[121]. A more recent study has suggested that the false positive non-responders could be reduced further, to decrease the need for FBS by 73%, by redefining an acceleration as 10 bpm for 10 s and considering whether the heart rate variation was normal before scalp stimulation[122].

A startle response also occurs with vibroacoustic stimulation, which has been used as an alternative, particularly when the membranes are intact[123]. This can produce a prolonged change in behavioural state and there have been some concerns that the accentuation of the sound, which occurs in utero, might be harmful, although there is no evidence for this[124].

The stimulation test is dependent on maturity[125] and is probably only appropriate after 32 weeks' gestation. This is in keeping with the ontogeny of sleep states. Stimulation during quiet sleep (unreactive CTG pattern) does not have the same response as stimulation during wakefulness or REM sleep (reactive CTG pattern), although it has been suggested this is merely a function of stimulus intensity[126]! The response also changes if the stimulus is presented repeatedly[127] and this phenomenon of habituation is being examined as a measure of higher, cortical brain function[126].

Stimulation testing has apparently reduced the need to rely on FBS[114] in some units in the USA, but it has been unclear how the non-responders have been managed, to separate those needing action from those which do not. The simplicity of the test has much to recommend it but an RCT now seems justified.

THE FETAL ELECTROCARDIOGRAM

FHR analysis may be particularly valuable for assessment of fetal condition when used in conjunction with analysis of the ECG, which may be obtained continuously from the same fetal clip[128]. The electrocardiogram (ECG) reflects the summation of electrical events within the myocardium as seen from the body surface. These are influenced by electromechanical, hormonal and metabolic events. Like the adult, the fetal ECG consists of P, QRS and T waves separated by the PR and ST intervals. The P wave represents atrial contraction; the PR interval, the conduction time from the atrioventricular node down the bundle of His; the QRS, ventricular contraction; and the ST waveform ventricular repolarization. Repolarization of the atria is obscured by the QRS complex.

Two portions of the ECG waveform have attracted particular study; the ST waveform and the relationship of the PR to PR interval. There is a substantial body of evidence from various groups, both observational and experimental, on numerous animal species including a randomized control trial in man that changes in the ST waveform of the fetal ECG occur in association with hypoxaemia and asphyxia[129]. Data on the PR/RR time constants are less clear and principally supported by one group, but may prove additionally useful in the future[130].

PR/RR RELATIONSHIPS

There are interrelationships between various time constants of the cardiac cycle to ensure the efficiency of the heart as a pump. There is usually a positive relationship between PR and RR interval in the adult and fetus, so that when the heart speeds up the PR shortens and vice versa. The sinoatrial (SA) node controls heart rate, under autonomic control, and the sensitivity of the atrioventricular (AV) node determines AV conduction times and thus PR interval. During hypoxaemia in sheep both with[131] and without acidosis[132] there was a parodoxical shortening of the PR interval with lengthening of the RR interval (bradycardia) – negative PR/RR. It is postulated that this occurs during hypoxia because the sensitivity of the AV node to circulating adrenaline is increased relative to the SA node so that the PR interval is shortened, whilst the RR interval is lengthened. Initially it was suggested, from observations in humans, that this reversal of the normal relationship of PR/RR ratio might identify heart rate decelerations which were hypoxaemic in origin from those that were not[133]. It was subsequently found that, whilst a consistently positive relationship was always associated with a normal outcome, 'any stress appeared to stimulate a switch to a negative relationship'[130]. There were also problems about expressing instantaneous beat-to-beat relationships over the course of labour, which have resulted in the use of some complicated mathematical derivatives over time. However, in a small RCT the use of these indices together with the CTG compared with CTG alone reduced the incidence of FBS[134]. It remains unclear whether there is a physiological basis to this. A more recent study of 618 normal-term fetuses has suggested the negative PR/RR ratio is a function of any bradycardia, whether hypoxaemic or haemodynamic in origin, and is a normal adaptive response to enable efficient atrial filling with the decreased venous return. The PR/RR was positive when there were no periodic changes in rate, was always positive with accelerations (shorter PR, shorter RR) and always negative (shorter PR, longer RR) when there was a bradycardia of more than 40 bpm from the baseline[135]. The P wave can disappear altogether with profound vagal bradycardia and then the PR interval cannot be measured[135,135a].

There clearly needs to be a better understanding of the physiology of these measurements before they can reasonably be used clinically and this requires further study.

THE ST WAVEFORM OF THE ECG

The process of repolarization of the myocardial cells is particularly sensitive to metabolic and ionic events about the cell. In the adult analysis of the ST waveform is useful to define the size and progress of myocardial infarcts and in the diagnosis of coronary insufficiency using the exercise ECG.

There is no doubt from the data of many animal studies[128,136] that ST waveform elevation, during fetal hypoxaemia, is related to anaerobic metabolism as evidenced by the production of lactate with the depletion of myocardial energy-rich substances of glycogen, creatinine phosphate and ATP[137,138]. During moderate hypoxaemia when some fetuses sustain aerobic metabolism there is no ST waveform elevation[139] and no substantial rise in catecholamine levels[140]. The ability of an individual fetus to maintain sufficient myocardial oxygen supply to maintain aerobic metabolism at a given pO_2 depends on the ability to increase coronary oxygen flow, by increased oxygen carriage and increased myocardial blood flow, balanced against myocardial oxygen consumption, which depends on the size of the myocardium and the workload on it. In the fetus, myocardial workload depends on the product of heart rate and blood pressure and is increased by circulating catecholamines.

If there is an imbalance between myocardial oxygen supply and consumption then anaerobic metabolism occurs with ST waveform elevation. The dynamics of this even in the same fetus have been demonstrated in a number of experiments in chronic fetal lambs by progressive decreases in maternal pO_2 during labour[141] and by repeated occlusions of either maternal aorta[142] or fetal cord[143].

As already discussed, many of the processes involved in these adjustments are beta-receptor mediated and so it is no surprise that elevation of the ST waveform has been produced by infusion of the beta-agonist isoprenaline and these changes and those produced during mild hypoxaemia were blocked by propranolol[144].

ST depression with negative T waves has been observed during hypoxia experiments in experimentally growth retarded guinea pigs whilst their normally grown littermates showed ST elevation[145]. Such runted fetuses have lower catecholamine levels and probably have depleted myocardial glycogen reserves and a blunted sympathoadrenal response. During hypoxia they are likely to have ineffective anaerobic metabolism and suffer the direct effect of oxygen lack in the deeper myocardial layers (endocardium) before the superficial layers (epicardium) to alter the sequence of repolarization to produce a negative ST waveform – the ischaemic pattern seen in the adult.

These data were used to design a clinical model of interpretation to use the ST waveform in combination with the CTG (Fig. 75.8) for fetal monitoring. This has been tested

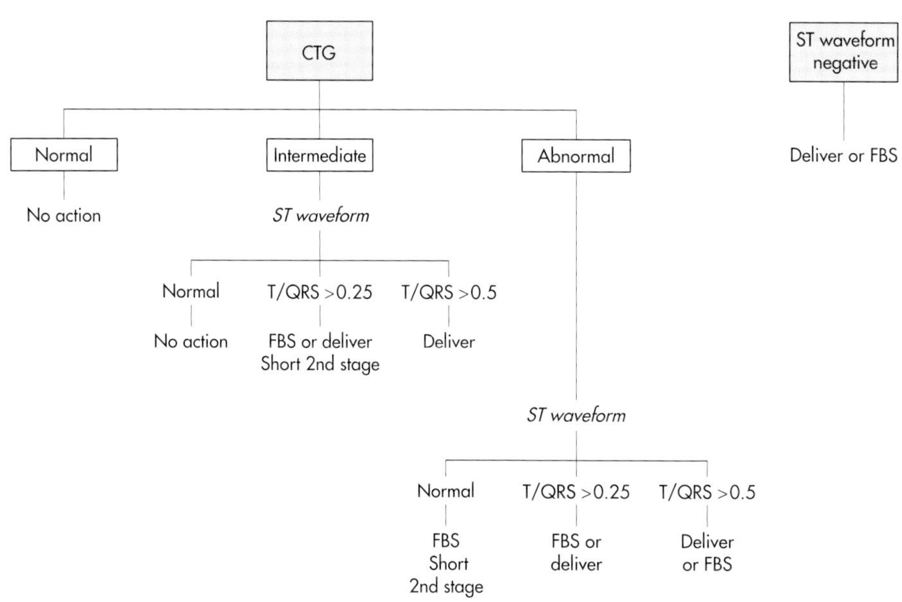

Fig. 75.8 Model of interpretation for use of CTG with ST waveform and fetal blood sampling.

against the CTG alone in a randomized trial of 2400 high-risk, near-term deliveries in Plymouth[146,147]. There was a highly significant reduction (46%) in operative deliveries for fetal distress in the ST + CTG arm (with no difference in operative deliveries for other reasons) together with a significant reduction in the use of FBS. There were no significant differences in the measures of neonatal outcome, but a trend to fewer low 5 min Apgar scores and less metabolic acidosis in the ST + CTG arm.

It does appear on the physiological and clinical evidence that CTG and ST waveform combinations may be used to differentiate the response of the healthy normoxic fetus from the healthy fetus suffering acute hypoxaemia and the chronically hypoxaemic or runted fetus (Fig. 75.1) by focusing on the most important mechanisms for the fetus to withstand asphyxia – increased myocardial blood flow and glycogenolysis. We can speculate that a fetus with maintained defence responses has normal heart rate reactivity and reacts to hypoxaemia with ST elevation, whereas a fetus with reduced ability has reduced heart rate reactivity and responds to hypoxaemia with ST depression.

Conclusions

Over the last couple of decades we have learnt a great deal about intrapartum monitoring and have a much better understanding of the physiological integrity and responses of the fetus. The relationship of possible monitoring strategies to the processes of hypoxaemia and asphyxia is much clearer and requires a thoughtful stepwise process of investigation dependent on individual need (Fig. 75.9). We can identify the certainly healthy fetus at the onset of labour and employ low-key monitoring strategies.

When we are concerned, continuous electronic fetal monitoring by the CTG will always be the principle means of surveillance; not only because it is a robust signal, which can be obtained non-invasively, but because it does give a wealth of information on the neurodevelopmental integration of the fetus and its response to changing haemodynamics. Cardiac output and therefore oxygen delivery is largely determined by heart rate. When the CTG is obtained by scalp clip there is the advantage of also obtaining continuous and complementary information from the fetal ECG, which provides direct information on the myocardium. Assessment of fetal reactivity and the response to stimulation at vaginal examination need to be part of an ongoing evaluation.

There is the real possibility that intermittent scalp sampling could be confined to a small number of fetuses where decision making remains uncertain and this may be more useful by lactate analysis done on a frequent sequential basis.

In the future, fetal pulse oximetry may provide additional, useful information though the relationship to the other variables is presently uncertain. As is evident from the experience

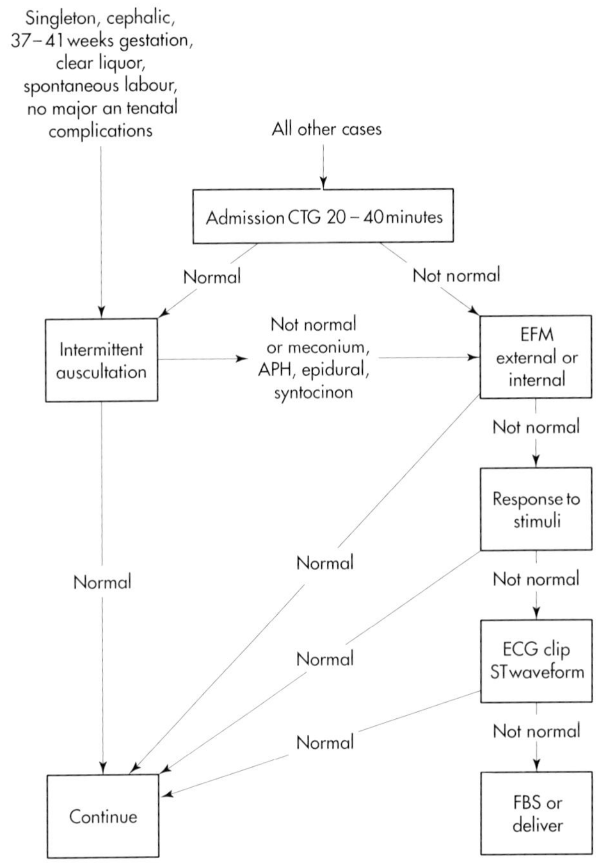

Fetal heart rate responses should be continuously assessed once electronic fetal monitoring (EFM) is commenced and the fetal ECG continuously assessed once the scalp clip is applied.

Fig. 75.9 Flow diagram for fetal monitoring based on the rationale of current evidence discussed in this chapter.

of EFM, widespread diffusion of a technology into clinical practice before efficacy and safety are determined can lead to misuse, misunderstanding, and unnecessary concerns regarding malpractice and litigation.

The real block to improved fetal monitoring today is human fallibility, not the need for another, yet to be proven, variable. Indeed, this problem already acts as a barrier to the implementation of new technology into clinical practice. For example, ST waveform analysis has not been promoted widely, despite the experimental background and findings of an RCT. It depends on pattern recognition and interpretation in conjunction with the CTG, which requires physiological understanding. In widespread use, inexperienced human interpretation of the data would probably repeat the past mistakes of CTG 'monitoring', and nothing would be gained.

It is difficult to see how this problem can be addressed other than by the use of expert systems for decision support but these will require very careful development and validation. The addition of stimulation testing or the ST waveform analysis algorithms to the rule base of a decision support system which has already been validated for CTG monitoring presents few new problems. Expert systems do offer opportunities for preprocessing complicated data, integrating information from different variables and presenting this to the clinicians, and possibly even the patient, in a way they can understand. In the meantime, complementary teaching/accreditation systems will be needed to educate clinicians on the information available from the different variables and to help effect change[147].

REFERENCES

1. Confidential Enquiry into Stillbirths and Deaths in Infancy (CESDI) *4th Annual Report Concentrating on Intrapartum Related Deaths 1994–95.* Maternal and Child Health Research Consortium, Chiltern Court, Baker Street, London NW1 5SD, 1997.
2. Hagberg B, Hagberg G, Olow I & von Wendt L. The changing panorama of cerebral palsy in Sweden. V. The birth year period 1979–82. *Acta Paediatr. Scand.* **78**, 283–290, 1989.
3. Pharoah POD, Cooke T, Cooke RWI & Rosenbloom L. Birthweight specific trends in cerebral palsy. *Arch. Dis. Child.* **65**, 602–606, 1990.
4. Nelson KB & Ellenberg JH. Antecedents of cerebral palsy. Multivariate analysis of risk. *N. Engl. J. Med.* **315**, 81–86, 1986).
5. Blair E & Stanley FJ. Intrapartum asphyxia a rare cause of cerebral palsy. *Paediatrics* **112**, 515–519, 1988.
6. Stanley FJ & Blair E. Why have we failed to reduce the frequency of cerebral palsy? *Med. J. Aust.* **154**, 623–626, 1991.
7. Cohn HE, Sachs EJ, Heymann MA & Rudolph AM. Cardiovascular responses to hypoxemia and acidemia in fetal lambs. *Am. J. Obstet. Gynecol.* **120**, 817–824, 1974.
8. Bocking AD, White SE, Homan J & Richardson BS. Oxygen consumption is maintained in fetal sheep during prolonged hypoxaemia. *J. Dev. Physiol.* **17**, 169–174, 1992.
9. Rosén KG. Intrapartum asphyxia. In *Fetal and Neonatal Neurology and Neurosurgery.* (eds M.I. Levene & R.J. Lilford) vol. **23**, pp. 389–404. London: Churchill Livingstone, 1995.
10. Rurak DW & Gruber NC. The effect of neuromuscular blockade on oxygen consumption and blood gases in the fetal lamb. *Am. J. Obstet. Gynecol.* **145**, 258–262, 1983.
11. Boddy K, Dawes GS, Fisher R, Pinter S & Robinson JS. Fetal respiratory movements, electrocortical and cardiovascular responses to hypoxaemia and hypercapnia in sheep. *J. Physiol. (Lond)* **243**, 599–618, 1974.
12. Natale RN, Clewlow F & Dawes GS. Measurements of fetal forelimb movements in the lamb in utero. *Am. J. Obstet. Gynecol.* **140**, 545–551, 1981.
13. Richardson BS, Carmichael L, Homan J & Patrick JE. Electrocortical activity, electrocular activity and breathing movements in fetal sheep with prolonged and graded hypoxemia. *Am. J. Obstet. Gynecol.* **167**, 553–558, 1992.
14. Rurak DW, Richardson BS, Patrick JE, Carmichael L & Homan J. Oxygen consumption in the fetal lamb during sustained hypoxemia with progressive acidemia. *Am. J. Physiology* **258**, 1108–1115, 1990.
15. Dawes GS, Mott JC & Shelley HJ. The importance of cardiac glycogen for the maintenance of life in foetal lambs and newborn animals during anoxia. *J. Physiol.* **146**, 516–538, 1959.
16. Shelley HJ. Glycogen reserves and their changes at birth. *Br. Med. Bull.* **17**, 137–143, 1961.
17. Mann LI. Effects of hypoxia on fetal cephalic blood flow, cephalic metabolism and the electroencephalogram. *Exp. Neurol.* **29**, 336–348, 1970.
18. Jones MD, Burd LI, Makowski EI, Meschia G & Battaglia FC. Cerebral metabolism in sheep: a comparative study of the adult, the lamb and the fetus. *Am. J. Physiol.* **229**, 235–239, 1975.
19. Levitsky LL, Fisher DE, Paton JB & Delannoy CW. Fasting plasma levels of glucose, acetoacetate, D-β-hydroxybutyrate, glycerol and lactate in the baboon infant: correlation and cerebral uptake of substrates and oxygen. *Pediatr. Res.* **11**, 198–202, 1977.
20. Bocking A, Gagnon R, Milne K & White S. Circulatory responses to prolonged hypoxemia in fetal sheep. *Am. J. Obstet. Gynecol.* **159**, 1418–1423, 1989.
21. Kitanaka T, Gilbert RD & Longo LD. Maternal responses to long-term hypoxemia in sheep. *Am. J. Physiol.* **256**, R1340–1347, 1989.
22. Robinson JS, Kingston EJ, Jones CT & Thorburn GD. Studies on experimental growth retardation in sheep. The effect of removal of endometrial caruncles on fetal size and metabolism. *J. Dev. Physiol.* **1**, 379–398, 1979.
23. Lagercrantz H & Bistoletti P. Catecholamine release in the newborn infant at birth. *Pediatr. Res.* **11**, 889–893, 1977.
24. Nylund L, Lagercrantz H & Lunell NO. Catecholamines in fetal blood during birth in man. *J. Dev. Physiol.* **1**, 427–435, 1979.
25. Lagercrantz H & Slotkin TA. The 'stress' of being born. *Sci. Am.* **254**, 100–107, 1986.
26. Keirse MJNC, Enkin M & Lumley J. Social and professional support during childbirth. In *Effective Care in Pregnancy and Childbirth* (eds I. Chalmers, M. Enkin & M.J.N.C. Keirse), pp. 805–814. Oxford: Oxford University Press, 1989.
27. Harrison KA. Childbearing, health and social priorities: survey of 22,774 consecutive hospital births in Zaria Northern Nigeria. *Br. J. Obstet. Gynaecol.* **92** (suppl. 5) 1–119, 1985.
28. Kaunitz AM, Spence C, Danielson TS, Rochat RW & Grimes DA. Perinatal and maternal mortality in a religious group avoiding obstetric care. *Am. J. Obstet. Gynecol.* **150**, 826–831, 1984.
29. Hon EH. Instrumentation of fetal heart rate and fetal electrocardiography. II. A vaginal electrode. *Am. J. Obstet. Gynecol.* **86**, 772–784, 1963.
30. Hon EH & Quilligan EJ. The classification of fetal heart rate. II. A revised working classification. *Conn. Med. J.* **31**, 779–784, 1967.
31. Beard RW, Filshie GM, Knight CA & Roberts GM. The significance of the changes in the continuous fetal heart rate in the first stage of labour. *J. Obstet. Gynaecol. Br. Commonw.* **78**, 865–881, 1971.
32. Paul RH & Hon EH. Clinical fetal monitoring. V. Effect on perinatal outcome. *Am. J. Obstet. Gynecol.* **118**, 529–533, 1974.
33. Lee WK & Baggish MS. The effect of unselected intrapartum fetal monitoring. *Obstet. Gynecol.* **47**, 16–520, 1976.
34. Renou P, Chang A, Anderson I & Wood C. Controlled trial of fetal intensive care. *Am. J. Obstet. Gynecol.* **126**, 470–476, 1976.
35. Haverkamp AD, Thompson HE, McFee JG *et al.* The evaluation of continuous fetal heart rate monitoring in high-risk pregnancy. *Am. J. Obstet. Gynecol.* **125**, 310–317, 1976.
36. Kelso IM, Parsons RJ, Lawrence GF *et al.* An assessment of continuous fetal heart rate monitoring in labor: A randomized trial. *Am. J. Obstet. Gynecol.* **131**, 526–531, 1978.
37. Haverkamp AD, Orleans M Langendoerfer S *et al.* A controlled trial of the differential effects of intrapartum fetal monitoring. *Am. J. Obstet. Gynecol.* **134**, 399–409, 1979.
38. Wood C, Renou P, Oats J *et al.* A controlled trial of fetal heart rate monitoring in a low-risk obstetric population. *Am. J. Obstet. Gynecol.* **141**, 527–534, 1981.
39. Neldam S, Osler M, Hansen PK, Nim J, Smith SF & Hertel J. Intrpartum fetal heart rate monitoring in a combined low- and high-risk population: a controlled clinical trial. *Eur. J. Obstet. Gynecol. Reprod. Biol.* **23**, 1–11, 1986.
40. MacDonald D, Grant A, Sheridan-Pereira M, Boylan P & Chalmers I. The Dublin randomized controlled trial of intrapartum fetal heart rate monitoring. *Am. J. Obstet. Gynecol.* **152**, 524–539, 1985.
41. Leveno KJ, Cunningham FG, Nelson S *et al.* A prospective comparison of selective and universal electronic fetal monitoring in 34.995 pregnancies. *N. Engl. J. Med.* **315**, 615–619, 1986.
42. Luthy DA, Shy KK, van Belle G *et al.* A randomized trial of electronic fetal monitoring in preterm labor. *Obstet. Gynecol.* **69**, 687–695, 1987.

43. Vintzileos AM, Antsaklis A, Varvarigos I, Papas C, Sofatzis I & Montgomery JT. A randomized trial of intrpartum electronic fetal heart rate monitoring versus intermittent ausculation. *Obstet. Gynecol.* **81**, 899–907, 1993.
44. Mahomed K, Nyoni R, Mulambo T, Kasule J & Jacobus E. Randomised controlled trial of intrapartum fetal heart rate monitoring. *Br. Med. J.* **308**, 497–500, 1994.
45. Herbst A & Ingemarsson I. Intermittent versus continuous electronic fetal monitoring in labour: A randomized study. *Br. J. Obstet. Gynaecol* **101**, 663–668, 1994.
46. Grant A. Monitoring the fetus during labour. In *Effective Care in Pregnancy and Childbirth* (eds I. Chalmers, M. Enkin & M.J.N.C. Keirse), pp. 846–882. Oxford: Oxford University Press, 1989.
47. Neilson JP & Grant AM. The randomised trials of intrapartum electronic fetal heart rate monitoring. In *Intrapartum Fetal Surveillance* (eds J.A.D. Spencer & R.H.T. Ward), pp. 77–93. RCOG Press, 1993.
48. Thacker SB, Stroup DF & Peterson HB. Efficacy and safety of intrapartum fetal monitoring: an update. *Obstet. Gynecol.* **86**, 613–620, 1995.
49. Westgate J, Harris M, Curnow JSH & Greene KR. Plymouth randomised trial of cardiotocogram only versus ST waveform plus cardiotocogram for intrapartum monitoring; 2400 cases. *Am. J. Obstet. Gynecol.* **169**, 1151–1160, 1993.
50. Windle WF. Asphyxial brain damage at birth, with reference to the minimally affected child. In *Perinatal Factors Affecting Human Development*, vol. 185, p. 214. Pan American Health Organisation Scientific Publication, 1969.
51. Berendes HW. Birth asphyxia and neurological deficit: report from the NINDB Collaborative Perinatal Study. In *Brain Damage in the Fetus and Newborn from Hypoxia or Asphyxia* (eds L.S. James *et al.*), p. 8. Columbus OH: Ross Laboratories, 1967.
52. Paneth N, Bommarito M & Stricker J. Electronic fetal monitoring and later outcome. *Clin. Invest. Med.* **16**, 159–165, 1993.
53. 26th RCOG Study Group. Recommendations arising from the 26th RCOG Study Group: intrapartum fetal surveillance. In *Intrapartum Fetal Surveillance* (eds J.A.D. Spencer & R.H.T. Ward), pp. 387–393. RCOG Press, 1993.
54. The American College of Obstetricians and Gynecologists. Committee Opinion Number 91: Utility of umbilical cord blood acid-base assessment, 1991.
55. Day E, Maddern M & Wood C. Auscultation of foetal heart rate: an assessment of its error and significance. *Br. Med. J.* **4**, 422–424, 1968.
56. Schifrin BS, Amsel J & Burdorf G. The accuracy of auscultatory detection of fetal cardiac decelerations: a computer simulation. *Am. J. Obstet. Gynecol.* **166**, 566–576, 1992.
57. Miller FC, Pearse KE & Paul RH. Fetal heart rate pattern recognition by the method of auscultation. *Obstet. Gynecol.* **64**, 332–336, 1984.
58. Strong TH & Jarles DL. Intrapartum auscultation of the fetal heart rate. *Am. J. Obstet. Gynecol.* **168**, 935–936, 1993.
59. Sandmire HF. Whither electronic fetal monitoring? *Obstet. Gynecol.* **76**, 1130–1134, 1990.
60. Guidelines for Perinatal Care, 3rd edn. ACOG, 1992.
61. Henderson-Smart D. Throwing the baby out with the fetal monitoring. *Med. J. Aust.* **154**, 576–578, 1991.
62. Wilson J & Schifrin BS. Is any pregnancy low risk. *Obstet. Gynecol.* **55**, 653–657, 1980.
63. Murphy KW, Johnson P, Moorcraft J, Pattinson R, Russell V & Turnbull A. Birth asphyxia and the intrapartum cardiotocograph. *Br. J. Obstet. Gynaecol.* **97**, 470–479, 1990.
64. Alessandri LM, Stanley FJ & Read AW. A case-control study of intrapartum, stillbirths. *Br. J. Obstet. Gynaecol.* **99**, 719–722, 1992.
65. Low JA, Galbraith RS, Muir D, Killen H, Karchmar J & Campbell D. Intrapartum fetal asphyxia: a preliminary report in regard to long term morbidity. *Am. J. Obstet. Gynecol.* **130**, 525–533, 1978.
66. Schifrin BS & Dame L. Fetal heart rate patterns – prediction of Apgar scores. *J. Am. Med. Assoc.* **218**, 1322, 1972.
67. Neilson JP. Cardiotocography during labour, an unsatisfactory technique but nothing better yet. *Br. Med. J.* **306**, 347–348, 1993.
68. Lee CY, DiLoreto PC & O'Lane JM. A study of fetal heart rate acceleration patterns. *Obstet. Gynecol.* **45**, 142–146, 1975.
69. Phelan JP, Cromartie AD & Smith CV. The nonstress test: the false negative test. *Am. J. Obstet. Gynecol.* **142**, 293–296, 1982.
70. Shenker L. Fetal cardiac arrhythmias. *Obstet. Gynecol. Surv.* **34**, 561, 1979.
71. Silber DL & Durnin RE. Intrauterine atrial tachycardia (associated with massive edema in a newborn). *Am. J. Dis. Child.* **117**, 722, 1969.
72. Van Der Horst RL. Congenital artrial flutter and cardiac failure presenting as hydrops at birth. *S. Afr. Med. J.* **44**, 1037, 1970.
73. McCue CM, Mantakus ME, Tingelstad JB & Ruddy S. Congenital heart block in newborns of mothers with connective tissue disease. Circulation **56**, 82, 1977.
74. Berube S, Lister G Jr, Toews WH, Creasy RK & Heymann MA. Congenital heart block and maternal systemic lupus erythematosus. *Am. J. Obstet. and Gynecol.* **130**, 595, 1978.
75. Michaelsson M & Engle MA. Congenital complete heart block: an international study of the natural history. *Cardiovasc. Clin.* **4**, 85, 1972.
76. Fusi L, Steer PJ, Maresh MJ & Beard RW. Maternal pyrexia associated with the use of epidural analgesia in labour. *Lancet* **1**, 1250–1252, 1989.
77. Nijhuis JG, Staisch KJ, Martin CB Jr. & Prechtl HFR. A sinusoidal-like fetal heart-rate pattern in in association with fetal sucking – report of 2 cases. *Eur. J. Obstet. Gynecol. Reprod. Biol.* **16**, 353–358, 1984.
78. Johnson P. Fetal distress or physiological response and adaptation? In *Fetal monitoring – Physiology and Techniques of Antenatal and Intrapartum Assessment* (ed. J.A.D. Spencer), pp. 31–32. Kent: Castle House, 1989.
79. Yambao TJ, Clark D, Ashby W & Abdul-Karim R. Sinusoidal fetal heart rate patterns: case reports and management. *Br. J. Obstet. Gynaecol.* **89**, 765–768, 1982.
80. Modanlou HD, Freeman RK, Ortiz O, Hinkes P & Pillsbury G Jr. Sinusoidal fetal heart rate pattern and severe fetal anaemia. *Obstet. Gynecol.* **49**, 537–541, 1977.
81. Verma U, Tejani N, Weiss RR, Chatterjee S & Halitsky V. Sinusoidal fetal heart rate patterns in severe Rh disease. *Obstet. Gynecol.* **55**, 666–669, 1980.
82. Spencer JAD & Johnson P. Fetal heart variability changes and fetal behavioural cycles during labour. *Br. J. Obstet. Gynaecol.* **93**, 314–321, 1986.
83. Sterman MB & Hoppenbrouwers T. The development of sleep-waking and rest-activity patterns from fetus to adult in men. In *Brain Development and Behaviour* (eds M.B. Sterman, D.J. McGinty & A.M. Adinolfi), p. 203. New York: Academic Press, 1971.
84. Visser GHA, Dawes GS & Redman CWG. Numerical analysis of the normal human antenatal fetal heart rate. *Br. J. Obstet. Gynaecol.* **88**, 792–802, 1981.
85. Dawes GS, Houghton CRS, Redman CWG & Visser GHA. Pattern of the normal human fetal heart rate. *Br. J. Obstet. Gynaecol.* **89**, 276–284, 1982.
86. Dreyfus-Brisac C. Ontogenesis of sleep in human prematures after 32 weeks of conceptional age. *Dev. Psychol.* **3**, 91–97, 1970.
87. Parmelee AH & Stern E. Development of states in infants. In *Sleep and the Maturing Nervous System* (eds C.D. Clements, D.P. Purpura & F.E. Mayer), p. 199. New York: Academic Press, 1972.
88. Prechtl HFR, Fargel JW, Weinmann HM & Bakker HH. Postures, motility and respiration of low-risk pre-term infants. *Dev. Med. Child. Neurol.* **21**, 23–27, 1979.
89. Nijhuis JG, Prechtl HFR, Martin CB Jr. & Bots RSGM. Are there behavioural states in the human fetus? *Early. Hum. Dev.* **6**, 177–195, 1982.
90. Dalton KJ, Dawes GS & Patrick JE. The autonomic nervous system and fetal heart rate variability. *Am. J. Obstet. Gynecol.* **146**, 456–462, 1983.
91. Miller FC & Paul RH. Intrapartum fetal heart rate monitoring. *Clin. Obstet. Gynecol.* **21**, 561–577, 1978.
92. Clewlow F & Dawes GS. The association between cardiac accelerations and movement in fetal sheep. *J. Dev. Physiol.* **7**, 281–287, 1985.
93. Dawes GS, Gardner WN, Johnston BM & Walker DW. Breathing in fetal lambs: the effects of brainstem section. *J. Physiol.* (Lond) **335**, 535–553, 1983.
94. Myers RE. Two patterns of perinatal brain damage and their conditions of occurrence. *Am. J. Obstet. Gynecol.* **112**, 246, 1972.
95. Bauer DJ. The slowing of the heart rate produced by clamping the umbilical cord in the fetal sheep. *J. Physiol.* **90**, 25p–27p, 1937.

96. Hon EH. The classification of fetal heart rate. 1. A working classification. *Obstet. Gynecol.* **22**, 137, 1963.
97. Yeh MN, Morishima HO, Niemann WH & James LS. Myocardial conduction defects in association with compression of the umblical cord. *Am. J. Obstet. Gynecol.* **121**, 951, 1975.
98. Donker DK, van Geijn HP & Hasman A. Interobserver variation in the assessment of fetal heart rate recordings. *Eur. J. Obstet. Gynecol. Reprod. Biol.* **52**, 21–28, 1993.
99. Trimbos JB & Keirse MJNC. Observer variability in assessment of antepartum cardiotocograms. *Br. J. Obstet. Gynecol.* **85**, 900–906, 1978.
100. Keith RDF, Beckley S, Garibaldi JM, Westgate JA, Ifeachor EC & Greene KR. A multicentre comparative study of 17 experts and an intelligent computer system for managing labour using the cariotocogram. *Br. J. Obstet. Gynaecol.* **102**, 688–700, 1995.
101. Hamilton E, Kimanani EK. Intrapartum production of fetal status and assessment of labour progress. In '*Analysis of Complex Data and Artificial Intelligence in Obstetrics* (eds A.M.Z. Chang & M.S. Rogers), Baillière's Clinical Obstetrics and Gynaecology (International Practice and Research), Vol. 8, No. 3, pp. 567–581. London: Baillière Tindall, 1994.
102. Keith RDF & Greene KR. Development, evaluation and validation of an intelligent system for the management of labour. In *Analysis of Complex Data and Artificial Intelligence in Obstetrics*, (eds A.M.Z. Chang & M.S. Rogers), Baillière's Clinical Obstetrics and Gynaecology (International Practice and Research), Vol. 8, No. 3, pp. 583–605. London: Baillière Tindall, 1994.
103. Greene KR. Intelligent fetal heart rate computer systems in intrapartum surveillance. *Curr. Opin. Obstet. Gynecol.* **8**, 123–127, 1996.
104. Siggaard-Andersen O. An acid base chart for arterial blood with normal and pathophysiological reference areas. *Scand. J. Clin. Lab. Invest.* **27**, 239–245, 1971.
105. Rosén KG & Murphy K. How to assess fetal metabolic acidosis from cord samples. *J. Perinat. Med.* **19**, 221–226, 1991.
106. Westgate J & Rosén KG. Acid base balance at birth. In *A Critical Appraisal of Fetal Surveillance* (eds H.P. van Geijin & F.J.A. Copray), pp. 595–603. Amsterdam: Elsevier, 1994.
107. Saling E. Neues Vorgehen zur Untersuchung des Kindes unter der Geburt – Einführung, Technik, Grundlagen. *Arch. Gynak.* **197**, 108–122, 1962.
108. Adamsons K, Beard RW & Myers RE. Comparison of the composition of arterial, venous and capillary blood of the fetal monkey during labor. *Am. J. Obstet. Gynecol.* **107**, 435–440, 1970.
109. Bowe ET, Beard RW, Finster M, Poppers PJ, Adamsons K & James LS. Reliability of fetal blood sampling. *Am. J. Obstet. Gynecol.* **107**, 279–287, 1970.
110. Towell ME. The rationale for biochemical monitoring of the fetus. *J. Perinat. Med.* **16** (Suppl 1), 49–54, 1988.
111. Nordstrom L, Ingemarsson I, Kublickas M, Persson B, Shimojo N & Westgren M. Scalp blood lactate: a new test strip method for monitoring fetal well-being in labour. *Br. J. Obstet. Gynaecol.* **102**, 894–899, 1995.
112. Westgren M, Kruger K, Ek S *et al.* Lactate compared with pH analysis at fetal scalp blood sampling: a prospective randomised study. *Br. J. Obstet. Gynaecol.* **105**, 29–33, 1998.
113. Wheble AM, Gillmer MDG, Spencer JAD & Sykes GS. Changes in fetal monitoring practice in the UK: 1977–1984. *Br. J. Obstet. Gynaecol.* **96**, 1140–1147, 1989.
114. Goodwin TM, Milner-Masterson L & Paul R. Elimination of fetal scalp blood sampling on a large clinical service. *Obstet. Gynaecol.* **83**, 971–973, 1994.
115. Westgate J & Greene KR. How well is fetal blood sampling used in clinical practice? *Br. J. Obstet. Gynaecol.* **101**, 250–251, 1994.
116. Van den Berg P, Schmidt S, Gesche J & Saling E. Fetal distress and the condition of the newborn using cardiotocography and fetal blood analysis during labour. *Br. J. Obstet. Gynaecol.* **94**, 72–75, 1987.
117. Steer PJ. Fetal scalp blood analysis current practice. In *Intrapartum Fetal Surveillance* (eds J.A.D. Spencer & R.H.T. Ward), pp. 127–138. London: RCOG Press, 1993.
118. Perkins RP. Perinatal observations in a high-risk population managed without intrapartum fetal pH studies. *Am. J. Obstet. Gynecol.* **149**, 327–334, 1984.
119. Clark SL & Paul RH. Intrapartum surveillance: the role of fetal scalp blood sampling. *Am. J. Obstet. Gynecol.* **153**, 717–720, 1985.
120. Clark SL, Gimovsky ML & Miller FC. Fetal heart rate response to scalp blood sampling. *Am. J. Obstet. Gynecol.* **144**, 706–708, 1982.
121. Clark SL, Gimovsky ML & Miller FC. The scalp stimulation test: a clinical alternative to fetal scalp sampling. *Am. J. Obstet. Gynecol.* **148**, 274–277, 1984.
122. Eliman A, Figueroa R & Tejani N. Intrapartum assessment of fetal well-being: A comparison of scalp stimulation with scalp blood pH sampling. *Obstet. Gynecol.* **89**, 373–376, 1997.
123. Smith CV, Nguyen HN, Phelan JP *et al.* Intrapartum assessment of fetal wellbeing: a comparison of fetal acoustic stimulation during the abnormal or equivocal biophysical profile. *Obstet. Gynecol.* **155**, 726–728, 1986.
124. Nyman M, Barr M & Westgren M. A four-year follow-up of hearing and development in children exposed *in utero* to vibro-acoustic stimulation. *Br. J. Obstet. Gynaecol.* **99**, 685–688, 1992.
125. Aladjem S, Vuolo K, Pazos R & Lueck J. Antepartum fetal testing: evaluation and redefinition of criteria for clinical interpretation. *Sem. Perinatol.* **5**, 145–154, 1981.
126. Leader LR & Bennett MJ. Fetal habituation and its clinical applications. In *Fetal and Neonatal Neurology and Neurosurgery* (eds M.L. Levene & R.J. Lilford), pp. 45–60. London: Churchill Livingstone, 1995.
127. Kuhlman KA, Burns KA, Depp R & Sabbagha RE. Ultrasound imaging of normal fetal response to external vibratory acoustic stimulation. *Am. J. Obstet. Gynecol.* **158**, 47–51, 1988.
128. Greene KR. The ECG waveform. In *Baillière's Clinical Obstetrics and Gynaecology*, (International Practice and Research). Vol. 1 (ed. M.J. Whittle), pp. 131–155. London: Baillière Tindall, 1987.
129. Greene KR & Westgate J. The fetal ECG with particular reference to the ST waveform. In *Intrapartum Fetal Surveillance* (eds J.A.D. Spencer & R.H.T. Ward), pp. 281–294. London: RCOG Press, 1993.
130. Symonds EM. The P wave and the PR interval. In *A Critical Appraisal of Fetal Surveillance* (eds H.P. van Geijn & F.J.A. Copray), pp. 381–387. Amsterdam: Elsevier, 1994.
131. van Wijngaarden WJ, de Haan HH, Sahota DS, James DK, Symonds EM & Hasaart THM. Changes in the PR time interval-fetal heart rate relationship of the ECG during fetal compromise in chronically instrumented sheep. *Am. J. Obstet. Gynecol.* **175**, 548–554, 1996.
132. Widmark C, Lindecrantz K & Rosén KG. Changes in the PR, RR intervals and ST waveform of the fetal lamb electrocardiogram with acute hypoxemia. *J. Dev. Physiol.* **18**, 99, 1992.
133. Murray HG. The fetal electrocardiogram: current clinical developments in Nottingham. *J. Perinat. Med.* **14**, 399, 1986.
134. van Wijngaarden WJ, Sahota DS, James DK *et al.* Improved intrapartum surveillance with PR interval analysis of the fetal electrocardiogram: A randomized trial showing a reduction in fetal blood sampling. *Am. J. Obstet. Gynecol.* **174**, 1295–1299, 1996.
135. Luizetti R, Erkkola R, Hasbargen U, Mattson LÅ, Thoulon JM & Rosén KG. European Community Multicentre Trial 'Fetal ECG Analysis During Labour': the P-R interval. *J. Perinat. Med.* **25**, 27–34, 1997.
135a. Pardi G, Tucci E, Udezo A & Zanini D. Fetal electrocardiogram changes in relation to fetal heart rate patterns during labour. *Am. J. Obstet. Gynecol.* **118**, 243, 1974.
136. Rosén KG, Greene KR, Hokegard K-G *et al.* ST waveform analysis of the fetal ECG – a potent method of fetal surveillance? A presentation of experimental and clinical data. In *Cardiovascular and Respiratory Physiology in the Fetus and Neonate*, Vol. 133, pp. 67–82. Colloque Inserm John Libbey Eurotex.
137. Rosén KG & Isaksson O. Alterations in fetal heart rate and ECG correlated to glycogen, creatine phophate and ATP levels during graded hypoxia. *Biol. Neonate.* **30**, 17–24, 1976.
138. Hökegård K-H, KarlssonK, Kjellmer I, Magno R & Rosén KG. Myocardial metabolism in relation to electrocardiographic changes and cardiac function during graded hypoxia in the fetal lamb. *Acta. Physiol. Scand.* **113**, 1–7, 1981.
139. Greene KR, Dawes GS, Lilja H & Rosén KG. Changes in the ST waveform of the fetal lamb electrocardiogram with hypoxaemia. *Am. J. Obstet. Gynecol.* **144**, 950–958, 1982.
140. Rosén KG, Dagbjartsson A, Henriksson B-A, Lagercrantz H & Kjellmer I. The relationship between circulating catecholamines and ST waveform in the fetal lamb electrocardiogram during hypoxia. *Am. J. Obstet. Gynecol.* **149**, 190–195, 1984.

141. Greene KR & Rosén KG. Long-term ST waveform changes in the ovine fetal electrocardiogram: the relationship to spontaneous labour and intrauterine death. *Clin. Phys. Physiol. Meas.* **10**, 33–40, 1989.
142. Widmark C, Hökegård K-H, Lagercrantz H, Lilja H & Rosén KG. Electrocardiographic waveform changes and catecholamine responses during acute hypoxia in the immature and mature fetal lamb. *Am. J. Obstet. Gynecol.* **160**, 1245–1250, 1989.
143. Watenabe T, Okamura K, Tanigawara S *et al.* Change in electrocardiogram T-wave amplitude during umbilical cord compression is predictive of fetal condition in sheep. *Am. J. Obstet. Gynecol.* **166**, 246–255, 1992.
144. Hökegård K-H, Karlsson K, Kjellmer I & Rosén KG. ECG changes in the fetal lamb during asphyxia in relation to beta-adrenoceptor stimulation and blockade. *Acta. Physiol. Scand.* **105**, 195–203, 1979.
145. Widmark C, Jansson T, Lindecrantz K & Rosén KG. ECG waveform changes, short term heart rate variability and plasma catecholamine concentrations in intrauterine growth-retarded guinea-pig fetuses in response to hypoxia. *J. Dev. Physiol.* **15**, 161–168, 1991.
146. Westgate J, Harris M, Curnow J & Greene KR. Randomised trial of cardiotocography alone or with ST waveform analysis for intrapartum monitoring. *Lancet* **340**, 194–198, 1992.
147. Beckley S, Stenhouse E & Greene KR. Evaluation of a computer-based teaching package for intrapartum monitoring. *J. Obstet. Gynaecol.* **17**(1), 18–19, 1997.

New optical methods of intrapartum fetal surveillance

76

P. O'Brien and D.M. Peebles

Introduction

The need for new methods of assessing fetal tissue oxygenation during labour has been highlighted by the shortcomings of current methods of intrapartum surveillance[1,2]. Continuous electronic fetal heart rate monitoring (EFM) was introduced into clinical practice without proper randomized controlled trials to show that it really did reduce fetal morbidity and mortality. Subsequent trials, including the influential Dublin randomized controlled trial of intrapartum fetal heart rate monitoring, found that EFM increases intervention rates, particularly that of caesarean section, with no improvement in neonatal outcome[3]. The fetal heart rate is an *indirect* indicator of fetal hypoxia and its specificity is low. Even when highly abnormal heart traces are identified, only 50% are associated with fetal acidosis and only 0.2% of these fetuses subsequently develop cerebral palsy, a false positive rate of 99.8%[4]. The concomitant use of fetal scalp blood sampling to measure pH and base excess has been shown to reduce intervention rates[4,5]. However, the procedure is invasive and often difficult and only provides an isolated measurement which often needs to be repeated to adequately define the trend of changing fetal pH. Moreover, the acid–base status of fetal blood is a poor predictor of long-term outcome[6].

Physiologically, both of these techniques have two disadvantages. First, neither directly measures fetal tissue oxygenation, but rather the size of the autonomic and anaerobic responses to hypoxia. Second, and perhaps most important, neither adequately addresses the consequences of fetal hypoxia, such as changes in cerebral perfusion and metabolism, both of which may determine long-term neurological outcome. It is now clear that the extent of cortical neuronal loss caused by hypoxia in the fetal sheep correlates better with the degree of hypotension than hypoxia[7].

In this chapter we will discuss two closely related optical methods of fetal monitoring, still in the development stage, which continuously and non-invasively quantify different aspects of fetal oxygenation. These are two adaptations of the original oximeters, pulse oximetry and near infrared spectroscopy (NIRS).

Theory

Oximetry is the measurement of haemoglobin oxygenation, based on the spectrophotometric absorption of specific wavelengths of light by a specimen of blood, either in vitro or in vivo. In 1935, Matthes built the first device that continuously measured the oxygen saturation of blood in tissue, using two wavelengths of light (one red, one green)[8]. This device was useful for following trends, but its bulky sensor rendered its use impractical. Important advances in non-invasive oximetry occurred during the second world war, stimulated by the need to monitor oxygenation in pilots flying at high altitudes in unpressurized cockpits[9].

PULSE OXIMETRY

A major breakthrough in non-invasive oximetry came during the mid 1970s when Takuo Aoyagi, a Japanese bioengineer, focused attention on the pulsatile change in light transmission due to the change in tissue arterial blood volume with each pulse. Pulse oximetry enables continuous measurements of arterial oxygen saturation and heart rate to be obtained. Since the early 1980s the technique has become widely used for monitoring both anaesthetic and neonatal patients, but it is only within the last 5 years that its use in obstetrics has been reported[10–12].

Pulse oximetry is based on the following two principles:

- The light absorption spectra of oxyhaemoglobin (HbO_2) and deoxyhaemoglobin (Hb) differ
- The assumption that the only pulsatile absorbance between the light source and the photodetector is that of arterial blood

Two wavelengths are employed, one in the red and one in the infrared part of the spectrum (generally 660 nm and 940 nm), to determine relative concentrations of HbO_2 and Hb. At both wavelengths, absorption occurs in skin, subcutaneous fat, and connective tissue (the non-pulsatile or DC component) as well as in the pulsatile vascular bed (pulsatile or AC component). The pulse oximeter measures the AC component of light absorbance at each wavelength and then divides this by the corresponding DC component; the resulting 'pulse-added' absorption is independent of the incident light intensity. By comparing the pulse-added absorption at both wavelengths, a ratio (*R*) is calculated as follows:

$$R = \frac{AC_{660}/DC_{660}}{AC_{940}/DC_{940}}$$

This ratio is then empirically calibrated against direct arterial blood S_aO_2 measurements obtained in volunteers using a CO-oximeter. The resulting calibration curve is stored in a digital microprocessor within the pulse oximeter and used to generate the pulse oximeter's estimate of arterial saturation.

NEAR-INFRARED SPECTROSCOPY

In 1977 Jobsis used a spectrometer which only analysed light absorption in the near infrared part of the spectrum (700–1000 nm) to measure changes in oxygenation within a cat brain[13]. Subsequently the technique has been used to measure cerebral oxygenation and haemodynamics in the neonatal brain[14–16], adult brain[17] and muscle[18]. More recently, several groups have adapted the technique to investigate the previously inaccessible fetal brain during labour[19,20].

NIRS is based on two physical principles. First, that biological tissue is relatively transparent to light in the near infrared region of the spectrum which means that with the use of modern light sources and detectors it is possible to transilluminate a substantial proportion of the head of the term fetus. Second, that brain tissue contains only a small number of light-absorbing compounds, called chromophores, whose concentrations are variable and whose optical properties change with oxygenation. These are oxyhaemoglobin (HbO_2), deoxyhaemoglobin (Hb) and oxidized cytochrome oxidase, the terminal member of the mitochondrial respiratory chain. Any *changes* in the amount of transmitted light will be accounted for by changes in the concentrations of these three chromophores.

Changes in light attenuation are related to changes in chromophore concentration by the Beer–Lambert law. This can be modified to describe optical absorption in a highly light-scattering medium such as brain, so that

$$OD = (acLB) + G$$

where OD is the tissue attenuation of light (units of optical density), *a* is the absorption coefficient of the chromophore (/mmol per cm), *c* is the concentration of chromophore (mmol/L), *L* is the distance between the point of light entry and exit (cm), *B* is a pathlength factor that takes account of the scattering of light in tissue, which causes the optical pathlength to be greater than *L*, and *G* is a factor related to the geometry of the tissue. If during a study *L*, *B* and *G* remain constant, changes in chromophore concentration can be calculated from changes in absorption. The absorption coefficients of HbO_2, Hb and cytochrome oxidase are known from in-vitro work[21] and a mean value for *B* of 4.99 (SD 0.45) has been obtained from previous studies in postmortem infants[22].

By summing changes in [HbO_2] and [Hb] it is possible to obtain changes in total cerebral haemoglobin concentration [Hb_{tot}]. If the large vessel haemoglobin concentration is known (e.g. from a cord blood sample) it is possible to convert changes in [Hb_{tot}] into changes in cerebral blood volume (CBV) in ml/100 g, assuming a cerebral/large vessel haematocrit ratio of 0.69[16].

Methods

PULSE OXIMETRY

Pulse oximeter sensors can be used in transmission mode (e.g. on the finger) or as a reflectance probe, with the photodiode and light-emitting diode placed next to each other. The latter method is the most feasible for intrapartum use and several reflectance probes have been designed. Direct contact with the skin is necessary to produce an adequate signal and various means of ensuring this have been employed including suction[12], a modified Copeland clip[23], a modified spiral electrode[24], an inflatable balloon on the maternal side of the sensor[25] and the Nellcor sensor which uses a 'fulcrum' modification to mechanically place the sensor surface against the fetal cheek.

A further modification necessary to adapt adult pulse oximeters for fetal use has been the range of haemoglobin saturation over which the machines are calibrated. Pulse oximeters for adult use are calibrated with blood from adult volunteers and do not therefore extend down to saturations of <60%, as might be seen in the fetus, for ethical and safety issues. Whilst attempts have been made to address this using animal studies and umbilical cord blood samples this aspect still gives rise to significant error (see 'Problems . . .').

NEAR-INFRARED SPECTROSCOPY

The principal components required for an NIRS system are a light source, a means of transmitting the light to and from the fetal head and a sensitive light detector[26] (Fig. 76.1). Most of the data presented in this chapter were collected using a commercially available prototype (NIRO 500, Hamamtsu Photonics, Japan), the details of which will be described briefly here. Semiconducting laser diodes are sequentially pulsed to produce light at four different wavelengths between 700 and 904 nm. The light is transmitted to the fetal head by a flexible

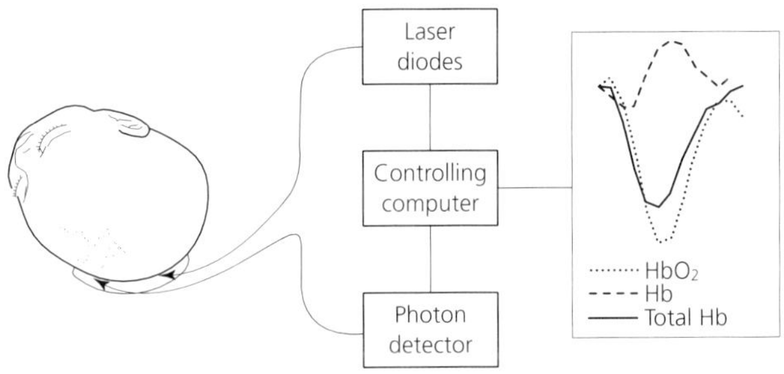

Fig. 76.1 A simplified diagram representing the near infrared spectroscopy apparatus. (Reprinted from *Contemp. Rev. Obstet. Gynaecol.* 1993; **5**, 124–129, with permission).

fibreoptic bundle (external diameter 5 mm) which passes through the cervix. After reflection through 90° by a glass prism, the light passes into the fetal head where it is attenuated by scattering and absorption. A similar fibreoptic bundle, placed between 3 and 4 cm from the point of light entry, receives the emerging light and conveys it to a photomultiplier tube. The ends of the two fibreoptic bundles (optodes) are held a fixed distance apart in a specially designed black silicone rubber moulding. This minimizes the possibility of artefact due to changes in the distance between the optodes. The moulding, in the form of a thin suction cup, also ensures stable measurements by maintaining good apposition of the optodes to the fetal scalp (Fig. 76.2). Following rupture of the membranes and at a minimum cervical dilation of 2 cm, the probe can easily be introduced through the cervix and applied against the fetal head where it is held in position by the continuous application of negative pressure as well as maternal tissue pressure. The exact position of the probe on the head is not critical as light is multiply scattered within the brain, but an attempt is made to situate the probe away from the face and ears.

Clinical studies

PULSE OXIMETRY

Pulse oximeters are cheap and widely available because of their use in adult and neonatal medicine. It has been suggested that oxygen saturation may be a more reliable indicator of fetal oxygenation than partial pressure of oxygen[12]. It was therefore logical to try to adapt the technique for intrapartum use. Published series suggest that pulse oximetry can provide a non-invasive, continuous measure of fetal scalp arterial oxygen saturation. The probe can be applied after 2 cm of cervical dilatation and measurements can be continued until delivery. Dildy *et al.* showed in 73 subjects that the percentage of time sensor contact was made with the skin progressively increased from 4 cm cervical dilatation (55%) to the second stage of labour (82%), presumably as a result of improved sensor application to the fetus as it descended the birth canal[27]. In this

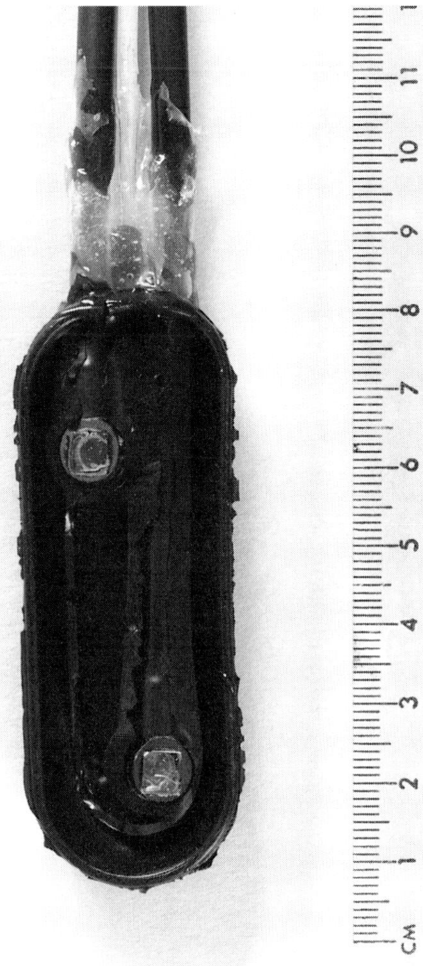

Fig. 76.2 The fetal probe developed at University College Hospital, London.

study saturation measurements (SpO_2) were obtained in 45% cases at 4 cm dilatation and 60% at 8–10 cm. These values are similar to those reported elsewhere.

When a reliable signal is obtained consistent data are produced. Initial studies suggested that the mean fetal SpO_2 during the first stage of labour ranged between 82% (SD 6%)[23] and 68% (SD13%)[12]. A later multicentre study including 291 women confirmed these findings with mean SpO_2 falling from 59% (SD 10%) in the first stage of labour to 53% (SD 10%) in the second stage[28] (Fig. 76.3). There was, however, a wide range of SpO_2 values and a lower limit of normal, defined as 2 SD below the mean, was 33% for the second stage of labour.

Fetal arteriolar oxygen saturation has been shown to change in a number of obstetric situations. McNamara *et al.* demonstrated an increase in SpO_2 when the mother was given oxygen; 27% and 100% oxygen given to women in normal labour with an epidural produced mean increases in SpO_2 of 7% and 11% respectively[29]. Luttkus and Dudenhausen related SpO_2 to fetal heart rate (FHR) patterns and showed

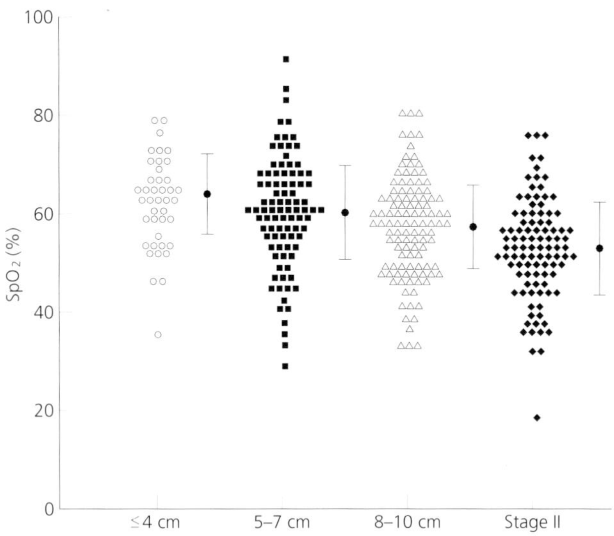

Fig. 76.3 Individual and mean (±SD) fetal SpO_2 values of a group of women with normal maternal and neonatal outcome plotted during progressive stages of labour. (Reprinted from *Am. J. Obstet. Gynecol.* 1994; **171**, 679–684, with permission.)

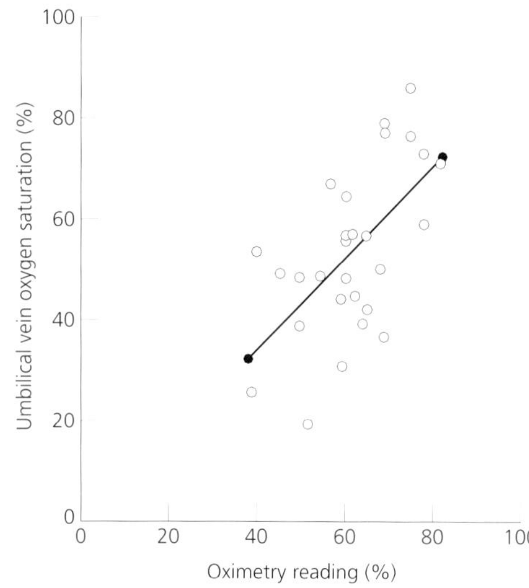

Fig. 76.5 The relation between the fetal pulse oximetry reading in the second stage of labour and umbilical cord venous oxygen saturation. (Reprinted with permission from *Br. J. Obstet. Gynaecol.* 1992; **92**, 735–738.)

that SpO_2 fell from a median value of 48% where the FHR was normal, to 39% during variable decelerations (Fig. 76.4)[30].

Fetal SpO_2 measured by pulse oximetry has been shown to correlate with accepted measures of neonatal outcome such as umbilical cord blood gas status. McNamara *et al.* monitored 37 fetuses just before delivery and demonstrated a close correlation between SpO_2 and umbilical vein SaO_2 ($r = 0.57, p = 0.001$) (Fig. 76.5) and pH ($r = 0.5, p = 0.02$)[31]. The correlation with fetal arterial blood was not so good (umbilical artery SaO_2, $r = 0.6, p = 0.6$). Luttkus *et al.* compared 51 SaO_2 measurements from fetal scalp blood analysis in human subjects to

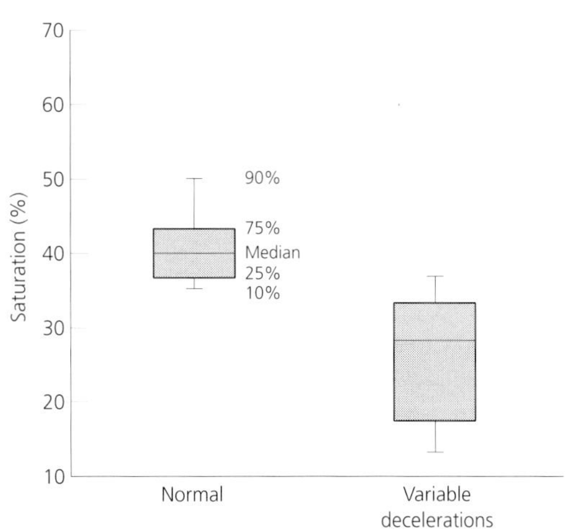

Fig. 76.4 Distribution of the saturation values in periods with 'normal' FHR pattern (left) and variable decelerations (right). (Reprinted from *Baillière's Clin. Obstet. Gynaecol.* 1996; **10**(2), 302.)

simultaneous SpO_2 readings; a correlation coefficient of 0.67 was obtained for values between 15% and 72%[32]. These findings confirm that the SpO_2 measured by pulse oximetry better reflects the oxygen saturation of blood delivered to the brain, rather than that leaving the brain, i.e. supply rather than consumption.

NEAR-INFRARED SPECTROSCOPY

Several centres are now using intrapartum NIRS as a research tool[19,20] and a total of approximately 300 fetuses have been studied. One-hundred-and-forty fetuses have been studied during labour at University College Hospital, London for periods lasting from 10 to 765 min. It is possible to commence measurements from an early stage of labour at 2 cm cervical dilatation and to continue in some fetuses until the time of delivery.

Satisfactory data have been obtained in approximately 65% of studies. The most common reason for failure to obtain interpretable data is the inability to transmit sufficient light through the fetal head with the result that no light reaches the receiving optode. One possible cause of this is poor skin contact, often caused by excessive movement of the mother. Another possible cause is loss of light through absorption by thick black hair, particularly in fetuses of Afro-Caribbean origin.

EFFECT OF UTERINE CONTRACTIONS ON CEREBRAL OXYGENATION

'Normal' uterine contractions, not associated with FHR decelerations, are associated with parallel changes in [HbO_2] and [Hb] and thus cerebral blood volume (CBV). These

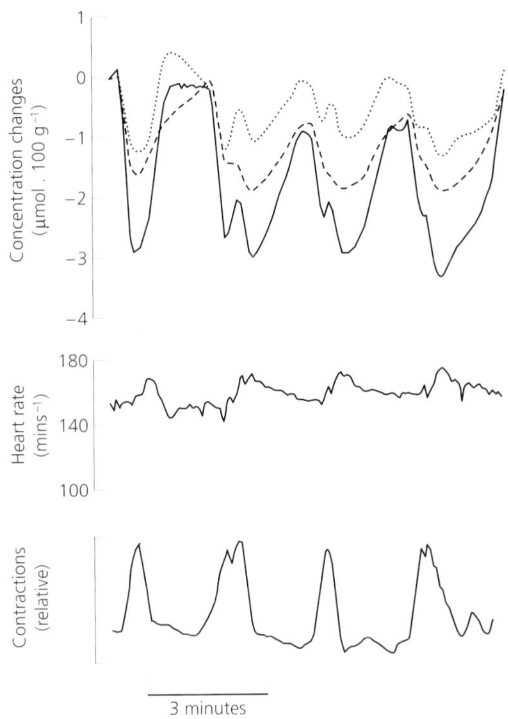

Fig. 76.6 Changes from an arbitrary baseline in the cerebral concentrations of HbO_2 (dotted line), Hb (dashed line) and Hb_{tot} (solid line) in the same fetus during two normal contractions. (Reprinted with permission from *MMRD Res. Rev.* 1997; **3**, 59–68.)

changes were first described in eight term fetuses[19]. In six of the eight studied with NIRS 'normal' uterine contractions were associated with a mean fall in cerebral total haemoglobin $[Hb_{tot}]$ concentration of 1.15 (SD 0.60) μmol/100 g, equivalent to a fall in CBV of 0.7 (SD 0.39) ml/100 g. Representative data from one fetus are shown in Fig. 76.6. These are sizeable concentration changes, representing a transient fall in CBV of about 30%, if normal neonatal values are assumed to apply during labour[16]. Conversely, in the remaining two fetuses $[HbO_2]$ and [Hb] increased with uterine contractions by similar amounts to the changes described above. It is likely that these changes reflect a balance between direct pressure effects causing head compression[33] and an obstruction of venous drainage, as might occur when the umbilical cord constricts the fetal neck[34]. A similar covarying pattern associated with uterine contractions has been described[35].

The effect of the frequency of uterine contractions on cerebral $[HbO_2]$ and [Hb] has been reported in 10 term infants[36]. Fig. 76.7 shows the relation between contraction interval, measured from peak to peak using external tocography, and the corresponding changes in $[HbO_2]$ and [Hb]. A highly significant relationship was found between contraction interval and cerebral oxygenation. It was apparent that $\Delta[HbO_2]$ was positively, and Δ[Hb] negatively correlated with the contraction interval. These data suggest that at short contraction intervals (less than 2 min) cerebral oxygenation will

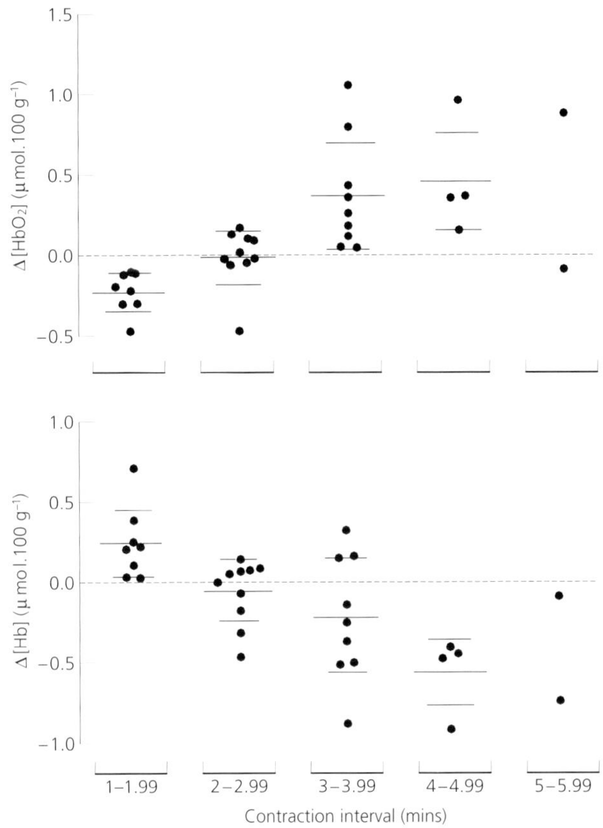

Fig. 76.7 Relations between contraction interval and changes in concentration of HbO_2 and Hb in 10 fetuses. Each point represents the mean value from an individual fetus: *n* was less than 10 for most time bands because not all fetuses had contraction intervals falling within all time bands. Group mean values ± SD are indicated. (Reprinted from *Contemp. Rev. Obstet. Gynaecol.* 1993; **5**, 124–129, with permission.)

tend to fall, while at longer contraction intervals it will rise. In seven fetuses it was possible to calculate a value for the interval at which brain oxygenation remained stable, which was 2.3 (SD 0.4) min. This is consistent with the reported frequency of four contractions every 10 min, considered to be normal during the active phase of labour[37].

The effect of oxytocin-induced uterine hyperstimulation on cerebral oxygenation in one fetus have been reported[38] and the data are shown in Fig. 76.8. Increasing fetal distress was associated with a reciprocal fall in $[HbO_2]$ and a rise in [Hb]. CBV rose by 1.2 ml/100 g. These changes are consistent with a period of brain desaturation which was presumably attributable to a fall in placental perfusion. The observed rise in CBV may have been due to vasodilation of the cerebral vasculature in response to increasing hypoxia.

LATE FETAL HEART RATE DECELERATIONS

Aldrich *et al.* described the changes in fetal cerebral oxygenation during contractions associated with late FHR decelerations and compared them with the changes during

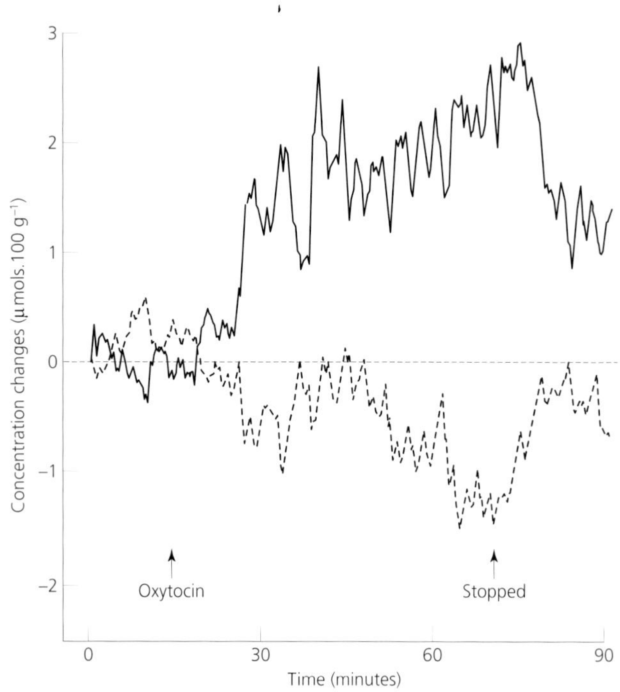

Fig. 76.8 Changes in the cerebral concentrations of HbO_2 (dotted line) and Hb (solid line) associated with uterine hyperstimulation caused by oxytocin infusion. (Reprinted from *Lancet* 1991; **338**, 254–255, with permission.)

contractions with no alteration of FHR in 10 fetuses during the first stage of labour[39]. They found that the changes occurring *during* contractions were quantitatively similar, regardless of the FHR changes. However, the changes *after* the contractions were different (Table 76.1). Late FHR decelerations were associated with a significantly greater fall in $[HbO_2]$ (0.52 versus 0.05 µmol/100 g) and a significantly greater rise in [Hb] (0.36 versus 0.09 µmol/100 g) *after* the contraction. The onset of cerebral deoxygenation coincided with the onset of the FHR deceleration. These data support the theory proposed by Myers *et al.* in 1973 to explain late FHR decelerations[40]. They proposed that the delay between the onset of a contraction and the onset of a late FHR deceleration is the time taken for the oxygen in the intervillous spaces to become depleted and for the bolus of desaturated blood to travel from the placenta to the fetus. Aldrich *et al.* also demonstrated the effects of obstetric manoeuvres such as active pushing[41], changing maternal position[42] and maternal oxygen administration on fetal cerebral oxygenation[43].

CALCULATION OF MEAN CEREBRAL OXYGEN SATURATION

Although NIRS records quantitative changes in concentration, these are changes from an *arbitrary* baseline. As a result, it is not possible to calculate the *absolute* cerebral concentration of HbO_2 and Hb. In order to establish a baseline at the start of a study, which can be compared with known values, it is necessary to define an absolute parameter, comparable with SpO_2 measured by pulse oximetry, which represents oxygenation. When $[HbO_2]$ and [Hb] change in the same direction in constant proportion to each other during a contraction, as in Fig. 76.3, the mean oxygen saturation of the blood entering or leaving the brain can be calculated[23] using the formula

$$SmcO_2 = \Delta[HbO_2] \times 100 / \Delta([HbO_2] + [Hb])$$

This value is assumed to reflect the mean saturation of blood within the cranial compartment ($SmcO_2$). Thus, if oxy- and deoxyhaemoglobin are present in equal amounts, $SmcO_2$ will be 50%. If it is assumed that $SmcO_2$ is not changing rapidly, measurements may be analysed over several contractions and a mean value obtained. From the data available so far, the normal range of $SmcO_2$ in healthy fetuses was 43% (SD 10%)[19]. This value represents an average saturation of haemoglobin in all vascular compartments but it is likely that the measurement is dominated by the cerebral venous compartment. SpO_2, reflecting the arterial side of the circulation, is therefore higher.

TABLE 76.1
Mean (SD) changes from baseline in $[HbO_2]$, [Hb], $[Hb_{diff}]$, $[Hb_{tot}]$ and fetal heart rate (FHR) during and after uterine contractions associated with no FHR alterations (control *n* = 10) and late FHR decelerations (*n* = 10)

	$\Delta[HbO_2]$ (µmol/100 g)		Δ[Hb] (µmol/100 g)		$\Delta[Hb_{tot}]$ (µmol/100 g)		$\Delta[Hb_{diff}]$ (µmol/100 g)		ΔFHR (bpm)	
	During	After	During	After	During	After	During	After	During	After
Control	−0.33 (0.30)*	−0.05 (0.21)	−0.20 (0.30)	0.09 (0.23)	−0.53 (0.50)*	0.03 (0.23)	−0.13 (0.36)	−0.14 (0.38)	−3.1 (3.2)	−1.3 (3.1)
Late	−0.44 (0.24)**	−0.52 (0.26)**	−0.29 (0.34)	0.36 (0.35)*	−0.73 (0.50)**	−0.17 (0.40)	−0.15 (0.33)	−0.87 (0.48)**	−8.5 (6.2)*	−11.9 (11.0)†

*$P < 0.01$; **$P < 0.001$; †$P < 0.02$ versus baseline (paired Student's *t* test within each group)

Reprinted from *Br. J. Obstet. Gynaecol.* 1995; **102**, 9–13, with permission.

CORRELATION BETWEEN $SmcO_2$ AND ACID–BASE STATUS AT BIRTH

Values for $SmcO_2$ in the 30 min immediately prior to delivery were obtained in thirty three fetuses studied by Aldrich *et al.*[44]. For each fetus the mean value for $SmcO_2$ was calculated over a 10 min period (two to five contractions) as close to the time of delivery as possible, and compared to each of the measurements obtained from umbilical artery and vein blood gas analysis immediately after delivery. There were strong positive correlations between $SmcO_2$ and measurements of pH in both umbilical vessels (Fig. 76.9) and a strong negative correlation between $SmcO_2$ and base deficit.

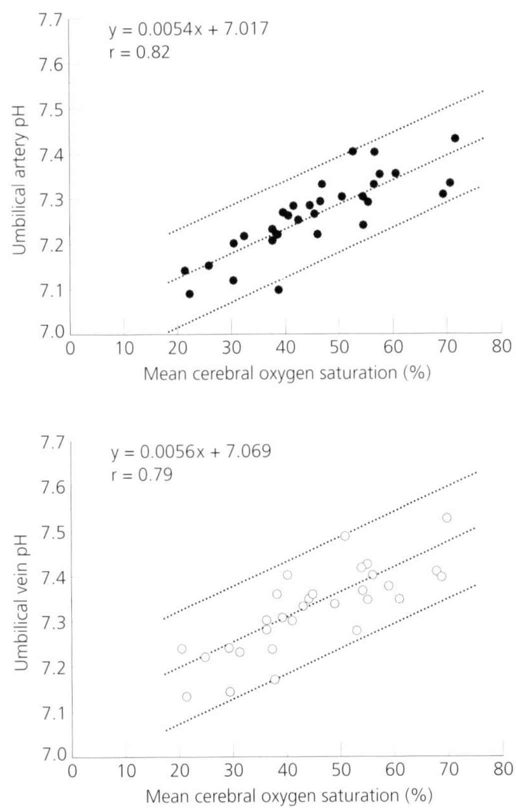

Fig. 76.9 The relation between fetal mean cerebral oxygen saturation within 30 min of delivery and umbilical artery and vein pH at birth. The regression line and 95% confidence interval of the data points are shown. (Reprinted from *Obstet. Gynecol.* 1994; **84**, 861–866, with permission.)

Physiological significance of outcome measures

Owing to the inaccessibility of the human fetus during labour it has not been possible to correlate SpO_2, $SmcO_2$ or $[Hb_{tot}]$ with any haemodynamic variables, other than heart rate, or histological outcome. The pathophysiological significance of these variables therefore remains unclear. Animal studies, mainly in the fetal sheep, have therefore been used both to validate intrapartum measurements and clarify the pathogenesis of perinatally acquired brain injury.

FETAL ARTERIOLAR OXYGEN SATURATION (SpO_2)

In order to calibrate pulse oximeters at the low ranges of saturation seen in the fetus it is necessary to use laboratory animals. Fetal SaO_2 is varied by controlling maternal FiO_2 or uterine blood flow. Using a pulse oximeter calibrated for fetal use Nijland *et al.* measured the standard deviation of the difference between simultaneous SpO_2 and blood SaO_2 values over an SaO_2 range of 18–100% and it was 5.4%[45,46]. This figure appears typical of other studies.

Similar studies have been designed to determine the 'critical' SpO_2 at which anaerobic metabolism occurs and lactic acidosis develops. Nijland *et al.* defined a value for SpO_2 of 30%, above which the fetus was able to maintain aerobic respiration and below which a metabolic acidosis developed[45]. This value is similar to the lower limit of the normal range (defined as 2 SD below the mean) described in the human fetus (see above).

However, follow-up studies in the human, supported by animal data, suggest that neither acid base status at birth nor degree of hypoxaemia are strongly associated with neurological outcome – the important endpoint[6,7]. One reason for this is that the normal fetal response to hypoxia is to redistribute cardiac output with an increase in blood flow, and preservation of oxygen and substrate delivery, to the brain, adrenals and heart at the expense of other tissues[47,48]. Only when this compensatory mechanism is overwhelmed, during severe asphyxia, and cerebral perfusion falls will neurological injury occur[49]. It is also worth noting that it is changing PaO_2 (not oxygen saturation or content) which stimulates the chemoreceptors, especially the carotid bodies, which initiate the rapid cardiovascular response to hypoxia[50]. This raises doubts about the use of measurements of SpO_2 to detect the fetus at risk of brain injury.

MEAN CEREBRAL OXYGEN SATURATION ($SmcO_2$)

The main advantage of $SmcO_2$ is that it is a direct measure of cerebral, rather than peripheral, oxygenation. However, so far there have been no attempts to validate this measurement in animal studies. As with SpO_2 there are theoretical concerns about the ability of measurements of $SmcO_2$ in isolation to detect fetuses at risk of hypoxic-ischaemic brain injury. Ideally, measurements of SpO_2 and $SmcO_2$ should not be mutually exclusive as they provide complementary information. Relative changes in SpO_2 (reflecting arterial saturation) and $SmcO_2$ (a predominantly venous signal), measured simultaneously, will reflect changes in oxygen extraction across the brain.

CHANGES IN TOTAL CEREBRAL HAEMOGLOBIN CONCENTRATION

The significance of a reduction in cerebral perfusion in the aetiology of hypoxic-ischaemic brain injury has been discussed. Of particular interest therefore is the relationship between changes in $[Hb_{tot}]$ (reflecting cerebral blood volume), measured by NIRS, and cerebral perfusion. To investigate this, fetal sheep in utero were chronically instrumented with NIRS probes, arterial and venous catheters, an ECG electrode and a transducer placed around a carotid artery to measure flow[51]. Typical fetal responses to 1 h of isocapnic hypoxia, induced by reduction of maternal $F_{i,o2}$, are shown (Fig. 76.10). Hypoxia was associated with a significant and rapid rise in carotid blood flow, arterial blood pressure and $[Hb_{tot}]$ (mean 2.27 ± 0.5 mmol/100 g). These changes were maintained during hypoxia. However, posthypoxia $[Hb_{tot}]$ fell independently of arterial blood pressure and carotid blood flow, which remained significantly elevated for the remainder of the experiment. The increase in $[Hb_{tot}]$, measured by NIRS during fetal hypoxaemia in this study is compatible with cerebral vasodilatation and suggests that changes in $[Hb_{tot}]$ will reflect changes in blood flow. However, the effect of changes in arterial and venous flow cannot be distinguished. Further studies will reveal whether NIRS can discriminate between fetal hypoxia associated with either cerebral vasodilatation or constriction.

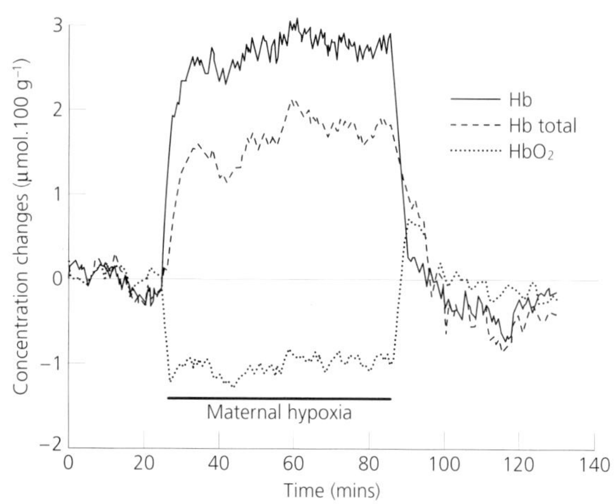

Fig. 76.10 Raw data from a sheep fetus showing the effect of 1 h of fetal isocapnic hypoxia (fetal PaO_2 reduced from 20 to 12 mmHg), induced by reducing maternal FiO_2, on the cerebral concentrations of HbO_2, Hb and total Hb. (Reprinted with permission from *MMRD Res. Rev.* 1997; **3**, 59–68.)

REDOX STATE OF CYTOCHROME OXIDASE

Cytochrome oxidase, the terminal enzyme of the mitochondrial electron transport chain, is responsible for more than 90% of oxygen consumption. It contains two haem iron and two copper redox centres and the redox state of these metals reflects changes in

- The supply of reducing equivalents to the respiratory chain
- The rate of ATP turnover
- The cellular oxygen concentration[52,53]

The redox state of cytochrome oxidase will therefore reflect oxygen delivery and metabolism at a cellular level. Of particular interest is the Cu_A centre of the enzyme. This has a characteristic absorption peak in the near infrared region that is sensitive to its redox state; the oxidized enzyme has a significantly greater absorbance at 830 nm than the reduced enzyme[21]. It is thus possible to detect changes in the Cu_A redox state in vivo by NIRS. Data from studies in animals show a close correlation between the redox state of Cu_A, measured by NIRS, and the concentration of high-energy phosphates, such as ATP, measured by nuclear magnetic spectroscopy[53,54]; if Cu_A becomes reduced the concentration of ATP falls. NIRS can therefore indirectly provide information about cellular energy status. At present the technique is not sensitive enough to reliably measure changes in Cu_A oxidation during labour; however, recent advances in technology (see 'Intensity-modulated optical spectroscopy' below) mean that this will become possible in the near future.

Sources of error

PULSE OXIMETRY

Monitoring of fetal SpO_2 has been encumbered by multiple technical obstacles. Firstly, haemoglobin oxygen saturation is measured in the arteriolar bed of the fetal scalp. This is an area particularly prone to pressure effects during labour[55] and loss of signal has been reported during uterine contractions. In addition scalp perfusion will be reduced in hypoxic fetuses who are peripherally vasoconstricted, thus reducing the size of the arterial signal in exactly those fetuses that one would wish to monitor accurately. Measurements from the fetal scalp may also be complicated by local tissue factors such as caput succedaneum which can cause a fall in oximeter readings[56]. For this reason the more recent fetal pulse oximeters are designed to be placed through the cervix, against the fetal cheek.

Another potential source of error arises from the fact that the size of the pulsatile AC signal is small compared with that of the non-pulsatile component. This means that if the weak AC signal is magnified automatically by the pulse oximeter to obtain a waveform, the non-pulsatile component will also be amplified, giving rise to increased levels of background noise. If an accurate SaO_2 is to be derived from the ratio of amplified absorbances against a background noise, it is important that the peaks of the AC waveform are accurately identified. This problem has been partly overcome by using the R wave of the fetal electrocardiogram (ECG) together with the pulsatile signal obtained by the photosensor. Saturation measurements are rejected if the two signals are not synchronous.

Inadequate sensor to skin contact may lead to a different type of artefact. A gap between probe and skin may be associated with a normal looking plethysmographic waveform, but a proportion of light from the LED will be reflected straight back from the skin surface. Because light in the infrared part of the spectrum permeates tissue better and is less absorbed by the air–skin interface than the visible red light, any increase in the amount of reflected light will affect the red/infrared ratio of the AC and DC components in a different way, resulting in an increase in the red/infrared ratio which is translated by the oximeter as a lower saturation value. Good apposition of probe to skin is therefore important and newer oximeter probes are designed to ensure good probe/skin contact. In addition, converting the LED at 660 nm with one emitting light in the infrared (735 nm) will reduce this source of error[46].

A mean level of oxygen saturation during early labour between 68% and 82% has been reported[12,23]. These are higher than would be expected. The healthy fetus at term is born with an umbilical vein blood oxygen saturation of between 40 and 70% and as umbilical vein blood mixes with deoxygenated blood from the inferior vena cava before entering the fetal carotid artery, scalp pulse oximetry readings should be lower. In adults, pulse oximetry readings have been found to be less accurate at low saturations (<70%)[57]. This is partly due to the difficulty in obtaining blood with low oxygen saturations from adult volunteers with which to generate the calibration curve used by the algorithm. This meant that the curve had to be extrapolated back from measurements in the range 70–100%. However, as described previously, modern pulse oximeters designed for fetal use are calibrated over a wide range of saturations using animal studies. Another source of inaccuracy at low oxygen saturations is the variation of the centre wavelength (± 15 nm) of different LEDs that emit light at 660 nm. Since the absorption spectra for Hb is relatively steep at this region and because Hb is present in increased concentration at low saturations, a slight shift in the centre wavelength of the LED can result in erroneous measurements. Improvement in LED quality and changing the lower wavelength from 660 to 735 nm has helped rectify this source of error.

NEAR-INFRARED SPECTROSCOPY

CHANGES IN INTEROPTODE SPACING

The application of the Beer-Lambert law assumes that the only variant to change during the course of the study is chromophore concentration (see Theory section). A change in optical pathlength (change in the term L, Beer–Lambert equation) may occur as a result of an alteration in optode separation due to a change in head shape or probe position during uterine contractions. The resulting alteration in light attenuation will be wrongly interpreted as a change in chromophore concentration.

Evidence that movement artefact may contribute to intrapartum NIRS measurements comes from a recently published case report by Hamilton *et al.*[58]. A fetus which had died as a result of a massive fetomaternal haemorrhage was studied by NIRS during labour. Changes in fetal cerebral $[HbO_2]$ and [Hb], of a similar order of magnitude to those seen in live fetuses, were observed during uterine contractions. In approximately two-thirds of contractions studied $[HbO_2]$ and [Hb] changed in opposite directions, whilst in the remaining third they changed in parallel. Hamilton *et al.* argued that because there was no possibility of a change in cerebral oxygenation in a dead fetus (whose oxygen saturation was presumably close to 0%), the apparent concentration changes recorded were likely to be due to movement artefact. They proposed that the similar changes previously described in live fetuses might also be solely due to movement artefact.

These findings have an important implication; that it is possible to obtain misleading data from the fetal brain due to artefact. However, the data shown above which describe a close correlation between changes in cerebral oxygenation and other parameters, such as fetal FHR and umbilical cord blood measurements, as well as expected fetal and placental physiology, suggest that the contribution of artefact may not be great. However, the only way to rigorously exclude the effect of changes in optical pathlength is to measure it continuously during the study, rather than assume that it remains constant.

INTENSITY-MODULATED OPTICAL SPECTROSCOPY

By measuring the phase shift between light entering and exiting the head, intensity-modulated optical spectroscopy (IMOS) can continuously record optical pathlength as well as light attenuation[24]. This allows continuous online correction for movement artefact in addition to conventional near infrared spectroscopy. Preliminary data have now been obtained from three fetuses during labour, using an intensity-modulated optical spectrometer designed and built by workers at University College, London[59]. The mean optical pathlength measured between contractions was 16.8 cm (range 15.5–17.2 cm) which is similar to that derived from $L \times B$ (3.5 × 4.39) in the Beer–Lambert equation. The maximum contraction-related change in pathlength was 6%. $SmcO_2$ was calculated for each contraction using pathlength-corrected and uncorrected data; there was no significant difference between the two calculations (Fig. 76.11). These findings suggest that while pathlength changes do occur during contractions, they are small and have no clinically significant effect on the calculation of changes in $[HbO_2]$ and [Hb].

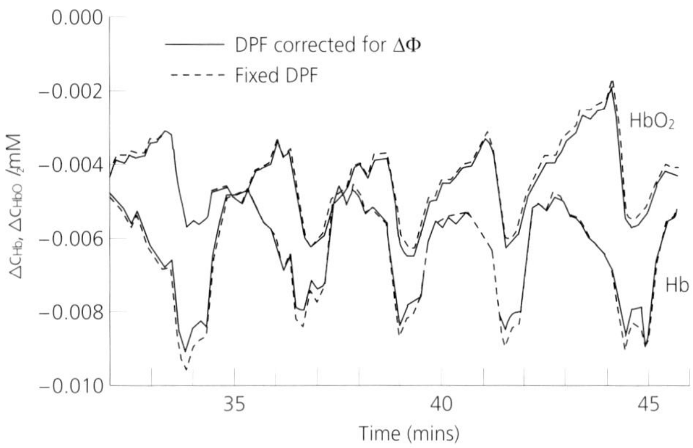

Fig. 76.11 Concentration changes in labour of fetal cerebral oxyhaemoglobin (HbO_2) and deoxyhaemoglobin (Hb), corrected (solid line) and uncorrected (dotted line) for optical pathlength changes. (Reprinted with permission from *MMRD Res. Rev.* 1997; **3** 59–68.)

Future developments

The observational studies described here suggest that both pulse oximetry and NIRS can provide information, in the majority of fetuses studied, about fetal oxygenation during labour. But before either technique can become incorporated into clinical practice developments are necessary in the following areas: technical, definition of suitable endpoints and clinical trials.

TECHNICAL

Many modifications, particularly in optode design and the choice of light emitting diodes, have resulted in improved oximeter performance. However, further refinements to overcome the problems of signal-to-noise ratio, motion artefact, impediments to light transmission (e.g. vernix and fetal hair) and calibration will make a significant different to the accuracy and reliability of intrapartum pulse oximetry.

The most significant advance in NIRS is the introduction of systems capable of continuous pathlength measurement, such as the fetal intensity modulated optical spectrometer described above. It is expected that the use of IMOS will become standard practice. The ability to correct continuously for any pathlength changes will improve accuracy, allowing interpretation of more subtle optical signals such as that derived from cytochrome oxidase, and improving the proportion of data which is interpretable.

Research continues into techniques aimed at measuring *absolute* concentrations of chromophores, as opposed to the changes from an arbitrary baseline measured with the present technology[60]. Absolute measurements of oxy-and deoxy-haemoglobin concentrations would allow calculation of oxygen saturation and cerebral blood volume instantaneously; it would not be necessary to wait for contractions suitable for calculating $SmcO_2$.

ENDPOINTS

In the absence of an absolute measure of chromophore concentration, $SmcO_2$ or SpO_2 are likely to remain individually the most useful clinical tools for the near future. Given the strong correlation between $SmcO_2$, SpO_2 and recognized parameters of fetal well-being demonstrated in the studies described above, it is conceivable that either value could be used in conjunction with CTG monitoring, perhaps replacing the need for fetal scalp blood sampling. It will first be necessary to establish, from observational studies in the human and animal, appropriate definitions of normality, both for absolute values as well as duration of hypoxia. Because of the complexity of the fetal response to hypoxia it is unlikely that any one variable in isolation will be sufficient to define the fetus at risk of hypoxic-ischaemic brain injury. A more physiological approach would be to assess simultaneously the metabolic (redox state of cytochrome oxidase) and cerebrovascular (changes in $[Hb_{tot}]$) consequences of changes in oxygenation (SpO_2 and $SmcO_2$. It is for this reason that no attempt is made here to determine whether NIRS or pulse oximetry is the better method of intrapartum surveillance; they are considered complementary techniques.

CLINICAL TRIALS

Obstetric intervention for fetal distress is common with up to 9% of babies delivered by caesarean section for this indication[61]. Conversely, the prevalence of poor neonatal outcome, attributable to intrapartum hypoxia ischaemia, is low with only 0.6/1000 live births having ischaemic encephalopathy[62]. This means that while trials which detect changes in intervention rates can be relatively small, they need to be much larger (40 000 to 80 000) to have sufficient power to detect changes in neonatal outcome[63]. This fact, combined with disillusionment stemming from the failure of EFM means that it is very difficult for any new method of intrapartum fetal surveillance to fulfil the necessary criteria for inclusion into clinical practice. Both NIRS and intrapartum fetal oxygen saturation monitoring are research tools which are continuing to clarify the pathophysiology of perinatal brain injury; more work needs to be done before their clinical potential is realized.

REFERENCES

1. Steer PJ & Carter MC. Cardiotocographs at a distance. *Br. Med. J.* **299**, 933–934, 1989.
2. Neilson J. Cardiotocographs during labour (editorial). *Br. Med. J.* **306**, 347–348, 1993.
3. MacDonald D, Grant A, Sheridan-Pereira M, Boylan P & Chalmers I. The Dublin randomized controlled trial of intrapartum fetal heart rate monitoring. *Am. J. Obstet. Gynecol.* **152**, 524–539, 1985.
4. Nelson KB, Dambrosia JM, Ting TY & Grether JK. Uncertain value of electronic fetal monitoring in predicting cerebral palsy. *N. Engl. J. Med.* **334**, 613–618, 1996.
5. Haverkamp AD, Orleans M, Langendoerfer S *et al.* A controlled trial of the differential effects of intrapartum fetal monitoring. *Am. J. Obstet. Gynecol.* **134**, 399–412, 1979.
6. Low JA, Muir D, Pater EA & Karchmar EJ. The association of intrapartum asphyxia in the mature fetus with newborn behaviour. *Am. J. Obstet. Gynecol.* **163**, 1131–1135, 1990.
7. Gunn AJ, Parer EC, Mallard CE, Williams CE & Gluckman PD. Cerebral histologic and electrocorticographic changes after asphyxia in fetal sheep. *Pediatr. Res.* **31**, 486–491, 1992.
8. Matthes K. Untersuchungen uber die Sauerstoffsattigungen des menschlichen Arterienblutes. *Arch. Exp. Pathol. Pharmac.* **179**, 698–711, 1935.
9. Millikan GA. The oximeter, an instrument for measuring continuously oxygen saturation of arterial blood in man. *Rev. Sci. Instrum.* **13**, 434–444, 1942.
10. Peat S, Booker M, Lanigan C & Ponte J. Continuous intrapartum measurement of fetal oxygen saturation. *Lancet* **ii**, 213, 1988.
11. Gardosi J, Carter M & Becket T. Continuous intrapartum monitoring of fetal oxygen saturation. *Lancet* **ii**, 692–693, 1989.
12. Johnson N, Johnson VA, Fisher J, Jobbings B, Bannister J & Lilford RJ. Fetal monitoring with pulse oximetry. *Br. J. Obstet. Gynaecol.* **98**, 36–41, 1991.
13. Jobsis FF. Noninvasive, infrared monitoring of cerebral and myocardial oxygen sufficiency and circulatory parameters. *Science* **198**, 1264–1267, 1977.
14. Wyatt JS, Cope M, Delpy DT, Wray S & Reynolds EOR. Quantification of cerebral oxygenation and haemodynamics in sick newborn infants by near infrared spectroscopy. *Lancet* **2**, 1063–1066, 1986.
15. Edwards AD, Wyatt JS, Richardson EC, Delpy DT, Cope M & Reynolds EOR. Cotside measurement of cerebral blood flow in ill newborn infants by near infrared spectroscopy. *Lancet* **2**, 701–702, 1988.
16. Wyatt JS, Cope M, Delpy DT *et al.* Quantitation of cerebral blood volume in newborn human infants by near infrared spectroscopy. *J. Appl. Physiol.* **68**, 1086–1091, 1990.
17. Fox EJ, Harme MH, Mitnick MH & Jobsis FF. Non-invasive monitoring of cerebral oxygen sufficiency during general anesthesia. *Anesthesiology* **57**, A160, 1982.
18. De Blasi RA, Alviggi I, Cope M, Elwell CE & Ferrari M. Noninvasive measurement of forearm consumption during exercise by near infrared spectroscopy. *Adv. Exp. Med. Biol.* **345**, 685–692, 1994.
19. Peebles DM, Edwards AD, Wyatt JS *et al.* Changes in human fetal cerebral hemoglobin concentration and oxygenation during labor measured by near-infrared spectroscopy. *Am. J. Obstet. Gynecol.* **166**, 1369–1373, 1992.
20. Doyle PM, O'Brien S, Wickramasinghe YABD, Houston R & Rolfe P. Near infrared spectroscopy used to observe changes in fetal cerebral haemodynamics during labour. *J. Perinat. Med.* **22**, 265–268, 1994.
21. Wray S, Cope M, Delpy DT, Wyatt JS & Reynolds EOR. Characterization of the near infrared absorption spectra of cytochrome aa_3 and haemoglobin for the non-invasive monitoring of cerebral oxygenation. *Biochim. Biophys. Acta.* **933**, 184–192, 1988.
22. Duncan A, Meek JH, Clemence M *et al.* Optical pathlength measurements on adult head, calf and forearm and the head of the newborn infant using phase resolved optical spectroscopy. *Phys. Med. Biol.* **40**, 295–304, 1995.
23. Gardosi J, Schram CM & Symonds EM. Adaptation of pulse oximetry for fetal monitoring during labour. *Lancet* **337**, 1265–1267, 1991.
24. Buschmann J, Rall G & Knitza R. Fetal oxygen saturation measurement by transmission pulse oximetry. *Lancet* **1**, 615, 1992.
25. Gardosi JO, Reed N & Sahota D. Fetal pulse oximetry with the balloon probe. In *Fetal Hypoxia During Labour* (ed. R. Knitsa) pp. 179–183. Darmstadt: Steinkopff, 1994.
26. Cope M & Delpy DT. A system for long term measurement of cerebral blood and tissue oxygenation in newborn infants by near-infrared transillumination. *Med. Biol. Eng. Comp.* **26**, 289–294, 1988.
27. Dildy GA, Clark SL & Loucks CA. Preliminary experience with intrapartum fetal pulse oximetry in humans. *Obstet. Gynecol.* **81**, 630–635, 1993.
28. Dildy GA, van den Berg PP, Katz M *et al.* Intrapartum fetal pulse oximetry: fetal oxygen saturation trends during labor and relation to delivery outcome. *Am. J. Obstet. Gynecol.* **171**, 679–684, 1994.
29. McNamara H, Johnson N & Lilford R. The effect on fetal arteriolar oxygen saturation resulting from giving oxygen to the mother measured by pulse oximetry. *Br. J. Obstet. Gynaecol.* **100**, 446–449, 1993.
30. Luttkus AK & Dudenhausen JW. Fetal Pulse Oximetry. *Baillière's Clin. Obstet. Gynaecol.* **10**(2), 295–306, 1996.
31. McNamara H, Chung DC, Lilford R & Johnson N. Do fetal pulse oximetry readings at delivery correlate with cord blood oxygenation and acidaemia? *Br. J. Obstet. Gynaecol.* **99**, 735–738, 1992.
32. Luttkus A, Fengler TW, Friedmann W & Dudenhausen JW. Continuous monitoring of fetal oxygen saturation by pulse oximetry. *Obstet. Gynecol.* **85**, 183–186, 1995.
33. Mann LJ, Carmichael A & Duchin S. The effect of head compression on FHR, brain metabolism and function. *Obstet. Gynecol.* **39**, 721–726, 1972.
34. D'Antona D, Aldrich CJ, Spencer JAD, Delpy D, Reynolds EOR & Wyatt JS. Effect of nuchal cord on fetal cerebral haemodynamics and oxygenation measured by near infrared spectroscopy during labour. *Eur. J. Obstet. Gynecol. Reprod. Biol.* **59**, 205–209, 1995.
35. O'Brien PMS, Doyle PM & Rolfe P. Near infrared spectroscopy in fetal monitoring. *Br. J. Hosp. Med.* **49**, 483–487, 1993.
36. Peebles DM, Spencer JAD, Edwards AD *et al.* Relation between frequency of uterine contractions and human fetal cerebral oxygen saturation studied during labour by near infrared spectroscopy. *Br. J. Obstet. Gynaecol.* **101**, 44–48, 1994.
37. Steer PJ. Abnormal uterine action. In *Obstetrics* (eds A. Turnbull & G. Chamberlain), pp. 783–792. Edinburgh: Churchill Livingstone, 1989.
38. Peebles DM, Edwards AD, Wyatt JS *et al.* Effect of oxytocin on fetal brain oxygenation during labour (letter). *Lancet* **338**, 254–255, 1991.
39. Aldrich CJ, D'Antona D, Spencer JAD *et al.* Late fetal heart decelerations and changes in cerebral oxygenation during the first stage of labour. *Br. J. Obstet. Gynaecol.* **102**, 9–13, 1995.
40. Myers RE, Mueller-Heubach E & Adamsons K. Predictability of the state of fetal oxygenation from a quantitative analysis of the components of late deceleration. *Am. J. Obstet. Gynecol.* **115**, 1083–1094, 1973.
41. Aldrich CJ, D'Antona D, Spencer JAD *et al.* The effect of maternal pushing on fetal cerebral oxygenation and blood volume during the second stage of labour. *Br. J. Obstet. Gynaecol.* **102**, 448–453, 1995.
42. Aldrich CJ, D'Antona D, Spencer JAD *et al.* The effect of maternal posture on fetal cerebral oxygenation during labour. *Br. J. Obstet. Gynaecol.* **102**, 14–19, 1995.
43. Aldrich CJ, Wyatt JS, Spencer JAD, Reynolds EOR & Delpy DT. The effect of maternal oxygen administration on human fetal cerebral oxygenation measured during labour by near infrared spectroscopy. *Br. J. Obstet. Gynaecol.* **101**, 509–513, 1994.
44. Aldrich CJ, D'Antona D, Wyatt JS, Spencer JAD, Peebles DM & Reynolds EOR. Fetal cerebral oxygenation measured by near infrared spectroscopy shortly before birth and acid-base status at birth. *Obstet. Gynecol.* **84**, 861–866, 1994.
45. Nijland R, Jongsma H & Nijhaus JG. Arterial oxygen saturation in relation to metabolic acidosis in fetal lambs. *Am. J. Obstet. Gynecol.* **172**, 810–819, 1995.
46. Nijland R, Jongsma H, Nijhaus JG *et al.* Reflectance pulse oximetry (RPOX): two sensors compared in piglets. *Am. J. Obstet. Gynecol.* **172**(1), 365, 1995.
47. Itskovitz J, LaGamma EF & Rudolph A. Effects of cord compression on fetal blood flow distribution and O_2 delivery. *Am. J. Physiol.* **252**, 100–109, 1987.

48. Giussani DA, Spencer JADS, Moore PJ, Bennet L & Hanson MA. Afferent and efferent components of the early cardiovascular response of the term sheep fetus to acute hypoxia. *J. Physiol.* **461**, 431–449, 1993.
49. Jensen A, Hohmann M & Kunzel W. Dynamic changes in organ blood flow and oxygen consumption during acute asphyxia in fetal sheep. *J. Dev. Physiol.* **9**, 41–55, 1987.
50. Hanson MA & Nijhuis JG. Pulse oximetry – physiological considerations. *Eur. J. Obstet. Gynecol. Reprod. Biol.* **72**, S3–S8, 1997.
51. Bennet L, Peebles DM, Edwards AD & Hanson MA. Cerebral haemodynamic changes in unanaesthetised fetal sheep measured by near infrared spectroscopy in acute hypoxia. *J. Physiol.* **479**, 24P, 1994.
52. Chance B & Williams GR. The respiratory chain and oxidative phosphorylation. *Adv. Enzymol.* **17**, 65–134, 1965.
53. Tamura M, Hazeki O, Nioka S, Chance B & Smith DS. The simultaneous measurement of tissue oxygen concentration and energy state by near infrared spectroscopy and nuclear magnetic spectroscopy. *Adv. Exp. Med. Biol.* **222**, 359–363, 1988.
54. Tsuji M, Naruse H, Volpe J & Holtzman D. Reduction of cytochrome aa3 measured by near infrared spectroscopy predicts cerebral energy loss in hypoxic piglets. *Ped. Res.* **37**, 253–259, 1996.
55. O'Connor MC, Hytten FE & Zanelli GD. Is the fetus scalped during labour? *Lancet* **ii**, 947–949, 1979.
56. Johnson N, Johnson VA, Bannister J & Lilford RJ. The effect of caput succedaneum on oxygen saturation measurements. *Br. J. Obstet. Gynaecol.* **97**, 493–498, 1990.
57. Jubran A. Pulse oximetry. *Contemp. Manag. Crit. Care.* **1**, 79–100, 1992.
58. Hamilton RJ, O'Brien PMS, Wickramasinghe YABD & Rolfe P. Intrapartum fetal cerebral near infrared spectroscopy: apparent change in oxygenation demonstrated in a non viable fetus. *Br. J. Obstet. Gynaecol.* **102**, 1004–1007, 1995.
59. Watson R, Kohl M, O'Brien P, Lawrence S, Delpy DT & Cope M. Fetal brain oxygenation during labor studied by frequency domain spectroscopy. *Biomed. Optic. Spectrosc. Diagn.* **3**, 117–122, 1996.
60. Matcher SJ & Cooper CE. Absolute quantification of deoxyhaemoglobin concentration in tissue by near infrared spectroscopy. *Phys. Med. Biol.* **39**, 1295–1312, 1994.
61. Thacker SB. Effectiveness and safety of intrapartum fetal monitoring. In *Fetal Monitoring* (ed. J.A.D. Spencer), pp. 211–217. Castle House Publications, 1989.
62. Ellenberg JH & Nelson KB. Cluster of perinatal events identifying infants at high risk for death or disability. *J. Pediatr* **113**, 546–552, 1989.
63. Mongelli M, Chung TKH & Chang AMZ. Obstetric intervention and benefit in conditions of very low prevalence. *Br. J. Obstet. Gynaecol.* **104**, 771–774, 1997.

The postmortem

S. Gould

77

Introduction

Despite advances in other forms of monitoring, the postmortem is still one of the most objective and valuable methods of providing insight into fetal life. The postmortem process has four overlapping and interconnected roles:

- Audit
- Education
- Research
- Diagnosis

While diagnosis is often the major focus of concern in individual cases, the full clinical benefits of audit, education and research result from the continual feedback of well-documented autopsy data over a prolonged period.

THE CONTRIBUTION OF THE AUTOPSY

The minimum recommended perinatal autopsy rate in the UK is 75%[1]. While perinatal autopsy rates do remain significantly higher than those of adults, this rate is becoming increasingly difficult to maintain, more so in some subcategories than others[2]. This is partly linked to the changing approach to fetal death where funerals even in the very immature are now common. In 1993, the national Confidential Enquiry into Stillbirth and Death in Infancy (CESDI) that covers England, Wales and Northern Ireland recorded an autopsy rate of 58%, with no requests for autopsy in 17% of cases[3].

Linked to this fall in autopsy rates is a clinical view and, regretfully, sometimes a misconception by some pathologists, that the autopsy is not likely to provide clinically useful information. This view may be a factor in the less than optimum conduct of some perinatal autopsies[4,5]. In a recent Welsh study, however, additional information was obtained in 26% of cases and a complete change in clinicopathological classification in 13%[5]. Even when the cause of death seemed understood clinically, there was either a change in diagnosis or new information in up to 21% of cases. Although the precise study populations were different, similar results have been recorded in other studies[6–8]. In neonates where diagnoses might be perceived as more secure, diagnosis may change in up to 10% with additional information in a further 17%[9].

Follow-up of termination after prenatal diagnosis is a specific area for audit, and fortunately one in which the role of the autopsy is widely recognized[10–12]; autopsy rates usually exceed 95%[10,11]. With improving quality of instrumentation, in experienced hands ultrasound provides an accurate diagnosis of major fetal pathology, sufficient to allow appropriate counselling for termination. Nevertheless, postmortem examination still provides more detail and identifies abnormalities that permit a more specific diagnosis and modifies genetic counselling. Important diagnostic refinements are identified in up to 40% of cases[10,11].

THE GOLD STANDARD?

In auditing fetal termination following prenatal diagnosis, a detailed fetal postmortem examination, including appropriate additional investigations, acts as a 'gold' standard against which prenatal diagnosis can be measured. However, it is necessary to recognize the postmortem's limitations. The general approach to abnormalities that may be difficult or impossible to verify post termination requires caution. Some isolated cerebral abnormalities, such as ventriculomegaly or posterior fossa 'cysts' in particular, are difficult. Maceration frequently leads to a soft, disrupted brain that can preclude adequate examination.

Further, the trend for earlier diagnosis and termination will pose additional problems. Examination of smaller and sometimes disrupted fetuses asks a difficult question of the pathologist[13]. For the obstetrician, additional techniques may need development to facilitate the continued role of postmortem fetal examination in genetic counselling and audit, especially in such a developing field[14]. The means to maintain a gold standard is a challenge for both clinician and pathologist.

The fetal and perinatal autopsy

As alluded to above, the fetal autopsy is not always viewed positively despite the evidence that it provides additional significant information in a high proportion of cases. This negative perception is partly linked to expectation. The greatest value will be extracted from fetal postmortem if both clinician and pathologist have a clear view of what can and, as importantly, what cannot be expected from the procedure.

This chapter is written primarily with the clinician in mind to help in extracting maximum benefit from the postmortem and the pathologist's report. Nevertheless, it is hoped that there is also sufficient here to aid the more general pathologist in structuring an approach to the fetal autopsy.

Much of this chapter will address the postmortem investigation of fetal death, but also the investigation of neonatal death where it provides information on fetal life. It is inappropriate to detail postmortem technique. Descriptions will be largely confined to the principles behind postmortem diagnosis rather than the details, particularly the histological, of pathological entities.

The diagnostic aspects of postmortem investigation will be considered in four parts:

- The process
- Basic assessment
- Pathological classification and diagnosis
- Pathology of the placenta

The process

For many, the postmortem refers to the procedure in which the body is dissected in the autopsy room. Especially in fetal medicine, it is important to view the term as a concept embracing far more than this. The postmortem investigation of fetal or early neonatal death is a multistage procedure and will often incorporate elements performed outside of the autopsy room that are every bit as important as those performed inside.

CONSENT

Consent for fetal autopsy will normally be obtained for all fetuses and babies over the age of 'viability' – that is greater than 24 weeks of gestation. However, it is now common practice and indeed recommended practice for consent to be obtained for examination of even previable fetuses less than 24 weeks of gestation[15].

Some parents may wish to have as much information as possible about the cause of their loss but are unhappy about aspects of the full autopsy. In these circumstances, consideration should be given for obtaining consent to a partial autopsy examination; a limited autopsy may be a more than adequate compromise. For instance, the head is often a sensitive area, so examination of the brain might be omitted; limited examination with biopsy of specific organs may also be an option.

Other concerns about the appearance of the body after autopsy and the scope for viewing also need to be addressed. Discussion with the parents by someone knowledgeable about the autopsy and the options is important in these circumstances. On occasions, the pathologist may be the most appropriate person to discuss the options available and clear lines of communication must exist between clinician and pathologist.

An occasional issue that arises at this stage is the question of fetal tissue, taken during the postmortem examination, for use in research. While one has to acknowledge there is a grey area, tissues taken for research purposes may require a specific protocol. In the UK, guidelines have been issued that recommend both special parental consent and approval by ethics committees[16] before tissue can be taken specifically for research.

TIMING OF THE AUTOPSY

Most fetal autopsies will be performed shortly after parental consent has been obtained. However, the change in the culture in dealing with fetal death is such that many parents will now wish to view the fetus or baby after delivery, possibly more than once. In general, a delay of 2–3 days between delivery and examination will not impair the quality of the autopsy significantly, particularly if the fetus is kept in cool surroundings, i.e. a fridge (not a freezer) between viewings.

Two more common situations, however, may be affected by delay. The first is the reduction in the chance of successful tissue culture for cytogenetic study. This problem can usually be side-stepped by taking a small skin/muscle biopsy from a less visible site, for instance in the axilla, as soon as possible. The main autopsy examination can follow later. The second problem is that delay may reduce the chance of identifying an infection with a specific organism due to postmortem overgrowth. Where this might be important, immediate surface cultures may help as well as culture of placental biopsy. More rarely, a metabolic disorder may be suspected and this will require prompt tissue and specimen sampling.

HISTORY

Perinatal autopsy requests should be accompanied by an adequate history, and in modern practice this is usually on a structured form. The importance of the history, as for any medical investigation, cannot be overstated. It should include details of past medical and past obstetric history, current pregnancy including investigations even if 'negative', the events leading to the death or diagnosis of fetal death and any specific questions the clinician wishes to ask the pathologist.

As important as the provision of a structured history is the ability of the pathologist to interpret the significance of the various elements. The pathologist should not only answer the specific questions asked by the clinicians including the obvious, if not always possible, definitive cause of death, but the questions implicit in the history.

Radiology

Radiology must be freely available to any pathologist performing fetal autopsy and, indeed, fetal autopsy should not be conducted where it cannot be obtained at all. In some circumstances, such as skeletal dysplasia, the X-ray is often the diagnostic investigation (Fig. 77.1). In the investigation of fetal abnormality, it can delineate additional skeletal abnormalities that will contribute to syndromic diagnosis. Negative information can also be of value, and may help in excluding some diagnoses where skeletal abnormality is a usual or common feature.

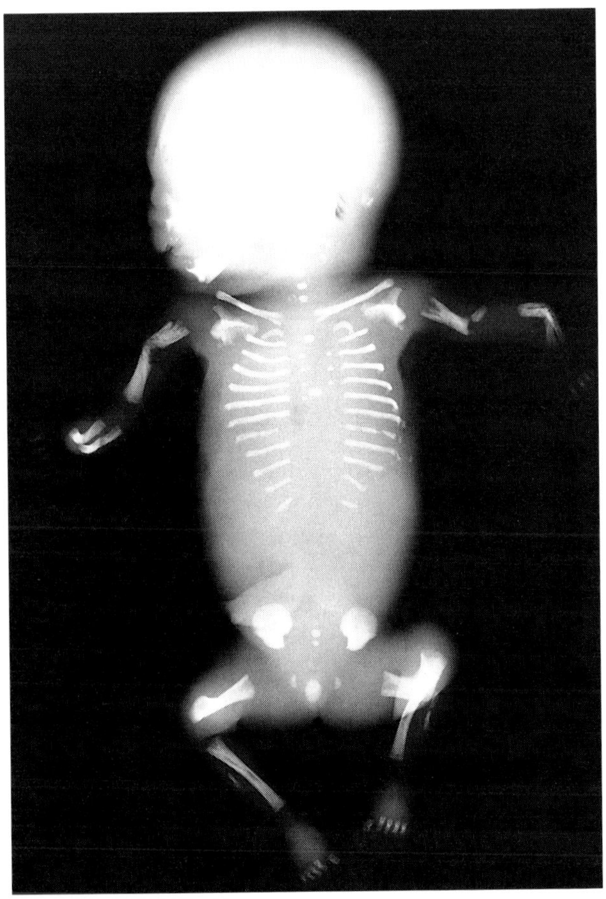

Fig. 77.1 Radiograph showing typical appearance of hypophosphatasia with patchy absence of ossification, for instance in the vertebral column. The prenatal differential diagnosis may include osteogenesis imperfecta and achondrogenesis; each diagnosis has its own implication for genetic counselling. Hypophosphatasia is an autosomal recessive condition, and specific testing for alkaline phosphatase activity of bone and sometimes other tissues taken at fetal examination may be required to confirm diagnosis.

Where congenital abnormality is not a particular question, X-rays can contribute to assessment of gestation as well as identify other pathology such as calcification in soft tissues.

PHOTOGRAPHY

All abnormal fetuses require photography for permanent record and should include lateral views. Verbal description of facial dysmorphism can be imprecise and cannot replace a photograph, especially if a referral opinion is required. It is our practice to take at least one photograph of every fetus autopsied, even if normally formed.

EXTERNAL AND INTERNAL EXAMINATION

Detailed descriptions of the external and internal autopsy procedures are beyond the scope of this chapter and are well described elsewhere[17,18]. Precise autopsy technique is not prescriptive as long as the appropriate answers are obtained. Besides an account of dysmorphic features as appropriate, all fetuses should have basic measurements recorded including crown–heel and crown–rump lengths, head circumference, foot length and weight. A comment on the presence and degree of maceration is vital (see below – estimation of period of fetal death).

Internal examination should include weighing of all major organs and this will require a balance with an accuracy of at least 0.1 g. The pattern of organ weights if they stray from the normal can provide valuable clues to the presence of underlying pathology.

Occasionally, a full examination of some organs usually the heart or brain, and possibly by a specialist pathologist may be considered necessary. While a different approach may be appropriate when there is a coroner's autopsy, both clinician and pathologist should be aware that whole organ retention is potentially a very sensitive area for parents and not a procedure for which they will have considered consent has been granted.

Where detailed examination of a congenital heart abnormality is required, it is preferable to maintain the lungs, or part of the lungs, in continuity with the heart to allow, amongst other aspects, examination of the pulmonary venous drainage. The heart is affected by autolysis to a far less extent than the brain, which softens quickly in the process of maceration. It may require considerable skill to retain the brain whole and occasionally it may be possible or preferable to fix in-situ. Alternatively it may be preferable to remove the brain under water to retain its form prior to fixation. Maceration should not discourage a full examination of the brain. Histology is often far better than might be anticipated from its macroscopic appearance.

HISTOLOGY

For most fetal autopsies, widespread tissue sampling for microscopic examination is mandatory. In the absence of a histological component to a perinatal autopsy report, the report can only be regarded as incomplete or provisional. Even in macerated fetuses, it will assist in assessing factors such as how long the fetus has been dead in utero, or the presence of a chronic intrauterine disease or infection.

In the presence of a clearly defined structural abnormality and/or chromosomal anomaly the contribution of histology to diagnosis may be limited. Occasionally, unsuspected structural liver or renal abnormalities can be missed and histology may confirm or expand macroscopic diagnosis (Fig. 77.2). This may have little implication for genetic counselling, for instance when subtyping adenomatoid malformation of the lung, but is vital when subcategorizing renal cystic disease into sporadic, autosomal recessive or dominant forms. In skeletal dysplasias, histology may assist in a specific diagnosis when radiology provides only a differential diagnosis.

Some syndromes may have characteristic histological aspects such as the enlarged adrenal cells (adrenocytomegaly) of Beckwith–Wiedemann syndrome. An awareness that some metabolic disorders can demonstrate dysmorphism should also encourage routine histology.

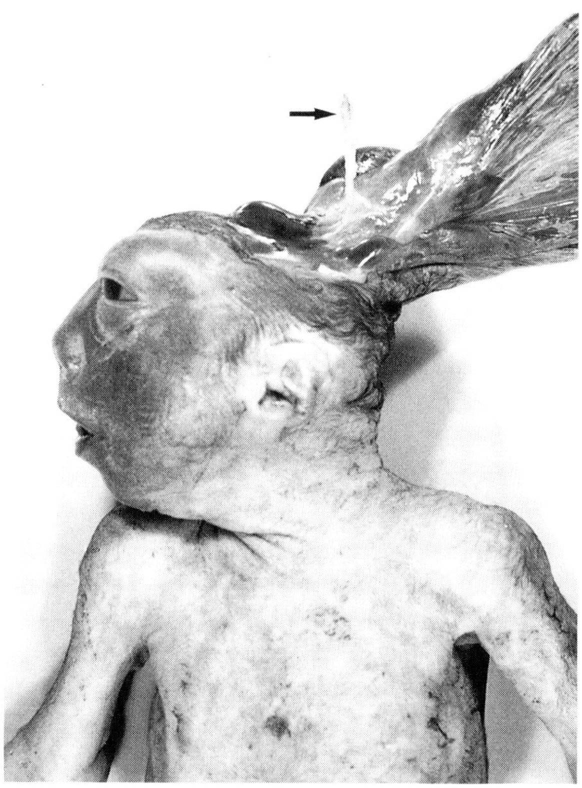

Fig. 77.2 Fetus terminated for anencephaly. In this case, a small attached piece of tissue (arrowed) was shown histologically to be amnion indicating that this slightly unusual appearance resulted from amniotic bands. This has a lesser recurrence risk than the usual anencephaly.

MICROBIOLOGY

An infective cause of fetal death is frequently high on the list of possible diagnoses. As a general rule, however, the role of microbiological studies is to assist in defining the organism causing infection, not to make the diagnosis of infection itself. In the absence of histological evidence of tissue inflammation, most isolates will be of dubious significance and likely to be postmortem overgrowth and contamination. There will be exceptions. For instance, Group B *Streptococcus* can cause overwhelming infection leading to death before significant inflammatory changes are found.

Selective sampling is appropriate. In the absence of specific clues (e.g. meningeal inflammation), blood and culture of lung biopsy is of value in fresh stillbirths and particularly so with intrapartum deaths. Lung biopsy in fetal death that may be associated with ascending infection may prove useful.

Placental swab or biopsy should supplement fetal specimens. The risk of spurious isolates is far greater if microbiological material is taken many hours after delivery in the postmortem room. Sampling below the amnion can reduce the risk of contamination or prompt sampling in the labour ward can be effective.

Virology is even less likely to be fruitful as a routine procedure and it is justified to sample when there are specific indications. Increasingly, it is possible to use techniques such as immunohistology or polymerase chain reaction on processed material to test for specific viruses rather than relying purely on culture or electron microscopy, the former being particularly difficult from postmortem samples.

CYTOGENETICS

For the investigation of fetal death, some protocols demand that fetal skin should be sent routinely for cytogenetic study, although it is a misconception to assume that, by itself, the presence of a karyotypic abnormality establishes a cause of fetal death. For most cytogenetic laboratories, receiving tissue for study when there is little or no indication that an abnormality is present, or maceration is advanced, is probably an inappropriate use of resources; yield from normally formed macerated fetuses will be extremely low both in terms of successful culture but also of an abnormal karyotype.

Nevertheless, thresholds for cytogenetic studies should be low and attempted in the presence of any minor abnormality, dysmorphic feature, hydrops or unexplained growth retardation. A small skin-with-muscle biopsy should be sent in appropriate tissue culture medium as soon after delivery as possible. Other tissues that may be of value include lung, gonad or placenta. The last has the advantage that it is a fetal tissue that has continued to receive a blood supply from the maternal circulation after death of the fetus itself. It is more likely to be viable than other tissues but has the disadvantage that, occasionally, maternal cells are cultured rather than fetal. Further, cytogenetic abnormality may be detected in the placenta but not in the fetus.

This may be of limited significance in many cases, but it is increasingly recognized that chromosomal abnormalities apparently confined to the placenta do have implications for an understanding of fetal loss. Trisomies of chromosomes 3, 9, 18 and 16 are the most common identified, the last often associated with severe intrauterine growth retardation. The fetal chromosome number may be normal but this is largely due to early post zygotic loss of one chromosome. In a proportion, uniparental disomy can be demonstrated[19,20].

In the presence of a high index of suspicion of cytogenetic abnormality or when confirmation of diagnosis post-termination is required, other techniques can be used. In our experience, fluorescent in-situ hybridization (FISH) can be a cost-effective mechanism, especially for confirmatory studies post termination, when looking for specific chromosomal abnormalities, such as trisomy 21 or 18. This will work in postmortem tissues despite maceration. Lung tissue is especially useful and results may be obtained quickly. FISH can also be used to examine mosacism and detection of more subtle chromosomal abnormalities[21].

METABOLIC STUDIES

Detecting metabolic abnormality following fetal autopsy is difficult without a high index of suspicion. Diagnosis is more likely to be made in certain circumstances such as previous family history, signs such as hydrops or sudden early neonatal death. A few storage disorders can be detected histologically in the placenta and even sometimes in macerated tissues. Fibroblasts should be cultured. These can be frozen for long term storage if necessary.

TISSUE STORAGE

Increasingly, facilities for storage of tissue and fluids are becoming a necessity. Even when the cause of death is not clear it is generally an inappropriate use of resource to instigate a full range of investigations immediately after the autopsy. Stored tissue becomes a resource for staged and directed investigation. The manner of storage will depend on the availability. In general, long-term tissue storage will require liquid nitrogen or a −70°C freezer, the former especially if histochemistry and retention of tissue morphology might be important. The more valuable tissues include brain, liver, skeletal muscle, kidney and heart. For a DNA archive, spleen can be frozen in a −20°C freezer.

Other specimens that may be considered include plasma and urine.

Basic assessment

In the introduction, it was stated that the postmortem would ideally conclude with a summary list of pathological findings and a specific diagnosis. This is achievable in a significant proportion of fetal postmortems, particularly in the presence of malformation, and neonatal deaths.

However, for many fetal cases a clear diagnosis with cause of death is not attainable. In these circumstances, simple descriptive reports with no conclusions or focus may be next to useless and will reinforce the impression that the investigation pointless. The clinician should expect the pathologist to provide, as far as possible, a minimum set of statements.

Even if they do not provide a clear cause of death, these statements will:

- Provide feedback as to the accuracy or otherwise of clinical understanding of the case
- Provide a more solid foundation for parental counselling and future pregnancy management

PRESENCE OF STRUCTURAL ABNORMALITY

A statement indicating a fetus is normally formed should be regarded as an important positive finding. Not only is it a statement about the present, but it allows more secure advice on future pregnancy risks.

ASSESSMENT OF GESTATION

The clinical estimate of gestation should be provided with all autopsy requests and whether this estimate is by dates, early ultrasound or both. The autopsy report should clearly indicate whether the fetal size and maturation is consistent with the stated clinical estimate of gestation.

There are many anthropometric charts detailing fetal weight, various external measurements, and organ weights and these should be routinely consulted by the pathologist[18,22,23]. Internal organ weights can be correlated with both fetal gestation and fetal weight. The presence of an internal consistency and agreement with clinical dates, will help to confirm gestation as well as help to exclude a chronic intrauterine disease process. Inconsistencies may be sufficient to question the clinical assessment of gestation.

Additional clues to gestation can be obtained from the gyral maturation of the brain. The complexity of gyral maturation progresses rapidly after 24 weeks of gestation and can be compared with standard illustrations. Some organs also show relatively consistent maturational changes that are useful in correlating with gestation and these include cerebellum, lung and kidney. The quality of assessment can require a certain amount of experience and can be influenced by the degree of tissue maceration.

It should be emphasized that no one measure can always be used as the indicator of gestation but, in general, greater reliance can be placed on assessment of the brain, particularly gyral maturation, than other measures. Although cerebral gyral maturation can be delayed in extreme circumstances, it will tend to be the last organ to be affected by such processes as growth retardation and chronic intrauterine stress (Fig. 77.3).

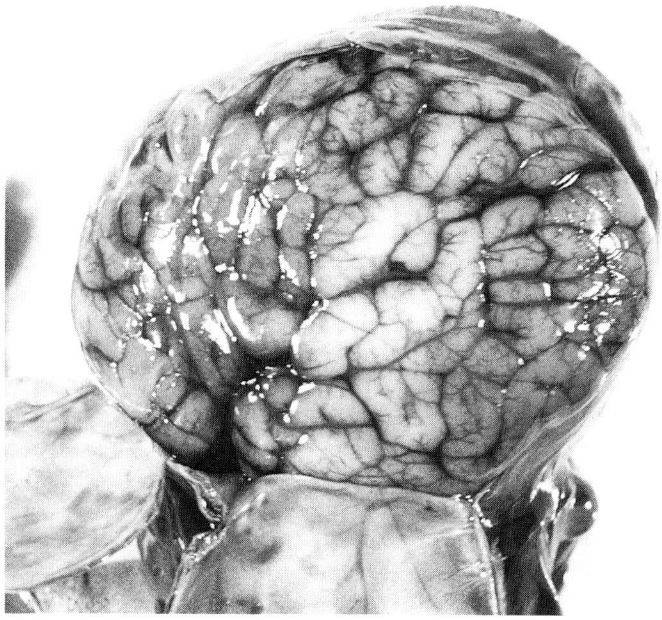

Fig. 77.3 External view of brain from a very macerated fetus weighing less than 1500 g. Clinical history suggested the baby was near term gestation. Gyral maturation here is mature indicating the presence of severe growth retardation rather than incorrect dates. Maceration does not preclude valuable inferences from brain examination.

ASSESSMENT OF MACERATION AND TIMING OF FETAL DEATH

Maceration is the progressive postmortem change in tissues that are immersed in water, the earliest changes of which start approximately 6 h after death. A conscious assessment of maceration and the degree of tissue autolysis by histology is required to enable some estimate of the time of fetal death. Clear discrepancies between the clinical and pathological estimates are rare but when they do occur, potentially very important clinically.

Determination of the time a fetus has been dead in utero from autopsy study is imprecise and some caution is required in any assessment. Both macroscopic appearances and tissue histology may be helpful[24–26]. Maceration occurs rapidly in utero but can be modified by other factors. Some skin changes are accelerated by the presence of hydrops, whereas maceration may be relatively slow in small growth-retarded fetuses. Depending when the assessment is made, allowances have to be made for the time between delivery and autopsy and the temperature at which the body is kept after delivery. This may affect the histological features especially; autolysis of tissues does not stop once delivery has taken place. Maceration may be associated with some weight loss.

ASSESSMENT OF MODE OF DEATH AND CHRONIC INTRAUTERINE STRESS

Particularly in the context of the macerated stillbirth, no specific cause of death may be identified. Death is often attributed to 'asphyxia', implying that the fetus has died due to a lack of oxygen delivery. Where there is evidence of a more chronic process, most obviously in the form of growth retardation, death has traditionally been attributed to 'placental insufficiency'. This is a potentially misleading phrase as it implies that the primary pathology lies within the placenta itself[27] and the label should be avoided.

Nevertheless, even in the absence of a specific diagnosis, the autopsy may still provide an indication as to whether there was a chronic intrauterine process and whether asphyxia, if it has occurred, was acute or more chronic.

At autopsy a simple but potentially useful element is a record of organ weights. A degree of caution is needed in the presence of severe maceration due to in utero weight loss but ratios of organ weights, rather than absolute values may still be of use. As discussed above, the pattern of organ weights may provide clues as to an intrauterine process. Thus:

- Small, relatively light thoracic and abdominal organs but normal brain weight is typical of asymmetric growth retardation. Liver/brain weight ratio is usually about 3:1 and a high ratio may suggest early 'malnutrition'
- A normal weight brain for gestation but heavy heart, liver and adrenals is typical of an infant of a diabetic mother
- Intrauterine infections and rhesus disease may give rise to a heavy liver, spleen and adrenals. The thymus may be small

Histological examination may supplement and help to verify the significance of these patterns. Lymphocyte depletion in a stressed thymus can be seen microscopically, often before weight loss can be detected. Fat in the adrenal fetal cortex may be a sign of severe chronic stress especially in the presence of severe maternal preeclamptic toxaemia (Fig. 77.4). Significant fat accumulation can normally be detected even in the absence of special stains.

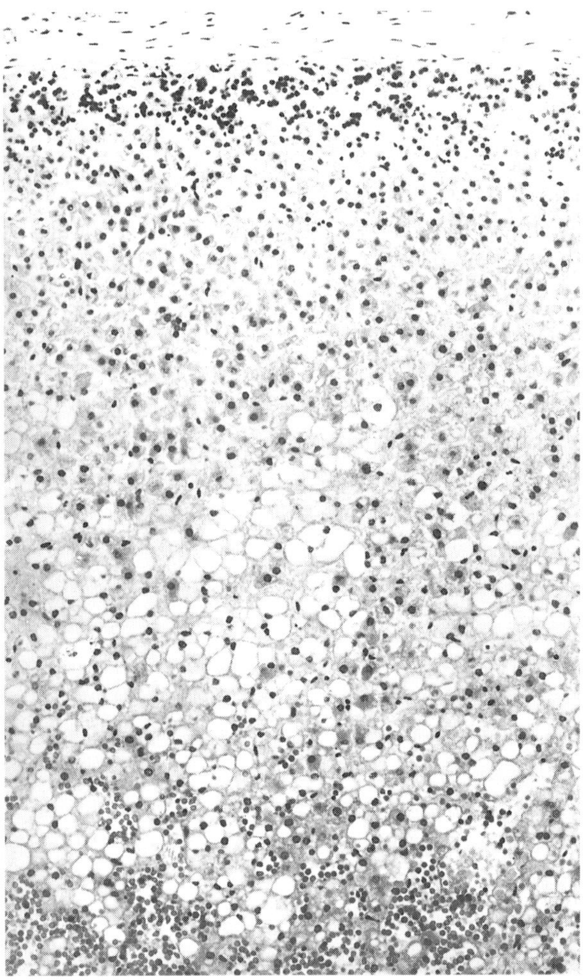

Fig. 77.4 Adrenal showing fat in fetal cortex. This is a good indicator for chronic intrauterine stress and is particularly associated with pre-eclamptic toxaemia.

EXTERNAL EXAMINATION ONLY

In the absence of autopsy consent, an external assessment of the fetus should still be made. Formal external examination is an opportunity to record fetal weights and measurement, assess gestation, the degree of maceration, and the presence of growth retardation or fetal dysmorphism (see above). Radiographs may contribute and where appropriate, placenta can be sent for cytogenetic study.

Although the conclusions may be less secure than following a full autopsy, the synthesis of all the external examination results may provide some indication as to the cause of fetal loss and the likelihood of other significant pathology.

Pathological diagnosis and classification

Where possible, a specific cause of death will be assigned to a fetal or neonatal loss over and above, or as part of, the basic assessment. While this might be possible immediately after the initial dissection, it should be stressed that it will usually require the collation of data from a variety of sources including a perinatal mortality meeting before such a specific diagnosis may be made.

Many classifications have been used to provide an overview of fetal loss. One approach is to classify fetal death, less by the immediate cause of death, than by the underlying aetiology; clinical criteria are used almost exclusively[28]. Other classifications use pathological data to classify by cause of death[29,30]. In 1980, Wigglesworth proposed a simple classification[31] that does not rely too heavily on postmortem data for use, but allows sensible modification of case description when postmortem data is available. The classification has been the subject of some minor modification[32] and is now used in an 'extended' version by CESDI.

It is beyond the scope of this chapter to detail all fetal and relevant neonatal pathology. Therefore, only the major subgroups will be discussed using the 'extended Wigglesworth' classification as a framework. It has a distinct advantage of simplicity and that it imposes a structure on thinking that is useful both clinically and pathologically.

CONGENITAL MALFORMATION

From the point of view of classification, congenital malformation is usually relatively straightforward bearing in mind one cannot always assume a causal relationship between the presence of a malformation and fetal death. The importance of a rigorous autopsy protocol including photography and radiology has already been discussed.

The value of a multidisciplinary approach to malformation[33] is worth restating. While this applies more obviously to the work-up of a diagnosis after the autopsy, in the context of prenatal diagnosis, it can be equally important pre-termination when it will help to ensure that special sampling or procedures are performed appropriately.

ASPHYXIA: ANTEPARTUM AND INTRAPARTUM

Asphyxia is probably one of the most widely applied labels in fetal medicine although, curiously, it is difficult to find a clear definition of the term. At the most basic level it implies that fetal gas exchange has been impaired and this leads to hypoxia, carbon dioxide retention and acidosis[34]. Whether it causes sufficient interference with normal function to result in permanent damage or death may depend on a host of other factors including the duration and severity of the asphyxia, and prior nutritional status of the fetus.

Much of obstetric focus has been on the detection of intrapartum asphyxia, with a view of reducing perinatal mortality and morbidity, the latter usually a consequence of cerebral damage. However, the clinical diagnosis of intrapartum asphyxia has proved far from straightforward and has even led Johnson[35] to question the term birth asphyxia. Examining criteria for diagnosis, he suggested that an objective definition might require evidence of fetal distress over a period of time, a low Apgar score and pH at birth, and evidence of postnatal central nervous system compromise.

Further, studies over recent years, primarily epidemiological, have suggested that a significant proportion of the morbidity, such as cerebral palsy, traditionally attributed to intrapartum asphyxia, may be initiated in the antepartum period[36–40]. Studies of the brains of stillborn infants and early neonatal deaths have shown cerebral damage with an antepartum origin in a significant proportion, and provide some pathological support for these conclusions[41–44]. Consequently, in addition to the diagnosis of asphyxia, the timing of the onset of the hypoxia forms a vital component of any pathological assessment.

Observation of either the acute or chronic changes of hypoxia within the fetus or infant forms the basis of the pathological diagnosis of asphyxia but does not imply, necessarily, an understanding of the underlying cause. Indeed, it will represent a final common pathway or mode of death of many fetuses and, particularly for macerated stillbirths, will be a category into which many will fall after other causes of death have been excluded.

The pathology of asphyxia is largely the same for both intrapartum and antepartum related deaths, hence they can be considered together. Differences in pathology are often more attributable to subsequent events. For instance, a longer survival time after severe hypoxia together with sequelae of intensive care will be a feature of intrapartum rather than antepartum asphyxiated babies. The brain and lung are usually the most important organs affected by asphyxia and the pathology will be discussed in more detail.

BRAIN

The fetal brain undergoes dramatic changes in the latter parts of gestation, both in growth and in development. Consequently, hypoxic-ischaemic insult will cause damage directly to formed brain but also has the potential to impair subsequent development.

As a general rule, the more vulnerable parts of the brain are those that are undergoing important changes at the time of the insult. These events may only have one chance to occur[45] although it is recognized that the immature brain may have a degree of plasticity.

Early insult is more likely to cause cerebral malformation. A specific association between a defined malformation and a hypoxic-ischaemic insult has not been made but malformation from a hypoxic insult is possible. For instance, significant neuronal migration occurring from periventricular tissues to their definitive site in the cortical plate still takes place up to midgestation. Some forms of migration defects and polymicrogyra may be of ischaemic aetiology[46,47].

The forms of brain damage that accompany both ante- and intrapartum asphyxia in later gestation are multiple. Only some of the underlying principles and major patterns of cerebral hypoxic-ischaemic injury are discussed.

White matter ischaemia

In the third trimester of gestation, hypoxic-ischaemic injury to the developing white matter is a particular feature. The susceptibility to, and pattern of, white matter injury is related to the interaction of three factors:

- The cellular components of the developing white matter. This period is marked by the process of myelination in the hemispheres and immature, very active oligodendrocytes have relatively high metabolic demands[48]
- The evolving vasculature of the white matter. Classical theories have always held that there are some areas of white matter that are relatively deficient in blood supply especially preterm. More recent study has cast doubt on some aspects of this attractive and plausible concept although it is still likely vascular distribution is important[49–51]
- A significant risk of systemic hypotension with low cerebral perfusion, particularly in the sick preterm infant

It should be stressed that neither of the first two factors are dependent on birth, but are a function of maturity and hence gestation. White matter damage is only more likely postnatally because of the circulatory disturbances to which the sick preterm infant is more susceptible.

There are two main patterns of white matter injury:

- *Periventricular leukomalacia (PVL)*[52]. The classic cerebral pathology of the preterm infant, it describes white matter necrosis close to the angles of the lateral ventricles (Fig. 77.5). Susceptibility to ischaemia of the periventricular white matter may be due to its being a boundary zone between major arterial blood supplies[50]. Because of its location and relationship to the long fibres of the internal capsule, it is of considerable interest as a possible underlying cause of some forms of cerebral palsy[39,53] such as spastic diplegia
- *White matter gliosis/perinatal telencephalic leukoencephalopathy*[54]. This describes a more diffuse process than PVL, in which there is a proliferation of hypertrophic astrocytes and infiltration of

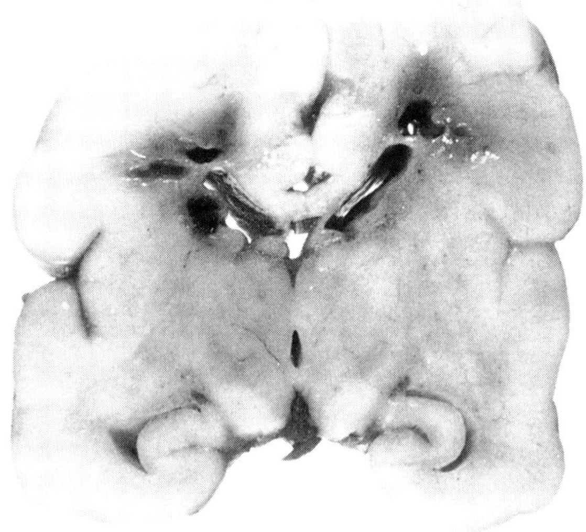

Fig. 77.5 Section of brain from extremely premature infant dying at few weeks of age. There is bilateral periventricular leukomalacia with clearly visible cysts superolateral to the angles of the lateral ventricles. Injury at this site may lead to damage of the long fibres of the internal capsule. Note that in very preterm brains, there is no distinction between grey and white matter due to the absence of myelination. On the left, there is residual old germinal layer haemorrhage. This size, it is of no significance.

macrophages, sometimes with evidence of individual cell necrosis. It has some overlap with PVL but without the necrosis. Personal experience shows this to be a not infrequent finding in the brains of stillborn infants. It is valuable as a marker of brain injury and with some reservations is probably largely attributable to hypoxic-ischaemic injury[43]. It can sometimes assist in dating the onset of obstetric problems into the antepartum period but it is not, in itself, a cause of death. Further, although it is intriguing to speculate about associations with impaired and delayed myelination[55] in survivors, it has not been correlated with any specific functional deficit

While white matter injury is found in term infants, it is more a feature of immaturity. Periventricular leukomalacia is more frequently seen between 28 and 32 weeks' gestation[53]. Antepartum white matter damage is identical to that seen in the preterm infant of similar corrected gestation and is well recorded pathologically[41–44].

Grey matter ischaemia

The susceptibility and response of the grey matter to injury is dependent on the interaction of multiple factors and can be summarized as:

- The quality of the hypoxic-ischaemic insult (s) such as the severity of the hypoxia, the length of time of the insult and the presence or otherwise of previous damage[56–58]
- Local factors intrinsic to the brain such as vascular distribution, regional metabolic demands and distribution of excitatory amino acid receptors[59–61]. These local factors may vary with gestation and the pattern of damage in the brain may vary significantly from case to case despite an apparently similar precipitating pathological event

While there is overlap, cortical injury with some predilection for the parasagittal cortex is more typical of the term infant than the preterm and may be accompanied by thalamic and basal ganglia necrosis. Broadly, two clinicopathological syndromes can be identified in term infants, both of which are reproducible in more 'pure' forms experimentally[56]. Partial, but more prolonged asphyxia is more likely to damage the cerebral cortex particularly in boundary zones such as the depths of sulci and parasagittal regions. Shorter periods of more total asphyxia may lead to basal ganglia damage and brain stem injury (Fig. 77.6). This may be due

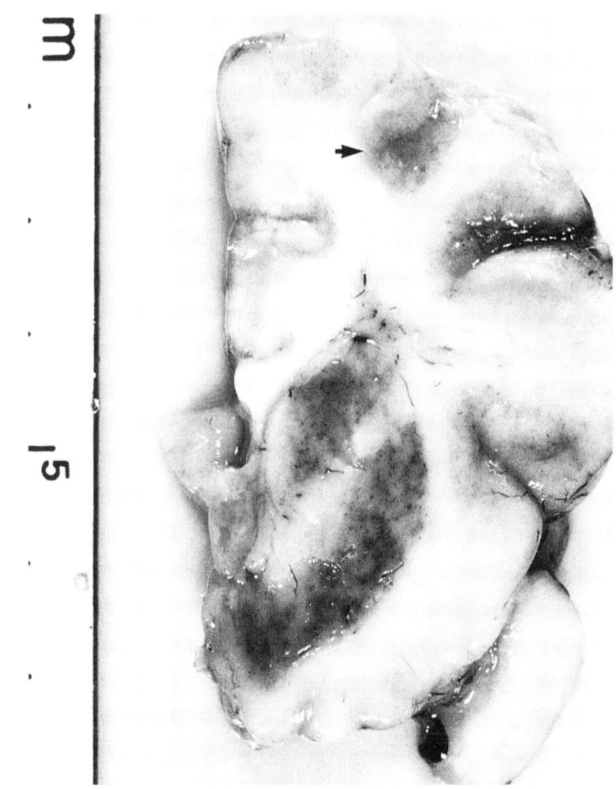

Fig. 77.6 Section of term baby dying at one day of age with severe hypoxic-ischaemic injury of the basal ganglia. This view shows the damaged head of the caudate and putamen with the internal capsule highlighted between them. Ischaemic brain around the depths of a sulcus, typical of severe acute cerebral damage at term, is arrowed.

to the higher metabolic demands of the latter and an inability for local vascular redistribution of cerebral blood flow to be effective.

Neuronal necrosis may affect the preterm basal ganglia, but a feature more typical of the immature brain is neuronal necrosis of the ventral pons and subiculum of the hippocampus. Typically this latter form of injury is associated with white matter damage as described above. The immature brain is unusual in that a hypoxic-ischaemic insult may give rise to injury relatively confined to the neuronal population.

Localized cerebral infarction

Despite a sometimes relatively localized pathology, the damage described above results largely from a more global asphyxial insult associated with a generalized fall in cerebral perfusion. In contrast, localized infarcts in the distribution of a major cerebral vessel with necrosis of both white and grey matter are less common. They are usually unilateral, more common in the distribution of the middle cerebral artery and with increasing gestation. In the long term, they may cavitate to form porencephalic cysts. Although there has been an assumption that these lesions are due to vessel occlusion such as from an embolus, in practice it is frequently impossible to be sure of their aetiology[59]. Infarction has been associated with traumatic delivery[62]. Despite the apparent destruction of a large volume of brain, for some infants there may be surprisingly little significant long-term clinical consequence. This suggests the immature brain may have a remarkable degree of adaptability[63].

LUNG

In-utero asphyxia may be associated with gasping and inhalation of amniotic fluid, and readily recognizable microscopically by the presence of fetal squames within the alveoli. It is a frequent observation in stillborn infants. Some amniotic fluid aspiration occurs fairly routinely and may be of little significance. Squames can frequently be observed in infants that die many weeks old of causes unrelated to birth asphyxia. However, when abundant, amniotic fluid inhalation in a stillborn infant acts as a good marker of acute hypoxia. Clearly in this context the pulmonary pathology is not the cause of death.

In the neonate, the most important pulmonary complication of asphyxia is meconium aspiration syndrome (MAS). Meconium is commonly released in the late third trimester and meconium stained liquor is found in up to 14% deliveries[64]. Release of meconium by itself is of little significance[65] and may simply be a sign of maturity. However, thick meconium may reflect oligohydramnios which in turn may be an indicator of more long standing fetal compromise and of more pathological importance[66,67].

There is considerable debate as to whether the aspiration of clinically significant volumes of meconium is a postnatal event and it is argued that meconium aspiration syndrome is due to antenatal inhalation[68–72]. There is experimental evidence that in utero gasping respiration causes little transfer of fluid down the airways and deep inhalation only occurs as the result of rhythmical breathing set up by more chronic hypoxia[73].

Meconium aspiration causes functional lung impairment due to: airway obstruction with distal pulmonary collapse; pneumothorax from a ball valve effect in obstructed airways; the bile salts in meconium may have a direct toxic effect on pulmonary pneumocytes[74]; inhibition of surfactant[75]; predisposition to infection[76]. The cumulative effect of meconium aspiration will be neonatal hypoxia. As oxygen is a major stimulant to normal postnatal dilatation of pulmonary vasculature, meconium aspiration is one of the more common associations of pulmonary hypertension of the newborn. There is a suggestion, but not universal agreement, that infants with MAS are born with a structurally abnormal pulmonary vasculature adding support to the concept that it is a condition reflecting long-standing hypoxia and is not just an acute phenomenon[77,78].

Macroscopically, acutely asphyxiated lungs show petechial haemorrhages over the pleural surface. When meconium aspiration has occurred, the lung may ooze meconium from the cut surface. Microscopically, meconium is recognizable as eosinophilic granular material admixed with squames and sometimes yellow meconium bodies. Acute inflammation may be present, which might reflect direct chemical irritation by the meconium but more likely from introduced infection[79]. Certainly, in the author's experience, stillborn lungs in which there is meconium rarely show any significant acute inflammatory reaction. Lungs may also show hyaline membrane disease possibly due to the direct acute hypoxic lung damage rather than the toxic effect of meconium.

OTHER TISSUES

In addition to the lung, acute asphyxia will also cause petechial haemorrhaging in the thymus and epicardial surface of the heart. Some features simply reflect heart failure, so severe congestion is common particularly in the liver, kidneys and adrenals. The liver may develop subcapsular haematomas that are at a risk of rupture.

Ischaemic injury to other organs can occur, although the underlying insult usually needs to be severe. Further, as survival for at least a number of hours is needed for morphological changes to become apparent, and autolysis may obscure subtle changes, they are more a feature of intra- rather than antepartum asphyxia. The heart may show focal infarction often involving papillary muscles and the adrenals may show complete or partial infarction[80]. Rarely, the liver may be affected. With the notable exception of the adrenal pathology, the other organ damage generally requires histology for confirmation of diagnosis.

TRAUMA: ANTEPARTUM AND INTRAPARTUM

Deaths directly attributable to trauma before the onset of labour are uncommon. The fetus is well protected in the amniotic cavity although direct injury is recorded[81]. More important are the effects of trauma on the placenta, which may separate prematurely[82,83].

Birth trauma is linked very closely to acute fetal asphyxia, often because it occurs in the setting of an attempted rapid delivery for fetal distress. Only the more common lesions likely to be associated with fetal death will be discussed here. A wider discussion of the pathology and associated factors is provided by Govaert[84].

TEARS OF THE TENTORIUM CEREBELLI

Tentorial tears are probably the most common intracranial traumatic lesion encountered by the pathologist. These lesions are often bilateral, situated close the midline and may extend into the vein of Galen or straight sinus causing massive haemorrhage. More usually, tears are incomplete and haemorrhage arises from small bridging veins to the cerebellum or small vessels in the tentorium itself. Tentorial tears are sometimes associated with falx tears.

In the author's experience, the possibility of a tentorial tear has rarely been considered clinically and the delivery, even in retrospect, not considered especially difficult. Most infants are thought only to have been asphyxiated, if clinically worse at birth than anticipated. The majority of tears occur in the context of either an instrumental delivery or caesarean section, although up to a fifth may occur during a spontaneous vaginal delivery[70].

For the pathologist, assigning death to trauma on the basis solely of a tentorial tear requires caution, if only for the potential medicolegal fallout. With current obstetric practice, the lesion is rarely so severe that death can be simply attributed to massive blood loss with compression of the cerebral structures from haematoma. However, the tears must be an indicator of significant cranial distortion that will have involved the brain itself. Tentorial tears are not inevitably fatal[85] and one estimate suggests that nearly 70% do not come to autopsy[84]. Assessing its significance requires a consideration of all the clinical and pathological evidence. It may even be inappropriate to try and disentangle the relative importance of asphyxia and trauma in an individual case.

OTHER TRAUMATIC LESIONS

Small linear fractures of the skull, usually the parietal bone, are not uncommon and are generally of little significance, and can occur during instrumental delivery or section. Depressed fractures are probably of predescent origin[86]. More extensive, sometimes comminuted fractures are fortunately rare and generally occur in the same setting as tentorial tears.

Soft tissue injuries are usually significant because of blood loss. Subaponeurotic haemorrhage following procedures such as vacuum extraction may hide a major and sometimes unsuspected blood loss. Tear of the liver capsule with intraperitoneal haemorrhage is associated with breech deliveries in particular.

IMMATURITY

For most deaths attributed to immaturity, from the perspective of the obstetrician, the infant autopsy may not be revealing. It is of importance, however, to identify possible causes of premature delivery and, as ascending infection or premature placental separation are potential contributing factors, it is vital that the placenta is examined from all premature births.

The deaths of the majority of infants reflect the immaturity of the lung – either because the lung cannot even start to support life ex utero or from hyaline membrane disease (HMD). Improved management of HMD including antenatal steroids and artificial surfactant therapy has significantly improved the outlook for immature babies[87,88].

A small proportion of very immature infants suffer cerebral complications of immaturity. The increased risk of ischaemic injury has already been discussed. The other major complication of extreme preterm birth is germinal layer with intraventricular haemorrhage (GLH/IVH). Immature cells destined to form glia persist on the lateral wall of the lateral ventricle up to approximately 34 weeks of gestation. This germinal layer is susceptible to haemorrhage due to its vascularity, lack of glial support for the vessels, relatively high blood flow, and tortuous venous drainage. Large haemorrhages may spread into the ventricle and involve the cerebral tissue lateral to the lateral ventricle (the same location as PVL – see above) (Fig. 77.7). Death may follow from particularly large haemorrhages or, in survivors, give rise to neurological disability.

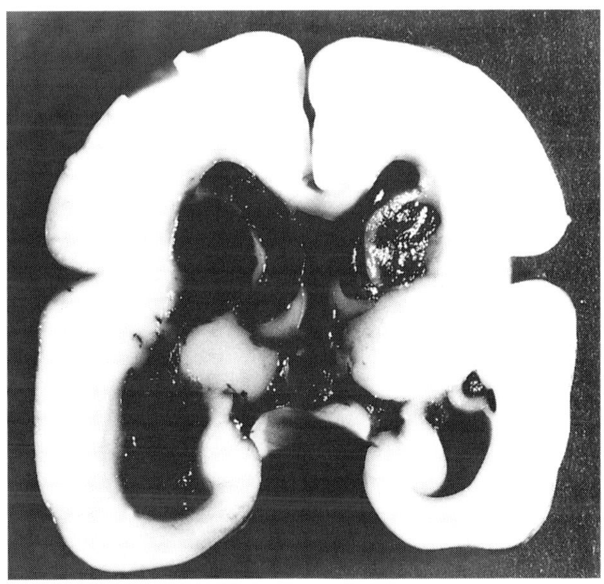

Fig. 77.7 Bilateral germinal layer and intraventricular haemorrhage in a 25-week gestation infant dying at 1 day of age. This typically occurs within the first couple of days after birth, rapidly decreases in incidence with increasing gestation and is unusual before birth.

INFECTION

Especially in fetal death, the major problem in categorizing infective cases is less one of diagnosing the presence of infection than deciding on whether infection is a primary or secondary phenomenon in the sequence of events leading to the death. While tissue or samples for culture can be important, the need for histology to establish or confirm diagnosis in cases of fetal death cannot be overstated.

ASCENDING INFECTION

Ascending infection is common and occurs in association with up to 20% of aborted fetuses. Its significance is not so much due to direct infection of the fetus than the precipitation of abortion or premature delivery[89,90]. In most cases, the main pathology is placental chorioamnionitis only (see below), but in some this will be associated with pulmonary inflammation. This involvement can justifiably be labelled pneumonia as studies have shown that the inflammatory infiltrate within the lung represents fetal reaction and not just aspirated cells[91].

Neonates may develop an early pneumonia as a result of ante- or intrapartum acquired infection from infected or colonized aspirated material such as amniotic fluid, blood or vaginal secretions[92]. Organisms include enteric bacteria, *Staphylococcus* or the Group B *Streptococcus* and, particularly with the last, infection may be so overwhelming that diagnosis will only be made at autopsy. The macroscopic pathology is non-specific and may resemble HMD. Occasionally a blood-stained effusion is present.

Although most bacterial infections are entirely non-specific in their macroscopic and microscopic appearance, listeria does show some specific characteristics. When disseminated, it forms small 1–2 mm diameter microabscesses in a wide variety of tissues including the placenta, liver, lungs and adrenals. In some cases it leads to a meningitis. The histology is characteristic but culture should be performed for confirmation[93].

VIRAL INFECTION

Viral infection is an uncommon cause of fetal or early neonatal death. By far the majority of fetuses are infected as a result of transplacental spread but infection acquired during delivery from maternal secretions is important in Herpes simplex, the enteroviruses such a Coxsackie or echovirus[94–96] and adenovirus[97].

Identifying a viral infection is normally possible histopathologically even in the presence of maceration although it may sometimes be difficult to specify the virus. When suspected, tissue culture may be performed although it is usually unsuccessful in intrauterine deaths due to autolysis. More recent techniques including polymerase-chain reaction and in-situ hybridization have started to allow specific diagnosis for some viruses even if the only material available is fixed embedded tissue.

The importance of maternal serological study and other prenatal studies[98] should not be overlooked. Where infection is suspected late in pregnancy, stored booking blood samples may provide a baseline result.

Presentation of viral infection to the pathologist is extremely varied. In-utero death is not uncommon, and there may be little maternal history. Macroscopic indications of an infection, particularly if obscured by severe maceration, may be minimal although features such as hepatosplenomegaly are more usual. Importantly some viral infections can present with growth retardation and malformation, most notably rubella and early varicella.

Viral infection, more notably cytomegalovirus (CMV) and parvovirus, is one of the more important causes of intrauterine or neonatal death associated with fetal hydrops[99]. In recent years, locally, parvovirus, which has a very characteristic histology, has been by far the most commonly recognized viral cause of second-trimester abortion, many of which are very macerated. Infection may not be suspected until histology is performed (Fig. 77.8).

Of the congenital infections presenting neonatally, CMV is the commonest although most are asymptomatic; if recognized late it may be difficult to distinguish between prenatally or postnatally acquired disease. The infections, at the severe end of the spectrum more likely to be seen by the pathologist, may present with growth retardation, hepatosplenomegaly, jaundice and evidence of cerebral damage. In this circumstance, histological diagnosis with the identification of the typical viral inclusions is usually straightforward.

Other infections acquired during delivery such as herpes or enterovirus may not present until the end of the first week of life. As far as the pathologist is concerned, the history may be that of a rapid onset, non-specific illness and rash. Macroscopic appearances may not be diagnostic of any one virus although the pattern of distribution of organ involvement is often suggestive. Occasionally, infection may present as sudden death with little or no preceding history.

SUDDEN INFANT DEATH SYNDROME (SIDS)

Undoubtedly, a few infants dying from SIDS show pathology that is likely to be of in-utero origin but the extent to which a less than optimum fetal existence is a risk factor for SIDS is very unclear. Premature birth increases the risk of SIDS. Hypoxia may be significant[100–102] and in some SIDS babies there is evidence of maturational delays that must be of long standing, particularly of the brain[103]. A recent study has suggested that the kidneys of SIDS infants show evidence of a developmental arrest that could only have a prenatal origin[104].

Pathology of the placenta

A key component in the autopsy of stillbirths and many neonatal deaths is the examination of the placenta. One needs

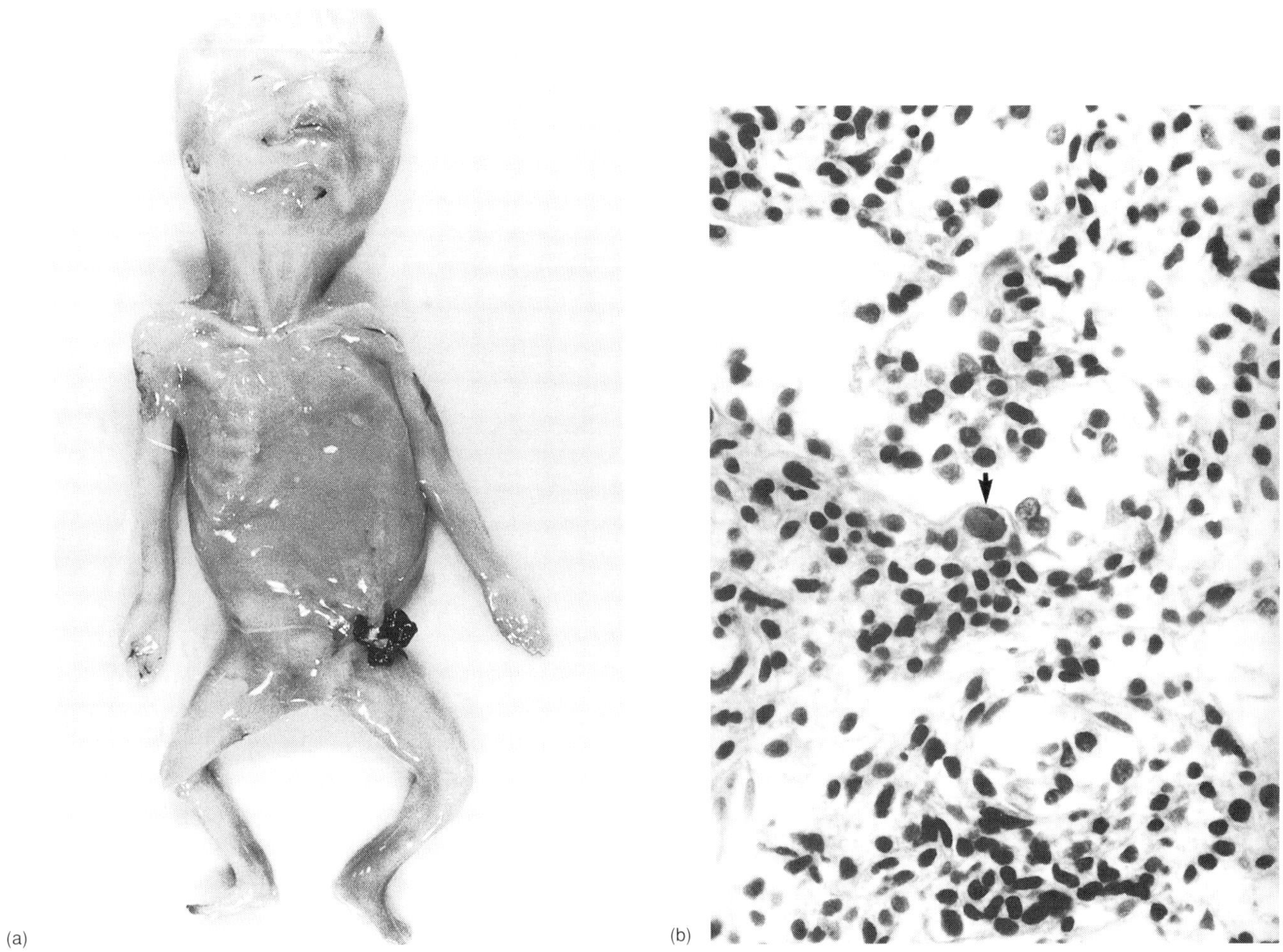

Fig. 77.8 (a) Macerated second-trimester abortion with parvovirus. Although this fetus does show slight oedema, it is not invariable. Histology is still valuable for diagnosis and viral inclusions such as those of parvovirus (b) (arrowed), are readily identifiable despite severe autolysis.

to be aware that placentae may show abnormality despite the birth of healthy infants at the end of an unremarkable gestation. Consequently, in the presence of an adverse clinical outcome, circumspection is needed as it is easy to ascribe undue significance to the mere presence of a placental abnormality. Nevertheless, there are clinically relevant lesions that, when placed in context with the clinical history, can provide insights into the cause of fetal mortality[105–107] or in some cases intrauterine related morbidity[108].

Despite the argument for all placentae to be examined[109], it will be beyond the resources of most pathology departments so there should be a clear policy on which placentae should be sent for pathological study.

As a minimum this should include those placentae:

- With any macroscopic abnormality, including membranes and cord
- From all fetal deaths and stillbirths
- From infants that have required resuscitation and admission to a neonatal unit, no matter how brief or for what reason
- Where there is any significant abnormal ante- or intrapartum process or event such as growth retardation or abruption
- Following preterm birth
- Multiple gestation

There are advantages in examining the placenta in the fresh state[108], although for the pathologist at least, it is becoming more difficult to justify the risks associated with infection from very bloody tissue. The placenta should be the subject of a systematic examination that inspects the membranes, cord, and maternal and fetal surfaces. Only the more commonly encountered placental entities with clinical relevance are described.

WEIGHT

Placental weight is extremely variable depending on the conditions under which it is performed. To assist standardization, the weight can be obtained after the cord and membranes have been trimmed and excess blood allowed to drain. Even under controlled conditions, term placentae may vary between 350 and 550 g (10th–90th centiles)[110]. Fox[111] has argued that placental weight is a largely valueless measurement. While it is probably true that, taken in isolation, it does not provide great insight into fetal life, excessively small or large placentae should alert the pathologist to the presence of more specific pathology.

A low placental weight may be associated with fetal malformation or poor uteroplacental blood flow, the latter often associated with maternal essential hypertension or preeclamptic toxaemia (PET). In the absence of severe congestion or attached clot, heavy placentae are most commonly associated with villous oedema or maternal diabetes mellitus. The former may occur together with any cause of fetal oedema and hydrops.

Maternal factors associated with a large placenta include anaemia and cyanotic heart disease. This may cause adaptive responses to hypoxia within the placenta that cause villous growth. Rare fetal congenital abnormalities associated with heavy placentae include Beckwith–Wiedemann syndrome.

MEMBRANES

MECONIUM STAINING

Meconium staining is relatively common near term. It is of little significance in isolation but its presence may act as a possible indicator of fetal aphyxia (see meconium aspiration – above). Macroscopically, the rapidity with which membranes stain is as much dependent on meconium concentration as length of exposure. However, with cautious interpretation, an indication of how long membranes have have been in contact with meconium can be obtained following histological study[112].

AMNION NODOSUM

Macroscopically visible as small 1–2 mm nodules on the surface of the amnion, histologically, the nodules comprise squamous debris. Amnion nodosum is associated with severe oligohydramnios that has been present for a number of weeks. Oligohydramnios of this severity may be due to urinary tract anomalies in the fetus and cause pulmonary hypoplasia[113].

CHORIOAMNIONITIS

Probably the most common significant lesion of the placenta, acute chorioamnionitis is almost invariably due to ascending infection. It may be found in the absence of any clinical signs and can occur despite intact membranes. Occasionally, there will be additional factors such as cervical cerclage.

Macroscopically, membranes with chorioamnionitis may be entirely normal although more florid infections turn the membranes opaque or yellow. In some cases, the inflammation is more apparent along the line of fetal blood vessels. The macroscopic and microscopic appearance is largely non-specific and provides no clue as to the infecting agent. However, in *Candida* infection[114,115] characteristic small yellow microabscesses can be discerned both on the surface of the placenta but more particularly within the substance of the cord.

Histologically, chorioamnionitis shows a non-specific acute inflammatory infiltrate that may be associated with membrane necrosis. Involvement of the cord (funisitis) or cord vessels (angiitis) is not infrequent and indicates that infection has been chronic enough to cause fetal reaction. Other than *Candida*, whose pseudohyphae are distinctive, the infecting organism confers no distinguishing microscopic characteristics.

The microbiology of the placenta is often difficult to interpret as isolation of vaginal colonizers is common. Naeye stresses that isolation of a single organism is possible in up to 70% of cases, but that care may be needed for culture of anaerobes[105,116]. Furthermore, unusual infections due to mycoplasma[117], *Chlamydia*[118,119] or ureaplasma[119,120,121] may be important in a proportion.

The major clinical consequence of chorioamnionitis is that it may precipitate labour and is an important factor in spontaneous abortion. In a proportion, pneumonia may be present in the fetus or aspiration of infected material may cause an early neonatal pneumonia (see above).

CORD

Cord length is routinely measured although as the pathologist often seems to receive only a part of the cord it can be an inaccurate measure when coming from the laboratory. Long cords (e.g. >100 cm at term) predispose to torsion and prolapse whereas short cords may be associated with birth asphyxia. A short cord may be significant because it interferes with vertex delivery but also reflect decreased movement by an already compromised fetus; movement 'stretches' the cord[122].

The significance of obstructed umbilical blood flow in fetal death is a frequent point of debate in perinatal mortality meetings. Extreme caution is required in attributing death of a macerated stillbirth to a true cord knot, nuchal entanglement or torsion found at delivery. Careful inspection for evidence of chronic compression both in the cord or underlying fetal part is necessary to assist in identifying a significant cord pathology[123–125]. With appropriate clinical evidence, however, intrapartum death or asphyxia may be less controversial and entanglement of twin cords in a monoamniotic pregnancy is well recognized (Fig. 77.9). Velamentously inserted cord, in addition to a greater risk of tearing, may also be at greater risk of obstruction. Cords with two vessels have an increased association with fetal malformation (25–50%) of any organ system.

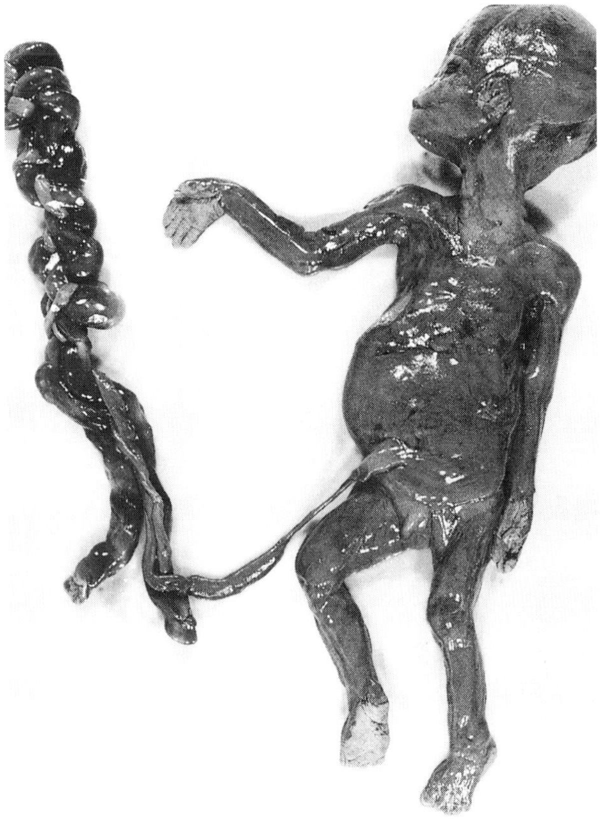

Fig. 77.9 Fetus, one of twins born at 21 weeks' gestation, whose death was associated with cord entanglement.

PLACENTAL SECTION

In addition to the careful inspection of the maternal and fetal surfaces, the placenta requires cutting into 0.5–1 cm slices for proper examination, a procedure not often carried out in the delivery suite. Omission leads to unhelpful descriptions of the placenta such as 'gritty and unhealthy', a phrase that not infrequently reflects the birth of a small and/or distressed baby as much as the state of the placenta.

RETROPLACENTAL HAEMORRHAGE

Premature placental separation encompasses acute retroplacental haemorrhage, i.e. abruption, and older, perhaps concealed, antepartum haemorrhage.

In older lesions, clear evidence of premature separation includes cavitation and compression of the overlying placenta; adjacent villi may be infarcted. In some cases, particularly when associated with preeclamptic toxaemia, the haemorrhage bulges into the placenta and is surrounded by a placental infarct that outlines the placental lobule. Strictly these haemorrhages are not retroplacental and have been labelled placental haematoma. Wigglesworth has postulated these lesions are generated following rupture of a maternal spiral arteriole that has undergone aneurysmal dilatation proximal to a thrombosis[126].

With acute placental abruption it may be difficult or impossible for the pathologist to distinguish between pathological, premature separation and normal separation. Histology may contribute by revealing decidual necrosis, reaction and old haemorrhage.

INFARCTION

The reliable diagnosis of infarction requires placental section as described above, otherwise infarction is both under- and overdiagnosed. Placental infarcts, due to ischaemic necrosis, outline the shape of the placental 'lobule', the functional unit of the placenta. Early infarcts may be difficult to identify in the fresh placenta when it will appear as a relatively localized area of intensely congested villi. It may be easier to diagnose after fixation and require histology for confirmation. More established infarcts will appear as a 'white' area of placenta with the base located on the maternal surface (Fig. 77.10).

Infarction is due to ischaemia and not surprisingly there is an association between placental infarction, reduced

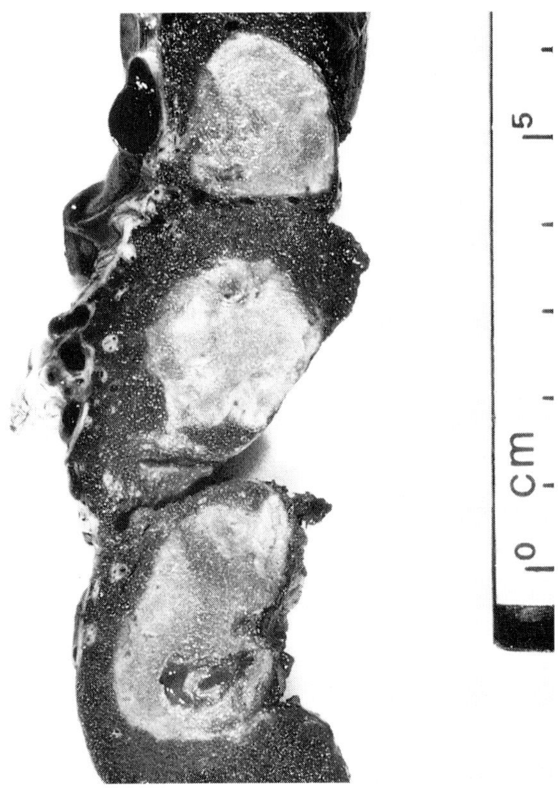

Fig. 77.10 Cut section of placenta demonstrating three well-established infarcts. Infarcts should show this typical outline of the placental lobule. Placental infarction is frequently misdiagnosed in the absence of placental section and the maternal surface only is examined.

uteroplacental blood flow, fetal morbidity[127] and mortality[122]. Nevertheless, the presence of an isolated infarct does not necessarily have any pathological significance. Because placental lobules receive blood from more than one maternal spiral arteriole, infarcts confined to the periphery of the placenta have less significance than those more centrally located. For the latter to occur, a greater reduction in uteroplacental blood flow is required.

It is difficult to define precisely the percentage of placental volume that needs to be infarcted before it can be considered of significance (and that ignores the difficulty of making any consistent estimate that does not involve morphometry). Probably less than 10% can be ignored particularly if the macroscopically normal placenta is also normal histologically. More than 30% infarction is commonly associated with stillbirth[128]. However, if the histology of the non-infarcted placenta shows features of ischaemia, then it is reasonable to interpret even a small volume of infarction as a more overt sign of generalized uteroplacental insufficiency.

MASSIVE PERIVILLOUS FIBRIN DEPOSITION

Occasionally, and more typically in placentae from preterm stillbirths, section of the placenta reveals a uniformly white and firm appearance, with little or no accentuation of placental lobules. Histologically this is associated with massive perivillous fibrin deposition. Some deposition of fibrin around villi is normal as term approaches and of no pathological significance. It is deposited predominantly in the areas of low maternal blood flow, i.e. around the margins of the lobule and subchorionic plate. However, massive perivillous fibrin deposition affects all parts of the placenta. The cause is unclear, although Rushton[129] speculates it reflects a diffuse trophoblastic injury. It is associated with fetal death, severe intrauterine growth retardation and may be recurrent.

CHORANGIOMAS

Chorangiomas are the commonest 'tumour' of the placenta, although strictly are vascular malformations. They affect at least 1% of placentae. Macroscopically, chorangiomas can appear as a localized mass of firm vascular tissue (Fig. 77.11) or may be paler and resemble an infarct. The majority, especially when small, are asymptomatic but chorangiomas can cause fetal hydrops probably secondary to high ouput cardiac failure. Sequestration may lead to thrombocytopenia. Recurrence in sequential pregnancies has been recorded[111].

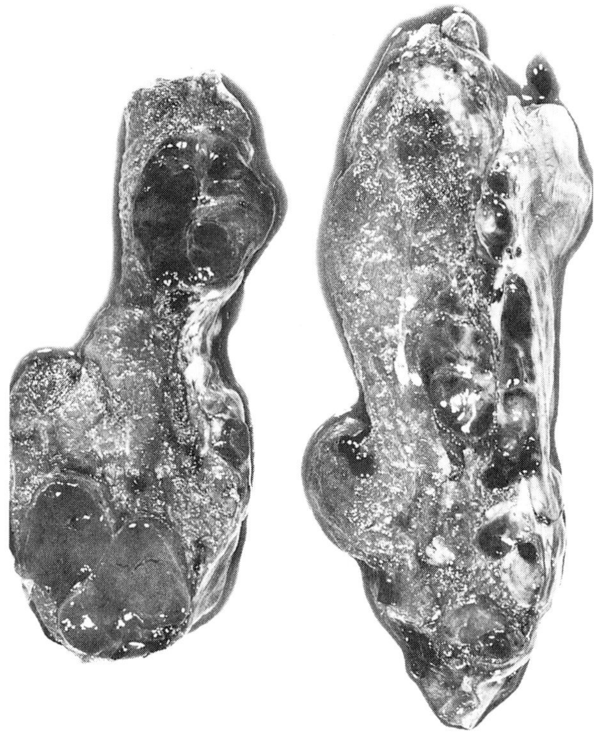

Fig. 77.11 Multiple placental chorangiomas with two large 'tumours'.

PLACENTAL HISTOLOGY

Placental examination is not complete without histology and this supplements the macroscopic appearances. Extreme caution is needed when searching for an explanation for fetal death when the only pathology is at the histological level. There is so much overlap between the histology of placentae associated with fetal death and placentae from normal deliveries, that it can only ever be taken in the context of the clinical and pathological findings as a whole.

ISCHAEMIA

Histological changes of placental ischaemia that reflect reduced uteroplacental blood flow does not imply, necessarily, the occurrence of fetal hypoxia. Many changes are not degenerative but a response to hypoxia; they are compensatory and therefore permit normal fetal oxygenation to continue. Some changes of ischaemia represent an exaggeration of features present in the ageing placenta; when this becomes clearly pathological can be very subjective[130].

More obvious lesions of ischaemia include small 'microinfarctions' represented by clusters of ischaemic villi. More diffuse villous change includes cytotrophoblastic hyperplasia, increased syncytial knots and smaller villi. Some of these are features of ageing. Hypoxia may be associated with a large placenta in which the villi are relatively immature for the gestation.

VILLITIS

Inflammation of the villi is a not uncommon histological observation and may be found in up to 13% of placentae[131,132]. The commonest pattern is where a few villi are affected by an infiltrate of lymphocytes and histiocytes. Occasionally, plasma cells are present. Villitis may be associated with maternal bloodborne infections, mainly viruses or toxoplasmosis.

However, the cause of by far the majority of villitis is not infective and its aetiology and significance remain a puzzle. Villitis of unknown aetiology may accompany intrauterine growth retardation[133–135] and, in a proportion of cases, has been associated with recurrent fetal loss[134].

MATERNAL SPIRAL ARTERIOLES

As a normal adaptive response in early gestation, maternal spiral arterioles are invaded by cytotrophoblast. Trophoblastic invasion leads to changes in the spiral arterioles, most notably a replacement of the normal muscular wall by fibrin and a lining of the vessel by trophoblastic cells[136]. This process facilitates dilatation and increased blood flow. Although not specific, this is defective in preeclamptic toxaemia[102]. Further, vessels may be affected by acute atherosis in which lipid-laden macrophages together with a round cell infiltrate are present in an arteriolar wall showing fibrinoid necrosis.

Occasionally, these changes can be detected in decidual segments of maternal spiral arterioles avulsed during placental separation[137] (Fig. 77.12). This failure of physiological change is also seen in some examples of early fetal loss[138]. Whether this represents a 'prodromal' phase of PET is not clear.

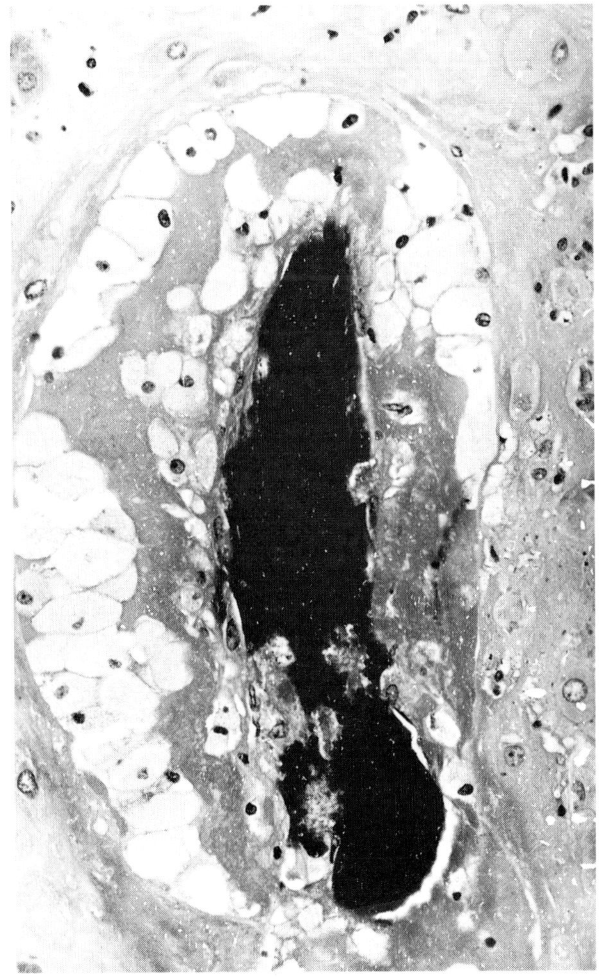

Fig. 77.12 Maternal spiral arteriole in decidua on placental surface. Mother was affected by severe preeclamptic toxaemia. Vessel shows an extensive infiltrate of foamy fat-laden macrophages in the wall. A mononuclear lymphoid infiltrate is also typical but not seen here.

REFERENCES

1. Joint Working Party of Royal College of Obstetricians and Gynaecologists and Royal College of Pathologists Report on fetal and perinatal pathology. London: RCOG, 1988.
2. Khong TY, Mansor FA & Staples AJ. Are perinatal autopsy rates satisfactory? *Med. J. Aust.* **162**(9), 469–470, 1995.
3. Confidential Enquiry into Stillbirths and Deaths in Infancy Annual Report, 1 January–31 December 1993, p. 53. Department of Health, 1993.
4. Rushton DI. West Midlands perinatal mortality survey, 1987. An audit of 300 perinatal autopsies. *Br. J. Obstet. Gynaecol.* **98**, 624–627, 1991.
5. Cartlidge PHT, Dawson AT, Stewart JH & Vujanic GM. Value and quality of perinatal and infant postmortem examinations: cohort analysis of 400 consecutive deaths. *Br. Med. J.* **310**, 155–158, 1995.
6. Porter HJ & Keeling JW. Value of perinatal necropsy examination. *J. Clin. Pathol.* **40**, 180–184, 1987.
7. Hagerstrand I & Lundberg LM. The importance of post-mortem examinations of abortions and perinatal deaths. *Qual. Assur. Health. Care.* **5**(4), 295–297, 1993.
8. Saller DN, Lesser KB, Harrel U, Rogers BB & Oyer CE. The clinical utility of the perinatal autopsy. *JAMA* **273**, 663–665, 1995.
9. Study Group Postmortem examinations in a statewide audit of neonatal intensive care unit admissions in Australia in 1992. *Acta Paediatr.* **85**, 865–869, 1996.
10. Brand IR, Kaminopetros P, Cave M, Irving HC & Lilford RJ. Specificity of antenatal ultrasound in the Yorkshire Region: a prospective study of 2261 ultrasound detected anomalies. *Br. J. Obstet. Gynaecol.* **101**(5), 392–397, 1994.
11. Clayton-Smith J, Farndon PA, McKeown C & Donnai D. Examination of fetuses after induced abortion for fetal abnormality. *Br. Med. J.* **300**, 295–297, 1990.
12. Chescheir NC & Reitnauer PJA. Comparative study of prenatal diagnosis and perinatal autopsy. *J. Ultrasound Med.* **13**(6), 451–456, 1994.
13. Klatt EC. Pathologic examination of fetal specimens from dilatation and evacuation procedures. *Am. J. Clin. Pathol.* **103**, 415–418, 1994.
14. Soothill PW & Rodeck CH. First-trimester fetal necropsy after ultrasound-guided aspiration [letter]. *Lancet* **343**(8905), 1096–1097, 1994.
15. Kohner N. Pregnancy loss and the death of a baby. Guidelines for Professionals. SANDS, 1996.

16. Polkinghorne J. Review of the guidance on the research use of fetuses and fetal materials. Cm 762, London: HMSO, 1989.
17. MacPherson TA & Valdes-Dapena M. The perinatal autopsy. In *Textbook of Fetal and Perinatal Pathology* (eds J.S. Wigglesworth & D.B. Singer) Vol. 1, pp. 93–122. Oxford: Blackwell Scientific Publications, 1997.
18. Keeling JW. The perinatal necropsy. In *Fetal and Neonatal Pathology*. (ed. J.W. Keeling), pp. 1–32. London: Springer-Verlag, 1992.
19. Kalousek DK & Barrett I. Confined placental mosaicism and stillbirth. *Paed. Pathol.* **14**, 151, 1994.
20. Kalousek DK, Langlois S, Barrett I *et al.* Uniparental disomy for chromosome 16 in humans. *Am. J. Hum. Genet.* **52**, 8–16, 1993.
21. Zahed L & Vekemans M. Use of in-situ hybridization in clinical genetics. *Paed. Pathol.* **11**, 497–505, 1991.
22. Stocker JT & Dehner LP (eds) Appendices. In *Paediatric Pathology*, pp. 1293–1397. Philadelphia: J.B. Lippincott, 1992.
23. Chambers HM, Knowles S, Staples A, Tamblyn M & Haan EA. Anthropometric measurements in the second trimester fetus. *Early Hum. Dev.* **33**(1), 45–59, 1993.
24. Genest DR, Williams MA & Greene MF. Estimating the time of death in stillborn fetuses: I. Histologic evaluation of fetal organs; and autopsy study of 150 stillborns. *Obstet. Gynecol.* **80**, 575–584, 1992.
25. Genest DR. Estimating the time of death in stillborn fetuses: II. Histologic evaluation of the placenta; a study of 71 stillborns. *Obstet. Gynecol.* **80**, 585–592, 1992.
26. Genest DR & Singer DB. Estimating the time of death in stillborn fetuses: III. External fetal examination; a study of 86 stillborns. *Obstet. Gynecol.* **80**, 593–600, 1992.
27. Ghidini A. Idiopathic fetal growth restriction: a pathophysiologic approach. *Obstet. Gynecol. Survey.* **51**, 376–381, 1996.
28. Cole SK, Hey EN & Thompson AM. Classifying perinatal death: an obstetric approach. *Br. J. Obstet. Gynaecol.* **93**, 1204–1212, 1986.
29. Machin GA. A perinatal mortality survey in South East London, 1970–1973: the pathological findings in 726 necropsies. *J. Clin. Pathol.* **28**, 428–434, 1975.
30. Naeye RL. Causes of perinatal mortality in the US Collaborative Perinatal Project. *JAMA* **238**, 228–229, 1977.
31. Wigglesworth JS. Monitoring perinatal mortality: a pathophysiological approach. *Lancet.* **ii**, 684–686, 1980.
32. Keeling JW, MacGillivray I, Golding J, Wigglesworth JS, Berry PJ & Dunn PM. Classification of perinatal death. *Arch. Dis. Child.* **64**, 1345–1351, 1989.
33. Craven CM, Dempsey S, Carey JC & Kochenour NK. Evaluation of a perinatal autopsy protocol: influence of the prenatal diagnosis conference team. *Obstet. Gynecol.* **76**, 684–688, 1990.
34. Agustsson P & Patel N. Intrapartum asphyxia and subsequent disability. *Baillière's Clin. Obstet. Gynaecol.* **2**, 167–186, 1988.
35. Johnson P. Birth asphyxia: should it be redefined or abandoned? In *Intrapartum Fetal Surveillance* (eds J.A.D. Spencer & R.H.T. Ward), pp. 157–180. RCOG Press, 1994.
36. Nelson KB & Ellenberg JH. Obstetric complications as risk factors for cerebral palsy or seizure disorders. *JAMA* **251**, 1843–1848, 1984.
37. Nelson KB & Ellenberg JH. Antecedents of cerebral palsy. Multivariate analysis of risk. *N. Engl. J. Med.* **315**, 81–86.
38. Blair E & Stanley FJ. , 1988) Intrapartum asphyxia: a rare cause of cerebral palsy. *J. Pediatr.* **112**, 515–519, 1986.
39. Kuban KCK & Leviton A. Medical progress: cerebral palsy. *N. Engl. J. Med.* **330**, 188–195, 1994.
40. Stanley FJ. The aetiology of cerebral palsy. Review article. *Early. Hum. Develop.* **36**, 81–88, 1994.
41. Ellis WG, Goetzmann BW & Lindenberg JA. Neuropathologic documentation of prenatal brain damage. *Am. J. Dis. Child.* **142**, 858–866, 1988.
42. Roland EH, Normal MG & Hill A. Antenatal periventricular white matter infarction. *Ann. Neurol.* **22**, 423, 1987.
43. Squier MV & Keeling JW. The incidence of prenatal brain injury. *Neuropathol. Appl. Neurobiol.* **17**, 29–38, 1991.
44. Murphy DJ, Squier MV, Hope PL, Sellers S & Johnson A. Clinical associations and time of onset of cerebral white matter damage in very preterm babies. *Arch. Dis. Child.* **75**, F27–F32, 1996.
45. Dobbing J & Sands J. Vulnerability of developing brain. IX. The effect of nutritional growth retardation on the timing of the brain growth-spurt. *Biol. Neonate.* **19**, 363–378, 1971.
46. Norman MG. Bilateral encephaloclastic lesions in a 26 week gestation fetus: effect on neuroblast migration. *Can. J. Neurol. Sci.* **7**, 191–194, 1980.
47. Volpe, J.J. Neuronal proliferation, migration, organization, and myelination. In *Neurology of the Newborn* (ed. J.J. Volpe), 3rd edn, pp. 43–92. W. Philadelphia: W.B. Saunders, 1995.
48. Leviton A & Paneth N. White matter damage in preterm newborns – an epidemiologic perspective. *Early Hum. Dev.* **24**, 1–22, 1990.
49. Moody DM, Bell MA & Challa VR. Features of the cerebral vascular pattern that predict vulnerability to perfusion or oxygenation deficiency: an anatomic study. *Am. J. Neuroradiol.* **11**, 431–439, 1991.
50. Paneth N, Rudelli R, Kazam E & Monte W. White matter damage: terminology, typology, pathogenesis. In *Brain Damage in the preterm Infant* (ed. N. Paneth), Clinics in Developmental Medicine vol. 131 pp. 99–118. London: Mac Keith Press, 1994.
51. Mayer PL & Kier EL. The controversy of the periventricular white matter circulation: a review of the anatomic literature. *Am. J. Neuroradiol.* **12**, 223–228, 1991.
52. Banker BQ & Larroche JC. Periventricular leukomalacia of infancy. *Arch. Neurol.* **7**, 386–410, 1962.
53. Perlman JM, Risser R & Broyles RS. Bilateral cystic periventricular leukomalacia in the premature infant: associated risk factors. *Pediatrics* **97**, 822–827, 1996.
54. Gilles FH & Murphy SF. Perinatal telencephalic leucoencephalopathy. *J. Neurol. Neurosurg. Psych.* **32**, 404–413, 1969.
55. van de Bor M, Guit GL, Schreuder AM, Wondergem J & Vielvoye GJ. Early detection of delayed myelination in preterm infants. *Pediatrics* **84**, 407–411, 1989.
56. Pasternak JF. Hypoxic-ischaemic brain damage in the term infant. Lessons from the laboratory. *Paed. Clin. N. Am.* **40**, 1061–1072, 1993.
57. Thordstein M & Kjellmer I. Cerebral tolerance of hypoxia in growth-retarded and approximately grown newborn guinea pigs. *Paed. Res.* **24**, 633–638, 1988.
58. Gluckman PD & Williams CE. When and why do brain cells die? *Dev. Med. Child. Neurol.* **34**, 1010–1021, 1992.
59. Volpe JJ. Hypoxic-ischaemic encephalopathy; neuropathology and pathogenesis. In *Neurology of the Newborn*, 3rd edn., pp. 279–313. Philadelphia: W.B. Saunders, 1995.
60. Lee HS & Choi BH. Density and distribution of excitatory amino acid receptors in the developing human fetal brain – a quantitative autoradiographic study. *Exp. Neurol.* **118**, 284–290, 1992.
61. Barkovich AJ. MR and CT evaluation of profound neonatal and infantile asphyxia. *Am. J. Neuroadiol.* **13**, 959, 1992.
62. Govaert P, Vanhaesebrouck P & de Praeter C. Traumatic neonatal intracranial bleeding and stroke. *Arch. Dis. Child.* **67**, 840–845, 1992.
63. Trauner DA & Mannino F. Brain reorganisation after injury in infancy. *Lancet* **347**, 1701, 1996.
64. Ostrea EM & Naqvi M. The influence of gestational age on the ability of the fetus to pass meconium in utero. *Obstet. Gynecol. Scand.* **61**, 275–277, 1982.
65. Miller FC, Sacks DA, Yeh S-Y *et al.* Significance of meconium during labour. *Am. J. Obstet. Gynecol.* **122**, 573–580, 1975.
66. Mitchell J, Schulman H, Fleischer A, Farmakides G & Nadeau D. Meconium aspiration and fetal acidosis. *Obstet. Gynecol.* **65**, 352–355, 1985.
67. Danielian PJ. Multiple parameters, including meconium. In *Intrapartum Fetal Surveillance* (eds J.A.D. Spencer & R.H.T. Ward), pp. 269–280. London: RCOG Press, 1993.
68. Wiswell TE, Tuggle JM & Turner BS. Meconium aspiration syndrome: have we made a difference? *Pediatrics* **85**, 715–721, 1990.
69. Katz VL & Bowes WA. Meconium aspiration syndrome: Reflections on a murky subject. *Am. J. Obstet. Gynecol.* **166**, 171–183, 1992.
70. Wiswell TE & Henley MA. Intratracheal suctioning, systemic infection and the meconium aspiration syndrome. *Pediatrics* **89**, 203–206, 1992.
71. Wiswell TE & Bent RC. Meconium staining and the meconium aspiration syndrome. Unresolved issues. *Ped. Clin. N. Am.* **40**, 955, 1993.
72. Goetzman BW. Meconium aspiration (editorial). *Am. J. Dis. Child.* **146**, 1282–1283, 1992.
73. Hooper SB & Harding R. Changes in lung liquid dynamics induced by prolonged fetal hypoxemia. *J. Appl. Physiol.* **69**, 127–135, 1990.

74. Oelberg DG, Downey SA & Flynn MM. Bile salt induced intracellular Ca accumulation in type 2 pneumocytes. *Lung* **168**, 297, 1990.
75. Moses D, Holm BA, Spitale P, Liu M & Enhorning G. Inhibition of pulmonary surfactant function by meconium. *Am. J. Obstet Gynecol.* **164**, 477–481, 1991.
76. Romero R, Hanaoka S, Mazor M *et al.* Meconium-stained amniotic fluid: a risk factor for microbial invason of the amniotic cavity. *Am. J. Obstet. Gynecol.* **164**, 859–862, 1991.
77. Perlman EJ, Moore GW & Hutchins GM. The pulmonary vasculature in meconium aspiration. *Hum. Pathol.* **20**, 701–706, 1989.
78. Murphy JD, Vawter GF & Reid LM. Pulmonary vascular disease in fetal meconium aspiration. *J. Pediatr.* **104**, 758–762, 1984.
79. Lauweryns J, Bernat R, Lerut A & Detournay G. Intrauterine pneumonia. An experimental study. *Biol. Neonate.* **22**, 301–318, 1973.
80. deSa DJ & Nicholls S. Haemorrhagic necrosis of the adrenal gland in perinatal infants: a clinico-pathological study. *J. Pathol.* **106**, 133–149, 1972.
81. Stafford PA, Biddinger PW & Zumwalt RE. Lethal intra-uterine fetal trauma. *Am. J. Obstet. Gynecol.* **159**, 485–489, 1988.
82. Oni OOA, Okpere EE, Tabowei O & Omu EA Severe road traffic injuries in the third trimester of pregnancy. *Injury* **15**, 376–378, 1984.
83. Eckford SD & Vyas S. Delayed placental abruption after road traffic accident. *J. Obstet Gynecol.* **15**, 186–187, 1995.
84. Govaert, P. Superficial haemorrhage. In *Cranial Haemorrhage in the term Newborn Infant.* Clinics in Developmental Medicine, vol. 129, pp. 16–85. Cambridge: Cambridge University Press, 1993.
85. Huang C-C & Shen E-Y. Tentorial subdural hemorrhage in term newborns: Ultrasonographic diagnosis and clinical correlates. *Pediatr. Neurol.* **7**, 171–177, 1991.
86. Strong TH, Feldman DB, Cooke JK, Greenspoon JS & Barton L. Congenital depression of the fetal skull. *Obstet. Gynecol. Survey* **45**, 284, 1990.
87. Jobe AH, Mitchell BR & Gankel JH. Beneficial effects of the combined use of prenatal corticosteroids and postnatal surfactant on preterm infants. *Am. J. Obstet. Gynecol.* **168**, 508–513, 1993.
88. Farrell EE, Silver RK, Kimberlin LV *et al.* Impact of antenatal dexamethasone administration on respiratory distress in surfactant treated infants. *Am. J. Obstet. Gynecol.* **161**, 628–633, 1989.
89. Zaaijman J, du T, Wilkinson AR, Keeling JW, Mitchell RG & Turnbull AC. Spontaneous premature rupture of the membranes: histology and neonatal outcome. *J. Obstet. Gynecol.* **2**, 155–160, 1982.
90. Drife J. Infection and preterm birth. *Br. J. Obstet. Gynaecol.* **96**, 1128–1132, 1989.
91. Grigg J, Arnon S, Chase A & Silverman M. Inflammatory cells in the lungs of premature infants on the first day of life; perinatal risk factors and origin of cells. *Arch. Dis. Child.* **69**, 40–43, 1993.
92. Isaacs D & Moxon ER. Pneumonia. In *Neonatal Infections* (eds D. Isaacs & E.R. Moxon), pp. 70–83. Oxford: Butterworth Heinemann, 1991.
93. Khong TY, Frappell J, Steel HM, Stewart CM & Burke M. Perinatal listeriosis. A report of six cases. *Br. J. Obstet. Gynecol.* **93**, 1083–1087, 1986.
94. Modlin JF. Perinatal echovirus infection: insights from a literature review of 61 cases of serious infection and 16 outbreaks in nurseries. *Rev. Inf. Dis.* **8**, 918–926, 1986.
95. Abzug MJ, Beam AC, Gyorkos EA & Myron J. Viral pneumonia in the first month of life. *Ped. Inf. Dis. J.* **9**, 882–885, 1990.
96. Toce SS & Keenan WJ. Congenital echovirus 11 pneumonia in association with pulmonary hypertension. *Ped. Inf. Dis. J.* **7**, 360–362.
97. Abzug MJ & Levin MJ. Neonatal adenovirus infection: four patients and review of the literature. *Pediatrics* **87**, 890–896, 1991.
98. Thorpe-Beeston JG & Nicolaides KH. Prenatal diagnosis and treatment. In *Congenital Perinatal and Neonatal Infections* (eds A. Greenough, J. Osborne & S. Sutherland), pp. 9–14. London: Churchill Livingstone, 1992.
99. Morey A, Keeling JW, Porter HJ & Fleming KA. Clinical and histopathological features of parvovirus B19 infection in the human fetus. *Br. J. Obstet. Gynaecol.* **99**, 566–574, 1992.
100. Naeye RL. Hypoxemia and the sudden infant death syndrome. *Science* **186**, 837–838, 1974.
101. Takashima S, Armstrong D, Becker LE & Huber J. Cerebral white matter lesions in sudden infant death syndrome. *Pediatrics* **62**, 155–159, 1978.
102. Esiri M, Urry P & Keeling JW. Lipid-containing cells in the brain in sudden infant death syndrome. *Dev. Med. Child. Neurol.* **32**, 319–324, 1990.
103. Kinney HC, Body BA, Finkelstein DM, Vawter GF, Mandell F & Gilles FH. Delayed central nervous system myelination in the sudden infant death syndrome. *J. Neuropathol. Exp. Neurol.* **50**, 29–48, 1991.
104. Hinchliffe SA, Howard CV, Lynch MRJ, Sargent PH, Judd BA & van Velzen D. Renal developmental arrest in sudden infant death syndrome. *Ped. Pathol.* **13**, 333–344, 1993.
105. Naeye RL. Functionally important disorders of the placenta, umbilical cord and fetal membranes. *Hum. Pathol.* **18**, 680–691, 1987.
106. Macpherson T. Fact and fancy. What can we really tell from the placenta? *Arch. Pathol. Lab. Med.* **115**, 672–681, 1991.
107. Kaplan C, Lowell DM & Salafia C. College of American Pathologists. Conference on the Examination of the Placenta: Report of the Working Group on the definition of structural changes associated with abnormal function in the maternal/fetal/placental unit in the second and third trimesters. *Arch. Pathol. Lab. Med.* **115**, 709–716, 1991.
108. Altshuler G. Some placental considerations related to neurodevelopmental and other disorders. *J. Child. Neurol.* **8**, 78–94, 1993.
109. Salafia CM & Vintzileos AM. Why all placentas should be examined by a pathologist in 1990. *Am. J. Obstet. Gynecol.* **163**, 1282–1293, 1990.
110. Naeye RL. Do placental weights have clinical significance? *Hum. Pathol.* **18**, 387, 1987.
111. Fox H. *Pathology of the Placenta.* London: W.B. Saunders, 1978.
112. Miller P, Coen RW & Benirschke K. Dating the time interval from meconium passage to birth. *Obstet. Gynecol.* **66**, 459–462, 1985.
113. Gould SJ. Pulmonary hypoplasia, hyaline membrane disease and chronic lung disease. In *Fetal Breathing* (eds M.A. Hanson, J.A.D. Spencer, C.H. Rodeck & D. Walters), pp. 214–238. Cambridge: Cambridge University Press, 1994.
114. Whyte RK, Hussain Z & De Sa DJ. Antenatal infections with Candida. *Arch Dis. Child.* **57**, 528–535, 1982.
115. Gravett MG, Hummel D, Eschenbach DA & Holmes KK. Preterm labor associated with subclinical amniotic fluid infection and with bacterial vaginosis. *Obstet. Gynecol.* **67**, 229–237, 1986.
116. Naeye RL. Acute bacterial chorioamnionitis. *Prog. Clin. Biol. Res.* **281**, 73–86, 1988.
117. Munday PE, Porter R, Folder PF *et al.* Spontaneous abortion, an infectious aetiology. *Br. J. Obstet. Gynaecol.* **91**, 1177–1180, 1984.
118. Gravett MG, Nelson P, DeRouen T, Chrichlow C, Eschenbach DA & Holmes KK. Independent associations of bacterial vaginosis and Chlamydia trachomatis infection with adverse pregnancy outcome. *JAMA* **256**, 1899–1903, 1986.
119. Lamont RF, Taylor-Robinson D, Wigglesworth JS, Furr PM, Evans RT & Elder MG. The role of mycoplasmas, ureaplasmas and chlamydiae in the genital tract of women presenting in spontaneous early preterm labour. *J. Med. Microbiol.* **24**, 253–257, 1987.
120. Quinn PA, Shewchuk AB, Shuber J *et al.* Serologic evidence of Ureaplasma urealyticum infection in women with spontaneous pregnancy loss. *Am. J. Obstet. Gynecol.* **145**, 245–250, 1983.
121. Cassell GH, Waites KB, Watson HL, Crouse DT & Harasawa R. Ureaplasma urealyticum intrauterine infection: role in prematurity and disease in newborns. *Clin. Microbiol. Rev.* **6**, 69–87, 1993.
122. Moessinger AC, Blanc WA, Marone PA & Polsen DC. Umbilical cord length as an indicator of fetal activity: experimental study and clinical implications. *Ped. Res.* **16**, 109–112, 1982.
123. Shepherd AJ, Richardson CJ & Brown JP. Nuchal cord as a cause of neonatal anaemia. *Am. J. Dis. Child.* **139**, 71, 1985.
124. Kiley KC, Perknis CS & Penney LL. Umbilical cord stricture associated with intrauterine fetal demise: a report of two cases. *J. Reprod. Med.* **29**, 110, 1984.
125. Glanfield PA & Watson R. Intrauterine fetal death due to umbilical cord torsion. *Arch. Pathol. Lab. Med.* **110**, 357, 1986.
126. Wigglesworth JS. The placenta in perinatal pathology. In *Major Problems in Pathology, Perinatal Pathology* (ed. J.S. Wigglesworth), Vol. 15, pp. 48–83. Philadelphia: W.B. Saunders, 1984.
127. Laurini R, Laurin J & Marsal K. Placental histology and fetal blood flow in intrauterine growth retardation. *Acta. Obstet. Gynecol. Scand.* **73**(7), 529–534, 1994.

128. Wigglesworth JS. Morphological variations in the insufficient placenta. *J. Obstet. Gynaecol Br. Commwlth.* **71**, 871–884, 1964.
129. Rushton DI. Pathology of the placenta. In *Textbook of Fetal and Perinatal Pathology* (eds J.S. Wigglesworth & D.B. Singer), vol. 1, pp. 161–220. Oxford: Blackwell Scientific Publications, 1991.
130. Khong TY, Staples A, Bendon RW *et al.* Observer reliability in assessing placental maturity by histology. *J. Clin. Pathol.* **48**, 420–423, 1995.
131. Mortimer G, MacDonald DJ & Smeeth A A pilot study of the frequency and significance of placental villitis. *Br. J. Obstet. Gynaecol.* **92**, 629–633, 1985.
132. Knox WF & Fox H. Villitis of unknown aetiology: Its incidence and significance in placentae from a British population. *Placenta* **5**, 395–402, 1984.
133. Russell P. Inflammatory lesions of the human placenta. III. The histopathology of villitis of unknown aetiology. *Placenta* **1**, 227–244, 1980.
134. Laberrere CA & Althabe OH. Chronic villitis of unknown aetiology in recurrent intrauterine fetal growth retardation. *Placenta* **8**, 167–174, 1987.
135. Salafia CM, Silberman L, Herrera NE & Mahoney MJ. Placental pathology at term associated with elevated midtrimester maternal serum alpha-fetoprotein concentration. *Am. J. Obstet. Gynecol.* **163**, 1064–1066, 1988.
136. Brosens I, Robertson WB & Dixon HG. The physiological response of the vessels of the placental bed to normal pregnancy. *J. Pathol. Bacteriol.* **93**, 569–579, 1967.
137. Khong TY, De Wolf F, Robertson WB & Brosens I. Inadequate maternal vascular response to placentation in pregnancies complicated by pre-eclampasia and by small for gestational age infants. *Br. J. Obstet. Gynaecol.* **93**, 1049–1059, 1986.
138. Khong TY, Liddell HS & Robertson WB Defective haemochorial placentation as a cause of spontaneous miscarriage: a preliminary study. *Br. J. Obstet. Gynaecol.* **94**, 649–655, 1987.

SECTION

10

The neonate

Adaptation and outcomes: the neonatal interface with fetal medicine

78

M.L. Chiswick

Introduction

In this chapter we will consider adaptation and outcomes as they are key elements in the continuum between fetal and extrauterine life. Perhaps the most robust test of fetal health is the quality of adaptation to extrauterine life. Three areas of adaptation – cardiorespiratory, thermoregulatory, and metabolic, exemplify those biological systems where major changes occur in the transition from fetus to newly born.

Adaptation within a particular biological system cannot be considered in isolation. First there is important interplay between systems. Thus, newborns who are subject to cold stress, even to a relatively modest degree, increase their metabolic rate and oxygen consumption at the expense of growth. Nursing newborns within the thermoneutral range thus allows calories to be used for growth rather than for maintenance of the central core temperature. Second, the fetal milieu or the state of preparedness modulates the quality of adaptation. For example, intrauterine hypoxia may impair the fall in pulmonary vascular resistance that normally occurs during transition and thereby promotes pulmonary hypertension and postnatal hypoxia. Third, many neonatal disorders can be attributed at their outset to a failure of adaptation, but subsequently become complicated by a chain of pathology that might culminate in brain damage (see later) or chronic disease. For example, prolonged survival of many extremely preterm babies with surfactant deficiency lung disease, itself a form of maladaptation, may be associated with the evolution of chronic lung disease, which is the culmination of many different insults to lungs that are anatomically, biochemically and immunologically immature.

As we learn more about the continuum between fetal and extrauterine life, it becomes difficult to locate appropriate outcomes to evaluate methods of fetal assessment and management. For example, the management of fetal growth retardation might be targeted at such diverse entities as the prevention of stillbirth, perinatal hypoxia, neonatal hypoglycaemia, neurodevelopmental disability in childhood, and hypertension in adult life. There are interactions between triggering intrauterine events, neonatal disease, and long-term outcome. Furthermore, it is likely that the intrauterine environment and fetal health *per se* predetermine long-term outcomes by ways that are not yet apparent to medical science.

Interventional preterm birth

Improved methods of investigating fetal health and better chances of survival of preterm babies has led to more interventional preterm births for both maternal and fetal reasons. The need to define with more precision the *balance of risk* between expediting delivery before term and leaving a fetus in the womb will remain a challenging problem until effective preventative or intrauterine treatment strategies are available for the common high-risk situations, including fetal growth retardation, antepartum hypoxia, and premature and prolonged rupture of membranes.

Advances in fetal assessment methodology might lead to a more robust approach towards intervention by preterm delivery. Joint obstetric and paediatric data-collecting systems need to be devised to facilitate the proper audit of interventional preterm birth as a basis for future decision-making. The current routinely collected statistics fall far short of our needs in this respect. In individual high-risk pregnancies it is readily apparent when an interventional preterm delivery has culminated in neonatal death due to complications of prematurity. In contrast, data on long-term neurodevelopmenal disability following interventional preterm delivery in high-risk pregnancies are more difficult to come by. The importance of this subgroup is that their study, particularly if supplemented by information from brain scans done soon after birth, might clarify the extent to which neuronal injury and disability are already determined before delivery.

The outcome measure of immediate concern to parents when extremely preterm birth is anticipated is survival. A request for information most commonly arises when spontaneous preterm labour has already supervened, or when interventional preterm delivery is a consideration. In effect, the parents pose the question: 'assuming that our baby will be born alive, what are the chances of him or her surviving?' Parents may be advised on the basis of national or local data on the survival rates at different gestational ages. While this is of some help, there are pitfalls. Many studies refer to survival rates only of babies admitted to neonatal units, excluding those who died on the delivery unit. Reliance on these figures will give an overoptimistic impression to parents.

The assessment of true survival rates of babies who are born alive at a given gestational age means using total live births at that gestational age as the denominator. A difficulty, especially when considering extremely preterm births, is that livebirths may be wrongly classified as stillbirths, and knowingly so. Again, this will lead to an overoptimistic impression of survival rates. There should be no confusion about what constitutes signs of life. They are the recognition of any degree of breathing (even a gasp), movement, or a heart beat detected by palpation or by auscultation. Of course, there are different emotional and practical implications for parents according to whether their baby is classified as a livebirth or stillbirth but these need to be dealt with by appropriate support rather than by distorting the facts. Choice is not permitted.

Finally, parents should be made aware that the chance of their baby surviving is very likely to be lower or higher than the mean survival rate. When providing information to parents based on epidemiological data then the degree of uncertainty of predictions should be acknowledged by indicating in simple terms the worst and best survival rates based on a range, or the 95% confidence interval when such data are available.

Brain damage and disability in preterm infants

Brain imaging, especially the use of cerebral ultrasound by the cot-side, has improved our understanding of the nature and topography of lesions associated with neurodisability. Similarly, technological developments including Doppler ultrasound, near-infrared spectroscopy, positron emission tomography and magnetic resonance spectroscopy, have allowed the estimation of indices such as cerebral blood flow, cerebral oxygenation and blood volume, and cerebral metabolism. This information has helped researchers propose models for the pathogenesis of cerebral lesions.

While we are still some way from effective forms of neuroprotection at tissue level, the focus of attention in preterm babies has quite properly been based on careful neonatal monitoring to minimalise perturbations in parameters such as blood pressure and blood gases, and to recognise early on signs of cardiorespiratory impairment before the downward spiral of deterioration occurs that in previous days culminated in babies being 'found collapsed' in their incubators.

The extent to which new and specific neuroprotection strategies applied postnatally might benefit preterm babies will remain unclear until we understand the contribution of cerebral insults in fetal life. Important areas that need further study include: antepartum hypoxic–ischaemic injury especially in twin pregnancies; the contribution of fetal malnutrition to neuronal injury; and the role of maternal and fetal infection in causing white matter damage.

The two most widely recognised types of cerebral damage in preterm babies are periventricular haemorrhage and periventricular leukomalacia.

PERIVENTRICULAR HAEMORRHAGE (PVH)

During the last decade, the incidence of PVH in babies born <32 weeks' gestation has fallen and is now probably around 25% with an increasing risk in babies at lower gestational ages. The origin of haemorrhage is within the germinal matrix, ventrolateral to the lateral ventricles, an area of primitive vessels with relatively thin walls and large lumens, poorly supported by surrounding glial tissue. The matrix is the site of proliferation of glial cell precursors and of neuronal precursors prior to their migration to the cerebral cortex. Involution of the matrix occurs in the final 16 weeks of gestation and is nearly complete by about 36 weeks, which helps to explain why PVH is more common in preterm babies, especially those born at less than 32 weeks' gestation.

Haemorrhage may be confined to the germinal matrix or blood may rupture through the overlying ependyma and enter the cavity of the ventricles. Small haemorrhages confined to the germinal matrix or to the ventricular cavities are not normally associated with adverse neurological outcomes. However, there is interest in the possibility that destruction of the germinal matrix by haemorrhage might lead to subtle impairments through loss of glial cell precursors destined to become oligodendroglia which contribute to myelination, and through loss of potential astrocytes which normally migrate to the cerebral cortex and contribute to its development.

Overt neurodevelopmental problems are likely with large haemorrhages that culminate in progressive ventriculomegaly and posthaemorrhagic obstructive hydrocephalus, and with haemorrhagic infarction of the white matter adjacent to the ventricles, a lesion that has a propensity to become cystic and communicate with the dilated ventricular cavity in the form of a porencephalic cyst. A range of disability may result from these lesions, especially cerebral palsy, epilepsy and learning impairment.

Probably half of all haemorrhages occur within 12 hours of birth, the remainder within four days. This timing is independent of gestational age. Ment *et al.*[1], using a beagle pup model, have shown that the risk period for haemorrhage corresponds with the time of postnatal induction of maturation of the germinal matrix, especially maturation of the basement membrane of endothelial cells. In addition to the vulnerability of the germinal matrix to haemorrhage, many factors have been implicated in provoking PVH, especially perturbations in cerebral blood flow around the time of birth and soon after. This probably explains the vulnerability of the preterm baby with unstable respiratory distress syndrome (surfactant-deficient lung disease). Although the use of surfactants has led to a decline in mortality from respiratory distress syndrome it is unclear whether it has been associated with protection against PVH in surviving babies, and more importantly with a reduction in PVH-related disability in childhood.

Many strategies have been used in clinical trials for the prevention of PVH[2], including the use of pharmacological agents such as ethamsylate, vitamin E, indomethacin and phenobarbitone, but none has been widely adopted because the results are unconvincing, or there are problems of safety yet to be resolved, or there is no clear evidence of protection against long-term neurodevelopmental disability. Based on first principles, the approach of the neonatal physician is to stabilise promptly the ill preterm baby, monitor vital signs and treat deviations and to give the baby 'a smooth ride' aiming to minimise handling and interventions that have been shown to cause perturbations in cerebral blood flow.

From an obstetric perspective, only glucocorticoids can be safely recommended antenatally for protection against PVH. The beneficial effect is probably through the reduction in the incidence of respiratory distress syndrome, but an effect independent of pulmonary maturation is possible. Further knowledge about the mechanisms of maturation of the germinal matrix microvasculature might allow the development of safe agents to promote acceleration before preterm birth. For example, indomethacin stimulates laminin and Type V collagen deposition in endothelial basement membranes of the germinal matrix[3].

PERIVENTRICULAR LEUKOMALACIA (PVL)

The characteristic site of hypoxic ischaemic brain damage in preterm babies is the periventricular white matter. Lesions causing impairments result in spastic cerebral palsy, including spastic diplegia. The reported incidence of PVL diagnosed by ultrasound in liveborn babies <32 weeks' gestation is probably between 5% and 20% and is certainly lower compared with PVH. The wide range reported is largely due to problems in defining the ultrasound appearances of PVL, especially confusion with non-cystic echo-densities and 'flares' which may be transient, and with 'periventricular haemorrhagic infarction'.

Although lesions can occur antenatally as evidenced by the appearance of well-developed cystic lesions on ultrasound scans done soon after birth, it has been considered that most lesions result from a hypoxic–ischaemic insult occurring postnatally with a peak frequency *after* the first week of life. The notion that most PVL is acquired postnatally as a result of hypotension in sick preterm babies has been challenged. Improved standards of neonatal monitoring and care have led to fewer babies suffering recurrent acute deteriorations in vital signs. Cystic PVL of postnatal origin tends now to occur in babies who have had a relatively benign neonatal course with no evidence of hypotension[4].

The origins and pathogenesis of PVL are more complex than was originally thought. There is an association between prolonged rupture of membranes, chorioamnionitis, and maternal infection on the one hand, and an increased risk of PVL in preterm babies on the other. Furthermore, chorioamnionitis is a risk factor for cerebral palsy in children who were born preterm[5,6]. Thus maternal infection might be the trigger for preterm birth, PVL and cerebral palsy. Dammann and Leviton[7] have recently proposed a unifying explanatory model for infection-induced PVL based on evidence that cytokines (interleukins IL-1β, IL-6 and tumour necrosis factor-α) have been found in three compartments (amniotic fluid, fetal circulation and the brain). They suggest that following maternal infection, cytokine production is stimulated in the uterus, amniotic fluid, placenta or in fetal blood. Cytokines can cross the blood–brain barrier (perhaps by first altering its permeability) and cause white matter damage either directly, or by inducing further cytokine production by microglia or astrocytes. It is well known that the occurrence of the more severe grades of PVH is associated with an increased risk of PVL. It is possible that cytokines in the intraventricular blood gain access to white matter and contribute to damage in that way.

There are many postulated mechanisms whereby cytokines may gain access to the brain parenchyma and cause tissue damage. The possible role of tumour necrosis factor as a cause of cerebral palsy in preterm births has been reviewed by Leviton[8]. One consideration is that future strategies designed to prevent preterm birth by the treatment of maternal infection may need to be supplemented by agents that interrupt the cytokine cascade.

HYPOXIC–ISCHAEMIC BRAIN DAMAGE IN TERM BABIES

Underlying the clinical manifestations of hypoxic–ischaemic brain injury in the newborn are disturbances in cellular biology that are currently attracting intense research interest, with the hope of developing effective neuroprotective strategies. The initial hypoxic insult is associated with primary cerebral energy failure as a result of impaired oxidative phosphorylation. Resuscitation at birth and restoring of the cerebral circulation and intracellular pH leads to recovery of energy stores. A proportion of babies who go on to develop hypoxic–ischaemic encephalopathy as outlined in Chapter 83, develop secondary cerebral energy failure after a variable latent period measured in hours. This is a reflection of mitochondrial dysfunction and the result of numerous disturbances in cellular function, culminating in neuronal apoptosis (programmed cell death) and necrosis (see Table 78.1).

TABLE 78.1
Summary of intracerebral pathological events following a damaging intrapartum hypoxic insult

- Primary cerebral energy failure (intrapartum hypoxic insult)
- Restoration of cerebral energy levels (resuscitation at birth)
- Postresuscitation biochemical changes including:
  - increased excitatory activity
  - accumulation of intracellular calcium
  - accumulation of toxic free radicals
  - enhanced cytokine expression
  - delayed increase in cerebral lactate
- Secondary cerebral energy failure (culmination of biochemical changes)
- Neuronal apoptosis (programmed cell death) and necrosis

In theory, there is a window of opportunity during the time interval between resuscitation and the development of secondary energy failure when neuroprotection is a consideration. Numerous experimental approaches to neuroprotection have been used in animal models, often with success depending on which particular measure of outcome is used. Experimental strategies have included the use of excitatory receptor blockage, calcium-channel blockers, antioxidants, cytokine inhibitors and inhibitors of apoptosis.

The use of controlled hypothermia is now attracting attention and has been the subject of recent reviews[9,10]. Animal experimental models have shown that mild-to-moderate hypothermia applied soon after an hypoxic–ischaemic insult to induce a reduction in core temperature ranging from 2 to 6°C for varying lengths of time (3 to 72 hours) is associated with a reduction in brain damage. The primary mechanism of the neuroprotective effect of cooling applied after the hypoxic–ischaemic insult is not clear. However, in a piglet experimental model a 4°C reduction in core temperature maintained for 12 hours was associated with a significant reduction in the extent of secondary energy failure[11,12]. The importance of this is that the magnitude of secondary energy failure as measured by magnetic resonance spectroscopy in babies with hypoxic–ischaemic encephalopathy is a useful predictor of neurodevelopmental outcome[13].

The practical problems in translating hypothermic neural rescue treatment to the cot-side has been summarised by Edwards and Azzopardi[14]. It is possible that hypothermia simply delays rather than prevents neuronal death. If that were the case, there might in the future be opportunities to use other neuroprotective treatment while hypothermia extends the therapeutic time window.

Ethical issues in the neonatal unit

The concept of a continuum between fetal and neonatal life is readily understood in terms of science and clinical practice. Yet attempts to apply a unified and coherent ethical code that spans intrauterine and extrauterine life presents many difficulties. The moral, philosophical, theological and legal concepts that impact on the moment of birth are academically stimulating but are of limited practical value in informing decision-making.

The use of assisted ventilation is central to the ethical problems that are posed in the neonatal period. This is understandable when we consider that the provision of warmth, and nutrition (including fluids) are *entitlements* in so far as even healthy newborns are dependent on a caregiver for their provision. In contrast, healthy newborns are expected to maintain their breathing and it is not a feature of their dependency. Assisted ventilation is not a treatment. Instead it is a way of supporting the life of a baby while the underlying cause of respiratory failure resolves. The concept behind the use of assisted ventilation is that the respiratory failure is potentially reversible, and that there is a reasonable chance of survival without the development of recognisable brain lesions that might lead to major disability.

When considering whether to start assisted ventilation, it may not be possible to decide whether respiratory failure is potentially reversible; even more difficult at the start is the prediction of a baby's chances of surviving without major disability. Therefore, from an ethical perspective, any neonatal physician who starts ventilation also has the responsibility of being receptive to the question of withdrawing support in certain circumstances.

In practice, there are two circumstances where withdrawal of life support is a consideration. The first is when the baby has already entered the process of dying, as indicated by multiple organ failure, and where the continuation of ventilation simply to prolong life is a pointless or futile exercise. Of course, clinical judgement is needed to define the point at which a baby may have entered the process of dying, but the principle is that further assisted ventilation will not save life, but will simply prolong it for hours, days, or possibly weeks.

The second circumstance is more controversial. Here we have to acknowledge that for some babies the continuation of assisted ventilation might well save life but only by further prolonged discomfiture of neonatal intensive care, and the likelihood that substantial neurodevelopmental or physical handicap will radically limit the child's ability to participate in human experience and will render him or her forever dependent on a caregiver for everyday living.

These decisions are never easy because of the difficulties in predicting the quality of life. There is an abundance of scientific literature indicating the proportion of babies with defined abnormalities on neonatal brain scans who have a very poor developmental outcome. This is helpful when discussing *risks*, but even when combined with other indices such as electroencephalograms, or the testing of visual and auditory evoked responses, a precise prediction of outcome *in individual babies* who are critically ill is not possible.

Whatever one's personal views on decision-making based on quality of life considerations, professionals have a duty to introduce the ethical issues to parents at an appropriate time and in a frank and informative way. In practice, it is likely to be a real issue for discussion only when there are severe abnormalities on a brain scan in a baby who is critically ill, especially if there are persistently abnormal neurological signs. One constraint is that there is often a limited window for withdrawing support in a critically ill baby who is dependent on assisted ventilation. By the time the medical facts are available, presented to the parents in an informative and reasoned way, and assessed by them, the baby's survival may no longer be dependent on assisted ventilation. In effect, the time for decision-making has passed because the baby will survive without ventilatory support.

The burden of decision-making around difficult ethical issues is something that neonatal physicians and nurses cannot escape, and they should not avoid the issues by placing the burden on parents: 'This is the problem – what do you want us to do?' Parents should know they are contributing to a joint decision, and the neonatal physician, after consulting with senior and experienced medical and nursing staff, should help parents toward this goal. A decision to withdraw support (or to continue) is one that often evolves over time following many discussions with parents led by the neonatal physician under whose care the baby was admitted, and who bore the responsibility (directly or indirectly) for starting life support.

There may be subtle issues surrounding decision-making for parents of babies who were born preterm by obstetric intervention where maternal or fetal health was compromised. In the former case, mothers may feel that they have sacrificed their baby's life for their own health; where interventional preterm birth resulted from poor fetal health a mother may find it difficult to come to terms with the notion that her consent for preterm delivery (to protect her unborn baby) resulted in her baby's death. Of course, these considerations arise whether or not death was bound up with an ethical decision to withdraw support. However, interventional preterm birth does add a new dimension to ethical decision making in the neonatal period.

REFERENCES

1. Ment LR, Stewart WB, Ardito TA & Madri JA. Germinal matrix microvasculature maturation correlates inversely with the risk period for neonatal: intraventricular hemorrhage. *Develop. Brain Res.* **84**, 142–149, 1995.
2. Vohr B & Ment LR. Intraventricular hemorrhage in the preterm infant. *Early Human Develop.* **44**, 1–16, 1996.
3. Ment LR, Stewart WB, Ardito TA, Huang E & Madri JA. Indomethacin promotes germinal matrix microvessel maturation in the newborn beagle pup. *Stroke* **23**, 1132–1137, 1992.
4. Perlman JM, Risser M & Broyles RS. Bilateral cystic periventricular leukomalacia in the premature infant: associated risk factors. *Pediatrics* **97**, 822–827, 1996.
5. Murphy DJ, Sellers S, MacKenzie IZ, Yudkin PL & Johnson AM. Case–control study of antenatal and intrapartum risk factors for cerebral palsy in very preterm singleton babies. *Lancet* **346**, 1449–1454, 1995.
6. Grether JK, Nelson KB, Emery III ES & Cummins SK. Prenatal and perinatal factors and cerebral palsy in very low birth weight infants. *J. Pediatrics* **128**, 407–414, 1996.
7. Dammann O & Leviton A. Maternal intrauterine infection, cytokines, and brain damage in the preterm newborn. *Pediatr. Res.* **42**, 1–8, 1997.
8. Leviton A. Preterm birth and cerebral palsy: is tumour necrosis factor the missing link? *Develop. Med. Child Neurol.* **35**, 553–558, 1993.
9. Toresen M & Wyatt J. Keeping a cool head, post-hypoxic hypothermia – an old idea revisited. *Acta Paediat.* **86**, 1029–1033, 1997.
10. Edwards AD, Wyatt JS & Thoresen M. Treatment of hypoxic–ischaemic brain damage by moderate hypothermia. *Archi. Dis. Childh.* **78**, F85–F88, 1998.
11. Thoresen M, Penrice J, Lorek A *et al.* Mild hypothermia following severe transient hypoxia–ischemia ameliorates delayed ('secondary') cerebral energy failure in the newborn piglet. *Pediatr. Res.* **5**, 667–670, 1995.
12. Amess PN, Penrice J, Lorek A *et al.* Mild hypothermia after transient hypoxia–ischemia reduces the delayed rise in cerebral lactate in the newborn piglet. *Pediatr. Res.* **41**, 803–808, 1997.
13. Roth SC, Baudin J, Cady E *et al.* Relation of deranged neonatal cerebral oxidative metabolism with neurodevelopmental outcome and head circumference at 4 years. *Develop. Med. Child Neurol.* **39**, 718–725, 1997.
14. Edwards AD & Azzopardi D. Hypothermic neural rescue treatment: from laboratory to cotside? *Arch. Dis. Childh.* **78**, F88–F91, 1998.

Cardiorespiratory adaptation to extrauterine life

79

N. Evans and D. Henderson-Smart

Introduction

In the minutes and hours after birth, vital changes must occur as the lungs take over the role of gas exchange from the placenta. Changes occur within the tissues and the blood vessels of the lungs, and within the heart. Respiratory and cardiovascular adaptation will be discussed separately. However, we must emphasise the extent of the interdependence of these changes, with changes occurring in one area being vital to changes in another. We will highlight not only the normal adaptation process but also the ways in which failure of these processes have important clinical consequences for the newborn infant.

Respiratory adaptation

Establishment of air breathing at birth is vital for the survival of mammals. The success of this change depends on a number of essential preconditions. These include adequate anatomical and biochemical development of the lungs, a change from lung liquid excretion *in utero* to absorption after birth, and breathing efforts that are both forceful and effective. Under certain clinical circumstances one or more of these components may be defective and respiratory failure can lead to asphyxia and even death. We consider here the factors that are important to ensure that conditions are optimal for the establishment and maintenance of air breathing at birth and describes the change in respiratory function during birth and early postnatal adaptation.

ANATOMICAL DEVELOPMENT OF THE LUNGS

A detailed account of the structural development of the lung has been given by Harding (Chapter 16) and others (Table 79.1)[1,2]. Important for an understanding of respiratory adaptation at birth is an appreciation of the stage of development of the lung at different gestational ages and that the lung is in a particularly rapid phase of development between 24 and 36 weeks' gestation. To undergo normal development, the lungs need space to expand, to be distended with lung liquid and probably to be physically distorted by fetal breathing efforts.

TABLE 79.1
Pulmonary anatomical and biochemical changes at different gestational ages

Parameter	Gestational age (weeks) 22–23	27–28	32–33	37–38
Average body weight (kg)	0.55	1.0	1.6	3.1
Lung structure				
Volume (ml/kg)	55	60	75	77
'Alveolar' surface area (m^2/kg)	0.55	0.8	1.06	1.7
Airspace wall thickness (μm)	3.7	2.6	1.8	1.5
Airspace (%)	<20	30	38	50
Amniotic fluid surfactant				
Lecithin/sphyngomyelin (L/S)	–	1.2	1.4	2.5
Phosphatidylglycerol (% total lipids)	0	0	0	2.2
Surfactant-associated protein A	–	20	20	50
Surfactant-associated protein B	–	0	5	50

Data from Hislop *et al.*[1], Langston *et al.*[2] and Froh and Ballard[6].

The most common structural abnormality of lung development is hypoplasia which is found in 15–20% of autopsies. It is not known what proportion of surviving infants also have a degree of lung hypoplasia that might contribute to disordered respiratory adaptation, since diagnosis in life is difficult. Experimentally, lung hypoplasia can be induced by producing a space-occupying lesion in the thorax such as a diaphragmatic hernia, by causing chest restriction through oligohydramnios, by chronically draining lung liquid through a tracheal cannula, by abolishing fetal breathing with phrenectomy or cervical cord transection, or by reduction in the amplitude of fetal breathing through the creation of an artificial flail chest.

Clinically, the main problems occur in association with congenital abnormalities of the thorax such as diaphragmatic hernia, cystic adenomatoid malformation, pleural effusions or rarely, asphyxiating thoracic dystrophy; or with prolonged oligohydramnios associated with prolonged rupture of the membranes from 20 to 24 weeks' gestation or renal agenesis. In extremely preterm birth (less than 28 weeks' gestation) anatomical limitations to pulmonary adaptation include primitive branching of the airways with respiratory bronchioles and saccules but no alveoli, a thick air–blood barrier to gas exchange and immature collagen and elastin-supporting elements in the interstitium. Apart from limiting postnatal adaptation in the short term, very early birth appears to interfere with the normal growth and differentiation of the lung, and is associated with chronic lung disease (CLD). Hypoplasia of the lungs has been found in pathological specimens from such infants who have survived to near term equivalent age. In childhood, preterm infants in general have a higher incidence of respiratory disorders[3] and those with a birth weight of less than 1 kg have altered respiratory function tests, even at eight years of age[4].

BIOCHEMICAL DEVELOPMENT OF THE LUNG

The most important substance required for postnatal pulmonary function is surfactant. It lowers surface tension at the air–liquid interface so the air space can be inflated with less effort and can remain inflated during expiration with minimal transpulmonary pressures. The development, composition, function and metabolism of surfactant has been reviewed by Harding and elsewhere by others[5–7]. The essential features of the development of surfactant secretion include its appearance at about 24 weeks' gestation and accelerated production as well as maturation of essential components at 34–36 weeks. The main components of mature surfactant are lipids (45% saturated phosphatidylcholine, 25% unsaturated phosphatidylcholine and 5% phosphatidylglycerol) that are responsible for lowering surface tension. Small (2%) but important components are the apolipoproteins (A, B, C, etc.) that are responsible for secretion, activation and metabolic recycling of the lipids. Surfactant is synthesised in the type II alveolar cells and the rate of maturation of most components is regulated by glucocorticoids. Thyroid hormones also regulate the production of some components of surfactant and there is synergism with glucocorticoids. Maturation can be accelerated antenatally by administering corticosteroids to the mother. Antenatal detection of surfactant immaturity is possible by examining its activity or concentration in amniotic fluid.

The most important function of surfactant is to assist in establishing and maintaining a functional residual capacity (FRC) which is important for continuing gas exchange (particularly oxygen) throughout the respiratory cycle. Although the most dramatic changes in pulmonary mechanics and gas exchange occur during the first minutes after birth, there are still considerable changes during the first day. In normal infants, the rise in FRC and fall in airways resistance is mostly completed in the first few hours of life. Compliance increases progressively over the first day and this is thought to be due in part to the removal of interstitial fluid (see below).

Immaturity or insufficiency of surfactant impairs the ability to establish a FRC at birth and to maintain it during the first days of life. This leads to the typical signs of the respiratory distress syndrome (RDS)[8] with marked costal recession and other signs of respiratory difficulty due to the high transpulmonary pressures required to inflate the lung with each breath (25–30 vs. 8–10 cm H_2O normally) and to maintain an FRC (5–10 vs. 2–3 cm H_2O normally). Immaturity of connective tissue in the lung interstitium probably also contributes significantly to lung stiffness. The ability to inflate the lung and maintain FRC is further compromised in the newborn, particularly if very preterm, by the low compliance of the chest wall. Strategies used to maintain FRC in these circumstances are expiratory laryngeal closure which is manifest clinically as an expiratory grunt, and limiting expiratory time by maintaining a high breathing rate. Both these are mediated via vagal feedback about lung volume to the brain stem.

The large and unequal forces applied across the lungs in infants with RDS lead to epithelial injury and consequent exudation of fluid and protein into the terminal air spaces. This further inactivates surfactant and leads to the formation of prominent hyaline membranes seen histologically in infants who die. The widespread atelectasis leads to the typical reticular granular chest X-ray appearance with prominent air bronchograms. The main disorder of gas exchange is ventilation/perfusion mismatching which leads predominantly to hypoxaemia. In very preterm infants, diminished respiratory drive and consequent inability to maintain alveolar ventilation in the face of a large mechanical load results in carbon dioxide retention and respiratory acidosis.

In most infants with RDS, surfactant synthesis appears to be adequate after 48–72 hours, respiratory failure abates and there is full recovery. Postnatal administration of surfactant via an endotracheal tube reduces the severity of RDS. Infants who have required a large amount of ventilatory support (positive pressure and oxygen) and those born before 28 weeks' gestation may progress to CLD. Surfactant deficiency can occur in other conditions where there is pulmonary epithelial injury with protein exudation, such as the 'shock lung syndrome' and pneumonia. Meconium aspiration also appears to be associated with surfactant dysfunction.

REGULATION OF LUNG LIQUID SECRETION AND ABSORPTION

Walters[9] and others have reviewed the physiological changes in lung fluid balance around birth. In fetal life fluid is actively excreted into the lumen, flows up the respiratory tract and is either swallowed or passes into the amniotic cavity. The rate of excretion has been measured at between 1 ml/kg/h in mid-gestation to 4 ml/kg/h in the late gestation fetal sheep.

Regulation of the escape of lung liquid by laryngeal and pharyngeal closure ensures that the lung is distended to a volume above the postnatal FRC. This distension appears to be vital for the development of the future airways, since experimental drainage leads to lung hypoplasia.

Active secretion is dependent on the Na^+,K^+-ATPase activity in the basolateral membrane of the epithelial cells which co-transports Cl^-. The latter then moves down an electrochemical gradient into the lumen, taking water with it. The switch to absorption commences during labour and is thought to be due to the opening of Na^+ channels in the apical membrane. This is stimulated by adrenaline-activated cAMP within the epithelial cell. It is thought that the surge of adrenaline that occurs during the latter part of labour halts net secretion. Cortisol and triiodothyronine appear to be important in priming the effect of adrenaline. After birth, absorption predominates and is essential for the maintenance of alveolar function. In addition to the mechanisms already mentioned this is probably assisted by the formation of a hydrophobic surfactant monolayer and the negative interstitial pressure, although the evidence for this is less clear.

During birth, the thorax and abdomen are compressed by the high pressures in the vagina and this probably contributes to emptying the lung of some of its liquid. The majority of the fluid is removed by absorption into the interstitial spaces and then via the venous circulation and lymphatics. While this occurs most rapidly within the first hour after birth, continued absorption over the next hours probably contributes to the rise in lung compliance over the first day of extrauterine life.

Infants who have been born by caesarean section without being exposed to labour and its surge of adrenaline often develop transient respiratory distress with the need for supplemental oxygen. It is thought that this reflects delayed clearance of lung liquid due to the switch to absorption occurring postnatally rather than in labour. The prevalence of cardiorespiratory maladaptation following caesarean section is influenced by the absence of labour as well as gestational age. Even near term, the rates of maladaptation at 37 weeks are seven times those at 39 weeks[10]. Clinical signs include tachypnoea, small increases in oxygen needs and non-specific streaky opacities on chest X-ray. This condition resolves spontaneously although, in a few infants, possibly due to inadequate oxygenation or a prenatal disposition, pulmonary hypertension complicates the picture and severe respiratory failure can occur. Accumulation of liquid in the interstitium and air spaces occurs as part of the pathophysiology of a number of disorders and further compromises pulmonary function. In RDS and CLD, both immaturity of cellular pumps and epithelial cell injury probably are involved. In heart failure, pulmonary vascular congestion is responsible.

REGULATION OF BREATHING EFFORTS

It is not the purpose here to examine in detail all the mechanisms that regulate breathing as these have been reviewed by others[11,12]. Rather, those aspects that appear important for the establishment of air breathing at birth and that are responsible for ensuring sustained breathing efforts during early postnatal adaptation, are reviewed.

The various control systems that regulate breathing are already present in fetal life. The central rhythm generator in the brain stem is capable of producing bursts of breathing movements that neurophysiologically resemble those seen after birth. Most of these are confined to active states, particularly rapid eye movement (REM) sleep and there are long periods without breathing which occur in quiet sleep. What changes at birth is the need to sustain breathing efforts to ensure a continued supply of oxygen and the removal of carbon dioxide.

Chemoreceptors, located in the carotid bodies to measure arterial levels of oxygen and carbon dioxide and in the brain stem to measure tissue levels, are the main sensors of mismatches in the supply and demand. Studies in fetal lambs indicate that breathing is augmented by elevated carbon dioxide and in human infants, this response has been shown to be present within the first 2 days of postnatal life. Responses to hypoxia differ in perinatal life from those in adult subjects. In the fetal animal, hypoxia immediately inhibits breathing, muscle tone and central nervous system activity. This response which reduces unnecessary metabolic work, is an appropriate defence in fetal life, when gas exchange is via the placenta. Soon after birth, hypoxia causes a transient increase then a reduction in breathing efforts. While this biphasic response is qualitatively similar to that seen in later life, the magnitude of the late reduction after a few minutes breathing, even a mildly hypoxic gas, is much greater in the newborn.

Chemoreceptors are essential in adult life but animals can still initiate postnatal breathing after arterial chemoreceptor denervation. Judging from the normal Apgar scores of infants with congenital central hypoventilation, central chemoreceptors also seem unnecessary for the initial establishment of breathing. It is only after the initial non-specific excitatory period is over and these infants go into quiet sleep that breathing fails and is unresponsive to the consequent respiratory acidosis. Of major importance to the stimulation of breathing efforts at birth are the non-specific stimuli such as pain, light and cold, that lead to arousal and non-specific stimulation of breathing. The surge of adrenaline release in late labour might also contribute to the aroused state. If regular breathing efforts fail and asphyxia ensues then autoresuscitative gasping occurs. This usually corresponds with significant acidosis and is generated by neurones in the brain stem that are distinct from those generating normal breathing.

The first breaths at birth in the majority of infants occur within 30 seconds of birth and are particularly forceful[13]. Negative intrapleural pressures of up to 100 cm H_2O have been recorded during the first breath (Table 79.2). These forceful manoeuvres are required to overcome the high-flow resistance and inertia of liquid within the airways and to inflate the lungs from their very low volume caused by the

TABLE 79.2
Mechanics of breathing during birth and the first breaths of air

	Birth canal pressure (cmH_2O)	Time to first breath	Length of first breath (s)	Oesophageal pressure (cmH_2O) Inspiratory	Oesophageal pressure (cmH_2O) Expiratory	Inspiratory volume (ml)	FRC (ml)
Median	128	10.5	0.58	−38.6	72	18.1	15.2
Range	88, 264	0.5, 31	0.29, 1.4	−28, −105	18, 115	6.5, 69	0, 32

After Vyas *et al.*[13].

vaginal squeeze. The first expiration is prolonged at about 4 s with large positive pressures due to active expiration against a closed larynx. This presumably assists in the distribution of gas throughout the lung and to formation of a gaseous FRC.

There are many factors that can influence respiratory adaptation at birth. Breathing efforts at birth can be reduced if the infant is immature or is neurologically abnormal due to intrauterine maldevelopment, to acute asphyxia or to maternal narcotic administration for analgesia during labour. Breathing may also fail because attempts are ineffective if there is a disorder of the respiratory pump that is congenital (e.g. diaphragmatic hernia) or acquired (e.g. RDS, meconium aspiration).

Failure to establish pulmonary gas exchange after placental function ceases results in hypoxaemia and acidosis which trigger a series of reflex defences to conserve oxygen and redistribute the supply to vital organs such as the heart and brain. These resemble the fetal response to hypoxia and include apnoea, hypotonia, vagal bradycardia and peripheral vasoconstriction. With severe acidosis gasping ensues. Some of these pathophysiological signs have been incorporated in the Apgar score which is used as a record of cardiorespiratory adaptation at birth. Knowledge of the physiological mechanisms helps guide the immediate care to the newborn infant who may need assistance with adaptation at birth[14], although not all interventions have been shown to be effective[15].

Even when there is no significant pulmonary disease, respiratory failure can occur due to lack of breathing efforts. This is manifest by episodes of apnoea and/or a rising P_{CO_2}. Detailed reviews are available concerning the pathophysiology[16,17] and treatment[18]. Apnoea occurring in the newborn infant after the period of respiratory adaptation at birth is defined as a pause in breathing of more than 20 s or a shorter pause associated with bradycardia or hypoxaemia. During apnoea rapid depletion of oxygen stores leads to hypoxaemia and reflex vagal bradycardia. Where the event is associated with an absence of breathing movements, this is defined as central apnoea. Where breathing movements continue without air flow, it is defined as obstructive and where there is a mixture of the two components with an initial central apnoea followed by obstructive efforts, this is called mixed apnoea.

Apnoea occurs more frequently in infants born at lower gestations and has become a greater clinical problem with the increased survival of very preterm infants. The specific reason for the higher incidence at lower gestational ages is not clear, although immaturity of the brain stem[19] and a reduction in ventilatory responses to carbon dioxide breathing and to respiratory loads has been documented in preterm infants with apnoea. The breathing and heart rate of infants born at less than 34 weeks' gestation are usually monitored to detect events that may warrant clinical attention. In addition to immaturity, various diverse factors that reduce the vigour of an infant, such as infection, hypoxaemia, metabolic disturbance or intracranial pathology, can reduce respiratory drive and aggravate apnoea. With maturation the episodes resolve and, while apnoea can recur around term equivalent age if there is an insult such as infection or general anaesthesia, there is no evidence that preterm infants with apnoea are at greater risk of sudden infant death than preterm infants in general[20].

Cardiovascular adaptation

Fetal survival is ensured by a circulation which diverts blood away from the lungs and towards the placenta. High resistance to blood flow through the fetal lungs is maintained by constriction of pulmonary arterioles which restrict flow to that which is sufficient to ensure lung growth and development. The ductus arteriosus allows blood to bypass the lungs and to return to the placenta while the oxygenated blood returning from the placenta is preferentially streamed by the ductus venosus across the foramen ovale to the left heart and hence the brain. In the immediate period after birth all this has to change. The pulmonary blood flow has to increase from 10 to 100% of the cardiac output from the right ventricle, the fetal channels have to close and the ventricles have to cope with the different demands which result from these changes. Failure of any component of this adaptation can have important clinical consequences for the newborn infant. How do these changes occur?

INCREASE IN PULMONARY BLOOD FLOW

The factors which control perinatal pulmonary blood flow are not completely understood. The available evidence points to an interplay of mechanical factors, changing levels of oxygen and endothelially-derived vasoactive mediators[21]. In fetal life, the highly muscular small pulmonary arterioles remain tightly constricted, partly due to external pressure from the fluid filled alveolar space but partly due to the vasoconstrictor effect of the relatively hypoxic fetal environment. In fetal lambs, decreasing the p_{O_2} will increase pulmonary vascular resistance[22] and increasing p_{O_2} causes a dramatic drop in resistance and resultant increase in pulmonary blood flow[23]. These effects probably occur through vasoactive mediators, with perinatal changes in pulmonary blood flow reflecting an intricate balance between vasoconstricting and vasodilating mediators.

Vasoconstrictors which may have a role in fetal life include leukotrienes which are produced in pulmonary arterial tissue. Leukotriene synthesis inhibition or receptor blockade increases fetal lamb pulmonary blood flow several times[24]. The effect of constrictors on the fetal pulmonary circulation is modulated by the constant production of vasodilators of which nitric oxide and prostacyclin are probably the most important. Nitric oxide is produced in the endothelial cell by the enzyme nitric oxide synthase causing the conversion of L-arginine to L-citrulline. Nitric oxide then diffuses to the smooth muscle cell where it causes an increase in the levels of cyclic GMP which in turn initiates muscle relaxation. Cyclic GMP is rapidly metabolised, so continuous production of endogenous nitric oxide is vital to maintainance of pulmonary vascular tone. Inhibition of nitric oxide synthesis in fetal lambs produces marked increases in pulmonary vascular tone, suggesting that basal nitric oxide production may be important in modulating pulmonary vascular tone in the fetus[25]. Prostacyclin is produced by the lung endothelial cells and causes vasodilation when infused into fetal lungs[26] but when production is inhibited, there is little effect on pulmonary vascular resistance[27], suggesting it's role may be more important postnatally. Endothelin is a vasoconstricting peptide which is also produced by the endothelial cell. The precise physiological role for this peptide is confused by the fact that there are two endothelin receptors which mediate opposite reactions. The vasoconstricting receptor (ET_A) is located on the smooth muscle cell but there is also a receptor on the endothelial cell (ET_B) which mediates vasodilation via the nitric oxide system. If endothelin is infused into fetal or neonatal lungs the initial response is vasodilation[28] but prolonged or repeated infusion causes vasoconstriction[29]. High circulating levels of endothelin in the fetal circulation[30] and the fact that ET_A receptor blockade reduces fetal pulmonary vascular resistance[31] suggest that it may have some role in the maintenance of fetal pulmonary vasoconstriction.

After delivery, in ovine studies, the pulmonary vascular resistance falls to 10% of fetal values and pulmonary blood flow increases accordingly within minutes of the onset of respiration[32]. Pressure is the product of flow and resistance and in the very early postnatal period the changes in these two parameters balance each other out so the early fall in pulmonary artery pressure is more gradual. Emmanouilides *et al.*[33] showed in catheterised healthy term infants that up to 6 hours of age systolic pulmonary artery pressure is similar to or slightly below systolic systemic pressure while diastolic pulmonary pressure falls more rapidly and is well below diastolic systemic pressure from the first postnatal hour. Mean pulmonary artery pressure continues to fall gradually over the first 48 hours of life. This slower postnatal fall in pulmonary artery pressure has been confirmed in echocardiographic studies of normal circulatory adaptation[34,35]. So postnatal change in pulmonary vascular resistance falls into an immediate rapid phase and a more gradual phase which lasts 48 to 72 hours. The factors which mediate this change probably relate to a shift in the balance between vasoconstrictors and vasodilators described above.

At birth, direct effects of gaseous lung expansion and increasing oxygen probably provide the primary stimuli for the arterioles to dilate. Ventilating animal fetal lungs without changing blood gases will cause some reduction in pulmonary vascular resistance but not to the extent seen in the newborn. This effect is partly due to a direct physical release of external pressure on the blood vessels but is also mediated by secondary release of vasoactive substances in response to physical forces associated with ventilation. Prostacyclin is produced by physical expansion of the lung and production by the lung increases after birth[32] and inhibition of synthesis attenuates the changes in pulmonary vascular resistance seen in response to physical forces[36]. So prostacyclin seems to play some role in the pulmonary blood flow changes seen with the onset of ventilation. However, several other vasoactive mediators have also been implicated, including other prostaglandins (D_2 and E_2), bradykinin, histamine, endothelin, angiotensin II and atrial natriuretic peptide[21]. The exact way all these relate to each other and to the postnatal changes remains unclear.

Increase in oxygen is vital for a complete postnatal fall in pulmonary vascular resistance. As described previously, fetal pulmonary arterioles will dilate dramatically when unventilated lungs are exposed to hyperoxic blood, a response which becomes more marked with advancing gestation[23]. The parallel rise through gestation in nitric oxide production by the endothelial cell would suggest that much of this effect might be mediated through the nitric oxide system[37]. In animals treated with a nitric oxide synthase inhibitor, there is a reduced vasodilatory response both to ventilation with oxygen and increased oxygenation without ventilation[38]. However, nitric oxide inhibition does not effect the immediate postnatal fall in resistance which may depend more on physical factors and the resultant release of mediators such as prostacyclin[21]. In conclusion, birth and the onset of respiration stimulates a shift in the balance of vasoactive mediators to facilitate vasodilatation and dramatic increases in postnatal pulmonary blood flow result.

In persistent pulmonary hypertension of the newborn (PPHN), these changes in the pulmonary circulation fail to occur and hypoxia results from a combination of right to left shunting within the lungs and through patent fetal channels. While this can be secondary to other insults such as asphyxia or meconium aspiration, in some babies there is no clear precipitating factor. There is speculation that endothelially-derived vasoactive mediators, particularly nitric oxide, may play a role in the development of this idiopathic PPHN. It is possible to produce a model of PPHN in fetal lambs by constricting the ductus arteriosus, after which endothelially derived vasodilation is impaired but arteriolar relaxation does occur in response to exogenous nitric oxide[39]. It is also possible in lambs to produce PPHN by chronically inhibiting nitric oxide synthesis *in utero*[40]. Inappropriate levels of constrictors may also play a role. High circulating endothelin levels are found in newborns with PPHN, thromboxane is increased in experimental models of PPHN and leukotrienes have been found in tracheal aspirates of newborns with PPHN. The exact way that these observations relate to the development of PPHN and the underlying precipitant of this condition is the subject of much ongoing research[21].

The identification of nitric oxide as an important component of pulmonary vasodilation has opened up a potentially major therapeutic breakthrough. Prostacyclin and tolazoline (an α-blocking vasodilator) will both cause pulmonary vasodilation when infused into infants with PPHN but the effects on oxygenation are often limited. This probably occurs for two reasons, firstly they also dilate the systemic circulation so systemic vascular resistance is reduced by the same extent as pulmonary moisture and secondly they will dilate all pulmonary vessels including those to unventilated parts of the lung thus potentially increasing intrapulmonary right-to-left shunting. Inhaled nitric oxide does not have these problems, specifically dilating up vessels in ventilated portions of lung and, because of rapid metabolism, not having any effect on the systemic circulation[29]. Nitric oxide causes improvements in oxygenation in most babies with PPHN and represents a major advance in the management of these potentially very sick babies[41].

CLOSURE OF THE DUCTUS ARTERIOSUS

The wall of the ductus arteriosus is mainly smooth muscle. In fetal life patency is maintained by circulating prostaglandins, particularly PGE_2 but also possibly prostacyclin[42]. Fetal PGE_2 levels are several times higher than adult levels and pharmacological inhibition of prostaglandin synthesis causes constriction of the fetal ductus arteriosius[43]. The latter is an important side effect of the antenatal tocolytic use of indomethacin. During the last trimester the sensitivity of the ductus to the dilating influence of prostaglandins diminishes and the sensitivity to the constrictor effects of oxygen increases[42]. So, at birth, the main stimulus for constriction is the increasing oxygen levels. At the same time the increased pulmonary blood flow increases the clearance of PGE_2, so reducing the dilatory stimuli.

Normal closure of the ductus arteriosus in term human newborns has been studied using echocardiography. While the term ductus constricts early, complete closure often takes a day or two. In a group of 18 term infants, only 1 case of a completely closed duct was observed on scans done within the first 20 hours, but all except 1 case had closed on scans done between 40 and 60 hours of age[34]. Lim *et al.*, using colour Doppler, showed that intermittent patency can persist for up to 5 days[44]. In healthy preterm babies, ductal closure occurs in much the same time frame as term babies[34,45]. In ventilated preterm babies, ductal closure can be delayed. However, even within this sicker group there is a wide spectrum of ductal constrictive pattern from those where there is minimal postnatal constriction to those where the duct completely closes very early[46]. The reason for this variation is not understood. Immaturity of the constrictive mechanism is part of the problem as the incidence of symptomatic patent ductus arterosus (PDA) has a close inverse relationship to gestation at birth[47]. This immaturity is probably compounded in some babies by the vasodilating influence of high circulating levels of PGE_2[48]. Between 30 and 40% of babies born before 30 weeks will develop a symptomatic PDA which requires medical or surgical closure[46,47]. The common shunt direction is left to right or from the systemic to pulmonary circulation[49]. The resulting increased pulmonary blood flow reduces lung compliance, increases vulnerability to pulmonary haemorrhage and increases the risk of chronic lung damage, while reduced systemic blood flow may contribute to ischaemic end organ injury particularly to the brain. In the small minority of preterm infants who have persistent pulmonary hypertension, the PDA is also a potential site for right-to-left shunting with resulting increased hypoxaemia[49]. Of preterm PDAs, 90% will close after treatment with a prostaglandin synthetase inhibitor, usually indomethacin; a few will need surgical closure[50].

CLOSURE OF THE FORAMEN OVALE

The foramen ovale, like the rest of heart, undergoes important structural changes during the last trimester. There are two components to the foramen ovale, the fossa ovalis, a muscular rimmed rounded hole in the secondary septum, and the thin foraminal valve which hangs like a curtain on the left side of the fossa ovalis. This foraminal valve tissue has excessive fullness and, *in utero*, balloons into the left atrium allowing an anterior opening for blood to shunt from right to left. The relative size of this anterior opening reduces through pregnancy, particularly in the last trimester[51].

After birth, the increased pulmonary venous return to the left atrium and the cessation of the placental venous return to the right atrium pushes the valve tissue back to the right against the rim of the fossa ovalis. Echocardiographically, it is possible to see that this valve tissue often prolapses through into the right atrium in the early postnatal period, hence the reason that left-to-right shunting occurs. Gradually the slackness disappears and the orifice is functionally sealed. The foramen ovale does not always structurally seal, often being probe-patent at adult autopsy. Shunting through an incompetent foramen ovale is a common normal finding in well, term infants. Hiraishi *et al.*[52] showed that, within an hour of birth, 92% of normal babies had a predominantly left-to-right atrial shunt detectable on colour Doppler. This shunting is transient in almost all babies but Hannu *et al.*[53] found that 1 (5%) infant of a group of 20 who had had newborn atrial shunts, still had a detectable shunt at one year of age. These shunts are invariably small and not of any haemodynamic significance. Atrial shunting in preterm infants had also been assumed to have little haemodynamic significance but structural and functional immaturity of the foramen ovale mean that left-to-right atrial shunting is more common in preterm babies[54,55]. About one-third of very preterm babies have large shunts which can persist for several weeks[54]. When exacerbated by the left-sided overload which results from a large ductal shunt, the volume of blood shunting left to right through an incompetent foramen ovale can be greater than that through a large PDA[55]. This shunting will have an additive haemodynamic effect to that of the ductal shunting on both the pulmonary and systemic circulations. As atrial shunting often persists for considerably longer than ductal shunting, it may have as much impact on long-term respiratory outcomes[54]. Like the ductus arteriosus, the foramen ovale is also a potential site for right-to-left shunting in PPHN[49].

CHANGES IN VENTRICULAR OUTPUTS

Within a very short space of time, the ventricles have to reverse their roles with the left ventricle having to take over the sole supply of the systemic circulation. In the fetal lamb, the right ventricular (RV) output is approximately 300 ml/kg/min and the left ventricular (LV) output 150 ml/kg/min. Within an hour of the onset of breathing, the RV output has increased to 400 ml/kg/min and the LV output has increased by over 100% to the same value[56]. Agata *et al.*[57] used Doppler echocardiography to study changes in the human LV output during the transition to extrauterine life. Prepartum LV output was 170 ml/kg/min; this increased to 327 ml/kg/min at one hour of age. There was little change in heart rate between these two time periods so most of the increase was accounted for by change in stroke volume. At 24 hours of age, the LV output falls back to 245 ml/kg/min. Much of the increase in LV output relates directly to the increase in pulmonary venous return due to the increase in pulmonary blood flow described above. Also unlike the lamb, the human ductus arteriosus takes a while to constrict and the resulting left-to-right shunt further increases the preload on the left side of the heart. As the duct constricts and closes so the preload is reduced, hence at 24 hours the LV output is lower than at one hour. Other factors probably also play a role in the heart's ability to increase its output postnatally. In fetal life the relative lack of compliance of the structures surrounding the heart imposes limitations on ventricular filling and hence the ability of the fetal heart to increase output in response to increase filling pressure. At birth, the filling of the lungs with air results in much of this restraint being removed and cardiac output can increase. Finally, the perinatal surge in catecholamine secretion will enhance myocardial contractility[56]. While these changes ensure good systemic blood flow in healthy term and preterm infants, cardiac output is often significantly compromised in newborns with respiratory distress. Approximately 30% of ventilated very preterm infants have very low early ventricular outputs[49]. These low outputs probably represent the combined effects of an immature myocardium, positive pressure ventilation and shunting from the systemic to the pulmonary circulation. Need for higher ventilatory pressures and larger left-to-right ductal and atrial shunts were significantly associated with lower ventricular outputs. There are also some data to suggest a relationship between these early low outputs and injury to end organs, particularly the brain[58].

Summary

Establishment of air breathing at birth is vital for the survival of mammals. Complex changes have to occur concurrently in the lungs and cardiovascular system within a short space of time. Structural and functional maturity of these organ systems is a vital precondition to the success of these changes. Failure of any component of this adaptation has important clinical consequences for the newborn infant.

REFERENCES

1. Hislop AA, Wigglesworth JS & Desai R. Alveolar development in the human fetus and infant. *Early Hum. Dev.* **13**:1–11, 1986.
2. Langston C, Kida K, Reed M & Thurlbeck WM. Human lung growth in late gestation and in the neonate. *Am. Rev. Respir. Dis.* **129**:607–613, 1984.
3. Rona RJ, Gulliford MC & Chinn S. Effects of prematurity and intrauterine growth on respiratory health and lung function in childhood. *Br. Med. J.* **306**:817–820, 1993.
4. Kitchen WH, Olinsky A & Doyle LW. Respiratory health and lung function in 8-year-old children of very low birth weight: a cohort study. *Pediatrics* **89**:1151–1158, 1992.
5. Hawgood S, Gluckman PD & Heymann MA (eds) The alveolar region. In *Perinatal and Pediatric Pathophysiology: A Clinical Perspective*, pp. 578–584. London: Arnold, 1992.
6. Froh DK & Ballard PL. Fetal lung maturation. In *Textbook of Fetal Physiology* (eds G.D. Thornburn & R. Harding), p. 168–185. Oxford: Oxford University Press, 1994.
7. Jobe AH & Ikegami M. Surfactant metabolism. *Clin. Perinatol.* **20**:683–696, 1993.
8. Greenough A & Roberton NR. Respiratory distress syndrome. In *Neonatal Respiratory Disorders* (eds A. Greenough & N.R. Roberton), pp. 238–279. London: Arnold, 1996.
9. Walters DV, Hanson MA, Spencer JAD, Rodeck CH & Walters D. (eds) Fetal lung liquid: secretion and absorption. In *Fetus and Neonate*, pp. 42–62. Cambridge: Cambridge University Press, 1994.
10. Morrison J, Rennie J & Milton P. Neonatal respiratory morbidity and mode of delivery at term: influence of timing of elective caesarean section. *Br. J. Obstet. Gynaecol.* **102**:101–106, 1995.

11. Henderson-Smart DJ. Regulation of breathing in the perinatal period: sleep and breathing. In *Lung Biology in Health and Disease*, 2nd edn. (ed. E. Lenfant), pp. 605–647. New York: Marcel Decker, 1994.
12. Bonora M & Boule M. Breathing during sleep in fetus and newborn. In *Fetus and Neonate* (eds M.A. Hanson, J.A.D. Spencer, C.H. Rodeck & D. Walters), pp. 42–62. Cambridge: Cambridge University Press, 1994.
13. Vyas H, Field D, Milner AD & Hopkin IE. Determinants of the first inspiratory volume and functional residual capacity at birth. *Pediatr. Pulmonol.* **2**:189–193, 1986.
14. Roberton NRC, Yu V (eds) Resuscitation of the Newborn Infant. In *Pulmonary Problems in the Perinatal Period and their Sequelae*, Vol. 1, pp. 1–26. Cambridge: Baillière Tindall, 1995.
15. Tyson JE, Sinclair JC, Bracken M (eds) Immediate care of the newborn infant. In *Effective Care of the Newborn Infant*, pp. 21–38. Oxford: Oxford University Press, 1992.
16. Henderson-Smart DJ, Beckerman RC, Brouillette RT & Hunt CE (eds) Apnea of prematurity. In *Respiratory Control Disorders in Infants and Children*, pp. 161–177. Baltimore, MD: Williams & Wilkins, 1992.
17. Glotzbach SF, Ariagno RL, Beckerman RC, Brouillette RT & Hunt CE (eds) Periodic breathing. In *Respiratory Control Disorders in Infants and Children*, pp. 142–160. Baltimore, MD: Williams & Wilkins, 1992.
18. Henderson-Smart DJ & Yu VYH (eds) Recurrent apnoea. In *Pulmonary Problems in the Perinatal Period and their Sequelae*, pp. 203–222. London: Baillière Tindall, 1995.
19. Henderson-Smart DJ, Pettigrew AG & Campbell DJ. Clinical apnea and brainstem neural function in preterm infants. *New Engl. J. Med.* **308**:353–357, 1983.
20. National Institutes of Health and Human Development. Consensus Development Conference on Infantile Apnea and Home Monitoring. *Pediatrics* **79**:292–299, 1987.
21. Fineman JR, Soifer SJ & Heyman MA. Regulation of pulmonary vascular tone in the perinatal period. *Annu. Rev. Physiol.* **57**:115–134, 1995.
22. Soifer SJ, Kaslow D, Roman C & Heymann MA. Umbilical cord compression produces pulmonary hypertension in newborn lambs: a model to study the pathophysiology of persistent pulmonary hypertension in the newborn. *J. Dev. Physiol.* **9**:239–252, 1987.
23. Morin FC, Egan EA, Ferguson W & Lundgren CEG. Development of pulmonary vascular response to oxygen. *J. Physiol.* **254**:H542–H546, 1988.
24. Soifer SJ, Loitz RD, Roman C & Heymann MA. Leukotriene end organ antagonists increase pulmonary blood flow in fetal lambs. *Am. J. Physiol.* **249**:H570–H576, 1985.
25. Moore P, Velvis H, Fineman JR, Soifer SJ & Heymann MA. EDRF inhibition attenuates the increase in pulmonary blood flow due to oxygen ventilation in fetal lambs. *J. Appl. Physiol.* **73**:2151–2157, 1992.
26. Cassin S, Winikor I & Tod ML. The effects of prostacyclin on the fetal pulmonary circulation. *Pediatr. Pharmacol.* **1**:197, 1981.
27. Morin FC, Egan EA & Norfleet WT. Indomethacin does not diminish the pulmonary vascular response of the fetus to increased oxygen tension. *Pediatr. Res.* **24**:696–700, 1988.
28. Bradley LM, Czaja JF & Goldstein RE. Circulatory effects of endothelin in newborn piglets. *Am. J. Physiol.* **259**:H1613–H1617, 1990.
29. Zeigler JW, Ivy DD, Kinsella JP & Abman SH. The role of nitric oxide, endothelin and prostaglandins in the transition of the pulmonary circulation. *Clin. Perinatol.* **22**:387–403, 1995.
30. Nakamura T, Kasai K, Konuma S, Emoto T, Banba N, Ishikawa M & Shimoda S. Immunoreactive endothelin concentrations in maternal and fetal blood. *Life Sci.* **46**:1045–1050, 1990.
31. Wong J, Fineman JR & Heymann MA. The role of endothelin-1 and of endothelin receptor subtypes in regulation of fetal pulmonary vascular tone. *Pediatr. Res.* **35**:664–670, 1994.
32. Leffler CW, Hessler JR & Green RS. The onset of breathing at birth stimulates pulmonary vascular prostacyclin synthesis. *Pediatr. Res.* **18**:938–942, 1984.
33. Emmanouilides GC, Moss AJ, Duffie ER & Adams FH. Pulmonary arterial pressure changes in human newborn infants from birth to 3 days of age. *J. Pediatr.* **65**:327–333, 1964.
34. Evans NJ & Archer LNJ. Postnatal circulatory adaptation in term and healthy preterm infants. *Arch. Dis. Childh.* **65**:24–26, 1991.
35. Skinner JR, Boys RJ, Hunter S & Hey EN. Non invasive assessment of pulmonary arterial pressure in healthy neonates. *Arch. Dis. Childh.* **66**:386–390, 1991.
36. Velvis H, Moore P & Heymann MA. Prostaglandin inhibition prevents the fall in pulmonary vascular resistance as a result of rhythmic distension of the lung in fetal lambs. *Pediatr. Res.* **30**:62–68, 1991.
37. Shaul PW, Farrar MA & Magness RR. Pulmonary endothelial nitric oxide production is developmentally regulated in the fetus and newborn. *Am. J. Physiol.* **265**:H1056–H1063, 1993.
38. Abman SH, Chatfield BA, Hall SL & McMurtry IF. Role of endothelium derived relaxing factor during transition of pulmonary circulation at birth. *Am. J. Physiol.* **259**:H1921–H1927, 1990.
39. McQueston JA, Kinsella JP, Ivy DD, McMurtry IF & Abman SH. Chronic pulmonary hypertension *in utero* impairs endothelium dependent vasodilation. *Am. J. Physiol.* **268**:H288–H294, 1995.
40. Fineman JR, Wong J, Morin FC, Wright L & Soifer SJ. Chronic nitric oxide inhibition *in utero* produces persistent pulmonary hypertension in newborn lambs. *J. Clin. Invest.* **93**:2675–2683, 1994.
41. Finer NN, Etches PC, Kamstra B, Tierney AJ, Peliowski A & Ryan GA. Inhaled nitric oxide in infants referred for extracorporeal membrane oxygenation: dose response. *J. Pediatr.* **124**:302–308, 1994.
42. Clyman RI. Ductus arteriosus: current theories of prenatal and postnatal regulation. *Semin. Perinatol.* **11**:64–71, 1987.
43. Coceani F & Olley PM. Role of prostaglandins, prostacyclin and thomboxane in the control of prenatal patency and postnatal closure of the ductus arteriosus. *Semin. Perinatol.* **4**:109–113, 1980.
44. Lim MK, Hanretty K, Houston AB, Lilley S & Murtagh EP. Intermittent ductal patency in healthy newborn infants: demonstration by colour Doppler flow mapping. *Arch. Dis. Childh.* **67**:1217–1218, 1992.
45. Reller MD, Rice MJ & McDonald RW. Review of studies evaluating ductal patency in the premature infant. *J. Pediatr.* **122**:S59–S62, 1993.
46. Evans N & Iyer P. Longitudinal changes in the diameter of the ductus arteriosus in ventilated preterm infants: correlation with respiratory outcomes. *Arch. Dis. Childh.* **72**:156–161, 1995.
47. Kluckow M & Evans N. Early echocardiographic prediction of symptomatic patent ductus arteriosus in preterm infants requiring mechanical ventilation. *J. Pediatr.* **127**:774–779, 1995.
48. Hammerman C, Strates E & Valaitis S. The silent ductus: its precursors and its aftermath. *Pediatr. Cardiol.* **7**:121–127, 1986.
49. Evans N & Kluckow M. Early determinants of right and left ventricular output in ventilated preterm infants. *Arch. Dis. Childh.* **74**:F88–F94, 1996.
50. Yu VYH. Patent ductus arterious in the preterm infant. *Early Hum. Dev.* **35**:1–14, 1993.
51. Patten BM, Sommerfield WA & Paff GH. Functional limitations of the foramen ovale in the human foetal heart. *Anat. Rec.* **44**:165–178, 1929.
52. Hiraishi S, Agata Y, Saito K, Oguchi K, Misawa H, Fujino N, Horiguchi Y & Yashiro K. Interatrial shunt flow profiles in newborn infants: a colour flow and pulsed Doppler echocardiographic study. *Br. Heart J.* **65**:41–45, 1991.
53. Hannu H, Pentii K, Hendrik E, Markku S & Illka V. Patency of the foramen ovale-does it influence haemodynamics in newborn infants? *Early Hum. Dev.* **20**:281–287, 1989.
54. Evans N & Iyer P. Incompetence of the foramen ovale in preterm infants supported by mechanical ventilation. *J. Pediatr.* **125**:786–792, 1994.
55. Evans N & Iyer P. Assessment of ductus arteriosus shunt in preterm infants supported by mechanical ventilation: effect of interatrial shunting. *J. Pediatr.* **125**:777–785, 1994.
56. Walker AM, Hanson MA, Spencer JAD & Rodeck CH (eds) Circulatory transitions at birth and the control of the neonatal circulation. In *Fetus and Neonate Physiology and Clinical Applications: The Circulation*, vol. 7, pp. 160–196. Cambridge: Cambridge University Press, 1993.
57. Agata Y, Hiraishi S, Oguchi K, Misawa H, Horiguchi Y, Fujino N, Yashiro K & Shimada N. Changes in left ventricular output from fetal to early neonatal life. *J. Pediatr.* **119**:441–445, 1991.
58. Evans N & Kluckow M. Early ductal shunting and intraventricular haemorrhage in ventilated preterm infants? *Arch. Dis. Childh.* **75**:F183–F186, 1996.

Thermal adaptation to extrauterine life

80

N. Rutter

Introduction

Man and the other mammals are homeotherms. They have the ability to control their body temperature within a narrow range in the face of a wide variety of environmental conditions. They achieve this by displaying a number of physiological and behavioural changes aimed at conserving or losing heat. The newborn is homeothermic too but physical, physiological and behavioural differences mean that conservation of heat is more difficult and the range of environmental conditions over which a normal body temperature can be maintained is smaller. The fetus has some homeothermic mechanisms but its size in relation to the mother and its position within her body mean that it is in effect poikilothermic. Thus its body temperature reflects the environmental temperature, namely that of its mother. If the mother's temperature is high, so will be the fetal temperature. If the mother's temperature is low, again so will be the fetal temperature. Adaptation from a state of poikilothermy to one of homeothermy has to take place quickly at birth.

Much information on the control of body temperatures in the newborn has been obtained from direct observation and study of the human as well as experimental animals. Understandably, most information on the control of body temperature *in utero* is derived from work in animals, in particular the ewe and fetal lamb. The newborn lamb is developmentally more advanced than the newborn infant and has more mature thermoregulatory mechanisms but the principles are the same. It is therefore likely that the findings can be applied to the human.

Fetal temperature

It might be assumed that fetal temperature is identical to that of the mother, and determined by the thermal environment provided by the amniotic fluid. However, it is consistently higher. Direct measurements in the human have been made at the time of elective caesarean section, induction of labour or during labour. The results are summarised in the Table 80.1[1–5]. The healthy fetus is about 0.5°C (0.2–0.8°C) warmer than its mother, depending on which maternal and fetal temperatures are measured. Amniotic fluid, fetal skin and fetal rectal temperatures are similar. This feto-maternal temperature gradient is present in the sheep[6], baboon[7] and rabbit[8] as well. It remains unchanged during the later stages of pregnancy. The gradient is unaffected by the presence of hypothermia in the mother but it widens during maternal fever[9]. The temperature of the fetus is always higher than that of the mother, regardless of maternal temperature.

The feto-maternal temperature gradient can be predicted on theoretical grounds. The fetus creates heat by metabolic activity and movement; this can only be dissipated to the mother if there is a downward temperature gradient from fetus to mother. In the newborn, the main site of dissipation of heat is from the surface of the skin. In the fetus it is via the placenta. It has been estimated in studies in sheep that 85% of heat produced by the fetal lamb is dissipated to the ewe via the placenta[10]. The remaining 15% is via the fetal skin, amniotic fluid and uterine wall. If assumptions are made for normal values of placental thermal diffusion capacity, fetal heat production and placental blood flow, a feto-maternal gradient of 0.3 to 0.6°C is predicted, similar to the measured difference[11].

FETAL THERMOREGULATION

Physiological mechanisms which after birth result in heat production or heat loss appear to be suppressed in the fetus. Sweating in response to a high environmental temperature occurs in the newborn from 36 weeks' gestation onwards but is absent *in utero*. Immersion in fluid suppresses sweating, a phenomenon known as anhydrohidrosis. Heat production from the oxidation of brown fat occurs in the newborn but

TABLE 80.1
Comparison of fetal and maternal temperatures in the human based on five studies

Study	Time of study	Patients (*n*)	Mean maternal temperature (°C)	Mean fetal temperature (°C)	Difference of mean temperatures (°C)
Wood and Beard[1]	In labour	8	36.7 (rectal)	37.6 (rectal)	0.9
Adamsons and Towell[2]	In labour	13	37.15 (colonic)	37.65 (rectal)	0.5
Walker *et al.*[3]	Elective LSCS*	4	37.15 (myometrium)	37.6 (skin)	0.45
	Labour	9	37.35 (rectal)	37.8 (scalp)	0.45
Mann[4]	At induction of labour	6	37.39 (rectal)	37.65 (intra-amniotic)	0.28
Macaulay *et al.*[5]	During labour	36	36.87 (uterine wall)	37.10 (skin)	0.23

*LSCS = lower segment caesarean section.

detailed experimental work in sheep suggests that it is suppressed *in utero*[12]. The potential for non-shivering thermogenesis is certainly present *in utero*, as it can be demonstrated immediately after birth. Cooling of the fetus and increasing the fetal oxygen tension to mimic postnatal existence do not result in non-shivering thermogenesis, but occlusion of the umbilical cord does. This suggests that the placenta secretes factors into the fetal circulation which inhibit the oxidation of brown adipose tissue to produce heat. It is postulated that placental prostaglandin E_2 and adenosine are the inhibitors.

THE EFFECTS OF A HIGH OR LOW FETAL TEMPERATURE

Since the fetal temperature is dependent on maternal temperature, maternal fever or hypothermia results in similar changes in fetal temperature. In early pregnancy during organogenesis, a link has been postulated between febrile illness in the mother and neural tube defects[13], in particular encephalocoele. A raised temperature of the embryo has been suggested as the cause of this possible association. In the second and third trimesters, the only effect of maternal hyperthermia or hypothermia appears to be on the fetal heart rate. There are isolated case reports of maternal hypothermia, either accidental or drug-induced, where a fetal bradycardia was noted which gradually resolved when the mother was rewarmed[14–16].

Deep hypothermia (cooling to below 30°C) is commonly used together with cardiopulmonary bypass in open heart surgery, but such surgery is not often necessary during pregnancy. In one reported case, a fetus at 21 weeks survived a maternal core temperature of 19°C for 37 min[17]. In a recent review of 69 cardiac operations performed on cardiopulmonary bypass in pregnancy, maternal mortality was 3% and embryo or fetal mortality was 20%[18]. There was a suggestion that the use of hypothermia increased the fetal loss, although it is difficult to separate the effect of hypothermia from poor placental perfusion during bypass. A raised maternal temperature can occur as a result of a febrile illness, in a hot environment such as a sauna, or after prolonged exercise. Apart from a possible teratogenic effect in early pregnancy[19], there is no evidence of any adverse effect on the fetus[20,21].

Fetal temperature during labour

The feto-maternal temperature gradient noted during pregnancy persists throughout labour (Table 80.1) to delivery[4]. There is some evidence that the gradient widens during labour, especially if prolonged. Epidural anaesthesia appears to exaggerate the normal increase in fetal temperature which occurs during labour. Macaulay *et al.*[22] measured fetal skin and maternal uterine wall temperature during 57 labours at term and estimated that 5% of fetuses reach a body temperature of 40°C by the end of a labour in which epidural anaesthesia is used. However, use of epidural anaesthesia is widespread and experience of its use extends over many years. No adverse effect of inadvertent fetal hyperthermia has been shown.

It was suggested some years ago that since most heat produced by the fetus is removed via the placenta, measurement of the feto-maternal temperature gradient would provide an indication of placental function and fetal wellbeing[11]. Theoretically, with failing placental function, the gradient would increase as heat removal is impaired. With increasing placental failure, fetal heat production would fall and the gradient would start to decrease. Finally, with fetal death, there would be no heat production and therefore no temperature gradient between mother and fetus. Macaulay *et al.*[5] have attempted to exploit this as a test of placental function. They rightly point out that although many fetuses develop a high body temperature during labour because of an increase in maternal temperature, some have an isolated rise. These are febrile fetuses who might have an underlying illness such as an intrauterine infection. Such a fetus would have a persistent tachycardia as a result of the fever, in the presence of a normal maternal temperature.

Thermoregulation adaptation at birth

Immediately after birth, the newborn infant must adapt to independent thermoregulation. Physical factors act to produce cold stress. The newborn produces heat by metabolic activity, a function of body weight. It loses heat by convection, radiation and evaporation from the skin, a function of surface area. The newborn has a low weight to surface area ratio, so heat production is low relative to heat loss. The smaller the infant the more unfavourable the ratio becomes and the greater the loss of heat relative to its generation. Thus the newborn infant is always at greater risk of hypothermia than overheating, and this risk is much greater for the small preterm infant.

HEAT PRODUCTION

The newborn produces heat as a by-product of cell metabolism and as a consequence of movement, in a similar way to a child or adult. In addition, it has a specialised organ of heat production, brown adipose tissue[23]. This tissue is situated subcutaneously between the scapulae, and deep within the body, particularly along the aorta. It has a rich blood supply. In response to catecholamines there is uncoupling of oxidative phosphorylation within the mitochrondria which releases energy as heat. The infant can more than double its resting heat production by this means[24]. This heat production, known as non-shivering thermogenesis (NST) is impaired in all newborn infants in the first few hours of life[25], in ill infants, especially those who are hypoxic or who have been asphyxiated, and in infants born to mothers who have been sedated with benzodiazepines, such as diazepam[26] and lorazepam[27].

Gunn and Gluckman[12] have demonstrated that NST is inhibited *in utero* by placental factors, including prostaglandin E_2[28] and adenosine[29]. This prevents brown adipose tissue from responding to the usual stimuli. Once the umbilical cord is occluded, this inhibition is removed[30]. The massive stimulation of cutaneous cold receptors by evaporative and convective cooling, and the increase in arterial p_{O_2} which occurs when breathing is established mean that NST is maximally stimulated in the newborn lamb[31]. It is likely that similar mechanisms result in the switching on of NST in the human newborn although the relative immaturity at the time of birth suggests that the magnitude of the response would be less.

Newborn body temperature

Mann[4] measured the rectal temperature of 50 spontaneous vertex deliveries at term and found a mean of 37.8°C (range 36.4 to 38.9°C). The mean maternal temperature was 37.3°C (range 36.1 to 38.7°C) and the mean neonatal maternal difference was 0.8°C (range 0.1 to 1.5°C). Similar findings were observed in three breech deliveries. If maternal temperature is raised, the newborn temperature will always be raised. If there is a raised newborn temperature at delivery in the absence of a raised maternal temperature, a febrile illness in the baby should be suspected.

The normal rectal temperature of the newborn beyond the first hours is 36.5 to 37.5°C regardless of weight or gestation. There is a fall in body temperature after birth because heat loss occurs readily from the skin rather than by the placenta. Mann[4] found that in a warm labour suite, a wrapped term infant experienced a fall in body temperature of 0.5°C in the first 15 min after birth. This is greater if the infant is small, exposed or asphyxiated. For example, a baby of less than 1 kg birthweight who is exposed in a cool room can experience a fall in body temperature of 1°C every five minutes.

Thermoregulation in the newborn[32]

Under steady-state conditions, heat production and heat loss are balanced and body temperature is stable. Heat production has previously been described. Heat loss can be increased or decreased by a number of physical, physiological and behavioural mechanisms. If heat loss exceeds production, body temperature falls until a new equilibrium is reached.

HEAT LOSS

PHYSICAL HEAT LOSS

Heat is lost by the processes of convection (from warm skin to cold air), radiation (from warm skin to cold surfaces) and evaporation of water. Conduction is a minor channel of heat loss.

PHYSIOLOGICAL HEAT LOSS

By diverting blood from the surface to the core, heat losses are reduced. Skin blood flow is an important determinant of heat loss in the newborn; even the most immature has the ability to regulate skin blood flow[33]. Sweating, which increases evaporative heat loss, can occur in the term infant in response to a warm environment[34]. However, in intensity and extent it is much less well developed than in the older infant or child. The preterm infant is unable to sweat in the newborn period[35]. Sweat glands are well developed by 22 weeks' gestation and are more densely distributed than in the child or adult since the number of glands is fixed in fetal life. The reduction or absence of sweating is therefore a result of functional immaturity of the sweating mechanism.

BEHAVIOURAL HEAT LOSS

The newborn infant has a limited capacity for behavioural thermoregulation. Some postural changes in response to cold or heat stress have been noted. For example, in a warm environment, the newborn will lie in an extended posture, maximising the exposed surface to increase heat loss. In a cold environment, a more flexed posture is adopted to reduce the exposed surface and reduce heat loss. More importantly perhaps, the hot or cold infant may wake up and cry, demanding a response from the mother. This behavioural thermoregulation is very important in the animal kingdom and underestimated in the human. The mother instinctively swaddles and cuddles her infant. A 3-kg infant held closely against a 70-kg mother now has a much larger thermal mass and a much reduced exposed surface for heat loss. Intervention by midwives and doctors prevents this form of thermoregulation.

THERMAL NEUTRALITY[36]

There is a zone of environmental temperature within which an infant's heat production is at a minimum, body temperature is in the normal range and there is no sweating. Fine thermoregulation is maintained by changes in skin blood flow, posture and activity. This is termed the 'thermoneutral range'. A very small preterm infant nursed naked has a higher and narrower thermoneutral range than a term infant. The effect of clothing is to lower and widen the range.

As the environmental temperature falls below the neutral range, heat production is increased by NST and body temperature remains normal (Fig. 80.1). Once heat production reaches a maximum level, further lowering of environmental temperature results in a fall in body temperature. If the environmental temperature increases beyond the neutral range, the infant sweats in an attempt to lose heat; when this is no longer effective, body temperature rises.

It is evident from this that a baby can be nursed in an environment which results in cold stress but no fall in body temperature. The body is expending energy on keeping warm rather than on growing. There is evidence from the pre-neonatal intensive care era that nursing preterm infants in a cold environment results in a higher mortality[37–40] and reduced growth[41,42]. Preterm infants who become hypothermic in the immediate newborn period are more likely to become ill and to suffer from long-term neurological sequelae or to die[43]. For these reasons, strenuous efforts should be made to prevent hypothermia at delivery and to nurse small babies in a warm neutral thermal environment.

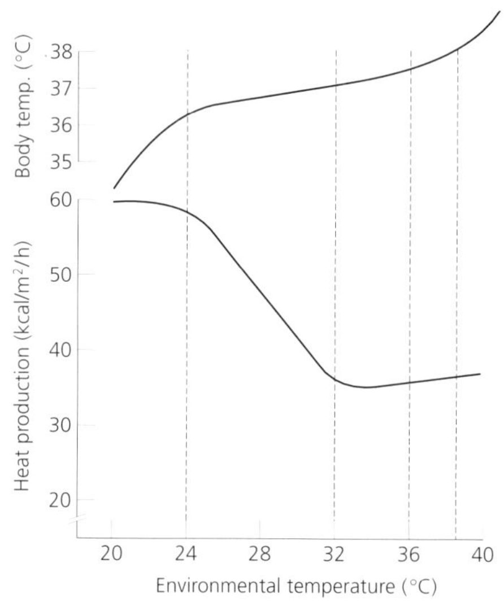

Fig. 80.1 The effect of environmental temperature on heat production and body temperature of a 1.9-kg infant of 34 weeks' gestation, nursed naked in surroundings of uniform temperature and moderate humidity. Between 32 and 36°C, heat production is minimal, there is no sweating and body temperature is normal (neutral thermal range). When the environmental temperature falls below 32°C, heat production increases by non-shivering thermogenesis, but below 24°C heat production has reached its maximum and body temperature rapidly falls. Above 36°C, the infant sweats, and above 38°C body temperature rises quickly[32].

The thermal environment of the newborn[32]

AT DELIVERY

Most delivery rooms and operating theatres are at a temperatures which are comfortable for clothed adults but too cold for naked infants, particularly if small or ill. Heat losses by convection, radiation and evaporation are high, exceeding the heat production. The ideal temperature of the room or theatre is about 25°C. The newly born infant should be dried at once with a warm towel. If resuscitation is necessary, supplementary heat should be from an overhead radiant heater. If the infant is going to spend some time within a cot in the delivery room, clothing, bedding and a supplementary heat source will prevent a fall in body temperature. Weighing, cleaning, bathing, care of the umbilical cord and the fixing of name-bands result in exposure, cold stress and a fall in body temperature. An infant is more likely to stay warm if held by the mother. Skin-to-skin contact, with covering of the baby's exposed skin, is an effective means of thermoregulation.

THE TERM INFANT

A newborn infant when dressed, wrapped and cot-nursed in a warm room is in a neutral thermal environment. The range of environmental temperatures the infant can tolerate is wide.

THE PRETERM INFANT

For reasons already explained, the small preterm infant is prone to cold stress. The risk of this is much greater if the infant is nursed naked, which may be necessary for access or observation. The infant therefore needs an alternative environment such as an incubator or radiant warmer. The required air temperature of the incubator may be as high as 37°C for a baby below 1 kg in the first few days of life.

THE VERY IMMATURE INFANT[44]

The extremely immature infant born at 26 weeks' gestation or earlier has a very unfavourable weight to surface ratio and requires a very high environmental temperature. The body temperature tends to drift up and down with the environmental temperature since thermoregulatory mechanisms are immature and swamped by high heat losses; the body therefore behaves like a poikilotherm. An additional and important heat loss is by evaporation from the skin. Epidermal development is poor[45], its barrier function is weak and transepidermal water loss is high[46]. Such infants are usually nursed in a highly humid environment in order to reduce water and evaporative heat loss from the skin[47].

REFERENCES

1. Wood C & Beard RW. Temperature of the human foetus. *J. Obstet. Gynaec. Brit. Cwlth.* **71**:768–769, 1964.
2. Adamsons K & Towell ME. Thermal homeostasis of the fetus and newborn. *Anesthesiology* **26**:531–548, 1965.
3. Walker D, Walker A & Wood C. Temperature of the human fetus. *J. Obstet. Gynaec. Brit. Cwlth* **76**:503–511, 1969.
4. Mann TP. Observations on temperatures of mothers and babies in the perinatal period. *J. Obstet. Gynaec. Brit. Cwlth.* **75**:316–321, 1968.
5. Macaulay JH, Randall NR, Bond K & Steer PJ. Continuous monitoring of fetal temperature by non-invasive probe and its relationship to maternal temperature, fetal heart rate and cord arterial oxygen and pH. *Obstet. Gynaecol.* **79**:469–474, 1992.
6. Gilbert RD & Power GG. Fetal and uteroplacental heat production in sheep. *J. Appl. Physiol.* **61**:2018–2022, 1986.
7. Morishima HO, Yeh M, Niemann WH, James LS. Temperature gradient between fetus and mother as an index for assessing intrauterine fetal condition. *Am. J. Obstet. Gynaecol.* **129**:443–448, 1977.
8. Hart FM & Faber JJ. Fetal and maternal temperatures in rabbits. *J. Appl. Physiol.* **20**:737–741, 1965.
9. Laburn HP, Mitchell D & Goelst K. Fetal and maternal body temperatures measured by radiotelemetry in near-term sheep during thermal stress. *J. Appl. Physiol.* **72**:894–900, 1992.
10. Gilbert RD, Schroder H, Kawamura T, Dale PS & Power GG. Heat transfer pathways between fetal lamb and ewe. *J. Appl. Physiol.* **59**:634–638, 1985.
11. Adamsons K. The role of thermal factors in fetal and neonatal life. *Pediatr. Clin. N. Am.* **13**:599–619, 1966.
12. Gunn TR & Gluckman PD. Perinatal thermogenesis. *Early Hum. Dev.* **42**:169–183, 1995.
13. Hunter AGW. Neural tube defects in Eastern Ontario and Western Quebec. *Am. J. Med. Gen.* **19**:45–63, 1984.
14. Rodis JF, Vintzileos AM & Campbell WA. Maternal hypothermia: an unusual complication of magnesium sulphate therapy. *Am. J. Obstet. Gynaecol.* **156**:435–436, 1987.
15. Jadhon ME & Main EK. Fetal bradycardia associated with maternal hypothermia. *Obstet. Gynecol.* **72**:496–497, 1988.
16. Tanaka M, Ikeda T, Suzuki T, Yakubo K & Fukuiya T. A case of fetal bradycardia and sinusoid-like fetal heart rate pattern associated with maternal hypothermia. *Fetal Diagn. Therapy* **10**:207–209, 1995.
17. Buffolo E, Palma JH, Gomes WJ *et al.* Successful use of deep hypothermic circulatory arrest in pregnancy. *Ann. Thoracic Surg.* **58**:1532–1534, 1994.
18. Pomini F, Mercogliano D, Cavalletti C, Caruso A & Pomiru P. Cardiopulmonary bypass in pregnancy. *Ann. Thoracic Surg.* **61**:259–268, 1996.
19. Milunsky A, Ulcickas M, Rothman KJ, Willett W, Jick SS & Jick H. Maternal heat exposure and neural tube defects. *JAMA* **268**:882–885, 1992.
20. Lotgering FK, Gilbert RD & Longo LD. The interactions of exercise and pregnancy: a review. *Am. J. Obstet. Gynecol.* **149**:560–568, 1984.
21. Sedgewick Harvey MA, McRorie MM & Smith DW. Suggested limits to the use of the hot tub and sauna by pregnant women. *Can. Med. Assoc. J.* **125**:50–53, 1981.
22. Macaulay JH, Bond K & Steer PJ. Epidural analgesia in labour and fetal hyperthermia. *Obstet. Gynecol.* **80**:665–669, 1992.
23. Hull D. The structure and function of brown adipose tissue. *Br. Med. Bull.* **22**:92–96, 1966.
24. Hey EN. The relation between environmental temperature and oxygen consumption in the newborn baby. *J. Physiol.* **200**:589–603, 1969.
25. Smales ORC & Kime R. Thermoregulation in babies immediately after birth. *Arch. Dis. Childh.* **53**:58–61, 1978.
26. Cree JE, Meyer J & Hailey DM. Diazepam in labour: its metabolism and effect on the clinical condition and thermogenesis of the newborn. *BMJ* **iv**:251–255, 1973.
27. Johnstone M & Whitelaw A. Effect of maternal lorazepam on the neonate. *BMJ* **282**:1973–1974, 1981.
28. Gunn TR, Ball KT & Gluckman PD. Withdrawal of placental prostaglandins permits thermogenic responses in fetal sheep brown adipose tissue. *J. Appl. Physiol.* **74**:998–1004, 1993.
29. Ball KT, Gunn TR, Power GG, Asakura H & Gluckman PD. A potential role for adenosine in the inhibition of nonshivering thermogenesis in the fetal sheep. *Pediatr. Res.* **37**:303–309, 1995.
30. Gunn TR, Ball KT & Gluckman PD. Reversible umbilical cord occlusion: effect on thermogenesis *in utero*. *Pediatr. Res.* **30**:513–517, 1991.
31. Gunn TR, Ball KT, Power GG & Gluckman PD. Factors influencing the initiation of nonshivering thermogenesis. *Am. J. Obstet. Gynecol.* **164**:210–217, 1991.
32. Rutter N. Temperature control and its disorders. In *Textbook of Neonatology*, 2nd edn. (ed. N.R.C. Robertson), pp. 217–231. Edinburgh: Churchill Livingstone, 1992.
33. Harpin VA, Chellapah G & Rutter N. The responses of the newborn infant to overheating. *Biol. Neonate* **44**:65–75, 1983.
34. Rutter N & Hull D. Response of term babies to a warm environment. *Arch. Dis. Childh.* **54**:178–183, 1979.
35. Harpin VA & Rutter N. Sweating in preterm babies. *J. Pediatr.* **100**:614–618, 1982.
36. Hey EN. Thermal neutrality. *Br. Med. Bull.* **31**:69–74, 1975.
37. Silverman WA, Fertig JW & Berger AP. The influence of the thermal environmental upon the survival of newly born premature infants. *Pediatrics* **22**:876–885, 1958.
38. Jolly H, Molyneaux P & Newell DJ. A controlled study of the effect of temperature on premature babies. *J. Pediatr.* **60**:889–894, 1962.
39. Day RL, Caliguiri L, Kamenski C & Erlich F. Body temperature and survival of premature infants. *Pediatrics* **34**:171–181, 1964.
40. Buetow KC & Klein SW. Effects of maintenance of normal skin temperature of survival of infants of low birth weight. *Pediatrics* **34**:163–170, 1964.
41. Glass L, Silverman WA & Sinclair JC. Effect of the thermal environment and cold resistance and growth of small infants after the first week of life. *Pediatrics* **41**:1033–1046, 1968.

The contribution of preterm birth to outcomes in children

82

N. Wood and N. Marlow

Introduction

Neonatal intensive care has been a major growth area in clinical medicine over the past twenty years as improving perinatal and neonatal care has resulted in the survival of children at gestations down to below 24 weeks. This chapter provides an overview of what the future may hold for very preterm survivors, with regards to impairments in neuromotor, sensory, cognitive, behavioural, developmental and psychological function, together with the longer term effects on the child. It remains important to address such issues as how children with problems are identified early, what problems they are likely to encounter, how they function with regards to their peer population and how morbidity may be minimised in this group.

Many studies have used birthweight as a marker of perinatal risk among the very preterm population. However, as the accuracy with which gestation is assessed has improved[1] it seems more appropriate to assess outcome on a gestational basis[2,3] and, within those groups, to consider the effect of restricted intrauterine growth, rather than persisting with the familiar birthweight groups (very low birthweight (<1501 g); extremely low birthweight (<1001 g) which comprise a mixture of appropriately grown very premature children and more mature but growth-restricted children. Where possible we will report studies which have used a gestational base but many of the descriptions of longer term outcomes are based on birthweight groupings.

Epidemiology

SURVIVAL

Survival rates at low gestations have increased dramatically since the 1980s with improvements in obstetric and neonatal care, in particular the now routine and well-validated use of antenatal steroids and artificial surfactant[4,5]. Studies which have reported survival rates by gestational age are summarised in Table 82.1. Survival beyond 27 weeks' gestation now exceeds 70%, and for many neonatal services will exceed 90%.

However, there is still debate as to whether there has been much change in survival at the limits of viability despite these measures. Survival rates for 23 to 26 weeks of gestation vary considerably within the literature, a result of differing population selection criteria, inclusion of outborn infants (only those in best condition are likely to be referred to tertiary units), and the individual experiences and beliefs of both neonatologists and obstetricians[7,38,39]. Reported rates of survival tending to be higher from North America. Figure 82.1 demonstrates the variation in reported rates of survival at 25 weeks' gestation, which are scattered widely around a mean of 43%, although common belief holds that survival without disability at this gestation is in excess of 50%. Survival at these low gestations across the UK and Eire in 1995 is currently the subject of the EPICure study[40]. This unique study is evaluating outcome for pregnancies which deliver at 20–25 weeks (inclusive) gestation across the whole range of maternity units and neonatal intensive care settings. Admission rates for births at 23, 24, 25 weeks' gestation were 22, 50 and 61%, respectively. Of these admissions, survival to expected date of delivery was reported in 28, 35 and 54% respectively (see Table 82.2).

DISABILITY

Changes in the incidence and prevalence of disability are difficult to identify; despite numerous studies, few are comparable due to differing population groups, methodology, statistical methods and assessment. The definitions of impairments, disabilities and handicap used also vary, often making the frequently used categories of 'mild', 'moderate' and 'severe' difficult to analyse. More recently, there have been

TABLE 82.1
Summary of studies reporting survival per gestational age

Study	Study Period	Survival at	Survival per gestational age (weeks) (percentage in parentheses) 22	23	24	25	26	27	28	29
Cartlidge[6]	1993–4	1 year	0/11	1/22 (5)	6/31 (19)	19/41 (46)	40/59 (68)	39/57 (68)	80/105 (76)	83/101 (82)
Gultom[7]	1992–4	Discharge		2/19 (11)	18/34 (53)	43/61 (70)	47/58 (81)	48/55 (87)		
Tin[8]	1991–4	One year	0/27	1/49 (2)	13/78 (17)	36/103 (35)	72/136 (53)	117/167 (70)		
Bohin[9]	1991–3	Discharge	0/6	1/37 (3)	27/95 (28)	38/104 (37)	73/132 (55)	132/186 (71)	181/227 (80)	199/230 (87)
Victorian Infant[10]	1991–2	2 years		5/52 (10)	21/63 (33)	51/88 (58)	71/98 (72)	77/100 (77)		
Hack[11]	1990–2	20 months	1/27 (4)	2/27 (7)	16/40 (29)	35/56 (63)	33/43 (77)	59/71 (83)		
Finnström[12]	1990–2	One year		4/47 (9)	25/90 (28)	59/110 (54)	94/133 (71)	62/85 (73)	45/63 (71)	37/46 (80)
Philip[13]	1990–2	Discharge			16/32 (50)	33/40 (83)	19/21 (90)	19/19 (100)	11/11 (100)	5/5 (100)
Katz[14]	1989–91	Discharge		0/21	5/11 (46)	14/22 (64)	18/25 (72)	31/35 (89)		
Gultom[7]	1989–91	Discharge		0/19	1/20 (5)	18/46 (39)	45/59 (76)	53/64 (83)		
Lefebvre[15]	1987–92	18 months		0/38	9/47 (19)	31/69 (45)	44/75 (61)	91/125 (73)	79/114 (69)	
Holtrop[16]	1988–91	Discharge		5/27 (19)	17/29 (59)	17/26 (65)				
Allen[17]	1988–91	6 months	0/22	6/36 (17)	19/54 (35)	31/39 (79)				
Tin[8]	1987–90	2 years	0/16	6/33 (18)	13/78 (17)	30/91 (32)	55/122 (45)	91/143 (64)		
Ferrara[18]	1986–90	Discharge			12/32 (38)	28/75 (37)	54/90 (60)	72/113 (64)		
Philip[13]	1986–9	Discharge			11/48 (23)	13/28 (47)	21/32 (66)	13/19 (69)	10/11 (91)	4/4 (100)
Wood[19]	1986–8	Discharge			1/10 (10)	9/21 (43)	24/30 (80)	20/24 (83)	21/24 (88)	29/32 (91)
Gultom[7]	1986–8	Discharge		0/19	0/20	12/27 (44)	28/49 (57)	52/71 (73)		
Nishida[20]	1984–90	Discharge		3/7 (43)	14/15 (93)	17/20 (85)	21/25 (84)	17/19 (89)	20/21 (95)	
EWP(England)[21]	1986	Discharge	0/1	1/6 (17)	2/15 (13)	3/11 (27)	5/10 (50)	5/14 (36)	11/17 (65)	
EWP(Germany)[21]	1986	Discharge	0/3	0/2	0/3	2/5 (40)	3/17 (18)	11/22 (50)	20/31 (65)	
Victorian Infant[22]	1985–7	5 years			10/86 (12)	31/109 (28)	54/121 (45)			
Ruys[23]	1985–7	Discharge			3/4 (75)	7/14 (50)	6/10 (60)	11/24 (46)		
Synnes[24]	1983–9	Discharge		9/56 (16)	46/108 (43)	88/160 (55)	111/177 (63)	144/188 (77)	192/222 (86)	
Eg-Anderson[25]	1984–7	Discharge			0/3	7/8 (88)	18/41 (44)	30/48 (63)	47/64 (73)	
EWP (Scotland)[21]	1985	Discharge	0/10	0/6	1/21 (5)	6/32 (19)	29/61 (48)	31/64 (48)	62/78 (79)	
Johnson[26]	1984–6	Discharge			5/60 (8)*	9/45 (20)	32/66 (48)	43/69 (62)	80/102 (78)	
Hack[11]	1982–8	20 months	1/29 (3)	3/37 (8)	8/51 (16)	42/80 (53)	49/82 (60)	59/82 (72)		
Cooke[27]	1980–9	3 years			8/64 (13)	46/111 (41)	73/180 (41)	117/191 (61)	200/277 (72)	
Tin[8]	1983–6	2 years	0/24	1/39 (3)	5/52 (10)	18/80 (21)	49/116 (42)	73/124 (59)		
Whyte[28]	1982–7	Discharge		12/55 (22)	54/114 (47)	114/175 (65)	165/224 (74)			
Philip[13]	1982–5	Discharge			5/34 (15)	11/32 (35)	23/43 (52)	16/22 (73)	18/22 (83)	6/6 (100)
Weissman[29]	1982–6	Discharge			5/40 (12)	2/27 (7)	8/19 (42)	22/33 (67)	35/50 (74)	
Gultom[7]	1983–5	Discharge		0/17	0/21	6/25 (24)	28/50 (56)	38/54 (70)		
POPS[30]	1983	Discharge			0/27*	7/48 (15)	29/77 (38)	56/103 (54)	90/136 (61)	134/171 (78)
Wariyar[31]	1983	2 years			1/19 (5)	6/23 (26)	12/27 (44)	13/30 (43)	26/40 (65)	
EWP (Netherlands)[21]	1983	Discharge	0/23	0/28	0/37	8/59 (14)	30/82 (37)	57/109 (52)	96/143 (67)	
Nwaesei[32]	1980–2	Discharge		0/7	1/10 (10)	5/13 (38)	6/13 (46)	13/17 (76)		
Milligan[2]	1979–82	Discharge		1/7 (14)	9/23 (39)	28/44 (64)	34/45 (76)	45/60 (75)	71/88 (81)	89/99 (90)
Yu[33]	1977–84	Discharge		2/28 (7)	13/40 (33)	11/44 (25)	35/62 (56)	63/87 (72)	68/95 (72)	
Kitchen[34]	1977–82	Discharge			2/27 (7)	11/54 (20)	36/80 (45)	47/67 (70)	76/98 (78)	
Herschel[35]	1977–80	28 days			2/7 (29)	3/28 (11)	17/38 (45)	23/38 (61)	23/25 (92)	
Dillon[36]	1977–80	Discharge			4/11 (36)	6/16 (38)	11/18 (61)	13/17 (76)		
Doyle[37]	1971–4	Discharge			0/29	0/36	4/33 (12)	8/42 (19)	26/53 (49)	
†Current typical survival rates (95% confidence intervals)			0.9% (0.0–5.0)	7.7% (5.4–10.7)	29.7% (26.4–33.1)	49.7% (46.5–53.0)	63.3% (60.4–66.2)	73.0% (70.5–75.5)	76.2% (72.3–79.8)	84.8% (80.9–88.3)

*Combined rate <24 weeks. †From cohorts whose mean period of study was 1988 or later.

attempts to standardise reporting of disability, as a measure of functional impairment, in very preterm populations at two years of age[41]. In a recent review of the literature published from 1960, 111 outcome studies were identified which had reported morbidity in very low birthweight (VLBW) cohorts, from which was derived a median prevalence of disability in 25% of survivors[42]. More recent studies suggest that, despite increasing survival, the overall incidence of disability has remained the same. The UK Northern Neonatal Network reported the outcome of children below 27 weeks' gestation in three time frames. Severe disability occurred in 15%, 28% and 27% during 1983–6, 1987–90, and 1991–4, respectively, when reviewed between one and two years of age[8]. In a North American VLBW population, Hack and colleagues

TABLE 82.2
EPICure survival data

Gestation (weeks)	Total births (including stillbirths)	Admissions for intensive care (%)	*Total births surviving to EDD (%)*	Admissions surviving to EDD (%)*
20	767	0	0	0
21	603	3 (0.5)	1 (0)	1 (0)
22	642	18 (3)	1 (0)	1 (0)
23	595	133 (22)	35 (6)	35 (26)
24	602	300 (50)	100 (18)	100 (33)
25	572	351 (61)	173 (32)	173 (49)
	3781	805 (21)	–	310 (41)

*The figures in these columns are derived from analysis of 94% of admissions (February 1997).

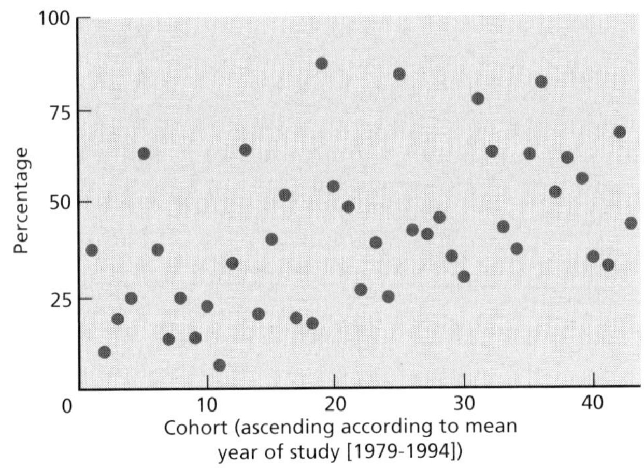

Fig. 82.1 Survival at 25 weeks' gestation: summary of 32 studies with a mean survival of 43% (95% confidence interval 37–50%).

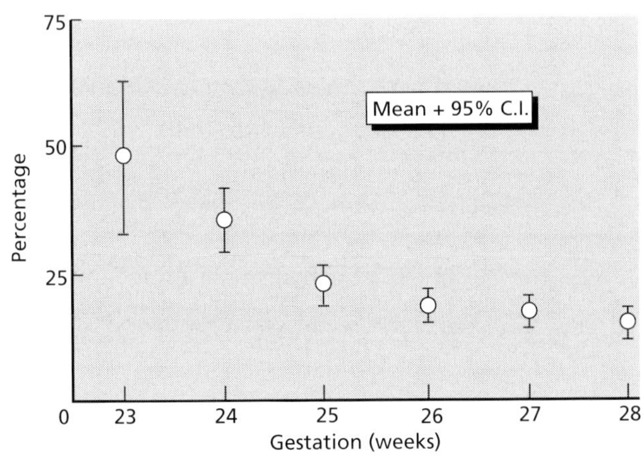

Fig. 82.2 Summary of reported rates of major disability from 15 studies[2,8,10,15,18,23–29,31–33].

have reported disability rates at 20 months of age of 33% and 31%, in 1982–8 and 1990–2, respectively[11]. La Pine and colleagues demonstrated stable VLBW disability rates at 19 months of age of 19%, 21% and 22% during 1977–80, 1983–5 and 1986–90, respectively[43]. Figure 82.2 summarizes reports of major disability rates at different gestational ages. The introduction of surfactant does not appear to have produced changes in short-term neurodevelopmental outcome despite reports of increased survival[44–48].

CEREBRAL PALSY

About half of all cases of cerebral palsy (CP) occur in children who were of low birthweight (<2500 g)[49], and the incidence of CP is 38 times higher in VLBW children compared to those born at term[42]. In a major review of outcome studies for VLBW children since 1960, the median prevalence of CP was 7.7% with little evidence of variation over time[42]. As most clinical conditions are recognisable by two years of age, CP is often chosen as an index measure of changes in perinatal or neonatal outcome, which allows early feedback to consider the relationship to care[41]. Definition of CP at 12 months may be relatively inaccurate[50] and follow up beyond the second year is desirable to determine prevalence of long-term disability. The prevalence of CP rises with decreasing gestational age and, like disability, must be considered when counselling parents anticipating a preterm birth, although many children with CP are not severely disabled.

Important CP registers, notably those from Mersey (UK), Western Australia and Sweden, have also evaluated time and birthweight-based changes in the prevalence of cerebral palsy. In the Mersey region of the UK, there were 1612 cases of CP identified in births between 1966 and 1989[49]. The birthweight specific prevalence of CP over this period is shown in Fig. 82.3. For children with birthweights between 1500 and 2499 g, there was an increase in prevalence from 4 per 1000 in the late 1960s to 12 per 1000 ten years later. Since then the rate has varied little. During the second half of the 1970s, the prevalence among VLBW children rose from 30 to 90 per 1000 survivors. In contrast to the stability of rates in the

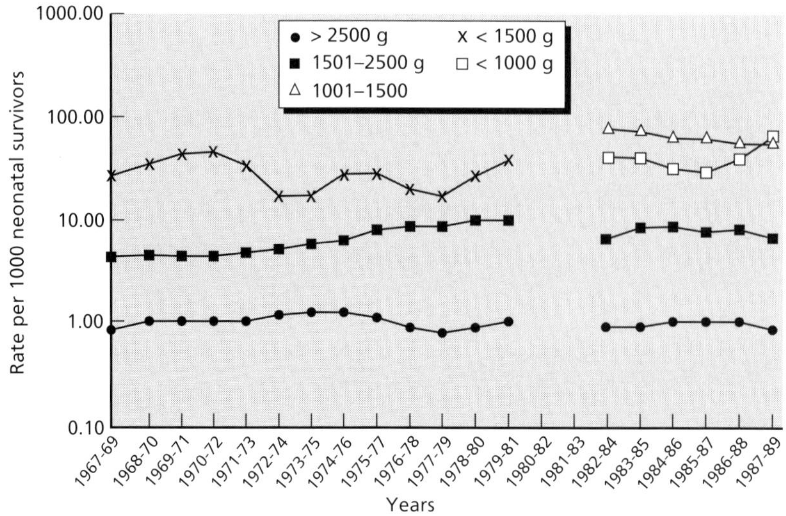

Fig. 82.3 Birthweight specific prevalence of cerebral palsy, Merseyside and Cheshire 1967–1989 (reproduced with permission from *Archives of Disease in Childhood*, the BMJ Publishing Group).

birthweight group 1000–1499 g, the prevalence among children <1000 g birthweight has continued to increase.

From the southern Sweden CP register, between 1987 and 1990, Hagberg and colleagues have reported a prevalence of 2.36 per 1000 livebirths, 0.98 per 1000 of which were preterm and 1.38 per 1000 term; gestational age specific prevalence of CP in this population was 80.32 per 1000 livebirths at <28 weeks, 53.51 at 28–31 weeks, 7.79 at 32–39 weeks and 1.35 over 36 weeks[51]. Prior to this last report, which implies a stable CP rate, Hagberg and colleagues had observed a steady small increase in CP rates, which has also been reported from Western Australia[52] and West Germany[53].

The relationship between CP, preterm birth and neonatal care is more difficult to establish. Over the period when intensive care is being established one might anticipate a rise in prevalence, while techniques become established and as mortality falls, facilitating survival of disabled individuals[54]; indeed, this may explain the rise in VLBW prevalence seen in the Mersey data during the late 1970s[55]. Once survival is near maximal and care optimised this should not rise further. Most neonatal services have seen a decline in the prevalence of intraventricular haemorrhage recently[56]. The possible translation of this into a decrease in the rate of CP may become obvious in the next few years. Alternatively, the previous relationship between ultrasound evidence of brain injury and CP may become less clear as may have happened in the Bristol population during the early 1990s (see Table 82.3; N. Marlow, unpublished data).

It is considered that the majority of impairments in very preterm children are acquired during the immediate perinatal or neonatal periods. Hagberg and colleagues evaluated the timing of causation carefully in their population. In their preterm group, 8% were considered to have a prenatal aetiology and 54% a perinatal one, as compared to 33% and 28%, respectively, in the term group[51]. A proposed list of aetiological factors is given in Table 82.4[57–61].

TABLE 82.3
Relationship of cerebral palsy and disability to neonatal ultrasound appearances, Bristol 1990–1993 (after N. Marlow)

	Absence of cerebral palsy		Cerebral palsy		Absence of disability		Disability, not severe		Severe disability	
Early ultrasound changes (week 1)	*n*	%	*n*	%	*n*	%	*n*	%	*n*	%
Normal	210	89.7	17	68	236	90.1	14	70	17	70.8
Small PVH	10	4.3	2	8	9	3.4	2	10	2	8.3
Large PVH	13	5.6	6	24	17	6.5	4	20	5	20.8
Late ultrasound appearances										
Normal	211	90.1	11	44	236	90.1	16	80	13	54.2
Mild changes	14	6.0	10	40	14	5.3	4	20	7	29.2
Cystic PVL	9	3.8	4	16	12	4.6	0	–	4	16.6

PVH = periventricular haemorrhage; PVL = periventricular leukomalacia

TABLE 82.4
Risk factors for cerebral palsy in the preterm infant (after adjustment for gestational age)

Maternal	High parity
Antenatal	Prolonged rupture of membranes Chorioamnionitis Other maternal infections *Pre-eclampsia associated with decreased risk* *Intrauterine growth retardation not associated with an increased risk*
Intrapartum	Caesarian section in labour *Delivery before labour associates with decreased risk*
Peri/neonatal	Large periventricular haemorrhage, intracerebral haemorrhage, or cystic periventricular leukomalacia Asystole or shock Confirmed bacteraemia Central nervous system infection Seizures Patent ductus arteriosus Blood transfusion Prolonged ventilation Pneumothorax Total parenteral nutrition Hyponatraemia

The issue of the timing of the cerebral insult which causes CP in relation to preterm birth, and therefore of its relationship to aspects of neonatal care, is far from clear and both CP and preterm birth may have similar aetiologies[52]. Blair and Stanley have investigated the relationship between growth restriction, prematurity and CP. The population attributable risk of CP is not increased where gestational age is below 34 weeks where birthweight falls below either the 3rd or 10th percentile. In contrast a birthweight below the 3rd percentile at 34–37 weeks is associated with a population attributable risk of 35.8% (95% confidence interval 17.6–58) compared with 11.3% (5.0–21) in those >37 weeks' gestation. There is thus interaction between antepartum events, premature birth and later risk of CP which may further complicate assessment of the impact of changes in perinatal care[62].

Definition of disability

Traditionally, terminology has followed the World Health Organization publication, International Classification of Impairment Disabilities and Handicap (ICIDH). This classification presented the model of:

Disease or disorder → impairment → disability → handicap

The definitions used in this, and the UK Children's Act, 1989 have become dated and are considered stigmatising. A Working Group of the British Association for Community Child Health and the Department of Health[63] has recently recommended a change in terminology. Because many people with disabilities object to the label 'handicap' with its associated negative public perception, the Working Group proposed the model of:

condition → impairment → disability → disadvantage ← discrimination ← environment

where

- *Condition* – disease or disorder or damage;
- *Impairment* – loss or abnormality of psychological or physiological or anatomical function due to underlying condition;
- *Disability* – restriction or lack of ability in expected human activity due to the underlying condition or impairment. The dimensions of disability may include some of the following list:

  1. *Locomotion*
  2. *Fine motor function*
  3. *Personal care*
  4. *Continence*
  5. *Hearing*
  6. *Vision*
  7. *Communication*
  8. *Learning*
  9. *Behaviour and social integration*
  10. *Physical health*
  11. *Consciousness*

  In each category, the disability level depends on the child's degree of functioning with or without assistance or aids, and/or the child's developmental skills as expected for age.

  Mild:

Older child:	some limitation present but able to function independently
Younger child:	functioning slightly behind the level expected for age

  Moderate:

Older child:	where aids and/or assistance may be required to perform tasks
Younger child:	functioning around two-thirds the level expected for age

  Severe:

Older child:	who is unable to perform tasks without aids and assistance most of the time
Younger child:	functioning around two-thirds the level expected for age

  Profound:

Older child:	completely dependent on carer to perform tasks

- *Disadvantage* – a person's disadvantage results from a combination of his impairment and discrimination imposed by norms and expectations of society.

For the young premature child, there is some consensus as to what comprises severe disability at two years[41]. Definition of cerebral palsy or neurological impairment is equally difficult but standardised schemes exist for recording and performing the neurological examination[64] and for recording central motor deficit[65]. The predictive validity of these schedules requires further elaboration.

Neuromotor function in premature children

CHILDREN WITH CEREBRAL PALSY

Cerebral palsy is the most common major motor disability associated with prematurity. Various classifications to categorise the impairment have been attempted (see Table 82.5[66]). Spastic diplegia with normal IQ (Little disease) has been classically associated with prematurity, since the first association with difficult deliveries[67] and preterm birth[68]. However, since the development of modern intensive care over the last twenty-five years, there has been an emergence of more complex types of cerebral palsy in the very preterm population[69]. Complex spastic hemiplegia is now the second most common disorder, followed by severe quadriplegia[51,55] which is usually associated with severe learning difficulties, and in whom up to 90% have epilepsy, 50% cortical blindness and bulbar palsies are frequent[51].

TABLE 82.5
Definition and classification of cerebral palsy*

Classification	Distribution of impairment
Spastic	
Diplegic distribution	Mono-, di-, tri-, quadriplegia
Hemiplegic distribution	
Dyskinetic	
Athetoid	
Ataxic	
Hypotonic	
Mixed	

*Definition: 'A disorder of movement and posture due to a defect or lesion in the immature brain'[66].

Within the preterm population, different antecedents may be found for the major types of CP[70–72]. In a multivariate analysis in a group of VLBW children with matched controls, infants with diplegia could be differentiated from non-impaired children on antenatal variables alone (preterm labour, amnionitis, smoking) whereas significant discrimination of infants with hemiplegia and quadriplegia required the addition of postnatal variables. For hemiplegia, antecedents comprised: an older mother, an at risk fetus (abnormal cardiotocogram, intrauterine growth restriction) and an infant with serious illnesses (hyaline membrane disease, pneumothoraces, ventriculoperitoneal shunt, fits, septicaemia). For quadriplegia: an ill mother; a chronic neonatal course (prolonged ventilation, necrotising enterocolitis, ventriculoperitoneal shunt); and severe changes on cranial ultrasound scan[72].

Amongst the various types of CP, it is well recognised that those with spastic hemiplegia or diplegia have a good potential for ambulation and may have less associated disability, in contrast to the majority of those with quadriplegia. This is reflected in studies of long-term survival for children with CP. In one study from Mersey Region of children with CP born 1966–84, 85% of full-term children survived to 20 years as opposed to 93% children born preterm. Children with quadriplegia had only 50% chance of 20-year survival and accounted for most of the excess risk[73].

CHILDREN WITHOUT CEREBRAL PALSY

In those survivors who do not have overt CP, it has long been recognised that there is a substantial group who suffer with more subtle motor and perceptual-motor difficulties. These children are often labelled as 'clumsy'. It is unclear whether this group represent the result of milder degrees of brain injury or of disordered brain maturation[74]. The prevalence of these difficulties appears to increase as gestational age decreases[75,76].

Poor motor skills are found frequently among school age VLBW children. In a longitudinal study of children with birthweights below 1251 g, motor impairment was assessed using the Test of Motor Impairment (TOMI-r)[77] or its successor, the Movement Assessment Battery for Children (Movement ABC)[78]. Over a range of tests of manual dexterity, balancing and ball skills, VLBW children had consistently higher scores than age- and sex-matched peers. At 6 years 75% of VLBW children had TOMI-r scores outside the 75th percentile for their peers[79]. By 12–13 years of age, using the Movement ABC 16 (34%) VLBW children scored in the 'significantly impaired' range and 8 (17%) had borderline scores compared to 3 (5%) and 2 (3.5%) controls respectively[80]. Jongmans and colleagues also observed that 54% of their VLBW cohort had abnormal or borderline scores on the Movement ABC, at 6 years of age[76].

Very preterm birth appears to produce a different spectrum of impairment to that found in unselected populations. Tracking of an individual's impairment scores from 6 years to 12–13 years was fairly consistent for the children in the non-impaired group at 6 years but among those with high impairments tracking was reliable in girls but less reliable in boys[80]. In contrast to studies of 'clumsy children', VLBW girls were found to have significantly higher overall impairment scores than VLBW boys, and on a wider variety of subtasks, particularly those involving dynamic balance, although both sexes found greatest difficulty with tasks of manual dexterity[80]. Elliman and colleagues reported significantly worse performance in tests of both fine and gross motor coordination in low-birthweight 7-year-olds, although girls tended to perform better than boys in fine motor tests[81].

The relationship between motor scores and educational performance is relatively weak. However, lack of motor impairment at 6 years had high negative predictive value for educational problems at 8 years, whereas high scores carry a 33% risk of poor performance[74]. The reasons for the relationship between fine motor and other difficulties is obscure. Although motor scores were associated with a small group of perinatal variables at 6 years, no association was found subsequently[74,80].

PREMATURITY AND LATERALITY

It is well documented that there exists an increased proportion of premature infants who show left hand or no lateral preference (non-right handedness)[82,83] but the pathogenesis and neurodevelopmental significance of this finding are unclear. The reported prevalence of left or non-right handedness in various VLBW and preterm populations ranges from 25 to 50%, compared to around 10% in the general population. Several theories have been advanced to explain this excess. Bakan proposed that all non-right-hand preference may be of pathological origin. If this is the case then there should be evidence of associated brain injury[84]. Annett suggested that very early delivery may somehow interrupt the progress of normal brain asymmetry, which she also considers to be under genetic control[85], and may have its origin in the second trimester[82]. Others have suggested that later lateral preferences may be modified by neonatal nursing practices[86]. Satz has proposed a model for predicting the proportion of hand preferences due to biological or pathological reasons[87].

An association between non-right preferences and neuropsychological impairment may reflect a pathological origin of this shift. In one study, lower IQ and increased frequency of articulation and language disorders was found in 4-year-old non-right-handed VLBW children[88]. In contrast, another investigation observed no cognitive differences between right and non-right-handed 8-year-old VLBW children, but a significant increase in neuroimpairment in the non-right handed[89]. In this study, males with impairments were more likely to be non-right-handed than unimpaired males (69% vs. 25%), but there were no differences in females. In a study of 137 VLBW children (gestation 24–35 weeks) at 12–13 years of age in mainstream school, on directly observed tasks 14 (10%) were left handed, 16 (12%) were mixed as compared to 11 (7%) and 10 (6%) of a matched comparison group[90]. There were no differences in the prevalence of foot or eye preferences or for crossed laterality. Handedness was examined in relation to motor skills, vision and cognitive outcome, which have all been noted to be poorer in these children. Manual dexterity scores and near vision were poorer in non-right-handed children. Overall motor scores in the borderline/impaired range were associated with 33% non-right preferences compared to 18% in the non-impaired group. Estimated IQ, reading, mathematical and spelling ability did not vary with hand preference.

Despite the concept of perinatal brain injury causing altered lateral preferences[84] no study has successfully associated specific perinatal variables with laterality[82,88–90]. In particular, the lateralisation of observed brain lesions using neonatal cerebral ultrasound could not be related to lateral preferences[83]. The excess of left and non-right preferences in this population remains unexplained at present.

NEUROLOGICAL AND DEVELOPMENTAL PROGRESS AFTER VERY PRETERM BIRTH

During the first two years, neuromotor functions develop rapidly. It has been long recognised that premature infants who seem to have a defined motor lesion over the first year can subsequently go on to have normal function[50,91]. There is evidence from animal models of plasticity in the developing brain, an ability to compensate for some brain lesions[92]. However, the unique deviant patterns of development seen in the preterm child may represent normal compensatory mechanisms (plasticity) following specific brain injury or 'catch up' following abnormal brain development outside the womb. Largo and colleagues, in reviewing the quality of motor performance as an expression of neurological integrity in three longitudinal studies[93], described three patterns of abnormal neurological influences on motor development:

1. Only severe impairment leads to a delay which is beyond the normal range. Most mildly impaired children attain each motor stage within the normal age range, for example, first movements through space were achieved before 9.5 months for 92% of preterm compared with 95% for term infants However, the achievement of motor milestones at the normal age does not exclude neurological impairment.
2. Neurological impairment affects the quality of posture and movements making them less smooth and economical, and limiting the variability of motor performance.
3. Neurological impairment may lead to deviant motor behaviour and deviant pathways of locomotion not usually seen in healthy children, for example rolling, snake-like movements or bridging.

TRANSIENT DYSTONIA

Neuromotor examination during the first two years of life correctly identifies most of those infants with major disabilities. However, it also identifies a group of individuals with transient abnormalities in muscle tone and neurological performance. Such infants present in a similar way to those who subsequently go on to develop cerebral palsy, but the neurological signs and dystonia resolve usually around the first birthday. The significance of this pattern of development is obscure, but it may be related to abnormalities detected on cerebral ultrasound[94]. Two studies have demonstrated neurodevelopmental delay, reduced cognitive scores and behavioural disorders following transient dystonia in VLBW populations at 3–6 years of age[95,96], and in one study a progression of dystonia via attention deficit disorders at 2 years to school problems has been described[91]. However, others have disputed the significance of these results, and failed to show any significant associations between transient dystonia and neurodevelopmental outcome at 5 years of age[97]. Dystonia has been associated with fine motor and locomotor problems, which may themselves be weak predictors of later educational and cognitive outcome[74]. The small numbers of infants available for study makes the differences observed difficult to assess.

Cognitive and behavioural problems

COGNITIVE AND EDUCATIONAL ISSUES

As the child develops, increasing intellectual challenges are encountered, exposing new patterns of impairment, not only in motor function but also in cognitive and language ability. Many children who perform normally on preschool developmental tests, which are often heavily motor-based, begin to experience difficulties as formal education begins. These difficulties may be further compounded by problems with motor coordination and behavioural disorders, and are influenced by social and environmental factors which may magnify impairments in vulnerable preterm or low birthweight children[98,99].

Since the 1940s preterm children have been recognised to be at cognitive disadvantage when compared to their term peers[100,101]. One major difficulty in the interpretation of studies of this area is the inclusiveness of the various populations studied. With a disability rate of up to 250 per 1000 children, population scores for cohorts of very preterm or VLBW survivors will be markedly disadvantaged compared to term children, where the disability rate may only be 2–3 per 1000. It is therefore important to be clear whether disabled children are included in the population studied, and that the performance of children without significant disability is reported separately. Parents and professionals must be aware of the relative prevalence of problems among this group when assessing information and need for follow up and support.

MAINSTREAM SCHOOLING

In the Liverpool longitudinal cohort, 58 of 72 (80.5%) children <1251 g birthweight born in 1980 were attending mainstream school at 8 years[74]. This is a similar order to reports from other parts of the UK[102], from the Dutch 1984 POPS cohort (81%)[103] and from North American 7-year-old VLBW cohorts (55–65%)[104–106]. The Liverpool cohort was assessed in terms of their school performance on standardised tests and by teacher assessment. Three times as many of the 53 VLBW children had scores below the 10th percentile in tests of reading, maths and spelling compared to a matched comparison group. Nearly half of VLBW children had difficulties in one or more subjects compared with 19% controls and 9 (18%) VLBW children were classified as 'failing' at school with problems in two or more areas, including 6 who had problems across all areas, compared to 4% controls. Similarly, in a Canadian population study of children of <1000 g birthweight only half were felt to have achieved normal academic achievement at 8 years[107]. The proportion of school failures dropped slightly when the Liverpool cohort was reassessed at 12–13 years[108]. In other studies special educational support is needed for between 48–57% children[103,107,109].

COGNITIVE SCORES

Assessing IQ scores in such populations is fraught with difficulty because of different populations, inclusion of disabled children, differences in test scores, availability of comparison groups and lack of correction for social mix. Many studies use relatively old scales of assessment and it is known that IQ scores drift upwards with time[110], making comparison to standardisation populations difficult.

Generally populations of preterm children without major disability have 5–10 point disadvantage when compared to their peers[74,107,109,111]. Of interest is that school performance may have a poor relation to the results of IQ tests. In the Liverpool study, there was much overlap of scores between children experiencing no difficulty (median 117, range 84–139), difficulty with one subject (median 105, range 82–139), two subjects (median 105.5, range 91–130) or three (median 101, range 97–122). As a whole, the study cases displayed a mean IQ within the normal range[74], a finding common with other studies with similar rates of academic difficulties[107,109].

The early prediction of learning difficulties may offer a window for preventative measures. MacKinlay and colleagues found significant association between poor motor scores on school entry and later school failure in the general population[112]. In the Liverpool cohort poor motor scores had a good negative predictive value but only 33% of those with poor scores subsequently failed at school two years later[74]. Academic performance remains hard to predict and is, as one might expect, highly related to social and environmental factors. The interactions between social factors and prematurity has not been well explored in this context. In America, the Infant Health and Development Program was set up to evaluate the effect of a special service intervention programme on cognitive, academic, behavioural and health outcome of premature (<37 weeks' gestation and <2500 g birthweight) infants. The newborns were randomised to either the intervention programme or normal paediatric follow up. Intervention occurred for the first three years of life, consisting of home visits, child development centre services and parent group meetings. At 3 years of age, the children in the intervention group had significantly higher intelligence test scores and receptive vocabulary test scores and lower scores of reported behavioural problems. When re-evaluated at 5 years and subsequently 8 years of age, there was attenuation of IQ effects with no significant overall differences in outcome measures between the two groups. There was, however, a modest intervention-related difference in cognitive and academic abilities seen in the heavier (2001–2500 g) infants. They were able to demonstrate a significant IQ difference between the children at 8 years of age as a function of maternal education, those children of mothers who had completed post-high school education having the highest IQ, whilst those children whose mother had less than 12 years of education had the lowest IQ. Again there were no differences between the intervention and follow-up groups except in the heavier infants[113].

INTERACTION WITH SOCIAL FACTORS

As development progresses, social and environmental factors begin to progressively influence childhood development. Older studies from Scotland and more recent work from Canada had confirmed that poor socio-economic status is associated with lower IQ in both preterm and term children. The observed interaction between birth weight, socio-economic status and IQ suggests that socio-economic status does not modify the relationship between birth weight and IQ. In other words, extremely low birthweight (ELBW) children from poorer socio-economic groups did not have a lower IQ than would be expected by the simple addition of the two effects[95,107].

BEHAVIOUR AND PSYCHOLOGICAL OUTCOMES

Most studies evaluating longer term outcomes have included behaviour checklists which demonstrate an excess of adverse behavioural traits among surviving VLBW children, reported by either parents or teachers. The finding of symptoms of attention deficit disorder, with or without hyperactivity (ADDH), seem to be the most consistent findings and has been recognised since the original studies of Drillien[95,114,115]. Even as toddlers, overactivity may be found more commonly among VLBW groups[114].

Later studies assessing the persistence or development of these traits are few, but persisting symptoms have been observed at 8 years[116] and into adolescence[117]. In non-VLBW populations, ADDH may translate into conduct problems in later childhood[118,119]. There are few data to inform outcome in the very preterm child, but there is a suggestion that the development of new traits may be less in VLBW children[116], although recently symptoms of anxiety and depression have been reported[120].

In the Liverpool study of children in mainstream school[121], self-completion and parental report questionnaires covering the areas of antisocial behaviour, anxiety, depression, hyperactivity and general behaviour were supplemented with the Child and Adolescent Psychiatric Assessment (CAPA)[122]. On the CAPA, 31 of 136 (23%) of the VLBW group met clinical criteria for ADDH compared to only 9 of 148 (6%) of their peers. The VLBW group scored more highly on screening inventories for anxiety and depression although the numbers with clinical criteria for disorders were small. No excess of conduct or oppositional disorders was found. Overall 38 of 136 (28%) VLBW adolescents met clinical criteria for any disorder compared to 15 of 148 (10%) of their peers (see Fig. 82.4), and the usual excess of males with behaviour or psychiatric symptoms found in most non-VLBW populations was not observed, suggesting a fundamental difference in the origin of such symptoms among VLBW children.

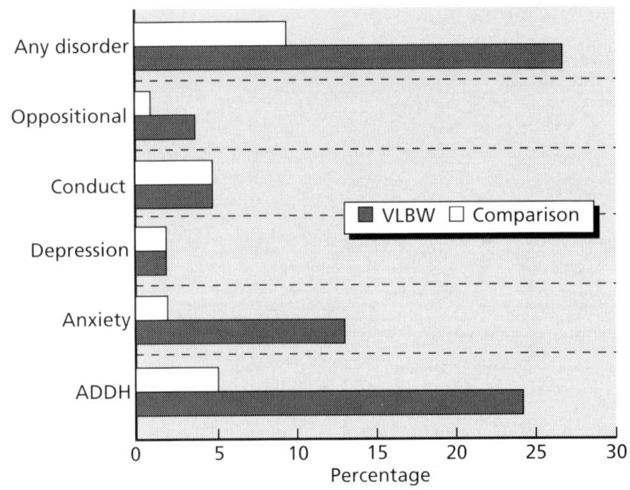

Fig. 82.4 Summary of psychiatric disorders among 136 VLBW children and 148 comparison children at 11–13 years (Botting *et al.*[121]). VLBW = Very low birthweight; ADDH = attention deficit disorder, with or without hyperactivity.

In a cluster analysis of cognitive and behavioural outcomes[123], 30% of the VLBW cohort were classified as 'normal' with good cognitive scores and no psychological morbidity, 42% had no psychological morbidity but lower than average cognitive scores, 18% had psychological morbidity with normal cognitive scores and 10% had a pervasive disorder with poor cognitive outcomes and high adverse scores on psychological questionnaires. Within this latter group the prevalence of ADDH was 75%.

Neurosensory impairments

HEARING

A significant permanent hearing loss (>50 dB HL) may be found in 0.5–4% VLBW children compared to 1–2 per 1000 live births in the general population[124]. There is, however, great variability in the tests used and threshold definitions for sensorineural hearing loss (SNHL) in the various studies. Little progress has been made in the understanding of the aetiology of SNHL in very preterm children since it was reviewed in 1985[69]. Potential candidates include hypoxia, apnoea, hyperbilirubinaemia, ototoxic drugs (e.g. aminoglycosides and frusemide), intrauterine infection, acoustic trauma, intracranial and haemorrhage. None has been satisfactorily identified as single causative agents. It is likely that a combination of factors (e.g. apnoea/hypoxia and hyperbilirubinaemia[125] or hyperbilirubinaemia and netilmicin or acidosis[124]) may be required to produce cochlear damage. All neonatal intensive care services should by now have established mechanisms for high-risk screening for SNHL before or soon after discharge from the neonatal unit.

Children without overt SNHL may also be at risk for poor speech discrimination[126] and it is likely that subtle hearing impairment may parallel the range of subclinical impairments described in other areas.

VISION

The visual pathway in the preterm infant can be damaged as a result of both ocular and cerebral pathology. Severe visual impairment or blindness may result from cicatricial retinopathy of prematurity (ROP) or from cortical loss; Fig. 82.5 gives a summary of the reported incidence of severe impairment by gestational age. Many more children will have less severe visual impairments from combinations of these and potentially other causes.

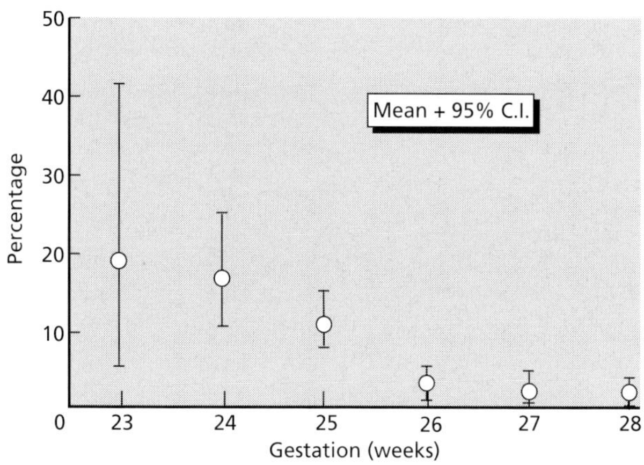

Fig. 82.5 Frequency of severe visual impairment (blind/sees light only) from six studies[15,24,25,27,28,32].

RETINOPATHY OF PREMATURITY

As the population of extremely preterm infants has increased so has the incidence of ROP. Surprisingly, the proportion of children with severe disease has not increased and may have fallen. Incidence and severity, however, still remain inversely proportional to gestational age. Retinal vascularistation progresses centrifugally from the optic disc to reach the margins of the retina around term. Interruption of this process after extremely preterm birth leads to disease close to the macula which is more active and of more serious import than that which may occur more peripherally in more mature babies. The aetiology is probably multifactorial, although the role of oxygen therapy seems without doubt. An initial vasoconstrictive phase, usually considered secondary to hyperoxia, is followed by a proliferative retinal recovery phase during which vascular overgrowth occurs at the margin of the advancing vascular border, which may be hastened by hypoxia[127]. Studies reporting reduction in ROP secondary to reduced oxygen administration also report increased rates of neurodisability[128].

ROP produces a continuous spectrum of disease, which is not easily classified. A pragmatic classification has been produced (the International Classification of Retinopathy of Prematurity (ICROP)[129,130]), which centres around describing the extent of the disease and its acuity. Disease which reaches a maximum stage of 2 or less usually resolves; the presence of 'plus' disease implies greater activity; stage 3 represents 'threshold' disease for treatment, although more active stage 2 'plus' disease in the extremely preterm infant may benefit from early intervention.

Among 4099 infants born weighing <1250 g and <32 weeks' gestation, 65.8% cohort developed ROP. 'Threshold' ROP was reached in 6.0% of the overall group, implying the need for treatment[131]. As gestational age at birth decreases so the prevalence of cicatricial ROP increases. Of 310 infants born <26 weeks' gestation, 13% required treatment for ROP[40]. A further study of 565 babies <32 weeks revealed that only 2.9% had serious sequelae of cicatrical disease at 2–3 years age[132]. However, a high prevalence of other ocular problems was found among the remainder. Significant refractive errors occurred in 81.3% of those with and 12.6% of those without cicatrical ROP. Strabismus was present in 12.5% of the full cohort. Prior to surgery, 10.6% had an esotropia and 2% an exotropia. Strabismus was also associated with cerebral palsy, being present in 51.9% of cases, 46.9% of those without cicatricial ROP. In 7 (1.3%) cases there was cortical blindness, all but one of whom had cerebral palsy. Of those without severe visual impairment, acuity of ≥6/9 was recorded in 424 (76%) and a further 18 had isolated refractive errors. Of those without cerebral palsy or ciciatricial ROP, 7.2% had strabismus of indeterminate origin, which is higher than the normal population average[132].

OTHER VISUAL MORBIDITY

Two studies have evaluated ocular and visual outcomes later in childhood among children without disabilities from populations born before widespread screening was practised. Dowdeswell *et al.* compared preterm children aged between 5 and 7.5 years with matched controls. In 36 children with no ocular or cerebral pathology, prematurity was associated with poorer contrast sensitivity and colour vision but no difference in acuity or stereopsis[133]. Powls *et al.* report similar findings in their cohort of 139 VLBW children aged 11–13 years in mainstream school. The whole range of subtle visual impairments were more common in the VLBW group compared to controls (63.5% vs. 36% respectively). Poor contrast sensitivity and strabismus were associated with poor motor skills and poor contrast sensitivity and visual acuity with lower IQ[134]. Impairments in contrast sensitivity and colour perception may have different aetiologies to the major impairments. It has been suggested that the exposure of preterm infants to 'blue' wavelength light (phototherapy lights and background ambient lights) in the neonatal nursery may lead to destruction of the blue cones in the retina and hence these later deficits[135,136]

Infants with abnormal neonatal cerebral ultrasound or magnetic resonance scans frequently have visual impairment[137]. Impaired acuity may be specifically related to ischaemic cerebral lesions[137,138], particularly where there are injuries to the optic radiation and/or occipitoparietal cortex[137], and is not a feature of children with posthaemorrhagic ventriculomegaly. The pattern and severity of a visual deficit cannot be predicted by imaging alone[137].

Growth

It is well recognised that many very premature infants grow poorly over the first few years and most studies report an excess of preterm infants with small size. The prognosis for final height, weight and head circumference seems less clear. There are varying opinions in the literature some predicting poor growth attainment[139,140], others normal outcome[141,142]. Few studies have evaluated final height, weight and head circumference attainment. In the Liverpool cohort study, 138 VLBW children were assessed at between 12 and 13 years old[143]. When compared to a term peer comparison group, the preterm group were significantly shorter, with a mean deficit of 4.1 cm. There was no difference in pubertal status between the two groups. There was a trend for growth in girls to be more affected than boys. The height of 7% of the VLBW group was <3rd centile and 22% <10th centile versus 2% and 9% in the comparison group, respectively. VLBW children had no disproportion between sitting and standing heights. A Tanner–Whitehouse 2 bone age was assessed in 70% of the VLBW group from a standard wrist X-ray, which was, on average, advanced from age-matched standards. Thus final height prediction, using the equations of Tanner and Whitehouse, indicated that the discrepancy with their peers would increase, 17% attaining height <3rd centile and 33% <10th centile as adults. Bone age was not calculated for the comparison group. Therapy with growth hormone is unlikely to be of benefit in this group.

In terms of weight, VLBW children were found lighter than their controls, with a mean difference of 2.5 kg. The difference was again more pronounced in girls but multivariate analysis indicated that height differences accounted for the weight discrepancy. This VLBW group was not, therefore, not disproportionately thin, an observation confirmed by similar skinfold thickness measures.

The VLBW children had smaller head circumferences than their peers, with a mean deficit of 0.47 cm, again greater in girls than boys. Small head circumference was associated with poorer scores in all measures of cognition and educational ability. This relationship between head growth and cognitive scores among older children attending mainstream school confirms the relationship between poor early head growth and developmental outcome[144,145]. Multiple regression analysis has shown that subnormal head growth at 8 months has an independently adverse effect on cognitive abilities at school age[145]. Dolichocephaly on the other hand, often seen in preterm children, has no effect on later IQ[144].

Respiration

CHRONIC LUNG DISEASE (BRONCHOPULMONARY DYSPLASIA)

Since bronchopulmonary dysplasia (BPD) was first described by Northway in 1967 following the introduction of mechanical ventilation[146], there has been a steady increase in the prevalence among survivors, but with an associated reduction in severity[147,148]. Much of this is due to increasing survival following extreme prematurity. Much of the variation in reported incidence relates to the definition of BPD. Traditionally, BPD is defined as a need for supplemental oxygen at 28 days postdelivery with typical chest X-ray changes. With increasing survival at very low gestation, it has been suggested that this may be considered as routine in this group and that it may be more appropriate to extend the age of definition to a gestational age of 36 weeks or term. In a recent report of a cohort of premature infants ≤32 weeks' gestation, chronic lung disease (the preferred term) was present in 19.6% at 28 days, 12.8% at 36 weeks and 4.2% required supplemental oxygen at least periodically at one year of age[149]. In the recent EPICure study, 10% of 310 survivors <26 weeks' gestation required home oxygen therapy at one year (N. Marlow, personal communication). The reduction in the prevalence of this condition among survivors is one of the important goals of modern neonatology.

GROWTH IN CHILDREN WITH CHRONIC LUNG DISEASE

Preterm children with chronic lung disease (CLD) are significantly shorter and lighter than matched gestational controls. In the one very long-term study, below average stature persisted into adulthood[150]. There may also be adverse consequences for head growth; Vohr and colleagues found that preterm children (born <1500 g with CLD) at 11 years of age had significant incidence of reduced (<10th centile) head circumference compared to matched preterm and full-term controls[151]. These findings were echoed when Vrlenich and colleagues reviewed their cohort of <1000 g children between 8 and 10 years of age[152]. Recently, one study of 12-year-old survivors found no height or weight discrepancy between CLD cases and matched preterm controls, although the proportion of CLD children who were underweight was higher[153].

RESPIRATORY FUNCTION AND ILLNESS

Pulmonary dysfunction is widely reported to persist into adolescence and beyond. Northway and colleagues demonstrated an obstructive pattern on respiratory function tests in 68% of their cohort of adolescents aged between 14 and 23 years, manifest as lower peak expiratory flow rate (PEFR), forced vital capacity (FVC), FEV_1, forced expiratory flow between 25 and 75% vital capacity (FEF_{25-75}) and maximal expiratory flow velocity at 50% of vital capacity (V_{max50}), compared to controls. A hyperreactivity response to either methocholine or isoproterenol (isoptenaline) was present in 52% (but no increase in family history of atopy). Hyperinflation was also more frequent, although there was no difference in total lung capacity between BPD cases and controls[150].

There has been concern about exercise ability and responses in children with CLD[150,154]. Exercise capacity in survivors of uncomplicated respiratory distress syndrome has shown to be normal or near normal[155]. In contrast, asymptomatic CLD survivors exhibit striking disturbances in their ventilatory response to exercise, manifest as inability to increase minute ventilation appropriately, leading to alveolar hypoventilation[154,156], although there is some doubt about aerobic capacity. It is unclear what the future holds for these children in later adulthood, for example whether they will be prone to chronic respiratory disease and have reduced exercise tolerance.

Pneumonia, asthma, bronchiolitis, bronchitis and otitis media all occur more frequently among CLD survivors[151,153]. Indeed 35% of the EPICure cohort required treatment for cough and wheeze over the first year (N. Marlow, unpublished data). Hospital readmission may be required for 50% of children in the first year, falling to 20% in the second[153,157,158].

Conclusions

Improvements in perinatal management and in neonatal intensive care have led to dramatic changes in survival for the smallest children. Although there remain concerns that this is accompanied with increasing rates of morbidity, there is little evidence for this as yet and rates of major disabling conditions such as cerebral palsy appear to have stabilised. Although the extremely preterm infant remains at risk of complex disabling conditions, there does appear to be an increasing population of non-disabled survivors. Such children are, however, still at risk of morbidity and disadvantage when compared to their peers, although on an individual basis, it is often difficult to ascribe this to prematurity *per se*. This increased burden of morbidity emphasises the need for longer term outcomes to be assessed as part of the study of perinatal interventions.

The goal of perinatal care must be to optimise the prognosis for the most immature survivors and calls for intervention to ameliorate non-disabling morbidity have been made[159]. As yet, the effects of developmental and behavioural interventions after discharge from neonatal services remain difficult to tease out from social influences on development, although there is early evidence of benefit for the smallest and biologically most vulnerable from one developmental education programme[160] but longer term projects have not shown persisting benefits[113]. Early identification of such impairments and targeted intervention may eventually be most effective means of achieving a further reduction in morbidity for this group.

REFERENCES

1. Keen DV & Pearse RG. Birthweight between 14 and 42 weeks' gestation. *Arch. Dis. Childh.* **60**, 440–446, 1985.
2. Milligan JE & Shennan AT. Perinatal intensive care: where and how to draw the line. *Am. J. Obstet. Gynecol.* **148**, 499–503, 1984.
3. Verloove-Vanhorick SP, Verwey RA, Brand R, Bennebroek Gravenhorst J, Keirse MJN & Ruys JH. Neonatal mortality risk in relation to gestational age and birthweight. *Lancet* **i**, 55–57, 1986.
4. Rennie JM, Wheater M & Cole TJ. Antenatal steroid administration is associated with an improved chance of intact survival in preterm infants. *Eur. J. Pediatr.* **155**, 576–579, 1996.
5. Soll RF & McQueen MC. Resipiratory distress syndrome. In *Effective Care of the Newborn* (eds J.C. Sinclair and M.B. Bracken), pp. 325–358. Oxford: Oxford University Press, 1992.
6. Cartlidge PH & Stewart JH. Survival of very low birthweight and very preterm infants in a geographically defined population. *Acta Paediatr.* **86**, 105–110, 1997.
7. Gultom E, Doyle LW, Davis P, Dharmalingam A & Bowman E. Changes over time in attitudes to treatment and survival rates for extremely preterm infants (23 to 27 weeks' gestational age). *Austral. NZ. J. Obstet. Gynaecol.* **37**, 56–58, 1997.
8. Tin W, Wariyar U & Hey E. Changing prognosis for babies of less than 28 weeks' gestation in the north of England between 1983 and 1994. *BMJ* **314**, 107–111, 1997.
9. Bohin S, Draper ES & Field DJ. Impact of extremely immature infants on neonatal services. *Arch. Dis. Childh. (Fetal. Neonatal)* **74**, F110–113, 1996.
10. The Victorian Infant Collaborative Study Group Outcome at 2 years of children 23 to 27 weeks' gestation born in Victoria in 1991–92. *J. Paediatr. Child. Health* **33**, 161–165, 1997.
11. Hack M, Friedman H & Fanaroff AA. Outcomes of extremely low birth weight infants. *Pediatrics* **98**, 931–937, 1996.
12. Finnström O, Olausson PO, Sedin G *et al.* The Swedish National Prospective Study on Extremely Low Birthweight Infants. Incidence, mortality, morbidity and survival in relation to level of care. *Acta. Paediatr.* **86**, 503–511, 1997.

13. Philip AG. Neonatal mortality rate: is further improvement possible? *J. Pediatr.* **126**, 427–433, 1995.
14. Katz VL & Bose CL. Improving survival of the very premature infant. *J. Perinatol.* **13**, 261–265, 1993.
15. Lefebvre F, Glorieux J & St-Laurent-Gagnon T. Neonatal survival and disability rate at age 18 months for infants born between 23 and 28 weeks of gestation. *Am. J. Obstetr. Gynecol.* **174**, 833–838, 1996.
16. Holtrop PC, Ertzbischoff LM, Roberts CL, Batton DG & Lorenz RP. Survival and short-term outcome in newborns of 23 to 25 weeks' gestation. *Am. J. Obstetr. Gynecol.* **170**, 1266–1270, 1994.
17. Allen MC, Donohue PK & Dusman AE. The limit of viability – neonatal outcome of infants born at 22 to 25 weeks' gestation. *New Engl. J. Med.* **329**, 1597–1601, 1993.
18. Ferrara TB, Hoekstra RE, Couser RJ *et al.* Survival and follow-up of infants born at 23 to 26 weeks of gestational age: effects of surfactant therapy. *J. Pediatr.* **124**, 119–124, 1994.
19. Wood B, Katz V, Bose C, Goolsby R & Kraybill E. Survival and morbidity of extremely premature infants based on obstetric assessment of gestational age. *Obstetr. Gynecol.* **74**, 889–892, 1989.
20. Nishida H. Outcome of infants born preterm, with special emphasis on extremely low birthweight infants. *Baillière's Clin. Obstetr. Gynaecol.* **7**, 611–631, 1993.
21. Working Group on the Very Low Birthweight Infant European Community collaborative study of outcome of pregnancy between 22 and 28 weeks' gestation. *Lancet* **336**, 782–784, 1990.
22. Doyle LW. Outcome to five years of age of children born at 24 to 26 weeks' gestational age in Victoria. The Victorian Infant Collaborative Study Group. *Med. J. Austral.* **163**, 11–14, 1995.
23. Ruys JH, Verloove-Vanhorick SP & Den Ouden AL. The viability of the preterm infant. *Eur. J. Obstetr. Gynecol. Reprod. Biol.* **33**, 31–37, 1989.
24. Synnes AR, Ling EW, Whitfield MF *et al.* Perinatal outcomes of a large cohort of extremely low gestational age infants (23 to 28 completed weeks of gestation). *J. Pediatr.* **125**, 952–960, 1994.
25. Eg-Anderson G. Prediction of outcome in 164 infants born after 24 to 28 weeks gestation. *Acta. Paediatr. Scand.* **360**, 56–61, 1989.
26. Johnson A, Townsend P, Yudkin P & Wilkinson AR. Functional abilities at age 4 years of children born before 29 weeks of gestation. *B.M.J.* **306**, 1715–1718, 1993.
27. Cooke RWI. Factors affecting survival and outcome at 3 years in extremely preterm infants. *Arch. Dis. Childh. (Fetal Neonatal)* **71**, F28–31, 1994.
28. Whyte HE, Fitzhardinge PM, Shennan AT, Lennox K, Smith L & Lacy J. Extreme immaturity: outcome of 568 pregnancies of 23 to 26 weeks' gestation. *Obstetr. Gynecol.* **82**, 1–7, 1993.
29. Weissman A, Jakobi P, Blazer S, Avrahami R & Zimmer EZ. Survival and long-term outcome of infants delivered at 24 to 28 weeks' gestation, by method of delivery and fetal presentation. *J. Perinatol.* **9**, 372–375, 1989.
30. Verloove-Vanhorick SP, Verwey RA, Ebeling M, Brand R & Ruys JH. Mortality in very preterm and very low birthweight infants according to place of birth and level of care: results of a national collaborative survey of preterm and very low birthweight infants in The Netherlands. *Pediatrics* **81**, 404–411, 1988.
31. Wariyar U, Richmond S & Hey E. Pregnancy outcome at 24 to 31 weeks' gestation: neonatal survivors. *Arch. Dis. Childh.* **64**, 678–686, 1989.
32. Nwaesei CG, Young DC, Byrne JM *et al.* Preterm birth at 23 to 26 weeks' gestation: Is active obstetric management justified? *Am. J. Obstetr. Gynecol.* **157**, 890–897, 1987.
33. Yu VYH, Loke HL, Bajuk B, Szymonowicz W, Orgill AA & Astbury J. Prognosis for infants born at 23 to 28 weeks' gestation. *B.M.J.* **293**, 1200–1203, 1986.
34. Kitchen WH, Ford G, Doyle LW *et al.* Cesarean section or vaginal delivery at 24 to 28 weeks' gestation: comparison of survival and neonatal and 2 year morbidity. *Am. J. Obstetr. Gynecol.* **66**, 149–157, 1985.
35. Herschel M, Kennedy J, Kayne H, Henry M & Cetrulo C. Survival of infants born at 24 to 28 weeks' gestation. *Obstetr. Gynecol.* **60**, 154–158, 1982.
36. Dillon WP & Egan EA. Aggressive obstetric management in late second-trimester deliveries. *Obstetr. Gynecol.* **58**, 685–690, 1981.
37. Doyle LW, Murton LJ & Kitchen WH. Increasing the survival of extremely immature (24 to 28 weeks' gestation) infants – at what cost? *Med. J. Austral.* **150**, 558–568, 1989.
38. Fenton AC, Field DJ & Clarke M. Attitudes to viability of preterm infants and their effect on figures for perinatal mortality. *B.M.J.* **300**, 434–436, 1990.
39. Haywood JL, Goldenberg RL, Bronstein J, Nelson KG & Carlo WA. Comparison of perceived and actual rates of survival and freedom from handicap in premature infants. *Am. J. Obstetr. Gynecol.* **171**, 432–439, 1994.
40. The EPICure Study Steering Group EPICure – the extremely preterm baby – a population based study of outcomes of babies born before 26 weeks gestation in the UK and Eire. *Proceedings of the Royal College of Paediatrics and Child Health Annual Meeting*. London, 1996.
41. Report of two working groups Disability and perinatal care: measurement of health status at two years. Oxford: National Perinatal Epidemiology Unit and Oxford Health Authority, 1995.
42. Escobar GJ, Littenberg B & Petitti DB. Outcome among surviving very low birthweight infants: a meta-analysis. *Arch. Dis. Childh.* **66**, 204–211, 1991.
43. La Pine TR, Jackson JC & Bennett FC. Outcome of infants weighing less than 800 grams at birth: 15 years' experience. *Pediatrics* **96**, 479–483, 1995.
44. Casiro O, Bingham W, MacMurray B *et al.* One-year follow-up of 89 infants with birth weights of 500 to 749 grams and respiratory distress syndrome randomized to two rescue doses of synthetic surfactant or air placebo. Canadian Exosurf Neonatal Study Group. Canadian Exosurf Neonatal Follow-Up Group. *J. Pediatr.* **126**, S53–60, 1995.
45. Courtney SE, Long W, McMillan D *et al.* Double-blind 1-year follow-up of 1540 infants with respiratory distress syndrome randomized to rescue treatment with two doses of synthetic surfactant or air in four clinical trials. American and Canadian Exosurf Neonatal Study Groups. *J. Pediatr.* **126**, S43–52, 1995.
46. Gerdes J, Gerdes M, Beaumont E *et al.* Health and neurodevelopmental outcome at 1-year adjusted age in 508 infants weighing 700 to 1100 grams who received prophylaxis with one versus three doses of synthetic surfactant. American Exosurf Neonatal Study Groups I and II. *J. Pediatr.* **126**, S26–32, 1995.
47. Gong A, Anday E, Boros S *et al.* One-year follow-up evaluation of 260 premature infants with respiratory distress syndrome and birth weights of 700 to 1350 grams randomized to two rescue doses of synthetic surfactant or air placebo. American Exosurf Neonatal Study Group I. *J. Pediatr.* **126**, S68–74, 1995.
48. Walther FJ, Mullett M, Schumacher R, Sundell H, Easa D & Long W. One-year follow-up of 66 premature infants weighing 500 to 699 grams treated with a single dose of synthetic surfactant or air placebo at birth: results of a double-blind trial. American Exosurf Neonatal Study Group I. *J. Pediatr.* **126**, S13–19, 1995.
49. Pharoah POD, Platt MJ & Cooke T. The changing epidemiology of cerebral palsy. *Arch. Dis. Childh. (Fetal Neonatal)* **75**, F169–173, 1996.
50. Nelson KB & Ellenberg JH. Children who 'outgrew' cerebral palsy. *Pediatrics* **69**, 529–536, 1982.
51. Hagberg B, Hagberg G, Olow I & van Wendt L. The changing panorama of cerebral palsy in Sweden. VII. Prevalence and origin in the birth year period 1987–90. *Acta. Paediatr.* **85**, 954–960, 1996.
52. Stanley FJ & Watson L. Trends in perinatal mortality and cerebral palsy in Western Australia, 1967 to 1985. *B.M.J.* **304**, 1658–1663, 1992.
53. Krageloh-Mann I, Hagberg G, Meisner C *et al.* Bilateral spastic cerebral palsy – a comparative study between South-West Germany and Western Sweden. II. Epidemiology. *Develop. Med. Child. Neurol.* **36**, 473–483, 1994.
54. Stewart AL, Reynolds EO & Lipscomb AP. Outcome for infants of very low birthweight: survey of world literature. *Lancet* **1**, 1038–1040, 1981.
55. Pharoah POD, Cooke T, Cooke RWI & Rosenbloom L. Birthweight specific trends in cerebral palsy. *Arch. Dis. Childh.* **65**, 602–606, 1990.
56. Ment LR, Oh W, Ehrenkranz RA, Philip AG, Duncan CC & Makuch RW. Antenatal steroids, delivery mode, and intraventricular hemorrhage in preterm infants. *Am. J. Obstet. Gynecol.* **172**, 795–800, 1995.
57. Krageloh-Mann I, Hagberg G, Meisner C *et al.* Bilateral spastic cerebral palsy – a collaborative study between South-West Germany and Western Sweden. III. Aetiology. *Develop. Med. Child. Neurol.* **37**, 191–203, 1995.

58. Murphy DJ, Sellers S, MacKenzie IZ, Yudkin PL & Johnson AM. Case-control study of antenatal and intrapartum risk factors for cerebral palsy in very preterm singleton babies. *Lancet* **346**, 1449–1454, 1995.
59. Murphy DJ, Hope PL & Johnson A. Neonatal risk factors for cerebral palsy in very preterm babies: case-control study. *BMJ* **314**, 404–408, 1997.
60. Nelson KB & Ellenberg JH. Predictors of low and very low birth weight and the relation of these to cerebral palsy. *JAMA* **254**, 1473–1479, 1985.
61. Amin H, Singhal N & Sauve RS. Impact of intrauterine growth restriction on neurodevelopmental and growth outcomes in very low birthweight infants. *Acta Paediatr* **86**, 306–314, 1997.
62. Blair E & Stanley FJ. Intrauterine growth and spastic cerebral palsy. *Am. J. Obstetr. Gynecol.* **162**, 229–237, 1990.
63. Report of the Working Group on Definitions of Disability in Childhood. Disability in childhood: towards nationally useful definitions. Part one: language definitions and recommendations. British Association for Community Child Health and Department of Health, 1994.
64. Amiel-Tison C & Stewart A. Follow up studies during the first five years of life: a pervasive assessment of neurological function. *Arch. Dis. Childh.* **64**, 496–502, 1989.
65. Evans PM, Johnson A, Mutch L & Alberman E. A standard form for recording clinical findings in children with a motor deficit of central origin [Letter]. *Develop. Med. Child. Neurol.* **31**, 117–129, 1989.
66. Bax M. Terminology and classification of cerebral palsy. *Develop. Med. Child. Neurol.* **6**, 295–297, 1964.
67. Little WJ. On the influence of abnormal parturition, difficult labours, premature birth, and asphyxia neonatorum on the mental and physical condition of the child, especially in relation to deformities. *Transcript Obstetric Soc. London* **3**, 293–344, 1862.
68. Freud S. Les diplegies cerebrales infantiles. *Revue Neurologique* **1**, 177–183, 1893.
69. Marlow N & Chiswick ML. Neurodevelopmental outcome in extremely low birth weight survivors. *Recent Adv. Perinatal Med.* **2**, 181–205, 1985.
70. Powell TG, Pharoah POD, Cooke RWI & Rosenbloom L. Cerebral palsy in low birthweight infants. I. Spastic hemiplegia: associations with intrapartum stress. *Develop. Med. Child. Neurol.* **30**, 11–18, 1988.
71. Powell TG, Pharoah POD, Cooke RWI & Rosenbloom L. Cerebral palsy in low birthweight infants. II. Spastic diplegia: associations with fetal immaturity. *Develop. Med. Child Neurol.* **30**, 19–25, 1988.
72. Cooke RWI. Cerebral palsy in very low birthweight infants. *Arch. Dis. Childh.* **65**, 201–206, 1990.
73. Hutton JL, Cooke T & Pharoah POD. Life expectancy in children with cerebral palsy. *BMJ* **309**, 431–435, 1994.
74. Marlow N, Roberts L & Cooke RWI. Outcome at 8 years for children with birth weights of 1250 g or less. *Arch. Dis. Childh.* **68**, 286–290, 1993.
75. Veen S, Ens-Dokkum M, Schreuder AM, Verloove-Vanhorick SP, Brand R & Ruys JH. Impairments, disabilities, and handicaps of very preterm and very-low-birthweight infants at five years of age. *Lancet* **338**, 33–36, 1991.
76. Jongmans M, Mercuri E, de Vries L, Dubowitz L & Henderson SE. Minor neurological signs and perceptual-motor difficulties in prematurely born children. *Arch. Dis. Childh. (Fetal Neonatal)* **76**, F9–14, 1997.
77. Stott DH, Moyer FA & Henderson SE. *Test of Motor Impairment (Henderson revision)*. Ontario: Brook Educational, 1984.
78. Henderson SE & Sugden D. *Movement Assessment Battery for Children*. London: Psychological Corporation, 1992.
79. Marlow N, Roberts BL & Cooke RWI. Motor skills in extremely low birth weight children at the age of six years. *Arch. Dis. Childh.* **64**, 839–847, 1989.
80. Powls A, Botting N, Cooke RWI & Marlow N. Motor impairment in children 12 to 13 years old with a birthweight of less than 1250 g. *Arch. Dis. Childh. (Fetal Neonatal)* **72**, F62–66, 1995.
81. Elliman AM, Bryan EM, Elliman AD, Walker J & Harvey DR. Coordination in low birth weight seven year olds. *Acta Paediatr. Scand.* **80**, 316–322, 1991.
82. O'Callaghan M, Burns Y, Mohay H, Rogers Y & Tudehope D. Handedness in extremely low birth weight infants: aetiology and relationship to intellectual abilities, motor performance and behaviour at 4 and 6 years. *Cortex* **29**, 629–637, 1993.
83. Marlow N, Roberts BL & Cooke RWI. Laterality and prematurity. *Arch. Dis. Childh.* **64**, 1713–1716, 1989.
84. Bakan P. Handedness and birth order. *Nature* **229**, 195, 1971.
85. Annett M. *Left, Right, Hand, Brain: The Right Shift Theory*. London: Erlbaum, 1985.
86. Konishi Y, Kuriyama M, Mikawa H & Suzuki J. The effect of body position on later postural and functional lateralities of preterm infants. *Develop. Med. Child. Neurol.* **29**, 751–757, 1987.
87. Satz P. Pathological left handedness; an explanatory model. *Cortex* **8**, 121–135, 1972.
88. Ross G, Lipper EG & Auld PA. Hand preference of four-year-old children: its relationship to premature birth and neurodevelopmental outcome. *Develop. Med. Child Neurol.* **29**, 615–622, 1987.
89. Saigal S, Rosenbaum P, Szatmari P & Hoult L. Non-right handedness among ELBW and term children at eight years in relation to cognitive function and school performance. *Develop. Med. Child Neurol.* **34**, 425–433, 1992.
90. Powls A, Botting N, Cooke RWI & Marlow N. Handedness in very-low-birthweight children at 12 years of age: relation to perinatal and outcome variables. *Develop. Med. Child Neurol.* **38**, 594–602, 1996.
91. Drillien CM, Thomson AJM & Burgoyne K. Low birthweight children at early school age: a longitudinal study. *Develop. Med. Child Neurol.* **22**, 26–47, 1980.
92. Wigglesworth JS & Pape KE. An integrated model for haemorrhage and ischaemic lesions in the newborn brain. *Early Hum. Dev.* **2**, 179–199, 1978.
93. Largo RH, Kundu S & Thun-Hohenstein L. Early motor development in term and preterm children. In *Motor Development in Early and Later Childhood: Longitudinal Approaches* (eds A.F. Kalverboor, B. Hopkins and R. Genze), pp. 247–285. Cambridge: Cambridge University Press, 1993.
94. de Vries LS, Dubowitz LM, Dubowitz V *et al.* Predictive value of cranial ultrasound in the newborn baby: a reappraisal. *Lancet* **ii**, 137–140, 1985.
95. Drillien CM. Abnormal neurological signs in the first year of life in low birthweight infants; possible prognostic significance. *Develop. Med. Child. Neurol.* **14**, 575–584, 1972.
96. Khadlikar V, Tudehope D, Burns Y, O'Callaghan M & Mohay H. The long term neurodevelopmental outcome for very low birth weight infants with 'dystonic' signs at 4 months of age. *J. Pediatr. Child Health* **29**, 415–417, 1993.
97. Sommerfelt K, Pedersen S, Ellertsen B & Markestad T. Transient dystonia in non-handicapped low-birthweight infants and later neurodevelopment. *Acta Paediatr.* **85**, 1445–1449, 1996.
98. Illsley R & Mitchell RG. *Low Birthweight: A Medical, Psychological and Social Study*. Chichester: John Wiley, 1984.
99. Sameroff AJ & Chandler MJ. Reproductive risk and the continuum of caretaking casuality. In *Review of Child Development Research, 1965* (ed. F.D. Horrowitz), pp. 187–244. Chicago: University of Chicago Press, 1975.
100. Gesell A & Armatruda CS. *Developmental Diagnosis: Normal and Abnormal Child Development*. New York: Hoeber, 1947.
101. Hess JH. Experience gained in a 30 year study of prematurely born infants. *Pediatrics* **11**, 425–434, 1953.
102. Lloyd BW, Wheldall K & Perks D. Controlled study of intelligence and school performance of very low birthweight children from a defined geographical area. *Develop. Med. Child Neurol.* **30**, 36–42, 1988.
103. Hille ETM, Den Ouden AL, Bauer L, van den Oudenrijn C, Brand R & Verloove-Vanhorick SP. School performance at nine years of age in very premature and very low birth weight infants: Perinatal risk factors and predictors at five years of age. *J. Pediatr.* **125**, 426–434, 1994.
104. Vohr BR & Garcia Coll CT. Neurodevelopmental and school performance of very low-birth-weight infants: a seven-year longitudinal study. *Pediatrics* **76**, 345–350, 1985.
105. Hack M, Taylor HG, Klein N, Eiben R, Schatschneider C & Mercuri-Minich N. School-age outcomes in children with birth weights under 750 g. *New Engl. J. Med.* **331**, 753–759, 1994.
106. Eilers BL, Desai NS, Wilson MA & Cunningham MD. Classroom performance and social factors of children with birthweights of 1250 g or less. *Pediatrics* **77**, 203–208, 1986.

107. Saigal S, Szatmari P, Rosenbaum P, Campbell D & King S. Cognitive abilities and school performance of extremely low birth weight children and matched term control children at age 8 years: A regional study. *J. Pediatr.* **118**, 751–760, 1991.
108. Botting N & Marlow N. Cognitive and educational outcome of very low birth weight children in early adolescence. *Develop. Med. Child Neurol.* **40**, 652–660, 1997.
109. Ross G, Lipper EG & Auld PA. Educational status and school-related abilities of very low birth weight premature children. *Pediatrics* **88**, 1125–1134, 1991.
110. Brand C. Intelligence testing: bryter still and bryter? *Nature* **328**, 110, 1987.
111. Halsey CL, Collin MF & Anderson CL. Extremely low birthweight children and their peers: a comparison of preschool performance. *Pediatrics* **91**, 807–811, 1993.
112. MacKinlay I, England A, Nash S, Sands J, Chesham I & Dobbing J. The predictive value of coordination testing. *Neuropediatrics* **12** (suppl.), 426, 1981.
113. McCarton CM, Brooks-Gunn J, Wallace IF *et al.* Results at age 8 years of early intervention for low-birth-weight premature infants. The Infant Health and Development Program. *JAMA* **277**, 126–132, 1997.
114. Astbury J, Orgill A & Bajuk B. Relationship between two-year behaviour and neurodevelopmental outcome at five years of very low birthweight survivors. *Develop. Med. Child Neurol.* **29**, 370–379, 1987.
115. The Scottish Low Birthweight Study Group The Scottish low birthweight study: II. Language attainment, cognitive status, and behavioural problems. *Arch. Dis. Childh.* **67**, 682–686, 1992.
116. Szatmari P, Saigal S, Rosenbaum P & Campbell D. Psychopathology and adaptive functioning among extremely low birth weight children at eight years of age. *Develop. Psychopathol.* **5**, 345–357, 1993.
117. Dunn HG, Ho HH & Schylzer M. Minimal brain dysfunction. In *Sequelae of Low Birthweight: The Vancouver Study* (ed. H.G. Dunn), pp. 97–113. Oxford: MacKeith Press, 1986.
118. Bird HR, Gould MS & Staghezza-Jaramillo BM. The co-morbidity of ADHD in a community sample of children aged 6 through 16 years. *J. Child Family Studies* **3**, 365–378, 1994.
119. Loeber R, Green SM, Keenan K & Lahey BB. Which boys will fare worse? Early predictors of the onset of conduct disorder in a six-year longitudinal study. *J. Am. Acad. Child Adolescent Psychiatry* **34**, 499–509, 1995.
120. Levy-Shiff R, Einat G, Mogilner MB, Lerman M & Krikler R. Biological and environmental correlates of developmental outcome of prematurely born infants in early adolescence. *J. Pediatr Psychol.* **19**, 63–78, 1994.
121. Botting N, Powls A, Cooke RWI & Marlow N. Psychiatric outcomes in teenage very low birthweight children. *J. Child Psychol. Psychiatr. Allied Disciplines* **38**, 931–941, 1997.
122. Angold A, Prendergast M, Cox A, Harrington R, Simonoff E & Rutter M. The Child and Adolescent Psychiatric Assessment (CAPA). *Psychol. Med.* **25**, 739–753, 1995.
123. Marlow N, Botting N, Powls A & Cooke RWI. Psychiatric outcomes in adolescent very low birthweight children. *Pediatr. Res.* **41**, 204A (Abstract), 1997.
124. Marlow ES. The Antecedents of Sensorineural Hearing Loss in Very Preterm Children. MSc Thesis. University of Manchester, 1997.
125. Abramovich SJ, Gregory S, Slemick M & Stewart A. Hearing loss in very low birthweight infants treated with neonatal intensive care. *Arch. Dis. Childh.* **54**, 421–426, 1979.
126. Doyle LW, Keir EH & Kitchen WH. Audiological assessment of extremely low birthweight infants: a preliminary report. *Pediatrics* **90**, 744–749, 1992.
127. Phelps DL & Rosenbaum AL. Effects of marginal hypoxemia on recovery from oxygen-induced retinopathy in the kitten model. *Pediatrics* **73**, 1–6, 1984.
128. Flynn JT. Retinopathy of prematurity. *Pediatr. Clin. North America* **34**, 1487–1516, 1987.
129. Committee for the Classification of Retinopathy of Prematurity An international classification of retinopathy of prematurity. *Arch. Ophthalmol.* **102**, 1130–1134, 1984.
130. Committee for the Classification of Retinopathy of Prematurity The classification of retinal detachment. *Arch. Ophthalmol* **105**, 906–912, 1987.
131. Palmer EA, Flynn JT, Hardy RJ *et al.* Incidence and early course of retinopathy of prematurity. *Ophthalmology* **98**, 1628–1640, 1991.
132. Pennefather PM, Clarke MP, Strong NP, Cottrell DG, Fritz S & Tin W. Ocular outcome in children born before 32 weeks gestation. *Eye* **9**, 26–30, 1995.
133. Dowdeswell HJ, Slater AM, Broomhall J & Tripp J. Visual deficits in children born at less than 32 weeks' gestation with and without major ocular pathology and cerebral damage. *Br. J. Ophthalmol.* **79**, 447–452, 1995.
134. Powls A, Botting N, Cooke RWI, Stephenson G & Marlow N. Visual impairment in very low birthweight children. *Arch. Dis. Childh. (Fetal Neonatal)* **76**, F82–87, 1997.
135. Abramov I, Hailine L, Lemerise E & Brown AK. Changes in visual functions of children exposed as infants to prolonged illumination. *J. Am. Optometric Ass.* **56**, 614–619, 1985.
136. Fielder AR, Moseley MJ & Ng YK. The immature visual system and premature birth. *Br. Med. Bull.* **44**, 1093–1118, 1988.
137. Pike MG, Holmstrom G, de Vries LS *et al.* Patterns of visual impairment associated with lesions of the preterm infant brain. *Develop. Med. Child Neurol.* **36**, 849–862, 1994.
138. Eken P, van Nieuwenhuizen O, van der Graaf Y, Schalij-Delfos NE & de Vries LS. Relation between neonatal cranial ultrasound abnormalities and cerebral visual impairment in infancy. *Develop. Med. Child Neurol.* **36**, 3–15, 1994.
139. Hack M, Merkatz IR, McGrath S, Jones PK & Fanaroff AA. Catch-up growth in very low birth weight infants. *Am. J. Dis. Childr.* **138**, 370–374, 1984.
140. Ross G, Lipper E & Auld PAM. Growth achievement of very low birth weight premature children at school age. *J. Pediatr.* **117**, 307–309, 1990.
141. Casey PH, Kraemer HC, Bernbaum JC *et al.* Growth patterns of low birth weight preterm infants: a longitudinal analysis of a large, varied sample. *J. Pediatr.* **117**, 298–307, 1990.
142. Kitchen WH, Doyle LW, Ford G & Callanan C. Very low birth weight and growth at age 8 years. I. Weight and height. *Am. J. Dis. Childr.* **146**, 40–45, 1992.
143. Powls A, Botting N, Cooke RWI, Pilling D & Marlow N. Growth impairment in very low birthweight children at 12 years: correlation with perinatal and outcome variables. *Arch. Dis. Childh. (Fetal Neonatal)* **75**, F152–157, 1996.
144. Kitchen WH, Doyle LW, Ford G, Callanan C, Rickards A & Kelly E. Very low birth weight and growth at 8 years. II: Head dimensions and intelligence. *Am. J. Dis. Childr.* **146**, 46–50, 1992.
145. Hack M, Breslau N, Weissman B, Aram D, Klein N, Borawski E. Effect of very low birth weight and subnormal head size on cognitive abilities at school age. *New Engl. J. Med.* **325**, 231–237, 1991.
146. Northway WH, Rosan RC & Porter DY. Pulmonary disease following respirator therapy of hyaline membrane disease. Bronchopulmonary dysplasia. *New Engl. J. Med.* **276**, 358–368, 1967.
147. Cooke RWI. Factors associated with chronic lung disease in preterm infants. *Arch. Dis. Childh.* **66**, 776–779, 1991.
148. Northway WH. Bronchopulmonary dysplasia: then and now. *Arch. Dis. Childh.* **65**, 1076–1081, 1990.
149. Farstad T & Bratlid D. Incidence and prediction of bronchopulmonary dysplasia in a cohort of premature infants. *Acta Paediatr.* **83**, 19–24, 1994.
150. Northway WH, Moss RB, Carlisle KB *et al.* Late pulmonary sequelae of bronchopulmonary dysplasia. *New Engl. J. Med.* **323**, 1793–1799, 1990.
151. Vohr BR, Coll CG, Lobato D, Yunis KA, O'Dea C & Oh W. Neurodevelopmental and medical status of low birth weight survivors of bronchopulmonary dysplasia at 10 to 12 years of age. *Develop. Med. Child Neurol.* **33**, 690–697, 1991.
152. Vrlenich LA, Bozynski ME, Shyr Y, Schork MA, Roloff DW & McCormick MC. The effect of bronchopulmonary dysplasia on growth at school age. *Pediatrics* **95**, 855–859, 1995.
153. Giacoia GP, Venkataraman PS, West-Wilson KI & Faulkner MJ. Follow up of school-age children with bronchopulmonary dysplasia. *J. Pediatr.* **130**, 400–408, 1997.
154. Bader D, Ramos AD, Lew CD, Platzker ACG, Stabile MS & Keens TG. Childhood sequelae of infant lung disease: exercise and pulmonary function abnormalities after bronchopulmonary dysplasia. *J. Pediatr.* **110**, 693–699, 1987.

155. Baraldi E, Zanconato S, Zorzi C, Santuz P, Benini F & Zacchello F. Exercise performance in very low birth weight children at the age of 7–12 years. *Eur. J. Pediatr.* **150**, 713–716, 1991.
156. Santuz P, Baraldi E, Zaramella P, Filippone M & Zacchello F. Factors limiting exercise performance in long-term survivors of bronchopulmonary dysplasia. *Am. J. Resp. Critical Care Med.* **152**, 1284–1289, 1995.
157. Koops BL, Abman SH & Accurso FJ. Outpatient management and follow up of bronchopulmonary dysplasia. *Clin. Perinatol.* **11**, 101–121, 1984.
158. Samuels MP & Warner JO. Bronchopulmonary dysplasia: the outcome. *Arch. Dis. Childh.* **62**, 1099–1101, 1987.
159. Davies P. Intervention. *Develop. Med. Child Neurol.* **33**, 283–284, 1991.
160. Marlow N & Robinson M. Post-discharge intervention for families with preterm babies. *Pediatr. Res.* **39**, 272A (Abstract), 1996.

The contribution of perinatal asphyxia in the term infant to outcomes in children

83

N. Marlow

Introduction

Most children who have neonatal symptoms attributable to perinatal hypoxia or asphyxia have no discernible impairment at follow up. Despite this, over the years, hypoxia occurring during the birth process has been cited in the causation of many outcomes, ranging from cerebral palsy, sensorineural hearing loss, behavioural difficulties, learning difficulty, left-handedness and even schizophrenia. Some of these associates are sustainable after careful consideration but others are not. Good longitudinal prospective studies which assess other than severely disabling conditions in this area are rare.

Similarly, most children with disability have not been asphyxiated at birth and perinatal hypoxia would appear to be a relatively uncommon cause of cerebral palsy[1–4]. From population studies[5,6], there appears to be consensus that only about 10% of cases of cerebral palsy are caused by intrapartum asphyxia. Nonetheless, this still represents a significant number of children who acquire their neurological impairment around the time of birth. Even in term infants with cerebral palsy, intrapartum events probably only account for 1 in 5 cases[6]. The 'gold standard' by which *significant* or damaging perinatal hypoxia is identified in the neonatal period is the presence of encephalopathy in the first few days after birth. Even encephalopathy may be a manifestation of conditions other than acute intrapartum hypoxia[7].

Because of these difficulties and the high likelihood of a normal outcome following 'asphyxia' identified by measures of condition made at birth, such as Apgar score and pH, the many studies of outcome have produced confusing and confounding results. One reason for this is that there is no single distinct neuropathological injury which may occur following acute intrapartum hypoxia, and appearances range from a global insult, with extensive swelling and necrosis, to more focal necrotic injuries[8] (Table 83.1). The pattern of injury probably relates to the differential effects of anoxia (acute total hypoxia) and hypoxia (chronic or partial hypoxia), to the time course of exposure of the fetus to a failure of oxygen delivery and to the individual vulnerability of each fetus[9]. To complicate issues, different animal models provide evidence of species differences in patterns of brain injury[10], making extrapolation of findings from such experiments to the human situation difficult. Furthermore, the pattern of injury appears different in the more immature fetus. Focal white matter injury, periventricular leucomalacia, occurs commonly in very preterm children post-hypoxia or ischaemia and will not be discussed further here. In the term infant, post-hypoxic neuronal necrosis more commonly affects grey or both grey and white matter.

TABLE 83.1
Patterns of brain injury following perinatal asphyxia

- Parasagittal cerebral injury
- Focal or multifocal neuronal necrosis
- Status marmoratus
- Selective neuronal necrosis
- Periventricular leucomalacia

In term post-hypoxic children, parasagittal neuronal necrosis is a frequent finding, resulting from cellular injury at the junction of territories between anterior, middle and posterior cerebral arteries[11]. Ulegyria, gyral sclerosis with widening of the sulci, which is also probably a 'watershed' injury, has been described particularly in the hippocampus, pre- and post-central gyri and occipital cortex[8]. Subcortical leucomalacia, with injury to both cortical and subcortical structures at the base of the sulci, may occur and is an injury which cannot be simply explained in vascular terms[12]. A marble-like appearance of the basal ganglia and thalamus due to abnormal myelination, status marmoratus, is classically associated with hypoxia and develops over several months. Bilateral thalamic involvement, usually as haemorrhage, is rare in autopsy specimens and associated with widespread brain injury. Thalamic injury may be seen in life and injuries to the basal ganglia may be found using a variety of cerebral imaging techniques[13] indicating that this is a frequent site for injury among post-hypoxic children. Brainstem injury may be found in association with basal ganglia lesions, and may be reflected in feeding and visual problems.

Generally, children with significant perinatal hypoxia will manifest usually reversible signs of tissue injury in other organs (Table 83.2), which reflect the redistribution of blood flow that occurs in response to hypoxia[14,15]. Of interest is the observation that neurological signs of encephalopathy may rarely coincide with signs of persistent pulmonary hypertension of the newborn, itself associated with perinatal and ongoing postnatal hypoxia, leading to the speculation that post-natal hypoxia may act in a protective fashion against further neurological injury[16]. It is prudent to seek evidence of non-CNS organ damage if perinatal hypoxia is suspected, not only for reasons of good clinical practice but also to differentiate those children in whom their encephalopathy may be due to other causes[7].

Hence, the outcome following perinatal hypoxia may not be completely predictable from clinical obstetric or neonatal measures and will reflect the pattern of underlying brain injury. Early studies seem to indicate that cerebral injury following hypoxia was an 'all-or-none' phenomenon, children either having evidence of severe neurological injury or surviving free of disability. The limitations of such a hypothesis will be discussed below.

TABLE 83.2
Specific organ damage following perinatal hypoxia defined at birth[14]

	Single organ involvement		Multiple organ involvement	
Infants with	Total† (*n* = 19)	Severe* (*n* = 11)	Total† (*n* = 40)	Severe* (*n* = 9)
CNS	14	2	38	5
Renal	3	3	27	8
Pulmonary	1	6	18	8
Heart	0	0	21	0
Gastrointestinal	1	0	20	1

Note: 30 infants had no organ injury.

†Hypoxic-ischaemic encephalopathy Stage 1 or 2. Oliguria; Inspired oxygen >0.4 for >4 h; heart murmur and ECG changes; gastric bleeding or vomiting
*Hypoxic-ischaemic encephalopathy Stage 3, Creatinine >110 μmol/l for >48 h; mechanical ventilation for lung disease; heart failure; necrotising enterocolitis or massive bleeding.

Major disability following perinatal hypoxia

The classic disabling condition associated with intrapartum hypoxia is cerebral palsy. This may be also associated with varying degrees of cognitive impairment, cortical visual loss, sensorineural hearing loss and seizures. In an eight-year follow up of 23 children with moderate or severe neonatal encephalopathy and disability, 13 had cerebral palsy, 10 severe/profound cognitive delay, 7 had a seizure disorder (5 multiply disabled), 6 had sensorineural deafness requiring amplification and 3 had visual loss (all multiply disabled)[17]. Such a pattern of outcomes would seem fairly typical.

Cerebral palsy most commonly comprises a spastic quadriplegia, which is usually severe and may have dystonic or athetoid features, although occasionally it may take the form of a hemiplegia. These children tend to have a protracted recovery from their initial illness with prolonged feeding problems. The neurological abnormality is often obvious at discharge from the neonatal service as hypo- or hypertonia, but may be manifest only as hypotonicity of the upper limb and shoulder girdle[17] and some children appear to have few signs. In those few who appear to make a good initial recovery, signs of evolving cerebral palsy develop over the first four months. Because of the likely associated disability, early referral for assessment of vision and hearing is important and the care for such children is best managed from within a multidisciplinary community child health service than from a hospital follow-up clinic.

A cerebral palsy in which athetosis predominates is also associated with intrapartum hypoxia and reflects the predilection for injury to the basal ganglia. These children may have an initial hypotonic phase during which signs of extrapyramidal movements evolve over the first year. In most children there are associated cognitive impairments. Rosenbloom[18] has argued that athetoid cerebral palsy without cognitive impairment may follow a period of acute anoxia and poor condition at birth, but with little neonatal sequelae. A further group have suggested that rarely the onset of athetoid cerebral palsy may be very delayed into the second decade[19].

Isolated severe cognitive impairment (IQ <70) has not been associated with perinatal hypoxia, but a variable degree of cognitive impairment is common among children with cerebral palsy. Visual loss is secondary to loss of central cortical connections, either as part of a brainstem injury or due to injury to the occipital cortex ('cortical blindness'), and it too is usually associated with other disability. Visual evoked potentials may be useful in the evaluation of vision[20].

Sensorineural hearing loss may be secondary to CNS injury or to direct damage to the organ of Corti during the hypoxic process. It is characterised by a bilateral high-frequency loss. In a series of elegant experiments, Jiang[21,22] has demonstrated differential effects of hypoxia on the brainstem and peripheral auditory systems. Central processing of the auditory signal may be depressed following hypoxia but generally recovers, making auditory brainstem responses (ABRs) poorly predictive for later abnormality. Peripheral auditory impairment may not recover. It is suggested that the peripheral auditory system may be one further site prone to hypoxic injury. Most children with auditory impairment following intrapartum hypoxia have other associated abnormalities, such as cerebral palsy, but in many studies there are individuals in which deafness is a sole impairment[23–25]. Deafness in the non-hypoxic population remains relatively rare and thus it seems likely, therefore, that sensorineural deafness is related to hypoxic injury, although some would dispute this, preferring to cite other potential aetiologies[17].

Epilepsy is by no means universal among survivors of severe perinatal hypoxia and is usually associated with other impairment. Occasionally seizure disorders may be severe and perinatal hypoxia is among the differential diagnoses in children with infantile spasms.

PREDICTION OF MAJOR DISABLING CONDITIONS

A number of studies have attempted to use a variety of neonatal measures to predict the likelihood of a poor outcome. Potential candidates include:

- Stage of neonatal encephalopathy
- Apgar score
- Fetal acidosis (pH or base excess measures)
- Time to onset of spontaneous breathing after birth
- Time to establish suckling feeds
- Neurological condition at discharge
- Neuroimaging
- Blood flow velocity studies
- Cortical evoked potentials

Clinical neurological observations

ENCEPHALOPATHY

Of clinical measures, the most powerful predictor remains the worst stage of encephalopathy observed in the child during the first week. In 1967, Prechtl categorised the abnormal neonatal neurological examination as three clinical pictures characterised by hyperalertness, lethargy or stupor, respectively[26]. These were refined into the commonly used three grades of encephalopathy as described by Sarnat and Sarnat in 1974[27]. Various attempts have been made to improve on these descriptions[28,29], but the original Sarnat grading appears robust and clear in its categorisation (Table 83.3). A meta-analysis of outcome following neonatal encephalopathy has recently been published[30] but it should be noted that small differences in the application of the grading may significantly modify the predictive value of the system[17].

STAGE 1 (MILD) ENCEPHALOPATHY

This includes hyperalertness, staring, normal or decreased motor activity, a low stimuli threshold and sympathetic responses. For the majority of children, this is a relatively transient phase with full recovery by one week, although the signs may persist[31]. It is agreed that all children in this category will be free of disability at follow up[17] and in long-term studies survivors appear to have normal cognitive and neuropsychological scores and growth[17]. In meta-analysis[30], the risk of mortality and morbidity in this group was close to zero (Table 83.4). In one study, a poor outcome has been reported in one

TABLE 83.3
Clinical staging of neonatal encephlopathy[27]

	Stage 1 (mild)	Stage 2 (moderate)	Stage 3 (severe)
Consciousness	Hyperalert	Lethargic	Stuporose
Neuromuscular control			
Muscle tone	Normal	Mild hypotonia	Flaccid
Posture	Mild distal flexion	Strong distal flexion	Intermittent decerebration
Stretch reflexes	Overactive	Overactive	Decreased/absent
Segmental myoclonus	Present	Present	Absent
Complex reflexes			
Suck	Weak	Weak/absent	Absent
Moro	Strong/low threshold	Weak; incomplete; high threshold	Absent
Oculovestibular	Normal	Overactive	Weak/absent
Tonic neck	Slight	Strong	Absent
Autonomic function	Generalised sympathetic	Generalised parasympathetic	Both systems depressed
Pupils	Mydriasis	Miosis	Variable; often unequal; poor light reflex
Heart rate	Tachycardia	Bradycardia	Variable
Bronchial and salivary secretions	Sparse	Profuse	Variable
Gastrointestinal motility	Normal or decreased	Increased/diarrhoea	Variable
Seizures	None	Common; focal or multifocal	Uncommon (excluding decerebration)

TABLE 83.4
Typical estimates of likelihood ratio (95% confidence interval) for the degree of encephalopathy as a predictor of outcome[30]

	Encephalopathy worst grade		
Outcome	Stage I (mild)	Stage 2 (moderate)	Stage 3 (severe)
Death vs. survival	0.09 (0.03, 0.30)	0.39 (0.21, 0.71)	10.98 (7.56, 15.94)
Severe vs. no handicap	0.10 (0.03, 0.28)	1.15 (1.19, 1.52)	15.60 (6.85, 35.70)
Death or severe handicap vs. no handicap	0.05 (0.02, 0.15)	0.94 (0.71, 1.23)	10.71 (6.71, 17.10)

child who was found to have severe spinal muscular atrophy[32]. The importance of accurate categorisation is demonstrated by the observation that inclusion of transient hypotonia or suppressed primitive reflexes in this group is associated with occasional adverse outcomes[17].

STAGE 2 (MODERATE) ENCEPHALOPATHY

This includes lethargy, decreased spontaneous movements and hypotonia, suppressed primitive responses and parasympathetic responses. Often children will show marked hypotonicity of the proximal upper limbs and shoulder girdle[17]. Some authorities consider this to be the last abnormal neurological sign to disappear in such children. Seizures may occur commonly in this grade. Indeed, some classifications suggest that a seizure automatically places the child into this category as a minimum[28], or that children with moderate encephalopathy and seizures are placed in a higher risk group (Stage 2b)[29]. Clinical experience suggests that children with a prolonged seizure disorder are at much higher risk than those with brief, easily-controlled seizures. About 1 in 5 children in this category will have a poor outcome and this risk is increased if the signs persist. In meta-analysis[30], the risk of death following moderate encephalopathy was 5.6%, the risk of handicap 20% and for a poor outcome (death or handicap) 24% (Table 83.4). For some children in this category, athetoid cerebral palsy may predominate[17], compared to children following more severe encephalopathy. Children in this group who are free of disability may have more subtle impairments at follow up (see below).

STAGE 3 (SEVERE) ENCEPHALOPATHY

Children in this category are flaccid, stuporose with absent primitive reflexes and often few seizures. There is marked respiratory depression. Care must be taken to differentiate the effects of hypoxia from those of anticonvulsant or sedative medication. Careful assignment of this category produces a group of children with high mortality and universal severe disability among survivors. Severe cognitive impairment is usual, the children are frequently dependent and life expectancy may be reduced. Some studies report 'normal' survivors in this category but difficulty in defining the effects of medication and a reduced emphasis on flaccidity and absence of primitive reflexes may account for this. In meta-analysis[30], the risk of death was 61%, of handicap 72% and for a poor outcome 78% (Table 83.4).

CONDITION AT BIRTH

Many studies have tried to predict outcome using measures made at birth or in the delivery room. Three recent studies have reviewed the outcome of successful resuscitation following apparent stillbirth[33–35]. Despite this being the highest risk group, in these three studies 43% children survived without major disability (95% confidence interval 31–55%). Within this group persistence of poor condition is associated with a worse outcome, one group suggesting a cut off of about 10 min. This is in keeping with the results of studies where late Apgar scores have been used as measures of persisting poor condition in population studies[30]. Following an Apgar score below 4 at 10 min, 38.6% died and 17.8% had neurological sequelae. In Nelson and Ellenberg's study (36), a similar Apgar score at 20 min was associated with 59% mortality and 57% severe morbidity. Time to spontaneous breathing may be related to the degree or duration of hypoxia and has been used as a predictor of outcome, defined as death or handicap, after periods of apnoea of 20 or 30 min[30]. These studies must be interpreted with caution as all are small studies and rarely population based. All have high rates of poor outcome in their reference groups. Death or disability is high in the extreme group (72%) compared to 12% in the group where breathing started before 30 min. A significant delay in the establishment of spontaneous respiration is associated with high risk of poor outcome.

Umbilical cord pH and other markers of acidosis (base excess, lactic acid concentrations) have been studied as predictors of outcome. Generally, they are considered poorly discriminative and, as with Apgar scores, it is the extremes of acidosis which are associated with poor outcome[37]. Cord pH values are often used as outcome measures for obstetric studies, citing evidence that the Apgar scores are unreliable. There are no data to support the contention that intermediate values of either acidosis or of Apgar scores are valuable as predictors of poor neurological outcome and it would seem that neither gives an adequate picture of fetal compromise for predictive purposes.

Neonatal neurological investigations

EARLY EEG RECORDINGS

For some years the EEG recorded early in the postnatal course has provided a good predictor of outcome. In meta-analysis of four studies performed between 1970 and 1984[30], severe EEG changes were associated with 95% risk of severe disability or death compared to 64% for moderately abnormal records and 3% for normal or mild abnormalities. Amplitude integrated, single channel EEG (cerebral function monitoring, CFM) also may be valuable in the prediction of outcome. In one Swedish study[38] continuous CFM activity over the first two days was associated with a normal outcome in all of 17 children, whereas burst suppression or paroxysmal activity was associated with adverse outcome in 20 of 21 children. More recently, the quality of the CFM trace made within the first 6 hours after birth has been shown to correctly identify outcome in 43 of 47 children (91.5%)[39]. Given the occasional difficulties in assessment of heavily sedated children after treatment of seizures, early EEG clearly has a place in the initial assessment of such children.

IMAGING: ULTRASOUND, COMPUTED TOMOGRAPHY (CT) AND MAGNETIC RESONANCE IMAGING (MRI)

Imaging has not been shown to be beneficial when performed in the first few days following birth. The early brain swelling that occurs obscures the impact of the hypoxic insult, whichever technique is used, although some early MRI appearances of significant injury may have now been recognised[40]. The appearance on ultrasound of bilateral thalamic haemorrhage carries a poor prognosis. Later evolution of ultrasound appearances, such as cortical atrophy and cystic leucomalacia, are poor prognosis signs, but the predictive value of an unremarkable scan is generally held to be low. However, in a recent comparison of ultrasound and MRI, Rutherford and colleagues correctly predicted outcome from ultrasound appearances in all but one of 40 patients, including 13 of 14 children with normal appearances[41].

Since the initial observations of Fitzhardinge and colleagues[42], CT has proven to be of great value in predicting outcome, and is more widely used than ultrasound. Based upon four studies, a meta-analysis of the predictive value of severe hypodensity or haemorrhage on CT gave a risk of death or handicap of 82% compared to 16% where patchy hypodensity or normal scans were found[30]. CT may be most useful when performed in the second postnatal week[42].

More recently, MRI has proved effective in defining a range of appearances associated with neonatal encephalopathy. MRI defines more lesions than either CT or ultrasound, but is also most useful if performed when the early swelling has subsided. Patchy white matter changes are not infrequent findings among normal survivors[43]. Where these changes are extensive or co-exist with atrophy of the basal ganglia or cysts, again prognosis is poor[43]. The pattern of brain injury on MRI may have some correlation with the preponderance of type of cerebral palsy and learning impairment in children with disabilities[44].

CORTICAL EVOKED POTENTIALS

The value of evoked cortical responses has recently been reviewed[20,45,46]. Transient abnormalities in the recordings of auditory brainstem responses following hypoxia make their use relatively restricted in the term infant in the prediction of either neurological or auditory outcome. In contrast, abnormalities in visual evoked potentials (VEPs) correlate well with neurological outcome and have some predictive validity for outcome, having an accuracy of 85–93% depending upon grouping. Absence of VEP or persisting abnormality over the first week is always associated with poor outcome. Median nerve somatosensory evoked potentials (SEPs) are more difficult to record but have similar accuracy in terms of positive and negative predictive power. Two recordings made at each end of the first week for VEP and SEP may prove the most accurate prediction on poor outcome.

OTHER MODALITIES

Prediction of outcome in asphyxia has been attempted with a range of biochemical investigations[47,48], none of which has proved successful in predicting disability. More recently magnetic resonance spectroscopy (MRS) has been used to identify children with secondary energy failure using phosphorus and proton spectroscopy. A low phosphocreatine:inorganic phosphorus ratio ($PCr:P_i$) ratio and a high P_i:ATP ratio are associated with adverse outcome[49] as is the persistence of cerebral lactate or a low *N*-acetylaspartate:choline ratio[50]. These techniques are most valuable in their contribution to understanding the pathophysiological changes which accompany asphyxia, although they provide potentially predictive investigations.

Doppler ultrasound measurement of flow velocity may be helpful in that low-resistance, high-flow patterns may be associated with poor outcome[51,52].

Children without major disability

For many years it was accepted that children who survived a major perinatal hypoxic event without major disability would develop normally. Indeed, on an individual basis it is difficult to ascribe problems in a child to such a history. In statistical terms, it is becoming apparent that there may be differences between populations of children who have and have not been exposed to perinatal hypoxia. These differences are, however, small and probably restricted to those survivors who have moderate or severe encephalopathy (the latter usually survive with major disability).

Population studies indicate that, in global terms, perinatal hypoxia is at best a weak associate of cognitive dysfunction[53]. Many of these studies used condition at birth or need for resuscitation as a marker for hypoxia, variables known to be poorly predictive of later major outcomes.

Many studies have compared cognitive outcome in hypoxia-exposed children to groups matched for social class and found little differences. Although there is some evidence that adverse neonatal events generally may be associated with lower cognitive scores, perinatal hypoxia seems to confer no additional deficit unless there are signs of a moderate or severe neonatal encephalopathy[17]. Similar conclusions are reached when academic pursuits are considered[23,54].

More subtle tests of psychological functioning have been applied in various studies. In those populations identified by birth condition, weak associations between asphyxia and vocabulary, perceptual-motor and perceptual-attention measures were found in one[54] but two further studies failed to demonstrate a significant effect[37,55]. In the more recent studies of Robertson and Finer[17], the moderate encephalopathy group without disability performed less well in comparisons with peer children, other non-asphyxiated neonatal unit admissions or those with mild encephalopathy. Overall IQ scores, using the Wechsler Pre-school and Primary Scales (1974), were slightly lower in the moderate group compared to mild encephalopathy or neonatal-matched groups, manifesting lower scores in four subgroups. This impairment was mainly manifest as deficits in auditory and memory related tasks rather than in motor or visually mediated items.

In the absence of major disability, there is little evidence that physical growth is impaired in children exposed to perinatal hypoxia[17]. Sexual maturation may be advanced in both disabled and non-disabled females[56] and physical growth, in particular head growth, is frequently poor in disabled children[17,57]. Early sexual maturation may be associated with poor adolescent growth but as yet no studies have reported data beyond 8 years of age.

Although a link between psychiatric disorder in later life and symptoms of hypoxia during birth has not been clearly demonstrated, there is a large body of evidence that genetically vulnerable individuals may develop schizophrenia following exposure to perinatal complications which are linked to hypoxia[58]. This work suffers from poor definition of perinatal factors and the linking together of disparate variables under the heading of 'obstetrical complications'.

Conclusions

In global terms, the contribution of perinatal hypoxia to the aetiology of major disabilities is relatively small. Perinatal hypoxia that does not cause significant neonatal neurological symptoms is most unlikely to lead to later disability or more subtle defects in functioning. Children who develop signs of a moderate or severe neonatal encephalopathy are at high risk of developing major disabling conditions, and in studies of populations of children following perinatal hypoxia, there is evidence of subtle impairment on tests of neurological functioning that appear to involve auditory and language function and memory. As yet, the expression of a homogeneous pattern of impairment following major or minor brain injury has not been identified. This is in keeping with the variety of brain lesions associated with perinatal hypoxia, which itself may account for differences in outcomes for children with similar degree of neonatal illness. Within the two more severe categories of neonatal encephalopathy, prediction of major disability may be enhanced by imaging and neurophysiological techniques, in conjunction with careful clinical neurological evaluation.

REFERENCES

1. Blair E & Stanley F. Intrapartum asphyxia: a rare cause of cerebral palsy. *J. Pediatrics* **112**, 515, 1988.
2. Grant A, Joy MT, O'Brien N *et al.* Cerebral palsy among children born during the Dublin randomised trial of intrapartum monitoring. *Lancet* **ii**, 1233, 1989.
3. Nelson KB. What population of cerebral palsy is related to birth asphyxia? *J. Pediatrics* **121**, 572, 1988.
4. Largo RH & von Siebenthal K. Brain damage in infancy: mostly not intrapartum. On the etiology of mental and neurologic handicaps. *Arch. Gynecol. Obstetr.* **256**(Suppl. 80), 1995.
5. Nelson KB & Ellenberg JH. Antecedents of cerebral palsy: multivariate analysis of risk. *New Engl. J. Med.* **315**, 81, 1986.
6. Yudkin PL, Johnson A, Clover LM & Murphy KW. Assessing the contribution of birth asphyxia to cerebral palsy in term singletons. *Paediatr. Perinatal Epidemiol.* **9**, 156–170, 1995.
7. Nichols MM. Perinatal asphyxia and other common causes of perinatal depression [Letter]. *Am. J. Dis. Childr.* **145**, 1325, 1991.
8. Levene MI. The asphyxiated newborn infant. In *Fetal and Neonatal Neurology and Neurosurgery*, 2nd edn. (eds M.I. Levene, R.J. Lilford, M.J. Bennett & J. Punt), pp. 405–425. London: Churchill Livingstone, 1995.
9. Hall DMB. Intrapartum events and cerebral palsy. *Br. J. Obstetr. Gynaecol.* **101**, 745–747, 1994.
10. Roohey T, Raju TN & Moustogiannis AN. Animal models for the study of perinatal hypoxic–ischemic encephalopathy: a critical analysis. *Early Hum. Develop.* **47**(2), 115–146, 1997.
11. Volpe JJ. *Neurology of the Newborn*, 2nd edn. Chicago: W.B. Saunders, 1993.
12. Barth PG, Valk J & Olislagers-de Slegte R. Aspect scanographique des zones corticales et sous-corticales dans les paralyses cerebrales. *J. Neuroradiol.* **11**, 65–71, 1984.
13. Voit T, Lemburg P, Neuen M, Lumenta C & Stork W. Damage of thalamus and basal ganglia in asphyxiated full-term infants. *Neuropediatrics* **18**, 176–181, 1987.
14. Martin-Ancel A, Garcia-Alix A, Gaya F, Cabanas F, Burgueros M & Quero J. Multiple organ involvement in perinatal asphyxia. *J. Pediatrics* **127**, 786–793, 1995.
15. Raivio KO. Neonatal organ damage due to ischemia reperfusion. *Biol. Neonate* **69**, 170–171, 1996.
16. Ballot DE, Rothberg AD, Davies VA, Smith J & Kirsten G. Does hypoxemia prevent brain damage in birth asphyxia? *Med. Hypotheses* **41**(4), 344–347, 1993.
17. Robertson CM & Finer NN. Long-term follow-up of term neonates with perinatal asphyxia. *Clin. Perinatol.* **20**(2), 483–500, 1993.
18. Rosenbloom, L. Dyskinetic cerebral palsy and birth asphyxia. *Develop. Med. Child Neurol.* **36**, 285–289, 1994.
19. Saint-Hilaire M-H, Burke RE, Bressman SB, Brin MF & Fahn S. Delayed-onset dystonia due to perinatal or early childhood asphyxia. *Neurology* **41**, 216–222, 1991.
20. Whyte HE. Visual-evoked potentials in neonates following asphyxia. *Clin. Perinatol.* **20**(2), 451–461, 1993.
21. Jiang ZD. Long-term effect of perinatal and postnatal asphyxia on

developing human auditory brainstem responses: peripheral hearing loss. *Int. J. Pediatr. Otorhinolaryngol.* **33**(3), 225–238, 1995.

22. Jiang ZD & Tierney TS. Long-term effect of perinatal and postnatal asphyxia on developing human auditory brainstem responses: brainstem impairment. *Int. J. Pediatr. Otorhinolaryngol.* **34**(1–2), 111–127, 1996.
23. D'Souza SW, McCartney E & Nolan M. Hearing speech and language in survivors of severe perinatal asphyxia. *Arch. Dis. Childh.* **56**, 245, 1981.
24. Halpern J, Hosford-Dunn H & Malachowski N. Four factors that accurately predict hearing loss in high risk neonates. *Ear Hearing* **8**, 21–25, 1987.
25. Das VK. Adverse perinatal factors in the causation of sensorineural hearing loss in young children. *Int. J. Pediatr. Otolaryngol.* **21**, 121–125, 1991.
26. Prechtl HF. Neurological sequelae of prenatal and perinatal complications. *BMJ* **4**, 763, 1967.
27. Sarnat HB & Sarnat MS. Neonatal encephalopathy following fetal distress: a clinical and electroencephalographic study. *Arch. Neurol.* **33**, 696, 1976.
28. Levene MI, Kornberg J & Williams THC. The incidence and severity of post-asphyxial encephalopathy in full-term infants. *Early Hum. Develop.* **11**, 21–28, 1985.
29. Amiel-Tison C & Ellison P. Birth asphyxia in the full-term newborn: early assessment and outcome. *Develop. Med. Child Neurol.* **28**, 671–682, 1986.
30. Peliowski A & Finer N. Resuscitation of the term infant at birth. In *Effective Care of the Newborn* (eds J.C. Sinclair & M.B. Bracken), pp. 253–255. Oxford: OUP, 1991.
31. Robertson CMT & Finer NN. Term infants with hypoxic–ischaemic encephalopathy: outcome at 3.5 years. *Develop. Med. Child Neurol.* **27**, 473, 1985.
32. Levene MI, Sands C, Grindulis H & Moore J. Comparison of two methods of predicting outcome in perinatal asphyxia. *Lancet* **i**, 67–69, 1986.
33. Jain L, Ferre C, Vidyasagar D, Nath S & Sheftel D. Cardiopulmonary resuscitation of apparently stillborn infants. *J. Pediatrics* **118**, 778–782, 1991.
34. Yeo CL & Tudehope DI. Outcome of resuscitated apparently stillborn infants: a ten year review. *J. Paediatr. Child Health* **30**(2), 129–133, 1994.
35. Casalaz D, Speidel BD & Marlow N. Outcome of resuscitation following apparent stillbirth. *Archiv. Dis. Childh.* **78**, 112–115, 1998.
36. Nelson KB & Ellenberg J. Apgar scores as predictors of chronic neurologic disability. *Pediatrics* **68**, 36–44, 1997.
37. Dennis J, Johnson A & Mutch L. Acid–base status at birth and neurodevelopmental outcome at four and one-half years. *Am. J. Obstetr. Gynecol.* **161**, 213, 1989.
38. Thornberg E & Ekstrom-Jodal B. Cerebral function monitoring: a method of predicting outcome in term neonates after severe perinatal asphyxia. *Acta Paediatr.* **83**(6), 596–601, 1994.
39. Hellstrom-Westas L, Rosen I & Svenningsen NW. Predictive value of early continuous amplitude integrated EEG recordings on outcome after severe birth asphyxia in full term infants. *Arch. Dis. Childh. (Fetal & Neonatal)* **72**, F38, 1995.
40. Rutherford MA, Pennock JM, Schweizo JE, Cowan FM & Dubowitz LMS. Hypoxic–ischaemic encephalopathy: Early magnetic resonance imaging findings and their evolution. *Neuropediatrics* **26**, 183–191, 1995.
41. Rutherford MA, Pennock JM & Dubowitz LMS. Cranial ultrasound and magnetic resonance imaging in hypoxic-ischaemic encephalopathy: a comparison with outcome. *Dev. Med. Child Neurol.* **36**, 813–825, 1994.
42. Fitzhardinge PM, Flomark O, Fitz CR & Ashby S. The prognostic value of computed tomography as an adjunct to the assessment of the term infant with postasphyxial encephalopathy. *J. Pediatrics* **99**, 777–781, 1981.
43. Rutherford MA, Pennock JM, Schweizo JE, Cowan, FM & Dubowitz LMS. Hypoxic–ischaemic encephalopathy: early and late magnetic resonance imaging findings in relation to outcome. *Arch. Dis. Childh. (Fetal Neonatal)* **75**, 145–151, 1996.
44. Yokochi K & Fujimoto S. Magnetic resonance imaging in children with neonatal asphyxia: correlation with developmental sequelae. *Acta Paediatr.* **85**(1), 88–95, 1996.
45. Taylor MJ. Evoked potentials in the neonatal period. In *Fetal and Neonatal Neurology and Neurosurgery*, 2nd edn. (eds M.I. Levene, R.J. Lilford, M.J. Bennett & J. Punt), pp. 179–189. Edinburgh: Churchill Livingstone, 1995.
46. deVries L. Somatosensory-evoked potentials in term neonates with postasphyxial encephalopathy. *Clin. Perinatol.* **20**(2), 463–482, 1993.
47. Ruth VJ & Raivio KO. Perinatal brain damage: predictive value of metabolic acidosis and the Apgar score. *BMJ* **297**, 24–27, 1988.
48. Ruth VJ, Autti-Ramo I, Granstrom ML, Korkman M & Raivio KO. Prediction of perinatal brain damage by cord plasma vasopressin, erythropoietin and hypoxanthine values. *J. Pediatrics* **113**, 800–815, 1988.
49. Azzopardi D, Wyatt JS & Cady EB. Prognosis of newborn infants with hypoxic ischaemic brain injury assessed by phosphorus magnetic resonance spectroscopy. *Pediatr. Res.* **25**, 445–451, 1989.
50. Groenendaal F, Veenhoven RH, van der Grond J, Jansen GH, Witkamp TD & de Vries L. Cerebral lactate and *N*-acetylaspartate/choline ratios in asphyxiated full-term neonates demonstrated *in vivo* using proton magnetic resonance spectroscopy. *Pediatr. Res.* **35**, 148–151, 1994.
51. Gray PH, Tudehope DI, Masel JP, Burns YR, Mohay HA, O'Callaghan MJ & Williams GM. Perinatal hypoxic-ischaemic brain injury: prediction of outcome. *Dev. Med. Child Neurol.* **35**(11), 965–973, 1993.
52. Levene MI, Fenton AC, Evans DH, Archer LNJ, Shortland DB & Gibson NA. Severe birth asphyxia and abnormal cerebral blood-flow velocity. *Dev. Med. Child Neurol.* **32**, 567–574, 1989.
53. Broman S. Perinatal anoxia and cognitive development in early childhood. In *Infants Born at Risk* (eds T. Field, A. Sostek & S. Goldberg), p. 29. New York: Spectrum Press, 1979.
54. Graham FK, Ernhart CB & Thurston D. *Development Three Years after Anoxia and other Potentially Damaging Neonatal Experiences*, p. 176(3) (whole no. 522). Psychological Monographs: General and Applied. Washington D.C.: American Psychological Association, 1962.
55. Thomson AJ, Searle M & Russell G. Quality of survival after birth asphyxia. *Arch. Dis. Childh.* **56**, 620, 1977.
56. Robertson CMT, Morrish DW, Wheeler HT & Grace MCA. Neonatal encephalopathy: an indicator of early sexual maturation in girls. *Pediatr. Neurol.* **6**, 102, 1990.
57. Shankaran S, Woldt E & Koepke T. Acute neonatal morbidity and long term central nervous system sequelae of perinatal asphyxia in term infants. *Early Hum. Develop.* **25**, 135, 1991.
58. Brixey SN, Gallagher BJ, McFalls JA Jr & Parmelee LF. Gestational and neonatal factors in the etiology of schizophrenia. *J. Clin. Psychol.* **49**(3), 447–456, 1993.

Appendix: Charts of fetal measurements

L.S. Chitty and D.G. Altman

Introduction

There are hundreds of published papers presenting charts (standards) of fetal measurements. Unfortunately many of these are methodologically unsound and thus of dubious value. The appropriate design and analysis of studies to derive reference centiles for fetal size is discussed in Chapter 71. More detailed descriptions can be found in the literature[1–3].

In this appendix, we present tables and charts of various measurements of fetal size derived from data collected in a prospective study which was designed expressly for the purpose of developing reference ranges[2,4–8]. In some cases these differ slightly from those presented previously[4], as a result of improvements to the modelling procedure. We also include charts derived from other data sets. In some cases (e.g. fetal haematological measurements) ideal study design is not possible as samples have to be collected opportunistically when assessment is made for a clinical indication. In these cases we have tried to include charts from studies with methodology as close as possible to the optimum. Where appropriate, we have added brief comments about methodological problems. For some measurements, because of inadequate documentation in published papers, we have been unable to produce suitable charts and tables although some data exist in the literature.

Tables and charts

The tables and charts in the following pages show 5th, 50th and 95th centiles for each measurement by exact gestational age. For those attributed to Chitty *et al.* (or Chitty and Altman) fractional polynomial regression models were used; details of the methods of analysis are described[1,2]. The dating charts show predicted gestational age (in weeks and days) by fetal size. For these charts only data up to approximately 35 weeks of gestation are included, i.e. biparietal measurement (BPD) <89 mm, head circumference <322 mm and femur length <67 mm[5]. The 5th and 95th centiles tabulated here are slightly narrower than those published before, because the earlier paper[5] included tabulations of 95% rather than 90% ranges.

It is important to note that there are two fetal size and dating charts for the BPD to account for the different methods of making this measurement. In one it was measured from the proximal echo of the fetal skull to the distal side of the border deep to the ultrasound beam (outer–outer) and for the other, it was measured from the proximal edge to the proximal edge of the deep border (outer–inner). The differences in measurement are small, but the user should take care to use the chart appropriate to his/her measurement technique. All circumference measurements[6–8] (and others presented here) were derived from the maximum diameters using the equation $\pi(d_1 + d_2)/2$ where d_1 and d_2 were the two diameters. As with the BPD charts, there are two charts for the dating and two size charts for fetal head circumference measurements to take account of the different methods of measuring the BPD, which is d_1 in the equation used to derive the circumference.

REFERENCES

1. Altman DG & Chitty LS. Design and analysis of studies to derive charts of fetal size. *Ultrasound. Obstet. Gynaecol.* **3**:378–384, 1993.
2. Altman DG & Chitty LS. Charts of fetal size: 1. Methodology. *Br. J. Obstet. Gynaecol.* **101**:29–34, 1994.
3. Royston P & Wright EM. How to construct 'normal ranges' for fetal variables. *Ultrasound Obstet. Gynecol.* **11**:30–38, 1998.
4. Chitty LS & Altman DG. Charts of fetal size. In *Ultrasound in Obstetrics and Gynaecology* (eds K Dewbury, H Meire & D Cosgrove), pp. 513–567. Edinburgh: Churchill Livingstone, 1993.
5. Altman DG & Chitty LS. New charts for ultrasound dating of pregnancy. *Ultrasound. Obstet. Gynecol.* **10**:1–18, 1997.
6. Chitty LS, Altman DG, Henderson A & Campbell S. Charts of fetal size: 2. Head measurements. *Br. J. Obstet. Gynaecol.* **101**:35–43, 1994.
7. Chitty LS, Altman DG, Henderson A & Campbell S. Charts of fetal size: 3. Abdominal circumference. *Br. J. Obstet. Gynaecol.* **101**:125–131, 1994.

8. Chitty LS, Altman DG, Henderson A & Campbell S. Charts of fetal size: 4. Femur length. *Br. J. Obstet. Gynaecol.* **101**:132–135, 1994.
9. Aoki S, Hata T & Kitao M. Ultrasonic assessment of fetal and neonatal spleen. *Am. J. Perinatol.* **9**:361–367, 1992.
10. Vintzileos AM, Neckles S, Campbell WA, Andreoli JW, Kaplan BM & Nochimson DJ. Fetal liver ultrasound measurements during normal pregnancy. *Obstet. Gynecol.* **66**:477–480, 1985.
11. Merz E, Wellek S, Bahlmann F & Weber G. Sonographische Normkurven des fetalen knöchernen Thorax und der fetalen Lunge. *Geburtsh. Frauenheilk.* **55**:77–82, 1995.
12. Robinson HP & Fleming JEE. A critical evaluation of sonar crown–rump length measurements. *Br. J. Obstet. Gynaecol.* **89**:926–930, 1982.
13. Nicolaides KH, Economides DL & Soothill PW. Blood gases, pH, and lactate in appropriate- and small-for-gestational-age fetuses. *Am. J. Obstet. Gynecol.* **161**:996–1001, 1989.
14. Arduini D & Rizzo G. Normal values of pulsatility index from fetal vessels: a cross-sectional study on 1556 healthy fetuses. *J. Perinat. Med.* **18**:165–172, 1990.
15. Bower S, Vyas S, Campbell S & Nicolaides KH. Color Doppler imaging of the uterine artery in pregnancy: normal ranges of impedance to blood flow, mean velocity and volume of flow. *Ultrasound. Obstet. Gynecol.* **2**:261–265, 1992.
16. Moore TR & Cayle JE. The amniotic fluid index in normal human pregnancy. *Am. J. Obstet. Gynecol.* **162**:1168–1173, 1990.
17. Nicolaides KH, Soothill PW, Clewell WH, Rodeck CH, Mibashan RS & Campbell S. Fetal haemoglobin measurement in the assessment of red cell isoimmunisation. *Lancet* **i**: 1073–1075, 1988.
18. Nicolini U, Fisk NM, Rodeck CH & Beacham J. Fetal urine biochemistry: an index of renal maturation and dysfunction. *Br. J. Obstet. Gynaecol.* **99**:46–50, 1992.
19. Hadlock FP, Harrist RB, Sharman RS, Deter RL & Park SK. Estimation of fetal weight with the use of head, body, and femur measurements – a prospective study. *Am. J. Obstet. Gynecol.* **151**:333–337, 1985.
20. Chitty LS, Campbell S & Altman DG. Measurement of the fetal mandible – feasibility and construction of a centile chart. *Prenat. Diagnos.* **13**:749–756, 1993.

LIST OF TABLES AND CHARTS

1. Biparietal diameter (outer–outer)

Weeks of gestation	Centiles (mm) 5th	50th	95th
12	16.0	19.7	23.4
13	19.8	23.5	27.3
14	23.4	27.3	31.2
15	27.1	31.0	35.0
16	30.7	34.7	38.8
17	34.2	38.3	42.5
18	37.7	41.9	46.1
19	41.1	45.4	49.7
20	44.4	48.8	53.3
21	47.6	52.2	56.7
22	50.8	55.5	60.1
23	53.9	58.7	63.4
24	57.0	61.8	66.6
25	59.9	64.8	69.7
26	62.7	67.8	72.8
27	65.5	70.6	75.7
28	68.1	73.4	78.6
29	70.7	76.0	81.3
30	73.1	78.6	84.0
31	75.5	81.0	86.5
32	77.7	83.3	88.9
33	79.8	85.5	91.2
34	81.8	87.6	93.4
35	83.7	89.6	95.5
36	85.5	91.5	97.4
37	87.1	93.2	99.3
38	88.6	94.8	100.9
39	89.9	96.2	102.5
40	91.1	97.5	103.9
41	92.2	98.7	105.2
42	93.1	99.7	106.3

Source: Chitty *et al.*[6]

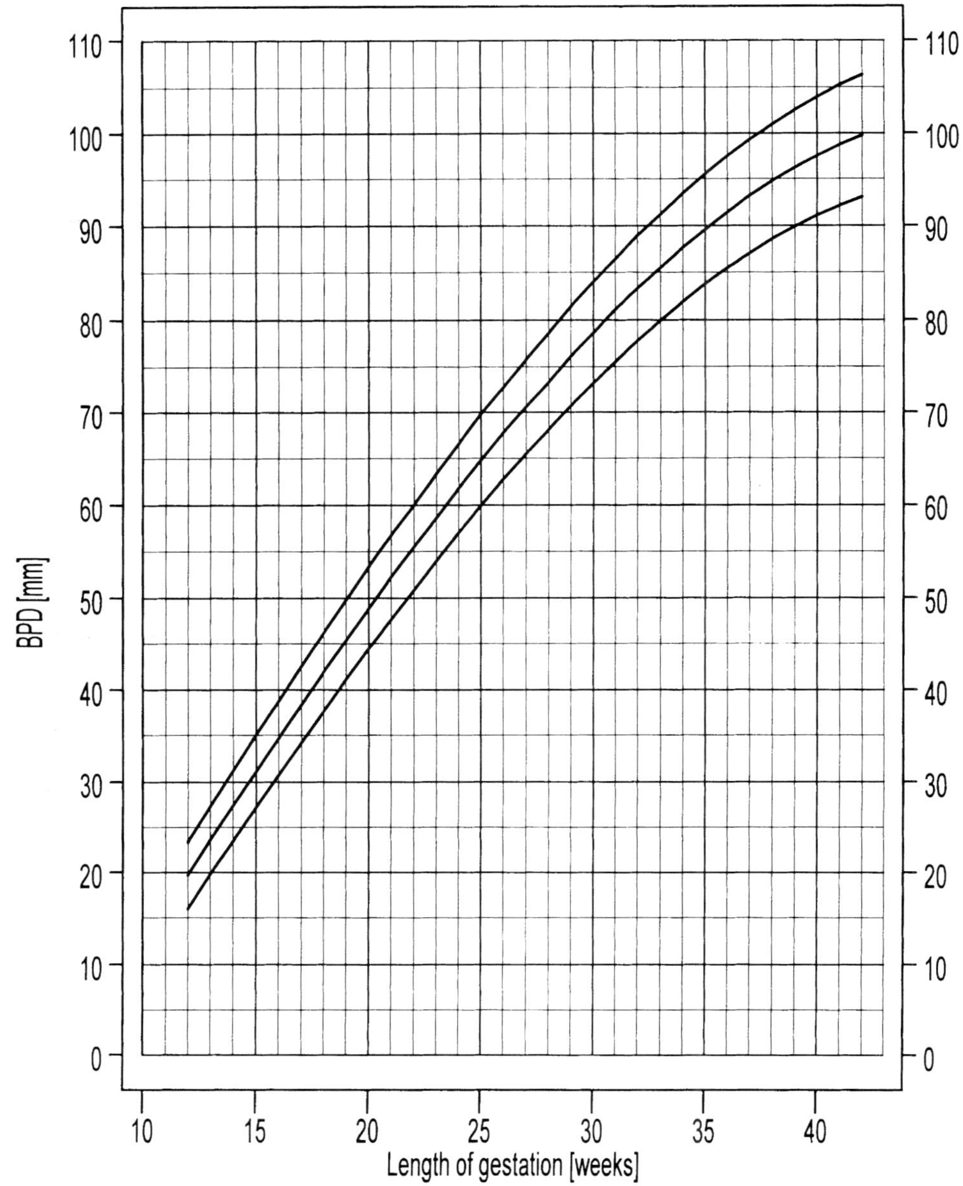

6. Head circumference/abdominal circumference ratio

Weeks of gestation	Centiles 5th	50th	95th
12	1.13	1.23	1.33
13	1.13	1.23	1.33
14	1.13	1.22	1.32
15	1.12	1.22	1.32
16	1.12	1.21	1.31
17	1.11	1.21	1.31
18	1.11	1.20	1.30
19	1.10	1.20	1.30
20	1.10	1.19	1.29
21	1.09	1.19	1.28
22	1.08	1.18	1.28
23	1.08	1.17	1.27
24	1.07	1.17	1.26
25	1.06	1.16	1.26
26	1.05	1.15	1.25
27	1.05	1.14	1.24
28	1.04	1.13	1.23
29	1.03	1.13	1.22
30	1.02	1.12	1.21
31	1.01	1.11	1.21
32	1.00	1.10	1.20
33	0.99	1.09	1.19
34	0.98	1.08	1.18
35	0.97	1.07	1.16
36	0.96	1.06	1.15
37	0.95	1.05	1.14
38	0.94	1.03	1.13
39	0.92	1.02	1.12
40	0.91	1.01	1.11
41	0.90	1.00	1.10
42	0.89	0.98	1.08

Source: Chitty and Altman (unpublished)

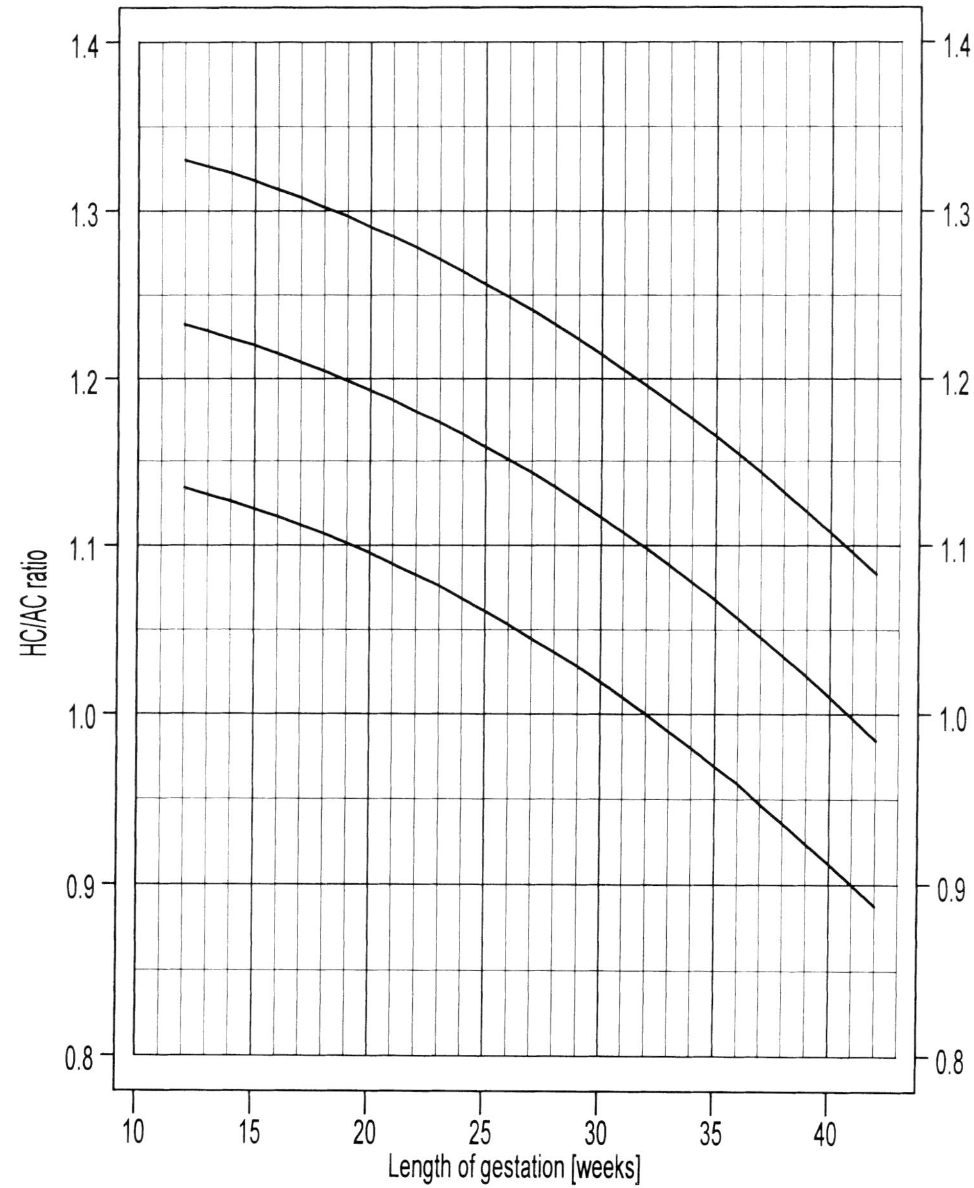

7. Femur length

Weeks of gestation	Centiles (mm) 5th	50th	95th
12	4.8	7.7	10.6
13	7.9	10.9	13.9
14	11.0	14.1	17.2
15	14.0	17.2	20.4
16	17.0	20.3	23.6
17	19.9	23.3	26.7
18	22.8	26.3	29.7
19	25.6	29.2	32.8
20	28.4	32.1	35.7
21	31.1	34.9	38.6
22	33.8	37.6	41.5
23	36.4	40.3	44.3
24	38.9	42.9	47.0
25	41.4	45.5	49.6
26	43.7	48.0	52.2
27	46.0	50.4	54.7
28	48.3	52.7	57.1
29	50.4	55.0	59.5
30	52.5	57.1	61.7
31	54.5	59.2	63.9
32	56.4	61.2	66.0
33	58.2	63.1	68.0
34	59.9	64.9	69.9
35	61.5	66.6	71.7
36	63.0	68.2	73.4
37	64.4	69.7	75.0
38	65.7	71.1	76.5
39	66.9	72.4	77.9
40	68.0	73.6	79.1
41	68.9	74.6	80.3
42	69.8	75.6	81.3

Source: Chitty *et al.*[8]

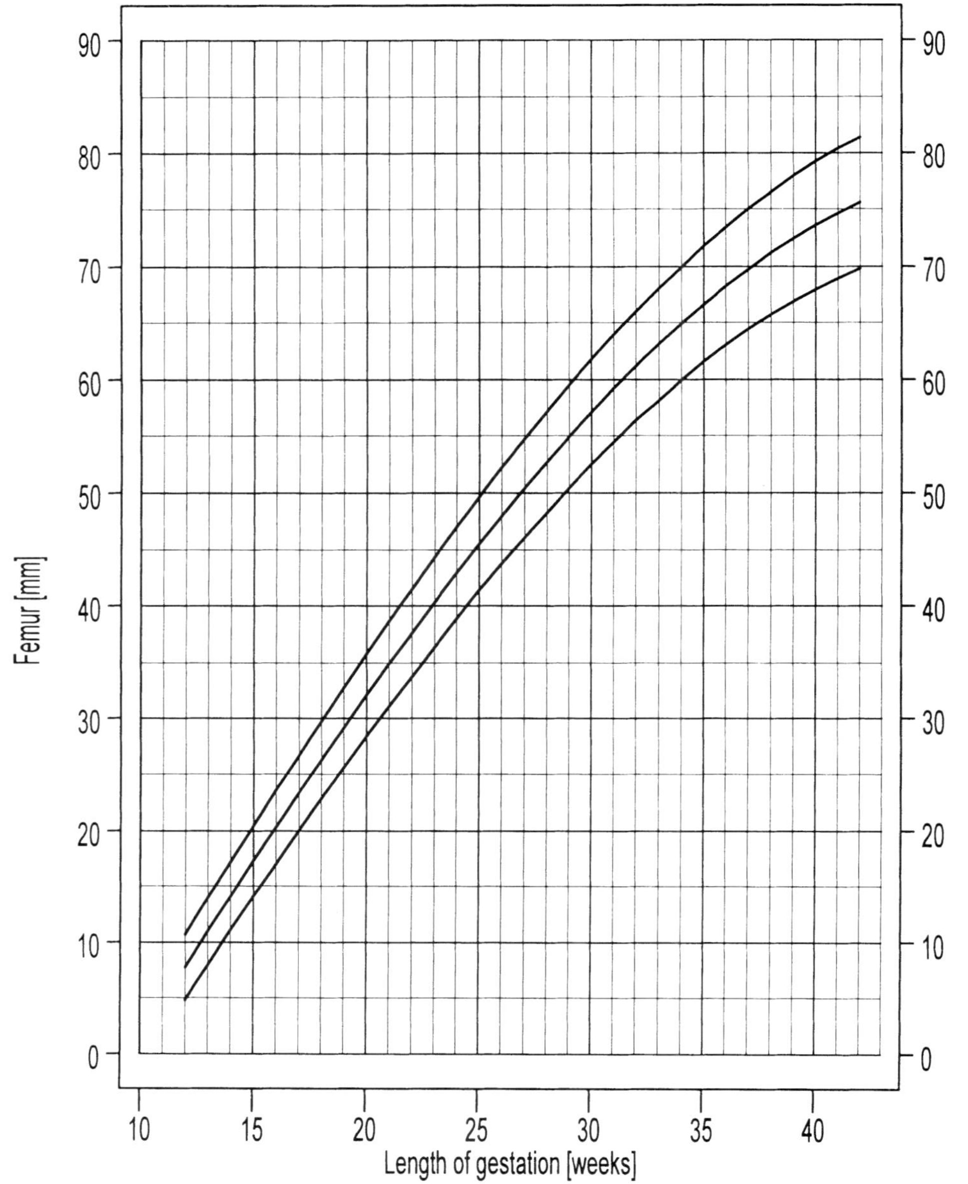

8. Humerus length

Weeks of gestation	Centiles (mm) 5th	50th	95th
12	4.1	7.1	10.1
13	7.6	10.7	13.8
14	11.0	14.1	17.2
15	14.1	17.3	20.6
16	17.2	20.4	23.7
17	20.1	23.4	26.7
18	22.8	26.2	29.6
19	25.4	28.9	32.4
20	28.0	31.5	35.0
21	30.4	34.0	37.6
22	32.7	36.3	40.0
23	34.8	38.6	42.3
24	36.9	40.7	44.6
25	38.9	42.8	46.7
26	40.9	44.8	48.7
27	42.7	46.7	50.7
28	44.4	48.5	52.6
29	46.1	50.2	54.4
30	47.7	51.9	56.1
31	49.2	53.5	57.7
32	50.6	55.0	59.3
33	52.0	56.4	60.8
34	53.3	57.8	62.3
35	54.6	59.1	63.6
36	55.7	60.3	64.9
37	56.8	61.5	66.2
38	57.9	62.6	67.4
39	58.9	63.7	68.5
40	59.8	64.7	69.6
41	60.7	65.6	70.6
42	61.5	66.5	71.5

Source: Chitty and Altman (unpublished)

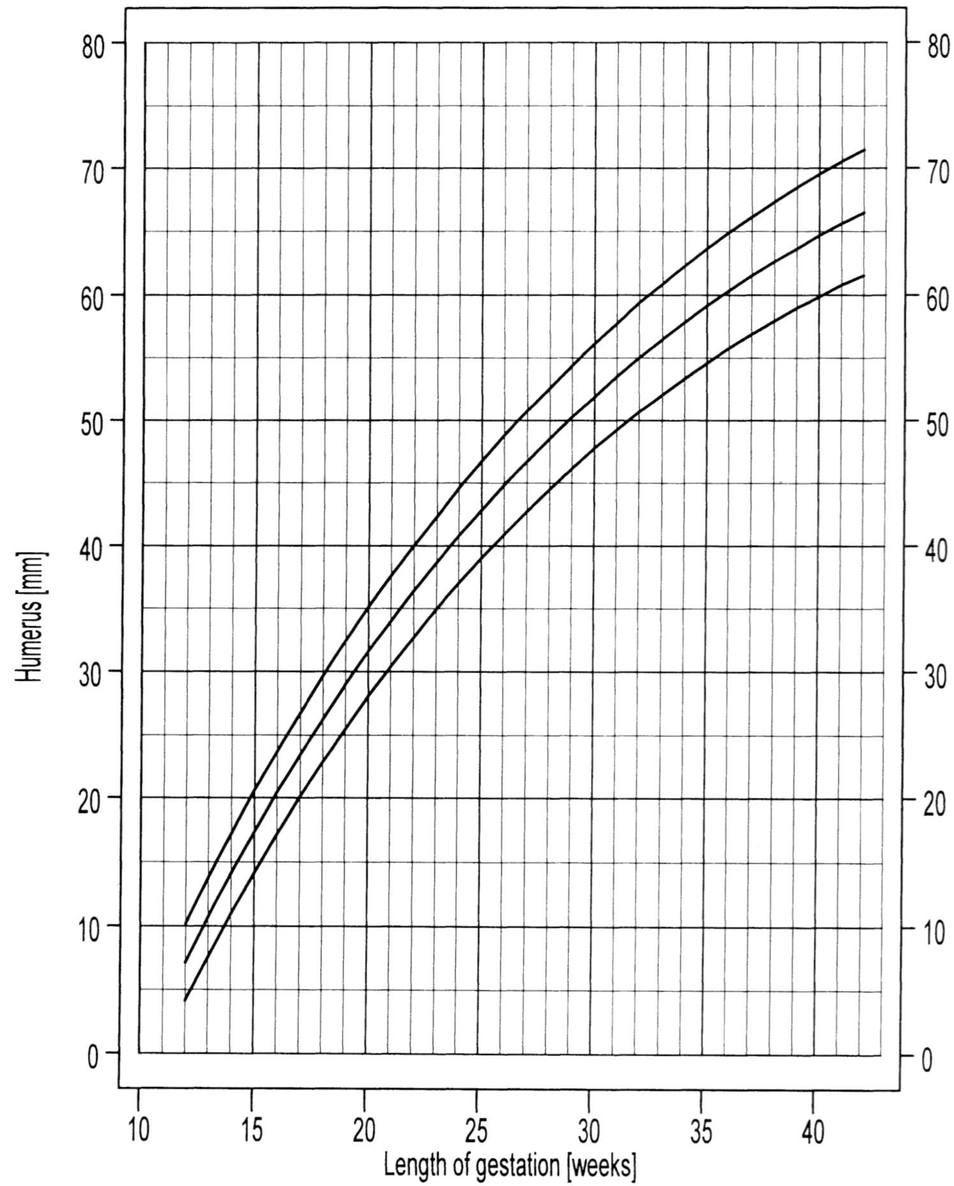

9. Radius length

Weeks of gestation	Centiles (mm) 5th	50th	95th
12	2.6	5.5	8.4
13	5.3	8.2	11.2
14	8.0	11.0	14.1
15	10.8	13.9	17.0
16	13.5	16.7	19.8
17	16.1	19.3	22.6
18	18.6	21.9	25.2
19	20.9	24.4	27.8
20	23.2	26.7	30.2
21	25.3	28.9	32.4
22	27.3	30.9	34.6
23	29.2	32.9	36.6
24	30.9	34.7	38.5
25	32.6	36.5	40.3
26	34.2	38.1	42.1
27	35.7	39.7	43.7
28	37.1	41.2	45.3
29	38.4	42.6	46.7
30	39.6	43.9	48.1
31	40.8	45.1	49.5
32	41.9	46.4	50.8
33	43.0	47.5	52.0
34	44.0	48.6	53.1
35	45.0	49.6	54.3
36	45.9	50.6	55.3
37	46.8	51.6	56.3
38	47.6	52.5	57.3
39	48.4	53.3	58.3
40	49.1	54.2	59.2
41	49.9	55.0	60.0
42	50.6	55.7	60.9

Source: Chitty and Altman (unpublished)

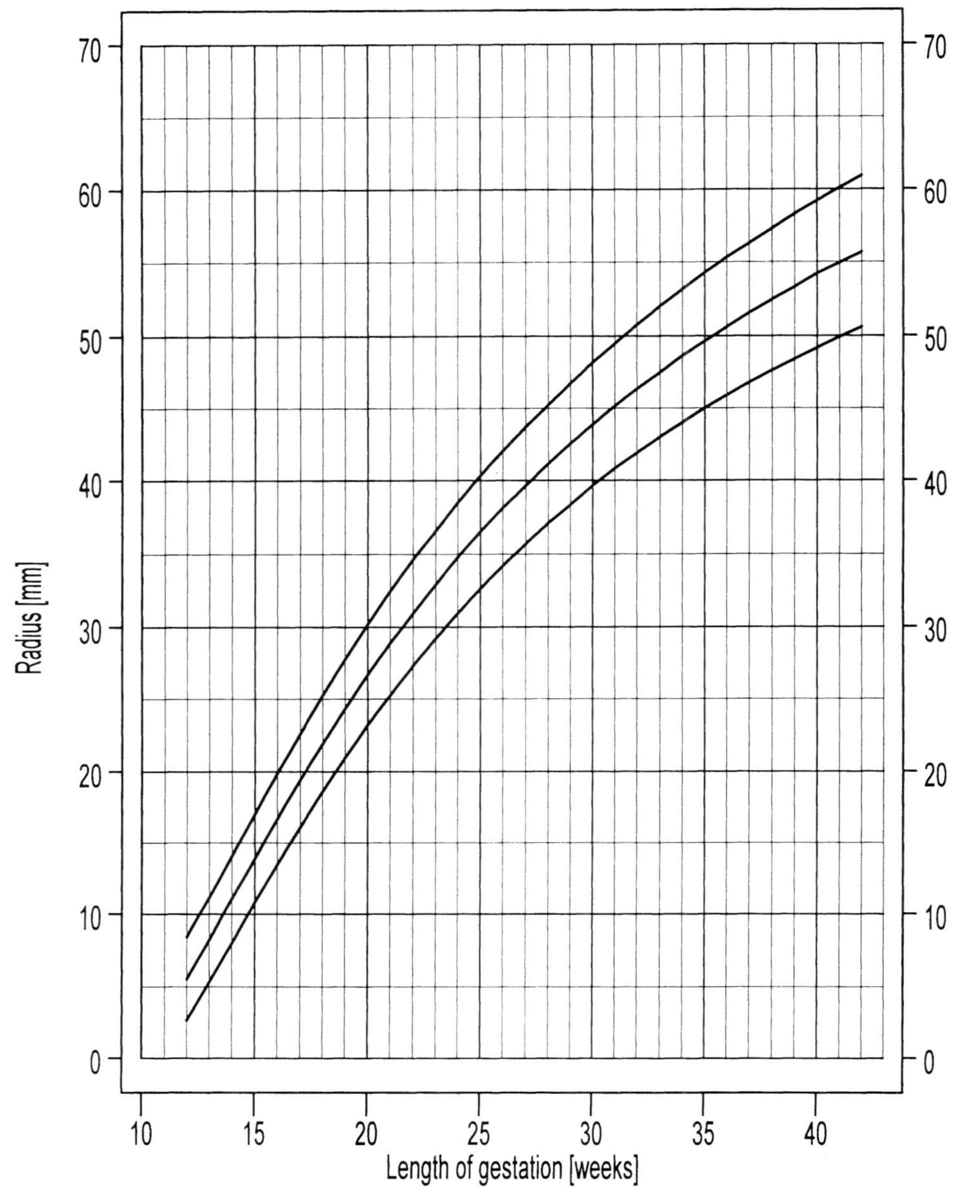

10. Ulna length

Weeks of gestation	Centiles (mm) 5th	50th	95th
12	4.4	7.3	10.3
13	6.6	9.6	12.7
14	9.3	12.4	15.5
15	12.1	15.3	18.5
16	15.0	18.2	21.5
17	17.8	21.2	24.5
18	20.6	24.0	27.5
19	23.3	26.8	30.3
20	25.8	29.4	33.0
21	28.3	32.0	35.6
22	30.6	34.4	38.1
23	32.8	36.6	40.5
24	34.9	38.8	42.7
25	36.9	40.9	44.9
26	38.8	42.8	46.9
27	40.5	44.7	48.9
28	42.2	46.5	50.7
29	43.8	48.2	52.5
30	45.3	49.8	54.2
31	46.8	51.3	55.8
32	48.2	52.7	57.3
33	49.5	54.1	58.8
34	50.7	55.4	60.2
35	51.9	56.7	61.5
36	53.0	57.9	62.8
37	54.1	59.1	64.0
38	55.1	60.2	65.2
39	56.1	61.2	66.4
40	57.0	62.2	67.5
41	57.9	63.2	68.5
42	58.8	64.1	69.5

Source: Chitty and Altman (unpublished)

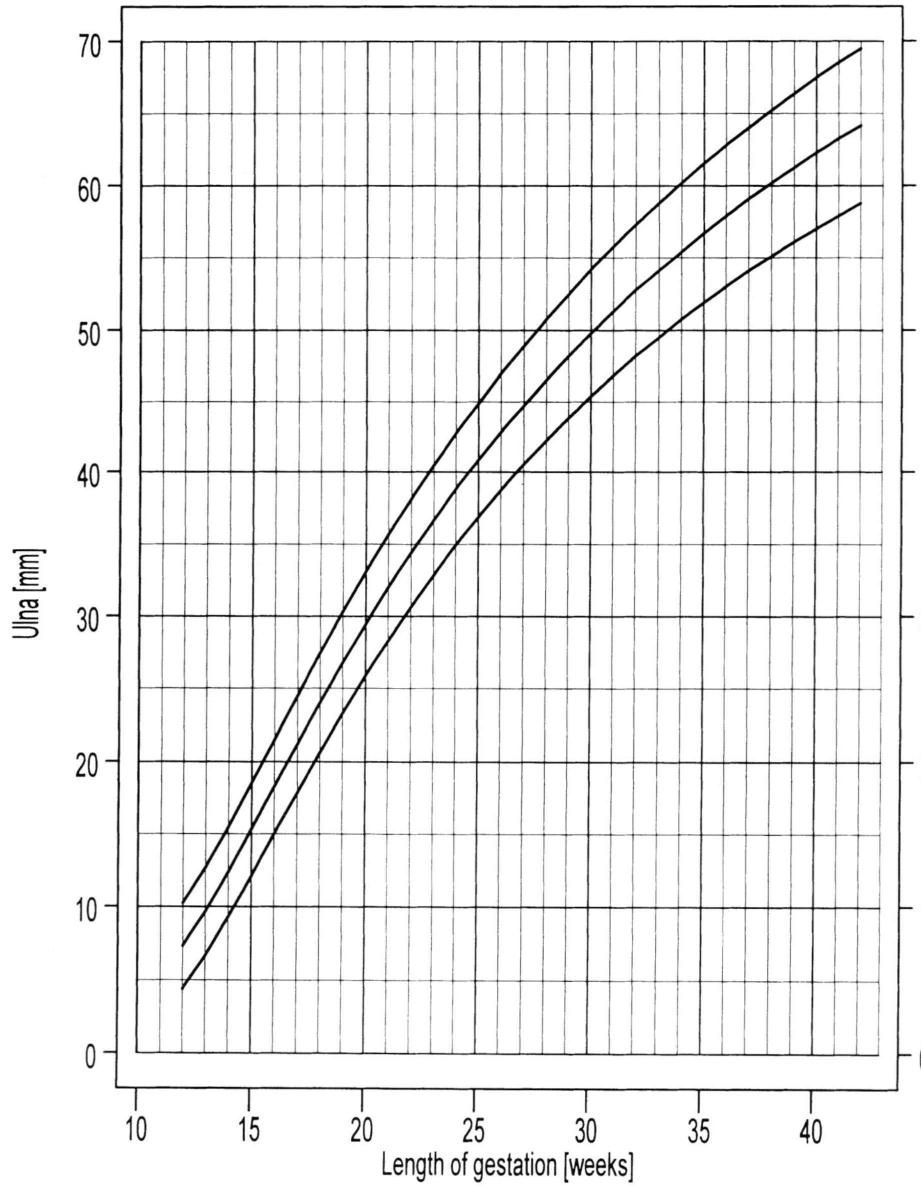

11. Tibia length

Weeks of gestation	Centiles (mm) 5th	50th	95th
12	4.8	7.6	10.4
13	6.3	9.2	12.0
14	8.4	11.4	14.4
15	11.0	14.1	17.1
16	13.8	16.9	20.1
17	16.6	19.9	23.1
18	19.5	22.8	26.1
19	22.3	25.7	29.1
20	25.0	28.5	32.0
21	27.7	31.2	34.8
22	30.2	33.8	37.5
23	32.6	36.4	40.1
24	35.0	38.8	42.6
25	37.2	41.0	44.9
26	39.3	43.2	47.2
27	41.3	45.3	49.4
28	43.2	47.3	51.4
29	45.0	49.2	53.4
30	46.7	51.0	55.3
31	48.3	52.7	57.1
32	49.9	54.4	58.8
33	51.4	55.9	60.5
34	52.8	57.5	62.1
35	54.2	58.9	63.6
36	55.5	60.3	65.1
37	56.7	61.6	66.5
38	57.9	62.9	67.8
39	59.0	64.1	69.1
40	60.1	65.2	70.4
41	61.2	66.4	71.6
42	62.2	67.4	72.7

Source: Chitty and Altman (unpublished)

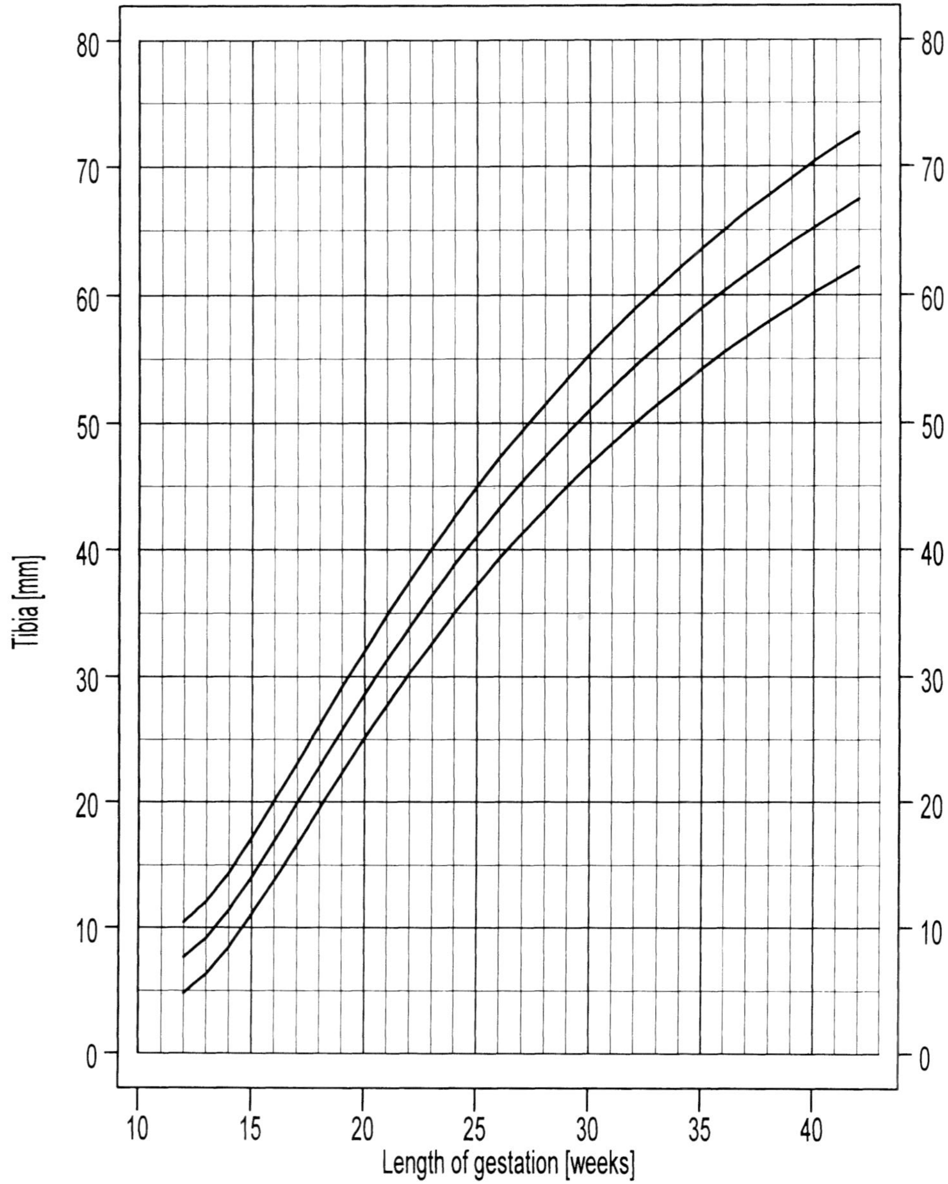

12. Fibula length

Weeks of gestation	Centiles (mm) 5th	50th	95th
12	4.0	6.8	9.6
13	5.6	8.5	11.4
14	7.9	10.8	13.8
15	10.5	13.5	16.6
16	13.3	16.4	19.5
17	16.1	19.3	22.5
18	18.9	22.2	25.5
19	21.7	25.1	28.5
20	24.4	27.9	31.3
21	26.9	30.5	34.1
22	29.4	33.1	36.8
23	31.8	35.5	39.3
24	34.0	37.9	41.7
25	36.2	40.1	44.0
26	38.2	42.2	46.3
27	40.2	44.3	48.4
28	42.0	46.2	50.4
29	43.8	48.0	52.3
30	45.4	49.8	54.2
31	47.0	51.5	55.9
32	48.5	53.1	57.6
33	50.0	54.6	59.2
34	51.3	56.1	60.8
35	52.6	57.5	62.3
36	53.9	58.8	63.7
37	55.1	60.1	65.1
38	56.2	61.3	66.4
39	57.3	62.5	67.7
40	58.4	63.6	68.9
41	59.4	64.7	70.1
42	60.3	65.8	71.2

Source: Chitty and Altman (unpublished)

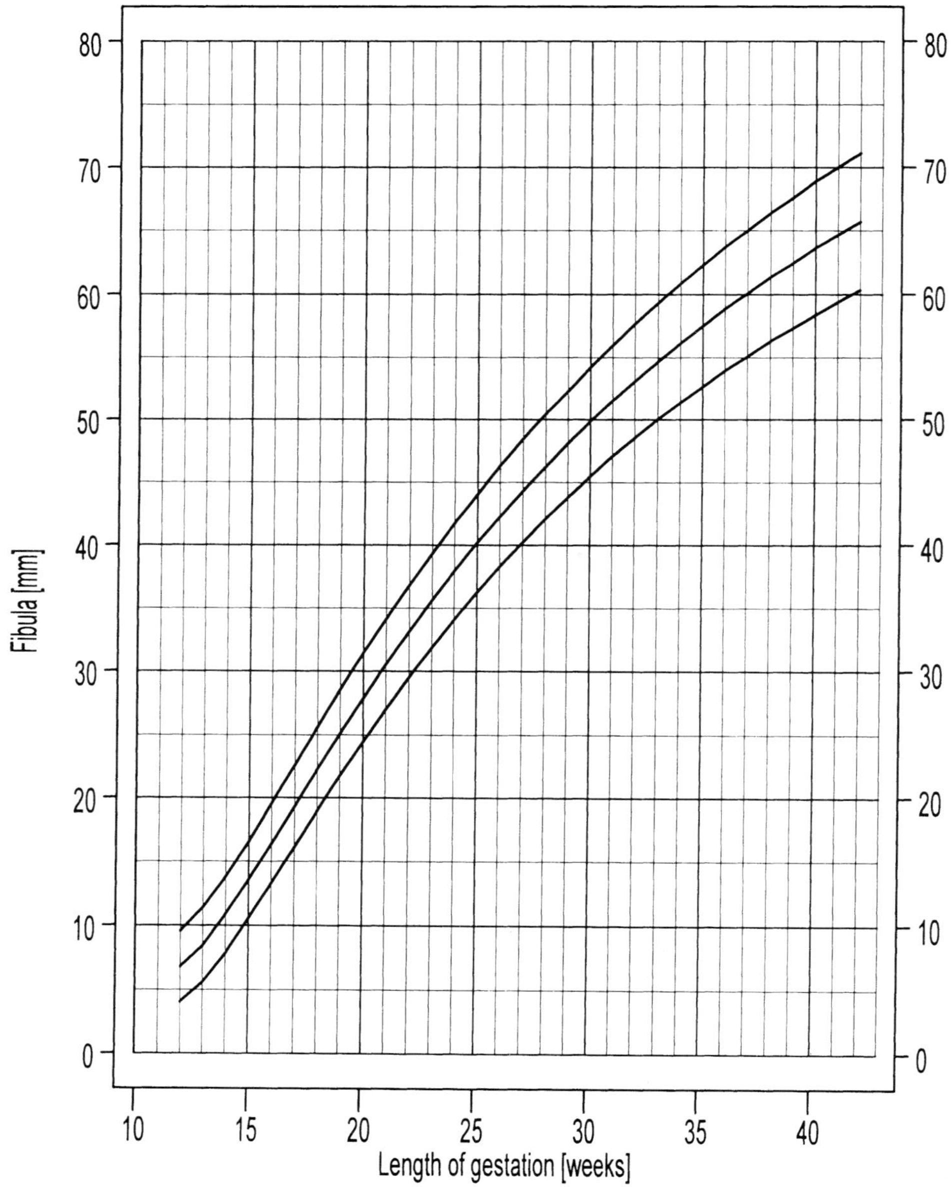

13. Foot length

Weeks of gestation	Centiles (mm) 5th	50th	95th
12	6.3	8.9	11.5
13	8.9	11.7	14.5
14	11.7	14.6	17.6
15	14.5	17.6	20.7
16	17.3	20.6	23.9
17	20.1	23.6	27.1
18	22.9	26.6	30.3
19	25.8	29.6	33.5
20	28.6	32.6	36.6
21	31.4	35.6	39.8
22	34.2	38.6	42.9
23	36.9	41.5	46.0
24	39.6	44.4	49.1
25	42.3	47.2	52.1
26	44.8	50.0	55.1
27	47.4	52.7	58.0
28	49.8	55.3	60.8
29	52.2	57.9	63.5
30	54.5	60.4	66.2
31	56.8	62.8	68.8
32	58.9	65.1	71.2
33	60.9	67.3	73.6
34	62.8	69.4	75.9
35	64.7	71.4	78.1
36	66.4	73.3	80.2
37	68.0	75.0	82.1
38	69.4	76.7	83.9
39	70.8	78.2	85.6
40	72.0	79.6	87.2
41	73.0	80.8	88.6
42	74.0	81.9	89.9

Source: Chitty and Altman (unpublished)

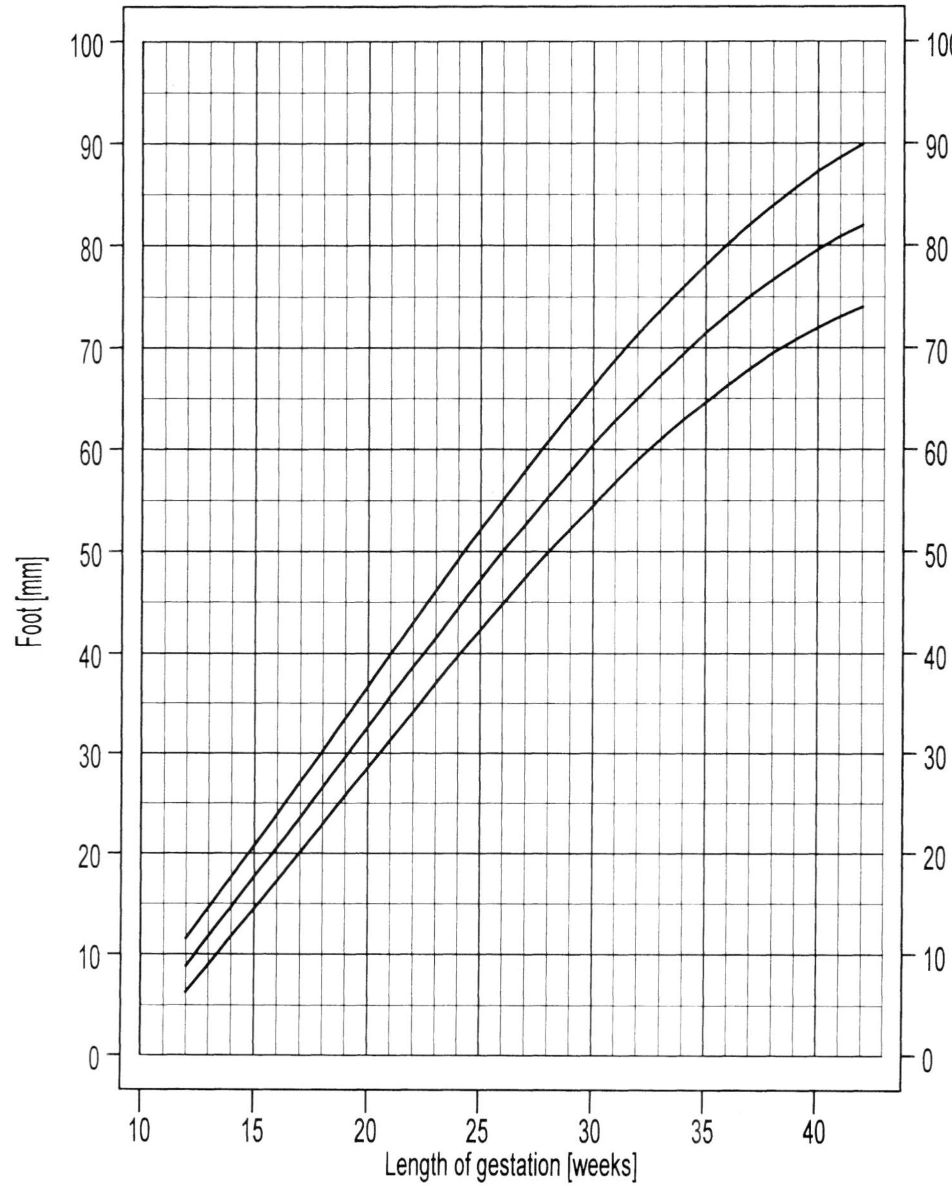

16. Internal orbit diameter

Weeks of gestation	Centiles (mm) 5th	50th	95th
12	4.8	5.7	6.9
13	5.6	6.8	8.1
14	6.4	7.7	9.3
15	7.2	8.7	10.5
16	7.9	9.6	11.5
17	8.6	10.4	12.5
18	9.3	11.2	13.5
19	9.9	11.9	14.3
20	10.4	12.6	15.2
21	11.0	13.2	15.9
22	11.4	13.8	16.6
23	11.9	14.3	17.3
24	12.3	14.8	17.9
25	12.7	15.3	18.4
26	13.1	15.7	19.0
27	13.4	16.1	19.4
28	13.7	16.5	19.9
29	14.0	16.9	20.3
30	14.3	17.2	20.7
31	14.5	17.5	21.1
32	14.8	17.8	21.4
33	15.0	18.0	21.7
34	15.2	18.3	22.0
35	15.4	18.5	22.3
36	15.6	18.7	22.6
37	15.7	19.0	22.8
38	15.9	19.1	23.1
39	16.0	19.3	23.3
40	16.2	19.5	23.5
41	16.3	19.7	23.7
42	16.5	19.8	23.9

Source: Chitty and Altman (unpublished)

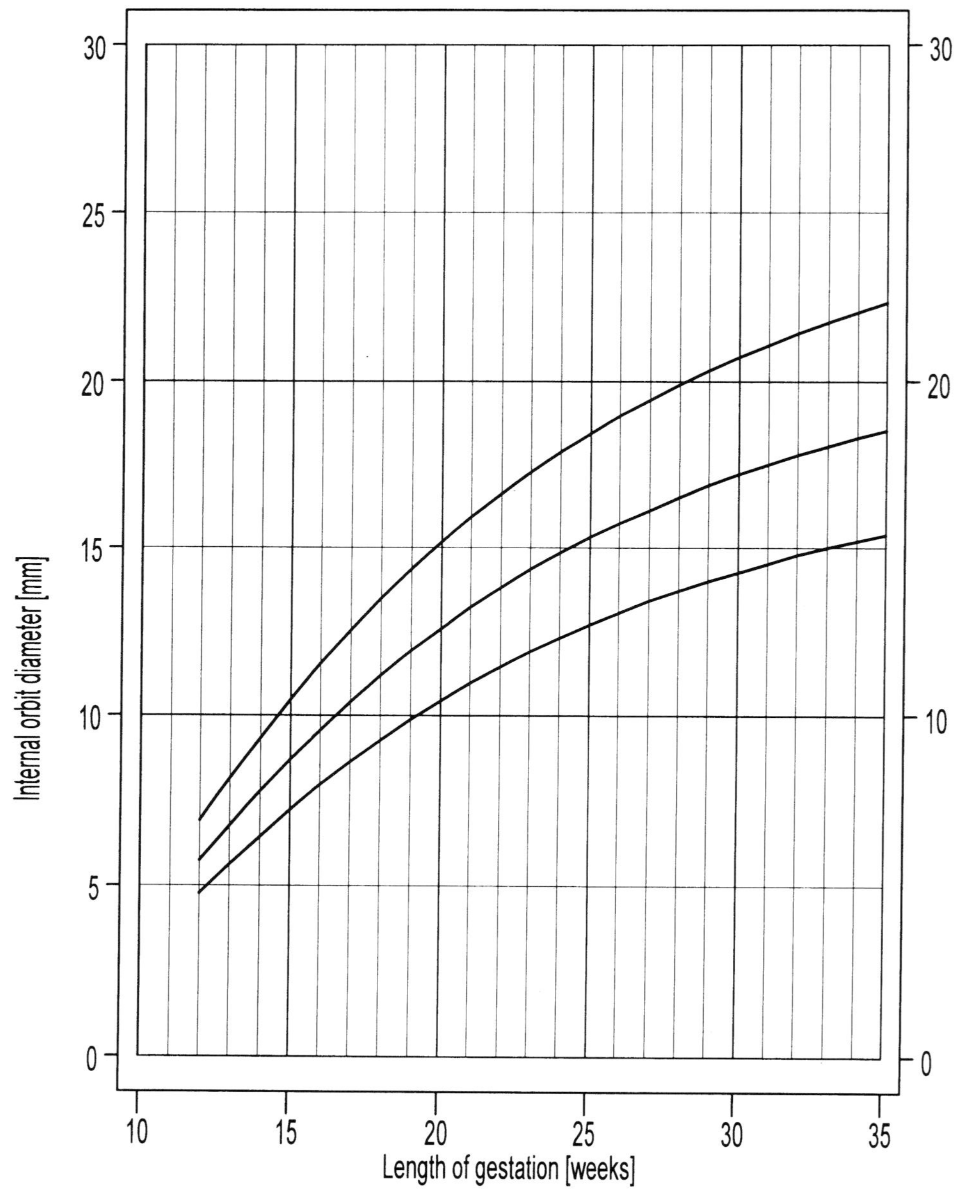

17. External orbit diameter

Weeks of gestation	Centiles (mm) 5th	50th	95th
12	12.0	13.3	14.7
13	14.2	15.6	17.3
14	16.3	18.0	19.9
15	18.4	20.3	22.4
16	20.5	22.6	25.0
17	22.5	24.8	27.4
18	24.5	27.0	29.8
19	26.4	29.1	32.1
20	28.2	31.1	34.4
21	30.0	33.1	36.5
22	31.7	35.0	38.6
23	33.3	36.8	40.6
24	34.9	38.5	42.5
25	36.4	40.2	44.4
26	37.9	41.8	46.1
27	39.3	43.3	47.9
28	40.6	44.8	49.5
29	41.9	46.3	51.1
30	43.2	47.6	52.6
31	44.4	49.0	54.1
32	45.5	50.3	55.5
33	46.6	51.5	56.8
34	47.7	52.7	58.2
35	48.7	53.8	59.4
36	49.7	54.9	60.6
37	50.7	56.0	61.8
38	51.6	57.0	62.9
39	52.5	58.0	64.0
40	53.4	59.0	65.1
41	54.2	59.9	66.1
42	55.0	60.8	67.1

Source: Chitty and Altman (unpublished)

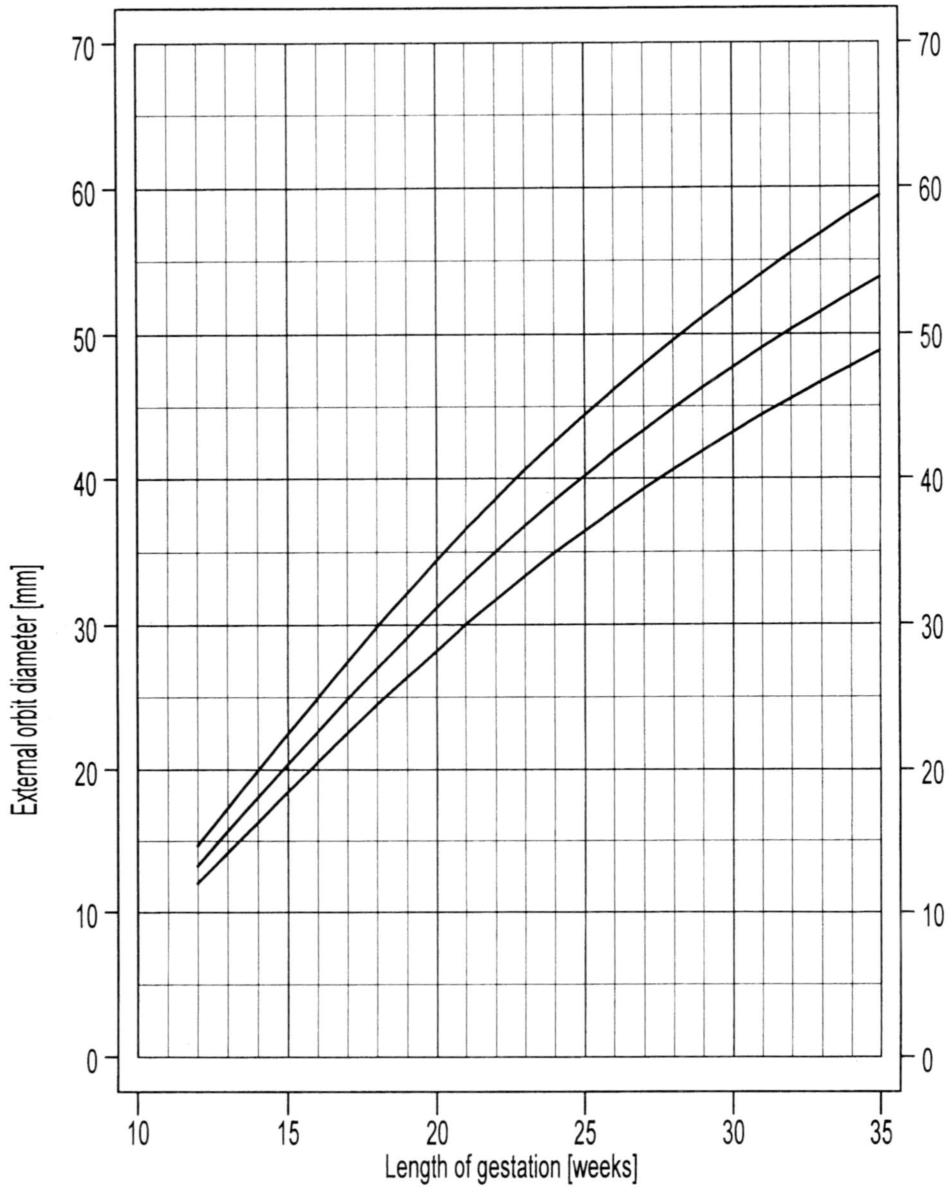

18. Posterior horn/hemisphere ratio

Weeks of gestation	Centiles (mm) 5th	50th	95th
12	0.50	0.61	0.71
13	0.46	0.56	0.67
14	0.42	0.52	0.63
15	0.39	0.49	0.59
16	0.36	0.45	0.55
17	0.33	0.42	0.52
18	0.30	0.39	0.49
19	0.28	0.37	0.46
20	0.25	0.34	0.43
21	0.23	0.32	0.41
22	0.21	0.30	0.39
23	0.20	0.28	0.37
24	0.18	0.26	0.35
25	0.17	0.25	0.33
26	0.16	0.23	0.31
27	0.15	0.22	0.30
28	0.14	0.21	0.28
29	0.13	0.20	0.27
30	0.12	0.19	0.26
31	0.12	0.18	0.25
32	0.11	0.18	0.24
33	0.11	0.17	0.23
34	0.10	0.16	0.22
35	0.10	0.16	0.22
36	0.10	0.16	0.21
37	0.10	0.15	0.21
38	0.10	0.15	0.20
39	0.10	0.15	0.20
40	0.10	0.15	0.20
41	0.10	0.15	0.20
42	0.11	0.15	0.20

Source: Chitty and Altman (unpublished)

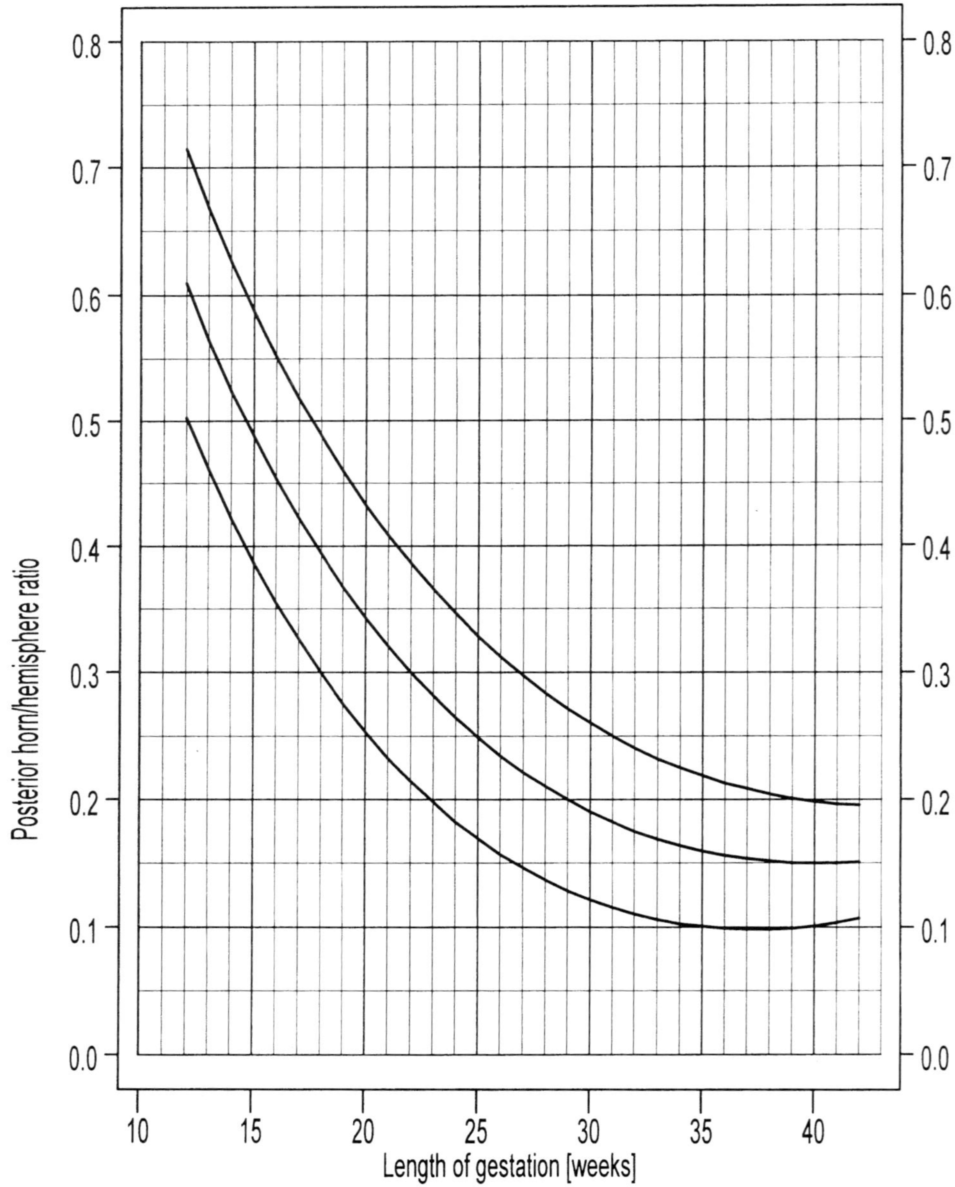

19. Kidney length

Weeks of gestation	Centiles (mm) 5th	50th	95th
12	5.2	6.3	7.7
13	6.4	7.8	9.4
14	7.7	9.3	11.3
15	9.0	11.0	13.3
16	10.5	12.7	15.4
17	11.9	14.5	17.6
18	13.4	16.3	19.8
19	15.0	18.2	22.1
20	16.5	20.0	24.3
21	18.0	21.8	26.5
22	19.5	23.6	28.7
23	20.9	25.4	30.9
24	22.3	27.1	32.9
25	23.7	28.8	35.0
26	25.0	30.4	36.9
27	26.3	31.9	38.8
28	27.5	33.4	40.5
29	28.6	34.7	42.2
30	29.7	36.0	43.8
31	30.7	37.2	45.2
32	31.6	38.3	46.6
33	32.4	39.4	47.8
34	33.2	40.3	48.9
35	33.9	41.1	50.0
36	34.5	41.9	50.9
37	35.1	42.6	51.7
38	35.6	43.2	52.4
39	36.0	43.7	53.1
40	36.3	44.1	53.6
41	36.6	44.5	54.0
42	36.9	44.8	54.4

Source: Chitty and Altman (unpublished)

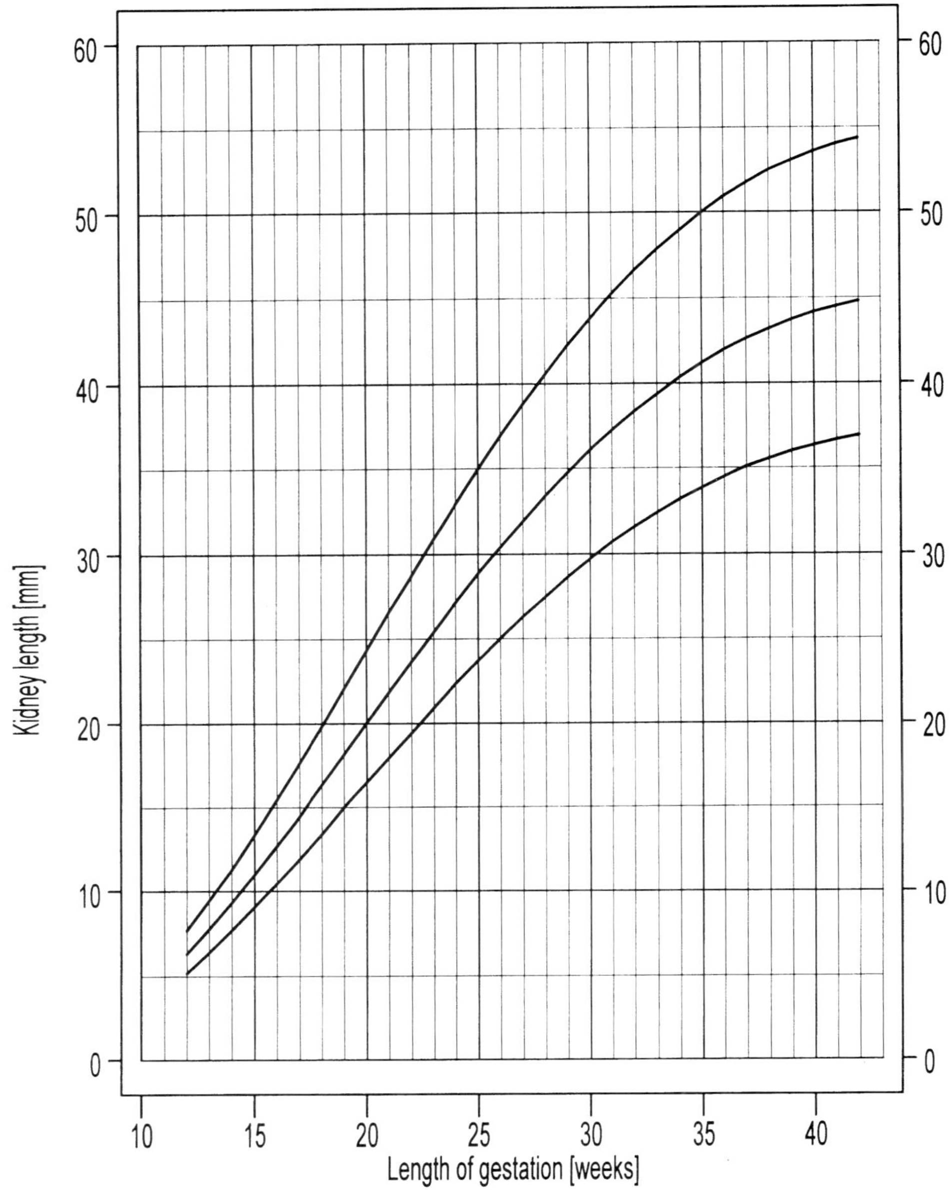

20. Spleen length

Weeks of gestation	Centiles (mm) 5th	50th	95th
20	11.1	15.2	19.2
21	13.0	17.0	21.0
22	14.8	18.8	22.8
23	16.6	20.6	24.6
24	18.4	22.4	26.4
25	20.2	24.2	28.2
26	21.9	25.9	30.0
27	23.6	27.6	31.7
28	25.3	29.3	33.3
29	26.9	30.9	34.9
30	28.4	32.5	36.5
31	29.9	33.9	38.0
32	31.3	35.3	39.4
33	32.6	36.6	40.7
34	33.8	37.8	41.9
35	34.9	38.9	43.0
36	35.9	39.9	44.0
37	36.8	40.8	44.8
38	37.5	41.6	45.6
39	38.1	42.2	46.2
40	38.6	42.6	46.7
41	38.9	43.0	47.0

Source: Aoki *et al.*[9]
Comment: Excluded birthweight <10th or >90th centile; SD taken as constant

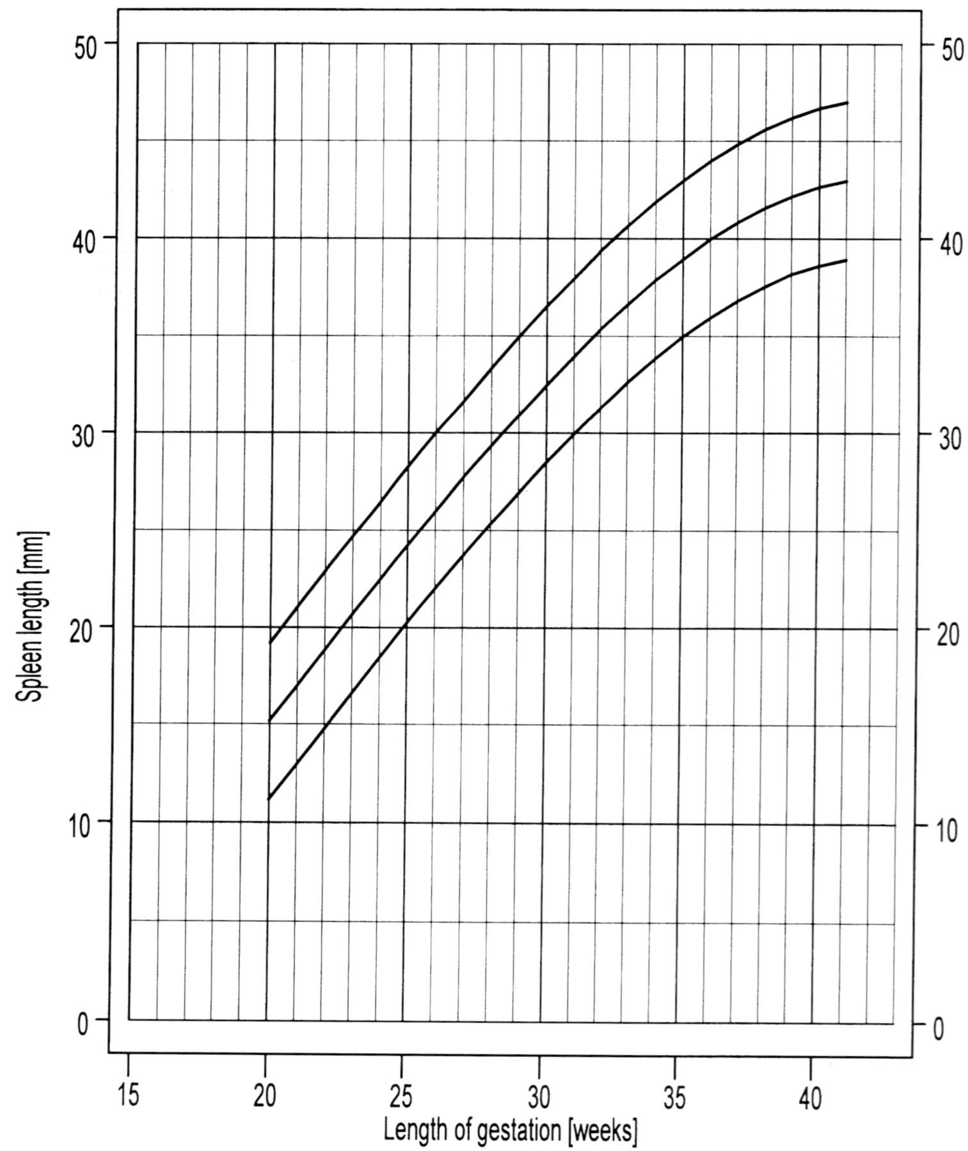

21. Liver length

Weeks of gestation	Centiles (mm) 5th	50th	95th
20	22.9	26.7	30.6
21	24.2	28.1	32.0
22	25.5	29.5	33.5
23	26.8	30.9	35.0
24	28.0	32.2	36.5
25	29.3	33.6	37.9
26	30.6	35.0	39.4
27	31.9	36.4	40.9
28	33.2	37.8	42.3
29	34.5	39.1	43.8
30	35.8	40.5	45.3
31	37.0	41.9	46.8
32	38.3	43.3	48.2
33	39.6	44.7	49.7
34	40.9	46.0	51.2
35	42.2	47.4	52.7
36	43.5	48.8	54.1
37	44.7	50.2	55.6
38	46.0	51.6	57.1
39	47.3	52.9	58.6
40	48.6	54.3	60.0
41	49.9	55.7	61.5

Source: Vintzileos *et al.*[10]
Comment: Excluded birthweight <10th or >90th centile and IUGR. Fetuses included more than once. Data reanalysed from tabulated means and SDs

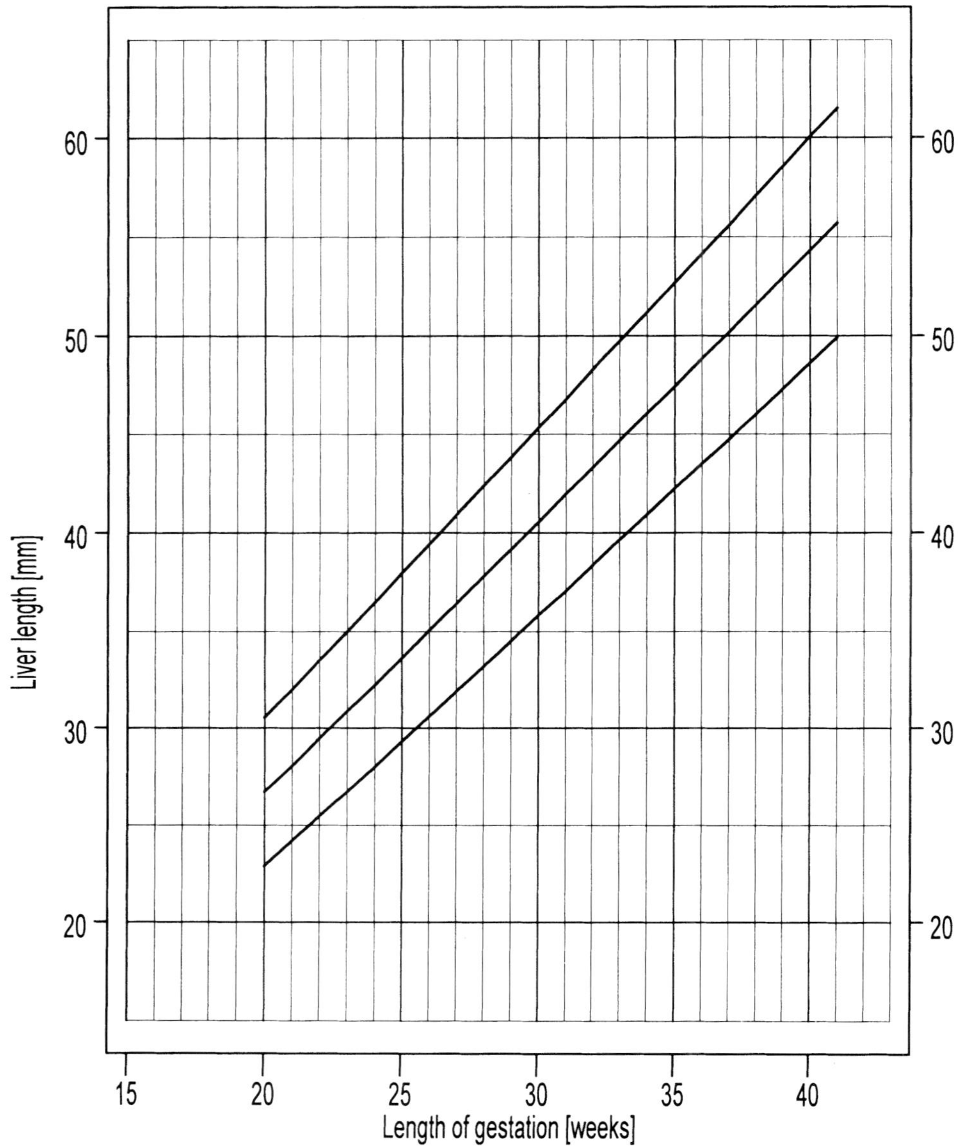

22. Thoracic circumference (derived from diameters)

Weeks of gestation	Centiles (mm) 5th	50th	95th
12	44	60	77
13	49	66	83
14	56	74	91
15	64	81	99
16	72	89	107
17	80	98	116
18	87	106	124
19	96	114	133
20	103	122	141
21	111	131	150
22	119	139	158
23	127	147	167
24	135	155	175
25	142	163	183
26	150	170	191
27	157	178	199
28	164	185	206
29	171	192	214
30	177	199	221
31	183	206	228
32	189	212	234
33	195	218	240
34	201	223	246
35	205	229	252
36	210	234	257
37	214	238	262
38	218	242	266
39	221	245	270
40	224	248	273
41	226	251	275

Source: Merz *et al.*[11]
Comment: Excluded IUGR

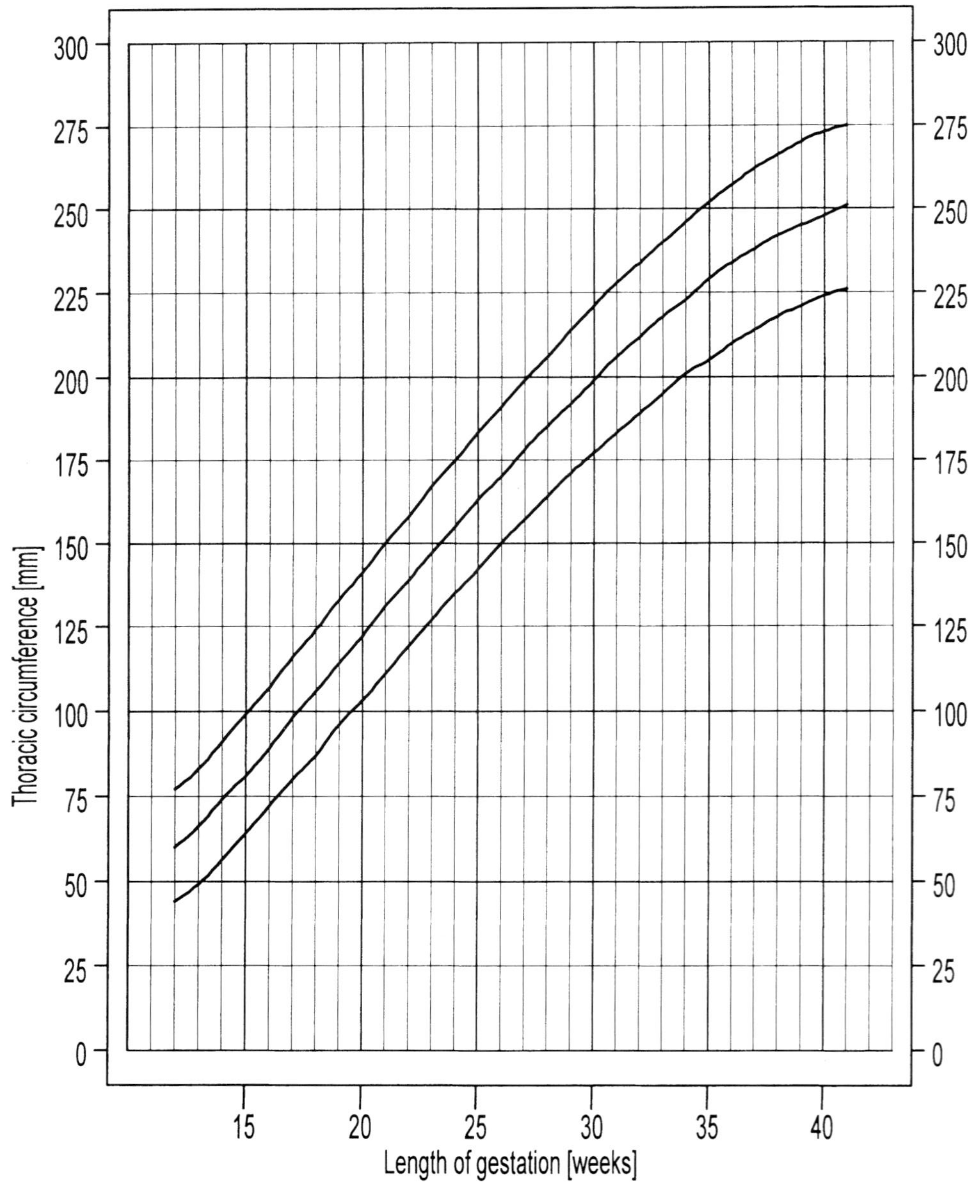

23. Biparietal diameter (outer–outer) – dating chart

BPD (mm)	Centiles (weeks + days) 5th	50th	95th
22	11 + 6	12 + 4	13 + 3
24	12 + 2	13 + 1	14 + 0
26	12 + 6	13 + 4	14 + 4
28	13 + 2	14 + 1	15 + 1
30	13 + 6	14 + 5	15 + 5
32	14 + 2	15 + 2	16 + 2
34	14 + 6	15 + 5	16 + 6
36	15 + 2	16 + 2	17 + 3
38	15 + 6	16 + 6	18 + 0
40	16 + 2	17 + 3	18 + 5
42	16 + 6	18 + 0	19 + 2
44	17 + 3	18 + 4	20 + 0
46	18 + 0	19 + 2	20 + 4
48	18 + 3	19 + 6	21 + 2
50	19 + 0	20 + 3	22 + 0
52	19 + 4	21 + 1	22 + 5
54	20 + 1	21 + 5	23 + 3
56	20 + 5	22 + 2	24 + 1
58	21 + 2	23 + 0	24 + 6
60	22 + 0	23 + 5	25 + 4
62	22 + 4	24 + 2	26 + 2
64	23 + 1	25 + 0	27 + 0
66	23 + 5	25 + 5	27 + 6
68	24 + 3	26 + 3	28 + 4
70	25 + 0	27 + 1	29 + 3
72	25 + 5	27 + 6	30 + 1
74	26 + 2	28 + 4	31 + 0
76	27 + 0	29 + 2	31 + 6
78	27 + 4	30 + 0	32 + 4
80	28 + 2	30 + 5	33 + 3
82	29 + 0	31 + 4	34 + 2
84	29 + 5	32 + 2	35 + 1
86	30 + 2	33 + 1	36 + 1
88	31 + 0	33 + 6	37 + 0
90	31 + 5	34 + 5	37 + 6

Source: Altman and Chitty[5]

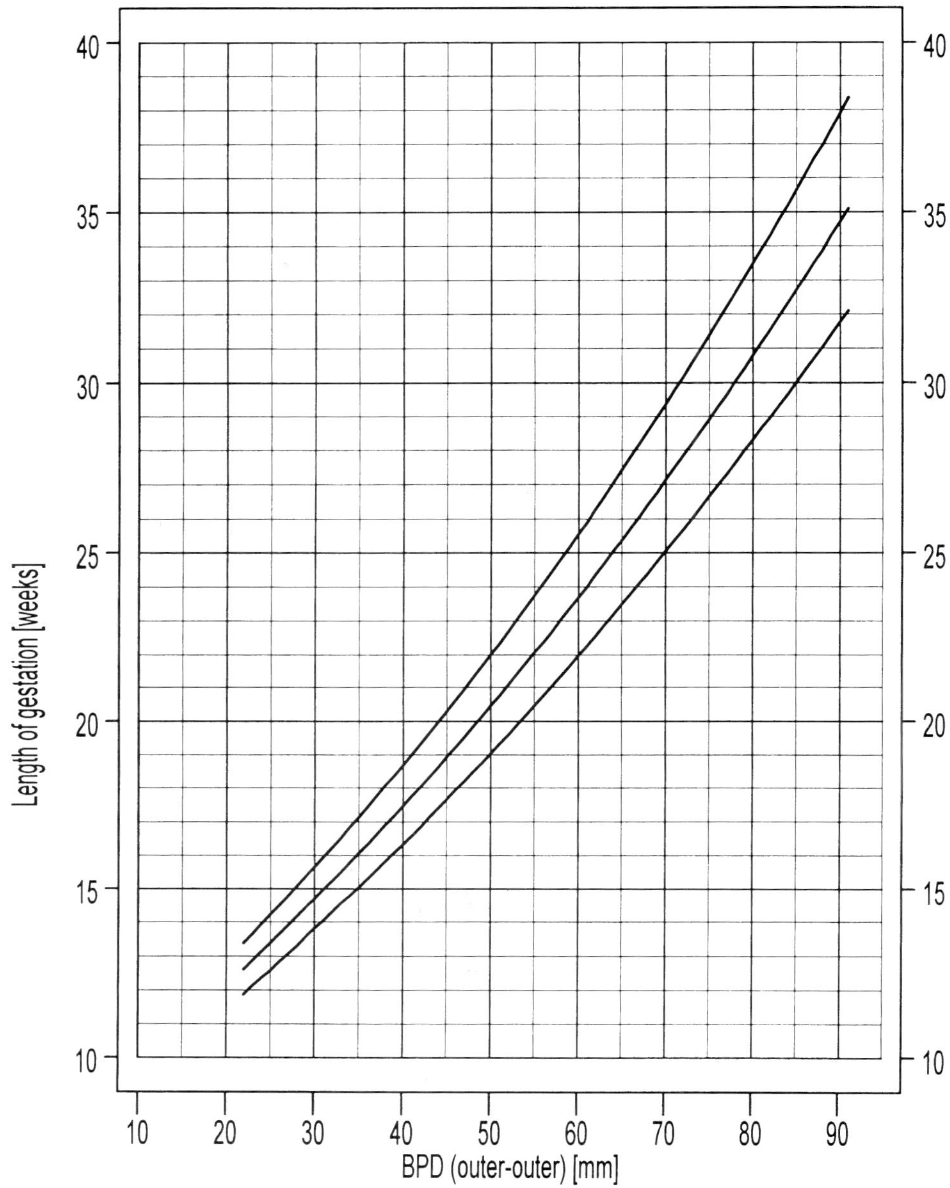

24. Biparietal diameter (outer–inner) – dating chart

BPD (mm)	Centiles (weeks + days) 5th	50th	95th
22	12 + 2	13 + 0	13 + 6
24	12 + 5	13 + 4	14 + 3
26	13 + 2	14 + 1	15 + 0
28	13 + 5	14 + 5	15 + 4
30	14 + 2	15 + 1	16 + 1
32	14 + 6	15 + 5	16 + 5
34	15 + 2	16 + 2	17 + 3
36	15 + 6	16 + 6	18 + 0
38	16 + 3	17 + 3	18 + 5
40	17 + 0	18 + 1	19 + 2
42	17 + 3	18 + 5	20 + 0
44	18 + 0	19 + 2	20 + 5
46	18 + 4	19 + 6	21 + 2
48	19 + 1	20 + 4	22 + 0
50	19 + 5	21 + 1	22 + 5
52	20 + 2	21 + 6	23 + 3
54	21 + 0	22 + 4	24 + 1
56	21 + 4	23 + 1	24 + 6
58	22 + 1	23 + 6	25 + 5
60	22 + 5	24 + 4	26 + 3
62	23 + 3	25 + 2	27 + 1
64	24 + 0	26 + 0	28 + 0
66	24 + 5	26 + 5	28 + 5
68	25 + 2	27 + 3	29 + 4
70	26 + 0	28 + 1	30 + 3
72	26 + 5	28 + 6	31 + 2
74	27 + 2	29 + 4	32 + 0
76	28 + 0	30 + 2	32 + 6
78	28 + 5	31 + 1	33 + 5
80	29 + 3	31 + 6	34 + 5
82	30 + 1	32 + 5	35 + 4
84	30 + 6	33 + 3	36 + 3
86	31 + 4	34 + 2	37 + 2
88	32 + 2	35 + 1	38 + 2

Source: Altman and Chitty[5]

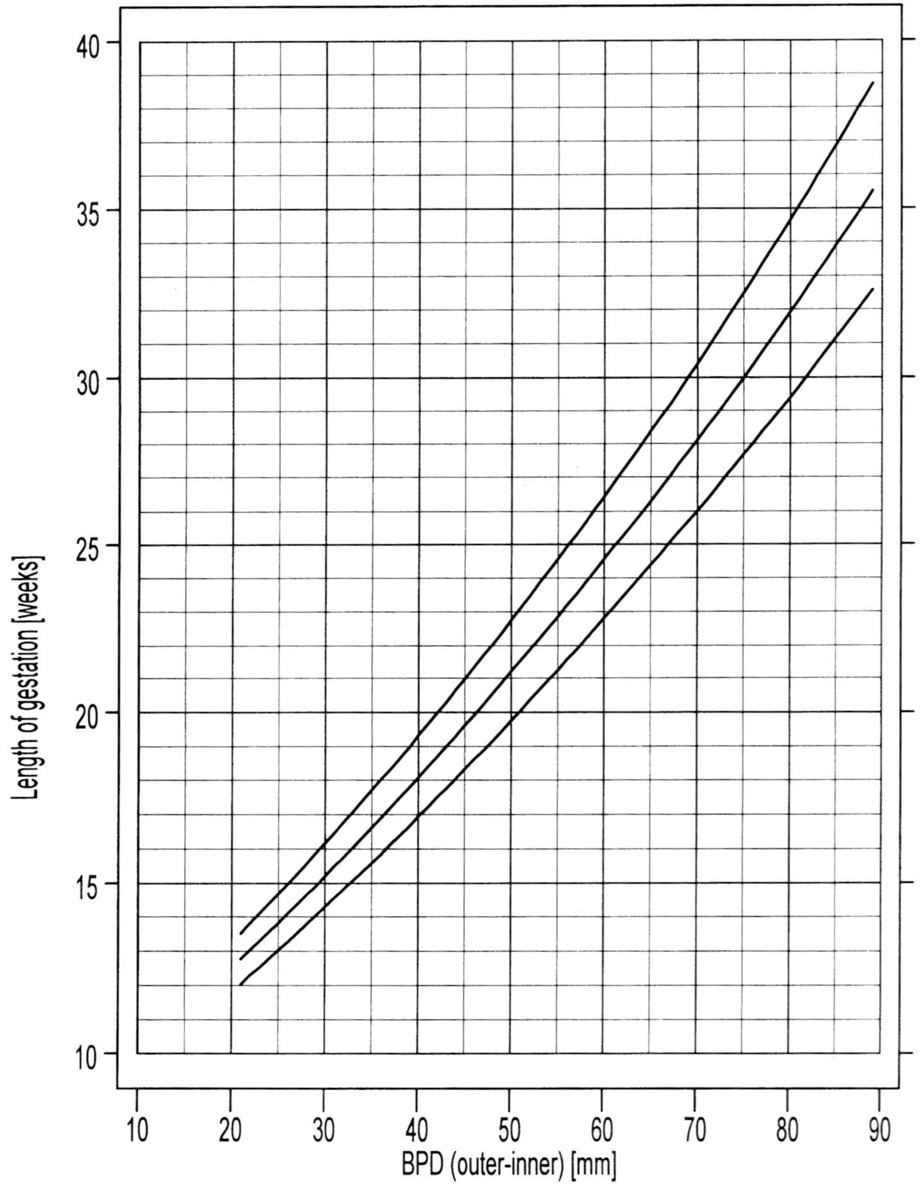

25. Head circumference (derived from diameters) – dating chart (a) using biparietal diameter outer–outer

Head circ. (mm)	Centiles (weeks + days) 5th	50th	95th
80	11 + 4	12 + 4	13 + 4
90	12 + 3	13 + 2	14 + 2
100	13 + 2	14 + 1	15 + 1
110	14 + 0	15 + 0	16 + 0
120	14 + 6	15 + 6	16 + 6
130	15 + 5	16 + 4	17 + 5
140	16 + 3	17 + 3	18 + 3
150	17 + 2	18 + 2	19 + 2
160	18 + 1	19 + 1	20 + 1
170	18 + 6	19 + 6	21 + 0
180	19 + 5	20 + 5	21 + 6
190	20 + 3	21 + 4	22 + 5
200	21 + 1	22 + 2	23 + 4
210	22 + 0	23 + 1	24 + 3
220	22 + 5	24 + 0	25 + 3
230	23 + 4	24 + 6	26 + 3
240	24 + 2	25 + 6	27 + 3
250	25 + 1	26 + 5	28 + 3
260	26 + 0	27 + 5	29 + 4
270	26 + 6	28 + 6	30 + 6
280	27 + 6	30 + 0	32 + 1
290	28 + 6	31 + 1	33 + 4
300	29 + 6	32 + 3	35 + 2
310	31 + 0	33 + 6	37 + 0
320	32 + 2	35 + 3	38 + 6

Source: Altman and Chitty[5]

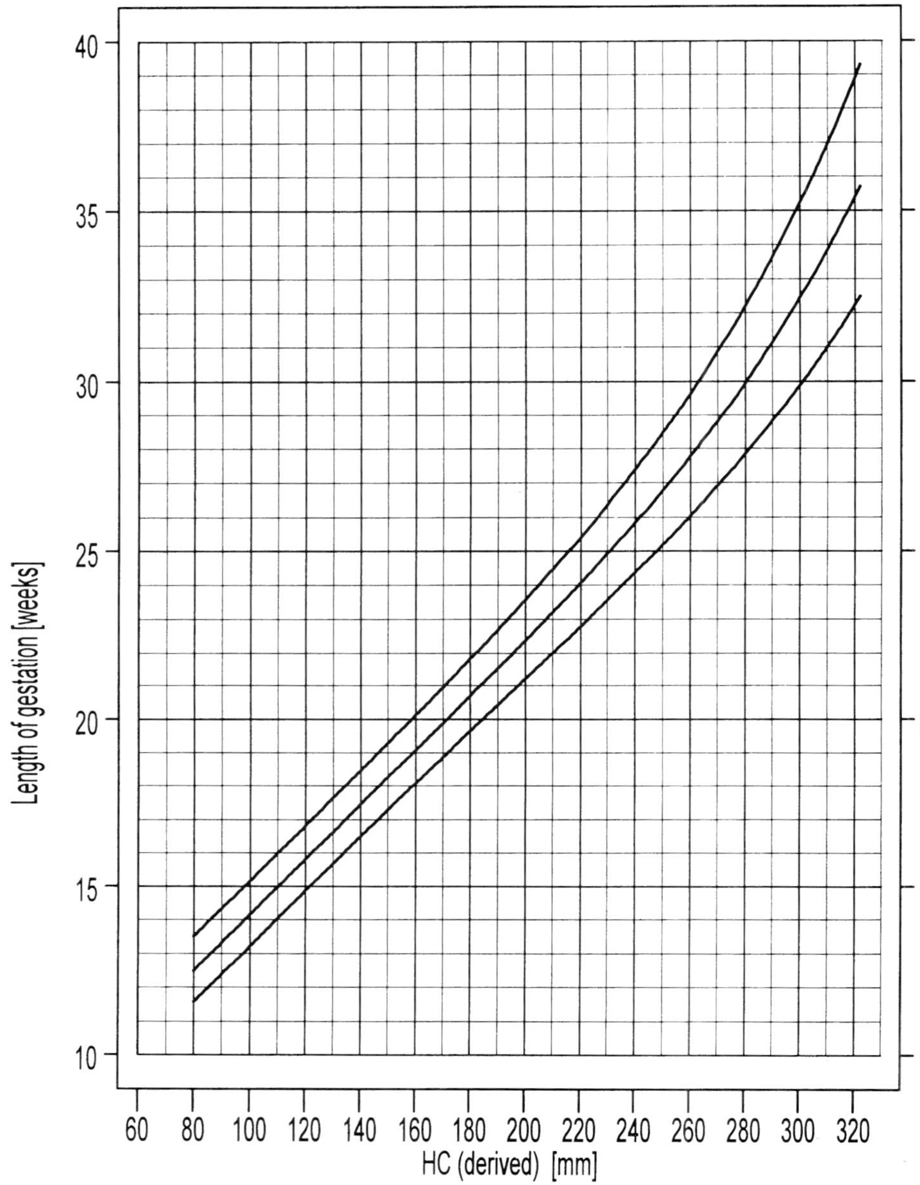

26. Head circumference (derived from diameters) – dating chart (b) using biparietal diameter outer–inner

Head circ. (mm)	Centiles (weeks + days) 5th	50th	95th
80	11 + 6	12 + 5	13 + 5
90	12 + 5	13 + 4	14 + 4
100	13 + 3	14 + 3	15 + 3
110	14 + 2	15 + 2	16 + 1
120	15 + 1	16 + 0	17 + 0
130	16 + 0	16 + 6	17 + 6
140	16 + 5	17 + 5	18 + 5
150	17 + 4	18 + 4	19 + 3
160	18 + 3	19 + 2	20 + 2
170	19 + 1	20 + 1	21 + 1
180	20 + 0	21 + 0	22 + 0
190	20 + 5	21 + 6	22 + 6
200	21 + 4	22 + 4	23 + 6
210	22 + 2	23 + 3	24 + 5
220	23 + 1	24 + 3	25 + 5
230	23 + 6	25 + 2	26 + 5
240	24 + 5	26 + 1	27 + 5
250	25 + 4	27 + 1	28 + 6
260	26 + 3	28 + 1	30 + 1
270	27 + 2	29 + 2	31 + 3
280	28 + 2	30 + 3	32 + 6
290	29 + 1	31 + 5	34 + 2
300	30 + 2	33 + 0	36 + 0
310	31 + 3	34 + 3	37 + 5
320	32 + 4	36 + 0	39 + 5

Source: Chitty and Altman (unpublished)

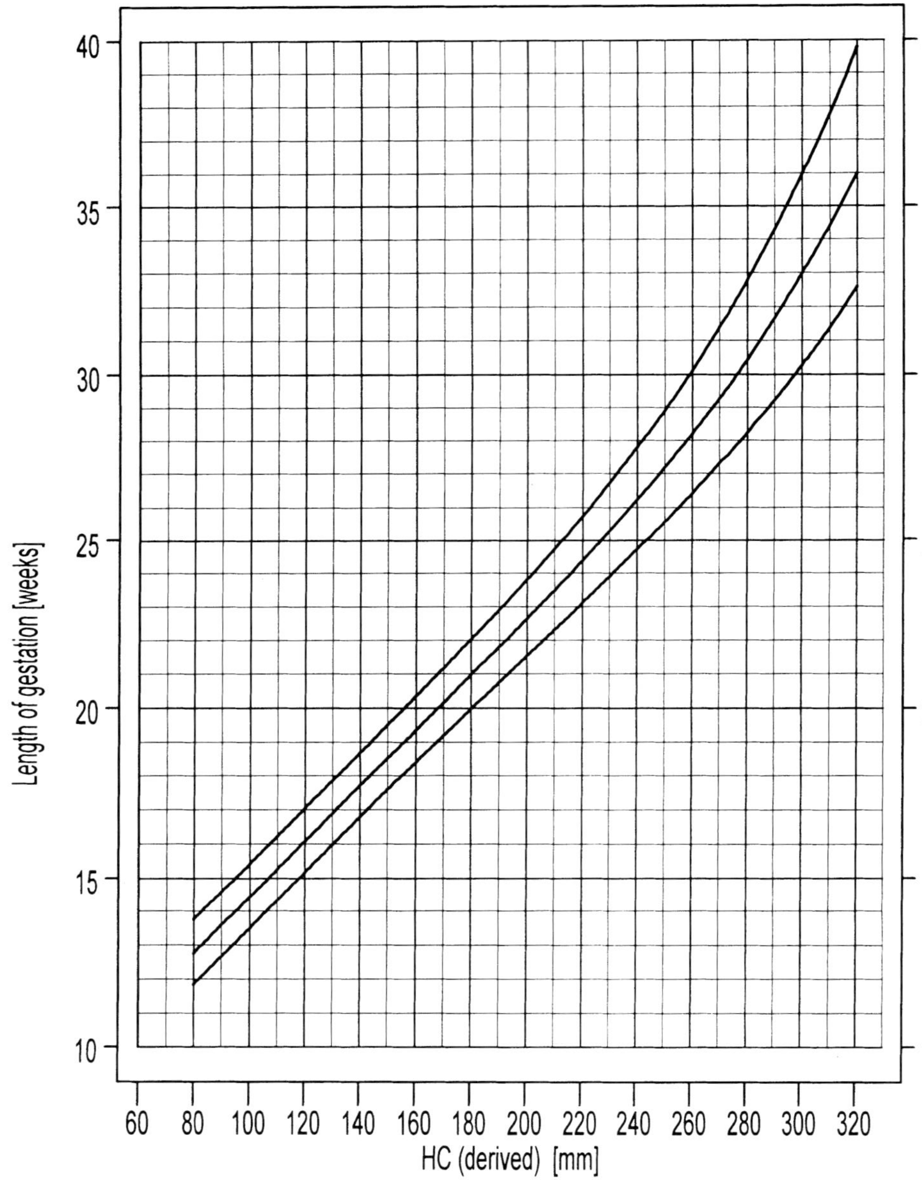

27. Femur length – dating chart

Femur (mm)	Centiles (weeks + days) 5th	50th	95th
10	12 + 2	13 + 0	13 + 5
12	12 + 6	13 + 4	14 + 2
14	13 + 2	14 + 1	15 + 0
16	13 + 6	14 + 5	15 + 4
18	14 + 3	15 + 2	16 + 2
20	15 + 0	16 + 0	17 + 0
22	15 + 4	16 + 4	17 + 4
24	16 + 1	17 + 2	18 + 2
26	16 + 6	17 + 6	19 + 0
28	17 + 3	18 + 4	19 + 5
30	18 + 0	19 + 2	20 + 4
32	18 + 5	20 + 0	21 + 2
34	19 + 2	20 + 5	22 + 0
36	20 + 0	21 + 3	22 + 6
38	20 + 5	22 + 1	23 + 5
40	21 + 3	22 + 6	24 + 4
42	22 + 1	23 + 5	25 + 3
44	22 + 6	24 + 3	26 + 2
46	23 + 4	25 + 2	27 + 1
48	24 + 2	26 + 1	28 + 1
50	25 + 1	27 + 0	29 + 0
52	25 + 6	27 + 6	30 + 0
54	26 + 5	28 + 5	31 + 0
56	27 + 4	29 + 5	32 + 0
58	28 + 3	30 + 4	33 + 0
60	29 + 2	31 + 4	34 + 1
62	30 + 1	32 + 4	35 + 2
64	31 + 0	33 + 4	36 + 2
66	32 + 0	34 + 4	37 + 3

Source: Altman and Chitty[5]

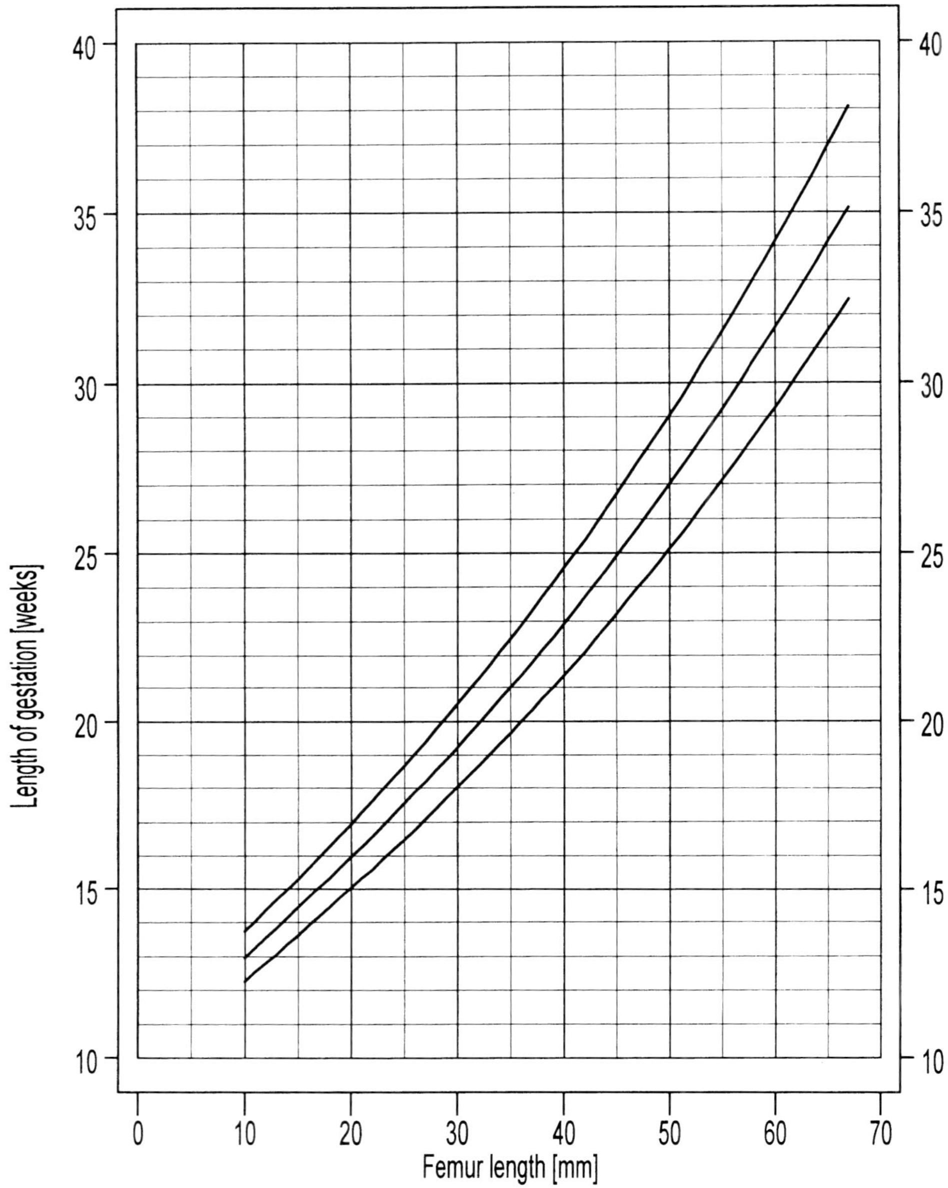

28. Transverse cerebellar diameter (TCD) – dating chart

TCD (mm)	Centiles (weeks + days) 5th	50th	95th
13	13 + 2	14 + 3	15 + 5
14	14 + 1	15 + 2	16 + 5
15	15 + 0	16 + 2	17 + 4
16	15 + 6	17 + 0	18 + 3
17	16 + 5	17 + 6	19 + 2
18	17 + 3	18 + 5	20 + 0
19	18 + 2	19 + 4	20 + 6
20	19 + 0	20 + 3	21 + 5
21	19 + 6	21 + 1	22 + 4
22	20 + 4	22 + 0	23 + 3
23	21 + 2	22 + 5	24 + 2
24	22 + 0	23 + 4	25 + 1
25	22 + 4	24 + 2	26 + 1
26	23 + 2	25 + 0	27 + 0
27	23 + 6	25 + 6	27 + 6
28	24 + 3	26 + 4	28 + 6
29	25 + 0	27 + 2	29 + 5
30	25 + 4	28 + 0	30 + 5
31	26 + 1	28 + 6	31 + 5
32	26 + 4	29 + 4	32 + 5
33	27 + 1	30 + 2	33 + 6
34	27 + 4	31 + 0	34 + 6
35	27 + 6	31 + 5	36 + 0
36	28 + 2	32 + 3	37 + 1

Source: Altman and Chitty[5]

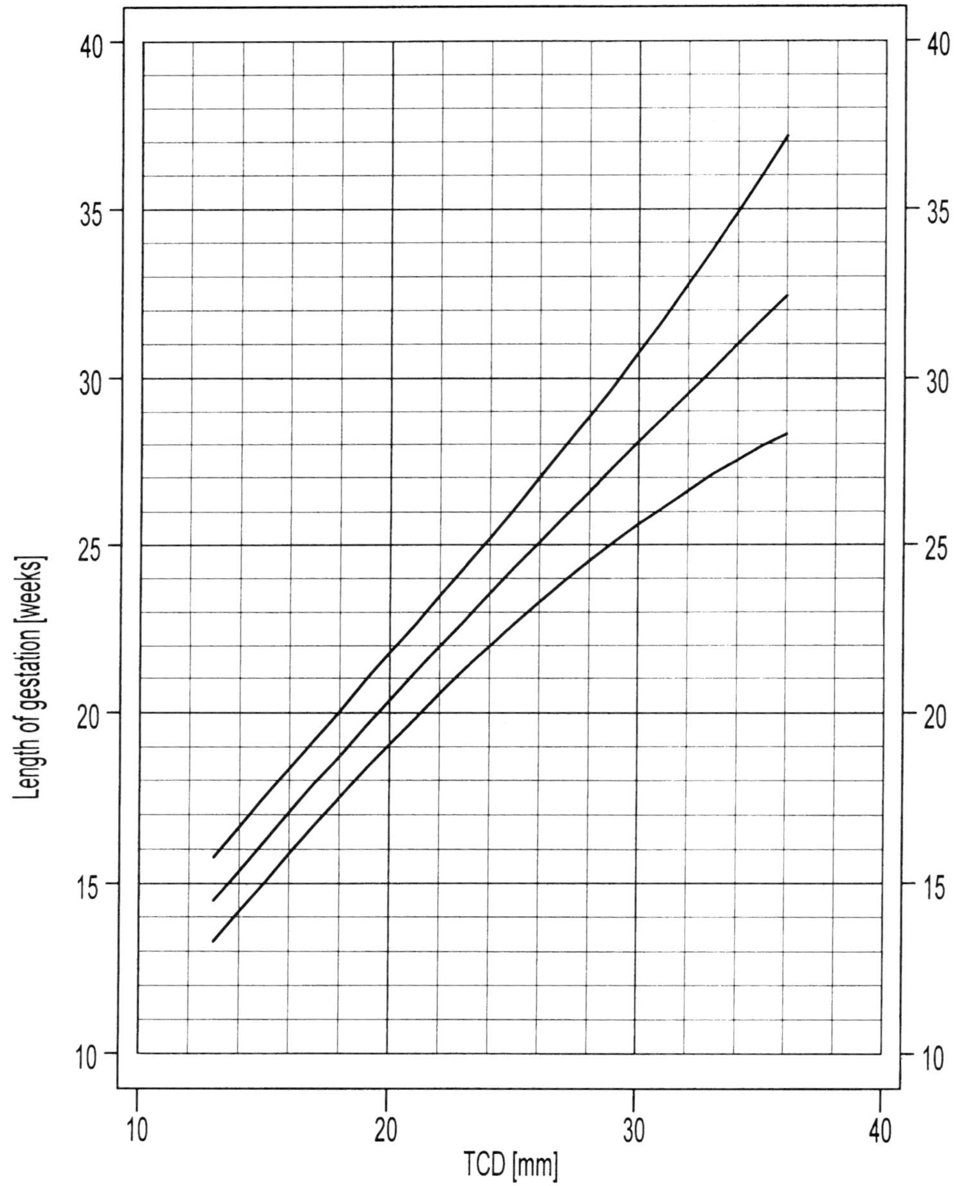

29. Crown–rump length – dating chart

Crown–rump length (mm)	Centiles (weeks + days) 5th	50th	95th
4	5 + 3	6 + 0	6 + 4
6	6 + 0	6 + 3	7 + 0
8	6 + 2	6 + 6	7 + 3
10	6 + 5	7 + 2	7 + 6
12	7 + 0	7 + 4	8 + 1
14	7 + 3	7 + 6	8 + 3
16	7 + 5	8 + 2	8 + 5
18	8 + 0	8 + 3	9 + 0
20	8 + 1	8 + 5	9 + 2
22	8 + 3	9 + 0	9 + 4
24	8 + 5	9 + 2	9 + 6
26	8 + 6	9 + 3	10 + 0
28	9 + 1	9 + 5	10 + 2
30	9 + 3	9 + 6	10 + 3
32	9 + 4	10 + 1	10 + 5
34	9 + 5	10 + 2	10 + 6
36	10 + 0	10 + 4	11 + 0
38	10 + 1	10 + 5	11 + 2
40	10 + 2	10 + 6	11 + 3
42	10 + 4	11 + 0	11 + 4
44	10 + 5	11 + 2	11 + 6
46	10 + 6	11 + 3	12 + 0
48	11 + 0	11 + 4	12 + 1
50	11 + 1	11 + 5	12 + 2
52	11 + 3	11 + 6	12 + 3
54	11 + 4	12 + 1	12 + 4
56	11 + 5	12 + 2	12 + 6
58	11 + 6	12 + 3	13 + 0
60	12 + 0	12 + 4	13 + 1
62	12 + 1	12 + 5	13 + 2
64	12 + 2	12 + 6	13 + 3
66	12 + 3	13 + 0	13 + 4
68	12 + 4	13 + 1	13 + 5
70	12 + 5	13 + 2	13 + 6
72	12 + 6	13 + 3	14 + 0
74	13 + 0	13 + 4	14 + 1
76	13 + 1	13 + 5	14 + 2
78	13 + 2	13 + 6	14 + 2
80	13 + 3	14 + 0	14 + 3

Source: Robinson and Fleming[12]

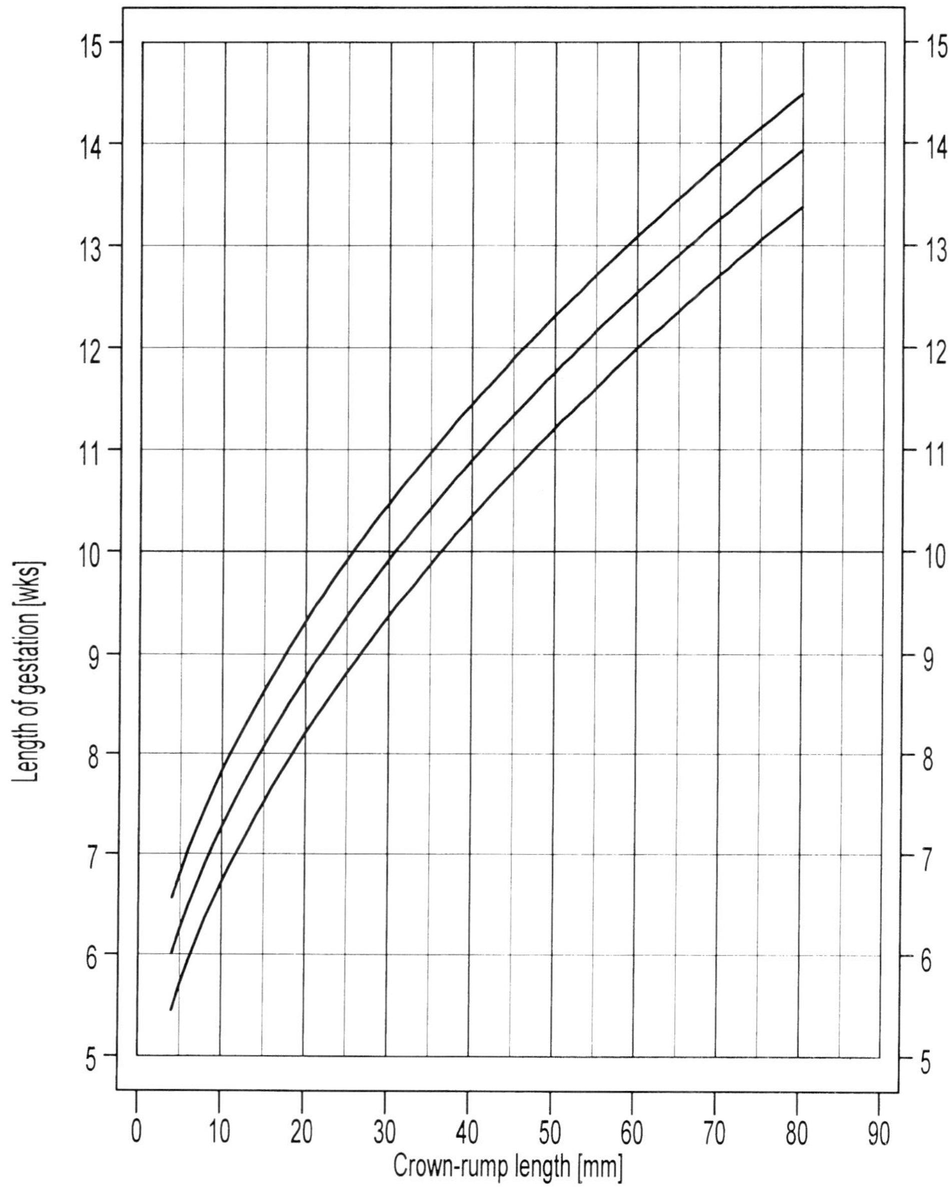

30. Umbilical vein Po_2

Weeks of gestation	Centiles (mm Hg) 5th	50th	95th
18	37.5	49.7	61.9
19	36.5	48.7	60.9
20	35.5	47.7	59.9
21	34.5	46.7	58.9
22	33.5	45.7	57.9
23	32.5	44.7	57.0
24	31.5	43.7	56.0
25	30.5	42.8	55.0
26	29.5	41.8	54.0
27	28.5	40.8	53.0
28	27.6	39.8	52.0
29	26.6	38.8	51.0
30	25.6	37.8	50.0
31	24.6	36.8	49.0
32	23.6	35.8	48.0
33	22.6	34.8	47.1
34	21.6	33.8	46.1
35	20.6	32.8	45.1
36	19.6	31.9	44.1
37	18.6	30.9	43.1
38	17.7	29.9	42.1

Source: Nicolaides *et al.*[13]
Comment: Model not fully specified; SD taken as constant

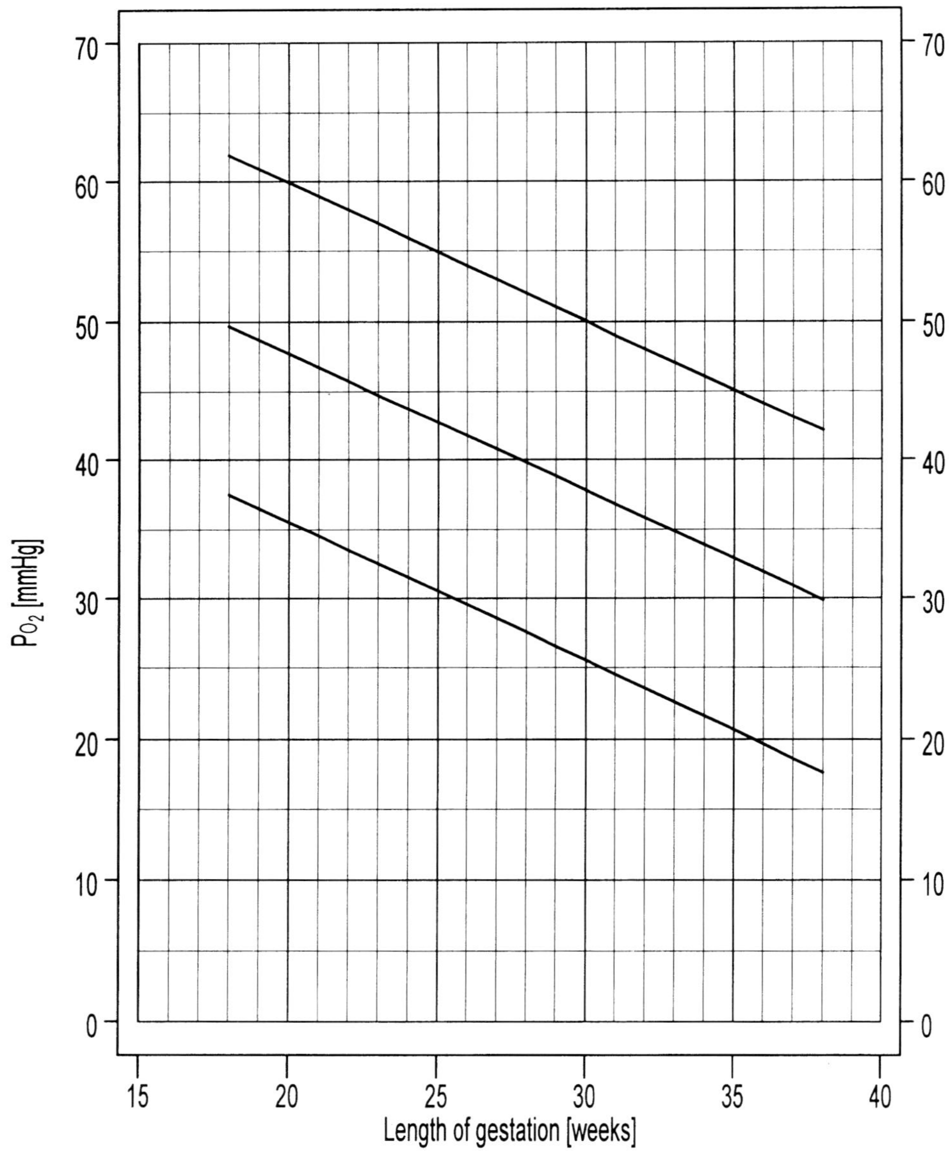

31. Umbilical vein P_{CO_2}

Weeks of gestation	Centiles (mm Hg) 5th	50th	95th
18	27.1	33.4	39.6
19	27.3	33.6	39.8
20	27.5	33.8	40.1
21	27.8	34.0	40.3
22	28.0	34.2	40.5
23	28.2	34.5	40.7
24	28.4	34.7	40.9
25	28.6	34.9	41.2
26	28.9	35.1	41.4
27	29.1	35.3	41.6
28	29.3	35.6	41.8
29	29.5	35.8	42.0
30	29.7	36.0	42.3
31	30.0	36.2	42.5
32	30.2	36.4	42.7
33	30.4	36.7	42.9
34	30.6	36.9	43.1
35	30.8	37.1	43.4
36	31.1	37.3	43.6
37	31.3	37.5	43.8
38	31.5	37.8	44.0

Source: Nicolaides *et al.*[13]
Comment: Model not fully specified; SD taken as constant

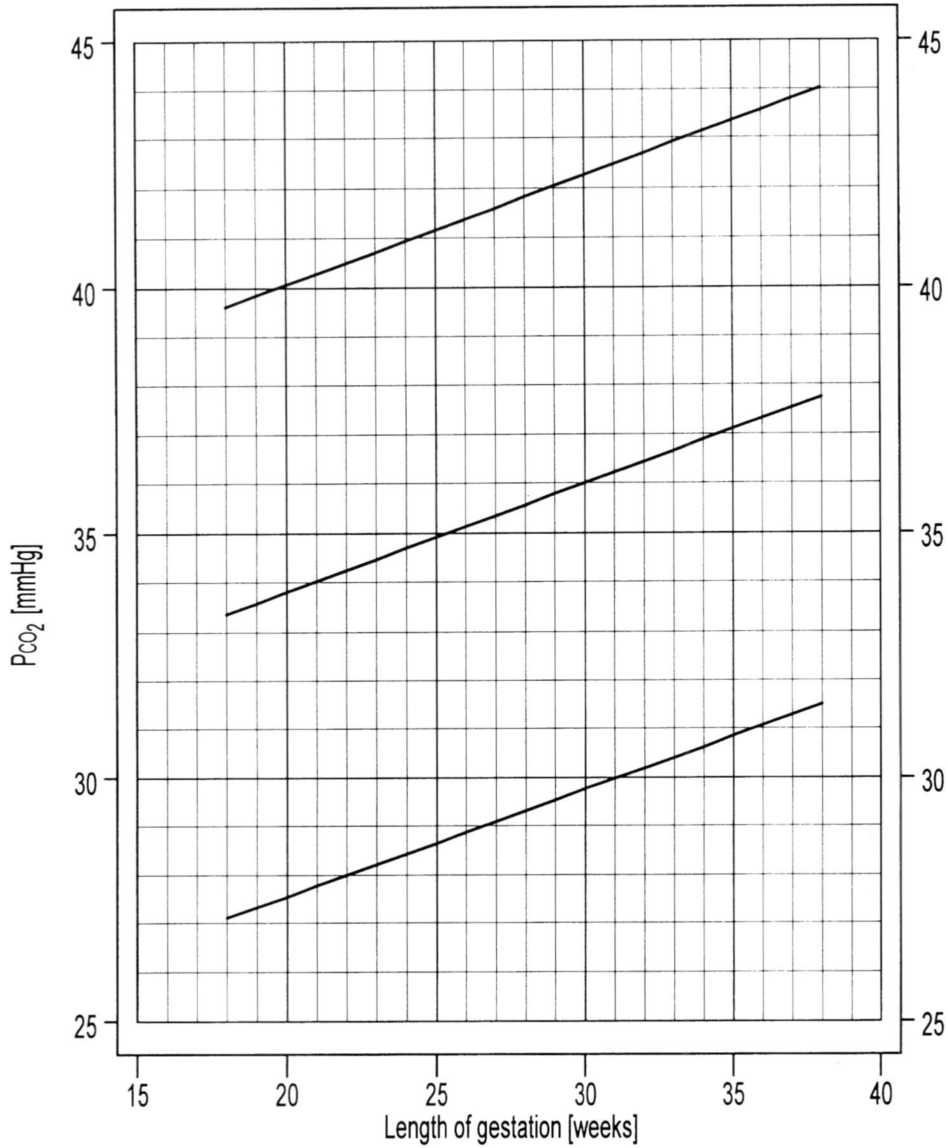

32. Umbilical vein pH

Weeks of gestation	Centiles 5th	50th	95th
18	7.38	7.42	7.47
19	7.38	7.42	7.47
20	7.37	7.42	7.47
21	7.37	7.42	7.46
22	7.37	7.42	7.46
23	7.37	7.41	7.46
24	7.37	7.41	7.46
25	7.36	7.41	7.46
26	7.36	7.41	7.45
27	7.36	7.41	7.45
28	7.36	7.40	7.45
29	7.36	7.40	7.45
30	7.35	7.40	7.45
31	7.35	7.40	7.44
32	7.35	7.40	7.44
33	7.35	7.39	7.44
34	7.35	7.39	7.44
35	7.34	7.39	7.44
36	7.34	7.39	7.43
37	7.34	7.39	7.43
38	7.34	7.38	7.43

Source: Nicolaides *et al.*[13]
Comment: Model not fully specified; SD taken as constant

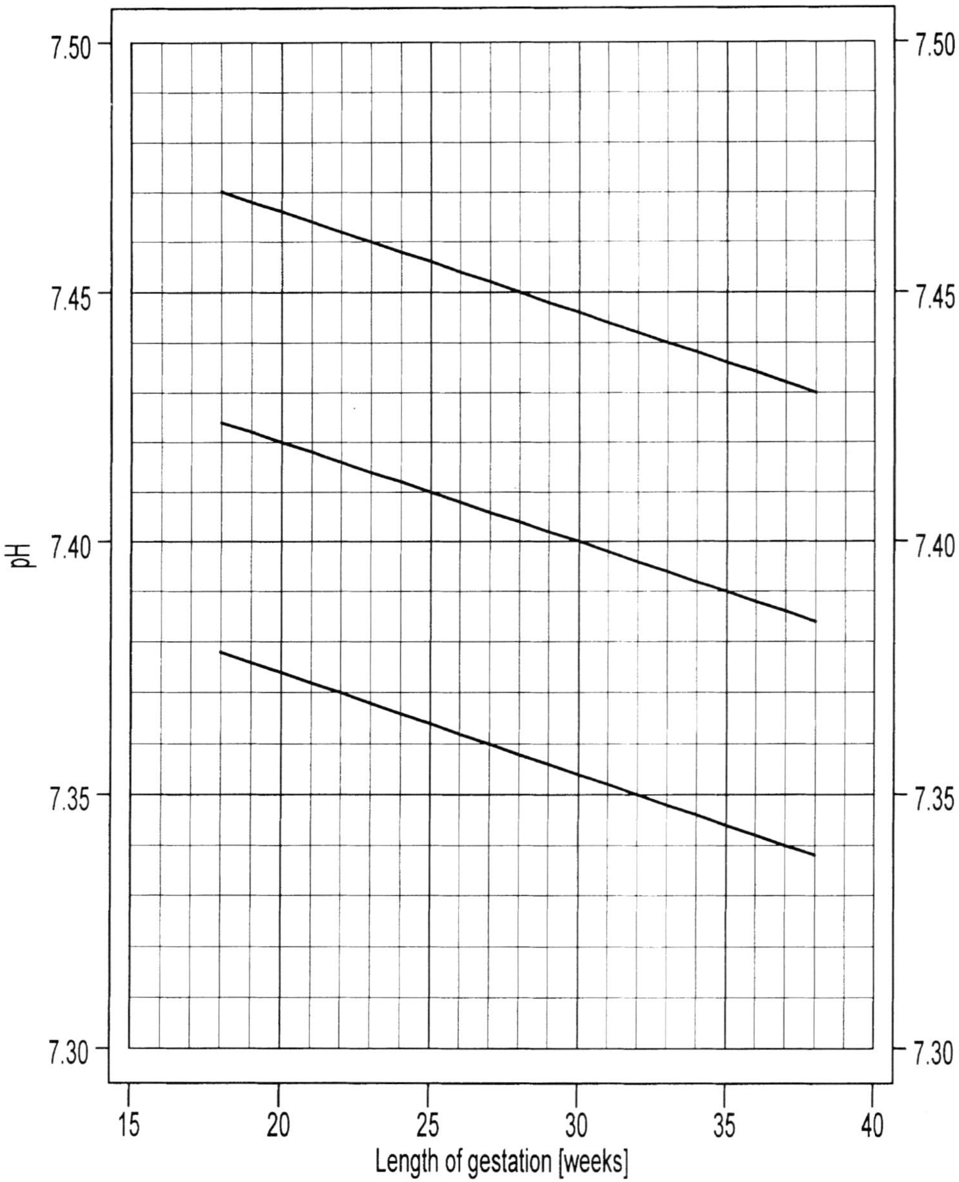

33. Umbilical artery pulsatility index

Weeks of gestation	Centiles 5th	50th	95th
20	1.04	1.54	2.03
21	0.98	1.47	1.96
22	0.92	1.41	1.90
23	0.86	1.35	1.85
24	0.81	1.30	1.79
25	0.76	1.25	1.74
26	0.71	1.20	1.69
27	0.67	1.16	1.65
28	0.63	1.12	1.61
29	0.59	1.08	1.57
30	0.56	1.05	1.54
31	0.53	1.02	1.51
32	0.50	0.99	1.48
33	0.48	0.97	1.46
34	0.46	0.95	1.44
35	0.44	0.94	1.43
36	0.43	0.92	1.42
37	0.42	0.92	1.41
38	0.42	0.91	1.40
39	0.42	0.91	1.40
40	0.42	0.91	1.40
41	0.42	0.92	1.41
42	0.43	0.93	1.42

Source: Arduini and Rizzo[14]
Comment: Excluded IUGR; SD taken as constant

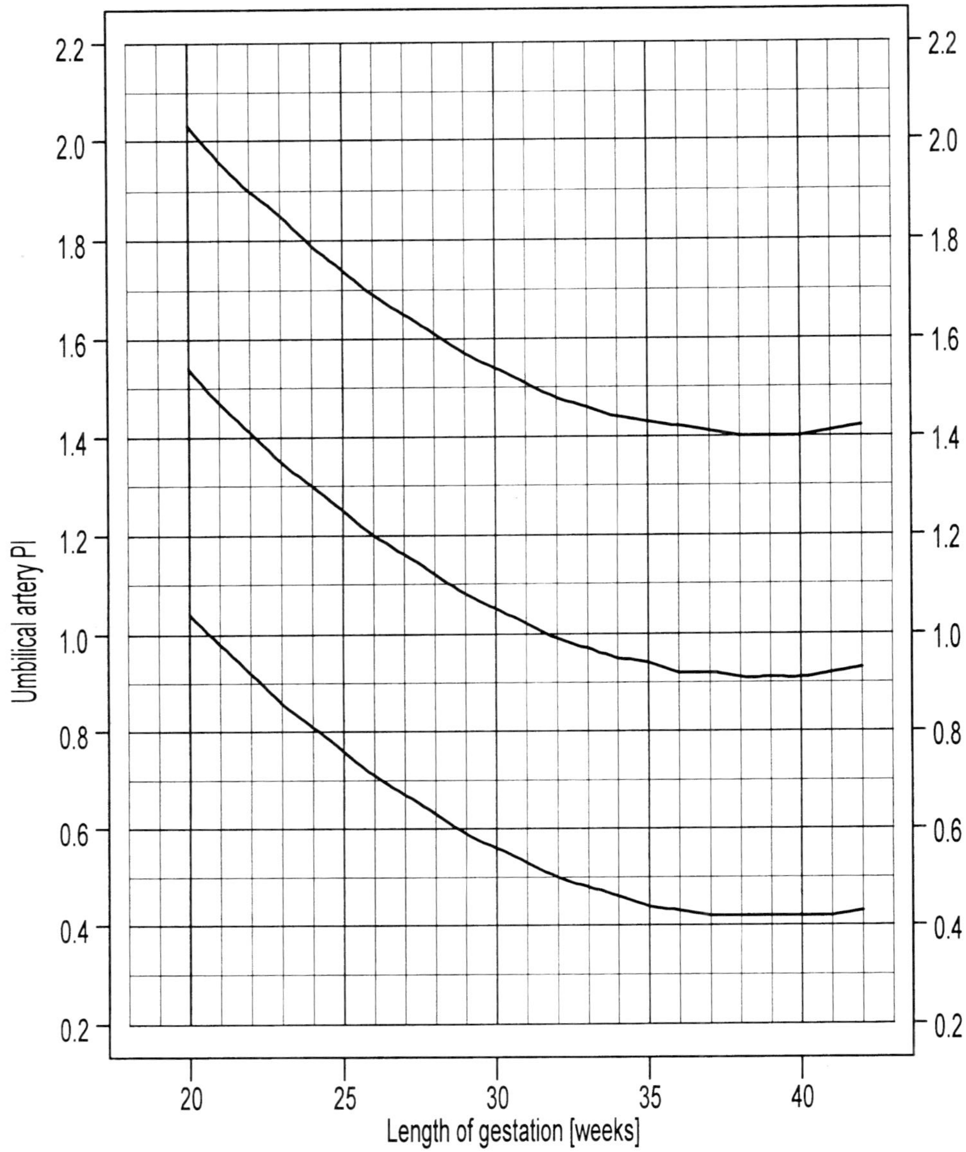

34. Descending aorta pulsatility index

Weeks of gestation	Centiles 5th	50th	95th
20	1.54	1.97	2.39
21	1.54	1.97	2.40
22	1.54	1.97	2.40
23	1.55	1.97	2.40
24	1.55	1.98	2.40
25	1.55	1.98	2.40
26	1.55	1.98	2.41
27	1.56	1.98	2.41
28	1.56	1.99	2.41
29	1.56	1.99	2.41
30	1.56	1.99	2.42
31	1.57	1.99	2.42
32	1.57	2.00	2.42
33	1.57	2.00	2.42
34	1.57	2.00	2.43
35	1.58	2.00	2.43
36	1.58	2.00	2.43
37	1.58	2.01	2.43
38	1.58	2.01	2.44
39	1.59	2.01	2.44
40	1.59	2.01	2.44
41	1.59	2.02	2.44
42	1.59	2.02	2.45

Source: Arduini and Rizzo[14]
Comment: Excluded IUGR; SD taken as constant

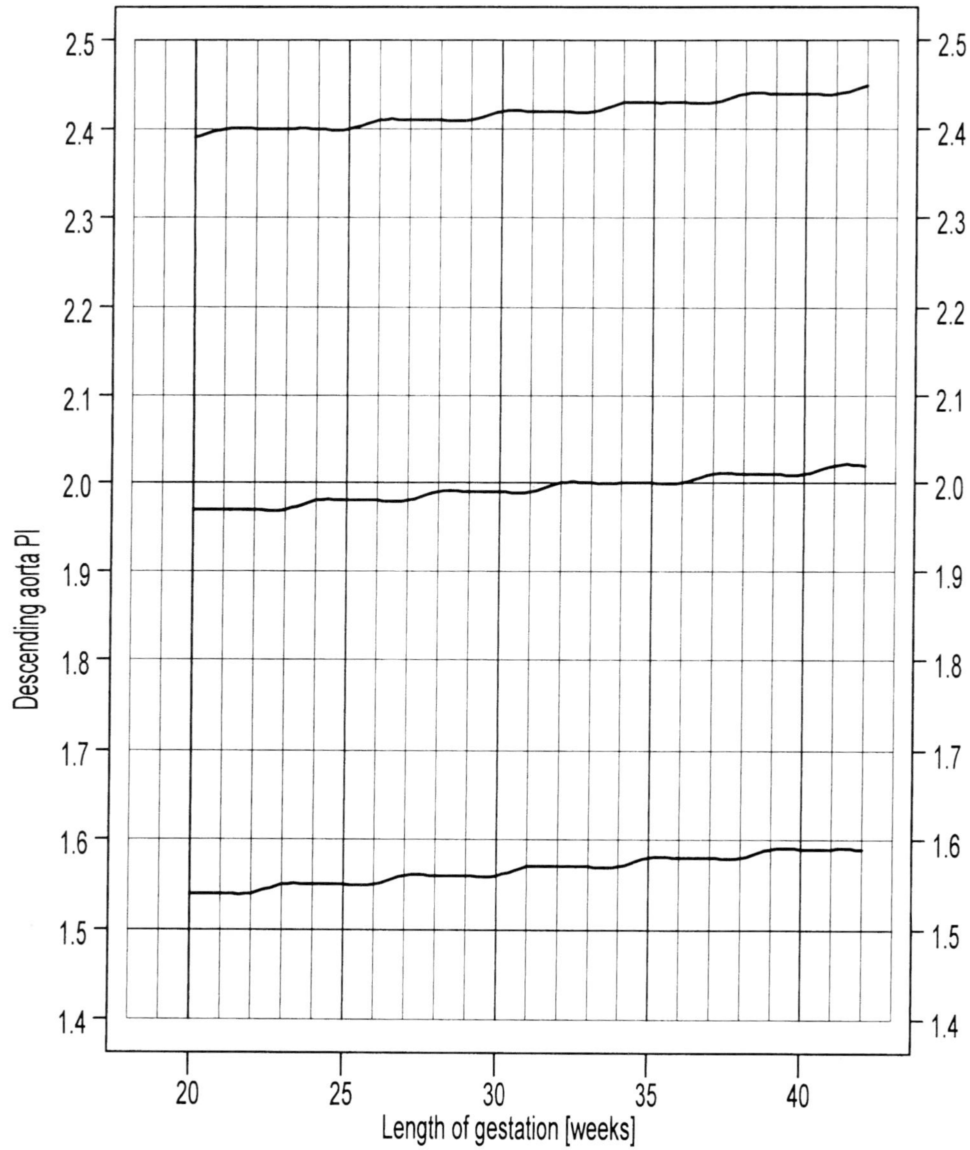

35. Renal artery pulsatility index

Weeks of gestation	Centiles 5th	50th	95th
20	1.61	2.52	3.43
21	1.59	2.50	3.41
22	1.57	2.48	3.39
23	1.55	2.46	3.36
24	1.54	2.44	3.34
25	1.52	2.42	3.32
26	1.50	2.40	3.29
27	1.48	2.38	3.27
28	1.46	2.35	3.25
29	1.44	2.33	3.23
30	1.42	2.31	3.20
31	1.40	2.29	3.18
32	1.38	2.27	3.16
33	1.36	2.25	3.14
34	1.34	2.23	3.12
35	1.32	2.21	3.10
36	1.30	2.19	3.08
37	1.28	2.17	3.06
38	1.25	2.15	3.04
39	1.23	2.13	3.02
40	1.21	2.11	3.00
41	1.19	2.08	2.98
42	1.16	2.06	2.96

Source: Arduini and Rizzo[14]
Comment: Excluded IUGR; SD taken as constant

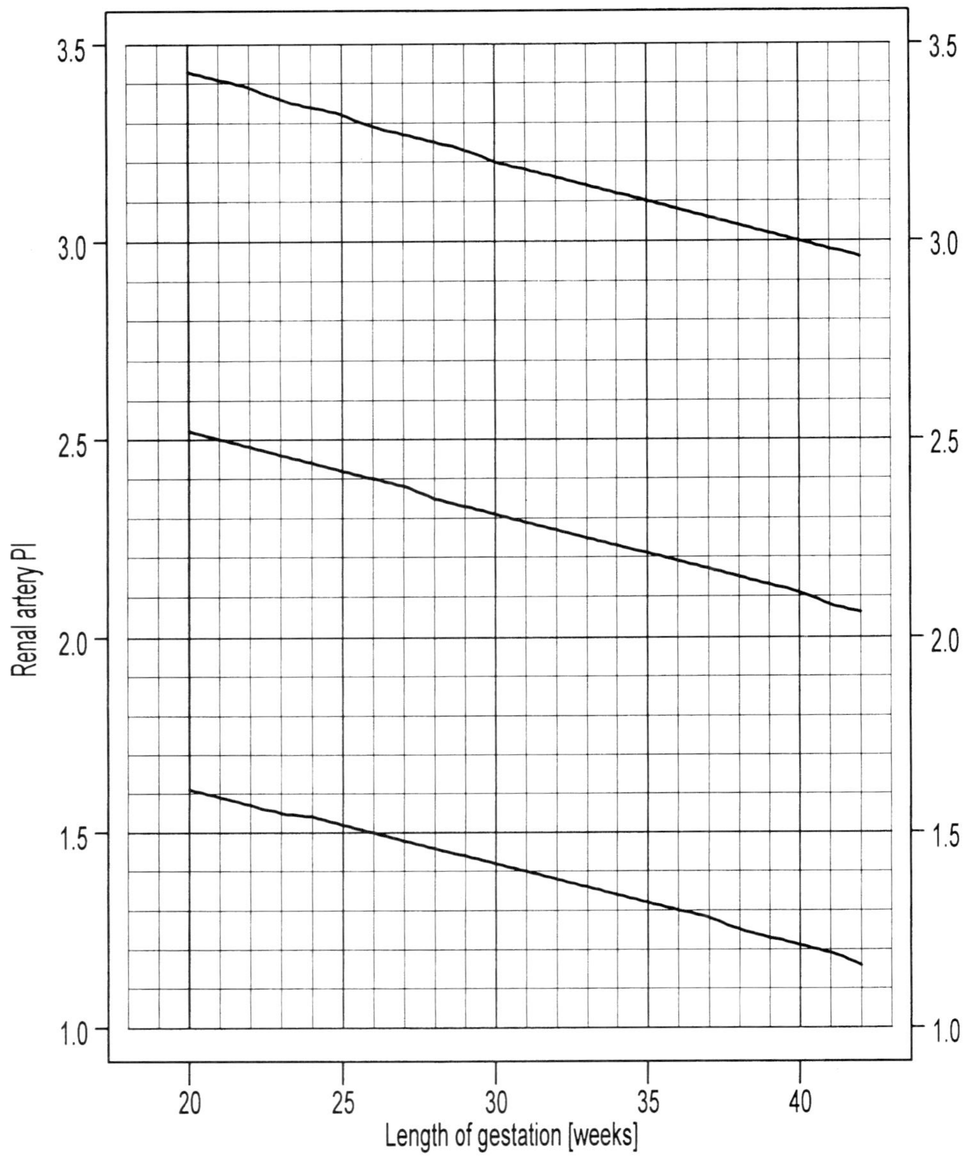

36. Internal carotid artery pulsatility index

Weeks of gestation	Centiles 5th	50th	95th
20	1.19	1.65	2.10
21	1.22	1.68	2.13
22	1.25	1.70	2.15
23	1.28	1.73	2.18
24	1.30	1.75	2.20
25	1.31	1.76	2.21
26	1.33	1.78	2.22
27	1.34	1.79	2.23
28	1.34	1.79	2.24
29	1.35	1.79	2.24
30	1.34	1.79	2.24
31	1.34	1.79	2.23
32	1.33	1.78	2.23
33	1.32	1.77	2.21
34	1.30	1.75	2.20
35	1.28	1.73	2.18
36	1.26	1.71	2.16
37	1.23	1.68	2.13
38	1.20	1.65	2.10
39	1.17	1.62	2.07
40	1.13	1.58	2.03
41	1.09	1.54	1.99
42	1.05	1.50	1.95

Source: Arduini and Rizzo[14]
Comment: Excluded IUGR; SD taken as constant

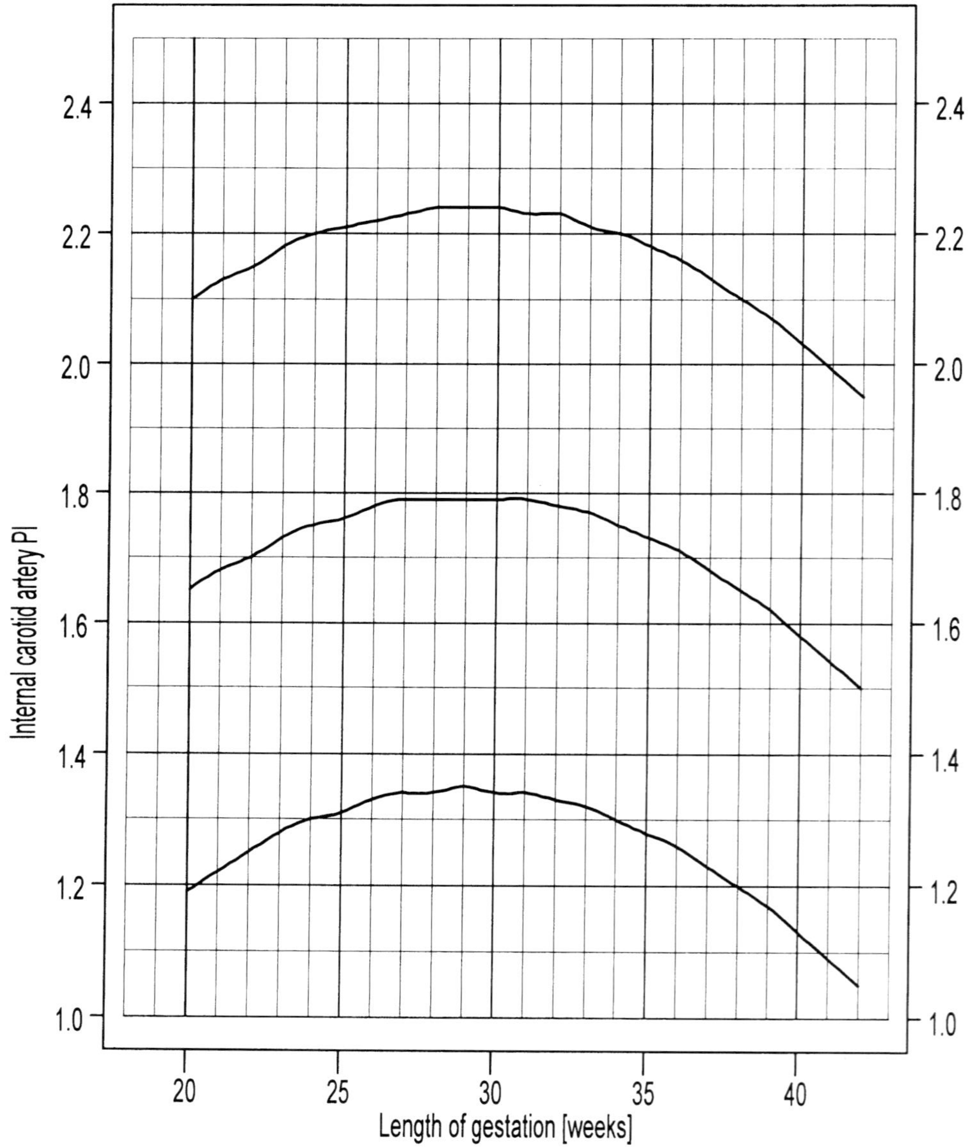

37. Middle cerebral artery pulsatility index

Weeks of gestation	Centiles 5th	50th	95th
20	1.36	1.83	2.31
21	1.40	1.87	2.34
22	1.44	1.91	2.37
23	1.47	1.93	2.40
24	1.49	1.96	2.42
25	1.51	1.97	2.44
26	1.52	1.98	2.45
27	1.53	1.99	2.45
28	1.53	1.99	2.46
29	1.53	1.99	2.45
30	1.52	1.98	2.44
31	1.51	1.97	2.43
32	1.49	1.95	2.41
33	1.46	1.93	2.39
34	1.43	1.90	2.36
35	1.40	1.86	2.32
36	1.36	1.82	2.28
37	1.32	1.78	2.24
38	1.27	1.73	2.19
39	1.21	1.67	2.14
40	1.15	1.61	2.08
41	1.08	1.55	2.01
42	1.01	1.48	1.94

Source: Arduini and Rizzo[14]
Comment: Excluded IUGR; SD taken as constant

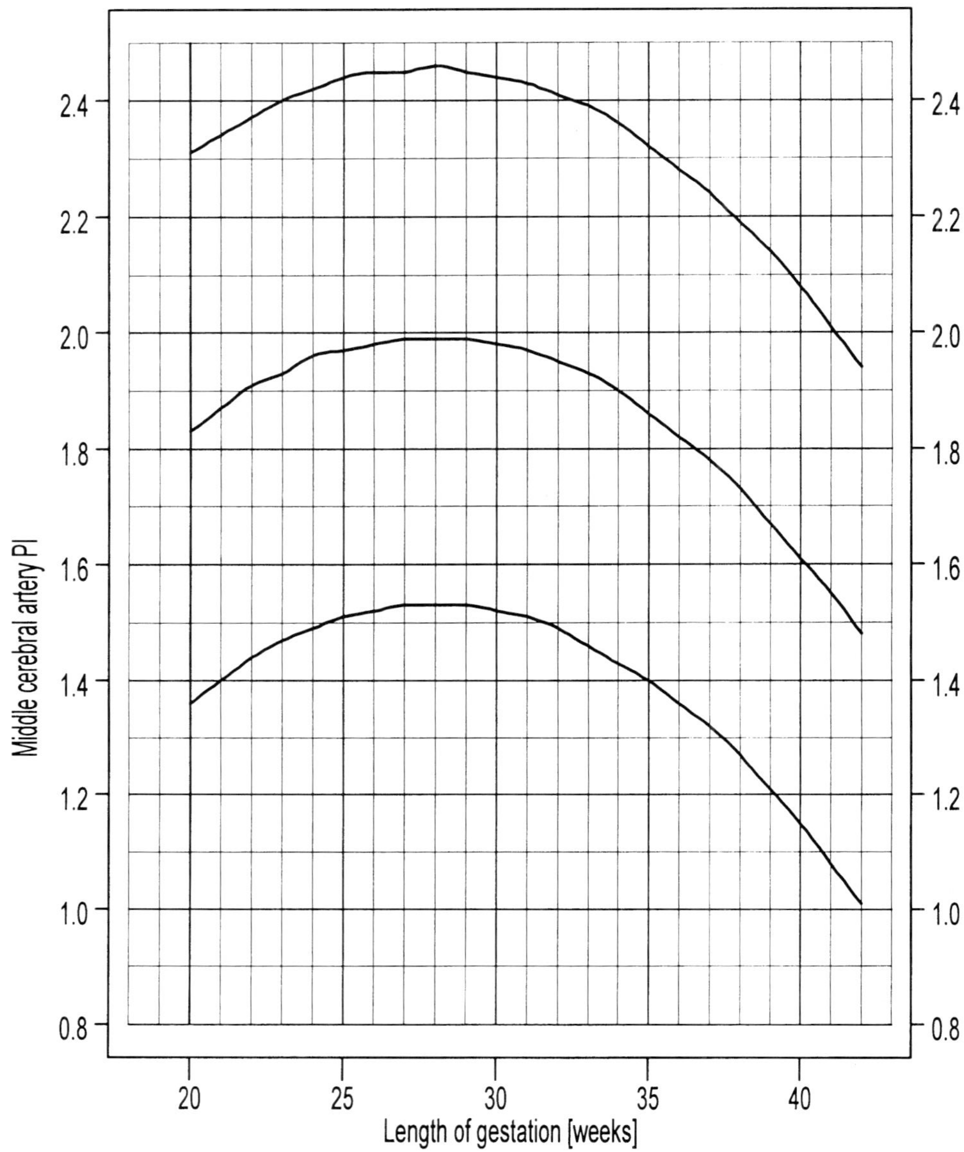

38. Non-placental uterine artery pulsatility index

Weeks of gestation	Centiles 5th	50th	95th
18	0.75	1.23	2.02
19	0.73	1.21	1.98
20	0.72	1.18	1.94
21	0.71	1.16	1.90
22	0.69	1.13	1.86
23	0.68	1.11	1.82
24	0.66	1.09	1.79
25	0.65	1.07	1.75
26	0.64	1.05	1.72
27	0.62	1.02	1.68
28	0.61	1.00	1.65
29	0.60	0.98	1.61
30	0.59	0.96	1.58
31	0.58	0.94	1.55
32	0.56	0.93	1.52
33	0.55	0.91	1.49
34	0.54	0.89	1.46
35	0.53	0.87	1.43
36	0.52	0.85	1.40
37	0.51	0.84	1.37
38	0.50	0.82	1.34
39	0.49	0.80	1.32
40	0.48	0.79	1.29
41	0.47	0.77	1.27
42	0.46	0.76	1.24

Source: Bower *et al.*[15]
Comment: Model not fully specified

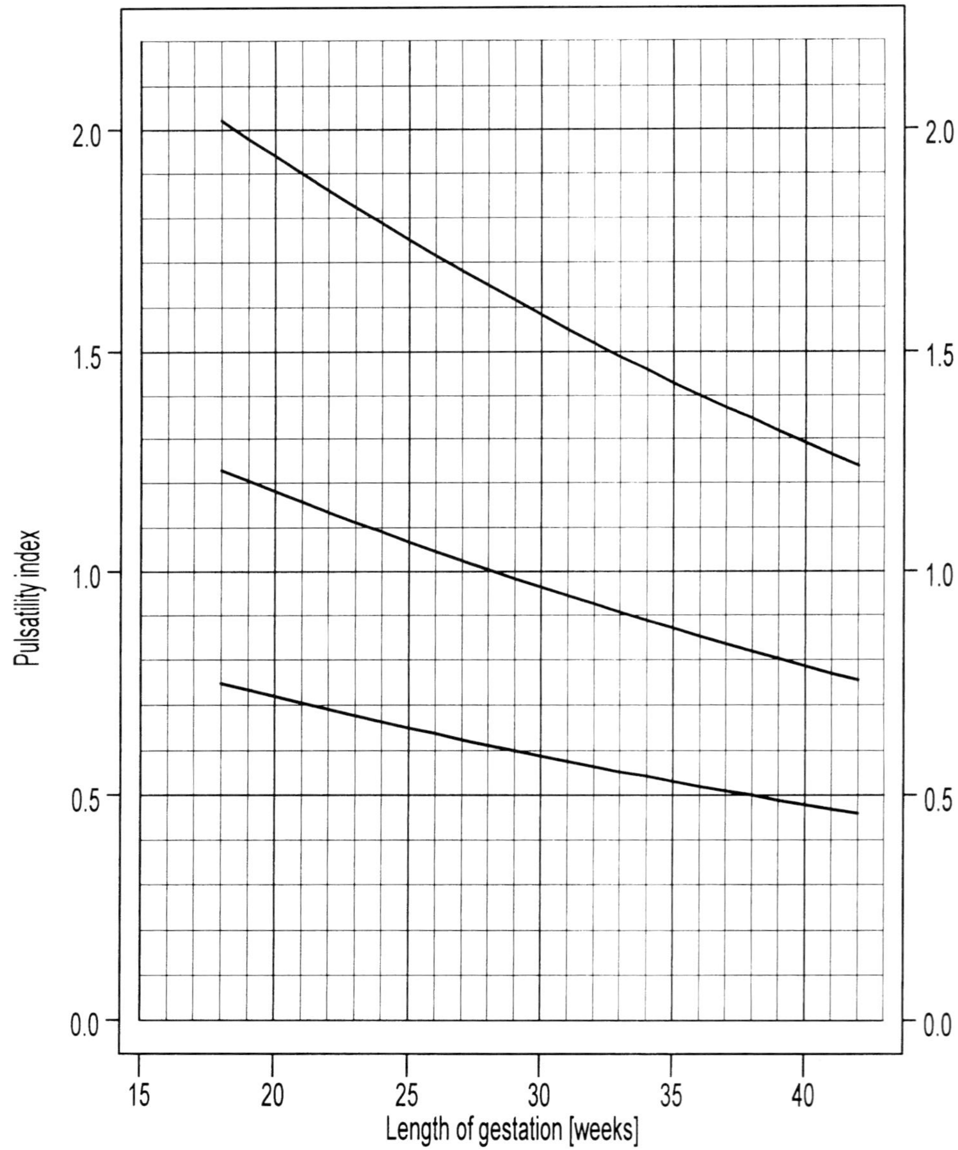

39. Placental uterine artery pulsatility index

Weeks of gestation	Centiles 5th	50th	95th
18	0.55	0.90	1.47
19	0.53	0.87	1.43
20	0.52	0.85	1.39
21	0.50	0.82	1.35
22	0.49	0.80	1.31
23	0.47	0.78	1.27
24	0.46	0.75	1.24
25	0.45	0.73	1.20
26	0.43	0.71	1.17
27	0.42	0.69	1.13
28	0.41	0.67	1.10
29	0.40	0.65	1.07
30	0.39	0.63	1.04
31	0.37	0.61	1.01
32	0.36	0.60	0.98
33	0.35	0.58	0.95
34	0.34	0.56	0.92
35	0.33	0.55	0.90
36	0.32	0.53	0.87
37	0.31	0.52	0.85
38	0.31	0.50	0.82
39	0.30	0.49	0.80
40	0.29	0.47	0.78
41	0.28	0.46	0.75
42	0.27	0.45	0.73

Source: Bower *et al.*[15]
Comment: Model not fully specified

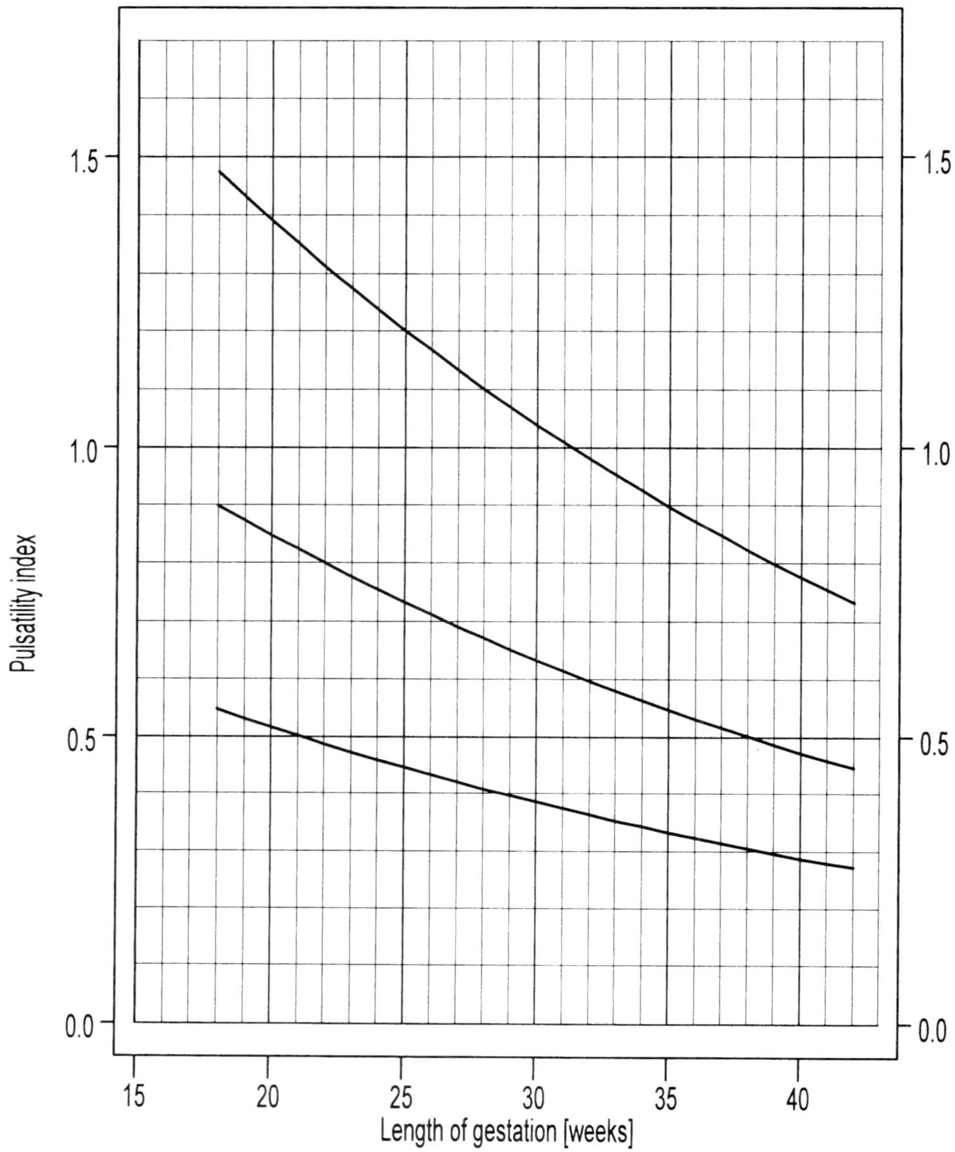

40. Amniotic fluid index

Weeks of gestation	Centiles (mm) 5th	50th	95th
16	79	121	185
17	83	127	194
18	87	133	202
19	90	137	207
20	93	141	212
21	95	143	214
22	97	145	216
23	98	146	218
24	98	147	219
25	97	147	221
26	97	147	223
27	95	146	226
28	94	146	228
29	92	145	231
30	90	145	234
31	88	144	238
32	86	144	242
33	83	143	245
34	81	142	248
35	79	140	249
36	77	138	249
37	75	135	244
38	73	132	239
39	72	127	226
40	71	123	214
41	70	116	194
42	69	110	175

Source: Moore and Cayle[16]
Comments: Excluded birthweight <10th or >90th centile. Model not fully specified

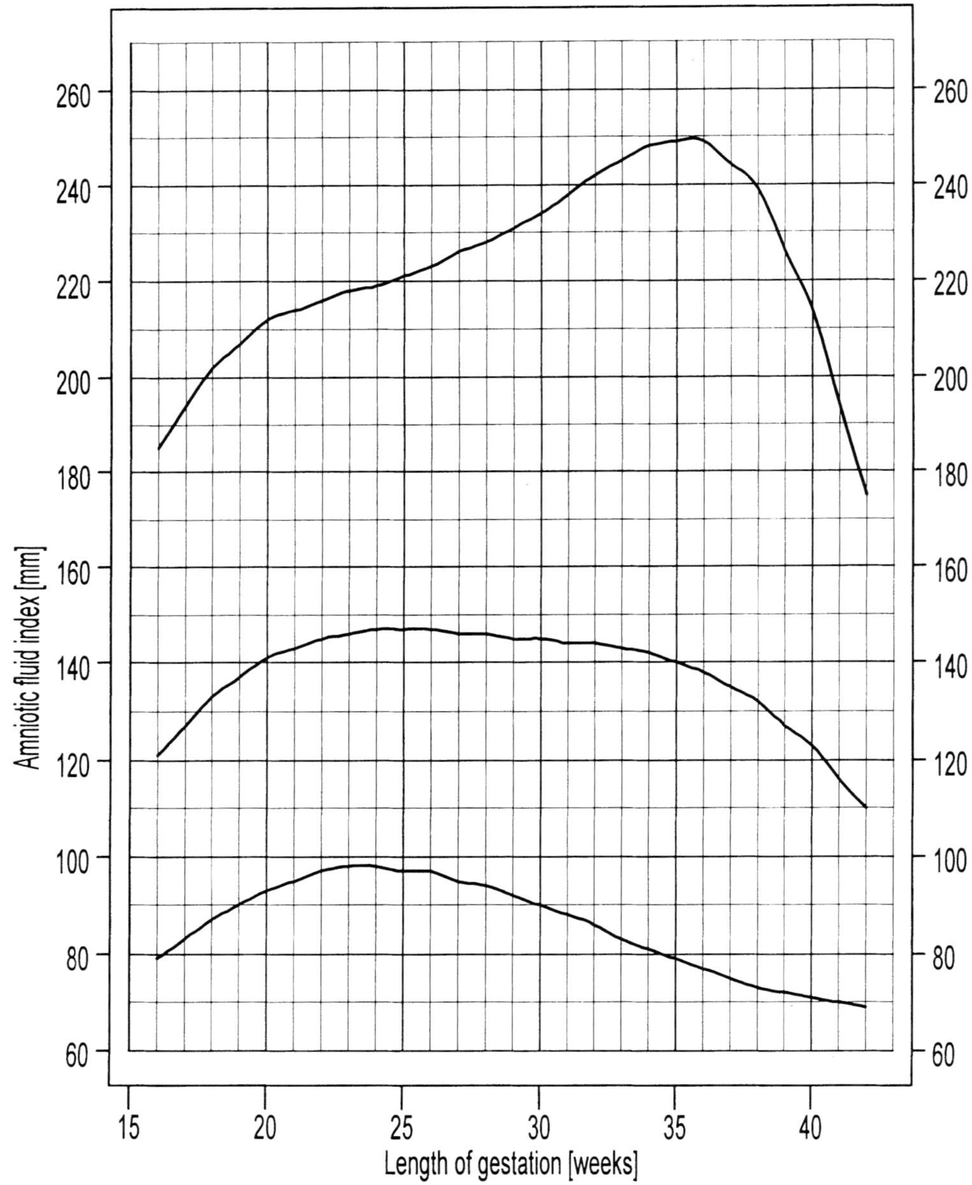

41. Fetal haemoglobin

Weeks of gestation	Centiles (g/dl) 5th	50th	95th
16	9.1	10.6	12.2
17	9.3	10.8	12.3
18	9.4	11.0	12.5
19	9.6	11.1	12.7
20	9.7	11.3	12.8
21	9.9	11.4	13.0
22	10.0	11.6	13.1
23	10.2	11.7	13.3
24	10.3	11.9	13.4
25	10.5	12.1	13.6
26	10.7	12.2	13.8
27	10.8	12.4	13.9
28	11.0	12.5	14.1
29	11.1	12.7	14.2
30	11.3	12.8	14.4
31	11.4	13.0	14.5
32	11.6	13.1	14.7
33	11.8	13.3	14.8
34	11.9	13.5	15.0
35	12.1	13.6	15.2
36	12.2	13.8	15.3
37	12.4	13.9	15.5
38	12.5	14.1	15.6
39	12.7	14.2	15.8
40	12.8	14.4	15.9

Source: Nicolaides *et al.*[17], Royston and Wright[3]

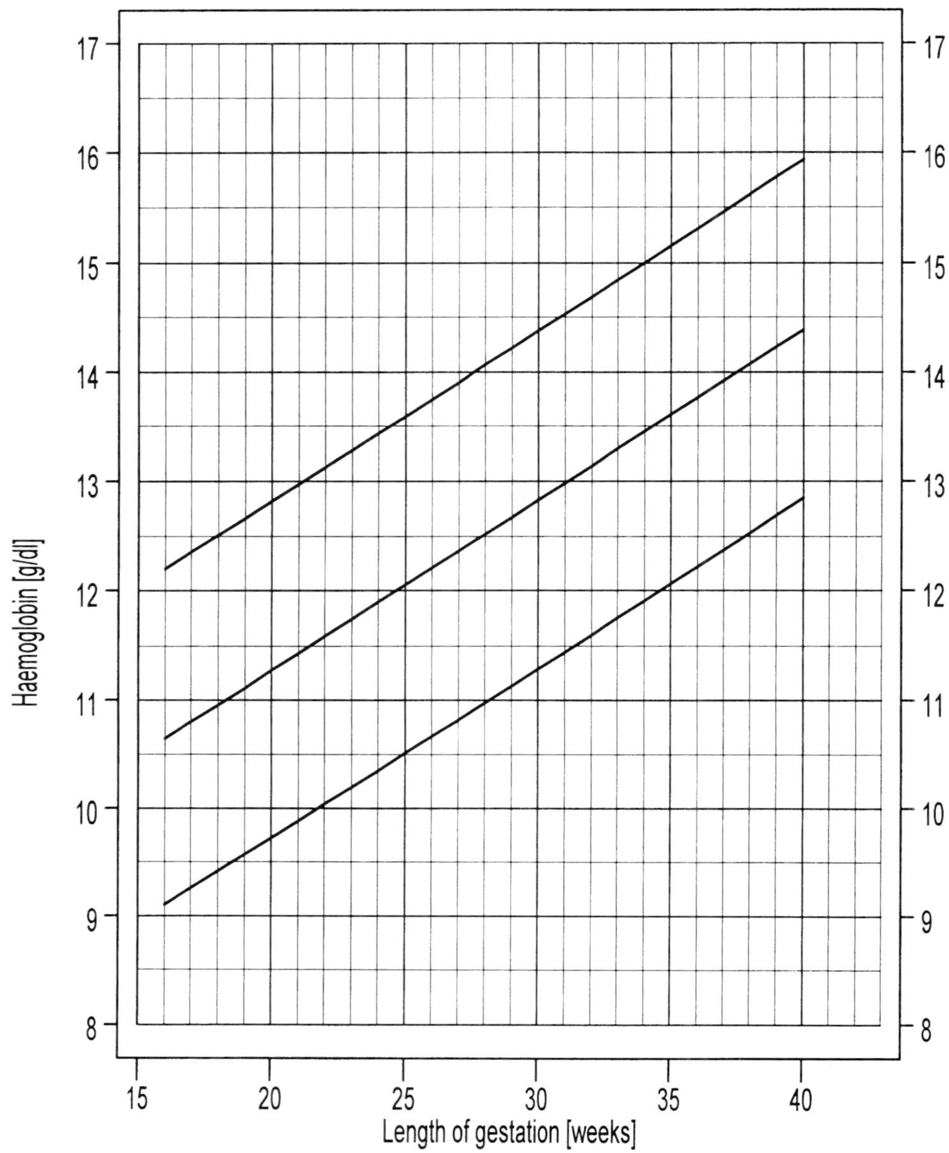

42. Fetal urinary sodium

Weeks of gestation	Centiles (mmol/l) 5th	50th	95th
18	70.6	87.0	107.1
19	62.8	77.3	95.2
20	56.4	69.5	85.6
21	51.3	63.2	77.8
22	47.2	58.1	71.5
23	43.9	54.0	66.5
24	41.2	50.8	62.5
25	39.2	48.3	59.5
26	37.7	46.4	57.2
27	36.6	45.1	55.6
28	36.0	44.4	54.7
29	35.8	44.1	54.3
30	36.0	44.4	54.6
31	36.6	45.1	55.6
32	37.7	46.4	57.1
33	39.2	48.2	59.4

Source: Nicolini *et al.*[18]
Comment: Based on sample of 26

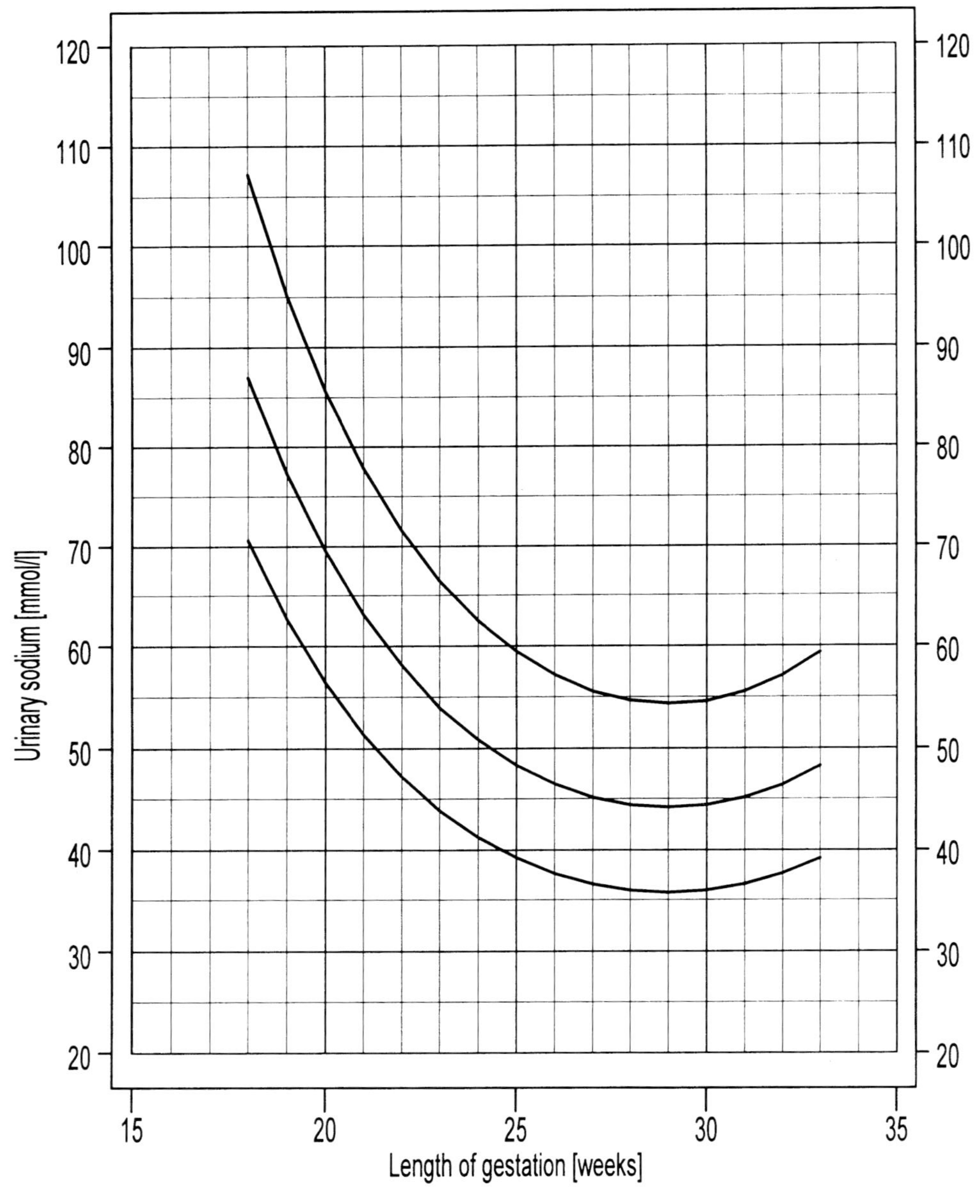

43. Fetal weight estimated from abdominal circumference and femur length

Femur length (mm)	Abdominal circumference (mm) 200	220	240	260	280	300	320	340	360	380	400
40	654	774	918	1087	—	—	—	—	—	—	—
42	689	813	960	1133	—	—	—	—	—	—	—
44	726	854	1004	1181	1389	—	—	—	—	—	—
46	765	896	1050	1231	1442	—	—	—	—	—	—
48	806	941	1099	1283	1497	1748	—	—	—	—	—
50	850	988	1149	1337	1555	1808	—	—	—	—	—
52	895	1037	1202	1393	1615	1871	2168	—	—	—	—
54	943	1089	1258	1452	1676	1936	2235	—	—	—	—
56	994	1144	1316	1513	1741	2003	2304	2650	—	—	—
58	1048	1201	1376	1577	1808	2072	2374	2721	—	—	—
60	1104	1261	1440	1644	1877	2143	2447	2795	—	—	—
62	1163	1324	1506	1713	1949	2217	2523	2870	3265	—	—
64	—	1390	1575	1786	2024	2294	2600	2948	3341	3787	—
66	—	1459	1648	1861	2102	2373	2680	3027	3419	3861	4360
68	—	1532	1724	1940	2182	2456	2763	3109	3498	3936	4428
70	—	—	1803	2021	2266	2540	2848	3193	3579	4012	4498
72	—	—	—	2107	2353	2628	2935	3279	3662	4090	4568
74	—	—	—	2196	2443	2719	3026	3367	3747	4170	4640
76	—	—	—	—	2537	2813	3119	3458	3834	4251	4713
78	—	—	—	—	2635	2910	3215	3551	3923	4333	4787
80	—	—	—	—	—	3011	3314	3647	4014	4418	4862

AC = abdominal circumference
FL = femur length
Source: Hadlock *et al.*[19]
Equation: $\log_{10}$ weight = 1.304 + 0.005281 × AC + 0.01938 × FL – 0.00004 × AC × FL

44. Fetal weight From abdominal circumference (AC) and femur length (FL) (in mm)

Weeks of gestation	Centiles (g) 5th	50th	95th
16	120	142	163
17	150	176	203
18	185	218	251
19	226	267	307
20	275	324	373
21	331	390	448
22	395	465	535
23	468	551	634
24	549	647	744
25	640	754	867
26	740	872	1003
27	850	1001	1152
28	968	1140	1312
29	1095	1290	1485
30	1231	1450	1669
31	1374	1618	1863
32	1524	1795	2066
33	1680	1978	2277
34	1840	2168	2495
35	2005	2361	2718
36	2172	2558	2945
37	2341	2757	3174
38	2511	2957	3403
39	2680	3156	3633
40	2848	3354	3860
41	3013	3549	4085
42	3176	3741	4305

Source: Hadlock *et al.*[19]
Comment: Related to gestation using Chitty *et al.*[6–8]
Equation: Log_{10} weight = 1.304 + 0.005281 × AC + 0.01938 × FL – 0.00004 × AC × FL
SD = 7.7% of weight
SD = standard deviation

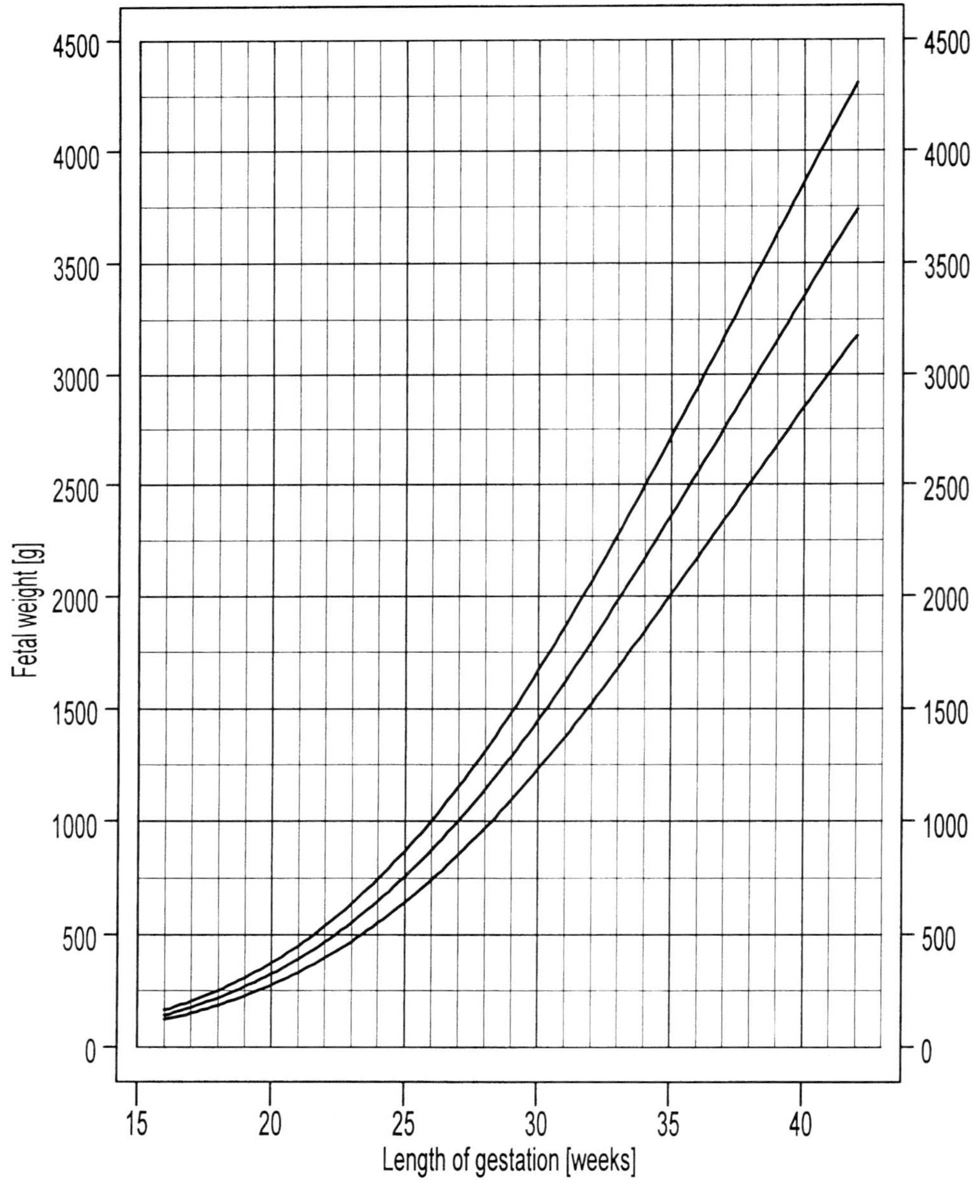

Index

Notes: 'fetal' is not used as an adjectival term – unless there is risk of confusion with 'maternal'. For example, these terms will be found: *fetal blood; maternal blood; development; growth*. Similarly, 'congenital' has been omitted as an adjectival term.